Michael A. Golden M.
April 5, 1982

To Mi[illegible]
With [illegible] for a
long + happy career in
surgery.

J. E. Murray
April 6, 1982

Plastic Surgery

Plastic Surgery Third Edition

EDITED BY

WILLIAM C. GRABB, M.D.
Professor of Surgery (Plastic Surgery)
and Head of the Section of Plastic Surgery,
The University of Michigan Medical School;
Staff Surgeon, University of Michigan Hospital,
Ann Arbor, Michigan

JAMES W. SMITH, M.D.
Associate Professor of Clinical Surgery,
Cornell University Medical College;
Associate Attending Surgeon, The New York
Hospital–Cornell Medical Center,
New York, New York

Foreword by
Reed O. Dingman, M.D., D.Sc.
Emeritus Professor of Surgery,
The University of Michigan Medical School,
Ann Arbor, Michigan

LITTLE, BROWN AND COMPANY
BOSTON

Published December 1979

Third Edition

Library of Congress Catalog Card No. 79-66922

ISBN 0-316-32269-5 (C)
ISBN 0-316-32268-7 (P)

Printed in the United States of America

HAL

Dedicated with love to our wives, Cozette and Nancy, and to the wives of all our co-authors.

Contents

Foreword by Reed O. Dingman ix
Preface xi
Contributing Authors xiii

I. GENERAL

1. **Basic Techniques of Plastic Surgery** 3
William C. Grabb

2. **Tissue Transplantation** 75
Noel Thompson

3. **Implantation Materials** 94
Ralph Blocksma and Silas Braley, Jr.

II. HEAD AND NECK

4. **Some Anomalies of the Head and Neck** 115
William C. Grabb

5. **Craniofacial Surgery** 131
Ian R. Munro

6. **Jaw Deformities and Temporomandibular Joint Disorders** 161
Melvin Spira

7. **Cleft Lip** 192
D. Ralph Millard, Jr.

8. **Cleft Palate** 205
Peter Randall

9. **Soft Tissue Injuries of the Face** 227
Richard C. Schultz

10. **Facial Bone Fractures** 242
Paul Natvig and Richard K. Dortzbach

11. **Reconstruction of the Scalp, Forehead, and Calvaria** 265
Thomas D. Rees and Richard J. Coburn

12. **Reconstruction of the Eyelids and Eyebrows and Correction of Ptosis of the Eyelid** 280
John C. Mustardé

13. **Reconstruction of the Ear** 299
Burt Brent

14. **Reconstruction of the Nose** 321
Ronald R. Cameron

15. **Reconstruction of the Facial Muscles, Lips, and Cheeks** 336
Bard Cosman and Jorge Niklison

16. **Primary Intraoral Tumors** 354
Dwight C. Hanna

17. **Radical Neck Dissection for Oral Cancer** 365
Lester M. Cramer and Norris K. Culf, Jr.

18. **Primary Tumors of the Salivary Glands and Neck** 391
John E. Hoopes

19. **Surgery of the Eyelids** 404
Salvador Castañares

20. **Cosmetic Surgery of the Aging Face** 410
James W. Smith

21. **Aesthetic Rhinoplasty** 424
George C. Peck

22. **Secondary Rhinoplasty** 434
Jack H. Sheen

23. **Deformities of the Ears** 440
Sten J. Stenström

III. SKIN AND ADNEXA

24. **Thermal Burns** 453
J. B. Lynch

25. **Radiation Injury and Electrical Burns**

Radiation Injury 484
Shattuck W. Hartwell, Jr.

Electrical Burns 489
Rex A. Peterson and John Gibney

26. **Basal Cell and Squamous Cell Carcinoma of the Skin** 497
Edward W. Gibson and Jorge Lopez-Garcia

27. **Malignant Melanoma** 511
Frederick R. Eilber, E. Carmack Holmes, and Donald L. Morton

28. **Hemangioma, Lymphangioma, and Arteriovenous Fistula** 518
Hugh G. Thomson

29. **Benign Growths and Generalized Skin Disorders** 530
Harvey A. Zarem and Allan L. Lorincz

30. **Hypertrophic Scars and Keloids** 552
Lynn D. Ketchum

31. **Tattoos** 559
Joseph Agris

IV. **HAND AND UPPER EXTREMITY**

32. **Fingertip Injuries, Amputations, and Infections of the Hand and Upper Extremity** 569
John M. Markley, Jr.

33. **Fractures and Joint Injuries of the Hand** 586
Richard G. Eaton and Richard A. Sperling

34. **Stiff Finger Joints** 598
Raymond M. Curtis

35. **Tendon Injuries in the Forearm and Hand** 604
James W. Smith

36. **Nerve Injuries in the Forearm and Hand** 618
James W. Smith

37. **Rheumatoid Arthritis of the Hand** 631
Jerome E. Adamson and Austin D. Potenza

38. **Dupuytren's Contracture** 637
John T. Hueston

39. **Tumors of the Hand** 641
James W. Smith and Randolph H. Guthrie

V. **MICROSURGERY**

40. **Introduction to Microsurgery** 653
Harry J. Buncke, Jr., and Zoltan Szabo

41. **Clinical Microvascular Surgery and Free Tissue Transfers** 660
Rollin K. Daniel

42. **Microsurgical Repair of Peripheral Nerves** 685
Hanno Millesi

43. **Replantation** 697
Graham D. Lister and Harold E. Kleinert

VI. **BREAST**

44. **Augmentation Mammoplasty** 719
James L. Baker, Jr.

45. **Reduction Mammoplasty and Correction of Ptosis of the Breast** 737
Paul K. McKissock

46. **Management of Benign and Premalignant Disease of the Female Breast** 760
Robert M. Oneal and William W. Blackburn, II

47. **Reconstruction of the Breast after Mastectomy** 785
Thomas D. Cronin

48. **Gynecomastia** 802
Bernard E. Simon

VII. **TRUNK AND LOWER EXTREMITY**

49. **Reconstructive Procedures of the Lower Extremity** 811
Luis O. Vasconez and John B. McCraw

50. **Pressure Sores** 818
B. Herold Griffith

51. **Lymphedema** 826
Timothy A. Miller

52. **Lipectomy** 838
Paule Regnault

VIII. **GENITALIA**

53. **Hypospadias, Epispadias, and Exstrophy of the Bladder** 855
Charles E. Horton, Charles J. Devine, Jr., Jerome E. Adamson, and James H. Carraway

54. **Injuries of the Male Genitalia** 869
Julius A. Howell

55. **Vaginal Agenesis** 873
Donald R. Laub and Bruce J. Dubin

56. **Gender Dysphoria** 883
Donald R. Laub and Bruce J. Dubin

Selected Reading List 901
Index 905

Foreword

This book, edited by William C. Grabb, M.D., and James W. Smith, M.D., is now in its third edition, the first having been printed in 1968 and the second in 1973. In the short period of eleven years *Plastic Surgery* has gained worldwide recognition as a comprehensive and accurate source of information on all aspects of plastic and reconstructive surgery. Because of the increased size and scope of their text, the authors have elected to drop "A Concise Guide to Clinical Practice" from the title. A larger format was necessary to accommodate the explosion of scientific information and new developments since the second edition.

Not only has there been exciting change in the attitudes, concepts and teaching of plastic and reconstructive surgery, but new authorities have emerged, requiring complete revision of the text. More than half of the authors are new collaborators in this work. Many new subjects have been included in the third edition, while some have been deleted.

Both editors are involved in administration, teaching, research, and patient care. They are active in writing, editing, and in the affairs of organized plastic surgery and are attuned to advances, progress, and changing concepts. This information forms the basis of frequent revisions which keep this book alive and current.

The editors have not lost sight of their original concept: to produce an inexpensive text with broad current coverage, written by aggressive, knowledgeable authorities in a readable, interesting, well-illustrated manner. This book has already had significant influence on the development of world plastic surgery and will continue as a living compendium of progress in the art.

Bill Grabb and Jim Smith with their great experience and ability have reached surgical maturity which is evident in this third edition.

Reed O. Dingman

Preface

Within the past several years we have entered a period in the history of plastic surgery in which there has been a great outpouring of new ideas – a future shock of information that is in such abundance that we cannot consume all of it and still have time for caring for patients and for living. There are now 23 journals relating to plastic surgery and a feast of excellent books, movies, sound-slide programs, videotapes, and symposia. It is our prediction that this future shock will gather momentum as we enter the next period in which in-depth research will receive well-deserved emphasis. This abundance of information will lead more plastic surgeons to become subspecialists in their areas of special interest.

Against this background we have pressed ahead in the third edition to include some information from all aspects of plastic surgery, keeping the same two main objectives: (1) to provide a current and succinct guide to clinical practice and (2) to make available an inexpensive text on the entire field of plastic surgery for the student, medical house officer, and practicing physician.

To keep the text in one volume we have eliminated parts of some chapters and combined others. To remain vital and current we have added or replaced approximately half of our contributing authors and have added ten chapters, including two entirely new sections on microsurgery and the breast. All other chapters have been rewritten or updated. With each subsequent edition we are determined to remain flexible, current, and concise.

As in the previous editions we wish to express what a joy it has been for us to put the book together – what a pleasure it has been to write, read, and edit the changing body of knowledge that makes up the specialty of plastic surgery.

We wish to acknowledge the authors of all articles included in the chapter references and the Selected Reading List, for this book, or any book, is a distillation of their contribution to our knowledge. In particular we extend our thanks to Lauralee Lutz and Richard Thirlby. The copyediting by Patricia H. Gross, the editorial supervision by Robert M. Davis, and the support by Fred Belliveau of Little, Brown and Company have been outstanding.

W. C. G.
J. W. S.

Contributing Authors

Jerome E. Adamson, M.D.
Professor of Plastic Surgery, Eastern Virginia Medical School; Chief of Plastic Surgery, DePaul and Medical Center Hospitals, Norfolk, Virginia
Chapters 37, 53

Joseph Agris, D.D.S., M.D.
Cora and Mading Department of Surgery, Division of Plastic Surgery, Baylor College of Medicine; Chief of Surgery, Texas Institute of Rehabilitation, Houston, Texas
Chapter 31

James L. Baker, Jr., M.D.
Chief of Plastic Surgery, Holiday Hospital, Orlando, Florida
Chapter 44

Ralph Blocksma, M.D.
Clinical Professor of Surgery, Michigan State University College of Human Medicine, East Lansing, Michigan; Chief, Plastic Surgery Division, Butterworth Hospital, Grand Rapids, Michigan
Chapter 3

William W. Blackburn, II, M.D.
Private Practice, Atlanta, Georgia
Chapter 46

Silas Braley, Jr., B.S.
Former Director, Dow Corning Center for Aid to Medical Research, Dow Corning Corporation, Midland, Michigan
Chapter 3

Burt Brent, M.D.
Assistant Clinical Professor and Research Adviser in Plastic Surgery, Stanford University Medical Center, Pala Alto, California
Chapter 13

Harry J. Buncke, Jr., M.D.
Associate Clinical Professor – Surgery, University of California Medical School; Co-director, Microsurgical Research Laboratory and Member of Surgical Staff, Ralph K. Davies Medical Center, San Francisco, California
Chapter 40

Ronald R. Cameron, M.D.
Assistant Clinical Professor of Surgery, George Washington University Hospital, Washington, D.C.; Attending Surgeon and Chief, Department of Surgery, Montgomery General Hospital, Olney, Maryland
Chapter 14

James H. Carraway, M.D.
Associate Professor of Plastic Surgery, Eastern Virginia Medical School; Chief of Plastic Surgery, Medical Center Hospitals, Norfolk, Virginia
Chapter 53

Salvador Castañares, M.S., M.D.
University of Southern California School of Medicine; Past Senior and Chief of Plastic Surgery Department, Plastic Surgery Division, Hospital of the Good Samaritan, Los Angeles, California
Chapter 19

Richard J. Coburn, D.M.D., M.D.
Senior Clinical Instructor, Department of Surgery, Mount Sinai School of Medicine of the City University of New York, New York, New York
Chapter 11

Bard Cosman, M.D.
Professor of Clinical Surgery, Columbia University; Attending Surgeon, Division of Plastic Surgery, Presbyterian Hospital, New York, New York
Chapter 15

Lester M. Cramer, D.M.D., M.D.
Attending Plastic Surgeon, Department of Surgery, Penrose Hospital, Colorado Springs, Colorado
Chapter 17

Thomas D. Cronin, M.D.
Clinical Professor, Plastic Surgery, Baylor College of Medicine; Attending and Director, Plastic Surgery Residency Program, St. Joseph Hospital, Houston, Texas
Chapter 47

Norris K. Culf, Jr., M.D.
Associate Director, National Board of Medical Examiners, Philadelphia, Pennsylvania
Chapter 17

Raymond M. Curtis, M.D.
Associate Professor of Plastic Surgery and Associate Professor of Orthopaedic Surgery, The Johns Hopkins Hospital; Chief, Division of Hand Surgery, The Union Memorial Hospital, Baltimore, Maryland
Chapter 34

Rollin K. Daniel, M.D., M.Sc., F.R.C.S. (C)
Associate Professor of Surgery, McGill University; Chief of Plastic Surgery, Royal Victoria Hospital, Montreal, Canada
Chapter 41

Charles J. Devine, Jr., M.D.
Chairman and Professor of Urology, Eastern Virginia Medical School; Attending Urologist, Medical Center Hospitals and DePaul Hospital, Norfolk, Virginia
Chapter 53

Richard K. Dortzbach, M.D.
Assistant Clinical Professor of Ophthalmology, University of Wisconsin Medical School, Madison, Wisconsin
Chapter 10

Bruce J. Dubin, M.D.
Acting Instructor of Surgery (Plastic and Reconstructive Surgery), Stanford University School of Medicine, Stanford, California
Chapters 55 and 56

Richard G. Eaton, M.D.
Associate Professor of Surgery, Columbia University College of Physicians and Surgeons; Co-Chief Hand Service, Roosevelt Hospital, New York, New York
Chapter 33

Frederick R. Eilber, M.D.
Associate Professor of Surgery, University of California, Los Angeles, School of Medicine, Los Angeles, California
Chapter 27

John Gibney, M.D.
Clinical Associate, Phoenix Plastic Surgery Residency, Phoenix, Arizona
Chapter 25

Edward W. Gibson, M.S., F.R.A.C.S.
Lecturer in Plastic Surgery, University of Sydney; Head, Department of Plastic Surgery, Royal Prince Alfred Hospital, Sydney, Australia
Chapter 26

William C. Grabb, M.D.
Professor of Surgery (Plastic Surgery) and Head of the Section of Plastic Surgery, The University of Michigan Medical School; Staff Surgeon, University of Michigan Hospital, Ann Arbor, Michigan
Editor; Chapters 1 and 4

B. Herold Griffith, M.D.
Professor of Surgery and Chief, Division of Plastic Surgery, Northwestern University Medical School; Senior Attending Plastic Surgeon: Northwestern Memorial Hospital, Children's Memorial Hospital, Rehabilitation Institute of Chicago, and Veterans Administration Lakeside Hospital, Chicago, Illinois
Chapter 50

Randolph H. Guthrie, M.D.
Associate Professor of Surgery, Cornell University Medical College; Associate Attending Surgeon, The New York Medical Hospital, New York, New York
Chapter 39

Dwight C. Hanna, M.D.
Chief, Division of Plastic Surgery, University of Pittsburgh School of Medicine; Western Pennsylvania Hospital, Pittsburgh, Pennsylvania
Chapter 16

Shattuck W. Hartwell, Jr., M.D.
Department of Plastic Surgery, Cleveland Clinic Foundation, Cleveland, Ohio
Chapter 25

E. Carmack Holmes, M.D.
Associate Professor of Surgery, Division of Oncology, Department of Surgery, University of California, Los Angeles, School of Medicine, Los Angeles, California
Chapter 27

John E. Hoopes, M.D.
Professor of Surgery (Plastic Surgery), The Johns Hopkins University School of Medicine; Plastic Surgeon-in-Charge, The Johns Hopkins Hospital, Baltimore, Maryland
Chapter 18

Charles E. Horton, M.D.
Chairman and Professor of Plastic Surgery, Eastern Virginia Medical School; Director, Eastern Virginia Graduate School of Medicine, Norfolk, Virginia
Chapter 53

Julius A. Howell, M.D.
Attending Surgeon, Section on Plastic and Reconstructive Surgery, Bowman Gray School of Medicine of Wake Forest University, Winston-Salem, North Carolina
Chapter 54

John T. Hueston, M.S., F.R.C.S., F.R.A.C.S.
Consultant Plastic Surgeon, Royal Melbourne Hospital, Melbourne, Victoria, Australia
Chapter 38

Lynn D. Ketchum, M.D.
Consultant to Hand Rehabilitation Center, Suburban Medical Center, Overland Park, Kansas
Chapter 30

Harold E. Kleinert, M.D.
Clinical Professor of Surgery, University of Louisville School of Medicine; Attending Surgeon, Jewish Hospital, Louisville, Kentucky
Chapter 43

Donald R. Laub, M.D.
Associate Professor of Surgery; Stanford University School of Medicine, Chief, Division of Plastic and Reconstructive Surgery, Stanford University Medical Center, Stanford, California
Chapters 55 and 56

Graham D. Lister, M.B., F.R.C.S.
Clinical Assistant Professor of Plastic Surgery, University of Louisville School of Medicine; Attending Surgeon, Jewish Hospital, Louisville, Kentucky
Chapter 43

Jorge Lopez-Garcia, M.D.
Department of Plastic Surgery, National University of Mexico, Ciudad Universitaria, Mexico City, Mexico; Attending Staff, Hospital Espanol de Mexico, Polanco, Mexico
Chapter 26

Allan L. Lorincz, M.D.
Professor of Medicine, University of Chicago/The Pritzker School of Medicine; Head, Section of Medicine, Los Angeles, Dermatology, University of Chicago Hospitals, Chicago, Illinois
Chapter 29

J. B. Lynch, M.D.
Professor and Chairman, Department of Plastic Surgery, Vanderbilt University School of Medicine, Vanderbilt University Medical Center; Professor and Chairman, Department of Plastic Surgery, Vanderbilt University Hospital, Nashville, Tennessee
Chapter 24

John M. Markley, Jr., M.D.
Clinical Assistant Professor, Section of Plastic Surgery, Department of Surgery, The University of Michigan Medical School; Primary Active Staff, St. Joseph's Mercy Hospital, Ann Arbor, Michigan
Chapter 32

John B. McCraw, M.D.
Associate Professor of Plastic Surgery, Eastern Virginia Medical School; Director, Plastic Surgery Residency Program, Eastern Virginia Graduate School of Medicine, Norfolk, Virginia
Chapter 49

Paul K. McKissock, M.D.
Assistant Clinical Professor, Department of Surgery, University of California, Los Angeles, School of Medicine, Los Angeles, California
Chapter 45

D. Ralph Millard, Jr., M.D.
Light-Millard Professor of Plastic Surgery and Chief, Division of Plastic Surgery, University of Miami School of Medicine, Miami, Florida
Chapter 7

Timothy A. Miller, M.D.
Associate Professor of Surgery/Plastic, University of California, Los Angeles, School of Medicine; Chief, Plastic Surgery, Wadsworth Veterans Administration Hospital, Los Angeles, California
Chapter 51

Hanno Millesi, M.D.
Professor of Plastic and Reconstructive Surgery, University of Vienna; Head, Department of Plastic and Reconstructive Surgery, Surgical University Clinic, Vienna, Austria
Chapter 42

Donald L. Morton, M.D.
Professor of Surgery and Chief, Division of Oncology, University of California, Los Angeles, School of Medicine, Los Angeles, California
Chapter 27

Ian R. Munro, M.A., M.B., B.Chir., F.R.C.S. (C)
Assistant Professor, Department of Surgery, University of Toronto Faculty of Medicine; Division of Plastic Surgery, Sunnybrook Hospital and The Hospital for Sick Children, Toronto, Canada
Chapter 5

John C. Mustardé, F.R.C.S.
Emeritus lecturer in Plastic Surgery, Glasgow University; Emeritus Consultant Plastic Surgeon, West of Scotland Plastic Surgery Unit, Canniesburn Hospital, Glasgow, Scotland
Chapter 12

Paul Natvig, D.D.S., M.D.
Associate Professor of Plastic and Reconstructive Surgery, The Medical College of Wisconsin, Milwaukee, Wisconsin; Chief of Plastic Surgery, Veterans Administration Hospital, Wood, Wisconsin
Chapter 10

Jorge Niklison, M.D.
Buenos Aires, Argentina
Chapter 15

Robert M. Oneal, M.D.
Clinical Associate Professor of Surgery (Plastic), University of Michigan Medical School; Staff Surgeon, University Hospital, University of Michigan Medical Center; Head, Department of Plastic Surgery, St. Joseph Mercy Hospital, Ann Arbor, Michigan
Chapter 46

George C. Peck, M.D.
Associate Professor of Plastic Surgery, Temple University School of Medicine, Philadelphia, Pennsylvania; Attending Plastic Surgeon and Director of Department of Plastic Surgery, Beth Israel Hospital, Passaic, New Jersey
Chapter 21

Rex A. Peterson, M.D.
Director, Phoenix Plastic Surgery Residency, Chief of Plastic Surgery, Arizona Children's Hospital, Good Samaritan Hospital and Maricopa County General Hospital, Phoenix, Arizona
Chapter 25

Austin D. Potenza, M.D.
Attending Plastic Surgeon, Sunrise Hospital, and Desert Springs Hospital, Las Vegas, Nevada
Chapter 37

Peter Randall, M.D.
Professor of Plastic Surgery, University of Pennsylvania, School of Medicine; Acting Chief, Division of Plastic Surgery, Hospital of the University of Pennsylvania, Philadelphia, Pennsylvania
Chapter 8

Thomas D. Rees, M.D.
Clinical Professor of Surgery (Plastic), New York University Medical Center, Chairman, Department of Plastic Surgery, Manhattan Eye, Ear, and Throat Hospital, New York, New York
Chapter 11

Paule Regnault, M.D.
Private practice, Montreal, Canada
Chapter 52

Kenneth Rothaus, M.D.
Chief Resident, Plastic Surgery, The New York Hospital – Cornell Medical Center, New York, New York
Selected Reading List

Richard C. Schultz, M.D.
Professor of Surgery and Chairman, Division of Plastic Surgery, Abraham Lincoln College of Medicine, University of Illinois; Chicago, Illinois; Head, Division of Plastic and Reconstructive Surgery, Lutheran General Hospital, Park Ridge, Illinois
Chapter 9

Jack H. Sheen, M.D.
Assistant Clinical Professor, Department of Surgery, Division of Plastic Surgery, University of California, Los Angeles, School of Medicine, Los Angeles, California
Chapter 22

Bernard E. Simon, M.D.
Clinical Professor of Surgery, Mount Sinai School of Medicine; Attending Surgeon and Chief of Division of Plastic Surgery, Mount Sinai Medical Center, New York, New York
Chapter 48

James W. Smith, M.D.
Associate Professor of Clinical Surgery, Cornell University Medical College; Associate Attending Surgeon, The New York Hospital – Cornell Medical Center, New York, New York
Editor; Chapters 20, 35, 36, and 39

Richard A. Sperling, M.D.
Fellow in Hand Surgery, The Roosevelt Hospital, New York, New York
Chapter 33

Melvin Spira, M.D.
Professor and Head, Division of Plastic Surgery, Baylor College of Medicine, Houston, Texas
Chapter 6

Sten J. Stenström
Professor of Plastic Surgery, University of Benghazi Medical School; Consultant Plastic Surgeon, Al-Jalaa Hospital, Benghazi, Libya
Chapter 23

Zoltan Szabo
Technical Director, Multidisciplinary Microsurgical Laboratory, Ralph K. Davies Medical Center, San Francisco, California
Chapter 40

Noel Thompson, M.S., F.R.C.S.
Consultant Surgeon, Regional Plastic Surgery Centre, Mount Vernon Hospital, Northwood, Middlesex, England
Chapter 2

Hugh G. Thomson, M.D., M.S., F.R.C.S. (C)
Associate Professor of Surgery, University of Toronto; Plastic Surgery Department, The Hospital for Sick Children, Toronto, Canada
Chapter 28

Luis O. Vasconez, M.D.
Professor of Surgery and Chief, Divison of Plastic Surgery, University of California, San Francisco, School of Medicine, San Francisco, California
Chapter 49

Harvey A. Zarem, M.D.
Professor of Surgery, University of California, Los Angeles, School of Medicine; Chief, Division of Plastic and Reconstructive Surgery, UCLA Medical Center, Los Angeles, California
Chapter 29

I

General

1

Basic Techniques of Plastic Surgery

WILLIAM C. GRABB

The techniques of plastic surgery are most often applied to the skin and soft tissues. In their most basic form they relate to the *excision of skin lesions, closure of skin wounds, skin grafts, flaps,* and *Z-plasty*.

EXCISION OF SKIN LESIONS

Factors in Obtaining a Fine Line Scar

The final appearance of the scar after the excision of a lesion depends on a great number of factors. Of importance are the use of atraumatic technique, the placement of the scar in the same direction as skin lines, the age of the patient, the region of the body, the type of skin, and such complicating factors as skin disorders and infection.

Atraumatic Technique

Careful handling of tissues is essential if one is to obtain a fine linear scar and maintain function. Skin and the subcutaneous tissues that have been crushed, dried by exposure to the air, damaged with hot sponges, or strangled by a suture under too much tension will undergo some degree of necrosis. The necrotic cells may serve as a culture medium for infection and at least will be replaced by scar.

The concept of care for skin and subcutaneous tissue should be a histological one [5]. All cells, whether of epidermal, fibrous, elastic, or fatty origin, are served by a network of blood vessels, lymphatics, and nerves. The simple crushing effect of a forceps or hemostat causes an appreciable amount of trauma to both cells and vessels, resulting in a loss of protoplasm, blood, and lymph into the interstitial spaces. Destroyed or damaged cells provide the substance on which organisms can multiply, create sepsis, and destroy more tissue. An atraumatic technique aids in minimizing this trauma. Sharp knives, scissors, needles, and skin hooks, as well as sutures of the proper size, swaged to a needle, are all important to this end.

Even the normal tremor of the surgeon's hand can be detrimental. Both the operator and his assistant should brace their elbows against their bodies (or the arm board in hand surgery) or brace their hands on the patient whenever possible to reduce this tremor. This is similar to the bracing which we do every day when we write at a desk.

Hot sponges have no place in atraumatic surgery. They increase not only capillary bleeding [26] but also, as the applied heat approaches 66°C. (the temperature produced by electric sponge basin warmers), the incidence of wound infection [16]. Such infections are probably the direct result of an increase in tissue necrosis caused by heat.

Skin Lines

Mature, fine linear scars result from excisions or incisions planned so that the final scar lies in, or parallel to, the adjacent skin lines. Borges [3] has written extensively about skin lines and has listed 36 descriptive terms in the literature, including changing dimension lines, dynamic facial lines, force lines, Langer lines, Kocher lines, and relaxed skin tension lines. It is my observation that scars are less conspicuous if they follow *any* skin line. If there are conflicting directions of two or more lines, it is preferable to follow the relaxed skin tension line. An example of this line can be seen on the volar surface of the forearm, where the skin lines formed between a wide pinch with thumb and forefinger are longitudinal when the elbow is extended, but horizontal with the elbow flexed and the skin *relaxed.* In areas without skin lines, such as the open plain of the cheek of a young person, scars can be especially noticeable.

As a practical matter, scars will be least conspicuous when the following factors are considered:

WRINKLE LINES (INCLUDING THE LINES OF FACIAL EXPRESSION AND THE RELAXED SKIN TENSION LINES). The wrinkle lines of the skin generally lie perpendicular to the long axis of the underlying muscles and are caused by the wrinkling that accompanies muscular contraction [14]. Wrinkle lines of the face, known as the *lines of expression* [12] (Fig. 1-1), develop in a rather predictable pattern and are frequently used as a criterion for judging a person's age. The lines of facial expression are accentuated with smiling, grimacing, frowning, pursing the lips, and closing the eyes tightly. If for some reason these active responses are not possible, the skin can be approximated passively with a wide pinch of the thumb and index finger in various directions (relaxed skin tension lines). In this way the most prominent ridges and furrows will be produced in the natural wrinkle lines of the skin. In most instances, these relaxed skin tension lines will be the same as the lines of facial expression. Wrinkle lines in many parts of the body can best be seen by having the patient flex or extend the part.

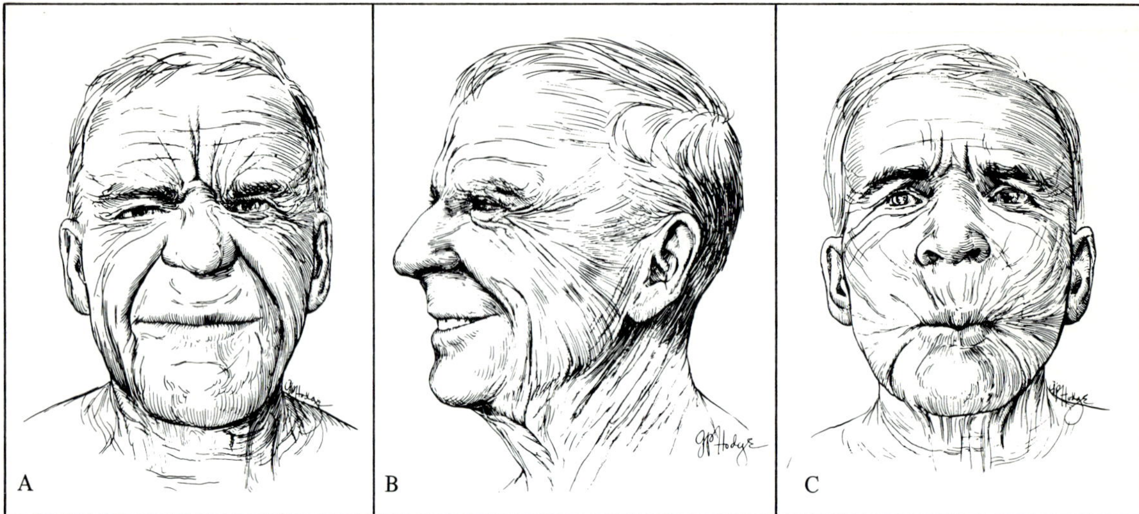

Fig. 1-1. Skin lines – the lines of facial expression, contour lines, and lines of dependency.

CONTOUR LINES. Contour lines are the lines of division at the juncture of body planes [20]. Examples are found at the juncture of the cheek with the nose, the cheek with the ear, the scalp with the ear, the skin of the lips with the vermilion (vermilion-cutaneous line), the cheek and neck skin in the submandibular region, and the juncture of the inferior aspect of the breast with the chest wall (inframammary fold). A favorite place to hide a scar is in the horizontal wrinkle line just under the chin, where it is usually out of sight.

LINES OF DEPENDENCY. The lines of dependency occur in older people due to the effect of gravity on loose skin and fatty tissue. The "turkey gobbler fold" in the submental region and the more laterally located jowl lines of the submandibular region are typical lines of dependency. The cross-hatching pattern of lines on the facial skin of elderly persons is partly due to the intersection of lines of dependency and lines of facial expression [20].

CONCEALING SCARS IN THE HAIR OF THE SCALP OR EYEBROW. This is an excellent way to camouflage a scar. Incisions in the lateral aspect of an eyebrow can be used for removing dermoid cysts from the lateral supraorbital rim and for internal wiring of fractures of the zygomaticofrontal suture line. The skin in this region is mobile, a factor that aids exposure even if the operative area does not lie exactly beneath the incision.

Scars located at the juncture of the scalp and facial skin are often poorly concealed because the fine hairs in this region are too short and sparse. However, in women this is not so much of a problem as the hair usually can be arranged to hide such scars. Scalp scars in men can be uncovered by progressing degrees of baldness.

In many areas of the body scars can be covered by clothing. This is particularly true for men, in whom scars on the lower neck, supraclavicular region, and extremities are covered by collars, shirts with sleeves, and trousers.

Age of the Patient

Children's scars can remain erythematous and hypertrophic for prolonged periods of time, and the final result may be less satisfactory under these circumstances. In general, such scars have a less desirable final appearance than scars of persons of middle age and older. A time lapse of two years or more is important to allow the normal process of maturation to alter the raised red scar into a flat white one.

Regions of the Body

Scars resulting from excisions or incisions in the eyelids, palms, soles, and in the vermilion or mucous membranes are usually finer and less conspicuous than those seen elsewhere [6]. This is especially true when contrasted with such areas as the sternal area, shoulder, and back. Before incisions are made in these areas, the patient should be warned that the scar will probably become hypertrophic. Particularly disappointing are scars of the sternal region in women, where a butterfly-shaped keloid often develops. When a keloid in this region is excised, a new and larger one may recur in its place. A further discussion of scars and keloids can be found in Chapter 29.

Length of Scar
In general the smaller the wound, the less disfiguring the scar will be. A long straight scar may contract, producing bowstringing and hypertrophy that would not occur with multiple small scars or a long scar composed of small segments running in different directions in an accordion-like fashion [3].

U-Shaped Scar
This scar is notorious in that it contracts to become a depressed groove circumscribing a bulging, convex circle of skin.

Angle of Wound to Skin Surface
The more oblique the incision to the skin surface is, the greater the width of the scar in the dermis. This dermal scar will then contract, causing the overlying skin to bulge. The thicker the skin, the greater is the deformity, so that while the scar is significant in the forehead, it is not a problem in the eyelid [3].

Type of Skin
Some patients have thick, oily skin which contains hypertrophied and overactive sebaceous glands. Wounds in this type of skin may heal with a very noticeable depressed scar. Skin with these characteristics may be present over the distal half of the nose, the middle portion of cheeks, and the forehead.

Skin Disorders
Patients who have abnormalities in their fibrous and elastic tissues often develop wide scars. Patients with this fibroelastic diathesis can usually be detected preoperatively by looking for hyperextensibility of the fingers or by pinching and elevating the skin over the back of the hand to demonstrate increased elasticity. The Ehlers-Danlos syndrome is a severe form of this fibroelastic disorder in which the skin heals very slowly and with a wide scar.

Methods of Excision
Lesions of the skin can be removed by elliptical, wedge, T, or circular excision.

Elliptical Excision
This is the technique most often used for excising skin lesions. Either a simple elliptical excision may suffice or multiple elliptical excisions (multiple excision technique) may be required, depending on the case.

The width of skin that can be excised varies enormously between young and old, between thin and corpulent, and of course in different regions of the body. The experienced plastic surgeon is continually, almost automatically, estimating this factor by noting the wrinkling and aging characteristics of the skin, by picking up the skin between his thumb and index finger, and by looking for the skin tension lines.

SIMPLE ELLIPTICAL EXCISION. Ideally, an ellipse (i.e., a "surgeon's ellipse" or lenticular configuration, for a true ellipse is rounded at each end rather than angular) should be planned so that its long axis parallels a wrinkle line, contour line, or line of dependency (Fig. 1-2), and ideally the long axis should be about four times as great as the short axis. If the long axis becomes too short, its sides form too great an angle with one another, and excess bunching of skin, known as a *dog ear,* will result when the wound is closed (Fig. 1-2A, 1-3A). A dog ear can also result if one side of the ellipse is much longer than the other (i.e., one side approaching a semicircle and the other side a straight line) (Fig. 1-3B). Dog ears tend to flatten over a period of several months but should be excised if they persist.

The dog ear resulting from the short, broad ellipse can be corrected simply by extending the ellipse to include the excess tissue (Fig. 1-3A). When it is due to one side of the incision being longer than the other, it can be corrected by making a short, right-angled

Fig. 1-2. Elliptical excision. If the ellipse is too short (A), dog ears (arrows) will form at the ends of the closed wound. The correct method is shown in B.

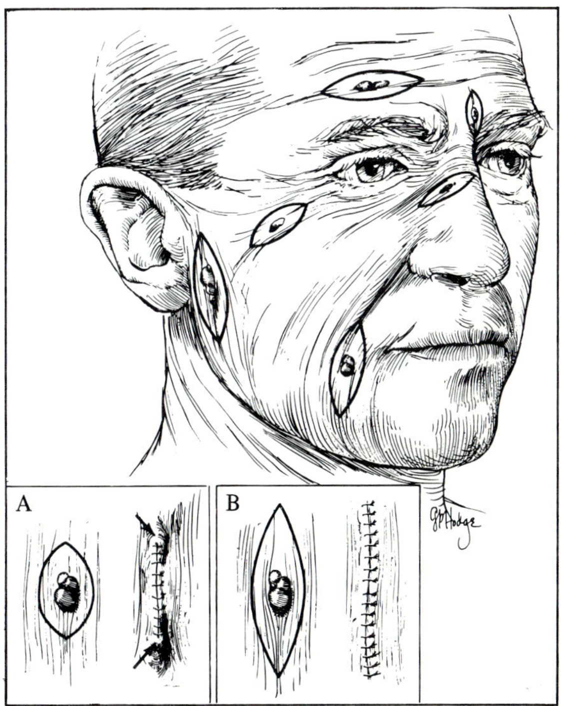

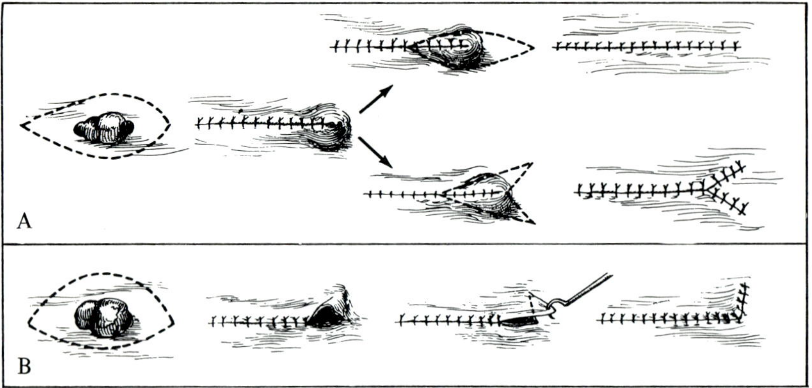

Fig. 1-3. A, two methods of removing a dog ear caused by making the elliptical excision too short. B, method of removing dog ear caused by making one side of the ellipse longer than the other.

incision at the end of the ellipse. The excess skin will overlap at the wound edge and can be trimmed away, permitting wound closure in the shape of an L (Fig. 1-3B).

Occasionally a scar curved slightly more than usual is needed to parallel closely a curved wrinkle, contour, or dependency line. This can be accomplished by increasing the curve on the side of the ellipse that most closely duplicates the curve of the skin line. The other side of the ellipse should be made as straight as possible. The skin must be distributed evenly in the closure of this wound to prevent a dog ear.

MULTIPLE EXCISION TECHNIQUE. This technique can be employed for the excision of certain larger skin lesions. The theory behind it is based on the fact that skin which has been placed on tension (i.e., following elliptical excision and wound closure) becomes looser over a period of months. This relaxation permits the remaining part of the lesion to be excised in multiple stages [17, 19]. Gibson and Kenedi [283] have noted that a certain amount of skin relaxation and stretch occur. There is a definite tendency at the time of a second excision for the wound to retract toward its original shape.

The technique of multiple excision has one of its greatest applications in the excision of non-hair-bearing areas (i.e., skin grafts or scars) of the scalp (Fig. 1-4). A well-planned procedure is necessary to avoid excising such a wide ellipse of tissue that the wound cannot be closed. In incising a large burn scar, for example, the initial incision can be made along one side, between the scar and normal tissue. The incision should be carried down to the loose areolar tissue beneath the galea aponeurotica. The scalp can then be undermined extensively at the level of the loose areolar layer and pulled medially over the portion to be excised. The scar should be marked with methylene blue along this line and then be excised. Closure of the wound is necessary before the procedure is repeated on the opposite side of the non-hair-bearing portion of the scalp. Several months should then be allowed to pass to permit the scalp to loosen up enough before further excision. Massage of the scalp during this interval may aid in loosening it. Anywhere from two to five operations may be required to move the non-hair-bearing area from the scalp, depending on its size.

The multiple excision technique has a more limited application for removing nevi, hemangioma, scars, radiation dermatitis, and other large lesions of the facial skin because distortion of the eyebrows, eyelids, nostrils, and lips may result from too extensive an excision adjacent to these structures, placing abnormal tension on them [21]. The lateral deviation of the nose toward a cheek where a lesion has been excised in multiple stages is not an uncommon sequela in children and young adults. In children, excessive serial excisions of skin overlying the malar prominence, nose, or chin may even retard the growth of bone in these regions. The lateral aspect of the cheek is the most favorable area of the face for employing the technique of multiple excision, as it is well away from eyelids, nose, and lips.

The use of the Z-plasty, rotation skin flaps, and skin grafts will increase the effectiveness of multiple excisions. The Z-plasty can be used to transpose normal tissue into a critical area, such as the lip, the nose, or an eyelid, and at the same time move pathological tissue to a position where it can be more easily excised at a subsequent stage. The Z-plasty can also be used to break up contracted lines of scar. Skin flaps may be rotated in from an adjacent area, such as the neck, in order to permit further excision of the lesion. Full-thickness skin grafts to the lower eye-

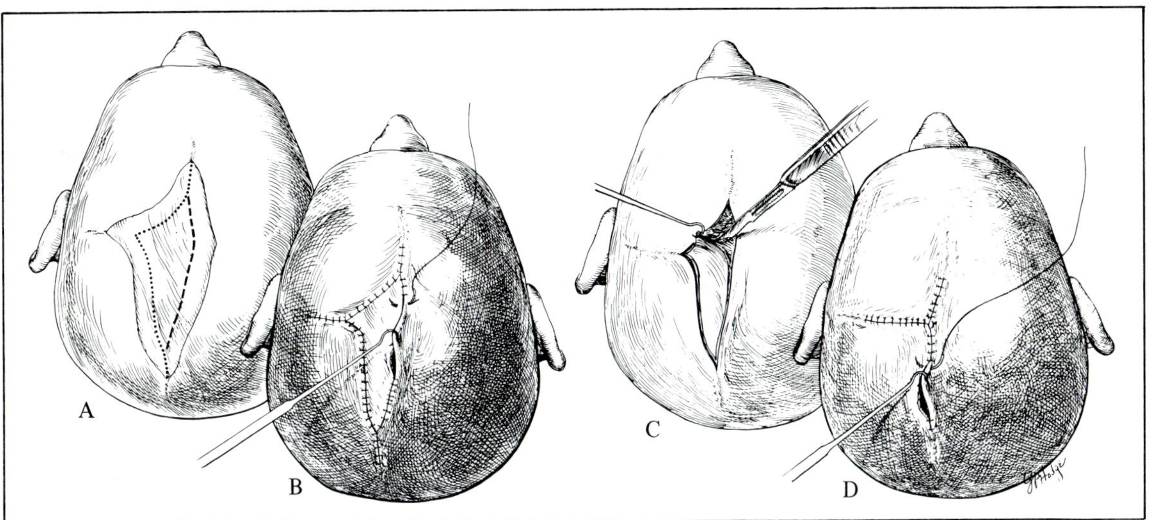

Fig. 1-4. Multiple excision technique. A and B, the first-stage excision. C and D, the second-stage excision several months later.

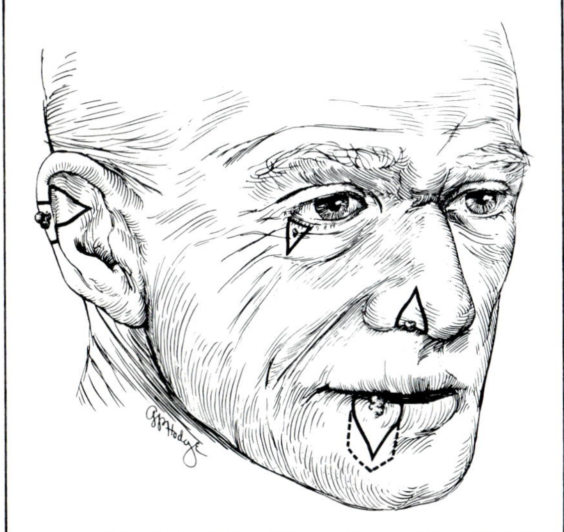

Fig. 1-5. Wedge excision. On the eyelid it may be possible to incise just below the lash line, removing only skin, though some lesions require the removal of the full eyelid thickness. On the ear, a notching of the helical rim can be prevented by stepping the limbs of the V at the helix. One-fourth the width of an eyelid or lower lip can be excised completely and simply closed without requiring any elaborate reconstruction.

lid, nasal tip, or lips can be utilized to supplement this procedure.

Wedge Excision

Lesions on, or adjacent to, such free margins of skin as the lips, nostril rim, eyelids, and ears can be excised in the shape of a wedge (Fig. 1-5). There is so much excess tissue in the lower lip that a third of its length can be removed by a wedge excision and the wound closed primarily. The upper lip is not as full as the lower, but primary closure is still possible when one-fourth or less has been excised. Larger defects of the upper lip can be reconstructed with a wedge-shaped Abbe flap from the lower lip. When the lesion of the lip margin is a squamous cell carcinoma, it is usually advisable to execute a block V excision (Fig. 1-5), in order to remove additional tissue in the path of lymphatic drainage. Closure of these wounds requires a careful realignment of the vermilion-cutaneous border.

The wedge excision of lesions of the nostril rim, if too large for primary closure, can be closed with a composite graft of similar size from the rim of the ear. Composite grafts will usually survive if all parts of the graft are within 1 cm. of the blood supply at the margins of the alar defect.

Lesions near the rim of the ear can be excised in the shape of a simple V or with the line of the V stepped at the helix to minimize the effect of scar contracture and to prevent notching at the helical rim following primary closure (Fig. 1-5).

T Excision

When the lesion lies adjacent to an anatomical obstruction such as the alar base, a T excision can be employed. The cross of the T lies in the alar-cheek

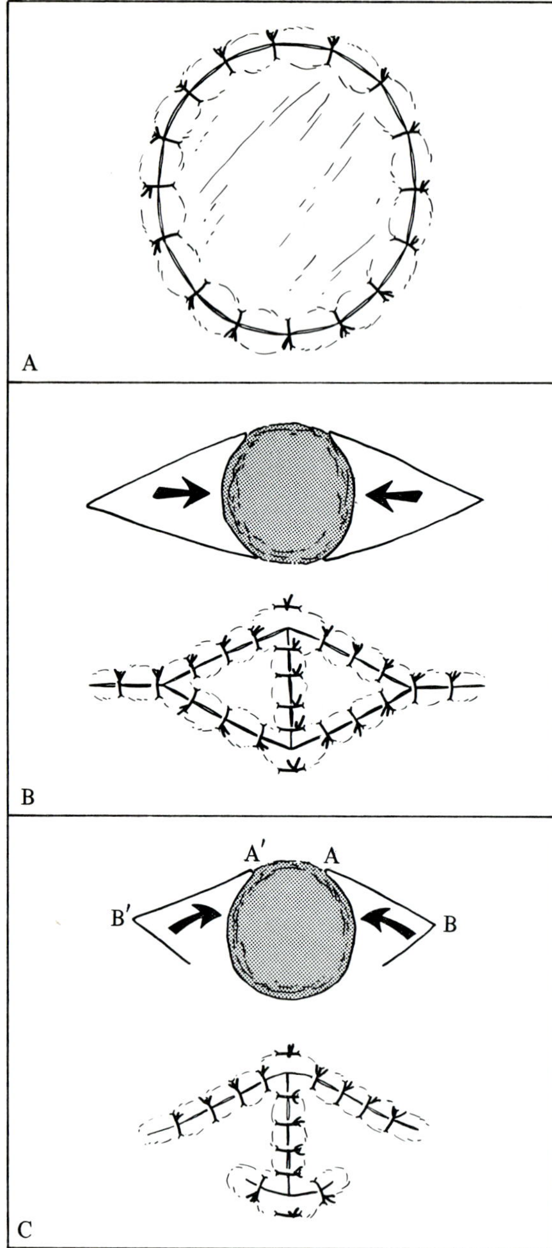

Fig. 1-6. Closure of wounds following circular excision. A, the most common way of closing a circular defect is with a skin graft. B, sliding triangular subcutaneous pedicle flaps can be advanced to close the circular defect; the triangular defect is closed in a V–Y fashion. C, transposition flaps based on a skin pedicle and rotated toward each other can also be used.

crease with the long arm of the T being two-thirds of an ellipse lying perpendicular to the alar base.

Circular Excision
Where the facial skin is closely applied to underlying cartilage, such as over the nasal tip or anterior surface of the auricle, lesions can be excised in a circular fashion and the defect closed with a full-thickness skin graft (Fig. 1-6A). This technique is also employed following the removal of some very large skin lesions on other parts of the body.

Local skin flaps can also be used to close the defect by following a circular excision. One ingenious method of closing a circular wound (e.g., up to 5 cm. diameter on the face of an adult and up to 2.5 cm. diameter on the lower leg) involves sliding subcutaneous pedicle skin flaps (Fig. 1-6B) [22, 24]. Typically, two triangular subcutaneous flaps are planned in the direction of the skin lines on either side of the circular defect. This gives the appearance of a large ellipse until the triangular flaps are advanced and sutured to each other, thus closing the circular defect. The triangular defects are each closed in a V-Y fashion. (Further information on subcutaneous skin flaps is provided in this chapter under the heading, Flaps.) Another local skin flap for this same purpose involves local transposition flaps, one on either side of the circular defect, which are based on a skin pedicle and rotated toward each other to meet and close the defect (Fig. 1-6C).

In planning for an elliptical excision, when there is some doubt as to the direction of the skin lines, a circular excision of the lesion can be employed. Then, by noting the longer axis of the defect created by adjacent skin tensions, the long axis of the ellipse can be determined.

Operative Techniques of Excising Skin Lesions

Instruments
Fine, sharp, single- and double-pronged skin hooks, sharp scissors, detachable knife blades (#11 and #15), and fine, sharp needles with the suture swaged on are the basic instruments needed for performing excisions with a minimum of trauma. A sturdy but light needle holder with smooth jaws and beveled joints is excellent for suturing and for instrument tying. A small, fine-toothed tissue forceps, such as the Brown-Adson, Thorpe, or Castroviejo forceps, should also be available.

Techniques of Excision

ELLIPTICAL EXCISION. The ellipse is outlined with methylene blue. Before beginning the excision, the surgeon and the assistant should place tension on the surrounding skin to stretch it out. This prevents false cuts and aids in following the lines of excision more accurately. The #15 blade is used to cut through the skin at right angles to its surface so that vertical margins can be approximated in the closure. The X-shaped "over cuts" at the ends of the ellipse can be prevented by starting the incision at the end of the ellipse. Undermining of the wound edges is usually advisable to facilitate wound closure without tension. With skin hooks at each end of the ellipse, undermining is carried out with a single sweep of the #15 blade in the superficial subcutaneous tissue. The edge of the ellipse should be undercut on either side for a distance approximating that of the transverse measurement of the ellipse. A two-layer closure is then carried out: the deep layer is approximated with inverted sutures of fine plain catgut, polyglycolic acid, or fine clear nylon; the skin edges are then approximated.

WEDGE EXCISION. After outlining the wedge with methylene blue, a #15 blade is used to incise only through the skin surface. The tissue is then held firmly on either side of the wedge so that a pointed #11 blade can be passed completely through the tissues, which are then cut with a sawing motion. The wound can be closed in three layers.

CIRCULAR EXCISION. This excision is carried out by simply incising the skin along the previously marked circle with the #15 blade.

Methods of Hemostasis

ELECTROSURGERY. An electrical current of high frequency (2–18 million cycles per second), relatively high amperage, and low voltage will coagulate the wall of a blood vessel to produce hemostasis, coagulation being caused by the heat of the current. Although a small amount of tissue is actually charred by the electrical current, there is no evidence that wound healing is more impaired by this technique than by the use of ligatures.

Electrosurgical techniques probably provide the most rapid and effective method for obtaining hemostasis of medium- and small-sized blood vessels. Trauma can be minimized and coagulation made more effective by bringing the active electrode of the electrosurgical unit into contact with a small hemostat or fine-tipped forceps which is accurately gripping the vessel. A fine-tipped electrode itself can also be used to touch the vessel. This latter method is especially helpful in obtaining the nearly absolute degree of hemostasis necessary in the recipient bed for a skin graft. Suction or frequent sponging aids in obtaining the dry field required for an effective electric current to pass into the tissues.

An understanding of the *physics of high-frequency currents* is helpful to the surgeon. Electrosurgery depends on the heating effect of certain electrical currents to produce thermocauterization. Electrical currents that oscillate at frequencies greater than a million times per second can be passed through the human body without causing the severe muscular contractions associated with low-frequency currents.

The dampened wave current produced by a spark gap is especially effective for electrosurgical coagulation. The nature of this dampened wave is such that each succeeding oscillation after the first diminishes until zero is reached. The condensers of the electrosurgical unit are then very rapidly recharged before they release another discharge of high-frequency current through the circuit [2, 13].

An electrosurgical unit may be either monoterminal or biterminal. A monoterminal unit, such as the Hyfercator, makes use of only an active electrode, with the patient being in circuit through the surrounding environment. Electrical currents from monoterminal units are adequate for obtaining hemostasis. The larger biterminal devices, such as the Bovie units, have both an active electrode and a broad inactive electrode, with the patient being placed in the circuit between them.

Self-contained coagulation units have been developed; equipped with a waterproof enclosed battery, they can be sterilized and used at the operating table as any other unit. Because of the explosion hazard, an electrosurgical unit should not be used in the presence of explosive anesthetic gases such as ether or cyclopropane.

The laser scalpel and the plasma scalpel are high energy scalpels that both incise and coagulate. These are still in an experimental stage [15].

LIGATURE. The ligation of blood vessels with fine suture materials is another way of effecting hemostasis. Bleeding vessels are clamped accurately with fine-pointed hemostats. A suture can be either simply tied about the vessel or, for a more secure ligation, passed on a needle through the immediately adjacent tissue before being tied.

Catgut sutures of sizes 4-0 and 5-0 are suitable for ligating small- and medium-sized vessels. Larger vessels should be tied with nonabsorbable sutures. Catgut sutures are preferred by many for ligating blood vessels and approximating deeper layers of tissue because their absorption minimizes the possibility of a late and prolonged reaction and extrusion of the suture.

PRESSURE AND TIME. Sustained pressure on the wound can effectively control capillary oozing. The pressure probably acts to occlude the capillaries until coagulation occurs. It is best to apply pressure for 5 minutes by the clock because there is usually a tendency to underestimate time elapsed. If the recipient bed for a skin graft continues to bleed uncontrollably, a pressure dressing may be applied for 24 to 48 hours before the skin is placed on the wound. This is termed *delayed skin grafting.*

CLAMPING AND TWISTING OF SMALL BLOOD VESSELS. Although this method avoids the introduction of foreign material into the wound, it is not truly reliable for hemostasis.

VASOCONSTRICTORS. Epinephrine continues to be the best vasoconstrictor for surgical procedures. The injection of epinephrine in a solution as dilute as 1 : 500,000 has been shown to provide excellent hemostasis if the surgeon is patient enough to wait several minutes until the first vasoconstrictive effect is manifest [9, 18]. Epinephrine solutions of 1 : 100,000 and 1 : 200,000 are commercially available in combination with local anesthetic agents, but more dilute solutions should be made up fresh because they are sensitive to oxidative degradation and a pH over 5.5. Epinephrine 1 : 500,000 can be prepared at the time of operation by adding a 1 ml. ampule of 1 : 1,000 epinephrine to 500 ml. of 5% dextrose in water (pH of 4.0). Large volumes of epinephrine solution are especially helpful in operations requiring a wide dissection of tissue. For example, I use 75 to 100 ml. of epinephrine 1 : 500,000 per breast when performing a reduction mammoplasty, and 50 to 75 ml. per side when performing a facelift.

Topical epinephrine (1 : 100,000) can be applied to an open wound on a moistened sponge to diminish bleeding from small vessels.

FIBRIN FOAM, GELATIN FOAM, AND MICROCRYSTALLINE COLLAGEN. These materials can be used as hemostatic agents, especially for packing a small cavity from which there is a constant oozing of blood. The fibrin foam is prepared from human fibrinogen and thrombin, while the gelatin foam is prepared from an absorbable gelatin. Small pieces of these foams are readily absorbed in the tissues with minimal reaction. Microcrystalline collagen is a white flourlike substance with remarkable hemostatic properties [1].

CLOSURE OF SKIN WOUNDS

Wounds can be closed with sutures, skin tapes, skin clips, or wound adhesives. These foreign materials act to hold the wound edges in approximation until the wound's tensile strength is increased to a degree sufficient to maintain wound closure without assistance.

Sutures

Type of Suture Material

Sutures are generally considered as being either absorbable (catgut and polyglycolic acid) or nonabsorbable (nylon, Dacron, polypropylene, silk, cotton, and stainless steel). They can also be judged in regard to their tensile strength, tissue reaction, pliability, knot-holding ability, capillary (or wick) action, and economy.

Sutures may be monofilament or have multiple filaments that are braided or twisted to form the suture. Nonabsorbable sutures may be coated with a medical grade of silicone (on silk), Teflon (on braided Dacron), or other synthetic materials to make them smoother or less reactive. The suture may have a cutting or noncutting needle swaged on one end, or it may have to be threaded through the eye of a needle in order to be used for wound closure.

With such a wide variation of suture materials, there is bound to be a difference of opinion as to which is the best. Those interested in rackets and rods are said to hold similar differences of opinion about strings and lines.

ABSORBABLE SUTURES. Sutures made of collagen or polyglycolic acid are capable of being digested by body enzymes. Thus they are frequently used as buried sutures to close the subcutaneous tissue layer or to repair mucous membranes. Because it is advantageous in children to be able to avoid the mechanical removal of skin sutures, absorbable sutures have also been used to suture skin grafts in place or to close skin wounds.

Catgut is the most common absorbable suture and is made from collagen of the submucosal layer of the small intestine of sheep and the serosal layer of the small intestine of cattle [47]. An extruded collagen suture has been developed by dispersing the collagen from flexor tendons of cattle and then extruding it to form a much more uniform, more pliable, and stronger suture [47].

A *plain catgut* suture will be absorbed faster than one that has been hardened by chromicization *(chromic catgut).* The smaller the caliber of the catgut, the faster it is absorbed. Because sutures in certain tissues (e.g., serous and mucous membranes) will be absorbed substantially faster than those in other tissues (e.g., muscle), it is difficult to specify an exact time for complete absorption. It is generally reported, though, as being between 2 weeks and 6 months [43].

Polyglycolic acid (Dexon) is a newer absorbable suture, made by the polymerization of the amino acid glycolic acid which is extruded and stretched to form fibers that are then braided to form the suture. This suture is stronger than catgut of comparable size, has greater knot security, and has an improved "feel" which more closely resembles linen thread. Little or no tissue reaction is produced by the suture, so that it is being used by some as an absorbable skin suture which disintegrates between the fourteenth and thirty-fourth days [11, 27]. This rather rapid disintegration is rated by some as a disadvantage when buried sutures are being relied on for tensile strength. While catgut is absorbed by phagocytosis as a part of its inflammatory response, polyglycolic acid undergoes enzymatic degradation, with little accompanying tissue reaction [42].

NONABSORBABLE SUTURES. Any of the organic sutures (silk or cotton), synthetic sutures (nylon, Dacron, or polypropylene), or metallic sutures (stainless steel) can be used to close the skin. These sutures are stronger and less reactive to the tissues than catgut; 4-0 monofilament nylon, Dacron, polypropylene, and stainless steel are excellent materials for a subcuticular suture because of their tensile strength, low frictional coefficient, and stiffness. Silk and cotton consistently show more tissue reaction than the synthetic sutures [36, 49]. Multifilament sutures are more reactive than the same material in a monofilament suture and are more likely to develop a discharging sinus in the skin wound [49, 104].

Silk, because of its great "knot holding" ability, is often advocated for suturing the mucous membranes and the tongue. It is also used to close the skin adjacent to the eye, as its pliability allows the suture ends to lie flat after the knot is tied. For tie-over dressings, silk is the suture material that is easiest to manage.

Avoiding Suture Marks in the Skin

Suture marks are the permanently imprinted scars of suture material on the skin surface (Fig. 1-7). The studies of Crikelair [32] on this subject are outstanding. Some of the factors that determine the severity of suture marks are the length of time a skin suture is left in place, tension, relationship of the suture to the wound edge, the region of the body, infection, and a propensity for keloid formation.

LENGTH OF TIME THAT A SKIN SUTURE IS LEFT IN PLACE. Crikelair [32] found that the largest suture marks invariably occurred when skin sutures were left in place for about 14 days. The size of the sutures and the needles used to insert them proved unimportant. In contrast, sutures removed within 7 days produced almost no permanent scar.

In the face, it is advisable to remove alternate skin sutures on the third postoperative day and the remaining ones on the fifth. Skin tape or fine mesh gauze and collodion can be used to support the area for several more days. On the extremities and anterior aspect of the trunk, sutures should be left in place for about 7 days to prevent wound disruption. On the back and on the feet, it is almost imperative that some sutures be retained for 10 to 14 days; for this reason, permanent suture marks may remain in the skin.

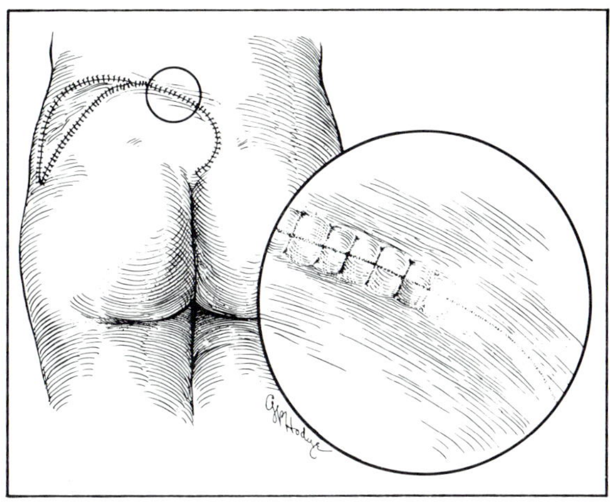

Fig. 1-7. Skin suture marks. The inset illustrates on the left the permanent scar caused by tying sutures too tightly, while there is no scarring on the right when sutures are tied under proper tension. (After Crikelair [32].)

TENSION. Skin suture marks (Fig. 1-7) are frequently caused by sutures tied too tightly or pulling laterally on the wound [32, 48]. It is important to learn to tie a suture just tight enough to approximate the wound edges, but no tighter. During the early postoperative period, edema causes tissues to swell, creating additional tension within the circle of each suture. Wound edges not quite in contact become further approximated in this way. Edges already in contact and under tension are further strangulated by postoperative swelling. The selected suture material should be just a little stronger than necessary to maintain closure of the wound. Fine sutures (4-0, 5-0, and 6-0) encourage closures with less tension than heavier ones.

Lateral pull on the wound results when a large segment of skin has been excised or when muscles are pulling at right angles to the wound. Much of this lateral pull can be eliminated by using subcutaneous sutures to take the tension off the skin and by placing the long axis of the excision parallel to the skin lines.

RELATIONSHIP OF THE SUTURE TO THE WOUND EDGE. When large bites of tissue are taken with the suture, larger suture marks can result because a larger segment of tissue will be subjected to the constricting effect of the suture. These marks can be avoided by keeping the sutures closer to the wound edge.

REGION OF THE BODY. Suture marks are fortunately not common on the face unless basic principles are violated or the skin is heavy with sebaceous glands. Skin suture marks almost never occur on the thin skin of the eyelids and mucous membranes. In contrast, the sternal area, trunk, and extremities (with the exception of the hands and soles of the feet) are common sites for these scars, unless the most precise operative techniques are followed.

INFECTION. Infection about a skin suture can lead to the formation of a suture mark. When such an infection develops, it is best treated by removal of the suture and application of warm moist dressings to the wound. This eliminates any constricting effect, removes the foreign body, increases circulation, and improves drainage. In a study of infection around sutures in experimental wounds (contaminated with *Staphylococcus aureus*), monofilament steel and nylon sutures demonstrated minimal reaction. In these wounds there was increasing reaction around other sutures in the following order: silk, Mersilene, Dexon, and catgut. Monofilament sutures induced less infection than braided sutures [25].

In contaminated experimental wounds, even buried monofilament nylon exerts a significant potentiation of infection as compared to no suture at all [7].

KELOID. In individuals susceptible to the formation of keloids, such a lesion may form at the site where a skin suture is placed. Additional information on this subject can be found in Chapter 30.

Buried Sutures

Both the subcutaneous and the deeper tissues should be sutured in order to obliterate dead space and remove tension from the site of skin repair. For this purpose, plastic surgeons have tried a variety of nonabsorbable and absorbable materials. Franch [39] showed that there were fewer wound infections (7.5 percent) where buried polyethylene (nonabsorbable) suture was used as compared with buried catgut (absorbable) sutures (14.4 percent). There is little doubt that the less foreign material (i.e., smallest size and fewest number of sutures) left in a wound, the more readily and soundly the wound will heal. One of the reasons for this was demonstrated nicely by Elek and Conen [33], who found in human volunteers that to produce a pustule required the intradermal injection of at least two million organisms of *S. pyogenes,* whereas in the presence of a buried suture only a hundred of these organisms were needed to produce a purulent lesion the size of an orange and a reaction so severe that they had great difficulty in finding further volunteers.

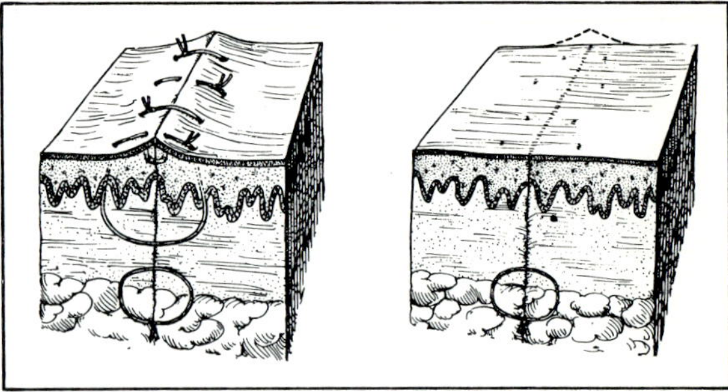

Fig. 1-8. Skin edges that are everted will gradually flatten to produce a level wound surface.

Eversion of Skin Edges

Skin edges that have been *everted* gradually flatten to produce a level wound surface (Fig. 1-8). By comparison, wounds with *inverted* edges will persist as a valley-like scar, trapping the shadows as light is cast across its surface. These shadows make the depressed scar even more noticeable.

Use of the vertical mattress suture (Fig. 1-8) is one effective method for everting the wound edges. The placement of buried sutures in the subcutaneous tissue is also important, because it provides a firmer foundation on which to evert the skin edges. Another way of assuring eversion of the skin edge is to make incisions so that the skin edges slightly overhang the perpendicular. In this way the skin everts automatically as the deeper layer is closed with buried sutures. Occasionally one or more Z-plasties (see Fig. 1-40) will break up a long linear depressed scar to permit eversion of its edges.

Scars crossing the inferior border of the mandible tend to become inverted. This tendency can sometimes be corrected by making an elliptical incision around the scar, denuding it of surface epithelium, undermining the wound edges, and then advancing and closing them over the central buttress of the denuded scar.

Closure of Wound Edges of Unequal Thickness

Occasionally wounds whose edges are of unequal thickness must be sutured. To equalize the two sides, a flap of subcutaneous tissue from the thicker side can be turned under the thinner side. It is best first to undermine both wound edges at the same depth in the superficial subcutaneous tissue. Then a subcutaneous tissue flap of the desired thickness can be advanced from the thicker side across and under the thinner, where it is sutured.

Operative Technique of Suturing Skin Wounds

METHODS OF WOUND SUTURE. Buried sutures aid in closing a wound in layers. The periosteum or perichondrium, the muscular fascia, and the subcutaneous tissue layer should each be closed by suture. It is wise to invert the suture in the subcutaneous layer so that the knot is tied deeply, away from the skin surface (Fig. 1-8).

Another method sometimes used for closing the subcutaneous tissue is the continuous alternating suture. The ends of this suture can be left permanently in the subcutaneous tissue or passed to the surface so that the suture can be removed after 2 or 3 weeks.

Skin sutures can be of several types:

1. The *simple interrupted suture* (Fig. 1-9A) should be inserted so that the needle enters the skin of the first side at an angle of 90 degrees *or greater.* Sufficient subcutaneous tissue is included to aid in eversion of the raw interface. As the needle passes through a comparable amount of subcutaneous tissue on the second side, it begins to angle back toward the wound edge. Ideally, the angle of exit for the needle is the same as its angle of entrance. If the same angle has been achieved, an identical volume of tissue is present within the suture on each side of the wound, and the result should be an exact approximation of the margins. The more accomplished a surgeon becomes in gaining equal amounts of skin and subcutaneous tissue from each side and in angling the needle, the less often will he need mattress sutures to aid in gaining symmetry. The closer the needle lies to the skin edge, the greater will be its effect in controlling the ultimate position of that edge. The number of sutures used in closing any wound will vary with the case, location of the repair, and

Fig. 1-9. Methods of skin suture. See text.

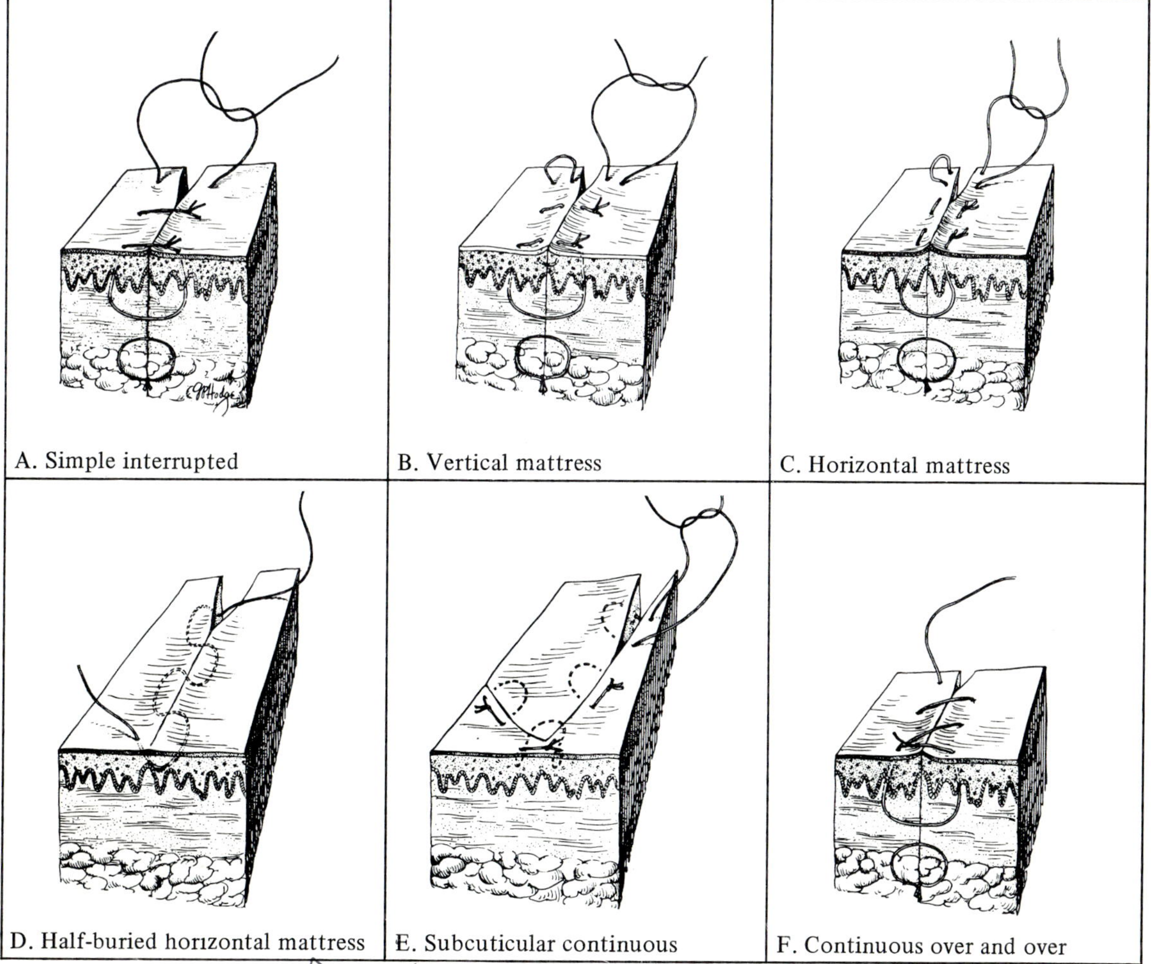

degree of accuracy required by the physician and his patient. In an area such as the face, sutures would probably be placed between 1 and 3 mm. apart and 1 to 2 mm. from the wound edge.

2. The *vertical mattress suture* (Fig. 1-9B) is used principally to assure eversion of skin edges and is unsurpassed for this purpose. A common technique in wound closure is to alternate a vertical mattress with a simple interrupted suture along the length of the wound.
3. The *horizontal mattress suture* (Fig. 1-9C) provides close approximation of the skin edges with some eversion. This can be helpful in closing skin wounds in the hand that are under tension.
4. The *half-buried horizontal mattress suture* (Fig. 1-9D) is very effective for closing the point of a V-shaped wound. The use of this suture often prevents necrosis of the tip of the V, which may follow the use of a simple interrupted suture. This suture is also advantageous for suturing a skin flap into place. The buried portion of the suture lies within the flap so that it effectively holds the flap in place, and yet the danger of damaging the skin by inserting sutures through it is avoided.
5. The *subcuticular* (intradermal) *continuous suture* (Fig. 1-9E) is a very practical and useful method of skin closure. The needle passes horizontally through the dermis, small bites being taken alternately on one side and then the other. As the suture is continued, care must be taken that it is maintained at the same level and that the entrance of each bite is backed up a little to prevent the entrance and exit on opposite sides from being opposite one another. When long wounds are closed by this method, it is well to pass the suture through the skin every 5 to 8 cm. to facilitate its removal. This suture can usually be left in place for 2 to 3 weeks. The tensile strength of 4-0 nylon makes it especially suitable for a subcuticular closure. A combination of the subcuticular closure and interrupted skin sutures gives both the excellence of approximation and a longer period of support to any wound.
6. The *continuous over-and-over suture* (Fig. 1-9F) is occasionally used for skin closure. A particular application is in closing scalp wounds where suture mark scars from the tension of this suture are covered by hair. It is also used for approximating incisions in the eyelids (6-0 silk), since this thin skin does not tend to show suture marks. However, because of the thinness of the skin, suture tracts become epithelialized if the eyelid sutures are not removed within 5 days. Small inclusion cysts which may appear 3 to 4 weeks following suture removal are another late manifestation of this epithelialization. This problem can be treated by either incision or excision of the cyst, depending on the circumstance.

KNOTS. Many of the sutures utilized for skin closure have needles which have been swaged onto the suture. Thus, this discussion is primarily concerned with using a needle holder to tie knots. It is best to have a smooth-jawed, lightweight needle holder with beveled joints so that sutures will not catch in it during the process of tying.

The knot most commonly used in surgery is the *square knot with an added half knot* [38]. Great care must be taken in placing the first portion of the square knot, for if the pull on each end of the suture is not equal, the knot will not lie flat but instead form a half hitch, which has no holding power. In the second phase of tying a square knot, the free ends must lie in opposite directions to prevent the knot from disrupting when the suture is cut. To avoid disruption it is wise to place an added half knot on top of the square knot. Then, even if the third knot were to come undone when the ends of the suture were held together, the underlying square knot should remain secure.

Catgut sutures are notorious for coming untied when located on the oral mucosa and tongue. One way to avoid this event is to substitute silk for the less-pliable catgut. Another way is to tie the catgut so that its knots lie inverted beneath the mucosal surface.

An interlocking slip knot [45] simplifies the removal of interrupted sutures after repair of a cleft lip and in areas where suture removal may prove difficult.

Skin Tape

Tapes which are adhered to the skin surface across a wound are satisfactory for the closure of skin wounds [35, 40, 50, 51]. Although this tape will hold the skin edges together without difficulty, buried sutures are essential to approximate deeper layers of tissue and to prevent inversion of the skin edges (Fig. 1-10).

Brunius [30] has shown in the rat that a more rapid healing of skin incisions occurred when a nonsuture technique (skin tapes alone) was used or when skin sutures were removed after 3 days of healing. This was thought to result from the more optimal tension across the wound, in addition to a lessened inflammatory reaction.

Microporous surgical adhesive tape (Steri-strip) has a backing of viscous rayon fibers coated with an adhesive acrylic copolymer of extremely high molecular weight. The rayon backing is formed of nonwoven random fibers, so that when the acrylic adhesive is applied by a selective process, a micro-

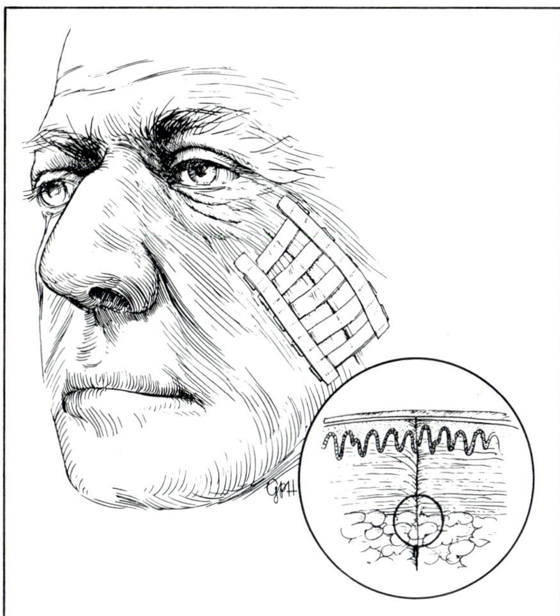

Fig. 1-10. Skin tapes. A buried suture is usually necessary to approximate the deeper layers of tissue.

porous face of adhesive is formed, rather than a solid, impervious sheet of adhesive. The tape is supplied in sterile strips, ¼ inch and ½ inch wide and 3 to 4 inches long. Ellenberg [34] noted that although this tape is pervious to sweat, it does not permit the passage through it of blood or purulent material.

The technique of applying these tapes is simple. In extensive wounds, the deeper layers should first be closed in layers by suture. The skin can then be cleaned and dried, acetone or alcohol being used to remove oily secretions from its surface if necessary. The tapes are applied perpendicular to the wound edge, first on one side and then on the other, so the edges can be pulled together.

These tapes do not stick to rubber gloves, nor does washing the skin around the wound with soap and water preoperatively lessen their holding power. However, if glue is used on the skin prior to applying the tape, even though the initial adhesion of the tape is strengthened, in a few days it will actually be weakened. Thus, such glues are contraindicated [40]. These skin tapes will usually stay firmly in place for 1 to 2 weeks, except in hirsute areas, where they may be pushed off by growing hair over a period of 5 to 7 days. On oily skin, the tape may also become loose in 7 to 9 days. Children have rubbed these tapes off on the third or fourth postoperative day [35]. In loose skin areas (e.g., eyelids, scrotum) or areas in constant motion (e.g., lips, anterior neck, antecubital and popliteal regions), these tapes frequently become loose.

Tape is especially advantageous for attaching a skin graft to such convex surfaces as an extremity or the trunk. Not only can it be applied and removed faster than suture material, but it also does away with the troublesome bleeding which can accompany the passage of a needle through the wound margin.

Some of the advantages of skin tape are as follows: it saves time in both application and removal, causes little or no skin reaction, avoids the possibility of skin suture marks, can be left in place for long periods beneath dressings or casts, and can be applied without an anesthetic; in addition the wound has greater tensile strength than sutured wounds [31]. Microporous surgical adhesive tape has the following disadvantages: it does not produce eversion of the skin edges, does not adhere to wet skin, will come off in about two-thirds of patients when they bathe, and can be removed prematurely by children or uncooperative patients. Ellenberg [34] evaluated skin tapes in over 300 patients and stated that the cosmetic appearance of the skin scar was inferior to wound closure by standard methods.

Molded plastic locking tabs attached to microporous tapes have been designed in such a way as to be drawn together from either side of the wound to permit rapid skin closure [10].

Skin Staples and Skin Clips

The skin stapler has been used by some surgeons to close the skin wound following face lift, mammoplasty, lipectomy, and skin grafts [23]. Skin clips presently available are the Michel clip with its objectionable large round teeth and the smaller, sharper-toothed Ethicon clip [29]. The Ethicon clips can be applied rapidly because they are loaded in a magazine and inserted with an applicator. The teeth of the clip should engage the skin with bites of equal size on each side before the instrument is squeezed to bring the edges into approximation. The edges of the clip are angled to provide slight eversion of the wound as this is done. Excessive pressure must be avoided in closing the applicator to ensure that the wound edges are not compressed excessively by the clips. These clips can be removed with a special clip remover that spreads the points of the clip and lifts it from the skin.

Wound Adhesives

Although wound adhesives have been available since 1956, they have still not been approved for general use in humans by the United States Federal Drug Administration. In 1977, only trifleuroisopropyl (manufactured by the 3M Company with the trademark MBR 4197) is approved by the FDA for investigation in humans [53]. The restriction on the cyanoacrylates in the United States is due to the development of fibrosarcomas in animals after large injections of these materials. In contrast surgeons in Germany, France, Switzerland, Canada, and Japan are using cyanoacrylates, such as methyl-2-cyanoacrylate and isobutyl-2-cyanoacrylate, for sealing vascular aneurysms, intestinal repairs, gynecological surgery, skin wound closure, and skin graft adhesion to the skin around an open wound [53].

When a wound adhesive is pressed into a thin film between surfaces to be joined, the polymerization, which occurs at room temperatures, is catalyzed by minute amounts of water from the air or the wound surface. Absolute hemostasis is required since excessive blood or other fluid will prevent adhesion [28, 37, 44].

This adhesive material is applied as a thin film between the cut edges of the skin or by spreading it over the skin surface. A firm bind is formed in from 30 seconds to 3 minutes. Ashley et al. [28] state that buried sutures are still necessary to close the deeper layers of tissue before applying adhesive to the skin. Application of the adhesive below the skin surface may create a barrier to healing.

When this material is used to hold a skin graft in place, it should be applied on the surrounding skin margin which is to be overlapped by this graft. Painting or spraying the adhesive on either the recipient bed or the raw surface of the graft will cause loss of the graft by preventing nutrients and capillary buds from entering the graft to nourish it [44]. Wound adhesives have been successfully used to immobilize plugs or strips of scalp used in hair transplantation [52].

SKIN GRAFTS

Wounds deficient in surface covering require closure by a skin graft or skin flap. Skin grafting is discussed in this section and the use of skin flaps in the following section.

DEFINITION. A skin graft is a segment of dermis and epidermis which has been completely separated from its blood supply and donor-site attachment before being transplanted to another area of the body, its recipient site. Skin grafts consist of the epidermis and a portion of the dermis if they are of the partial-thickness type (split-thickness skin graft). The complete thickness type (full-thickness skin graft) contains the epidermis and all of the dermis. All such grafts contain varying portions of the sweat glands, sebaceous glands, hair follicles, and capillaries of the skin, depending on their thickness (Fig. 1-11).

Rudolph and Klein [127] have prepared a comprehensive review of the healing processes in skin grafts.

Types of Skin Grafts

Skin grafts can be classified as autografts, allografts (homografts), or xenografts (heterografts) (see Chapter 2 as well as later in this chapter under the headings, Split-Thickness Skin Grafts and Full-Thickness Skin Grafts; information on the dermis graft is also included in Chapter 2).

Split-Thickness Skin Grafts

Autografts of skin, cut at the split-thickness level, are the most popular and useful of all skin grafts. They contain the epidermis and a portion of the dermis. The split-thickness graft is further subdivided, depending on the amount of dermis included. These subdivisions are: *thin* split-thickness skin grafts (Thiersch or Ollier-Thiersch grafts), *intermediate* (medium) split-thickness skin grafts, and *thick* split-thickness skin grafts (three-quarter thickness grafts) (Fig. 1-11).

The thickness of the graft is a very relative thing, as the actual thickness of the skin varies with the age, sex, and the region of the body [81, 141]. Skin tends to be thinner in infants than in adults, with adult skin being 3.5 times thicker than that of the newborn. By the age of 5 years though, the skin thickness of the child is essentially the same as the adult [91]. The skin is thinner in women, especially in the dermal layer, than in men. Measurements by Southwood [141] of epidermal and dermal thickness in various age groups, sexes, and sites indicate that the skin varies from about 17 to 150 thousandths of an inch in thickness. It is thickest on the soles of feet and palms of the hands and thinnest over the eyelids and in the postauricular area. To impart some idea of the much greater contribution of the dermis to the thickness of the skin, the dermis is calculated to be 20 times thicker than the epidermis on the lateral thigh of a male adult (Fig. 1-11).

Surgeons tend to refer to skin grafts as being either thin, intermediate, or thick grafts, depending on the setting of the dermatome (10 to 25 thousandths of an inch), the translucency of the graft, and the bleeding pattern of the donor site. The setting of a dermatome or skin graft knife should always be checked by sighting the distance between the blade and the drum of the dermatome which comes in contact with the skin surface as the graft is cut. The translucency of a skin graft will vary from the thin split-thickness graft, with its translucent tissue-paper appearance, to that of the thick split-thickness graft, which is nearly opaque. The pattern of bleeding at the donor site also varies from a high intensity of fine bleeding points with the thin graft to a lower intensity of bleeding from larger points with the thick split-thickness skin graft [109].

The thinner a skin graft, the more the interface of fibrous tissue between the dermis and the recipient

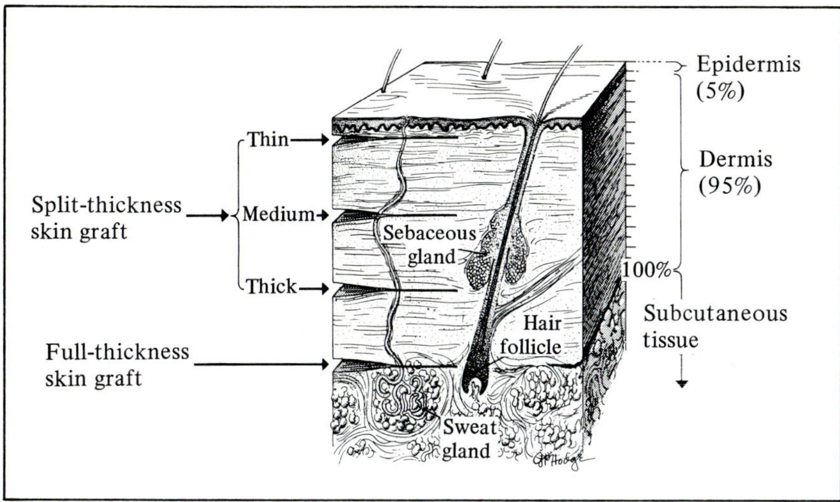

Fig. 1-11. Skin graft thickness. The thickness of the epidermis and dermis varies in different areas of the body. This drawing is characteristic of the lateral thigh skin of the adult.

site contracts during the first few months after transplantation. The thick split-thickness skin graft contracts less than an intermediate-thickness graft, whereas the full-thickness graft contracts hardly at all.

The thin split-thickness skin graft is more likely to survive on its recipient site because it can survive very well during the phase of plasmatic absorption and can wait longer for vascularization. It should also be noted that skin from a more vascular donor site will become vascularized more rapidly [137].

The thin split-thickness skin graft taken from a hirsute donor site will not have hair growing in it following transplantation, whereas the thick split-thickness and full-thickness graft will usually contain some hair follicles to permit the growth of hair.

The donor site for a thin split-thickness skin graft reepithelializes more rapidly than that for a thick split-thickness skin graft. The donor site of a full-thickness skin graft does not reepithelialize because no accessory skin structures remain.

Tissue-cultured skin grafts have been grown experimentally. In the rabbit 1 square centimeter of skin will grow on tissue culture to 50 square centimeters over a 1- to 3-week period [89].

Full-Thickness Skin Grafts

A full-thickness skin graft (Wolfe graft) contains the epidermis and entire thickness of dermis from the site of origin (Fig. 1-11). Following transplantation, this free graft will more closely resemble normal skin in color, texture, hair growth, and failure to contract than split-thickness skin. This is one reason why it is often selected for resurfacing on the face. The usual full-thickness skin graft is relatively small so that its donor site can be closed by undermining and approximating the wound edges.

A full-thickness skin graft plus 2 or 3 mm. of subcutaneous fat can be grafted if the skin is flagellated prior to transplantation [144]. Using a 1-foot-long thick rubber tube, the graft donor area is beaten until it is red and mild bruising begins to appear. The graft of skin with 2 to 3 mm. of fat attached is excised rapidly and sutured in the recipient site. Sweeney [144] reported that 23 out of 28 of these skin-fat composite grafts survived in patients and gave results in most cases comparable to those of flap repairs.

Uses of Skin Grafts

Skin grafts can be used to close any wound in the body which has a blood supply sufficient to produce the growth of granulation tissue. The most notable exceptions are cortical bone denuded of its periosteum, cartilage denuded of its perichondrium, tendon denuded of its paratenon, and nerve denuded of perineurium.

Most skin grafts are used to serve as permanent coverage for a wound, although in some instances a split-thickness skin graft is applied temporarily to a wound to aid in controlling or eliminating infection or to cover some vital structure. Later, when infection has disappeared and the wound has become smaller because the split-thickness skin graft has contracted, it can be replaced with a skin flap or full-thickness graft to provide more stable and cosmetically acceptable coverage.

Split-thickness skin grafts are durable if they have a good blood supply and have a good padding of subcutaneous tissue or muscle between the skin and bony pressure points. Although some surgeons maintain that a full-thickness skin graft or a skin flap is needed on the pressure areas of the plantar surface of the foot or the sites of decubitus ulcers, I do not believe this is necessary if there is sufficient soft tissue padding.

Facial Wounds

Full-thickness skin grafts obtained from the preauricular, postauricular, or supraclavicular regions are commonly used to close intermediate-sized defects resulting from the excision of basal cell or squamous cell carcinoma of the face. These grafts most closely resemble facial skin. Moderately thick split-thickness skin grafts from the scalp also provide a good color match for facial skin replacement.

The large wounds that follow orbital exenteration or maxillectomy are most often closed with split-thickness skin grafts from the thigh or abdominal wall. Deficiencies of skin in the lower eyelid can be repaired very nicely with full-thickness skin grafts of postauricular origin. Grafts of split-thickness skin should be utilized in the upper eyelid, however, because this skin must be sufficiently pliable and thin to permit folding and unfolding as the lids open and close. One excellent donor site for split-thickness skin which fills these requirements is the medial aspect of the upper arm.

Composite grafts often are the best for closing defects of the alar rim. The ear is an ideal donor site for composite grafts, containing a piece of cartilage sandwiched between two pieces of skin.

For surfacing large areas of burn on the face, it is frequently necessary to use split-thickness skin grafts and accept a cosmetically poor result. The shiny, stiff, scarred skin that results from this invariably imparts a masklike appearance to the face.

Flexor Surfaces

When skin grafts have to be applied to the flexor surfaces of the neck, fingers, palm, wrist, elbow, axilla, toes, ankle, or knee, they may require special care to prevent the development of a late contracture. When these sites lie adjacent to such major joints as the shoulder or knee, it may be necessary to splint the part in extension for about 2 or 3 months, although for the anterior portion of the neck 6 months of splinting is probably best in order to prevent contracture [69]. During the period of splinting, the strong contracting force subsides as the fibrous tissue in the wound matures. Extension splints on the extremities should be removed at least once a day in order to put the joints through their full range of motion, thus minimizing joint stiffness.

Treatment of Burns

Split-thickness skin autografts are preferred for replacing the skin lost from burned surfaces. When thin split-thickness skin grafts are used, a new "crop" of skin can be taken from the same donor site about every 2 to 3 weeks. Gillman et al. [78] state that 15 or 16 days is the best time to take a second thin split-thickness skin graft.

Stored viable allografts of split-thickness skin are a second choice for closure of burn wounds when a sufficient amount of skin autograft is not available. These grafts are only temporary covering and will be rejected in a few weeks. When possible, it is best to excise and replace them with autografts before the onset of the necrosis of rejection with its bacterial contamination and infection. Another method for using allografts is to apply alternate strips of autograft and allograft skin about 2.5 cm. in width. As the allografts begin to thin and undergo resolution after several weeks, the 2.5-cm. rectangles are replaced by ingrowing epithelium from the autografts lying on either side.

Because of the great depth of destruction caused by some electrical and radiation burns, skin grafts often are not sufficient for resurfacing the wound, and a skin flap must be utilized. For additional information regarding thermal, radiation, and electrical burns see Chapters 24 and 25.

Closure of Donor Sites of Skin Flaps and Full-Thickness Skin Grafts

A split-thickness skin graft may be necessary to close the donor site of a large skin flap or a large full-thickness skin graft when the wound margins cannot be approximated sufficiently to gain primary closure.

Mucosal Replacement

Split-thickness skin grafts serve well as replacements for the mucosa of the mouth, pharynx, nose, vagina, and urinary bladder when there has been a large loss of lining. However, split-thickness skin so utilized tends to contract during the first 3 to 6 months, so that unyielding molds or prostheses must be used during this period. Skin grafts used for mucosa replacement are altered somewhat in their characteristics, but they do not undergo metaplasia to become mucosa, since skin is too highly differentiated. Because hair follicles transplanted with skin continue to grow hair, grafts used for a mucosal replacement should ideally be either of medium thickness or from a non-hair-bearing area.

Conjunctiva of the eyelids and nasal mucosa are best replaced with a split-thickness graft of oral mucosa taken from the lower lip with the Castroviejo electrical dermatome. Mucosa is preferable to skin for conjunctival replacement, since the keratinized layer of the latter often causes corneal irritation. Either mucosa or skin can be used in the reconstruction of nasal lining, but many prefer the latter because of its stability and resistance to trauma.

Closure of Exposed Dura, Pericardium, Pleura, and Peritoneum

Split-thickness skin grafts will survive on dura, pericardium, pleura, and peritoneum, and can be used for either temporary or permanent wound closure. Skin grafts will also grow on areas in the abdominal cavity denuded of peritoneum, and on liver, spleen, and kidney [84]. Wounds that contain a large blood vessel, especially if it has been stripped of its surrounding adventitia, are more safely closed with an immediate skin flap.

When additional operations on deeper structures are contemplated, such as placing a bone graft between the dura and its overlying skin graft, the skin graft should first be replaced with a skin flap. It is a well-established principle that operations on deeper structures covered only with a skin graft should be delayed until the graft has been replaced with a skin flap. This is because of the high risk of necrosis and failure to heal of an incised and undermined skin graft.

Millard et al. [111] have shown experimentally in the rat and dog that a split-thickness skin graft can be sutured into the margins of an abdominal wall defect (e.g., an omphalocele) and that it will survive, effectively sealing off the abdominal cavity from the outside. Attachment of the omentum, small bowel, and liver to the underside of the graft provided blood supply to the graft.

Overgrafting Unstable Scars, Tattoos, Nonhairy Pigmented Nevi, and Thick Split-Thickness Skin Graft Donor Sites

Hynes [88] introduced the technique of overgrafting. The epidermis is removed with either a knife or a dermabrader, following which the skin graft is applied to the resulting vascular dermal bed. In this way, layer after layer of dermis can be built up over such unstable scars as are found over the anterior tibia and other bony prominences. For best results, the scar should be allowed to mature each time for 3 to 6 months before another layer is added. By using this overgrafting technique, the skin flap, with its greater investment in time and expense, can often be avoided.

Tattoos and large, non-hair-bearing pigmented nevi can sometimes be removed and yet a thin network of dermis be left behind in the base of the wound. Skin grafts placed on this bed have a better blood supply than they would on the underlying fat. Care must be taken, however, not to leave nevus cells behind, for they will be visible through the graft. These cells can even grow through the graft and give it a speckled look. If tattoo pigment is left in the bed, it can also be seen through a skin graft.

Thompson [146] has shown that the donor sites of thick split-thickness skin grafts heal more rapidly and with less scarring when they are overgrafted with thin split-thickness skin grafts. In such an overgrafted wound, any epidermal cysts which might persist tend to undergo dissolution within a year, except for the less than 4 percent which require removal. A few sweat glands and an occasional hair follicle will continue to function. The sweat glands may discharge their secretions to the surface, but are usually absorbed into the local circulation. Hairs will appear on the surface of the skin if a follicle in the graft and its shaft fortuitously lie over a follicle in the deeper host tissue.

Donor Sites

The color, texture, vascularity, thickness, and hair-bearing nature of skin varies markedly from one area of the body to another. In general, the nearer the donor site is to the recipient site, the more closely will the skin match. Skin grafts to the face from above the clavicle will retain their natural blush state, whereas those from below the clavicle will take on a yellowish or brownish hue.

Postauricular Skin

The postauricular surface of the ear and adjoining mastoid area (Fig. 1-12) serve as excellent sources for grafts of full-thickness skin which match the skin of the face. Its color and texture are similar to that of facial skin.

Grafts as large as 2 X 2 cm. can be removed, and yet the donor sites be closed by obliterating the depth of the postauricular sulcus. The entire area of postauricular skin from the helical rim to the hairline over the mastoid can be utilized for a full-thickness skin graft and this large donor site closed with a split-thickness skin graft. When reconstruction of a nasal defect requires skin and cartilage, it is possible to include a portion of the conchal cartilage along with the full-thickness graft, or even to take skin, cartilage, and skin through the entire thickness of the external ear, then split the cartilage into two layers to provide a "banana split" for use as lining of the nasal alae [72]. Postauricular skin sometimes has a highly vascular "pinkish" appearance for as long as 3 to 6 months after operation. This ultimately subsides to give an agreeable color match.

Supraclavicular Skin

The supraclavicular region (Fig. 1-12) serves as a larger donor area for either full-thickness or split-thickness grafts of skin for the face. The color match

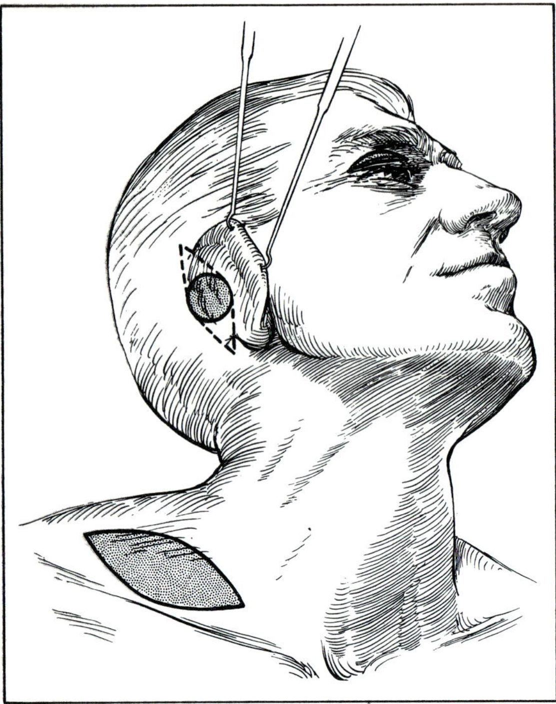

Fig. 1-12. Common donor sites for full-thickness skin grafts to the face are the postauricular, upper eyelid, and supraclavicular regions. The entire area of postauricular skin from the helical rim to the hairline over the mastoid can also be excised and resurfaced with a split-thickness skin graft.

and texture of this skin are nearly as good as those of the postauricular skin. Sufficient skin can be removed from this donor site to cover such units as an entire forehead, nose, cheek, upper lip, or chin. When grafting is performed in such units, the junctures can be hidden in the hair margins or along contour lines of the face.

Edgerton and Hansen [74] have described a technique for removing split-thickness skin grafts from the supraclavicular region. The skin is first ballooned up with several hundred milliliters of normal saline solution. The needle used for this injection should not be introduced through any area of the skin which must later be covered with dermatome cement because the leaking of saline solution from the puncture site will interfere with the dermatome's adherence to the skin. Grafts 0.012 to 0.014 inch thick and as large as 4 X 8 inches in area can be removed by this technique.

In women, the supraclavicular area may prove objectionable as a source of split-thickness skin grafts because subtle but permanent changes will be found in the character of the skin. For this reason, some surgeons prefer a donor site high on the lateral chest wall in women.

Preauricular Skin

A good color match for white facial skin can be obtained by using an ellipse of full-thickness skin from just in front of the superior helical juncture with the cheek. About a 1-cm. width of skin can be removed from this hairless area while still permitting primary closure of the donor site.

Upper Eyelid Skin

The upper eyelid (Fig. 1-12) is occasionally used as a donor site when a small, thin graft of full-thickness skin is needed for another lid. Only a narrow ellipse of skin can be removed without deforming the donor eyelid, although in older patients the skin is looser and a wider graft can be obtained.

Antecubital and Inguinal Region Skin

The antecubital flexor crease serves as an excellent donor site for grafts of full-thickness skin for the finger, hand, or face. Although only a relatively small ellipse of skin can be removed if the wound is to be closed primarily, the proximity of this area to the fingertip makes it a common donor site for skin grafts to the finger.

The flexor crease of the inguinal region has also been used in children as a source of full-thickness skin for denuded areas between the fingers following the division of a syndactylism. The later growth of pubic hair can be avoided by using only the lateral inguinal skin.

Hand Skin

Split-thickness skin grafts can be taken from the ulnar aspect of the hypothenar area for resurfacing of skin avulsion on the fingers [116]. Full-thickness skin grafts can be taken very readily from this same area (up to 2.5 cm. wide and 3 cm. long) [99].

Scalp

Split-thickness skin grafts can be taken from the scalp with the freehand knife or an electric dermatome. This is an especially welcome source of skin in an extensively burned patient. Crawford [68] reported that very little hair growth was noted in the grafted skin, but hair growth in the scalp donor site was essentially normal. The skin also has a good color match to facial skin.

Prepuce and Labia Majora

The preputial skin, removed by circumcision, is occasionally used when a graft of thin full-thickness skin is needed. The pigmentation of this skin and that of the labia majora makes them ideal replacements for the areolar and nipple area of the breast.

Areola
The areola can be partially removed from one breast and grafted to a reconstructed breast by a variety of areola-sharing operations, as described in Chapter 47. The full thickness of the nipple will not survive as a graft.

Abdominal Wall, Buttock, and Thigh
These are the most common donor sites for split-thickness skin grafts. The grafts from these large donor areas often become yellowish, light brown, or dark brown in color. Pontén [120] has shown that thinner grafts tend to be darker than those of greater thickness. The pigmentation of a skin graft is increased even more by its exposure to the ultraviolet rays of the sun, and it will persist for much longer periods than the usual suntan. Control of these gradations of pigmentation in grafted skin is one of the future challenges in plastic surgery.

When possible, grafts should be removed from the abdomen, buttock, or high posterior aspect of the thigh, where any permanent change in the skin of the donor site can be hidden by a bathing suit or shorts. Care should be taken not to include the hair-bearing areas of the pubis. Bony prominences should be avoided because it is difficult to remove grafts of split-thickness skin from these areas with any of the instruments currently available. In severe burns, where large amounts of skin may be required, any area of skin on the body, including the scalp, can be used as a donor site. Only such specific areas as the areola and nipples should be avoided.

The average blood loss from the donor site after a 10 × 20 cm. split-thickness skin graft has been removed was determined by Robinson [124] to be 46 ml. This amount can be reduced appreciably if a vasoconstrictor in low concentration is applied topically to the raw surface of the donor area – i.e., 5 drops of epinephrine 1 : 1,000, in an ounce of saline solution.

Requirements for Survival of a Skin Graft
In order for a skin graft to take it must have a vascular recipient bed, contact of skin graft and recipient bed, and proper preparation of any granulation tissue. The experimental work of Clemmesen [62] on the healing of skin grafts is outstanding.

Vascular Recipient Bed
A skin graft requires a sufficiently good blood supply in its recipient site for survival. A quantitative estimate of this need used by some surgeons is that the blood supply should be ample enough to support the growth of granulation tissue. This does not imply that the skin graft has to be placed on granulation tissue but rather that it has to be placed on a vascular bed. The only exception to this rule is the *bridging phenomenon* [109], whereby that portion of a skin graft overlying a small avascular area may survive. This phenomenon is based on the fact that collateral vessels connect the skin graft in the avascular area to the vascularized graft and serve as a network for transporting both an initial plasmatic circulation and a later ingrowth of capillary buds to nourish this area. In ideal circumstances this collateral circulation will bridge a gap of 0.5 cm. from any one margin. In the rabbit, if the square avascular defect is 1 cm. on a side, an average of 85 percent of a full-thickness skin graft will survive. Preparing the recipient bed 48 hours in advance will increase the survival of the graft an additional 2 mm. on each side. Of importance is the fact that split-thickness skin grafts of the same size on a similar-sized avascular defect became necrotic [80].

It is sometimes possible to apply the principle of the bridging phenomenon in successfully covering a denuded tendon or nerve with a skin graft. If the tendon or nerve has a diameter of 1 cm. or less and the recipient bed for the skin graft on either side is good, it may be possible to cover the area with a single, continuous skin graft carefully fitted to the contour of the area. This ensures maximal contact between the skin graft and the recipient bed adjacent to the less vascular area. Also worthy of emphasis is the fact that the area being bridged through this indirect process requires a longer period of time to regain vascularity than areas overlying good recipient beds. Covering exposed tendons and nerves with skin grafts protects them from the detrimental effects of exposure and can for long periods prevent them from undergoing autolysis and death. Another example of the bridging phenomenon is found in the vascularization of composite grafts (skin, cartilage, and skin) such as those used in the reconstruction of nasal alae (see Chapter 14). Composite grafts of skin-cartilage-skin of the monkey's external ear have been demonstrated to have a much increased survival (88 percent complete survival as compared to 22 percent complete survival in unprepared controls) by preparing the recipient wound 10 or 11 days in advance. Preparation involves simply excising the epithelium from the recipient wound, which leads to an increased number of vessels in the wound margin for inosculation with the graft vessels [107].

Smahel [135] demonstrated in the rat that the recipient bed could be "prepared" by first creating the wound and covering it temporarily with a skin graft. Then 2 days later the permanent graft is placed on the wound. This skin graft becomes revascularized and healed at a definitely faster rate than normal due to a reduction of the stage of plasmatic imbibition.

COMPARATIVE VASCULARITY OF RECIPIENT BEDS. Cortical bone denuded of periosteum, cartilage denuded of perichondrium, and tendon denuded of paratenon are avascular on their external surfaces and cannot be expected to nourish a skin graft placed in contact with them. Neither will any of the body's *stratified squamous epithelial surfaces* support the growth of a skin graft.

Heavily irradiated tissue is a relatively poor recipient bed for skin grafts because it has a poor blood supply. *Fat* has fewer blood vessels than dermis, fascia, and most other tissues, and thus should be considered among the less desirable recipient beds. *Long-standing granulation tissue* also serves as a poor bed for skin grafts because it becomes fibrotic, less vascular, and infected, as do the exposed surfaces of *chronic ulcers. Arteriosclerotic changes* in the blood vessels of the foot and ankle in older patients and diabetic patients make these regions poor recipient beds. In general, recipient beds having limited circulation will require a long period for the completion of vascularization of a skin graft and consequently require longer immobilization and aftercare than do grafts placed on beds of greater vascularity.

COMPARATIVE VASCULARITY OF SKIN GRAFTS. Thin split-thickness skin grafts have a more abundant network of capillaries on their undersurface than do thick split-thickness or full-thickness grafts. This fine network of terminal vessels is located in the superficial dermis, whereas slightly larger vessels are located in the deep dermis. In overgrafting a scarred recipient bed, Hynes [87] has taken advantage of this more favorable capillary network lying in the superficial dermis by reversing the surface of the dermis graft. Thus the deeper surface of the dermis graft is placed in the more superficial position. It is this deeper surface that is initially covered with a split-thickness skin graft. Often the initial graft of split-thickness skin will not take, but 1 to 2 weeks later, when the dermis is well vascularized, a second split-thickness skin graft can be applied to close the wound.

VASCULARIZATION OF SKIN GRAFTS. Smahel [136] as well as Rudolph and Klein [127] has written extensively on this subject. Vascularization occurs as follows:

1. *Plasmatic imbibition.* Almost immediately after a skin graft comes into contact with the underlying bed it begins to absorb a plasma-like fluid from it. This fluid is absorbed into the spongelike structure of the capillary network by capillary action, providing a state of in vivo tissue culture [57, 58, 60, 66]. On microscopic examination it can be observed that this fluid lying in the endothelial-lined spaces of the graft contains a few erythrocytes. While this process continues, a fibrin network is also being formed between the graft and the recipient bed to hold the graft in place. The plasma-like fluid appears to be absorbed into the graft (plasmatic imbibition) over the first 48 hours, causing its weight to gradually increase (20 percent increased weight in 24 hours and 30 percent increased weight in 48 hours) [61]. At the 48-hour point, blood flow begins in the graft, and the plasma-like fluid is carried away. The pink color that some grafts attain during the first 12 hours after transplantation probably results from the accumulation of red blood cells drawn into the capillaries of the graft by the plasmatic circulation [64].
2. *Inosculation of blood vessels.* During the first 48 hours after grafting, vascular buds grow in the intervening fibrin network that binds the skin graft to its recipient site [61, 63, 126, 139]. There are two different views as to what happens next; one view is that there is a random *inosculation of the vascular buds from the bed with both arteries and veins in the graft,* following which the blood enters the graft vessels moving to and fro in a sluggish manner until the fourth to seventh day, when true circulation occurs in the graft. The other view is that the *vascular buds grow into the graft,* even inside some of the old graft vessels, forming an entirely new vascular network [136]. There is a great deal of evidence supporting the first viewpoint [136]. Haller and Billingham [83], for example, found the vascular pattern in the healed grafts in the hamster cheek pouch to be the same as before grafting. They also observed that blockage of the graft vessels by injecting them with silicone rubber solution prior to grafting was followed by necrosis of the graft.

The development of anastomoses between bed and graft, and the flow of blood into the vessels of the graft, have an inhibiting effect on further proliferation of the vascular buds [136]. If there is a hematoma or seroma separating the graft from its bed, this inhibiting effect is slower in occurring, so that proliferation of granulation tissue continues and connective tissue infiltration into the dermis will occur to varying degrees [136].

Concurrent with these events in the hemic circulation, continuity of the lymphatic systems in the bed and graft is being restored. Scothorne [130], Psillakis [121], and Oden [114] have shown that lymphatic drainage from the graft is established by the fourth or fifth postoperative day, when graft lymphatics connect with recipient bed lymphatics.

Contact of the Skin Graft and the Recipient Bed
Good contact between a skin graft and its recipient bed is essential for vascularization of a graft and its survival. The thin fibrin network that begins to form almost immediately between the graft and its bed seems to serve as a glue to hold the surfaces together and prevent one from slipping on the other.

FACTORS PREVENTING PROPER CONTACT BETWEEN THE GRAFT AND ITS RECIPIENT BED. These factors include *improper tension* on the graft, a collection of *fluid* beneath it, and *movement* between the graft and its bed. It is important that a proper degree of *tension* exist in a skin graft once it has been sutured into place. If the tension is insufficient, wrinkles result that never become revascularized because of a failure to be in proper contact with the recipient bed. This same lack of contact results when a graft is stretched too tightly: acting like a drum head, the graft will not dip properly into the recesses of the recipient bed.

Blood, serum, and *purulent material* may separate the skin graft from its bed, prevent vascularization, and thus cause loss of the graft. The chance of a hematoma beneath a graft can be greatly decreased by careful hemostasis of even the smallest bleeding points. Much of the bleeding will stop spontaneously over a period of 5 or 10 minutes so that the stages of the operation should be planned in such a way that this time can be consumed in taking the skin graft. The use of a fine-tipped electrocautery is unexcelled for obtaining absolute hemostasis.

A delay of 24 to 48 hours before applying the skin graft is definitely indicated when oozing of blood from the bed persists. The wound can simply be dressed with a pressure dressing that is not removed until the time of delayed grafting. This decision to delay the application of a skin graft is often a difficult one to make, but it is usually a very wise one.

Capillary buds race against time to revascularize the graft before the cells undergo autolysis and death ensues. When a hematoma only 0.5 mm. thick is present, the time required for capillary buds to grow through the added thickness of the clot might be only 12 hours, and if the maximal allowable time for vascularization has not been exceeded, the graft will survive in these areas, even though it is vascularized 12 hours later than other areas. When, however, the clot is 5 mm. thick, the vascularization process will be delayed by 120 hours. At body temperature, most grafts will not survive this long a delay before revascularization, and so when the maximal allowable time for vascularization has been exceeded, autolysis begins.

Inspection of the graft on the second postoperative day should be carried out in all instances, except when a tie-over dressing is used. At this time the skin graft over any fluid collection can be incised and the fluid expressed. This should be repeated at least daily until there is no further fluid collection. This simple technique has saved many grafts that would otherwise be lost. When a tie-over dressing is used, Randall [123] suggests inserting all sutures around the margin of a graft, but tying only one of the two long ends of each suture over a stent. Then, two or three days postoperatively, the stent is removed and any fluid collections removed. The graft is then pressed back against its bed and the remaining sutures tied over a new stent. The moistened cotton-tipped applicator can be very useful in removing a small, discrete hematoma lying away from the graft margin.

Littlewood [101] has demonstrated that a split-thickness skin graft, elevated from its bed by a seroma, will become epithelialized on its dermal surface by the fourth day after grafting. Because of this, the elevated portion of any graft usually will not take after 4 days unless the epithelium is curetted from its undersurface.

Movement between the graft and its bed damages the capillaries growing into a graft and prevents proper revascularization. When a skin graft is applied to the extremities, splinting should be used to immobilize the adjacent joints. Skin grafts on the trunk can best be protected by keeping the patient at bed rest and in a position that prevents distortion or tension on the graft. Either a *tie-over dressing technique or complete exposure of the graft* is the most satisfactory way to treat the graft itself. It is especially difficult to immobilize skin grafts on the face because of the movement of the facial muscles. A tie-over dressing that immobilizes the graft in its bed as a unit is a very effective way of handling the problem.

Preparation of the Open Wound
A sharp distinction must be made between the recipient bed created just before a graft is applied and one which has been an open wound for a number of days. The important aspects in the evaluation of an open wound are its blood supply and quantitative bacteriology.

BLOOD SUPPLY. Almost all open wounds have sufficient blood supply to give nourishment to connective tissue and to provide the capillaries that combine to make up granulation tissue. Even irradiated tissues will produce granulations, although at a much slower rate than normal. Only bare bone and bare cartilage will not produce granulation tissue.

QUANTITATIVE BACTERIOLOGY. Robson and Krizek [98, 125] have written extensively on this subject. They have demonstrated that all wounds containing more than 100,000 (10^5) bacteria per gram of tissue are infected to such a degree that a skin graft will not take on this surface. Furthermore, evidence is lacking to support the *exogenous* source of bacteria as the etiologic agent. However, there is overwhelming evidence to document *endogenous* sources due to: (1) direct contact of bacteria from within the body with the edges of the incision, and (2) bacteria present at a distant site in the body entering the wound through the blood stream. It has long been known that injury to any tissue will cause the localization in that tissue of microorganisms present in the blood stream. The open wound in this case is a *locus minoris resistentiae.*

A rapid (30 minute) slide technique has been used clinically for several years to determine the number of bacteria in tissue taken by a skin punch or scalpel from the open wound [98, 125]. Wounds with less than 10^5 bacteria per gram of tissue and a good blood supply should support the growth of a skin graft.

The former designation of bacteria as *pathogenic* or *saphrophytic* should be discontinued in light of our present knowledge that any bacteria present in sufficient numbers will cause a clinical infection. The beta-hemolytic streptococcus is an exception to the rule using 10^5 bacteria per gram of tissue as a dividing line, since this organism will cause a clinically significant infection in much lower numbers. The presence of this organism will cause dissolution of a skin graft, and it is therefore a contraindication to skin grafting.

There are 10^3 *Staphylococcus, Streptococcus,* and other bacteria per gram of tissue deep in the skin of each of us. But as long as there is a normal balance between host resistance and the bacteria, there is no clinical infection. In an open wound, *time* is an important factor. The *golden period* is that period of hours for the initial inoculum in the wound to reach 10^5 bacteria per gram of tissue. Foreign bodies in the wound enhance wound sepsis.

The removal of bacteria from the wound is best accomplished by mechanical debridement and the pulsating jet lavage. It is our practice to remove granulation tissue by scraping the wound with the back of a knife handle prior to applying a skin graft. In most instances, complete hemostasis can be effected with the electrocautery and the graft applied immediately. If bleeding cannot be controlled, a pressure dressing is applied and skin grafting is postponed for 24 to 48 hours. Perforating or meshing the graft, or even using postage-stamp-size grafts, will allow for the inevitable wound exudate to drain to the surface without lifting the graft off its bed.

Biological dressings (such as skin allografts and fresh amniotic membranes) placed on the granulating wound and changed every 24 hours have been shown to achieve a marked reduction of the bacterial flora in an open granulating wound [98]. Systemic antibiotics will fail to alter the quantitative level of bacteria in the granulating wound. There is also abundant evidence to indicate that systemic antibiotics begun *more than 3 or 4 hours after wounding* are of no value. On the other hand, topical antibiotics have been shown to decrease bacterial growth in the open wound.

In wounds where skin allografts or autografts will take, biopsies of the underlying tissue obtained 24 hours after placing the graft on the wound will reveal no organisms, whereas prior to grafting there were large numbers of bacteria [133].

Skin autografts, allografts, or xenografts, soaked in 1 million units of aqueous penicillin and 1 gm. of streptomycin for 15 minutes before grafting onto an infected wound, have reportedly led to a dramatic increase in the ability to obtain a sterile wound [55]. In standardized contaminated rabbit wounds, control skin grafts did not alter the bacterial count in 96 percent of the wounds by the fourth postoperative day. But by soaking the skin grafts in the antibiotic solution, only 8 percent of the wounds were still contaminated by the fourth postoperative day. Soaking the graft for 15 minutes in a 5% neomycin solution has also been reported to provide an increased graft take (71 percent take of treated grafts as compared with 47 percent take of untreated grafts) [147].

Cutting the Skin Graft

Cutting the Split-Thickness Skin Graft

Three basic types of instruments have been designed for removing a graft of split-thickness skin from its donor site: the knife, the drum-type dermatome, and the electrical dermatome (Fig. 1-13). The choice of instrument usually depends on the surgeon's past experience; knives are generally more popular with the surgeons of Great Britain and the Continent, whereas dermatomes are favored in North America. The principle on which all of these instruments are based is that of a sharp blade moving back and forth to cut a piece of skin whose thickness is controlled by a calibrated setting on the instrument or by the surgeon himself.

KNIFE. Some knives, such as the Humby knife, have an adjustable roller that controls the thickness of the skin graft, whereas others, such as the Blair knife and Ferris-Smith knife, are simply long cutting blades with a handle at one end and no adjustable roller to control graft thickness. A Weck blade or even an

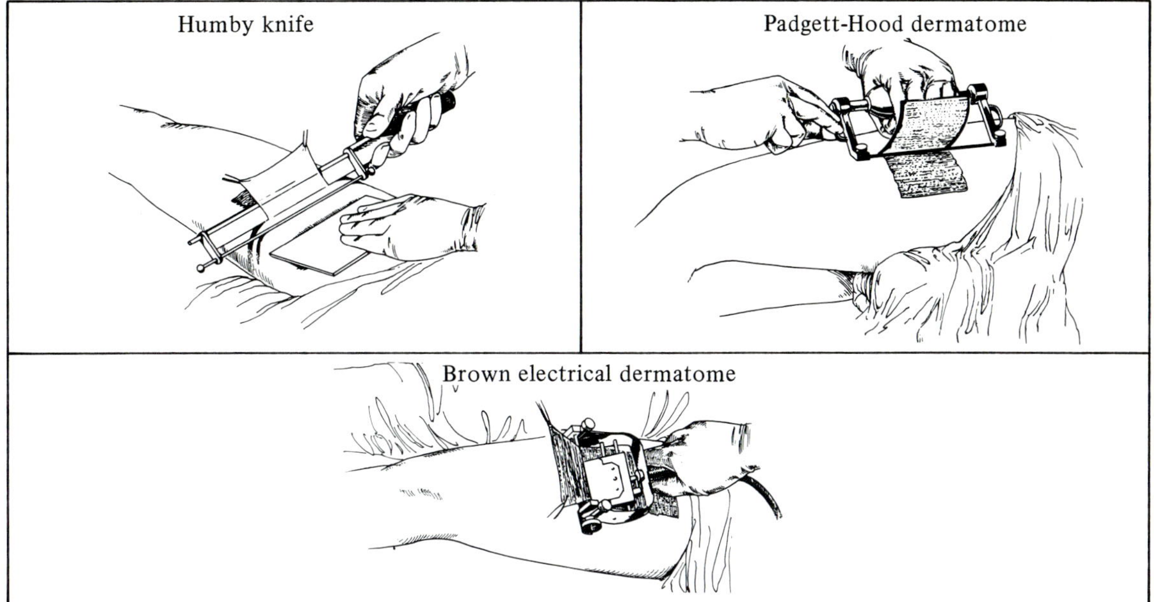

Fig. 1-13. Instruments for cutting split-thickness skin grafts.

ordinary razor blade can be used to take narrower skin grafts.

With the Humby knife (Fig. 1-13), modified by Bodenham, Braithwaite, and Marcks, the actual thickness can be measured with shims which are included in the set, or the surgeon can learn to set the desired thickness by sighting between the blade and the roller. The thickness of a graft can also be checked from time to time as it is being cut, by observing its translucency and the bleeding pattern of the donor site.

Long but narrow grafts of split-thickness skin can be obtained more easily from the thigh if they are cut in a *longitudinal* direction. The buttock or arm can serve in a similar fashion as donor sites. The abdomen is less satisfactory as a donor site for skin grafts cut with a knife because there is no underlying bony or cartilaginous framework to support it.

The cutting of a split-thickness graft with a Ferris-Smith knife requires that the donor skin be flat and under some tension. An assistant can aid in holding the skin behind the knife stationary, flat, and under some tension with the edge of a sterile board or some other flat instrument. The operator advances a second board or a suction cup just in front of the knife to flatten and stretch out the skin for cutting. If the skin is lubricated with petrolatum or mineral oil, the efficiency of the suction is increased and the knife will glide more smoothly. The suction block is applied to the skin just before the graft is cut. Any longer contact will produce ridges in the skin and make the cutting more difficult. The knife blade is beveled at an angle of about 30 degrees to the skin margin for the first several strokes of the blade. Once the knife has passed through the surface of the skin, the blade is rotated backward until it nearly parallels the skin surface. As the blade continues back and forth with long, effortless strokes, little attention should be given to the forward motion of the knife. Any attempt to force the knife forward most often results in altering the depth of the cut, making it either too deep or so superficial that its continuity is disrupted. Probably one of the most important prerequisites for the cutting of a successful graft is a sense of self-assurance on the part of the surgeon.

Knives that have been fitted with an adjustable roller are used in the same way as the Ferris-Smith knife. The roller attachment has the important advantage of ensuring that the depth of the knife blade will not change significantly from its predetermined setting during the cutting of the skin graft.

Furnas [76] has described a method of gluing the epithelial surface of large pieces of skin and subcutaneous tissue (e.g., following avulsion or excision of congenital lymphedematous skin from the lower leg) to a glass plate, and then, with a free-hand #20 or 21 knife blade on a bent handle, cutting a split-thickness skin graft from this giant piece of tissue. Ross and Gibson [126] have accomplished the same thing with a 12-inch-long blade held on a rigid framework at a fixed angle and at an adjustable distance from the part of the framework in contact with the skin.

Snow [140] has described the use of an unmodified Schick injector razor and blade for taking a split-thickness skin graft 0.012 to 0.014 inch in thickness and 1¼ inches wide. Shoul [132] modified a Gillette safety razor by simply filing out the central strut of the safety guard and by using another blade with the cutting edge broken off as a shim. Each shim increases the space between the cutting blade and the safety guard, so that with three shims a graft 0.012 inch thick and 1.25 inches wide can be cut. Goulian [82] has modified the Weck straight razor by adding a fixed handle, by removing two struts from the blade protector, and by modifying the blade protector, so that the razor can be preset at the factory to cut at 0.008, 0.0010, or 0.012 inch in thickness and 1.25 inches wide.

DRUM TYPE OF DERMATOME. This type of dermatome is known for its ability to cut a skin graft of a uniform thickness. The *Padgett-Hood dermatome* (Fig. 1-13), which is the prototype of the drum dermatomes, comes in three sizes: the baby model, which cuts 3 X 8 inch grafts; the standard model, which cuts 4 X 8 inch grafts; and the giant size, which can cut a graft as large as 4 X 16 inches. It works on the principle of fixing the outer surface of the skin to one-half of a metal drum and then moving a rotating blade back and forth close enough to the surface of the drum to cut off a partial thickness of skin at the desired level. The knife blade, which is disposable, can be adjusted with a calibrated dial so that its cutting edge will lie at any desired level between 0.005 and 0.050 inch from the surface of the drum. All settings should be checked either by eye or with a measuring shim to be certain that the blade is the desired distance away from the drum before the graft is taken. Before inserting the disposable blade into the carrier arm it is necessary to insert a thin metal strip (adapter) to keep the blade far enough from the drum. The original blades for this instrument were thicker and thus did not require the addition of a metal adapter strip.

The Padgett-Hood dermatome requires either a dermatome cement (Padgett-Hood dermatome cement, Reese compound, or Evo-stik "impact" household adhesive) or a removable dermatome tape to make the skin adhere to the drum. The donor site is best prepared by applying a layer of dermatome cement to the skin, removing the cement with acetone, and then reapplying a second thin layer of cement. While the dermatome is still resting on its special stand, a thin layer of cement is also applied to the surface of the drum. The cement should be allowed to dry for *3 minutes* in order to be most effective. Meanwhile, petrolatum or mineral oil can be applied to the metal axis on which the blade moves back and forth, and to the surface of the blade which will come into contact with the skin.

Skin grafts can be cut more readily with the Padgett-Hood dermatome in a *circumferential* direction, around the thigh. The drum can be pressed down firmly onto the skin to obtain the desired degree of adherence before gently rotating it to draw the skin up so that it can be incised with the blade. The blade swings back and forth as the drum is rotated. Care must be taken to press the drum against the skin as it is rotated to maintain a constant degree of thickness and width. If the blade should cut into the skin beyond the edge of the drum, the skin can be gently retracted away with a hemostat. When necessary, the thickness of the graft can be changed during cutting simply by moving the calibrated dial. When the graft is completely cut, it can be removed from the drum by attaching small hemostats to each of its corners. The addition of glove powder or blood to the epidermal surface of the graft will neutralize any adhesive still on its surface, or the adhesive can be rubbed off with a gauze sponge.

A drum type of dermatome makes it possible to cut skin grafts to fit an exact pattern. An outline of the graft required can be drawn on the skin and then dermatome cement applied within the boundaries. Petrolatum or mineral oil is applied to the skin outside the pattern to be certain it does not adhere to the drum. Thus only the skin within the pattern adheres to the drum and is removed. Another technique for obtaining a graft of a given configuration is to apply the pattern upside down to the cut surface of a skin graft before the graft is removed from the drum. The skin can then be cut to this pattern with a knife.

Two other drum-type dermatomes were designed by Reese and Schuchardt. The *Reese dermatome* is more elaborate and precise than the Padgett-Hood dermatome. The distance between the blade and the drum is adjusted by inserting a shim of the desired thickness adjacent to the blade in its carrying arm. A tape containing an adhesive on its surface is fixed to the drum. The *Schuchardt dermatome* adheres to the skin without adhesives. The graft is removed by a to-and-fro motion of a knife blade, which is adjusted with thumbscrews to give the desired thickness.

ELECTRICAL DERMATOME. Motor-driven dermatomes allow the surgeon to rapidly remove long strips of skin, 8 cm. or less in width, from almost any site on the trunk or extremities. This saves a great deal of time in the grafting of patients with extensive burns. Another advantage of the motor-driven unit is that satisfactory grafts can be cut even by the less experienced surgeon.

The *Brown electrical dermatome* (Fig. 1-13) is equipped with a disposable knife blade that moves back and forth like the blade of a haircutter. A long, sterile cable, serving as the drive shaft, runs between the dermatome and its unsterile motor, which is taped to a stool or table adjacent to the donor site. A foot pedal activates the motor.

The thickness of the skin graft can be controlled by adjusting two calibrated knobs on either side of the instrument. This actually alters the pitch of the blade. Because the instrument can fall out of proper alignment, it is important to close the knobs down completely and use this reading as the zero point on each side. Once both sides are set, it is best to double-check by holding the instrument up to the light to see that the aperture between the blade and the instrument is the same on either side. The desired width of the graft can then be obtained by making an inward or outward adjustment of the shoelike attachment on either side of the dermatome.

Sterile mineral oil, applied to the donor site, will lubricate it so that the instrument can move forward smoothly. After the skin has been steadied, the dermatome blade is set in motion and the instrument placed on the donor site so that its flat undersurface lies at a slightly downward angle. A moderate but constant pressure is required as the dermatome moves steadily forward to keep it from jumping or skipping over the skin. As the graft begins to appear on the upper surface of the blade, the graft can be lifted by an assistant to ensure that it is of the proper thickness and to prevent it from bunching near the blade. After this initial maneuver, it is not usually necessary to continue to withdraw the skin cut by the dermatome.

Skin grafts are usually taken from the extremities in a *longitudinal* direction. Because multiple grafts of uniform thickness can be taken from a limb without wasting any space between adjoining donor sites, it is possible to "strip" an extremity of nearly its entire potential donor capability and yet know that it will heal with uniformity.

One disadvantage of the electrical dermatomes is that they can break down and require factory adjustment. For this reason, it is wise to have a second instrument available. It should also be emphasized that these instruments are not calibrated as accurately as the drum dermatomes, and, therefore, do not cut grafts of a desired thickness as precisely. Thus, for cutting thick split-thickness skin for such important areas as the face, when the graft must be wide and of an exact and consistent thickness, a drum-type dermatome is commonly used.

Other electrical dermatomes include the Padgett, the Stryker, and the Castroviejo dermatomes. The *Padgett electrical dermatome* has its motor in the handle of the instrument. The *Stryker dermatome* is similar to the Brown dermatome and uses a cable to connect it to the motor. The *Castroviejo dermatome* was designed primarily for cutting split-thickness grafts of mucosa from the inner surfaces of the lips and cheeks with a small razor blade. Shims are used to regulate the thickness of the grafts. A razor blade in a spring-wound safety razor handle, with a blade with the cutting edges removed for a shim, has been used for cutting narrow (4 cm.) strips of skin [56].

Anesthesia of the skin graft donor site can be obtained by refrigeration. Howie [85] described the use of crushed ice in several polyethylene bags, which were held firmly on the skin of the thigh with an elastic wrap for 45 minutes. Analgesia, which lasted for 15 to 20 minutes after removing the ice, was confirmed by testing with a needle.

Cutting the Full-Thickness Skin Graft

Full-thickness grafts contract so little that it is important to cut them to fit into the recipient site as exactly as possible. When such lesions as a hemangioma, nevus, or foreigh body tattoo are to be removed, the size of the defect and its contour are evident before the operation. This makes it practical to prepare an exact pattern for the full-thickness graft before the excision. Such preparation eliminates the possibility of making the pattern too large, an error that will almost invariably accompany the making of an imprint of the defect after the excision has been carried out. This occurs because the skin edges around the margin of the defect retract as soon as the opposing skin tension is gone. The specimen, of course, is not suitable for a pattern since it contracts as soon as it is removed.

In many instances it will be impossible to ascertain the size of the defect before surgery – either because the extent of the excision could not be determined beforehand, as in the case of malignancy, or because scar contracture disguises the true size of the defect. Under these circumstances, it is far better to carry out the excisional surgery before attempting to determine the size of the full-thickness graft which will be needed.

Many materials have been suggested for patterning the defect: exposed x-ray film, vinylite, lead sheet, jaconet, oil silk, cloth toweling, rubber dam, and aluminum sheet. Transparent pliable substances which do not stretch and yet can be sterilized by either autoclaving or soaking in a solution without distorting their outline are the best. An outline of the defect can be made with methylene blue and either imprinted on the patterning material with pressure or cut to the desired size and shape. If the area is irregular, it is best to maintain proper orientation of both the pattern and the graft to the defect by marking each of them with corresponding symbols or dots. It is also important to identify which side of the pattern will correspond to the epidermal surface of the graft and which one represents the dermal side. Without sufficient attention to this point, the pattern can be mistakenly turned over and a useless mirror image of the defect obtained.

Full-thickness skin grafts are cut with either a #15 or a #10 knife blade. It is helpful when the skin of the donor site is irregular in its surface contour to distend the skin by injecting either a saline or an anesthetic solution beneath the dermal layer. This aids in the surgical separation of the dermis from the underlying fat. If epinephrine (Adrenalin) is added to the solution, the line of incision between dermis and subcutaneous tissue can be visualized even more clearly.

The skin is incised just to the depths of the dermis, along the outline of the pattern (Fig. 1-14). Fine sutures of atraumatic silk can be inserted into the margins of the graft at the points where the identifying marks are located. Skin hooks are used for counteraction. The graft, under tension, is turned back over the operator's index finger and removed under direct vision, with care to minimize the amount of fat left on it. Another method is to tense the graft in a plane almost parallel to the wound surface and cut blindly with an oscillating gesture in the plane immediately beneath the dermis. Seeing or feeling the tip of the blade through the thickness of the skin will serve as a guide to keep the proper level.

After the graft has been cut, the epidermal surface of the graft is stretched over the surgeon's index finger and the residual fat is usually removed with small, curved sharp scissors (Fig. 1-14C). However, the graft will survive with some fat still left in place. The donor area is closed in most instances by converting the defect to an elliptical shape, undermining the wound edges, and approximating them by suture. If the defect is too large to permit primary suture, a split-thickness graft can be applied.

All of the postauricular skin and the adjacent non-hair-bearing mastoid skin can be used as a full-thickness skin graft and this large donor area covered with a split-thickness skin graft.

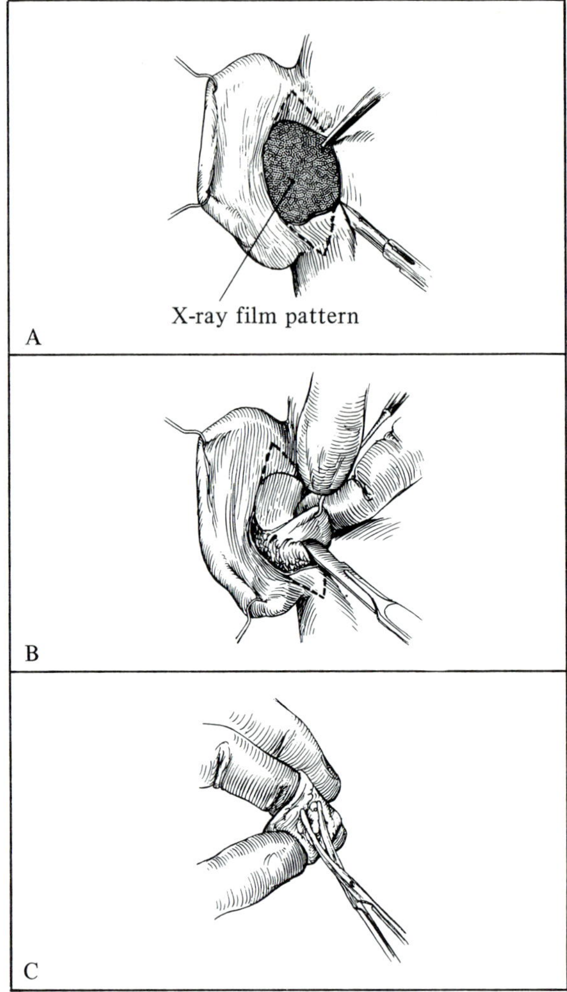

Fig. 1-14. Technique for cutting a full-thickness skin graft. Excess fat should be trimmed away as shown in C.

Application and Care of Skin Grafts

The basic techniques for applying split-thickness and full-thickness skin grafts are the same. It is important to *remove any clot* from the recipient bed before applying the graft. As the graft is being sutured into place, a cotton applicator stick can be twisted beneath the graft to remove any remaining clots that can be seen through the translucent graft.

If a tourniquet has been used during the preparation of the graft recipient site, a bulky compression dressing should be placed over the skin graft before releasing the tourniquet.

When it is not possible to obtain absolute hemostasis of the recipient bed, a common occurrence following the excision of a burn scar, it is sometimes worthwhile to *delay* applying the skin graft. The wound is simply covered with a pressure dressing that contains a layer of nonadherent material (nylon, rayon, Telfa) on the wound surface. The dressing is removed 24 to 48 hours later and coagulated blood is removed from the recipient bed, which should now be dry. Skin grafts obtained at the initial operation can be stored by placing them back on the donor site temporarily or by refrigeration at 4°C. and then later applied without anesthesia if they are simply laid on the wound without fixation, or fixed to the surrounding skin with skin tape or glue. Delayed grafting more than compensates for the additional time involved, because it usually ensures success and a better functional and cosmetic result.

When the defect to be closed with a skin graft has been created by excising a nevus, scar, or other closed wound, the skin graft is usually applied in a sheet. But when the wound has been open and thus is infected, it is usually wiser to allow for drainage through the skin graft. This is accomplished with a *mesh grafting device* or by cutting the graft into *postage-stamp-sized pieces.* The Tanner-Vandeput cutting machine, the Michigan Research Corporation mesh expander, and the Concept mesh expander are all designed to produce multiple uniform slits in the graft, approximately 1 mm. apart [104]. When the graft is pulled on the bias, numerous diamond-shaped openings appear. These openings will epithelialize, and, particularly when the long axis of the perforations are placed parallel to the skin lines, the mesh graft pattern will not give a cosmetically displeasing appearance. Though these mesh grafting devices were designed to expand the graft to cover up to three times its unexpanded area, we have found them most useful in providing multiple drainage points for serum, blood, and the products of low-grade infections.

An alternative to expanding a graft to increase the area covered is the relay graft [138]. Strips of split-thickness skin, 3 to 6 mm. wide, are placed on the recipient bed so that they are 5 to 10 mm. apart. In about a week, when epithelial growth from these strips is good, the strips are picked up and moved to the next recipient site without anesthesia. These strips have been moved as many as four times. The space where the skin strips have been removed will gradually epithelialize from the adjacent new epithelium.

In the skin grafting of concave defects, there must be sufficient skin to cover completely the depths of the wound, rather than only enough to bridge the skin like a drum head from the wound margins. A tie-over dressing is often helpful. Occasionally, it is useful in covering concave defects to cut a pie-shaped triangle out of a circular piece of skin and then close the triangle so as to form the skin into a cone.

Fixation of Skin Grafts

SUTURES. Suturing is the method most often used for approximating a skin graft to the margins of a wound. Such sutures may be either interrupted, continuous, or both. The interrupted sutures, if their ends are left long, may be tied over a bulky cotton dressing to aid in immobilizing the graft (Fig. 1-15).

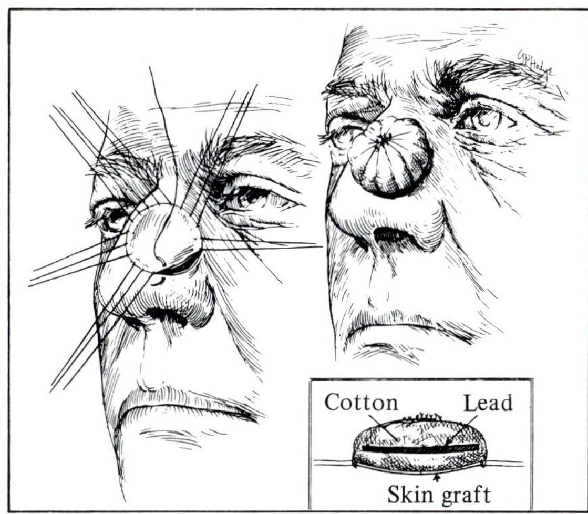

Fig. 1-15. Tie-over dressing for skin grafts.

Nonabsorbable sutures are preferred, although in children absorbable material is worthwhile in order to avoid the need for removal of the sutures.

A three-point suture may prove helpful in attaching the skin graft to a thick-edged wound. This suture is placed through the graft about 4 or 5 mm. from its edge, then woven in and out of the subcutaneous tissue of the wound margin, and finally through the skin, where it is tied [92]. If the margin is actually a skin flap, it is wise to anchor the graft to the recipient bed as well (see Fig. 1-26). In this way, any blood beneath the flap will be less likely to extend underneath the skin graft.

SKIN TAPES AND ADHESIVES. Microporous surgical adhesive tape (Steri-strip) or a single thickness of fine mesh gauze fixed with collodion adhesive can be used to secure a skin graft to the margin around the bed. The tapes are usually positioned across the wound margin in a radial fashion.

Dermatome cement or methyl-2-cyanoacrylate can also be used to hold the graft to the skin margins. The adhesive is applied to the skin surrounding the recipient wound. The undersurface of the graft should be dried before it is applied so the portion that comes into contact with the glue will remain adherent. The overlapping wound edge will not survive and can be debrided away later. The methyl-2-cyanoacrylate should not be applied except in a droplet size between the graft and the actual recipient bed, because nutrients cannot penetrate this adhesive barrier, and the graft will fail. McGibbon and Paletta [108] advocate using a spider-like device made from soldering together two or three draftsman's compasses with alligator clips on the points to stretch the graft out and hold it for the 10 to 20 seconds that are required for the methyl-2-cyanoacrylate to bond the graft to the recipient site.

Skin tapes and adhesives are especially helpful in grafting chronic ulcerations of the lower extremity, as the ulcers are usually surrounded by a thin, atrophic skin which bleeds easily and does not hold sutures well.

NO EXTERNAL FIXATION. The fibrin that normally forms between the skin graft and its recipient site rapidly binds the two surfaces together. Within a few minutes of application, most grafts have become adherent to the bed. While this bond is not strong enough to withstand significant trauma, it is effective enough to hold either large, thin grafts or thicker ones the size of a postage stamp to the wound. The tendency for large, thick, split-thickness skin grafts to retract makes this technique less satisfactory for their application to granulating wounds. The easiest way to eliminate this problem is to suture the graft at its four corners under its normal tension to the skin *beyond* the margin. This is another way to solve both bleeding at the thin margins of scar epithelium and the tendency not to hold well.

It has proved unnecessary to apply plasma or thrombin to the recipient bed for fixation of the graft. The fibrinogen and enzyme system which convert it to fibrin are already in ample supply in the wound [109].

Dressing of Skin Grafts

TIE-OVER DRESSING. This is one of the most satisfactory methods for immobilizing skin grafts (Fig. 1-15). It is especially useful on the face and neck, where the movements of the muscles of facial expression can make graft immobilization so difficult.

The tie-over dressing contains a nonadherent gauze next to the graft surface. Over this, a bolus of saline-soaked cotton is placed and the sutures tied to hold firm pressure on the graft. A piece of sheet lead cut to the pattern of the skin graft can be sandwiched in the cotton dressing to prevent bunching inward of the graft as the sutures are tied over the cotton (Fig. 1-15).

If the margin around the recipient bed remains dry and odorless, the tie-over dressing can be left in place for 5 to 7 days. If there is any question about whether fluid will collect beneath the graft, one of the tie-over sutures can be left untied initially, but tied after inspection of the graft in 1 or 2 days [123]. The edges of the tie-over dressing should be inspected daily for evidence of infection beneath the graft. If any is found, the dressing should be removed, the wound cultured, and saline dressings begun.

EPITHELIAL INLAY (STENT). This technique is good for applying a skin graft to the labial or buccal sulcus, orbital cavity, external auditory canal, inner surface of the nose, and vagina. Contact with the recipient bed is maintained by wrapping the graft about a preformed mold of acrylic, dental modeling compound, silicone, or similar material (Fig. 1-16). After the recipient bed has been created, an impression of it can be taken with acrylic or similar material. The mold or stent is allowed to harden before the skin graft is wrapped around it, with the raw surface to the outside. The graft can be trimmed, and sutured or glued to itself. It may be advisable to form a second mold or stent before tying the one covered with the skin graft into place. The second mold can serve as a model for making a more permanent splint of lighter weight which can be substituted when the skin graft is first inspected about 7 days later. Any extra skin beyond the edge of the defect which was not revascularized will be dry and tissue-paper thin and can be easily trimmed off at this time. It is important not to leave these grafts unsplinted for more than short periods of time because the cavity quickly becomes obliterated as the graft contracts. Permanent units can be hollowed out to make them lighter. In the nose, an airway can be placed through the center of the mold for the patient's comfort.

In the mouth it may be advantageous to fix the epithelial inlay mold to the teeth, to permit prolonged splinting of the graft during the period of graft contracture (Fig. 1-16). Often the molds can be fashioned preoperatively to the approximate size and then altered to fit exactly at the time of operation. Skin grafts applied to mucosal areas seem to have an especially marked propensity to contract, so that splinting must often be maintained for 3 to 6 months. Skin grafts applied to the periosteum of the maxilla or mandible, on the contrary, do not contract.

Fig. 1-16. Epithelial inlay mold of dental compound to hold a split-thickness skin graft in the labial sulcus.

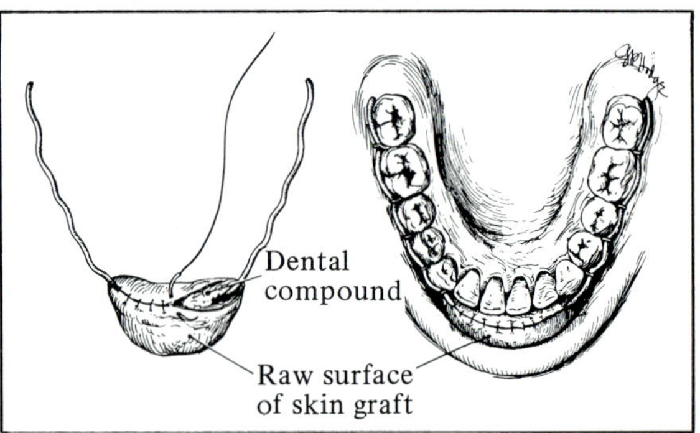

PRESSURE DRESSING. This dressing is often useful for immobilizing grafts on an extremity. After the non-adherent dressing and flattened gauzes have been applied to a graft, padding of gauze, cotton waste, or cotton is applied on top of the graft and held in place by an elastic tape (Elastoplast) or an Ace bandage. The graft as well as the joints on either side of it should be immobilized with a plaster or aluminum splint.

OPEN METHOD. Leaving the graft open or exposed can be especially useful in such areas as the face, neck, and trunk, where the movement of muscles in the base of the wound might shear the graft from its bed if a pressure dressing were used. It is also an effective way of applying postage-stamp-sized grafts to granulating wounds and observing them. Contact from clothing and bed coverings can be prevented by keeping a wire cage or a cardboard box over the exposed grafts. This facilitates inspection of the graft and permits the removal of any fluid which has collected beneath it. The open technique of skin grafting should not be used in any patient (child or adult) whose willingness or ability to cooperate is in doubt.

Postoperative Care of Skin Grafts

REMOVAL OF HEMATOMAS AND SEROMAS. As a rule any skin graft suspected of harboring a collection of fluid beneath it should be inspected on the second postoperative day and the fluid, if present, evacuated. This treatment must be repeated every day until there is no further fluid beneath the graft. The exception to this rule can be found in sterile wounds where a tie-over dressing has been applied to an absolutely dry recipient bed under ideal circumstances. If neither odor nor fever is present and a sense of confidence prevails, the dressing change can be delayed for 5 to 7 days.

It is easy to recognize a hematoma or seroma beneath skin grafts because of the translucency of the graft. The #11 knife blade is good for incising the graft, the fluid being removed by either the pressure of a gauze sponge or the use of a sterile cotton applicator stick. Blood clots not expressed with pressure alone can be removed by twirling the cotton applicator and wrapping the clot around it.

Skin grafts adhere quite strongly to a proper recipient site, gaining their greatest adherent strength in the first 8 hours after grafting, and then they continue to gain in adherent strength more slowly with each subsequent 24 hours [119]. Careful dressing changes will not dislodge them.

CARE OF THE INFECTED SKIN GRAFT. Most infections arising in the area beneath the graft usually do not cause temperature elevations during the first 24 hours following operation. The high spike of temperature which comes this soon is usually caused by pulmonary or renal pathology. Low-grade fever, odor, or redness around the margins of the graft between the second and fourth postoperative day support the diagnosis of infection.

When a patient complains of increased pain in the grafted site a few days after operation, this usually indicates that there is a wound infection. The opposite is also true, that a daily decrease of soreness in a grafted wound indicates that the graft has taken.

Local wound care should include debridement of any necrotic tissue in the wound and frequent moist saline soaks. *Mechanical cleanliness* is essential to good wound care.

When the predominant bacteria are *group A beta-hemolytic streptococci (S. pyogenes)*, the skin graft may be totally lost. To prevent a further loss of grafts, additional skin should not be applied until this organism has been eradicated with systemic penicillin or one of its modifications. Infections with *Pseudomonas aeruginosa (P. pyocyanea)* are less deleterious to a graft and may result in the loss of only portions of it. The British Medical Research Council Burn Research Unit recommends the use of topical polymyxin for the treatment of this infecting agent [109].

HYPERBARIC OXYGEN. In a clinical study of 48 patients, there was evidence that twice daily whole body exposure to two atmospheres absolute of hyperbaric oxygen for 3 days increased the take of split-thickness skin grafts. Of the treated group, 84.2 percent had permanent graft survival, whereas 62.7 percent of the control had graft survival; this was a statistically significant difference [117].

Immobilization Period for Skin Grafts

IMMOBILIZATION TO PREVENT CONTRACTION OF THE SKIN GRAFT. All skin grafts are contracted to varying degrees as the scar tissue between the skin graft and its recipient bed matures. This process begins about 10 days after the graft is applied and may continue for as long as 6 months [69, 110]. Thick split-thickness skin grafts on convex and rather fixed surfaces will contract less than thin grafts on surfaces that are concave and more mobile. Full-thickness skin grafts usually show little or no tendency to contract.

SPLINTING OF THE GRAFTED AREA. Skin grafts are known to be contracted more rapidly and to a greater degree on certain areas on the body than at other locations. For example, the anterior aspect of the neck, oral mucosa, nasal lining, and vagina require

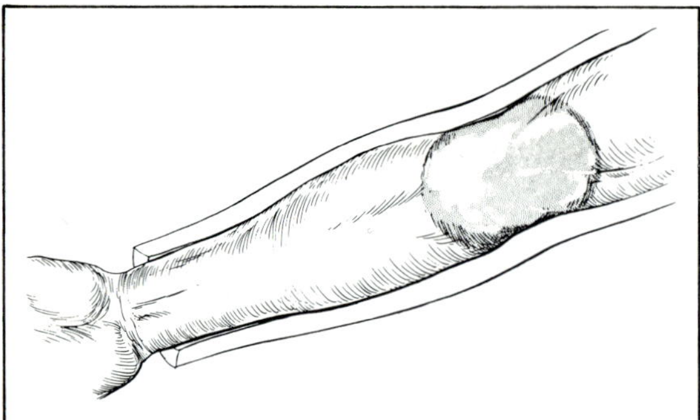

Fig. 1-17. Extension splint to prevent contracture of skin graft in the antecubital region.

splinting for periods up to 6 months; the axilla, flexor surface of fingers, and popliteal, antecubital (Fig. 1-17), and postauricular regions must be splinted for periods of 2 to 3 months. The splint may need to be only intermittently applied during the day or at night during the last 1 or 2 months. Lightweight splints for all of these regions can be made and applied at the time of operation. When joints are involved, it may be advisable to remove the splints daily and put the part through a full range of motion.

The degree to which a graft contracts can sometimes be diminished by making suture lines follow the lines of neutrality (e.g., the midlateral line of the finger or extremity). Late contracture of straight-line scars can be altered by incising adjacent skin and inserting darts of skin graft to alter the line of scar.

IMMOBILIZATION OF SKIN GRAFTS OF THE LOWER EXTREMITY. Skin grafts on the lower extremity or in relatively avascular areas (e.g., irradiated tissue) may require a longer time than usual before becoming completely revascularized and stable [123]. The many factors present in these cases do not allow for any hard-and-fast rule as to either the period of immobilization or the rapidity with which mobilization can be accomplished once it has been started.

One fundamental point that should be observed following the skin grafting of lower-extremity ulcers is that the process which causes the ulcer should be eliminated, if possible, before ambulation has begun. Otherwise, the repair which might seem satisfactory with the extremity elevated and at rest is very likely to fail. Venous disorders are common in the area of the malleoli. When perforating veins become incompetent, this area can be subjected to the entire weight of the column of blood within the vena caval system. Arterial disorders can have a similar deleterious effect on the local circulation. Recurrent infections can be followed by massive amounts of fibrosis and ischemia.

Traditionally, patients with skin grafts on the lower extremity have been kept at bed rest for 1 or 2 weeks before being allowed to dangle their legs and then ambulate. Bodenham and Watson [59] have successfully ambulated 25 patients with lower limb grafts by 48 hours postoperatively. Their program is to suture the skin edge to the deep fascia with a continuous catgut suture, suture the graft in place with a few sutures, dress the wound, including a 2.5-cm. foam pad over the graft, and wrap the leg with an elastic bandage. Ambulation is started 24 to 48 hours postoperatively, beginning with a 15-meter walk and progressing by 1 week to walking freely about the ward. Dressings are left in place until the third to fifth day, at which time the graft is inspected, any hematomas removed, and the complete dressing reapplied. When the graft is over a joint, immobilization of this joint with plaster is advised. Patients are discharged at 2 to 3 weeks postoperatively.

Storage of Skin Grafts

A simple and very effective way to store a split-thickness skin graft is to *replace it on the donor site.* The graft can then be removed easily and without anesthesia up to 10 days; from 10 to 14 days removal is with increasing difficulty and pain. Such grafts have been removed from their storage site on the thigh up to 24 days later. Split-thickness skin grafts stored in this manner have been "prepared" so that they remain pink when placed on their new recipient site. They have a definitely higher rate of take compared with grafts stored in saline at 4°C. [97, 131].

Split-thickness skin can be *refrigerated* as long as 21 days and still be used for grafting. Sterile conditions should be maintained while the graft is being covered with a gauze sponge moistened with saline or Ringer's solution and placed in a sterile jar or rubber glove. It should be refrigerated at 4°C., a temperature provided by any standard household refrigeration unit. No additional steps are necessary to prepare the graft for use. Several additional points are worth mentioning: (1) Actual immersion of the skin in solution during the period of storage is not advisable because it tends to macerate the skin. (2) The longer a graft is stored, the less likely are its chances of being successfully revascularized when applied to the recipient area. (3) The viability of a skin graft can be maintained for longer periods when it is stored in Hank's tissue culture fluid, which contains plasma and neomycin [75].

Freeze-dried skin that has been stored at room temperature for long periods of time can still take on the recipient site for a few weeks before being rejected [118].

Care of the Donor Site

After the split-thickness skin graft has been removed from a donor site, it heals by a process of reepithelialization. Epithelial cells from the remains of pilosebaceous units (hair follicles and sebaceous glands) and the sweat glands migrate across the surface until they unite with one another. Anatomically, pilosebaceous units do not extend into the subcutaneous tissue, whereas the sweat glands do. A donor site from which a thick split-thickness skin graft has been removed will heal more slowly than one from which a thin graft has been removed. On the average, the donor site of a thin split-thickness skin graft will heal within 10 days, whereas that of a medium-thick skin graft will heal in 10 to 21 days. The donor area of a thick graft will require 21 to 56 days for healing [65]. The dermis itself is inactive and shows no evidence of regeneration. Thus, the portion of the dermis removed with the graft is a net loss to the skin [129].

Donor sites require a proper amount of attention to gain early healing and to prevent them from becoming infected. When an open draining area is to be grafted, it may be advisable to prepare the donor site, remove the graft from it, and dress the area before exposing the infected or contaminated recipient site.

Fine-mesh cotton gauze continues to be the simplest, most effective split-thickness skin graft dressing. A study was performed comparing cotton gauze either impregnated with petroleum jelly, scarlet red, xeroform, or Aquaflo, or left plain in some 50 patients, and it was demonstrated that the rate and quality of healing was the same regardless of the dressing used. An adjacent area left undressed healed at the slowest rate [77].

Split-thickness skin allografts have been shown to be detrimental as a skin graft donor site dressing, in that they produce a rejection reaction leading to a full-thickness wound rather than the healed wound which was intended [112]. Porcine xenografts in one study [138] were shown to have no advantage over fine-mesh gauze as a donor site dressing.

The nonadherent dressing on the donor site will dry on exposure to air for a day or two. Drying can be hastened with a heat lamp or with an electrical hair dryer. As epithelialization continues, the dressing will come away from the donor site in about 2 weeks. This process can be aided by soaking in a tub of water. Once it is completely exposed, the donor site can be lubricated with either lanolin or cocoa butter.

Increased temperature of the skin surface increases the rate of donor site epithelialization. Elevation of the skin temperature from the normal 34° to 36°C. up to about 40°C. causes a marked increase in the rate of epithelialization. Above 40°C. the growth is sharply reduced, and at 44°C. there is cell death [79].

Delay in healing of the skin graft donor site may be due to the removal of an excessively thick split-thickness skin graft or to infection. When the delay in healing is due to the removal of a thick graft, it is best to actually graft the donor site with a thin split-thickness skin graft from another site. When infection is the major factor in a donor site's failure to heal, it will usually require treatment with moist saline dressings. These should be changed frequently (at least every 4 hours).

Characteristics of Grafted Skin

Skin that has been transplanted from one region to another will maintain most of its original characteristics, with the exception that sensation and sweating in the graft will more closely resemble that of the recipient site.

Contraction of Grafted Skin

Skin grafts undergo two types of contraction, primary and secondary.

PRIMARY CONTRACTION. The elastic fibers of a skin graft cause it to diminish in size as soon as it has been cut. This can easily be overcome by stretching the graft as it is sutured into place. Since elastic fibers are located in the dermis, thicker grafts with a thicker dermis will contract more than thin grafts. Davis and Kitlowski [70] found that full-thickness skin grafts shrank primarily 41 percent in surface area, whereas thin split-thickness grafts shrank only 9 percent.

SECONDARY CONTRACTION. Maturation of the scar tissue lying between a skin graft and its recipient bed causes the skin graft to contract, permanently decreasing its surface area [122]. This secondary contracture is of greater importance than primary contracture. It is influenced by the following factors:

1. The *thicker a skin graft,* the less its tendency to undergo secondary contraction; full-thickness skin grafts show little or no evidence of contracture.
2. The *more rigid the recipient bed,* the less a skin graft contracts; grafts on the periosteum of bone contract less than grafts on more mobile areas and flexor surfaces.
3. *Complete take* of a skin graft also decreases its degree of contracture; areas of partial loss of a skin graft heal by contraction and epithelialization from the surrounding skin.

Secondary contraction begins about the tenth day after grafting and continues up to 6 months [69, 110]. The contracting force exerts a steady, unrelenting pull on the wound and can easily overcome even the efforts of strong muscles to prevent it. Occasionally the surface of the skin graft will become wrinkled.

Splinting of the skin grafted area is a principal means of preventing contraction (Fig. 1-17). Darts into the surrounding normal skin are also helpful.

Not all skin graft contraction is detrimental. In some areas, such as in the fingertip, a skin graft for replacement of avulsed skin will shrink up to 50 percent, thus pulling more normal tactile skin over the area.

Color of Grafted Skin

Skin grafts and flaps from above the clavicles tend to retain their natural blush shade, while those from below the clavicle take on a yellow or brownish hue with no vestige of red coloration. Full-thickness skin grafts from the eyelid, postauricular, and supraclavicular regions have a good color and texture match with the skin of the face. Although these grafts are initially redder than the facial skin, they will usually become paler over a period of months.

A major disadvantage of split-thickness skin grafts from the thigh or abdomen is their yellow, pale brown, and dark brown colors, which match poorly on the face and other exposed areas. Pontén [120] reports that thinner split-thickness skin grafts from the same donor site are usually darker than thicker ones, making them even less desirable.

Hyperpigmentation of skin grafts is due to the stimulation of melanophores by both hormones and the ultraviolet rays from the sun [113]. It may become less pronounced over a long time. Mir y Mir [113] has demonstrated that dermabrasion will lighten the color of hyperpigmented skin grafts. The effect is more permanent if enough time has passed for the graft to become reinnervated. Lopez-Mas et al. [103] found that by taking a split-thickness skin graft from a previously used skin graft donor site, the color match of the previously decolorized skin was retained. No severe hyperpigmentation was observed even on prolonged sun exposure.

Prevention of hyperpigmentation by keeping the grafted skin out of direct sunlight and by applying sunscreen creams that filter out the ultraviolet rays will be of assistance. It is more difficult to apply cosmetics to the smooth shiny surface of a split-thickness skin graft than to normal skin.

Accessory Skin Structures in Grafted Skin

Any accessory skin structures (i.e., hair follicles, sebaceous glands, and sweat glands) transplanted with a skin graft will continue to function, but if not included in the graft, these accessory structures do not regenerate. For practical purposes, only in full-thickness and thick split-thickness skin grafts will hair growth, sebaceous gland function, and sweating be retained, for these are the only grafts thick enough to include the pilosebaceous apparatus and sweat glands [67, 102, 120].

Hair growth can be preserved in full-thickness skin grafts containing functioning hair follicles, and the technique is useful in eyebrow reconstruction and in covering bald areas of the scalp with hair [92, 95, 115]. Hair-bearing scalp also can be transplanted successfully with skin punches as large as 12 mm. in diameter or strips of scalp up to 5 mm. in width. Some of the fat which contains hair follicles should be left attached. Characteristically the transplanted hairs are shed within 3 weeks, and a new growth of hair begins in 8 to 10 weeks.

Sebaceous secretion is destroyed by transplantation except in full-thickness and some thick split-thickness skin grafts, where function will return after several months. Thus, skin grafts must be lubricated with lanolin, cocoa butter, or other creams to prevent dryness and crusting in the early postoperative period.

Sweating is destroyed by transplantation except in grafts of full-thickness and some thick split-thickness skin. Its eventual return somewhat parallels that of sensory innervation, which is a prerequisite to sweat gland activity [120]. In the palms, soles of the feet, and axillae, sweating is stimulated by emotion, whereas over the rest of the body (including the axillae), it is related to body temperature. Following transplantation, the sweating pattern of a graft is determined by where it is located. Thus a thick skin graft taken from the abdominal wall and transplanted to the palm will be controlled by emotional, rather than thermal, stimuli [120, 142].

Sensation of Grafted Skin

When there is no dense scarring in the bed to prevent nerve fibers from penetrating the graft, its final sensation will approximate that of the surrounding skin [86, 120, 143]. On the fingertip, Sturman and Duran [143] demonstrated that two-point discrimination in a split-thickness skin graft averaged 5 mm., whereas on the corresponding finger of the opposite normal hand it was 3 mm. The skin graft donor site area on the forearm averaged 33 mm. In a cross finger flap the two-point discrimination is similar to that of a split-thickness skin graft.

The final return of sensibility in skin grafts placed on a scarred recipient bed, granulation tissue from bone, or in an area of deep tissue destruction (e.g., full-thickness burns) will always be less than in those skin grafts overlying more favorable recipient sites. The four sensory modalities (i.e., pain, touch, heat, and cold), if they return, follow the pattern of the recipient site. Sensation begins to return 3 weeks after grafting and must be considered to have reached its maximum after 1½ to 2 years [86]. At first there is hyperalgesia, but over a period of months a more normal sensation returns. By the use of electrophysiological techniques it has been shown that initially the sensory fibers to a skin graft are unmyelinated, and they become increasingly myelinated with time [145].

Durability of Grafted Skin
In general, thick split-thickness skin grafts that have regained sensation are durable. They function very well on the palms of the hands and soles of the feet when there is sufficient soft tissue between the graft and the underlying bone for padding.

Growth of Grafted Skin
Skin grafts grow in a manner paralleling the growth of the total body surface. Both split-thickness and full-thickness skin graft growth has been studied in growing rats, where grafts were placed on 300-square-millimeter defects and measured over a 3-month period. Following an initial stage of graft shrinkage, there was a secondary phase of growth at the same rate as the growth of the total body surface [96]. Tension was shown to be the greatest influence on growth. Similar growth was shown to occur in skin flaps [96].

FLAPS

Our choices for reconstruction of external body parts has greatly expanded in the past decade. To our 450-year-heritage of skin flaps has been added (1) the muscle flap plus a skin graft, (2) the omental flap plus a skin graft, and (3) the myocutaneous flap. These newer types of flaps have in common the fact that they are arterialized tissues possessing a longitudinal artery and will thus survive to a greater length (Fig. 1-18).

Wounds too extensive to permit primary repair by suturing can be closed by a skin graft or a flap. Although *the skin graft is often the simpler of the two methods and should be considered first,* there are cases where a flap is required or may be more desirable. Flaps are usually required for covering recipient beds with poor vascularity; for reconstructing the full thickness of the eyelids, lips, ears, nose, and cheeks; for padding body prominences; and when it is necessary to operate through the wound at a later date to repair underlying structures. Flaps, however, have some disadvantages in that they are bulky in appearance, may carry hair into non-hair-bearing areas, and may require multiple operations with long periods of hospitalization. Expressions usually conveyed by the facial muscles can be masked by the thickness and bulkiness of skin flaps used in facial reconstruction.

We will now consider the various types of flaps available to us: skin, muscle, omental, and myocutaneous flaps.

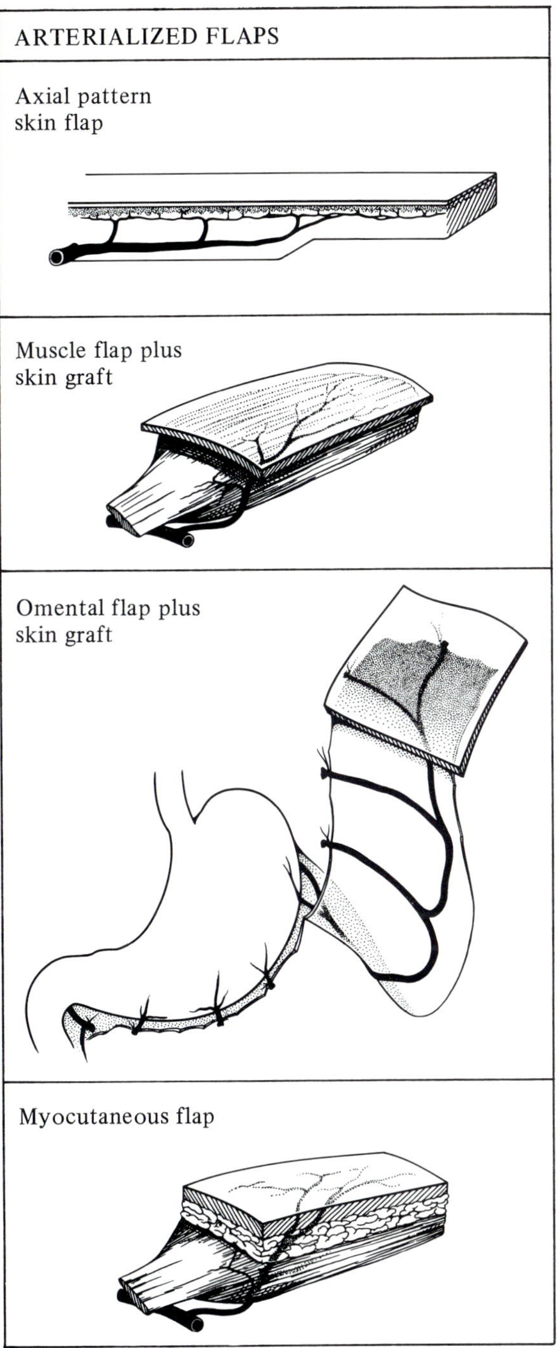

Fig. 1-18. Arterialized flaps survive to a greater length than flaps that do not include a longitudinal artery. For example, an axial pattern skin flap will survive to about 50 percent greater length than a random pattern skin flap.

SKIN FLAPS

Definition

A skin flap consists of skin and subcutaneous tissue that is moved from one part of the body to another with a vascular pedicle or attachment to the body being maintained for nourishment. This vascular attachment can be changed from one part of the flap to another as the flap is transplanted to a new area, and can even be changed from one supplying segmental vessel to another by microvascular anastomosis. The word *flap* should be used to denote a tongue of tissue, whereas *pedicle* is used to denote its base or stem. Thus the term "pedicle flap" is redundant.

Fundamental Principles

Although the principles for the planning, developing, and transfer of skin flaps have grown empirically over a period of centuries, during the past few years these principles have been altered and strengthened by experimental studies. The investigations of Milton [225, 226], Myers and Cherry [235, 236], and Daniel and Williams [176] are especially outstanding.

These principles are as follows:

1. Think of using a *skin graft* first. Our progression in choosing the type of skin coverage should be from skin graft, to local skin flap, to distant skin flap – from the simple to the most complex.
2. Plan skin flaps carefully: begin at the recipient site to outline the tissue requirements; make a pattern of them and carry out, in an assimilated fashion, the steps required in transferring the needed tissue from the donor area to the recipient site; and be sure to add extra length on the pattern to allow for the thickness of casts and bandages and for tissue contraction.
3. The length of a rectangular single pedicle or bipedicle skin flap is dependent on the perfusion pressure in the blood vessels of the flap. It has been demonstrated experimentally that flaps made under similar conditions of blood supply survive to the same length regardless of width [225]. Increasing the width of a flap will not increase the surviving length (Fig. 1-19). The design of a skin flap of safe dimensions must take into account knowledge of the anatomy of the arteries and veins supplying the skin, and the perfusion pressure through these vessels to nourish the tissue. Favorable factors, learned by experience, which permit us to make a longer flap are:
   a. The presence of *large blood vessels (direct cutaneous artery and vein) coursing in the longitudinal axis of the flap* (i.e., an axial pattern flap). Arterial skin flaps such as this survive to 50 percent greater length than flaps based on the musculocutaneous artery–perforator artery–dermal-subdermal plexi of vessels alone (i.e., a random pattern skin flap) [176, 227]. Thus an arterialized flap has the advantage of providing a great length of skin for immediate coverage, as opposed to a delayed random pattern flap (Fig. 1-18).
   b. Location of the flap in the *head and neck* where the vascularity is excellent.
   c. Transfer of the flap is *delayed.* Skin flaps that are delayed will survive to somewhere between 60 [226] and 100 percent [176] greater length than undelayed flaps based on the musculocutaneous artery–perforator artery–dermal-subdermal vascular plexi [226].
   d. The flap is designed as a *bipedicle* rather than a single pedicle flap.
   e. Younger patients, and those without diabetes and arteriosclerosis, probably have a flap survive to a greater length.
4. Transfer of the flap should be delayed when there is a question of its viability; most flaps should be delayed about 1 to 1½ weeks before being transferred.
5. When dividing the base of a cross leg flap or one base of a bipedicle flap, or the third side of a delayed flap which was initially delayed by two parallel incisions and undermining, it is best done in two or three stages, each 2 or 3 days apart.
6. In planning flaps below the knee and in areas of scar or radiation therapy, especially in elderly patients, caution is advisable because diminished vascularity is a frequent finding. Experimentally, it has been shown that pig skin which has recently received intensive x-ray radiation continues to support a skin flap of almost the same length as a control, but beginning 5 to 6 weeks after radiation there is a definite reduction in the surviving length of the flap [246].

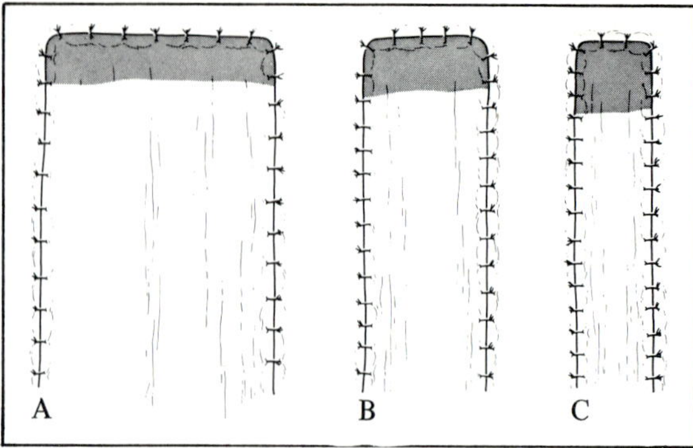

Fig. 1-19. Drawing of experimental skin flaps of varying width. Note that the flaps survive to approximately the same length, regardless of width.

7. In most regions, the blood supply to the skin flap is via the dermal-subdermal plexus of blood vessels (random pattern skin flap).
8. Excessive tension, kinking, pressure, hematoma, and infection in the flap should be avoided, but if present, they should be treated promptly.

Blood Supply of the Skin

Anatomy

Daniel and Williams, and others, have underlined the importance of the skin's blood supply in the planning of a skin flap. An understanding of the anatomy of these vessels will permit us to change our emphasis from "how a flap is moved" to "what vessels supply it" [176]. The major vessels from the aorta are the segmental, anastomotic, and axial arteries. These then give off perforator-musculocutaneous or perforator-direct cutaneous arteries which supply the dermal-subdermal plexus of the skin. The two main anatomical patterns of blood supply to the skin of importance to a surgeon planning a skin flap are (1) the pattern in which the large artery from the aorta or major vessel *lies deep to the muscle* and sends up perforator-musculocutaneous branches to the dermal-subdermal plexus in the skin (most of the skin is supplied by this pattern of vessels); (2) the pattern in which a direct cutaneous artery comes off from the large artery, by way of a short perforator artery, to *lie superficial to the muscle* and supply the dermal-subdermal plexus (Fig. 1-20). Because the long direct cutaneous arteries are in the lower portion of the subcutaneous tissue, a flap that can be designed so as to include such an artery will survive to an approximately 50 percent greater length than a flap supplied by the perforator-musculocutaneous pattern of vessels [224].

SEGMENTAL, ANASTOMOTIC, AND AXIAL ARTERIES. These large vessels in the trunk and extremities course deep to the muscles and give off a number of vessels, including those to the skin. Embryologically, there are some 30 rows of dorsal *segmental* branches from the aorta whose dorsal rami supply the spinal cord and whose ventral rami become the intercostal and lumbar arteries. A longitudinal ventral *anastomosis* exists between these parallel rows and develops into the internal mammary and epigastric arteries. *Axial* arteries to the extremities (e.g., brachial a., femoral a.) come off of the aorta, or major branches of the aorta, and lie deep to the muscles proximally and more superficially distally [176].

In general, these segmental, anastomotic, and axial arteries have the following characteristics: (1) they are major arteries which are in continuity with the

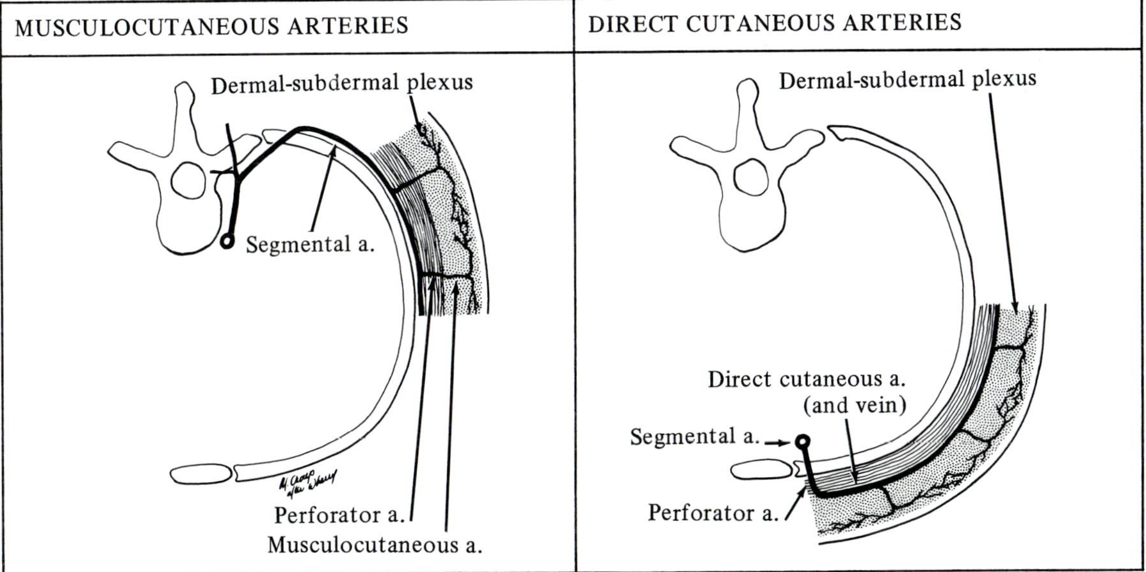

Fig. 1-20. The two anatomical patterns of blood supply to the skin. The important difference between them is the level at which the longitudinally oriented artery lies, with the longitudinal segmental, anastomotic, or axial artery lying beneath the muscle *and the longitudinal direct cutaneous artery lying* deep in the subcutaneous tissue. *The former is the predominant blood supply to the skin and is the type of blood supply to a random pattern skin flap. The latter is the blood supply to the axial pattern skin flap, which can be planned to a greater length because of the inclusion of this artery in the flap.*

aorta in regard to perfusion pressure, (2) they *course deep to the muscle,* and (3) they are accompanied by a single large vein and often a peripheral nerve [176].

PERFORATOR-MUSCULOCUTANEOUS AND PERFORATOR-DIRECT CUTANEOUS ARTERIES. These vessels arise from a segmental, anastomotic, or axial vessel and carry the blood to the skin. They can be described as follows:

1. *Perforator-musculocutaneous arteries* (providing blood supply for random pattern skin flaps) arise from segmental, anastomotic, and axial vessels, with the perforator portion passing perpendicularly through muscle to exit in the subcutaneous tissue where its name changes to the musculocutaneous artery (Fig. 1-20). This musculocutaneous artery then terminates in the spider-like dermal-subdermal plexus of the skin. Thus, a random pattern flap after being elevated is supplied by perpendicular musculocutaneous arteries at its base and then longitudinally via the dermal-subdermal plexus. Venous drainage is via the same route plus the readily visible subdermal venous network. These vessels are the predominant blood supply to the skin of the human body [176].
2. *Perforator–direct cutaneous arteries* (providing blood supply for axial pattern flaps) parallel the skin for long distances [176, 220]. These arteries, which supply the *dermal-subdermal plexus* directly, lie in the subcutaneous tissue close to the muscle fascia (Fig. 1-20). Venous drainage is by way of the associated named subdermal vein, the paired venae comitantes, and the dermal venous plexus. A listing of the *named* direct cutaneous arteries in the body must include (1) superficial temporal a. (the vascular supply for a variety of forehead and scalp flaps); (2) posterior auricular a.; (3) occipital a.; (4) supraorbital a.; (5) supratrochlear a.; (6) facial a.; (7) a grouping consisting of the anterior perforators of the internal mammary a. (the arteries of the deltopectoral flap, see Fig. 1-22); (8) perforating branches of the deep epigastric arcade (the arteries of the transverse abdominal flap) [160]; (9) lateral (long) thoracic and (10) superior thoracic arteries (providing blood to the upper end of a thoracoepigastric flap); (11) superficial inferior epigastric a. (providing blood to the lower end of a thoracoepigastric flap); (12) superficial circumflex iliac (the artery of the groin flap, see Fig. 1-22); (13) superficial external pudendal a.; (14) dorsal artery of the penis [176]; and (15) the dorsalis pedis artery.

Hill, Brown, and Jurkiewicz [198] have pointed out that the subdermal vascular plexus extends uninterrupted across the midline as in other areas of the body. Therefore the midline need no longer be considered a barrier to the design of flaps, as demonstrated by the fact that the transverse abdominal flap, the lumbodorsal rotation flap, and the transverse lumbosacral back flap are quite safe.

Classification of Skin Flaps According to Their Blood Supply

Later in this chapter, skin flaps are classified according to where they are moved. Another way of classifying flaps is according to their blood supply.

1. *Random pattern skin flaps (cutaneous flaps).* These flaps receive their blood supply from segmental, anastomotic, or axial arteries which lie deep to the muscle, sending perpendicular perforator-musculocutaneous arteries at the flap's base to the interconnecting dermal-subdermal plexus of the skin. Thus they derive their blood supply through the cutaneous dermal-subdermal plexus (Fig. 1-21). Surviving length of such a flap is related to the vessels' perfusion pressure [176]. Thinning of these flaps is safe as long as a small amount of fat remains to protect the dermal-subdermal plexus. These flaps can be made longer (50 to 100 percent) by the delay procedure, as will be discussed subsequently. Most skin flaps are of this type.
2. *Axial pattern flaps (arterial or arterialized flaps).* These flaps receive their blood supply through a direct cutaneous artery which arises from a segmental, anastomotic, or axial artery, often by way of a short perforator artery. The length of such a flap is related to the length of the direct cutaneous artery included in the flap, plus additional more distal skin supplied by the dermal-subdermal plexus (Fig. 1-21). Thus an arterial flap consists of a proximal arterial pedicle and a more distal cutaneous portion [176]. The arterial pedicle must include the full thickness of subcutaneous tissue because the direct cutaneous artery courses close to the underlying muscular fascia, but the cutaneous portion can be thinned, leaving only a little fat to protect the dermal-subdermal plexus (Fig. 1-22B). Axial pattern flaps can be made even longer by the delay procedure. These arterialized skin flaps (Fig. 1-21) can be further subdivided into the following:
   a. *Peninsular flaps.* These flaps have a direct cutaneous artery and vein and a bridge of skin and subcutaneous tissue at their base. Examples are the deltopectoral (Fig. 1-22A) and groin flaps (Fig. 1-22B).
   b. *Island flaps.* Such flaps are connected to their base by a direct cutaneous artery and vein, with

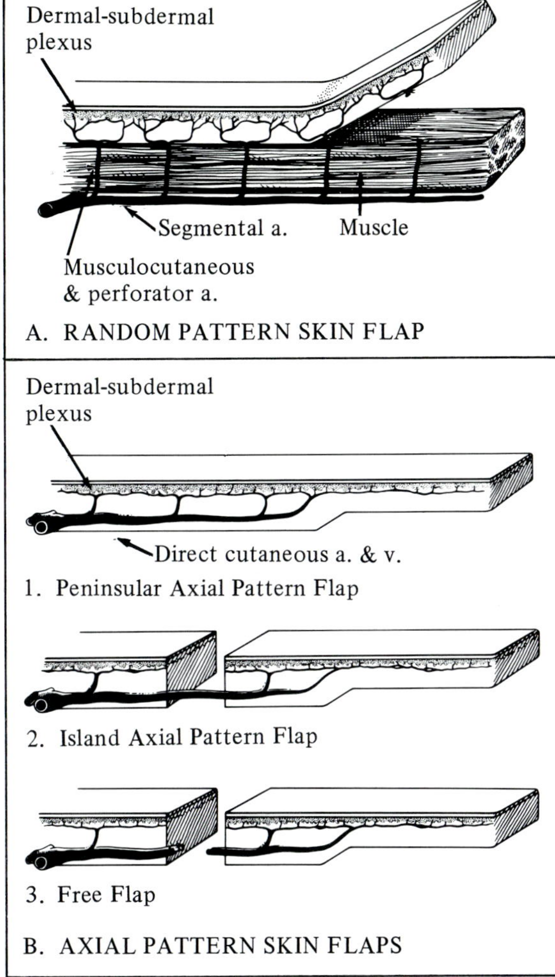

Fig. 1-21. Classification of skin flaps according to their anatomical blood supply. A, random pattern flaps. *These have a segmental, anastomotic, or axial artery and vein coursing deep to the muscle and giving off perforator-musculocutaneous vessels to the dermal-subdermal plexus of the skin. These perforator-musculocutaneous vessels enter the base of the flap, supplying the blood to the plexus in a relatively small area of skin. The dermal-subdermal plexus, however, has a vast interconnection of different size vessels in the dermal and perifollicular layers, which carry the blood supply to the random pattern flap. B,* axial pattern flaps. *These have direct cutaneous vessels lying subcutaneously, just above the muscular fascia that supply the dermal-subdermal plexus. There is adequate perfusion pressure to support not only the arterial pedicle but also an additional random pattern portion of the flap. The* peninsular flap *has an artery, a vein, and skin in continuity, at its base, whereas an* island flap *is connected to the body by only an artery and a vein. The* free flap *is an island flap with the vessels divided prior to being moved so that the vessels can be joined by microvascular techniques to segmental vessels.*

no skin bridge. Examples are the neurovascular island flap of the finger and the superficial temporal artery island flap. Converting a peninsula arterial flap into an island flap provides a greater flexibility in rotating the flap about its pivot point [176]. Another variation is to place a split-thickness skin graft directly on the direct cutaneous artery and vein, such as has been done with the superficial temporal artery and vein [183]. This technique transforms a thinner hairless skin graft into a vascularized flap. After incising the hair-bearing scalp on three sides in the distribution of the superficial temporal vessels and folding the scalp on itself, a skin graft is placed on these vessels. Twenty-one days later the skin graft is raised as a vascularized flap and used to cover the cartilage framework for an external ear reconstruction.

c. *Free flaps.* The perfection of microvascular surgery has enabled the transfer of free axial pattern skin flaps from a distant site in one operation (Fig. 1-21). Donor sites for free skin flaps include the ileofemoral island flap [174], lateral forehead island flap [239], deltopectoral island flap, a scalp flap nourished by the superficial temporal vessels [193], and a neurovascular free flap from the medial arm [175]. Recipient sites include the face, scalp, ankle, and hand. The anatomy of free flap donor sites has been detailed by Taylor and Daniel [269]. Much additional information on free flaps is included in Chapter 41.

Serafin et al. [255] have reported on their experience with free arterialized skin flaps for lower extremity reconstruction, as opposed to a cross leg flap or a jump flap. Although they reported only a 58 percent success rate with 17 free flaps, 77 percent success rate with 18 cross leg flaps, and 33 percent success with 6 jump flaps, it was their opinion that with increased experience survival statistics on microvascular free flaps will improve to make this the method of choice. They indicated that free flaps have the advantage of decreasing the total time of immobilization and hospitalization, as well as decreasing the number of operations and costs. In our opinion the free flap

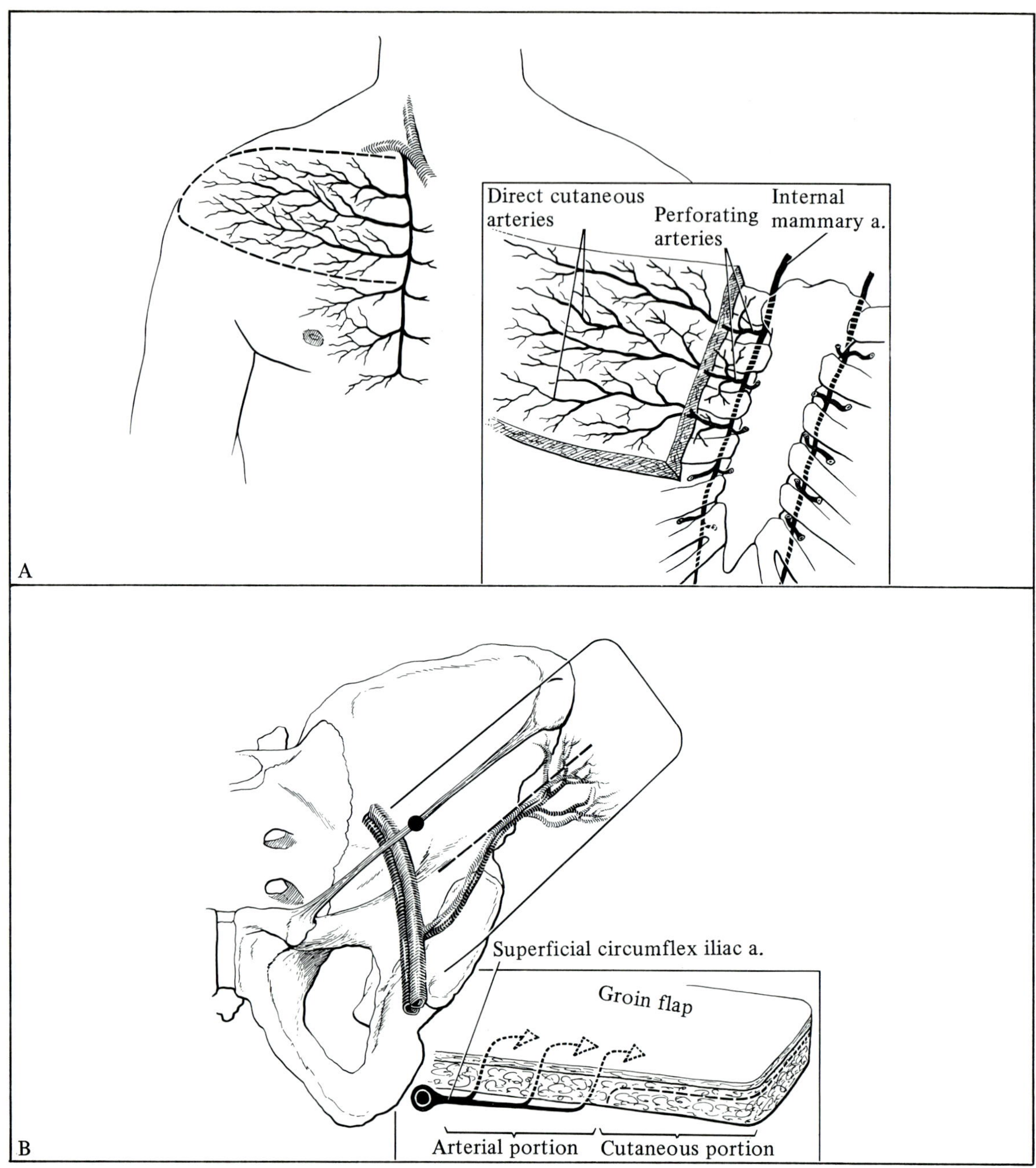

Fig. 1-22. Examples of axial pattern skin flaps based on direct cutaneous arteries and veins which take advantage of the fact that flaps based on such vessels survive to a 50 percent or more greater length than flaps based on the musculocutaneous-perforator-dermal-subdermal plexus of vessels. A, the deltopectoral (Bakamjian) flap *is based medially on the second, third, and fourth anterior perforator arteries of the internal mammary artery. The second perforator is the largest and most important. The superior margin of the flap follows the underlying clavicle, whereas the inferior margin runs laterally at a level approximately three fingerbreadths above the nipple (in the recumbent male), and the lateral margin can extend*

is still near the bottom of the list of choices for wound closure.

Man's ingenuity has added a variety of *composite tissues* to the list of body parts that can be moved as free flaps. These tissues include the following: dermafat compound free flap from the buttock to the breast [187], muscle flaps, myocutaneous gracilis flap to the forehead [195], omental free flap to the scalp, and a free osteocutaneous flap of the ninth rib and its overlying skin [183].

Uses of Skin Flaps

The following four categories include many of the indications for using skin flaps: (1) closure of wounds with a poor vascular bed, (2) reconstruction of facial features (eyelids, eyebrows, lips, ears, nose, and cheeks), (3) providing padding over bony prominences, and (4) permitting operation through the flap on underlying structures.

Closure of Wounds with a Poor Vascular Bed

WOUNDS OVERLYING THE TIBIA. Wounds of the lower extremity often have poor circulation and may require a skin flap, muscle flap, or myocutaneous flap for closure. Where cortical bone is exposed in the bed of a wound and lacks periosteal covering, the permanent pedicle blood-carrying flap described by Brown and McDowell [159] should be considered. It adds an additional supply of blood to the poorly vascularized recipient site because the original pedicle is preserved. When local tissues do not provide a satisfactory donor source for this type of flap and more distant tissues are to be transferred, it is important to excise sufficient surrounding scar so that the margins of the flap can be sutured to healthy tissues in order to obtain a satisfactory blood supply.

When the cortical surface of the tibia is removed, it may be possible to get a skin graft to survive on the cancellous bone or on the granulations which form. Because these grafts often are not stable enough to ensure against recurrent ulceration, a skin flap should be considered as a primary procedure, or as a secondary procedure after the wound has been closed with a skin graft.

Muscle and myocutaneous flaps have a major role in lower extremity reconstruction. Chapter 49 includes information on these flaps.

WOUNDS OVERLYING BARE BONE, CARTILAGE, TENDON, OR NERVE. Bone, cartilage, tendon, and nerve will not have sufficient circulation of their own to support a skin graft unless they are covered by the vascular envelope of periosteum, perichondrium, paratenon, or epineurium. A skin flap usually is necessary to gain a closed wound of sufficient stability. Even on healthy periosteum, skin grafts often will not withstand repeated trauma and must be replaced by a skin flap. Nerves should be covered by muscle, fat, or subcutaneous tissue to protect them from trauma.

OPEN CAVITIES. Open wounds of the chest, skull, or maxilla can be closed by a local permanent blood-carrying pedicle flap. A skin graft can be applied to the undersurface of the flap in any region where it bridges a cavity.

Reconstruction of Facial Features

Chapters 11 through 15 are concerned with reconstruction of the scalp, forehead, eyebrows, eyelids, ears, nose, lips, and cheeks. Skin flaps play an essential role in the reconstruction of these facial structures.

Padding over Bony Prominences

Skin flaps play a very important role in the treatment of pressure sores and those fingertip injuries in which all soft tissues have been lost. The principles of treating pressure sores are discussed in Chapter 50.

An injury of the fingertip with loss of skin and tactile pad may be treated with a skin flap to maintain finger length and restore proper padding. Treatment of fingertip injuries is discussed more fully in Chapter 32.

Operation through a Skin Flap on Underlying Structures

A skin graft will withstand only minimal degrees of undermining, manipulation, and wound retraction, and it has always been taught that it is not sufficiently stable for secondary operations on underlying nerve, tendon, artery, bone, or cartilage. Any wound of this type should first be closed with a skin flap and

---

to the lateral or even posterolateral aspect of the shoulder without being delayed. B, the groin flap *is based medially, and the outline of the flap has a* central axis *which lies between a mark made 2.5 cm. below the midpoint (solid black circle) of a line connecting the pubic tubercle and the anterior superior iliac spine, and 2.5 cm. below the anterior superior iliac spine. The flap is then made 7.5 to 10 cm. wide and can extend 2.5 to 5.0 cm. lateral to the anterior superior iliac spine [221]. All axial pattern skin flaps have an arterial and a cutaneous (random pattern) portion. The level of undermining of the arterial portion should include all the subcutaneous tissue so as to include the artery, whereas in the cutaneous portion only enough subcutaneous tissue to protect the subdermal plexus need be retained.*

allowed to mature before operation on these underlying structures is undertaken.

When an avulsion of overlying skin is accompanied by the division of such deeper structures as blood vessels, nerves, or tendons, the underlying structures can be repaired and the wound closed immediately with a skin flap.

Other Uses of Skin Flaps
The skin flap, if transferred with its nerve supply intact, will *restore sensation* to an area where it is needed. This technique has been particularly useful in providing sensation to anesthetic areas such as the ulnar aspect of the tip of the thumb or radial aspect of the index finger. An island of skin from the area of the tactile pad on the ulnar side of either the middle or the ring finger and based on one neurovascular bundle is utilized for this purpose [247].

Whole digits, based on their neurovascular pedicles, can be moved from one part of the hand to another. For example, the thumb can be reconstructed from an index finger by shortening and rotating it at the same time as it is transferred to the thumb position.

Composite skin flaps containing bone or cartilage are sometimes used in reconstruction. The bone or cartilage can be inserted beneath the skin flap a few weeks before the flap is to be transferred, or the flap can actually be developed so as to include the clavicle or iliac bone.

Requirements for Survival of a Skin Flap
When designing and transferring skin flaps, one's preoccupation should always be on the survival of the flap, with care taken that it has a sufficient inflow of arterial blood and outflow of venous blood to remain viable. Among matters that must be considered are the *size and location of the flap* that can be supported by the available blood supply, *delaying* the flap to increase its blood supply, and *maintaining* the blood supply present in the flap.

Size and Location of the Flap
There is no rule, no formula, no proportion of length to width for the safe design of a skin flap.

In designing a skin flap the following information can be helpful: (1) the presence of *large blood vessels* (direct cutaneous arteries and veins) coursing in the longitudinal axis of the flap permits the construction of a longer flap; (2) a flap designed in the *head and neck region* where the vascularity is greatest can be of more precarious design than in less vascular regions; (3) *delaying* a skin flap increases its blood supply and thus increases its surviving length; (4) a *bipedicle* skin flap will survive to a greater length than a single pedicle skin flap; and (5) *younger patients* have a better blood supply to their tissues and thus will probably have safe flaps of greater length than elderly patients.

Milton [225] has demonstrated experimentally in the pig the fallacy of the concept that the viable length of a skin flap depends on the width of its pedicle. Rather he showed that *flaps made under similar conditions of blood supply survive to the same length regardless of the width* (Fig. 1-19). Snell [258] has challenged this conclusion by showing in the pig that random pattern flaps with a narrower base (less than 3.0 cm.) will have a surviving length that increases with their width.

Planning of a skin flap so that a large artery and vein enter in through the base of the flap will definitely increase its surviving length. Milton [227] has demonstrated in the pig that the surviving length of skin flaps based on a direct cutaneous artery and vein is 50 percent greater than that of a skin flap based on the musculocutaneous artery–perforator artery–dermal-subdermal plexus.

The vascular supply within a segment of skin varies from area to area, but in general it decreases from the head down to the foot. Single pedicle flaps of greater length can be designed with greater safety in the head and neck region than around the ankle, where it is usually necessary to delay the flap. Collateral circulation across the midline of the body is poor on the trunk. This is especially true over the anterior aspect of the chest, where flaps extending across the midline are prone to become necrotic.

Decisions on the location of a flap or its dimensions must take into account other variables in blood supply. Arteriosclerotic changes will decrease the arterial supply of blood to the skin. Such pathological alterations in circulation must be considered in both the design and the execution of flaps in older patients [170]. If trauma, infection, or radiation has resulted in scarring or extensive fibrosis of the skin and subcutaneous tissue, it can also alter the blood supply of a region and the efficiency of its collateral circulation.

Delaying the Flap
The term *delaying a flap* is frequently used in the field of reconstructive surgery to indicate that the flap is being developed and transferred in more than a single stage to ensure its safety.

At this writing, although we have a better understanding of the mechanism of skin flap delay, there is a lack of agreement on all the details. Reinisch [251] believes that delay occurs by sympathectomizing the arteriovenous anastomoses of the skin. Finseth et al. [185, 186] believe that vascular smooth muscle relaxation (i.e., vasodilatation) augments the blood flow to the nutritional capillary bed of the skin, producing the delay phenomenon.

An early observation that stimulated Reinisch's

interest was that temperature readings on the skin surface of freshly raised long skin flaps were as warm at the distal end of the flap that would eventually die as they were at the base of the flap. With this preliminary finding that circulation exists in the end of the flap destined to become necrotic, he continued his investigation. One of his series of experiments on freshly raised flaps in pigs demonstrated that the circulation beyond the fluorescein-stained viable proximal portion of the flap exists in large arterio-venous channels and not in the small nutrient capillaries of the skin. Fifteen-micron microspheres injected intraarterially do not become trapped in the capillary bed of the skin of the distal flap, as they are circulating from artery to vein and out of the flap by passing through the large-diameter open arteriovenous shunts. If this blood had been able to circulate through the capillary bed of the skin, the spheres would have been trapped in the capillary bed (microspheres larger than 10 microns become permanently trapped in the first capillary bed they enter).

Arteriovenous shunts are incompletely understood precapillary communications between the arterial and venous circulations; when dilated their internal diameter ranges between 50 and 150 microns. Reinisch believes that as these shunts are innervated by the sympathetic nervous system, denervation (e.g., surgically delaying a skin flap) causes them to dilate and remain dilated for 10 to 14 days. After this length of time they acquire tonicity and constrict, as a result either of disuse atrophy or of denervation hypersensitivity to endogenous circulating catecholamines [251, 252].

Pharmacological delay [185, 252] and electrical delay [252] have also been shown to be effective in delaying a skin flap.

Finseth et al. [185, 186] maintain that precapillary sphincter and ateriolar vasodilatation is a principal factor resulting in the augmentation of nutritional capillary blood flow, as opposed to a parallel increased arteriovenous shunt blood flow. They reasoned from Poiseuille's law (which states that flow in a tube varies as the fourth power of the vessel radius) that precapillary vasodilatation alone can account for the observed augmentation of nutritional (capillary) blood flow, considering the density distribution of precapillary sphincters (10,000 to 15,000 per square centimeter of skin) compared to arteriovenous shunts (20 to 25 per square centimeter of skin) and their relative diameters (10-micron diameter of precapillary shunt as compared with approximately 50-micron diameter of arteriovenous shunt). For example, if there is a 1-micron dilatation of each of these vessels, the proportional amounts of blood distributed to the capillaries are considerably increased.

Finseth et al. [185, 186] also demonstrated that devascularization (that is, ligation of arterial or venous vessels to an island flap) and sympathectomy without devascularization will produce the delay phenomenon. Thus, both ischemia and sympathectomy appear to be significant factors.

Finseth states (in a personal communication, 1977) that he is still not certain how vasodilatation accounts for the delay phenomenon, nor why delay maneuvers must be maintained over a given time period to obtain greater surviving length of a skin flap.

Vasodilation with isoxsuprine, a long-acting smooth muscle relaxing agent that dilates the precapillary sphincter and arteriole, has been demonstrated to produce the delay phenomenon in rats [185]. Isoxsuprine was given to rats intraperitoneally daily for 15 days before raising neurovascular island skin flaps, and it was continued for 7 days postoperatively. Flaps in the treated rats survived to twice the length (30 cm.) of control flaps (14 cm.). These flaps had grossly visible vasodilatation of the capillary bed which could be seen on the skin surface.

Clinically we prefer delaying the flap by incision on the two parallel sides and undermining (Fig. 1-23), then *dividing the third side in two or three stages,* 2 or 3 days apart, beginning 7 days following the initial procedure. Such staging can usually be carried out under local anesthesia, on an outpatient basis. Often the first incision across the end of the flap consists of dividing one-half of the remaining intact skin and resuturing it, while the second stage consists of division of the one-quarter or even the remaining one-half of intact skin. Though time consuming, these staged incisions give us assurance that when the flap is finally moved it should remain viable.

Milton [226] determined experimentally in the pig that after delaying a flap as described above there

Fig. 1-23. Delay of a random pattern skin flap. Initially the flap is incised on its two parallel sides and the area of the flap is undermined. Seven days following this initial procedure, division of the third side is begun and is continued in stages usually 2 or 3 days apart. The flap is then moved 2 or 3 days after completion of this division of the third side.

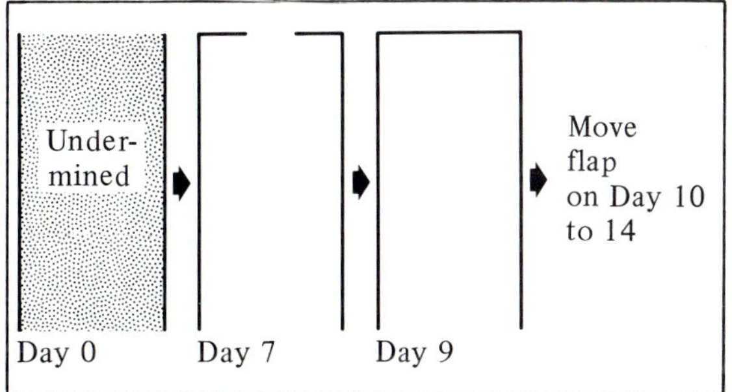

was an increase in surviving length of approximately 60 percent. Myers and Cherry [236] demonstrated an increase in length after delay of 80 percent, whereas Daniel and Williams demonstrated a 100 percent increase [176].

Myers [234] maintains that in most areas of the body a flap of any width over 3.0 cm. will survive for at least 5.0 cm. Thus a bipedicle flap 9.0 cm. long is safe, and when the third side is divided in stages, the entire flap will survive. If a longer flap is needed, a *double delay* procedure can be done. At the first operation, two in-line 9.0-cm. bipedicle flaps are raised with a 2.0-cm. bridge between them. One week later this bridge is incised in such a way as to join the two 9.0-cm. bipedicle flaps, creating a bipedicle flap 20.0 cm. long. After another 7 to 10 days this flap can be raised and *at least 13.0 cm. will survive* from either end. The fluorescein test should be used to determine the surviving length, with the nonfluorescing tissue being excised. Brent [158] has described the double delay of a narrow (14 mm.) flap that eventually survives to a safe length of 12 cm. for use in reconstructing the helical rim.

When one end of the flap is divided and transplanted, it usually takes 4 to 5 days before venous connections can be demonstrated by microangiography to have developed between the flap and recipient site. Arterial anastomoses are not seen for 7 days. The number of arterial and venous connections increases rapidly during the second week [274]. Myers and Cherry [234a] showed in the rabbit that the maximal surviving length of experimental skin flaps occurred at 8 to 10 days after delay. There was even a definitely increased survival at 4 days, reaching the maximum at 8 to 10 days, then falling off. There was still a definitely increased survival up to 21 days, the longest delay time studied. Hoffmeister [199], after studying the rates of radioactive sodium (^{24}Na) clearance, suggested that a flap that had been delayed by incising on three sides and undermined could best be transferred about 2 to 4 weeks after being developed.

Goetz [189, 190] has studied by plethysmography the amount of blood flowing through normal skin under various circumstances. During rest the flow is 15 ml. per minute for 100 cc. of tissue, and with full vascular dilatation it is 90 ml. per minute; however, the skin only needs a flow of 1 to 2 ml. per minute to provide nutrition for 100 cc. of tissue. Burton [163] has also emphasized that the primary purpose of the blood supply to the skin is for thermoregulation (90 to 97 percent) and not nutrition (3 to 10 percent). It is fortunate that such a low rate of flow will sustain the skin, for Hoffmeister has shown that there is a profound drop in the circulatory efficiency of a flap immediately following incision and undermining.

The use of a tourniquet or rubber-shod clamp across the base of a flap in an attempt to increase its vascular supply is not as effective as incising and undermining. Temporarily clamping the flap produces only a transient reactive hyperemia.

TESTS OF CIRCULATION. Various tests of the circulation in a skin flap have been developed to aid in determining when the pedicle of a direct flap can be divided, if a flap which has been elevated will survive, and the earliest time that a delayed flap can be moved safely. Creech and Miller [172] have written extensively on the many tests of skin flap viability.

There has been a trend toward earlier division of the pedicle of direct flaps. For example, the vermilion-bordered lip flap (Abbe flap) can be divided at 8 days [256], and the cross finger flap at 12 to 14 days. Klingenström and Nylén [209] have demonstrated in three large, tubed bipedicle flaps from the anterior chest or abdomen, five cross leg flaps, and two cross finger flaps that the flaps could be divided in 7 to 14 days. Some of the bipedicle and cross leg flaps were divided in two stages, 3 days apart. More evidence for earlier division has been added by Tauxe et al. [268], who followed the disappearance rate of radioactive pertechnetate from 44 flaps after injecting it adjacent to the site of the planned flap division, with both the flaps' blood supply unoccluded and then occluded at this end. When the blockage of outflow of the radioactive material was down to 80 percent of the occluded value, the flap could be safely divided. Although many of the flaps could be divided by 10 days or so, two flaps in radiated tissue were not ready for division until 42 and 45 days.

The intravenous fluorescein test, a measure of the perfusion of tissues, is the best clinical test to predict skin flap viability at the time of operation. For this test, 20 ml. of 5% sodium fluorescein is injected rapidly intravenously about 20 minutes after the flap has been raised. The almost immediate yellow fluorescence of the patient's epithelial surfaces is noted with an ultraviolet light in a darkened room. Areas of spotty fluorescence can be stroked with a hemostat, and if a yellow line appears where the flap was stroked, the skin will survive. Myers [231–233] has used this method for predicting the adequacy of blood supply to the skin of anterior chest skin flaps for closure following radical mastectomy. In some 65 cases there was a definite correlation of fluorescence (yellowish-green color in ultraviolet light) with skin survival and nonfluorescence (purplish-blue color) with skin necrosis. Areas of nonfluorescence have an impaired blood supply and will go on to necrosis; such areas should be excised. Goode and Linehan [191] report a similar finding in 20 patients with radiated neck skin who had a Y incision for radical neck dissection. In the 9 patients who showed definite nonfluorescent areas, 6 had this area excised, and there was no subsequent necrosis, whereas necrotic skin developed in the predicted area in the other 3 patients. These authors were not as successful in predicting skin viability in nonirradiated neck flaps, as there were false negatives due to the distal end of the flap not taking up the dye, but remaining viable. One anaphylactic reaction to intravenous fluorescein has been reported, with pruritus and partial respiratory obstruction successfully treated by intramuscularly administrated 1 : 1,000 epinephrine [212]. Thorvaldsson and Grabb [272] have similarly reported on the reliable evaluation of the viability of 19 skin flaps in their patients by using this test.

The *Doppler flowmeter* can be used to monitor flow in even the small arteries of an arterialized flap. This instrument can also be used to map out the course of vessels in the axial pattern skin flap.

Other tests of circulatory efficiency include the following:

1. The *histamine wheal test* is a simple method of evaluating circulation in a skin flap. The rate of skin wheal formation in the flap is compared to wheal formation in a control area of skin [119].
2. Injection of a radioisotope into the flap with its rate of disappearance from the flap being compared with that from a control area on the opposite side of the body [156, 195, 199, 268].
3. The absorption of atropine from the flap as evidenced by tachycardia, inability to focus on newsprint, and dryness of the mouth [201].
4. The photoplethysmograph, which utilizes changes in the amount of light reflected by tissues to normal pulsatile blood flow, has been successfully used to determine the proper time for moving of a delayed or distant skin flap [197, 270].
5. Determination of the temperature of the flap by thermography using an infrared scanner in a controlled environment [157, 243, 271].
6. The saline wheal test, which has the disadvantage of requiring an hour to execute, has an indistinct end point [264].
7. Use of a thermocouple to measure skin temperature, a method which is probably too imprecise for clinical use [182, 277].

Maintaining the Blood Supply of the Flap

Once a skin flap with an adequate blood flow has been moved to its recipient site, it should survive unless there is *tension, kinking, pressure, hematoma,* or *infection* in the flap. Each of these conditions can be treated.

Tension may develop in a local flap if it is stretched tightly in order to reach the furthest extent of the wound. Blanching of the skin along the line of greatest tension (the line between the pivot point and that part of the flap most distant to it) may be seen in rotation, transposition, and interpolation of flaps if they are stretched too tightly (see Figs. 1-25, 1-28, 1-34). Sundell [266] showed that a small tensile force (25 gm.) was sufficient to lead to venous congestion and partial flap necrosis unless the tension was released within 4 hours. This tension can be relieved by returning the flap to its site of origin by a tiny incision with a #11 blade through the skin at right angles to and in the center of the blanched zone (see Fig. 1-27) [283], skin grafting the flap donor site rather than approximating the wound edges, or back cutting a short segment of the base of the flap, starting at the pivot point (see Figs. 1-25, 1-28). Whatever the technique used for releasing tension in the flap, it is probably necessary that it be carried out within 4 hours after its onset.

Kinking is most likely to occur in tubed pedicle flaps. This can be corrected by proper repositioning or immobilization, so that there is no acute angulation of the flap.

Pressure may be either external or internal in origin. External pressure from too tight a dressing or a compression of the flap by the patient's position can be easily corrected. Internal pressure, by contrast, is usually harder to correct if it results from including too much fatty tissue in a tubed pedicle. Milton [226] has studied the problems of enclosing enough fat in the tubed arterial flap to preserve the vessels without strangling the circulation by too much tension. It has been calculated that edema causes flaps to increase in weight by 35 percent in the first 24 hours. Allowing for this percentage of swelling, Milton calculated that the width must be at least 17 times the thickness of the tubed flap to prevent pressure necrosis. Patterson and Cherry [245] in their studies in the pig noted that strangulation of the blood supply occurred only when the width of the flap was less than four times the thickness of the flap.

Hematoma in a flap should be treated by returning the patient to the operating room, evacuating the clotted blood, and obtaining absolute hemostasis. The internal pressure caused by hematoma can cause necrosis of the flap.

Infection in a skin flap in the early postoperative period may be disastrous. Because of its decreased blood flow, a recently elevated flap may be capable of supplying or supporting only its basic metabolic needs [190], and will be unable to provide the increased flow needed for an inflammatory reaction. Thus, an infection which might be of little consequence in normal tissue can readily destroy the poorly vascularized tissue of a skin flap. Treatment should consist of proper drainage, frequent wet-dressing changes, and antibiotics.

Myers [234] has discovered that some of the skin flaps which became necrotic a few days after operation had become infected with an anaerobic organism, *Bacteroides aeruginosa*. He found that the diagnosis of this infection could be made by shining an ultraviolet light on the flap and noting a visible red fluorescence from the organisms.

Epinephrine is not detrimental to flaps raised primarily, but the surviving length of a delayed flap will be impaired by epinephrine [249].

DESPERATION MEASURES TO IMPROVE THE CIRCULATION IN A FLAP. A great deal of effort has been devoted to finding ways in which a skin flap with vascular insufficiency can be salvaged. Unfortunately, most of the methods described are of limited clinical value for improving the compromised circulation of a flap. They never serve as a substitute for proper planning.

Postural assistance to venous outflow from the flap may be of some benefit. If the base of a tubed flap is placed in a dependent position, gravity may aid the flow of venous blood from a flap [202, 204]. *Leeches* have been employed to remove venous blood from a flap [180, 204]. *Alternating pressure* by blood pressure cuffs attached to an automatic intermittent venous occluder can force blood in and out of the flap every 2 minutes [202]. *Returning the flap to its recipient site* probably has its most sound application when there is tension on the flap. None of these measures have been properly evaluated with suitable controls.

Cooling the flap to a surface temperature between 0° and 20°C. within 4 hours of operation reduces the severity of necrosis in experimental skin flaps, but does not prevent it [282]. Such extreme cooling of flaps has not been adopted clinically, although fans have been used by many in hopes of decreasing the metabolic needs of a flap. *Low-molecular-weight dextran* has been infused intravenously in an unsuccessful effort to improve circulation by decreasing the intravascular aggregation of blood cells [192, 241], although one study showed a beneficial effect of intravenously administered dextran, as well as mannitol [266]. *Hyperbaric oxygen* has been used with both no success and definite success for improving the salvage rate of experimental skin flaps [56, 151, 205, 219].

Complamin, which has a fibrinolytic effect, was not helpful [151]. *Dimethyl sulfoxide,* which has been shown to increase the length of survival of skin flaps in one series [149], was not effective in three other series [151, 210, 235]. *Histamine iontophoresis* has been ineffective [179, 228]. *Systemic hypertension* produced vascular augmentation of experimental skin flaps according to one group [207], but a subsequent study failed to show any increased surviving length of skin flaps [228]. *Negative suction drainage* through polyethylene tubing beneath the flap decreased interstitial flap tissue pressure 30 percent on the average and seemed to have a beneficial effect on flap survival [266].

When a portion of a skin flap has definitely become necrotic, it is best to excise that portion immediately. Infection in necrotic tissue that is left in place will only act to spread the extent of tissue loss.

Planning of a Skin Flap

The proper planning of a flap is essential to the success of the operation. All possible sites and orientations for the flap should be considered to be certain that the most suitable one is selected. Wet dressings may be required to clean a dirty wound, and it may be best to first obtain a closed wound with a skin graft before applying the skin flap.

Planning of the flap in reverse is probably the most important part of the operation. A pattern of the defect is transferred onto a piece of cloth toweling (Fig. 1-24). The steps in the operative procedure are carried out in reverse order, using this pattern until the donor site is reached. It is important that the pattern is cut to include the base of the flap and that it is made a little longer and wider than needed. The pattern is then tried again, being certain each time it is shifted that the base is held in a fixed position and not allowed to shift with the flap. The *final pattern should be larger than needed,* particularly in its length. In this way undue tension and kinking can be avoided. It is easier to trim a flap which is a little large than to add to one which is too small.

Planning of a transposition or rotation flap requires special attention to ensure that the line of greatest tension from the pivot point to the most distal part of the flap is of sufficient length (Fig. 1-25; also see Fig. 1-28). The outlining of flaps to be transferred from a distance should also be done with an additional margin of reserve in length, so that the pedicle will not be kinked or under tension during transfer. Such decisions as to which arm to use as a carrier are also made at this time and in the same reverse fashion.

All planning should be done at a time prior to operation when all of the possible sites and orientations of the flap can be considered adequately. The final pattern can then be sterilized for use in the operating room.

Classification of Skin Flaps and Their Operative Technique

Skin flaps can be classified as to their anatomical blood supply: random pattern skin flaps supplied by

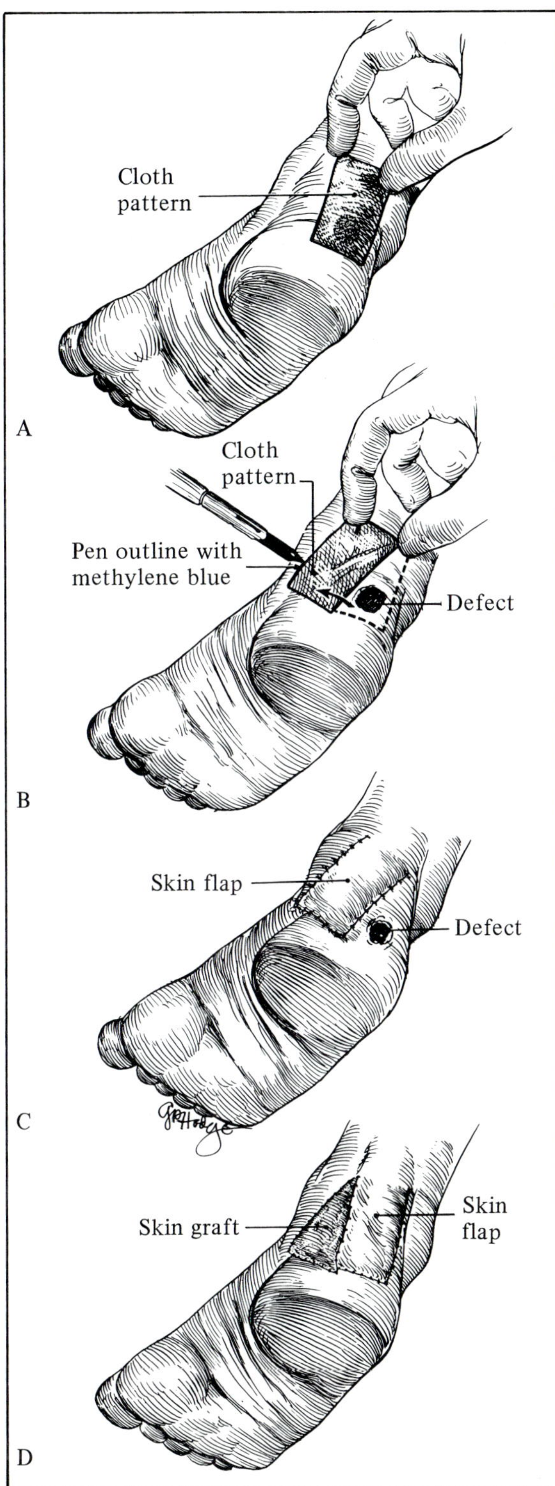

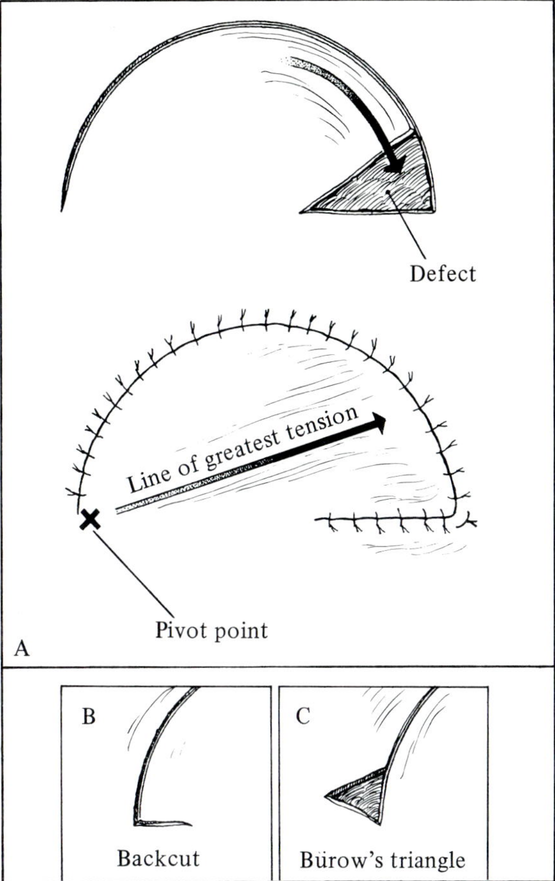

Fig. 1-25. Rotation flap. A back cut or a Bürow's triangle can be used if the flap is under too much tension, although proper planning should make this unnecessary.

Fig. 1-24. Planning a skin flap in reverse to cover a defect over the Achilles tendon. A and B, with a cloth pattern the steps of the flap transposition are carried out; the base of the flap should be held firmly in place. C, the flap is delayed because of the relatively poor blood supply of the foot and the excessive length-to-width ratio of this flap. D, 3 weeks later the flap is transposed.

the musculocutaneous artery—perforator artery—dermal-subdermal plexus, and axial pattern skin flaps supplied by direct cutaneous arteries to the dermal-subdermal plexus. Skin flaps can also be classified as to where they are moved. This latter classification includes local skin flaps, distant skin flaps, and variations on the theme – free flaps, the crane principle, and compound flaps.

Local Skin Flaps

Local flaps contain tissues lying adjacent to the defect which usually match the skin at the recipient site in color, texture, hair, and thickness. Such flaps require fewer operative stages and a shorter period of hospitalization than flaps from a distance.

Local flaps are usually *open* and are applied directly to the recipient site without leaving the subcutaneous surface of the pedicle exposed. These flaps may be *closed* or lined by applying a split-thickness skin graft to the undersurface of the flap or folding the flap on itself.

Local skin flaps are of two types: (1) flaps that rotate about a pivot point (rotation, transposition, and interpolation flaps) and (2) advancement flaps (single pedicle advancement, V-Y advancement, Y-V advancement, and bipedicle advancement flaps).

It bears mention that all of these local flaps are more easily executed in the older patient, whose skin is looser and will give in to a change in location more easily.

FLAPS THAT ROTATE ABOUT A PIVOT POINT. Rotation, transposition, and interpolation flaps all have in common a *pivot point,* and an *arc* through which the flap is rotated. The *radius* of this arc is the line of greatest tension of the flap. The realization that these flaps can only be rotated about the pivot point is important to their planning.

The *rotation flap* is a semicircular flap of skin and subcutaneous tissue that rotates about a pivot point into the defect to be closed (Fig. 1-25) (examples of rotation flaps are included in Chapters 11 and 50). Its donor site can be closed by a skin graft or by direct suture of the wound.

The line of greatest tension in a rotation flap extends from the pivot point outward in the direction indicated in Figure 1-25. Careful preoperative planning in reverse ensures that rotation of the flap into the defect will be accomplished without excessive tension.

When the donor site is closed with a split-thickness skin graft, a tie-over dressing may prove advantageous; it permits pressure to be maintained on the skin graft without putting pressure on the skin flap. Sutures for the tie-over dressing should not be placed in the flap, but rather through the bed for the skin graft adjacent

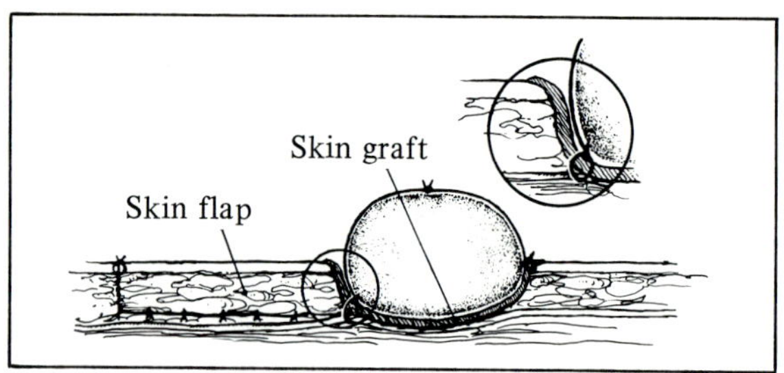

Fig. 1-26. The skin flap donor site can be closed with a split-thickness skin graft which is held in place with a tie-over dressing. The tie-over sutures should be inserted through the base of the wound, rather than the edge of the flap.

to the flap. These sutures are placed through the graft so that the edge of the graft can be approximated to the edge of the flap (Fig. 1-26). The donor site is rarely closed by primary suture because so often this places excessive tension on the flap itself.

A flap that is too tight along its radius can be released by making a short *back cut* from the pivot point along the base of the flap (Fig. 1-28B). Since this back cut decreases the blood supply to the flap, its use requires some degree of caution. In some flaps it will be possible to selectively back cut only the tissue responsible for the tension, without reducing the blood supply to the flap. Examples of this selective cutting are found in the galea aponeurotica of the scalp and in areas over the trunk where the fascia within the thick subcutaneous layer can be divided. The necessity for a back cut may be an indication of poor planning.

A triangle of skin (Bürow's triangle [162]) can be removed from the area adjacent to the pivot point of the flap to aid its advancement and rotation (Fig. 1-25C). This is of only modest benefit in decreasing tension along the radius of the flap.

Gibson and Kenedi [283] have shown that the initial pull to stretch skin will permit considerable stretching with little force. With continued force, the stretching decreases rapidly and then finally very little stretching will be produced by markedly increased force. This increased force produces blanching of the skin along the line of greatest tension, which they have been able to relieve by a tiny incision through the skin at right angles to, and in the center of, the blanched zone (Fig. 1-27). Up to 60 percent more force can be absorbed by this simple technique. The incision is small, penetrating the dermis with little risk of damaging the dermal-subdermal plexus of a cutaneous skin flap.

A dog ear forms at the pivot point with rotation, transposition, and interpolation flaps. In most

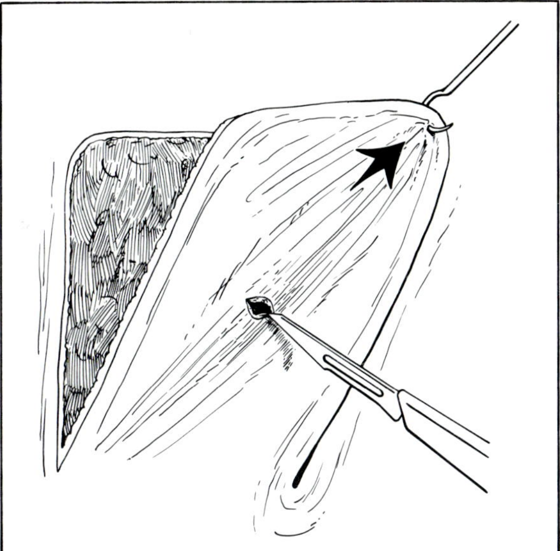

Fig. 1-27. Blanching along the line of greatest tension in a tightly stretched skin flap can be relieved by a tiny incision with a #11 knife blade at right angles to, and in the center of, the blanched zone. It should be emphasized that proper planning of the flap would have prevented the blanching.

patients it flattens out and becomes inconspicuous after several months but if it persists, a second operation may be necessary to remove the redundant tissue.

The *transposition flap* is a rectangle or square of skin and subcutaneous tissue which also is rotated about a pivot point into an immediately adjacent defect (Fig. 1-28) (examples of transposition flaps are included in Chapter 11). This fact necessitates that the end of the flap adjacent to the defect be designed to extend beyond it (Figs. 1-29, 1-33). Then, as the flap is rotated, with the line of greatest tension as the radius of the rotation arc, the advancing tip of the flap will be sufficiently long. A short back cut can also be carried out in these flaps if they are too tight along the line of greatest tension (Fig. 1-28B).

The flap donor site can be closed by skin grafting, by direct suture of the wound, or by a secondary flap from the most lax skin at right angles to the primary flap. An example of this last technique is the *bilobed flap* (Fig. 1-30) [178]. The key to a successful bilobed flap is an area of loose skin to permit the direct closure of the secondary flap defect [178]. Pinching the skin between the examiner's fingers will help in finding the loosest skin, such as in the glabellar area and lateral to the eyelids.

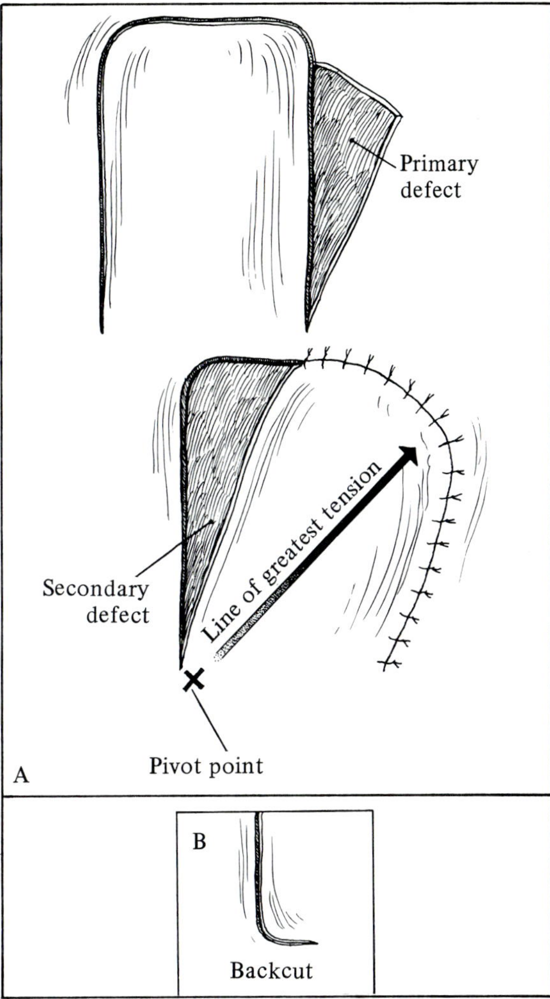

Fig. 1-28. Transposition flap. The secondary defect is often closed by a skin graft. A back cut can be used if the flap is under too much tension.

In the Z-plasty, another example of the transposition flap, each of two adjacent triangular skin flaps is rotated into the defect left by the other flap (see Fig. 1-40). An extensive discussion of the Z-plasty is included later in this chapter.

The *Limberg flap* is another transposition flap that the surgeon can draw from his quiver of techniques to close a skin defect. This flap, like the bilobed flap and the Z-plasty, depends on the looseness of adjacent skin, which can be located by pinching various areas of skin between thumb and forefinger. Fortunately the majority of patients requiring local skin flaps are in the older age group and therefore have looser skin. A

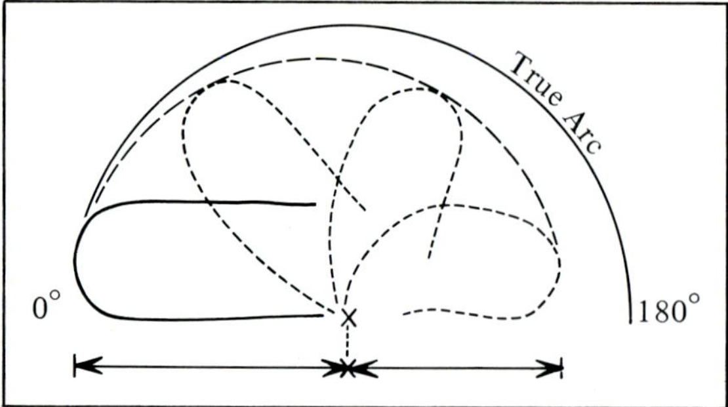

Fig. 1-29. A skin flap rotated about a pivot point will become shorter in effective length the further it is rotated. Planning with a cloth pattern is most helpful in designing such a flap.

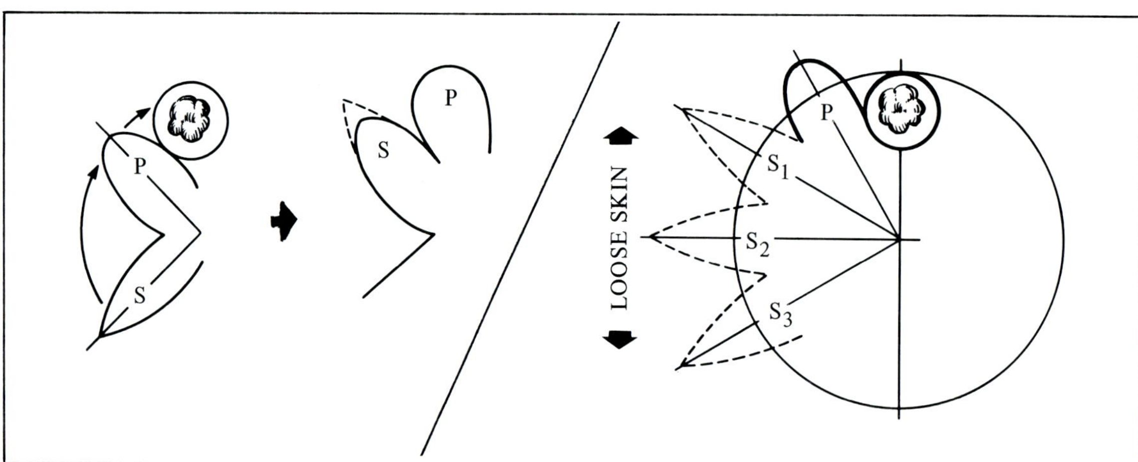

Fig. 1-30. The bilobed flap. After the lesion at the top is excised, the primary flap (P) is transposed into the initial defect. The secondary flap (S) is then transposed into the defect left after the primary flap has been moved. The primary flap is slightly narrower than the defect caused by the excision of the initial lesion, and the secondary flap is narrower than the primary flap. In order for the bilobed flap to be successful, the secondary flap must come from an area of loose skin, so that the defect remaining after moving this secondary flap can be closed by approximation of the wound edges. Three possible choices for the secondary flap (S_1, S_2, S_3) are depicted.

Limberg flap is suitable only for the closure of rhomboid defects with angles of 60 and 120 degrees [203, 214]. The Limberg flap has sides of the same length as the short axis of the rhomboid defect. The planning of such a flap is illustrated in Figures 1-31 and 1-32. In one series of 35 Limberg and Dufourmentel flaps, mostly in the face, all had satisfactory results, although there were 3 partial sloughs, 1 minimal wound separation, and 1 flap donor site in the scalp that was too tight to close by direct suture and thus required a skin graft [203].

The *Dufourmentel flap* is similar, except that it can be used for rhomboids with angles up to 90 degrees [203, 214]. Its planning is more complex; since a rhomboid with an angle of 90 degrees can be converted to one with angles of 60 and 120 degrees by additional skin excision, we prefer to use the Limberg flap.

When thickness is desirable for the purposes of padding, the entire subcutaneous layer can be included with the flap. In other cases only sufficient fat to restore a contour may be desired. Sometimes, when a relatively thin flap of sufficient length is needed, the thickness near its base can be increased so that additional perforating vessels to this area of skin might also be included for additional assurance of its circulation. Once such a flap has been developed, it is important that adequate hemostasis be achieved both on the undersurface of the flap and in the bed. Atraumatic technique is important to the success of these flaps, and skin hooks should be used for handling and rotating the flap to its new site. It may prove desirable to attach the underside of the flap to its bed with a few fine catgut sutures to obliterate a potential dead space. This must be done carefully, however, so that circulation of the tip of the flap will not be altered. Half-buried horizontal mattress sutures or simple interrupted sutures can be used for approximating the skin margins. Large flaps should be drained with a catheter connected to suction if there is a reason to believe that fluid might accumulate beneath the flap. Pressure must be kept off the flap.

An *interpolation flap* consists of skin and subcutaneous tissue which is rotated in an arc about a pivot point into a *nearby, but not immediately adjacent, defect.* The pedicle of this flap must therefore pass over or under the intervening tissue (Fig. 1-34).

A good example of this type of flap is the sickle flap, in which forehead skin based on the temporal vessels is utilized for facial reconstruction [237]. The deltopectoral (Bakamjian) flap (see Fig. 1-22A) is a very useful interpolation flap for head and neck

Fig. 1-31. Planning of a Limberg flap. The rhomboid defect must have 60- and 120-degree angles. The flap must be planned in an area of loose skin so that direct closure of the wound edges is possible. The short diagonal BD (which is also the same length as each side) is extended by its own length to point E. The line EF is drawn parallel to CD and of the same length. After the flap margins have been incised, the flap is transposed into rhomboid defect.

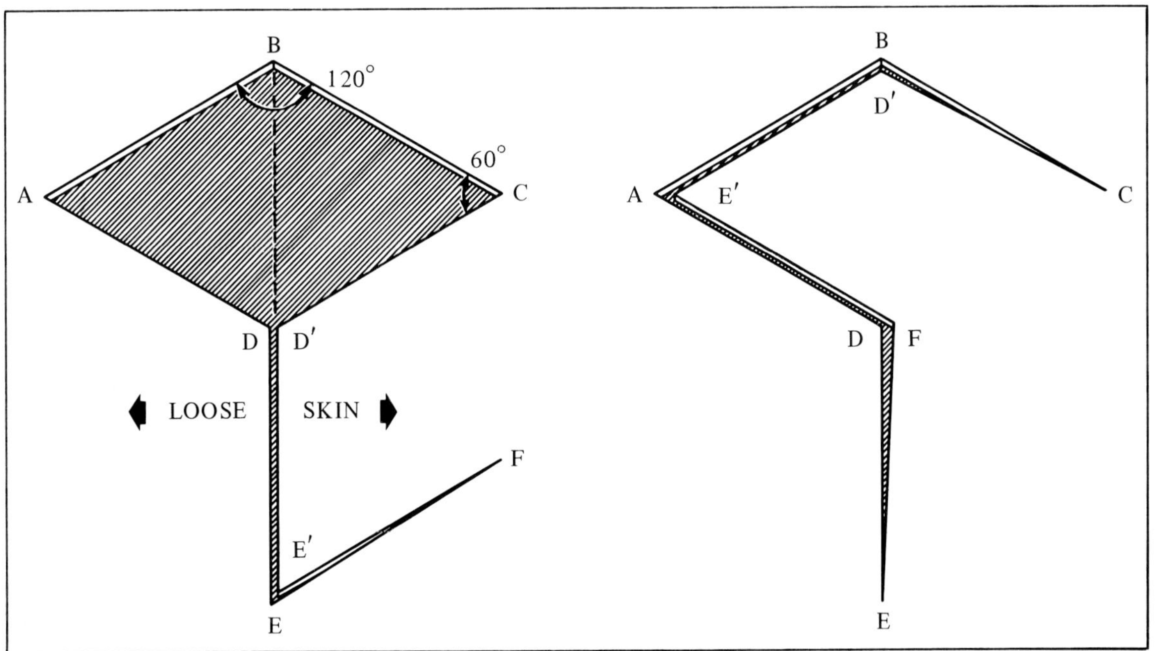

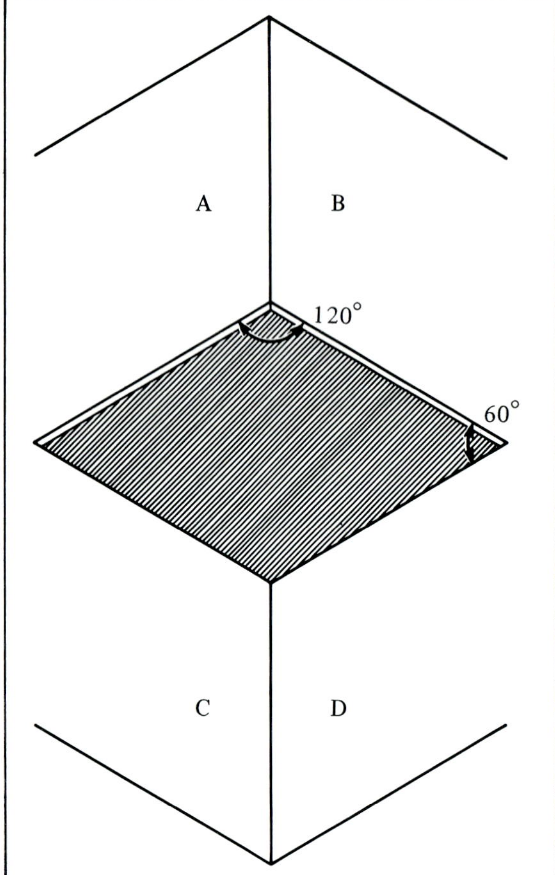

Fig. 1-32. There are four Limberg flaps available for any rhomboid defect with a 60- and a 120-degree angle.

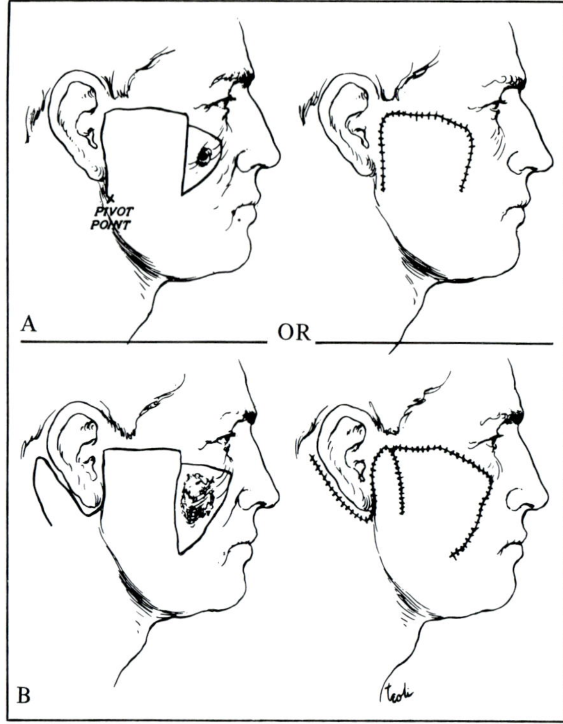

Fig. 1-33. Transposition flap which can be used to close defects on the anterior cheek. A, small defects can be closed by a single transposition cheek flap which follows the skin lines. B, large defects can be closed by a double transposition flap which uses a flap of postauricular skin to close the cheek flap donor site.

reconstruction. In these examples of interpolated flaps, the pedicle of the flap passes across the surface of the intervening skin. The exposed portion of the pedicle may be closed with a skin graft, but this is usually unnecessary.

The *island flap* is another type of interpolation flap, in which an island of skin with its neurovascular pedicle (in the hand) or an arteriovenous pedicle (in the face) is transferred through a tunnel beneath the skin and sutured into its new position. Additional information on island flaps is included in Chapters 14 and 32.

ADVANCEMENT FLAP. All the advancement flaps are moved directly forward into a defect without any rotation or lateral movement. Modifications are the single pedicle advancement, the V-Y advancement, the Y-V advancement, and the bipedicle advancement flaps.

The *single pedicle advancement flap* (sliding or French flap) is a rectangular- or square-shaped flap of skin and subcutaneous tissue which is stretched forward. Advancement is accomplished by taking advantage of the elasticity of the skin (Fig. 1-35A) and by excising Bürow's triangles lateral to the flap (Fig. 1-35B). These triangular excisions help to equalize the length between sides of the flap and adjacent wound margins. Pantographic expansion further aids the advancement, as Stark [261] has described, by back cutting each side of the wide base so that these cuts will open up as a V when the flap is advanced (Fig. 1-35C).

Converse [166] has utilized a "1-2" type of advancement which deliberately places the flap under tension initially. Two to 3 weeks later it is released by transecting its base, and the resulting defect is covered

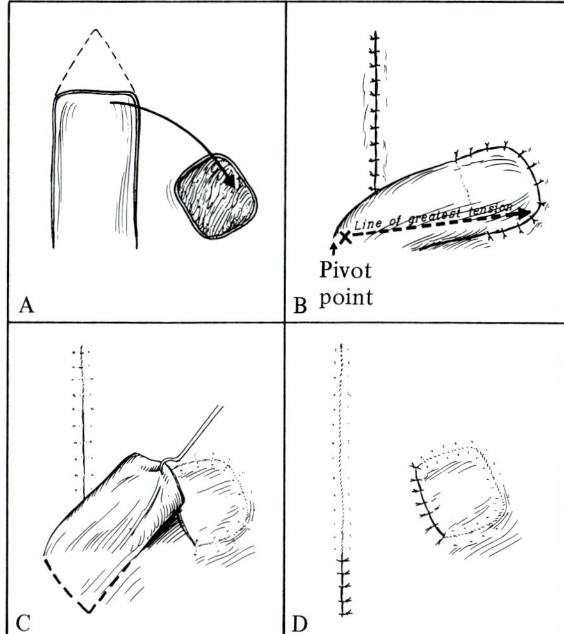

Fig. 1-34. Interpolation flap. A and B, skin flap is rotated into the nearby defect with the pedicle passing over the intervening skin. C and D, 3 weeks later, after the distal end of the flap has gained its new blood supply, the pedicle is excised.

with a skin graft. This technique is employed primarily in the head and neck, where the vascularity is sufficient to ensure survival of skin even under high degrees of tension.

The *V-Y advancement* technique has numerous applications. It is not an advancement in the same sense as the forward movement of a skin flap just described. Rather a V-shaped incision is made in the skin, after which the skin on each side of the V is advanced and the incision closed as a Y (Fig. 1-36). This V-Y technique can be used to lengthen such structures as the nasal columella, eliminate minor notches of the lip, and, in certain instances, close the donor site of a skin flap.

The *Y-V advancement flap* is just the opposite to the V-Y advancement. Y-V flaps are usually used in a serial arrangement to release skin scar contractures, such as occur with Dupuytren's contracture. As can be seen in Figure 1-37, the advancement is obtained in a direction perpendicular to the axis of the scar contracture. In multiple Y-V flaps, the number of these flaps should be about four, the advancing angle should be about 90 degrees, and the maximum length of the straight limb of the Y should be determined by the amount of lateral give, but

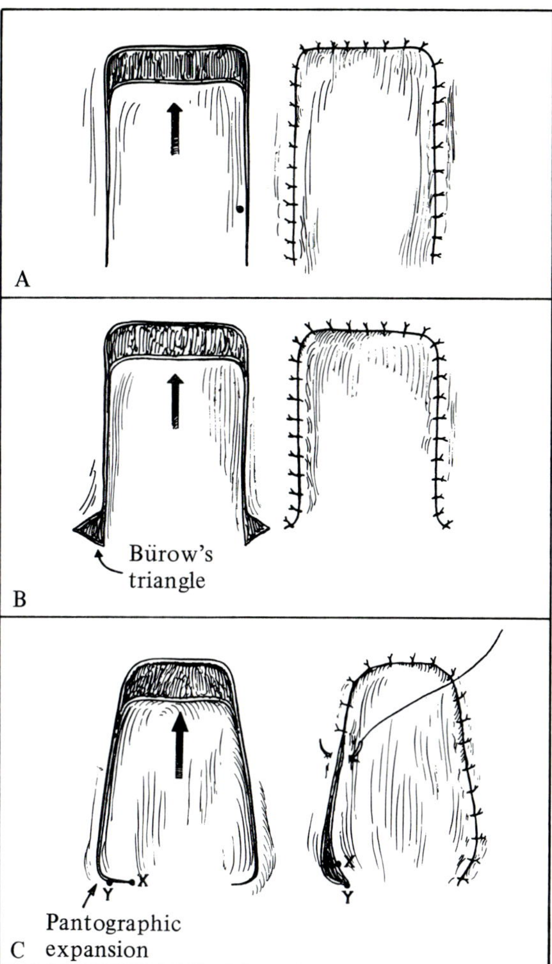

Fig. 1-35. Single pedicle advancement flaps. A, advancement by taking advantage of the skin's elasticity; B, advancement by excising Bürow's triangles of skin laterally to equalize the length of the flap and the adjacent wound edge; and C, pantographic expansion.

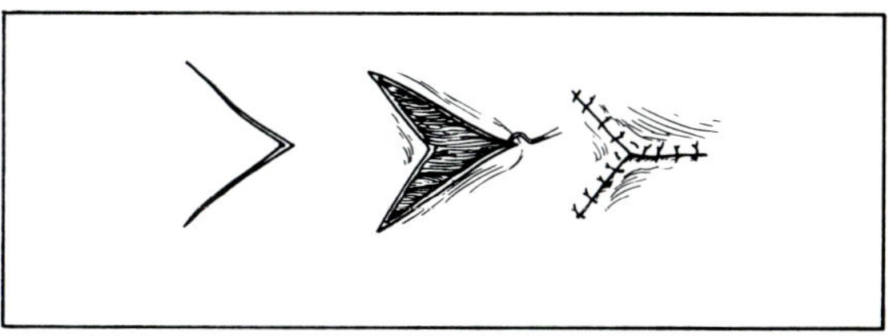

Fig. 1-36. V-Y advancement. It is the skin on each side of the V that is actually advanced.

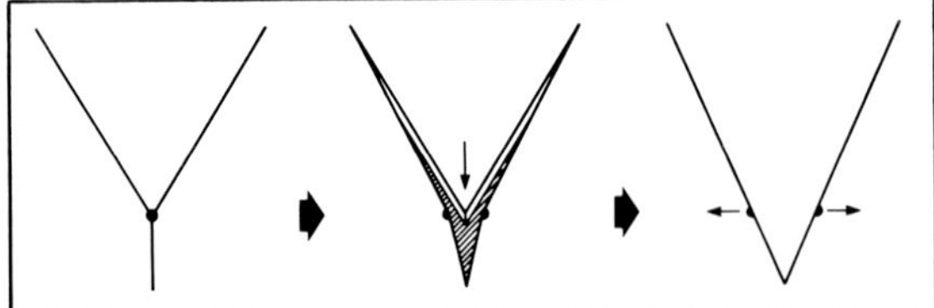

Fig. 1-37. The Y-V advancement flap.

should not exceed one-third of the length of the side (Fig. 1-38) [155]. The theoretical gain is 1.4 times the straight limb of the Y.

The *bipedicle advancement flap* can be constructed by simply making an incision parallel to the long axis of a defect. The skin between the incision and the defect is undermined and advanced into the defect; the donor site is closed with a skin graft. Advancement of such flaps is facilitated by curving the relaxing incision so that its concave side is toward the defect. One useful application of this technique is the bipedicle advancement of skin and subcutaneous tissue from the upper forehead and scalp into a mid-forehead defect. The skin graft used to surface the donor site is covered by combining adjacent hair over it. This graft can often be removed later by the technique of multiple excision.

Advancement flaps have the limitation of aiding the closure of defects only of short length, because tension decreases the flow of blood in the flap. Patients in the older age groups have looser skin, which increases the extent to which these flaps can be advanced.

Distant Skin Flaps

Flaps can be constructed at a distance from the defect and then transferred to it, either *directly* (e.g., by raising a skin flap on the chest wall and positioning the defect on a hand under the flap) or *indirectly* (e.g., by raising a skin flap on the anterior aspect of the trunk and then using the wrist as a carrier to transfer it to surface a large defect on the face).

DIRECT FLAPS FROM A DISTANCE. Direct flaps are usually of the open type and can be constructed and transferred in a single stage.

Direct flaps are usually obtained from or transferred to an extremity, because the mobility of the extremity is an important advantage in this surgery. Some examples of direct flaps from a distance are (1) direct flaps from the trunk, (2) direct flaps from an upper extremity, and (3) direct flaps from a lower extremity.

1. *Direct flaps from the trunk* are usually transferred to the upper extremity. White [276] has described a V-shaped flap from the relatively hairless area on the lower anterior chest wall, a site which has a relatively thin subcutaneous layer (Fig. 1-39). The base of the flap, if placed laterally, will take advantage of the better blood supply, but should not cross the midline medially. If the upper or lower limb of the V incision is extended for a distance equal to the width of the flap's base, the flap can be rotated 180 degrees to facilitate primary closure of the donor site. The flap is sutured directly into the defect on the upper extremity. To keep the elbow from protruding, White believes that the flap for the right hand should be taken from the left side of the chest and vice versa. Elastoplast or a similar adhesive dressing is sufficient initially to hold the arm to the side, but the area between the arm and the chest must be padded carefully. After 10 to 14 days the immobilizing dressing may be discontinued. Two and one-half weeks after the initial operation, the base of the pedicle can be divided under local anesthesia. It may be divided all at once if the base of the flap is not to be used for part of the resurfacing. If the base is needed, the base may be divided in two stages with 2 or 3 days between the stages.

Larger rectangular flaps can be elevated from the anterior aspect of the trunk and transferred directly to the upper limb. The donor site is usually closed with a skin graft and a tie-over dressing is used to hold it in place. In these cases the base of the pedicle also can be divided after 2½ weeks in two or three stages, a few days apart.

2. *Direct flaps from an upper extremity* are most often used for repairing the contralateral upper extremity (cross arm flap) or the face. The cross arm flap is advantageous for closing defects on the hand and fingers because it provides thin skin with a minimum of subcutaneous tissue. A flap with either a single pedicle or a bipedicle is raised from the relatively hairless area on the flexor surface of the forearm or the anterior surface of the upper arm. Single pedicle flaps should be based proximally. Though the injured hand is joined to the opposite forearm or upper arm, the free hand can still be moved through a range of positions from the head to the perineum without too much difficulty. The flap can be divided at its base in one or two stages beginning at 2 or 2½ weeks.

For small defects on the fingers, a cross finger flap is often very satisfactory. See Chapter 32 for further information on these flaps.

The use of a skin flap from the upper arm for nasal reconstruction was first described by Tagliacozzi in 1597 [267]. Proximally based flaps can be elevated and transferred in a single stage. When there is enough nasal skin available, it should be turned down as an inner lining for the flap. Additional information is included in Chapter 14.

3. *Direct flaps from a lower extremity* are most often used on the opposite leg to provide stable coverage of exposed tendon or bone on the foot, ankle,

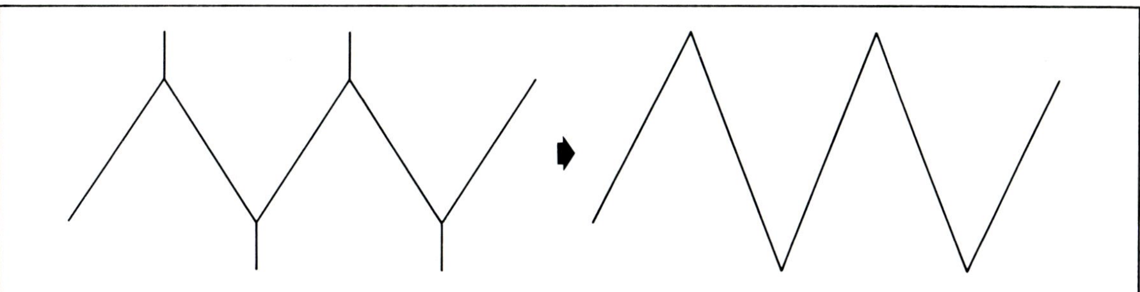

Fig. 1-38. *Multiple Y-V advancement flaps.*

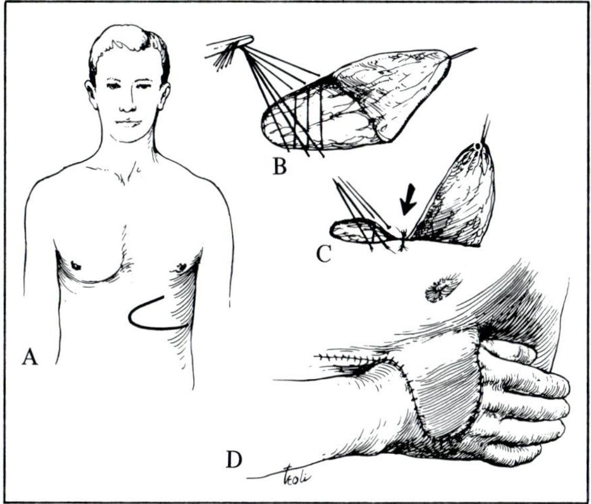

Fig. 1-39. Direct skin flap from the lower anterior chest wall to an upper extremity. The lateral incisions are staggered at the base of the flap to permit rotation of the flap 180 degrees and primary closure of the flap donor site. The length of the longest side of the flap is designed to be longer than the shorter side by the same distance as the width of the base of the flap, as measured directly across from the end of the shorter limb.

lower leg, and knee. The calf is used most frequently as the donor site, and when planned with a wide base, this flap can be transferred directly to the opposite extremity.

In the child, the lower extremity may be limber enough to permit a skin flap to be applied directly to the foot from the dorsum of the upper thigh or buttock [229]. Sharp flexion of the knee is required to permit the use of this direct flap from a distance.

Further information on direct flaps to the lower extremity is included in Chapter 49.

With the advent of muscle flaps, myocutaneous flaps, and free flaps, the cross leg flap is gradually becoming of only historical interest.

INDIRECT FLAPS FROM A DISTANCE. These rather seldom used flaps are transferred to a distant site by a *carrier* (e.g., the wrist) or by *migration*. Such flaps are almost always tubed and are usually transferred to their new site by using the wrist as a carrier. If they are moved by the technique of migration, they travel only a distance equal to the length of the flap at each stage, whereas each operation causes further scarring of the end of the flap. Methods of migration are by *waltzing* (i.e., the ends of the flap are alternately moved laterally one step at a time), by the *caterpillar method* (i.e., one end of the flap is moved up close to the other so that the flap is doubled on itself at the first stage, following which the other end is moved forward as far as possible to migrate the flap), or by *tumbling* the flap (i.e., the flap is moved in the same fashion as an athlete tumbles head over heels). Some examples of these indirect flaps are (1) indirect flaps from the trunk, (2) indirect flaps from the neck, and (3) indirect flaps from a lower extremity.

1. *Indirect flaps from the trunk* can supply great amounts of tissue to any part of the body. The anterior surface of the trunk is the preferred site for forming large skin flaps.

A *tubed arterial skin flap* of the anterior abdominal wall is usually formed along the vascular axis between the inguinal and axillary regions. This rarely used thoracoepigastric flap gains its name from the thoracoepigastric vein (lateral thoracic and superficial epigastric veins), which extends in most patients from the axilla to the groin and is included in the flap. The arterial supply in the inguinal region is provided from the superficial inferior epigastric artery, and in the axillary region it comes from the superior thoracic and long thoracic arteries. This vascular supply has been well described by Webster [275].

A *marsupial flap* can be moved by a carrier to any part of the body in a series of operations, but it does not have any great advantage over the tubed flap. Cuthbert [173] has provided a very good description of this flap.

2. *Indirect flaps from the neck* are frequently used in reconstructing defects of the nose, lips, or auricle. This donor site has much in its favor because the color and texture of the skin are satisfactory, and the flap can be migrated without the need of a carrier. In men a portion of the resulting scar will be covered by a shirt collar.

Most bipedicle tubed flaps on the neck are developed with their long axis in the direction of the flexion creases [263]. The donor site can be closed by direct suture when the defect is not too wide. Neck flaps of this type are either transferred directly or waltzed up to the face in one step, or in two steps about 3 weeks apart, depending on the case. Because of the excellent vascularity of this skin, the end of the flap to be transferred can be divided and moved in one operation. Subsequent moves often require staged cutting of the end of the flap.

3. *Indirect flaps from a lower extremity* are constructed on the anterior aspect of the thigh as tubed bipedicle flaps for transfer to the opposite lower leg. They serve mainly to cover traumatic defects located along the anterior tibia. The donor site on the thigh is usually closed with a skin graft.

Skin Flaps Utilizing Expansion of Adjacent Skin, the Crane Principle, and Compound Flaps

Expansion of Adjacent Skin by Inflatable Subcutaneous Silicone Bag

An inflatable silicone bag can be gradually filled with saline to stretch the overlying skin [249]. Once the skin is sufficiently stretched, the device can be removed and the skin spread to the adjacent recipient site, such as a decubitus ulcer, a denuded tibial bone, or a defect left after a tattoo removal; this technique may also be used in reconstruction of the breast after radical mastectomy. First an empty silicone bag of the appropriate size is placed in the subcutaneous tissue, and then saline is injected by needle every 3 to 5 days over a 3- or 4-week period, through a buried reservoir connected to the bag by a tube with a one-way valve.

A self-inflating subcutaneous silicone bag has also been devised to expand the overlying skin [152]. This device contains sodium chloride crystals in the collapsed bag, so that when it is placed subcutaneously the osmotic pressure differential on either side of the silicone membrane will draw fluid into the bag, thus expanding it.

The Crane Principle

Subcutaneous tissue can be carried in a skin flap to cover bare bone, tendon, cartilage, or other structures. In this technique, the skin and a very thin layer of subcutaneous tissue are returned to the flap donor site after 7 days. The subcutaneous tissue left at the recipient site will be vascular enough to nourish a split-thickness skin graft after an additional 5 days. The principal advantage in doing this is to decrease the period of limb immobilization, such as would be involved in a cross leg flap [223].

Compound Flaps
Skin flaps which carry along with them immediately contiguous muscle, bone, or cartilage fall in this category. A tubed flap of skin overlying the clavicle can be elevated in stages; the flap contains a sagitally split strip of clavicular bone with the clavicular periosteum between the bone and the overlying skin left intact. This compound flap can then be transferred to reconstruct the mandible [258]. Compound myocutaneous flaps are discussed later in this chapter, as well as in Chapter 49.

Pedicled Pericranium as Base for Skin Grafts
Saunders [253] has described the use of a flap of pericranium elevated from the skull through a small skin incision and moved to cover avascular defects of the frontal bone or medial canthal region. At the same operation, a full-thickness supraclavicular skin graft was applied to the vascular flap of pericranium.

Characteristics of Skin Flaps Postoperatively

Color and Texture
The skin of a flap, even after transfer, maintains its original color and texture with little or no change. This is why skin flaps of head or neck origin are best for facial reconstruction. Skin flaps from such distant sites as the abdomen will continue to maintain characteristics of abdominal skin following transfer to the face.

Bulkiness
Pedicled tissue from the trunk, because it is too thick or has an excess of fat, may not compare favorably at all with the original tissue. This is especially true in the face, where the skin normally is thin enough to allow the underlying movements of facial muscles to register expression. It is also true in the hands, where the contours are complex, and on the fingers, where the clearance between parts may be small. The bulkiness in a flap may be further increased if the patient gains weight, for the flap will continue to respond as though the tissue were still on the trunk.

Aggressive thinning of the flap at the time it is first developed, to remove subcutaneous tissue, preserving only the subdermal plexus at the junction of dermis and subcutaneous tissue, will prevent much of this bulkiness. Use of the *fat flip flap* secondarily involves the turning over upon itself of a flap of fatty tissue from beneath the skin flap so that it lies immediately beneath the thinner surrounding skin.

Hair Growth and Sebaceous Secretion
Hair growth and sebaceous secretion will continue to have the same characteristics in a skin flap as they did at their original site.

Sensation and Sweating
Sensation and sweating, lost immediately after the transfer of a flap, usually return sometime between 6 weeks and 3 years later [217]. These functions tend to acquire the characteristic pattern of the recipient site, in much the same manner as occurs in a skin graft. Sensation returns by the ingrowth of nerve fibers from surrounding skin and also from the recipient bed.

Sturman and Duran [265] have demonstrated on the tip of a reconstructed finger that the two-point discrimination of skin grafts, cross finger flaps, and palmar flaps is close to that of the normal fingertip. Abdominal pedicled tissue transferred to the fingertip does not develop good two-point discrimination, presumably because of the excess fatty tissue.

When pedicled tissue is applied to a recipient area that has been the site of extensive tissue destruction, there rarely is good return of sensation and sweating. Scar tissue in the bed as well as along the junction between adjacent skin and the flap tends to block reinnervation.

Sweating, because of its dependence on the sympathetic nervous system, is usually restored at the same rate as pain, temperature, and touch sensation. McGregor [220] estimates that 70 to 80 percent of the sweat glands in a flap regain their function.

Durability
A flap containing a good layer of fat will usually provide bony prominences with a durable cover. The principal disadvantage is that for a long time following operation the flap is anesthetic, so that prolonged pressure can result in a painless ischemia of the tissues and a pressure sore. Occasionally a neurovascular flap may help maintain some sensation at the point of pressure.

Growth
A skin flap will grow in proportion to body growth, a fact which has been demonstrated in growing rats observed over a 3-month period [94]. Though initially there was a reduced growth rate, this was followed by growth which was faster than the growth of the total body surface.

Muscle Flaps Plus Skin Grafts

Another type of arterialized flap is the muscle flap which is transferred with its intact neurovascular bundle into an adjacent recipient site and then is covered with a split-thickness skin graft (Fig. 1-18).

These long muscle flaps have proved to be a valued addition to the tissues available for reconstruction in the lower extremity, trunk, and face.

Chapter 49 provides information on these flaps, including details on the anatomy of the musculotendinous units, as well as their sites of innervation and blood supply. Some of the commonly used *muscle flaps in the lower extremity* are derived from the gastrocnemius, soleus, flexor digitorum longus and brevis, abductor hallucis, and abductor digiti minimi muscles [273]. The split-thickness skin graft which is placed on the muscle at the initial procedure will have a better chance of taking if it has been meshed. Functional deficits caused by the loss of these muscles have been minor [273].

Ger [188], who pioneered the use of muscle flaps, has confidence in their application for the *treatment of decubitus ulcers.* The upper half of the gluteus maximus muscle can be rotated for coverage of a sacral ulcer, while the lower half is rotated into the defect of an ischial ulcer. The rectus femoris or vastus lateralis muscles can be transposed into a trochanteric ulcer defect. Split-thickness skin grafts are then placed on the muscle at the initial procedure. The recurrence rate of these decubitus ulcers, as reported by Ger, was dramatically low. Additional information is included in Chapter 50.

The *temporalis muscle flap* has an important role in the reconstruction of operative defects in the upper face [154]. This broad, fan-shaped muscle receives its nerve and blood supply (from branches of the internal maxillary artery) on its deep surface near its coronoid insertion. Therefore all or part of the muscle can be detached from the side of the skull and rotated over the zygoma into the orbit, or over exposed dura, after which a skin graft can be applied.

Pers and Medgyesi [248] have extended the use of muscle flaps to repair the chest wall (serratus anterior m.), to cover femoral vessels (sartorius and adductor longus m.), for filling the retropubic cavity following surgical removal of the bladder (gracilis m.), to control urinary or anal incontinence (gracilis m.), for closure of vesicovaginal fistulas (gracilis m.), and to restore the contour of the anterior axillary fold (latissimus dorsi m.).

Omental Flaps Plus Skin Grafts

The greater omentum is another type of arterialized flap which can be transposed extraperitoneally to a recipient site on the body surface and covered with a skin graft (Fig. 1-18) [177, 183]. The omentum ranges in length from 14 to 34 cm. and in width from 20 to 46 cm. [177]. There are three ways to lengthen the omentum progressively: (1) detachment from the transverse colon – 2 to 12 cm. of lengthening obtained; (2) detachment from the stomach with division of the left (or right) gastroepiploic vessels – lengthening so that the omentum can reach the sternal angle in all cases; (3) division of the omentum by an L-shaped cut near the middle portion of the omental attachment to the stomach as described by Das [177], so that in all cases the omentum would reach to the vault of the skull or to the midleg, although some width will be lost [177].

The greater omentum is a ready source of coverage for chest wall defects, axillary defects, and an exposed carotid artery.

Myocutaneous Flaps

Flaps of muscle and their attached overlying skin are another type of arterialized flap which can be used for reconstruction on the surface of the body (Fig. 1-18). Hueston and McConchie [200] used such a flap of skin and pectoral muscle based on the shoulder to close a full-thickness defect of the upper anterior chest wall. If the muscle remains attached at its base and runs the full length of the flap, the blood supply through numerous musculocutaneous arteries augments the skin's blood supply, thus providing a very safe flap. The sternocleidomastoid muscle and its overlying skin have been put to work in a similar manner for facial reconstruction [153, 215]. O'Brien [238] has carried an island of skin attached to the underlying lower end of the sternocleidomastoid muscle, which then serves as the vascular pedicle in moving the skin to reconstruct the lower lip in one operation.

Myocutaneous flaps have been found most useful in lower extremity reconstruction. Orticochea [242] used the gracilis muscle and its overlying skin as a cross leg flap to cover a defect of the opposite ankle. Some of the myocutaneous flaps that have been used clinically involve the following muscles: gracilis, sternocleidomastoid, upper part of the trapezius, latissimus dorsi, lower portion of the sacrospinalis, upper rectus abdominis (island flap), lower rectus abdominis (island flap), thoracoepigastric, upper half of the sartorius, lower half of the sartorius, rectus femoris, and biceps femoris [218]. McCraw and Vasconez detail their extensive experience with these lower extremity myocutaneous flaps in Chapter 49.

Z-PLASTY

DEFINITION. The Z-plasty is simply a technique by which two triangular flaps are interchanged, one for another.

Geometrical Principle of the Z-Plasty

The Z-plasty geometrically consists of a central limb and two limbs (Fig. 1-40) which are positioned so that they resemble the letter Z. The *limbs of the Z must*

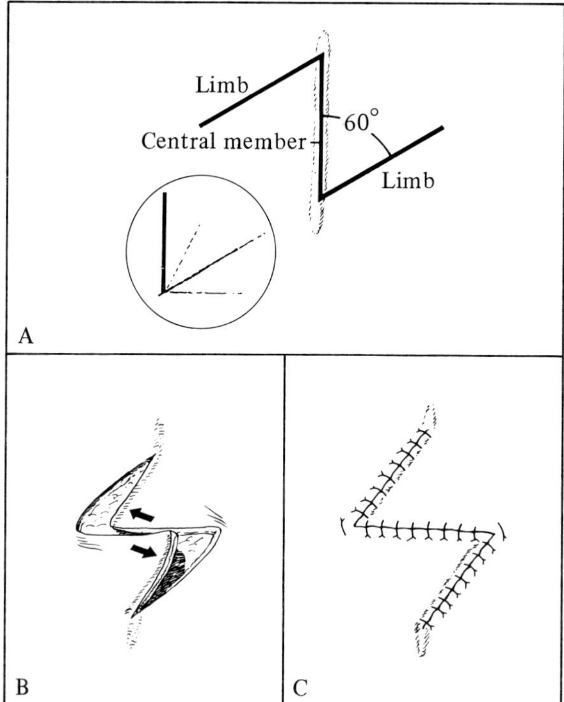

Fig. 1-40. *The classic 60-degree-angle Z-plasty. Inset shows method of finding the 60-degree angle by first drawing a 90-degree angle, then dividing it in thirds by sighting. The limbs of the Z must be equal in length to the central member.*

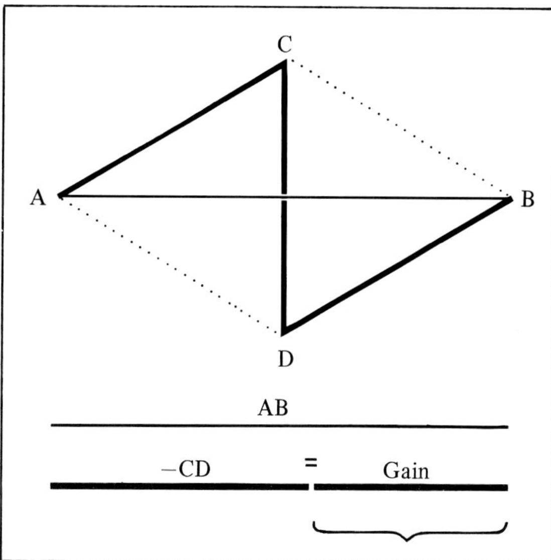

Fig. 1-41. *Calculating the* theoretical *gain in length of the Z-plasty. The theoretical gain in length is the difference in length between the long diagonal and the short diagonal. In actual practice the gain in length has varied from 45 percent less to 25 percent more than calculated geometrically, due to the biomechanical properties of the skin [283, 284].*

always be equal in length to the central member and should extend outward from it at *an angle which can vary between 30 and 90 degrees. In the classic Z-plasty this angle is 60 degrees.* Clinical experience has repeatedly shown that 60 degrees is the largest angle that will permit the transposition of the triangular flaps while obtaining the maximal increased length in the direction of the central member. At the completion of the Z-plasty, the Z has been rotated 90 degrees and reversed (Fig. 1-40).

Gain in Length

In the Z-plasty, the gain in length in the direction of the central member has been calculated mathematically (Table 1-1).

A means by which the theoretical gain in length can be determined in any Z-plasty is illustrated in Figure 1-41. However, it should be emphasized that the theoretical gain in length is based on geometry and studies with paper models. In contrast, the biomechanical properties of skin causing its tension to vary from loose to elastic to taut prevent surgery from being honed to such an exact science as mathematics. Grabb [284] reported on results obtained by measuring in 20 patients the actual gain in length of 60 degree–60 degree angled Z-plasties, as opposed to the theoretical gain in length. The actual gain in length was measured with a ruler and the theoretical gain in length was determined as in Figure 1-41. In 8 of the Z-plasties the actual and theoretical gain in length were the same. In 10 of the Z-plasties the actual gain in length was 15 to 45 percent less than the theoretical gain (15 percent less in 4 patients, 25 percent less in 4, and 45 percent less in 2). In 2 of the Z-plasties, the gain in length was 10 to 15 percent more than the theoretical gain. Gibson and Kenedi [283] measured

Table 1-1. Z-plasty, Angles, and the Theoretical Gain in Length

Angles of Z-plasty	Theoretical Gain in Length
30°–30°	25 percent
45°–45°	50 percent
60°–60°	75 percent
75°–75°	100 percent
90°–90°	120 percent

the theoretical and actual gain in length in 4 Z-plasties in human beings. The actual gain in length was either less (14 and 16 percent less) or more (7 and 27 percent more) than calculated. Furnas and Fischer [282] have shown in experimental studies of Z-plasties on the skin of the trunk in dogs that the actual gain in length was always less than the theoretical gain. In a 60-degree-angle Z-plasty, the actual gain in length was 28 percent less than calculated for a Z with 8-cm. limbs (73 percent theoretical gain minus 45 percent actual gain equals 28 percent less). As the limb length decreased, the actual gain in length decreased, so that for a Z-plasty with 1-cm. limbs it was 45 percent less than calculated.

In order to transpose the flaps of a Z-plasty, the skin in the base of these flaps must be loose or elastic enough to be pulled over into its new position. When the skin is contracted in a direction perpendicular to the central member of the planned Z, then it may be impossible to do a Z-plasty. This occurs particularly following the skin grafting of a burned extremity, where the skin is often very tight.

The skin on the face varies from loose to taut in alternate areas. For example, the skin is loose just lateral to the eye and between the eyebrows; it is taut on the cheek and on the forehead. In a Z-plasty, one of the ideal factors in planning is to be able to base the flaps in an area of loose skin [283].

Fig. 1-42. The theoretical *gain in length of the Z-plasty calculated for angles of 30, 45, and 60 degrees. In actual practice the gain in length depends also on the varying degrees of rigidity or looseness of the skin which is being transposed in order to provide the increased length.*

Variation of Angle Size and Length of the Central Member

In planning a Z-plasty the *size of the angle* created by the central member and each arm, and the actual *length of the central member,* are the only two factors which can be varied. It is important to reemphasize that the length of the limbs of the Z should always remain equal to the length of the central member.

ANGLE SIZE. A greater *percentage gain* in length is to be expected as the angle of each limb of the Z-plasty is increased (Fig. 1-42) [288]. The *force* required to transpose the Z-plasty flaps and pull them into their new position will increase as the tip angle increases. On the trunk of the dog, the tension needed to close a 90 degree–90 degree angle and 8 cm. limbed Z-plasty is approximately ten times that needed to close a 30 degree–30 degree and 8 cm. limbed Z-plasty [282].

The angle of the limbs from the central member can vary from 30 degrees to 90 degrees, and it is not necessary that both angles be the same. Some examples of Z-plasties with varying angle sizes are illustrated in Figure 1-43.

LENGTH OF CENTRAL MEMBER. The greater the length of the central member, the greater will be the actual gain in length accomplished by the Z-plasty (Fig. 1-44). This naturally follows because it has already been demonstrated that the length to be gained is a percentage of the length of the central member.

In actual practice the amount and looseness of the tissue on either side of the central member available for flaps limit the length of the central member. Also, the scar resulting from a very large Z-plasty is

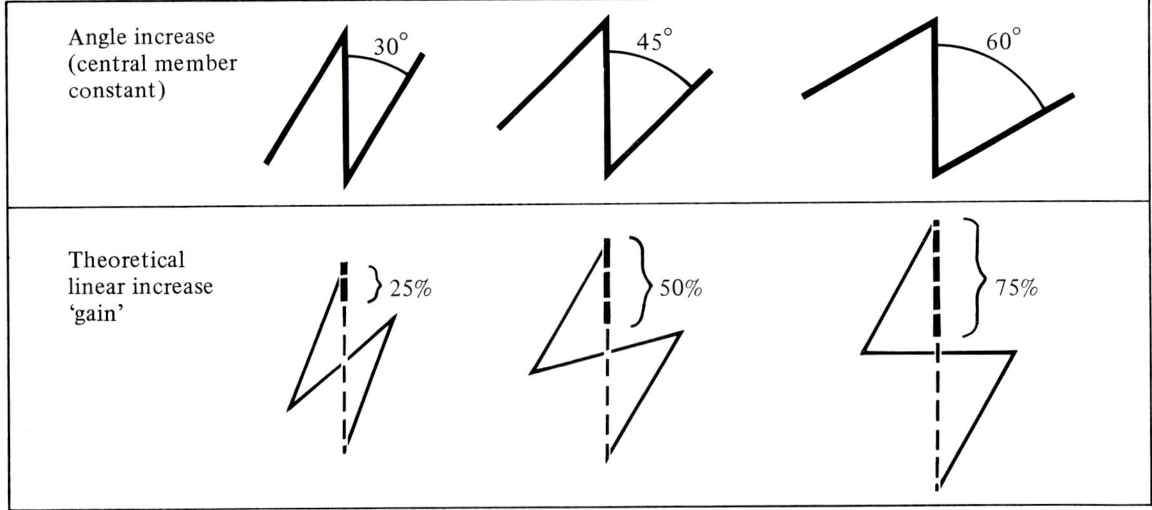

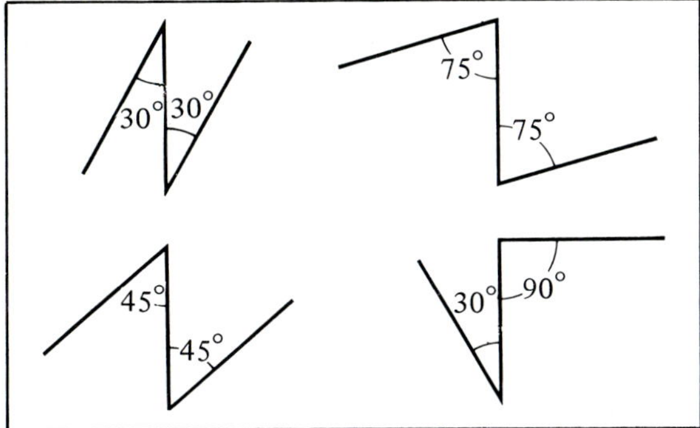

Fig. 1-43. Examples of Z-plasties with varying angle sizes.

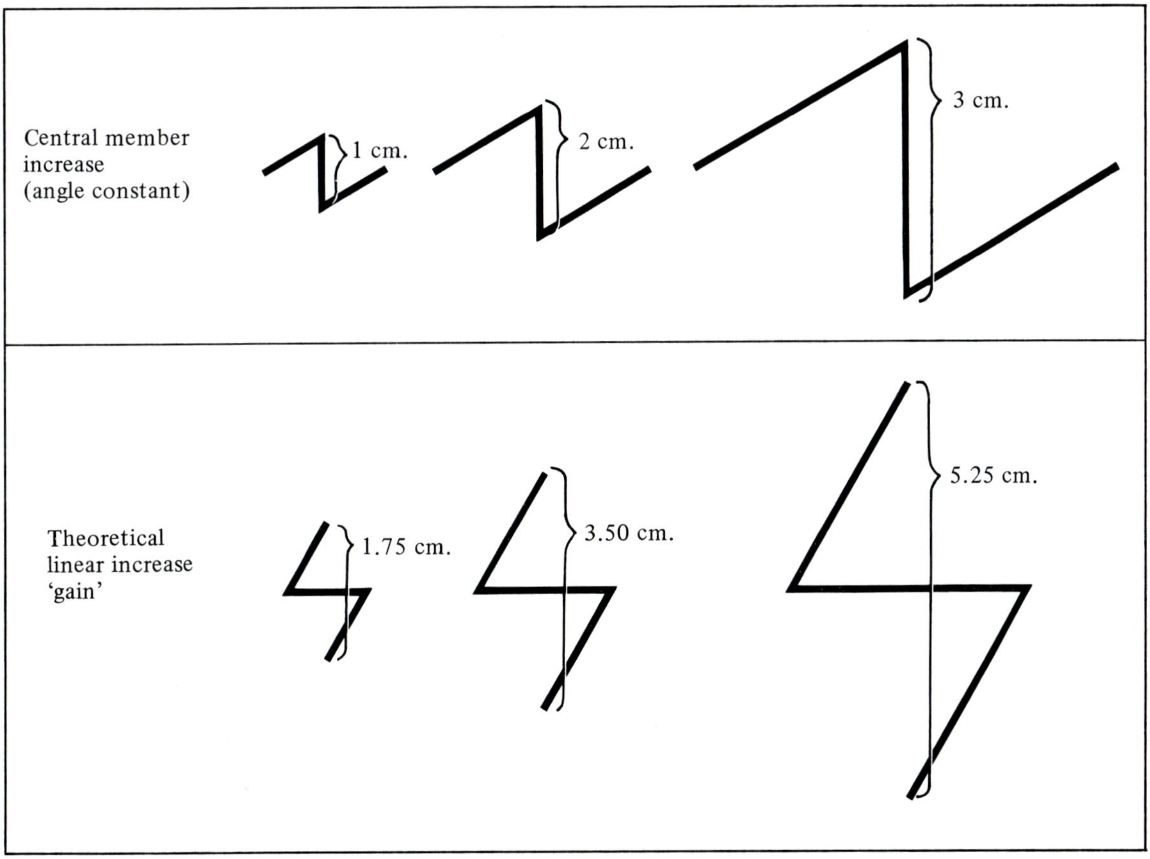

Central member increase (angle constant)

1 cm.

2 cm.

3 cm.

Theoretical linear increase 'gain'

1.75 cm.

3.50 cm.

5.25 cm.

Fig. 1-44. The greater the length of the central member, the greater the gain in length accomplished by the Z-plasty.

usually more noticeable than the one resulting from a series of smaller Z-plasties. Cosmetically, it is preferable on such areas as the face to keep the central member of the Z relatively short.

Multiple Z-plasties

Any number of Z-plasties can be designed in series (see Fig. 1-51A for an example of a multiple Z-plasty). However, it has been demonstrated in experiments in the dog that more length can be gained by making one Z-plasty with a long central member than by making multiple Z-plasties whose central member lengths collectively add up to the same total length. For example, a single 60 degree–60 degree angled 8 cm. limbed Z-plasty provided an actual gain in length almost twice that for a series of eight 60 degree–60 degree angled 1 cm. limbed Z-plasties [282]. Despite this fact, there is a place for the multiple Z-plasty when there is not sufficient tissue for a large Z and also when the cosmetically superior appearance of a series of small Z's versus one large Z is a factor.

Four-Flap Z-plasty

In this variation on the theme, a 90 degree–90 degree angled Z-plasty is designed and then each flap is subdivided into 45 degree angled flaps. This design permits a greater gain in length (124 (percent) with less tension on the flaps (Fig. 1-45).

The four-flap Z-plasty is particularly effective in correcting web space contractures in the hand [294]. Flaps with angles as large as 120 degree–120 degree have been subdivided into 60 degree angled flaps for the four-flap Z-plasty.

Six-Flap Z-plasty

In this variation, an additional 45 degree-angle flap is tacked on to each end of a 45°, 45°, 45°, 45° four-flap Z-plasty [289]. After the three 45 degree-angle flaps have been incised at each end of the central member, all six flaps are transposed in the way that one interlocks one's fingers from the right and left hand. That is, one uses first a flap from one end of the central member, then a flap from the opposite end, and so on. The six-flap Z-plasty provided a theoretical gain in length in the direction of the central member of 180 percent.

Like the four-flap Z-plasty, the six-flap Z-plasty can be carried out in a stepwise fashion, by first incising the 90 degree-angle Z-flaps. If enough length is *not* gained by transposing these flaps, and transverse tension is not too great, then the 90 degree flaps can be divided into 45 degree flaps for a four-flap Z-plasty. This can be temporarily sutured; if still more length is needed, 45 degree-angle flaps can be added on to each end of the central member, thus creating a six-flap Z-plasty.

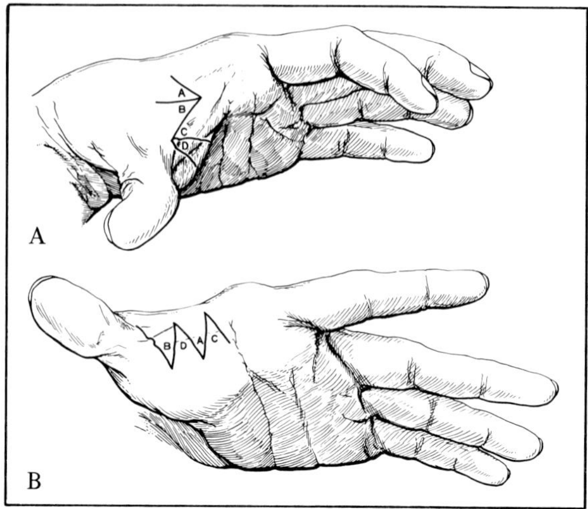

Fig. 1-45. Four-flap Z-plasty. Each flap of a 90 degree–90 degree angled Z-plasty has been divided into two 45 degree-angle flaps (A and B, C and D). These four flaps are then easily transposed to provide a greater lengthening of the central member than could be accomplished by a typical 60 degree–60 degree angled Z-plasty.

Five-Flap Y-V Advancement and Z-Plasty

This combination of flaps has been described as being very effective in releasing transverse contractures of the dorsum of the interdigital web spaces and in other concave regions of the body (Fig. 1-46). The hypertrophic scar does not need to be excised, but rather can be incised. Once the tension on this scar is released, it will gradually involute [290].

Z-plasty Across Webs

Furnas and Fischer [282] have demonstrated that when a Z-plasty is plotted on a web, each of the triangular flaps lies on a different plane, and the two planes meet along the crest of the web at an angle (peak angle) (Fig. 1-47). After transposition, the two flaps occupy two entirely new planes and the web is converted into a cleft. If the peak angle happens to be ideal (71-degree peak angle for a 60 degree–60 degree angled Z-plasty), the flaps after transposition will lie easily in the new cleft. If the peak angle is narrower than ideal, the tips of the flap will overhang the defect and the lower edge of the flap will not meet the lower edge of the defect without tension. If the peak angle is wider than ideal, the Z-plasty flaps will need to be pulled under tension into their new position.

Method of Planning So That the Completed Z-plasty Is Properly Situated

The central member of the completed Z-plasty should

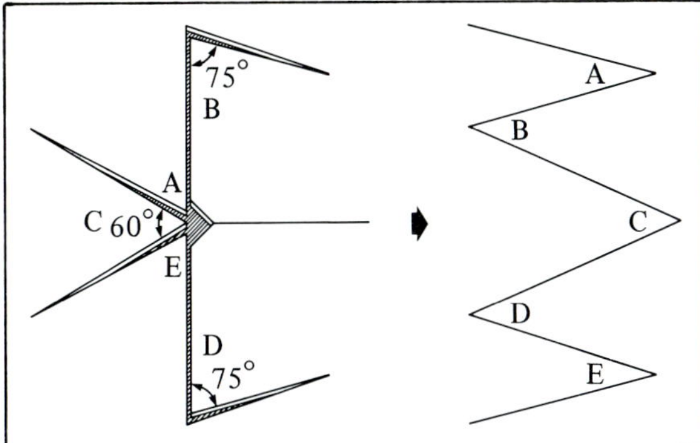

Fig. 1-46. Five-flap Y-V advancement and Z-plasty. The central flap (C) is advanced in a Y-V fashion. The flaps of the two Z-plasties on each side of the central flap are transposed.

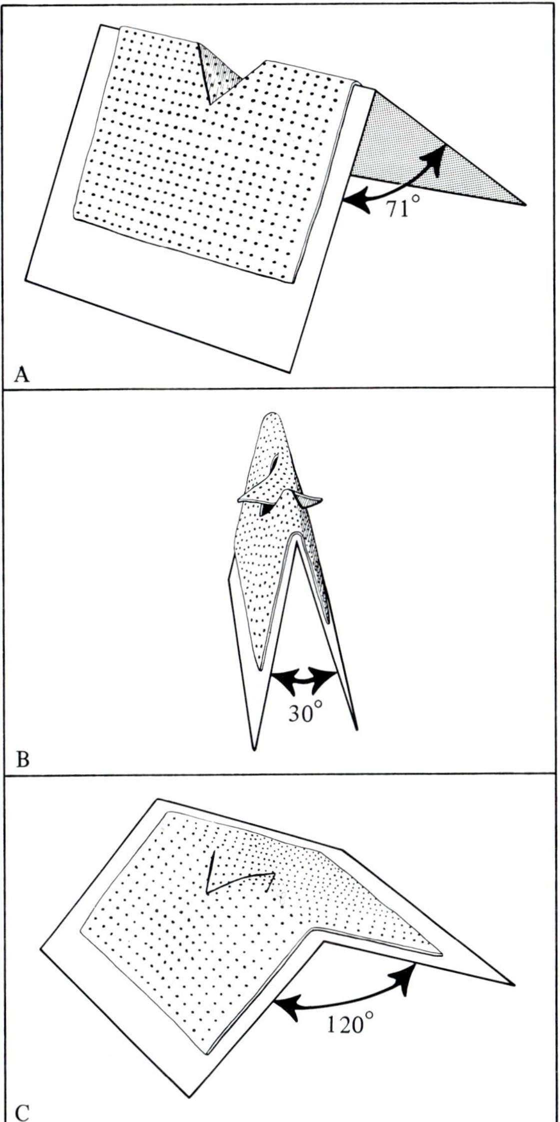

Fig. 1-47. Z-plasty on webs. A, with a peak angle of 71 degrees, the flap of a 60 degree–60 degree angled Z-plasty lies easily in the cleft formed after tranposition of the flaps. B, with a peak angle of 30 degrees the tips of the 60 degree–60 degree angled Z-plasty flaps overhang redundantly and will not meet the deepest part of the cleft without tension. C, with a peak angle of 120 degrees, the Z-plasty flaps can only be pulled into the cleft under tension.

lie in the same direction as the skin lines whenever practicable. For example, this central member should finally lie in a direction parallel to the nasolabial fold whenever a Z-plasty is carried out in the region of this fold. In this manner, the direction of a scar can be changed to correspond to the direction of the skin lines.

Figure 1-48 illustrates the method of planning so that the central member of the completed Z-plasty lies in the direction of the skin line. This method can be used whenever the smallest angle between the scar and the skin line is more than 30 degrees. Fundamentally this method of planning takes advantage of the fact that the central member and limbs of the Z-plasty must be of equal length.

The length of the central member along the scar must first be selected. This may be the entire length of the scar or a portion of it, depending on the size of the Z-plasty desired. The central member must be drawn so that its midpoint lies on the skin line. A triangular flap is then constructed so that the length of each limb is the same length as the central member and so that the end of each limb falls on the skin line. A protractor can be used for this purpose.

Though this technique is effective in placing the central member of the completed Z-plasty in the proper direction, it does triple the length of the scar and adds two lines which are oblique to the direction of the skin lines. In the best results the eye will visualize the unconnected scars which form the limbs of the Z with the central member of the Z being indiscernible.

Uses of the Z-Plasty

The Z-plasty has three major uses: (1) to increase the length of the skin in a desired direction, (2) to change the direction of a scar so that it will lie in the same

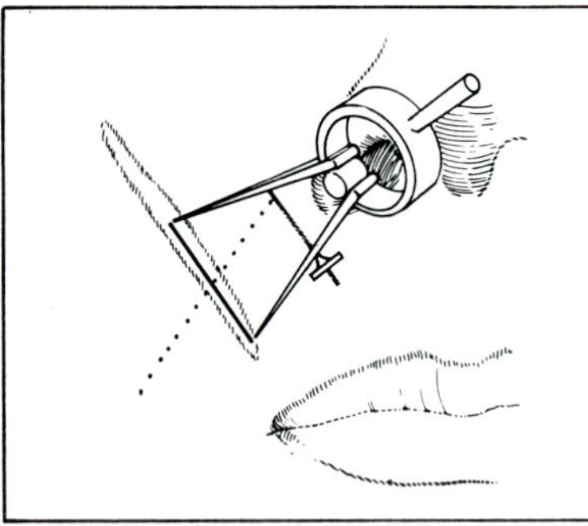

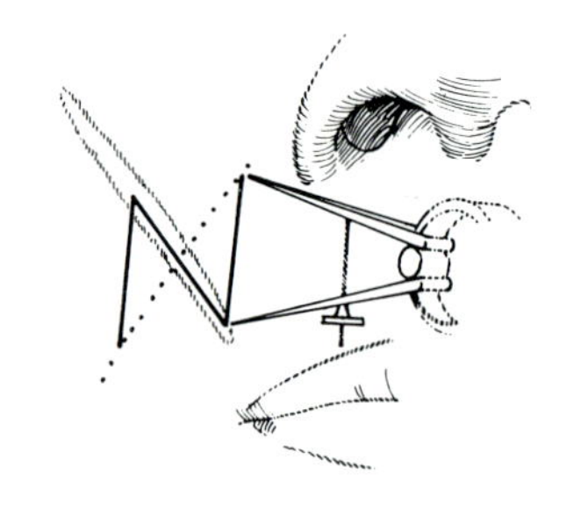

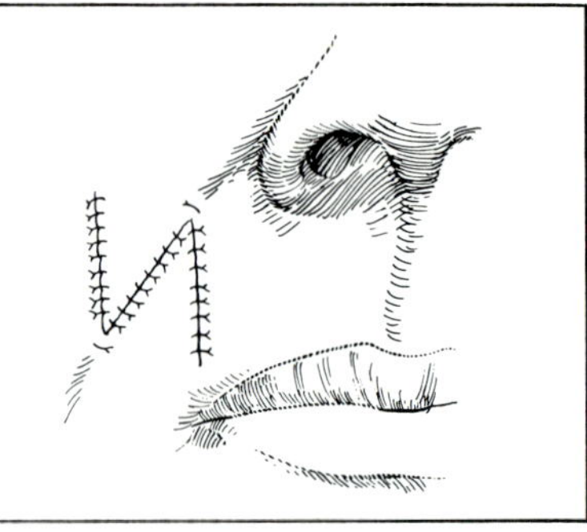

Fig. 1-48. Siting the Z-plasty so that the central member of the completed Z-plasty will lie in the direction of the nasolabial fold. See text for the method of planning.

direction as the skin lines, and (3) to rotate the axis of the tissue included in the Z-plasty flaps.

Increasing the Length of the Skin in a Desired Direction

Most Z-plasties are used for this purpose.

LENGTHENING SCAR CONTRACTURES. Examples of scar contractures which can be lengthened by means of the Z-plasty are as follows:

Scars that cross flexion creases of the axilla, elbow, fingers, knee, or neck often contract and produce a bowstring type of scar which may limit extension. If the scar is a linear one and the adjacent skin is not burned or damaged, one or more Z-plasties can be performed to lengthen it. Clinical judgment is important in knowing when a contracture is too extensive for Z-plasty and must be released and skin grafted in order to obtain the maximal improvement.

In burn-scar contractures, the adjacent skin may have decreased vascularity due to the injury, making it a poor site for a Z-plasty. There is always the risk that the tips of these densely scarred flaps will not survive [280]. In order to minimize this, the width of the flaps near their tips can be maintained by curving the limbs of the Z-plasty incision (Fig. 1-49). Spina [291] has even advocated delaying the flaps of the Z-plasty in tissues with a poor blood supply. Wilkinson and Rybka [293] have demonstrated in the guinea pig that the incidence of necrosis of the tips of Z-plasty flaps was reduced from 20 percent to 0 percent by the use of skin tapes or wound adhesives rather than sutures. Another difficulty encountered in performing a Z-plasty in skin that has been burned is that the tightness and loss of elasticity make transposition of the flaps more difficult. For these reasons, the Z-plasty in skin scarred by burns must be approached with caution.

Scars or congenital skin webs that cross a concave surface will invariably bridge the concavity. They can be lengthened and made to conform to the concave surface by placing a Z-plasty in the deepest part of the concavity. Examples of this type of problem are scars that lie transversely across the junction between the nose and the cheek or those that cross the slight hollow of the submandibular region. Pterygium colli is the classic example of a congenital skin web that can be corrected by a Z-plasty [281].

U-shaped scars are often elevated in the center because of the action of the contracting scar. Such scars in the face are unsightly. They can be improved by breaking the contracting line of the scar with one or two Z-plasties at or near the bottom of the U (Fig. 1-50). Attempts at correction of the U-shaped scar by only trimming the excess tissue from beneath the elevated skin are usually unsatisfactory. Occasionally very small U-shaped scars can be removed by elliptical excision of the entire scar.

It is unwise to perform a Z-plasty in any of these cases as a primary procedure. The tissue that will make up the flaps of the Z-plasty has usually been traumatized at the time of injury, so that the blood supply at this time may be precarious.

Circular scars of the extremities or body orifices can be released by a Z-plasty. Constricting scars of the arms or legs have traditionally been released in two stages, with a Z-plasty being carried out on about half the circumference of the scar in each stage [281, 292]. Congenital annular bands and grooves can be treated in a similar fashion. Circular contractures at orifices, such as the external auditory canal, the urethra, colostomy openings, and vesicostomy openings, can be released (or prevented) by a series of Z-plasties around the opening. These can be performed in one operative procedure.

CLEFT LIP REPAIR. All of the techniques for repair of unilateral or bilateral cleft lip, with the exception of the straight line repair, make use of the Z-plasty. In this way the shortened lip at the cleft can be lengthened. Chapter 7 includes a complete discussion of cleft lip repair.

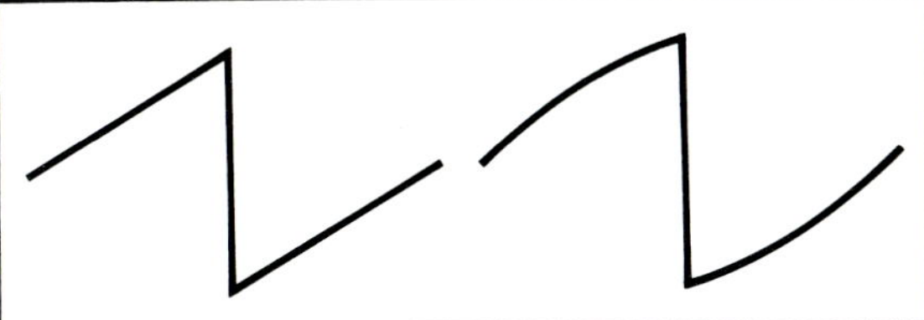

Fig. 1-49. The Z-plasty flaps can be broadened by curving the limbs of the Z. This may decrease the likelihood of skin slough in burn-scarred tissue.

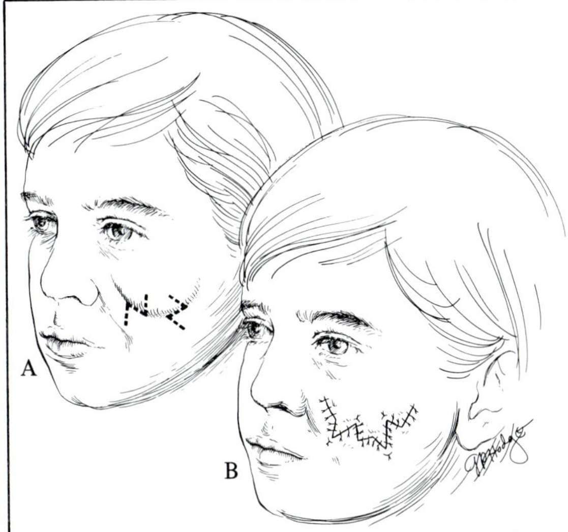

Fig. 1-50. The fullness of the tissue encompassed by a U-shaped scar can best be improved by two Z-plasties near the bottom of the U.

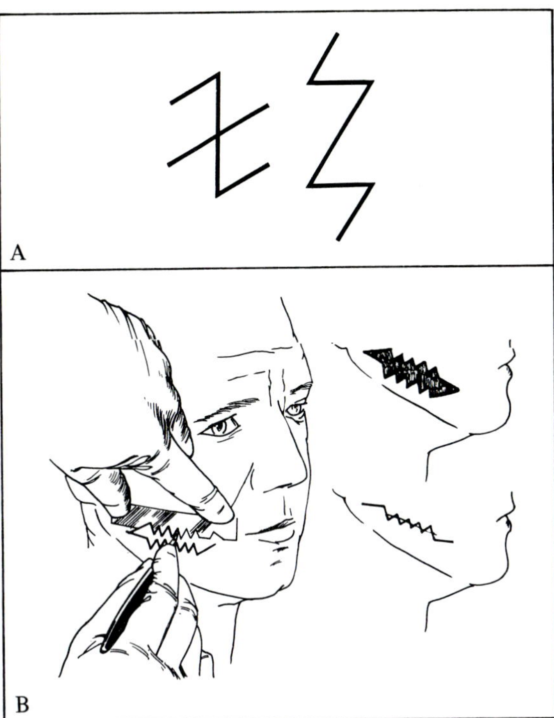

Fig. 1-51. Methods of changing the direction of a scar. A, multiple Z-plasties can be planned so that the central member of the completed Z-plasties will lie in the direction of the skin lines. B, the W-plasty can also be used to break up a long scar that does not lie in the direction of the skin lines.

Changing the Direction of the Scar

Long scars on the face, except for those which lie in or adjacent to a skin line, are usually conspicuous. The line of scar can be changed by breaking it with a series of Z-plasties so situated that the central member of the Z lies in the same direction as the skin lines (Fig. 1-48). Thus the eye visualizes a series of unconnected short scars representing the limbs of the Z with the central member of the Z being indiscernible, or a running Z scar which, though longer than the original straight line scar, is less noticeable. It is a rare long linear scar that does not cross a skin line at some point and that cannot be improved by breaking it up with one or more Z-plasties.

The W-plasty has been described by Borges [278, 279] as another method of changing the direction of a linear scar. This method simply involves excising the scar in multiple small triangles which are so situated that they will interdigitate (Fig. 1-51B). A special metal instrument with the pattern of these triangles (or W's) cut into it is of great assistance in making the triangles of equal size. Though the W-plasty changes the direction of the linear scar, it would only be by chance that one of the limbs of the W would lie in the same direction as the skin lines. However, usually one of them is close to this direction. As a W-plasty will not lengthen a contracted scar line, it is best to use the Z-plasty for this purpose.

Both the Z-plasty and the W-plasty have the additional attribute of breaking up a linear scar into an accordion-like scar that has some degree of elasticity to it. This permits the facial skin to be more mobile in its contribution to facial expressions.

Both of these techniques have to their detriment the fact that they more than double the length of the scar; thus they should be used only rarely in revising scars.

Rotation of Tissue in Z-plasty Flaps

This is a borderline use of the Z-plasty and could very

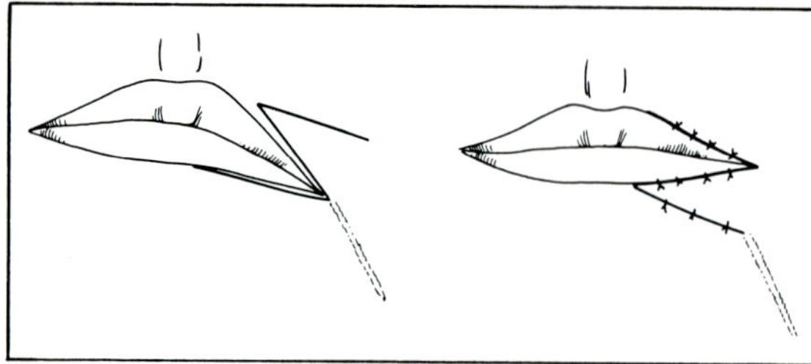

Fig. 1-52. By means of a Z-plasty, the scarred depressed corner of the mouth can be rotated into its normal position.

easily be included in the discussion of local rotation skin flaps. When necessary, the disfigured corner of the mouth or end of the eyebrow can be rotated into a more normal direction by use of the Z-plasty (Fig. 1-52).

The Z-plasty can also be an effective adjunct to the multiple excision procedure. Tissue which is to be removed (e.g., nevus) can be included in one of the triangular flaps of the Z-plasty and thus have its axis rotated to facilitate excision in a direction where there is greater relaxation of the skin.

Operative Technique of the Z-plasty

The following is a description of the operative steps for performing a *classic 60 degree–60 degree angled Z-plasty* to lengthen the skin along a line of scar contracture. The central member of the Z is first drawn on the line of scar (remember that in general it is best to keep the size of the Z small on the face for cosmetic reasons).

The limbs of the Z are laid out at each end of the central member. The limbs should be the same length as the central member and should be at a 60-degree angle with the central member. The 60-degree angle can be drawn by first making a 90-degree angle and then dividing it by sight into thirds (Fig. 1-40), or by using a precut 60-degree pattern. A means of checking the accuracy of this drawing is to connect the free ends of the arms of the Z with a straight line. In the classic Z-plasty, this straight line will be perpendicular to, and pass through, the midpoint of the central member.

The triangular flaps of the Z can then be incised. The scar which makes up the central member can be excised in an elliptical fashion if it is not too wide. The flaps should be thick enough to include some of the subcutaneous tissue. Hemostasis is obtained with electrocautery or ligature. The flaps must be handled with skin hooks in order to preserve their viability.

The *triangular flaps can then be transposed.* This is emphasized, as occasionally the flaps are mistakenly sutured back in their original position. Simple interrupted sutures with fine nonabsorbable suture material can be used. At the tips of the flap a half-buried horizontal mattress suture is very effective.

REFERENCES

Excision of Skin Lesions

1. Abbott, W. M., and Austen, W. G. Effectiveness and mechanism of collagen induced hemostasis. *Surgery* 78:723, 1975.
2. Blech, G. B. *Clinical Electrosurgery.* New York: Oxford Press, 1938.
3. Borges, A. F. *Elective Incisions and Scar Revision.* Boston: Little, Brown, 1973.
4. Borges, A. F., and Alexander, J. E. Relaxed skin tension lines, Z-plasties on scars, and fusiform excision of lesions. *Br. J. Plast. Surg.* 15:242, 1962.
5. Bunnell, S. An essential in reconstructive surgery – "atraumatic" technique. *Calif. State J. Med.* 19:204, 1921.
6. Crikelair, G. F. Skin suture marks. *Am. J. Surg.* 96:631, 1958.
7. deHoll, D., Rodeheaver, G., Edgerton, M.T., and Edlich, R. F. Potentiation of infection by suture closure of dead space. *Am. J. Surg.* 127:716, 1974.
8. Fischi, R. A. A flap for naso-labial defects, or "saving the dog-ear." *Br. J. Plast. Surg.* 22:351, 1969.
9. Grabb, W. C. Personal communication, 1977.
10. Hasson, H. M., Nicoloff, D., Ford, C. R., Lazarus, H., O'Donoghue, J., and Powell, J. R. New sutureless technique for skin closure. *Arch. Surg.* 111:83, 1976.
11. Hermann, J. B. Changes in tensile strength and knot security of surgical sutures in-vivo. *Arch. Surg.* 106:707, 1973.
12. Kazanjian, V. H., and Converse, J. M. *The Surgical Treatment of Facial Injuries* (2nd ed.). Baltimore: Williams & Wilkins, 1959.
13. Kelly, H. A., and Ward, G. E. *Electrosurgery.* Philadelphia: Saunders, 1932.
14. Kraissl, C. J. The selection of appropriate lines for elective surgical incisions. *Plast. Reconstr. Surg.* 8:1, 1951.
15. Link, W. J., Incropera, F. P., and Glover, J. L. Plasma scalpel: Comparison of tissue damage and wound healing with electrosurgical and steel scalpels. *Arch. Surg.* 111:392, 1976.
16. McDowell, A. J. Wound infections resulting from the use of hot wet sponges. *Plast. Reconstr. Surg.* 23(1):168, 1959.
17. Morestin, H. La réduction graduelle des difformités tégumentaires. *Bull. Soc. Chir. Paris* 41:1233, 1915.

18. Siegel, R. J., Vistnes, L. M., and Iverson, R. E. Effective hemostasis with less epinephrine. *Plast. Reconstr. Surg.* 51:129, 1973.
19. Smith, F. *Plastic and Reconstructive Surgery, A Manual of Management.* Philadelphia: Saunders, 1950.
20. Stark, R. *Plastic Surgery.* New York: Hoeber Med. Div., Harper & Row, 1962.
21. Steffensen, W. H., and Worthen, E. F. Limitations of multiple excision. *Am. J. Surg.* 95:237, 1958.
22. Szymonowski, J. von. *Handbuch der operativen Chirurgie.* Brunswick: Frederich Viewig und Sohn, 1870.
23. Thompson, D. P., and Ashley, F. L. Use of stapler in skin closure. *Am. J. Surg.* 132:136, 1976.
24. Trevaskis, A. E., Rempel, J. Okunski, W., and Rea, M. Sliding subcutaneous-pedicle flaps to close a circular defect. *Plast. Reconstr. Surg.* 46:155, 1970.
25. Varma, S., Ferguson, H. L., Breen, H., and Lumb, W. V. Comparison of seven suture materials in infected wounds – an experimental study. *J. Surg. Res.* 17:165, 1974.
26. Willman, V. L., and Hanlon, C. R. The influence of temperature on surface bleeding: favorable effects of local hypothermia. *Ann. Surg.* 143:660, 1956.

Closure of Skin Wounds

27. Anascombe, A. R., Hira, N., and Hunt, B. The use of a new absorbable suture material (polyglycolic acid) in general surgery. *Br. J. Surg.* 57:917, 1970.
28. Ashley, F. L. Stone, R. S., Polak, R., Berman, O. D., and Delabar, M. Further studies involving wound closure with a rapidly polymerizing adhesive. *Plast. Reconstr. Surg.* 31:333, 1963.
29. Brown, A. M. A new surgical skin clip for wound approximation. *Industr. Med. Surg.* 30:232, 1961.
30. Brunius, U. Wound healing impairment from sutures. *Acta. Chir. Scand.* Suppl. 395, 1968.
31. Brunius, U., and Ahren, C. Healing during the cicatrization phase of skin incisions closed by non-suture technique. *Acta. Chir. Scand.* 135:289, 1969.
32. Crikelair, G. F. Skin suture marks. *Am. J. Surg.* 96:631, 1958.
33. Elek, S. D., and Conen, P. E. The virulence of *Staphylococcus pyogenes* for man. A study of the problems of wound infection. *Br. J. Exp. Pathol.* 38:573, 1957.
34. Ellenberg, A. H. Surgical tape wound closure: A disenchantment. *Plast. Reconstr. Surg.* 39:625, 1967.
35. Emmett, A. J. J., and Barron, J. N. Adhesive suture strip closure of wounds in plastic surgery. *Br. J. Plast. Surg.* 17:175, 1964.
36. Everett, W. G. Suture materials in general surgery. *Prog. Surg.* 8:14, 1970.
37. Fischl, R. A. An adhesive for primary closure of skin incisions. *Plast. Reconstr. Surg.* 30:607, 1962.
38. Flinn, R. M. Knotting in medicine and surgery. *Practitioner* 183:322, 1959.
39. Franch, P. Surgical wound infections. *Universitetsforlaget* (Aarhus), 1970.
40. Gibson, E. W., and Poate, W. J. The use of adhesive surgical tape in plastic surgery. *Br. J. Plast. Surg.* 17:265, 1964.
41. Golden, T., Levy, A. H., and O'Connor, W. T. Primary healing of skin wounds and incisions with a threadless suture. *Am. J. Surg.* 104:603, 1962.
42. Hermann, J. B., Kelly, R. J., and Higgins, G. A. Polyglycolic acid sutures. *Arch. Surg.* 100:486, 1970.
43. Jenkins, H. P., Hrdina, L. S., Owens, F. M., and Swisher, F. M. Absorption of surgical gut: III. Duration in the tissues after loss of tensile strength. *Arch. Surg.* 45:74, 1942.
44. Jesse, R. H., Jr., Anderson, B. C., and Healey, J. E., Jr. Fixation of split-thickness skin grafts with adhesive. *Plast. Reconstr. Surg.* 33:272, 1964.
45. Lucid, M. L. The interlocking slip knot. *Plast. Reconstr. Surg.* 34:200, 1964.
46. Madsen, E. T. An experimental and clinical evaluation of surgical suture materials. *Surg. Gynecol. Obstet.* 97:73, 1953.
47. Miller, J. M., Zoll, D. R., and Brown, E. O. Clinical observations on use of an extruded collagen suture. *Arch. Surg.* 88:167, 1964.
48. Myers, M. B., and Cherry, G. Functional and angiographic vasculature in healing wounds. *Ann. Surg.* 36:750, 1970.
49. Postlethwait, R. W. Long term comparative study of nonabsorbable sutures. *Ann. Surg.* 171:892, 1970.
50. Skoog, T. Porous tape in wound closure, skin grafting and wound dressing. *Acta Chir. Scand.* 126:383, 1963.
51. Weisman, P. A. Microporous surgical tape in wound closure and skin grafting. *Br. J. Plast. Surg.* 16:379, 1963.
52. Wilkinson, T. S. Tissue adhesive as an adjunct in hair transplantation. *South. Med. J.* 67:1408, 1974.
53. Wilkinson, T. S. Personal communication, 1977.

Skin Grafts

54. Alexander, J. W., Wheeler, L. M., Rooney, R. C., McDonald, J., and MacMillan, B. G. Clinical evaluation of Epigard, a new synthetic substitute for homograft and heterograft skin. *J. Trauma* 13:374, 1973.

55. Allen, H. E., Edgerton, M. T., Rodeheaver, G. T., Prusak, M. P., Kurtz, L., and Edlich, R. Skin dressings in the treatment of contaminated wounds. *Am. J. Surg.* 126:45, 1973.
56. Aulenbacher, C. E., and Monafo, W. W. New spring wound dermatome for skin grafting under local anesthesia. *Am. J. Surg.* 118:131, 1969.
57. Birch, J., and Branemark, P. I. The vascularization of a free full thickness skin graft: I. A vital microscopic study. *Scand. J. Plast. Reconstr. Surg.* 3:1, 1969.
58. Birch, J., and Branemark, P. I. The vascularization of a free full thickness skin graft: II. A microangiographic study. *Scand. J. Plast. Reconstr. Surg.* 3:11, 1969.
59. Bodenham, D. C., and Watson, R. The early ambulation of patients with lower limb grafts. *Br. J. Plast. Surg.* 24:20, 1971.
60. Clemmesen, T. The early circulation in split skin grafts. *Acta Chir. Scand.* 124:11, 1962.
61. Clemmesen, T. The early circulation in split-skin grafts. Restoration of blood supply to split-skin autografts. *Acta Chir. Scand.* 127:1, 1964.
62. Clemmesen, T. Experimental studies on the healing of free skin autografts. *Dan. Med. Bull.* Suppl. 14, 2:1, 1967.
63. Converse, J. M., and Ballantyne, D. L., Jr. Distribution of diphophopyridine nucleotide diaphorase in rat skin autografts and homografts. *Plast. Reconstr. Surg.* 30:415, 1962.
64. Converse, J. M., Ballantyne, D. L., Jr., Rogers, B. O., and Raisbeck, A. P. "Plasmatic circulation" in skin grafts. *Transplant. Bull.* 4:154, 1957.
65. Converse, J. M., and Robb-Smith, A. H. T. The healing of surface cutaneous wounds; its analogy with the healing of superficial burns. *Am. Surg.* 120:873, 1944.
66. Converse, J. M., Uhlschmid, G. K., and Ballantyne, D. L., Jr. "Plasmatic circulation" in skin grafts – the phase of serum imbibition. *Plast. Reconstr. Surg.* 43:495, 1969.
67. Conway, H. Sweating function of transplanted skin. *Surg. Gynecol. Obstet.* 69:756, 1939.
68. Crawford, B. S. An unusual skin donor site. *Br. J. Plast. Surg.* 17:311, 1964.
69. Cronin, T. D. The use of a molded splint to prevent contracture after split skin grafting on the neck. *Plast. Reconstr. Surg.* 27:7, 1961.
70. Davis, J. S., and Kitlowski, E. A. The immediate contraction of cutaneous grafts and its cause. *Arch. Surg.* 23:954, 1931.
71. Dingman, R. O. Personal communication, 1972.
72. Dingman, R. O., and Walter, C. Use of composite ear grafts in correction of short nose. *Plast. Reconstr. Surg.* 43:117, 1969.
73. Eade, G. G. The relationship between granulation tissue, bacteria, and skin grafts in burned patients. *Plast. Reconstr. Surg.* 22:42, 1958.
74. Edgerton, M. T., and Hansen, F. C. Matching facial color with split thickness skin grafts from adjacent areas. *Plast. Reconstr. Surg.* 25:455, 1960.
75. Feller, I. A., and DeWeese, M. S. The use of stored cutaneous autografts in wound treatment. *Surgery* 44:540, 1958.
76. Furnas, D. W. Freehand technique for cutting one-piece split-skin grafts from avulsed or excised skin and fat. *Plast. Reconstr. Surg.* 39:497, 1967.
77. Gemberling, R. M., Miller, T. A., Caffee, H., and Zawacki, B. Dressing comparison in the healing of donor sites. *J. Trauma* 16:812, 1976.
78. Gillman, T., Penn, J., Bronks, D., and Roux, M. A re-examination of certain aspects of the histogenesis of healing cutaneous wounds. *Br. J. Surg.* 43:141, 1955.
79. Gimbal, N. S., and Farris, W. Skin grafting. *Arch. Surg.* 92:554, 1966.
80. Gingrass, P. J., Grabb, W. C., and Gingrass, R. P. Rat skin autografts over silastic implants: A study of the bridging phenomenon. *Plast. Reconstr. Surg.* 55:65, 1975.
81. González-Ulloa, M., Stevens, E., Alveres, F. G., and Leonelli, F. Espesor cutaneo; reporte de nuestro estudio microscopico. *Cir. Cir.* 24:455, 1956.
82. Goulian, D. A new economical dermatome. *Plast. Reconstr. Surg.* 42:85, 1968.
83. Haller, J. A., and Billingham, R. E. Studies of the vascularization in free skin grafts. *Ann. Surg.* 166:896, 1967.
84. Horton, C., Georgiade, N., Campbell, F., Masters, F., and Pickrell, K. The behavior of split thickness and dermal skin grafts in the peritoneal cavity. *Plast. Reconstr. Surg.* 12:269, 1953.
85. Howie, C. C. M. Refrigeration anesthesia for donor sites. *Br. J. Anaesth.* 43:616, 1971.
86. Hutchison, J., Tough, J., and Wyburn, G. Regeneration of sensation in grafted skin. *Br. J. Plast. Surg.* 2:82, 1949.
87. Hynes, W. The reversed dermis graft. *Br. J. Plast. Surg.* 7:97, 1954.
88. Hynes, W. The treatment of scars by shaving and skin grafting. *Br. J. Plast. Surg.* 10:1, 1957.
89. Igel, H. J., Freeman, A. E., Broeckman, C. R., and Kleinfeld, K. A new method of covering large surface area wounds with autografts: Application of tissue culture expanded autograft. *Arch. Surg.* 108:724, 1974.
90. Jackson, D. M., Lowbury, E. J. L., and Topley, E. Chemotherapy of *Streptococcus pyogenes* infection of burns. *Lancet* 2:705, 1951.

91. Kazanceva, N. D. Growth characteristics of skin thickness in children and its significance in free skin grafts. *Acta Chir. Plast.* (Praha) 11:71, 1969.
92. Kazanjian, V. H., and Converse, J. M. *The Surgical Treatment of Facial Injuries* (2nd ed.). Baltimore: Williams & Wilkins, 1959.
93. Kikuchi, I. Studies on the pressure dressing in full thickness skin grafting: II. Observations on rabbit skin autografts. *Kumamoto Med. J.* 23:65, 1970.
94. Kikuchi, I., and Omori, M. Demonstration of leaking vessels under skin grafts. *Plast. Reconstr. Surg.* 45:66, 1970.
95. Kirschbaum, J., and Rider, H. The surgical treatment of baldness. *Med. Times* 91:1037, 1963.
96. Koehnlein, H. E., and Deitrich E. E. Influence of different tensions on growth of skin grafts. *Surg. Forum* 26:562, 1975.
97. Kraft, R. O. Personal communications, 1971.
98. Krizek, T. J., and Robson, M. C. Evolution of quantitative bacteriology in wound management. *Am. J. Surg.* 130:579, 1975.
99. Lie, K. K., Magargle, R. K., and Posch, J. L. Free full-thickness skin grafts from the palm to cover defects of the fingers. *J. Bone Joint Surg.* [Am.] 52:559, 1970.
100. Liedberg, N., Kuhn, L. R., Barnes, B. A., Reiss, E., and Amspacher, W. Infection in burns: II. The pathogenicity of streptococci. *Surg. Gynecol. Obstet.* 98:693, 1954.
101. Littlewood, A. H. M. Seroma: An unrecognized cause of failure of split-thickness skin grafts. *Br. J. Plast. Surg.* 13:42, 1960.
102. Lofgren, L. Recovery of nervous function in skin transplants with special reference to sympathetic functions. *Acta Chir. Scand.* 102:229, 1951.
103. Lopez-Mas, J., Ortiz-Monasterio, F., de Gonzales, M. V., and Olmedo, A. Skin graft pigmentation: A new approach to prevention. *Plast. Reconstr. Surg.* 49:18, 1972.
104. MacMillan, B. G. The use of mesh grafting in treating burns. *Surg. Clin. North Am.* 50:1347, 1970.
105. Maris, F., Jurkovic, I., Kohut, P., and Suchanek, A. Re-innervation of free and flap skin grafts. *Acta Chir. Plast.* (Praha) 5:57, 1963.
106. Masson, J. K. Exposure in free split-thickness skin grafts. *Arch. Surg.* 82:342, 1961.
107. McCollum, M. S., and Grabb, W. C. Increasing the incidence and the size of successful experimental composite ear grafts by advance preparation of the recipient bed. *Plast. Reconstr. Surg.* 60:759, 1977.
108. McGibbon, B., and Paletta, F. X. The skin "spider." *Plast. Reconstr. Surg.* 47:299, 1971.
109. McGregor, I. A. *Fundamental Techniques of Plastic Surgery* (2nd ed.). Edinburgh: Livingstone, 1962.
110. McIndoe, A. H. The treatment of hypospadias. *Am. J. Surg.* 38:176, 1937.
111. Millard, D. R., Piggott, R., and Zies, P. Free skin grafting of full-thickness defects of abdominal wall. *Plast. Reconstr. Surg.* 43:569, 1969.
112. Miller, T. A. The deleterious effect of split-skin homograft coverage on split-skin donor sites. *Plast. Reconstr. Surg.* 53:316, 1974.
113. Mir y Mir, L. The problem of pigmentation in the cutaneous graft. *Br. J. Plast. Surg.* 14:303, 1961.
114. Oden, B. Microlymphangiographic studies of experimental skin autografts. *Acta Chir. Scand.* 121:219, 1961.
115. Orentreich. N. Autografts in alopecias and other selected dermatological conditions. *Ann. N. Y. Acad. Sci.* 83:463, 1959.
116. Patton, H. S. Split-skin grafts from hypothenar area for fingertip avulsions. *Plast. Reconstr. Surg.* 43:426, 1969.
117. Perrins, D. J. D. Influence of hyperbaric oxygen on the survival of split skin grafts. *Lancet* 1:868, 1967.
118. Perry, V. P. A review of skin preservation. *Cryobiology* 3:109, 1966.
119. Polk, H. C., Jr. Adherence of thin skin grafts. *Surg. Forum* 17:487, 1966.
120. Pontén, B. Grafted skin – observations on innervation and other qualities. *Acta Chir. Scand.* Suppl. 257, 1960.
121. Psillakis, J. M. Lymphatic vascularization of skin grafts. *Plast. Reconstr. Surg.* 43:287, 1969.
122. Ragnell, A. The secondary contracting tendency of free skin grafts. *Br. J. Plast. Surg.* 5:6, 1952.
123. Randall, P. Problems in skin grafting. *Surg. Clin. North Am.* 40:1629, 1960.
124. Robinson, D. W. Blood loss from donor sites in skin grafting procedures. *Surgery* 25:105, 1949.
125. Robson, M. C., Krizek, T. J., and Heggars, J. P. Biology of Surgical Infections. In Ravitch, M. M. (Ed.), *Current Problems in Surgery.* Chicago: Year Book Medical Publishers, 1973.
126. Ross, D. S., and Gibson, T. A new dermatome for preparing large free skin grafts. *Med. Electron Biol. Eng.* 3:403, 1965.
127. Rudolph, R., and Klein, L. Healing processes in skin grafts. *Surg. Gynecol. Obstet.* 136:641, 1973.
128. Salisbury, R. E., Wilmore, D. W., Silverstein, P., and Pruitt, B. A. Biologic dressings for skin graft donor sites. *Arch. Surg.* 106:705, 1973.
129. Sawhney, C. P., and Subbaraju, G. V. Healing of donor sites of split skin grafts – an experimental study in pigs. *Br. J. Plast. Surg.* 22:359, 1969.

130. Scothorne, R. J. Lymphatic repair and the genesis of homograft immunity. *Ann. N. Y. Acad. Sci.* 73:673, 1958.
131. Shepard, G. H. The storage of split-skin grafts on their donor sites. *Plast. Reconstr. Surg.* 49:115, 1972.
132. Shoul, M. I. Skin grafting under local anesthesia using a new safety razor dermatome. *Am. J. Surg.* 112:959, 1966.
133. Shuck, J. W., Pruitt, B. A., Jr., and Moncrief, J. A. Homograft skin for wound coverage. *Arch. Surg.* 98:472, 1969.
134. Smahel, J. The revascularization of free skin autograft. *Acta Chir. Plast.* (Praha) 9:76, 1967.
135. Smahel, J. Free skin transplantation on a prepared bed. *Br. J. Plast. Surg.* 24:129, 1971.
136. Smahel, J. The healing of skin grafts. *Clin. Plast. Surg.* 4:409, 1977.
137. Smahel, J., and Clodius, L. The blood vessel system of free human skin grafts. *Plast. Reconstr. Surg.* 47:61, 1971.
138. Smahel, J., and Ganzoni, N. Relay transplantation: A new method of expanding a free skin graft. *Plast. Reconstr. Surg.* 28:49, 1975.
139. Smith, J. W., Ringland, J., and Wilson, R. Vascularization of skin grafts. *Surg. Forum* 15:473, 1964.
140. Snow, J. W. Safety razor dermatome. *Plast. Reconstr. Surg.* 41:184, 1968.
141. Southwood, W. F. W. The thickness of the skin. *Plast. Reconstr. Surg.* 15:423, 1955.
142. Stark, R. B. *Plastic Surgery.* New York: Hoeber Med. Div., Harper & Row, 1962.
143. Sturman, M. J., and Duran, R. J. Late results of finger-tips injuries. *J. Bone Joint Surg.* [Am.] 45:289, 1963.
144. Sweeney, N. V. Composite grafts of skin and fat. *Br. J. Plast. Surg.* 26:72, 1973.
145. Terzis, J. K. Functional aspects of reinnervation of free skin grafts. *Plast. Reconstr. Surg.* 58:142, 1976.
146. Thompson, N. A clinical and histological investigation into the fate of epithelial elements buried following the grafting of "shaved" skin surfaces. *Br. J. Plast. Surg.* 13:219, 1960.
147. Zietkiewicz, W. Influence of antibacterial defense of skin grafts on the degree of graft taking. *Pol. Med. J.* 7:863, 1968.

Flaps

148. Adams, W. M., Jr., Wisner, H. K., Larson, D. L., Lynch, J. B., and Lewis, S. R. Steinmann pin fixation of extremities for cross-leg flap. *Plast. Reconstr. Surg.* 44:364, 1969.
149. Adamson, J. E., Horton, C. R., Crawford, H. H., and Ayers, W. T., Jr. The effects of dimethyl sulfoxide on the experimental pedicle flap: A preliminary report. *Plast. Reconstr. Surg.* 37:105, 1966.
150. Alms, M. Skeletal fixation for the cross leg pedicle flap. *Can. Med. Assoc. J.* 89:419, 1963.
151. Arturson, G., and Khama, N. N. The effects of hyperbaric oxygen, dimethyl sulfoxide, and Complamin on the survival of experimental skin flaps. *Scand. J. Plast. Reconstr. Surg.* 4:8, 1970.
152. Austad, E. Personal communication, 1977.
153. Bakamjian, V. A technique for primary reconstruction of the palate after radical maxillectomy for cancer. *Plast. Reconstr. Surg.* 31:103, 1963.
154. Bakamjian, V. Y., and Souther, S. G. Use of temporal muscle flap for reconstruction after orbitomaxillary resections for cancer. *Plast. Reconstr. Surg.* 56:171, 1975.
155. Baker, G. C., and Watson, H. K. The mathematical principles in the use and design of serial Y-V advancements. Paper presented at Plastic Surgery Senior Residents Conference, New Orleans, 1976.
156. Barron, J. N., Veall, N., and Arnott, D. G. The measurement of the local clearance of radioactive sodium in tubed skin pedicles. *Br. J. Plast. Surg.* 4:16, 1952.
157. Bloomenstein, R. B. Viability prediction in pedicle flaps by infrared thermometry. *Plast. Reconstr. Surg.* 42:252, 1968.
158. Brent, B. The acquired auricular deformity: A systematic approach to its analysis and reconstruction. *Plast. Reconstr. Surg.* 59:475, 1977.
159. Brown, J. B., and McDowell, F. *Skin Grafting* (3rd ed.). Philadelphia: Lippincott, 1958.
160. Brown, R. G., Vasconez, L. O., and Jurkiewicz, M. J. Transverse abdominal flaps and the deep epigastric arcade. *Plast. Reconstr. Surg.* 55:416, 1975.
161. Buncke, H. J., Furnas, D., Gordon, L., and Achauer, B. M. Free osteocutaneous flap from a rib to the tibia. *Plast. Reconstr. Surg.* 59:799, 1977.
162. Bürow, A. Zur Blepharoplastik. *Monatsschr. Med. Augenh. Cir.* 1:57, 1838.
163. Burton, A. C. Physiology of Cutaneous Circulation. Thermoregulatory Functions. In Rothman, R. (Ed.), *The Human Integument.* Washington, D.C.: American Association for the Advancement of Science, 1959.
164. Champion, W. M., McSherry, C. K., and Goulian, D. Effect of hyperbaric oxygen on the survival of pedicled skin flaps. *J. Surg. Res.* 7:583, 1967.
165. Constant, E., and Grabb, W. Steinmann pin fixation of tibiae for cross leg flap. *Plast. Reconstr. Surg.* 41:179, 1968.
166. Converse, J. M. *Reconstructive Plastic Surgery.*

Philadelphia: Saunders, 1964.
167. Converse, J. M., and Wood-Smith, D. Experiences with the forehead island flap with a subcutaneous pedicle. *Plast. Reconstr. Surg.* 31:521, 1963.
168. Conway, H. Notes on cutaneous healing in wounds. *Surg. Gynecol. Obstet.* 66:140, 1938.
169. Conway, H., Stark, R. B., and Joslin, D. Cutaneous histamine reaction as a test of circulatory efficiency of tubed pedicles and flaps. *Surg. Gynecol. Obstet.* 93:185, 1951.
170. Corso, P. F. Variations of the arterial, venous and capillary circulation of the soft tissues of the head by decades as demonstrated by the methyl methacrolate injection technique, and their application to the construction of flaps and pedicles. *Plast. Reconstr. Surg.* 27:160, 1961.
171. Crawford, B. S. The management of tube pedicles. *Br. J. Plast. Surg.* 18:387, 1965.
172. Creech, B. J., and Miller, S. H. Evaluation of Circulation in Skin Flaps. In Grabb, W. C., and Myers, M. B. (Eds.), *Skin Flaps.* Boston: Little, Brown, 1975.
173. Cuthbert, J. B. The "marsupial" skin flap. *Br. J. Plast. Surg.* 2:125, 1949.
174. Daniel, R. K., and Taylor, I. Distant transfer of an island flap by microvascular anastomoses. *Plast. Reconstr. Surg.* 52:111, 1973.
175. Daniel, R. K., Terzis, J., and Schwarz, G. Neurovascular free flaps. *Plast. Reconstr. Surg.* 56:13, 1975.
176. Daniel, R. K., and Williams, H. B. The free transfer of skin flaps by microvascular anastomoses. *Plast. Reconstr. Surg.* 52:16, 1973.
177. Das, S. K. The size of the human omentum and methods of lengthening it for transplantation. *Br. J. Plast. Surg.* 29:170, 1976.
178. Dean, R. K., Kelleher, J. C., Sullivan, J. G., and Baibeck, G. J. Bilobed Flaps. In Grabb, W. C., and Myers, M. B. (Eds.), *Skin Flaps.* Boston, Little, Brown, 1975.
179. DeHaan, C. R., and Stark, R. B. Changes in efferent circulation of tubed pedicles and in the transplantability of large composite grafts produced by histamine iontophoresis. *Plast. Reconstr. Surg.* 28:577, 1961.
180. Derganc, M., and Zdravic, F. Venous congestion of flaps treated by application of leeches. *Br. J. Plast. Surg.* 13:187, 1960.
181. Dingwell, J. A., and Lord, J. W. The fluorescein test in the management of tubed (pedicle) flaps. *Bull. Johns Hopkins Hosp.* 73:129, 1943.
182. Douglas, B., and Buchholz, R. The blood circulation in pedicle flaps. *Ann. Surg.* 117:692, 1943.
183. Dupont, C., and Menard, Y. Transposition of the greater omentum for reconstruction of the chest wall. *Plast. Reconstr. Surg.* 49:263, 1972.
184. Finseth, F. Personal communication, 1977.
185. Finseth, F., and Adelberg, M. Prevention of skin flap necrosis by vasodilator pharmacologic agents. *Plast. Reconstr. Surg.* 61:738, 1978.
186. Finseth, F., and Cutting, C. An experimental neurovascular island flap for the study of the delay phenomenon. *Plast. Reconstr. Surg.* 6:412, 1978.
187. Fujino, T., Harishina, T., and Aoyagi, F. Reconstruction for aplasia of the breast and pectoral region by microvascular transfer of a free flap from the buttock. *Plast. Reconstr. Surg.* 56:178, 1975.
188. Ger, R., and Levine, S. A. The management of decubitus ulcer by muscle transposition. *Plast. Reconstr. Surg.* 58:419, 1976.
189. Goetz, R. H. The diagnosis and treatment of vascular diseases. *Br. J. Surg.* 37:146, 1949.
190. Goetz, R. H. The rate and control of the blood flow through the skin of the upper extremities. *S. Afr. J. Med. Sci.* 8:65, 1963.
191. Goode, R. L., and Linehan, J. W. The fluorescein test in postirradiation surgery – a preliminary report. *Arch. Otolaryngol.* 91:526, 1970.
192. Grabb, W. C., and Oneal, R. The effect of low molecular weight dextran on the survival of experimental skin flaps. *Plast. Reconstr. Surg.* 30:649, 1966.
193. Harii, K., Ohmori, K., and Ohmori, S. Successful clinical transfer of ten free flaps by microvascular anastomoses. *Plast. Reconstr. Surg.* 53:259, 1974.
194. Harii, K., Ohmori, K., and Sekiguchi, J. The free musculocutaneous flap. *Plast. Reconstr. Surg.* 57:294, 1976.
195. Hauser, W. H., Tauxe, W. N., Owen, C. A., Jr., and Lipscomb, P. R. Determination of the vascular status of pedicle skin grafts by radioactive tracer studies. *Surg. Gynecol. Obstet.* 112:625, 1961.
196. Hayes, H. Cross-leg flaps after the age of fifty. *Plast. Reconstr. Surg.* 30:649, 1962.
197. Hayes, J. E., Robinson, D. W., Schloerb, P. R., and Masters, F. W. A simple method of testing the circulation of pedicle flaps. *Surg. Forum* 18:516, 1967.
198. Hill, H. L., Brown, R. G., and Jurkiewicz, M. J. The transverse lumbosacral back flap. *Plast. Reconstr. Surg.* 62:177, 1978.
199. Hoffmeister, F. S. Studies on timing of tissue transfer in reconstructive surgery. *Plast. Reconstr. Surg.* 19:283, 1957.
200. Hueston, J. T., and McConchie, I. H. A compound pectoral flap. *Aust. N. Z. J. Surg.* 38:61, 1968.
201. Hynes, W. A simple method of estimating blood

flow with special reference to the circulation in pedicled skin flaps and tubes. *Br. J. Plast. Surg.* 1:159, 1948.

202. Hynes, W. The "blue flap": A method of treatment. *Br. J. Plast. Surg.* 4:166, 1951.
203. Jervis, W., Salyer, K. E., Vargas Busquets, M., and Atkins, R. W. Further applications of the Limberg and Dufourmental flaps. *Plast. Reconstr. Surg.* 54:335, 1974.
204. Kazanjian, V. H., and Converse, J. M. *The Surgical Treatment of Facial Injuries* (2nd ed.). Baltimore: Williams & Wilkins, 1959.
205. Kernahan, D. A., and Littlewood, A. H. M. Experience in the use of arterial flaps about the face. *Plast. Reconstr. Surg.* 28:207, 1961.
206. Kernahan, D. A., Zingg, W., and Kay, C. W. The effect of hyperbaric oxygen on the survival of experimental skin flaps. *Plast. Reconstr. Surg.* 36:19, 1965.
207. Ketchum, L. D., Ellis, S. S., Robinson, D. W., and Masters, F. W. Vascular augmentation of pedicled tissue by combined histamine iontophoresis and hypertensive perfusion. *Plast. Reconstr. Surg.* 39:138, 1967.
208. Kiehn, C. L., and Des Prez, J. D. Effects of local hypothermia on pedicle flap tissue: I. Enhancement of survival of experimental pedicles. *Plast. Reconstr. Surg.* 25:349, 1960.
209. Klingenström, P., and Nylén, B. Timing of transfer of tubed pedicles and cross flaps. *Plast. Reconstr. Surg.* 37:1, 1966.
210. Koehnlein, H. E., and Lemperle, G. Experimental studies on the effect of dimethyl sulfoxide on pedicle flaps. *Surgery* 67:672, 1970.
211. Kubacek. V. Transposition of flaps in the face on a subcutaneous pedicle. *Acta Chir. Plast.* (Praha) 2:108, 1960.
212. LaPiana, F. G., and Permer, R. Anaphylactoid reaction to intravenously administered fluorescein. *Arch. Ophthalmol.* 79:161, 1968.
213. Letterman, G. S., Schurter, M., and Prandoni, A. G. Prophylactic anticoagulation in the cross-leg flap procedure. *Plast. Reconstr. Surg.* 27:520, 1961.
214. Lister, G. D., and Gibson, T. Closure of rhomboid skin defects: The flaps of Limberg and Dufourmental. *Br. J. Surg.* 25:300, 1972.
215. Littlewood, M. Compound skin and sternomastoid flaps for repair in extensive carcinoma of the head and neck. *Br. J. Plast. Surg.* 20:403, 1967.
216. Manchot, C. *Die Hautartenian des menschlichen Körpers.* Leipzig: Vogel, 1889.
217. Maris, F., Jurkovic, I., Kobut, P., and Suchanek, A. Re-innervation of free and flap skin grafts. *Acta Chir. Plast.* (Praha) 5:57, 1963.
218. McCraw, J. B., Dibbell, D. G., Horton, C. E., Carraway, J. H., and Adamson, J. E. Clinical definition of independent myocutaneous vascular territories. Paper presented at the meeting of the American Association of Plastic Surgeons, Atlanta, 1976.
219. McFarlane, R. M. The treatment of ischemic pedicle flaps with hyperbaric oxygen. Personal communication, 1968.
220. McGregor, I. A. The regeneration of sympathetic activity in grafted skin as evidenced by sweating. *Br. J. Plast. Surg.* 3:12, 1950.
221. McGregor, I. A., and Jackson, I. T. The groin flap. *Br. J. Plast. Surg.* 25:3, 1972.
222. McLean, D. H., and Buncke, H. J. Autotransplant of omentum to a large scalp defect, with microsurgical revascularization. *Plast. Reconstr. Surg.* 49:268, 1972.
223. Millard, D. R. The crane principle for the transport of subcutaneous tissue. *Plast. Reconstr. Surg.* 43:451, 1969.
224. Milton, S. H. The Survival of Experimental Pedicled Skin Flaps. Ph.D. thesis, 1967.
225. Milton, S. H. Pedicled skin flaps: The fallacy of the length : width ratio. *Br. J. Surg.* 57:502, 1970.
226. Milton, S. H. The tubed pedicle flap. *Br. J. Plast. Surg.* 22:53, 1969.
227. Milton, S. H. Experimental studies on island flaps: I. The surviving length. *Plast. Reconstr. Surg.* 48:574, 1971.
228. Milton, S. H., and Corbett, J. L. Failure to increase the survival of experimental flaps by histamine and hypertension. *Plast. Reconstr. Surg.* 43:235, 1969.
229. Mladick, R. A., Pickrell, K. L., Thorne, F. L., and Royer, J. R. Ipsilateral thigh flap for total plantar resurfacing. *Plast. Reconstr. Surg.* 43:198, 1969.
230. Murray, J. F., Ord, J. V. R., and Gavelin, G. E. The neurovascular island pedicle flap. *J. Bone Joint Surg.* [Am.] 49:1285, 1967.
231. Myers, M. B. Wound tension and vascularity in the etiology and prevention of skin sloughs. *Surgery* 56:945, 1964.
232. Myers, M. B. Prediction and prevention of skin sloughs in radical cancer surgery. *Pacific Med. Surg.* 75:315, 1967.
233. Myers, M. B. Investigation of Skin Flap Necrosis. In Grabb, W. C., and Myers, M. B. (Eds.), *Skin Flaps.* Boston: Little, Brown, 1975.
234. Myers, M. B. Personal communication, 1977.
235. Myers, M. B., and Cherry, G. Enhancement of survival in devascularized pedicles by the use of phenoxybenzamine. *Plast. Reconstr. Surg.* 41:254, 1968.

236. Myers, M. B., and Cherry, G. Mechanism of the delay phenomenon. *Plast. Reconstr. Surg.* 44:52, 1969.
237. New, G. B., and Erich, J. B. *The Use of Pedicle Flaps in Plastic Surgery of the Head and Neck.* Springfield, Ill.: Thomas, 1950.
238. O'Brien, B. A muscle-skin pedicle for total reconstruction of the lower lip. *Plast. Reconstr. Surg.* 45:395, 1970.
239. O'Brien, B., Morrison, W. A., Ishida, H., MacLeod, A. M., and Gilbert, A. Free flap transfers with microvascular anastomoses. *Br. J. Plast. Surg.* 27:220, 1974.
240. Omer, G., Day, D. J., Ratcliff, H., and Lambert, P. Neurovascular cutaneous island pedicles for deficient median nerve sensibility. New technique and results of serial functional tests. *J. Bone Joint Surg.* [Am.] 52:1181, 1970.
241. Oneal, R. M., Knode, R. E., Grabb, W. C., and Dingman, R. O. The effect of low molecular weight dextran on the survival of skin flaps in pigs vascularized either by a single artery and vein or by a subdermal plexus. *Plast. Reconstr. Surg.* 40:595, 1967.
242. Orticochea, M. The musculo-cutaneous flap method: An immediate and heroic substitute for the method of delay. *Br. J. Plast. Surg.* 25:106, 1972.
243. Parker, G. M. Personal communication, 1965.
244. Patterson, T. J. S. The survival of skin flaps in the pig. *Br. J. Plast. Surg.* 21:113, 1969.
245. Patterson, T. J. S., and Cherry, G. Personal communication, 1972.
246. Patterson, T. J. S., Berry, R. J., and Wiernik, G. The effect of x-radiation on the survival of skin flaps in the pig. *Br. J. Plast. Surg.* 25:17, 1972.
247. Peacock, E. E., Jr. Reconstruction of the hand by the local transfer of composite tissue island flaps. *Plast. Reconstr. Surg.* 25:298, 1960.
248. Pers, M., and Medgyesi, S. Pedicle muscle flaps and their applications in the surgery of repair. *Br. J. Plast. Surg.* 26:313, 1973.
249. Radovan, C. Personal communication, 1976.
250. Reinisch, J. F. The effect of local anesthesia with epinephrine on skin flap survival. *Plast. Reconstr. Surg.* 54:324, 1974.
251. Reinisch, J. F. Pathophysiology of skin flap circulation. *Plast. Reconstr. Surg.* 54:585, 1974.
252. Reinisch, J. F. The Role of Arteriovenous Anastomoses in Skin Flaps. In Grabb, W. C., and Myers, M. B. (Eds.), *Skin Flaps.* Boston: Little, Brown, 1975.
253. Saunders, W. H. Pedicled pericranium as base for skin grafts. *Laryngoscope* 78:1088, 1968.
254. Schechter, G. L., Biller, H. F., and Ogura, J. H. Applications of the autotransplanted vascular pedicle skin flap. *Surg. Forum* 20:474, 1969.
255. Serafin, D., Georgiade, N. G., and Smith, D. H. Microsurgical composite tissue transplantation for reconstruction of defects of the distal lower extremity: A comparison with older methods. *Plast. Reconstr. Surg.* 62:527, 1978.
256. Smith, J. W. Clinical experiences with the vermillion bordered lip flat. *Plast. Reconstr. Surg.* 27:527, 1961.
257. Smith, P. J., Foley, B., McGregor, I. A., and Jackson, I. T. The anatomical basis of the groin flap. *Plast. Reconstr. Surg.* 49:41, 1972.
258. Snell, P. M. The pig as an experimental model for skin flap behavior: A reappraisal of previous studies. *Br. J. Plast. Surg.* 30:1, 1977.
259. Snyder, C. C., Bateman, J. M., Davis, C. W., and Warden, G. D. Mandibulo-facial restoration with live osteocutaneous flaps. *Plast. Reconstr. Surg.* 45:14, 1970.
260. Stark, R. *Plastic Surgery.* New York: Hoeber Med. Div., Harper & Row, 1962.
261. Stark, R. B. The pantographic expansion principle as applied to the advancement flap. *Plast. Reconstr. Surg.* 15:222, 1955.
262. Stark, R. B., and Kaplan, J. M. Cross-leg flaps in patients over 50 years of age. *Br. J. Plast. Surg.* 25:20, 1972.
263. Steiss, C. F. Utilization of the tube pedicle in the reconstruction of facial defects. *Plast. Reconstr. Surg.* 4:545, 1949.
264. Stern, W. G., and Cohen, M. B. The intracutaneous salt solution wheat test. *J.A.M.A.* 87:1355, 1926.
265. Sturman, M. J., and Duran, R. J. Late results of finger-tip injuries. *J. Bone Joint Surg.* [Am.] 45:289, 1963.
266. Sundell, B. Studies on the circulation of pedicle skin flaps. *Ann. Chir. Gynaecol. Fenn.* Suppl. 53, 133:1, 1963.
267. Tagliacozzi, G. *De Curtorum Chirurgia per Insitionern.* Venetus: G. Bindonus, 1597.
268. Tauxe, W. N., Simons, J. N., Lipscomb, P. R., and Hamamato, K. Determination of vascular status of pedicled skin flaps by used radioactive pertechnetate (99 m/Tc). *Surg. Gynecol. Obstet.* 130:87, 1970.
269. Taylor, G. I., and Daniel, R. K. Anatomy of several free flap donor sites. *Plast. Reconstr. Surg.* 56:243, 1975.
270. Thorne, F. L., Georgiade, N. G., Wheller, W. F., and Mladick, R. A. Photoplethysmography as an aid in determining the viability of skin flaps. *Plast. Reconstr. Surg.* 44:279, 1969.
271. Thorne, F. L., Georgiade, N. G., and Mladick, R. The use of thermography in determining viability of pedicle flaps. *Arch. Surg.* 99:97, 1969.

272. Thorvaldsson, S. E., and Grabb, W. C. The intravenous fluorescein test as a measure of skin flap viability. *Plast. Reconstr. Surg.* 53:576, 1974.
273. Vasconez, L. O., Bostwick, J., and McCraw, J. Coverage of exposed bone by muscle transposition and skin grafting. *Plast. Reconstr. Surg.* 53:526, 1974.
274. Velander, E. Vascular changes in tubed pedicles: An animal experimental study. *Acta Chir. Scand.* Suppl. 322:1, 1964.
275. Webster, J. P. Thoraco-epigastric tubed pedicles. *Surg. Clin. North Am.* 17:145, 1937.
276. White, W. L. Flap grafts to the upper extremity. *Surg. Clin. North Am.* 40:389, 1960.
277. Winsten, J., Manalo, P., and Barsky, A. Studies on the circulation of tubed flaps. *Plast. Reconstr. Surg.* 28:619, 1961.

Z-plasty

278. Borges, A. F. Improvement of antitension-lines scar by the "W-plasty" operation. *Br. J. Plast. Surg.* 12:29, 1959.
279. Borges, A. F. The W-plastic versus the Z-plastic scar revision. *Plast. Reconstr. Surg.* 44:58, 1969.
280. Davis, J. S. Present evaluation of the merits of the Z-plasty operation. *Plast. Reconstr. Surg.* 1:26, 1946.
281. Dingman, R. O. Some applications of the Z-plasty procedure. *Plast. Reconstr. Surg.* 16:246, 1955.
282. Furnas, D. W., and Fischer, G. W. The Z-plasty: Biomechanics and mathematics. *Br. J. Plast. Surg.* 24:144, 1971.
283. Gibson, T., and Kenedi, R. M. Biomechanical properties of skin. *Surg. Clin. North Am.* 47:279, 1967.
284. Grabb, W. C. Personal communication, 1977.
285. Jayapathy, B., Huffmann, W. C., and Lierle, D. M. The Z-plasty procedure – some mathematic considerations and application to cleft lip. *Plast. Reconstr. Surg.* 26:203, 1960.
286. Limberg, A. A. *Mathematical Principles of Local Plastic Procedures on the Surface of the Body.* Leningrad: Medgis, 1946.
287. Limberg, A. A. *Planning of Local Plastic Operations on the Body's Surface: Theory and Practice.* Leningrad: Medgis, 1963.
288. McGregor, I. A. *Fundamental Techniques of Plastic Surgery* (2nd ed.). Edinburgh: Livingstone, 1962.
289. Mir y Mir, L. The six-flap Z-plasty. *Plast. Reconstr. Surg.* 52:625, 1973.
290. Russo, M. Brûlures dorsalis graves de la main. *Ann. Chir.* 29:1015, 1975.
291. Spina, V. "Z" plasty. *Rev. Paul. Med.* 36:347, 1950.
292. Stevenson, T. W. Release of circular constricting scars by Z flaps. *Plast. Reconstr. Surg.* 1:39, 1946.
293. Wilkinson, T. S., and Rybka, F. J. Experimental study of prevention of tip necrosis in ischemic Z-plasties. *Plast. Reconstr. Surg.* 47:37, 1971.
294. Woolf, R. M., and Broadbent, T. R. The four flap Z-plasty. *Plast. Reconstr. Surg.* 49:48, 1972.

Tissue Transplantation

NOEL THOMPSON

Plastic surgery in its day-to-day practice is fundamentally concerned with the transplantation of tissues, and its future development is likely to depend to an important degree on the successful contribution of its technical resources to the battery of measures designed to breach the biological barrier involved in transplanting tissue from one individual to another.

CLASSIFICATION

Free grafts or transplants may be classified according to the terminology introduced by Snell [11] in 1964: (1) an *isograft* (synonyms: isogenic graft, syngeneic graft) is a graft between genetically identical individuals – that is, a graft within inbred strains, between identical twins, or between F_1 hybrids produced by crossing inbred strains; (2) an *autograft* (synonyms: autogenous graft, autogenic graft) is a graft transferred from one place to another on the same individual; (3) an *allograft* (synonyms: homograft, allogenic graft) is a graft between genetically disparate individuals of the same species, a graft between outbred strains; (4) *xenograft* (synonym: heterograft) is a graft between members of different species.

Tissue to be transplanted to an anatomically similar site (e.g., a skin graft to replace an area of skin loss) is referred to as an orthotopic transplant or orthograft; if otherwise, it is heterotopic.

Transplants are usually free grafts – that is, they are totally detached from the host during transfer and consequently have all vascular and nervous connections severed from the outset. A pedicle transplant (or flap) remains attached to the host and carries an intact blood supply at all stages during transfer. Occasionally the free graft need only act as a scaffolding to be invaded by host tissues which thereby restore lasting tissue continuity at the graft site, in which case the graft need not be viable; more usually the graft is required to survive and function by developing direct vascular connections with the host. In organ transplantation, a direct vascular anastomosis between host and graft is performed at the time of transfer, a method being more widely adopted with the current development of microsurgical techniques. Finally, transplants may be subdivided as viable or nonviable, fresh or preserved.

ALLOGRAFTS

For the individual to survive in an inimical environment populated by potentially injurious agents in the form of bacteria and viruses capable of producing disease, it is essential that the host has the means of promptly recognizing protein foreign to itself, and also the power of rapidly rejecting it. The mechanism involved is that of immunity. The invading agent exciting the immune reaction is the antigen, and as a result of the immune process, certain tissues in the host respond by producing other protein (usually globulin) agents – antibodies – which resist the invading foreign protein. The antibody, with the assistance of complement, then unites with, precipitates, or otherwise inactivates the protein antigen in preparation for its subsequent rejection. In rare cases the host may permit the antigen to remain in the body unmolested, a condition referred to as immunological tolerance, which is exemplified by the normal presence in the human being of certain viruses and bacteria that do not cause disease. It is noteworthy that the antigens and antibodies concerned in the allograft reaction have never been isolated or positively identified [4].

The host responds to allografts with the same reaction that would apply to any other foreign antigen. The allograft survives for an initial period of days or weeks, but thereafter, depending on the tissue used and the site to which it is transplanted, it becomes necrotic and is either shed or replaced by fibrous tissue or the creeping substitution of host cells. Allograft destruction is the consequence of an immunological reaction referred to as the *allograft rejection.*

Xenografts are destroyed in the same way as allografts, but the rejection process is usually much more precipitate and fulminating in character, and achieved in a much shorter time.

The Allograft Reaction

The allograft reaction (Fig. 2-1) depends on there being a means of communication between the transplanted cells and the reactive immunological centers of the host. Thus skin transplanted to an orthotopic site is usually rejected in 5 to 15 days.

The transplant undergoes a series of changes manifested first in its vascular system and terminating in the progressive and complete disintegration of the graft. The blood vessels become engorged, blood flow ceases, and interstitial edema appears. The mitochondrial elements of the cytoplasm disappear [43], and the graft becomes invaded within 2 to 5 days by mononuclear cells resembling small lymphocytes,

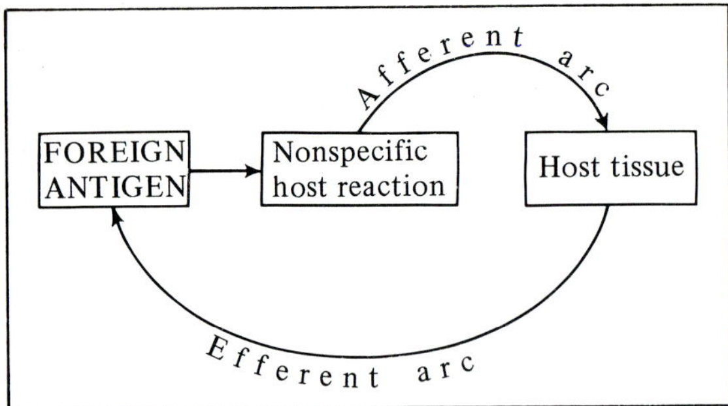

Fig. 2-1. Fundamental principles involved in the immune response.

later supported by plasma cells in limited numbers, which become replaced by polymorphonuclear leukocytes and macrophages as necrosis of the graft supervenes. This leukocytic infiltration is the most characteristic histological feature in the rejection process.

Changes also appear in the regional lymph nodes draining the graft site [41], which enlarge as a result of active proliferation of lymphoid cells in response to stimulation by antigens deriving from the allograft. Since specific reactivity appears first in the regional lymph nodes draining the graft site, it appears that a regional immunological reaction precedes the general hypersensitivity that ensues. As is to be expected in such an acquired immunological response by the host to transplantation antigens, a latent interval of a few days is required for the buildup of host antibodies, during which period the transplant appears to be accepted; also, a subsequent repetition of the grafting procedure between the same subjects results in accelerated and much more violent rejection of the second transplant – the so-called second-set reaction [23]. Since this reaction follows the transfer of different tissues from the same donor, it appears that the transplantation antigens initiating the reaction are for the most part common to all tissues of the individual. In some persons the second-set reaction may be so intense that the repeated graft may remain white and inert from the outset (white-graft reaction), undergoing necrosis without ever having acquired a blood supply from the host [38]; in such cases, therefore, vascular obstruction producing ischemia predominates over the cellular response seen in first-set allografts.

Transplantation antigens appear to be located in the insoluble lipoproteins of plasma membranes, and also possibly in the internal membranous structures of cells (e.g., lysosomes). Although nonvital extracts of cells possess immunological potency, this is far inferior to the potency of the living cells from which the extract is made.

The specificity of the antigens involved in the allograft reaction is genetically determined, and the mendelian location of the genes controlling these antigens has been established by grafting tissues between mice of different pure strains. Within each strain the mice accept grafts from each other, and, therefore, must be homozygous for the genes concerned with transplantation. If, for example, the parental strains differ by a single gene, one strain being A and the other B (Fig. 2-2), then crossing the strains gives a first familial generation (F_1) of constitution AB in which the parental strains are codominant; the F_1 progeny carry both types of transplantation antigen, and will, therefore, accept grafts from either parent. On mating the F_1 generation, out of the four possible combinations into which the original genes can be paired in the F_2 progeny, half will carry the codominant susceptibility genes of both parental stocks (and so will be heterozygous AB) and one-quarter each will be homozygous for one histocompatibility gene or the other (AA or BB). Thus three out of four of the F_2 generation accept parental strain grafts. If, instead of one locus with a pair of allelic genes, there were n loci, then the proportion of the F_2 generation accepting parental strain grafts would be $(3/4)^n$; by this means the number of loci controlling transplantation antigens can be estimated.

There are at least 20 such loci in the mouse, but, of these, one in particular (the H-2 locus) is of the greatest importance because the strength of its transplantation antigens elicits intense allograft reactions. These antigens are distributed over the cell surface and are especially plentiful on lymphoid cells. In man there is also one locus producing strong allograft reactions: it is the human leukocyte antigen (HL-A) system, the human equivalent of the H-2 system of mice. The HL-A system and the ABO group (long known in red blood cells) constitute the only two histocompatibility (or H) systems of antigens identified in man. Since HL-A antigens are richly present on human leukocytes (also platelets, fibroblasts, and most organ tissues) but absent from red cells, their presence is detected either by leukocyte agglutination (involving mainly polymorphs), or by cytotoxic tests carried out on leukocytes obtained from the peripheral blood. Of these, the lymphocytotoxic test is probably the more reliable.

Further evidence supporting the immunological concept of allograft rejection was obtained when it was shown that the actively acquired immunity developed by an animal receiving an allograft could be passively transferred to a third animal by inoculating the latter with lymphoid cells derived from the regional nodes draining the graft site in the recipient animal. Since such specific sensitivity could not be

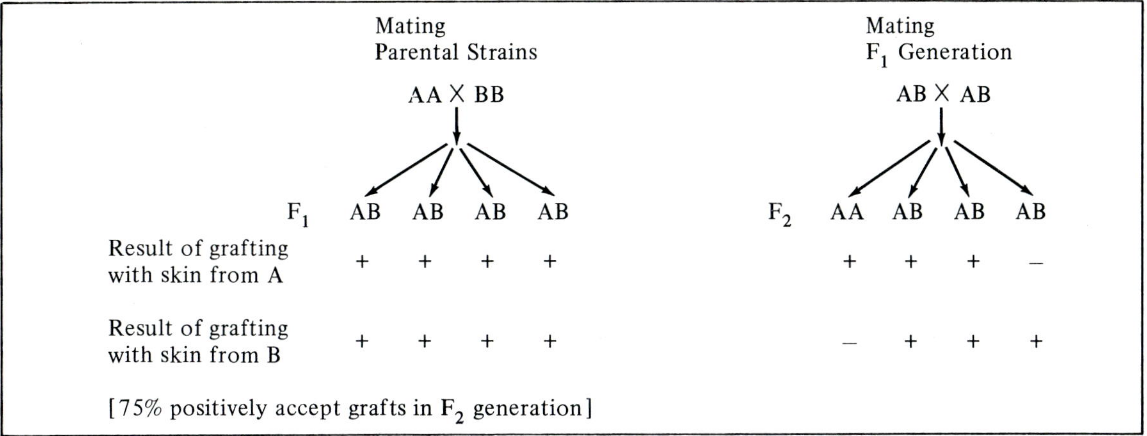

Fig. 2-2. Inheritance of genes controlling transplantation antigens. A and B genes, at the same genetic locus, express the corresponding transplantation antigens. The pure strains are homozygous for AA and BB, respectively.

transferred by serum, this constituted a clear demonstration of the importance of cellular rather than humoral antibodies in the process of allograft rejection. Such an adoptive transfer of immunity was demonstrated first in tumor allografts, but it was subsequently confirmed in allografts of normal tissues [16, 35]. It has successfully followed the transfer of cells of the lymphoid series from the spleen [33], thoracic duct lymph [27], and the peripheral blood stream [20] of the allografted animal. This transfer of immunity is not achieved by the transfer of cell-free plasma alone and has now been confirmed as occurring in human beings in the same manner [29]. The transplantation antigens are genetically determined, and apparently exist in all nucleated cells of the individual.

Although Gorer [25] has shown that cytotoxic humoral antibodies acting against donor cells can be demonstrated in host serum after the allograft rejection crisis, these must be regarded as of minor importance (except in grafts inoculated as suspensions of cells in ascites tumours, or normal or malignant lymphoid cells) in precipitating rejection of the transplant. This is demonstrated by the indefinite survival, even as a second-set allograft, of allografts removed from all contact with host cells by being enclosed in a fine membrane permeable only to tissue fluids and not to cells before burial in host tissues [45]. Further evidence that cellular rather than humoral antibodies are concerned in the rejection of allografts is confirmed by the survival of allografts immersed in the cell-free fluid of the anterior chamber of the eye, where they are protected against cellular invasion, and also by the appearance of plasma cells and lymphocytes of host derivation in allografts immediately before rejection.

If the large antigenic molecules are actually liberated from the allograft to reach the regional lymph nodes after traversing the intervening lymphatic pathways, it might be expected that allografts contained in a cell-permeable filter chamber might release the relevant antigens to sensitize the host; however, this apparently does not occur experimentally. There is increasing evidence that the cells of the lymphoid series transport the transplantation antigens from the allograft to the regional lymph nodes of the recipient animal, and subsequently carry the host antibodies to the allograft, which becomes destroyed as a consequence of the ensuing antigen-antibody reaction. Although the central importance of cells in mediating the allograft rejection response is accepted, it is not known whether the cells concerned act by virtue of their own inherent specificity or achieve this from adherent humoral antibody produced by other cells. Since sensitivity can be detected only after 2 or 3 days, at a time when vascular and lymphatic continuity between graft and host has become established, it seems likely that these channels might assist the passage of antigen in either a free or an intracellular state.

Immunological Enhancement

On exposure to solid or dissociated cellular allografts, humoral isoantibodies result – hemagglutinins, hemolysins, leukocyte agglutinins, and cytotoxins.

In solid tissue allografts, rejection is mediated largely by cellular rather than humoral immunity: the latter at best plays a minor supporting role. However, in the interesting phenomenon known as *immunological enhancement* (Fig. 2-3), preliminary immunization, by producing a high titer of serum antibodies,

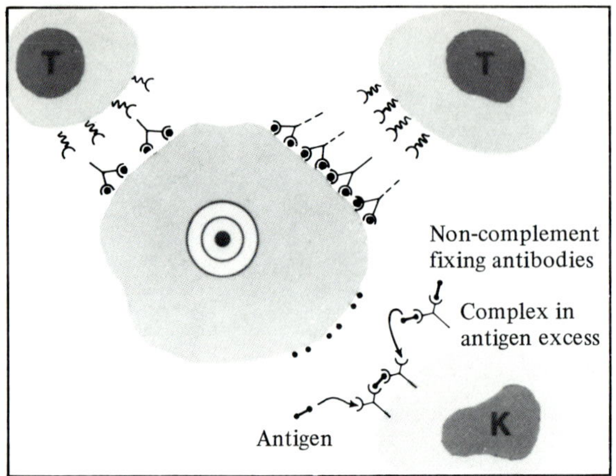

Fig. 2-3. Enhancement, showing the possible mechanisms involved. The central target cell is under attack by two T lymphocytes above (the chief source of which is the thymus) and by a K cell below (a lymphoreticular immune cell) having specific receptors to bind it to the antibodies coating the target cell. The target cell is protected from aggressor cells by antibody masking the surface antigens; if these antibodies are capable of fixing complement, the target cell is killed (see left, above) but if non-complement-fixing antibodies predominate then the T lymphocytes (see right, above) are unable to attack. Below, the aggressor K cell is prevented from attack by having its antibody-antigen complexes blocked by free or complexed antigen present in the serum.

actually weakens the animal's capacity to react against tissue allografts from the same donor. This preliminary immunization is either active, by inoculation with nonvital cell-free extracts from a donor strain, or passive, by the transfer of immune serum. It is important that although the humoral response to the inoculation of nonviable tissue extracts is good, there is no cellular response – an important factor in establishing enhancement, rather than sensitization in the host animal. The phenomenon is chiefly manifested in tumor allografts, but is present to some degree in rabbits receiving skin allografts after preliminary inoculation with donor epidermal cells or leukocytes. The phenomenon is explained by the high titer of serum antibodies, which presumably block the immunological response to the donor graft by uniting preferentially with transplantation antigens of the graft or by inhibiting the response of the host lymphoid centers [42].

Role of the Lymphocyte in the Allograft Reaction

Lymphocytes are the only cells capable of immune competence, which involves the ability to recognize an antigen and to create a specific immune response against it. There are two kinds of immune-competent lymphocytes, B lymphocytes and T lymphocytes; indistinguishable morphologically, they have differing surface immunoglobulins and abilities to fix complement. They probably derive from the same primitive mesenchymal stem cell, but have different immunological roles. The T lymphocytes are developed in the thymus, are released into the circulation to migrate to spleen and lymph nodes, and are responsible for cell-mediated immunity. In birds, the B lymphocytes are developed in the bursa of Fabricius (a lymphoid organ attached to the large intestine proximal to the cloaca). No such bursa exists in mammals, but in both species the B cells end by populating the bone marrow; by the circulation they ultimately reach the spleen and lymph nodes, where they are involved in the synthesis of circulating antibody and develop into the plasma cell series.

More recently [37] a third subpopulation of lymphocytes, termed K (or killer) cells, has been described. Normally the target cell is destroyed either by direct combination of antibody with the surface antigens of the cell (thereby promoting phagocytosis), or by activation of the complement system (which results in direct membrane damage). However, the K cell is able to kill, in nonspecific fashion, target cells that have been coated with antibody. In this situation, specific antibody is able to attach to a cell carrying the corresponding antigen without the cell being destroyed, usually because the antibody is unable to fix complement. But if K cells are then added to the antibody-coated cells, the latter are destroyed by an extracellular mechanism in a quite nonspecific fashion, without phagocytic activity.

Evidence implicating the small lymphocyte as having a central role in allograft rejection [26] may be listed as follows:

1. Lymphocyte depletion in animals diminishes the effectiveness of allograft rejection. Neonatal thymectomy results in later reduction of the number of lymphocytes normally present in lymph nodes, spleen, and blood, and may be associated with an impaired capacity to reject allografts. This capacity to reject allografts can be restored by grafts of neonatal thymus or isogenic adult spleen, and lymphoid cells, which also serve to reconstitute the animals' lymphoid tissue [34]. It is clear that the thymus is a chief center for the differentiation of new immunologically competent cells.
2. In rodents the responsible agent for graft-versus-host reaction is known to be the small lymphocyte, indicating the strong possibility that the response of normal animals to allografts may be

initiated by the same cell. Animals failing to destroy allografts because of their immunological tolerance can be shown to be deficient in small lymphocytes.

3. The manner in which antigens from vascularized grafts reach the host lymphoid cells is not precisely known, but it seems likely to be through the draining lymphatics to the regional lymph nodes, since allografts tend to survive in sites without lymphatic drainage, such as the brain and the hamster cheek pouch. The graft antigens probably are transported there by lymphocytes initially carried to the graft by the blood stream.
4. Specific immunological tolerance to skin allografts produced in fetal or neonatal mice by the injection of adult cells into the immature animal is abolished by the subsequent injection of normal lymphoid cells from a normal adult member of the same strain, as demonstrated by the prompt rejection of the formerly tolerated allograft. Moreover, the speed of rejection of the allograft is accelerated if the transferred lymphoid cells are derived from the regional lymph nodes of an animal which has already been immunized with skin of the same strain as donor-strain skin [17].
5. Although there is slight evidence that soluble antibody may be concerned in allograft destruction, it seems probable that activated lymphoid cells enter the blood stream from the regional lymph nodes, penetrate the graft from the vascular circulation, and thereafter cause its destruction in some unknown way. Thus blood leukocytes and lymph node cells from skin-allografted mice cause destruction of skin allografts when transferred to tolerant mice which had hitherto tolerated their grafts [16]. It is certain that skin allografts are invaded by considerable numbers of cells that originated from the regional lymph nodes.

The Clonal Selection Theory

The central problem in transplantation biology is concerned with the exact mechanism by which a foreign protein antigen elicits an antibody from the cells of the reticuloendothelial system [4]. Burnet's [1] clonal selection theory, although far from proved, has an attractive simplicity and serves to make it easier to think effectively about a complex mass of experimental results and observations. Burnet has underlined the necessity for an acceptable theory of immunology to explain three aspects of the immune reaction.

1. Recognition: How is it that the immune system is able to distinguish between its own proteins as "self" and harmless, and all other proteins as "nonself" and potentially injurious?
2. Tolerance: How can an animal learn, under certain circumstances, to allow certain foreign tissues or organisms to survive within it?
3. Memory: How can an animal, many weeks or even years after exposure to a foreign antigen, still react with increased force following a second exposure to the same antigen, with unique recognition of its former adversary?

In this concept, a clone is a colony of cells having similar characteristics because they result from the initial division of a single cell. The cell concerned is a member of the reticuloendothelial system – probably a lymphocyte developing from a primitive mesenchymal stem cell – which becomes capable of producing antibody in response to antigenic stimulation. The developing embryo is believed to have many millions of clones or colonies of such cells. When the cells are very immature they are destroyed in the presence of an appropriate antigen, but later in fetal or early postnatal development a critical point is reached when, instead of being killed by antigenic contact, the clone begins to react more strongly and is stimulated to proliferate (with or without a change of morphological type) or be converted to the plasma cell form, with its capacity for active synthesis and liberation of antibody.

Thus at birth all clones capable of producing antibodies against circulating "self" proteins have been destroyed in their immature phase, leaving alive only those clones capable of reacting against foreign protein, a process that is termed *clonal selection.* If a foreign protein is introduced before the clones have reached maturity, then those clones capable of reacting against this foreign antigen are destroyed, so that in later life a further encounter with the same antigen will result in the latter being recognized as "self," even though originally foreign.

Prolongation of Allograft Survival

The factors involved in extending the survival period of allografts are:

SELECTION OF TISSUE TRANSPLANTED. Avascular tissues such as cornea and cartilage survive for indefinite periods unless they become vascularized, which would allow invasion of the graft by host cells.

IMMUNOLOGICAL INACCESSIBILITY OF THE ALLOGRAFT. The cerebral cortex and the anterior chamber of the eye allow extended survival of allografts inserted into them. In the case of the brain the transplant apparently fails to elicit an immune response because of the absence of any true lymphatic system to drain graft antigens to a regional lymph node system where antibody formation might follow. This view is supported by the failure of the intracerebral transplant to survive if the host animal has been previously immunized by a graft to an alternative, antigenically effective site. In the case of the anterior chamber of the eye, it seems that the immunological reaction is blocked by the inability of antibodies to reach the transplant, since this transplant survives only in any already immunized host if it remains nonvascularized. It has been recognized that the connective tissue of the cheek pouch of the hamster acts as an immunological barrier preventing the egress of graft antigens into the reactive host centers [20]. As yet no other examples of this insulating effect of connective tissue are known.

SPECIFIC IMMUNOLOGICAL TOLERANCE. A tolerance may exist to allografts from a particular donor; an example of this is seen in nonidentical twins showing blood chimerism. (A chimera is an animal organism containing two or more healthy living tissues of different genetic origin). Owen [36] showed that in cattle twins, due to their common placental circulation in utero, a successful intercolonization of bone marrow cells resulted in each twin carrying blood cells of two different blood groups. Skin allografts exchanged between two such animals attain permanent survival, since the operation merely results in the superimposition of an experimental skin chimerism upon the natural blood chimerism already existing. It is now known that such chimerism may also occur in sheep and chickens, and has several times been reported in man. It seems clear that an infusion of nucleated cells through the placental circulation (which occurs at a stage of development when the immunological defense mechanisms are too immature to be able to recognize the invading antigens as foreign) results in permanent acceptance not only of these cells but of all future tissue allografts from the same source.

AGAMMAGLOBULINEMIA. In human beings agammaglobulinemia has been reported as resulting in successful acceptance of skin allotransplants.

UREMIA, HODGKIN'S DISEASE, PREGNANCY, AND ADVANCED NEOPLASIA. In all these conditions, prolongation of allograft survival may occur, probably as a result of the toxic and debilitated state of the patient.

Methods of Prolonging the Survival of Allografts

Attempts to prolong the survival of allografts are directed either to the nonspecific suppression of the allograft reaction by the use of immunosuppressive agents, or to establishing a specific transplantation tolerance to allotransplants from a particular donor. Purified histocompatibility antigens are slowly becoming available, so that in the future, with continued low dosage of antigens combined with other immunosuppressive measures (such as antilymphocyte globulin), a specific and advanced state of tolerance may be achieved.

IMMUNOSUPPRESSIVE AGENTS. Ionizing irradiation applied to the entire subject before exposure to foreign antigens effectively inhibits the response to transplantation or to other antigens. The chief difficulty in its use lies in giving a sufficiently high dosage to suppress the allograft reaction without simultaneously depressing bone-marrow function to a level of fatal pancytopenia precipitating generalized infection and hemorrhages. The subsequent transplantation of allograft bone marrow or spleen cells may do something to combat this by establishing a state of irradiation chimerism in the recipient animal, enabling it to accept transplants of other tissues from the same donor. Alternatively, the combination of irradiation and drug therapy may be used to decrease the effective therapeutic dose of each agent. Irradiation chimerism has very limited application to man because of the obvious risks implicit in using a lethal dose of irradiation, and also because of the danger that a graft-versus-host reaction (see p. 82) might develop following acceptance of the hemopoietic graft. However, irradiation chimerism has been used in human cases of leukemia. It should also be pointed out that the susceptibility of lymphoid cells to x-rays is such that sublethal irradiation greatly increases the efficiency of a given dose of antigen in inducing specific transplantation tolerance in adult animals. In renal allografts, irradiation is used clinically as a treatment for suspected rejection. It is directed specifically at the transplanted organ (usually in three applications of totalling 450 roentgen) in a dosage calculated to be lethal to attacking host lymphocytes but not to the parenchymal cells of the kidney.

A series of chemical agents have been claimed to assist in the suppression of the allograft immunological reaction. Of these, the first used were the corticosteroids, but these have been followed by a succession of alkylating agents (nitrogen mustards), antimetabolites (methotrexate, 6-mercaptopurine, azathioprine, cyclophosphamide), and antibiotics (actinomycin C).

Cortisone was the first drug used, and it effectively prolonged the survival time of skin allografts in rabbits even when merely applied locally to the graft. It may inhibit antigen uptake, since it impairs phagocytic function and may delay lymphatic regeneration between graft and host. The effectiveness of cortisone in man is very much less certain, although it may potentiate other drugs or enhance the effect of x-ray irradiation; it helps to reverse rejection crises, probably by its antiinflammatory effect on graft rejection mechanisms.

The effect of immunosupressive drugs varies from species to species, and is often complicated by their capacity to inflict ancillary damage on hemopoietic tissue and intestinal epithelium. Knowledge of their mode of action is incomplete, but many of these drugs inhibit cell mitosis either primarily (nitrogen mustard) or by interfering with the synthesis of deoxyribonucleic acid (DNA). The antimetabolites inhibit biochemical reactions by competing with natural metabolites for the appropriate enzyme sites, which results in inhibition of nucleic acid synthesis.

The basis of most immunosuppressive programs is azathioprene used in combination with steroids. At first both are applied in high dosage, with subsequent reduction to maintenance levels that are continued permanently.

Antilymphocytic serum (ALS) is a more recent addition to immunosuppressive therapy, introduced by Woodruff and Anderson in 1963 [46, 47]. It is produced in animals of another species by injecting into them lymphoid cells from animals of the species in which it is to be used. Thus ALS for use in mice is normally prepared by injecting mouse lymphoid cells into rabbits, and ALS for human use is produced from horses with the resulting serum collected and the globulin fraction isolated. If given to an animal which has been sensitized by graft rejection, it can erase the memory of the primary contact with antigen so that if the animal is subsequently challenged with a second graft from the same donor, it will respond with a first-set, not a second-set, reaction. In addition, unlike other immunosuppressive agents it lacks unwanted side effects, is harmless and nontoxic, and acts more against cellular than against humoral immunities. It appears to act selectively against the thymus-derived population of long-lived lymphocytes in the recirculating pool. It is used as an adjunct to the battery of immunosuppressive procedures used in man in organ transplants, contributes to the treatment of certain rejection crises, and may assist in the induction of tolerance. Regrettably, ALS, together with more general forms of immunosuppressive therapy, has the disadvantage of increased incidence of cancer in the patients treated.

Grafts exchanged between outbred populations of animals usually manifest a wide variation in rejection times, usually extended by immunosuppressive therapy. The survival time in the majority is often doubled, constituting a significant experimental result which is, however, of minor clinical importance. Those grafts surviving longest may be preserved alive for many months by such therapy, indicating the possibility of a major clinical advance if reduplicated in human subjects. The spread in rejection times is attributable to the varying degree of antigenic compatibility between donor and host, so that the results of immunosuppressive therapy might be appreciably improved by a practicable method of assessing relative compatibility between donor and host before allograft transfer. Since the allograft reaction appears to be a quantitative expression of the genetic difference between donor and host, a relatively weak reaction between individuals who are relatively antigenically compatible might be suppressed to a significant degree by irradiation or drug therapy. A graft surviving under the protection of an immunosuppressive drug may be rejected very gradually when medication ceases; indeed, in cases where a high degree of host-donor antigenic compatibility exists it apparently may not be rejected at all. It is also of interest that allotransplant kidneys in both animals and man may have the process of rejection halted and even reversed, at least temporarily, by the use of immunosuppressive therapy.

INDUCTION OF SPECIFIC IMMUNOLOGICAL TOLERANCE TO ALLOTRANSPLANTS FROM A SPECIFIC DONOR. This can be achieved experimentally in many animals. The discovery of erythrocyte chimerism in cattle led to the experimental injection of red cells into immature animals. Success followed when it was found that the injection of adult cells into fetal mice while still in utero resulted in the latter accepting, after birth, skin grafts from the donor strain but not from other strains. It has been subsequently shown that many species, including mice, can achieve induced tolerance by such a maneuver even when it is carried out very shortly after birth, while the immaturity of the central immunological mechanism exists (in most animals this period amounts to 14 days after birth). That this acquired tolerance is due to a central failure of immunological response is shown by the total absence of circulating antibodies directed against the allograft antigens, as well as by the restoration of reactivity against the allograft on transferring to the recipient animal lymphoid cells from a normal adult member of the same strain.

The creation of acquired transplantation tolerance in newborn animals is much more difficult when genetic diversity between donor and recipient is great. Under these circumstances in mice the dosage of injected spleen cells may need to be increased 20 times, as compared with mice in which the genetic barrier is relatively weak. When the genetic barrier between donor and recipient is very weak, transplantation tolerance can be induced even in adult animals by using a large dose of foreign antigen [32]. Inevitably such tolerance is specific and in no way prevents the host from reacting normally against unrelated antigens. Where the tolerance-inducing antigen is in the form of viable cells, the host becomes a cellular chimera of its own and donor cells, and the tolerant state is permanent.

When one applies experimental findings in animals to human beings, certain basic rules appear applicable when seeking to establish specific allotransplantation tolerance. Thus, it appears desirable to avoid preliminary sensitization to any of the allograft antigens before operation; genetic similarity between host and donor should be as close as possible; the tolerance-inducing antigen should not produce a graft-versus-host reaction or elicit a transplantation immunizing reaction.

The Graft-Versus-Host Reaction

When animals are injected with adult lymphoid cells which lack antigens present in the host, the animal may fail to reject the graft; the graft may then attack immunologically the transplantation antigens in the host cells.

Most tissue allotransplants contain immunologically competent cells – that is, cells of the lymphoid series capable of producing antibodies when stimulated by a foreign antigen. An allograft which is not rejected by the recipient animal may therefore produce antibodies against its new host, resulting in deterioration and usually death of the latter.

It is possible that graft-versus-host reactions occur in subclinical degree in all cases of allotransplantation, but are obliterated by the intensity of the opposing reaction of the host, so that they become discernible only when:

1. The host reaction is immunologically immature, as in the embryo and the newborn (runt disease).
2. The host reaction is depressed artificially either by exposure to ionizing irradiation (secondary disease) or antimetabolite drugs, or by removal of the thymus soon after birth.
3. The graft is from a homozygous parental donor (AA) to a host that is the first-generation hybrid offspring (AB) between the donor strain and a dissimilar homozygote (BB). The graft does not possess any antigens foreign to the host, which cannot therefore reject the graft; it is plain, however, that the graft can react immunologically against the host antigens deriving from the BB parent of the hybrid.

The injection of adult splenic cells into newborn or embryo chickens and mice results after a week or so in runt disease in the form of wasting or failure to grow, involution of lymphoid tissue, diarrhea, dermatitis, and death from infection, often after many months. Although there is atrophy of lymph nodes and thymus, there is a characteristic enlargement of liver and spleen, presumably as a result of host reactivity. If fetal instead of adult splenic cells are injected, the incidence of runt disease is greatly reduced because of the immunological immaturity of the transplanted cells at this early stage of development. The intensity of the reaction may be gauged by the mortality in animals, by a weight-gain assay, or by the degree of splenomegaly expressed as a ratio of spleen to body weight.

Evidence exists to indicate that graft-versus-host reactions might well constitute a considerable obstacle to the production of specific immunological tolerance in man. However, while some authorities believe that experimental sensitization by allograft transplantation in man may rarely be justified because of the danger of establishing preliminary conditions favoring onset of this syndrome, others believe the dangers may have been overstated in the past, since the early cellular infiltration of the renal cortex in human kidney allotransplants is now known not to represent proliferations of donor cells in the graft but is largely the result of host cells, as demonstrated by labeling host leukocytes with tritiated thymidine.

Attempts to control the reaction in mice have met with some success, either by administration of the antimetabolite drug methotrexate, or by the injection of normal adult recipient strain spleen cells shortly after the foreign splenic cells; adult cells from animals already immunized to the donor strain exert even better protection against subsequent runt disease.

Since it is now accepted that immunologically competent cells can be exchanged between mother and fetus across the placenta, it is possible that maternal small lymphocytes entering the fetal circulation can cause runt disease if not promptly rejected. This condition has also been reported in infants with hereditary thymic dysplasia after attempts to reconstitute their immunological capacity by bone marrow allografts have been made. The intrauterine transfusion of Rh-sensitized fetuses has resulted in cases of runt disease, but this can be avoided by removing all viable lymphocytes from the blood transfused, before use.

Donor Selection and Antigenic Tissue Typing

Tissue Typing

Antibodies against antigens of the HL-A (human leukocyte antigen) system can be detected in the sera of patients who have received multiple blood transfusions, but these antibodies were often polyvalent and recognized many different antigens. For grouping purposes, monospecific reagents are essential. The discovery by van Rood [40] that multiparous women may become immunized by fetal products did much to solve this problem, since a woman who has been pregnant will form antibodies only against antigens carried by her husband but absent from her (provided she has never received a blood transfusion). Sera from human volunteers immunized by means of skin or leukocyte allografts are of equal merit. Approximately 100 such sera were tested against a panel of leukocyte samples from randomly selected donors. Using computer analysis, the results obtained with each serum were compared with those obtained from every other serum. These sera were then tested in population and family studies for monospecificity. More than 20 different leukocyte antigens have now been recognized; most of these belong to the HL-A system, in which more than 30 different alleles have been identified, of which 5 have been shown by skin-grafting experiments to be identified as transplantation antigens. The clinical importance of HL-A antigens is clear from the demonstration that skin grafts exchanged between siblings with identical HL-A-type antigens survive significantly longer than grafts exchanged between unmatched sibling controls. Refinement of techniques has resulted in the production of monospecific sera, by absorption of unwanted antibodies. This serological approach, combined with the study of family inheritance, has defined at least 2 – and probably 3 – major subloci of the HL-A system. If every individual is presumed to have 4 antigens, then a match in which all 4 antigens are detected is likely to have a high rate of success clinically, but in practice only about 75 percent of typings fall into this group. The undetected antigens in the remaining 25 percent may be mismatched, or newly identified antigens may in future be demonstrated to be composed of more than one antigen, causing wrong interpretations of matching procedures. The importance of accurate matching of tissues between donor and recipient is shown in Figure 2-4, illustrating the late results of renal transplantation.

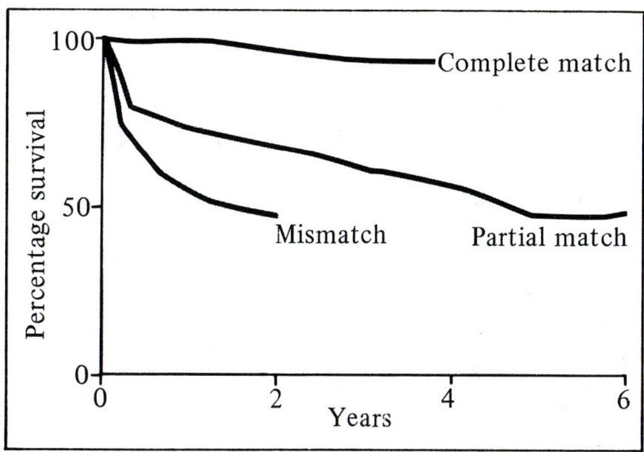

Fig. 2-4. Survival of renal transplants in relation to HL-A matching. Complete match *(siblings) consists of cases in which all HL-A antigens are identical;* partial match *(siblings and parent to child) involves cases where the antigens on one chromosome only are identical;* mismatch *(unrelated) occurs in cases in which all the HL-A antigens are different.*

Histocompatibility Tests

The problem of successful clinical allografting would be ideally solved only if donor and recipient were matched so completely that the latter had no foreign transplantation antigens with which to contend. Since matching of unrelated individuals with regard to their HL-A antigens alone is excessively difficult (leaving aside the enormous number of other determinants of transplantation antigens) this objective is unlikely to be achieved. However, where antigenic differences are of minor degree and the immunological barrier correspondingly weak, it is possible to induce immunological tolerance, which, although limited, is clinically significant. Of biological tests calculated to assist the selection of the most compatible donor for a given recipient, the following are in current use.

THE MIXED LEUKOCYTE CULTURE (MLC) TEST. As a result of the independent investigations of Bain, Vas, and Lowenstein [15], and Bach and Hirschorn [13], the in vitro demonstration of an immunological response has been developed, based on the visible changes occurring in blood lymphocytes on exposure to HL-A incompatible cellular isoantigens, which for convenience are usually viable leukocytes. When the leukocytes from two normal unrelated donors are placed in a mixed culture for several days, some of them become transformed into large basophilic, blast-like cells taking up tritiated thymidine and undergoing mitosis. But when both donors have identical HL-A alleles, there is no significant uptake of tritiated thymidine. Although the test as described allows two-directional reaction of the lymphocytes between the donors, it can be made unidirectional by incubation of the potential donor's lymphocytes with mitomycin C (which prevents replication of DNA in cells treated, and so prevents taking up of radioactive thymidine) before admixture with the recipients cells, thus inhibiting mitotic activity in the potential donor lymphocytes. The MLC test thus affords a reliable means of selecting HL-A compatible donors for given recipients.

LYMPHOCYTE-DEPENDENT ANTIBODY (LDA) TEST. This test is based on the release of the isotope ^{51}Cr from labeled target cells after incubation with antibody and effector lymphocytes (in the absence of complement), as compared with the activity released by control mixtures having no serum or lymphocytes.

It is more sensitive than the conventional mixed leukocyte culture test [31].

CELL-MEDIATED LYMPHOLYSIS (CML) TEST. Among the genes controlling immune responsiveness are those responsible for the production of lymphocyte-activating determinants (Lad, also called lymphocyte-dependent antibodies, or LDA), which are surface products leading to lymphocyte activation in the mixed lymphocyte culture test [30]. These Lad elements are not identical with HL-A specificities, though closely linked on the same chromosome and usually genetically transmitted together. In the CML test (Fig. 2-5), if lymphocytes from donor B react against A in a one-way MLC test because of differences in Lad, the transformed lymphoblasts are cytotoxic for A cells, provided that there are HL-A incompatibilities between them. Thus matching for Lad seems likely to prove more critical than HL-A compatibility.

The difficulties of accurate tissue typing are in great part due to the extreme polymorphism of the HL-A system, since different individuals have different combinations of antigens associated with each HL-A allele. In one study of 500 mixed cultures from unrelated donors, not one identical pair was found. The limitations of the various matching procedures described above are due to these factors:

1. Family donors alone provide a readily available source of HL-A compatible antigens.
2. Means of preservation of cadaveric organs for a period of months will be necessary to provide major compatibility between donor and host.
3. Matching procedures are specific for the particular combination of host and donor tested only, and provide no information facilitating selection of alternative compatible individuals.

Thus the future of successful tissue typing is likely to involve serologically based leukocyte typing, using monospecific serums. It is to be hoped that one day individuals may be typed for histocompatibility antigens with the same ease that at present obtains in the identification of blood group factors.

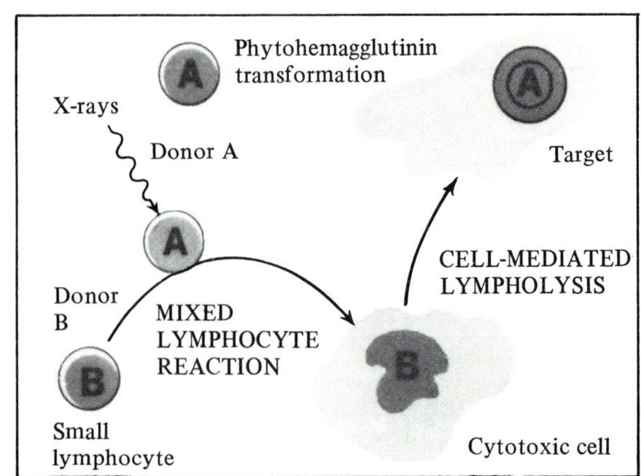

Fig. 2-5. Cell-mediated lymphocytic test. Stage 1: Mixed lymphocyte reaction indicating difference in Lad. The lymphocytes of donor B divide and are transformed into killer cells on recognizing Lad on A, but the lymphocytes of A are incapable of reacting because they have been blocked by X-irradiation. Simultaneously other A lymphocytes are transformed into blasts with phytohemagglutinin and labeled with isotope ^{51}Cr, to act as targets in stage 2. Stage 2: Cytotoxic reaction depending on HL-A differences. An excess of transformed B lymphoblasts will be cytotoxic for labeled A target cells, as disclosed by release of chromium. (After I. M. Roitt, Essential Immunology *(2nd ed.). Oxford, England: Blackwell, 1974.)*

Allografts of Clinical Importance

Only a limited number of tissues are of value to the plastic surgeon as allografts. Isogenic transplants have obvious biological advantages for use as allografts, but are inevitably limited in practice by the relative rarity of identical twins, which occur only once in about 300 pregnancies.

Bone

Cadaveric allografts of bone have been used, but are greatly inferior to autograft bone, and should be applied only if the latter is not available, since they invariably show markedly inferior survival. Allograft bone is best preserved by freeze-drying. Preliminary deproteinization and decalcification add little to its experimental survival.

Claims have recently been made for the successful use of xenograft bone, as an "antigen-free" calf bone in the form of the Kiel bone graft in Europe and Boplant in the United States. The calf bone is cleaned with detergents and freeze-dried to remove antigenic proteins, including all vascular and marrow material, and vacuum-sealed as nonvital grafts consisting of mineral-bone elements from which all protein and fat have been removed. Such a graft acts as a scaffolding for replacement by host bone. In subperiosteal position it has been used with success in ununited fractures, but is uniformly unsuccessful when used in nasal bridge reconstruction [58]. Attempts to increase osteogenic capacity in Kiel bone by impregnating it with autologous bone marrow [63] still leave a graft far inferior to autogenous bone.

Skin

Skin is more antigenic than most tissues, in that even small antigenic differences result in rejection of the graft by the host. It has its chief application in the treatment of patients suffering from extensive burns, where its use may be lifesaving. In such patients, survival of the allografts is fortunately prolonged beyond the ordinary limits obtained in normal individuals, with survival extending for 21 days or even longer. The reasons for such prolonged survival are uncertain but probably arise from three causes [39]:

1. The chance sharing of tissue transplantation antigens by randomly selected unrelated individuals.
2. Antigen competition, where the immune response to any one antigen is impaired by the additional injection of a second competing antigen.
3. Immunological paralysis, in which massive doses of antigen appear to overwhelm the immune response and abolish antibody formation both then and on subsequent exposure to the same antigen.

It is to be noted that the burned tissues constitute a major source of potentially antigenic protein bodies of great variety, absorbed into the circulation. The use of skin from multiple donors results in extended survival of the grafts, possibly on the basis of antigen competition noted above.

Allograft skin may be obtained fresh from human volunteers (usually a relative) and used without delay, or stored for subsequent use after being taken from recent disease-free cadavers under full aseptic precautions. Stored skin may be freeze-dried as a nonviable graft, or kept in the viable state after treating with glycerol in saline solution for 30 minutes and slowly frozen in solid carbon dioxide at a temperature of −79°C. When needed for use, it is thawed to body temperature as rapidly as possible. Such a deep-frozen graft behaves like a fresh allograft when applied to the host; a freeze-dried graft, being nonviable, does not of course constitute a vital biological dressing, but remains adherent to the recipient site for about 14 days.

Allografts of skin at present have their chief clinical application as a temporary biological dressing. Stored for up to 2 weeks at 4°C., they can be expected to take successfully, but they should be changed every 48 to 96 hours. Once the graft takes, its later removal is accompanied by excessive bleeding, while removal after 7 to 10 days is accompanied by the phenomena of graft rejection (inflammation and necrosis). Used in this way as a biological dressing, it results in decrease in bacterial flora and improved wound healing [28]. Using careful matching procedures, including tissue typing, allografts have been applied following the excision of massive burns in children, together with continuous azathioprine administration, resulting in increased survival of patients without the expected serious complications from infection [21].

Cartilage

Cartilage is an avascular tissue consisting of a homogenous matrix of chondromucoprotein which is immunologically inert and so does not elicit an allograft reaction even when the host has been previously sensitized against the donor. Vital cartilage cells (chondrocytes) live in this matrix and actively metabolize sulfur, as can be demonstrated in experiments using a labeled isotopic form of this element. Allograft cartilage can therefore be used with success as a graft which survives as a vital tissue; in man it has been shown to be metabolically active 2 years after transplantation and populated by surviving chondrocytes [22]. Earlier experimental evidence that allograft cartilage not only survived in young rabbits but grew with the host animals has not been confirmed [44].

The usual donor sites of cartilage grafts in plastic surgery are from the rib costal cartilages, and more rarely from the ear. Allografts or xenografts (ox cartilage) of dead cartilage killed by formalin, boiling, or prolonged storage in thimerosal (Merthiolate) usually demonstrate an advanced degree of absorption within 2 years, and are no longer used clinically.

Fat

Fat cells are not used as allotransplant material, since they are invariably replaced by host fibrous tissue with such considerable loss of bulk as to render fat allografts clinically useless.

Fascia

Fresh allograft fascia does not survive, merely serving as a scaffold into which host cells grow. The process of host cell replacement is increased by using preserved fascia, either freeze-dried, irradiated, or preserved in a chemical medium, when the graft may be completely replaced by host tissue after 60 days [74]. Freeze-dried allograft fascia used clinically and biopsied 6 years after insertion has the histological appearance of normal fascia [75]. Since the patient's own fascia is readily available, however, most surgeons prefer to use autogenous fascial grafts.

AUTOGRAFTS

Lyndon Peer [7] has stressed that most autografts may be expected to survive as living transplants and retain their normal structure when transferred to an anatomically favorable site. Cartilage as an avascular tissue receives nourishment and excretes waste products of metabolism by diffusion of fluid to and from the surrounding host tissues, but vascular tissues survive by this means only for the few days required before they acquire a blood supply from adjacent host vessels. Such cellular survival in transplants may be limited by the size of the graft, so that the central cells may undergo avascular necrosis before vascular penetration has occurred. This occurs characteristically in cortical or massive bone grafts, where the necrotic central graft material may be replaced by "creeping substitution" of host tissue of the same type. With this exception, and with the exception of peripheral nerve grafts, it is likely that most, if not all, other autografts survive from the outset and are not replaced by host tissues.

Autografts of Clinical Importance

Skin

The free skin graft is the simplest and most economical (in tissue used and in treatment period required) method available for resurfacing extensive areas of skin loss. Such a free graft is totally detached from its donor site before transfer to the recipient site, and so is completely deprived of all blood and nerve supply at the time of transplantation.

The thinnest free skin graft (or Thiersch graft), which can be cut by a graft knife freehand or by dermatome, must always include the entire thickness of epidermis together with a minimal amount of the underlying superficial dermis. A full-thickness skin graft includes the entire thickness of epidermis and dermis, with the subcutaneous fat trimmed from its undersurface in order to allow its revascularization from host vessels in the bed on which it is laid.

The character and appearance of a skin graft are affected by its thickness. Because of its thickness and because of the minute residual islands of fat on its deep surface which interfere with revascularization, survival of the full-thickness graft is less certain, but its final appearance approximates more closely the appearance of normal skin in texture, color, and resilience. On the other hand, the split-thickness graft may be expected to take with much greater certainty due to its greater accessibility for, and smaller bulk of tissue awaiting, revascularization from host vessels; its final appearance, however, is paler and less matt, and it has a quality of resilience correspondingly less than that of normal skin. It is the bulk of dermis transplanted in the skin graft that affords protection against trauma and limits contraction of the graft after transfer.

Inevitably, healing of the donor site from which the graft is taken is increasingly prolonged with increased thickness of the graft taken. Donor sites of full-thickness skin grafts too extensive to be closed by direct approximation of wound edges must themselves be treated by the application of a suitable split-thickness graft from elsewhere.

Successful transfer of a skin graft (referred to as "take" of the graft) depends on rapid and complete revascularization of the graft from the recipient bed – which, in turn, depends on the presence of an adequate supply of host vessels in the bed, adequate fixation of the graft, absence of collections of blood or serum beneath the graft, and of course, absence of infection. Thus, scars from which all epithelium has been shaved, clean wounds, and healthy granulation tissue may provide a sufficiently vascular bed for successful graft take. Fat, having a poor blood supply, takes grafts poorly, and bare cortical bone, articular cartilage, or tendon stripped of paratenon may be expected to fail to nourish adequately any skin graft applied to them. Many skin grafts take on a pink color in 12 to 24 hours after grafting [50] but there is no true circulation of blood and the color may be attributed to the presence of red blood cells washed into the graft vessels by the entering transudate from the host bed, or to increased translucency from the resultant edema of graft tissue. Using a transparent chamber on the ear of the mouse [56], active blood flow occurs in 3 days and becomes brisk and unidirectional by the fifth day. Development of the vascular plexus into a mature complex of capillaries, arterioles, and venules occurs by 6 to 8 days after transplantation. Classically, the clinical vascularization of a skin graft is regarded as occurring primarily through the direct anastomosis of vessels within the graft to underlying host vessels, to be later reinforced by the ingrowth of new host vessels into the graft. It may, however, be true that the most important factor is the ingrowth of new host vessels through the preexisting graft vessels, which act merely as nonviable conduits [56]. The sensory reinnervation [52] of full-thickness skin grafts is less complete than in skin flaps, and is least in split-thickness grafts. The sensory return is greatest at the periphery of the graft and decreases toward the center, and its pattern resembles that of the donor skin rather than the recipient site.

Additional information on skin grafts is included in Chapter 1.

Dermis

If a thin split-thickness skin graft is taken and discarded, and from its donor site all residual cutaneous tissue is carefully removed with the least possible adherent subcutaneous fat, this free graft consists of dermis, with its contained truncated epithelial appendages – sweat glands, hair follicles, and sebaceous glands. Such a dermal graft has its maximum bulk when taken from the site of the thick skin of the buttock, submammary fold, or lateral aspect of upper arm or thigh. When inserted beneath the skin of the host, it serves as a useful means of correcting deficient contours, as in the saddle nose, depressed scars, or deficient facial outlines from any cause. Its bulk is increased by doubling the dermis on itself. If it is inserted as a lipodermal graft with attached subcutaneous fat, the dermal surface in contact with host tissues derives a blood supply from the latter with such rapidity that it acts as a vascularizing membrane for the fatty elements, thereby greatly limiting subsequent absorption of fat cells.

Care must be taken to prevent hematoma formation in the bed of the graft, which otherwise may fail to take as a free graft, with ensuing necrosis and progressive absorption. Where there is a successful take, about 80 percent of the bulk of the graft should be maintained permanently. The use of antibiotics has virtually eliminated infection as a significant complication, allowing uncomplicated degeneration of epithelial elements present, and ensuring successful survival of at least 90 percent of dermis grafts [53].

HISTOLOGICAL CHANGES IN DERMIS GRAFTS. In human beings, these histological changes have been studied repeatedly [51, 53], with essentially confirmed results. The pilomotor muscles and sweat gland units apparently survive permanently, the latter as actively secreting glands whose secretion is not discharged from the severed ducts, but is apparently resorbed internally into the vascular circulation of the graft [54]. The sebaceous glands and hair follicles form epidermoid cysts, which ultimately rupture and undergo phagocytosis by giant and mononuclear cells, with complete late replacement by fibrous tissue over a period of 1 to 2 years. The collagen, elastic, and reticulin fibers of the dermal tissue seemingly survive intact permanently [53], providing a unique, supple, and well-vascularized tissue of great tensile strength, quite different from ordinary fibrous tissue.

Injectable Collagen

Human and bovine collagen can be made soluble by controlled proteolytic digestion [50a]. At colder temperatures this material is a viscous liquid, which then forms into a firm gel on warming to 37°C.

When injected through a 30-gauge needle into the intradermal or subdermal plane, this collagen was helpful in correcting concave contour defects of the face such as seen in patients with severe acne vulgaris. The initial clinical trial of this material in 28 patients followed for 3 to 18 months has been reported to provide lasting and substantial correction [50a].

Bone

STRUCTURE OF BONE. Bone consists of calcareous material in a complex crystalline form deposited in a fine organic matrix of collagen fibers. Characteristically bone has a dense, thin outer layer of compact or cortical bone and an inner core of bone marrow; the cancellous bone between these layers consists of a spongework of bony trabeculae interlaced with marrow tissue. The basic structural unit of bone is the osteon, consisting of concentric rings of lamellae surrounding a central haversian canal, containing minute blood vessels and nerve fibrils. Between the lamellae are minute oval cavities, lacunae, each containing a living bone cell or osteocyte, which is linked to neighboring similar cells by fine protoplasmic processes traversing fine canals called canaliculae. Osteocytes are derived from bone-forming cells, the osteoblasts, and retain the capacity to resume osteoblastic function if the need should arise for bone repair.

Each bone is ensheathed in a tough external membranous envelope, the periosteum, whose deepest layer adjoining the bone consists of a vascular loose connective tissue that contains cells capable of becoming active osteoblasts – the osteogenetic layer.

Osteoblasts producing new bone may therefore derive from the periosteum or the endosteum haversian canals and marrow cavity). The osteoblast, the bone-forming cell concerned with growth and the production of new bone in repair, probably arises from a primitive mesenchymal cell which, under conditions where bone absorption is taking place, can also fuse with its fellows to produce a multinucleated giant cell, the osteoclast; when their work of absorption is ended, osteoclasts may either revert to osteoblasts or the reticular cells of bone marrow, or undergo degeneration and die.

THE FATE OF FREE BONE GRAFTS IN MAN. When bone grafts are transferred to a heterotopic site in contact with soft tissues only, the bone grafts always undergo absorption and replacement by fibrous tissue, with the exception of grafts of nasal, septal, or turbinate bones, which for some unknown reason apparently survive [62]. The following account therefore refers only to orthotopic bone grafts placed in direct contact with host bone.

Cortical bone grafts are rarely used, since they contain few osteoblasts and only some of these osteoblasts survive because of their inaccessibility to tissue fluids for the early preservation of their nutrition. The period of immobilization required is longer than for cancellous bone if union to host bone is to be obtained, and ultimately the entire graft is replaced by host bone. Cancellous bone grafts are therefore usually preferred; when increased strength is required, a cortical strip may be left on one aspect of the graft. The most usual donor sites of cancellous bone grafts in plastic surgery are the iliac crest and the ribs, and there is general agreement that the most effective bone transplant in clinical practice is the fresh autogenous cancellous bone graft.

It was formerly believed that all cancellous bone grafts, like cortical bone grafts, died and underwent creeping substitution from host cells, with the graft merely acting as an inert scaffolding to be slowly absorbed and completely replaced by host bone. Surgical technique [57] was directed chiefly toward accurate carpentry of the graft and the preparation of precise mortised joints between graft and host, with no thought for the damage done to vital cells by power saws and drills. It is now accepted, however, that the transplantation of bone as a living tissue is desirable to harness the osteoblasts of periosteal and endosteal origin in the graft to the function of active bone regeneration. To ensure such cell survival, it is necessary to prepare a fully vascularized bed for the graft, so that, by direct anastomosis of host and graft blood vessels, circulation is restored to the graft within a few days, assisted in cancellous grafts by subsequent capillary penetration from the host bone [61, 62]. Under such circumstances many of the graft osteocytes survive to maintain the calcified matrix and, by conversion to active osteoblast form, clothe the graft trabeculae with a fresh layer of osteoid tissue from which new bone can invade those parts of the graft where osteocytes have failed to survive. At the same time, along with host osteoblasts, they act to unite host bone with grafted bone where the two meet. The graft in its final consolidated form is probably the result of the combined activity of surviving graft bone cells assisted by host cells at the point of graft-host junction and at points in the graft where graft cells have failed to survive.

Cancellous bone grafts require immobilization as well as contact with living host bone if they are to persist and establish bony union with the host. Under the stress of subsequent function the graft will survive and its shape and structure undergo modification according to the physical demands made upon it. The importance of functional stress in perpetuating the graft is demonstrated by the frequency with which autogenous cancellous bone grafts, applied to host bone as simple onlay grafts to restore bony contours, undergo slow and progressive absorption [7].

The growth of bone grafts in contact with bone can occur only by the increased deposition of bone on that surface of the graft having contact with soft tissue. Such appositional bone growth is generally accepted as occurring in bone grafts in growing children.

The split-rib autogenous bone graft has been successfully reintroduced by Longacre [60] and his colleagues. It has the advantages of easy availability, rapid regeneration of bone at the donor site for subsequent repeated use, and ready application in children, without the possibility of damage to growing epiphyses. Because the rib is split, its contained cancellous bone is placed in contact with vascular host tissues, allowing early revascularization of the graft and assisting survival of osteocytes that introduce early bone regeneration. Although for the most part the graft is replaced by new bone, the process is exceptionally rapid.

Much recent evidence has stressed the importance of the periosteal membrane in the regeneration of bone. In the repair of maxillary clefts, mucoperiosteal flaps have shown greater capacity for bone regeneration than autogenous bone grafts, both in animals [59] and in human beings [66]. In an investigation of bone onlay grafts to the jaw in dogs, only those grafts with intact periosteum showed consistent survival [67], while in onlay iliac bone grafts to the nasal bones in rabbits, the grafts survived better if the periosteum was applied as a separate periosteal graft to cover the bone graft [68]. The beneficial role of periosteum in osteogenesis has been further demonstrated in rabbits by consistent bone production resulting from the application of free grafts of tibial periosteum to the cleft between the mandibular arches [65], and in human subjects a similar result followed from the application of free tibial periosteal autografts to congenital maxillary clefts [64].

Cartilage

Cartilage constitutes one of the more frequently used autogenous transplants buried in the tissues, because of its ready availability, high survival rate, ease of technical manipulation, and capacity to survive heterotopic transplantation, even to sites where it is not subjected to functional stress – unlike bone.

The most commonly used autogenous cartilage graft is that taken from the costal cartilages, but cartilage from the external ear, septal cartilage, and nasal cartilage may all be successfully transplanted.

Cartilage is an avascular tissue consisting of a fibrous matrix in which chondromucoprotein is deposited by the activity of chondroblasts, which in adult cartilage are seen as chondrocytes enclosed in small spaces of lacunae scattered throughout the matrix. The chondrocytes are vital cells, nourished by diffusion of tissue fluids through the matrix. The cartilage is enclosed in a connective tissue sheath, the perichondrium. Chondrocytes are living cells and survive transplantation, as shown by their being stained in long-standing cartilage grafts by supravital stains [71], and by their continuing to metabolize sulfate injected in isotope-labeled form [69].

The hyaline cartilage of the lower rib cartilages may be removed from the donor site in considerable amount without creating any disability. It takes readily as a free graft in subcutaneous sites to restore defective nasal or facial contours, provided that contact of graft and host bed is preserved without intervening hematoma in order that the nutritional requirement of the graft may be met. Absorption of cartilage autografts is more frequently observed in children than in adults [7].

Since the rib cartilages act as a spring to assist restoration of the thoracic cage to neutral position during respiration, the matrix is in a state of varying tension. When costal cartilage is shaped for insertion as a free graft, carving must be executed according to the principle of balanced cross section [69] whereby stresses must be symmetrically balanced throughout the length of the graft if late warping of the transplant is to be avoided. In simple terms this involves removing equal amounts of cartilage from each aspect of the graft, or alternatively removing appreciably less than half the thickness of the graft from one aspect only at any one level. If these simple rules are observed, delayed curvature of the graft can be avoided. In practice the limitation imposed is slight, provided careful selection of an appropriately shaped costal cartilage is made when inspecting those available at the donor site. Cartilage killed by boiling, formalin, or irradiation does not warp, but is subject to progressive absorption over the years.

According to Peer, the available evidence indicates that cartilage isotransplants do not grow with the child, when used in young patients [72].

Perichondrium can be successfully transplanted as a free graft; it has been taken from costal cartilage and used to regenerate normal articular cartilage in osteoarthritic joints in the thumb [70].

Fat

Fat cells offer a readily available tissue for subcutaneous implantation to reconstruct the deficient contours of such areas as face and breast, but they have the disadvantage of losing one-third to one-half of their bulk during the months following transplantation. Free fat grafts are no longer used in clinical practice [73].

The absorption of adipose cells in considerable numbers in free fat grafts may be appreciably limited by using a graft of combined dermis and subcutaneous fat (the dermafat graft). The dermis serves to establish an early host-graft vascular anastomosis, rapidly restoring blood circulation to the poorly vascularized adipose tissue. Such a composite graft may be expected to lose not more than 20 percent of its total bulk; it offers one of the most effective means of restoring defective surface contours by autogenous transplantation [53]. Such grafts are most effective when thcy arc of limited size, and they are now replaced in augmentation mammoplasty by synthetic materials.

Fascia

This tissue, taken from the iliotibial tract of fascia lata of the thigh by a suitable fascial stripper, is used chiefly for the support of paralyzed facial musculature, but other surgical specialties find it useful in the repair of hernias, defects of the chest wall or cerebral dura mater, and joint ligaments, as well as in the reconstruction of heart valves.

Blood circulation in fascial grafts is restored within about 3 days of transfer by direct anastomosis between host and graft vessels. Although there is no absolute certainty that the graft may not undergo creeping replacement by host fibroblasts, most authorities consider that the transplant survives intact; the fibroblasts of the fascia remain viable and are not replaced by host cells [7].

Muscle

Although the erector pili muscles of buried dermis grafts survive, these are of visceral muscle and of no clinical importance [53].

The Abbe flap or lip-switch operation affords an example of successful skeletal muscle transplantation, where the vascular supply is preserved intact throughout, and nervous reinnervation takes place before muscle degeneration can occur. That such transplanted muscle retains its contractile power has been shown by histochemical staining of active motor endplates [92], and by electromyography [87].

It is an accepted practice in treating exposed bones, particularly in crushing and avulsion injuries of the lower limb, to use a transposition of muscle bellies as local pedicled flaps in which the vascular supply is kept intact; a split-skin graft is applied direct to the muscle flap in a one-stage repair [85, 93]. Such methods have largely replaced the cross leg skin flap in the treatment of these injuries (see Chapter 49).

A musculocutaneous flap is a composite flap which includes a muscle with preserved blood and nerve supply, together with its overlying skin, transposed to an adjacent defect. The overlying skin is supplied by perforating musculocutaneous vessels. Muscles used in this way are the sternomastoid [76], and gracilis and latissimus dorsi [94, 95].

Following upon the successful transplantation of skeletal muscle with microsurgical anastomosis of vein, artery, and nerve at the recipient site in animals [88], the method has been applied clinically to restore movement in cases of facial paralysis by transplanting the gracilis muscle to the face with microneural suture to trigeminal motor nerve axons [83].

The transplantation of skeletal muscle as a free graft has recently become established, though only in muscles of limited size [79, 82, 89]. There are three prerequisites for success:

1. The muscle selected must be transplanted as a complete anatomical entity by transferring the entire muscle belly intact after subperiosteal stripping of its origin and including its tendon of insertion with the transplant, in order to include the entire muscle fibers which run the whole length of the muscle [7].
2. The muscle must be denervated 2 weeks prior to transfer in order to increase its vascularity and establish an economical metabolic level enabling the transplant to survive the initial 3 days of ischemia and total anoxia following transplantation, while direct vascular anastomoses are established between graft and host at the recipient site [84, 86]. It is now known that denervation of white skeletal muscle is rapidly followed by a change in its constituent enzymes, resulting in the replacement of its anaerobic glycolytic metabolism by an oxidative and lipolytic form, requiring an increased blood supply, and resulting in greatly reduced metabolic requirements.
3. The free muscle graft must be applied in direct contact with normal innervated skeletal muscle at the recipient site, so that "muscular neurotization" of the transplant by the ingrowth of axons from the normal host muscle can occur. The outgrowing motor axons spread most rapidly where they enter the endoneurial tubes of the degenerated nerves in the transplant, but can also spread along denervated muscle fibers, which they can then penetrate to form motor end-plates [77].

By using the palmaris longus muscle of the forearm and the extensor digitorum brevis muscles of the foot as free grafts to the face, successful reanimation of the mouth and eyelids in cases of unilateral facial paralysis has been reported [80, 90, 91] and the same muscles have been transplanted into the posterior pharyngeal wall as a pharyngoplasty in cleft palate patients [90], to the external vesical sphincter in congenital bladder neck defect, to the bilateral cleft lip to restore muscular continuity, and to the anal canal in cases of fecal incontinence [78, 81, 90].

REFERENCES

General

1. Burnet, M. *The Integrity of the Body.* Cambridge, Mass.: Harvard University Press, 1962.
2. Castro, J. E. *Immunology for Surgeons.* Lancaster, England: M.T.P. Press, 1976.
3. Medawar, P. B. *The Uniqueness of the Individual.* London: Methuen, 1957.
4. Moore, F. D. *The Give and Take of Tissue Transplantation.* New York: Simon & Schuster, 1972.
5. Munster, A. M. *Surgical Immunology.* New York: Grune & Stratton, 1976.
6. Najarian, J. S., and Simmons, R. L. *Transplantation.* Philadelphia: Lea & Febiger, 1972.
7. Peer, L. A. *Transplantation of Tissues,* Vols. 1 and 2. Baltimore: Williams & Wilkins, 1955, 1959.
8. Rapaport, F. T., and Dausset, J. *Human Transplantation.* New York: Grune & Stratton, 1968.
9. Roitt, I. M. *Essential Immunology* (2nd ed.). Oxford, England: Blackwell, 1974.
10. Russell, P. S., and Monaco, A. P. *The Biology of Tissue Transplantation.* Boston: Little, Brown, 1964.
11. Snell, G. D. The terminology of tissue tramsplantation. *Transplantation* 2:655, 1964.
12. Woodruff, M. F. A. *The Transplantation of Tissues and Organs.* Springfield, Ill.: Thomas, 1960.

Allografts

13. Bach, F., and Hirschorn, K. Lymphocyte interaction: A potential histocompatibility test in vitro. *Science* 143:813, 1964.
14. Bain, B., Lowenstein, L., and MacLean, L. D. The in vitro Mixed Leukocyte Reaction and Initial Studies in Its Application as a Test for Histocompatibility. In *Histocompatibility Testing.* Report of a Conference and Workshop sponsored by the National Academy of Sciences and National Research Council. Washington, D.C., 1965.
15. Bain, B., Vas, M. R., and Lowenstein, L. The development of large immature mononuclear cells in mixed leukocyte cultures. *Blood* 23:108, 1964.
16. Billingham, R. E., Brent, L., and Medawar, P. B. Quantitative studies on tissue transplantation immunity: II. Origin, strength and duration of actively and adoptively acquired immunity. *Proc. R. Soc. Lond.* [Biol.] 143:58, 1954.
17. Billingham, R. E., Brent, L., and Medawar, P. B. Quantitative studies on tissue transplantation immunity: III. Actively acquired tolerance. *Philos. Trans. R. Soc. Lond.* [Biol.] 239:357, 1956.
18. Billingham, R. E., and Silvers, W. K. Studies on Cheek Pouch Skin Homografts in Syrian Hamster. In Wolstenholme, G. E. W., and Cameron, M. P. (Eds.), *Ciba Foundation Symposium on Transplantation.* Boston: Little, Brown, 1962.
19. Billingham, R. E., and Silvers, W. K. *The Immunobiology of Transplantation.* Englewood Cliffs, N.J.: Prentice-Hall, 1971.
20. Billingham, R. E., Silvers, W. K., and Wilson, D. B. Further studies on adoptive transfer of sensitivity to skin homografts. *J. Exp. Med.* 118:397, 1963.

21. Burke, J. F., May, J. W., Albright, N., Quinby, W. C., and Russell, P. S. Temporary skin transplantation and immunosuppression for extensive burns. *N. Engl. J. Med.* 290:269, 1974.
22. Gibson, T., Davies, W. B., and Curran, R. C. The long-term survival of cartilage homografts in man. *Br. J. Plast. Surg.* 11:177, 1958.
23. Gibson, T., and Medawar, P. B. The fate of skin homografts in man. *J. Anat.* 77:299, 1943.
24. Goldsmith, K. L. G. Donor selection and compatibility typing. *Br. Med. Bull.* 21:162, 1965.
25. Gorer, P. A. Some recent work on tumor immunity. *Adv. Cancer Res.* 4:149, 1956.
26. Gowans, J. L. The role of lymphocytes in the destruction of homografts. *Br. Med. Bull.* 21:106, 1965.
27. Gowans, J. L., McGregor, D. D., and Cowen, D. M. The Role of Small Lymphocytes in the Rejection of Homografts of Skin. In Wolstenholme, G. E. W., and Knight, J. (Eds.), *The Immunologically Competent Cell: Its Nature and Origin.* Boston: Little, Brown, 1963.
28. Krizek, T. J. Biologic Dressings. In Krizek, T. J., and Hoopes, J. E. (Eds.), *Symposium on Basic Science in Plastic Surgery.* St. Louis: Mosby, 1976.
29. Lawrence, H. S., Rapaport, F. T., Converse, J. M., and Tillet, W. S. Homograft Sensitivity in Human Beings. In Wolstenholme, G. E. W., and Cameron, M. P. (Eds.), *Ciba Foundation Symposium on Transplantation.* Boston: Little, Brown, 1962.
30. Lightbody, J., Bernoco, D., Miggiano, V. C., and Cepellini, R. Cell mediated lympholysis in man after sensitization of effector lymphocytes through mixed leukocyte cultures. *G. Batteriol. Virol. Immunol.* 64:243, 1971.
31. McClellan, I. C. M. Antibody in the induction and inhibition of lymphocyte toxicity. *Transplant. Rev.* 13:67, 1972.
32. McKhann, C. F. Transplantation studies of strong and weak histocompatibility barriers in mice: II. Tolerance. *Transplantation* 2:620, 1964.
33. Medawar, P. B. Immunology of Transplantation. *The Harvey Lectures 1956–1957.* New York: Academic Press, 1958.
34. Miller, J. F. A. P. The thymus yesterday, today and tomorrow. *Lancet* 2:1299, 1967.
35. Mitchison, N. A., and Dube, O. L. Studies on the immunological response to foreign tumor transplants in the mouse: II. The relation between hemagglutinating antibody and graft resistance in the normal mouse and mice pretreated with tissue preparations. *J. Exp. Med.* 102:179, 1955.
36. Owen, R. D. Immunogenetic consequences of vascular anastomoses between bovine twins. *Science* 102:400, 1945.
37. Perlmann, P., Perlmann, H., and Wigzell, H. Lymphocyte mediated cytotoxicity in vitro: Induction and inhibition by humoral antibody and nature of effector cells. *Transplant. Rev.* 13:91, 1972.
38. Rapaport, F. T., and Converse, J. M. The immune response to multiple-set skin homografts: An experimental study in man. *Ann. Surg.* 147:273, 1958.
39. Rapaport, F. T., Converse, J. M., Horn, L., Ballantyne, D. L., and Mulholland, J. H. Altered reactivity of skin homografts in severe thermal injury. *Ann. Surg.* 159:390, 1964.
40. Rood, J. J. van, and Eernisse, J. G. The detection of transplantation antigens in leucocytes. *Semin. Hematol.* 5:187, 1968.
41. Scothorne, R. J. Studies on the response of the regional lymph node to skin homografts. *Ann. N.Y. Acad. Sci.* 64:1028, 1957.
42. Snell, G. D. Immunological enhancement. *Surg. Gynecol. Obstet.* 130:1109, 1970.
43. Thompson, N. The role of succinic dehydrogenase and sulfhydryl groups during epidermal rejection in skin homografts: A preliminary histochemical study in rats. *Transplant. Bull.* 30:1, 1962.
44. Walia, I., Peer, L. A., Bernhard, W. G., and Gordon, H. Does growth occur in young rabbit ear cartilage grafts transplanted in young rabbits? *Plast. Reconstr. Surg.* 29:259, 1962.
45. Weaver, J. M., Algire, G. H., and Prehn, R. T. The growth of cells in vivo in diffusion chambers: II. The role of cells in the destruction of homografts in mice. *J. Natl. Cancer Inst.* 15:1737, 1955.
46. Wolstenholme, G. E. W., and O'Connor, M. Antilymphocytic Serum. *Ciba Foundation Study Group No. 29.* London: Churchill, 1967.
47. Woodruff, M. F. A., and Anderson, N. F. Effect of lymphocyte depletion by thoracic duct fistula and administration of antilymphocytic serum on the survival of skin homografts in rats. *Nature* 200:702, 1963.

Skin and Dermis

48. Converse, J. M., and Ballantyne, D. L. Distribution of diphosphopyridine nucleotide diaphorase in rat skin autografts and homografts. *Plast. Reconstr. Surg.* 30:415, 1962.
49. Converse, J. M., and Robb-Smith, A. H. T. The healing of surface cutaneous wounds: Its analogy with the healing of superficial burns. *Ann. Surg.* 120:873, 1944.
50. Hynes, W. The early circulation in skin grafts with a consideration of methods to encourage their survival. *Br. J. Plast. Surg.* 6:257, 1954.
50a. Knapp, T. R., Kaplan, E. N., and Daniels, J. R. Injectable collagen for soft tissue augmentation.

Plast. Reconstr. Surg.* 60:398, 1977.
51. Peer, L. A., and Paddock, R. Histological studies on the fate of deeply implanted dermal grafts: Observations on sections of implants buried from one week to one year. *Arch. Surg.* 34:268, 1937.
52. Pontén, B. Grafted skin: Observations on innervation and other qualities. *Acta Chir. Scand.* [Suppl.] 257, 1960.
53. Thompson, N. The subcutaneous dermis graft: A clinical and histologic study in man. *Plast. Reconstr. Surg.* 26:1, 1960.
54. Thompson, N. Tubular resorption in human eccrine sweat glands: Based on a histochemical study of buried autogenous dermis grafts in man. *Clin. Sci.* 19:95, 1960.
55. Thompson, N. A clinical and histological investigation into the fate of epithelial elements buried following the grafting of "shaved" skin surfaces. *Br. J. Plast. Surg.* 13:219, 1961.
56. Zarem, H. A. Transplantation of the Skin. In Krizek, T. J., and Hoopes, J. E. (Eds.), *Sympo sium on Basic Science in Plastic Surgery.* St. Louis: Mosby, 1976.

Bone

57. Albee, F. H. *Bone-Graft Surgery.* Philadelphia: Saunders, 1915.
58. Bell, R. An Interim Report on the Use of Kiel Bone in the Correction of Nasal Deformities. In *Symposium on Bone Grafting Materials.* Eastbourne, England: Armour Pharmaceutical Co., 1966.
59. Engdahl, E. Bone regeneration in maxillary defects. *Scand. J. Plast. Reconstr. Surg.* Suppl. 8, 1972.
60. Longacre, J. T. Transplantation of Bone. In Converse, J. M. (Ed.), *Reconstructive Plastic Surgery,* Vol. 1. Philadelphia: Saunders, 1964.
61. Mowlem, R. Editorial. *Br. J. Plast. Surg.* 4:231, 1952.
62. Peer, L. A. The fate of autogenous human bone grafts. *Br. J. Plast. Surg.* 3:233, 1951.
63. Plenk, H., Hollmann, K., and Wilfert, K. H. Experimental bridging of osseous defects in rats by the implantation of Kiel bone containing fresh autologous marrow. *J. Bone Joint Surg.* 54:735, 1972.
64. Ritsila, V., Alhopuro, S., Gylling, U., and Rintala, A. The use of free periosteum for bone formation in congenital clefts of the maxilla: A preliminary report. *Scand. J. Plast. Reconstr. Surg.* 6:57, 1972.
65. Ritsila, V., Alhopuro, S., and Rintala, A. Bone formation with free periosteum: An experimental study. *Scand. J. Plast. Reconstr. Surg.* 6:51, 1972.
66. Skoog, T. The use of periosteum and Surgicel for bone restoration in congenital clefts of the maxilla. *Scand. J. Plast. Reconstr. Surg.* 1:113, 1967.
67. Thompson, N., and Casson, J. A. Experimental onlay bone grafts to the jaws. A preliminary study in dogs. *Plast. Reconstr. Surg.* 46:341, 1970.
68. Thompson, N., and Lewis, A. W. The role of free periosteal grafts in improving the survival of autogenous onlay bone grafts to the facial bones in rabbits. *Chir. Plastica* (Berlin) 3:243, 1976.

Cartilage

69. Gibson, T., and Davis, W. B. The distortion of autogenous cartilage grafts: Its cause and prevention. *Br. J. Plast. Surg.* 10:257, 1958.
70. Ohlsen, L., Fuente, A. de la, Johansson, S., and Skoog, T. Reconstruction of articular cartilage. *Transactions of the Sixth International Congress of Plastic and Reconstructive Surgery.* Paris: Masson, 1976.
71. Peer, L. A. Experimental observations on the growth of young human cartilage grafts. *Plast. Reconstr. Surg.* 1:108, 1946.
72. Peer, L. A. Transplantation of Cartilage. In Converse, J. M. (Ed.), *Reconstructive Plastic Surgery,* Vol. 1. Philadelphia: Saunders, 1964.

Fat

73. Hoopes, J. E. Dermis-Fat Grafts. In Krizek, T. J., and Hoopes, J. E. (Eds.), *Symposium on Basic Science in Plastic Surgery.* St. Louis: Mosby, 1976.

Fascia

74. McGregor, J. C., and Lindop, G. B. M. The behaviour of cialit stored and freeze-dried human fascia lata in rats. *Br. J. Plast. Surg.* 27:155, 1974.
75. Snyderman, R. K., Ego-Acquirre, E., and Starzynski, T. E. The ultimate fate of freeze-dried fascia: Experience with its use in the correction of facial paralysis. *Plast. Reconstr. Surg.* 38:219, 1966.

Muscle

76. Bakamjian, V. A technique for primary reconstruction of the palate after radical maxillectomy for cancer. *Plast. Reconstr. Surg.* 31:103, 1963.
77. Erlacher, P. Direct and muscular neurotization of paralyzed muscles. Experimental research. *Am. J. Orthop. Surg.* 13:22, 1915.
78. Freilinger, G., Holle, J., and Mamoli, B. Free muscle transplants for anal sphincter reconstruction in pigs. *Chir. Plastica* (Berlin) 2:133, 1974.
79. Gruber, H., Freilinger, G., Holle, J., and Mayr, R. Motor end-plates in autologous muscle transplants. *Experientia* 30:1191, 1974.

80. Hakelius, L. Transplantation of free autogenous muscle in the treatment of facial paralysis. *Scand. J. Plast. Reconstr. Surg.* 8:220, 1974.
81. Hakelius, L. Free autogenous muscle transplantation in two cases of total anal incontinence. *Acta Chir. Scand.* 141:69, 1975.
82. Hakelius, L., Nystrom, B., and Stalberg, E. Histochemical and neurophysiological studies of autotransplanted cat muscle. *Scand. J. Plast. Reconstr. Surg.* 9:15, 1975.
83. Harii, K. In Fisch, U. (Ed.), *Facial Nerve Surgery.* Birmingham, Alabama: Aesculapius, 1977. P. 258.
84. Hogan, E. L., Dawson, D. M., and Romanul, F. C. A. Enzymatic changes in denervated muscle: II. Biochemical studies. *Arch. Neurol.* 13:274, 1965.
85. Pers, M., and Medgyesi, S. Pedicle muscle flaps and their application in the surgery of repair. *Br. J. Plast. Surg.* 26:313, 1973.
86. Romanul, F. C. A., and Hogan, E. L. Enzymatic changes in denervated muscle: I. Histochemical changes. *Arch. Neurol.* 13:263, 1965.
87. Smith, J. W. The anatomical and physiologic acclimatization of tissue transplanted by the lip-switch technique. *Plast. Reconstr. Surg.* 26:40, 1960.
88. Tamai, S., Komatsu, S., Sakamoto, H., Sano, S., Sasauchi, N., Hori, Y., Tatsumi, Y., and Okuda, H. Free surgical transplants in dogs with microsurgical neurovascular anastomoses. *Plast. Reconstr. Surg.* 46:219, 1970.
89. Thompson, N. Investigation of autogenous skeletal muscle free-grafts in the dog. With a report on a successful free graft of skeletal muscle in man. *Transplantation* 12:353, 1971.
90. Thompson, N. A review of autogenous skeletal muscle grafts and their clinical applications. *Clin. Plast. Surg.* 1:349, 1974.
91. Thompson, N., and Gustavson, E. H. The use of neuromuscular free autografts with microneural anastomosis to restore elevation to the paralysed angle of the mouth in cases of unilateral facial paralysis. With an analysis of late results of muscle grafts in the treatment of 103 cases of facial hemiparesis. *Chir. Plastica* (Berlin) 3:165, 1976.
92. Thompson, N., and Pollard, A. C. Motor function in Abbé flaps: A histochemical study of motor reinnervation in transplanted muscle tissue of the lips in man. *Br. J. Plast. Surg.* 14:66, 1961.
93. Vasconez, L. O., Bostwick, J., and McCraw, J. Coverage of exposed bone by muscle transposition and skin grafting. *Plast. Reconstr. Surg.* 53:526, 1974.
94. Vasconez, L. O., and McCraw, J. B. The Use of Muscle in Plastic and Reconstructive Surgery. In Krizek, T. J., and Hoopes, J. E. (Eds.), *Symposium on Basic Science in Plastic Surgery.* St. Louis: Mosby, 1976.
95. Woods, J. E., Irons, G. B., and Masson, J. K. Use of muscular, musculocutaneous, and omental flaps to reconstruct difficult defects. *Plast. Reconstr. Surg.* 59:191, 1977.

3

Implantation Materials

RALPH BLOCKSMA AND SILAS BRALEY, JR.

Autogenous tissue has always been considered the best implantation material. It should continue to be utilized wherever feasible in preference to synthetic materials. However, there are certain situations in which autogenous tissue is not available or will not give a good result. Autogenous bone, cartilage, derma-fat, and fascia require surgical assault on the body at positions distant from the primary repair area. Once obtained, they often must be shaped at operation instead of prior to it, thus prolonging the procedure. After implantation, there is the possibility of absorption, and often undesirable scar formation eventuates. Furthermore, only limited amounts of donor tissue are usually available. For these reasons there have been many attempts over the years to utilize alloplastic materials for subdermal implantation.

In general, the body's protective mechanism against the intrusion of foreign materials is so good that very few have been found acceptable. In the past, certain metals have been used, especially in orthopedics, but the problem of successful soft tissue replacement has continued to plague the surgeon.

Since most uses in plastic surgery involve replace- of soft rather than hard tissue, the materials available to the plastic surgeon have been seriously restricted, and most attempts at extensive soft tissue replacement in the past have failed to give adequate correction.

TISSUE SUBSTITUTES

Properties of Ideal Substitutes

The properties of an ideal soft tissue substitute were defined by Scales [1] in 1953. This ideal tissue substitute is:

1. Not physically modified by soft tissue.
2. Not capable of inciting an inflammatory or foreign body reaction.
3. Not capable of producing a state of allergy or hypersensitivity.
4. Chemically inert.
5. Noncarcinogenic.
6. Capable of resisting strain.
7. Capable of fabrication in the form desired.
8. Capable of sterilization.

General Precautions Regarding Substitutes

Some precautionary measures which a surgeon desiring to utilize allopathic materials should follow are:

1. *Secure complete description* regarding medical acceptability of a material before surgical use. Remember that generic names can be misleading. The term *polyvinyl,* for instance, can be applied to materials made from polyvinyl alcohol, polyvinyl chloride, polyvinyl butyral, or even polyvinylidine chloride, all of which are quite different. It also can vary from a hard, brittle material to a rubbery one to a foam. It is not sufficient to describe a given implant material as "the same as another." The fact that an investigator reported the use of "polyvinyl" or "polyethylene" in a particular implant means only that his particular lot of material was or was not acceptable in that particular application. The next surgeon wishing to utilize that material would do well to convince himself that what he has is exactly the same formulation that was used previously. Even if the material is identical, however, there is no guarantee that it will be satisfactory in the new application, since problems of stiffness and tissue erosion vary in different parts of the body.
2. *Secure a pure material* that is quality controlled by the manufacturer for medical purposes. One should remember that most plastics and rubbers contain many ingredients other than the basic polymer. These can include catalysts, activators, plasticizers, antioxidants, and antiozidants, as well as almost infinite variation in kinds and amounts of such reagents. In some cases, these additives exceed in volume the basic polymer. The formulations of the plastics are usually of a proprietary nature, and unless a full and complete history of acceptable implantation of a given formulation is obtained, the material should not be introduced into the body.
3. *Avoid chemical sterilization* of the implant wherever possible, since many allopathic materials are capable of absorbing sterilizing liquids and gases. These can subsequently cause severe reactions when the implant is placed in the tissues.

Safeguards

Observe safeguards in surgical techniques:

1. Shape the implant to avoid sharp corners and edges.
2. Bury the implant as deeply as possible under the skin and subcutaneous tissue.

3. Avoid tension in the adjacent tissues or tension against the overlying cutaneous coverage.
4. Place the incision line as far from the implant as possible.
5. Handle the implant with instruments to avoid soiling with glove powder, lint, or fingerprints during and subsequent to the preparation period.
6. Utilize the proper stiffness of material – it should be as soft as is consistent with the application. Do not use any hard material for soft tissue replacement.

Basic to the successful use of any implantation material, therefore, is the development of a conservative implantation philosophy. The utilization of an inert foreign body subcutaneously requires:

1. A comprehensive knowledge of the material, its properties and limitations.
2. An intimate knowledge of the literature relating to any given implant material.
3. Mastery of the particular surgical technique, with emphasis on minimal trauma to tissue in the implantation of foreign materials.

Materials Available

An exhaustive summary of implant materials available is beyond the scope of this chapter. In the past, a host of substances have been tried: ivory, various organic rubbers, amber, silver, gold, platinum, paraffin, and xenogeneic bone are a few examples. Certain of these materials are still in use; others have been abandoned entirely. Some of the more modern materials include polyvinyl alcohol–formaldehyde sponge (Ivalon), polyethylene sponge, polyvinyl chloride, polystyrene, polyurethanes, silicones, and others, all with varying degrees of success. Some of these are no longer available. Ivalon, for instance, has been discontinued. Some of these are available in forms specifically for medical purposes, others only as industrial materials.

The acceptability of these allopathic materials is as varied as the materials themselves. Some have immediately caused intense foreign body reaction; others took longer periods to develop such reaction. Most were too hard for soft tissue replacement. Open-cell foams, which initially were soft, were found to permit ingrowth of tissue and subsequent contracture and hardening. Other materials would drift; still others deteriorated and were absorbed. A few seem to be satisfactory. Grau [4] has prepared an exhaustive bibliography of materials used for implant purposes for the surgeon who wishes to investigate the history of this subject in more detail.

At the present time, the following substances have been found to be the most acceptable for implant purposes.

Metals

VITALLIUM.* These are nonferrous alloys furnished in two types – castable and wrought. The approximate constituents of these are given in Table 3-1. The remaining constituents are small proportions of iron, manganese, and other metals. Many bone replacements are available as fabricated parts from the manufacturer, as well as plates, bolts, screws, and so forth, all finely developed for the surgeon's specific use. Specially cast parts are also available. ASTM (American Society for Testing Materials) Specification F-54† covers castable chrome-cobalt alloys for subdermal implantation.

STAINLESS STEEL. Several kinds of stainless steel have been used for implant purposes, but recent ASTM specifications F-55T and F-56T set standards for optimal formulations. These call for a stainless steel containing 17 to 20 percent chromium, 10 to 14 percent nickel, and 2 to 4 percent molybdenum.

Textiles

TEFLON‡, CLOTH FORM. This is a polymer of tetrafluoroethylene.

$$\left[\begin{array}{c} \text{F} \quad \text{F} \\ | \quad\; | \\ -\text{C}-\text{C}- \\ | \quad\; | \\ \text{F} \quad \text{F} \end{array}\right]_x$$

It can be made into straight weaves, tricots (knits), and felt.

PROPLAST.§ Proplast is a highly porous material prepared from Teflon fluorocarbon polymer and carbon fibers.

DACRON.‡ This is a polyester fiber made from polyethylene terephthalate.

*Available from Austenal Co., Surgical Products, 224 East 39th Street, New York, N.Y. 10016.
†Available from American Society for Testing and Materials, 1916 Race Street, Philadelphia, Penn. 19103.
‡Available from E. I. Du Pont de Nemours & Co., Inc., 1007 Market Street, Wilmington, Del. 19801.
§A registered trademark of Vitek, Inc., Houston, Tex., and is available from Dow Corning Co., Midland, Mich. 48640.

Table 3-1. Main Constituent of Castable and Wrought Vitallium

Type of Vitallium	Chromium (%)	Cobalt (%)	Molybdenum (%)	Nickel (%)	Tungsten (%)
Castable Vitallium	29	63	6	–	–
Wrought Vitallium	20	52	–	10	15

$$\left[-\overset{\displaystyle H}{\underset{\displaystyle H}{\overset{|}{\underset{|}{C}}}}-\overset{\displaystyle H}{\underset{\displaystyle H}{\overset{|}{\underset{|}{C}}}}-O-\overset{\displaystyle O}{\overset{\|}{C}}-C_6H_4-\overset{\displaystyle O}{\overset{\|}{C}}-O- \right]_x$$

Next to Teflon, this is probably the least reactive of all textile fibers and is available in many weaves, tricots, and felts. It is very widely used for sutures, cardiac patches, and vascular prostheses. It is known in Europe as Terylene. The solid form is called Mylar.

Plastics

METHYLMETHACRYLATE. This is a clear, hard polymer made of the methyl ester of methacrylic acid.

$$\left[-\overset{\displaystyle H}{\underset{\displaystyle H}{\overset{|}{\underset{|}{C}}}}-\overset{\displaystyle CH_3}{\underset{\displaystyle \underset{\underset{\displaystyle O-CH_3}{|}}{C=O}}{\overset{|}{\underset{|}{C}}}}- \right]_x$$

One widely known brand is called Plexiglas.* Methylmethacrylate is available from a number of plastic manufacturers either as the monomer with catalyst, or as the plastic itself. It has been used for skull plates, jaws, chins, and other hard tissue uses. Recently it has been used rather extensively in orthopedic surgery as a cement in reconstruction of the total hip.

TEFLON, SOLID FORM. Teflon is a polymer of tetrafluoroethylene.

$$\left[-\overset{\displaystyle F}{\underset{\displaystyle F}{\overset{|}{\underset{|}{C}}}}-\overset{\displaystyle F}{\underset{\displaystyle F}{\overset{|}{\underset{|}{C}}}}- \right]_x$$

Teflon is probably one of the least reactive of available materials. It has been widely used in the textile form for vascular prostheses and in the solid form for various uses where hardness and stiffness are needed. It will creep – that is, it will flow very slowly under constant stress, at room temperature, so it should not be used where such flow could cause problems.

POLYURETHANE. This is a diisocyanate polymer.

$$\left[-O-R-O-\overset{\displaystyle O}{\overset{\|}{C}}-\overset{\displaystyle H}{\overset{|}{N}}-R'-\overset{\displaystyle H}{\overset{|}{N}}-\overset{\displaystyle O}{\overset{\|}{C}}- \right]_x$$

It can be in solid or foam form. Etheron† is a commonly used polyurethane foam. The foam form has been most widely used by plastic surgeons, although solvent solutions of the polymer are available from which solid parts can be made. Because of the wide variety of formulations, it should not be assumed that all polyurethanes are acceptable as implant materials.

POLYETHYLENE. Polyethylene is a polymer of ethylene.

$$\left[-\overset{\displaystyle H}{\underset{\displaystyle H}{\overset{|}{\underset{|}{C}}}}-\overset{\displaystyle H}{\underset{\displaystyle H}{\overset{|}{\underset{|}{C}}}}- \right]_x$$

Marlex‡ is a widely used surgical grade. It has been used as an implant in the nose, orbital floor, and chin. In the woven form, it has served to reinforce hernia repairs.

Fluids

Soft tissue augmentation by the use of fluid injection has been tried many times in the past. Of historical interest are the now discredited paraffin injections.

Silicone fluids have been used as injectable prostheses with considerable success. This use of the silicone fluids has been termed by the Federal Food and Drug Administration a "drug use." Hence, silicone fluids used in this manner must follow the Food

*Available from Rohm and Haas Co., Independence Mall W 1, Philadelphia, Penn. 19105.

†Available from Robbins Instruments Company, 2 North Passaic Avenue, Chatham, N. J. 07928.

‡Available from Phillips Petroleum Company, 16-C1 Phillips Building, Bartlesville, Okla. 74004.

and Drug protocol for investigation of a "new drug," and at the time of this writing they are not generally available for clinical augmentation.

Elastomers (Rubbery Materials)
Since plastic surgery is concerned primarily with soft tissue manipulation, soft rubbery materials have been those most needed by the plastic surgeon. Until the advent of medical grade silicone rubber, however, there was no material of this type that could be safely used as a permanent replacement for soft tissue. Because of the wide use of silicones, and because medical grades are produced specifically for the plastic surgeon,* they are discussed at length in the following section.

THE SILICONES
The silicones are a large family of chemically related materials and can take many forms. They can be watery or oily liquids, or they can be very rubbery materials almost indistinguishable from natural rubber. The rubbery, or elastomeric, silicones are available in the form of sponge, blocks of varying hardness, adhesives, and gels.

Most of the medical grade silicones are composed of long chains of dimethylsiloxane units strung together. These have the following formula:

$$\left[\begin{array}{l} CH_3 \\ | \\ -Si\quad -O \\ | \\ CH_3 \end{array} \right]_x$$

The medical silicone nomenclature is as follows:†

Dow Corning Silicone Fluid
Dow Corning Medical Fluid (MDX 44-011)

Viscosities from 20 to 100,000 centistokes are available; the clinical preference is for a viscosity of 350 centistokes.

Silastic Silicone Rubber
Heat-Vulcanizing
 Soft – Silastic 370 Medical Grade Elastomer
 Medium – Silastic 372 Medical Grade Elastomer
 Hard – Silastic 373 Medical Grade Elastomer
Room-Temperature-Vulcanizing (RTV)
 Solid – Silastic 382 Medical Grade Elastomer
 Foam – Silastic 386 RTV Foam Elastomer

Silastic Silicone Adhesives
Silastic Medical Adhesive Silicone Type A
Hollister Medical Adhesive‡

Available Forms of Medical Grade Silicone

Silicone Fluids
The formula for the silicones shown above indicates a silicone fluid having x number of units in the chain. As x increases in the silicone fluid, viscosity of the fluid increases. If there are 130 units in the chain, for instance, the viscosity is 350 centistokes (a centistoke is a measurement of viscosity; the viscosity of water at standard conditions is 1 centistoke). These are clear, limpid fluids that do not change their properties with aging, temperature change, or exposure. Table 3-2 shows the variation in viscosity as the average number of dimethylsiloxane units in the polymer chains increases.

Silicone Rubber
Silicone rubber is made from extremely high-viscosity silicone fluid to which very pure and very fine particle size (0.02 micron) silica has been added to increase the tensile strength. The resultant putty-like raw material is vulcanized by the use of dichlorobenzoyl peroxide. This vulcanizing agent is activated by heat and changes the mass to a true rubber. The process of vulcanization is also referred to as a cross-linking process. A silicone fluid can be compared to a mass of spaghetti, where each strand of spaghetti (each polymer chain) is independent and can be readily separated. If, however, these are tied together (i.e., cross-linked), the strands or chains no longer can be separated readily, and the mass is like a fish net. Careful control of the cross-linking between the silicone polymer chains produces a silicone rubber.

There are *two major types* of silicone rubber used for medical purposes. The *heat-vulcanized* types (described above) are most commonly used since they are strong and tough. These are supplied in the already vulcanized form by the manufacturer. The *room-temperature-vulcanizing* (RTV) types can be used where heat cannot be tolerated. They produce a relatively weak silicone rubber, but they do not require, nor do they produce, large amounts of heat during the vulcanization process, so it is possible to set them up in direct contact with living tissue. The RTV silicone rubbers used in medicine are supplied in the raw state as viscous liquids. When the operator adds the catalyst, stannous octoate, the silicone

*Available from Medical Products Division, Dow Corning Co., Midland, Mich. 48640. Silastic is their trade name for silicone rubber, both industrial and medical grades, and is not a generic term for all silicone rubber. The various forms of Silastic silicone rubber made specifically for medical purposes are listed on pp. 97, 98, 100, and 102.
†Unspecified silicones for research purposes are available upon special request from the Dow Corning Center for Aid to Medical Research, Midland, Mich. 48640.
‡Hollister, Inc., 211 E. Chicago Ave., Chicago, Ill. 60611.

Table 3-2. Relation of Polymer Size to Viscosity of Silicone Polymers

No. of Dimethylsiloxane units	Viscosity (Centistokes)	Similar to
2	0.65	Water
10	26.0	
70	100.0	SAE 10 oil
130	350.0	SAE 35 oil
160	500.0	
200	1,000.0	
550	12,000.0	Very thick honey
3,000	10,000,000.0	Almost imperceptible flow

polymer cross-links to a rubber in a few minutes. It should be noted that silicone fluids will not vulcanize with the addition of the catalyst; it is effective only on the RTV liquid rubbers.

Silicone Adhesives
There are two types of silicone adhesives currently available: *Silastic Medical Adhesive Silicone Type A* is a self-curing adhesive. It is available in collapsible tubes and has the consistency of Vaseline. It requires approximately 24 hours to acquire its full adhesive properties, and when fully cured is a silicone rubber itself. This curing is achieved by the reaction of the polymer with the moisture in the air, causing the evolution of approximately 6% acetic acid (vinegar contains about 4% acetic acid). This adhesive is used to attach Dacron and Teflon cloth to silicone rubber prostheses so that there can be fibrous tissue ingrowth into the cloth to anchor the prosthesis. It can also be used to attach silicone rubber to itself and to such materials as stainless steel, certain plastics, wood, glass, and most metals. It does not adhere well to polyethylene, to unetched solid Teflon, or to living tissue.

Hollister Medical Adhesive is a pressure-sensitive adhesive – that is, it does not set up to a rubber but rather stays permanently sticky, like adhesive tape. It is used for adhering external prostheses (colostomy bags, ears, noses) to the skin surface. It cannot be used for adhering subdermal tissues together but will adhere to skin and to almost all alopathic materials.

Clinical Advantages of Medical Grade Silicones
The past years of intensive application of the silicones to medical usage have demonstrated several primary reasons for their acceptability as implant materials [2].

THE SILICONES ARE HEAT STABLE. Silastic silicone rubber and silicone fluids can be autoclaved or dry-heat sterilized with impunity. Variations of temperature within the body will not cause either the silicone rubber to become soft or brittle, or the viscosity of the silicone fluid to be changed.

THE SILICONES ARE TIME STABLE. The medical grade fluids do not evaporate or turn gummy, and silicone rubber does not deteriorate with time. Samples of silicone rubber exposed to the weather for more than 15 years in the South Florida Testing Station show no significant change. There are no plasticizers to be leached out and cause change in consistency.

VERSATILITY. The silicones may be used in the rubbery state, either as a solid or as a sponge; can be shaped at the operating table or used as prefabricated parts shaped to a moulage; and can be used as an injected liquid which will (in the case of the RTV rubber) or will not (in the case of the silicone fluids) become rubbery after injection. The versatility of these materials constitutes a challenge to the plastic surgeon.

NO ADHERENCE. Almost nothing will stick to a silicone except certain other silicones. Because the silicones are excellent insulation, they can develop a static charge on their surface and hence may attract and hold dust, dirt, and lint. If fixation to a body tissue is desired, a porous material such as Dacron can be adhered to the prosthesis, or perforations can be made through it to permit fixation by the subsequent ingrowth of fibrous tissue.

THE SILICONES ELICIT MINIMAL TISSUE REACTION. Properly prepared, the medical grade silicones elicit less tissue reaction than almost any other nonautogenous material. Histological studies following implantation of various types of medical grade Silastic silicone rubber subcutaneously implanted in rats have shown only a thin, delicate capsule surrounding the implant and virtual absence of heavy fibroblastic activity [3, 6]. Similar results are reported after injection of silicone fluid. If physical trauma causes exposure of a small segment of Silastic silicone elastomer, some operators have found it possible to trim away a small piece of the silicone and simply clean and suture the wound. It is true of Silastic implants generally that exposure after implantation does not in all cases require total removal of the implant, since secondary infection seems to occur only rarely.

THE SILICONES ARE NOT ATTACKED OR ALTERED BY THE BODY. There is no indication that any living organism can dissolve or metabolize a silicone. Almost all organic material can be altered in some manner by the body, either by solution, metabolism, phagocytic attack, or other means. Certain polyurethanes, for instance, were thought to be useful for artificial heart valves and artificial hearts, but after 2 years in the tissues, they deteriorated beyond usefulness. Leininger [5] reports no change in tensile strength or elongation of very thin films of silicone rubber after 17 months of implantation in animals.

Handling Silastic Silicone Rubber

It should be remembered that, although medical grade Silastic silicone rubber elicits less foreign body reaction than almost any other allopathic material in existence, foreign material on its surface or dissolved in it can cause tissue reaction which is mistakenly attributed to the silicone itself. Since silicone rubber tends to develop a static charge on its surface, it can attract and hold lint and dust. Fingerprints on the surface and oils or cold sterilizing solutions and gases dissolved in the silicone can also cause tissue reaction.

In preparing a silicone rubber prosthesis for implantation, it should first be washed thoroughly in a pure soap solution (Ivory soap has proved to be satisfactory), using distilled water to reduce soap-curd formation, and then rinsed very thoroughly in distilled water. The person handling the prosthesis should wear rubber gloves that have had the powder rinsed off. The prosthesis should then be sterilized by autoclaving under standard conditions or by dry-heat sterilization at 200°C. for 1 hour. Do not use detergents for washing silicone rubber since detergents can absorb into the silicone and are very difficult to remove. If ethylene oxide gas is used for sterilization, it can be absorbed into the rubber, so that extreme care must be taken to remove it before the rubber is implanted.

Solid blocks of silicone rubber can be shaped to size by carving a block of suitable density on a wooden board after carefully divesting the gloves of powder. The soft Silastic silicone elastomer is most easily handled, and shapes with ease using a #11 or #15 Bard-Parker blade. The Brown-Adson tissue forceps holds the implant most securely during the carving. A pattern of the defect prepared from exposed x-ray film prior to the surgery may be helpful.

Room-temperature-vulcanizing silicone rubber can be cast into molds and shaped prior to operation or can be carved at operation. Many prefabricated implants are now available; they all require sterilization.

Toxicity of Silicones

There are literally thousands of different silicones, manufactured by a number of different companies. A few of these silicones have been tested for medical purposes and subsequently have been manufactured for this purpose; these are the subject of this discussion. There are, however, other silicones, both of the fluid and rubber types, that have been tested and have been found to be very toxic. The vast majority of the silicones have never been tested for medical purposes and should be considered suspect.

It cannot be overemphasized that only medical grade silicones, manufactured under medical conditions, and with a long history of implantation, should be used for surgical purposes.

Carcinogenicity of Silicones

Extensive laboratory and clinical studies have established the advantageous properties, limitations, and many reconstructive surgical applications for medical grade silicone rubber implants. All synthetics, however, raise presently unanswerable questions with respect to the absolute safety of long-term implantation in human beings [7, 8, 10].

There have been no substantiated reports of cancer caused by implanted polymers in human beings. Harris [11] reports no neoplasms in 16,660 cases of breast augmentations with various implant materials. De Cholnoky [9] reports 7 cases of breast cancer in a survey of 10,941 patients, subsequent to augmentation mammoplasty, but concludes that they "apparently had no relation to the previously introduced prostheses." Over 500,000 persons now have had silicone rubber hydrocephalus shunts installed since 1955; at least 50,000 persons are living with synthetic heart valves; many thousands of bands encircling the globe for repair of detached retinas have been installed, as have been many thousands of arterial prostheses. In no case has there been a report of cancer caused by these implants. Oppenheimer et al. [13] and Hueper [12] report the formation of cancer in laboratory animals in conjunction with many implant materials. Their work was done on cancer-prone animals, and the relationship of this work to human cancer induction is questioned by many.

OPERATIVE TECHNIQUES FOR IMPLANTATION MATERIALS

A description of the uses and operative procedures

for the insertion of subcutaneous implantation materials does not imply that the authors necessarily approve of these procedures or utilize them extensively in their own practice. It should be underscored that autogenous tissue wherever possible should be utilized in preference to a synthetic substance. However, the sites where synthetic materials have been successfully used as substitutes for soft and bony tissue continue to grow in number. Some of these are listed below.

Face

Nose

The advantages of silicone rubber for nasal repair are the same as those in other parts of the body: silicone rubber is easily available, is easy to shape and to sterilize, and is not absorbed; its use reduces the number of operative procedures. The disadvantages are likewise those encountered in other implantations [33], namely, the dangers of exposure and infection.

Teflon and Silastic silicone rubber have been utilized successfully in the correction of saddle nose deformity. Rhinoplasty implants have been prefabricated of Silastic 370 Medical Grade Elastomer in three sizes to fit varying degrees of saddle nose deformity. These parts can also be carved by the surgeon from blocks of Silastic. The soft grade of block (Silastic 370 Medical Grade Elastomer) has proved to be the most satisfactory for this use since it has reduced, but not eliminated, the problem of erosion that sometimes can occur with the harder blocks. Introduction of the implant is usually through an intercartilagenous incision in the patient's left nasal fossa, with the skin in the depressed area undermined to form a pocket for the reception of the appropriate implant. As an alternative, a vertical midcolumellar incision can also be used. The implant should be handled only by forceps after autoclaving, and a light intranasal packing can be left in position for about 48 hours after its insertion. Some operators prefer to adhere a Dacron backing to a silicone rubber rhinoplasty implant, so that subsequent tissue growth into the textile material will immobilize it. Many variations in technique have been reported [14–41]. The lack of tissue reaction can be a disadvantage when the silicone is in an area of stress, since a protective layer of heavy fibrous tissue is not laid down. The more delicate subdermal tissues are squeezed against the implant and thus can be destroyed, leading to exposure of the implant. This exposure has been noted in tight skin over the dorsum and at the tip of the nose, particularly when efforts are made to form a more pointed nose from a flat one, usually by trying to lengthen the columella.

Some surgeons in attempting to do this have used an L-shaped prosthesis, others have used two separate implants, one along the dorsum and one in the columella. In either case, a piece of Dacron felt* or tricot* attached to the prosthesis directly under the tip of the nose, combined, of course, with care to minimize the stresses as much as possible, will help to reduce this erosion.

More recently Proplast has been favored by many investigators for contour restoration when a firm material is acceptable [49]. It is not intended for use in areas where there is insufficient underlying bone or tissue to prevent collapse of the implant from external pressure. In block form Proplast can be carved to shape; it is stabilized by tissue ingrowth rather than by circumferential fibrous encapsulation.

Chin

To correct moderate degrees of micrognathia, a self-carved or commercially prepared implant of soft Silastic 370 Medical Grade Elastomer is preferable, in our experience, to other implant materials. Prefabricated chin implants are now available to fit the normal curvature of the mandible. Dacron felt is supplied with the implant, to be used at the option of the operator for fixation. These implants are firm enough to maintain contour and flexible enough to permit their introduction through a small incision.

Safian recommends a submental incision about 3 cm. in length to permit undermining the fat pad over the chin for the creation of a pocket to receive the implant. Tissues along the margin of the mandible remain attached to form a shelf on which the implant rests and so prevent it from slipping downward [59]. The implant rests on the periosteum of the mandible. Millard [54] and others recommend insertion through an incision in the inferior buccal sulcus. Splinting with adhesive tape helps prevent dislocation of the implant following its introduction into the pocket.

Probably a wider variety of materials have been successfully used for augmentation mentoplasty than in almost any other part of the body. This is attributable to the following facts: erosion through the skin is not the problem that it can be elsewhere, softness is not necessary, and the skin covering is usually fairly generous.

Teflon [44, 45] has been reported to be successful for mental augmentation. Rubin reports an astonishing 21-year follow-up in the use of polyethylene [58] while Rish [55, 56], Weinstein [62], and Pitanguy [54] and others have used the acrylics.

Silicone rubbers have been reported on widely [42, 43, 46, 47, 50, 53, 55, 59–62].

The advantages of silicone rubber over other mate-

*Available upon request from Dow Corning Center for Aid to Medical Research, Midland, Mich. 48640.

rials for chin augmentation seem to be primarily (1) its ease of carving to adjust to individual variations, (2) its easy sterilization, and (3) the ready availability of a grade manufactured specifically for implantation purposes. Both the buccal and the submental approach have been used, and each has its advocates and denigrators.

The attachment of Dacron tricot and felt* serves to supply an artificial stroma for tissue ingrowth and reduces motion of the implant. It has been suggested that holes punched through the device will also serve this purpose.

Robinson and Shuken [57] reported in 1969 on bone resorption under both acrylic and Silastic chin implants. One excellent retrospective study showed that over half of 85 patients who received solid silicone rubber chin implants were found to have some absorption of bone beneath the implant [48]. It appears that bone absorption is less when the implant is placed over the hard bone of the lower mandible rather than over alveolar bone, and it is *preferable* that it be placed *superficial* to the periosteum [52].

Ears

Cronin [63] has reported favorably on the utilization of a Silastic otoplasty prosthesis to serve as a supporting framework in total and subtotal ear reconstruction. This prosthesis, produced commercially, has membrane-like fenestrations which can readily be cut away to allow for greater tissue fixation. It may also be trimmed easily for adaptation to ears that are smaller.

At the initial operation the implant is placed under a flap of postauricular skin. At a second stage, the implant is carried forward by posterior dissection, with great pains taken not to expose the Silastic framework at any point. A thick split-thickness skin graft is utilized to cover the posterior surface of the reconstructed ear.

In a follow-up study in 1968 Cronin, Greenberg, and Brauer [64] reported on 19 congenital microtias and 11 patients with complete traumatic auricular losses repaired by the use of the Silastic otoplasty prosthesis. In half the cases, they used a prosthesis to the helix of which Dacron cloth had been attached. The purpose of the cloth was to serve as an artificial stroma into which fibrous tissue would grow.*

Of 15 patients with the cloth attached to the prosthesis, there were 3 exposures, whereas in 15 patients without the cloth there were 5. All the exposures (except in 1 patient who had not returned) were subsequently repaired either by closure or by removal and subsequent replacement. The authors felt that the cosmetic results were excellent and that a minimum of procedures was needed.

In 1969 Edgerton [66] reported 16 successes out of 18 uses of a silicone rubber ear prosthesis. He also reported both success and failure in the use of Teflon and polyethylene prostheses. In 1969 Curtin, Bader, and Ellenby [65] reported the use of the Silastic otoplasty prosthesis to which Dacron mesh had been attached. They reported only 3 failures out of 42 patients and felt that the device should be a definite consideration in many cases of reconstruction of the external ear, with caution used in the selection of each candidate and in each surgical state.

In 1972 Monroe [68] reported on the use of the Silastic otoplasty prosthesis in 10 cases of congenital microtias, 5 ears reconstructed after burns, and 2 after trauma. Fourteen of these prostheses had been in place for 1½ to 5 years, and 3 were thus far incomplete. Exposure again is the main complication, 1 device having been exposed for 3 months. All, including the latter, were either snipped and closed, or removed and later replaced successfully. Monroe felt that a delay of 2 to 3 months before bringing out the ear contributed to success.

Lynch, Pousti, and Doyle [67] reported on 46 patients in whom 56 ears had been rebuilt with a silicone rubber prosthesis. Again exposure was the chief complication; 25 percent of the congenital implants, 50 percent of the post-traumatic implants, and 70 percent of the postburn implants required removal. They stated that although the procedure is not condemned, it should not be routinely employed in post-traumatic patients and not be used as frequently as cartilage in congenital deformities.

In summary, the consensus at the time of writing seems to be that in selected patients, particularly those in whom the possibility of future trauma is low, a silicone rubber ear armature has the advantage over autogenous cartilage in that it is easily available, it has good architecture, it is easy to sterilize, it reduces the number of operative procedures, it is not absorbed, and most complications can be managed.

The major disadvantage has been exposure, with its concomitant problems. Exposure of a silicone implant, however, is not inevitably followed by the problems experienced with other implant materials,

*Those interested in this use of an artificial stroma of Dacron are advised of the following points: be certain that the Dacron cloth is attached to the prosthesis in such a manner that the interstices of the cloth are open to permit tissue ingrowth. If Dacron tricot is used, it can simply be sewed onto the helix, or it can be "spot-welded" in place with Silastic Medical Adhesive Silicone Type A. Dacron felt has also been used, with attachment by means of the Silicone Adhesive Type A. Both types of textile are available upon request from the Dow Corning Center for Aid to Medical Research, Midland, Mich. 48640.

not even with autografts, and efforts at recovery have proved to be surprisingly effective. In some cases the rubber can be snipped away and then covered again with adjacent skin. Infection has been successfully handled with antibiotics. Should these procedures fail, the removal and subsequent replacement of the prosthesis has been successful, and is worthy of consideration.

Orbit

Dacron, Teflon, and Silastic silicone elastomer have all been used successfully in the immediate reconstruction of the floor of the orbit after fracture [70]. Synthetic implant materials are particularly useful in treatment of the "blow-out" fracture, as described by Converse and Smith [69]. A transverse incision is made over the inferior orbital rim and deepened through the orbicularis muscle to expose the periosteum of the floor of the orbit, which is incised and elevated. A piece of Silastic may be carved to the desired shape and thickness, and wedged firmly into position beneath the periosteum. The hard, medium, and soft blocks of silicone rubber have all been used for this application with the particular variety, as well as its size and shape, being determined by the desire of the surgeon and the degree of deformity requiring correction. This approach is also useful in old depressed malar fractures where there is loss of support of the orbital contents and diplopia. In such cases a larger block of soft Silastic is utilized. In recent years we have preferred Teflon felt in correction of blowout orbital fractures because of the ease with which it is shaped and inserted, and because of its excellent tissue tolerance.

Fine caliber Silastic tubing has been utilized in dacryocystorhinostomy repairs, acting as an inner splint to facilitate healing of the lacrimal duct system [72].

Malar Complex

A moderate degree of depression of the malar may be corrected with a thin strip of soft Silastic block. It is introduced into a pocket over the periosteum through a small incision in one of the lateral wrinkle lines of the eye. Great care must be exercised to eliminate any irregularities in the prosthesis and to make it smooth. There is little subcutaneous fat in this area, and imperfections may become apparent through the overlying skin. In large malar defects, a prefabricated Silastic 382 RTV substitution can be made with the help of a preoperative facial moulage. Such prosthetic appliances should be accurately positioned and held with internal wire fixation [71]. They also can have Dacron fabric attached to allow fibrous tissue ingrowth.

Silicone sponge should be avoided since it changes contour with fibrous tissue invasion. A similar criticism has been applied to Proplast in some cases. The simplest and most effective malar area augmentation has been Dow Corning silicone fluid (MDX 44-011), implanted by injection [92].

Superior Maxilla

In correction of the hypoplastic superior maxilla, or the "dish pan face" secondary to fractures of the middle third of the facial bone, augmentation by silicone implantation is feasible. Under local or general anesthesia, a curved incision is made within the lateral alar fold. A pocket is formed extending under the adjacent check structures and medially under the floor of the nose. Great care must be exercised not to violate the mucosal lining of the floor of the nose, especially in those patients who have had a cleft lip repair. We have used horseshoe-shaped prostheses carved from blocks of Silastic silicone elastomer, inserted through the buccal sulcus. If there is a dental appliance in the superior buccal sulcus, pressure between the appliance and the Silastic implant must be avoided to prevent damage to the mucosal tissue, with formation of a fistula and exposure of the prosthetic material.

Skull

Depressions of the skull secondary to surgery or trauma may include loss of the outer table of bone, both tables of bone, or both tables of bone and the dura. Sheets of Silastic-coated Dacron have been utilized by Taheri [78] and Wallace [79] to replace the dura. Full-thickness defects have long been filled by Vitallium and stainless-steel [75], although recently methyl methacrylate has been used very successfully [180], especially by neurosurgeons, in the closure of bone flap defects.

Laub et al. [72] have described the accurate reconstruction of traumatic bony contour defects of the periorbital area with prefabricated Silastic silicone elastomer. This gives the advantage of reduced heat transfer compared with the metal, and of less shattering compared with the plastic.

A variety of innovative approaches have been described that utilize several acceptable implant materials [71, 73, 74, 76, 77].

Mandible

Teflon and Silastic silicone elastomer have been used to replace the entire lower jaw after a resection for carcinoma [82]. However, such implants may be purely temporary in their usefulness since erosion can occur when dentures are inserted. The compression between the external and internal appliances puts great strain upon the mucosa. Brown et al. [82] have inserted blocks of Silastic into the glenoid area to maintain motion following the resection of the temporomandibular joints for bilateral ankylosis. Movement of tissues or of the implant itself often speeds its ejection from the site, but removal of the implant at a later date in such cases does not seem to affect jaw movements. Marlex 50 has also been used as a replacement for the mandibular condyle [88].

A large number of devices have been utilized successfully for partial jaw defects, full jaw defects, and bridging gaps, utilizing prefabricated devices made of silicone rubber, tantalum mesh, stainless-steel frameworks, chrome cobalt alloys, and others. In some instances, autogenous bone grafts have been used in conjunction with these devices [81–90]. Swanson et al. [90] have successfully combined silicone prefabricated implants with autogenous bone grafts to replace major mandibular losses. A total of 13 patients were treated in this way; extrusion of the implant occurred in 3 of these patients. The bone grafts are inserted through a tunnel to encourage faster vascularization. Bony union has been observed to occur between graft and mandible, with the prosthesis providing the necessary contour.

Skin and Subcutaneous Tissue

Dow Corning Medical Fluid of 350 centistokes viscosity has proved extremely useful in the treatment of defects that could not be improved before except by complicated surgical procedures.

Silicone fluid appears to meet the criteria for an alloplastic material because it is chemically and physically inert; it is extremely simple to use; it is nonantigenic, noncarcinogenic, nontoxic, and locally and systemically nonreactive; it does not change with time, heat, or pressure; it does not support bacterial growth; it is available in sterile form; and it is relatively inexpensive. However, in spite of its intriguing potential for unique usefulness, the possible consequences of releasing silicone fluid for unrestricted use are worrisome. In the United States, final approval for the clinical injection of medical silicone fluid has not been given by the federal Food and Drug Administration pending the evaluation of clinical trials by a limited number of investigators working in cooperation with the Dow Corning Corporation. The original injection committee, which was composed of eight surgeons, was organized in 1965 by the Dow Corning Corporation at the direction of the FDA. Supplies of sterilized purified liquid silicone called MDX 44-011 at 350 centistokes viscosity were made available only to this group of investigators. In 1967 the material was withdrawn and all supplies were withheld until March, 1969, when a new IND was instituted and supplies again were made available to the same investigators. In 1976 the IND was terminated, and at the time of this writing the American Society of Plastic and Reconstructive Surgeons is cooperating with the Dow Corning Company and the FDA in an expanding program that includes a much larger number of investigators. It should be emphasized that in no case was silicone fluid permitted for augmentation of the breast, and in all cases a complete laboratory screening (including complete blood count, hemoglobin, urinalysis, and SMA-12) was required before injection and at intervals thereafter. To the date of this writing, no untoward systemic results have been reported, and tissue tolerance in general has been excellent [91, 92, 95, 96].

Silicone fluid is mainly useful in the treatment of serious facial deformities that cannot be corrected satisfactorily by surgical procedures. I have treated over 50 cases of hemifacial atrophy (Romberg's disease) with uniformly satisfactory results. Facial lipodystrophy, first and second branchial arch deformities, and some post-traumatic and postoperative facial deformities lend themselves well to injection treatment. In those cases where scleroderma and associated pigmentation changes in the skin are present, a good result may be more difficult to obtain. The success of injection therapy is limited to some extent by the degree to which the soft tissues can be stretched by the injectant. In cases where the skin is stretched tight over bone, the results are less satisfactory. I have utilized the material successfully in superior maxilla hypoplasias in adults secondary to radical cleft palate pushback surgery in infancy that resulted in the characteristic "flatface deformity." My use of the material has included defects secondary to nasal fractures, postradiation facial deformity, receding chin, subcutaneous atrophy secondary to facial acne, oral and perioral deformities secondary to an alveolar ridge resorption and rhytidies. I no longer favor the use of silicone fluid to obliterate wrinkling of the skin, frown lines, or nasolabial fold lines, and my experience indicates that injecting silicone fluid into the eyelid areas is contraindicated. Experience has shown that facial tissues accept the cautious implantation of small quantities of silicone fluid introduced at intervals, but utilization in the upper extremities has limited application and in the lower extremities is contraindicated [93].

The technique for using silicone fluid is as follows [91, 92]. After an adequate skin preparation, 1% lidocaine (Xylocaine) is injected with sparse subcutaneous infiltration. Block anesthesia is utilized wherever possible. Injections of the Dow Corning Medical Fluid are given subcutaneously with a #23 or 27 needle, using a standard tuberculin syringe, in amounts diminishing from about 10 ml. initially to 1 ml. as the final contour develops, at biweekly intervals, or longer, according to convenience. Care is taken to inject only small quantities in one place, using a "fanning-out technique." In this way, large cystic spaces are prevented, and patients are encouraged to massage the area gently either by hand or with a vibrator to help disperse this material. The patients usually report a slight swelling in the area for 2 to 4 days, but discomfort is minimal. Apparently the dimethylpolysiloxane fluid is dispersed into numerous small droplets in the adipose and subdermal tissue. Histologically, there is very limited inflammatory response.

Over a period of 16 years, all patients on whom I used MDX 44-011 have been pleased or satisfied with the results, with the greatest enthusiasm shown by those patients with the most significant deformities. Soft tissue augmentation that had formerly required extensive surgery could be accomplished swiftly and with relative simplicity and freedom from pain. I was conservative in using the fluid, limiting the amount to a few milliliters during each injection episode, although the initial treatment involved injecting as much as 12 ml. in severe cases. Most adults will tolerate the injection of silicone fluid without any anesthesia at all, although frequently a block of the supraorbital, infraorbital, or mental nerves will be helpful. Infiltrating the tissues with anesthetic agent prior to injection disguises the deformity and makes accurate sculpturing difficult. In my experience the largest total amount of silicone fluid deposited for the correction of severe hemifacial was 95 ml. After 6 years, this patient has exhibited no untoward reaction to the silicone and has enjoyed a remarkable improvement in appearance.

Tissue response as reported by the Dow Corning investigators has been excellent. Immediately following multiple needle insertion and vigorous massage, patients experience slight burning and discomfort, but practically none require any analgesic. The initial reaction subsides generally within 24 to 72 hours and in no case have I seen any inflammatory reaction. Edgerton et al. [103] have described a severe granulomatous reaction in a lower extremity following extensive injection of the fluid, and Wilkie [97] has described a late development of granuloma in the face. All of these cases responded to treatment with antibiotics, antihistamines, or cortisone. It should be emphasized, however, that no reaction should be credited to dimethylpolysiloxane itself until the following are known: the exact source of the material, the technique of injection, the exact amount injected, and the identity of the injector. Experience with the Sakurai silicone fluid from Japan has demonstrated convincingly that small amounts of contaminate can produce catastrophe [94, 95]. It is my view that extensive use of contaminated or commercial silicone fluid injected by unauthorized and inexperienced physicians in completely contraindicated portions of the body (e.g., the breast) has created an environment of unwarranted suspicion in regard to pure medical grade silicone fluid. Eventually I anticipate a clear delineation of indications for this material, and it will assume its rightful place as a valuable adjunct in the treatment of severe facial deformity.

Pharynx

In cases of velopharyngeal incompetence with nasal emission in speech where the palate is too short to close the velopharyngeal orifice completely, a posterior pharyngeal implant may be effective in improving speech. After animal experimentation to prove the safety of silicones used [108], a variety of Silastic silicone rubber implants have been buried into the posterior pharynx, with encouraging speech results in correcting rhinolalia, but with a high percentage of rejections [98, 99]. A survey was conducted by the authors in which 378 surgeons participated to gain a broader perspective on the use of various implantation materials in the posterior pharynx [100]. Conclusions drawn from this survey in our experience are as follows:

1. Patients most likely to benefit from a posterior pharyngeal implant met the following criteria:
   a. Soft palate relatively mobile with good levator function.
   b. Lateral pharyngeal motion normal.
   c. Nasal emission in speech minimal.
   d. Closure failure does not exceed 3 to 4 mm.
   e. Younger patients were better candidates than older ones.
   f. Intelligence normal or above normal.
2. To ensure proper selection of patients who could be benefited, preoperative evaluation studies should be *complete.* Decisions regarding the degree and type of incompetence can best be made with the assistance of the oral cleft team.
3. Implants should be placed at the level of maximal potential for soft palate impact, usually just above the atlas promontory. The incision should be large enough to admit the implant, but as small as possible. Hess et al. [105] preferred a 2-cm. transverse incision into which they placed homogenous cartilage. It is essential that the pocket should be deep enough, well underneath the muscle and above the prevertebral fascia. The velum should be carefully retracted and an atraumatic technique used.
4. Virtually all autogenous tissues used in the posterior pharynx have shown a high rate of absorption, with good speech results reported by some authors despite the obvious absorption of the implant [105]. Of the inert materials used, virtually all showed a significant rejection percentage, with solid silicone rubber implants showing

approximately 50 percent rejection rate [100]. It is nevertheless evident that while synthetic implants have a high erosion rate, they are more effective over the long term because of the late absorption rate of tissue implants.

5. The most effective inert material placed in the posterior pharynx to date with the least percentage of loss is Teflon paste, supplied by the Ethicon Corporation to investigators under the trade name DTFE [106]. The Teflon paste is a 50 percent suspension of 50- to 100-micron particles of polytetrafluoroethylene in glycerine. Although the material has the consistency of toothpaste, it will pass through a 17-gauge needle attached to a special Brunning syringe. Among the first to use this technique, Ward [111, 112] recommends the formation of a hump or ridge across the posterior pharynx confining the Teflon paste to the submucosa and superior constrictor muscle. It is prevented from progressing along the prevertebral fascia inferiorly by pressing a tongue depressor or similar broad curved retractor against the body of the first cervical vertebrae. The quantity of material injected varies from 2 to 30 cc. per injection, although our experience in injecting this material indicates a need for caution in injecting amounts above 5 cc.

Bluestone et al. [101] have cautioned that Teflon paste is effective only in small-sized velopharyngeal deficits where the gap between the pharynx and soft palate is not over 3 mm. Our own experience confirms this observation and a decision to utilize Teflon has been based on preoperative inspection with the Taub oral panendoscope in all cases. It has been especially helpful in those cases where leakage in the gutters continues after pharyngeal flap, and reduction in the lateral ports must be accomplished to eliminate nasal emission in speech. It should be emphasized that Teflon paste for injection continues under FDA regulation at the time of this writing, and a final conclusion regarding its usage cannot yet be reached.

To date in our series of 70 patients in whom we have utilized Teflon paste in the posterior pharynx, we have seen four complications. The first was an acute streptococcus pharyngitis which subsided within 4 days after treatment with antibiotics. This has lead us subsequently to use prophylactic antibiotics concurrent with each pharyngeal implant. The second was an area of ulceration in the posterior pharynx with exposure of a portion of the implant and requiring surgical excision. In this patient normal speech was maintained. In two other patients 3 and 4 years after injection, a granuloma-like foreign body reaction was evidenced by a gradually increasing mass in the posterior pharynx requiring surgical excision. In each case, recovery was without incidence. Other investigators have made similar observations [107, 109, 110].

Brauer [102] reports excellent results with retropharyngeal implantation of "silicone gel pillows."

Neck

Esophageal reconstruction has been attempted with some measure of success by replacement with a silicone rubber tube to which a Dacron skirt has been welded at each end for attachment purposes [104]. This procedure is at present still in the research stage.

Breasts

A great variety of materials have been utilized for mammary augmentation, but the silicones provide the best inert material for this purpose. Early experiences with Silastic silicone rubber sponge [103] and with Etheron and Ivalon sponges were successful only temporarily because the creeping invasion of the sponge with fibrous tissue made them increasingly firm. This problem was partially corrected by the development of the Edwards Teflon-silicone [117] and the Pangman polyurethane-silicone [119] breast implants. In both these implants, a silicone layer forms a barrier to tissue ingrowth into the sponge. Ashley uses a thin sponge cover on a silicone gel–filled silicone rubber bag [113, 114].

I prefer to use the Dow Corning silastic mammary prostheses without Dacron fixation patches, exercising conservatism in regard to size. Cronin and Gerow [115] first utilized a contoured silicone rubber bag containing a very soft gelatinous silicone gel for breast augmentation and it has, in our opinion, stood the test of time with modifications. The use of this prosthesis has generally resulted in breasts with pleasing contours and with softness comparable to the young adult breast [116]. Also available are silicone mammary prostheses which are implanted as unfilled sacks and then inflated with saline to the desired size. These inflatable prostheses have a distinct advantage in treating breast asymmetry, and it is possible to insert them with minimal scar [118, 119, 122]. Cases of accidental deflation have been reported.

To reduce scarring, it is also possible to insert the mammary prosthesis through a small incision along the inferior margin of the nipple areola. The most common early complication of augmentation mammoplasty is hematoma, and the most frequent late complication is firmness of the operated breast [121]. Treatment of these complications, together with a summary of indications for augmentation mammoplasty and technique for insertion of breast prostheses, is presented in Chapter 44.

Chest

For minor deformities of the chest, the use of a Silastic rubber implant is useful. The correction of *pectus excavatum* by the subcutaneous implantation of catalyzed Silastic 382 RTV has been described by Murray [125]. Since long-accepted methods for correcting pectus excavatum have required extensive exposure and an operation of considerable magnitude, the use of the inert preformed Silastic silicone rubber certainly presents a less complicated method for correcting the funnel chest deformity where there are no associated medical problems [124]. Also, in another approach, through a small transverse incision, a pocket is formed in the region of the deformity, into which is poured the catalyzed Silastic 382 RTV silicone rubber. The material sets up to a rubbery subcutaneous solid, which is virtually free from any reaction in the tissue and gives an adequate cosmetic effect. The silicone gel utilized in the Cronin prosthesis has also been inserted for the correction of combined chest wall and breast deformities [123]. Ultimately, small silicone rubber gel "pillows" covered with Dacron may be found useful in correcting such chest deformities as pectus excavatum and congenital absence of pectoralis muscles.

Although we have used injectable silicone fluid for mild cases of pectus excavatum, our best result has been achieved with the use of Silastic 382 RTV silicone rubber introduced through a very small incision after the addition of stannous octuate catalyst. The catalyzed Silastic sets up under direct vision and can be gently molded to the desired contour. If the procedure is done in two stages, creating the pocket first and then introducing the gel at a separate surgical procedure, the dangers of hematoma can be averted [127].

Genitalia

Testicular Prostheses

These prostheses are available in the form of prefabricated Silastic 370 ovules for those patients who have had orchidectomy [133]. The insertion of one of these devices into a pocket in the scrotum produced through a high scrotal incision is relatively simple. Oversized testicles are available by special order through the manufacturer. Silicone gel–filled testicular prostheses are now available in four sizes and are said to yield a more natural consistency after implantation [131, 133, 134].

Lash [130] and Pearman [132] have devised operations for organic impotence that involve the insertion of a specially prepared Silastic 372 rod along the dorsum of the penis into a pocket specially prepared for this purpose.

Urethral Reconstruction

Reconstruction of the urethra by replacement throughout its length with a silicone rubber tube has been reported by de Nicola [128]. We have reconstructed the membranous urethra over a silicone rubber tube after winding a thick split-thickness skin graft, raw surface out, in spiral fashion around the tube and securing it firmly with sutures prior to its insertion. A skin-lined tube results. In one case in which we performed this operation, there was normal urinary function continuing after 3 years. Silastic prostheses have been used successfully for the control of urinary incontinence in the male and for repair of urethral strictures [129, 134]. Polytef by injection has also been utilized in a urethroplasty for correction of urinary incontinence [126].

Extremities

Bones and Joints

The past few years have seen much work on the replacement of both bones and joints. The chrome-cobalt alloys and 316L stainless steel have been used to make a wide variety of prostheses for use with, or in place of, bone; examples include femoral heads, plates, screws, wire, and rods. High-density polyethylene has been used for constructing the acetabulum. Its application to this use, plus the development of methacrylate "cement" to lock the acetabulum in place, has permitted the orthopedic surgeon to perform many successful total hip replacements. Methacrylate and Teflon have been used to construct femoral heads, but have proved to be unsatisfactory because of the high stresses encountered.

Brannon [135] and Flatt [138] have designed metal hinge prostheses that insert into the medullary canals of the articulating phalanges for complete joint replacement in the hand.

Niebauer et al. [140] and Swanson [142] have developed finger joint prostheses of silicone rubber. The motion takes place within the rubber. Thousands of these rubbery prostheses have been used for the repair of hands affected with rheumatoid arthritis. Swanson reports the correction of deformity in 97 percent of 3,409 metacarpophalangeal joints operated on in 211 clinics. The range of motion achieved was from 4 to 57 degrees.

Kessler and Axer [139] report on arthroplasty of the first carpometacarpal joint, and Swanson reports on the replacement of the trapezium to achieve the same repair of this joint [143]. Swanson also reports on the replacement of the carpal lunate and scaphoid [141], a great toe prosthesis for repair of bunions [144], and prostheses for the ulnar [136] and radial heads [137].

Tendons

Experimental tendons made of Silastic silicone rubber and containing Dacron sutures or ribbon have been tested. These have been successful for short-time function. Numerous other forms of Silastic silicone rubber tubes and rods have also been investigated for this purpose, but long-term failures have been encountered due to breakdown at the anastomotic site. Other investigators [146] have used Silastic silicone rubber tubes or rods to create new tunnels. Subsequently, the rods are removed and replaced with autogenous tendon, thus reducing the incidence of adhesions in badly traumatized areas. The use of these rods aids in the retention of function by permitting motion during the healing period. An excellent technique for the use of silicone rods in the formation of tendon sheaths, with subsequent tendon grafting, has been described by Gaisford, Hanna, and Richardson [147].

Ashley et al. [145] have reported on the use of Silastic silicone rubber sheeting to reduce adhesions at the sites of anastomoses of the autogenous tendon replacement. The sheeting is placed around the area and removed when healing is complete.

Nerves

Amputation neuromas of peripheral nerves have been excised and the nerve inserted into a small-diameter Silastic silicone rubber tube that has one end closed with a glued-on piece of the same material, thus successfully preventing recurrence of the neuroma [148]. A flexible, thin-walled silicone tubular sheath has been designed to provide uniform nonconstricting nerve encasement in peripheral nerve repair. This cuff serves as an immediate pseudoepineurium around the repaired nerve, and appears to aid in the longitudinal alignment of neural regenerating components and limit ingrowth of adjacent scar tissue at the nerve repair site. About a dozen sizes of the Ducker-Hayes design are commercially available for use in peripheral nerve neurorrhaphy [149, 150].

REFERENCES

General

1. Scales, J. T. Discussion on metals and synthetic materials in relation to soft tissues; tissue reaction to synthetic materials. *Proc. R. Soc. Med.* 46:647, 1953.

Materials Available

2. Blocksma, R., and Braley, S. The silicones in plastic surgery. *Plast. Reconstr. Surg.* 35:366, 1965.
3. Grabb, W. C., and Dingman, R. O. Unpublished data presented at the Annual Meeting of the Plastic Surgery Research Council, Spring, 1964.
4. Grau, H. R. Bibliography of foreign substance implants in reconstructive surgery. Addendum No. 2. *Plast. Reconstr. Surg. Trans. Bull.* 29:113, 1962.
5. Leininger, R. I., Mirkovitch, V., Peters, A., and Hawks, W. A. Change in properties of plastics during implantation. *Trans. Am. Soc. Artif. Intern. Organs* 10:320, 1964.
6. Speirs, A. C., and Blocksma, R. New implantable silicone: An experimental evaluation of tissue response. *Plast. Reconstr. Surg.* 31:166, 1963.

Carcinogenicity of Implants

7. Brown, J. B. Editorial: Studies of silicones and Teflon as subcutaneous prostheses. *Plast. Reconstr. Surg.* 28:86, 1961.
8. Brown, J. B., and Ohlwiler, D. A. Evaluation of silicones as tissue substitutes. *The Bulletin,* Dow Corning Center for Aid to Medical Research 2:1, 1960.
9. De Cholnoky, T. Augmentation mammoplasty: Survey of complications in 10,941 patients by 265 surgeons. *Plast. Reconstr. Surg.* 45:573, 1970.
10. Dunaif, C. B., Stubenbord, W. T., and Conway, H. Observations on subcutaneously implanted polyetherurethane sponge in mice. *Surg. Gynecol. Obstet.* 117:454, 1963.
11. Harris, H. I. Survey of breast implants from the point of view of carcinogenesis. *Plast. Reconstr. Surg.* 28:81, 1961.
12. Hueper, W. C. Cancer induction by polyurethane and polysilicone plastics. *J. Natl. Cancer Inst.* 33:1005, 1964.
13. Oppenheimer, B. S., Oppenheimer, E., and Stout, A. P. Sarcomas induced in rodents by imbedding various plastic films. *Proc. Soc. Exp. Biol. Med.* 79:366, 1952.

Nose

14. Aufricht, G. Rhinoplasty and the face. *Plast. Reconstr. Surg.* 43:219, 1969.

15. Barry, W. B. Experimental observations upon reconstruction of the nasal dorsum. *Laryngoscope* 75:1320, 1965.
16. Beekhuis, G. J. Silicone rubber implants in nasal reconstructive surgery. *Laryngoscope* 74:1405, 1964.
17. Beekhuis, G. J. Use of silicone rubber in nasal reconstructive surgery. *Arch. Otolaryngol.* 86: 114, 1967.
18. Caronni, E. P. A new method to correct the nasolabial angle in rhinoplasty. *Plast. Reconstr. Surg.* 50:33, 1972.
19. Cipcic, J. A. Silicone implant correction of facial deformities. *Laryngoscope* 78:4, 1968.
20. Craig, R. D. The correction of facial contour defects by precision-made Silastic implants. *Br. J. Plast. Surg.* 28:67, 1975.
21. Farrior, R. T. Implant materials in restoration of facial contour. *Laryngoscope* 76:934, 1966.
22. Farrior, R. T. Synthetics in head and neck surgery: With particular reference to silicone. *Arch. Otolaryngol.* 84:82, 1966.
23. Freeman, B. M., Biggs, T., and Beall, A. Injectable Silastic in deformities of the facial skeleton. *Arch. Surg.* 90:166, 1965.
24. Freeman, B. S. Proplast, a porous implant for contour restoration. *Br. J. Plast. Surg.* 29:158, 1976.
25. Janeke, J. B., and Shea, J. J. Proplast implants used in otology and in facial reconstructive surgery. *S. Afr. Med. J.* 50:781, 1976.
26. Janeke, J. B., Komorn, R. N., and Cohn, A. Proplast in cavity obliteration and soft tissue augmentation. *Arch. Otolaryngol.* 100:24, 1974.
27. Khoo, B. C. Augmentation rhinoplasty in the Orientals. *Plast. Reconstr. Surg.* 34:81, 1964.
28. Khoo, B. C. Some aspects of plastic (cosmetic) surgery in Orientals. *Br. J. Plast. Surg.* 11:60, 1969.
29. Marshall, A., and Withers, B. T. Silastic as dorsal transplant for saddle nose deformity: A preliminary report. *Eye Ear Nose Throat Monthly* 47:40, 1968.
30. Millard, D. R. Alar margin sculpturing. *Plast. Reconstr. Surg.* 40:337, 1967.
31. Morani, A. D. Surgery of facial trauma. Review of principles of treatment. *Int. Surg.* 46:391, 1966.
32. Patterson, C. N. Reconstructive septonasoplasty. *Arch. Otolaryngol.* 84:457, 1966.
33. Rees, T. D. Nasal plastic surgery in the Negro. *Plast. Reconstr. Surg.* 43:13, 1969.
34. Rhodes, R. D., III. Restoration of facial defects with individually prefabricated silicone prostheses. *Plast. Reconstr. Surg.* 43:201, 1968.
35. Riggs, R., and Wilson, J. W., Jr. Relapsing polychondritis: Report of a case. *Laryngoscope* 77: 534, 1967.
36. Rise, E., Huffman, W., and VerVais, P. Silicone nasal implants: A pilot study on dogs. *Plast. Reconstr. Surg.* 36:231, 1965.
37. Safian, J. Progress in nasal and chin augmentation. *Plast. Reconstr. Surg.* 37:446, 1966.
38. Stark, R. B., and Frileck, S. P. Conchal cartilage grafts in augmentation rhinoplasty and orbital floor fracture. *Plast. Reconstr. Surg.* 43:591, 1969.
39. Stellmach, R. Reconstruction of facial contours with Silastic. *Fortschr. Kiefer Gesichtschir.* 12: 141, 1967.
40. Uchida, J. I. A design for a prosthesis in augmentation rhinoplasty: The projection method. *Plast. Reconstr. Surg.* 33:485, 1964.
41. Vinas, J. Surgical experiences with silicone rubber implants. Presented at the meeting of Uruguayan Society Plastic Surgeons, October 1962.

Chin

42. Bayne, H. R. Pseudoretrognathia: Evaluation and treatment. *Dent. Dig.* 72:112, 1966.
43. Bell, W. H. Correction of the contour-deficient chin. *J. Oral Surg.* 27:108, 1969.
44. Brown, J. B., Fryer, M. P., and Ohlwiler, D. A. Study and use of synthetic materials, such as silicones and Teflon, as subcutaneous prostheses. *Plast. Reconstr. Surg.* 26:264, 1960.
45. Brown, J. B., Fryer, M. P., Ohlwiler, D. A., and Kollias, P. Dimethylpolysiloxane and halogenated carbons as subcutaneous prostheses. *Am. Surg.* 28:146, 1962.
46. Calderwood, R. G. Polydimethylsiloxane implants in oral surgery. *J. Oral Surg.* 26:33, 1968.
47. De Moura Andrews, J. Inclusoes de silicone: Estudo experimental e clinico. *Escola Paul. Med.*, 1966.
48. Friedland, J. A., Coccaro, P. J., and Converse, J. M. Retrospective cephalometric analysis of mandibular bone absorption under silicone rubber chin implants. *Plast. Reconstr. Surg.* 57:144, 1976.
49. Merrin, M. L., Parkes, M. L., and Kamer, F. M. Proplast chin augmentation. Presented at the Second International Symposium on Plastic and Reconstructive Surgery of the Head and Neck, Chicago, June 1975.
50. Meyer, R. A., Behrig, J. D., Funk, E. C., and Beder, O. E. Restoring facial contour with implanted silicone rubber. *Oral Surg.* 24:598, 1967.
51. Millard, D. R. Unpublished data presented at the meeting of the American Society of Plastic and Reconstructive Surgery, Philadelphia, October 1965.
52. Parker, M. Avoiding bone absorption under plastic chin implants. *Arch. Otolaryngol.* 98:101, 1973.

53. Parkes, M. L. Chin implants with a newer plastic compound. *Arch. Otolaryngol.* 74:429, 1962.
54. Pitanguy, I. Augmentation mentoplasty. *Plast. Reconstr. Surg.* 42:5, 1968.
55. Rish, B. B. Alloplastic materials in the creation of facial contour. *Arch. Otolaryngol.* 72:212, 1960.
56. Rish, B. B. The esthetic-plastic profile. *Proc. Penn. Acad. Ophthalmol. Otolaryngol.* 18:79, 1965.
57. Robinson, M., and Shuken, R. Bone resorption under plastic chin implants. *J. Oral Surg.* 27:116, 1969.
58. Rubin, L. R., Bromberg, B. E., and Walden, R. H. Long term human reaction to synthetic plastic. *Surg. Gynecol. Obstet.* 132:603, 1971.
59. Safian, J. Silastic chin implant. *The Bulletin* 14-085, Medical Products Division, Dow Corning Corp., 1965.
60. Scheunemann, H. Kinnkonstruktion mit Silastik in Combination mit einem fromgebenden Kirschner-Draht. *ZWR.* 79:3, 1970.
61. Serson, D. A new technique of chin augmentation. *Plast. Reconstr. Surg.* 46:406, 1970.
62. Weinstein, I. R., and Veiner, A. Chin implant. *Dent. Surg.* 44:45, 1968.

Ear

63. Cronin, T. D. Use of a Silastic frame for total and subtotal reconstruction of the external ear: Preliminary report. *Plast. Reconstr. Surg.* 37:399, 1966.
64. Cronin, T. D., Greenberg, R. L., and Brauer, R. O. Follow-up study of Silastic frame for reconstruction of external ear. *Plast. Reconstr. Surg.* 42:6, 1968.
65. Curtin, J. W., Bader, K. F., and Ellenby, J. E. Improved techniques for the successful reconstruction of the external ear. *Plast. Reconstr. Surg.* 44:372, 1969.
66. Edgerton, M. T. Ear construction in children with congenital atresia and stenosis. *Plast. Reconstr. Surg.* 43:373, 1969.
67. Lynch, J. B., Pousti, A., and Doyle, J. E. Experience with Silastic ear implants. *Plast. Reconstr. Surg.* 49:283, 1972.
68. Monroe, C. W. Experience with the silicone ear prosthesis: A report of 17 ears on 15 patients. *Plast. Reconstr. Surg.* 49:428, 1972.

Orbital Floor

69. Converse, J. M., and Smith, B. Enophthalmos and diplopia in fractures of the orbital floor. *Br. J. Plast. Surg.* 9:265, 1957.
70. Lipschultz, H., and Ardizone, R. The use of silicone rubber in the immediate reconstruction of fractures of the floor of the orbit. *J. Trauma* 3:563, 1963.

Skull

71. Brown, J. B., Fryer, M. P., and Lu, M. Polyvinyl and silicone compounds as subcutaneous prosthesis. *Arch. Surg.* 68:744, 1954.
72. Laub, D. R., Spohn, W., Holderness, H., Lash, H., and Crowley, L. Accurate preoperative fabrication of subcutaneous and bony implants with Silastic MDX 4-4515 and MDX 4-4516: Technique and results. *Bull. Prosthet. Res.* 206, Spring 1970.
73. Maniscalco, J. E., and Garcia-Bengochea, F. Cranioplasty: A method of prefabricating alloplastic plates. *Surg. Neurol.* 2:339, 1974.
74. Schenck, N. L., Tomlinson, M. J., and Ridgley, C. D. Experimental evaluation of a new implant material in frontal sinus obliteration. *Arch. Otolaryngol.* 102:524, 1976.
75. Scott, M., Wycis, H., and Murtagh, F. Long term evaluation of stainless steel cranioplasty. *Surg. Gynecol. Obstet.* 115:453, 1962.
76. Segall, B. S. The construction and implantation of a silicone rubber cranial prosthesis. *J. Prosthet. Dent.* 31:184, 1974.
77. Shaw, R. C., and Thering, H. R. Reconstruction of cranial defects. *Clin. Plast. Surg.* 2:539, 1975.
78. Taheri, Z. E. Silicone dura substitute. *The Bulletin,* Dow Corning Center for Aid to Medical Research 5:4, 1963.
79. Wallace, W. E. Prosthesis for dural defects. *The Bulletin,* Dow Corning Center for Aid to Medical Research 2:1, 1960.
80. Woolf, J. I., and Walker, A. E. Cranioplasty, collective review. *Surg. Gynecol. Obstet.* 81:1, 1945.

Mandible

81. Bear, S. E., et al. Experimental use of stainless steel wire mesh in mandibular defects. *J. Oral Surg.* 31:348, 1973.
82. Brown, J. R., Fryer, M. P., Kollias, P., Ohlwiler, D. A., and Templeton, J. B. Silicone and Teflon prostheses, including full jaw substitution: Laboratory and clinical studies of Etheron. *Ann. Surg.* 157:932, 1963.
83. Habal, M. B., and Chalian, V. A. Prefabricated silicone subdermal mandibular implants: Observations and problems related to their application. *J. Biomed. Mater. Res.* 10:529, 1976.
84. Hartwell, S. W., Jr., and Hall, M. D. Mandibular condylectomy with silicone rubber replacement. *Plast. Reconstr. Surg.* 53:440, 1974.
85. Kent, J., Lavelle, W., and Dolan, K. D. Condylar reconstruction: Treatment planning. *Oral Surg.* 37:489, 1974.
86. Leake, D., Murray, J. E., Habel, M. B., and Swanson, L. T. Custom fabrication for mandibular reconstruction. *Oral Surg.* 33:879, 1972.
87. McQuarrie, D. G. Immediate functional restora-

tion of the mandible after surgical treatment of advanced oral cancer: A simple prosthesis. *Arch. Surg.* 102:447, 1971.

88. Pennisi, V. R., Shapiro, R. L., Boucher, J. H., Pickens, G. E., and Shadish, W. R. Marlex 50 as a replacement for the mandibular condyle. *Plast. Reconstr. Surg.* 35:212, 1965.
89. Schechter, L., and Pories, W. Partial mandibular replacement with a silicone strut. *Am. J. Surg.* 113:846, 1967.
90. Swanson, L. T., Habal, M. B., Leake, D. L., and Murray, J. E. Compound silicone-bone implants for mandibular reconstruction. Development and application. *Plast. Reconstr. Surg.* 51:402, 1973.

Injection

91. Ashley, F. L., Thompson, D. P., and Henderson, T. Augmentation of surface contour by subcutaneous injections of silicone fluid: A current report. *Plast. Reconstr. Surg.* 51:8, 1973.
92. Blocksma, R. Experience with dimethylpolysiloxane in soft tissue augmentation. *Plast. Reconstr. Surg.* 48:564, 1971.
93. Edgerton, M. T., and Wells, J. H. Indications for and pitfalls of soft tissue augmentation with liquid silicone. *Plast. Reconstr. Surg.* 58:157, 1976.
94. Kagan, H. D. Sakurai injectable silicone formula. *Arch. Otolaryngol.* 78:53, 1963.
95. Rees, T. D. Silicone Injection Therapy. In Rees, T. D., and Wood-Smith, D. (Eds.), *Cosmetic Facial Surgery*. Philadelphia: Saunders, 1970.
96. Rees, T. D., Ashley, F. L., and Delgado, J. P. Silicone fluid injections for facial atrophy: A ten-year study. *Plast. Reconstr. Surg.* 52:118, 1973.
97. Wilkie, T. F. Late development of granuloma after liquid silicone injections. *Plast. Reconstr. Surg.* 60:179, 1977.

Pharynx

98. Blocksma, R. Correction of velopharyngeal insufficiency by Silastic pharyngeal implant. *Plast. Reconstr. Surg.* 31:268, 1963.
99. Blocksma, R. Silicone implants for velopharyngeal incompetence: A progress report. *Cleft Palate J.* 1:72, 1964.
100. Blocksma, R., and Bradley, S. Current status of retropharyngeal implantation for velopharyngeal insufficiency. *Plast. Reconstr. Surg.* 44:242, 1969.
101. Bluestone, C. D., Musgrave, R. H., and McWilliams, B. J. Teflon injection pharyngoplasty – status 1968. *Laryngoscope* 4:558, 1968.
102. Brauer, R. O. Retropharyngeal implantation of silicone gel pillows for velopharyngeal incompetence. *Plast. Reconstr. Surg.* 51:254, 1973.
103. Demergian, V. Experience with the newer subcutaneous implant materials. *Surg. Clin. North Am.* 43:1313, 1963.
104. Fryfogle, J. D., Cyrowski, G. A., Rothwell, D., Rheault, G., and Clark, T. Replacement of the middle third of the esophagus with a silicone rubber prosthesis: An experimental and clinical study. *Dis. Chest* 43:464, 1963.
105. Hess, D. A., Hagerty, R. F., and Mylin, W. K. Velar motility velopharyngeal closure and speech proficiency in cartilage pharyngoplasty: An eight year study. *Cleft Palate J.* 5:153, 1968.
106. Lewy, R., Cole, R., and Wepman, J. Teflon injection in the correction of velopharyngeal insufficiency. *Ann. Otol. Rhinol. Laryngol.* 74:3, 1965.
107. Rubin, A. J. Misadventures with injectable polytef (Teflon). *Arch. Otolaryngol.* 101:114, 1975.
108. Speirs, A. C., and Blocksma, R. New implantable silicone: An experimental evaluation of tissue response. *Plast. Reconstr. Surg.* 31:166, 1963.
109. Sturim, H. S. Bleeding complication with pharyngeal flap construction in humans following Teflon pharyngoplasty. *Cleft Palate J.* 11: 292, 1974.
110. Walsh, F. M., and Castelli, J. B. Polytef granuloma clinically simulating carcinoma of the thyroid. *Arch. Otolaryngol.* 101:262, 1975.
111. Ward, P. H. Uses of injectable Teflon in otolaryngology. *Arch. Otolaryngol.* 87:637, 1968.
112. Ward, P. H., and Wepman, W. M. Pharyngeal implants for reduction of air space in velopharyngeal insufficiency: An experimental study. *Ann. Otolaryngol.* 73:443, 1964.

Breast

113. Ashley, F. L. A new type of breast prosthesis: Preliminary report. *Plast. Reconstr. Surg.* 45: 421, 1970.
114. Ashley, F. L. Further studies on the natural-Y breast prosthesis. *Plast. Reconstr. Surg.* 49:414, 1972.
115. Cronin, T. D., and Gerow, F. J. Augmentation Mammaplasty: A New "Natural Feel" Prosthesis. In Transactions of the Third International Conference of Plastic Surgery. Amsterdam: Excerpta Medica, 1964.
116. Cronin, T. D., and Greenberg, R. L. Our experiences with the Silastic gel breast prosthesis. *Plast. Reconstr. Surg.* 46:1, 1970.
117. Edwards, B. F. Teflon-silicone breast implants. *Plast. Reconstr. Surg.* 32:519, 1963.
118. Mutou, Y. Augmentation mammaplasty with the Akiyama prosthesis. *Br. J. Plast. Surg.* 23:1, 1970.

119. Pangman, W. J. A new mammary prosthesis for breast augmentation. Data sheet, Codman & Shurtleff, Inc., Boston, 1965.
120. Tabari, K. Augmentation mammaplasty with Simaplast implant. *Plast. Reconstr. Surg.* 44:468, 1969.
121. Williams, C., Aston, S., and Rees, T. D. The effect of hematoma on the thickness of pseudosheaths around silicone implants. *Plast. Reconstr. Surg.* 56:194, 1975.
122. Wilson, C. A. Experiences with Arion's Simaplast inflatable prosthesis. *South. Med. J.* 62:1107, 1969.

Pectus Excavatum

123. Krause, J. L., Jr., Crikelair, G. F., and Cosman, B. The Cronin implant in the treatment of combined chest wall and breast deformities. *Plast. Reconstr. Surg.* 44:536, 1969.
124. Masson, J. K., Payne, W. S., and Gonzalez, J. B. Pectus excavatum: Use of preformed prosthesis for correction in the adult. *Plast. Reconstr. Surg.* 48:599, 1970.
125. Murray, J. F. Correction of pectus excavatum by synthetic subcutaneous implant. Presented at the meeting of the American Society of Plastic and Reconstructive Surgeons, Philadelphia, October 1965.

Genitalia

126. Berg, S. Polytef augmentation urethroplasty: Correction of surgically incurable urinary incontinence by injection technique. *Arch. Surg.* 107: 379, 1973.
127. Braley, S. The chemistry and properties of medical grade silicones. *J. Macromol. Sci. Chem.* A4:529, 1970.
128. de Nicola, R. R. Permanent artificial (silicone) urethra. *J. Urol.* 63:168, 1950.
129. Heller, E. Surgical repair of urethral strictures with a silicone rubber patch. *J. Urol.* 94:576, 1965.
130. Lash, H. The os penis implant. Presented at the meeting of the American Society of Plastic and Reconstructive Surgeons, Philadelphia, October 1965.
131. Lattimer, J. K. *Bulletin 51-108,* Medical Products Division, Dow Corning Corp., 1972.
132. Pearman, R. O. Insertion of a Silastic penile prosthesis for the treatment of organic sexual impotence. *J. Urol.* 107:802, 1972.
133. Prentiss, R.,Boatwright, D., Pennington, R., Hohn, W., and Schwartz, M. Testicular prosthesis: Materials, methods and results. *J. Urol.* 90:208, 1963.
134. Watkins, J. K., Straffon, R. A., and Poutasse, E. F. A medical Silastic prosthesis for the control of urinary incontinence in the male *Cleve. Clin. Q.* 31:157, 1964.

Extremities

135. Brannon, E. W. Experiences with finger joint prosthesis. *J. Bone Joint Surg.* [Am.] 41:87, 1959.
136. *Bulletin* 51-006A, Medical Products Division, Dow Corning Corp., June 1971.
137. *Bulletin* 51-007A, Medical Products Division, Dow Corning Corp., June 1971.
138. Flatt, A. E. Restoration of rheumatoid finger joint function. *J. Bone Joint Surg.* [Am.] 43: 753, 1961.
139. Kessler, I. I., and Axer, A. Silicone implant for arthroplasty of the first carpometacarpal joint. *Plast. Reconstr. Surg.* 47:252, 1971.
140. Niebauer, J. J., Shaw, J. L., and Doren, W. W. Silicone-Dacron hinge prosthesis: Design evaluation and application. *Ann. Rheum. Dis.* 28:56, 1969.
141. Swanson, A. B. Silicone rubber implants for replacement of carpal scaphoid and lunate bones. *Orthop. Clin. North Am.* 1:299, 1970.
142. Swanson, A. B. Flexible implant arthroplasty for arthritic finger joints: rationale, technique and results of treatment. *J. Bone Joint Surg.* [Am.] 54:435, 1972.
143. Swanson, A. B. Disabling arthritis at the base of the thumb. *J. Bone Joint Surg.* [Am.] 54:456, 1972.
144. Swanson, A. B. Implant arthroplasty for the great toe. *Clin. Orthop.* 85:75, 1972.

Tendon Sheaths

145. Ashley, F. L., McConnell, D. V., Polak, T., Stone, R. S., and Marmor, L. An evaluation of the healing process in avian digital flexor tendons and grafts following the application of an artificial tendon sheath. *Plast. Reconstr. Surg.* 33:411, 1964.
146. Bassett, C. A. L., and Carroll, R. E. Formation of tendon sheath by silicone rod implants. *J. Bone Joint Surg.* [Am.] 45:884, 1963.
147. Gaisford, J. C., Hanna, D. C., and Richardson, G. S. Tendon grafting: A suggested technique. *Plast. Reconstr. Surg.* 38:302, 1966.

Nerves

148. Campbell, J. B. Nerve sheath curbs phantom pain. Paper presented at the meeting of the American Association of Neurologists, May 1965.

149. Ducker, T. B., and Hayes, G. T. A comparative study of the technique of nerve repair. *Surg. Forum* 18:443, 1967.
150. Ducker, T. B., and Hayes, G. T. Experimental improvements in the use of Silastic cuffs for peripheral nerve repair. *J. Neurosurg.* 28:582, 1968.

II

Head and Neck

4

Some Anomalies of the Head and Neck

WILLIAM C. GRABB

Cleft lip and cleft palate, which will be discussed in the following two chapters, are the most common congenital anomalies of the head and neck. This chapter will discuss several others of special interest to the plastic surgeon. These other anomalies are often found together, occurring in specific groupings, so that they are usually referred to as syndromes.

These congenital anomalies can have either a hereditary or an environmental basis. In *most cases* though, the anomaly is caused by an environmental agent interacting with a genetically determined predisposition, so that both factors are important.

Neel [11] has pointed out that the empirical risk for the inheritance of most carefully studied congenital anomalies is between 3 and 5 percent. Thus when we see a child with a rare facial anomaly syndrome whose empirical risk has not been calculated from the pedigrees of a large number of similar patients and there is no known teratogenic agent and no similar anomaly in either family, we can tell the parents that as a rule of thumb there is a 3 to 5 percent chance that they will have another child with this facial anomaly.

No effective classification of these congenital facial anomalies has been devised. Karfik [5] has proposed a classification involving only the rare congenital facial clefts. Information on the treatment of many of these facial anomalies is included in Chapter 5.

HEMIFACIAL MICROSOMIA

(First and second branchial arch syndrome; craniofacial microsomia; oral-mandibular-auricular syndrome; otocraniocephalic syndrome; auriculobranchiogenic dysplasia; necrotic facial dysplasia; intrauterine facial necrosis; otomandibular dystosis; hemignathia and microtia syndrome; and unilateral facial agenesis)

The hemifacial microsomia syndrome is made up of a constellation of congenitally malformed facial structures which arise from the first and second branchial arches, the intervening first pharyngeal pouch and first branchial cleft, and the primordia of the temporal bone. The complete syndrome is not usually fully expressed, though in its fullest expression a patient with this syndrome would exhibit the following (Fig. 4-1):

1. Unilateral or bilateral underdevelopment of the external ear, middle ear, mandible, zygoma, maxilla, temporal bone, facial muscles, muscles of mastication, palatal muscles, tongue, and parotid gland.
2. Macrostomia.
3. First branchial cleft sinus.

Incidence

Males were affected with this syndrome more commonly than females (63 males and 39 females) in one large study [3]. An incidence of this syndrome of *1 in 5,642 births* has been suggested [3] after finding 7 infants with this syndrome in 39,492 hospital births. This ranks the first and second branchial arch syndrome as the second most common facial anomaly syndrome, with cleft lip and/or cleft palate being first.

Etiology

Heredity

The hemifacial microsomia syndrome is inherited only rarely. An abbreviated pedigree of 102 persons with this condition revealed that there were only 4 cases in which either a sibling or a parent was affected with the syndrome. Interestingly enough, all but 1 of the patients had macrostomia along with other facial anomalies included in the first and second branchial arch syndrome [3].

The information from these pedigrees suggests that there is no simple mode of inheritance of this syndrome. Based on the study of 102 persons with the syndrome [3], there would be an empirical risk of 2 percent that subsequent affected children would be born to parents who have a child with this syndrome.

Chromosome studies in persons with this syndrome have shown no indication of abnormal chromosomes segregating in these families [3].

Krampitz [7], Kunkel [8], and Roosa [12] have also described instances of inheritance of the first and second branchial arch syndrome.

Environment

Kleinsasser and Schlothane [6] have reported that the first and second branchial arch syndrome is the second most common malformation resulting from thalidomide ingestion during pregnancy. This malformation occurred in approximately 3,000 children born between January 1959 and July 1962; these children usually had bilateral involvement of facial structures.

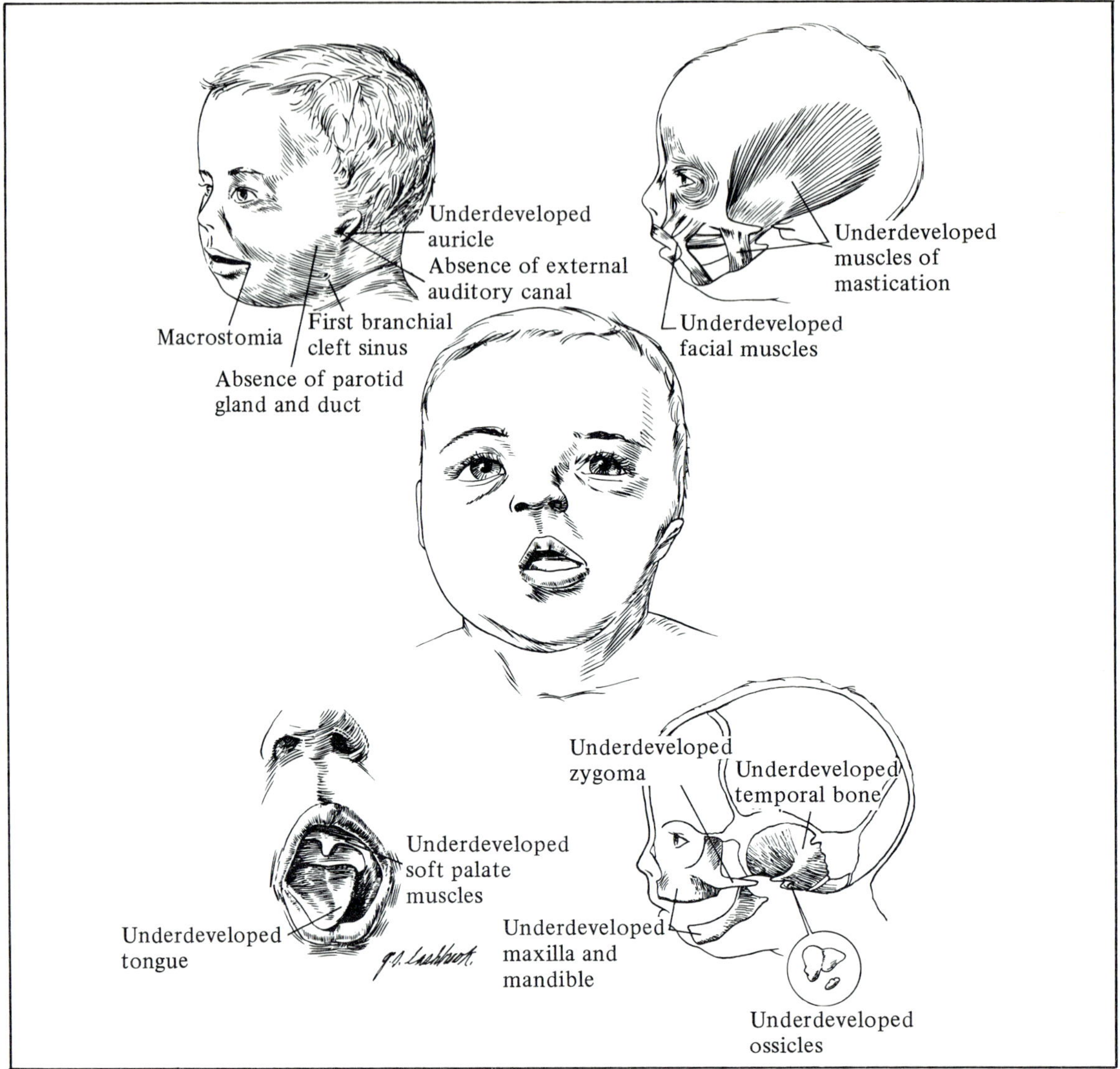

Fig. 4-1. Hemifacial microsomia. Only when the syndrome is fully expressed are all the anomalies illustrated present. This syndrome is usually unilateral.

There are no other reported teratogenic agents that produce this syndrome.

Physical Characteristics

In this syndrome malformations occur in facial structures arising from the first two branchial arches, the intervening first pharyngeal pouch and first branchial cleft, and the primordia of the temporal bone. Though most affected persons will have unilateral facial anomalies, about 10 percent will have bilateral facial anomalies, with one side of the face being more severely affected than the other.

Specific Anomalies

AURICULAR ANOMALIES. These range in degree from an auricle that is only slightly smaller than normal down to one that is represented by two tags of skin. Commonly there is a vertical remnant of skin and cartilage, including a rudimentary lobule.

EXTERNAL AUDITORY CANAL ANOMALIES. The canal is usually absent, but in some instances it is cone-shaped, ending at a rudimentary tympanic membrane.

MIDDLE EAR ANOMALIES. These deformities range from a minimally underdeveloped malleus, incus, or stapes to a complete fusion of the malleus and incus (first branchial arch), and a stapes (second branchial arch) that is represented by a separated ball of bone. The severity of the middle ear anomalies is generally in proportion to the degree of external ear underdevelopment. Patients have a conduction-type hearing loss which ranges between 25 and 70 decibels [3].

MANDIBULAR ANOMALIES. These anomalies vary from a minimal underdevelopment of the condyle to an absence of the ascending ramus and condyle, with underdevelopment of the horizontal ramus. The glenoid fossa of the temporal bone may be underdeveloped or absent. Characteristically, the mandibular deformities are severest in the condylar region and progressively less severe nearer the midline.

MAXILLA AND ZYGOMA UNDERDEVELOPMENT. Varying degrees of underdevelopment of these facial bones may occur, but they have never been seen to be completely absent.

TEMPORAL BONE UNDERDEVELOPMENT. Physical examination and dissections of autopsy material have shown that any part of the temporal bone other than the petrous portion that houses the inner ear may be underdeveloped. The inner ear probably escapes underdevelopment because of its separate origin from the auditory placode.

FACIAL MUSCLE, MASTICATORY MUSCLE, AND PALATAL MUSCLE UNDERDEVELOPMENT. Paresis and decrease in bulk of any of the muscles belonging to these muscle groups can occur.

UNDERDEVELOPMENT OF THE TONGUE. Unilateral hypoplasia of the tongue may be present.

ABSENCE OF THE PAROTID GLAND. The patients with this syndrome may have absence of a functioning parotid gland.

MACROSTOMIA. Persons with macrostomia also usually have an absence of the parotid gland, as well as of the sinuses and remnants of cartilage in the cheek. These are all related to an abnormal fusion of the primordia of the upper and lower jaws.

FIRST BRANCHIAL CLEFT SINUS. This sinus extends from the external auditory canal downward and forward adjacent to the parotid gland and lies either medial or lateral to the facial nerve. Its course continues downward posterior to the angle of the mandible to open inferior to the body of the mandible halfway between the anterior border of the sternocleidomastoid muscle and the midline of the neck. A generous portion of the parotid gland must usually be excised during the removal of this sinus tract.

Associated Anomalies

Some of the other congenital anomalies found in conjunction with the first and second branchial arch syndrome and their incidence in one large series [3] are as follows:

1. Anomalies of the vertebrae and/or ribs (11 out of 102 persons). The vertebral anomalies may consist of hemivertebrae, fusion of vertebrae, spina bifida, and scoliosis.
2. Anomalies of the eye and/or eyelid (10 out of 102 persons). These consisted of epibulbar dermoid, microphthalmia, bilateral eyelid ptosis, coloboma of the upper eyelid, and strabismus.
3. Cleft lip and/or cleft palate (7 out of 102 persons).

This syndrome does not appear to have as strong an association with the malformations of the genitourinary tract as certain other auricular anomalies [4, 14].

Treatment

Auricular Anomaly

The treatment of this anomaly for males is different from that for females. The microtic ear of a boy can be either constructed with autogenous tissues or replaced with a prosthetic ear, as discussed in Chapter 13. A girl does not necessarily need correction of the auricular anomaly because it can be covered so easily by either long hair or proper hair styling. If the lobule tends to show beneath the hair, it can be placed in a more normal position posteriorly by transposing it with a postauricular flap of skin.

Bony Anomalies

ONLAY GRAFTS. The most practical method of correcting a unilateral underdevelopment of the mandible is by onlay grafts of autogenous bone or preserved cartilage. Implants such as medical grade silicone of the solid type can also be used. Longacre et al. [11, 12] have described the technique of removing alternate ribs from the patient and then splitting these ribs lengthwise to provide additional bone. Two or three ribs, such as the sixth, eighth, and tenth ribs, can be removed at one operation, being careful to leave alternate ribs to prevent respiratory distress. The periosteum of these ribs is left in pace to encourage bony regeneration, thus providing an unlimited supply of bone. Longacre has used a rib regenerated from the same bed as often as five times.

Cartilage allografts preserved by irradiation [2] have also been used effectively as onlay grafts for the mandible. They have shown no signs of resorption when in good contact with bone and become readily fixed to it by the fibrous tissue.

Because of the deviation of the mandible toward the affected side, the normal body of the mandible often appears to be severely flattened. Thus the grafts are usually placed over the normal body of the mandible; however, when there is marked mandibular underdevelopment, grafts to both sides are required. These grafts are usually inserted onto the body of the mandible through a submandibular incision 3 or 4 cm. long. The pocket for the graft can be dissected with long curved scissors, with care taken to stay close to bone. Fixation of the graft by means of fine wire sutures passed through holes drilled in the bone is often carried out.

This mandibular deformity is commonly corrected at the age of 16 years when the mandible has nearly reached its full growth. Longacre [9, 10] reported on the reconstruction of the facial bones with onlay split-rib grafts in young children (ages 3 to 5 years) with first and second branchial arch syndrome. As these children grow older, additional grafts are required to build out the underdeveloped facial bones so that they will correspond to the increasing size of the bone structure on the normal side of the face.

Converse [1] has written extensively on this subject. Other operative procedures are included in Chapter 5.

Paresis of Facial, Masticatory, and Palatal Muscles

FACIAL MUSCLES. These muscles usually have some degree of function, so fascial sling operations to support the affected side of the face are unnecessary.

MUSCLES OF MASTICATION. No treatment of these unilateral paretic muscles is indicated as they, along with the normal muscles on the unaffected side, are strong enough to permit mastication.

PALATAL MUSCLES. In no instance has velopharyngeal insufficiency due to the unilateral paresis of the palatal muscles been reported.

Macrostomia

Macrostomia can be corrected at any time. Stark and Saunders [13] excise the excess tissue from the oral aperture and then close it in layers. When the macrostomia is large, a Z-plasty of the skin will improve the appearance of the scar. This Z can be outlined on the skin after the wound has been temporarily sutured. To position the commissure properly requires care, and it is advisable to insert a triangular flap or mucosa into this angle to prevent its obliteration by progressive scar contracture. Longacre [10] chooses to mark out the Z-plasty flaps, one from the upper lip and one from the lower lip, prior to the repair of the macrostomia.

TREACHER COLLINS SYNDROME

(Mandibulofacial dysostosis, Berry syndrome, Franceschetti-Zwahlein-Klein syndrome, bilateral facial agenesis)

The Treacher Collins syndrome is an uncommon hereditary syndrome that is seen in any degree of severity ranging from the complete form to the incomplete form to the abortive form [15, 16–20]. The *complete form* (Fig. 4-2) is characterized by:

1. Antimongoloid (downward and outward) slant of the palpebral fissures.
2. Notching of the lateral lower eyelids.
3. Deficient or absent eyelashes of the medial two-thirds or three-fourths of the lower eyelids. The punctum lacrimale and meibomian glands of the lower lids may also be absent.
4. Underdevelopment of the facial bones, particularly the zygoma and mandible.
5. Underdevelopment of the external and middle ears, and very rarely the inner ear.
6. Macrostomia, a high palate, and abnormal dentition with malocclusion.
7. Atypical tongue-shaped projections of the hairline (sideburns) onto the cheek.

The *incomplete form* may be evidenced by only two or three of the above physical characteristics.

Fig. 4-2. Treacher Collins syndrome (mandibulofacial dysostosis).

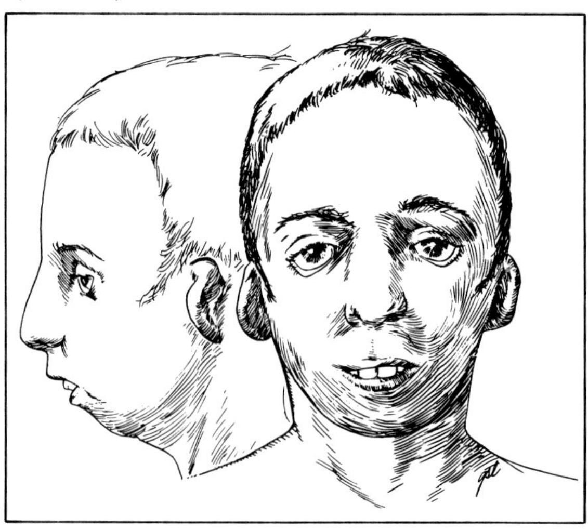

There may be only a bilateral underdevelopment of the zygoma, bilateral notching of the lateral lower eyelids, and deficiency of the medial lower eyelashes. Other incomplete forms will be evidenced by a bilateral antimongoloid slant of the palpebral fissures, notching of the lateral eyelids, and underdevelopment of the zygoma or mandible or both. Though the external ear may be normal or only slightly underdeveloped, patients may have some deafness due to the middle ear anomalies.

The *abortive form* is characterized by deformities of only the eyelids and palpebral fissures. These cases are quite rare.

The unilateral form of Treacher Collins syndrome as described by Franceschetti and Klein [16] is in actuality the first and second branchial arch syndrome [3, 18], though there may be rare exceptions. There is generally no impairment of mentality in persons with this syndrome.

Etiology

Treacher Collins syndrome has a strong hereditary component in its etiology. It is transmitted by an irregularly dominant gene. This gene has weak penetrance in some instances, thus resulting in incomplete or abortive forms of the anomaly. Succeeding generations may show increasing evidence of the syndrome, with progression from the abortive to incomplete to complete forms in each generation. The anomalies may become so marked that children in later generations will die in infancy; the gene thus has a lethal or sublethal component at least in some instances.

Children with the Treacher Collins syndrome may be born into families in which no one has this syndrome. In these cases, the condition may result from the action of an environmental factor on the developing embryo or from a mutation.

Treatment

Eyelid Anomalies

The *Kuhnt-Szymanski operation* which is commonly used for the correction of atonic ectropion can be used to correct the notching of the lateral lower eyelid. In this procedure the lower eyelid is split along the grey line of the lid margin and the skin and orbicularis oculi muscle layer are separated from the tarsal plate. This incision is carried laterally so that the skin can be pulled in this direction and a triangle of skin and muscle removed. A corresponding triangle of tarsal plate and conjunctiva is then removed from the middle portion of the lid, and the incisions are closed. A variety of operations including skin flaps from the lateral upper eyelid and a tarso-conjunctival flap from the upper lid have been described [19].

Bone or cartilage grafts or Silastic implants to the infraorbital rim will also help to prevent the antimongoloid slant of the palpebral fissures [20]. The external canthal ligament can also be disinserted and reattached to the periosteum more superiorly to elevate the external canthus.

Cilia grafts or scalp-hair grafts can be used to provide eyelashes, but they are not very satisfactory. False eyelashes trimmed to the proper length can be glued to the lower lid margin.

Other Facial Anomalies

The treatment of the other facial anomalies is the same as that discussed previously under the first and second branchial arch syndrome.

CROUZON'S SYNDROME

(Craniofacial dysostosis,
hereditary craniofacial dysostosis)

Crouzon's syndrome is a rare hereditary congenital anomaly that is characterized by premature closure of the cranial sutures (premature cranial synostosis); it resembles other types of premature cranial synostosis, such as Apert's syndrome and simple cranial synostosis. It may be difficult to distinguish between these deformities. Crouzon's syndrome and Apert's syndrome may even occur together [22].

The physical characteristics of Crouzon's syndrome are typically as described below, although an individual patient will not necessarily show each characteristic (Fig. 4-3):

Fig. 4-3. Crouzon's syndrome (craniofacial dysostosis).

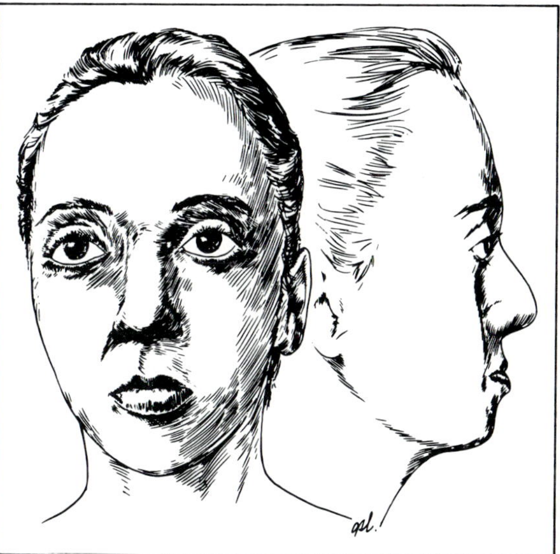

1. Deformity of the skull. Most authors describe a high prominent forehead and ridged saggital suture as characteristic of this syndrome. The cranium often is shortened in the anteroposterior length and widened in the transverse diameter, though there is no definite cranial shape because it depends on whether the coronal, saggital, or lambdoidal suture becomes synostosed first [22]. As in any cranial synostosis the skull may be oxycephalic (tower shaped), scaphycephalic (boat shaped), trigonocephalic (wedge shaped), or plagiocephalic (asymmetrical shaped).
2. Exophthalmos and hypertelorism; the orbit is usually shallow.
3. Maxillary hypoplasia with a relative mandibular prognathism.
4. Parrot's beak nose.
5. A high arched palate, external divergent strabismus, optic nerve involvement, nystagmus, mental deficiency, bilateral atresia of the external auditory canal, and partial anodonia.

A combination of these deformities gives these persons a froglike appearance when seen in full face (Fig. 4-3).

Etiology

An autosomal dominant inheritance has been demonstrated, though sporadic cases without a hereditary background do occur.

Treatment

Treatment of Crouzon's syndrome is discussed in Chapter 5. The parrot's beak nose is a nasal deformity that can be corrected by rhinoplasty at the age of 16 years, or thereafter.

APERT'S SYNDROME

(Acrocephalosyndactylia, acrodysplasia, akrokraniodysphalangie, sphenakranio-syndaktylie)

Apert's syndrome is a rare syndrome of congenital anomalies that is very closely related to Crouzon's syndrome. One of the principal differences between the two is that persons with Apert's syndrome have syndactyly or other hand anomalies. Characteristics of the syndrome are:

1. Deformity of the skull. Typically this is a tower-shaped skull (oxycephaly) with a broad forehead, though any of the skull deformities due to premature closure of the cranial sutures may occur.
2. Exophthalmos and hypertelorism.
3. Maxillary hypoplasia and relative mandibular prognathism in some cases.
4. Hand anomalies – usually varying degrees of syndactyly. Other anomalies of the hand (e.g., polydactyly, clinodactyly) have also been reported [23].

Etiology

The exact etiology of this syndrome is not known. Of 41 cases of Apert's syndrome reviewed by Cometta et al. [21] in only 10 was there a family history of this syndrome. When inherited, it is probably due to a recessive gene.

Treatment

Treatment of the abnormal facial features in Apert's syndrome is the same as that described for Crouzon's Crouzon's syndrome (see Chapter 5).

MEDIAN FACIAL DEFECTS ASSOCIATED WITH MEDIAN CLEFT LIP

Two distinct and separate syndromes of facial anomalies are associated with median cleft lip: (1) syndrome of median cleft lip with orbital hypotelorism, and (2) median cleft face syndrome with hypertelorism [27]. While the child with the former syndrome will probably die in infancy, the child with the latter syndrome will have a normal life expectancy.

MEDIAN CLEFT LIP WITH ORBITAL HYPOTELORISM

(Holoprosencephaly, arhinencephaly, median facial dysgenesis)

In this rare syndrome, there are congenital anomalies of structures arising from the primitive forebrain and the frontonasal process of the face (Fig. 4-4). There are no reported survivals beyond infancy of patients with the fully developed syndrome, though less severely affected persons will survive [26, 27].

Characteristics of the syndrome are the following:

1. Median complete cleft lip with absent premaxilla and prolabium.
2. Underdeveloped flat nose with absent columella, septal cartilage, and nasal bones.
3. Orbital hypotelorism.
4. Mongoloid slant of the eyes.
5. Fusion of eyebrows in midline.
6. Sparse frontal hair.
7. Forebrain is formed by a single large central ventricle with little cerebral cortex, as the olfactory tracts and bulbs are absent, and the head usually transilluminates as it is largely fluid-filled [26].
8. The frontal bones may be keel-shaped (trigonocephaly).
9. A cleft palate may be present.

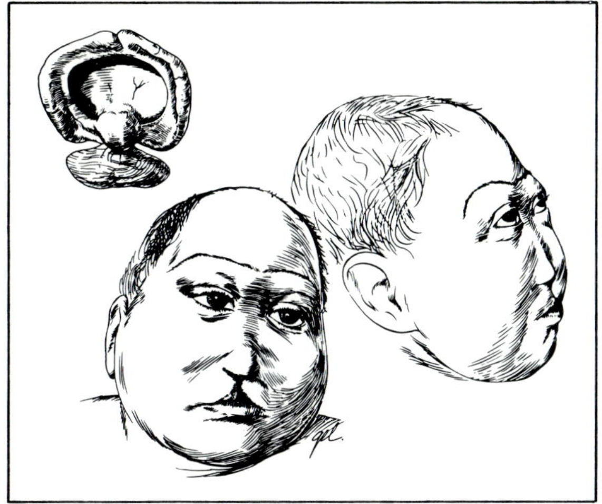

Fig. 4-4. Holoprosencephaly with cleft lip. Inset illustrates the forebrain with its single large central ventricle and thin cerebral cortex.

There is a positive correlation between the severity of the median facial and forebrain defects, so that by looking at the face it is possible to predict the external form of the brain (Fig. 4-5).

Brucker et al. [26] have pointed out that the congenital anomalies of cyclopia (one central eye) and cebocephaly (monkey head) are closely related to this deformity. They propose that the term *median cerebrofacial dysgenesis* be used to describe this entire group of midline face-brain anomalies.

Etiology

Underdevelopment and agenesis of structures of the median portion of the face and forebrain have no known etiology in human beings. Binns et al. [24] have shown in sheep that ewes which feed on a poisonous weed, *Veratrum californicum,* are likely to produce lambs with arhinencephaly, cyclopia, and cebocephaly.

Treatment

Since life is usually limited to a few months in those

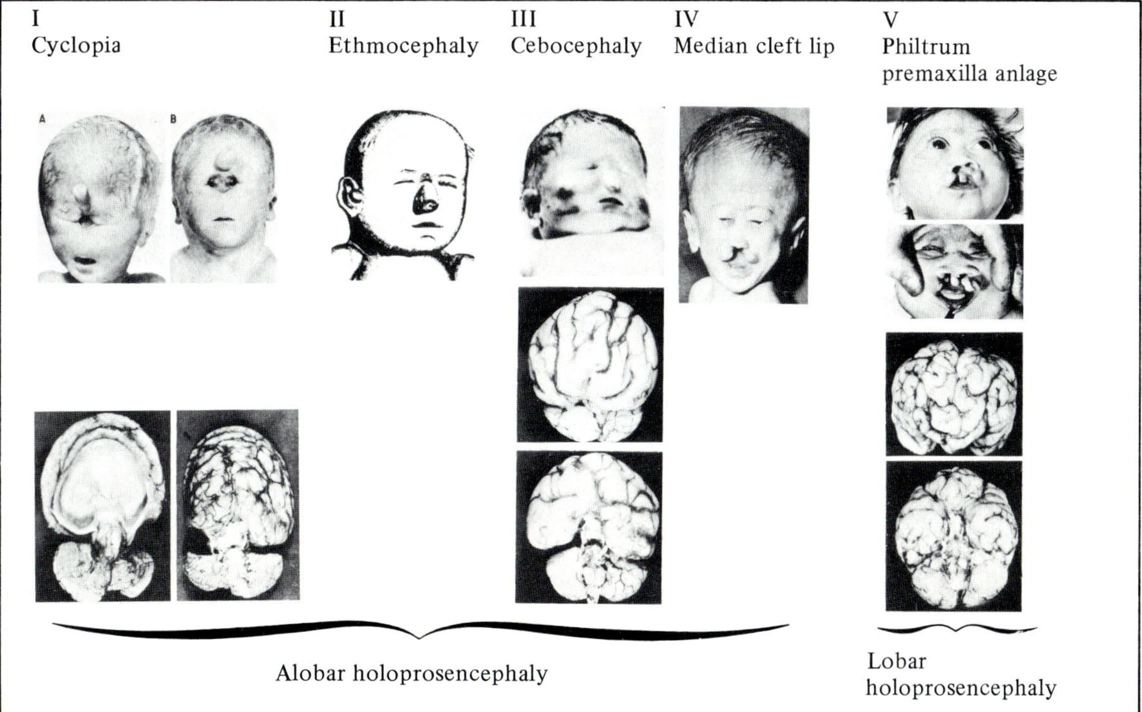

Fig. 4-5. Diagnostic facies of holoprosencephaly and parallelism with the external form of the brain. (Reproduced, with permission, from C. J. Kurlander, W. De Myer, and J. A. Campbell, Radiology *88:473, 1967.)*

infants with the fully developed syndrome, extensive treatment is not realistic. In less severely deformed infants the wide midline cleft lip can be closed with a triangular flap type of cleft lip closure.

MEDIAN CLEFT LIP WITH HYPERTELORISM

(Median cleft face syndrome)

There is a spectrum of severity in median cleft lip with hypertelorism that extends from the less severe hypertelorism alone to the most severe form with median cleft lip and palate, and bifid nose, as well as hypertelorism and cranium bifidum occultum (Fig. 4-6). Usually there are no significant extracephalic anomalies. Most patients with median cleft lip and palate have premaxillary tissue, even though it is cleft. The median cleft face syndrome has not been reported as having been inherited [27].

Some of the anatomical deformities of this syndrome and their treatment will be discussed separately.

Hypertelorism and Telecanthus

Hypertelorism is defined as an increased breadth between the eyes, as measured by an increased interpupillary distance. *Telecanthus* is an increased breadth between the medial canthi. Either of these conditions may be congenital (e.g., the hypertelorism associated with the bifid nose and the telecanthus of blepharophimosis) or traumatic (e.g., the hypertelorism of a severe naso-orbital fracture with lateral displacement of the medial orbital walls along with the globe and the telecanthus of a less severe naso-orbital fracture with splaying of the nasal bones, frontal processes of the maxilla, lacrimal bones, and ethmoid air cells). Telecanthus commonly occurs with hypertelorism, but not vice versa [29].

Webster and Deming [31] have pointed out the differentiation between "true hypertelorism" and "false hypertelorism." In the true form there is an increased interpupillary distance, whereas the false form is actually an optical illusion, created by the wide spacing of facial features (especially the eyebrows) adjacent to the eyes.

Etiology

Hypertelorism is probably due to an arrest in embryonic development. Embryologically the orbital axis moves anteriorly from an angle of 180 degrees in the second month of fetal life to 71 degrees at birth. Any interference with this anterior rotation of the orbital axis could produce hypertelorism [23, 30].

Occasional reports of inheritance of this anomaly have appeared, but it usually occurs sporadically [23, 34].

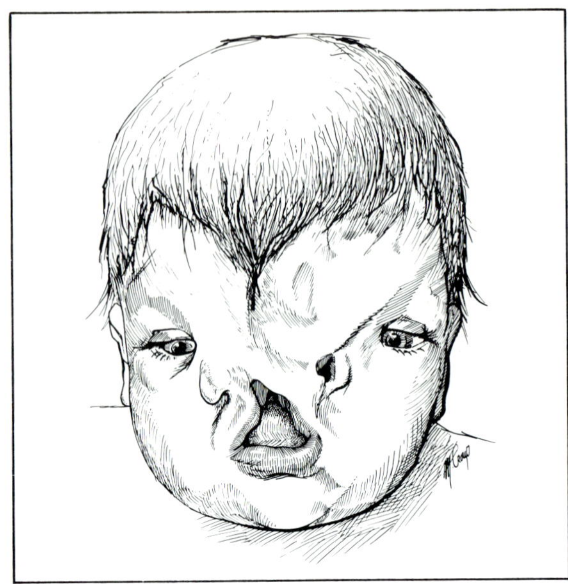

Fig. 4-6. Median cleft lip with orbital hypertelorism. Notice the low V-shaped hairline, cranium bifidum occultum, bifid nose, and median cleft palate. This represents the most extreme form of this anomaly [27].

Treatment

DIRECT APPROACH. This is described in Chapter 5.

INDIRECT APPROACH. Medial advancement of the inner portion of both eyebrows by a generous Y-V advancement can create an optical illusion to minimize the appearance of hypertelorism [30]. The thickened subcutaneous tissue of the lateral nasal walls can also be excised to suggest narrowing of the interorbital distance.

MEDIAN CLEFT LIP AND BIFID NOSE

Median clefts of the upper lip are often associated with some form of bifid nose and hypertelorism. The physical characteristics of this rare anomaly are as follows:

1. Median cleft of upper lip which is widest at the vermilion margin of the lip.
2. Bifid nose. The cleft of the upper lip may extend up the columella to involve the nasal tip. When this occurs the columella and nasal tip are wide. If the cleft of the nasal tip is extensive, widening of the nasal bridge and hypertelorism may be present. The nasal bones are never cleft.
3. Premaxilla and teeth. The central incisors may have a wide space between them. The upper labial

frenulum and nasal spine of the maxilla may be duplicated. A complete cleft of the premaxilla may be present. The secondary palate is not cleft.
4. Hypertelorism.

Median clefts of the lower lip are very rare and not found in association with upper lip clefts. The mandible and anterior portion of the tongue may also be bifid in patients with median cleft of the lower lip.

Etiology

Median clefts of the lip and bifid nose are the result of a persistence of the paired origins of the medial nasal process and the globular process.

Treatment

The cleft of the lip and nose can be approximated after the margins have been freshened and prepared for suture. A triangular flap will be of value, as the lip needs to be lengthened. An ellipse of skin and subcutaneous tissue can be excised in a vertical direction from the midline of a bifid nose. The ellipse may even be extended to include the skin of the midline of the forehead to narrow the distance between the eyebrows in more severe cases. Through this exposure the nasal bones also can be narrowed by osteotomy and the upper lateral and alar cartilages from each side sutured to each other in the midline [25, 30].

LATERAL AND OBLIQUE FACIAL CLEFTS

Lateral Facial Cleft

This very rare cleft extends from the commissure of the mouth laterally and upward across the cheek to above the auricle. It may be a shallow furrow throughout or extend into the oral cavity as a complete fissure to the anterior border of the masseter muscle after which it continues as a furrow. The muscles of mastication, as well as the maxilla, zygoma, and auricle, may be underdeveloped. This anomaly is due to failure of fusion of the maxillary and mandibular processes of the first branchial arch.

Oblique Facial Cleft

On the basis of a study of 43 cases, Boo-Chai [32] has subdivided these clefts into three subdivisions. (1) *Naso-ocular cleft,* which can extend from the lip through the lateral nose to the lower eyelid, extends more deeply to involve the maxilla (cleft runs between the central and lateral incisors) and medial bony orbit, and then ends in the temporal region. (2) *Oro-ocular cleft* can be of the medial or lateral type. The medial type of fissure can extend from the lip (usually lateral to the peak of the cupid's bow) along the nasolabial fold, ending in the medial canthal region or the lower eyelid medial to the infraorbital foramen. The rarer, more lateral type of fissure extends from the angle of the mouth upward to the orbit, ending in the lateral canthus or in a coloboma in the midlateral portion of the lower eyelid. When the maxilla is involved, the cleft begins between the cuspid and first molar tooth (bicuspid teeth are absent in the primary dentition). (3) *Mixed group of oblique facial clefts.*

Treatment usually consists of one or several Z-plasties to bring tissue into the cleft. Eyelid colobomas can have their edges excised and the defect closed.

PIERRE ROBIN SYNDROME

The elements of this syndrome are *micrognathia or retrognathia,* and *glossoptosis* with *obstruction of the airway.* An *incomplete cleft of the palate* is usually, but not always, present. The physical characteristics of the syndrome are:

1. Micrognathia or retrognathia. There is a posterior displacement of the chin due to hypoplasia of the mandible (micrognathia) or to posterior positioning of a normal-sized mandible (retrognathia).
2. Glossoptosis. Because of retroposition of the chin, the tongue falls backward and its base impinges against the posterior pharyngeal wall and the epiglottis, causing inspiratory obstruction in a ball-valve fashion. Children can often maintain an airway when crying and straining, but when they are relaxed or sleeping the airway may become obstructed. Diagnosing this type of respiratory obstruction may be difficult and should be based upon the infant's ability to breathe normally when asleep or resting [42]. Feeding may also prove difficult and accentuate respiratory difficulties. The tongues of these infants may appear either large or small in size [41].
3. Cleft palate. When a palatal cleft is present, it is incomplete. There may actually be no cleft, but simply a high palatal vault. Cleft lip is rarely seen with this syndrome [36].

Etiology

The Pierre Robin syndrome may be due either to *external pressure* on the anterior mandible during uterine life so that growth is retarded or to *inherent lack of growth potential* in the mandible. In the former, the pressure most likely results from a sharp flexion of the head on the chest, preventing forward growth of the mandible; it is probably this group of patients whose mandibles attain normal size in later years. In the latter case, the lack of growth potential may or may not be associated with a generalized failure of normal craniofacial growth. Though individual case histories have shown a familial tendency toward this being an inherited trait, larger series have not strongly supported this thesis [42].

Randall et al. [42] have studied cephalometric roentgenograms of 18 patients between 6 and 24 months of age with Pierre Robin syndrome. Two-thirds of them had mandibles smaller than normal (micrognathia) and one-third had mandibles of normal size, but in a posterior position (retrognathia). A study of older children who had this syndrome revealed that the growth of the mandible can range from persistent underdevelopment to normal development.

Treatment

The treatment of these infants is aimed at *preventing airway obstruction, aspiration, and respiratory infections.* Methods of treatment, in order of increasing severity, are positioning of the patient, obturator, tongue-to-lip adhesion, and tracheotomy.

Positioning

Placing the child in the prone position with the head slightly lower than the feet will permit the tongue and jaw to fall forward. Maintaining this position for a few weeks, except during periods of feeding, may allow sufficient growth to eliminate the respiratory obstruction.

Feeding can be carried out with the child held bolt upright with the jaw held forward so that there is less tendency for the tongue to fall backward. Gavage feeding can also be employed if the infant tends to aspirate repeatedly.

Obturator

Pielou [39], Pielou and Allen [40], and Cookson and Hall [33] have described the successful use of an obturator that fits into the palate, then curves downward, with a distal flange that holds the tongue forward. This flange has a degree of curvature which approximates that of hyperextended thumb. Two wings extend back outside the cheek to facilitate taping the appliance in place.

Tongue-to-Lip Adhesion

This operation is indicated for any of the following reasons: inability of the infant to breathe easily while resting or sleeping (these infants must cry and struggle in order to breathe and may die of exhaustion), periods of cyanosis, pneumonia, and failure to gain weight. There is sound evidence of the efficacy of the tongue-to-lip adhesion operation. Douglas [35] reported only one death (a premature infant) in 31 patients operated on by him and others, while there was a 65 percent mortality in 21 patients who did not have the tongue-to-lip adhesion operation. Kiskadden and Dietrich [38] reported no deaths in 10 patients operated on and a 30 percent mortality in 15 patients treated without this operation. Gunter and Wakefield [37] have reported a dramatic reduction in morbidity and length of stay in the hospital by using this operation. It should be mentioned that there may be other congenital anomalies, such as congenital heart disease, that are the primary cause of death in these infants.

When it is recognized that the tongue-to-lip adhesion operation is necessary, it is best to hold the tongue forward with a large traction suture or to leave an indwelling nasotracheal tube in place while preparations are made for operation, ideally within the next 24 hours.

OPERATIVE TECHNIQUE. The operative technique of tongue-to-lip adhesion has been described by Douglas [34] and effectively modified by Routledge [43] and Randall [41]. The technique is shown in Figure 4-7.

The operation can be carried out under local or general anesthesia. General anesthesia is preferable, either an oral or a nasal endotracheal tube being inserted with the infant awake. This requires the skills of an experienced anesthesiologist.

The traction suture through the body of the tongue can be utilized for 7 to 10 days and the tongue-to-lip adhesion maintained for 10 to 18 months. Gavage feeding should be used for 7 to 10 days.

Fig. 4-7. A, tongue-to-lip adhesion operation. B, horizontal incisions below the tip of the tongue and in the lower lip mucosa are made, after which the lower edges of each wound are sutured together. C, the traction suture of heavy silk is passed through the body of the tongue and tied over a button near the base of the tongue and under the chin. D, the upper edges of the tongue and lower lip are then sutured together. (After P. Randall. In J. M. Converse [Ed.], Reconstructive Plastic Surgery *[2nd ed.]. Philadelphia: Saunders, 1964.)*

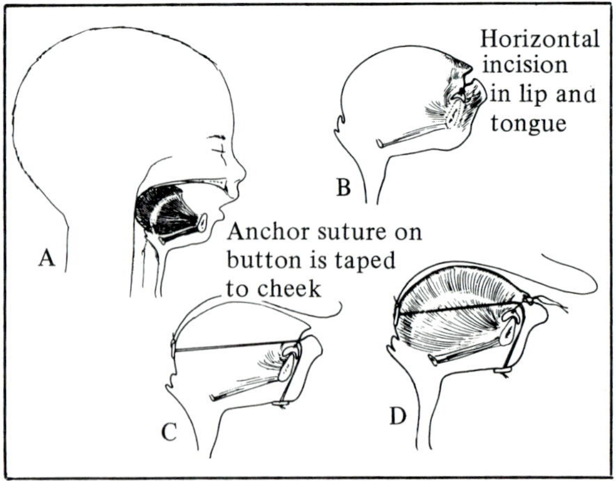

Tracheotomy

A tracheotomy should be used only in those rare cases where advancing the tongue forward either by a temporary traction suture or by tongue-to-lip adhesion does not relieve the airway obstruction.

It is difficult to remove a tracheotomy from any infant until the age of 8 to 10 months, which means that continuous hospitalization or careful home care is almost always necessary.

INFANTILE CORTICAL HYPEROSTOSIS

(Caffey-Silverman syndrome, Caffey's disease, Smyth's syndrome)

Infantile cortical hyperostosis is a rare, self-limiting disease of children that is characterized by the sudden onset of fever and marked irritability, followed by soft tissue swelling and roentgenographic evidence of periosteal new bone formation – particularly of the mandible. The usual age at which symptoms first appear is 2 to 4 months; no case has been reported which had its onset after 5 months of age. Swelling of the body and ramus of the mandible at the site of new bone formation gives a cherubic appearance to the child. These swellings and other manifestations of the disease usually regress completely within 3 to 9 months, though intermittent swelling for as long as 7 years has been reported [44]. Roentgenographic evidence of the disease may be present for 18 to 24 months after its onset. At least 150 cases have been described.

Etiology

A definite cause is not known, though hereditary factors play a definite role in some cases. Holman [44] noted a hereditary history in 3 of 33 cases.

Treatment

In the mild cases, treatment has been symptomatic. In severely ill patients, patients with pleuritis, and patients with bony deformity, treatment with *corticosteroids* is indicated. The response to this treatment is dramatic, with resolution of the signs and symptoms in a few days. The steroids must be continued with tapering doses over several months, or severe exacerbations will occur. The entire clinical picture can reappear if the dosage of steroids is dropped too rapidly [44]. Three deaths have been reported in children with this disease, but none of them occurred in the corticosteroid-treated group.

FIBROUS DYSPLASIA OF THE JAWS

(Monostotic fibrous dysplasia)

Fibrous dysplasia of the jaws is a rare condition in which the bone of the mandible or maxilla expands because of a diffuse involvement with a partially calcified osteoid material. The swelling usually becomes evident in late childhood or in the young adult, but arrests itself spontaneously with skeletal maturation [45].

The mandible may protrude on either the lingual or the buccal surface. The bone may be smooth or nodular and is covered by mucosa. Any portion of the maxilla may expand with this slow-growing tumor, and the process may extend into the zygoma.

Roentgenograms will usually show irregular radiolucent areas, often with islands of well-calcified bone. In some cases a more radiopaque ground-glass appearance is seen.

This monostotic type of fibrous dysplasia is different from polyostotic fibrous dysplasia (Albright's disease) in which several bones in various parts of the body are involved with fibrous displasia and cysts. Polyostotic fibrous dysplasia in addition is characterized by café au lait spots on the skin and precocious puberty in the female [44].

Etiology

A definite cause of monostotic fibrous dysplasia is unknown, but it is thought to be of congenital origin.

Treatment

Contouring of the overgrown soft bony tissue with a hand chisel or motor-driven saw is the treatment of choice. Resection of the mandible is definitely not indicated. This contouring of the tumor will improve the cosmetic appearance; the fibrous osteoma will spontaneously stop growing with skeletal maturation, usually in the late teens. The operation may have to be repeated in some instances [45].

MÖBIUS SYNDROME

(Congenital facial diplegia, congenital nuclear aplasia or agenesis, congenital oculofacial paralysis, congenital abducens-facial paralysis)

The Möbius syndrome is a rare congenital syndrome that is characterized by bilateral facial and abducens nerve paralysis. It may be inherited; however, in the vast majority of patients there is no known etiological factor. Over 125 cases have been reported [46]. The physical characteristics are:

1. Facial paralysis. From birth these patients have paralysis of the facial muscles; the paralysis is usually bilateral, but may be asymmetrical. The lower face is often not paralyzed.
2. Lateral rectus muscle paralysis. The patients are usually cross-eyed due to an inability to abduct the eyes beyond the midline because of this paralysis.

3. Other anomalies. Thirty percent of these children have club foot, 15 percent have pectoral muscle aplasia or hypoplasia, and 20 percent have brachial muscle aplasia or hypoplasia. Anomalies of the hands are not uncommon. The third, fifth, and last four cranial nerves may also be involved.

KLIPPEL–FEIL SYNDROME

(Congenital synostosis of cervicothoracic vertebrae, brevicollis)

The Klippel-Feil syndrome is a congenital anomaly characterized by shortness of the neck and fusion of all or some of the cervical vertebrae into a solid mass so that the head seems to sit directly on the thorax. Motion of the neck is limited, and the skin in the posterolateral region of the neck is held out by the trapezius muscle so that it forms a web. This web can be released by means of a Z-plasty [47]. Another method of treatment is to excise a wide elipse of skin from the posterior midline of the neck. The effectiveness of this procedure can be determined preoperatively by grasping this skin between the examiner's fingers.

In an occasional instance this syndrome is inherited, probably by an autosomal dominant gene with poor penetrance and variable expression.

BRANCHIAL CYSTS, SINUSES, AND FISTULAS

Brachial cysts, sinuses, and fistulas are epithelial-lined tracts in the lateral aspect of the neck that are due to persistence of embryonic remnants of the second and occasionally the third branchial cleft or pouch (or both). A *branchial cyst* occurs when this tract, which is closed at both ends, becomes filled with fluid secretions. An *external branchial sinus* opens on the skin along the anterior border of the sternocleidomastoid muscle, usually below the level of the thyroid cartilage. The small slitlike opening will often have a drop of serous or purulent fluid at its orifice. An *internal branchial sinus* opens in the posterior tonsillar pillar, just behind the tonsil. These internal sinuses are not commonly found, probably because they rarely give rise to symptoms. A *branchial fistula* has both an external and internal opening. Wilson [50] reported that between 75 and 80 percent of all these tracts were branchial cysts, making them more common than branchial sinuses or fistulas.

The lining of branchial fistulas is stratified squamous epithelium in the major part of the tract, but the inner portion is generally columnar or ciliated columnar. Cysts are usually lined by squamous epithelium. All tracts have lymphoid tissue along their wall.

The branchial cysts commonly lie on the surface of the carotid sheath deep to the anterior border of the sternocleidomastoid muscle. Large cysts occasionally extend upward toward the base of the skull or inward toward the pharyngeal wall.

A hereditary factor is believed to be present in some patients with branchial cyst, sinus, and fistula. Fischer [49] found evidence of heredity in 21 out of 100 cases.

Treatment

Treatment consists of complete excision of the branchial cyst, sinus, or fistula in those cases where there is no evidence of an acute infectious process in the tract. Methylene blue can be injected into the orifice of the sinus or fistula prior to operation to assist in its identification and complete removal.

The first step is to excise elliptically around the orifice of the tract, after which the entire tract can be dissected upward, utilizing two or three transverse or "step ladder" incisions, one above the other, paralleling the direction of the skin lines of the neck.

Wilson [50] has described in extensive detail the relationships of the tract to the adjacent carotid artery; internal jugular vein; digastric and stylohyoid muscles; and vagus, hypoglossal, and spinal accessory nerves. If the tract has an internal opening it can be excised and the defect in the posterior tonsillar pillar closed. A catheter can be inserted in through the neck wound and attached to suction for drainage for 2 or 3 days before removing it.

Branchial cysts, sinuses, and fistulas may become infected. If an abscess is present, its treatment is usually by incision and drainage. Once the infection has been controlled, the remnants can later be excised.

Rarely *branchiogenic carcinoma* can arise from these embryonic remnants in the lateral aspect of the neck. Treatment consists of excision of the primary lesion and radical neck dissection on the same side. Carp and Stout [48] reported on 4 men, all over the age of 40, who had branchiogenic carcinoma. A preponderance of males has also been reported in other series.

THYROGLOSSAL DUCT CYSTS AND FISTULAS

A thyroglossal duct cyst is a soft movable mass in or near the midline of the anterior aspect of the neck, over or just below the hyoid bone. When there is an opening on the skin or at the base of the tongue at the foramen cecum, it is called a thyroglossal duct fistula. The terms *fistula* and *sinus* are usually considered to be synonymous. While the cyst or fistula usually occurs in the midline, at or above the thyroid cartilage, it may occur anywhere between the foramen cecum of the tongue and the suprasternal notch. Thyroglossal duct cysts or fistulas are most commonly noted in children, though they can occur in patients of any age [51]. Sistrunk [52] reported an incidence of 1:2,800 in 86,000 consecutive patients examined.

This group of cysts and fistulas are remnants of the *embryonic thyroglossal duct.* Normally the median lobe of the thyroid gland develops from the ventral surface of the pharyngeal primordium along the midline. It originates at the level of the first branchial pouch, where it is connected to the pharynx by a stalk known as the thyroglossal duct. The duct normally loses its connection with the pharynx (foramen cecum of the base of the tongue) as the median lobe of the thyroid migrates downward. In its descent it may pass superficial or deep to the hyoid bone, or even pass through it to eventually lie anterior to the thyroid cartilage.

The usual signs and symptoms of thyroglossal duct anomalies are swelling or the presence of a fistulous opening in the midline of the neck. Infection is not uncommon. If a cyst is infected, it should be incised and drained to control the infection before surgical removal.

The lining of thyroglossal duct cysts and fistulas may be stratified squamous, columnar, or transitional epithelium. Ectopic thyroid tissue may be seen on histological examination to lie adjacent to the wall of the cyst or fistula.

Treatment

Sistrunk's [52] operative technique for removing these cysts and fistulas is an excellent method of treatment. Dilute methylene blue can be injected into the cyst or fistula prior to operation so that any lateral branches, which are occasionally present, can be identified and removed. Through a 5-cm. horizontal incision at the level of the hyoid bone, the skin and platysma muscle are reflected. The cyst or fistula is dissected up to the hyoid bone, where a 0.6-cm. segment of the midhyoid bone is removed. The remainder of the tract is removed as a core 0.6 cm. in diameter, the excision following a line between the hyoid bone and the foramen cecum of the tongue (an angle of 45 degrees upward and backward from the hyoid). The finger of an assistant, inserted into the mouth so that outward pressure can be placed on the foramen cecum, is of great assistance. Following excision, the ends of the hyoid bone can be approximated by sutures through the tissues attached to the bone. The operative site should be drained with a catheter connected to suction.

PROGRESSIVE FACIAL HEMIATROPHY

(Romberg's disease, Parry-Romberg syndrome, progressive hemifacial atrophy, facial trophoneurosis)

Even though progressive facial hemiatrophy is probably not a congenital anomaly of the face, it seems most appropriate to include material about this facial deformity here, rather than to devote a separate chapter to this subject. Although this disorder is known as progressive facial hemiatrophy, the term *progressive hemifacial atrophy* is more correct [55].

Clinical Course and Physical Characteristics

Progressive facial hemiatrophy characteristically starts in the paramedian area of the face (an area one or two fingerbreadths wide next to the midline) with *atrophy of the subcutaneous fatty tissue* (Fig. 4-8). This is the cardinal sign of the disorder, there being no case of progressive hemiatrophy in which the subcutaneous tissue is not involved [59]. The overlying *skin,* the underlying *facial muscles,* and in some instances the *bone* and *cartilage* of the face and skull may become atrophied. *Atrophy* of the *ipsilateral side of the tongue* may occur. The *loss of hair* of the eyebrows and anterior scalp in the paramedian area commonly occurs early in the course of the disorder. *Epilepsy* involving the contralateral side of the body occurs late in the clinical course of some patients with progressive facial hemiatrophy. *Inflammatory processes involving the eye* are frequent.

The progressive hemiatrophy usually has its onset in the adolescent or young adult. Beer [54] found that in 75 percent of 109 cases the disease began before the twentieth year. The atrophy progresses slowly, but is usually limited to one side of the face, although a few bilateral cases have been reported. The atrophy usually reaches its maximum in 2 to 12 years, but it may stop at any time leaving only minimal deformity [58].

Fig. 4-8. Progressive facial hemiatrophy. The markers point to the regions of most pronounced atrophy in this patient.

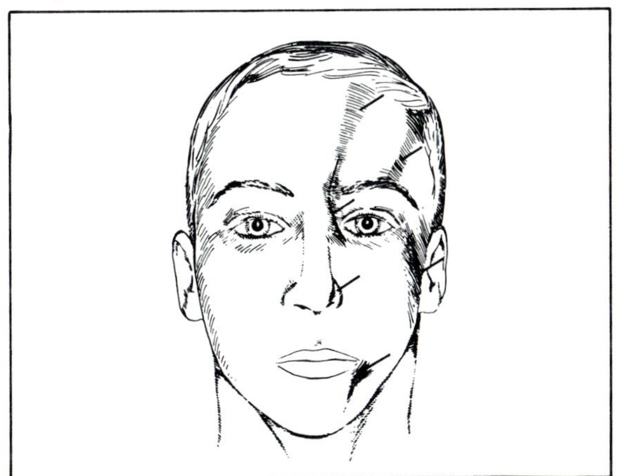

The atrophy may be confined to the area of distribution of one of the branches of the trigeminal nerve, or it may occasionally transgress the boundaries of the face to involve the ipsilateral neck, shoulder, arm, trunk, and even leg.

The *skin* frequently has a brownish yellow color, but in more severe cases, it often appears brownish gray. Histologically there is thinning of the epidermis and atrophy of the adnexal structures, a microscopic picture difficult to differentiate from localized scleroderma [58]. The *facial muscles* decrease in bulk but continue to function. The *bone and cartilage* of the face are underdeveloped to a degree directly related to the age of onset of the hemiatrophy. Since the facial bones do not reach 90 percent of their adult size until the patient is 12 or 13 years of age, the onset of hemiatrophy during childhood causes the most severe bony atrophy [58].

Etiology

There is no proved cause for this disorder. Rogers [58] has carefully reviewed the various hypotheses and concluded that a *sympathetic nervous system cause* is the most likely one. It seems that the factor affecting the sympathetic nervous system is acting at a central level, perhaps in the diencephalon. Rogers has evaluated 772 cases of facial hemiatrophy and found no statistically significant evidence of a hereditary component.

Moss and Crikelair [56] report that unilateral cervical sympathectomy in month-old rats produces changes similar to progressive facial hemiatrophy. Histologically they found a fairly constant decrease of fatty tissue, while all other structures remained unchanged.

Treatment

Dimethylpolysiloxane Fluid Injections

Dimethylpolysiloxane fluid is a liquid form of silicone (Dow Corning Medical Fluid 360, of 350 centistoke viscosity); when injected beneath the skin it has produced a *dramatic improvement* in the appearance of these patients [57]. Ashley, Rees and their coworkers [53] have used this treatment in 11 patients with progressive facial hemiatrophy. Using a sparse infiltration of 1% lidocaine (Xylocaine) to obtain anesthesia, a #18 needle on a three-ring Luer-Lok syringe is used to inject the Dow Corning Medical Silicone Fluid 360 at weekly or biweekly intervals. The fluid is injected on several occasions just beneath the skin, being careful to fan out the injections and to deposit only small quantities in one place to prevent large cystic spaces. As much as 10 ml. of this fluid can be used for the initial injection, while 1 ml. or less may be all that is required for the final injections to fill small areas of depression. Follow-up examinations over 8 years have shown no migration or decrease in soft tissue bulk. This continues to be the best method of treatment, and at this time (1979) it is under evaluation by about 20 plastic surgeons in the United States. See Chapter 3 for more information on this method of treatment.

Grafts and Flaps

Any grafts (bone, cartilage, dermis, fat, fascia) placed in the atrophied side of the face while the degree of facial hemiatrophy is still increasing will probably be partially absorbed, owing to the same unknown factors that cause this disorder. After the active process has subsided, this is less likely to occur [58].

Skin flaps, especially tubed abdominal flaps, do not appear to undergo absorption when transferred to the atrophied side of the face to restore lost bulk [58].

REFERENCES

First and Second Branchial Arch Syndrome

1. Converse, J. M., McCarthy, J. G., Wood-Smith, D., and Coccaro, P. J. Craniofacial Microsomia. In Converse, J. M. (Ed.), *Reconstructive Plastic Surgery* (2nd ed.). Philadelphia: Saunders, 1977.
2. Dingman, R. O., and Grabb, W. C. Cartilage homografts preserved by irradiation. *Plast. Reconstr. Surg.* 28:562, 1961.
3. Grabb, W. C. The first and second branchial arch syndrome. *Plast. Reconstr. Surg.* 36:485, 1965.
4. Hilson, D. Malformation of ears as sign of malformation of genito-urinary tract. *Br. Med. J.* 2:785, 1957.
5. Karfik, V. Proposed classification of rare congenital cleft malformations in the face. *Acta Chir. Plast.* 8:163, 1966.
6. Kleinsasser, O., and Schlothane, R. Ear deformities among thalidomide embryopathies. *Z. Laryngol. Rhinol. Otol.* 43:344, 1964.
7. Krampitz, R. Uber einige seltenese formen von Missbildungen des Gehörorgans. *Z. Ohrenh.* 65:44, 1912.
8. Kunkel, O. Microtia in a mother and three children. *H.N.O.* 8:80, 1959.
9. Longacre, J. J., deStefano, G. A., and Holmstrand, K. E. The early versus the late reconstruction of congenital hypoplasias of the facial skeleton and skull. *Plast. Reconstr. Surg.* 27:489, 1961.
10. Longacre, J. J., deStefano, G. A., and Holmstrand, K. E. The surgical management of first and second branchial arch syndromes. *Plast. Reconstr. Surg.* 31:507, 1963.
11. Neel, J. V. The meaning of empirical risk figures for disease or defect. *Eugen. Q.* 5:41, 1958.
12. Roosa, S. *Treatise on the Disease of the Ear.* New York: Wood, 1891.

13. Stark, R. B., and Saunders, D. E. The first branchial syndrome. The oral-mandibular-auricular syndrome. *Plast. Reconstr. Surg.* 29:229, 1962.
14. Vincent, R. W., Ryan, R. F., and Longenecker, C. G. Malformation of ear associated with urogenital anomalies. *Plast. Reconstr. Surg.* 28:214, 1961.

Treacher Collins Syndrome

15. Debusmann. Familiare kombinierte Gesichtsmissbildung in Bereich des ersten Viszeralbogens. *Arch. Kinderheilk.* 120:133, 1940.
16. Franceschetti, A., and Klein, D. The mandibulofacial dysostosis: A new hereditary syndrome. *Acta Ophthalmol.* (Kbh.) 27:144, 1949.
17. Gorlin, R. J., and Pindborg, J. J. *Syndromes of the Head and Neck.* New York: McGraw-Hill, 1964.
18. Rogers, B. Berry–Treacher Collins syndrome. *Br. J. Plast. Surg.* 17:109, 1964.
19. Rogers, B. O. Mandibulofacial Dysostosis. In Converse, J. M. (Ed.), *Reconstructive Plastic Surgery* (2nd ed.). Philadelphia: Saunders, 1977.
20. Snyder, C. C. Bilateral facial agenesia (Treacher Collins syndrome). *Am. J. Surg.* 92:81, 1956.

Crouzon's Syndrome and Apert's Syndrome

21. Cometta, F., Juillard, E., and Rosselet, P. À-propos d'un cas d'aerocephalo-syndactylie. syndactylie. *Ophthalmologica* 120:72, 1950.
22. Gorlin, R. J., and Pindborg, J. J. *Syndromes of the Head and Neck.* New York: McGraw-Hill, 1964.
23. Rogers, B. Embryology of the Face and Introduction to Craniofacial Anomalies. In Converse, J. M. (Ed.), *Reconstructive Plastic Surgery* (2nd ed.). Philadelphia: Saunders, 1977.

Median Facial Defects Associated with Median Cleft Lip

24. Binns, W., Anderson, W. A., and Sullivan, D. J. Cyclopian-type malformations in lambs. *Am. J. Vet. Res.* 137:515, 1960.
25. Boo-Chai, K. The bifid nose. *Plast. Reconstr. Surg.* 36:626, 1965.
26. Brucker, P. A., Hoyt, C. J., and Trusler, H. M. Severe cleft lip with arrhinencephaly. *Plast. Reconstr. Surg.* 32:527, 1963.
27. De Myer, W. Median Cleft Lip. In Grabb, W. C., Rosenstein, S. W., and Bzoch, K. R. (Eds.), *Cleft Lip and Palate – Surgical, Dental, and Speech Aspects.* Boston: Little, Brown, 1971.
28. Gorlin, R. J., and Pindborg, J. J. *Syndromes of the Head and Neck.* New York: McGraw-Hill, 1964.
29. Mustardé, J. C. *Repair and Reconstruction in the Orbital Region.* Baltimore: Williams & Wilkins, 1966.
30. Walker, D. G. *Malformations of the Face.* Edinburgh: Livingstone, 1961.
31. Webster, J. P., and Deming, E. G. The surgical treatment of the bifid nose. *Plast. Reconstr. Surg.* 6:1, 1950.

Lateral and Oblique Facial Clefts

32. Boo-Chai, K. The oblique facial cleft. *Br. J. Plast. Surg.* 23:352, 1970.

Pierre Robin Syndrome

33. Cookson, A., and Hall, B. D. Use of obturators in the early management of a case of Pierre Robin syndrome (Pielou's method). *Dent. Pract.* 18:264, 1968.
34. Douglas, B. The treatment of micrognathia associated with obstruction by a plastic procedure. *Plast. Reconstr. Surg.* 1:300, 1946.
35. Douglas, B. A further report on the treatment of micrognathia with obstruction by a plastic procedure: Results based on reports from 21 cities. *Plast. Reconstr. Surg.* 5:113, 1950.
36. Gorlin, R. J., and Pindborg, J. J. *Syndromes of the Head and Neck.* New York: McGraw-Hill, 1964.
37. Gunter, G. S., and Wakefield, A. R. Early management of the Pierre Robin syndrome. *Cleft Palate J.* 7:495, 1970.
38. Kiskadden, W. S., and Dietrich, S. R. Review of the treatment of micrognathia. *Plast. Reconstr. Surg.* 12:364, 1953.
39. Pielou, W. D. Non-surgical management of Pierre Robin syndrome. *Arch. Dis. Child.* 42:20, 1967.
40. Pielou, W. D., and Allen, A. The use of an obturator in the management of the Pierre Robin syndrome. *Dent. Pract.* 18:169, 1968.
41. Randall, P. The Robin Anomalad: Micrognathia and Glossoptosis with Airway Obstruction. In Converse, J. M. (Ed.), *Reconstructive Plastic Surgery* (2nd ed.). Philadelphia: Saunders, 1977.
42. Randall, P., Krogman, W. M., and Jahina, S. Mandibular Growth in Pierre Robin Syndrome. In *Transactions of the Third International Congress of Plastic Surgeons.* Amsterdam: Excerpta Medica, 1963.
43. Routledge, R. T. The Pierre Robin syndrome: A surgical emergency in the neonatal period. *Br. J. Plast. Surg.* 13:204, 1960.

Infantile Cortical Hyperostosis

44. Holman, G. H. Infantile cortical hyperostosis: A review. *Q. Rev. Pediatr.* 17:24, 1962.

Fibrous Dysplasia of the Jaws

45. Thoma, K. H. *Oral Surgery* (5th ed.). St. Louis: Mosby, 1969.

Möbius Syndrome

46. Gorlin, R. J., and Pindborg, J. J. *Syndromes of the Head and Neck.* New York: McGraw-Hill, 1964.

Klippel-Feil Syndrome

47. Gorlin, R. J., and Pindborg, J. J. *Syndromes of the Head and Neck.* New York: McGraw-Hill, 1964.

Branchial Cysts, Sinuses, and Fistulas

48. Carp, L., and Stout, A. P. Branchial anomalies and neoplasms. *Ann. Surg.* 87:186, 1928.
49. Fischer, G. Historische Notiz zur angeborluen Halsfistel. *Deutsch. Z. Chir.* 2:570, 1873.
50. Wilson, C. P. Lateral cysts and fistulae of the neck of developmental origin. *Ann. R. Coll. Surg. Engl.* 17:1, 1955.

Thyroglossal Duct Cysts, Sinuses, and Fistulas

51. Brauer, R. O. Congenital Cysts and Tumors of the Neck. In Converse, J. M. (Ed.), *Reconstructive Plastic Surgery* (2nd ed.). Philadelphia: Saunders, 1977.
52. Sistrunk, W. E. The surgical treatment of cysts of the thyroglossal tract. *Ann. Surg.* 71:121, 1920.

Progressive Facial Hemiatrophy

53. Ashley, F. L., Rees, T. D., Ballantyne, D. L., Galloway, D., Machida, R., Grazer, F., McConnell, D. V., Edgington, T., and Kiskadden, W. An injection technique for the treatment of facial hemiatrophy. *Plast. Reconstr. Surg.* 35:640, 1965.
54. Beer, M. Bertrag zur Kenntnis der Hemiatrophia facialis progressiva. *Inaugural Dissertation.* Konigsberg i br.: Krause and Ewerlein, 1898.
55. Gorlin, R. J., and Pindborg, J. J. *Syndromes of the Head and Neck.* New York: McGraw-Hill, 1964.
56. Moss, M. L., and Crikelair, G. F. Progressive facial hemiatrophy following cervical sympathectomy in the rat. *Arch. Oral. Biol.* 1:254, 1959.
57. Rees, T. D. Silicone fluid injections for facial atrophy – a ten year study. *Plast. Reconstr. Surg.* 52:118, 1973.
58. Rogers, B. Rare Craniofacial Deformities. In Converse, J. M. (Ed.), *Reconstructive Plastic Surgery.* Philadelphia: Saunders, 1977.
59. Wartenberg, R. Progressive facial hemiatrophy. *Arch. Neurol. Psychiatry* 54:75, 1945.

5

Craniofacial Surgery

IAN R. MUNRO

WARNING

This chapter is an outline of the principles and techniques of orbitocraniofacial surgery. It must not be used as a reference for undertaking the surgery. These procedures should be limited to regional teams handling a population of 20 to 30 million people, in order to provide enough new cases each year to enable continual experience and make the operations facile and as safe as possible [34, 36, 54]. The presence of a large pediatric team is essential. The descriptions in this chapter outline only salient features of the deformities and some methods of osteotomy for correction. The detail is *not sufficient* to permit any plastic surgeon to perform these operations *without further training;* plastic surgeons need extra training in order to become full-time "hard tissue" or craniofacial surgeons [54].

The "jig-saw" procedures described on pp. 150–152 are exceptionally hazardous and should be undertaken only by considerably experienced craniofacial surgeons and neurosurgeons, and a neuroanesthetist must also be present.

HISTORICAL BACKGROUND

Corrective surgery for maxillofacial deformities began its main development during World War I, since a large amount of bone and soft tissue facial destruction resulted from trench warfare. World War II produced the "guinea pigs" who survived disastrous burns of the face (and hands). These two wars provided basic techniques for the *replacement* of missing bone, soft tissue, and skin of the face. In the late 1940s and in the 1950s, attempts were being made to ameliorate some of the congenital upper facial deformities [32, 50]. Gillies was the first to demonstrate that adequate correction could only be achieved by actually repositioning displaced parts of the skeletal framework [22]. However, it has taken the work of Paul Tessier and his violation of hitherto accepted "facts" in the late 1960s to demonstrate that most skeletal deformities of the face and calvarium are now correctable – or at least can be significantly improved [51–60].

Tessier proved two facts and, consequently, destroyed two myths of facial surgery. Large segments of the facial and cranial skeleton can be completely denuded of their blood supply, be repositioned, and yet completely survive. His second, and more drastic, breakthrough was in establishing that the eyes themselves can be translocated horizontally or vertically over considerable distances without impairing vision. These two principles have enabled the development of modern orbitocraniofacial surgery to the level of a new surgical specialty [36, 54].

Craniofacial surgery has enabled the correction of severe deformities of the skull and face and has also facilitated the correction of associated soft tissue problems; most of these severe congenital deformities are extremely rare. The planning of reconstruction and assessment of the deformity must be extremely detailed, since the potential complications of this surgery are numerous and can be disastrous. The principles of the surgery are, however, simple: (1) First, correct the bone, then the soft tissue. (2) The skeleton must be adequately and completely exposed. (3) Bone segments can be mobilized as desired and moved in virtually any direction. (4) Completely rigid fixation must be achieved by direct wiring of fragments. (5) Additional autogenous bone grafts of rib and ilium are needed to enhance stability, fill defects, and produce smooth contours.

TYPES OF DEFORMITY

The majority of skeletal deformities of the skull are now correctable by craniofacial techniques. In addition, many of the associated soft tissue deformities, such as the bifid nose in orbital hypertelorism or the antimongoloid palpebral fissure of Treacher Collins syndrome, are more easily and completely corrected after the underlying skeleton has been correctly aligned.

The following can now be considered for treatment: oxycephaly; turricephaly; brachycephaly; plagiocephaly; craniostenosis (all types); orbital hypertelorism; orbital dystopia; anophthalmic orbit; Crouzon's syndrome; Apert's syndrome; craniofacial microsomia; Treacher Collins syndrome; midface retrusion or asymmetry; some cases of deformity from tumor, trauma, or radiation; and soft tissue problems related to these conditions.

PLANNING: THE TEAM APPROACH

Craniofacial surgery is technically the most complex of all surgical specialties. It is akin to cardiac surgery in magnitude; however, unlike patients undergoing cardiac or neurological surgical procedures, patients with craniofacial deformities will not die if they are not operated upon. Hence, preparation for this kind of surgery must be extremely detailed. The four main complications that always remain a realistic possibility are *death, blindness, brain damage,* and disastrous *infection,* including meningitis and osteomyelitis of a major part of the skull. In order to minimize these risks, regional or national teams must be large and particularly experienced in the pediatric aspect of their specialty.

Members of the Team

Craniofacial Surgeon

The craniofacial surgeon performs a detailed examination of the entire skull, face, orbits, eyes, and oral cavity, and estimates the asymmetry and relative importance of each area of deformity. The initial evaluation includes the consideration of the different types of operation that may be necessary and the referral of the patient to any other members of the team appropriate for the magnitude of surgery considered. The craniofacial surgeon *must warn the patients and parents* of the type of surgery being considered and its inherent risks.

Neurosurgeon

A complete neurological examination should include olfaction; the likelihood of craniostenosis; the presence of hydrocephalus or intracranial skeletal anomalies (see p. 136); and previous intracranial surgery.

Otolaryngologist

Many patients have associated anomalies of the external and middle ear, nose and upper respiratory airway. Tracheotomy may be indicated prophylactically or, in some cases, it may be mandatory.

Pediatric Anesthetist

Craniofacial surgery is routinely the most prolonged of all types of elective surgery. Small children and infants are not adults on a smaller scale, and thus different instruments, techniques, and considerations are necessary. Profound hypotension and sometimes hypothermia must be maintained for many hours; measurement of blood loss is difficult. It is essential to monitor blood gases, urinary output, temperature, blood pressure via arterial line, heart sounds, and lung inflation. In addition, it is necessary to humidify inspired gases, warm transfused blood, monitor blood coagulation during surgery, and shrink brain size without the use of lumbar cerebrospinal fluid drainage [14, 40].

Neuroradiologist

Cephalometric and plain radiographs of the skull are not adequate for intracranial or orbital surgery. Polytomography in three planes – anteroposterior, lateral, and basal – enables precise measurement of one deformed area compared to another. Particular deformities should be looked for in the shape of the medial orbital walls, in the relation of the lateral orbital walls to the middle cranial fossa, level of the cribriform plate, and in the rotation of the cranial base (cranioscoliosis).

Computerized transaxial tomography will demonstrate cerebral disorders, such as hydrocephalus or small encephaloceles. In addition, the position of the eye and periorbital contents related to the orbital walls is shown. The cranial volume can also be calculated [19].

Neuroophthalmologist

The examination should include: external measurements of outer canthal distance, inner canthal distance (and also anteroposterior and vertical asymmetry), interpupillary distance, palpebral fissure length and width, and exophthalmometry; ocular balance; vision, including visual acuity, cycloplegic refraction, and color vision; visual fusion, including the degree of stereopsis and the visual fields; the ocular globe, fundi, and media; sensual and visual reaction; and orthoptic mensuration.

Pedodontist

The patient must be completely free of caries, including incipient caries. The planning and manufacture of occlusal splints are important, even for infant dentition.

Orthodontist

Cephalometric analysis, dental models, and an unusual appreciation of facial configuration are needed. It is important to plan the precise amount of movement of maxilla or mandible, or both, to *produce a normal face.* Production of a normal occlusion must remain secondary to the external contour of the face.

Geneticist

The diagnosis of the syndrome should be ascertained where possible, and the parents or patient counseled about the inheritance pattern.

Psychiatrist and Social Worker

The psychiatrist measures the level of intelligence and determines the effect of the deformity on the patient, parent, siblings, and peers. He warns of the psychological, as well as physical, implication of the operation and determines the best age for the procedure (increased evidence points toward operation as early as possible). The social worker provides support in the period before, during, and after the operation, helping prevent the patient or parent from having unrealistic expectations from the surgery and *reemphasizing* the dangers of the operation.

Speech Pathologist
In addition to routine examination, nasal air flow studies, speech cephalometrics, and video fluoroscopy are needed. Articulation errors related to dentition and the aesthetic aspects of speech must be determined. The speech pathologist estimates the possibility of converting hyponasality to normality and the likelihood of producing hypernasality as a result of maxillary advancement.

Audiologist
The audiologist performs a routine check in all patients with cleft lip or palate, in those with Crouzon's or Apert's syndrome, and in other patients as indicated.

Medical Artist
Life-size photographs should be used to produce drawings of the ideal face for the patients. Measurements of soft tissue correction are needed. When the initial drawings are unrealistic in patients with severe deformities, compromise drawings can be made.

Anthropologist
Although an anthropologist is not strictly necessary for most types of craniofacial surgery, external measurements of the face and calvarium have three purposes. (1) Certain skull measurements can be used to calculate the intracranial volume. (2) Asymmetries of the face may be revealed that are not otherwise obvious. (3) Records of the growth of the face and progressive distortion prior to the operation, as well as the effect of surgery immediately and on a long-term basis, can be used to improve future planning.

Craniofacial Conference
The timing of the operation and the type of procedure to be performed should be discussed and planned for each patient. In addition, *all patients* should have *repeat* examinations by all appropriate members of the team at *1 year, 2 years,* and *4 years,* as well as every 2 years thereafter until growth is completed.

In addition, all craniofacial patients should be routinely admitted to the same ward in the hospital and the same operating room and nurses should be used.

SURGICAL EXPOSURE OF THE SKULL AND FACIAL BONES
The entire skeleton of the skull can be exposed and osteotomized by incisions that leave no visible mark on the face.

The Meisterschnitt Exposure
An incision is made from immediately in front of one ear, over the region of the coronal suture to the other ear. The scalp is then peeled forward at the subgaleal level to the superior orbital rims or posteriorly as far as the inion. In this plane, it can be continued over the temporalis fascia to the zygoma, zygomatic arch, and capsule of the temporomandibular joint. The periosteum is then incised high over the frontal bone. Very sharp flat periosteal elevators* then strip sharply in the cambium layer down to the superior orbital rim. The superior orbital neurovascular bundle passes through a canal or foramen at the orbital rim and must be dissected out with a fine osteotome if necessary. The orbital roof is stripped posteriorly to the level of the lateral margin of the superior orbital fissure. On the medial orbital wall, the anterior ethmoidal vessels are divided. The lacrimal sac is stripped from its fossa, except where the nasolacrimal duct passes through its canal. Laterally, if it is necessary to mobilize the temporalis muscle, this can be stripped subperiosteally for its anterior two-thirds. The periosteum over the lateral orbital wall curving laterally over the zygoma and zygomatic arch is incised, and these areas are stripped. The lateral orbital wall is stripped to the inferior orbital fissure. From this approach, the orbital floor, inferior orbital rim, zygoma, and anterior maxilla can be stripped medially as far as the inferior orbital foramen. *No traction* should be placed on the periorbital envelope during these procedures. Malleable brain retractors *pressed against bone* can facilitate exposure. For the Le Fort III osteotomy, subperiosteal stripping can continue down the posterior maxilla to the pterygomaxillary fissure, which can be stripped by feeling although it cannot be visualized. Medially, after the orbit has been stripped, dissection can continue over the nasal bones to the upper lateral cartilages and to the medial inferior orbital rim and adjacent maxilla.

Transconjunctival Exposure
After distention of the conjunctiva by saline, an incision is made in the inferior fornix immediately below the tarsal plate level; the incision is then continued by blunt dissection in front of the orbital septum to the inferior orbital rim. *The cornea must be protected* while the incision is being made. The periosteum at the rim is divided, connecting the already exposed orbital floor, anterior maxilla, zygoma, and inferior orbital nerve.

Exposure of Oral Cavity

Upper Exposure
An incision high in the upper buccal sulcus, well clear

*Walter Lorenz, 9850 Interstate Center Drive, Jacksonville, Florida 32218.

of the reflection from the gingiva from one maxillary tuberosity to the other, around the anterior nasal spine, permits subperiosteal stripping of the entire maxilla, laterally to the pterygoid plates and superiorly to the inferior orbital rim. The lateral nasal wall mucosa and nasal floor can be stripped as necessary.

Converse has described an extension of midface degloving when no nasotracheal tube is in place [2]. If a standard rhinoplasty intercartilaginous incision extended through membranous septum is added, it can be extended into the upper buccal sulcus exposure allowing the end of the nose and upper lip to be lifted more extensively. This is rarely necessary and sometimes causes late nasal constriction from the circumferential incision within the nose.

Lower Exposure

Staying well lateral in the lower buccal sulcus, the entire anterior mandible (i.e., body and ascending ramus to the level of the sigmoid notch) can be stripped subperiosteally; care should be taken to avoid the mental nerve.

The mandibular condylar head region can be exposed via the Meisterschnitt approach or separately via a preauricular approach.

The Medial Canthal Ligament

Subperiosteal stripping from the Meisterschnitt approach detaches the medial palpebral tendon when extended down to the lacrimal sac, making its secondary identification for repositioning very difficult. If the palpebral tendon is put on a stretch by pulling at the lateral canthus, it can be felt as a tight cord medially beneath the skin [21]. A 4-mm. skin incision directly over this cord will permit exposure by scissor dissection; the medial palpebal tendon is marked with a suture and the periosteal attachment is incised medially, permitting easy identification later. This is best done at the beginning of the surgery prior to the scalp peeling.

Protection of the Eye

The eyelids should be kept closed by a suture placed through the upper and lower gray line throughout surgery to prevent inadvertent corneal abrasion.

BONE GRAFTS

Ribs

Bone grafts from the ribs are used best for contour defects of the orbital rims or forehead, or for producing a zygomatic arch. An oblique incision is made from the anterior to the posterior axillary line, with the patient on the side. Diathermy is used to cut muscle, and then the underlying rib is stripped subperiosteally from the costochondral junction posteriorly to the angle, using long retractors for exposure. Through this relatively short incision it is possible to remove four ribs easily: two adjacent ribs can be removed, the next rib is left intact, and two more are removed. After removing the ribs, the surgeon should fill the incision with saline, and Valsalva's maneuver is performed. If a pleural leak is present, as shown by the appearance of bubbles, the pleura should be sutured and a chest drain inserted through an intercostal space – not through rib periosteum. If each rib periosteum is precisely sutured, the rib will regrow with a smooth contour.

Iliac Bone

Children

The iliac bone does not have an epiphysis, but a cartilaginous apophysis. The skin incision should be well below the iliac crest and more horizontal, in the line of a mini-bikini. The skin is retracted medially. The perichondrium of the apophysis is exposed. Holding this between the thumb and a finger of one hand, the apophysis is split with a scalpel. This allows subperiosteal stripping of the ilium inferiorly to just above the acetabulum and posteriorly as far as necessary. The anterior superior iliac spine and the crest 1 cm. posterior to it should be left and the lateral cutaneous nerve of the thigh avoided. After removal of as much full-thickness bone as necessary, the split apophysis can be sutured with Dexon suspended from the intact crest anteriorly and posteriorly. Progressive wound closure in watertight layers obviates the need for any drainage. No hip deformity will occur and the site can be reused 1 year later. If necessary, both iliac bones can be taken simultaneously. Although there is more bone in the posterior ilium, it is usually not convenient to place the patient prone on the table.

Adults

To prevent a depression deformity, the periosteal muscle attachment should be left on the iliac crest. The periosteum is incised at the lateral margin of the crest, and the lateral ilium is stripped subperiosteally. A 15-mm. osteotome is passed horizontally through the ilium 10 to 15 mm. below and parallel to the iliac crest. Anteriorly (again well posterior to the spine) and posteriorly, the osteotome is passed obliquely through the iliac crest, producing a bevel. The crest can then be pushed medially, and a medial subperiosteal dissection of ilium is performed. After full-thickness bone is removed, the crest is repositioned firmly on each bevel and the periosteum is sutured. This prevents any noticeable deformity and permits rapid bone regeneration.

ORBITAL HYPERTELORISM

Orbital hypertelorism involves an increased distance between the medial orbital walls as measured at the dacryon. There is always an associated increased distance between the lateral orbital walls. The normal interorbital distance (IOD) is 23 to 28 mm. in adults. Tessier has classified orbital hypertelorism into Type I, 30 to 34 mm.; Type II, 35 to 39 mm.; and Type III, 40 mm. or greater [57]. The medial orbital walls can be of four shapes, as shown in Figure 5-1; Types C and D are more difficult to correct adequately because of the difficulty of decreasing the maximum width. In addition, the measurement of IOD at the dacryon is not the greatest distance in these types. These deformities can be visualized and measured only on basal tomography. The shape of the medial orbital wall can also vary, as seen on progressive tomograms taken from the superior to inferior orbital rim; this will influence the type and success of the operation. Seventy percent of the adult IOD is reached by the age of 2 years in the normal person [29]. Thus, correction for severe deformities can be considered from the age of 2 years and older (although it has been performed on younger children in very large pediatric hospitals). In the majority of cases, the optic canals are normal in distance apart. However, occasionally they are wider apart, and this is usually associated with an increase in the width of the cribriform plate. Orbital hypertelorism is always secondary to another deformity, such as craniostenosis, anterior encephalocele, facial clefting, or frontonasal dysplasia. The underlying condition must be identified prior to the operation.

Correction of Hypertelorism

Extracranial Approach

MEDIAL WALL OSTEOTOMY. This is accomplished via a Meisterschnitt approach or midline nasal incision (Fig. 5-2). A central segment of bone is removed and the medial walls are repositioned together with the medial palpebral ligament. This was the first procedure described and is largely ineffective [50].

SUBCRANIAL ORBITAL CORRECTION. This procedure (Fig. 5-3) can be used when the deformity is not severe (i.e., in Tessier Type I or II), when the cribriform plate is high (i.e., above the level of the frontonasal suture), and when there is no associated frontal deformity (e.g., in encephalocele). It is efficient only for corrections of up to 1 cm. IOD. (Some cases of mild hypertelorism with an inner canthal distance of up to 38 mm. and a normal nose can be quite attractive; *these do not need correction.*)

Intracranial Approach (Frontal Bar)

The orbit can be considered as a box with the eye inside. To reposition the eye adequately, it is necessary to move the box (Figs. 5-4 and 5-5). This tech-

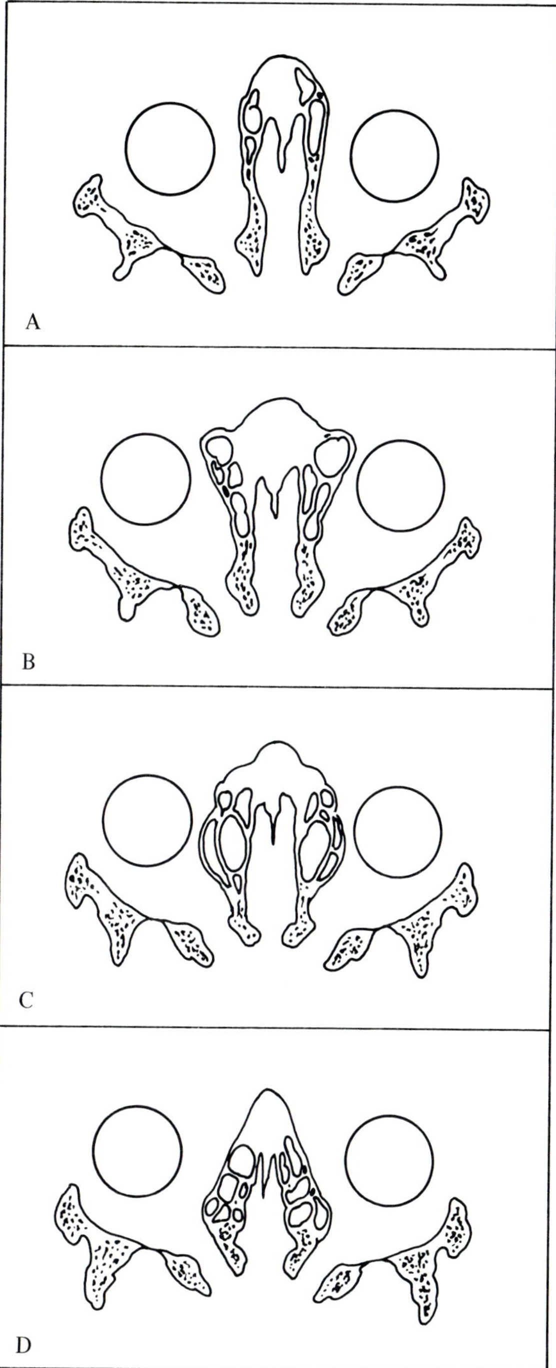

Fig. 5-1. Types of medial orbital wall deformity in orbital hypertelorism. Type A, medial orbital walls parallel; Type B, wedge-shaped posteriorly; Type C, oval; and Type D, wedge-shaped anteriorly.

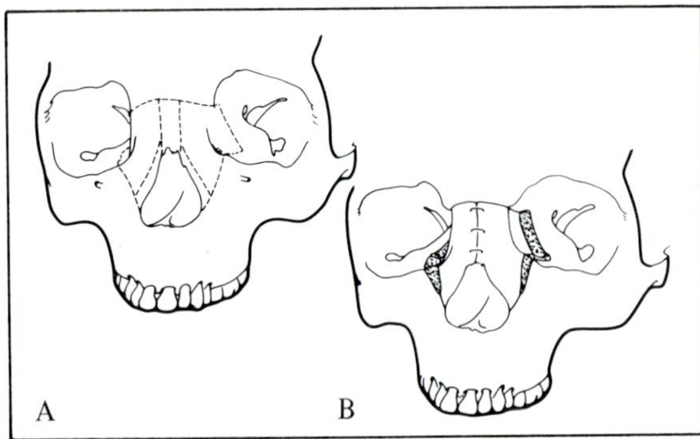

Fig. 5-2. Extracranial osteotomy through the medial orbital wall. A, bone cuts. B, medial repositioning and insertion of bone grafts has been performed.

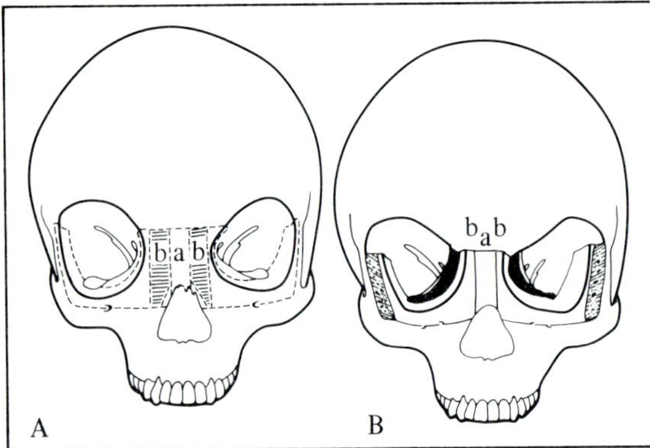

Fig. 5-3. Subcranial orbital osteotomy. A, the frontonasal cut is below the cribriform plate. Segments b are removed and the lateral orbital wall is split. B, the bottom U of the orbit is migrated medially. If the nasal root is very deformed, segment a can be removed as an alternative and an iliac bone graft used to reconstruct the nose. Iliac bone grafts are inserted laterally.

nique is needed for severe cases, in known anterior intracranial disorders (such as frontal or nasal encephalocele or meningocele), or when the cribriform plate is shown on anteroposterior radiographs to be below the level of the frontonasal suture.

SURGICAL TECHNIQUE. The first steps in this procedure are to garner the necessary iliac bone grafts and to expose and identify the medial canthal ligaments. Most patients will have excess skin on the nose and often the nose is of an abnormal shape. Through a midline nasal incision, dissect subperiosteally over the nasal bones and extend the dissection laterally

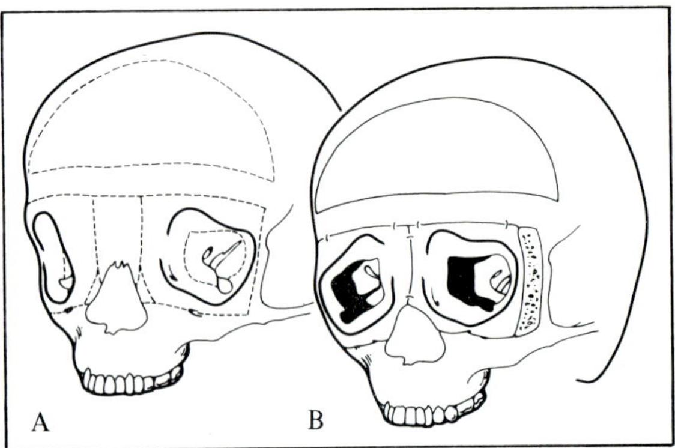

Fig. 5-4. Intracranial orbital hypertelorism correction with intact frontal bar. A, the central nasofrontal region is removed, and the lateral orbital wall is split in the plane of the wall. The margins of the piriform fossa are removed so that with medial transmigration, nasal obstruction will not occur. B, after medial repositioning, iliac bone grafts are inserted into the lateral orbital split.

over the anterior maxilla. Dissect subperichondrally the upper and lower lateral cartilages.

Through the Meisterschnitt approach, strip the frontal bone and all orbital walls, zygoma, medial zygomatic arch, and lateral maxilla. Using a right-angled nitrogen-powered saw, the medial anterior maxilla is cut horizontally via the nose into the antrum. The lateral part of the maxilla is cut from the coronal incision. The lateral orbital wall is split in its plane with a power saw for the lower two-thirds. The medial part of the lateral orbital wall is cut at right angles to join the splitting incision. This cut joins the inferior orbital fissure posterolaterally. The lateral orbital floor is cut into the antrum with an osteotome (the inferior orbital canal should be avoided). At this point, two parallel lines 1 cm. apart are marked 1 cm. above the superior orbital rim. The neurosurgeon then performs a bifrontal craniotomy and frees extradurally the frontal lobes over the orbital roof to the pterion and lesser wings of the sphenoid. Medially, freeing is taken to the cribriform plate margin. Three anomalies commonly occur that are not apparent on preoperative radiographs: very small tongues of dura pass in the region of the foramen cecum to the root of the nose; stalagmites of bone grow up from the orbital roof invaginating the dura of the frontal lobes; and sometimes there is a spur or sail-like projection of bone posteriorly from the metopic suture invaginating into the sagittal sinus. The craniofacial surgeon then measures the interdacryon distance and calculates the amount of bone to be removed (this amount depends on the age of the patient and the shape of the medial orbital walls as seen on basal tomography). The true facial midline is marked on the frontal bar. The horizontal cut of the frontal bone abcve the orbits is made. The orbital roof is cut either from within the orbit with a right-angled saw or via the intracranial route with a 20-degree attachment on a nitrogen-powered burr. The orbital roof cut is immediately in front of the lesser sphenoid wing from the pterion to the margin of the cribriform plate. It then passes anteriorly and around the cribriform plate at the foramen cecum. A rectangular, or triangular, segment of orbital roof is removed beside the cribriform plate. The lateral orbital split is completed where it enters the anterior fossa. The central nasofrontal segment of bone is removed with the saw and the medial orbital wall osteotomy connects that of the roof and floor. The orbital box should now be completely free and capable of being moved medially by fingertip pressure only. The frontal bar ensures correct horizontal and anteroposterior repositioning of the orbit. Complete medial positioning is prevented by the margin of the piriform fossa, which is removed by a saw; the anterior and middle ethmoid sinuses, which are removed by a rongeur; and the nasal septum. Subperiosteal and subperichondral dissection now permits removal of as much bony nasal septum and posterior cartilaginous septum as necessary. The mucosa in this area is also removed and the nose converted to a unichannel in this area. The medial canthal ligament is identified and a monofilament wire or nylon suture is passed first through it and then through an ipsilateral drill hole and similar contralateral hole. The nasal mucosa is repaired, particularly in the nasal root. The orbital boxes are then wired to each other and to the frontal bar, ensuring symmetry by the previous mark on the frontal bar. A wide hole is made into the nasofrontal region with a burr. The dura is checked for bleeding and tears. Then the frontal bone is wired into place. Custom-fitted bone grafts are inserted and wired into the lateral orbital walls. The scalp is sutured. An iliac (or rib) graft is shaped and pegged into the hole in the frontonasal region and tied over with wire sutures as a cantilever. The medial canthal tendon is pushed into the drill holes, and the suture is tightened over the nasal bone graft. Anomalies in the nasal cartilages are then corrected as necessary and these cartilages are sutured together over the cantilever bone graft. Finally, excess skin of the nose is removed, which is best done through an S-shaped excision. When this is sutured, there is skin lengthening and a straight midline scar. A Z-plasty at the nasofrontal region also lengthens skin and tightens this area, but leaves a stigmatizing scar. The nasal subcutaneous area is then sutured together, pressed against the nasal bones and bone graft, and the skin is sutured. This technique obviates the necessity of external canthal buttons to hold the skin in tightly. If skin excision has been correctly judged, no epicanthal folds will occur. Finally, a dressing is applied to the head, but *not to the face or eye,* and the eyelid sutures are removed. The patient is awakened and *visual acuity is confirmed* by the patient on the table.

Postoperative management includes monitoring the neurological vital signs and the use of steroids, anticonvulsants, and antibiotics (started preoperatively); *no analgesics should be used.*

VARIATIONS. When the lateral orbital wall is very thin, a coronal cut is made from temporal fossa into the lateral orbit (Fig. 5-5). This cut must be anterior to the middle cranial fossa. Before scalp closure, the anterior two-thirds of the temporalis is stripped subperiosteally from its origin, divided vertically, advanced, and sutured to the lateral orbital wall. This prevents an hour-glass hollow appearing in this area.

INTRACRANIAL APPROACH (FRONTAL SPUR). Occasionally, in the presence of a frontal encephalocele or congenital absence of bone, it is not possible to leave the frontal bar (Figs. 5-6 and 5-7). In these cases, a lateral spur should be left long enough to guide the position of the medial orbital movement. If no guideline is present, there is great danger of placing one orbit higher than the other or anterior to the other. Judgment of the facial midline also becomes very difficult.

Fig. 5-5. Intracranial orbital hypertelorism correction with intact frontal bar. A, when the lateral orbital wall is very thin, it must be cut posteriorly from the temporal fossa into the orbit. The osteotomy must be anterior to the middle cranial fossa. Superiorly, it enters the anterior fossa. B, postoperative appearance with bone grafts in the lateral cut.

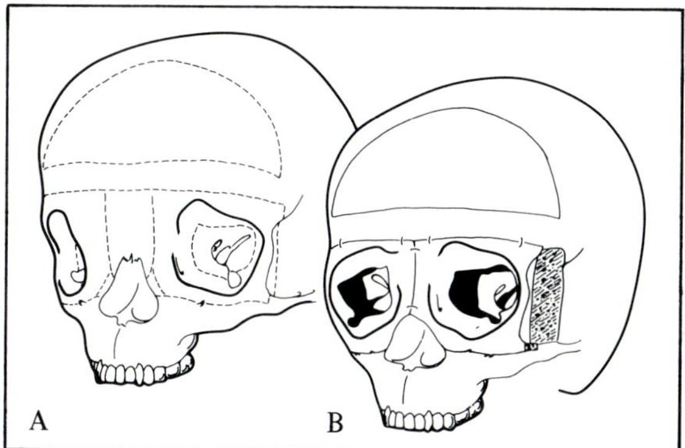

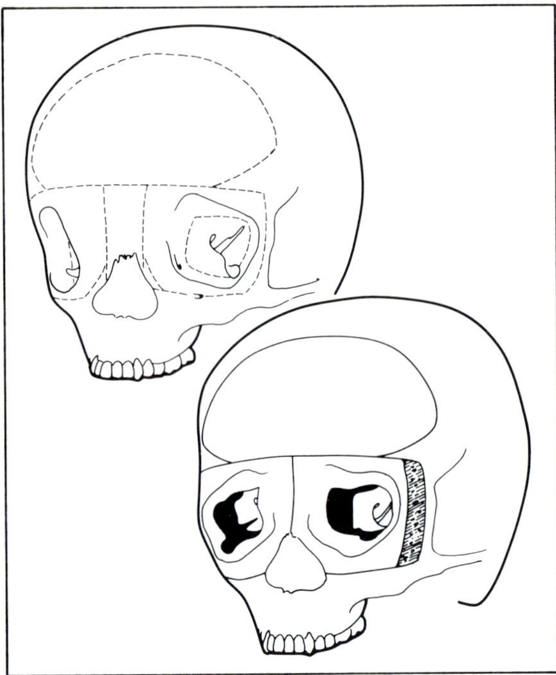

Fig. 5-6. Intracranial orbital hypertelorism correction with frontal spur and with the lateral orbital wall split.

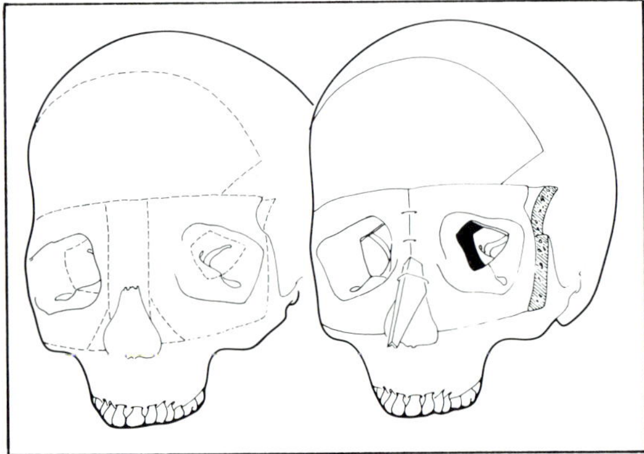

Fig. 5-7. Intracranial orbital hypertelorism correction with frontal spur and with the lateral orbital wall intact. This also shows a cantilevered rib graft split and pegged into the midline.

Complications

ANESTHESIA. Anesthetic complications are numerous, but basically related to inexperience with the procedure. They include inadequate fluid and blood replacement, inability to shrink the brain completely to allow safe retraction of the frontal lobes, failure to prevent the oculocardiac reflex, and oversedation (so that the patient is not immediately awake and alert at the end of the procedure).

NEUROSURGICAL. Bone anomalies in the midline increase the danger of opening the sagittal sinus. It is very rare for these patients to have a completely normal inner skull. Failure to repair dural tears may cause a postoperative leak of cerebrospinal fluid (which is best treated by continuous external lumbar drainage until the leak stops spontaneously).

PLANNING. Some complications result from the failure to diagnose the deformity correctly. Asymmetry preoperatively is very common. Lateral canthal dystopia may occur; the lateral canthi must be horizontally realigned prior to scalp closure. Inadequate correction may involve the failure to remove enough central bone (more must be removed than is theoretically necessary due to rotation of the posterior medial orbital wall laterally), the failure to make the inner orbital wall cuts posterior to the globe of the eye, or the failure to position the medial canthal tendon correctly into the drill hole.

ORBITAL DYSTOPIA

Symmetrical lateral displacement of each orbit in orbital hypertelorism is relatively uncommon. More often, one orbit is displaced laterally, or rotated laterally, more than the other. The standard operation is modified to correct these problems. Occasionally, a facial cleft can cause unilateral orbital displacement; thus, only one "box" needs to be repositioned. If one orbit is at a different vertical height than the other, a suitable amount of bone above the superior rim can be used to raise the orbit; conversely, a block from the anterior maxilla and zygoma will permit lowering. If there is an antimongoloid (or mongoloid) position to the orbit, appropriate wedges superiorly (or inferiorly) will allow horizontal realignment. In these cases, particular care must be given to realign the canthal levels correctly.

TREACHER COLLINS SYNDROME

Most of the external deformities in the Treacher Collins syndrome (Fig. 5-8) are due to underlying skeletal deficiencies. There are varying degrees of severity from mild to severe. In the mild cases there is hypoplasia of bone, whereas in the severe deformity

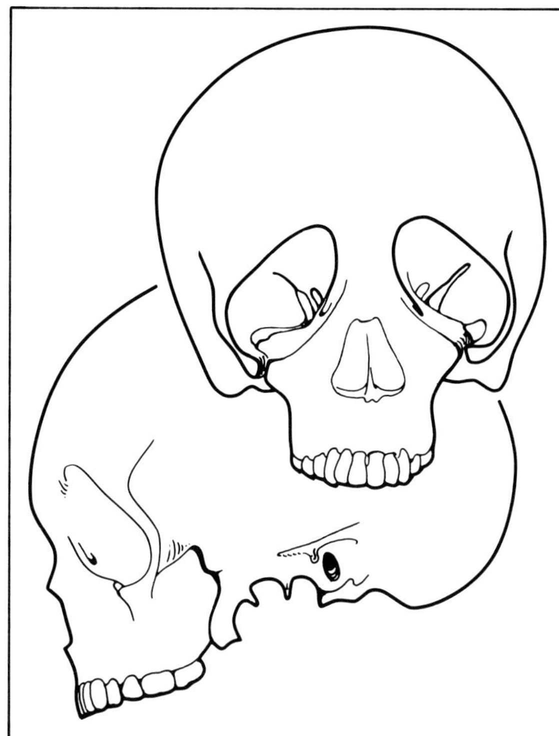

Fig. 5-8. Treacher Collins upper facial skeletal deformity. The orbits slope obliquely. There is a cleft through the inferior orbital rim. The lateral orbital wall is severely hypoplastic. The zygoma and zygomatic arch are absent.

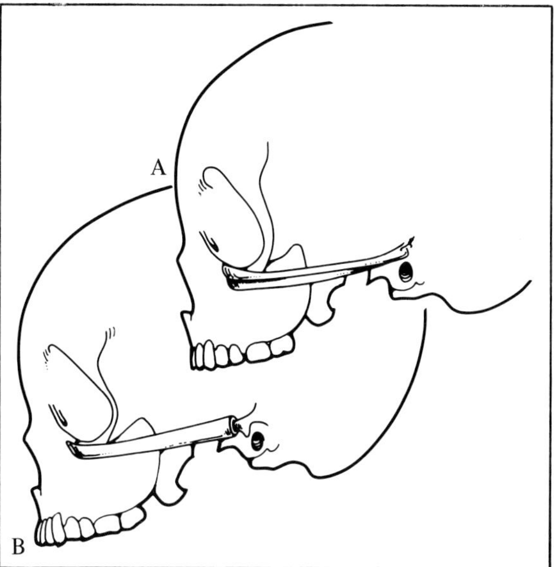

Fig. 5-9. Rebuilding the zygomatic arch. A, one or two split ribs can be laid over the inferior orbital rim and passed backward to be attached to a small flap of elevated temporal bone. B, if there is a residual part of the zygomatic process of the temporal bone, an intact rib can be pegged over this and brought forward; it is then beveled to blend with the inferior orbital rim.

there is actual absence of bone. The most stigmatizing deformity is the periorbital area. The ear deformity, if present, is more easily covered by the patient. In the most severe cases, there is a marked antimongoloid slope to the palpebral fissures, coloboma of the lower eyelids (absence of eyelashes in the medial two-thirds of the lower eyelids), and cheek depression. The antimongoloid slope is associated with hypoplasia of the lateral superior orbital rim. Severe hypoplasia of the lateral orbital wall will extend even as far back as the greater wing of the sphenoid. The zygoma may be extremely small or even absent. The zygomatic arch may be completely absent, or there may be a residual spur of the zygomatic process of the temporal bone. The maxilla lateral to the inferior orbital foramen may be hypoplastic, and its contribution to the zygomatic buttress may be absent. The entire orbit is oblique, sloping downward and laterally; this is due to lowering of the lateral part of the orbital roof and rim and lowering of the lateral orbital floor, made worse by absence of the zygomatic part of the floor. In addition, three facial clefts may be present: through the zygomatic arch (if present), at the frontozygomatic suture level, and at the inferior orbital rim (usually just lateral to the maxillozygomatic suture line). When the zygoma is absent, the inferior orbital fissure is exposed laterally. Additional skeletal deformities include anomalies of the external and middle ear, a short anterior cranial base with an acute angle, loss of the nasofrontal angle, and a short down-curved mandible.

Surgical Technique (Upper Face)

For simple hypoplasia of the cheek buttress due to hypoplasia of the zygoma and absence or clefting of the zygomatic arch, the deficiency can be reconstituted by split or intact ribs (Fig. 5-9).

Tessier Technique

In the Tessier technique (Fig. 5-10), three or four full-length ribs are usually necessary. The Meisterschnitt approach is used, with subperiosteal dissection of the entire periorbita except medially. This allows rotation of the periorbita to correct the antimongoloid slope after skeletal correction. Freeing the periosteum

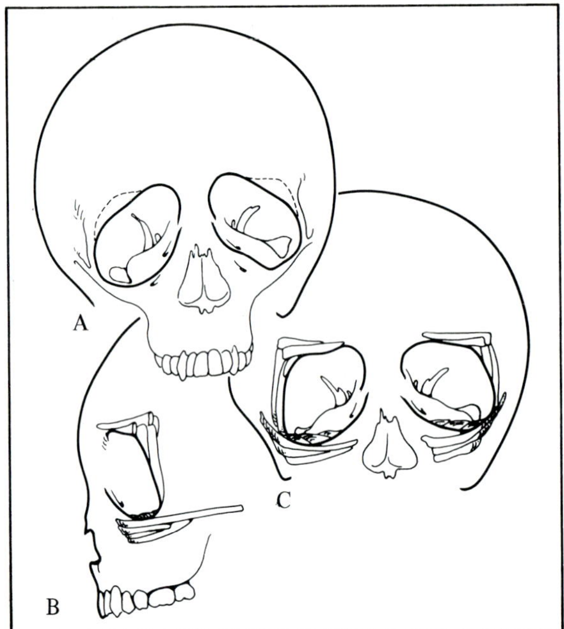

Fig. 5-10. Total periorbital correction of Treacher Collins syndrome (Tessier technique). Upper left, A, the lateral superior orbital rim is enlarged by burring out the bone (beware of entering the anterior cranial fossa). B, C, onlay split ribs, dove-tailed at the corners, are placed over the lateral superior orbital rim and frontal bone, lateral orbital wall, inferior orbital rim, maxilla, and zygoma and zygomatic arch. Further grafts are placed in the lateral orbital floor to raise it.

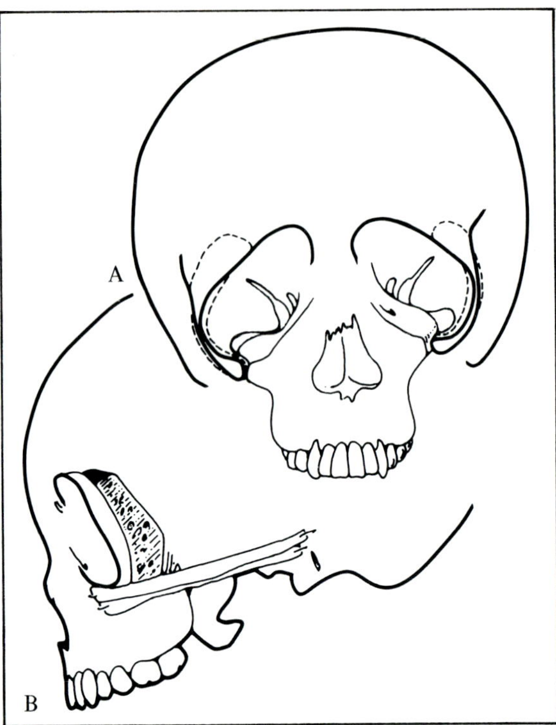

Fig. 5-11. Variation of the Tessier technique for periorbital correction. A, the residual and posteriorly displaced lateral orbital wall and lateral superior orbital rim are osteotomized. B, they are then advanced and rotated outward and buttressed forward with a block of iliac bone. Additional rib grafts are applied as shown, with augmentation of the orbital floor and superior rim as in Fig. 5-10 if necessary.

from the bone cleft (complete or incomplete), and then reconstituting the bone, is often all that is necessary to correct the lower eyelid coloboma that has been caused by a tethering of the eyelid through to the periosteum in the clefting.

The lateral superior orbital rim may be sloping downward as well as posterolaterally. The frontal bone of the rim can be burred to enlarge and lift this area. However, slightly more posteriorly, the orbital roof is very thin and could only be lifted by an intracranial approach, which is rarely necessary. Split ribs (if a large correction is necessary, the ribs can be used intact) are placed over the lateral frontal bone, down the lateral orbital wall, and over the anterior maxilla, zygoma, and zygomatic arch. Dove-tailing, or interlocking, a horizontal with a vertical strut at each corner provides increased stability. Additional rib grafts are placed in the lateral orbital floor to raise it. The grafts are wired to each other and to the underlying skeleton. If a significant orbital wall advancement is performed, the temporalis should be advanced. The lateral canthal ligament should now be firmly reattached to the lateral orbital wall via a drill hole to correct the antimongoloid slope permanently.

VARIATION. A large amount of rib grafts is needed for the above technique. I have thus found it logical to cut and advance the residual lateral superior rim and orbital wall and buttress it forward with iliac bone, giving further support by attaching it to the rib grafts, forming the zygoma and zygomatic arch (Fig. 5-11).

Surgical Technique (Lower Face)

Many patients have severe retrognathia and apertognathia. The latter is associated with a reversed Spee's curve and marked antigonal notching. When the mandible is not short in length, the anterior mandible can be rotated upward (Fig. 5-12A, B). If there is true retrognathia, the mandible can be advanced forward

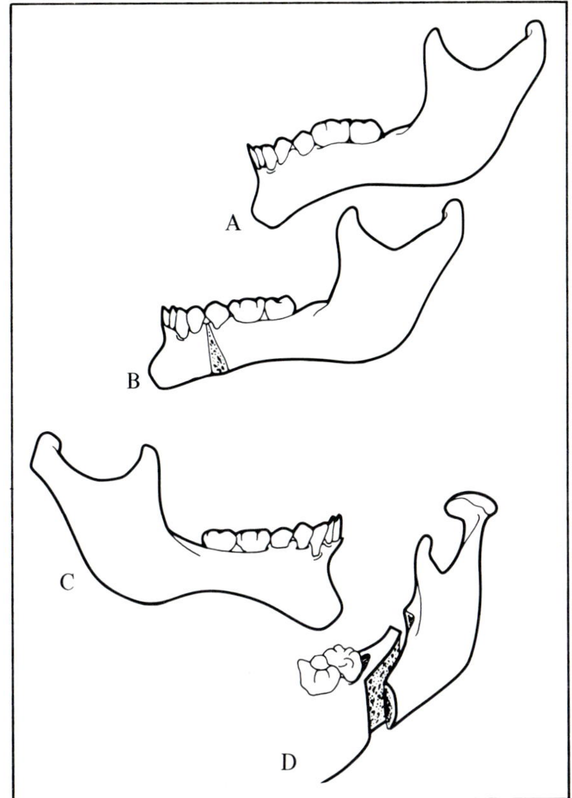

Fig. 5-12. Correction of mandible deformity in Treacher Collins syndrome. A, B, to correct the reversed Spee's curve, the anterior mandible must be osteotomized at the appropriate level (usually between the first and second bicuspid teeth); it is then rotated upward and a wedge-shaped iliac graft is inserted. C, D, for simple retrognathia with a flat occlusal plane, an Obwegeser–Dal-Pont sagittal split of the mandible can be used for advancement.

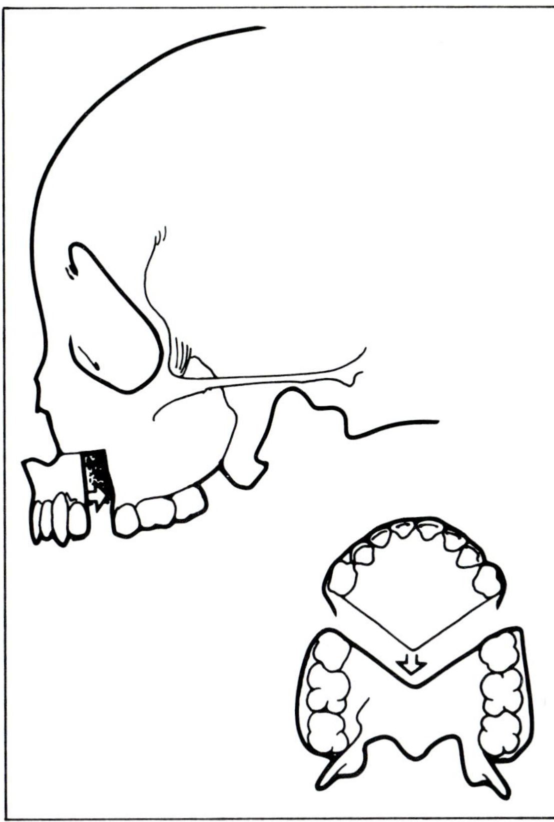

Fig. 5-13. Wassmund procedure. One upper bicuspid tooth is extracted, and the bone is resected through alveolus, hard palate, and lower maxilla, with a horizontal osteotomy through the anterior nasal septum and lower piriform margin. The segment is then recessed and fixed into a predesigned occlusal splint, and transosteotomy wires are inserted at the piriform margin.

and rotated upward by a sagittal splitting of the ascending ramus via the intraoral approach (Fig. 5-12C, D). Sometimes it may be necessary to level the occlusal plane as well; the two procedures can be performed simultaneously through the intraoral approach, provided that adequately designed occlusal splints of cast metal or acrylic are made available.

Many patients appear to have a protrusive anterior lower maxilla, although cephalometric measurement usually shows it to be in the correct place. A better facial profile may thus be designed by utilizing a Wassmund (or Wunderer) technique to recess the anterior maxilla (Fig. 5-13). This procedure should be done simultaneously with the mandibular repositioning and can be done in the same operation as the upper face correction.

Complications

Complications are usually due to inadequate correction at the primary operation. Bone graft resorption is variable and unpredictable. Therefore, slight overcorrection should be achieved, because it is easier to remove excess bone a year later than to add more bone. Advancing the lateral orbital wall causes less of a problem with resorption and makes it easier to produce a smooth contour. In spite of the fact that the zygomatic arch was reconstructed in the absence of a periosteal envelope, the grafts are still present after many years.

Relapse and recurrence of the sloping palpebral fissure may result from (1) inadequate correction of the oblique orbital skeleton, (2) inadequate rotation of the periorbita, (3) inadequate fixation of the lateral canthal ligament to its new position, or (4) inadequate freeing of tethered periosteum in a complete or incomplete cleft.

ANOMALIES OF THE CENTRAL FACE

Perinasal Osteotomy

Isolated cases of severe nasal shortening and flatness and perinasal retrusion may occur, sometimes associated with maxillonasal dysplasia of Binder [1]. If the occlusion is normal, there are two alternative principles: (1) augmentation by synthetic or autogenous implants as an L-shaped strut down the nose, with additional implants around the margins of the piriform aperture, or (2) moving the basal bone and cartilaginous skeleton. When the nasal advancement is large (e.g., 10 mm.) and the nasal length must be significantly increased (e.g., 6 to 8 mm.), onlay procedures tend to fail from either rapid resorption or erosion through the skin. If the basal skeleton is repositioned, much greater and more permanent correction can be achieved.

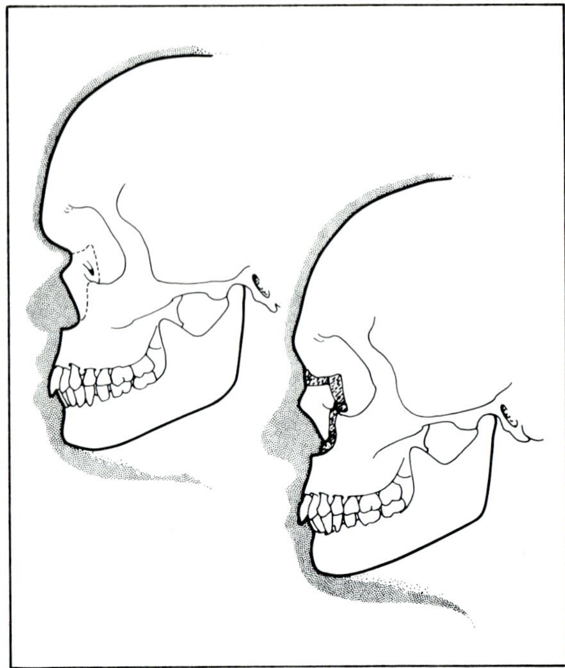

Fig. 5-14. The perinasal osteotomy and advancement with stabilization by iliac grafts.

The root of the nose can be exposed via a variety of skin incisions: (1) directly over it, or (2) by the Meisterschnitt approach. The nasal bones are stripped subperiosteally, the upper lateral cartilages are stripped subperichondrally, and then the mucosa beneath the nasal bones is undermined, permitting the lengthening and caudal transposition of the cartilages. The perinasal skeleton is then osteotomized as shown in Figure 5-14, or alternatively the lateral cut can be brought anterior to the lacrimal fossa to avoid having to reattach the medial palpebral ligaments. The osteotomy around the piriform fossa can be as lateral as necessary to correct the flatness. The caudal horizontal cut must be at the level of the nasal floor, or higher, depending on the roots of the teeth as shown on a panoramic (Panorex) radiograph. The entire skeleton is then advanced and maintained with iliac bone grafts.

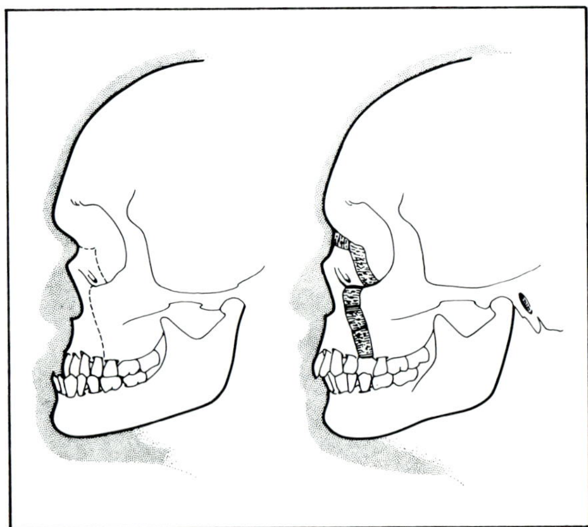

Fig. 5-15. Nasomaxillary osteotomy.

Nasomaxillary Osteotomy

For perinasal flatness and anterior maxillary retrusion, the central face can be advanced as shown in Figure 5-15. This can be approached through a nasal skin incision and buccal sulcus approach, via a complete midface degloving, or through the scalp and upper buccal sulcus. However, this procedure will disrupt the maxillary dental arch, creating a dental gap that will require a dental plate or bridgework. It would be more sensible to use a Le Fort II osteotomy

Zygoma and Anterior Maxillary Osteotomy (Tripartite Osteotomy Type II)
The zygoma and anterior maxillary osteotomy (Fig. 5-16) would logically be used to advance the cheek and inferior orbital rim and to recess the anterior maxilla. However, advancement of both would be better achieved by the winged Le Fort II osteotomy, since that would not disrupt the dental arch.

Le Fort II Maxillary Osteotomy
The Le Fort II maxillary osteotomy (Fig. 5-17) is indicated for retromaxillism with a Class III malocclusion and a small nose. This procedure is needed in some cleft lip and palate cases and in some patients with maxillonasal dysplasia of Binder.

SURGICAL TECHNIQUE. Subperiosteal exposure is through an upper buccal sulcus incision combined with a nasal root skin incision or a sulcus and Meisterschnitt approach to prevent scarring. Since a tracheostomy is rarely indicated and a nasotracheal anesthetic tube is in place, a midface degloving is not possible. The horizontal cut nasofrontal osteotomy is made with a saw; the remaining cuts are best made with a fine burr or a side-cutting rotating saw on a drill handpiece. The osteotomy between the maxillary tuberosity and pterygoid plates is made with a fine curved pterygoid osteotome. The nasal septum is divided by a curved osteotome passed downward and backward from the nasofrontal region to the posterior nasal spine. It is important for this osteotome to be driven downward more than backward initially in order to avoid the cribriform plate. The maxilla is then advanced using disimpaction forceps and wired into occlusal position over an acrylic wafer precisely designed for the required occlusion. Iliac bone grafts are inserted at the nasofrontal region, medial orbital walls, and anterior maxilla, and they are wired into position. Wedge-shaped grafts are inserted into the pterygoid osteotomy. Additional fixation is provided by circumzygomatic wires fixed to the maxillary or mandibular arch bar.

Le Fort II Maxillary Osteotomy (Winged)
If the patient has flatness extending more laterally on the face, the osteotomy can be extended laterally as necessary to include the orbital floor, inferior orbital rim, medial zygoma, and zygomatic buttress (Fig. 5-18). These areas can be best approached by extending the subperiosteal dissection from the upper buccal sulcus upward and laterally to give exposure. After stripping the periorbita from the orbital floor, malleable brain retractors should be inserted prior to making the osteotomy. Bone grafts will be needed in all areas except the orbital floor (see under the heading Le Fort III Maxillary Advancement).

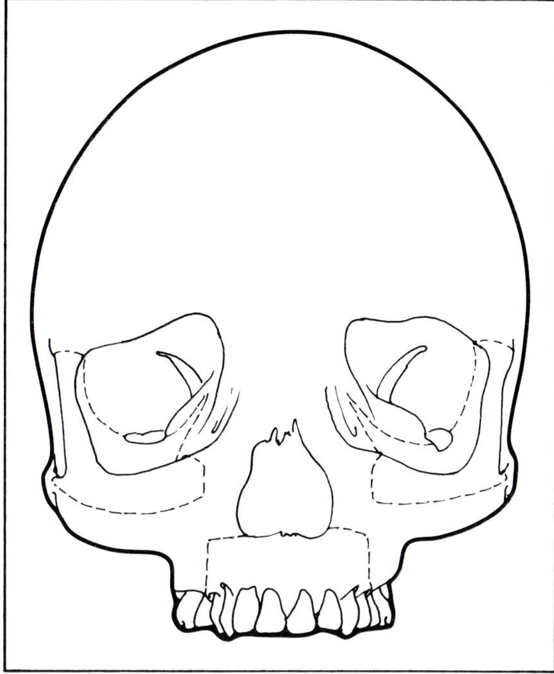

Fig. 5-16. Zygoma and anterior maxilla osteotomy (this is also termed a tripartite osteotomy Type II).

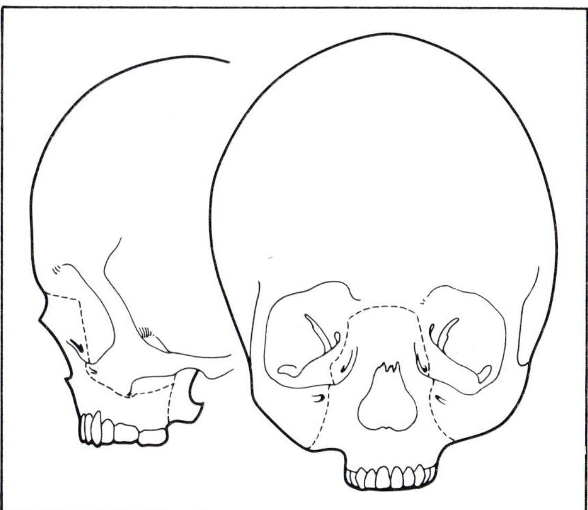

Fig. 5-17. Le Fort II maxillary advancement. The osteotomy runs across the nasofrontal suture, behind the lacrimal fossa, across the inferior orbital rim, downward to join the horizontal cut of a Le Fort I osteotomy, and backward to join the vertical pterygomaxillary disjunction.

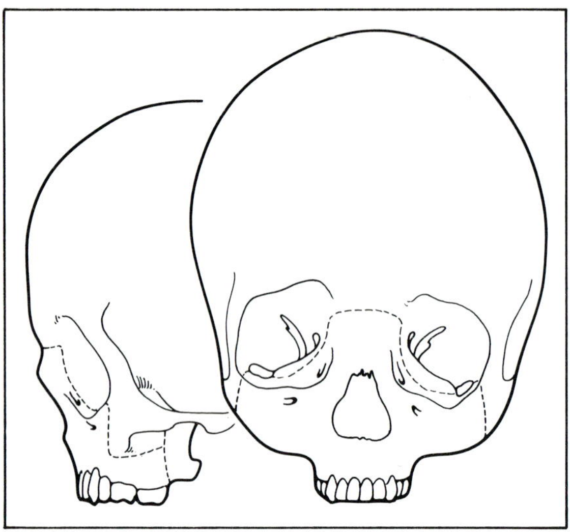

Fig. 5-18. Le Fort II maxillary osteotomy (winged). The inferior orbital rims and medial zygoma are included for advancement.

Tripartite Osteotomy (Type I)

The tripartite osteotomy (Type I) has been described for advancement of the cheek and orbital walls. For further orbital expansion, this segment can be moved laterally as well as forward (Fig. 5-19). The nasomaxillary segment can be advanced a different amount. This procedure still has the disadvantage of creating a gap in the dental arch. A similar and easier correction can be achieved by using a Le Fort I and III osteotomy simultaneously, which does not disrupt the dental arch (see p. 145).

CROUZON'S AND APERT'S SYNDROMES

Crouzon's syndrome and Apert's syndrome have similar craniofacial deformities of varying expressivity. Both have an autosomal dominant pattern of inheritance. Apert's patients differ from patients with Crouzon's syndrome by having syndactyly of the hands and feet and, in many cases, a decreased level of intelligence. Many Crouzon's patients are well above average in intelligence. The skull nearly always has bilateral coronal synostosis, but other sutures are

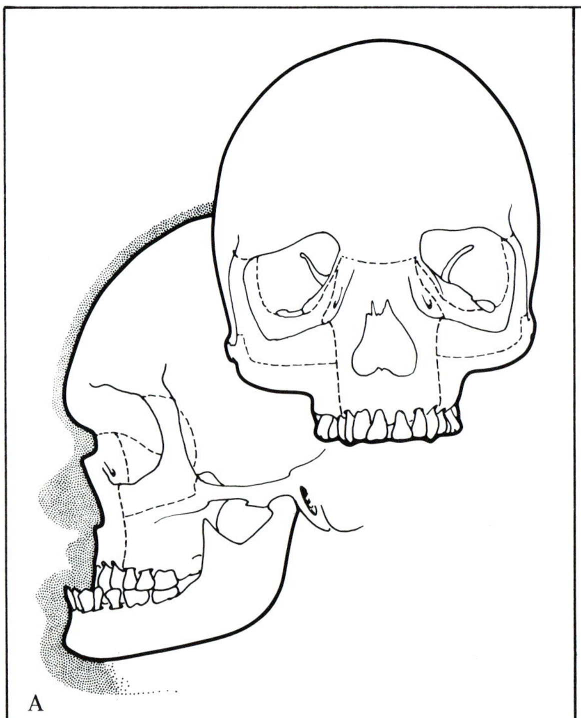

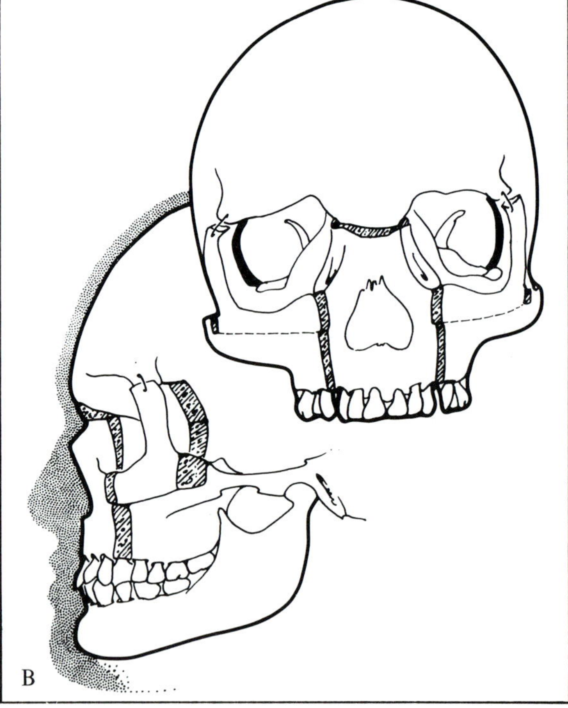

Fig. 5-19. Tripartite osteotomy (Type I). A, the lines of osteotomy are shown. B, the orbital wall, rim, and zygoma are advanced forward and laterally if necessary, and the nasomaxillary complex can be advanced a different amount.

often involved, including the sagittal, lambdoid, parietal, frontosphenoidal, and frontoethmoidal sutures. The maxillas and zygomas are hypoplastic. The combination of basal skull stenosis, underdevelopment of the zygoma and maxilla, and often a compensatory bulging of the middle cranial fossa into the orbit produces a very shallow orbit that does not grow adequately. The eye and periorbital contents are unaffected and grow at a normal rate, causing progressive protrusion of the eyeballs until they rest outside (anterior) to the orbital rims, giving rise to the term *exorbitism.* In this situation, the cornea is easily subject to abrasion and the eye may prolapse through the eyelids, which then become trapped behind it and rapidly cause blindness. In addition, the nose is small and short with a characteristic "parrot-beak" shape. There is usually a moderate degree of orbital hypertelorism. The palate is high arched and its mucosa thickened by infiltration with mucopolysaccharides. There is progressively disproportionate growth between maxilla and mandible, causing a worsening Class III malocclusion. In some cases, the maxilla is so far posterior that it almost rests on the base of the skull. The soft palate is then hanging low down in the pharynx and the patient has hyponasality. Growth of the tonsils and adenoids in the first 2 years of life causes increasing respiratory obstruction.

Treatment of the craniostenosis is discussed on pp. 154-155.

Le Fort III Maxillary Advancement

Standard Le Fort III Maxillary Advancement

In the standard version of the Le Fort maxillary advancement (Fig. 5-20), the amount of occlusal advancement, inferior orbital rim, and lateral orbital wall advancement is determined in advance and an occlusal wafer provided. After iliac grafts have been collected, the entire procedure can be performed through a Meisterschnitt approach. The forehead, entire periorbita, orbital rims, nasal root, zygoma, and posterior maxilla to the pterygomaxillary junction are stripped subperiosteally. The frontozygomatic suture is cut horizontally. The lateral orbital walls are cut in the coronal plane. Basal tomograms will determine the amount of bulging of the sphenoid wing into the orbit and the distance from this to the anterior border of the lateral orbital wall is measured. If this distance is very short, a burr hole should be placed prophylactically into the middle cranial fossa and a pack inserted extradurally in front of the temporal lobe. The zygoma is cut vertically at its junction with the arch. Osteotomes are passed across the orbital floor. This can usually be done through the Meisterschnitt approach, but a transconjunctival approach can increase visualization. The frontonasal

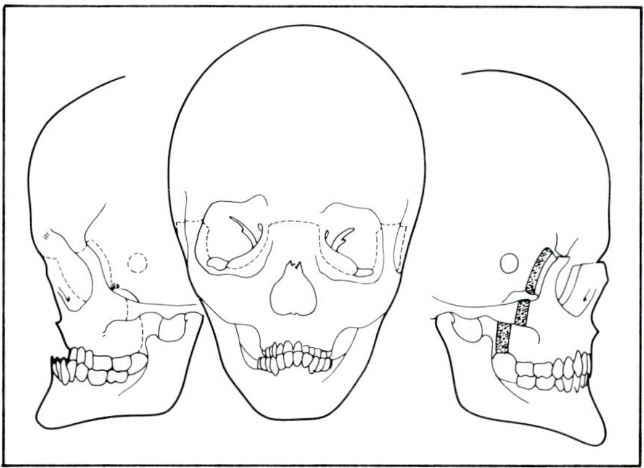

Fig. 5-20. Le Fort III maxillary advancement (standard). The maxilla is cut and advanced as shown. Wire fixation is at the frontonasal, frontozygomatic, and zygomatic osteotomy. In addition to those bone grafts shown, it is usually necessary to insert grafts at the frontonasal osteotomy.

suture is cut with a saw horizontally and the medial orbital walls are cut posteriorly. The pterygomaxillary fissure is cut from above with a fine curved osteotome. Another curved osteotome is then passed downward and backward from the frontonasal osteotomy to the posterior nasal spine dividing the nasal septum. The maxilla is advanced and wired into occlusion. Wires are inserted at the frontonasal and frontozygomatic osteotomies and bone grafts are wired into these places as well as the lateral orbital wall and the zygomatic cut. Wedge-shaped grafts are inserted into the pterygomaxillary separation. Because the skin and periorbita are still united and the skin has been advanced, the periorbita should be incised superiorly, medially, and laterally, and if necessary, inferiorly. No bone grafts need to be inserted into the orbital wall medially or inferiorly – prolapse of the periorbita into the antrum does not occur in spite of this gap.

As in all cases of periorbital stripping, the patient should have a head bandage, but *no eye bandage,* and should be awakened and have the *visual acuity* checked while still on the operating table. Young patients having this procedure should always have a tracheostomy. In larger patients (adolescents or adults), a nasotracheal tube can be used with these *precautions:* (1) care should be taken to avoid cutting the anesthetic tube while making the osteotomy in the nasal septum, and (2) the tube must be inserted well through the vocal cords to just above the carina. At the time of maxillary advancement, the forehead and mandible must be held to prevent neck flexion because this, combined with sudden maxillary advancement, can cause the anesthetic tube to ride suddenly upward through the larynx.

SELF-RETENTION. In order to provide greater stability, the frontozygomatic osteotomy can be beveled upward and backward. If the horizontal and vertical distances of this bevel are long, it will enter the anterior cranial fossa; hence a burr hole and packing must be inserted to protect the dura and frontal lobe. Then, if the lateral walls are rocked from side to side during advancement, the posterior spur of the bevel can be brought anteriorly to the zygomatic process of the frontal bone for increased stability and wiring. If good pterygoid and other grafts are inserted, there is then no need, theoretically, to wire the patient into occlusion.

Le Fort III Osteotomy with Split Lateral Wall

The zygomatic cut shown in Figure 5-20 sometimes results in the fracturing of the zygomatic arch during fixation; hence, there is a loss of stability for inserting a bone graft in this area. If the lateral orbital wall is thick enough, it can be split in its plane, as shown in Figure 5-21, and the cut continued down through the zygoma, leaving an intact posterolateral rim of orbital wall and zygomatic arch for the insertion of bone grafts.

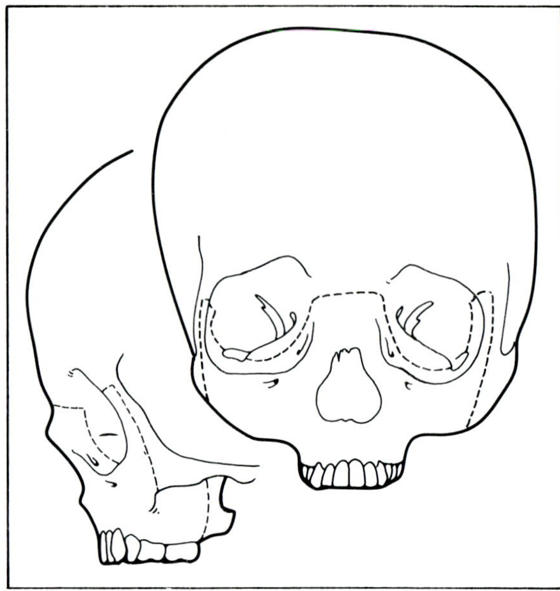

Fig. 5-21. Le Fort III maxillary advancement with lateral orbital wall split.

Le Fort III Maxillary Advancement with Zygomatic Step Cut

Tessier originally described a step cut in the zygoma (Fig. 5-22), which gives increased stability for bone grafting. However, separate grafts must be inserted in the lateral orbital wall and the lower vertical osteotomy of the zygoma. There is little advantage in this procedure.

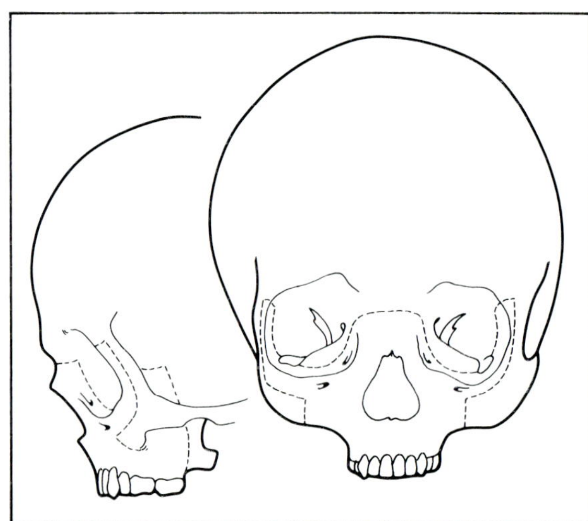

Fig. 5-22. Le Fort III maxillary advancement with zygomatic step cut.

Le Fort III Maxillary Advancement with Anterior Open Bite

Many patients with Crouzon's or Apert's syndrome have an anterior open bite because the anterior maxillary occlusal plane is tilted upward. As the maxilla is advanced forward and downward to close the open bite, the incisors act as a hinge point or fulcrum. Thus, the nasal root is at the end of a long arm and will advance much further (Fig. 5-23). When this area is bone grafted and stabilized with wires, the nasofrontal angle is lost, producing a characteristic deformity of a prominent long nose. Secondary rhinoplasty to deepen this angle is not easy because of the wires and the solid bone graft. Detailed planning can predict the amount of correction needed at each area and a variation in the surgery can prevent the need for secondary correction.

Le Fort III Maxillary Advancement with Frontal Spur and Forehead Rib Grafts

Some patients have recession of the superior orbital rim. In these cases, the lateral wall osteotomy can be continued upward and medially into the lateral superior orbital rim (Fig. 5-24). The two lateral wings

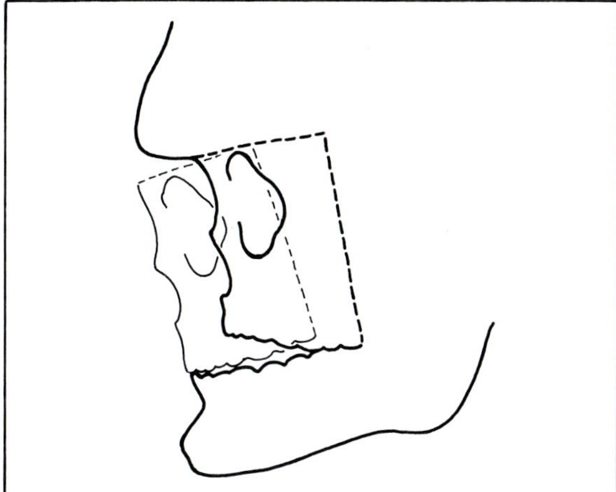

Fig. 5-23. Le Fort III maxillary advancement with anterior open bite. As the maxilla is advanced forward and downward, the nasal root may project too far.

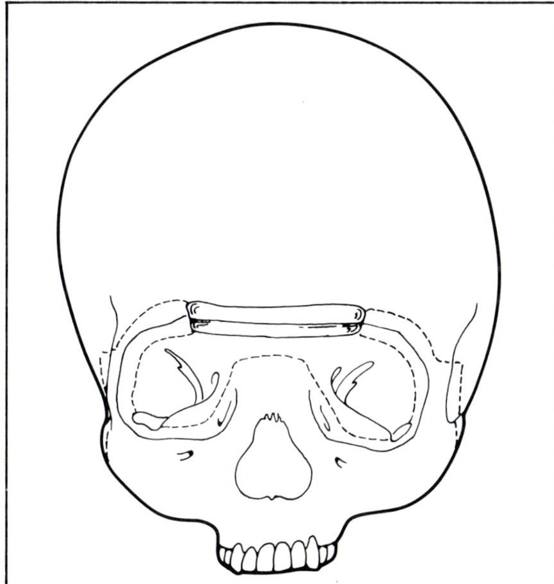

Fig. 5-24. Le Fort III maxillary advancement with frontal spur and forehead rib grafts.

are then advanced with the maxilla, and the contour is smoothed by inserting rib grafts behind them and extending across the midline of the glabella. These rib grafts must be progressively beveled upward to produce a smooth contour. This procedure is dangerous because there is little margin of error in the vertical cut down through the frontal bone into the orbital roof. The anterior fossa is easily entered. A burr hole can be used laterally and packing inserted. However, this has to be done over a long distance and is not without hazard, particularly if the patient had a coronal craniectomy in infancy. In addition, it is difficult to produce a smooth blending of superior rim into the forehead. There is often an unsightly atavistic bulge in this area.

Forehead Advancement Plus
Le Fort III Maxillary Advancement

The exophthalmometer was originally used to decide on the amount of advancement of the orbit rims needed. However, this is not the key area, and if the orbit is rotated laterally in the presence of associated hypertelorism, the measurement is erroneous. It is more important to assess the relationship of the eyebrow (hence, superior orbital rim) to the cornea; this should be approximately 15 mm. in front of the cornea. Similarly, the skin of the cheek at the level of the inferior orbital rim is 5 to 10 mm. in front of the cornea in most people. In addition, many patients with these syndromes have brachycephaly from incomplete treatment of the coronal synostosis.

SURGICAL TECHNIQUE. After exposure, a standard Le Fort III osteotomy (Fig. 5-25) is performed. The neurosurgeon performs a standard bifrontal craniotomy, but the dural reflection must be continued laterally over the pterion, with packs inserted in front of the temporal lobe (if necessary, a burr hole can be inserted through the greater wing of the sphenoid to ensure complete protection). The dural dissection must also continue backward into the middle cranial fossa inside the squamous temporal bone. The orbital roof, superior orbital rims, and a lateral tongue-in-groove cut is then made as shown. The forehead is then removed, and the Le Fort III advancement is performed and wired into place for occlusal correction. The lateral orbital wall and inferior rim are advanced as much as necessary, then the forehead is replaced and advanced as much as necessary to produce the correct eyebrow-corneal relationship and to produce a normal nasofrontal angle. Wiring of the tongue-in-groove spur to the remaining skull gives great stability, and the Le Fort III osteotomy is wired at the frontozygomatic and frontonasal region. Bone grafts are inserted into all defects, except inside the orbital walls. This reproduces a stable skull. The bifrontal craniotomy is repositioned and additional grafts are provided as needed to fill the defect created. In Figure 5-25, the vertical height of the orbit has been increased and the face and nose lengthened by pushing the maxilla downward and inserting bone blocks between it and the advanced forehead. This

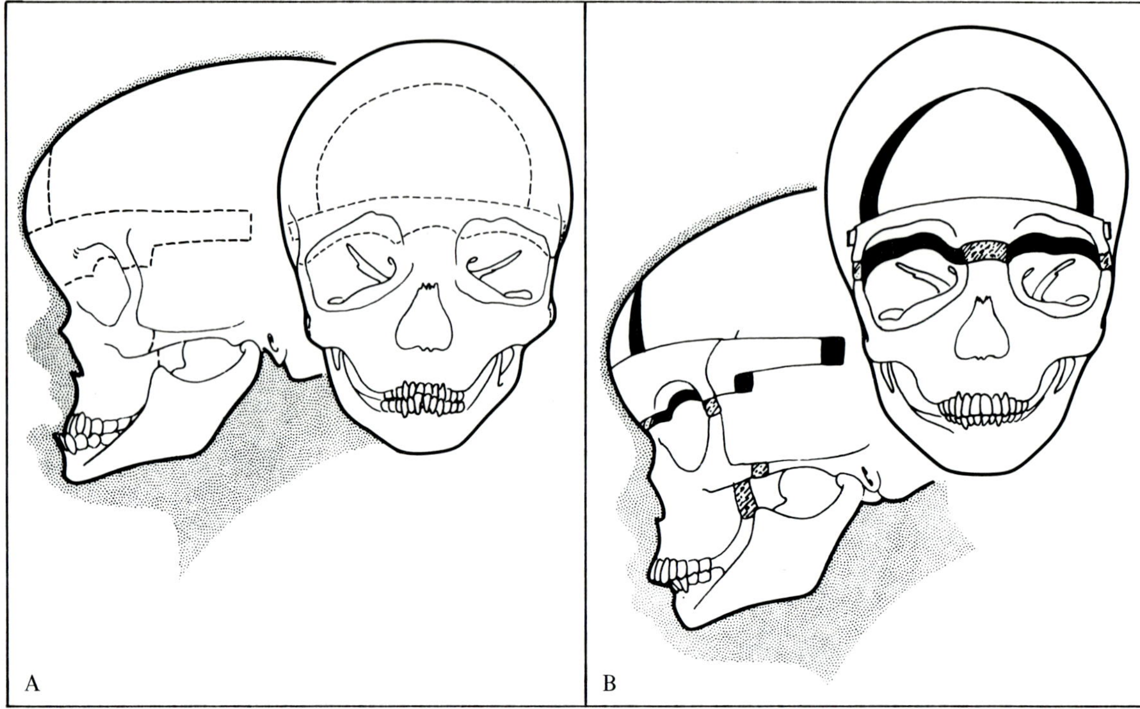

Fig. 5-25. Forehead plus Le Fort III maxillary advancement. A, the forehead, frontal bone, and maxilla are osteotomized as shown. The tongue-in-groove slide of sphenoid and temporal bone on the side of the skull is made long enough for the lateral spur to be wired to intact skull in the advanced position. The bone grafts used to fill the gaps behind it are not shown. B, the maxilla is not only advanced, but also lowered to increase the vertical height of the orbits and maxilla and to lengthen the nose.

procedure produces a much better facial contour (without the need for a secondary operation) in many cases. If there is associated oxycephaly or plagiocephaly, additional procedures are needed (see page 149–152).

Combined Le Fort III and I Osteotomy

The Le Fort III osteotomy is an en bloc advancement of the midface. It should be remembered that the amount of advancement needed to correct the occlusion is not necessarily the same as that needed to correct the nasal root or the amount of inferior orbital rim advancement. If there is an anterior open bite, the problem is compounded (see Fig. 5-23). When the relationship of the superior orbital rim to the cornea is satisfactory, an alternative procedure is to combine an upper Le Fort III advancement with a Le Fort I advancement (Fig. 5-26). This allows the nasal root to be advanced as needed for correction in this area. The inferior orbital rim can be advanced more or less than this amount, depending on the amount of cheek correction and rim correction related to the cornea (usually more than for the nasal root). Below this, a Le Fort I osteotomy is cut. It can be moved forward and, if necessary, tilted downward to correct the apertognathia. Bone grafts are then applied to the horizontal gap between the two lines of osteotomy, to provide solid fixation.

Combined Le Fort III and I Osteotomy and Subcranial Hypertelorism Correction

Many cases of Crouzon's and Apert's syndrome have a Tessier Type I or II degree of orbital hypertelorism. If the level of the cribriform plate is above the nasofrontal suture, the split Le Fort III and I procedure can be combined with subcranial hypertelorism correction (Fig. 5-27). Usually, these patients have a reasonable shape to the nose, but the nose is simply retruded. In these cases, parasagittal segments of bone are removed on either side of the nose. The U of the orbit can then be transposed medially at the same time as it is advanced (and tilted if necessary) to correct the relationship of inferior orbital rim to the cornea. The central nasal segment is advanced as needed for nasal profile correction, and the Le Fort I is used to correct the occlusion and lower midface.

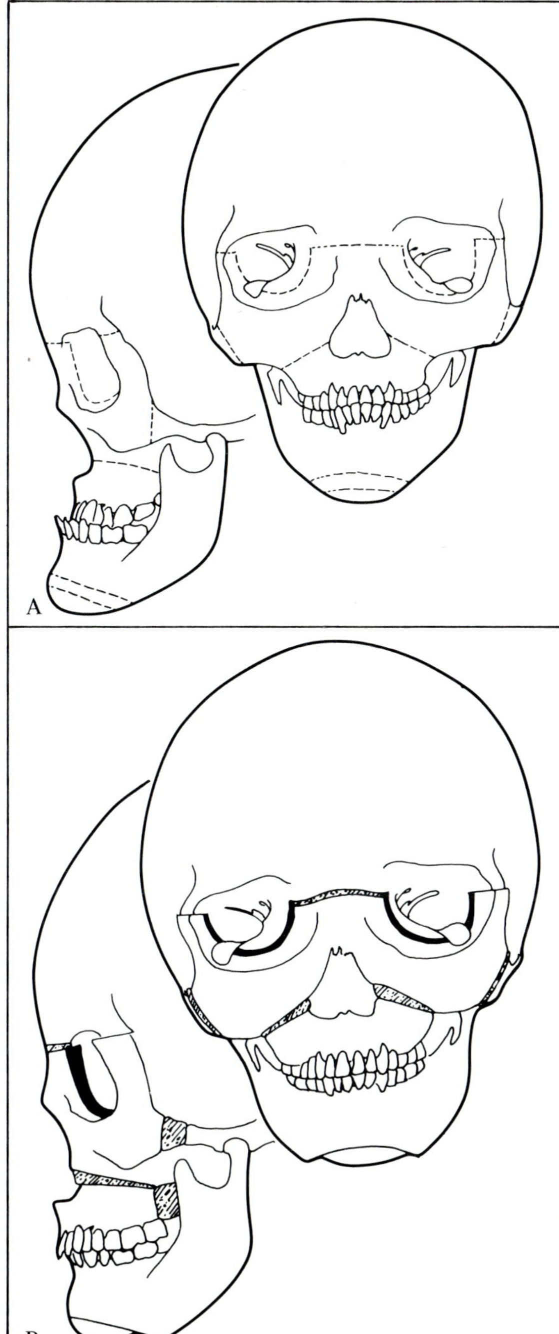

Fig. 5-26. *Combined Le Fort III and I osteotomy. A, the upper part of a Le Fort III osteotomy is cut as shown. A horizontal Le Fort I is cut below this and advanced to the correct occlusion. The segment is removed from the chin. B, the nasal root is advanced to produce a good frontonasal angle. The inferior rims and central maxilla are hinged further outward and bone grafts are applied to produce the normal convexity.*

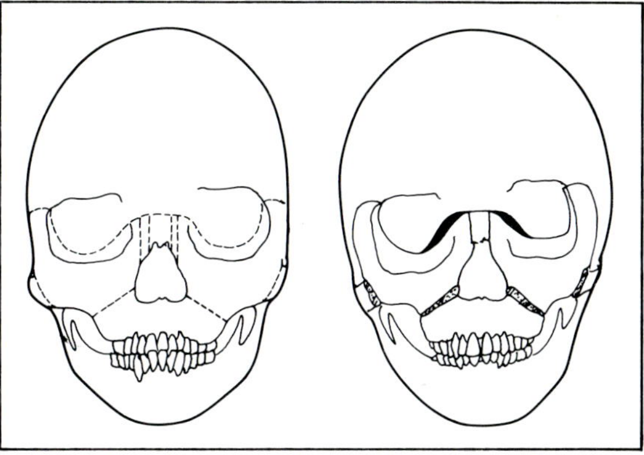

Fig. 5-27. Combined Le Fort III and I osteotomy and subcranial hypertelorism correction. After mobilization of the split Le Fort III and I, parasagittal segments are removed from the nose, allowing medial migration of the orbital rim as well as advancement.

TOTAL CRANIAL VAULT RESHAPING

The Jig-saw Procedures

The techniques for total cranial vault reshaping, known as the "jig-saw" procedures, are *extremely hazardous*, as stated in the warning at the beginning of the chapter. These three techniques illustrate principles that can be varied according to the type of deformity needing to be corrected. The preoperative cranial capacity and the *predicted* cranial capacity must be estimated prior to the operation to ensure that there is no decrease in cranial volume. In most cases, the cranial volume is found to be smaller than normal; after the operation, the cranial volume is usually enlarged and is then normal.

Jig-saw Type I: Forehead Advancement and Anterior Cranial Vault Reshaping

Untreated anterior craniostenosis may produce a recession of the forehead to such a degree that there is exorbitism related to the superior orbital rim, even though the relationship of the globe to the inferior orbital rim; the face; and occlusion are all normal. There usually is a high anterior skull, but the posterior skull has a normal shape. The osteotomy must be designed to advance the superior orbital rim and lateral orbital wall, as well as tilt the forehead from a posterior sloping one to an upright one. The cranial vault is removed in segments as shown in Figure 5-28A. The forehead segment is then replaced with a

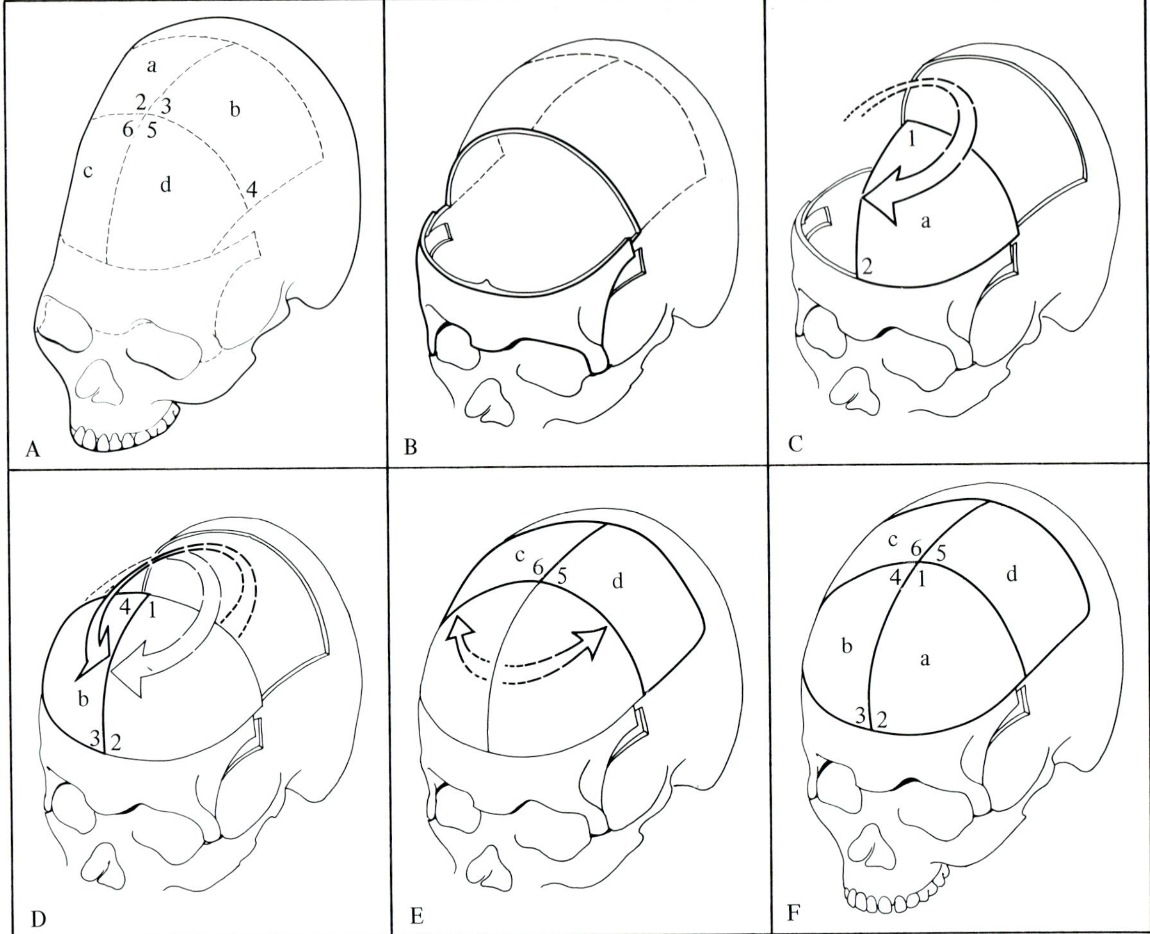

Fig. 5-28. Jig-saw procedure Type I, with forehead advancement and anterior cranial vault reshaping. This procedure is applicable to a severely receding forehead and anterior oxycephaly. A, the osteotomy cuts are made as shown. B, the frontal bone (a and b) is removed and the forehead tilted to advance the lateral walls and the superior orbital rim, and to produce a normal frontonasal angle and an upright forehead. C, D, E, the vault of the skull (frontal and parietal bone, or c and d) is removed. By transposition and rotation as shown, each segment is replaced to produce a normal forehead shape and cranium. F, final result after all the segments are wired back into position.

hinge action at the junction of the lateral orbital wall and the inferior orbital wall. The frontal bone is made vertical. This advances bone at the nasofrontal region, producing a normal nasofrontal angle. Because the skull tends to narrow as one proceeds from caudal to cephalic, the tongue-in-groove lateral strut can be placed lateral to the intact spur of squamous temporal and sphenoid bone and wired to it (Fig. 5-28B). The segments a, b, c, d can be removed, rotated, and repositioned as shown to produce a normal contour (Fig. 5-28C, D, E, F). Defects created in the lateral part of the greater sphenoid wing are filled with iliac bone grafts to give additional support for holding the forehead segment anteriorly. The temporalis muscle must also be advanced.

Jig-saw Type II: Lowering Cranial Vault, Forehead Advancement, and Reshaping

After incomplete treatment of infants with craniostenosis, particularly sagittal synostosis, severe oxycephaly may occur. Often this is associated with forehead flattening and other irregularities. In Figure 5-29A, moderate forehead recession is associated with a concavity of the upper frontal bone, a very high forehead, and extreme oxycephaly. In order to lower the vault of the skull, a compensatory expansion of the cranial volume must be performed elsewhere to prevent compression of the brain. Figure 5-29A shows the standard tongue-in-groove technique for a straightforward advancement of the lower frontal bone and superior orbital rim. The central frontal bone is concave and can be removed and used for bone grafts elsewhere. The upper frontal bone can then be lowered and attached to the advanced forehead, producing a lower and normal-shaped forehead. Severe oxycephaly usually shows marked digital impressions on the plain skull radiographs. Removal of the bone over the sagittal sinus in these cases is extremely difficult and dangerous because of the irregular inner table over the sinus. A central sagittal strip of bone is left intact but divided posteriorly (Fig. 5-29B). The skull is often wider anteriorly than posteriorly. The parietal bones can be removed intact. The sagittal bone strip is then bent forward and wired to the new position of the frontal bone. By replacing the parietal bones on the opposite side of the head in the opposite direction, the position of the maximum cranial width is altered and the cranial vault is widened as well as lowered by judicious trimming of bone (Fig. 5-29C). As much as 16 mm. of lowering has been achieved by this method.

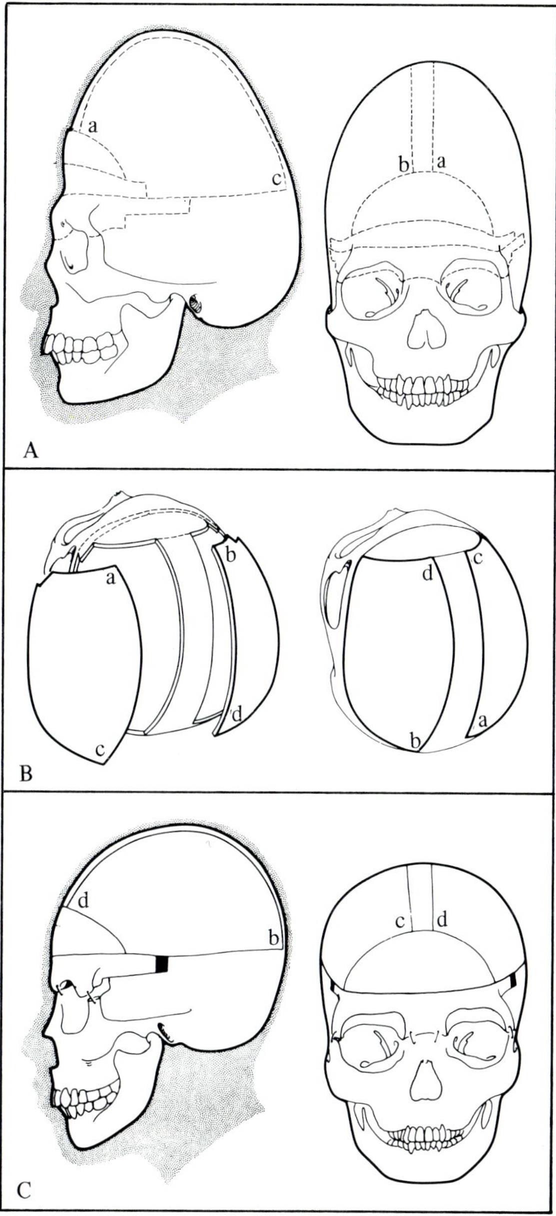

Fig. 5-29. Jig-saw procedure Type II, with forehead advancement and cranial vault lowering. A, recession of frontal bone and concavity, with extreme oxycephaly. The frontal bone is cut into three segments. A bone strip is left over the sagittal sinus. A posterior craniotomy is performed at the level of the junction of the lambdoid and sagittal sutures. B, after the forehead is corrected and the sagittal strip aligned, the parietal bones are removed, reversed, and replaced. C, the final shape with lowering of oxycephaly.

Jig-saw Type III: Forehead and Upper Maxillary Advancement, Cranial Vault Lowering, and Correction of Plagiocephaly

Some cases of craniostenosis, if incompletely treated, can produce bizarre shapes of simultaneous oxycephaly and plagiocephaly and can change the shape of the upper face. This can result in a normal lower face and occlusion, but exorbitism and extreme recession of the forehead. The osteotomy cuts depicted in Figure 5-30A show the lateral orbital wall and inferior orbital rims being mobilized separately from the central nasal segment. It is easier to handle this area as a unit as in an upper Le Fort III osteotomy, with the nose and orbital rims being handled as a single unit.

The forehead and frontal bone are first removed and then the upper Le Fort III segment is mobilized (Fig. 5-30B). The forehead is advanced and the upper Le Fort III is hinged forward to meet it. The advancement at this stage (Fig. 5-30B, right) may be so great that the scalp cannot be closed due to the tremendous increase in volume; hence, the remainder of the procedure must be completed. A central strip of bone over the sinus is left intact and the parietal bones are removed. The central bone can now be tipped downward and forward to match the frontal bone, but it can also be tilted sideways to place it in the true skull midline (Fig. 5-30C). The parietal bones are then replaced, but to allow for the relative differences in size, a wedge is removed from one side and replaced on the other. All defects shown in Figure 5-30D are filled with iliac bone grafts.

Discussion of Cranial Vault Surgery

The three jig-saw procedures described demonstrate the principles that can be used. The Meisterschnitt

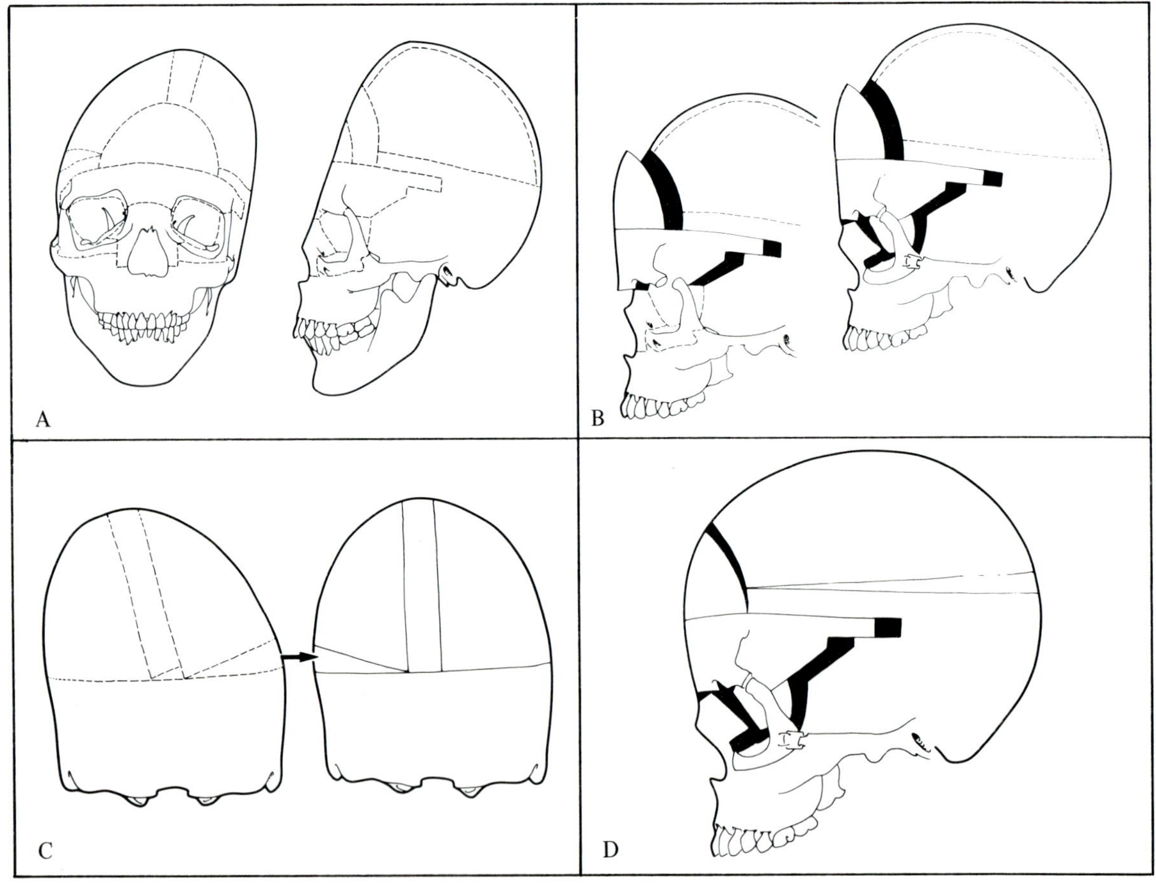

Fig. 5-30. Jig-saw procedure Type III, with forehead and upper maxillary advancement, cranial vault lowering, and correction of plagiocephaly. A, the lines of osteotomy. B, on left, the forehead is advanced with the tongue-in-groove technique; on right, the lateral orbital walls, inferior orbital rims, upper maxilla, and nose are hinged forward. C, the central strip of bone is left intact over sagittal sinus and the parietal bones are removed. The central strip is uprighted and brought forward. The parietal bones are replaced, but a wedge is removed on one side and replaced on the other. D, final shape; the zygomatic arch is lengthened by a full-thickness rib.

approach peeled forward and backward is often adequate, but exposure can be facilitated by a midline incision through the posterior skin flap. The shape of the skull dictates the procedure to be used. The basic principles are as follows: (1) a decrease in one dimension must be compensated for by an increase in another dimension; (2) the vault of the skull can be divided into as many segments as necessary to produce a normal contour; and (3) all segments should be wired back together, and defects should be filled with bone grafts wired into position. This produces a strong stable skull to protect the brain against minor trauma and will also achieve rapid early bony reunion.

TOTAL CORRECTION OF APERT'S SYNDROME
Some patients with Apert's (and occasionally Crouzon's) syndrome have forehead recession, exorbitism, hypertelorism, and a retrodisplaced maxilla. Simultaneous correction is possible, although this is the most complex and difficult of all combined osteotomies because of the multiple segments that must be advanced in different planes of space; these segments must then be restabilized and bone grafts applied. Because the skeletal exposure can be made complete by the simultaneous use of the Meisterschnitt and the upper buccal sulcus approaches, it becomes possible to correct all deformities at the same time. This procedure is extremely difficult on the very young child because the skeleton is small and soft. In addition, the transverse maxillary cut must be made high through the antrum to avoid the unerupted secondary dentition. This is feasible since hypertelorism correction is often performed in the very young child). Intermaxillary fixation of the primary dentition is also extremely difficult unless special techniques and splints are available.

Surgical Technique
The operation (Fig. 5-31) is best performed from the lowest position on the face first, then progressively worked cephalically. For ease of understanding, it will be described from cephalic to caudal. The upper frontal bone is removed in two segments (Fig. 5-31B). The horizontal cut for forehead advancement is made 1 cm. above the superior orbital rim. The tongue-in-groove spur is made at the lower rather than upper part of the frontal advancement segment. (The skull sides are more parallel over the squamous temporal region than they are over the lateral frontal bone.) In order to tilt the forehead into a more vertical position, a bevel is cut on the side of the skull at the level of the advanced tongue-in-groove. This produces increased stability and self-retention (Fig. 5-31B, C). The central segment between the orbits is removed and the orbital boxes are mobilized. They can be transposed medially to correct the hypertelorism and, at the same time, advanced to correct the exorbitism. They can also be rotated in such a way that the inferior orbital rim can be advanced either more or less than the superior rim depending on the amount of midface and eyebrow advancement needed. The Le Fort I osteotomy is now cut below this. The zygomatic arch and lateral inferior segment of zygoma are best left intact as a stable buttress for fixation. Many of these patients have developed a vertical macrogenia by adolescence. After the Le Fort I advancement, a horizontal segment is removed from the anterior mandible below the level of the mental foramen and the inferior segment can be brought upward and forward if an advancement is also needed. In performing a genioplasty repositioning, it is best to remove an intervening segment of bone. If the lowest part of the chin is removed, a square chin will be

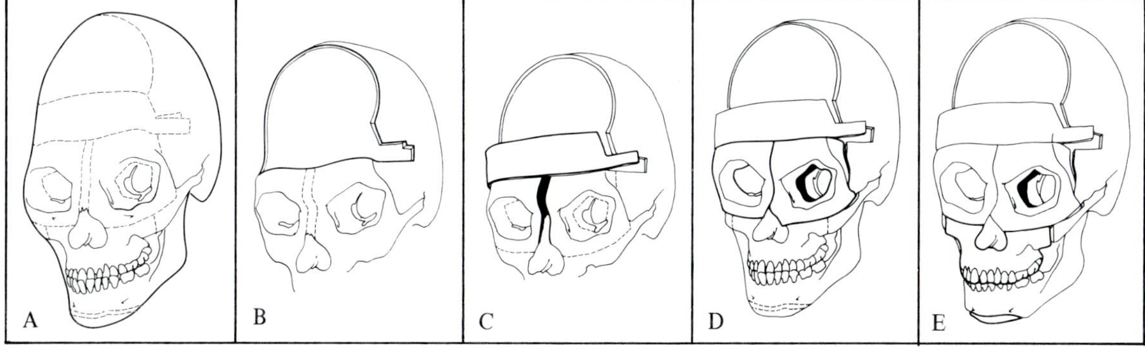

Fig. 5-31. Simultaneous correction of forehead recession, exorbitism, hypertelorism, malocclusion, and macrogenia. A, the osteotomies. B, removal of frontal bone in two sections. C, the forehead is advanced and tilted upright; the central segment between orbits is removed. D, the orbits are transposed medially and advanced forward. E, Le Fort I maxillary advancement and vertical reduction genioplasty. (The frontal bone is subsequently replaced, which is not shown.)

produced unless the edges are well rounded. In addition, cancellous bone is exposed inferiorly; when the periosteum reattaches to this, the overlying soft tissues are more firmly attached, preventing their normal mobility until a new cortex is produced (this may take a year or more to occur).

In some of these patients, there may be associated oxycephaly and plagiocephaly. If these are present or if the forehead advancement is extensive (20 mm. or more), it may be necessary to lower and reshape the cranial vault at the same operation in order to achieve scalp closure.

The greatest problem in this surgery, in addition to the extensive number of osteotomies, is the fixation of each part to other parts, as well as the numerous bone grafts that must be wired into position to maintain stability of the whole unit.

SURGERY FOR CORONAL SYNOSTOSIS

Stenosis of a cranial suture produces a fusion and obstruction of growth in that area with compensatory growth in the opposite plane. Thus, sagittal synostosis prevents growth in the lateral plane of the skull, but permits growth in the anteroposterior plane as well as vertically (if the parietal suture is not affected), producing oxycephaly. Coronal synostosis results in brachycephaly, a wide but short skull. The principle of craniostenosis surgery is to remove the affected suture in the first few weeks of life, preventing early refusion by the placement of an inert substance such as Silastic sheeting over the sectioned margins, and allowing the rapidly expanding brain to produce remodeling of the skull. Even if the coronal suture is removed adequately, not all patients will develop a normal skull shape. Some patients have a characteristic recession of the lateral superior orbital rim, even though the upper frontal bone has grown forward to the normal position. This has been demonstrated to be caused by an associated stenosis at the base of the skull involving the frontoethmoidal and frontosphenoidal suture [30]. In order to permit growth, these sutures must be released and the superior rim of the orbit advanced [23].

Surgical Technique

In the operation to correct coronal synostosis (Fig. 5-32), the coronal suture is removed in the usual way, but it must be extended down to include the pterion. The frontal bone is removed, but the superior orbital rim is left intact. An osteotomy is then made across the orbital roof from pterion through the region of the frontosphenoidal suture, then anteriorly beside the cribriform plate through the frontoethmoidal suture to the superior orbital rim. Laterally, a cut is made through the frontozygomatic suture. The orbital rim can now be hinged forward (together with the

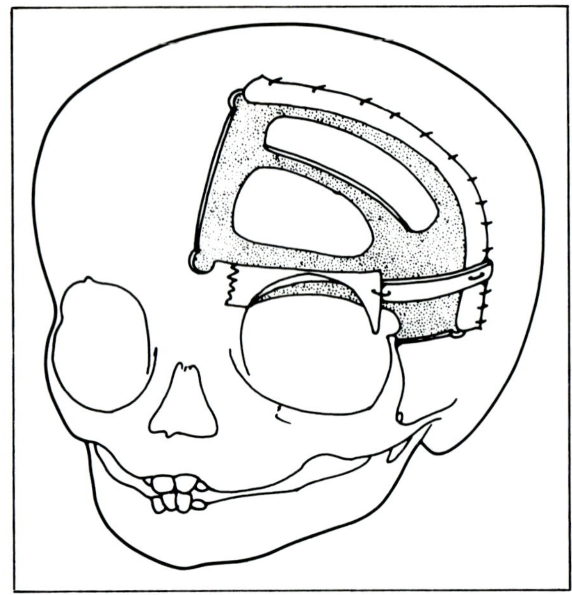

Fig. 5-32. Coronal craniectomy and superior orbital rim advancement in infancy.

orbital roof). Either the medial part can be cut or a green stick fracture can be produced. Silastic sheeting is fixed over the posterior part of the craniotomy and a segment of the coronal suture is used as a lateral strut to hold the superior rim forward at the lateral margin. This osteotomy can be extended downward to include the lateral orbital wall and lateral inferior orbital rim, if necessary. However, in children younger than 3 months old, the frontozygomatic suture is a soft fibrous union, making it difficult to prevent comminutions of the lateral orbital wall. Finally, residual pieces of frontal bone are laid back over the dura. Because this procedure is performed in the very young infant, there is no need to use extra bone grafts to fill all the defects. New cranium regenerates very quickly in these infants and it will be contoured by the expanding brain.

Coronal Craniectomy in Crouzon's and Apert's Syndromes

Patients with Apert's or Crouzon's syndrome usually have bilateral coronal synostosis, which produces the characteristic brachycephaly. They may have other types of craniostenosis as well, which may produce a variety of different shapes. It has been proposed that the midface hypoplasia in these two syndromes may be due to basal skull stenosis fusing the maxillary growth. If this is true, early release of the basal skull sutures (frontoethmoidal and frontosphenoidal) may permit normal forward growth of the face. However,

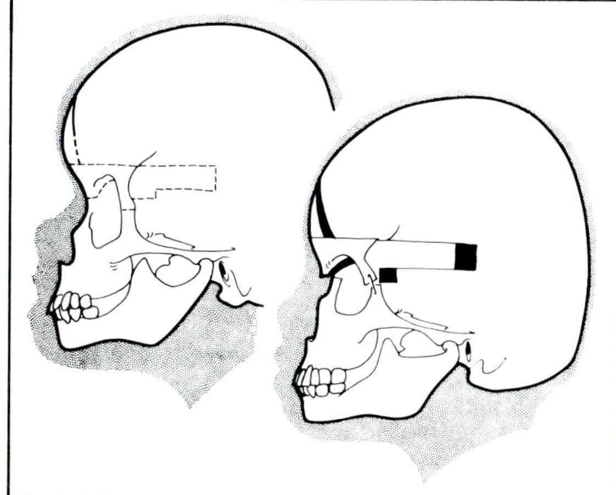

Fig. 5-33. Superior orbital rim advancement in infancy.

this has not yet been proved. Figure 5-33 shows a tongue-in-groove technique that can be utilized to advance the superior orbital rims alone in infancy. This is usually associated with a simultaneous coronal craniectomy; hence, the frontal bone coronal osteotomy would be more posterior than is shown in the illustration. Often, these patients' skulls narrow so much anteriorly that the lateral spur will not slide forward inside the groove, but passes lateral to this plane. The soft skull of the very young infant can allow the lateral spur either to be bent medially to permit fixation or to be removed as a separate segment and utilized as a strut (as in Fig. 5-32). This procedure corrects for a time the exorbitism seen in some very young infants with Crouzon's syndrome. Patients will have to be followed for 10 to 15 years to know whether this technique can prevent the "stenosis of the midface" by releasing the basal skull sutures. There may be, however, a true genetic influence on the growth of the midface, in which case basal skull stenosis is not the prime cause of midfacial growth.

ANOPHTHALMIA AND CONTRACTED EYE SOCKET

The presence of the eye globe within the orbit during the first 2 years of life is the prime reason for normal orbital expansion. In anophthalmia, either congenital or iatrogenic, the orbit remains extremely small. If a ball prosthesis is placed inside the orbit in early infancy and replaced serially with larger sizes, the orbit can be expanded so that an adequate ocular prosthesis can be fitted. If this has not been done, it is necessary to expand the orbital wall surgically, to enable prosthetic fitting. A procedure has recently been described by Marchac and co-workers [33], utilizing an intracranial approach to expand the orbital size.

EXTENSIONS OF CRANIOFACIAL PRINCIPLES

The principles of correction of congenital craniofacial skeletal deformities have allowed more effective treatment of acquired deformities, including trauma, radiation, and tumors.

Trauma

In major trauma, the skeleton can be exposed either through the lacerations that were caused by the injury or through the incisions previously described (Surgical Exposure of the Skull and Facial Bones [p. 133]). Because the methods used in congenital deformities are so effective, they can be utilized in acute trauma. Each displaced segment of bone should be repositioned and wired progressively to other segments until fixation against uninvolved skeleton is reached. This may involve multiple small pieces. If segments of bone are missing, or complete stability is not achieved, free primary bone grafting can be used at the initial operation. Although this may make the operation more prolonged, a better final result is produced than is possible by attempting to correct deformities at a later operation.

In the late treatment of acquired deformities, correction is more difficult. Minor contour irregularities are best treated by onlay autogenous bone grafting (some surgeons prefer inert materials, but these always have potential long-term complications). If the skeletal deformity is severe, segments should be osteotomized, repositioned, and buttressed with bone grafts. In malunited fractures, it is usually found that a fibrous rather than bony union has occurred. It is difficult to achieve osteotomies along the elective lines described for congenital deformities, since ignoring the original fracture lines may cause the fractures to reopen after the periosteum over them has been removed to permit visualization [26]. Thus, it often becomes necessary to reproduce the original fractures, mobilize the segments to the correct position, wire them together, and stabilize them with bone grafts.

In either acute or late correction of traumatic deformities, it is possible to eliminate the use of external skeletal fixation by adhering to the underlying principles of adequate exposure of all fractures, direct wire fixation, and further stabilization by free autogenous bone grafts if needed.

Tumors

Some cases of benign tumor such as neurofibroma or fibrous dysplasia may cause significant skeletal deformity. A few advanced cases of squamous or basal cell carcinoma may involve extensive areas of bone. In selected cases, it is possible to completely remove large segments of the skull (e.g., frontal bone and orbital walls) and then primarily reconstruct them to prevent some of the horrendous iatrogenic deformities that have been created in the past.

CRANIOFACIAL MICROSOMIA

Congenital facial asymmetry has two etiologies. (1) Basal skull stenosis of the frontoethmoidal and frontosphenoidal sutures, with or without coronal synostosis, can distort the frontal bone, orbit, upper maxilla, and nose, but these patients always have a normal lower face with horizontal occlusal plane and a normal-sized mandible. (2) Intrauterine hemorrhage, as demonstrated by Poswillo [48a], produces craniofacial microsomia and has variable expressivity varying from minor mandibular asymmetry through to absence of ascending ramus, severe occlusal tilt, absence of zygomatic arch, orbital dystopia, flattening of squamous temporal bone and skull base, hypoplasia or absence of muscles of mastication and parotid gland, and variable types of microtia.

Surgical Technique

1. With a horizontal occlusal plane and minor mandibular flatness, the face can be augmented by subperiosteal onlay grafts of rib from the intraoral route. The chin can be moved to the midline by a transposition genioplasty. Through an anterior lower vestibular mucosal incision, the mandible is exposed below the level of the mental foramina. The bone is cut horizontally and moved sideways to the facial midline and fixed by direct wiring. Wedges of bone may be removed or added to tilt the chin point if necessary. In these cases, it is necessary to leave as much periosteal attachment anteriorly as possible so that the soft tissues move the same amount as the bone.
2. When there is an occlusal tilt to the involved side, the oral commissure is elevated and the lower face flattened. The mandible and lower maxilla are hypoplastic, but are also rotated backward. The teeth are usually already in good occlusal contact which should not be disturbed. Thus, it is necessary to move the lower maxilla and mandible at the same time (Fig. 5-34). The hinge point of the Le Fort I osteotomy should not be at the opposite zygomatic-maxillary buttress, but in the region of anterior nasal spine, thus preventing elongation of the

Fig. 5-34. The lower maxilla and mandible are moved at the same time.

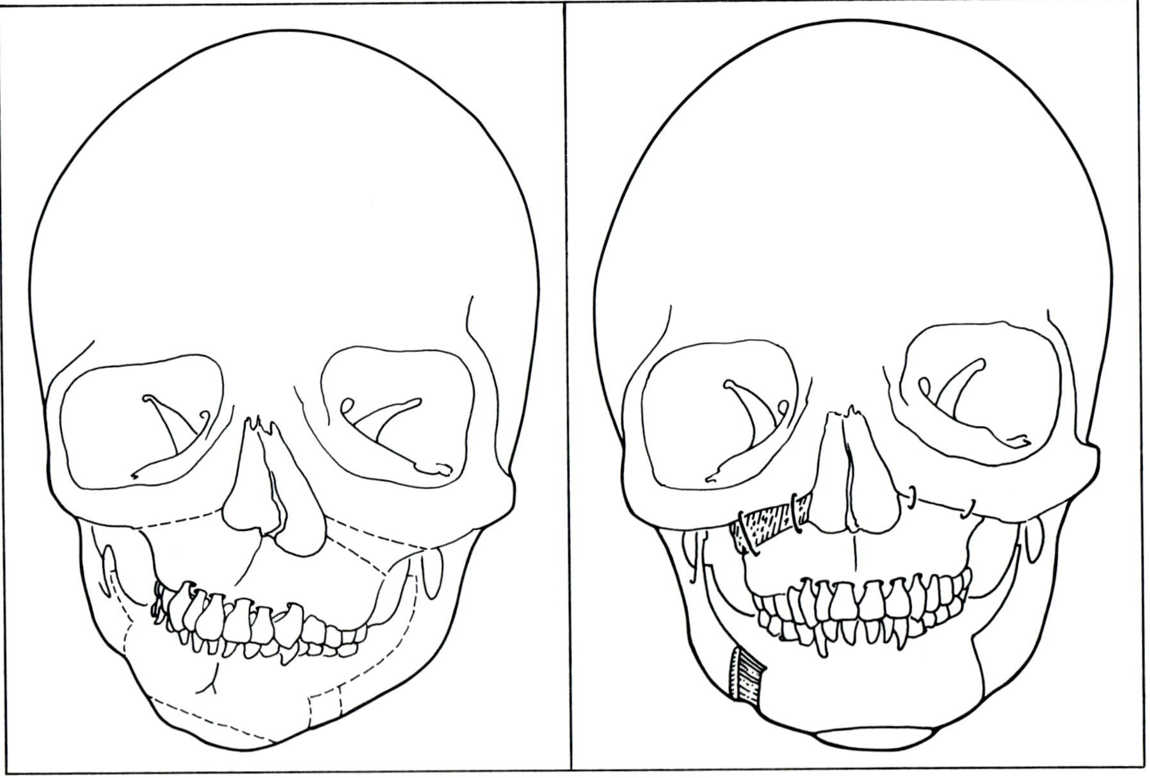

uninvolved side. In addition to lowering the maxilla and mandible, they need to be rotated forward to produce symmetry. The elevated oral commissure is corrected automatically by leveling maxilla and mandible.

3. The mandibular ascending ramus may be so hypoplastic that the condyle is vestigial or may be completely absent. In either case, there is no temporomandibular articulation. The body and ramus, if present, are also rotated medially in relation to the base of the skull and the teeth may be tipped lingually. The glenoid fossa is flat or absent. The ascending ramus can be reconstructed with a rib graft with adjacent costal cartilage still attached. Exposure can be via a submandibular skin incision or through a combined preauricular and intraoral exposure which minimizes external scarring. The rib graft is wired directly to the residual mandible at the angle and the cartilage articulates in the glenoid fossa (bone to bone articulation may cause ankylosis). When the mandible is significantly displaced medially, the graft must be angled laterally and a new glenoid fossa constructed lateral to the temporal process of the zygomatic arch. If the teeth are tilted lingually, an osteotomy of the mandible through the symphysis allows lateral rotation of the body and rotation of the teeth to a vertical position. If this procedure is done early in life, the maxillary alveolar bone is allowed to develop and prevents an occlusal tilt due to secondary maxillary hypoplasia. If the maxilla is already involved, a Le Fort I osteotomy and osteotomy of the opposite mandible must be included to equalize the face (Fig. 5-35).
4. More severe cases of craniofacial microsomia have an absent zygomatic arch and glenoid fossa and flatness of the squamous temporal region. This can be corrected after the manner of Obwegeser [46]. At the first stage, a coronal incision is used and rib grafts are placed subperiosteally on the temporal bone and covered by the temporalis muscle. The zygomatic arch is constructed from rib and a glenoid fossa built from costal cartilage (Fig. 5-36). The lower maxilla and mandible are treated as in No. 3 at a second stage. Cases of ankylosis have occurred where the two procedures are performed at the same stage.
5. In the most extreme form of craniofacial microsomia, the orbit is lower. This should be elevated as in orbital dystopia at the first stage, together

Fig. 5-35. Le Fort I osteotomy and osteotomy of the opposite mandible.

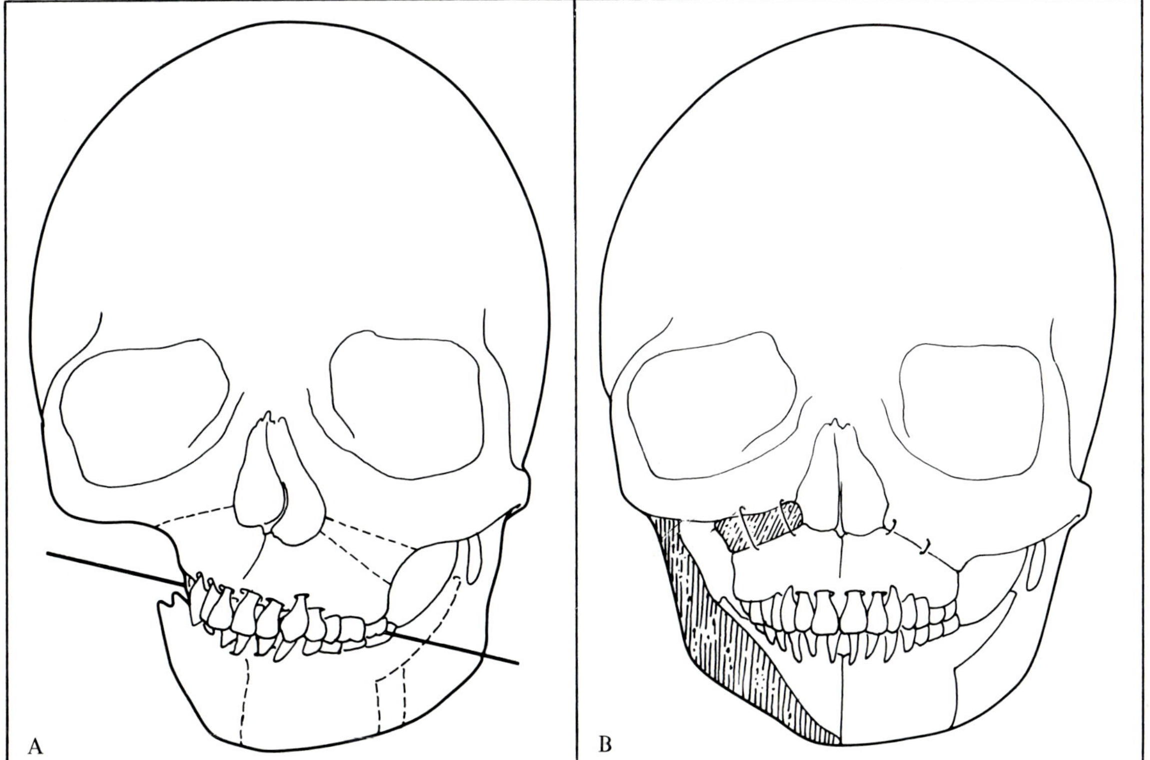

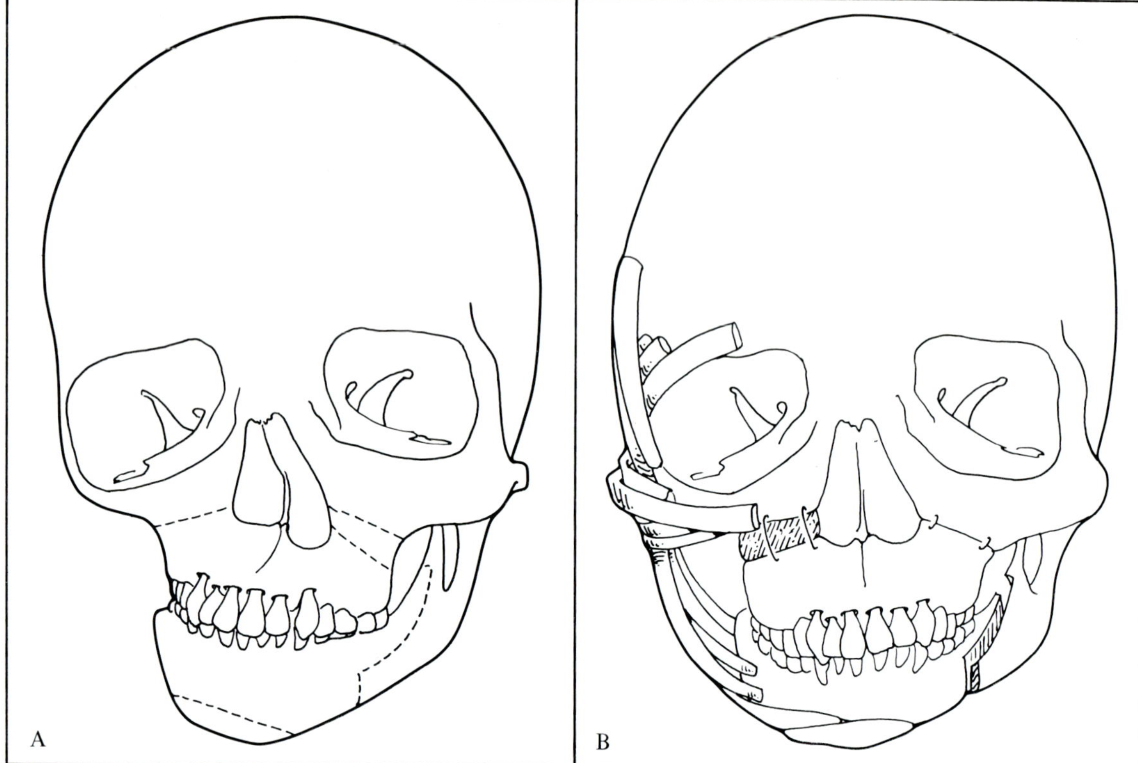

Fig. 5-36. The zygomatic arch is constructed from rib and a glenoid fossa built from costal cartilage.

with zygomatic and temporal reconstruction. If the eye remains lowered, the face always looks deformed, even if the lower face is symmetrical. Conversely, once the eyes and orbit are corrected, the lower facial deformity becomes minimized.

Soft Tissue Correction

Even though perfect skeletal symmetry is achieved, the face may still have some flatness. The soft tissues can be augmented by free dermis grafts or dermal fat grafts transferred on a pedicle via a wrist carrier. However, the fate of these is unpredictable. It is now more logical to rebuild the primary deficiency of muscle and fat by free microvascular transfer.

REFERENCES

1. Binder, K. H. Dysostosis maxillo-nasalis, ein arhinencephaler Missbildungskomplex. *Dtsch. Zahnärztl. Z.* 17:438, 1962.
2. Casson, P. R., Bonanno, P. C., and Converse, J. M. The midface degloving procedure. *Plast. Reconstr. Surg.* 53:102, 1974.
3. Converse, J. M. Surgical elongation of the traumatically foreshortened nose. The perinasal osteotomy. *Plast. Reconstr. Surg.* 47:539, 1971.
4. Converse, J. M., McCarthy, J. G., Wood-Smith, D., and Coccaro, P. J. Craniofacial Surgery. In Converse, J. M. (Ed.), *Reconstructive Plastic Surgery* (2nd ed.). Philadelphia: Saunders, 1977.
5. Converse, J. M., Horowitz, S. L., Valauri, A. J., and Montandon, D. The treatment of nasomaxillary hypoplasia. A new pyramid nasoorbital maxillary osteotomy. *Plast. Reconstr. Surg.* 45: 527, 1970.
6. Converse, J. M., Ransohoff, J., Matthews, E. S., Smith, B., and Molenaar, A. Ocular hypertelorism and pseudohypertelorism. *Plast. Reconstr. Surg.* 45:1, 1970.
7. Converse, J. M., and Smith, B. An Operation for Congenital and Traumatic Hypertelorism. In Troutman, R. C. (Ed.), *Plastic and Reconstructive Surgery of the Eye and Adnexa.* Melbourne: Butterworth, 1962.
8. Converse, J. M., and Telsey, D. Tripartite osteotomy of the midface for orbital expansion and correction of the deformity in craniostenosis. *Br. J. Plast. Surg.* 24:365, 1971.
9. Converse, J. M., and Wood-Smith, D. An atlas and classification of mid-facial and craniofacial oste-

otomies. *Transactions of the Fifth International Congress of Plastic and Reconstructive Surgery.* Melbourne: Butterworth, 1971.

10. Converse, J. M., Wood-Smith, D., and McCarthy, J. G. Report on a series of 50 craniofacial operations. *Plast. Reconstr. Surg.* 55:3, 1975.
11. Converse, J. M., Wood-Smith, D., McCarthy, J. G., and Coccaro, P. J. Craniofacial surgery. *Clin. Plast. Surg.* 1:499, 1974.
12. Dal-Pont, G. Retromolar osteotomy for the correction of prognathism. *J. Oral Surg.* 19:42, 1961.
13. Edgerton, M. T., Jane, J. A., and Berry, F. A. Craniofacial osteotomies and reconstruction in infants and young children. *Plast. Reconstr. Surg.* 54:13, 1974.
14. Edgerton, M. T., Jane, J. A., Berry, F. A., and Fisher, J. C. The feasibility of craniofacial osteotomies in infants and young children. *Scand. J. Plast. Reconstr. Surg.* 8:164, 1974.
15. Edgerton, M. T., Jane, J. A., Berry, F. A., and Marshall, K. A. New surgical concepts resulting from cranio-orbito-facial surgery. *Ann. Surg.* 182: 228, 1975.
16. Edgerton, M. T., Udvarhelyi, G. B., and Knox, D. L. The surgical correction of ocular hypertelorism. *Ann. Surg.* 172:473, 1970.
17. Epker, B. N., and Wolford, L. M. Middle-third facial osteotomies: Their use in the correction of acquired and developmental dentofacial and craniofacial deformities. *J. Oral Surg.* 33:491, 1975.
18. Epstein, F. J., Wood-Smith, D., Converse, J. M., Benjamin, V., Becker, M. H., and Ransohoff, J. Radical one-stage correction of craniofacial anomalies. *J. Neurosurg.* 42:522, 1975.
19. Fitz, C. R. Craniofacial anomalies – the radiological work-up. Personal communication, 1977.
20. Fleming, J. P. Improvement of the face in Crouzon's disease by conservative operations. *Plast. Reconstr. Surg.* 47:560, 1971.
21. Furnas, D. W., and Bircoll, M. J. Eyelash traction test to determine if the medial canthal ligament is detached. *Plast. Reconstr. Surg.* 52:315, 1973.
22. Gilles, H., and Harrison, S. H. Operative correction by osteotomy of recessed malar maxillary compound in a case of oxycephaly. *Br. J. Plast. Surg.* 3:123, 1950.
23. Hoffman, H. J., and Mohr, G. Lateral canthal advancement of the supraorbital margin. *J. Neurosurg.* 45:376, 1976.
24. Hogeman, K. E., and Willmar, K. On Le Fort III osteotomy for Crouzon's disease in children. *Scand. J. Plast. Surg.* 8:169, 1974.
25. Jabaley, M. D., and Edgerton, M. T. Surgical correction of congenital midface retrusion in the presence of mandibular prognathism. *Plast. Reconstr. Surg.* 44:1, 1969.
26. Jones, W. D., Whitaker, L. A., and Murtagh, F. Applications of reconstructive craniofacial techniques to acute craniofacial trauma. *J. Trauma* 17:339, 1977.
27. Kawamoto, H. K. The kaleidoscopic world of rare craniofacial clefts: Order out of chaos (Tessier classification). *Clin. Plast. Surg.* 3:529, 1976.
28. Kusher, J., Alexander, E., Davis, C. H., and Kelly, D. L. Crouzon's disease (craniofacial dysostosis). Modern diagnosis and treatment. *J. Neurosurg.* 37:434, 1972.
29. Laestadius, N. D., Aase, J. M., and Smith, D. W. Normal inner canthal and outer orbital dimensions. *J. Pediatr.* 74:465, 1969.
30. Latham, R. A., Hoffman, H. J., and Munro, I. R. Structure of cranial sutures in craniosynostosis. Presented at the Third International Congress on Cleft Palate and Related Craniofacial Anomalies, Toronto, June 1977.
31. Littlewood, M., and Maisels, D. Reconstructive surgery in the intracranial approach to malignant disease. *Proc. R. Soc. Med.* 63:681, 1970.
32. Longacre, J. J., De Stefano, G. A., and Holmstrandt, K. The early versus late reconstruction of congenital hypoplasias of the facial skeleton. *Plast. Reconstr. Surg.* 27:489, 1961.
33. Marchac, D., Cophignon, J., Archard, E., and Dufourmentel, C. Orbital expansion for anophthalmia and micro-orbitism. *Plast. Reconstr. Surg.* 59:486, 1977.
34. McCarthy, J. G. The concept of a craniofacial anomalies center. *Clin. Plast. Surg.* 3:611, 1976.
35. Munro, I. R. The ugly face – deformity not defectiveness. Advances in facial rehabilitation. *Can. Fam. Physician J.* 19:57, 1973.
36. Munro, I. R. Orbitocraniofacial surgery: The team approach. *Plast. Reconstr. Surg.* 55:170, 1975.
37. Munro, I. R. The correction of severe facial deformity. *Can. Med. Assoc. J.* 113:531, 1975.
38. Munro, I. R. Pre-operative Planning in Orbital Surgery. In Tessier, P., and Salyer, K. E. (Eds.), *Symposium on Plastic Surgery in the Orbital Region.* St. Louis: Mosby, 1976.
39. Munro, I. R. Craniofacial surgery – a change of face. *Can. Med. Assoc. J.* 117:210, 1977.
40. Munro, I. R., and Davies, D. W. The anesthetic management and perioperative care of patients undergoing major facial osteotomies. *Plast. Reconstr. Surg.* 55:50, 1975.
41. Munro, I. R., Salyer, K. E., Whitaker, L. A., and Jackson, I. Difficulties and problems to be solved in the approach to craniofacial malformations. *Birth Defects* 11:315, 1975.
42. Murray, J. E., and Swanson, L. T. Midface osteotomy and advancement for craniostenosis. *Plast.*

Reconstr. Surg. 41:299, 1968.
43. Murray, J. E., Swanson, L. T., and Cohen, M. Correction of midfacial deformities. *Surg. Clin. North Am.* 51:341, 1971.
44. Murray, J. E., Swanson, L. T., Strand, R. D., and Hricko, G. M. Evaluation of craniofacial surgery in the treatment of facial deformities. *Ann. Surg.* 182:240, 1975.
45. Murray, J. E., Swanson, L. T., Strand, R. D., and Hricko, G. M. Reconstructive surgery for major craniofacial deformities. *Surg. Clin. North Am.* 56:495, 1976.
46. Obwegeser, H. L. The indications for surgical correction of mandibular deformity by the sagittal splitting technique. *Br. J. Oral Surg.* 1:157, 1964.
47. Obwegeser, H. L. Surgical correction of small or retrodisplaced maxillae – "the dish-face deformity". *Plast. Reconstr. Surg.* 43:351, 1969.
48. Peterson, S. J., and Pruzansky, S. Palatal anomalies in the syndromes of Apert and Crouzon, *Cleft Palate J.* 11:394, 1974.
48a. Poswillo, D. Otomandibular deformity; pathogenesis as a guide to reconstruction. *J. Maxillofac. Surg.* 2:64, 1976.
49. Rogers, B. O. Surgical treatment of mandibulofacial dysostosis. *Clin. Plast. Surg.* 3:653, 1976.
50. Schmid, E. Surgical Management of Hypertelorism. In Longacre, J. J. (Ed.), *Craniofacial Anomalies: Pathogenesis and Repair.* Philadelphia: Lippincott, 1968.
51. Tessier, P. Osteotomies totales de la face. Syndrome de Crouzon. Syndrome d'Apert, Oxycephalies. Scaphocephalies. Turricephalies. *Ann. Chir. Plast.* 12:273, 1967.
52. Tessier, P. Dysotoses Cranio-faciales. Osteotomies Totales de la Face. *Transactions of the Fourth International Congress of Plastic and Reconstructive Surgery.* Amsterdam: Excerpta Medica, 1969.
53. Tessier, P. Definitive plastic surgical treatment of the severe facial deformities of craniofacial dysostoses – Crouzon's and Apert's diseases. *Plast. Reconstr. Surg.* 48:419, 1971.
54. Tessier, P. The Scope and Principles: Dangers and Limitations and the Need for Special Training in Orbitocranial Surgery. In *Transactions of the Fifth International Congress of Plastic and Reconstructive Surgery.* Melbourne: Butterworth, 1971.
55. Tessier, P. Total osteotomy of the middle third of the face for faciostenosis or for sequelae of Le Fort III fractures. *Plast. Reconstr. Surg.* 48: 533, 1971.
56. Tessier, P. Traitment des dysmorphies faciales propres aux dysostoses craniofaciales (D.C.F.) maladies de Crouzon et d'Apert. *Neurochirurgie* 17:295, 1971.
57. Tessier, P. Orbital hypertelorism: I. Successive surgical attempts. Materials and methods. Causes and mechanisms. *Scand. J. Plast. Reconstr. Surg.* 6:135, 1972.
58. Tessier, P. Orbital hypertelorism: II. Definitive treatment of orbital hypertelorism by craniofacial osteotomies. *Scand. J. Plast. Reconstr. Surg.* 7:39, 1973.
59. Tessier, P. Experiences in the treatment of orbital hypertelorism. *Plast. Reconstr. Surg.* 53:1, 1974.
60. Tessier, P., Guiot, G., Rougerie, J., Delbert, J. P., and Pastoriza, J. Osteotomies cranio-naso-orbito-faciales pour hypertelorisme. *Ann. Chir. Plast.* 12:103, 1967.
61. Van Der Meulen, J. C. The pursuit of symmetry in craniofacial surgery. *Br. J. Plast. Surg.* 29:85, 1976.
62. Wassmund, M. Lehrbuch der praktischen Chirurgie des Mundes und der Kiefer, Vol. 1. Leipzig: Meusser, 1935.
63. Webster, J. P., and Deming, E. G. Surgical treatment of the bifid nose. *Plast. Reconstr. Surg.* 6:1, 1950.
64. Whitaker, L. A., Munro, I. R., Jackson, I. T., and Salyer, K. E. Problems in craniofacial surgery. *J. Maxillofac. Surg.* 4:131, 1976.
65. Whitaker, L. A., and Randall, P. The developing field of craniofacial surgery. *Pediatrics* 54:571, 1974.
66. Wood-Smith, D., and Dey, D. L. Australian experience in craniofacial surgery for facial deformity. *Aust. N.Z. J. Surg.* 44:382, 1974.
67. Wunderer, S. Die prognathieoperation mittels frontal gestieltem Maxillafragment. *Ost. Z. Stomatol.* 59:98, 1962.

6

Jaw Deformities and Temporomandibular Joint Disorders

MELVIN SPIRA

The emphasis in this chapter is on the developmental deformities of the mandible and maxilla, and on disorders of the temporomandibular joint. Post-traumatic deformities of the jaws are also included. Congenital deformities of the jaws are discussed in Chapters 4 and 7.

DEVELOPMENTAL DEFORMITIES

Malocclusion

Malocclusion is a common feature of the various developmental jaw deformities. The diagnostic key to malocclusion lies in the relationship most often found between the mesiobuccal cusp of the upper first molar and the mesiobuccal groove of the lower first molar, with a normal overjet and overbite of the teeth. The prefix *mesio-* refers to that portion of the tooth closest to the midline space between the central incisor teeth, whereas the prefix *disto-* refers to that position on the horseshoe-shaped dental arch farthest from the midline, i.e., in the region of the last molar tooth. *Mesio-* and *disto-* thus refer to approximately anterior and posterior directions. *Mesioclusion* describes the condition in which the teeth of the mandibular arch are located mesially to their opposite numbers in the maxillary arch, whereas *distoclusion* is the reverse condition. Where there is abnormal horizontal protrusion of the incisor edges or cusps of the upper teeth over the lower teeth, the condition is referred to as *overjet.* When the disparity from "normal" exists in a vertical direction, it is called *overbite.* Angle's classification [1] of malocclusion is most commonly used, with the basic occlusal relationships shown in Figure 6-1, together with their associated facial disharmonies [4].

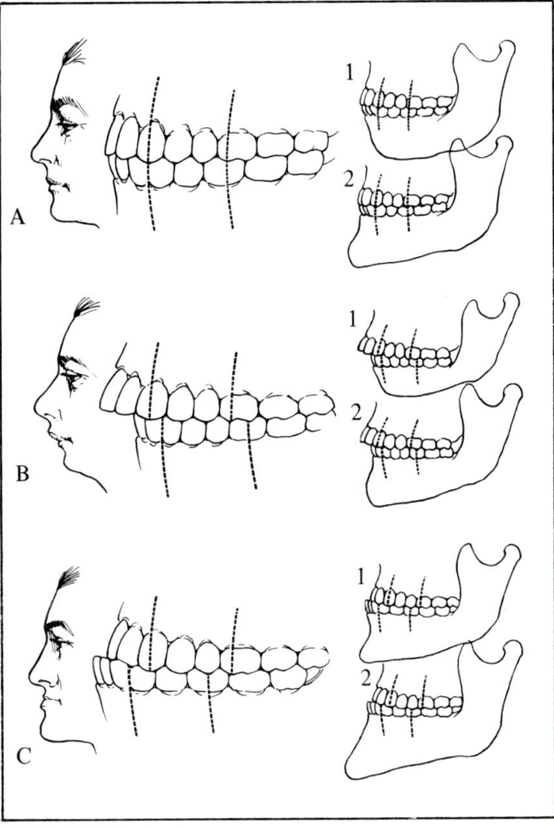

Fig. 6-1. Angle's classification of malocclusion. A, Class I. Normal mesiodistal relationship of the dental arches; the mesiobuccal cusp of the maxillary first molar tooth interdigitates with the mesiobuccal groove of the mandibular first molar (neutroclusion). There may be varied forms of individual tooth malocclusions, especially in the anterior maxillary region. A1, microgenia – an abnormal small mentum. No malocclusion. A2, macrogenia – an abnormally large mentum. B, Class II. Retrognathia or distoclusion. B1, retrognathia associated with micrognathia. B2, the mandible is of relatively normal size but is retruded. C, Class III. Prognathism – protrusion of the mandible with teeth in mesioclusion. C1, prognathism associated with a mandible of normal size. C2, prognathism associated with an abnormally large mandible (macrognathia).

True lateral skull radiographs (cephalograms) are essential for the accurate diagnosis and treatment of most jaw deformities. Cephalometric studies sufficiently accurate for clinical use can be made by varying the technique, using a standard machine [2]. A soft-density profile, which may be made by the standard double-exposure technique, with or without barium paste outline, is an additional aid in the analysis.

The significant angles in a cephalometric analysis and their normal range are presented in Figure 6-2. These are described in detail by Hinds and Kent [3]. Abnormalities or variations in the angles SNA and SNB directly relate to the diagnosis of mandibular

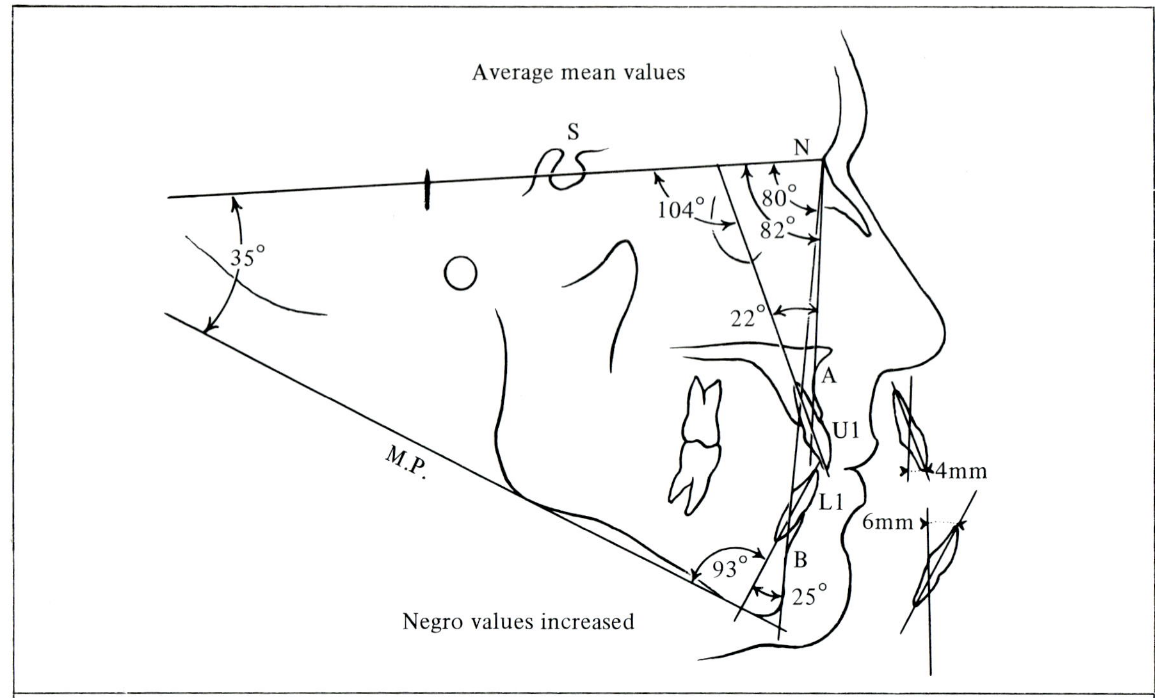

Composite cephalometric analysis						
	Normal Values		Mandibular		Maxillary	
Measurement	Mean	Range	Prognathism	Retrognathia	Protrusion	Retrusion
SNA	82°	70° – 85°			↑	↓
SNB	80°	76° – 84°	↑	↓		
ANB	2°	0° – 4°	↓	↑	↑	↓
MP-SN	35°	30° – 40°	↑	↑		
U1-SN	104°	100° – 110°			↑	
U1-NA	22°	15° – 29°			↑	↓
L1 -MP	93°	87° – 99°	↓	↑	↑	↓
L1 -NB	25°	18° – 32°	↓	↑	↑	↓
U1 to NA	4 mm.	0–8 mm.			↑	↓
L1 to NB	6 mm.	2–10 mm.	↓	↑		

Fig. 6-2. Composite cephalometric analysis for surgical use. The measurements on the left in the table refer to the lines connecting points in the drawing of the cephalogram – for example SNA *refers to the line from sella turcica* (S) *to nasion* (N) *and the line from nasion to supspinale* (A). *These limbs meet to form the* SNA *angle. The average mean values of the angles of the cephalogram drawing are for Caucasians. Generally the angles for Negroes are increased. Additional information is included in Figure 6-3.*

and maxillary prognathism and/or retrognathia and are particularly diagnostic when the anterior dental analysis is within normal range relative to angulation and height of the teeth. Conversely, abnormal inclinations, particularly of the anterior teeth, in the face of essentially normal SNA–SNB angles may be seen in pseudoprognathism or bimaxillary protrusion (buck-tooth deformity).

A commonly seen malocclusion, the typical Class II buck-tooth deformity, is cited as an example of how treatment may vary. When malocclusion is the only deformity present, treatment is usually orthodontic. Where maxillary protrusion is present, extractions, combined with surgical set-back of the involved maxillary segments, may be necessary. In the presence of micrognathia, an advancement osteotomy of the mandible, usually with a bone graft inserted into the operative defect, is required to restore both form and function. The orthodontic approach is usually inadequate for the correction of the basic facial deformity of this condition.

In addition to the cephalometric analysis, the bony configuration of both mandible and maxilla, as well as the soft tissue profile, must be considered in the diagnosis of all developmental jaw deformities [5]. The height of the upper and lower lips with reference to the incisor edges is important in planning treatment [6] (Fig. 6-3), since deficiencies in lip length can often be improved by a new refinement in orthognathic surgery, surgical repositioning in the vertical plane.

Fig. 6-3. A, classical bony landmarks. B, Minnesota integumental profile with soft tissue points: a, *frontal;* b, *subnasal;* c, *superior labial sulcus;* d, *labrale superius;* e, *stomion;* f, *labrale inferius;* g, *inferior labial sulcus;* h, *pogonion;* i, *menton.*

Underdevelopment of the Mandible

Micrognathia is characterized by a hypoplastic retruded mandible, with the teeth in distoclusion (Class II malocclusion). It must be differentiated from pure *microgenia,* in which localized underdevelopment of the anterior, or mental, portion of the mandible results in a retruded chin without significant malocclusion. An entirely different surgical approach is required for correction of each of these deformities. Micrognathia should also be distinguished from pure *retrognathia* (see Fig. 6-1), in which retrusion of a relatively normal-sized mandible causes deformity.

In micrognathia, in addition to the finding of a hypoplastic mandible, there may be accentuation of the antegonial notch and the angle of the jaw may be displaced posteriorly. This deformity may be congenital in origin (e.g., in branchial arch deformities, Pierre Robin syndrome, and Treacher Collins syndrome), or it may be acquired. Rarely is it caused by infection, birth trauma, old untreated fractures, osteomyelitis, rheumatoid arthritis (which affects the condylar growth center), rickets, cretinism, or radiation sequelae. In most instances the etiology is unknown.

Cephalometric radiographs, photographs, and dental casts are mandatory for accurate appraisal of

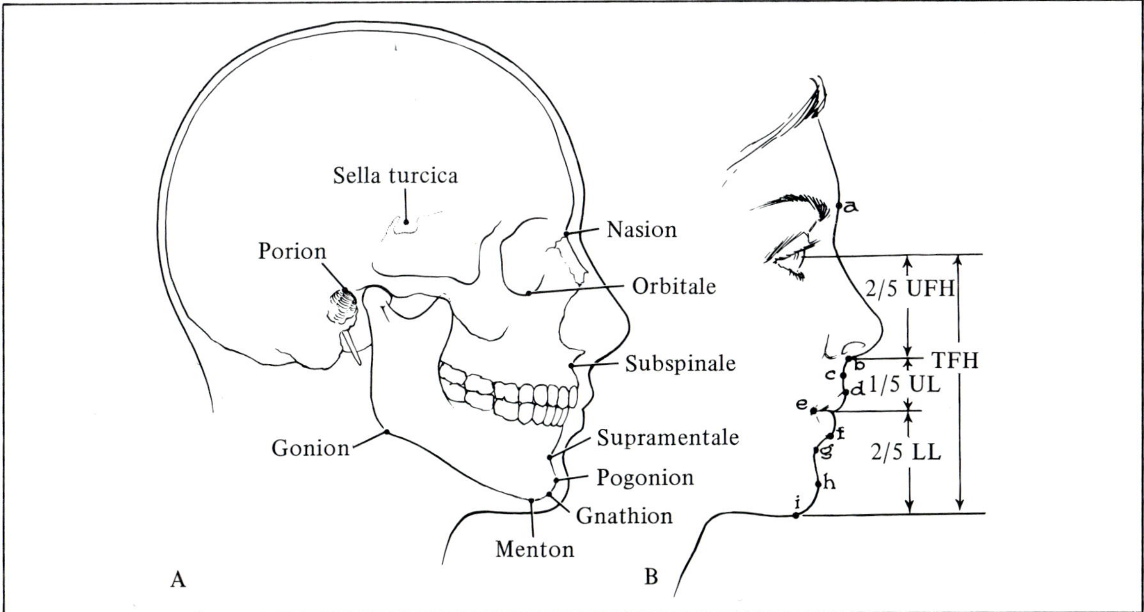

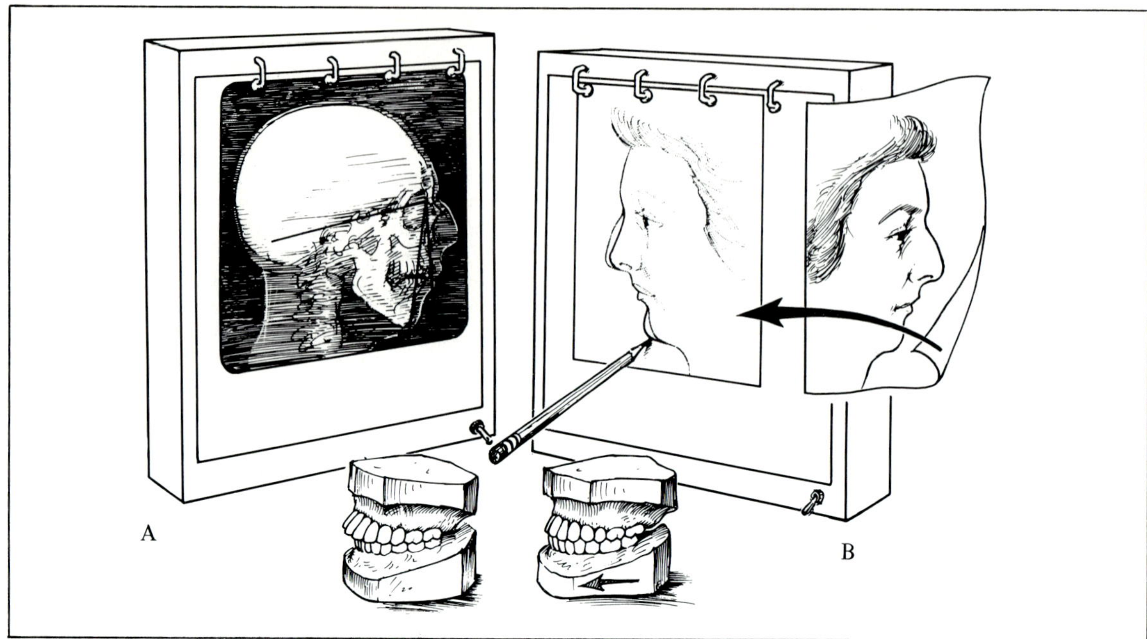

Fig. 6-4. Composite illustration of various aids to treatment planning. After analysis of the reversed photograph on viewbox, the necessary profile correction can be drawn on the photo. The dental casts and radiographs are very helpful in planning any operative procedure on the jaws.

any jaw deformity in order to determine the surgical approach required. Dental impressions are taken, poured in dental stone, and mounted on an articulator. Realignment of the teeth in proper occlusion by dental cast repositioning, or sectioning, dictates the degree and amount of correction necessary [3]. The improvement in profile will be a reflection of the change in occlusal relationship and can be visualized by studying lateral photographs (Fig. 6-4). Where a severe overbite and/or overjet exists, orthodontic treatment must precede surgery. Preoperative grinding of the teeth may be indicated, but in the absence of gross tooth-cusp interference, this occlusal adjustment is generally made after the operation. Surgical treatment to correct displacement of less than one-half the width of one cusp is rarely indicated.

When there are missing and/or malrotated teeth in either arch, preoperative construction of an occlusal acrylic wafer splint will assist in guiding the mandible into its new position and help maintain it with the aid of intermaxillary fixation.

Operative Correction of Retrognathia, Micrognathia, and Microgenia

RETROGNATHIA. The mandible is of relatively normal size but retruded, with the teeth in distoclusion. An osteotomy may be accomplished through an extraoral, intraoral, or combined approach, either through the body or the ramus of the mandible (Fig. 6-5). If a convenient edentulous area presents in a segment of the alveolar arch or an anterior open bite is present, a step osteotomy with preservation of the inferior alveolar nerve is suggested (Fig. 6-5B). If there is a full complement of teeth, I prefer to use a vertical oblique or modified C-shaped osteotomy in the ramus [7, 8] (Fig. 6-5C). In sliding-type osteotomies, direct bony contact of the repositioned segments over a distance of at least 2 cm. is highly desirable [6]. The sagittal split osteotomy, as described by Trauner and Obwegeser [14] and modified by Dal Pont [10], has the advantage of providing wide, excellent medullary contact of bone, promoting bony union and permitting great versatility in correcting a number of defects (see Fig. 6-9). Orthodontic consultation in preoperative planning is invaluable.

OPERATIVE TECHNIQUE OF THE VERTICAL OBLIQUE (C-SHAPED) OSTEOTOMY OF THE RAMUS. Arch bars or orthodontic bands for intermaxillary fixation are applied. With the patient under general nasal endotracheal anesthesia, an inframandibular or retromandibular incision is made to strip the masseter away from the lateral side of the ramus. The medial pterygoid is detached from the inner aspect, fully exposing the posterior body and the ramus of the mandible. The osteotomy lines are outlined as shown in Figure 6-5C with bur holes or with an oscillating air-driven

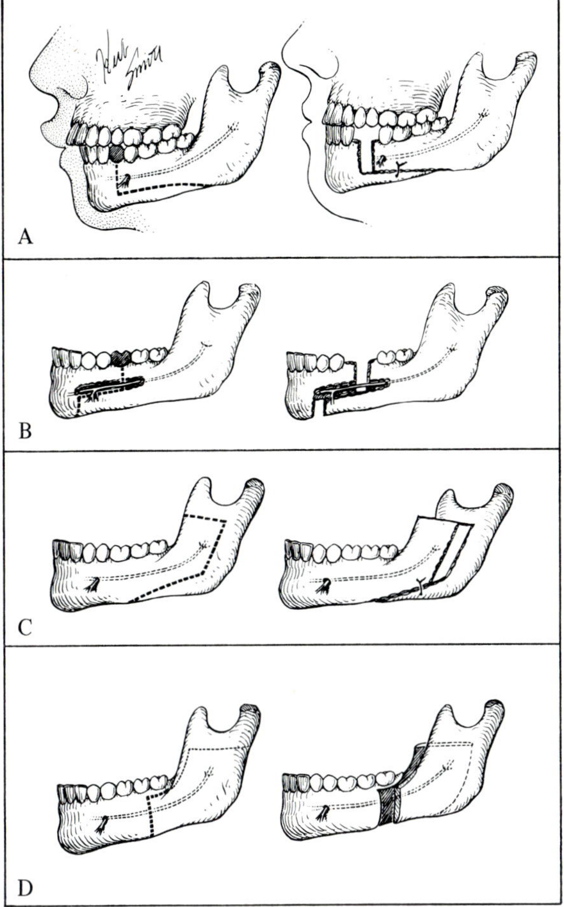

Fig. 6-5. Operative correction of retrognathia. A, sliding osteotomy of the body of the mandible with the vertical cut anterior to the mental foramen. If the first bicuspid is not absent it may require extraction. A rectangular-shaped iliac bone graft is often inserted into the mandibular defect. B, step osteotomy through the body of the mandible. The first molar was extracted in this case. Two rectangular-shaped bone grafts can be inserted in the mandibular defects. Care should be taken to avoid sectioning the alveolar nerve. C, vertical oblique (modified C-shaped) osteotomy of the ramus of the mandible. The vertical component is similar to a subcondylar ramus osteotomy with the inferior oblique and superior horizontal components added to give greater apposition of bone. Frequently, an interpositional bone graft is employed to hasten union. D, Dal Pont's modification of Obwegeser's technique for an offset sagittal splitting of the ramus and body of the mandible. This technique provides a greater surface of bony contact, obviating the need for bone graft (see Fig. 6-9).

saw, avoiding the inferior alveolar artery and nerve. The separation is completed with an osteotome. With the segments separated, the desired forward movement is accomplished and intermaxillary fixation secured so it establishes the predetermined new occlusion. A 26-gauge stainless-steel interosseous wire loop, passed through bur holes on either side of the osteotomy lines, approximates and fixates the segments. Care is taken not to move the posterior fragment forward, which would dislocate the condyles. When an advancement of 1 cm. or more is needed, a wedge bone graft is inserted in the ramus defect to promote better and more rapid healing. The endotracheal tube is left in place until the patient is awake. The period of intermaxillary fixation depends on the length and extent of bony continuity between the segments on either side of the oblique osteotomy. When bony continuity is tenuous, 8 to 10 weeks of fixation may be necessary to avoid displacement and open bite; the minimum fixation period is 6 weeks. Removing the intermaxillary fixation wires, the examiner can test for springiness at the osteotomy site by manipulating the segments with the fingers. X-ray studies are of no help in determining the strength of the bony union.

The sagittal split osteotomy is described under Mandibular Prognathism.

MICROGNATHIA. The mandible is hypoplastic and retruded, with a more severe degree of malocclusion than that noted in the retrognathic mandible. To correct this, an osteotomy usually must be combined with bone grafting to ensure bony union, restoration of contour, and an acceptable occlusion [9]. Occasionally, the degree of correction is limited by the availability of soft tissue, a salient point in planning.

Various operative techniques can be used to correct micrognathia, including the previously described technique for retrognathia, i.e., C osteotomy. When an occlusal pattern can be reestablished in patients with the less severe type of deformity in this category (i.e., those who have adequate teeth with a moderately retruded hypoplastic mandible), the osteotomy is best performed through the ramus, with an iliac bone graft inserted into the defect. Sagittal splitting of the ramus appears to reduce the need for bone grafts at the osteotomy site; however, the incidence of difficult-to-control hemorrhage has been reported as greater with the sagittal splitting technique, as has the incidence of mandibular hypoesthesias [15]. When protrusion to a new normal position cannot be obtained by advancement osteotomy alone, as in the severe "bird-face" deformity with missing teeth, the addition of a bone graft to the region of the symphysis will improve the profile. Later, utilization of intraoral skin grafts may be necessary to deepen the buccal sulcus and provide an adequate denture-bearing area (see information on vestibuloplasty under heading of Preprosthetic Surgery).

On occasion, particularly in the older person with an edentulous mandible, atrophy may result in loss of vertical dimension; inferior border rib grafting for augmentation of such a mandible may be necessary, both as a preliminary step to ridge augmentation for preprosthetic surgery and in an effort to achieve a more aesthetic dimension to the face [12].

MICROGENIA. In this deformity only a small retruded chin is seen. Treatment is primarily directed toward augmentation in the area of the mental symphysis. Preoperative profile studies of the patient's photographs will help determine whether the microgenia is absolute or relative. In the latter case, a rhinoplasty, incorporating reduction in size of the nose, will either obviate the need for or reduce the degree of augmentation of the chin. Conversely, increasing the chin projection improves the profile in many patients undergoing a reduction rhinoplasty.

Correction is accomplished by means of either a sliding horizontal osteotomy or an onlay or inlay "sandwich" implant, utilizing autogenous, homologous, or alloplastic materials [13]. Bone grafting is laborious and is associated with an increased morbidity and late resorption; it is now the method of choice only in conjunction with sliding osteotomy to provide both additional lateral body and mental symphyseal contour. Solid or closed cell sponge Silastic, Proplast, acrylic, or Ivalon implants are easily formed, commercially available, well tolerated, and used most commonly. They are frequently inserted through a submental incision, although the intraoral route is gaining in favor since oral contamination of the implants, especially the silicones, has proved to be a relatively insignificant factor (Fig. 6-6). Robinson and Shuken [11] have pointed out the drift of the prosthesis distally, resulting in a pressure-type erosion of the anterior mandible that in some instances may end with embedment of the implant well within the bone. In my experience, excessive augmentation appears to encourage this backward drift or migration. The phenomenon appears self-limiting, and tooth injury is rare. A clinical observation is that it is seen less frequently in minimal augmentations when the implant is properly placed over the periosteum.

OPERATIVE TECHNIQUE FOR AUGMENTATION OF THE MENTAL SYMPHYSIS. Under local anesthesia, an extraoral approach, with a short transverse incision placed well back in the submental region, probably is used most commonly (Fig. 6-6D). A supraperiosteal pocket is created, dissected *just large enough* to accommodate the prosthesis. Use of a commercially available preformed silicone rubber implant, fixed deep with a single mattress suture of 4-0 Dacron to the midline raphe, is my preference for this correction. The implant may be tailored to provide adequate contour. A two-layer closure, with an adequate pressure dressing, is sufficient to prevent movement. When employing the intraoral route to insert the implant, the incision is created so as to leave an adequate cuff of mucosa in the labial sulcus for closure. After the operation, the patient is kept on a liquid diet for 48 hours, and systemic antibiotics are given for 5 days.

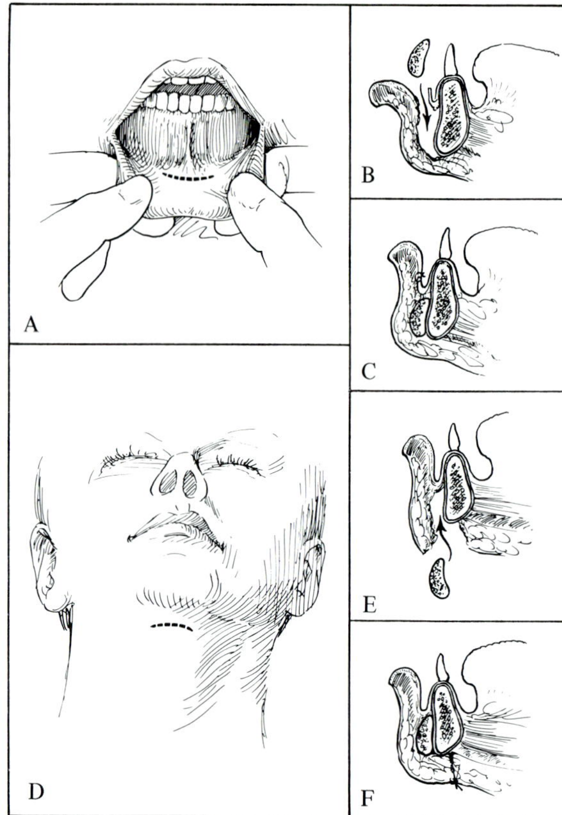

Fig. 6-6. Operative technique for the correction of microgenia by augmentation of the mental symphyseal region. A, B, C, intraoral approach. When making the incision an adequate cuff of mucosa is maintained to facilitate a layered closure. The implant is placed in a pocket developed over the periosteum and not directly on bone. D, E, F, submental approach.

A variety of segmental sliding advancement osteotomies, with or without additional onlay or interpositional bone grafting, have been described (Fig.

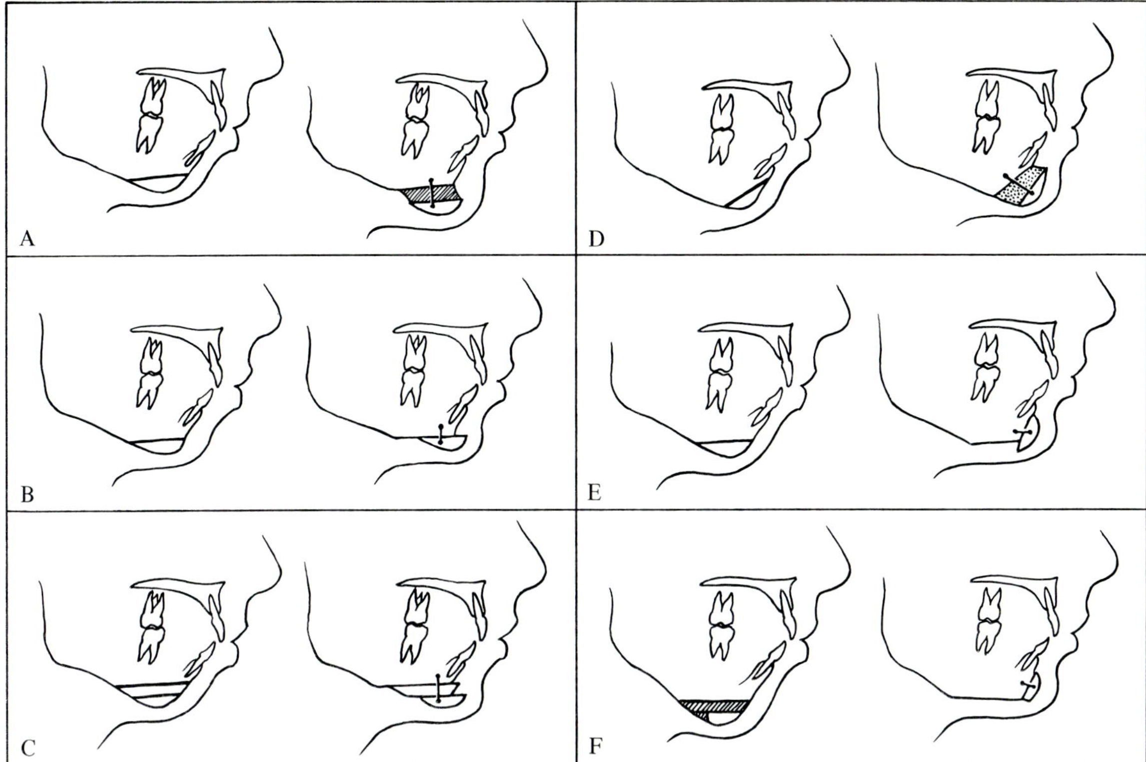

Fig. 6-7. A–F, a variety of osteotomies with and without bone grafting employed in the treatment of a hypoplastic chin (microgenia). The drawing on the left shows the preoperative condition and the drawing on the right the postoperative.

6-7). These osteotomies are particularly useful when the mandible is of reasonably normal size or when the anterior mandible is elongated vertically. Utilizing an intraoral degloving procedure, following appropriate osteotomy, the bony excess can be slid forward or rotated upward, or both, so as to serve both as a sliding osteotomy procedure and as an onlay bone graft. Occasionally, an interpositional bone graft is employed in a frontal split osteotomy in order to maintain reasonable contour to this area and at the same time provide additional downward and forward projection.

Overdevelopment of the Mandible

Mandibular Prognathism

Idiopathic enlargement of the mandible causing prognathism is a relatively common deformity. Characteristically, this enlargement is accompanied by mesioclusion (Class III malocclusion) (see Fig. 6-1C). Although the deformity is usually bilateral and asymptomatic, a unilateral overgrowth may occur; the etiology may be idiopathic, or the condition may result from hyperplasia of the mandibular condyle. Etiological factors in many cases are obscure, though a hereditary factor is common. Prognathism occasionally manifests itself late in life, being associated with pituitary dysfunction (acromegaly) or Paget's disease. True mandibular prognathism must be differentiated from relative prognathism, pseudoprognathism, and macrogenia. *Relative prognathism* is simply the appearance of prognathism in a person with a normal mandible and an underdeveloped middle one-third of the face. Most commonly it occurs in patients with congenital craniofacial growth abnormalities (cleft palate, cranial dysostosis). *Macrogenia* is mandibular overdevelopment confined to the chin and the anterior segment of the body of the mandible. Cephalometric studies assist in differentiating between these entities (see Fig. 6-2).

Orthodontics has an important role in the management of prognathism because malocclusions without gross facial deformity or imbalance may be amenable to orthodontic treatment alone. Invariably, preoperative orthodontics can correct individual malrotations and improve arch alignment to facilitate the planned surgical procedure.

The surgical treatment of mandibular prognathism

requires preoperative analysis and planning similar to that required for retrognathia. The basic surgical procedure to correct a prognathism involves some type of osteotomy, of either the ramus or the body of the mandible with or without an ostectomy (Fig. 6-8). On articulated dental casts, the occlusion can be improved by removing a measured section of the lower cast (ostectomy of the body), or simply by moving the lower dental cast posteriorly (osteotomy of the ramus). The choice of the operative site and amount of setback required are decided by the degree of realignment needed to obtain a satisfactory occlusal relationship. If the patient possesses an adequate complement of teeth and a mandible of normal width in comparison with the maxillary segment, then osteotomy of the ramus is the method of choice. When there is an anterior open bite or a disparity in mandibular width, or when teeth are missing, especially in the bicuspid area, ostectomy of the body may be indicated. Frequently, either approach may be successfully utilized. Approaching through the ramus has the advantage of safety to the teeth and inferior alveolar nerve, as well as technical ease in performing the operation with minimal complications. The ostectomy of the body is performed as a one-stage operation, with the cuts being either entirely vertical or stepped. Ostectomy of the body is particularly effective for the correction of apertognathia and laterognathism in the presence of a functional molar relationship. Good bony contact facilitates union, allowing shorter periods of immobilization. The historical background and a number of variations of either method are described by Hinds and Kent [3]. Complications that are occasionally seen with any of the operative approaches include both temporary and permanent paresthesias, persistent occlusal disharmony, nonunion, and open bite [15]. Although more rapid, the older method of using a Gigli saw through an external approach for the subcondylar osteotomy is attended by more complications, particularly regression, than the more tedious body or ramus technique.

Surgical procedures for prognathism are occasionally indicated in an edentulous mouth, particularly if the jaw relationship is so malposed as to preclude construction of stable dentures.

Independent of the technique chosen, intermaxillary arch bar-wire fixation is planned. Cap splints, a prosthetic appliance, or both, may be employed if the number of teeth is limited. Remounting articulated dental models in their improved position preoperatively will point out the need for the grinding of major cusp interferences, although ideally these adjustments are made postoperatively, after bony union. When the cusp interdigitation is poor, the use of an acrylic bite plate or "wafer," constructed preoperatively and set between the upper and lower teeth at the time of operation, will accurately guide the surgeon and help maintain the new relationship. From the variety of procedures available, three are described in the following sections. If ostectomy of the body is planned, the teeth at the site of the ostectomy are removed several weeks before the operation.

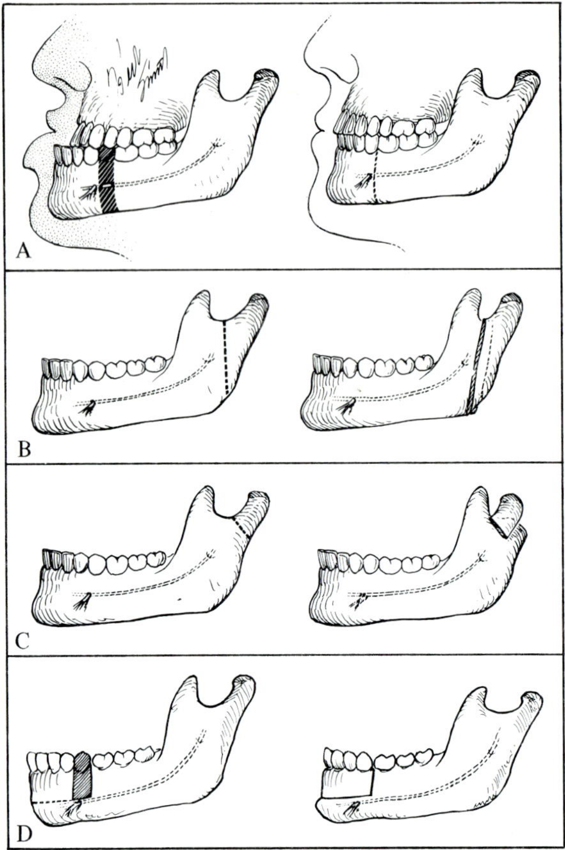

Fig. 6-8. Operative correction of prognathism. A, mandibular body ostectomy. The second bicuspid or first molar is usually extracted and a predetermined segment of bone removed. B, vertical subcondylar osteotomy. The osteotomy is made between the sigmoid notch and the mandible angle posterior to the inferior alveolar artery and nerve. This is the preferred method. C, external blind osteotomy using the Gigli saw. This method is rarely used. D, anterior segmental ostectomy.

OPERATIVE TECHNIQUE FOR OSTECTOMY OF MANDIBULAR BODY. Ostectomy of the body by a one-stage intraoral approach, as proposed by Converse et al. [16] and modified from the original Dingman [17] procedure, is as follows: with the patient under general nasal endotracheal anesthesia, an incision is made in the buccal sulcus and the mucoperiosteum is reflected superiorly, giving access to the outer surface of the mandible. The alveolar canal is exposed, using a large dental bur. With the inferior alveolar nerve under direct visualization, a predetermined vertical segment of mandible is outlined in step fashion for removal. (Metal templates of the proper size of the mandibular segment to be removed are most helpful at this point; these templates are made preoperatively at the time of sectioning of the articulated dental casts.) The step should be made in such a manner that the posterior fragment will be pulled upward by the muscles of mastication into good bony contact with the anterior fragment (Fig. 6-8). Through-and-through bur holes are made with a contra-angle drill or an oscillating saw is used, great care being taken not to injure the roots of adjacent teeth. With an osteotome, the ostectomy is completed, and the bone removed. By decompressing the lateral inferior alveolar canal wall, the nerve may be retracted laterally to avoid crush injury during setback. The procedure is repeated on the opposite side and the mucoperiosteum closed in a single layer. Interosseous wiring, below the levels of the root apices, secures the fragments. This new union is then maintained by intermaxillary fixation, with a 6-week immobilization period. Varying degrees of injury to the nerve are common; sensory return, however, is usually complete, although lip paresthesia lingers for months.

OPERATIVE TECHNIQUE FOR OSTEOTOMY OF MANDIBULAR RAMUS. Osteotomy of the ramus can be performed a number of ways. The vertical subcondylar osteotomy (Fig. 6-8B) as described by Hinds [18] is preferred. Arch bars are applied with additional stabilization secured by an anterior circummandibular wire around the lower bar and a nasal spine wire around the upper bar. The lateral surface of the ramus of the mandible is exposed through a submandibular or retromandibular incision, avoiding the ramus mandibularis of the facial nerve. The insertion of the masseter muscle is detached and reflected superiorly. Exposure of the operative site is complete when there is visualization of the sigmoid notch, facilitated by the use of a Young prostatic, Aufricht nasal, or Obwegeser retractor. Using a round dental bur or an oscillating saw, cuts are made through the inner and outer cortical plates in a line extending from the sigmoid notch to a point just above the angle. The lingula is avoided, and great care is taken not to injure the inferior alveolar nerve and artery. With an osteotome, bone division is completed, separating the ramus. The posterior fragments are then permitted to slide laterally so that the muscle pull from the lateral pterygoid will hold them against the anterior fragment. Next, attention is directed to the opposite side, where a similar procedure is performed. The assistant who is working on the mouth then adjusts the body of the mandible to its new retroposition, occluding the teeth by wiring together the previously placed arch bars. The posterior fragment is then rechecked, care being taken to ensure that this segment lies lateral to and in good contact with the anterior body portion. Any bony prominence is smoothed with a rongeur and closure is effected in a routine fashion. Wire fixation of the sectioned fragments is unnecessary.

When marked recession is needed, detachment of the medial pterygoid insertion may facilitate the setback and reduce the tendency toward an open bite postoperatively. Rarely, in the severe cases, either sectioning the base of the coronoid process or removing the coronoid process may be necessary to permit the desired retrusion. Occasionally, an additional loop of 24-gauge stainless-steel circummandibular wire placed about the symphysis and attached to the nasal spine will be necessary to reinforce the intermaxillary fixation and prevent an open bite. In the usual case, intermaxillary fixation is maintained for 6 weeks. The development of an open bite following removal of fixation is a distressing complication that may require reapplication of fixation for an additional period of up to several weeks.

SAGITTAL SPLIT TECHNIQUE. The following is a description of Dal Pont's [10] modification of Obwegeser's sagittal split of the mandible. With the patient under general nasal endotracheal anesthesia, an intraoral incision is made, beginning high over the pterygoid mandibular raphe and extending into the buccal vestibule to the first molar. Employing a heavy periosteal elevator, the lateral posterior inferior border of the mandible is exposed by the reflection of a mucoperiosteal flap, detaching the lower insertion of the masseter muscle. The upper half of the medial side of the ramus is then exposed above the lingula. The pterygomasseter muscular sling attachment to the inferior and posterior border of the mandible and angle must be stripped completely using a special curved periosteal elevator (Obwegeser). Excellent exposure following reflection of the soft tissues medially from the mandible can be achieved by slipping an Obwegeser or similar channel-type retractor into and around the posterior border of the ramus. With a reciprocating saw, the first cut is made medially above the lingula. The second cut is made with a #8 round bur, creating a series of holes from the first cut down along the anterior border of

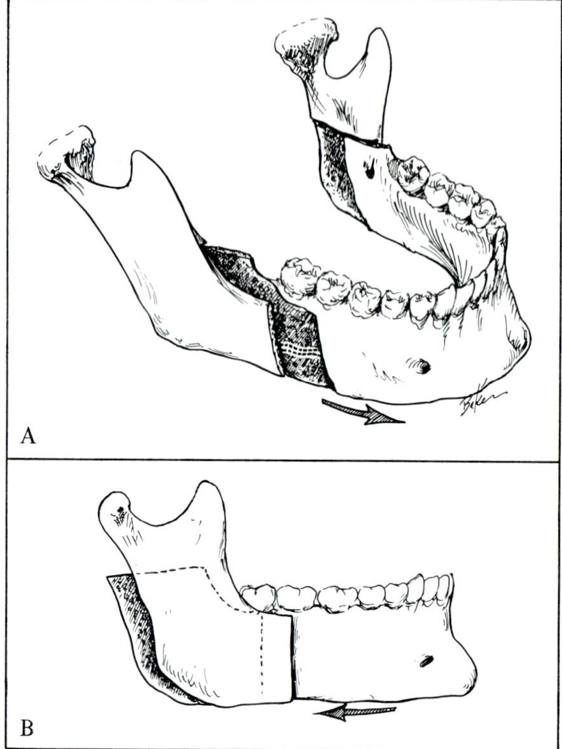

Fig. 6-9. The Dal Pont modification of Obwegeser's sagittal split technique, which can be employed for either (A) retrognathia or (B) prognathism.

the ramus, across the retromolar area, and onto the buccal side of the mandible opposite the third molar (Fig. 6-9). The third cut extends from the third molar region to the inferior border of the mandible on the outer or lateral surface of the mandible. All cuts are made *just through the cortical plane to, but not into, medullary bone.* Two or three osteotomes, placed close to and following the inner surface of the lateral plane, are used to complete the sagittal split. Great care is taken not to injure the inferior alveolar neurovascular bundle. The position of the condyle and lateral ramus with the coronoid process remains unchanged while the body of the mandible is moved distally (posteriorly), resetting the jaw in the preoperatively planned position. The fragments are stabilized with a single circumferential wire of 26-gauge stainless steel. Intermaxillary fixation is carried out in a routine fashion. The sagittal split osteotomy has the advantage of providing a large area of bony contact, which facilitates healing, and it can be employed as a versatile procedure – in prognathism, retrognathia, or apertognathia. In addition to being the most technically difficult orthognathic surgical procedure of the mandible, the sagittal split technique has the disadvantages of hemorrhage, infection, and a high incidence of temporary and permanent alveolar nerve involvement, as well as occasional bone resorption [15].

SUBAPICAL ALVEOLAR SURGERY. Occasionally the overall jaw relationship is satisfactory, but there is protrusion of the alveolar process resulting in malocclusion. Orthodontic treatment will usually be satisfactory; however, a surgical setback of the involved segment employing a mandibular subapical osteotomy is suitable (Fig. 6-8D). The procedure is performed intraorally, the second bicuspids are extracted and subjacent alveolar bone removed. A transverse osteotomy cut 5 mm. below the apexes of the teeth anterior to the ostectomy will permit distal movement of the anterior alveolar segment; that segment is stabilized with either a splint or interdental wiring. Intermaxillary fixation is not needed [5]. Essentially the same procedure is performed on the maxilla for bimaxillary protrusion.

Macrogenia

Overdevelopment of the chin, or macrogenia, is characterized by elongation, protrusion, or both, of the chin. It is frequently associated with prognathism, but it may also occur as a separate entity, in which case the occlusal relationship is usually normal.

When macrogenia occurs alone, a transverse ostectomy of the mental symphyseal region to remove the enlarged portion of bone will correct the deformity (Fig. 6-10). When macrogenia and prognathism occur together, a reduction in size of the mental region is carried out following one of the mandibular setback operations described previously.

When true prognathism and maxillary hypoplasia have been ruled out, bony resection of the chin through an intraoral approach should be planned. The amount to be removed is determined preoperatively with the aid of a true lateral skull x-ray and profile photographs.

OPERATIVE TECHNIQUE OF TRANSVERSE OSTECTOMY OF THE MENTAL SYMPHYSEAL REGION. The operation is performed through the mouth under local mandibular block anesthesia. The mental prominence is exposed through an incision in the labial buccal sulcus from molar to molar, well away from the alveolar process. The mucoperiosteum is elevated and, together with the lower lip and soft tissue of the chin, shifted down and under the chin, thus degloving and exposing the anterior mandibular border. With a motor-driven saw, a transverse osteotomy is made at a predetermined level to correct the elongation or pro-

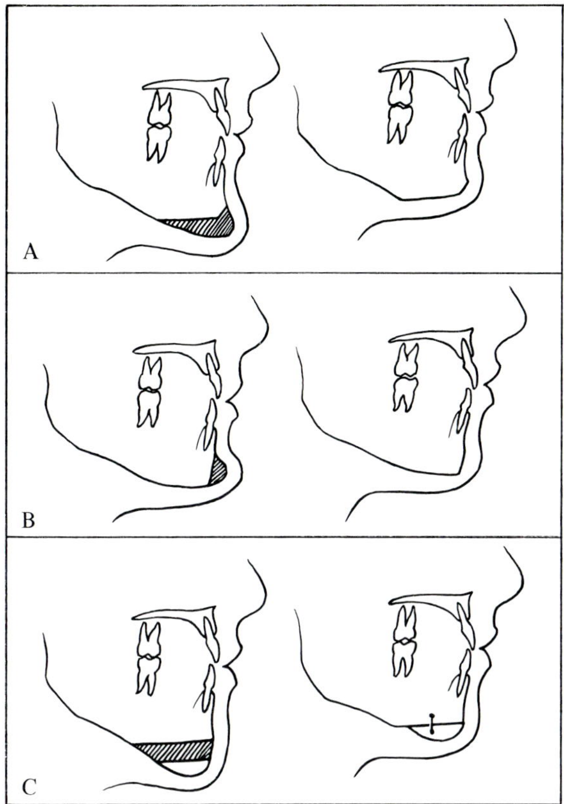

Fig. 6-10. A, B, C, three procedures employed in the treatment of macrogenia. The drawing on the left shows the preoperative appearance and the planning for operation. Drawing on the right depicts the postoperative appearance.

trusion of the chin. Occasionally, the lower segment may be repositioned and wired in place, depending on the desired contour. Following the rongeuring of sharp corners and the replacement of the soft tissue, the wounds are closed and a pressure dressing applied.

LATEROGNATHISM. Mandibular laterognathism, or asymmetry, is most commonly due to unilateral underdevelopment, agenesis (arrest of growth), or overdevelopment of the mandible. It may also be due to malunited mandibular fractures, unilateral loss of a part of the mandible, or mandibular tumors [20].

Hemifacial and bilateral facial microsomia (craniofacial microsomia) is a common cause of mandibular laterognathism. Onlay bone grafts have been employed over the hypoplastic mandible as early as the age of 3 years, in an effort to promote soft tissue and bony growth on the involved side. More recently, alloplastic (silicone block) grafts have also been introduced. In an attempt to induce active growth, a metatarsal bone graft to replace a missing or severely hypoplastic condyle has been described. These techniques and others are described by Converse et al. [19a]. Effective aesthetic and functional reconstruction necessitates staged surgical, orthodontic, and prosthodontic treatment. Timing is important. Treatment can commence about the age of 9 years, with the patient in the mixed dentition stage. A bilateral mandibular ramus osteotomy is performed to permit rotation, inferior displacement, and advancement of the mandible to a midline horizontal plane (see Fig. 6-5). Iliac crest bone grafts are used to bridge the gaps at the osteotomy sites as indicated. The procedures vary considerably, depending on the degree of mandibular hypoplasia. Osteotomy of the noninvolved side is necessary so as not to disturb condylar function. A bite block to fill in the gap in the interocclusal space on the involved side (a gap left by movement of the mandible) is used and maintained with intermaxillary fixation for 8 weeks. Orthodontic therapy is commenced following healing, aimed at taking advantage of maxillary and mandibular growth to maintain functional occlusion and an alignment that is as close to normal as possible. The goal is to level the mandible (and thus the lower face) and keep it at the midline. The second surgical stage is performed several years later, during adolescence, and is directed at correcting position and contour abnormalities of both the mandible and maxilla, as well described by Converse et al. [19a] in 1973. Simple anterior mandibular osteotomy (see Fig. 6-7) and onlay bone grafts may be all that is needed; however, because of continued growth disparity, repeat vertical osteotomies of the ascending rami may be indicated. In addition, simultaneous Le Fort I (simple transverse) maxillary osteotomy (as shown in Fig. 6-12) is performed, also with bone grafting, to correct both hypoplasia and the abnormal horizontal tilt. Not infrequently soft tissue augmentation is also needed to restore midfacial and lower facial contour on the affected side. Resorption of autogenous bone grafts and recurrence of the deformity are not uncommon. Full and permanent correction is difficult both to achieve and to maintain. Following secondary surgery, orthodontic treatment is usually required to refine the occlusion. There is always the possibility of interfering with an already reduced potential for full growth by early surgery in the mandible. When present, the condylar growth center should not be violated during its growth stage by the operation.

The classification and treatment of the soft tissue and jaw deformities associated with bilateral facial microsomia were well described by Converse et al.

[19b] in 1974. The treatment of these disorders requires modified vertical osteotomies (C-shaped and sagittal split, as shown in Fig. 6-9), usually combined with interpositional bone grafts. In addition, it is frequently necessary to perform either horizontal advancement osteotomies or procedures to lengthen the mandible body, or both. Again, orthodontic work done before the operation is needed for proper dental occlusal alignment to facilitate the repositioning affected during the osteotomy. Soft tissue deficits may limit the desired amount of bone correction obtainable and provide a deleterious force, promoting bone resorption and regression. Overcorrection at the time of surgery is hence desirable.

Unilateral overdevelopment of the mandible can occur with or without unilateral hyperplasia of the mandibular condyle [19]. *Hyperplasia of the mandibular condyle* with the condylar head showing progressive enlargement is relatively uncommon and has no known cause. The condylar neck and ascending ramus may be elongated also. Histologically, there is evidence of active cartilage and bone formation in the condyle. Treatment should consist of condylectomy after the affected side of the mandible has attained its expected normal size. Operations directed solely at the body or ascending ramus of the mandible should be discouraged, since continued enlargement of the condyle may be expected.

Unilateral overdevelopment of the mandible without hyperplasia of the mandibular condyle is closely related to mandibular prognathism. Treatment is by means of ostectomy of the mandibular body or ramus, as described under the heading of Mandibular Prognathism. In the surgical correction, it may be necessary to remove a segment of bone from the body of the mandible on the affected side and perform a simple vertical osteotomy through the body on the other side to allow the bone ends on the affected side to be brought into apposition [20].

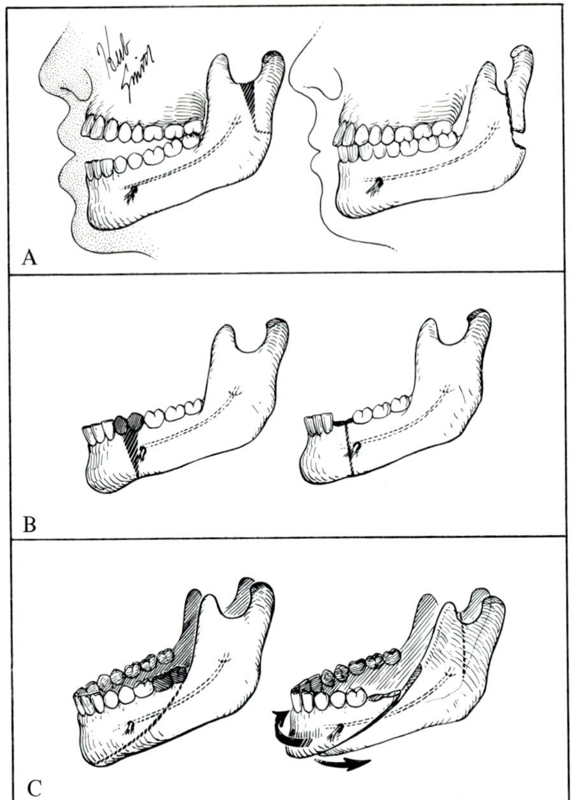

Fig. 6-11. Operative correction of apertognathia (open bite). A, sliding ostectomy and osteotomy for correction when the entire dental arch is involved. B, wedge ostectomy for anterior open bite. One or two teeth may need to be extracted. C, sliding body osteotomy combined with subcondylar vertical osteotomy, used to correct open bite in a mandible that is both retrognathic and laterognathic.

Apertognathia (Open Bite)

In apertognathia, the teeth fail to occlude anteriorly when the jaws are closed. The deformity is usually idiopathic or developmental but is sometimes seen following malunion of mandibular fractures and surgical respositioning of the mandible. It may accompany varying degrees of prognathism and laterognathism or may be associated with micrognathia and displacement of the premaxillary segments of the maxilla.

Treatment is predicated on the proper analysis of the deformity. The most common method used to correct the fixed deformity when the condition is associated with overdevelopment of the mandible involves a bilateral wedge resection of the mandibular body [21]. The operative procedures involve modifications of previously described techniques (Fig. 6-11).

Benign Masseteric Hypertrophy

Benign masseteric hypertrophy is a condition of unknown cause involving a unilateral or bilateral painless hypertrophy of the masseter muscle. The diagnosis is based on the facial contour over the ramus and a characteristic posteroanterior x-ray finding of a marked prominence or hyperostosis of the mandibular angle (gonion). When the condition is unilateral in nature, the various differential diagnoses include local soft tissue and parotid gland tumors. An excellent review of all facets of this condition is given by Bloem and Van Hoot [22].

Treatment of benign masseteric hypertrophy is directed toward removal of the offending, but histologically normal, muscle and bone. The resection is via an intraoral or extraoral route. Hyperostotic bone is excised, together with enough of the medial portion of the masseter muscle to restore contour. A postoperative pressure dressing is mandatory if hematoma is to be avoided.

Underdevelopment of the Maxilla

Developmental deformities of the maxilla in this category are usually the result of cleft lip and cleft palate defects, manifesting themselves as hypoplasia and collapse of the maxillary alveolar arches, with varying degrees of malocclusion [24]. Maxillary hypoplasia with retrusion related to craniofacial dysostosis is discussed below. Pure idiopathic hypoplasia of the middle one-third of the face, the classic "dishface" deformity, is rare without congenital defect or history of injury, surgery, radiation, or other type of trauma.

Treatment is generally dictated by the findings, after establishment of the cause and nature of the deformity. Often it is necessary to rule out a relative retroposition of the maxilla secondary to mandibular prognathism. When retrusion and collapse of the maxilla are secondary to cleft palate, treatment is usually directed toward restoration of an acceptable occlusion, using orthodontic methods. In the severe cases, osteotomy of the maxilla, with or without bone graft, may be necessary. Pure maxillary hypoplasia, in the absence of overt malocclusion, may be corrected with onlay rib grafts inserted through the mouth via an incision in the labial sulcus [29]. Infrequently, the deformity is localized in the premaxillary segment under the nose; correction is made at the time of rhinoplasty and submucous resection, either by utilizing a portion of the resected nasal septum or by implanting materials through the incision in the membranous septum adjacent to the columella. While autografts of bone cartilage are preferred, preserved irradiated cartilage and alloplastic materials may be equally effective in this area.

OPERATIVE TECHNIQUE FOR CORRECTING MAXILLARY HYPOPLASIA AND RETRUSION WITHOUT CLEFT PALATE. With the patient under general nasal endotracheal anesthesia, the mucosa in the floor of the nose is elevated on either side of the septum and both cartilaginous and bony portions of the latter are transected at the level of the nasal floor but not removed. Associated severe septal deformity may necessitate an intraoral intubation initially. After division of the septum, extubation and reinsertion of the endotracheal tube through the nose can be accomplished. Incisions are then made in the lateral buccal sulcus subperiosteally to expose the lateral and anterior segments of the alveolar arch. Osteotomies are performed above the level of the apexes of the teeth from the piriform aperture anteriorly to the maxillary tuberosity posteriorly. The maxillary sinuses are entered as the dissection is kept below the level of the mucosa (Fig. 6-12A). Next, a posteriorly based palatal flap is developed and elevated so that a transverse palatal osteotomy can be made anterior to the greater palatine foramina. This cut is continued to each medial side of the alveolar arch segments, joining the lateral osteotomies and mobilizing sufficiently to create a "free floating" maxilla. The incisions are closed with 4-0 chromic catgut; anterior repositioning is carried out, aligning the occlusion in a predetermined relationship with intermaxillary fixation [25]. Several variations in the position of the palatal cuts are used. These vary from a site just behind the incisive foramen [30] to separation of the tuberosity from the pterygoid plates. Ideally, autogenous bone blocks are placed posteriorly between the tuberosities and pterygoid plates to aid in preventing late regression.

Immediate postoperative airway problems may be avoided if the nasal endotracheal tube is left in place until the patient is fully reactive. A simple head dressing with chin-strap immobilization is sufficient, and there is no need for a plaster head-cap or cranial frame fixation. Muscle tone will maintain the rest position of the mandible without the need for cranial attachment. Intermaxillary fixation is maintained for 6 to 8 weeks, or longer if union is not clinically demonstrable by attempted manipulation of the maxilla with the intermaxillary wires removed.

Correction of the short face syndrome [23] employs a transverse maxillary osteotomy (Le Fort I) with interpositional bone grafting to correct the deformity in either dentulous or edentulous patients.

OPERATIVE TECHNIQUE FOR CORRECTING MAXILLARY RETRUSION AND COLLAPSE ASSOCIATED WITH CLEFT PALATE. A combined orthodontic and surgical approach has been advocated for these cases. Ideally, orthodontic realignment of malpositioned teeth is achieved as an initial step. A newer approach involves corticotomy by vertical cuts through the outer maxillary alveolar bone, permitting more rapid expansion with an orthodontic appliance. Either the surgical approach outlined above, or one of the others such as that described by Obwegeser [31], may be utilized. Consideration must be given to the insertion of bone grafts into any of the osteotomy defects that are wider than 2 or 3 mm. Split-rib bone grafts are used most frequently and are maintained in place by closure of the mucoperiosteal flaps over them. Additional onlay rib grafts may be used to restore anterior maxillary contour. Intermaxillary fixation is applied and maintained as described above.

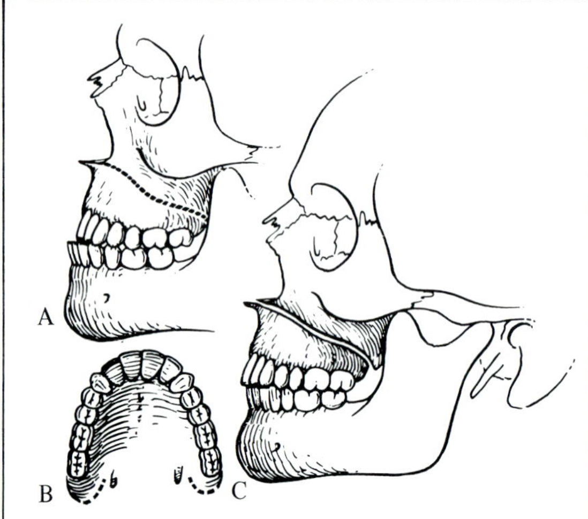

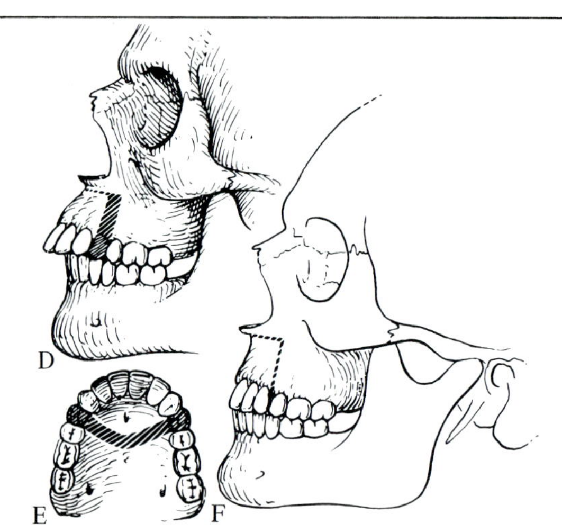

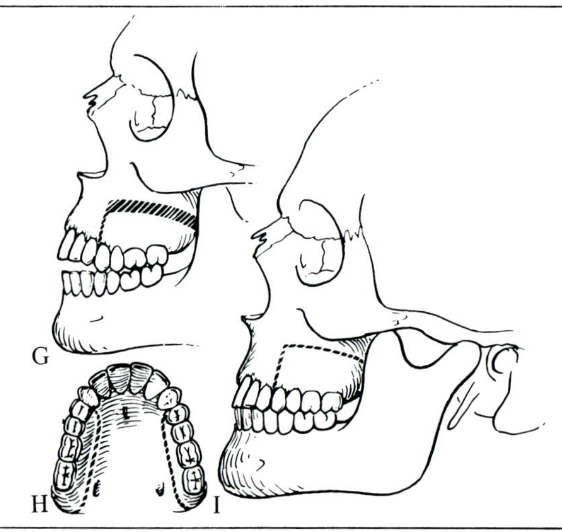

Overdevelopment of the Maxilla

Frequently overdevelopment of the maxilla is confined to the anterior alveolar segment and is associated with the Class II malocclusion commonly referred to as the "bucktooth deformity." Correction is generally effected by orthodontic methods, usually involving extraction of the upper first bicuspids, orthodontic repositioning of the teeth, and the wearing of a retaining appliance. Although this method is safe and effective in youngsters, the fixed deformities of adults respond slowly to this form of treatment. Ostectomy of the anterior maxilla after the extraction of both upper first bicuspid teeth has proved to be a rapid and effective solution to the problem [27] (Fig. 6-12D, E, F). Often a great deal of functional and cosmetic improvement will be obtained in a patient who otherwise would not have been treated or who would have had all the protruding teeth extracted and replaced with a denture [28].

PREOPERATIVE PLANNING. This should include soft tissue profile studies, a cephalometric analysis and mock surgery on stone study models. Observing the relationship of the upper lip line to the maxillary incisors becomes important when the lip is short, since it is often desirable to move the premaxillary segment upward as well as posteriorly. Cephalometric studies quantitate the position and angle of the maxillary incisors relative to the anterior extent of the maxilla and the occluding mandibular teeth.

The base of the maxillary stone model is notched, and indexes are made of both occlusal and base surfaces. Then a mock ostectomy is performed on the models, and, with the premaxillary segment in the desired position, a second set of occlusal and base indexes are made in the stone. Transfer of the model segments from the preoperative to postoperative

Fig. 6-12. Operative correction of maxillary overdevelopment and underdevelopment. A, B, C, underdevelopment of the maxilla can be corrected by a transverse osteotomy of the maxilla above the apexes of the teeth. The tooth-bearing portion of the maxilla can be slid forward and held by intermaxillary fixation. Transfacial wiring may be required for stability. D, E, F, overdevelopment of the anterior maxilla in the adult can be corrected by extraction of both upper first bicuspids and ostectomy of a wedge of anterior maxilla. The new posterior position of the maxilla is held by intermaxillary fixation or a maxillary splint. G, H, I, overdevelopment of the posterior, tooth-bearing portion can be corrected by ostectomy above the apexes of the teeth as shown. Many variations of these procedures are employed.

occlusal or base position in the indexes should demonstrate the amount of bone to be removed.

Frequently, maxillary protrusion is associated with the overeruption of lower incisors. Therefore, the premaxillary segment cannot be moved posteriorly to eliminate the excessive overbite unless the overerupted lower incisors are corrected by preoperative orthodontic leveling of the lower arch (incisal grinding) or lowered by alveolar osteotomy.

OPERATIVE CORRECTION OF ANTERIOR MAXILLARY PROTRUSION. When osteotomies are performed through a tooth socket, a vertical incision one tooth posterior to the osteotomy site is recommended. Subperiosteal "tunneling" on the palate will permit adequate exposure for the removal of palatal bone, combined with a midline incision to facilitate the joining of the palatal bone cuts. Bony cuts and resections are made with appropriate drills, saws, or chisels. Great care must be taken to avoid injuring the roots of adjacent teeth. The removal of horizontal bone is limited only by the distance between the apex of the incisor roots and the floor of the nose. Adequate bone must be resected with the original cuts to accomplish the planned setback, since it is difficult to remove bone once the premaxillary segment has been mobilized. Using an acrylic splint wired to all of the teeth in the arch, the segments may be immobilized without intermaxillary fixation [26]. Splint fixation is maintained for 6 to 8 weeks. Following this procedure, Hawley-type retainers are inserted and worn for another 3 months.

Provided that there is no direct injury to the roots, viability of both pulp and bone is maintained, but response to nerve stimulation from electric pulp testers does not return for 3 to 6 months.

POST-TRAUMATIC DEFORMITIES

The most common post-traumatic jaw deformities are due to malunion of the mandible or maxilla. Gross facial disharmony, open bite, micrognathia, asymmetry, and fibrous union may accompany the malunion. While seen more frequently following untreated facial fractures, nonunion may result from inadequate immobilization, especially with fractures at the mandibular symphysis.

Post-traumatic Deformities of the Mandible

A malpositioned, healing fracture of the mandible can often be treated within 3 to 6 weeks of the injury by arch bar fixation and intermaxillary elastics if reasonable bony alignment can be achieved. This immobilization should be maintained for a minimum of 6 to 8 weeks. Residual minor occlusal discrepancies can be corrected by selective grinding of the teeth. The edentulous, deformed, but well-healed mandible will require no surgical correction if dentures can be constructed over the bony irregularity. A prosthesis with a plumper may restore adequate contour to the lower face and make bone grafting unnecessary. This approach is preferred in the elderly patient who has a thin, atrophic mandible, since the attempt at a difficult type of reconstruction is fraught with complications.

Gross malunion of the mandible following healing should be treated by open reduction at the old fracture site, interosseous wiring of bony fragments, and intermaxillary fixation. If the post-traumatic deformity is accompanied by loss of bone length, an osteotomy to separate the bone ends, a bone graft to bridge the defect, and prolonged intermaxillary fixation are required (Fig. 6-13). Dental impressions will permit construction of articulated models to assess the degree of deformity. Usually such injuries are accompanied by the loss of several, and in some cases almost all, of the teeth. The preparations for postoperative fixation should therefore be made preoperatively. Radiographic analysis will determine the availability of local bone to permit alignment in continuity.

OPERATIVE TECHNIQUE FOR CORRECTING GROSS MALUNION OF THE MANDIBLE. Under general nasal endotracheal anesthesia, the old fracture site is exposed through the local scar or through a new inframandibular incision. Previous trauma of the site may make it difficult to identify the mandibular ramus of the facial nerve; a nerve stimulator can be helpful in this dissection. Using the motor-driven saw, cuts are made along the healed fracture site, completing the division without fragmentation. This division may be made in such a way as to permit a sliding osteotomy procedure similar to that used in the treatment of developmental deformities (see Fig. 6-5).

Depending on the number of remaining teeth, the site of injury, and the patient's age, the original amount of bone loss may preclude realignment without a bone graft. Good contact over a distance of 2 cm. or more should be obtained. If good bony contact cannot be obtained, then an autogenous appropriately carved segment of iliac crest or rib graft with the cortical surface present on one side may be inserted into the defect. The graft is mortised into either side of the mandibular defect, partially decorticating the recipient site to ensure rapid vascularization and union (Fig. 6-13A). Local interosseous fixation, along with intermaxillary fixation, generally will be adequate when small segments are grafted and when the mandible is heavy enough to permit mortise wedging of the inlaid bone. When longer defects are to be spanned, the preoperative construction of a tantalum tray has been found to be efficacious, serving to maintain the graft in position and to fix it solidly to the remaining bone [34]. This method, when combined with intermaxillary fixation, presents the optimal conditions for rapid healing. Titanium, Vitallium, or chrome cobalt alloy hollow-mesh trays filled with autogenous marrow from the iliac crest have also been employed for this purpose [38]. In most cases, the alloplastic tray is eventually removed, although it can be left in place until bony union occurs, even in the presence of drainage postoperatively. An alternate technique involves the use of onlay plates of Vitallium or stainless steel either wired or screwed into the involved segments [41, 44]. Skewer fixation of the iliac crest or rib grafts (Fig. 6-13) on a Kirschner wire has proved successful in the reconstruction of the symphyseal area [32].

Postoperative jaw fixation is no problem when teeth are present in sufficient quantity for application of arch bars and intermaxillary wires. When teeth are few in number and widely spaced, cap splints or similar prostheses should be constructed preoperatively to make fixation absolute. In the edentulous mandible, the use of a tray or a modification of the Gunning-type splint is recommended to immobilize the mandible. Denture bases, with bite blocks keyed appropriately, are used as intraoral splints. Metal lugs, as hooks, are incorporated in the dentures, permitting the subsequent placement of intermaxillary elastics to maintain fixation. Transfacial circumferential wiring around the malar arches is used to fix the upper denture to the skull while circummandibular wires stabilize the lower denture. Care should be taken to place the wires well away from the graft junctions. The prosthodontist consultant will afford the surgeon great assistance in determining the most effective method for immobilization. Fixation or immobilization is maintained generally 6 to 8 weeks.

In the reconstruction of large defects of the body or ramus of the mandible, the bone graft must be large enough to permit proper carving, must possess a respectable cortical plate on one surface, and should ideally resemble in character the bone to be replaced. Bone from the iliac crest meets these requirements very well, but free rib grafts do not. An advancement in bone grafting this area occurred with the experimental [36] and clinical [42] publication of techniques employing transfer of an island rib graft to reconstruct the mandible. A new era in reconstructive surgery at this site was ushered in by the introduction of a rib transplantation reconstruction employing microvascular anastomotic techniques [39, 40]. These newer methods show great promise of obviating two pitfalls in bone grafting – early loss through infection and late resorption.

In reconstructing the mandible following trauma with the loss of a long segment of bone, the availability of healthy soft tissue to cover the graft is a prime consideration. To attempt reconstruction with a bone graft in the presence of dense, thick scar tissue or worse yet, where infection lingers, is to court disaster. Resurfacing the site with local or distant skin flaps, obtained either extraorally or intraorally, must precede bone grafting. Excision of adherent scar and advancement of local flaps is the preferred method of repair, especially in the male where the absence of beard over the chin and cheek area is more noticeable and more difficult to camouflage. The amount of correction possible is often limited by the availability of soft tissue to cover the graft without tension. Any type of reconstructive procedure should be delayed until all induration from previous surgical treatment has resolved, and the scars have become soft and mature. This period of waiting should be at least 3 months.

Post-traumatic Deformities of the Maxilla

Deformity of the maxilla following trauma is characterized by a "floating" maxilla when seen early and later by the "dishface" deformity if proper reduction and immobilization have not been obtained. This deformity is not unusual when the patient either is edentulous or has only a few teeth. Occasionally the patient's general condition is so precarious that local treatment of the maxillofacial injury cannot be undertaken until late.

There are three principal methods of treating malunited maxillary fractures. In the patient who has an edentulous maxilla or only a few maxillary teeth, correction of minor degrees of retrusion can be accomplished by construction of a denture with a plumper to restore contour to the upper lip and cheeks. When adequate dentition exists, fibrous union of the malunited fracture is usually strong enough by 3 or 4 weeks after injury that refracture cannot be accomplished by the usual manipulation of the maxilla. Within a period of roughly 1 to 6 months after injury, an upper impression tray that contains compound can be used to gain control of the maxilla and break up the fibrous union [33]. The soft compound in the tray is forced over the teeth and then cooled so as to harden the compound. A wooden block placed on the tray can be struck with a mallet to free the malunited maxilla. The tray with the hardened compound can be removed by striking it in such a direction as to free it from the teeth. When the malunion of the maxilla is so solid that this technique is ineffective, a transverse osteotomy of the maxilla as previously described (see Fig. 6-12) will be necessary.

Utilization of the Rowe disimpaction rocking forceps is a useful adjunct in disimpacting an osteotomized maxilla.

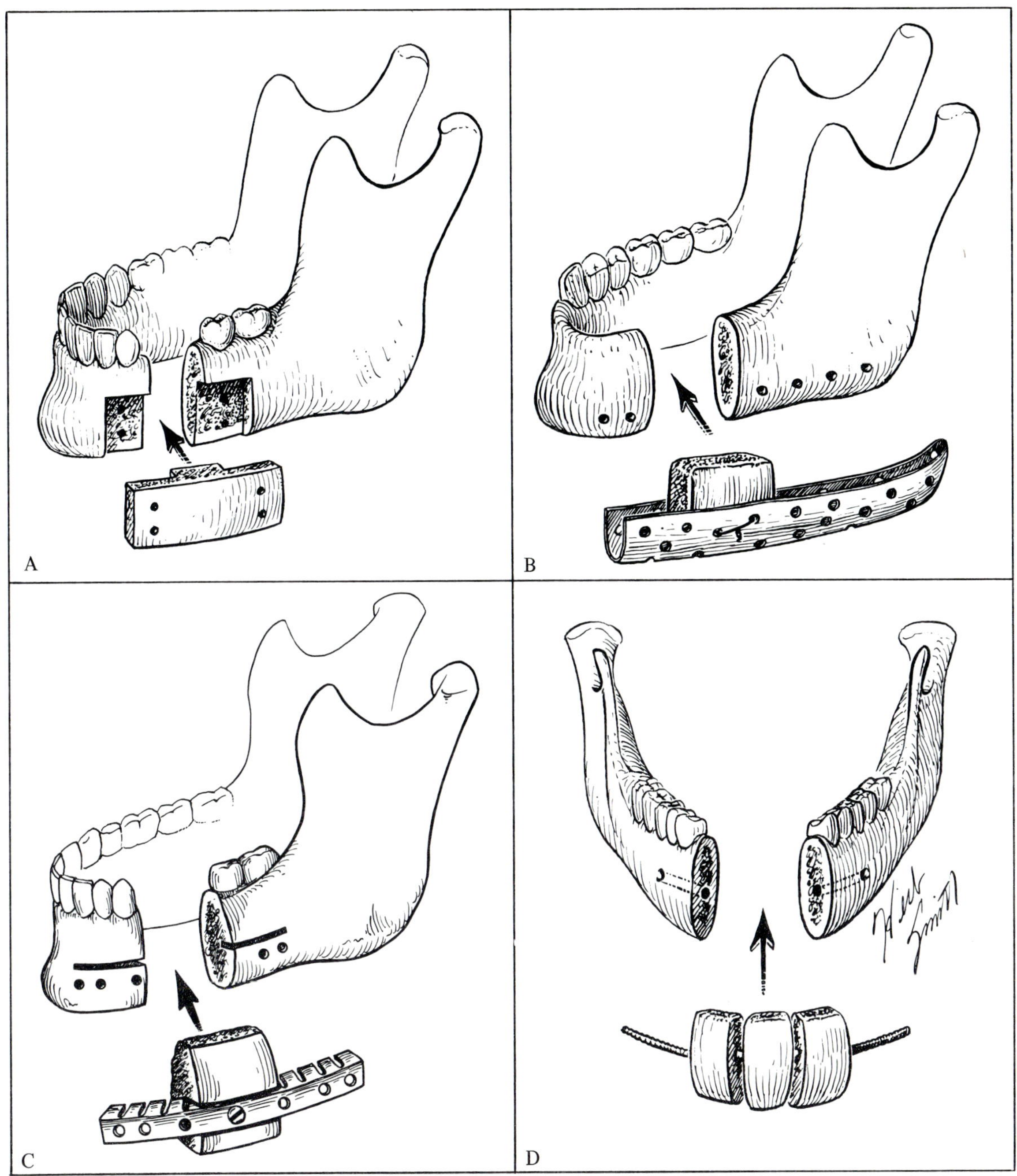

Fig. 6-13. Methods of bridging mandibular defects with bone grafts. A, the iliac bone graft is mortised into either side of the mandibular defect after partially decorticating the recipient site. Interosseous fixation is accomplished with a 26-gauge stainless-steel wire. B, longer defects can be bridged by a bone graft held in place with a tantalum or other alloplastic tray. C, an onlay plate is screwed into either side of defect with bridge of autogenous bone. D, reconstruction of symphyseal area is accomplished by either multiple bone grafts or a rib graft skewered on a Kirschner wire to hold the bone in place.

Preprosthetic Surgery

Not infrequently, irregularities in the alveolar ridge, protuberences in the form of tori (hyperostotic tuberosities of the maxilla), or bony undercuts make the construction and fitting of dentures difficult. The most frequently performed procedure in preprosthetic surgery is the alveoplasty [45], which includes the excision of bony projections and undercuts, followed by minimal recontouring of the alveolar process. While usually performed with the removal of teeth, it can frequently be done later. An incision is made, under local anesthesia, on the crest of the alveolar process, extending one tooth in front of and in back of the area of bony surgery, or equivalent length of alveolar process. A full-thickness mucoperiosteal flap is reflected and the alveolar ridge is contoured with a rongeur. Final smoothing is carried out with a bone file or bur. Excess mucosa is excised and interrupted sutures of 4-0 black silk or an absorbable suture material is employed in the closure. There are many variations in this type of surgery.

Palatine tori are removed through a midline incision directly over the torus, with careful reflection of the mucoperiosteum over the bony prominence as well as the adjacent palate. A #6 round bur is employed to drill into the torus in a cross-hatch fashion to serve as a guide for the depth of removal of the remaining bone, which is removed with either an osteotome or a large acrylic-type bur. Care must be taken not to fracture the palate shelf, which is quite thin. The torus linguales on the lingual side of the mandible near the bicuspid region can frequently be removed with a simple tap of an osteotome. These have a more polypoid configuration and the underlying cortical bone is thicker and will not fracture.

Vestibuloplasty is employed to create a larger alveolar base to support dentures. Vestibuloplasties can generally be divided into four groups: (1) vestibuloplasty with the use of local mucosa, to reposition the labial and buccal mucosa at a higher level, which is not practical in the mandible because of the usual shortage of mucosa; (2) vestibuloplasty with secondary epithelization, which also is more useful on the maxilla, and only when there is sufficient height to the alveolar ridge (when it is used on the mandible, regressions or relapses are too common); (3) vestibuloplasty with skin grafting (mandible); and finally (4) vestibuloplasty with free grafts of mucosa. These are reviewed by Steinhauser [46].

The prime goal in reconstructive surgery is restoration, both of form and of function. Severe traumatic deformities frequently leave the patient edentulous. Following union of a bone graft to the mandible, an adequate buccal and lingual sulcus must be provided if dentures are to be worn. It is common for the alveolar ridge to be completely obliterated, especially after extensive initial bone loss. Creation of a sulcus in which flanges of a denture can lie generally necessitates an intraoral skin graft.

OPERATIVE TECHNIQUE FOR RECONSTRUCTING THE MANDIBULAR SULCUS WITH A SKIN GRAFT (VESTIBULOPLASTY). Under general nasal endotracheal anesthesia, the site of the absent sulcus is opened widely, carrying the dissection down almost to the lower border of the mandible. Hemostasis by cautery must be absolute. Previously removed from a hairless donor site, a thick split-thickness skin graft (0.018 to 0.020 inch) is used for the new lining. Split-thickness mucosa, taken with the Castroviejo dermatome, is excellent tissue for use in resurfacing when only a small amount of epithelium is needed. Its usefulness is limited by its availability and the difficulties that arise in removing it from donor areas in the lips and cheeks. More recently, the use of a free graft of palatal mucosa instead of a split-thickness skin graft has been employed [32]. It has proved to be as good as, or better than, buccal mucosa and better than split-thickness skin for vestibuloplasty. The graft is maintained in position by being glued with dermatome cement to a preformed prosthesis or by direct suturing to the edges of the defect, also using a prosthetic appliance, to which dental compound has been added to overcorrect the soft tissue defect created for the graft (Fig. 6-14). Overcorrection must be emphasized if the permanent sulcus is to be of adequate depth, since some graft shrinkage is difficult to prevent. Ten days later, the temporary compound stent prosthesis is removed and immediately replaced with a more permanent prosthesis providing maintenance and security of position in the newly created sulcus. Here, the time interval is most critical; a delay of only a few hours will allow graft contraction to begin, making replacement of the conformer difficult. The prosthesis should be left in place for 3 to 6 months to minimize contraction of the skin graft.

When extremely large areas are involved, another approach to immobilization of the skin graft is the suturing of the graft to the soft tissue portion of the bed, leaving the peripheral sutures long enough to be tied over a bolus-type dressing.

Summary of Principles of Reconstruction of Post-traumatic Jaw Deformities

The salient principles in the reconstruction of post-traumatic jaw deformities are as follows:

1. Maturation of all injured tissues should precede reconstruction. When infection or severe trauma has caused the defect or has intervened during the reconstruction, a waiting period of 3 to 6 months is mandatory before beginning a new surgical effort.

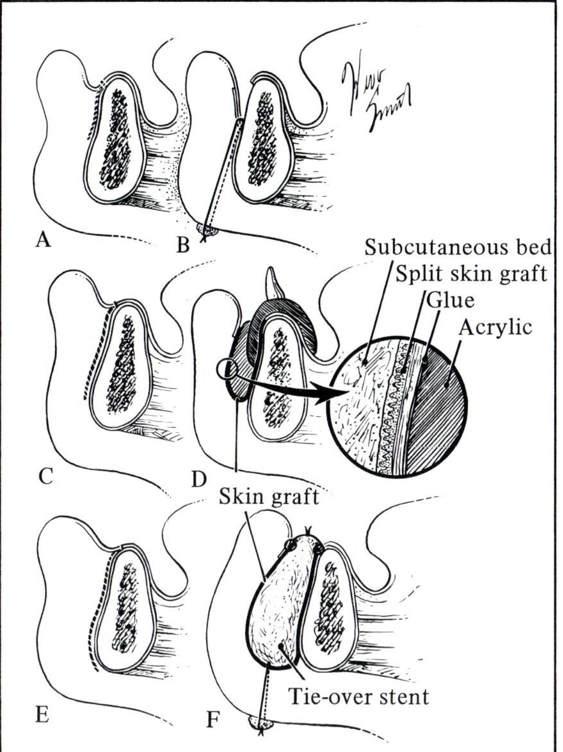

Fig. 6-14. Methods of creating a mandibular buccal and lingual sulcus. A, B, small segments of the obliterated sulcus can be reconstructed by incising the mucoperiosteum and reattaching it at the bottom of the new sulcus with a submandibular retention suture. The exposed alveolar bone will become reepithelized from the surrounding mucosa. C, D, the obliterated sulcus can be incised almost down to the lower border of the mandible and skin grafted. In this instance, the thick split-thickness skin graft is glued, dermis side out, to a preformed prosthesis. To counteract the late contracture of the skin graft it is important to overcorrect the depth of the sulcus and leave a semirigid conformer in place for 3 to 6 months. E, F, another method of skin grafting the sulcus utilizes a mold of dental compound to which a split-thickness skin graft is glued, dermis side out. The sulcus has been purposely overcorrected to allow for skin graft shrinkage. The temporary stent is held in place by a submandibular retention suture.

2. Adequate soft tissue cover, both extraoral and intraoral, must be present in order to permit adequate restoration of bone contour. It is imperative that provision be made for a well-vascularized bed for bone graft and wound closure without tension.
3. Autograft bone is preferred to allograft, xenograft, or alloplastic material. This is especially true in any area subject to stress. It is used when available and can be taken without materially increasing morbidity.
4. When the restoration of function, or form and function, is of prime importance, iliac bone is preferred. When contour only is involved, large defects can be corrected most effectively with onlay rib grafts, including homologous and heterologous bone, and the new alloplastic materials.
5. Fixation and immobilization are of prime importance in successful bone grafting.
6. As shrinkage of a skin graft inside the mouth can be anticipated, a conformer must be maintained in place for at least 3 months if the effect of surgery is to be permanent.
7. The late effects of radiation at the site of the proposed reconstruction will have a deleterious effect on reconstructive efforts.
8. The transfer of free composite grafts of skin, muscle, or bone, employing microvascular surgical techniques, should be considered in select cases.

TEMPOROMANDIBULAR JOINT DISORDERS

The temporomandibular joint is a ginglymoarthrodial (hinged-gliding) joint, formed by the articulation of the condyloid process of the mandible with the glenoid fossa and articular eminence of the squamous portion of the temporal bone (Fig. 6-15). Each temporomandibular joint actually consists of two separate synovial cavities contained within a common capsule and separated by a thin fibrocartilaginous articular disc, the meniscus. This disc, covering the condylar head, conforms to the shape of the condyle and to the glenoid fossa. The capsule is lax enough to permit a wide variety of condylar movements. Its forward wall is weakest but strength is gained from the accessory ligaments (temporomandibular, sphenomandibular, and stylomandibular), which assist in stabilizing the joint. The nerves of the temporomandibular joint are derived from the auriculotemporal and masseteric branches of the mandibular nerve, the fifth cranial nerve; the arteries are derived from the internal maxillary and superficial temporal branches of the external carotid.

The tendon of the superior belly of external pterygoid muscle is the only one that physically forms part of temporomandibular articulation. This muscle penetrates the articular capsule to insert into the vascularized anterior margin of the articular disc,

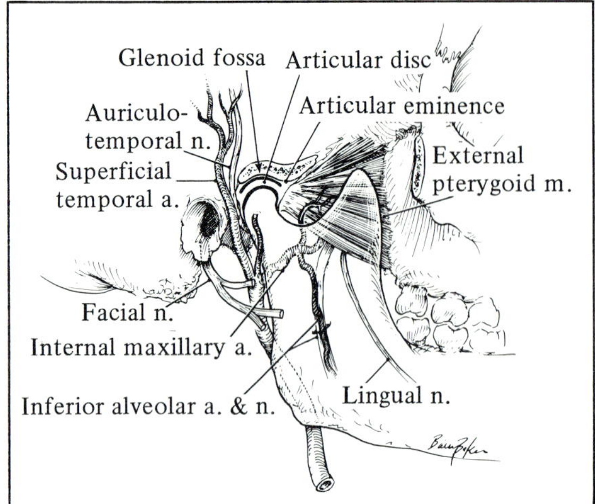

Fig. 6-15. The anatomy of the temporomandibular joint.

drawing the disc forward when it undergoes contraction [48].

The temporomandibular joint is a complex anatomical entity subjected to repeated stresses not only during chewing, but also during speech, respiration, straining, deglutition, and emotional responses. Its major function of mastication combines the simultaneous action of many muscles and ligaments.

The following terms are frequently used in describing the relationship between the positions of the mandible, occlusion of the teeth, and the temporomandibular joint.

1. *Occlusal position.* The position of the mandible when the occlusing teeth are in contact, that is, when the teeth are articulating with each other.
2. *Rest position.* The position maintained by the constant tone of the opposing muscles of mastication and the cervical musculature. When the mandible is not functioning, its rest position is constant and unalterable. (This is related to the freeway space.)
3. *Freeway space.* The 2- to 3-mm. space that is present between the maxillary and mandibular teeth when the mandible is in the rest position.
4. *Centric position.* The position of the lower jaw when the condyle is in its most comfortable retruded position in the joint with the articulating teeth and musculature in balance. Ideally, the occlusal position coincides with the centric position.

There are two basic movements of the mandible: one the *rotary* or hinge movement, a rotation of the mandible around a horizontal axis passing through the center of the condyles, as when the mandible moves from the centric or the occlusal position to the rest position; and secondly a *translatory,* or forward, sliding movement, in which a sliding of the mandibular head and disc along temporal bone occurs, as when the mandible moves from the rest position to full opening.

Clinical Evaluation of the Temporomandibular Joint
The history should include symptoms, their location and duration, the circumstances surrounding onset, any aggravating or relieving factors, previous consultations, diagnosis and treatment rendered and its effects, and emotional considerations, as well as significant medical and dental history. Physical examination should begin with specific attention to asymmetry. Mandibular movements, including opening, closing, lateral, and protrusive movements, should be observed; any limitation in range of motion or in mouth opening (or both) and any deviation present during opening and protrusive movements should be noted. Next, the temporomandibular joints should be inspected, checking for condylar motion and tenderness, both by digital palpation over the temporomandibular joint areas and with the middle finger through the auditory meatus. Employing a stethoscope, the examiner should check for the presence of abnormal sounds, including clicking and crepitation. Following this, the muscles of mastication should be observed and palpated, particularly with reference to size and the presence or absence of painful areas within the musculature. Bimanual palpation, both intraorally and extraorally, is important. A cursory dental examination should be carried out with specific attention to the state of oral hygiene, status of the occlusion, missing teeth, abnormality in arch form, and the presence or absence of caries and soft tissue pathology [46].

When pain is a symptom, it is important to determine aspects such as its location or sensation, its duration, specific description, any changes in intensity or character of pain with time, the response to drugs taken for pain, and the relationship of the pain to jaw function, time of day, and possible trauma to the face.

Radiography of the temporomandibular joint requires visualization of the joint structures from various aspects; a number of techniques are employed. The most commonly used view is a transcranial lateral–oblique used to visualize the joint components from their lateral aspect. Ideally, the joint is taken in terminal occlusion, the rest position, and maximum opening. The transorbital or anteroposterior technique seen with a modified Towne view visualizes the lateral medial aspects and the articulating surface of the condyle when the x-ray is taken with the mouth open. The submental vertex view is employed primarily in cases of trismus or extremely limited mandibular opening. The panoramic technique (Panorex) gives an overall view of the maxillomandibular region, and it should be a standard view in all problems involving any portion of the mandible and its contiguous structures. Finally, tomography is the ultimate refinement in radiographic procedures of the temporomandibular joint [49]. In evaluating the x-rays, the position, size, shape, and movement of the condyle can be noted, together with the presence or absence of focal erosions of the condyle, glenoid fossa, or articular eminence as well as the presence or absence of calcific deposits, spurs, fracture, or neoplasm. The width of the joint space is also important.

The Temporomandibular Joint Syndrome

The temporomandibular joint syndrome or the *myofacial pain dysfunction syndrome* (MPDS), originally referred to as Costen's syndrome [51], is the most common extracapsular disorder of the temporomandibular joint and is, in fact, the most common temporomandibular joint problem seen by the physician. The main symptom of MPDS is a generally unilateral pain that is located within the muscle(s) of mastication, in the neck muscles, or in and around the ear, or a combination of these locations. This pain, often poorly defined, is rarely constant and is frequently present intermittently for months or even years. There may be limitation of mandibular motion and deviation of the mandible to the side of affliction on opening. Joint noises may or may not be present; clicking or crepitation may be an intracapsular symptom of an extracapsular disorder. Ear symptoms including tenderness and a vague sensation of fullness may be present. Not uncommonly, there is evidence of stress, anxiety, or nervousness that can be uncovered by a careful and considerate historian. Oral habits, particularly excessive yawning, nervous jaw motion, and bruxism, may all aggravate the symptoms. Occlusal abnormalities, resulting in either sudden or extensive changes in centric position, may be secondary to occlusal alterations following extractions or due to imperfect dental restorations. Masticatory efforts frequently exacerbate pain; on rare occasions, a history of a psychophysiological disorder such as chronic colitis or gastrointestinal ulcer may be present. Most of the patients I have seen with MPDS are unmarried females between 20 and 30 years old.

In addition to bruxism, a history may be elicited of such activities as fingernail, lip, or cheek biting, or pipe smoking, all involving the lateral pterygoid muscle in a protrusive or lateral protrusive mandibular repositioning, resulting in chronic spasm of this muscle and pain [50]. *It cannot be too strongly stressed that the physician must rule out all intracapsular temporomandibular joint disorders before a diagnosis of myofacial pain dysfunction syndrome is made.* Trauma not involving fracture; infection, usually intraoral; otologic causes including otitis media or external otitis; and neoplastic problems including parotid gland tumor, nasopharyngeal tumor, neuroma, and intracranial lesions may cause symptoms similar to MPDS and must be ruled out. Conservative, nonoperative treatment is indicated for patients with MPDS, as described later in this chapter.

Disorders of the Temporomandibular Joint

Osteoarthritis of the temporomandibular joint is a degenerative disease that usually follows internal derangement after either chronic or acute trauma, particularly in older patients. In the chronic degenerated joint (degenerative osteoarthritis), there is softening, roughening, and cracking of the meniscus and the articular cartilages. Blood fills the cracks and may undermine the cartilage, separating it from the bone; the cartilage may become fractured or worn away, with exposure of subcondylar bone. Erosion of the articular tubercle and marginal proliferation of the condylar head as osteophytes may also appear. The articular discs may become grooved, ridged, fractured, and later disappear. The symptoms of clicking and crepitation experienced clinically may be due to actual tears in the joint structure, resulting in the formation of scar tissue. This condition is usually accompanied by chronic, long-standing pain in the affected joint, with varying degrees of mandibular dysfunction, resulting from an inadequate functional occlusion. Radiographically, in addition to the observations already described previously, the joint space may be completely obliterated. Therapy is similar to that for MPDS and is discussed in a later section.

Rheumatoid arthritis is a systemic disease with an earlier onset than osteoarthritis, although it may occur from very early childhood to old age. Its specific etiology is unknown; however an abnormal immune response and a yet unidentified viable agent have been demonstrated as part of the disease. Joint involvement is characterized by an early synovitis with extensive synovial fluid production and subsequent inflammatory pannus formation with granulation tissue overgrowth on the cartilage. The articular surfaces of the bones become eroded, after which there may be a progression to a fibrous or bony ankylosis. The disease is unpredictable, but it is commonly characterized by progressive symptomatology and intermittent periods of disease activity. The condyles of both joints are affected, simultaneously displaying marked decalcification with resorption that increases as the disease progresses. As years pass, retrognathic relationship with an anterior open bite between the jaws develops as a result of the loss of condylar support and contracture of the masseter musculature [54]. While no drug or treatment regimen can effect a cure, salicylates, indomethacin, phenylbutazone, gold compound, and corticosteroids can afford measures of relief and possible remission. Chewing gum to maintain joint motion is often helpful. When apertognathia or ankylosis has occurred, the treatment of choice is operative (see Operative Management of Temporomandibular Joint Disorders).

Congenital intracapsular disorders, resulting in either agenesis or hypoplastic condyle, are discussed in Chapter 4.

Primary *bacterial* infections within the joint are rare; however, such systemic diseases as gonorrhea, syphilis, tuberculosis, typhoid fever, dysentery, pneumonitis, influenza, scarlet fever, and measles can result in *infectious arthritis.* Joint inflammation may be secondary to extension of local lesions involving the middle ear, mastoid processes, parotid gland, or even the teeth. Even more rarely, infectious arthritis may follow direct trauma when a penetrating wound has caused bacterial contamination.

The general local treatment, which is the same as the management of any infection, includes specific antibiotic therapy, the application of moist heat, rest, and the control of pain. If extensive bone necrosis is produced, osteomyelitis may result, leading to the subsequent formation of a sequestrum. Physical therapy in the form of selective jaw movements and progressive increase in diet may be necessary to overcome the tendency to ankylosis following such joint infections.

Tumors of the temporomandibular joint are rare, and the detection of both benign and malignant neoplasms depends primarily on the radiographic examination. Enlargement of the condyle secondary to hyperplasia, a chondroma, or an osteoma (osteochondroma) constitutes the largest group of tumors originating primarily in the temporomandibular joint. Other benign tumors include myxoma and fibrous dysplasia; the even rarer malignant tumors that have been reported include multiple myeloma, fibrosarcoma, and chrondrosarcoma of the condyle. Treatment is operative [54].

Functional disorders are primarily either subluxations or dislocations. *Subluxation* describes the condition that occurs when the condyle moves over the articular eminence during open excursion but returns to the glenoid fossa with closure. In many patients the condyle may move as much as 5 mm. anteriorly to the summit of the eminence when the mouth is opened; however, subluxation is considered only if accompanied by symptoms such as transitory locking or clicking in the terminal opening position [52]. Pathologically, there frequently is an abnormal capsular laxity, inordinate jaw movement secondary to muscular incoordination, or a combination of the two factors. When pain is present, it is usually secondary to muscle spasm. Treatment is primarily conservative; analgesics, rest, and local heat may be used when pain is a problem following recurrent subluxation. Sclerosing solutions such as Sylnasol and sodium morrhuate may be injected into the joint to scar the capsule, reduce its laxity, and restrict mandibular motion.

When there is a derangement that is not self-reducing between the articulating components of the temporomandibular joint, it is referred to as a *dislocation.* Occasionally, patients are seen with a history of repeated mandibular dislocation. Dislocations treated prior to the onset of severe muscle spasm can usually be reduced by pressing the mandible downward to position the condyle below the eminence and then posteriorly to relocate it within the glenoid fossa (Fig. 6-16). Usually analgesia or anesthesia is not necessary; however, a general anesthetic is occasionally necessary to relieve muscle spasm in order to permit treatment. With repeated bouts of dislocation, operative treatment is usually necessary as subsequently described in this chapter.

Fractures of the condyle and subcondyle areas are discussed in Chapter 9.

Nonoperative Management of Temporomandibular Joint Disorders

Seventy-five to 95 percent of all patients who present with symptoms of joint pain or with a functional impairment (or with both) can be controlled by various combinations of such nonoperative methods as rest; medications, including analgesics, sedatives, antispasmodics, and ataractic muscle relaxants; physiotherapy, including diathermy, ultrasound, exercise, and massage; occlusal adjustments or equilibration; anesthesia; joint instillations, including anesthetic solutions, sclerosing agents, steroids, and hyaluronidase; and finally psychiatric counseling.

REST. The patient with an acutely painful temporomandibular joint syndrome is encouraged to rest by limiting speaking, by inaugurating a liquid diet, and by stifling yawns. When there has been an acute strain, hematoma, or capsular tear, immobilization is indicated. This can be accomplished by the use of two opposing Ivy loops and intermaxillary elastic traction for 7 to 10 days. In cases where there has been dislocation with "locking," immobilization for 3 weeks is recommended.

MEDICATIONS. Analgesics to relieve pain, sedatives or ataractics to decrease cortical excitability, and antispasmodics or muscle relaxants to decrease muscle

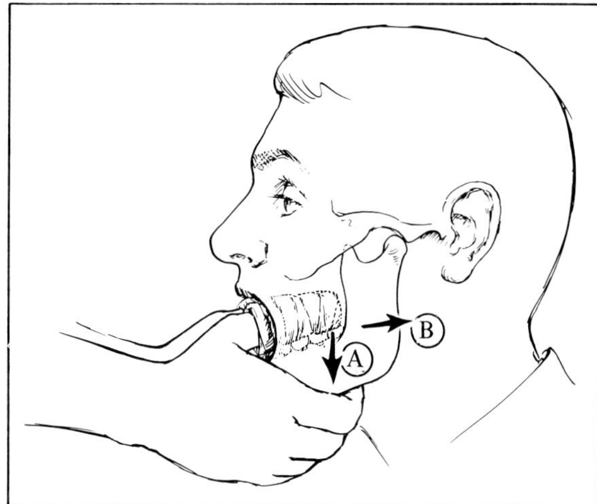

Fig. 6-16. Reducing the dislocated mandible. See text for further details.

tension and excitable foci are very valuable ancillary agents to treatment, in both acute and chronic situations. Diazepam (Valium) has proved exceptionally helpful.

PHYSICAL THERAPY. The frequent application of moist heat can be an effective form of physiotherapy during acute exacerbations. Shortwave or microwave heat applications have also been reported as effective in palliation of pain. Ultrasound is useful if local heat relieves pain [67]. The physical therapy prescription should be written to include the application of heat to the temporomandibular joint area for 10 minutes followed by ultrasound for 4 minutes at 0.5 watts, increasing to 1.5 watts per square centimeter as tolerated. Usually a course of ten treatments over a 2-week period is given. Ultrasound therapy, even in the chronic condition complicated by scarring, can be helpful. Exercises, including active stretching, reflex relaxation, and assistive stretching, as recommended by Schwartz [47], are rewarding. After these exercises have been mastered, the patient can be taught to use hingelike motions of the mandibular joint without any forward movement and made to recognize consciously the mandibular pathways so that he may prevent lateral shifting and incoordinated movements. The local application of rubefacients and other counterirritants has also been of some limited help.

OCCLUSAL ADJUSTMENTS. These should be carried out by a dentist who is familiar with this condition and treatment. Frequently, a preliminary step includes construction of a diagnostic bite plane appliance intended to eliminate proprioceptive stimulation caused by occlusal cusp interference and to aid in restoring proper muscle balance. A night guard can be constructed to support occlusion and reduce joint trauma in cases of bruxism. Occlusal therapy may include occlusal adjustments by selective grinding and maxillary and mandibular posterior-fixed restorations. Corrective occlusal or prosthetic techniques should not be begun before attempting treatment by the conservative measures outlined above [47].

ANESTHESIA. In a situation evolving from muscle spasm, local anesthesia is the single most important aspect of therapy. An injection of 2% lidocaine into the muscles of mastication at sites of intramuscular spasms is very effective. By palpation the areas of spasm can be sharply localized and injected to give immediate relief. The most common spasm involves the combined origins of the external and internal pterygoids just behind the maxillary tuberosity on the sphenoid bone. A refrigerant such as ethyl chloride or Freon sprayed onto the overlying skin can break up muscle spasms and may be diagnostic as well as therapeutic. Sometimes a direct intraarticular injection of 2 ml. of 2% lidocaine may be helpful in interrupting the pain cycle when other methods have failed. Anesthetizing the nerve endings within and around the articular disc occasionally will dramatically eliminate the pain for long periods. Injection therapy may be repeated as often as needed. Intraarticular injection of steroids in combination with a local anesthetic is reserved for treatment of persistent joint symptoms unresponsive to conservative treatment measures; it is also employed in the treatment of recurrent rheumatoid synovitis, in which situation it can be reliably effective.

PSYCHIATRIC COUNSELING. The physician can begin psychiatric treatment by providing emotional support, including listening to the patient with sincere interest and offering a calm approach with reassurance and firm direction. Advising the patient to be aware of oral habits (e.g., bruxism) and to reduce habit activity may be sufficient to control muscle dysfunction. Several patients have been observed with temporomandibular joint symptomatology, with associated psychiatric problems.

Operative Management of Temporomandibular Joint Disorders

In my experience, fewer than 15 percent of the patients with temporomandibular joint disorders require surgical treatment. The anesthesia of choice is general anesthesia administered nasally through an endotracheal tube. Blind nasal intubation in patients with ankylosis may be necessary under heavy premedication;

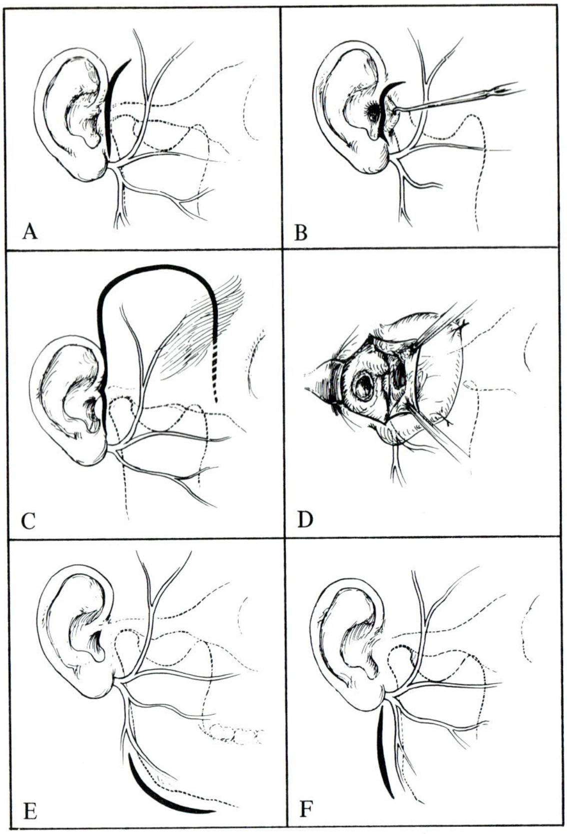

Fig. 6-17. Surgical approaches to the temporomandibular joint: A, preauricular; B, endaural; C, temporal flap; D, postauricular; E, submandibular; F, retromandibular.

however, a tracheostomy set must be available for immediate use. A variety of incisions have been advocated for operative approach to the temporomandibular joint (Fig. 6-17). This surgical area is small, frequently deep, and in close proximity to several important structures, including the facial nerve. Difficulties previously encountered by surgeons are attested to by the variety of operative approaches described.

Temporomandibular Joint Incisions (After Laskin [53])

PREAURICULAR INCISION. This 4-cm. hockey stick–shaped incision is the most commonly employed and permits the best exposure and the least amount of tissue undermining; it should not endanger the facial nerve. It is the incision of choice for most surgical procedures on the joint. The superficial temporal artery and vein are ligated and divided and the posterior portion of the zygomatic arch exposed. The parotid gland is retracted anteriorly, and by sharp dissection, the posterior one-third of the masseter fibers originating from the zygomatic arch permit wide exposure of the joint.

SUBMANDIBULAR OR RISDON APPROACH. This approach is employed for exposure of the superior portion of the ramus and condylar neck and is particularly useful in cases of extracapsular ankylosis. Direct injury to or excessive traction on the ramus mandibularis can result in nerve damage. This approach is not recommended for surgery on the temporomandibular joint itself.

RETROMANDIBULAR INCISION. This incision lies parallel to and about 1 cm. behind the posterior border of the ascending ramus of the mandible. The scar is acceptable, and this approach has the advantage over the submandibular or Risdon approach in that it does not necessitate complete elevation of the masseter muscle, and the ramus mandibularis of the facial nerve is easier to avoid.

FACIAL-ENDAURAL INCISION. This is a more sophisticated approach that decreases the danger of facial nerve injury and leaves a less discernible scar, but limits exposure.

POSTAURICULAR INCISION. This incision is carried completely through the cartilaginous auditory canal and the entire area is reflected anteriorly to expose the joint from behind. External auditory stenosis and infection secondary to necrosis of the ear cartilage are possible complications of the postauricular incision, as well as of the facial-endaural and purely endaural approaches. None of these incisions is advised.

TEMPORAL FLAP. This may be necessary in severe cases of extracapsular temporomandibular joint ankylosis with involvement of such structures as the zygomatic arch or the coronoid processes, and it may even be combined with an intraoral pterygomandibular raphe incision for maximum exposure in the more difficult cases.

Operative Techniques

The techniques of surgical management of the temporomandibular joint disorders are discussed in this section, although the great majority of the patients with signs and symptoms of internal joint derangement are now classified as patients with myofacial pain dysfunction syndrome, and pure operative management is generally contraindicated.

MENISECTOMY. This controversial procedure has been strongly advocated by some [65] as the procedure of choice to deal with symptoms of pain, noise, trismus, and locking. Others deprecate the procedure, describing improvement of the signs only, but not of symptoms, and in many instances, the persistence or subsequent recurrence of pain and limitations of motion and crepitation [62]. The joint capsule is exposed through a preauricular incision; the mandible is protruded, moving the condyle anteriorly, to facilitate exposure. The capsule is incised and the meniscus excised from its strong attachments on all sides. Bleeding is frequently a problem and is best controlled by retruding the mandible temporarily and packing the area. Because premature occlusion of the molars on the affected side may occur postoperatively, employment of a polyethylene cap over the condyle to replace the vertical height lost by removal of the meniscus has been described by Hanson and De Shazo [61].

ARTHROPLASTY. Arthroplasty is another rarely employed procedure that is useful when small exostoses are present over the condylar head. The surface of the condyle is simply smoothed over its articular surface [58].

CONDYLECTOMY. Like arthroplasty, high condylectomy is performed through a preauricular approach; the cut in the condyle is made *above* the attachment in the lateral pterygoid muscle and the remaining portion of the condyle is recontoured.

LOW CONDYLECTOMY. The condylar neck and condyle are removed at the level of the sigmoid notch or slightly above it, but *below* the attachment of the lateral pterygoid muscle (see description under Operative Procedures for Ankylosis). In all operations for internal derangement, postoperative care is important. Treatment is begun 2 days after surgery and the patient progresses to a nearly normal diet by the end of the first week. Both active and passive jaw exercises are encouraged as soon as the pain has decreased enough; physiotherapy is frequently a useful adjunct.

In my experience, whenever a condylectomy is performed, replacement with either a preformed alloplastic condyle [35] or a small modified Silastic implant (of the type usually used for chin augmentation) should be employed in order (1) to maintain joint space without loss of vertical dimension, which may result in secondary occlusal dysfunction, and (2) to prevent secondary limitations of motion and alkylosis because of late scarring (Fig. 6-18).

Patients who have undergone condylectomy for rheumatoid arthritis are much more likely to develop ankylosis than are patients with simple degenerative osteoarthritis.

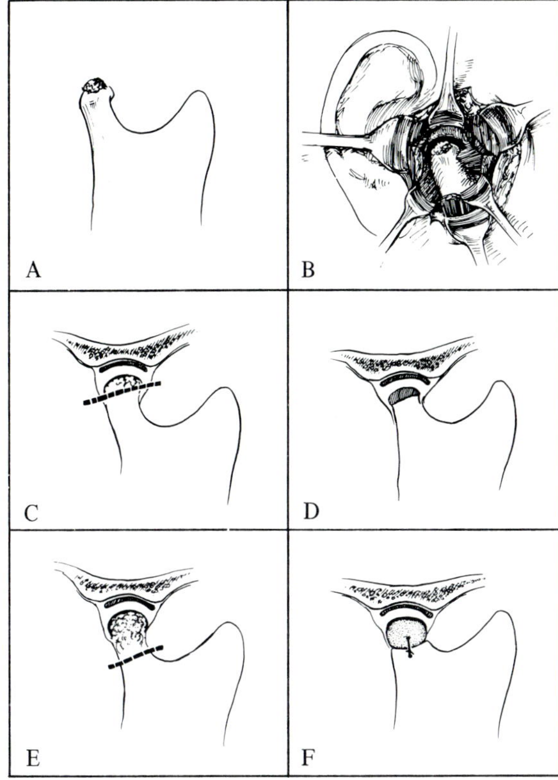

Fig. 6-18. Surgical management of the temporomandibular joint disorders. A, B, excision of exostosis. C, D, condylotomy. E, F, condylectomy with alloplastic replacement of resected condylar head.

OPERATIONS FOR HYPERMOBILITY SYNDROMES. In subluxation, the condyle head moves anterior to the articular eminence during full opening; such movement may be accompanied by momentary locking or clicking in the terminal opening position. Surgical treatment is indicated only if the signs continue even when the patient avoids opening. Utilization of sclerosing solutions by injection will result in sufficient tightening of the joint capsule and adjacent ligaments to obviate the necessity for any direct surgical intervention. While habitual temporomandibular joint dislocation should be treated conservatively initially, surgery should be considered when nonoperative methods fail to control the dislocation.

A reefing *capsulorrhaphy* (a procedure in which the capsular tissue is shortened) is an integral part of most operations for hypermobility of the joint. Fastening the mandible using fascia lata suspension through drill holes between the condylar neck and temporal bone is not generally effective on a long-term basis. If the fascial suspension is stretched and the etiological factors persist, recurrence of the problem is more likely.

There are three types of *anterior blockage operations* aimed at preventing mechanical anterior dislocations of the condyle: (1) intracapsular tuberculum plasty (increasing the height of the tubercle by bone grafting anterior to the joint); (2) osteotomy of the mandible (tilting the tubercle downward and filling in the defect with bone graft chips); (3) antepositioning of the meniscus (bringing the meniscus down and forward over the condyle). These procedures are rarely employed.

According to Laskin [66], "the common factor in all of the above procedures is that they are all intra-articular operations and may probably result in a degree of capsular fibrosis which limits mandibular excursion and prevents subluxation and/or dislocations." The utilization of sclerosing agents is probably preferable.

Another operation for hypermobility syndromes is the *external pterygoid myotomy.* Sectioning of the insertion of the lateral pterygoid muscle through a preauricular approach close to the neck of the condylar process is a successful procedure with long-lasting results [55]. A piece of Silastic sheeting may be wired over the neck of the condyle where the external pterygoid inserts; this acts as a safeguard against reattachment of the muscle and recurrence of the problem (Fig. 6-19).

In bilateral dislocation, the first procedure should involve operating only on the painful side. The contralateral joint will probably be cleared of symptoms by the reduced mobility, which will obviate a further operation.

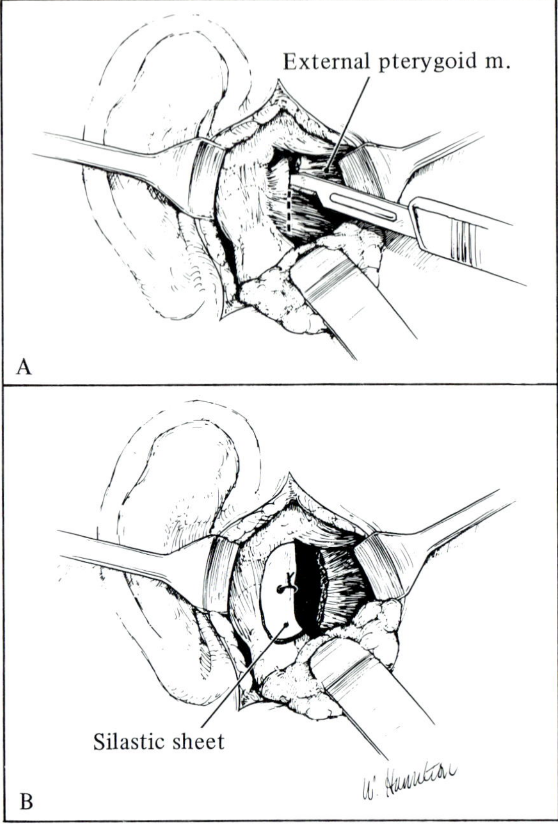

Fig. 6-19. Technique for external pterygoid myotomy for treatment of recurring subluxation and/or dislocation. (After Laskin [66].)

Temporomandibular Joint Ankylosis

Ankylosis may be defined as stiffening or fixation of the joint; when applied to the temporomandibular joint, ankylosis indicates some interference with normal mobility of the jaws. It may vary from minimal restriction of motion that does not interfere with function to a complete, or almost complete, inability to open the jaws. One may divide ankylosis at the temporomandibular joint into true and false ankylosis.

In *true ankylosis,* commonly referred to as intra-articular ankylosis, there is a bony, fibrous, or scarred union between the articular surfaces of the joint. The result is extreme limitation of mandibular opening; only rarely is complete immobility of the joint seen. The most common cause of true intraarticular ankylosis is trauma, either direct or indirect, causing injury of the condylar head and/or meniscus, with or without fracture. The other principal cause of true ankylosis is infection, which may be blood-borne (e.g., osteomyelitis, meningitis) and may also result from direct extension of the infection from the adjacent sites, including otitis media, mastoiditis, and osteomyelitis of the temporal bone. Finally, true ankylosis may be caused by direct disease involvement of the joints such as is seen occasionally in rheumatoid arthritis.

The other principal category of ankylosis is commonly called *false ankylosis,* or extraarticular ankylosis; the joint surfaces of the temporomandibular joint are not involved. Ankylosis of this type is usually unilateral and is rarely complete; it is exemplified by the type of ankylosis that is seen in (1) fractures of the malar arch with lockage of the coronoid process of the mandible, (2) cicatricial bony adhesions of the coronoid processes of the mandible where the sigmoid notch approximates the arch to the adjacent temporal bone, or even (3) a frank bony fusion of the ramus without condylar involvement with the infratemporal surface of the maxilla.

During the physical examination, one can usually differentiate extracapsular from intracapsular ankylosis. In extracapsular or false ankylosis, the articular surface of the temporomandibular joint is usually not involved and movement of the condyle is palpable on forced opening. In true ankylosis, mandibular protrusion is usually not possible; in addition, pain is absent on forced opening. In false ankylosis the reverse is true; a degree of protrusion may be possible and pain is usually present on forced opening. X-ray examination is essential. In addition to routine forced open and closed x-ray studies of the temporomandibular joint, the panoramic (Panorex) view and, most important, tomography studies are employed to outline the site of ankylosis.

Treatment

One can state that the treatment of all true ankylosis of the temporomandibular joint is operative. The utilization of such devices as fancy splints, mouth openers, rubber band arrangements, and springs is generally a waste of time and is ineffectual, as is forced opening and manipulation of the jaws with the patient under general anesthesia. On the other hand, there are patients with extracapsular, extra-articular ankylosis in whom the ankylosis is secondary to fibrosis or immobility caused by muscle spasms; in these cases one might consider forced manipulation.

The following general principles [63] should be adhered to:

1. Surgical treatment should be instituted as soon as possible, particularly in the young, if growth deformities are to be minimized.
2. In severe cases, tracheotomy to facilitate the administration of anesthesia and postoperative airway control should be considered.
3. The surgical approach to the joint area of ankylosis must provide adequate exposure even to the extent of utilizing the classic Webber-Ferguson incision.
4. Surgical lysis of fibrotic tissue, followed by forced opening and/or simple osteotomy in the case of ankylosis secondary to bony union, is inadequate and is usually followed by recurrence.
5. Wide release, with removal of at least 1 cm. of involved tissue with the interposition of appropriate local tissue, an autogenous graft, or an alloplastic implant, is necessary if recurrence is to be prevented. In the child, maintenance of ramus height is important and consideration should be given to replacement, employing either a costochondral or metatarsal growth center [57, 59] or an artificial joint [64].
6. The cooperation of the patient is necessary to maintain the surgical result.
7. The degree of jaw opening obtained at surgery is rarely improved upon. At best, in most cases it diminishes slightly.
8. Muscle derangements – permanent shifts of position in the jaw with resultant malocclusion include cross bite, and open bite relationships – are complications that can usually be prevented. It is essential that appropriate prosthetic devices be utilized, combined with adequate and long-term postoperative care.

OPERATIVE TECHNIQUES FOR ANKYLOSIS. Surgical approaches are described under the heading Temporomandibular Joint Incisions. In addition, the Webber-Ferguson approach, which lays back the entire cheek, is occasionally necessary in severe cases of extraarticular ankylosis. Finally, a separate intraoral exposure may be useful in some cases of extracapsular ankylosis.

Two basic operations are employed in the treatment of ankylosis: a *condylectomy* and *osteoarthrotomy*. Excision of the condyle involves the following steps: With the patient under general nasal endotracheal anesthesia, the field is exposed, usually through a preauricular angulated vertical incision. The posterior part of the masseter muscle is detached and downward retraction is employed to expose the joint capsule. A vertical incision is made into the periosteum at the neck of the condyle, exposing the joint to confirm the diagnosis. Osteotomy is then performed, with care being taken to protect the medial vessels located next to the joint (internal maxillary artery) and the pterygoid plexus of veins. The mandible is moved to confirm an adequate release, followed by removal of the condyle and adjacent capsular ligaments. A joint arthroplasty (utilization of a prosthetic condyle, or similar space maintainer) is carried out as indicated (as described under Postoperative Care). Drainage and closure are routine.

True total anatomical joint reconstruction is rarely necessary. Although unilateral condylectomy in the adult will cause displacement of the jaw toward the operated side, this usually is compatible with acceptable function of the lower jaw and produces minimal deformity. The only indications for the use of joint transplants are in (1) unilateral condylectomy in a child or (2) the reconstruction of congenital deformities associated with the first and second branchial arch syndromes. Joint reconstruction is also advocated in bilateral condylectomy in adults. The utilization of metallic prosthetic joints is controversial. Many early successes have been failures over a long-term period. Free half-joint transplants, employing a growth center for either an autogenous metatarsal or costochondral junction, have been employed [57, 59]. Theoretically, growth should be anticipated; however, while function is frequently adequate, anticipated growth has been disappointing.

When there is bony ankylosis of the condyle and

fusion of the adjacent ramus of the mandible to the base of the skull, it can be treated by an osteoarthrotomy. The osteoarthrotomy may be either a gap arthroplasty or an interpositional arthroplasty, 1 to 1.5 cm., and the space is left open; in the interposition arthroplasty less bone is removed than with the gap arthroplasty, and either autogenous muscle, dermis fat, fascia lata, or cartilage is interposed to prevent the fragments from uniting. Alloplastic materials in a variety of forms and shapes have been employed. Generally, reconstruction involves the use of only autogenous grafts in the young, while alloplastic materials are considered in older patients. A clever operation, which employs a turndown of temporalis muscle fibers and fascia interposed between the cut bony edges, has been described by Converse [56]. Georgiade [60] has reported successful use of a dermal fat graft over the osteotomy site in the treatment of ankylosis.

Steps in the osteoarthrotomy procedure include: Under general anesthesia, wide surgical exposure, usually extraoral but occasionally intraoral, is used either alone or in combination with an external approach. In the event that endotracheal intubation cannot be performed because of ankylosis, anatomical variations, or other problems, a temporary tracheotomy should be carried out as an initial procedure. By sharp dissection, all involved fibrous tissue and bone are removed. The adequacy of release is confirmed by passive movement of the mandible in all directions. Either a gap or an interpositional arthroplasty is performed. Joint motion is reconfirmed when the interpositional arthroplasty is completed. Drainage and closure are routine. The patient is encouraged to start active motion as soon as swelling and pain permit, usually by the third postoperative day (Fig. 6-20).

POSTOPERATIVE CARE. If a gap arthroplasty has been performed, it is essential that the patient wear a splint in order to prevent scar contraction and subsequent malocclusion and cross bite. If the operation is performed bilaterally in one procedure, it is likely that an open bite will result. The use of a splint to raise or open the bite increases the gap between the bone edges so that after healing is complete, there is slack that allows the teeth to be brought into occlusion when the splint is removed.

Devices such as tongue blade exercises or commercially available exercisers should be employed; if there is a tendency to malocclusion, night intermaxillary fixation should be employed. Functional treatment must be carried out over a period of at least a year to achieve optimum results. There is a tendency to open bite formation in some patients, and an acrylic monoblock occlusal "splint" must be placed between the last molars with strong elastics to the anterior part and even a chin strap to prevent formation of open bite. Complications include severe hemorrhage at the time of surgery, injury to the facial nerve, and early postoperative pain. Later, the most common complication is recurrence of the problem.

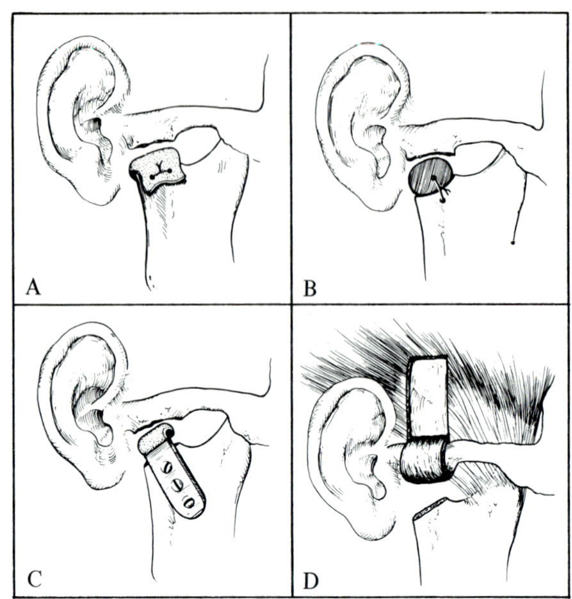

Fig. 6-20. Several techniques employed in the treatment of ankylosis of the mandible following ostectomy. A, dermis overlay. B, silicone rubber interpositional graft. C, prosthetic condyle. D, temporalis fascia–muscle flap to prevent reoccurrence of ankylosis.

ACKNOWLEDGMENT

I would like to express my appreciation to Dr. Lester Cramer, who wrote the chapter on the temporomandibular joint in the two previous editions of this text, for allowing me to borrow freely from his fine original script.

REFERENCES

Occlusion and Growth

1. Angle, E. H. Classification of malocclusion. *Dental Cosmos* 41:248, 1899.
2. Bean, L. R., Kramer, J. R., and Khouw, F. E. A simplified method for taking radiographs for cephalometric analysis. *J. Oral Surg.* 28:675, 1970.
3. Hinds, E. C., and Kent, J. N. *Surgical Treatment of Developmental Jaw Deformities.* St. Louis: Mosby, 1972.

4. Salzmann, J. W. *Practice of Orthodontics.* Philadelphia and Montreal: Lippincott, 1966.
5. Sarnat, B. G., and Robinson, I. B. Surgery of the mandible. *Plast. Reconstr. Surg.* 17:27, 1956.
6. Waite, D. E., and Worms, F. W. Orthodontic and Surgical Evaluation and Treatment of Maxillomandibular Deformities. In Irby, W. B. (Ed.), *Current Advnaces in Oral Surgery.* St. Louis: Mosby, 1974.

Micrognathia and Microgenia

7. Caldwell, J. B., and Amaral, W. J. Mandibular micrognathia corrected by vertical osteotomy in the rami and bone graft. *J. Oral Surg.* 18:3, 1960.
8. Caldwell, J. B., Hayward, J. R., and Lister, R. L. Correction of retrognathia by vertical "L" osteotomy: A new technique. *J. Oral Surg.* 26:259, 1968.
9. Converse, J. M. Micrognathia. *Br. J. Plast. Surg.* 16:197, 1963.
10. Dal Pont, G. Retromolar osteotomy for correction of prognathism. *J. Oral Surg. Anesth. Hosp. Dent. Serv.* 19:42, 1961.
11. Robinson, M., and Shuken, R. Bone resorption under plastic chin implants. *J. Oral Surg.* 27:116, 1969.
12. Sanders, B., and Cox, R. Inferior border rib grafting for augmentation of the atrophic edentulous mandible. *J. Oral Surg.* 34:897, 1976.
13. Spira, M. Surgery of the Chin. In Whitaker, L. (Ed.), *Educational Foundation Symposium – Surgery of Jaw Deformity.* Philadelphia: Mosby, 1978.
14. Trauner, R., and Obwegeser, H. L. The surgical correction of mandibular prognathism and retrognathia, with consideration of genioplasty. *J. Oral Surg.* 10:677, 787, 899, 1957.

Prognathism

15. Behrman, S. J. Complications Associated with Orthognathic Surgery. In Irby, W. B. (Ed.), *Current Advances in Oral Surgery.* St. Louis: Mosby, 1974.
16. Converse, J. M., Horowitz, S. L., and Wood-Smith, D. Deformity of the Jaws. In Converse, J. R. (Ed.), *Reconstructive Plastic Surgery.* Philadelphia: Saunders, 1964.
17. Dingman, R. O. Surgical correction of developmental deformities of the mandible. *Plast. Reconstr. Surg.* 3:124, 1948.
18. Hinds, E. L. Correction of prognathism by subcondylar osteotomy. *J. Oral Surg.* 16:209, 1963.

Laterognathism

19. Bruce, R. A., and Hayward, J. R. Condylar hyperplasia and mandibular asymmetry: A review. *J. Oral Surg.* 26:281, 1968.
19a. Converse, J. M., Horowitz, S. L., Coccaro, P. J., and Wood-Smith, D. The corrective treatment of the skeletal asymmetry in hemifacial microsomia. *Plast. Reconstr. Surg.* 52:268, 1973.
19b. Converse, J. M., Wood-Smith, D., McCarthy, J. G., Coccaro, P. J., and Becker, M. H. Bilateral facial microsomia. *Plast. Reconstr. Surg.* 54:413, 1974.
20. Dingman, R. O., and Grabb, W. C. Mandibular laterognathism. *Plast. Reconstr. Surg.* 31:564, 1963.

Apertognathia

21. Caldwell, J. B. Developmental Deformities of the Jaws. In *Krugers Textbook of Oral Surgery.* St. Louis: Mosby, 1964.

Benign Masseteric Hypertrophy

22. Bloem, J. J. A. M., and Van Hoot, R. M. Hypertrophy of the masseter muscles. *Plast. Reconstr. Surg.* 47:138, 1971.

Maxillary Deformities

23. Bell, W. H. Correction of the short face syndrome: Vertical maxillary deficiency. A preliminary report. *J. Oral Surg.* 35:110, 1977.
24. Converse, J. M., Horowitz, S. L., and Wood-Smith, D. Surgical orthodontic correction in the bilateral cleft lip. *Cleft Palate J.* 1:153, 1964.
25. Converse, J. M., and Shapiro, H. H. Treatment of developmental malformations of the jaws. *Plast. Reconstr. Surg.* 10:473, 1952.
26. Kent, J. N., and Hinds, E. C. Management of dental facial deformities by anterior alveolar surgery. *J. Oral Surg.* 29:13, 1971.
27. Kent, J. N., and Spira, M. The Buck Tooth Deformity. In *Proceedings of the First International Symposium on Plastic and Reconstructive Surgery of the Face and Neck,* Vol. 1. Stuttgart: George Thieme, 1972.
28. Kole, H. Surgical operations on the alveolar ridge to correct occlusal abnormalities. *J. Oral Surg.* 12:277, 413, 515, 1959.
29. Longacre, J. J., and DeStefano, G. A. Further observations of the behavior of autogenous split-rib grafts in the reconstruction of extensive defects of the cranium and face. *Plast. Reconstr. Surg.* 20:281, 1957.
30. Mohnac, A. M. Maxillary osteotomy in management of occlusal deformities. *J. Oral Surg.* 24:305, 1966.
31. Obwegeser, H. Surgical Correction of Maxillary Deformities. In Grabb, W. C., Rosenstein, S. W., and Bzoch, K. R. (Eds.), *Cleft Lip and Palate.* Boston: Little, Brown, 1971.

Post-traumatic Deformities of the Mandible

32. Converse, J. M. *Kazanjian and Converse's Surgical Treatment of Facial Injuries* (3rd ed.). Vol. 2. Chapter 24, Deformities of the Jaws. Baltimore: Williams & Wilkins, 1974.
33. Dingman, R. O., and Natvig, P. *Surgery of Facial Fractures.* Philadelphia: Saunders, 1964.
34. Hinds, E. C., Spira, M., Sills, A. J., Jr., and Galbreath, J. C. Use of tantalum trays in mandibular surgery. *Plast. Reconstr. Surg.* 32:439, 1963.
35. Irby, W. B. Techniques for Application of Alloplastic Materials in Reconstructive Surgery or Corrective Surgery of the Jaws. In Irby, W. B. (Ed.), *Current Advances of Oral Surgery.* St. Louis: Mosby, 1974.
36. Ketchum, L. C., Masters, F. W., and Robinson, D. W. Mandibular reconstruction using a composite island rib graft. *Plast. Reconstr. Surg.* 53:471, 1974.
37. Leake, D. L. An interim report on osseous contour reconstruction using alloplastic materials and particulate bone grafting. *Int. J. Oral Surg.* 3:286, 1974.
38. Leake, D. L., and Rappaport, M. Mandibular reconstruction: Bone graft induction in an alloplastic tray. *Surgery* 72:332, 1972.
39. McKee, D. Microvascular rib transposition for reconstruction of the mandible. Presented at the Annual Meeting of the American Society of Plastic and Reconstructive Surgeons, Montreal, 1971.
40. Ostrup, L. T., and Fredrickson, J. M. Distant transfer of a free living bone graft by microvascular anastomoses. *Plast. Reconstr. Surg.* 54:274, 1974.
41. Spiessl, B., Prien, J., and Schmoker, R. Anatomic Reconstruction and Functional Rehabilitation of Mandibular Defects after Ablative Surgery. In Spiessl, B. (Ed.), *New Concepts in Maxillofacial Bone Surgery.* Berlin and New York: Springer, 1976.
42. Strauch, B., Bloomberg, A. E., and Lewin, M. L. An experimental approach to mandibular replacement: Island vascular composite rib grafts. *Br. J. Plast. Surg.* 24:334, 1971.
43. Swanson, L. T., Habal, M. B., Leake, D. L., and Murray, J. E. Compound silicone bone implants for mandibular reconstruction. *Plast. Reconstr. Surg.* 51:402, 1973.
44. Topf, J. S. The three dimensional mandibular bone plate. *J. Oral Surg.* 34:364, 1976.

Preprosthetic Surgery

45. Starshak, T. J. *Preprosthetic Oral Surgery.* St. Louis: Mosby, 1971.
46. Steinhauser, E. M. Vestibuloplasty – Skin Grafts. *J. Oral Surg.* 29:777, 1971.

Temporomandibular Joint Disorders: General Considerations

47. Schwartz, L. *Disorders of the Temporomandibular Joint.* Philadelphia: Saunders, 1959.
48. Sicher, H. Functional Anatomy of the Temporomandibular Joint. In Sarnat, B. G. (Ed.), *The Temporomandibular Joint* (American Lecture Series). Springfield, Ill.: Thomas, 1951.
49. Updegrave, W. J. Interpretation of temporomandibular joint radiographs. *Dent. Clin. North Am.* 10:567, 1966.

Temporomandibular Joint Syndrome

50. Alderman, M. M. Disorders of the Temporomandibular Joint and Related Structures. In Burket, L. W. (Ed.), *Oral Medicine.* Philadelphia: Lippincott, 1971.
51. Costen, J. B. A syndrome of ear and sinus symptoms dependent upon disturbed function of the temporomandibular joint. *Ann. Otolaryngol.* 43:1, 1934.
52. Lamont-Havers, R. W. Arthritis of the temporomandibular joint. *Dent. Clin. North Am.* 10:621, 1966.
53. Laskin, D. M. Diseases of the Mandibular Joint. In Hayward, J. R. (Ed.), *Oral Surgery.* Springfield, Ill.: Thomas, 1976.
54. Sarnat, B. G., and Laskin, D. M. *Diagnosis and Surgical Management of Diseases of the Temporomandibular Joint.* Springfield, Ill.: Thomas, 1962.

Treatment of Temporomandibular Joint Disorders

55. Boman, K. A new operation for luxation in the temporomandibular joint. *Acta Chir. Scand.* 99:96, 1949.
56. Converse, J. M. *Kazanjian and Converse's Surgical Treatment of Facial Injuries* (3rd ed.). Chapter 26, Temporomandibular Ankylosis. Baltimore: Williams & Wilkins, 1974.
57. Dingman, R. O., and Grabb, W. C. Reconstruction of both mandibular condyles with metatarsal bone grafts. *Plast. Reconstr. Surg.* 34:441, 1964.
58. Dingman, R. O., and Grabb, W. C. Intra-articular temporomandibular joint arthroplasty. *Plast. Reconstr. Surg.* 38:179, 1966.
59. Entin, M. A. Transplantation of Autogenous Bone and Joints in Man. In Wallace, A. B. (Ed.), *Transactions of the International Society of Plastic Surgeons, Second Congress, 1959.* Baltimore: Williams & Wilkins, 1960.
60. Georgiade, N. G. Disturbances of the Temporomandibular Joint. In Converse, J. M. (Ed.), *Reconstructive Plastic Surgery* (2nd ed.), Vol. 3. Philadelphia: Saunders, 1977.
61. Hanson, W. C., and DeShazo, B. W. Silastic reconstruction of the temporomandibular joint arthroplasty. *Plast. Reconstr. Surg.* 43:388, 1969.

62. Henny, F. A., and Baldridge, O. L. Condylectomy for the persistently painful joint. *J. Oral Surg.* 15:24, 1957.
63. Husted, E. Surgical diseases of the temporomandibular joint. *Acta Odontol. Scand.* 14:119, 1957.
64. Kent, J. N., Homsy, C. A., Gross, B. D., and Hinds, E. C. Pilot studies of a porous implant in dentistry and oral surgery. *J. Oral Surg.* 30:608, 1972.
65. Kiehn, C. L., and DesPrez, J. D. Meniscectomy for internal derangement of temporomandibular joint. *Br. J. Plast. Surg.* 15:199, 1962.
66. Laskin, D. Surgical Management of Diseases of the Temporomandibular Joint. In Hayward, J. R. (Ed.), *Oral Surgery.* Springfield, Ill.: Thomas, 1976.
67. Mahan, P. E. Differential diagnosis of craniofacial pain and dysfunction. *Alpha Omegan,* Dec. 1976, p. 43.

7

Cleft Lip

D. RALPH MILLARD, JR.

In order to transform a cleft lip and its associated nasal deformity into a natural-looking structure, it is essential first to define the normal. A careful, detailed study of what is present in each case is necessary before it is possible to utilize to the best advantage what we *have* to make what we *want.*

ANATOMY

Normal Lip Anatomy

The normal nose has a straight columella of adequate length backed by a straight septum (Fig. 7-1A). Symmetrical alar arches are supported by equivalent alar cartilages and rest on equally balanced alar bases. Equal nasal floors are bounded by nostril sills. The normal upper lip, with its intact orbicularis oris musculature, has a philtrum with a pair of curved column prominences bounding a central dimple hollow. The gently curving cupid's bow with its midline vermilion tubercle is highlighted by a white skin roll along its upper mucocutaneous junction. The natural position of the lips places the loose upper lip, with eversion of its lower portion, over and slightly in front of the lower lip (Fig. 7-1A).

Cleft Lip Anatomy

Each cleft lip deformity varies, but in broad generalities the lip-nose distortion can be divided into the categories of unilateral incomplete cleft with nasal deformity, unilateral complete cleft with nasal deformity (Fig. 7-1B), bilateral incomplete cleft with or without adequate columella, bilateral cleft complete on one side and incomplete on the other (Fig. 7-1C), bilateral complete cleft with inadequate columella (Fig. 7-1D), and the rare median clefts. Whether or not there is an alveolar defect or associated postalveolar palate cleft (or both) is also important. Maxillary and premaxillary prosthodontic and orthodontic manipulation, alveolar bone grafting, and palate closure and lengthening are not discussed in this chapter, but are included in Chapter 8.

OPTIMUM TIME FOR CLEFT LIP CLOSURE

Of course the cleft in the lip can be closed at any time from the first day of life, but the rule of "over ten" is advocated. When the infant is over 10 weeks in age, over 10 pounds (45.4 kg.) in weight, and over 10 gm. in hemoglobin, not only is the condition more suitable for surgery, but also the lip and nose tissues have increased in size to facilitate the detailed surgery. Thus the age of *3 months* has been set as the most favorable time for the initial lip surgery.

The condition of the *bony platform* also influences the time of surgery. If the alveolar and hard palate cleft is associated with distortion of the maxillary components, then orthodontia is indicated to stimulate growth and instigate a shifting into better alignment. When no presurgical orthodontia is available, the cleft is complete, and the alveolar gap is wide, then a simple, adhesion-type lip procedure is used as early as the first 2 to 3 weeks of age to act as a moderate molding device on the maxillary elements. This satisfies the parents' concern, as something positive has been done, and they are then willing to wait until the child is 6 months old for the definite lip and nose surgery.

In *bilateral clefts* when the premaxilla is jutting far forward of the maxillary components, earlier lip closure (in the first week) has the advantage of constructing a muscle band across the premaxillary prow to retard its further protrusion. Here orthodontia may be necessary to prevent medial collapse of the lateral maxillary segments. If the prolabium is extremely small, then an adhesion-type lip closure is carried out on both sides simultaneously. In time this will help to mold the projecting premaxilla but will also stretch the small prolabium to larger proportions, so that a forked flap can be spared.

ANESTHESIA FOR CLEFT LIP CLOSURE

Endotracheal anesthesia is administered through an oral tube coming out and over the midline of the lower lip, with absolutely no distortion to the soft tissues of the mouth. In addition, an anesthetic solution carrying epinephrine 1 : 100,000 is infiltrated into the areas where hemostasis with hemostats is not as effective. This includes the upper labial sulcus, where the soft tissues will be cut free from the maxilla, and the floor of the nose. Minimal local anesthetic is injected into the actual lip so as to avoid the resultant distortion, particularly when the bleeding at this site can easily be controlled with small hemostats applied directly to the coronary vessels.

Of course, when endotracheal anesthesia is not available or, owing to the patient's condition, is contraindicated, sedation and local infiltration with 1% lidocaine (Xylocaine) will allow surgery; however, this approach is not conducive to accurate and detailed surgery.

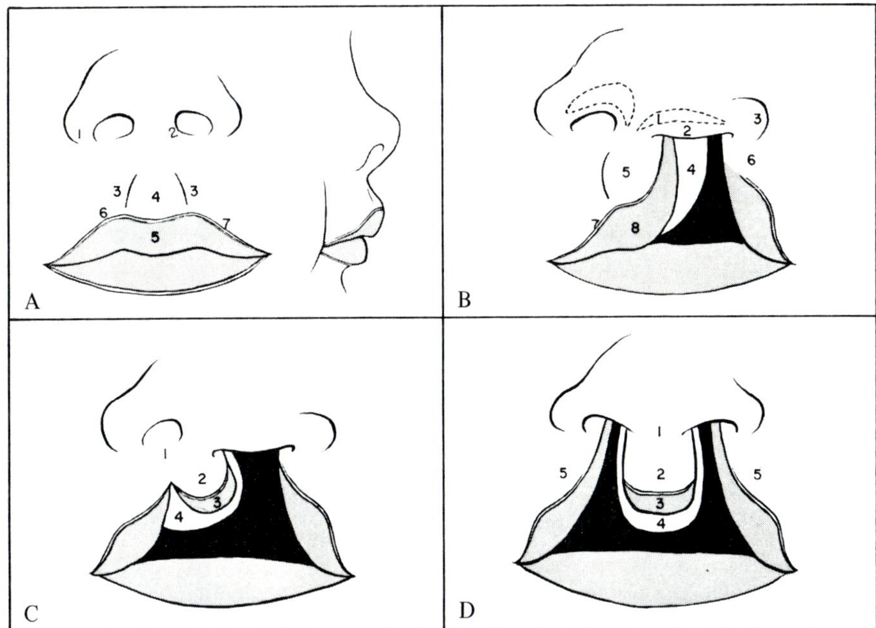

Fig. 7-1. Normal lip and cleft lip anatomy. A, normal lip front and profile. 1, *alar base;* 2, *nostril sill;* 3, *philtrum column;* 4, *philtrum dimple;* 5, *vermilion tubercle;* 6, *arch of cupid's bow;* 7, *white skin roll of mucocutaneous junction. B, unilateral complete cleft of the lip and alveolus.* 1, *dislocated alar cartilage;* 2, *alar web;* 3, *alar base (flared);* 4, *alveolus;* 5, *non-cleft component with two-thirds cupid's bow and philtrum dimple;* 6, *lateral lip cleft component;* 7, *white skin roll of the mucocutaneous junction;* 8, *vermilion mucosa. C, bilateral cleft of the lip showing incomplete (right) and complete (left) clefts.* 1, *Simonart's band;* 2, *prolabium;* 3, *prolabium vermilion;* 4, *premaxilla.* D, *bilateral complete cleft of the lip.* 1, *short columella;* 2, *prolabium;* 3, *prolabium mucosa;* 4, *premaxilla;* 5, *lateral lip elements.*

UNILATERAL CLEFT LIP

In a unilateral cleft of the lip with nasal deformity, there are varying degrees of absence of tissue as well as actual distortion. The vital primary action is to visualize what is normal and to shift these tissues into a normal position. Clefts, among other deficiencies, have an inherent vertical shortness along each side involving both the lip and the nose. The failure of mesodermal penetration, which would have forced the lip to fill out, has left the potential lower portion of the lip actually retaining its high attachment to the nose on either side of the cleft. The noncleft side shows a twisted distortion with lack of vertical length from the height of the arch of the ala to the height of the arch of the cupid's bow at the mucocutaneous junction. Equally distorted on the cleft side may be the short columella and the flattened alar arch, with its cartilage displaced and its flaring base attached to intact lip musculature. A compensation in all this distortion is the presence of two-thirds of a cupid's bow, one column prominence of the philtrum, and a dimple hollow. This component is in a deceptive position up near the columella, having never been forced downward by mesoderm ingrowth. For many years clefts of the lip have been repaired with the use of techniques that completely ignored the normal landmarks. Once these important features have been destroyed they are lost forever, and the ultimate result for the patient must fall short of ideal.

Methods of Unilateral Cleft Lip Closure

Straight Line Closure

Simple paring of the lip cleft edges and closure destroys natural landmarks in the lower two-thirds of the lip. Long considered to be a conservative approach, this procedure actually turns out to be destructive. Yet direct straight line closure of the upper one-third of wide clefts [15, 24, 31] is a means of temporarily evading a difficult issue without destroying landmarks. It also achieves early molding of the maxilla, thus rendering the second procedure somewhat less difficult. Only in bizarre examples is this indicated, and even then the true long-term advantages have been questionable.

Quadrilateral Flap
The quadrilateral flap of Hagedorn, popularized by LeMesurier [16], creates an artificial cupid's bow by advancing this flap across the lower border of the lip. The long-term follow-up studies of this technique show good results in many of the lips, but inadequate nasal correction. Many of these lips have a lopsided cupid's bow, are too long on the cleft side, and are flat and relatively tight along the free border. This technique has its greatest value in providing after operation a loose lip where the original landmarks have already been destroyed; then, the construction of an artificial cupid's bow is desirable.

Triangular Flap

MIRAULT-BLAIR-BROWN METHOD. The Mirault-Blair-Brown [5] approach, turning a triangle flap from the cleft side in the lower one-third of the lip, breaks the straight line closure but destroys natural landmarks and does not achieve a cupid's bow, a natural line for the scar, or an economical nasal correction. When executed by experts, the first impression of the early result is favorable, but the eventual criticism must be the inartistic disregard for natural landmarks.

TENNISON-RANDALL METHOD. The Tennison Z-plasty [39], marked with the aid of a stencil, transposes a triangular flap slightly higher than in the Mirault-Blair-Brown approach. The popularity of this general approach was greatly enhanced by the clear mathematical design charted by Randall [30] (Fig. 7-2). In principle, there is preservation of the cupid's bow by an interdigitation in the lower one-third of the lip. This positions the cupid's bow but breaks the gentle natural curve of the philtrum column on the scar side, places the tension in the lower portion of the lip, shows some disregard for the dimple hollow, and forces excision of tissue to correct the wide nasal flaring. Results are good when measurement has been accurate, and the scars are perfect. Secondary correction of this design is even more difficult than in the quadralateral flap approach.

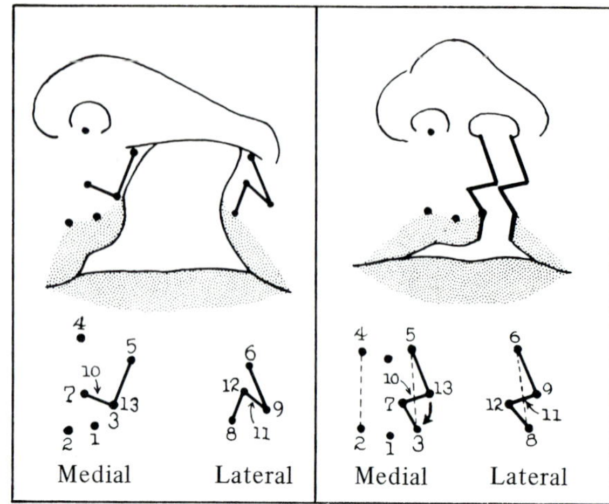

Fig. 7-2. Mathematical design used in the Tennison-Randall method. 1. *midpoint of the mucocutaneous junction;* 2, *superior peak of the cupid's bow on the noncleft side;* 3, *superior peak of the cupid's bow on the cleft side;* 4, *base of the columella on the noncleft side;* 5, *base of the columella on the cleft side;* 6, *this point has the same relationship to the ala on the cleft side as point* 4 *has to the ala on the noncleft side. Line* 3-7 *extends at about right angles to line* 5-3*;* 10, *about the midpoint of line* 3-7*;* 8, *placed on the mucocutaneous junction where the mucocutaneous ridge starts to disappear;* 4-2 *minus* 5-10 *equals the width of the triangular flap* 8-11. *Pick point* 9 *so that* 6-9 *equals* 5-13*; then sketch the triangular flap so that:* 5-10 *plus* 11-8 *equals* 4-2, *and lines* 9-12, 8-12, *and* 3-7 *are all equal (move point* 9, 12, *or* 7, *if needed). (Reproduced, by permission, from P. Randall,* Plast. Reconstr. Surg. *23:331, 1959.)*

Rotation-Advancement
The rotation-advancement method [18, 20, 22], although it can be measured accurately, is usually executed with a free eye and hand in a "cut as you go" approach. This probably is the main reason why many surgeons hesitate to use the method initially. In principle, however, it offers the complete or partial answer to many of the objections noted in other methods, and in practice it does work. If positioning the lower one-third of the lip to the correct position (Tennison) is desirable, it seems that lowering the entire cupid's bow and dimple component (rotation) is better, particularly when this opens a gap into which the lateral lip element carrying the flared alar base can be inserted (advancement). This simple double action achieves natural conformity, with a cupid's bow, dimple, and symmetrical alar bases and nasal floors, along with the maneuvering of the scars so that they are hidden in the nasal creases and shadows or along a natural philtrum column line.

In the incomplete cleft, Simonart's band, when needed, can be used in the advancement flap. In the complete cleft, when tension is a vital factor, it is directed where it will do the most good – that is, over the maxilla and across the flaring nasal base so that not only is the maxilla molded but the gaping nasal deformity is corrected. This relative tension high in the lip avoids the usual tightness of the free border of the upper lip and in fact forces its natural eversion.

Operative Technique for the Rotation-Advancement Closure

Technique for Complete Unilateral Cleft Lip Closure
There is a vestige of a cupid's bow and philtrum dimple in all unilateral clefts, but, as in the normal lip, bow strength and dimple depth vary. With portions of the normal lip and nose missing it is important to throw nothing away and make the best of what is present.

First visualize the cupid's bow. Starting at the peak on the noncleft side, measure to the midline, which is at the center of the tubercle, and mark these points on the mucocutaneous junction line with methylene blue (Fig. 7-3A). The distance between these two points will determine the third point along the mucocutaneous junction line, which indicates the future cupid's bow peak on the cleft side. Mark it. (Another guide to the position of the cleft side point marking the arch of the cupid's bow is the measurement on the normal side from the arch of the bow to the commissure. If this distance is transposed on the cleft side with the cleft element under slight stretch, then it is possible to know exactly how far out laterally the cleft element can be pared and where the lateral point of the cupid's bow arch must be set.) From this point, freshen with the scalpel up along the cleft edge, curving under the columella base and extending to the midline through the full thickness of the lip (Fig. 7-3B). The actual extent of this rotation incision can be misleading owing to the slant of the columella and the deviation of the septum. What seems to reach the midline may actually be found short of the mark when the columella has been straightened and the cupid's bow and dimple component rotated down into normal position. The extent of the rotation incision is adequate only when the cupid's bow is resting symmetrically in a normal position. In an occasional case the rotation incision will have to extend slightly beyond the midline to achieve this. As long as it *does not transgress past the base of the columella* there should be no repercussion. Surgical freeing of the lip from the maxilla in the labial sulcus even on the noncleft side is important. *Promiscuous rotation, with the incision extending into the lip on the normal side, obviously will result in a lip abnormally long in the vertical axis.* This must be avoided.

An aid in rotation is a backcut at the end of the incision [24]. This reduces the need for extension into the normal side, and is often used to advantage. The triangle excision of the Recamiers [32], although not considered sufficient for adequate rotation, could be an adjunct when the normal side is too long vertically. Yet their Veau-type vertical straight line scar is considered a disadvantage, as the normal philtrum column has a gentle medial curve.

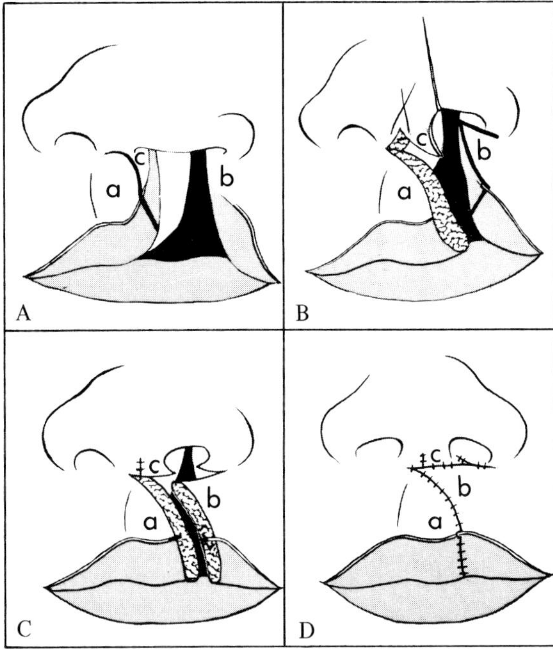

Fig. 7-3. Rotation-advancement method in complete unilateral cleft of the lip. A, the rotation incision is marked so that cupid's bow–dimple component (a) *will rotate down into normal position; flap* c *will advance into columella and then form nostril sill. B, flap* a *has dropped down, flap* c *has advanced into the columella, and flap* b *has been marked. C, flap* b *is being advanced into the rotation gap; the white skin roll flap is interdigitated at the mucocutaneous junction line. D, the scar is maneuvered into strategic position where it is hidden at the nasal base and floor, philtrum column, and interdigitated at the mucocutaneous junction.*

The portion of the rotation incision that runs under the columella base not only allows the cupid's bow and dimple component to drop but enables the shortened columella to lengthen on the cleft side. If a hook is placed in the height of the nostril arch on the slumped side and is lifted until the arches match, a defect will appear at the base of the columella on the cleft side (Fig. 7-3B). This raw area indicates the potential increase in columella length. Maintenance of this lengthening is possible by advancing flap c up into the columella defect similar to a modified one-sided forked flap, or by rotating the tip of flap c around into the depth of the cutback of the rotation gap. There can be sufficient tissue in flap c to accomplish this and still swing across the nostril floor to provide the medial portion of the nostril sill. Holdsworth [13] suggests that at this point one should continue the dissection and free the medial alar crus all the way to the tip to reduce the tether and to aid in the elevation of the slumped tip, thus facilitating the better advancement of flap c.

In the wake of the rotation incision there is left a rotation gap. If this gap is filled adequately, the normal position of the cupid's bow and dimple will be retained. In incomplete clefts, Simonart's band can be included in the advancement flap from the lateral lip element. In complete clefts the lateral lip element will vary in its size. When this component is deficient, as it usually is with severely wide clefts, this lateral flap can be increased by extension into the excess skin of the stretched nasal vestibule (Fig. 7-3B). Whether the lateral flap b includes Simonart's band, vestibule skin, or merely the lateral lip element, its advancement into the rotation gap fills this gap and maintains the normal position of this element of the cupid's bow. Furthermore, this advancement carries with it the flaring alar base, positioning it in the desired symmetry (Fig. 7-3C). Wide freeing of the lateral lip element from the maxilla is important, and the adequacy of this dissection is determined when flap b is moved into the rotation gap with no resultant tension noted by a fingertip feeling along the maxilla under the lip. Further scalpel freeing is carried from the labial sulcus up into the nasal vestibule, freeing the adherent alar base from its attachment to the maxilla. This will allow the base of the ala to come up and forward with flap b.

Recent improvements have added two adjuncts: (1) The upper lateral cleft edge mucosa is salvaged as a flap with its base above, to be transposed into the vestibular defect formed when the alar base is released from the maxilla. (2) More dependable tying-in of the flaring alar base is achieved by denuding its tip or cutting a subcutaneous pedicle from its undersurface and using this extension to be tethered to the septum with a 4-0 Vicryl suture.

The distance from the height of the rotation incision to the peak of the cupid's bow on the cleft side is measured accurately along the side of the lateral cleft element. The vermilion is trimmed off by this exact amount along with a small amount of skin, when expendable, to produce a concave line to fit the convexity of the noncleft edge. A 1 X 2 mm. skin flap of the mucocutaneous white skin roll is preserved (Fig. 7-3C). A notch for this tiny flap is prepared in the mucocutaneous junction at the edge of the noncleft side. This interdigitation of the white skin roll interrupts the red of the scar running into the red of the vermilion. The purpose of this white flap turned across the linear scar at the mucocutaneous junction line is to counteract by camouflage the impression of a notch contracture should there be a spreading of the scar at this point.

Closure is begun by placing a hook in the depressed alar arch and lifting so that flap c advances up into the columella where it is fixed with 6-0 silk sutures (Fig. 7-3B). Then the muscle and subcutaneous tissue in the point of flap b are sutured into the depth of the rotation gap. This is the key suture of 4-0 Vicryl, and once it is correct all other sutures are merely a matter of detail. Two or three 4-0 chromic catgut sutures are used to approximate muscle to muscle. These sutures should bring the skin edges together so close that there is no need for tension with the 6-0 silk in the skin. This will ensure a fine scar; 4-0 chromic catgut sutures are used in the nostril floor, 6-0 chromic catgut approximates the vermilion edges in a straight line closure, and finally a 7-0 silk fixes the white roll flap into the opposite notch (Fig. 7-3D). Suturing of the posterior mucosa is postponed until the last. In certain cases where the cleft has been wide and the lateral components small, advancement has caused some attenuation of the vermilion border along the cleft side. This can be corrected at a later date with a V-Y posterior mucosal advancement or a V-Y posterior "rolldown" (Fig. 7-4). In some cases it has been found advantageous to bolster this weak vermilion during the primary procedure.

With the relative tightness of the lip in the upper portion, there exists an excess of mucosa in the lower part of the noncleft side. This can be taken from along the edge as a transposed mucosal flap with its base distal near the tubercle. Then the thin, attenuated vermilion on the cleft side can be incised posteriorly and hinged down and forward to fill out the red border. Into this gap the transposed flap can be sutured with 6-0 catgut (Fig. 7-5). The remaining closure of the posterior mucosa will be completed with 4-0 chromic catgut.

Any remaining alar web overhanging the nostril arch will be excised and closed by a "roll-in" with 6-0 silk sutures (Fig. 7-3C, D).

Technique for Incomplete Unilateral Cleft Lip Closure

Incomplete clefts represent less missing tissue and usually less overall distortion, and thus require important differences in the economy of the technique. In general principle, the approach is the same but the essential perfection of the result in a less difficult deformity depends on the accuracy of detail in the execution. Usually the shortness on the noncleft side will require a surprisingly radical release by the rotation incision and a slight back cut. Here again, it may pass the midline as far as the base of the columella, but it must not enter the lip on the normal side. Flap c is used to lengthen the columella and form

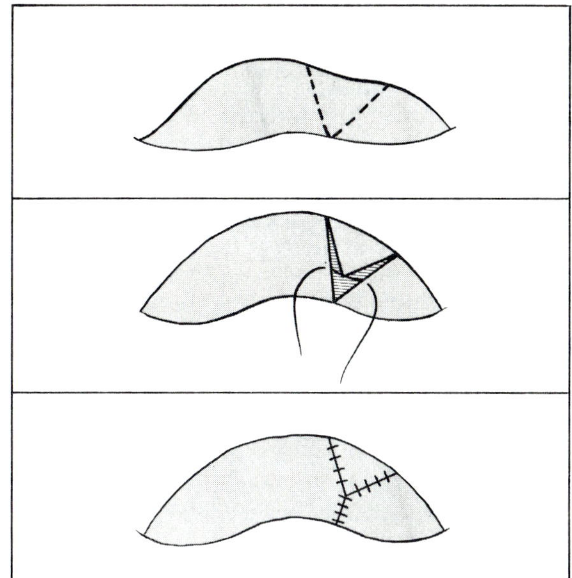

Fig. 7-4. *Upper lip turned up presenting posterior view. Secondary posterior V-Y rolldown of mucosa fills out a free-border vermilion defect.*

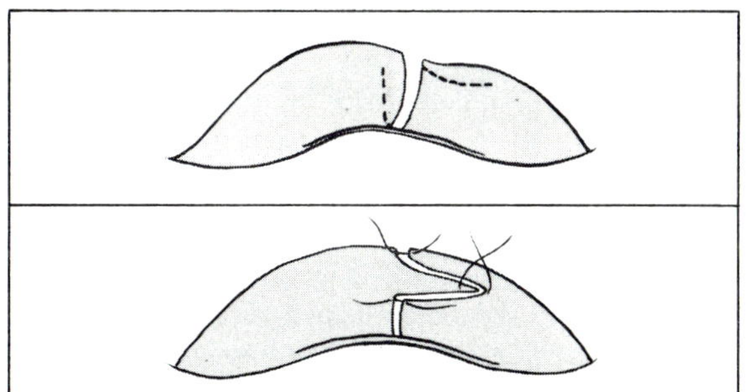

Fig. 7-5. *Upper lip turned up presenting posterior view. Primary or possibly secondary use of a posterior mucosal transposed flap fills out a free-border defect.*

nostril sill as needed. Flap b includes as much of Simonart's band as is required, preferably only that amount that has muscle within it (Fig. 7-6A, B). Advancement of flap b into the rotation gap must achieve two goals in addition to its primary function of filling the rotation gap: it should (1) position the alar base in exact symmetry with its opposite mate and (2) balance the lateral lip element to complement the cupid's bow and dimple component.

In some incomplete clefts the nasal distortion may be minor and the nasal floor and position of the alar base may be nearly normal. In these cases the amount

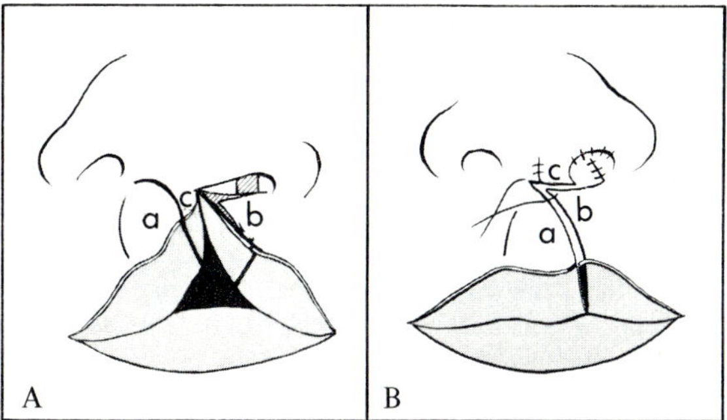

Fig. 7-6. *A, incomplete unilateral cleft of the lip with rotation of flap* a *and advancement of flap* b *is marked. Flap* c *will lengthen the columella and then form a portion of the nostril sill. Simonart's band can be trimmed and a wedge excised from the nostril floor as necessary. B, alar web is excised, flap* b *moving in to fill the rotation gap of flap* a; *interdigitation of the mucocutaneous junction is executed.*

of advancement of flap b must be guarded, and the use of Simonart's band can reduce the extent of advancement required. Of course, the wedge excision from the floor of the nose will vary with each case and in some may be avoided completely. If the advancement seems to restrict the nostril slightly, no wedge is excised. Maintenance of an intact nasal floor will, in time, help to offset the nostril discrepancy.

Occasionally in the incomplete cleft, the lateral lip element is bulky or longer vertically than its counterpart carrying the cupid's bow and dimple. When the repair was made by other methods this presented a technical difficulty, but in the rotation-advancement technique it is possible to reduce flap b along its upper margin so that it can be patterned to fit into the rotation gap and present symmetry along its free border. The white skin roll interdigitation and the posterior mucosal flaps are of course all available and useful in the incomplete cleft.

Secondary Revisions in Unilateral Cleft Lip

Following the rotation-advancement approach, revision can vary from minor trimming of the mucosa to excision of the entire scar of union and repeating, with correction, the complete operation. Mucosal trimming of the free edge of vermilion can be carried out on the cleft side or the normal side for the sake of symmetry. Where there is a notching or a thinning this can be corrected by the various mucosal "rolldowns" and transposition already described. When there has been insufficient rotation of the medial element or inadequate advancement of the lateral element, then mere scar excision will allow more radical revision toward an improved result. The simplicity of secondary correction is one of the advantages of this approach.

When the primary repair was a straight line closure resulting in only partial loss of the normal landmarks, the rotation-advancement principle can be of value in positioning what remains of the cupid's bow and at the same time advancing the alar base into symmetry with that on the opposite side. The relative tightness in the upper lip will tend to evert the lower portion. When the primary straight line closure has destroyed all vestige of a cupid's bow but there is more than adequate tissue in the horizontal dimension along the free border, the Hagedorn-LeMesurier quadrilateral flap can be used to make an artificial cupid's bow. If the free border is tight, the quadrilateral flap cannot be spared.

The postoperative upper lip without a cupid's bow and tight along its free border is seen following certain straight line closures or with modifications of the Mirault principle. Tissue is inadequate in the horizontal dimension; the only solution is to bring in new tissue from a distance. Here the Sabattini-Stein-Estlander-Abbe flap can be of benefit. The tendency has been to insert this flap into the unilateral position of the old postoperative scar. When there is no cupid's bow and no philtrum dimple, there is a better way to use the Abbe flap [25]. For the moment forget the previous off-center scar and split this tight lip in the middle as high as the lip is tight. This may be only one-third or two-thirds of its vertical height. Into this defect, which usually is not wide, fit a philtrum-shaped full-thickness flap from the middle of the lower lip. It has been noted that a dimple is often present in this central position and, when transposed to the upper lip, gives the pleasing semblance of a cupid's bow and dimple [25]. Once the tension of the lip has been released, more effective revision of the previous unilateral scar can be accomplished secondarily.

Secondary correction of the unilateral cleft lip nose again depends on the primary lip surgery. Following the rotation-advancement approach, minor excision of the web across the alar rim will be satisfactory until the nose has matured, at which time the strong alar cartilage from the normal side can be used as an onlay over the depressed side to improve symmetry. When the primary lip surgery does not lengthen and straighten the columella or position the alar base, more radical nasal correction may be indicated. This can be carried out primarily as advocated by Berkeley [1] or as secondary procedures in the mature nose as described by Musgrave and Dupertius [28a], Reynolds and Horton [33], and Millard [26].

BILATERAL CLEFT LIP

The complete answer to bilateral cleft lip has not been conceived. Of the many honest surgical efforts to surmount the multiple difficulties, only a few can be discussed in any detail. Although the asymmetry seen in the unilateral cleft is not usually seen in these defects, the difficulty here is the bilateral absence of parts plus the severe symmetrical distortion of what is present. Bilateral clefts, in addition to the actual clefts and the absence of a cupid's bow remnant, also have a varying degree of vertical shortness in what is referred to embryologically as the frontonasal component, which is measured from a position at the nasal tip to the midinferior point of the free border of the prolabium of the upper lip. The discrepancy may lie in the prolabial length, the columella length, or a combined shortness in both. Because of this shortness, an age-old tug-of-war continues to be waged in which the prolabium is being pulled from both below and above. Some surgeons drag the prolabium down into the lip, with little regard for the sanctity of the nasal tip, whereas others haul it up into the columella, suturing the lip together tightly beneath it. Each maneuver has its strong advocates, which ensures that neither will be crowned the undisputed winner. A primary compromise with respect for both the lip and the nose is advocated.

Operative Technique for the Rotation-Advancement Closure

Technique for the Incomplete Bilateral Cleft Lip Closure

In bilateral incomplete clefts, the columella can be nearly of adequate length, the nasal tip near normal position, and the premaxilla within the maxillary arch. The discrepancy in vertical frontonasal length lies in the shortness of the prolabium. One common approach toward correction of this discrepancy has been the use of variously shaped skin flaps from the lateral lip elements which, when brought together under the lower border of the prolabium, bolster this short center component [12]. This approach produces a lip that is too long in its vertical dimension, often tight horizontally, and with unnatural cross scars in the lower middle lip, which spoil any attempt at a philtrum effect. This approach should be *condemned,* as it has been responsible for many unacceptable results that, in addition, are extremely difficult to correct secondarily.

Application of the rotation-advancement principle in this deformity has been described, and it produces acceptable results [21, 23]. When the columella is of normal length, the prolabium can be retained in toto in the lip as a philtrum. This is achieved by freshening one edge of the prolabium and curving the incision under the base of the columella just short of the midline. One-half of the free border vermilion is turned down to line the cupid's bow. The advancement flap

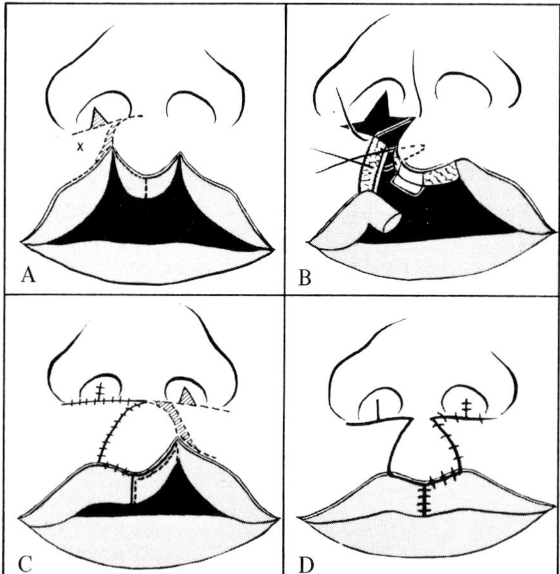

Fig. 7-7. Bilateral incomplete cleft of the lip. A, first-stage lateral flap (x) *is advanced between the columella and prolabium. A wedge is excised from the nasal floor. Lateral lip vermilion and one-half of the prolabium vermilion are turned down as flaps. B, mucosa and muscle of lateral lip element are advanced half way under the prolabium. C, lateral vermilion flap overlaps the turndown vermilion of the prolabium to form one-half of the cupid's bow. Second stage is marked on the opposite side. D, advancement and vermilion overlap are completed on the second side.*

from the lateral lip element on this side has its edge freshened by the turning down of a thick vermilion flap (Fig. 7-7A). The lateral flap x is advanced into the rotation gap and the lateral vermilion flap is used to overlap the turndown vermilion flap of the prolabium to form one-half of the cupid's bow. A wedge is excised from the nasal floor if indicated (Fig. 7-7B). One month later a similar procedure is carried out on the opposite side (Fig. 7-7C, D). Since this approach was originally described, certain modifications have been instituted.

Advancement of the lateral flaps so that they interdigitate even slightly between the columella base and the prolabium can be responsible ultimately for a lip that is too long vertically. It is better in most instances that these flaps come to within a millimeter or so of each other, thus preserving undivided a small strand of original columella-prolabium junction. This ensures a more natural and attractive vertical shortness. Of course, when the prolabium is truly diminutive, joining the lateral flaps tip to tip above it may be indicated.

The absence of muscle in the prolabium justifies lateral advancement of the mucosa and muscles posterior to the prolabium. In this type of cleft the prolabium is freed from the premaxilla on the side of the first rotation-advancement flap, and the lateral mucosa and muscle elements can be sutured under it to the midline (Fig. 7-7B). One month later a similar procedure is carried out on the opposite side so that there is a posterior join in the midline of mucosa and, when possible, muscle flaps from the lateral lip elements. The prolabium is then used as a philtrum, and the lateral vermilion flaps form the cupid's bow.

Preservation of the vermilion of the prolabium as lining rather than as visible cover is preferred because of the usual discrepancy in color match. The white roll of the mucocutaneous junction, when present on the prolabium, of course can be retained.

Technique for the Complete and Incomplete Bilateral Cleft Lip Closure

When the bilateral cleft is complete on one side and incomplete on the other, there is not only bilateral deficiency but asymmetry of distortion (Fig. 7-1C). Adaptation of the rotation-advancement principle again is advocated in two stages, the complete cleft being rotated and advanced for closure first in order to use the blood supply to the prolabium through the incomplete cleft. If the columella has unilateral shortness, flap c (Fig. 7-3B) is available for lengthening. One month or more later the opposite side is rotated and advanced to achieve symmetry.

Technique for the Complete Bilateral Cleft Lip Closure

Complete bilateral clefts pose three additional problems that are not usually encountered in incomplete clefts: (1) a protruding premaxilla, (2) inadequacy or absence of the columella, and (3) the fact that the sole source of blood supply to the prolabium is through the columella and premaxilla.

TREATMENT OF THE PROTRUDING PREMAXILLA. When the cleft is complete bilaterally, the premaxilla is attached to the face only by the septum and columella. The premaxilla, when unattached to the maxilla, may protrude on a septal stalk for varying distances out in front of its usual position in the alveolar arch. There is justified controversy as to what to do with this jutting premaxilla.

If the premaxilla is well in the arch, then by turning mucosal flaps a fibrous union can be achieved, and this can be solidified with a bone graft.

For patients with a protruding premaxilla, the conservative approach which merely freshens the edges of the soft tissue cleft and joins the lateral lip elements to the sides of the prolabium early (1 week) is still popular. This completes a band across the cleft which will tend to restrict further projectile growth of the "uninhibited" premaxilla-septal component. Some advocate bandage harness pressure to the premaxilla as a means of restraint [2]. This seems ineffective when compared with actual soft tissue closure across the clefts. When the premaxilla deviates markedly to one side, closure of the lip cleft on the opposite side will soon pull the premaxilla into the midline. Then the other cleft can be closed.

Prior to early surgery and thereafter, the prosthodontic bite plate of Burston [7] is advocated to stimulate hypertrophy and growth of the retarded maxillary components, and, in fact, force and maintain these elements laterally to prevent collapse.

In spite of prolonged orthodontic treatment and early lip closure, there are certain protruding premaxillas that end up too prominent. Such cases come under consideration for a surgical pushback. Monroe [28] gives the 8-year follow-up results of the Cronin-type [9] resection of the midvomer with an incision in the cartilage to the root of the nose. This technique allegedly allows a straight setback, and, by avoiding the epiphyseal line immediately behind the premaxilla, avoids growth retardation of the middle third of the face. Even Burston [8] admits that in certain cases a delayed (8 months of age) sliding osteotomy may be indicated. Cronin [11] prefers early external pressure and orthodontia, but when this fails or the patient is seen too late (8 months of age), he still advocates premaxilla pushback in a slightly undercorrected position.

TREATMENT OF THE SHORT COLUMELLA. In complete bilateral clefts, the prolabium may or may not be short, but the discrepancy in vertical frontonasal length is often seen in the inadequacy or absence of columella. To use the entire prolabium as columella lifts the nasal tip but is unacceptable, as it leaves the lip without a philtrum. To incorporate the prolabium in the lip has obvious labial advantages, but in the process it pulls the nasal tip flat. Some of the alternatives are:

1. Closure of the bilateral lip cleft in one or two stages and then lengthening of the columella several months later with a forked flap [21, 23].
2. Closure of the lip early and delay for several years (5 years) before lengthening the columella by the Cronin [9], the forked flap method [19], or Brauer's [4] alar web flaps.
3. Closure of the bilateral lip clefts along with a forked flap columella lengthening all in one early operation; this approach is not advocated.
4. Closure of one side of the bilateral lip cleft with partial columella lengthening at the same time by the Skoog [38] method.
5. Closure of the lip in one stage but with the forked flap banked and the mucosa or muscle approximated behind the prolabium. At a second stage undertake the columella lengthening with the banked fork tissue. (See Banking the Forked Flap, p. 202.)

The fourth of these compromises may be broken down into three parts to simplify what may seem to be a complicated procedure. It is actually a combination of principles ingeniously combined by Skoog into a two-stage procedure for bilateral clefts (Figs. 7-8, 7-9). He originally combined the rotation-advancement principle in the upper lip with the triangle flap in the lower lip for unilateral clefts [37]. For bilateral clefts he has added a transverse transposed flap of lateral prolabium based above to be inserted across the base of the columella, similar in principle to the flap described by Marcks et al. [17] for secondary columella lengthening. From the cases published this approach shows promise and may gain in popularity. Yet from experience with bilateral clefts, among the advantages two disadvantages seem likely: (1) there is limitation in the amount of possible columella lengthening; and (2) the double lengthening of the prolabium may end up with an upper lip that is too long in its vertical dimension.

LATERAL MUSCLE AND MUCOSA INSERTED BEHIND THE PROLABIUM. Initial side-to-side closure of the lateral lip elements to the prolabium is responsible for stretching of the prolabium. This can be explained by the fact that there is no musculature in the prolabium, and therefore when the strong active lateral muscle elements are attached to each side, the pull on the subcutaneous component is effective. Owing to this enlargement by traction, the prolabium is soon capable of supplying lateral forked flaps for early columella lengthening. According to Schultz [36], Browne [6], and Trusler et al. [40], if in this primary closure the prolabium is freed from the premaxilla, and the mucosa and muscle of the lateral lip elements are sutured together behind the prolabium, a more functional lip is formed. This intact muscle band will exert a far more effective restraining power on the premaxilla (Fig. 7-10A, B, C).

With the lateral muscles incorporated behind the prolabium, there will not be the stretch of this component and extra tissue for a forked flap will not be so readily available. This will require a delay of several years before execution of the forked flap. The advantages of this approach seem to outweigh any delay in columella lengthening.

PRIMARY FORKED FLAP. This approach has been

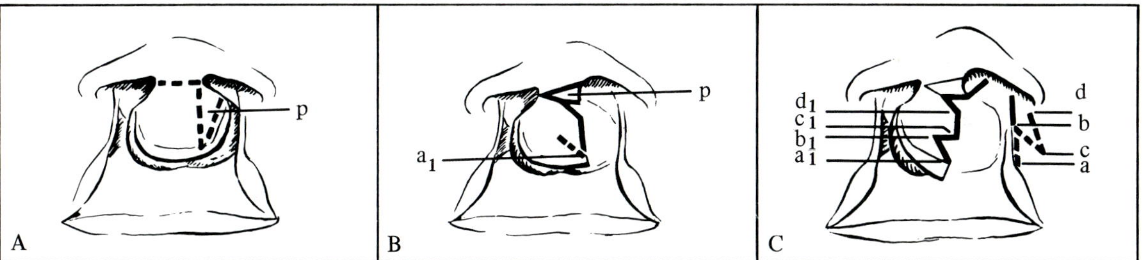

Fig. 7-8. Skoog's method. The diagrams show reconstruction of the columella utilizing prolabial tissue (A and B), and design for repair of the cleft lip (B and C). In C, point a *will be sutured to point* a_1, b *to* b_1, *etc. (Courtesy of T. Skoog.* Plast. Reconstr. Surg. *35: 34, 1965.)*

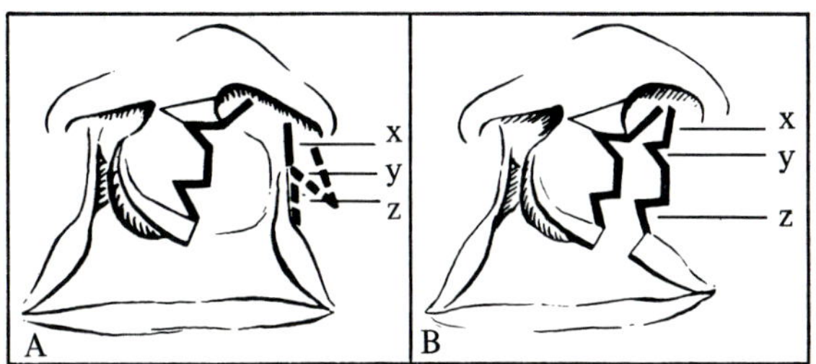

*Fig. 7-9. Skoog's method. The diagrams illustrate how the flaps (*y *and* z*) formed from the lateral border of the cleft are used for elongation of the lip and for shaping and repositioning of the alar base. (Reproduced, by permission, from T. Skoog,* Plast. Reconstr. Surg. *35:34, 1965.)*

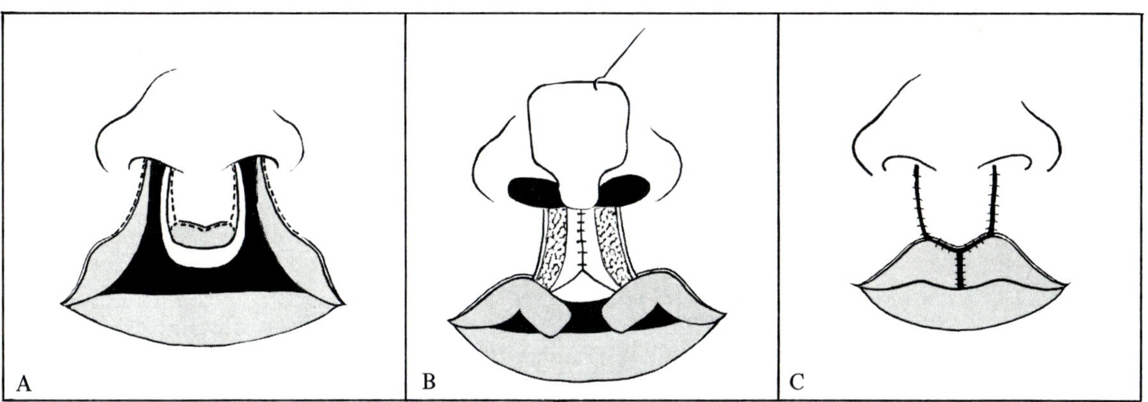

Fig. 7-10. Lateral muscle and mucosa are inserted behind the prolabium. A, the lateral lip elements are freshened by turndown of the vermilion flaps. Sides of the prolabium are freshened and the inferior vermilion turned down. B, the prolabium is freed from the premaxilla. Mucosa of the lateral lip elements are sutured together. C, the prolabium is replaced and the lateral vermilion flaps overlap the turndown or the prolabium vermilion to complete the first stage.

discontinued in complete clefts as there is some danger to the prolabial blood supply, and there seems to be gradual lengthening in vertical dimension of the upper lip.

BANKING THE FORKED FLAP. It seems that the best plan is to cut the forked flaps from the sides of the prolabium and leave them free. The muscle and mucosa of the lateral lip elements are brought together behind the prolabium, and the lateral mucosa is used to overlap the prolabium mucosa. The forks are then sutured to the alar base flaps or in whisker position for banking. Months or years later these forks can be moved up into the columella in a motion similar to the Cronin nasal floor and alar base rotation, but with more tissue now available. This avoids having to go back onto the lip to get the forked flap (Fig. 7-11A, B, C, D, E).

SECONDARY FORKED FLAP. Details of the forked flap technique for lengthening the columella secondarily may be helpful. When the prolabium is wide it forms an unnatural philtrum, and if the columella is also short the forked flap lengthens the columella and reshapes the prolabium in one action.

With the columella as the base, the prongs of the forked flap are marked so as to reduce the prolabium-to-philtrum dimensions and at the same time include the bilateral scars and varying amounts of the lateral lip element, depending on the specific requirements (Fig. 7-12A). A membranous septal incision will free the short columella, and when this incision is carried up over the septal tip, the nasal tip will rise free. For further correction the incisions are extended a short distance bilaterally through mucosa and cartilage in the anterior vestibule. The two prongs of the fork are then sutured together in a midline seam with 6-0 silk. To avoid the typical kinked notch in the columella just below the tip, the posterior edges of the upper 1 cm. of forked flap are not sutured to the lining of the septum or vestibule but are merely rolled loosely and sutured gently into a tube (Fig. 7-12B, C). The remaining portion of the forked flap is fixed with sutures to the membranous septum in corrected position. This tubing ensures a lift to the nasal tip and avoids the necessity of bone or cartilage props in the columella.

The lateral lip elements are then advanced medially to the reduced prolabium and sutured. It has been found helpful to advance the vermilion flaps along the inferior border of the prolabium toward the midline, which increases the tubercle when needed. Otherwise the excess vermilion is excised in the middle (Fig. 7-12C, D). If the upper lip is short vertically, then Poupard's modification [29], using Webster's crescentic perialar cheek excisions [41], will add to

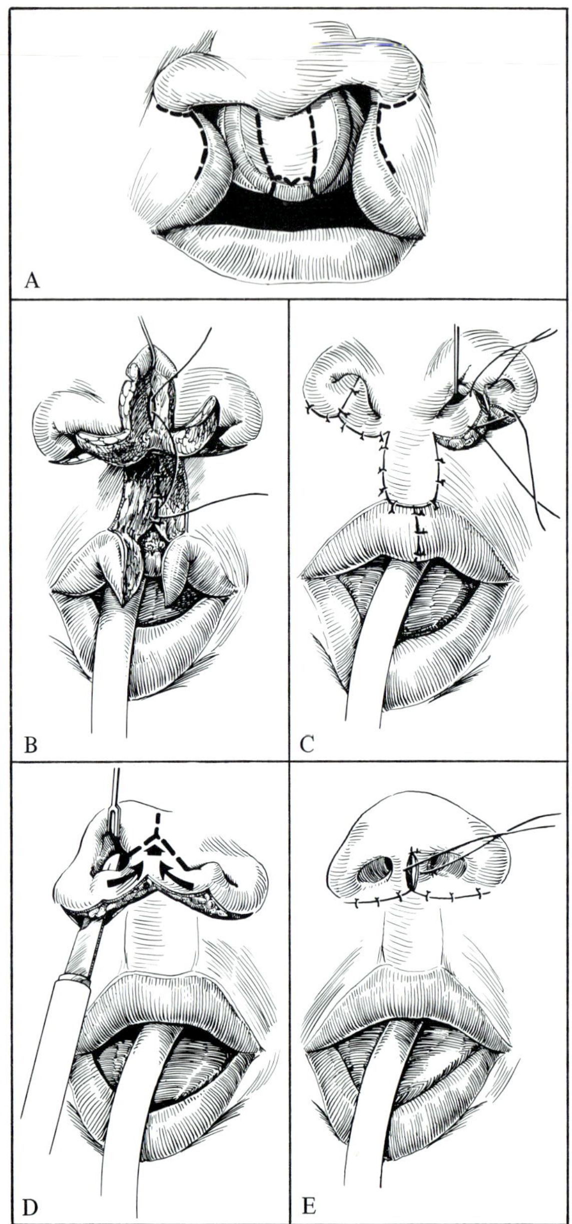

Fig. 7-11. Banking the forked flap. A, prolabial markings outline the shaped philtrum, turndown flap of prolabial vermilion, and first stage of forked flap; circumalar markings outline the alar base flaps; lateral lip markings outline the freshening of edges by turndown of vermilion flaps. B, suturing of vertical partial-thickness slit in the rear of the prolabium picks up the dermis and takes a bite in the periosteum of the premaxilla. The suture is left untied while the posterior mucosa and the muscle of the lateral lip elements are

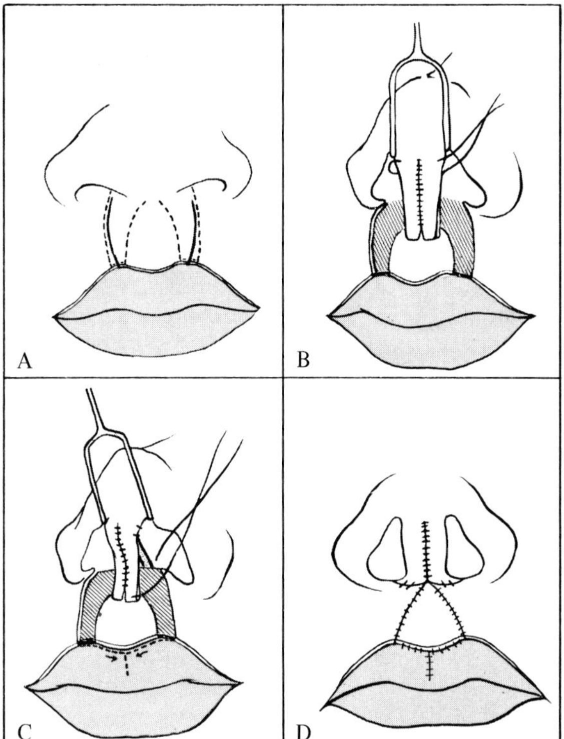

Fig. 7-12. Secondary forked flap. A, second-stage forked flap incorporates bilateral scars and lateral portions of the prolabium to lengthen the columella. Membranous septal incision is carried over the tip of the septum to release the depressed nasal tip and allow columella lengthening. B, flaps are sutured together down the middle; then the upper one-third is tubed gently on itself. C, upper portion of the forked flap has been tubed gently. The inferior portion is being sutured to the membranous septum. Medial advancement of vermilion flaps along the inferior border of the prolabium has been marked. D, columella has been lengthened and the prolabium reduced to philtrum dimension.

Fig. 7-11 (Continued)
sutured together behind the prolabium. C, at right, fork is sutured end-on to the alar base flap; raw undersurfaces of both flaps are approximated to take up slack. D, at 1 year in incomplete clefts or 5 years in complete clefts, the strap-flaps of the forked flap and the alar base flap in continuity are joined in front by an inverted V *incision and behind by a membranous septal incision carried over the tip of the septum* (broken line). *E, after deep subcutaneous closure with 5-0 catgut, closure with 6-0 silk favorably places future scars. (After Millard [27].)*

lip length, though one should be aware of ending up with a lip that is unattractively long.

Secondary Revisions in Bilateral Cleft Lip

Secondary revisions in bilateral cleft lip can vary from minor mucosal trimming to radical release of the entire lip. The most common postoperative deformities are tightness of the lip in the horizontal dimension and too great length of the lip in the vertical dimension. Tightness is released by midline division of the full thickness of the upper lip and the filling of this defect with a composite flap from the middle of the lower lip. An upper lip too long vertically can be shortened either along its free border or along the base of the nose.

The commonest postoperative secondary nasal deformity is the short columella. Once this is corrected the associated nasal discrepancies are improved simultaneously or can be corrected with minor surgery. Various methods already mentioned are available to lengthen the columella, including the forked flap, which has been discussed in detail. When the upper lip is tight and the columella is short, then the prolabium is moved into the columella and the midline Abbe flap is transposed from the lower lip to form a new philtrum.

POSTOPERATIVE CARE AFTER THE CLEFT LIP CLOSURE

Antibiotic ointment is applied generously to all skin suture lines immediately after surgery, and such application is continued three times daily until the fifth postoperative day. This will protect the suture holes from contamination of nasal discharge. The sutures are removed on the fourth postoperative day. A Logan bow, with strong inward tension to the cheeks, applied after surgery will counteract crying and thus aid in early healing. Arm restraints are applied before the baby comes out of the anesthesia; these, along with the Logan bow, are maintained for 2 weeks. Feeding is carried out with a spoon, cup, or asepto syringe with a short-sleeve extension of the catheter. The baby is allowed to go home on the fifth postoperative day, and that type of feeding is continued at home.

REFERENCES

1. Berkeley, W. The cleft lip nose. *Plast. Reconstr. Surg.* 23:567, 1959.
2. Brauer, R. O., and Cronin, T. D. Maxillary orthopedics and anterior palate repair with bone graftings. *Cleft Palate J.* 1:31, 1964.
3. Brauer, R. O., Cronin, T. D., and Reaves, E. L. Early maxillary orthopedics, orthodontia and alveolar bone grafting in complete clefts of the palate. *Plast. Reconstr. Surg.* 29:625, 1962.
4. Brauer, R. O., and Foerster, D. W. Another

method for lengthening the columella in the double cleft patient. *Plast. Reconstr. Surg.* 38:27, 1966.
5. Brown, J. B., and McDowell, F. Small triangular flap operation for the primary repair of single cleft lips. *Plast. Reconstr. Surg.* 5:392, 1950.
6. Browne, D. Harelip. *Ann. R. Coll. Surg. Engl.* 5:169, 1949.
7. Burston, W. R. The early orthodontic treatment of cleft palate conditions. *Dent. Pract.* (Bristol) 9:41, 1958.
8. Burston, W. R. Personal communication, 1964.
9. Cronin, T. D. Surgery of the double lip and protruding premaxilla. *Plast. Reconstr. Surg.* 19:389, 1957.
10. Cronin, T. D. Lengthening columella by use of skin from nasal floor and alae. *Plast. Reconstr. Surg.* 21:417, 1958.
11. Cronin, T. D. Personal communication, 1965.
12. Federspiel, M. N. *Harelip and Cleft Palate.* St. Louis: Mosby, 1927.
13. Holdsworth, W. G. Personal communication, 1965.
14. Johanson, B., and Ohlsson, A. Die Osteoplastik bei Spätbehandlung der Lippen-Kiefer-Gaumenspalten. *Arch. Klin. Chir.* 295:876, 1960.
15. Johanson, B., and Ohlsson, A. Bone grafting and dental orthopaedics in primary and secondary cases of cleft lip and palate. *Acta Chir. Scand.* 122:112, 1961.
16. LeMesurier, A. B. A method of cutting and suturing the lip in the treatment of complete unilateral clefts. *Plast. Reconstr. Surg.* 4:1, 1949.
17. Marcks, K. N., Trevaskis, A. E., and Payne, N. J. Elongation of columella by flap transfer and Z-plasty. *Plast. Reconstr. Surg.* 20:466, 1957.
18. Millard, D. R., Jr. A Primary Camouflage in the Unilateral Harelook. *Transactions of the International Society of Plastic Surgeons* (First Congress). Baltimore: Williams & Wilkins, 1957.
19. Millard, D. R., Jr. Columella lengthening by a forked flap. *Plast. Reconstr. Surg.* 22:454, 1958.
20. Millard, D. R., Jr. A radical rotation in single harelip. *Am. J. Surg.* 95:318, 1958.
21. Millard, D. R., Jr. Adaptation of the Rotation-Advancement Principle in Bilateral Cleft Lip. *Transactions of the International Society of Plastic Surgeons* (Second Congress). Edinburgh: Livingstone, 1960.
22. Millard, D. R., Jr. Complete unilateral clefts of the lip. *Plast. Reconstr. Surg.* 25:595, 1960.
23. Millard, D. R., Jr. A primary compromise for bilateral cleft lip. *Surg. Gynecol. Obstet.* 111:557, 1960.
24. Millard, D. R., Jr. Composite lip flaps and grafts in secondary cleft deformities. *Br. J. Plast. Surg.* 17:22, 1964.
25. Millard, D. R., Jr. Refinements in rotation-advancement cleft lip technique. *Plast. Reconstr. Surg.* 33:26, 1964.
26. Millard, D. R., Jr. The unilateral cleft lip nose. *Plast. Reconstr. Surg.* 34:169, 1964.
27. Millard, D. R., Jr. Closure of bilateral cleft lip and elongation of columella by two operations in infancy. *Plast. Reconstr. Surg.* 47:324, 1971.
27a. Millard, D. R., Jr. *Cleft Craft: The Evolution of Its Surgery,* Vols. 1 and 2. Boston: Little, Brown, 1976, 1977.
28. Monroe, C. W. Recession of the premaxilla in bilateral cleft lip and palate. *Plast. Reconstr. Surg.* 35:512, 1965.
28a. Musgrave, R. H., and Dupertius, S. M. Revision of. the unilateral cleft lip nose. *Plast. Reconstr. Surg.* 25:223, 1960.
29. Poupard, B. Sequelles de guele de loup. *Ann. Chir. Plast.* 8:112, 1963.
30. Randall, P. A triangular flap operation for the primary repair of unilateral clefts of the lip. *Plast. Reconstr. Surg.* 23:331, 1959.
31. Randall, P. A lip adhesion operation in cleft lip surgery. *Plast. Reconstr. Surg.* 35:371, 1965.
32. Recamier, J., and Recamier, M. Bec-de-lievre unilateral total. *Ann. Chir. Plast.* 8:1, 1963.
33. Reynolds, J. R., and Horton, C. E. An alar lift procedure in cleft lip rhinoplasty. *Plast. Reconstr. Surg.* 35:377, 1965.
34. Schmidt, E. Die Annäherung der Kieferstumpfe bei Lippen-Kiefer-Gaumenspalten: Ihre schädlichen Folgen und Vermeidung. *Fortschr. Kiefer Gesichtschir.* 1:37, 1955.
35. Schuchardt, K. Die Entwicklung der Lippen-Kiefer-Gaumenspalten-Chirurgie unter besonderer Berücksichtigung asthetischer und functioneller Momente. *Arch. Klin. Chir.* 295:850, 1960.
36. Schultz, L. W. Bilateral cleft lips. *Plast. Reconstr. Surg.* 4:311, 1949.
37. Skoog, T. A design for the repair of unilateral cleft lips. *Am. J. Surg.* 95:223, 1958.
38. Skoog, T. The management of the bilateral cleft of the primary palate (lip and alveolus). *Plast. Reconstr. Surg.* 35:34, 1965.
39. Tennison, C. W. The repair of unilateral cleft lip by the stencil method. *Plast. Reconstr. Surg.* 9:115, 1952.
40. Trusler, H. M., Bauer, T. B., and Tondra, J. M. The cleft lip–cleft palate problem. *Plast. Reconstr. Surg.* 16:174, 1955.
41. Webster, J. P. Crescentic perialar cheek excision for upper lip flap advancement. *Plast. Reconstr. Surg.* 16:434, 1955.

8

Cleft Palate

PETER RANDALL

ANATOMY

Major Components

The palate (Fig. 8-1) is composed of the bony or hard palate anteriorly and the soft palate posteriorly. The alveolus borders the hard palate. Anteriorly and centrally the hard palate consists of the premaxilla, which gives rise to incisor teeth; the premaxilla extends posteriorly to the incisive foramen. The major portion of the hard palate is made up of the paired maxillas. Posterior to the maxillas are the palatine bones.

The major blood supply comes through the major palatine foramen. A secondary blood supply comes through the lesser palatine foramen and incisive foramen. The sensory nerves reach the palate through these foramina and from the nasal side of the soft palate by way of the posterior palatine nerve [14]. The soft palate is densely attached to the posterior edge of the palatal bones by the palatal aponeurosis. The major musculature consists of two slinglike muscles: (1) the levator palati muscles, which pull the palate upward and backward, and (2) the tensor palati muscles, which course around the hamulus process of the sphenoid bone and function as their name implies. Other pairs of muscles contributing to speech and swallowing include the palatoglossus, the palatopharyngeus, the stylopharyngeus, and the superior pharyngeal constrictors. The innervation of the levator palati is by way of the pharyngeal plexus. The tensor palati are innervated by way of the mandibular division of the trigeminal nerve [4, 22].

Prepalatal and Palatal Clefts

Clefts usually follow the lines of fusion so that anterior to the incisive foramen the cleft diverges between the maxilla and the premaxilla. They usually traverse the alveolus between the lateral incisor and the canine teeth. There may be some variation in the location of the cleft in the alveolus. In addition, rarely one will see a midline cleft of the anterior structures [2, 28].

Those structures anterior to the incisive foramen (including the alveolus, lip, nasal floor, and alar cartilages) are called the *prepalatal structures* or the structures of the primary palate. Those posterior to the incisive foramen are called the *palatal structures* or those of the secondary palate. These two areas are embryologically distinct [19, 32].

Clefts in the alveolus are usually associated with clefts in the lip. Without the restraining forces of the intact orbicularis oris muscle, the cleft alveolar segments are most often displaced outward from the normal position, causing an anterior flaring of the premaxilla in a unilateral cleft and often a marked protrusion in the bilateral cleft. The lateral maxillary segment is also usually laterally displaced prior to lip repair, but after lip repair it is compressed medially and may be in a crossbite position. In addition, it is usually lacking in the vertical height as well. The teeth adjacent to the cleft are likely to be angled into the cleft and are frequently distorted in their size and shape.

In unilateral clefts, the vomer is almost always attached to the maxilla on the noncleft side for its entire length. In bilateral clefts of the prepalatal and palatal structures, it is unattached laterally, and this is also the case in palatal clefts extending to the incisive foramen.

One of the most important anatomical distortions seen in cleft palate is in the musculature of the soft palate. Kriens and the Dicksons have stressed again the findings of Victor Veau that the levator palati muscles, instead of being directed toward the midline, are oriented in a more longitudinal direction, and are inserted not only along the posterior edge of the bony palate but often along the medial edge of the cleft as well (Fig. 8-2) [7, 8, 22, 25].

Even in a submucosal cleft with most of the soft palate mucosa intact but with a dehiscence of the underlying muscles in the midline, this abnormal placement of muscle can be seen as two longitudinal ridges in the soft palate on either side of the midline. Ideally, this abnormal attachment and orientation of the levator muscles should be corrected if they are to be expected to function normally.

The tensor palati muscles are also abnormal with little or no tissue found medial to the pterigoid hamulus. At times, fibers seem to bypass the hamulus altogether. Reconstruction of the tensor muscles does not seem to be important so far as speech is concerned. However, both the tensor and the levator palati muscles also insert along the eustachian tubes. Malfunctioning of the eustachian tubes is usually a significant finding in children with palatal clefts [8, 22, 31].

Soft Palate Movement and Speech

The *major action* of the soft palate during speech (Fig. 8-3) consists of a rapid and voluntary, though subconscious, motion of the palate upward and back-

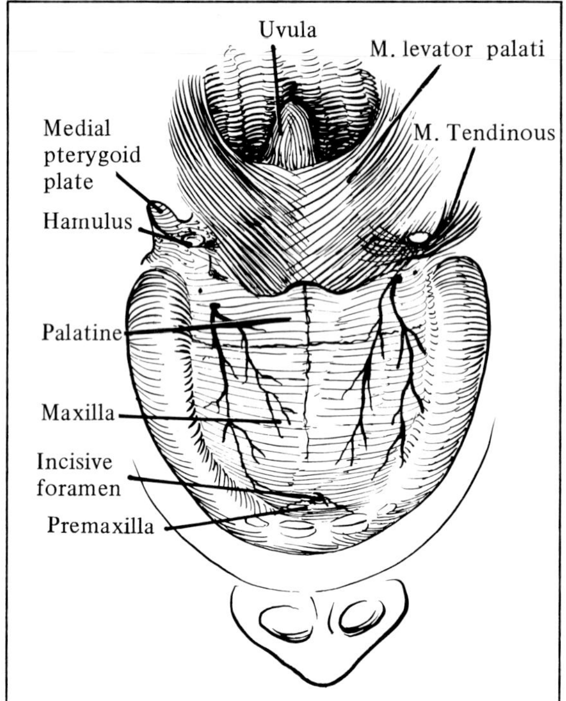

Fig. 8-1. Normal palatal structures. The incisive foramen is the dividing point between clefts of the prepalatal structures and those of the palatal structures.

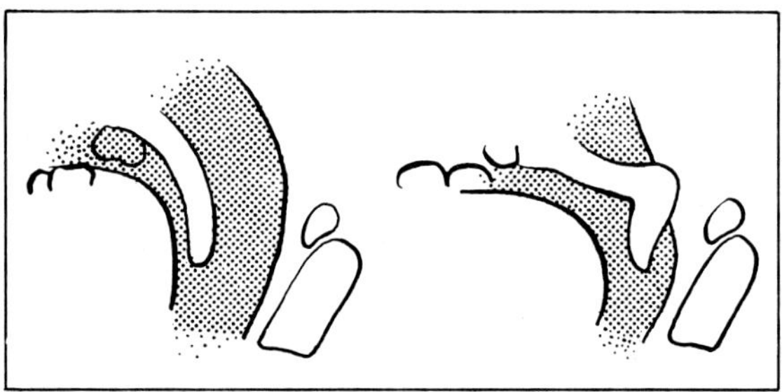

Fig. 8-3. Outline of the posterior pharynx, the soft palate, and the tongue in sagittal cross section. At rest (left), the palate hangs free. Normal velopharyngeal closure (right) is achieved mostly by the levator palati muscles pulling the middle one-third of the palate upward and backward; firm contact is made at about the level of the adenoid pad.

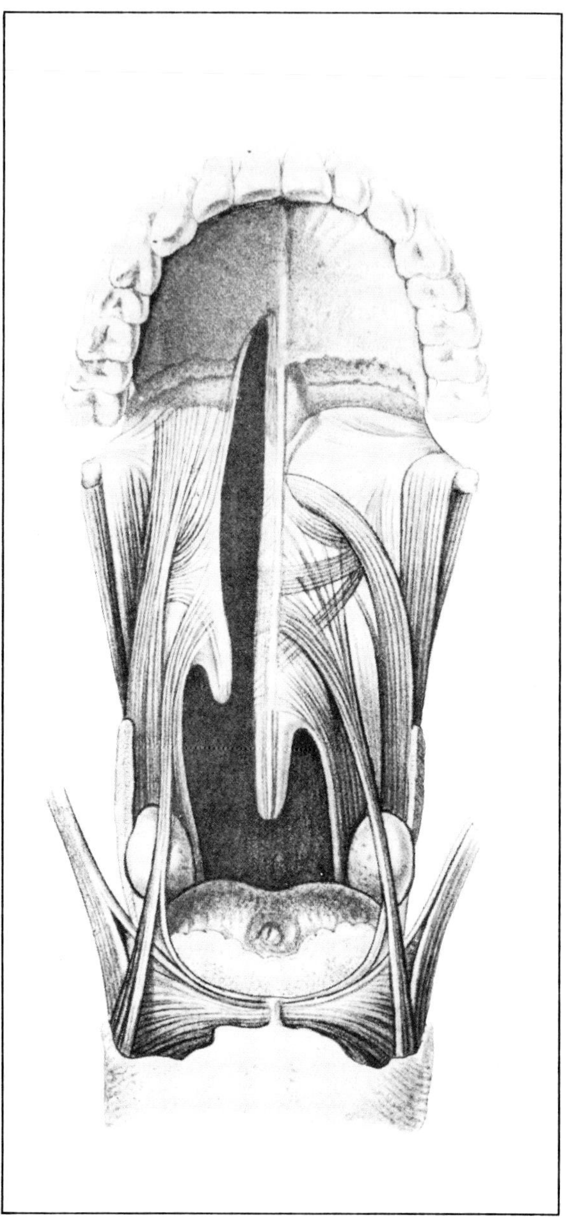

Fig. 8-2. Schematic drawing by Victor Veau showing the muscles of the normal palate on the right and the anatomy seen in cleft palate on the left. Note particularly in the cleft the more longitudinal direction of the levator palati muscle and its attachment not only to the posterior edge of the palatal bone but also along the edge of the bony cleft. (From Veau [33].)

ward, producing intimate contact with the posterior pharyngeal wall at the level of the adenoid pad [91]. This is called *velopharyngeal closure.* The major muscles for achieving velopharyngeal closure are the paired levator palati muscles. They are unusual in that they are very efficient, contract rapidly, and fatigue slowly [5]. Velopharyngeal closure is also aided by most of the constrictor muscles in the velopharyngeal area. Skolnick has shown that there is considerable variation in the way velopharyngeal closure is achieved, even in the normal person [31]. The motion appears to be truly sphincteric, with the greatest action being achieved by the levator palati. The terms *velopharyngeal competence* and *velopharyngeal incompetence* refer respectively to the presence or absence of velopharyngeal closure [13].

The Production of Normal Speech
Normal speech requires a competent *speech mechanism,* plus adequate *hearing* and *intelligence.* So many factors go into speech production, and there is so much variation under normal conditions, that it is difficult to define "normal speech." Complete or nearly complete velopharyngeal closure is needed. All *consonant sounds* in the English language, with the exception of the "nasal consonants" of "m," "n," and the "ng" sound, require the building up of intraoral air pressure. The sudden release of pressure produces an explosive sound or a "stop plosive" consonant, such as "p," "t," and "d." At the end of a word (the terminal position), the air stream is abruptly stopped, as in the word "stop." The production of sound by friction produces the consonants called *continuants;* when voiced as in "v" and "z" they are called *fricatives,* whereas the more silent continuants are subclassified as *sibilants,* such as "s" and "sh" [93, 96, 98].

Cleft Palate Type of Speech
Vowel sounds when produced by patients with velopharyngeal incompetence take on a nasal quality that is called *hypernasality,* in contrast to the *hyponasality* heard in obstructed conditions, such as choanal atresia, obstructing hypertrophied adenoids, or a simple "cold in the nose."

Consonants when enunciated by patients with velopharyngeal incompetence are frequently distorted by inadequate pressure and/or by the sound of air leakage into the nose, which is called *nasal escape.* Patients may *omit* these sounds, or *substitute* sounds such as those produced by building up pressure behind the glottis, producing a plosive called a *glottal stop.* The word "daddy" then becomes "ah-ee," with the consonants omitted or close to "ga-gee" with the glottal stop.

Good speech requires not only a capable mechanism, adequate hearing, and intelligence, but also a home and school environment where good speech is heard. A higher percentage of children with cleft palates will develop normal speech if an *adequate mechanism is provided before formal speech develops* than if a child first learns incorrect speech due to an incompetent palate. Even though a subsequent procedure provides an adequate speech mechanism, it is usually difficult for a patient who is accustomed to hearing his own incorrect speech to feel comfortable when hearing himself produce normal speech, simply because "normal speech" sounds so different to him. This often presents a considerable problem. Some patients, however, do avoid this difficulty completely [93].

In *testing speech,* it should be noted that a patient with borderline velopharyngeal incompetence can often put enough extra effort into his speech that no hypernasality or articulatory errors are made. Under these circumstances, poor speech would probably be heard when the patient is more relaxed (as in conversational speech) or when he is fatigued. The collaboration of a competent *speech pathologist* to help evaluate postoperative surgical results is extremely helpful. *Speech* is the *most important function to consider* in cleft palate repair, though few surgeons have had any training in speech pathology.

EMBRYOLOGY AND ETIOLOGY OF PALATAL CLEFTS

Prepalatal Clefts

In theory the prepalatal clefts are caused by a *lack of mesodermal development.* Stark [32] has described three mesodermal islands, one central and two lateral, which ordinarily develop and fuse. Lack of development of one or more of these mesodermal islands leaves an unstable condition, with ectoderm of the skin in contact with ectoderm of the oral mucosa, and a complete or incomplete breakdown occurs at this point [11, 12, 28].

This theory explains the various types of lateral clefts that are seen, depending on whether one or both lateral mesodermal islands fail to develop. In addition, it explains the unusual midline cleft. The severe midline defect as seen in arrhinocephaly, consisting of a severe midline loss of lip and columella, could be due to a failure of all three mesodermal islands to develop.

This theory also explains the usual involvement of the ala nasi cartilages along with the lip, and the associated defects of the alveolus, in all prepalatal clefts. In addition, such a lack of mesodermal development explains the hypoplasia seen in the adjacent maxillary structures.

Palatal Clefts

The palatal structures are present in a 7-week-old embryo as two shelves that lie in an almost vertical position with their medial edges alongside of the tongue. Normally, the tongue drops downward and the shelves rotate upward to the horizontal position and fuse from anterior to posterior to form the intact palate by 12 weeks [32]. Whether the cleft condition is a result of the two halves never coming together or of an imperfect union and subsequent separation is open to some question [21]. Experimentally, it has been shown that in rodents, the right palatal shelf reaches the horizontal position before the left one, thus leaving the left side vulnerable to interruption or interference in its normal development for a longer period of time than the right. This may explain the more frequent occurrence of unilateral clefts on the left than on the right side [12].

Production of Palatal Clefts

Experimental clefts have been produced by a number of conditions, such as deficiencies of vitamin A, riboflavin, folic acid, pantothenic acid, and nicotinic acid. They have also been produced by an excess of vitamin A, fasting, hypoxia, nitrogen mustard, nucleic acid antagonists, corticosteroids, ACTH, irradiation, the loss of amniotic fluid, and a number of other agents [6, 18, 29, 34, 35, 36].

Though the *etiology in man is not known, heredity* has been shown to play a significant part. The most frequent type of cleft in man (left unilateral cleft of the palate and prepalate) is predominantly seen in males with a rather high hereditary background, whereas the second most frequent type of cleft (cleft palate alone) is predominantly seen in females with a fairly low hereditary background, thus suggesting entirely different causes. Since the defect is a frequent one, it is probably easily produced in man and is likely to have a number of causes. A distinction should be made between those with a prepalatal cleft (with or without an accompanying palatal cleft) and those with only a palatal cleft. They are quite different in respect to their inheritability and their sex distribution.

Woolf et al. [37] have stated that in their series "there is a statistically significant increase of [cleft lip and cleft palate] in the relatives of a patient with [cleft lip and palate], but the frequency of [cleft palate alone] in these relatives is the same as in the general population." The same relationship exists in the families of patients with cleft palate alone. A number of monozygotic twins with discordant anomalies have been described, which would indicate that a slight *environmental difference* can alter the degree of manifestation or penetration of the anomaly [30].

Incidence

The incidence of various types of clefts has been reported by Veau [33]. The overall incidence of clefts in the general population is reported by Fogh-Andersen [10] as 1 in 665 and by Ivy [16] as 1 in 762 live births, placing it second only to club feet among congenital anomalies reported on birth certificates. Brogan and Woodings [3] report a recent decrease in the incidence of clefts in western Australia, while Fogh-Andersen feels there is a slight increase in Scandinavia. In general, there seems to be a greater incidence in Orientals as compared with Caucasians, and a decreased incidence in blacks. Fogh-Andersen [10] has found that the chances of cleft lip occurring in the child of parents, of whom one has a cleft, is about 2 percent. This increases to 14 percent if there is already a sibling with a cleft lip. If two normal parents have a child with a cleft lip, there is said to be a 4.5 percent chance that subsequent siblings will have the deformity. Similar figures have been reported by Woolf et al. [37].

Classification of Clefts

The incisive foramen has been mentioned as the dividing point between the prepalatal clefts (clefts of the primary palate) and the palatal clefts (clefts of the secondary palate). (See Fig. 8-1.) This separation is made because embryologically these two types of clefts are different, and because they can occur either separately or together [32, 33].

Prepalatal clefts involve the anterior palate, the alveolus, the lip, the nostril floor, and the ala nasi. They are either unilateral or bilateral though, rarely, they can occur in the midline. A further subdivision is made depending on whether they are *complete* or *incomplete* (total or subtotal), which depends on whether the structures involved are completely separated or incompletely separated. Even more explicitly the cleft can be described as being 1/3, 2/3, or 3/3 complete, with added notes concerning rotation, protrusion, and measurements of the amount of separation between the involved parts [15, 19].

Palatal clefts (posterior to the incisive foramen) are also classified as *complete* or *incomplete* (total or subtotal), depending on whether they extend all the way through the soft palate and the hard palate to the incisive foramen or only part of the way. (The most rudimentary form of cleft palate is the bifid uvula.) Again a more explicit classification describes the cleft as involving 1/3, 2/3, or 3/3 of the soft palate and also the hard palate. *Palatal clefts* are *considered* to be *midline clefts,* but a note should be made of those patients with hard palate involvement, describing any attachment of the vomer to either the right or left maxillary bone. Further notes should describe *submucosal clefts* when they are recognized.

Certain combinations of clefts occur more frequently than others. The *most frequent* (aside from the bifid uvula) is a left unilateral complete cleft of the palate and the prepalatal structures. The *second most common* is a midline cleft of 3/3 of the soft palate and part of the hard palate without a cleft in the prepalatal area. Bilateral clefts of the prepalatal area are usually accompanied by bilateral palatal clefts, and incomplete clefts in one area usually accompany incomplete clefts in the other. However, virtually any combination of clefts can occur. The hard palate posterior to the incisive foramen is almost never cleft without a 3/3 cleft of the soft palate.

Bifid Uvula

Interestingly, the most frequent cleft is really the bifid uvula, which was reported by Meskin in 2 percent of the population [24, 26, 27]. Most of the time, this is an incidental finding and is not associated with velopharyngeal incompetence or any other problems. However, it can be inherited as a palatal cleft, and should serve as a warning that the palate may indeed be close to velopharyngeal incompetence so that an adenoidectomy might produce incompetence.

Submucosal Cleft

A bifid uvula may also be part of a complex known as a submucosal cleft with dehiscence of the levator muscles, displacement of the orientation of the levator muscle into a more longitudinal direction, a short anteroposterior dimension of the palate, and even a submucosal cleft in the posterior third of the bony palate. Usually, if these are present, the midportion of the posterior third of the soft palate has a very thin appearance on examination. This is easily demonstrated at operation, if an elevator is placed behind the palate. On gagging, the displaced levator palati muscles stand out in their abnormal position. One might also be able to palpate a notch in the posterior edge of the hard palate instead of the usual tubercle.

Pierre Robin Syndrome

In clefts extending no farther anteriorly than the incisive foramen, the *mandible* may be *retropositioned* or structurally small (or both). Under these conditions, a ball-valve type of respiratory obstruction due to glossoptosis can occur. This is the *Pierre Robin syndrome,* and though it is often associated with a cleft palate, this is not an essential part of the syndrome (see Chapter 4).

GENERAL CARE OF PATIENT WITH CLEFT PALATE

Neonatal Period

Four points are to be emphasized in the treatment of young infants with clefts of the palate: (1) feeding, (2) maintenance of an airway, (3) middle ear disease, and (4) the possibility of other abnormalities.

Feeding

Feeding in a child with a cleft palate is usually difficult because of the *inability to develop suction,* even though the infant may make sucking movements. Since swallowing should not be affected, adequate nutrition is possible when milk or soft food is delivered to the posterior part of the oral cavity. An abundance of breast milk may make breast feeding practical; otherwise, milk should be given in such a way that suction is not needed. Artificial nipples can have the holes made larger so that the milk will drip freely from an inverted bottle, or they can be attached to a Brecht-type feeder with a bulb syringe. Plastic bottles that can be squeezed are also useful. It is helpful to hold the infant at about 45 degrees above the horizontal so that the milk will flow to the back of the mouth, with minimal regurgitation into the nose. More air than usual is swallowed, and feeding will take longer than the average time.

In the matter of feeding, it is important to urge the *mother* to *take an active part,* and to help regardless of how difficult the feedings might be. The mother can be expected to be timid at first but soon learns the little tricks that are needed. In time, she should feel more expert than anyone else in the feeding of her child. At this point, the baby is more dependent on his mother for survival than on any other person. In a simple, subtle way a strong, healthy mother-to-child relationship is begun. Advice from an experienced nursery nurse is very helpful, but care should be taken that she does not "take over" the complete feeding of the child. This is the parent's responsibility, and it should begin as soon as possible [41].

Maintenance of an Airway

Breathing can be a problem, particularly if the chin is retropositioned ("short chin," "micrognathic," "undershot jaw"). The effectiveness of the genioglossus muscle is lost and the tongue falls backward, partly or completely blocking the airway on inspiration (the Pierre Robin anomalad – see Chapter 4) [50].

Middle Ear Disease

The middle ear space, even in the neonatal period, is usually not properly aerated if the child has a cleft palate. Examination with an office otoscope is difficult because the infant is usually squirmy, the auditory canal is tiny, and in the infant the eardrum is much more horizontal than in older children. A thorough examination with an *operating microscope under a general anesthetic will reveal abnormal fluid behind the eardrum in about 90 to 100 percent of these infants.* Usually, this fluid is very thick but sterile; however, in older children, evidence of prolonged infection is often encountered. Examination by an otologist is carried out with an operating microscope, and a diagnostic myringotomy is done virtually whenever a child with a cleft palate undergoes a general anesthetic. Malfunction of the eustachian tube appears to be the most likely cause of this problem, so the myringotomy incision is usually kept open with a small Silastic tube or button, which allows equalization of air pressure through the eardrum rather than by way of the eustachian tube. Otolaryngological consultation and follow-up is obviously helpful. Children with cleft palate used to have about a 40 to 50 percent incidence of *permanent hearing loss* in the range of 30 to 40 decibels in one or both ears. With careful attention to ear problems, this incidence has improved greatly [48, 53, 124].

Other Congenital Abnormalities

Other congenital abnormalities occur more frequently in the cleft palate population than in the average infant. The incidence can be as high as 30 percent. A very complete history and physical examination, with the usual laboratory studies, should be carried out. The history should include an inquiry about other clefts and deformities in the family, and any known illness or problems in the early months of pregnancy [17, 20].

Questions from Parents

Most parents of children with cleft palate will ask if there is a *known cause* and whether or not the condition *could have been prevented.* They may ask what chance there is of a cleft occurring in subsequent children. What can be done about the deformity? When can it be done? How much will it *cost*? Will the child be able to *speak* correctly? These queries should be answered simply, directly, and honestly, but reassuringly. Even if they are not asked, they probably should be raised because if the answers are not supplied by a competent person, they are likely to be volunteered by a less experienced person.

Parents are told that in most cases, the *exact cause* of the cleft is *not known* and that in some families it appears to be an inherited trait, whereas in others it is not. In the absence of a significant family history, it has been helpful to describe the cleft as an *accident in development.* This description seems to convey a realistic appreciation of something that can be slight or severe and something that can happen to anyone with or without known reason. In addition, it also implies that some conditions can be corrected virtually completely, and others will always leave some stigmata of the "damage."

Parents are told that there is *nothing known that can prevent* the occurrence of clefts under most circumstances and that nothing could have been done during the pregnancy that was not done, nor was anything done that should not have been done. Despite this reassurance, a deep guilt complex frequently will remain.

In the *absence of a strong family history of clefts,* parents are told that having had one child with a cleft, the likelihood of another being born with the same deformity is greater than in the general population. This increased likelihood, however, is probably so small that it should not interfere with plans to have more children, nor should it interfere with their child's plans to grow up, get married, and have a family, except that the child with a cleft should not marry another person with a cleft.

The general *time schedule* of steps for correcting the defect is discussed. If appropriate, the cost of treatment, the expected coverage from insurance, the approximate duration of hospitalization, and the availability of cleft palate clinic facilities are explained. Articles written for lay consumption can be very helpful and can be obtained from the American Cleft Palate Educational Foundation* [41, 44, 93].

GENERAL TIMETABLE OF CARE

The Alveolar Cleft and Hard Palate

The alveolar cleft and hard palate cleft can probably be closed at any time prior to 4 or 5 years of age depending on priorities. These priorities include the ease of surgery, the effect of an anterior opening on speech, the plans to move alveolar segments during this time, the ease and effectiveness of maintaining obturation with a dental "shell," and decisions regarding early bone grafting or closure with a so-called "boneless bone graft." Reports conflict greatly as to the effect of the timing of these procedures on the eventual dental occlusion and on speech [69, 75–77, 79–81, 87].

At the present time, I close the alveolar cleft with a buccal sulcus mucosal flap and the hard palate with a vomer flap. This is done at the time of the initial lip repair if the cleft is not wide and at the time of the palatal repair if it is wide. In my experience, delay has led to considerable difficulty in maintaining prosthetic obturation and has also caused difficulties with anterior articulation of speech, but it has not avoided the malocclusion problems.

*The American Cleft Palate Educational Foundation, 331 Salk Hall, University of Pittsburgh, Pittsburgh, PA 15261.

The Soft Palate

The soft palate is closed before the age of 24 months. I have usually preferred 12 to 18 months of age, and more recently patients have been operated on at 3 to 6 months of age. As pointed out by Schweckendick and Slaughter, this might hold a real advantage in the functional development of the speech mechanism. In addition, since closure of the soft palate appears to have a favorable effect on the ubiquitous incidence of middle ear disease, early closure has been beneficial in this regard too. Children who have their soft palates closed after the onset of formal speech will usually have poorer speech than those in whom surgery is completed before the development of speech patterns [51].

A *dental prosthesis* is another way to achieve closure of the soft palate, and is advised for those patients with unusually wide defects when there is a paucity of soft tissue. A dental prosthesis is also advised in older patients whose soft palate tissues have atrophied through disuse beyond the point of surgical salvage, in patients whose palates have been badly mutilated through poor surgery, and in patients with other medical problems severe enough to contraindicate a surgical procedure [54]. The appliance must be made with great care, however, and when used in small children, it must be altered as the child grows. An appliance usually depends on stable dentition for anchorage, though occasionally a satisfactory restoration with a speech bulb can be made for the edentulous patient. Should an adult lose his teeth and no longer be able to retain a prosthesis, a difficult situation can exist because such adults, who have not had soft palate surgery, generally have considerable atrophy of the soft palate remnants. Surgery under these conditions has a high incidence of failure, even when combined with a posterior pharyngeal flap. In general, *speech has been better* in a higher percentage of patients when the cleft has been closed *surgically* rather than by a *dental prosthesis.*

TREATMENT OF THE ANTERIOR PALATAL CLEFT

When clefts of the prepalatal structures occur, the alveolus is always involved. With minimal *incomplete clefts,* this may be merely delayed eruption of the teeth adjacent to the cleft. As the severity of the cleft increases, so does the incidence of these teeth being maldeveloped or distorted in growth and position [23]. In addition, the underlying alveolus is likely to be underdeveloped and malpositioned.

Alveolar Bone Grafts

Much attention has been directed toward controlling the shifting of the alveolar segments, and also to molding the shape of these segments [56–67, 69, 75–76]. The use of *bone grafts* to stabilize these structures and to replace deficiencies in bony bulk was enthusiastically received at first.

Because of disappointment in the wake of initial enthusiasm for bone grafts, few surgeons are undertaking this sort of "primary bone grafting" and prefer to reserve the use of bone grafts for the care of deficiencies in older children [75]. Careful work and study by Nylen and co-workers [76] and Nordin [75] on cases done since 1953 and a somewhat smaller series reported by Rosenstein [81a] show very good results with early bone grafting. Rehrmann and co-workers [79, 80] in Dusseldorf, as well as Jolleys and Robertson [69] in Manchester, England, in comparing a group of cleft palate children treated with and without bone grafting in a randomized series, have each shown a slight but appreciable restriction of growth as the result of early bone grafting. Furthermore, Pruzansky [77, 78] and Harding and Mazaheri [64, 71] have pointed out that few of these patients need much in the way of expansion anyway; thus early maxillary orthodontics and primary bone grafting are not being done routinely in our clinics [70].

None of the bone grafting techniques seems to help to make up for the *lack of vertical height* of the bony structures adjacent to the cleft. It has been pointed out, however, that the *addition of bone,* particularly at the nostril base in the form of *onlay grafts,* does *improve the facial distortion* that results from a bony deficiency in this area.

In general, *several premises* can be stated:

1. *Movement of alveolar segments* can be achieved in the infant with relative *ease,* and in the older patient and adult to a more limited extent, by a variety of dentures, braces, and expansion prostheses.
2. *Bone grafts* can be used in the mouth with even less than ideal mucosal coverage and with demonstrable survival. Flaps of periosteum can be used as "boneless bone grafts."
3. *After maxillary segments are moved* to new positions by "maxillary orthopedics," these segments have a tendency to drift back toward their original positions, unless some means of maintaining the new position is provided. Changes with age, and discomfort from the eruption of teeth in the infant and with the mixed dentition, can make the wearing of dentures difficult, and the need for changes in the prosthesis frequent.

Dental Occlusion

RETAINING DENTURE. A simple retaining denture made from an impression taken at the time of lip closure will do much to prevent the collapse and shifting of the alveolar arches.

Study casts of the upper jaw made at the time of lip closure allow the dentist to make his impressions with an endotracheal tube in place. Serious airway obstruction can occur in small infants from the use of ungainly impression trays and semisolid impression material unless the impression is done by those having experience in this technique. The head down position can be helpful if an endotracheal tube is not used [67].

EXPANSION DENTURE. Should the lateral maxillary segment be found to be medially placed so that collapse of the upper arch has already occurred, it can be expanded into a more lateral position by the use of *gradual changes in the denture.* The anterior portion of this prosthesis can be cut out to allow the pressure of the lip to move the premaxilla into position.

These expansion dentures are usually worn continuously and are held in place with the aid of a denture powder or paste. Haggerty and, more recently, Georgiade [61–63] have been enthusiastic about mounting metal pins to these prostheses. The pins seat into the maxillary bone to hold the prostheses in place. Though apparently successful, with a few reported drawbacks, they have not been widely adopted. They are removed for cleaning several times a day. At first, the infant can be expected to object violently to the apparatus, and may tolerate it only for short periods. However, infants usually adapt very quickly, and it is more than likely that the infant will become extremely unhappy when the denture is removed, particularly during feeding times. Dentures must be checked frequently and altered or remade as teeth erupt and changes occur. Though simple in principle, they require close and competent dental attention.

A split denture with a jackscrew can be made when the *lateral maxillary* segment is *already collapsed.* The maxilla is then gradually expanded to its proper position. The newly made denture is inserted within a week or less after lip closure since further delay can allow sufficient shifting of the alveolar arch segments to require a new impression being made. When the denture is well accepted, the jackscrew is opened about one-quarter of a turn, three to seven times per week. When fully expanded, the jackscrew is covered with plastic and the expansion denture is then used as a retaining denture.

These expansion techniques are particularly popular in patients with severe complete bilateral clefts. They are often combined with elastic bands on head caps or special prostheses designed to move the protruding premaxilla posteriorly and to reposition it within the maxillary arch.

In patients with severe bilateral clefts, I feel that it is wrong to move the protruding premaxilla back into the upper dental arch. The most severe growth deficiency in these children is in the anteroposterior direction. The most severe facial deformity is a retruded middle third of the face when these children are grown. For this reason, I prefer to keep the premaxilla in a protruding position, expecting the face to catch up with it in time. This is a distracting appearance in the young child, and when it is severe in the school years I will compromise this stand and move it back or trim the protruding labial plate. As these children grow, they seem to have less of the "dished in" facial appearance formerly seen, and the likelihood of a severe Class III malocclusion appears to be much less imminent [73, 74]. The same dental expansion techniques can be carried out in older children and adults, but with increasing age, the movement of bony tissue becomes more difficult [72].

TREATMENT OF PALATAL CLEFTS

Preoperative Considerations

Any elective surgical procedure should be postponed if the child is not in good health and not free from an acute respiratory infection. With an open cleft palate, however, it is virtually impossible in some patients to be completely free from tenacious mucus or even mucopurulent material in the nasopharynx. *Unless an acute inflammatory process* is found, these conditions have not led to operative complications. As mentioned previously, pathological changes in the middle ear are usual. Preoperative antibiotics may be indicated in the rare individual who continues to run a low-grade fever despite repeated attempts to avoid infections [41].

Routine culture of the nasopharynx is practiced in some clinics preoperatively, but I do not find this necessary. Examination of the hemoglobin level, white blood cell count, and routine urinalysis have been sufficient. In particularly difficult cases in older children or adults, crossmatching for a possible blood transfusion is done. Patients are admitted the day before surgery.

Anesthesia

Endotracheal anesthesia probably has been one of the greatest assets to cleft palate surgery. In infants and children it must be handled with even greater skill than in adults. If an experienced anesthesiologist is not available, anesthesia can be administered by insufflation, with a heavy silk suture to hold the tongue forward and with *constant vigilance* to keep the airway clear. This is a poor second choice, but is preferable to inexpert handling of an endotracheal tube.

Operative Considerations

Equipment

The child is positioned at the very end of the table with hyperextension of the neck. This extended position is aided by taking the foot mattress off the usual operating-room table and placing it under the trunk and shoulders.

Intravenous fluids are administered routinely during surgery with an attempt to supply about half of the daily feeding requirement while the patient is asleep. A proper *mouth gag* is essential. It should provide a wide opening of the mouth, fixation of the endotracheal tube, and retraction of the corners of the mouth. The Dingman gag* is particularly good. The Russell-Davies modification of the Kilner, and the Dott, are also good. *Suction* is essential. An *instrument table* placed several inches over the chest allows ready access to a variety of instruments, and permits the anesthesiologist to reach his anesthetic apparatus.

The surgical instruments should include a variety of knife blades, such as the Bard-Parker #15 blade for making incisions, the #11 blade for excising cleft margins, and the #12 blade for reaching out-of-the-way places. The long knife handle is useful. Large and small scissors should be available. Forceps for handling tissues should have teeth, such as those found on the Brown forceps and on the Brown-Addison forceps.† Dural hooks are used to handle the palatal tissues when possible, thus preventing the bruising caused by thumb forceps. I use a Freer septal elevator, a Joseph nasal elevator, the flat palate elevator, the right-angle palate elevator, and the L-shaped palate elevator.†

A small dental "spoon" is helpful as a periosteal elevator in difficult-to-reach areas. Small chisels and a small bone drill are needed at times. A small right-angle knife – Cronin [38, 39] – and a septal knife† are useful in obtaining mucosal flaps from the floor of the nostril; a needle holder (Randall-Brown)† with a hole in the jaws to allow end-on positioning of the needle is useful for suturing in the posterior pharynx.

Closure of the Hard Palate

If the cleft extends through the alveolus, and the palate is closed in two separate steps, it is possible to carry out a lengthening procedure and to avoid the junction of four flaps in the center of the hard palate. When done simultaneously, this has led to a higher instance of fistulas in this area. As noted previously, the alveolar and hard palate clefts can be closed at the time of lip closure, prior to the closure and lengthening of the soft palate, or at the same time as soft palate closure, or closing may be postponed until about 3 to 5 years of age [39].

VOMER FLAP TECHNIQUE. The vomer flap is made by elevating a broad based flap from the cleft side of the vomer, with the base placed superiorly. The lines of incision are injected with a dilute solution of epinephrine (1% lidocaine with epinephrine 1 : 100,000). As little as 1 to 3 ml. of this solution is used, thus distorting the tissues to a minimal degree. At least 7 minutes (by the clock) must be allowed after the injection of this solution for satisfactory hemostasis. The incision in the vomer is carried down to cartilage and bone (Fig. 8-4), and then raised widely by blunt dissection. A second flap of palatal mucosa is raided from the lateral side of the cleft. Slightly more mucosa can be obtained by incising through nasal mucosa down to the nasal side of the palatal shelf and reflecting the mucosa off the edge of the cleft and then off the oral side of the bony cleft. These two flaps are overlapped and secured with through-and-through vertical mattress sutures of 5-0 chromic catgut. The alveolar cleft is closed by raising a pedicle of mucosa and submucosa from the buccal sulcus, and rotating it through the alveolar cleft so as to overlap the anterior edge of the vomer flap. The edges of this buccal flap are sutured to flaps elevated from the edge of the alveolar cleft [40]. The oral side of the vomer flap is left raw; it soon granulates and epithelializes. This operation can be done simultaneously on both sides of a bilateral cleft.

The vomer flap closure is easy, quick, and causes little displacement of tissue. If the cleft is extremely wide, it may be necessary to raise lateral mucosal flaps from the adjacent palate by making an incision at the junction of the palate and gingiva to aid in the closure. Small perforations through the palate in the region of the alveolar ridge are difficult to keep clean, and even though they can be covered by a dental prosthesis, closure with autogenous tissue is preferred, if feasible.

Bone Grafting

After the vomer flap is well healed, a bone graft can be inserted if desired, though I do not do this. In older children I will use a bone graft to stabilize a "floating" premaxilla in bilateral clefts, or as an onlay graft to augment the maxilla under a retruded ala nasi. A pocket is formed between the oral and nasal coverings in the alveolar cleft, and the dissection is carried posterior into the palatal cleft. I prefer rib. The bone is used either as chips or as a wedge plus chips [68]. An *onlay graft* to the *maxilla* can be done at the same time.

A number of *other techniques* have been described which provide mucosal flaps *at the time the bone graft* is done. These flaps can be similar to those illustrated in Figure 8-4; an alternative method is to raise a large flap of vomerine mucosa with its base placed anteriorly. This flap is folded upon itself so that the

*Padgett Instrument Co., 3953 Broadway, Kansas City, Mo. 64111.

†Storz Instrument Company, 3365 Tree Court Industrial Drive, St. Louis, Mo. 63122.

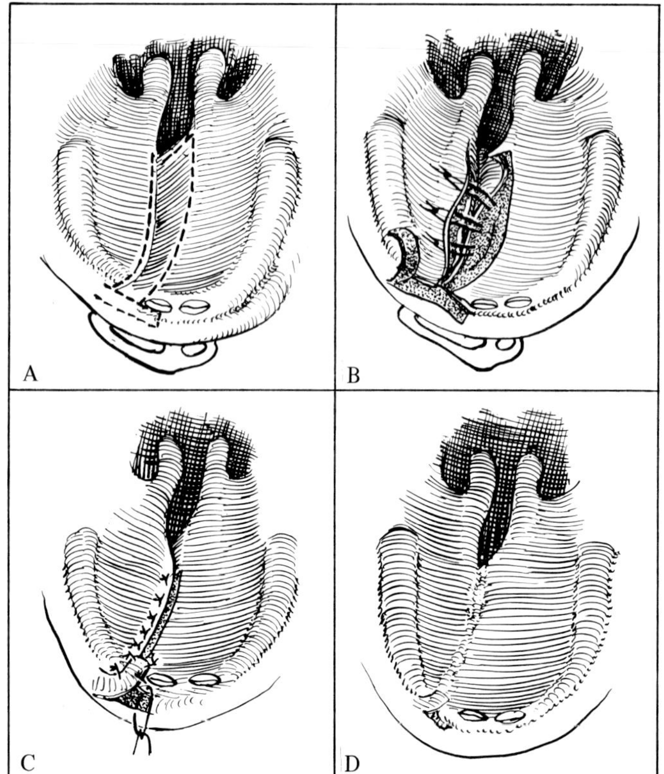

Fig. 8-4. Closure of the alveolar cleft and hard palate cleft by means of a flap of mucosa from the buccal sulcus and another from the vomer. These are interdigitated. The oral side of the vomer flap must granulate and epithelialize. This operation can be done at the time of lip closure or at the time of soft palate closure, or it can be delayed until the child is older, obturating the cleft with a dental "shell" or prosthesis.

base forms the nostril lining and the tip forms the oral lining. Another technique is to slide the mucosa of the nostril floor over the cleft, removing the inferior turbinate and using its mucosa if need be [55, 57, 58, 61, 66, 75, 76, 82–88]. These latter procedures do not allow much opportunity to lengthen the soft palate at the time of soft palate closure. Skoog has preferred a "boneless bone graft" consisting of a large pedicle flap of maxillary periosteum, which is rotated into the alveolar cleft and sutured around a packing of Surgicel.

Closure of the Soft Palate

The *most important* aspect of soft palate closure is the achievement of a *structure which is supple, and moves easily, quickly, and far* enough to *achieve velopharyngeal competence. Its action should be as quick, effortless, and automatic as a blink.* The surgery needed to achieve this end should probably be as careful as that needed on the eyelid.

Kriens [44] has pointed out the malpositioning of the levator palati muscles in the child with a cleft and noted that they insert into the posterior edge of the hard palate in a position which is about 75 degrees out of line with their position in the normal palate. Dickson's [7, 8] excellent study of the anatomy of these abnormal structures has been very useful, noting extension of the muscular insertion along the bony cleft margin. Kriens advocated an *intravelar veloplasty* to correct this malposition, and to help reconstruct the levator mechanism. He uses an end-on approximation in the midline [44]. I feel that the intravelar veloplasty is a very significant improvement in soft palate repair but have preferred to dissect out the levator muscles sufficiently to allow considerable overlapping of the free ends; this technique will be described in detail under the heading Intravelar Veloplasty and Palate Lengthening Technique [49].

Most surgeons prefer a technique for closure of the soft palate which includes lengthening of the palate as well as careful approximation of the cleft margins. Adequate relaxation of the palatal tissue is achieved by lateral relaxing incisions so that closure is completed under *virtually no tension* at all, and mucosa is provided for complete coverage of the nasal side of the repair.

INTRAVELAR VELOPLASTY AND PALATE LENGTHENING TECHNIQUE. The lines of incision are injected with a dilute solution of epinephrine (as noted under Closure of the Hard Palate). The incision is started at about the level of the anterior tonsillar pillar and extended to the lateral side of the posterior maxillary tubercle (Fig. 8-5). It is continued around the posterior maxillary tubercle and forward midway between the palatal vessels and the gingiva. In most cases the incision is *angled posteriorly from the premolar teeth to the posterior edge of the hard palate.* In patients with *clefts* through the *soft palate only, a horseshoe-shaped incision* is made by extending the lateral incisions around anteriorly from one side to the other. This incision is *not carried farther anteriorly* than the *incisive foramen* so as to leave an appreciable amount of mucosa behind the incisor teeth; otherwise, premature eruption of the permanent incisors and contraction of the anterior dental arch is likely to occur.

The *incisions are carried down to bone,* and blunt dissection is used to elevate the palatal flaps between bone and periosteum. The *major palatine vessels* are identified and *isolated.* The dissection is carried out carefully around the greater palatine foramen, and the *palatine vessels are stretched* out of their canals with a blunt instrument (Fig. 8-5). They are carefully preserved. About 1 cm. of length can be obtained by this stretching maneuver, but additional length can be achieved by chiseling off the posterior wall of the major palatine foramen or by dissecting the vessels for a short distance off of the cephalad side of the palatal flap. The edges of the cleft are usually incised, but if the tissues are hypoplastic, the cleft margins are excised.

Blunt dissection with scissors or the index finger is carried down *lateral* to the *pterygoid hamulus* and *lateral* to the *pharyngeal wall.* The oral mucosa of the cleft just anterior to the posterior edge of the hard palate is held by a hook. Scissors are used to dissect along the oral side of the levator muscle, which is quite easy because the mucosa and submucosa on the soft palate are quite thick.

Again using a hook on the nasal mucosa, the dissection is started between the mucosa and the bone. A small "spoon" elevator and then scissors are used extending back between muscle and nasal mucosa. The muscle is then cut free from its attachment to the bony palate and, with great care, dissected away from the nasal mucosa. This mucosa is very thin at this point and the dissection is quite difficult. By so doing, a good flap of the levator muscle is usually obtained, allowing repositioning in the transverse direction and suturing with considerable overlap [49]. If the dissection is difficult, the muscles can be approximated end-to-end in their new (retroplaced) position as suggested by Kriens [44]. The hamulus process is fractured if the closure would otherwise be tight. Occasionally, the levator muscles will be found to be very atrophic. Under these conditions, it can hardly be expected that they will be able to achieve good velopharyngeal closure. I think this is a direct indication to construct a superiorly based posterior pharyngeal flap "primarily" at the same operation.

A large Z-plasty as described by Stark [52] is used to lengthen the nasal mucosa. Another method is to elevate the mucosa from the floor of the nostril as described by Cronin [54]. I have not had any experience with use of the "island flap" for nasal lining [45, 46]. In this technique a sizable piece of anterolateral palatal tissue is cut free with its attached major palatine vessels and is rotated onto the raw nasal surface of the palate for coverage. I have not been able to justify the drastic reduction in blood supply to this dynamic tissue without further evidence of improvement in the end results.

The nasal mucosa is closed with interrupted 5-0 chromic catgut, with the knots being placed on the nasal side. The two levator muscles are then sutured in an overlapped position, using 4-0 chromic catgut. Closure of the oral mucosa is completed mostly with vertical mattress sutures of 5-0 chromic catgut to prevent inversion of the wound edges (5-0 chromic catgut). Simple over-and-over sutures can be used in addition if need be.

The sutures are tied just tightly enough to approximate the cleft margins but not so tight as to cause strangulation of tissue, which would inevitably lead to excess scar. Approximation of the cleft margins should require little or no tension; if it does, then further undermining and relaxation are needed. Further relaxation can be achieved by fracture of the hamulus process with a finger or blunt elevator. Though it has been reported that this could exert an adverse effect on the incidence of middle ear disease, an extensive study by Noone et al. [47] in a series of cases, all of which had one hamulus process fractured and the other not (chosen alternately), failed to reveal any significant difference in regard to middle ear disease.

In older children and in children whose palates are unusually short, the *primary closure* and lengthening of the soft palate are combined with a *posterior pharyngeal flap* procedure. Packing in the lateral incisions is usually not needed unless there is persistent bleeding, or if it is desired to pack along the medial pterygoid plate to prevent reattachment of the separated superior pharyngeal constrictor muscle, or if it is felt advisable to relieve tension still further

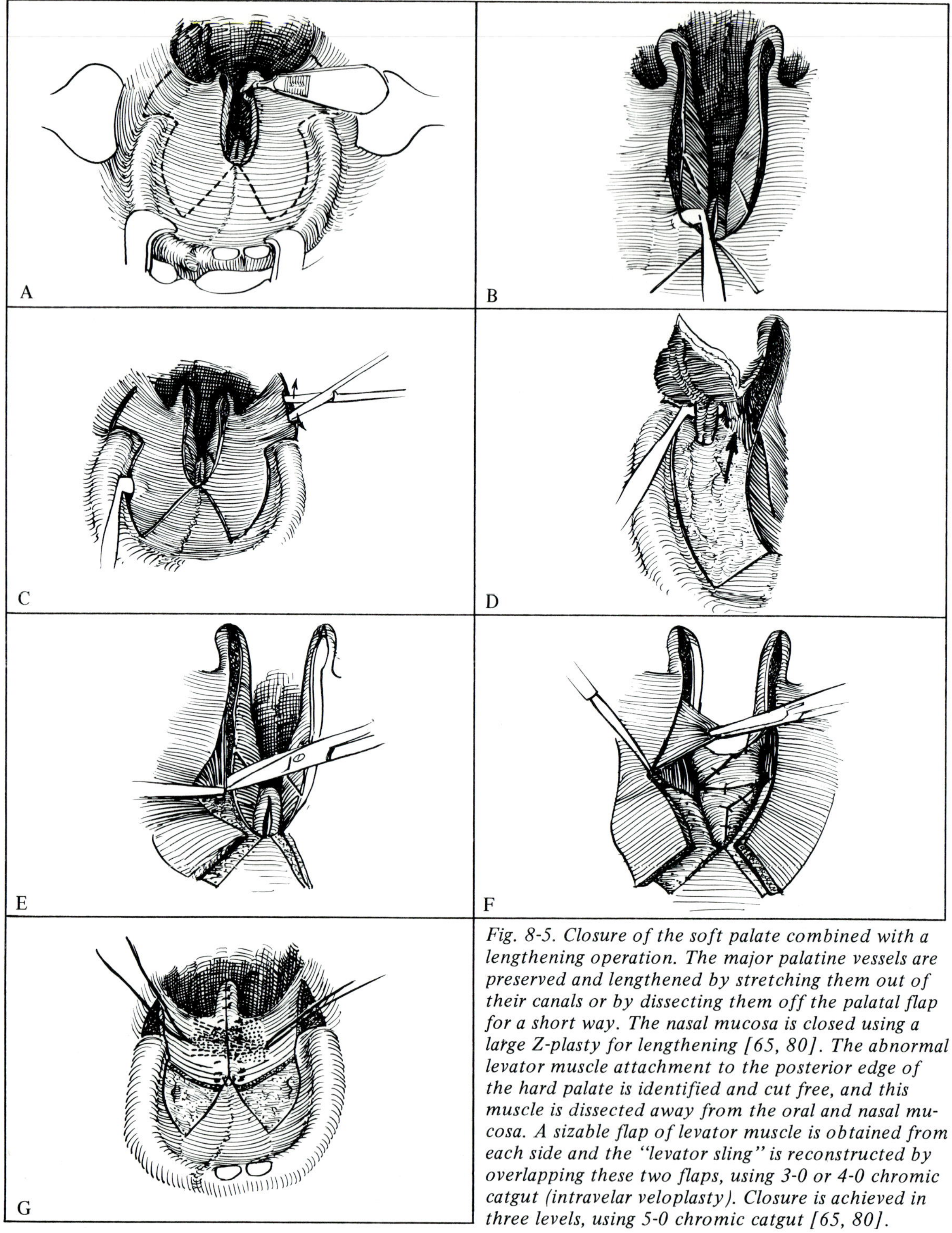

Fig. 8-5. Closure of the soft palate combined with a lengthening operation. The major palatine vessels are preserved and lengthened by stretching them out of their canals or by dissecting them off the palatal flap for a short way. The nasal mucosa is closed using a large Z-plasty for lengthening [65, 80]. The abnormal levator muscle attachment to the posterior edge of the hard palate is identified and cut free, and this muscle is dissected away from the oral and nasal mucosa. A sizable flap of levator muscle is obtained from each side and the "levator sling" is reconstructed by overlapping these two flaps, using 3-0 or 4-0 chromic catgut (intravelar veloplasty). Closure is achieved in three levels, using 5-0 chromic catgut [65, 80].

on the suture line.

In patients with a *short mandible,* a heavy silk suture for retraction of the tongue and a nasotracheal tube can be good precautions to maintain the airway after extubation. *Blood transfusion* is usually not needed, but in older patients, or in prolonged operations, it should be considered. The blood loss is measured during the operation, and when it approximates 10 to 15 percent of the circulating blood volume, replacement is advised [42].

As noted earlier, abnormal collections of fluid have been encountered in the middle ear when a diagnostic myringotomy has been done with the aid of an operating microscope at the time of the palatal surgery. An excellent opportunity to prevent irreversible middle ear injury is available at this time, and such an opportunity should not be overlooked.

Postoperative Care

Clear liquids are given by mouth for about 24 to 48 hours, starting as soon as the child is completely awake from the anesthetic. Thereafter, any liquids and mechanically semiliquid foods may be given, such as milk, junket, custard, gelatin, ice cream, and any pureed foods. Antibiotics and sedation are not used routinely. Elbow splints are used for restraints. Sucking and blowing actions are avoided. The patient is discharged from the hospital in 3 to 5 days, or when the temperature is within normal range, and the oral intake is good. The semiliquid diet, restraints, and avoidance of sucking and blowing actions are continued for about 3 weeks after discharge. Food is offered by cup. If a spoon is used, it is handled by an adult and not by the patient [41].

Three weeks after discharge, the operative site should be well healed, and most of the catgut sutures should have disappeared so that the patient can be allowed to return to normal activity with no limitations on diet. At this point, it is stressed that the child should be brought up as normally as possible, and that the parents must be particularly careful not to provide special attention or limitations unless necessary for other reasons. The parents are urged to talk with their child, and to begin *speech stimulation* with picture books and magazines. Gentle *sucking and blowing exercises,* using whistles, mouth organs, soap bubble pipes, and drinking straws, are carried out several times daily as long as they do not become a chore. *No attempt is made to correct speech errors* at this early age, but attention is directed toward developing a vocabulary, and an outgoing, uninhibited personality, which can be of great help later if speech therapy is needed [92, 93, 96].

Follow-up Care

Return Visits

The patient is seen at yearly intervals, or more frequently if desired. Careful attention is focused on the condition of the palate, the appearance of the ear drums, the hearing acuity and history of ear infections, the condition and position of the teeth, and most importantly on the development of speech. The coordinated efforts of a cleft palate team, which can be helpful in the preoperative decisions, are particularly useful in directing the postoperative care.

Ear Problems

Persistent middle ear effusions are frequent and can lead to hearing impairment, repeated infection, and permanent damage. The ears are examined and audiometric testing is carried out regularly. Examination with a pneumatic otoscope is essential to check the mobility of the drum. Retraction of the drum and cholesteatoma may also be found. With persistent effusion, recurrent infection, or progressive middle ear disease (retraction), myringotomies are done, and general anesthesia is used. The middle ear space is evacuated and plastic tubes or prostheses are placed in the myringotomy openings. The ear canals must be kept dry to avoid infection occurring through the tubes. Children with chronic ear disease should be checked frequently (every few months), particularly during the ages of increased respiratory infection. Audiometric examinations provide a further measure of middle ear infection. *Conservative treatment* is aimed at *preventing permanent changes* and requires close attention [1, 38, 43, 95]. Removal of the tonsils and adenoids is advocated by some for repeated ear infections, yet the bulk of adenoid tissue can be exceedingly important for adequate velopharyngeal competence, particularly if the soft palate is short and its excursion is limited by scar. For this reason, adenoidectomy is not done unless all other methods fail to prevent continued middle ear disease.

On the other hand, if the tonsils are huge, they can cause significant obstruction to the airway postoperatively. I do not hesitate to do a tonsillectomy (not an adenoidectomy) at the time of the soft palate surgery or at the time of a posterior pharyngeal flap under this condition. Some prefer to do this as a separate procedure prior to the palatal surgery.

Speech Problems – Velopharyngeal Incompetence

Though the problems associated with cleft palate are many, the remaining remarks are concentrated on *speech* because, without question, it is the *most important function to be considered.* The surgeon interested in cleft palate surgery should develop a facility for handling children that will encourage relaxed conversational speech at the time of their office follow-up visits. A gentle approach, a conversational tone with parents, the availability of children's picture books, or a school lunchbox full of plastic toys can go a long way in bringing out conversational speech in a young child. Unless the surgeon can do this and evaluate his own results, he is missing the most important measure of his ability and a considerable portion of his own reward. The collaboration of a *competent speech therapist or speech pathologist* is needed for more detailed documentation of information and advice relative to therapy.

A *high percentage* of the patients will develop "normal" speech without evidence of hypernasality, nasal emission, or articulation disorders due to the cleft palate (see p. 207). A *hypernasal tone* is usually the first indication of *velopharyngeal incompetence.* It is often accompanied by *distortion of sibilant* sounds in conversational speech and in simple test words and phrases [89, 90, 92, 93, 96]. Direct observation will reveal the length, flexibility, and the excursion of the palate. If the patient can be induced to say "kah, kah," a good view of the soft palate in motion can be obtained [97, 108]. The presence of scarring, dehiscence, or fistulas should be noted. The excursion of the lateral pharyngeal wall and the presence or absence of Passavant's pad (a forward bulging of the posterior pharyngeal wall) can also be noted. This overactive use of the superior pharyngeal constrictor muscles usually indicates a soft palate that is not achieving full excursion. Direct examinations, however, reveal little concerning the contour of the nasal side of the soft palate, the size of the adenoid tissue, and the ability of the levator palati muscles to approximate the two (see Fig. 8-3).

The simple use of fogging on a hand mirror held under the nose during speech, the blowing away of a piece of tissue placed under the nose, and the observation of "nasal grimacing" are of help in testing for nasal escape [89, 93]. The ability to build up pressure and pronounce the letter "p" repeatedly with the use of a paper "paddle," as advocated by Bzoch to demonstrate this ability or inability, is helpful. Oral panendoscopy, pressure gauges, spirometer tests, sound spectrographic analyses, and instruments for measuring nasal airflow can also aid in the study of velopharyngeal closure, although children in the 2- to 4-year-old age group usually cannot cooperate sufficiently for these tests.

Lateral static x-rays and *cinefluorographic and video techniques* do a far better job of demonstrating the presence or absence of velopharyngeal incompetence. These studies can show whether the patient is achieving velopharyngeal closure consistently; velopharyngeal closure occasionally; closure, but only by virtue of a very active superior pharyngeal constrictor muscle or by the help of a large volume of adenoid tissue; or no kind of velopharyngeal closure [94, 102, 114, 117]. Skolnick has described several anteroposterior views that are helpful in pointing out the level of the maximal lateral pharyngeal wall excursion [118, 119].

In general, if *velopharyngeal competence* can be demonstrated, and *speech distortions are present* due to *incompetency,* such a patient should be given *speech therapy* to see if he can be taught to use his palate properly. If closure is borderline and speech is good to excellent, further surgery is difficult to justify.

As experience is gained with examination techniques, it becomes evident that two postoperative conditions are especially common:

1. Velopharyngeal closure can be achieved but barely so; this might be called "touch closure," the soft palate barely touching the posterior pharyngeal wall.
2. Velopharyngeal closure can be achieved only by marked action of the superior pharyngeal constrictors (seen on the x-rays as an obliteration of the air shadow with the nasal side of the soft palate at a distance of 2 to 3 mm. from the posterior pharyngeal wall or by a definite forward movement of the posterior pharyngeal wall).

If speech is poor under these conditions, and remains so after competent speech therapy, *such patients are usually good candidates for a secondary surgical procedure.* Furthermore, it seems warranted to be extremely critical of the speech in these patients, when studies demonstrate only borderline velopharyngeal closure. The reason is that even though speech distortions are slight, a secondary surgical procedure has usually brought the level of speech well within the normal range in such cases. In addition, it has allowed these children to articulate with so much less effort that the patient will frequently become appreciably more relaxed and happier as a result [115].

Obviously, if there is *marked velopharyngeal incompetence,* there is *little reason to attempt even a trial period of speech therapy,* and a great deal can be gained by providing a competent palatal mechanism at the earliest possible age.

Velopharyngeal incompetence is seen in a number of conditions in the absence of clefts of the palate. This may be the result of a congenitally short palate, deficiencies in neuromuscular action, a congenitally large nasopharynx (often associated with cervical spine anomalies), and deficiencies due to ablative surgery and trauma. Many of the tests for palatal incompetence and the techniques for correcting incompetence are applicable to these patients [116]. In most patients, if marked incompetence is present, it can be demonstrated by the age of 3 to 5 years. Occasionally it can be verified at the age of 2 or 3 [117, 119].

SECONDARY PALATAL PROCEDURES

Palatal Fistulas

Palatal fistulas are bothersome because they permit leakage of fluid into the nose, the packing of food particles into crevices producing uncleanliness, and the leakage of air into the nose causing articulation distortions, particularly with sibilant sounds. These speech distortions are usually not great.

Closing a palatal fistula can be among the most difficult of all surgical techniques. Each failure and the scarring it produces makes additional attempts more difficult. In general, the tissue adjacent to a palatal fistula, particularly in the region of the hard palate, is *not elastic.* Closure must be achieved with the complete excision of the *epithelium of the fistula,* though occasionally this tissue can be used as turnover flaps to aid in the closure. *Complete relaxation* of the adjacent tissue is absolutely necessary, so that closure can be achieved without tension and preferably with the use of a fine surgical suture (such as 5-0 chromic catgut). In the region of the *hard palate,* this usually requires raising a surprisingly *large adjacent pedicle flap* and freeing it to the extent that it can literally fall or drop into place without tension. During the dissection, care must be taken to preserve the blood supply because it is usually limited at best. *All sutures must be tied loosely* to prevent strangulation and necrosis. Occasionally in the soft palate area, relaxation incisions are adequate, but usually a formal repair is required. Closure in two layers is preferred if possible, but it is not always necessary or feasible. The closure of palatal fistulas is a good example of a big operation being needed for a small defect.

THE TREATMENT OF VELOPHARYNGEAL INCOMPETENCE

Posterior Pharyngeal Flap

The use of a posterior pharyngeal flap is discussed in detail in this section. Other types of palatopharyngoplasties and palatal lengthening procedures may be more popular elsewhere, but I have found their results to be disappointing. My experience with these other techniques is also insufficient to discuss them in detail.

The *superiorly based posterior pharyngeal flap* is the pharyngoplasty most favored in the United States and Canada (Fig. 8-6). It can be raised with sufficient length to reach even the shortest soft palate and its base is located near the usual site of velopharyngeal closure so that as it contracts, it tends to pull the soft palate in this direction. To attach such a flap usually requires reopening the soft palate repair. It is located at a high level where there may be less superior pharyngeal constrictor motion, and it is almost impossible to reach if the lateral openings are found to be too large or too small. It is often difficult, even on x-ray examination, to tell the difference between superiorly and inferiorly based flaps, as each tends to approach the same point during the healing process.

The *Inferiorly based posterior pharyngeal flap* is constructed more easily than the superiorly based flap. It has the advantages of acting somewhat as a sounding board to direct the airstream into the mouth, it may well be located at a level where the greatest amount of lateral pharyngeal wall motion takes place, its construction does not require opening the soft palate repair, and it lends itself well to secondary procedures that may be needed to make the lateral openings larger or smaller [101, 111, 113, 122].

Retrospective studies by Skoog [87] and Hamlen [103], and a prospective study by Whitaker, Randall, and co-workers [122], have failed to show appreciable differences between the superiorly and inferiorly based flap. Accordingly, I usually prefer the superiorly based flap, but if exposure is difficult, if the patient is in poor condition, or if the palate is so mobile that one would be reluctant to make a through-and-through incision in the soft palate, I would prefer to use the inferiorly based posterior pharyngeal flap. On the other hand, if the space to be bridged is great, a superiorly based flap must be used, or the palate would have to be lengthened at the same operation. If the x-ray examination described by Skolnick [118] shows the maximal lateral pharyngeal wall motion to be "high" rather than "low," the superiorly based flap should be better, and vice versa. If the amount of incompetence is very slight but with good palatal movement, in all likelihood, any method of secondary palatal correction should have a good result [113, 122, 123].

The technique for the posterior pharyngeal flap requires endotracheal anesthesia, a good mouth gag, and a local injection with 1% lidocaine with epinephrine 1 : 100,000. An incision is made longitudinally through the mucosa on each side of the posterior pharyngeal wall at its junction with the lateral pharyngeal wall (Fig. 8-6), thus constructing a very wide flap. When the flap is used as a primary posterior pharyngeal flap in conjunction with primary closure of the cleft palate, I usually prefer to make the flap only one-half to two-thirds the total width of the posterior pharynx. Each incision is carried down through the pharyngeal constrictor muscle to the prevertebral fascia by blunt scissor dissection, and then medially along the prevertebral fascia, either by curved scissors or by a palate elevator, until the dissection from the opposite side is reached, thus raising a flap of mucosa and the superior pharyngeal constrictor muscle. If the flap is to be based superiorly, it is cut across transversely about as far as one can

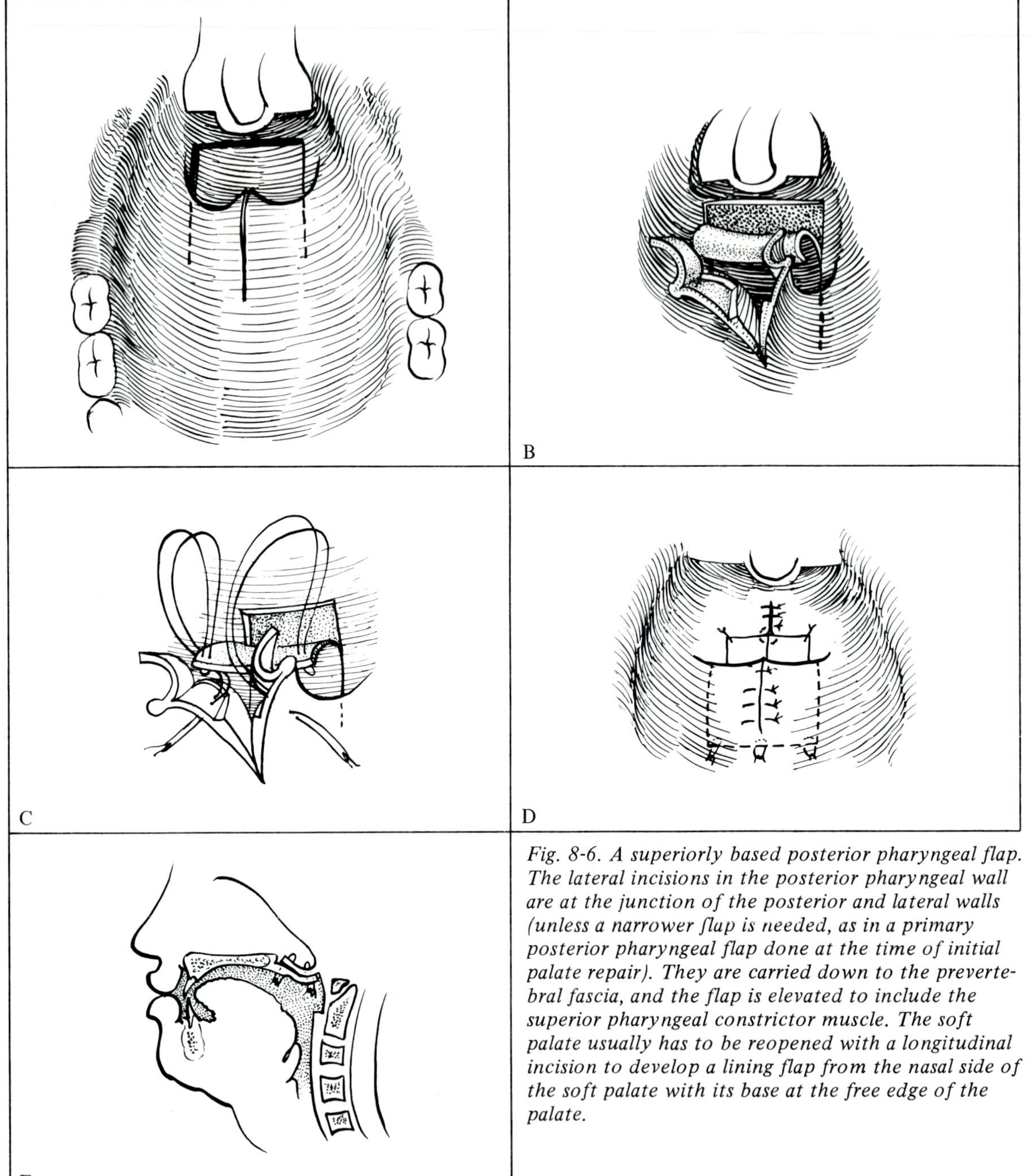

Fig. 8-6. A superiorly based posterior pharyngeal flap. The lateral incisions in the posterior pharyngeal wall are at the junction of the posterior and lateral walls (unless a narrower flap is needed, as in a primary posterior pharyngeal flap done at the time of initial palate repair). They are carried down to the prevertebral fascia, and the flap is elevated to include the superior pharyngeal constrictor muscle. The soft palate usually has to be reopened with a longitudinal incision to develop a lining flap from the nasal side of the soft palate with its base at the free edge of the palate.

reach down the pharynx. If it is to be based inferiorly, the palate is retracted and the flap cut across just below the adenoid pad. The lateral margins of the donor area are approximated with interrupted 3-0 chromic catgut, and if this approximation tends to pull the edges away from the prevertebral fascia, the sutures can include prevertebral fascia to obliterate this dead space. A needle holder with a hole in the jaws to allow "end-on position of the needle" (Randall-Brown needle holder*) can be very helpful under these conditions. Some surgeons prefer to leave the donor site open.

Occasionally, the soft palate will be loose enough so that it can be everted and a satisfactory flap of mucosa raised from the nasal side of the soft palate. More usually, the *incision* in the midline of the *soft palate* must be reopened and nasal mucosal flaps elevated on either side to line the underside of the posterior pharyngeal flap. Closure is achieved with a through-and-through 3-0 chromic catgut suture holding each corner and a third one through the center of the flap. The edges of the flap are sutured to the recipient site with simple 3-0 chromic catgut. The turnover lining flaps of nasal mucosa are held in place with 5-0 chromic catgut and the palate closed in layers with 4-0 or 5-0 chromic catgut. The lateral openings should be about the size of the tip of an average curved hemostat. This flap can survive even when sutured under a slight amount of tension, *but with undue tension it is doomed to failure.* Most authors who favor the superiorly based flap stress that its insertion should be "high" and close to the posterior edge of the hard palate [112, 113].

In patients with *scarred posterior pharyngeal walls,* and in those whose palates are long, the Trauner procedure has been helpful. The soft palate is displaced posteriorly until it touches the posterior pharyngeal wall. At this point a transverse incision is made in both surfaces, and the soft palate is fixed to the posterior pharyngeal wall with through-and through sutures [121].

Three steps are suggested to ensure an adequate airway postoperatively. If a child is small,if the mandible is short, or if bleeding has been a problem, it is probably wise to insert a nasopharyngeal airway, either at the time the posterior pharyngeal flap is sutured into place or at the end of the operation. If difficulty is encountered in passing such a tube, a small tube can be passed first and used as a guide. This can even be placed in a retrograde manner if need be. Secondly, a tongue suture of heavy (0 or #1) silk can be placed. A deep bite should be taken far back in the tongue, a big loop tied, and the ends taped loosely to the cheek. If it is necessary to retract the tongue, it must be held by hand. Taping it in the retracted position cannot be relied on. Finally, if the tonsils are huge, they should be removed at the beginning of the operation since the nasopharyngeal space will be constricted by the surgical procedure.

*Storz Instrument Company, 3365 Tree Court Industrial Drive, St. Louis, Mo. 63122.

Other Operations for Velopharyngeal Incompetence

PALATAL LENGTHENING. Various lengthening operations when used alone have been disappointing in overcoming velopharyngeal incompetence. A lengthening procedure combined with repositioning and reconstruction of the levator muscles has gained popularity in the United States and may be worthwhile if these steps were not taken at the time of the initial palatal repair.

POSTERIOR PHARYNGEAL AUGMENTATION. The *insertion of retropharyngeal implants* of various kinds to build the posterior pharyngeal wall forward is another approach to the problem of velopharyngeal incompetence. This is particularly valuable when the incompetence is very small (2 to 3 mm. gap in lateral cephalometric x-rays) and the excursion of the soft palate is good. Shredded Teflon in glycerine seems to be the most reliable material, but these patients must be selected carefully and this material loses about 50 percent of its initial volume after absorption of the glycerine [100].

The *Hynes pharyngoplasty,* which is designed to augment the posterior pharynx with bilateral superiorly based mucosal and salpingopharyngeal muscle flaps, is held in more favor in the British Isles than in the United States. Though it obviously achieves good results in the hands of many surgeons and does have contractility, it has the drawback of providing the least amount of excursion at the midpoint posteriorly where the most amount of correction is needed. It is a good procedure when a small amount of improvement is needed [106, 107]. The flaps, as described by Hynes, when inserted into the soft palate, as described by Moore [110] and Sullivan [120], are also effective, although concomitant series comparing this technique with others have not been forthcoming.

Lateral pharyngeal flaps, as described by Kapetansky [109], appear to preserve more of the superior pharyngeal constrictor muscle, but this technique requires the separation of the levator muscles at the site of inset of the flaps. This would appear to be a disadvantage. Approximation of the posterior tonsillar pillars apparently provides significant speech improvement but does not seem to improve the function at the level of the levator muscle.

From the number and variety of secondary palatopharyngoplasties started over 100 years ago by Passavant and Rosenthal, it is apparent that there are many ways to improve palatal function. It should be noted that there are also a number of ways in which the mechanism can be deficient, so that in studying these patients, the possible cause for the incompetence should be looked for.

Postoperative Care Following Treatment of Velopharyngeal Incompetence
Postoperatively, these patients are handled in much the same way as those with primary cleft palate repairs. Antibiotics are seldom used, and if healing progresses rapidly, the time schedule is accelerated. Postoperative changes in speech have been fascinating. Some patients achieve immediate and lasting "normal" speech, whereas a few may show only slight improvement. Hypernasality has almost always been diminished or obliterated. Some patients have shown initial improvement, apparently due to postoperative swelling and blood-clot formation, which is then followed by a degeneration almost to the preoperative level. Usually these patients will continue to have poor speech until the operative area becomes comfortable and the tissues soft and pliable. When the patient becomes aware of how to use this newly constructed mechanism, a gradual and steady improvement in speech should be observed. With these patients the addition of *speech therapy* can be very helpful.

Many *older patients,* however, have been so accustomed to hearing their voice with hypernasal characteristics and articulatory distortions that speech produced in a nonnasal manner with good crisp articulation will sound distinctly abnormal to them. Under these conditions, it is difficult to teach these patients to speak normally even though they may possess the mechanisms to do so. The "overcorrection" of the problem with very small lateral ports, as described by Hogan [104, 105], can be useful under these conditions even if the openings have to be made larger at a later date. A tape recorder to allow the patient to hear his own voice as others hear him can be helpful.

Occasionally these posterior pharyngeal flaps produce hyponasal speech because the lateral openings are too small. This is usually due to edema and is transient. If it should persist, the lateral openings should be made larger by the Z-plasty technique. Rarely the openings are too large and have to be made smaller by a reverse Z-plasty technique.

Palatal Prostheses and Orthodontia

When a *postoperative cleft palate is so scarred* that secondary cleft palate procedures have failed or would seem very likely to fail, the use of a *prosthesis* is usually indicated. Under these conditions, the skill of a good prosthodontist is tremendously appreciated. It should be recognized that such conditions are far from ideal for a good prosthetic result, and it is unjustified to criticize the poor result with a prosthesis when such unsatisfactory conditions prevail. The time-honored Gillies-Fry procedure and the use of an external skin-tube pedicle or a pedicle preferably of tissue from the tongue or nasal septum may be an occasional alternate procedure [45, 47].

A pharyngeal prosthesis is advocated by some as a preliminary step to secondary palatal surgery. It is used to stimulate contraction of the superior pharyngeal constrictor muscle, thus presumably improving the function of this muscle postoperatively. A forked pharyngeal prosthesis can be useful after a posterior pharyngeal flap in those patients with persistent postoperative hypernasality and lack of superior pharyngeal constrictor activity. It functions as a temporary obturator, again stimulating superior pharyngeal constrictor action [99].

An alternative procedure is to construct a *palatal lift prosthesis* if the soft palate can be elevated to touch the posterior pharyngeal wall. This simply holds the palate upward and backward into a more closed position. Though causing tension and pressure on the palate, at times the prosthesis can be gradually reduced and even removed without losing the degree of palatal competence.

Routine dental care in patients with cleft palates is extremely important because there is an increased tendency to develop dental caries, and because many of these patients require orthodontia. Unless teeth are sound, orthodontic procedures cannot be carried out. There has been considerable enthusiasm, as noted previously, for shifting alveolar segments either prior to the eruption of teeth, or in infants with deciduous teeth. The *shifting of individual teeth,* however, is usually postponed until eruption of the permanent dentition, at which time the replacement, or repositioning of missing, malpositioned, or deformed teeth is carried out.

The *overall care* of patients with cleft palates is a *continuing care* concerned with *many different factors* and requiring observation throughout the formative and early adult years. The *cooperative efforts of a number of specialists* are usually needed.

REFERENCES

Anatomy, Embryology, Etiology, and Classification

1. Bluestone, C. D. Eustachian tube obstruction in the infant with cleft palate. *Otol. Rhinol. Laryngol.* 29:Suppl. 2, 1971.
2. Brescia, N. J. Anatomy of the Lip and Palate. In Grabb, W. C., Rosenstein, S. W., and Bzoch, K. R. (Eds.), *Cleft Lip and Palate.* Boston: Little, Brown, 1971.

3. Brogan, W. F., and Woodings, T. L. A decline in the incidence of cleft lip and palate in Western Australia, 1963 to 1972. *Med. J. Aust.* 2:8, 1974.
4. Broomhead, I. W. The nerve supply of the muscles of the soft palate. *Br. J. Plast. Surg.* 4:1, 1951.
5. Calnan, J. The error of Gustav Passavant. *Plast. Reconstr. Surg.* 13:275, 1954.
6. Cohlan, S. Q. Excessive intake of vitamin A as a cause of congenital anomalies in the rat. *Science* 117:535, 1953.
7. Dickson, D. R. Anatomy of the normal velopharyngeal mechanism. *Clin. Plast. Surg.* 2:235, 1975.
8. Dickson, D. R., and Dickson, W. M. Velopharyngeal anatomy. *J. Speech Hear. Res.* 15:372, 1972.
9. Fara, M., and Dvorak, J. The Musculature of Cleft Lip and Palate. In Converse, J. M. (Ed.), *Reconstructive Plastic Surgery* (2nd ed.). Philadelphia: Saunders, 1977.
10. Fogh-Andersen, P. *Inheritance of Harelip and Cleft Palate,* NYT Nordisk Forlag. Copenhagen: A. Busck, 1942.
11. Fraser, F. C. Etiology of cleft lip and palate. *Am. J. Hum. Genet.* 22:125, 1970.
12. Fraser, F. C. Etiology of Cleft Lip and Palate. In Grabb, W. C., Rosenstein, S. W., and Bzoch, K. R. (Eds.), *Cleft Lip and Palate.* Boston: Little, Brown, 1971.
13. Fritzell, B. The velopharyngeal muscles in speech. *Acta Otolaryngol.* [Suppl.] (Stockh.), 1969. P. 250.
14. Gray, H. *Anatomy of the Human Body* (28th ed.), Goss, C. M. (Ed.). Philadelphia: Lea & Febiger, 1966.
15. Harkins, C. S., Berlin, A., Harding, R. L., Longacre, J. J., and Snodgrasse, R. M. A classification of cleft lip and cleft palate. *Plast. Reconstr. Surg.* 29:31, 1962.
16. Ivy, R. H. Modern concept of cleft lip and cleft palate management. *Plast. Reconstr. Surg.* 9:121, 1952.
17. Jordan, R. E., Kraus, B. S., and Neptune, C. M. Dental abnormalities associated with cleft lip and/or palate. *Cleft Palate J.* 3:22, 1966.
18. Kalter, H., and Warkany, J. Experimental production of congenital malformations in strains of inbred mice by maternal treatment with hypervitaminosis A. *Am. J. Pathol.* 38:1, 1961.
19. Kernahan, D. H., and Stark, R. B. A new classification for cleft lip and cleft palate. *Plast. Reconstr. Surg.* 22:435, 1958.
20. Kitamura, H., and Kraus, B. S. Visceral variations and defects associated with cleft lip and palate in human fetuses: A macroscopic description. *Cleft Palate J.* 1:99, 1964.
21. Kraus, B. S. Some aspects of the anatomy of normal and cleft palate development in man. Presented at meeting of the American Cleft Palate Association, Los Angeles, April 1964.
22. Kriens, O. Anatomy of the velopharyngeal area in cleft palate. *Clin. Plast. Surg.* 2:261, 1975.
23. Krogman, W. M. The problem of cleft palate face. *Plast. Reconstr. Surg.* 14:370, 1954.
24. Lindemann, G., Riis, B., and Sewerin, I. Prevalence of cleft uvula among 2,732 Danes. *Cleft Palate J.* 14:226, 1977.
25. Maue-Dickson, W. Cleft lip and palate research: An updated state of the art: II. Anatomy and physiology. *Cleft Palate J.* 14:270, 1977.
26. Meskin, L. H., Gorlin, R. J., and Isaacson, R. J. Abnormal morphology of the soft palate: I. The prevalence of cleft uvula. *Cleft Palate J.* 1:342, 1964.
27. Meskin, L. H., Gorlin, R. J., and Isaacson, R. J. Abnormal morphology of the soft palate: II. The genetics of cleft uvula. *Cleft Palate J.* 2:40, 1964.
28. Patten, B. M. Embryology of the Palate and Maxillofacial Region. In Grabb, W. C., Rosenstein, S. W., and Bzoch, K. R. (Eds.), *Cleft Lip and Palate.* Boston: Little, Brown, 1971.
29. Peer, L. A., Strean, L. P., Walker, J. C., Jr., Bernhard, W. G., and Peck, G. C. Study of 400 pregnancies with birth of cleft lip-palate infants: Protective effect of folic acid and vitamin B_6 therapy. *Plast. Reconstr. Surg.* 22:442, 1958.
30. Randall, P. A triangular flap operation for the primary repair of unilateral clefts of the lip. *Plast. Reconstr. Surg.* 23:331, 1959.
31. Skolnick, M. L. Velopharyngeal function in cleft palate. *Clin. Plast. Surg.* 2:285, 1975.
32. Stark, R. B. The pathogenesis of harelip and cleft palate. *Plast. Reconstr. Surg.* 13:20, 1954.
33. Veau, V. *Division Palatine.* Paris: Masson, 1931.
34. Walker, B. E. The association of mucopolysaccharides with morphogenesis of the palate and other structures in mouse embryos. *J. Embryol. Exp. Morphol.* 9:22, 1961.
35. Walker, B. E., and Crain, B., Jr. Effects of hypervitaminosis A on palate development in two strains of mice. *Am. J. Anat.* 107:49, 1960.
36. Warkany, J., Roth, C. B., and Wilson, J. G. Multiple congenital malformations: A consideration of etiologic factors. *Pediatrics* 1:462, 1948.
37. Woolf, C. M., Woolf, R. M., and Broadbent, T. R. Genetic and nongenetic variables related to cleft lip and palate. *Plast. Reconstr. Surg.* 32:65, 1963.

General Patient Care and Primary Palatal Procedures

38. Cronin, T. D. Method of preventing raw area on nasal surface of soft palate in push-back surgery. *Plast. Reconstr. Surg.* 20:474, 1957.
39. Cronin, T. D. Pushback Palatorrhaphy with Nasal Mucosal Flaps. In Grabb, W. C., Rosenstein, S. W., and Bzoch, K. R. (Eds.), *Cleft Lip and Palate.* Boston: Little, Brown, 1971.

40. Dunn, F. S. Results of the vomer flap technic used in surgery of the cleft palate during the past eleven years. *Am. J. Surg.* 92:825, 1956.
41. Grabb, W. C. General Aspects of Cleft Palate Surgery. In Grabb, W. C., Rosenstein, S. W., and Bzoch, K. R. (Eds.), *Cleft Lip and Palate.* Boston: Little, Brown, 1971.
42. Holdsworth, W. G. *Cleft Lip and Palate* (3rd ed.). London: Heineman, 1963.
43. Hotz, M., Gnoinski, W., and Nussbaumer, H. Early maxillary orthopedics in cleft lip and palate cases. Presented at the Third International Congress on Cleft Palate and Related Craniofacial Anomalies. Toronto, June 1977.
44. Kriens, O. B. Fundamental anatomic findings for an intravelar veloplasty. *Cleft Palate J.* 7:27, 1970.
45. Millard, D. R., Jr. Wide and/or short cleft palate. *Plast. Reconstr. Surg.* 29:40, 1962.
46. Millard, D. R., Batstone, J. H. F., Heycock, M. H., and Bensen, J. F. Ten years with the palatal island flap. *Plast. Reconstr. Surg.* 46:540, 1970.
47. Noone, R. B., Randall, P., Stool, S., Hamilton, R. W., and Winchester, R. A. The effect on middle ear disease of fracture of the pterygoid hamulus during palatoplasty. *Cleft Palate J.* 10:23, 1973.
48. Paradise, J. L., and Bluestone, C. D. On the universality of otitis media in fifty infants with cleft palate. *Pediatrics* 44:35, 1969.
49. Randall, P. Muscle Reconstruction in Cleft Palate Repair. *Transactions of the Sixth International Congress of Plastic and Reconstructive Surgery.* Paris: Masson, 1976.
50. Randall, P. The Robin Anomalad: Micrognathia and Glossoptosis with Airway Obstruction. In Converse, J. M. (Ed.), *Reconstructive Plastic Surgery* (2nd ed.). Philadelphia: Saunders, 1977.
51. Slaughter, W. B., and Pruzansky, S. The rationale for velar closure as a primary procedure in the repair of cleft palate defects. *Plast. Reconstr. Surg.* 13:341, 1954.
52. Stark, D. B. Nasal lining in partial cleft palate repair. *Plast. Reconstr. Surg.* 32:75, 1963.
53. Stool, S., and Randall, P. Unexpected ear disease in cleft palate patients. *Cleft Palate J.* 4:99, 1967.

Bone Grafting and Maxillary Orthopedics

54. Adisman, I. K. Cleft Palate Prosthetics. In Grabb, W. C., Rosenstein, S. W., and Bzoch, K. R. (Eds.), *Cleft Lip and Palate.* Boston: Little, Brown, 1971.
55. Backdahl, M., Nordin, K. E., Hylen, B., and Strombeck, J. D. Bone Grafts to the Maxillary Defect in Cleft Lip and Palate by the Method of Backdahl and Nordin. *Transactions of the Third International Congress of Plastic Surgery* (1963). Amsterdam: Excerpta Medica, 1964.
56. Brauer, R. O., and Cronin, T. D. Maxillary orthopedics and anterior palate repair with bone grafting. *Cleft Palate J.* 1:3, 1964.
57. Brauer, R. O., and Cronin, T. D. Maxillary Orthopedics and Bone Grafting in Cleft Palate. In Converse, J. M. (Ed.), *Reconstructive Plastic Surgery.* Philadelphia: Saunders, 1964.
58. Burston, W. R. The Pre-surgical Orthopaedic Correction of the Maxillary Deformity in Clefts of Both Primary and Secondary Palate. *Transactions of the International Society of Plastic Surgeons* (Second Congress). Edinburgh: Livingstone, 1960.
59. Burston, W. R. The early orthodontic treatment of alveolar clefts. *Proc. R. Soc. Med.* 58:767, 1965.
60. Friede, H., and Johanson, B. A follow-up study of cleft children treated with primary bone grafting: I. Orthodontic aspects. *Scand. J. Plast. Reconstr. Surg.* 8:88, 1974.
61. Georgiade, N. C. Varying concepts in bone grafting of alveolar palatal defects. *Cleft Palate J.* 1:43, 1964.
62. Georgiade, N. C. The management of premaxillary and maxillary segments in the newborn cleft palate patient. *Cleft Palate J.* 7:411, 1970.
63. Georgiade, N. C., and Latham, R. A. Maxillary arch alignment in the bilateral cleft lip and palate infant, using the pinned coaxial screw appliance. *Plast. Reconstr. Surg.* 56:52, 1975.
64. Harding, R. L., and Maxaheri, M. Growth and spatial changes in the arch in bilateral cleft lip and palate patients. *Plast. Reconstr. Surg.* 50:591, 1972.
65. Hellquist, R. Jaw orthopedic and orthodontic treatment for cleft lip and palate patients in the Uppsala region of Sweden. *Scand. J. Plast. Reconstr. Surg.* 4:11, 1970.
66. Hotz, R. (Ed.). *Early Treatment of Cleft Lip and Palate.* Berne: Hans Huber, 1964.
67. Jacobson, B. N., and Rosenstein, S. W. Early maxillary orthopedics: A combination appliance. *Cleft Palate J.* 2:369, 1965.
68. Johansen, B., and Ohlsson, A. Bone grafting and dental orthopaedics in primary and secondary cases of cleft lip and palate. *Acta Chir. Scand.* 122:112, 1961.
69. Jolleys, A., and Robertson, N. R. E. A study of the effects of early bone-grafting in complete clefts of lip and palate – 5 year study. *Br. J. Plast. Surg.* 25:229, 1972.
70. Matthews, D., Chir, M., and Broomhead, I. Early and late bone grafting in cases of cleft lip and palate. *Br. J. Plast. Surg.* 23:115, 1970.
71. Mazaheri, M., Harding, R. L., and Nanda, S. The effects of surgery on maxillary growth and cleft

width. *Plast. Reconstr. Surg.* 40:22, 1967.

72. McNeil, C. K. *Oral and Facial Deformity.* London: Pitman, 1954.
73. Monroe, C. W., Griffith, B. H., and McKinney, P. Surgical recession of the premaxilla and its effect on maxillary growth in patients with bilateral clefts. *Cleft Palate J.* 7:784, 1970.
74. Monroe, C. W., and Rosenstein, S. W. Maxillary Orthopedics and Bone Grafting in Cleft Palate. In Grabb, W. C., Rosenstein, S. W., and Bzoch, K. R. (Eds.), *Cleft Lip and Palate.* Boston: Little, Brown, 1971.
75. Nordin, K-E. Bone Grafting to the Alveolar Process Clefts following Orthodontic Treatment of Secondary Cleft Palate Deformity. *Transactions of the International Society of Plastic Surgeons* (First Congress). Baltimore: Williams & Wilkins, 1957.
76. Nylen, B., Korlof, B., Arnander, C., Leanderson, R., Barr, B., and Nordin, K-E. Primary early bone grafting in complete clefts of the lip and palate: A follow-up study of 53 cases. *Scand. J. Plast. Reconstr. Surg.* 8:79, 1974.
77. Pruzansky, S. Pre-surgical orthopedics and bone grafting for infants with cleft lip and palate: A dissent. *Cleft Palate J.* 1:164, 1964.
78. Pruzansky, S., and Aduss, H. Arch form and the deciduous occlusion in complete unilateral clefts. *Cleft Palate J.* 1:411, 1964.
79. Rehrmann, A. Bone Grafting in Cleft Palate Repair. In Gibson, T. (Ed.), *Modern Trends in Plastic Surgery.* London: Butterworth, 1964.
80. Rehrmann, A., Koberg, W. R., and Koch, H. Long-term postoperative results of primary and secondary bone grafting in complete cleft of the lip and palate. *Cleft Palate J.* 7:207, 1970.
81. Ritsila, V., Alhopuro, S., Gylling, U., and Rintala, A. The use of free periosteum for bone formation in congenital clefts of the maxilla. *Scand. J. Plast. Reconstr. Surg.* 6:57, 1972.

81a. Rosenstein, S. W., and Jacobson, B. N. Early maxillary orthopedics: a sequence of events. *Cleft Palate J.* 4:197, 1967.

82. Schmid, E. Die aufbanende Kieferkamplastik. *Os. Z. Stomatol.* 51:582, 1954.
83. Schmid, E. Die Osteoplastik bei Lippen-Kiefer-Gaumenspalten. *Langenbecks Arch. Klin. Chir.* 295:868, 1960.
84. Schuchardt, K., and Pfeifer, G. Primary and secondary operations for cleft palate. *J. Int. Coll. Surg.* 38:237, 1962.
85. Schuchardt, K., Pfeifer, G., and Kriens, O. Primary Osteoplasty in Patients with Cleft Lip Alveolus and Palate. *Transactions of the Fourth International Congress of Plastic and Reconstructive Surgery* (1967). Amsterdam: Excerpta Medica, 1969.
86. Schultz, R. D. A survey of European and Scandinavian bone grafting procedures for cleft palate deformities. *Cleft Palate J.* 1:188, 1964.
87. Skoog, T. *Plastic Surgery.* Philadelphia: Saunders, 1974.
88. Stellmach, R. Primare Knochenplastik bei Lippen-Kiefer-Gaumenspalten am Sauglingunterbesunderer Berucksichtigung der Transplantatdeckung. *Langenbecks Arch. Klin. Chir.* 292: 865, 1959.

Speech

89. Bzoch, K. R. Articulation proficiency and error patterns in pre-school cleft palate and normal children. *Cleft Palate J.* 2:340, 1965.
90. Bzoch, K. R. Etiological Factors Related to Cleft Palate Speech. In Grabb, W. C., Rosenstein, S. W., and Bzoch, K. R. (Eds.), *Cleft Lip and Palate.* Boston: Little, Brown, 1971.
91. Calnan, J. S. Movement of the soft palate. *Br. J. Plast. Surg.* 5:286, 1953.
92. McWilliams, B. J. Speech and language problems in children with cleft palate. *J. Am. Med. Wom. Assoc.* 21:1005, 1966.
93. Morley, M. E. *Cleft Palate and Speech* (6th ed.). Edinburgh: Livingstone, 1966.
94. Nylen, B. O. Cleft palate and speech. *Acta Radiol.* [Suppl.] (Stockh.) 203, 1961.
95. Shelton, R. L. Oral Sensory Function in Speech Production. In Grabb, W. C., Rosenstein, S. W., and Bzoch, K. R. (Eds.), *Cleft Lip and Palate.* Boston: Little, Brown, 1971.
96. Spriesterbach, D. C., and Morris, H. L. Speech Problems of Patients with Cleft Lip and Palate. In Converse, J. M. (Ed.), *Reconstructive Plastic Surgery* (2nd ed.). Philadelphia: Saunders, 1977.
97. Spriestersbach, D. C., and Sherman, D. (Eds.). *Cleft Palate and Communication.* New York and London: Academic, 1968.
98. Wise, C. W. *Applied Phonetics.* Englewood Cliffs, N.J.: Prentice-Hall, 1957.

Follow-up Care and Secondary Palatal Procedures

99. Blakely, R. W. The rationale for a temporary speech prosthesis in palatal insufficiency. *Br. J. Disord. Commun.* 4:134, 1969.
100. Bluestone, C. D., Musgrave, R. H., McWilliams, B. J., and Crozier, P. A. Teflon injection pharyngoplasty. *Cleft Palate J.* 5:19, 1968.
101. Bzoch, K. R. Clinical studies of the efficiency of speech appliances compared to pharyngeal flap surgery. *Cleft Palate J.* 1:275, 1964.
102. Calnan, J. S. Diagnosis, prognosis and treatment of "palato-pharyngeal incompetence" with special reference to radiographic investigations. *Br. J. Plast. Surg.* 8:265, 1956.

103. Hamlen, M. Speech changes after pharyngeal flap surgery. *Plast. Reconstr. Surg.* 46:437, 1970.
104. Hogan, V. M. Clarification of surgical goals and cleft palate, speech and introduction of the lateral port control (LPC) pharyngeal flap. *Cleft Palate J.* 10:31, 1973.
105. Hogan, V. M. A biased approach to the treatment of velopharyngeal incompetence. *Clin. Plast. Surg.* 2:319, 1975.
106. Hynes, W. The results of pharyngoplasty by muscle transplantation in "failed cleft palate" cases, with special reference to the influence of the pharynx on voice production. *Ann. R. Coll. Surg. Engl.* 13:17, 1953.
107. Hynes, W. Pharyngoplasty by muscle transplantation. *Br. J. Plast. Surg.* 3:128, 1956.
108. Hynes, W. The examination of imperfect speech following cleft palate operations. *Br. J. Plast. Surg.* 10:114, 1958.
109. Kapetansky, D. I. Bilateral transverse pharyngeal flaps for repair of cleft palate. *Plast. Reconstr. Surg.* 52:52, 1973.
110. Moore, F. T. A new operation to cure nasopharyngeal incompetence. *Br. J. Surg.* 47:424, 1960.
111. Morris, H. L., and Spriestersbach, D. C. The pharyngeal flap as a speech mechanism. *Plast. Reconstr. Surg.* 39:84, 1967.
112. Owsley, J. Q., Creech, B. J., and Dedo, H. H. Poor speech following the pharyngeal flap operation: Etiology and treatment. *Cleft Palate J.* 9:312, 1972.
113. Owsley, J. Q., Jr., Lawson, L. I., Miller, E. R., and Blackfield, H. M. Experiences with the high attached pharyngeal flap. *Plast. Reconstr. Surg.* 38:232, 1966.
114. Randall, P. Surgery for Cleft Palate. In Goldwyn, R. M. (Ed.), *The Unfavorable Result in Plastic Surgery.* Boston: Little, Brown, 1972.
115. Randall, P. Surgery and speech. *Surgery* 56:810, 1964.
116. Randall, P., Bakes, F. P., and Kennedy, C. Cleft palate-type speech in the absence of cleft palate. *Plast. Reconstr. Surg.* 25:484, 1960.
117. Randall, P., O'Hara, A. E., and Bakes, F. P. A simplified x-ray technique for the study of soft palate function in patients with poor speech. *Plast. Reconstr. Surg.* 21:345, 1958.
118. Skolnick, M. L. Videofluoroscopic examination of the velopharyngeal portal during phonation in lateral and base projections: A new technique for studying the mechanism of closure. *Cleft Palate J.* 7:803, 1970.
119. Skolnick, M. L. Velopharyngeal function in cleft palate. *Clin. Plast. Surg.* 2:285, 1975.
120. Sullivan, D. Bilateral pharyngoplasty as an aid to velopharyngeal closure. *Plast. Reconstr. Surg.* 27:31, 1961.
121. Trauner, R., and Doubek, F. I. A new procedure in velopharyngeal surgery for secondary operations on too short soft palates: II. The speech results compared with other surgical or prosthetic methods. *Br. J. Plast. Surg.* 8:291, 1956.
122. Whitaker, L. A., Randall, P., Winchester, R., and Graham, W. P. A prospective and randomized series comparing superiorly and inferiorly based posterior pharyngeal flaps. *Cleft Palate J.* 9:304, 1972.
123. Williams, H. B., and Woolhouse, F. M. Comparison of speech improvement in cases of cleft palate after two methods of pharyngoplasty. *Plast. Reconstr. Surg.* 30:36, 1962.
124. Yules, B., and Chase, R. A. Secondary Techniques for Correction of Palatopharyngeal Incompetence. In Grabb, W. C., Rosenstein, S. W., and Bzoch, K. R. (Eds.), *Cleft Lip and Palate.* Boston: Little, Brown, 1971.

9

Soft Tissue Injuries of the Face

RICHARD C. SCHULTZ

Facial injuries deserve special attention because of their enormous functional and aesthetic significance. Although facial injuries can logically be divided into soft tissue injuries and facial bone fractures, each form of injury interrelates and bears on the approach to management of the other. (Facial bone fractures are discussed in Chapter 10.)

INITIAL CARE OF THE PATIENT

Triage, the sorting of patients according to the seriousness of their injuries for priorities of treatment, also applies to the individual patient with multiple injuries. Victims of multiple injury must always be viewed with the following priorities [31]: First a clear airway is ensured, then hemorrhage is controlled, shock is treated, and associated injuries are evaluated; only then are facial injuries diagnosed and treated.

Clear Airway

Blood, dentures, or vomitus can fully or partially obstruct the upper airway, resulting in an extremely agitated or nearly lifeless patient. These obstructions can usually be cleared quickly by sweeping a finger deeply into the mouth and oral pharynx [33]. Aspiration and tracheostomy are never as prompt, effective, or informative as use of a finger can be in these circumstances. Partially aspirated foreign bodies or occluding edema from a fractured larynx or trachea requires prompt surgical attention, but only after the mouth and oral pharynx have been cleared [36]. The condition of a patient with an airway problem stemming from uncontrolled facial hemorrhage or grossly displaced facial tissue can often be dramatically improved simply by sitting him upright [31]. When patients with facial injuries make violent efforts to sit up or to thrust the head forward, they should be allowed to do so, as they almost invariably are exhibiting a protective reflex to maintain the upper airway. Strapping or forcibly holding prone a patient with extensive facial injuries could result in his death [33].

Control Hemorrhage

Although hemorrhage from facial wounds can appear alarming, it is seldom of such magnitude as to be the sole cause of systemic shock, except in the case of close-range shotgun wounds [13, 14]. Extensive arterial hemorrhage from facial wounds usually results from injury to the external maxillary artery, the superficial temporal artery, or the angular artery [32]. Hemorrhage from these arteries can almost always be controlled by direct pressure to the wound. Ligation of the vessel can then be done directly through the wound. The most dangerous aspect of facial hemorrhage is the possibility that it might obstruct the upper airway [31]. Also, if the patient swallows large amounts of blood, gastric irritation and vomiting may result, thus further complicating the management of the patient [23].

Treat Shock

Shock is only occasionally caused by facial injury alone. Penetrating or avulsing ocular injuries may initiate the shock syndrome through pain and apprehension [12]. Extensive facial injuries, even including facial bone fractures, seldom cause great pain. When a patient with facial injury is found in shock, associated injuries should be suspected and evaluated as the cause [28].

Evaluate Associated Injuries

Once a clear airway is ensured and hemorrhage and shock have been controlled, consideration is given to associated injuries before undertaking treatment of the facial injuries themselves [34]. Patients do not die from facial injuries, but patients with facial injuries do die from associated injuries [29].

DIAGNOSIS OF FACIAL INJURIES

A comprehensive diagnosis and classification of facial injuries should be made before initiating definitive treatment [33].

Observation of a facial injury logically begins with the surface for indications of soft tissue injuries. Eyelids should always be opened to look for associated ocular injury [7, 9, 19].

The types of soft tissue injuries are [33]: contusion with or without hematoma; abrasion; accidental tattoo (numerous small particles embedded in dermis); retained foreign bodies; puncture; laceration (which is subdivided into simple, beveled, tearing, and burst or stellate type); avulsion flap (undermined laceration); and avulsion injury (loss of tissue).

After life-threatening problems have been resolved, soft tissue injuries amenable to repair under local anesthesia are usually treated first. One exception is the close-range shotgun wound of the face [33]. Such a complex facial injury with tissue loss and extensive fractures can seldom be treated immediately, since these patients are usually poor candidates for a general anesthetic.

When definitive care must be postponed, the simplest type of accurate tissue approximation will help promote a better end result. If necessary, soft tissue injuries can wait without repair up to 24 hours without compromising the final result, provided that bleeding has been controlled and the wounds have been properly cleaned and dressed [36]. Systemic antibiotics are advisable when significant delay in soft tissue repair is anticipated.

Documentation of Injury

Proper records of facial injuries should include diagnosis of type, anatomical location, and, in the case of soft tissue injury, measurements. In addition, a photograph of every extensive facial injury should be taken before definitive treatment begins [36]. Such a record of injury can subsequently prove invaluable in understanding and explaining secondary problems and the nature of final healing (as well as be useful in the event of medicolegal problems) [33].

PREPARATION FOR TREATMENT OF SOFT TISSUE INJURIES

Attempting to repair extensive soft tissue injuries of the face in a corner of the emergency room with inadequate light and without assistance invites frustration and second-rate results. Such injuries should be repaired in the operating theater with the help of at least a scrub nurse and a circulating nurse.

When a penetrating injury extends through the scalp, beard, or moustache, the hair should be shaved around the wound to facilitate suturing – but the eyebrow should *never* be shaved [36]. The shape and periphery of the eyebrow provide a valuable landmark for accurate repair. Once an eyebrow has healed with misalignment of its edge, it becomes exceedingly difficult to correct.

ANESTHESIA

For a reasonably cooperative patient, local anesthesia is unquestionably preferable for the repair of most soft tissue injuries [24], both from the standpoint of safety and in terms of ultimate patient comfort, since victims of acute trauma often arrive in the emergency room with their stomachs filled with food, alcohol, or blood. In addition, local anesthesia allows the surgeon far greater access to the face. When possible, the patient's comfort can be significantly enhanced under local anesthesia by supplemental oral, intramuscular, or intravenous sedation with promethazine (Phenergan), diazepam (Valium), or meperidine (Demerol).

For most extensive soft tissue facial injuries, my choice of agent is 1% lidocaine (Xylocaine) with epinephrine (1 : 100,000). Where only small quantities of solution should be injected, such as into the eyelids, a 2% solution is preferred. The discomfort of the injection can be minimized by introducing it through the cut edge of the wound rather than through the adjacent intact skin [3].

The sensory nerve distribution to the face lends itself fairly well to local nerve block anesthesia. In common practice, there are five areas on the face that are amenable to local block anesthesia: (1) supraorbital, (2) nasal, (3) infraorbital, (4) maxillary (the second division of the trigeminal nerve), and (5) mandibular (the third division of the trigeminal nerve). Maxillary and mandibular blocks require the most technical skill and are the most difficult to achieve.

Cocaine (5% solution) is still the best topical anesthetic agent available for nasal mucous membranes. It is introduced into the nose on cotton pledgets, cotton dental rolls, or cotton-tipped applicators.

When soft tissue injuries are being repaired in small children and local anesthesia is used, authoritative assurance can often make the patient cooperative. If not contraindicated by associated injuries, a combination of narcotic and tranquilizing drugs given by injection (varying the dosage according to weight and age) [33] will help achieve a cooperative patient in about 15 minutes. The sedative mixture may be composed of meperidine (Demerol) 50 mg. (1 ml.), promethazine (Phenergan) 12.5 mg. (0.5 ml.), and chlorpromazine (Thorazine) 12.5 mg. (0.5 ml.); the dosage is 1.5 ml. for an 18-kg. child and 2 ml. for a 27- to 45-kg. child.

When the child continues to be agitated, comfortable physical restraint is appropriate. This can be provided by a skillful assistant if the repair can be done quickly. When more time is needed, the patient's trunk and extremities can be "mummied" with an ordinary sheet. When it is necessary to restrain all extremities, the head, and the torso, an infant restraining board with Velcro straps is more suitable [33].

When general anesthesia becomes necessary, for example when the repair involves multiple injuries, a brief preinduction discussion with the anesthestist is appropriate. This will facilitate both the selection of compatible anesthetic agents (if the surgeon intends to inject a solution containing epinephrine for purposes of hemostasis) and the positioning of the anesthetic equipment.

TREATMENT OF SOFT TISSUE INJURIES

Contusion (with or without Hematoma)

Contusion is a bruising injury caused by blunt trauma. It seldom results in serious injury to the skin, and cleaning and observation are usually sufficient treatment. However, this type of injury can be associated with an underlying hematoma.

Small hematomas of the face will often spontaneously resorb; those that become encapsulated, however, usually require surgical treatment. Left untreated, such hematomas form permanent subcutaneous scar deformities. Proteolytic enzyme preparations given systemically have not proved helpful in reducing hematomas in my experience.

When still in the "currant-jelly" stage, a hematoma is best evacuated by incision [21]. As further liquefaction takes place, aspiration with a large-bore needle (18 gauge or larger) may be possible.

Abrasion

Abrasion injuries are best treated by cleaning with mild, nonirritating soap. It is usually best to leave abrasions uncovered, but when the pain is significant, the abrasion may be protected from the air by a thin layer of antibiotic ointment, such as bacitracin (Neosporin). The injury may also be covered with a light, serum-absorbent dressing, such as cellulose acetate gauze, which is then covered with ordinary cotton dressing gauze. Such dressings should be removed after 1 or 2 days. Healing is usually prompt, leaving no apparent residual scar unless the abrasion approaches third-degree depth or becomes infected.

Accidental Tattoo

Small dermal-embedded particles must be removed promptly from an abrasion before they become tissue fixed, which usually occurs within 12 hours. If the area involved does not lend itself well to treatment under local anesthesia, general anesthesia must be used. Scrubbing with a stiff, sterile scrub brush and mild soapsuds, if done early, will be adequate to remove most tattooing foreign bodies. When grease or oil is present in or about the wound, it can usually be dissolved and removed by small amounts of ether, acetone, or xylol.

Once foreign particles have become fixed in the tissues, a formal surgical abrasion is necessary [11]. If the area is extensive, the procedure should be planned under general anesthesia. It is best done with power equipment, either electric or air driven.

With all methods of abrasion, including scrubbing, care must be taken not to penetrate the deep dermal layers, or permanent scarring will result. Occasionally, when isolated foreign bodies are deeply embedded, a scalpel blade can be used as a spud to tease out or to excise these particles individually.

The dressing applied over a surgical abrasion should be absorptive but nonadherent. Cellulose acetate gauze is ideal for this purpose.

When left untreated, accidental tattoos result in permanent, unattractive discoloration in the skin. Additional material on this subject is included in Chapter 31.

Retained Foreign Bodies

Retained foreign bodies are larger than the particles that cause accidental tattoos and should routinely be removed from the face, with the exception of metal fragments from missiles. (Bullets or missile fragments usually are sterile when they enter the face and commonly penetrate deeply [13]. If there is minimal reaction, more harm is often done by attempting to remove them than by leaving them in place.) Glass, ornamental metal, wood splinters, and dental fragments all require removal.

Failure to remove foreign bodies originating in the mouth can lead to severe cellulitis and subsequent abscess formation [25].

Puncture

Puncture wounds of the face are uncommon; these small wounds must alert one to the possibility of injury to deeper structures. Swelling about puncture wounds is most often due to hematoma. However, arteriovenous fistula may form following puncture wounds, particularly in the parotid and preauricular regions.

Graphite fragments from lead pencils, paint chips, rust particles, and wood splinters are the commonest foreign bodies implanted by puncture. These must be removed to prevent infection, scar formation, and pigmentation. The puncture wound itself must sometimes be excised to achieve the best healing.

The possibility of pathogenic inoculation requires prophylactic treatment for tetanus and early follow-up examination [35].

Simple Laceration

Laceration is the most common form of facial injury [33]. Repair should be undertaken only after underlying structures have been put in order. The time lapse between injury and repair is important in terms of the possibility of infection and the choice of repair techniques. After observing the effects of varying time intervals between injury and repair, I have concluded that, with the exception of animal bites and accidental tattoos, most soft tissue wounds of the face, properly cleaned and dressed, can await primary repair for up to 24 hours without serious risk of infection and without jeopardizing the final aesthetic result [28].

Wound toilet consists of cleaning, irrigation, and debridement. Tissue that is devitalized must be cut away, regardless of its location or its former importance [26]. Although debridement should be conservative, it must be adequate. Ragged, severely contused wound edges should be conservatively excised to provide perpendicular skin edges that will heal primarily with a minimum of scar [30]. Closely parallel lacerations can be converted to a single wound by excising the intervening skin bridge, thus facilitating repair and reducing scar formation.

Displaced tissue should be returned to its original position. Only occasionally is there an indication for immediately changing the direction of a wound by Z-plasty or for making tissue allowance for scar contracture at the time of primary wound repair.

SUTURING. Muscular and subcutaneous tissue is best closed with plain catgut suture to minimize dead space and the accumulation of blood and serum [36]. In the event of infection, the more rapid resorption of plain catgut suture proves to be an advantage. Similarly, interrupted sutures of 5-0 or 6-0 nylon are ideal for skin closure; if hematoma or pocketing of serum or pus occurs, one or two sutures can be removed to permit drainage leaving the remainder of the repair intact.

REMOVAL OF SUTURES. Facial wounds have the advantage of a rich vascular supply, which contributes to early healing. Where the skin is thin, as in the eyelids, sutures may be removed in 3 or 4 days; elsewhere on the face they may be left 4 to 6 days. Sutures in the ears may often be left in place 10 to 14 days with definite advantage when there has been injury to underlying cartilage, since scars over divided ear cartilage tend to thicken and spread when sutures are removed too early. Suture scars on the ears are not usually noticeable.

Avulsion Flap

The avulsion flap is an undermined laceration that can be one of the most disfiguring of all soft tissue injuries (Fig. 9-1). Broad, tangentially located scar tissue in the dermis and subcutaneous tissue interferes with free circulation of venous blood and lymph to adjacent skin. The resulting venous engorgement and lymphedema swell the flap and partially contribute to the spreading and subsequent depression of the peripheral scar. Further, as the scar contracts, the avulsion flap tissue which is bordered by it assumes a heaped-up appearance [33].

It is important, therefore, to minimize the thin, beveled portion of these flaps (Fig. 9-2). If the flap is small and the location is fortunate, it can be totally excised, which solves the problem [30]. When avulsion flaps are larger or involve features, a more conservative approach to repair must be taken. The thinnest peripheral portions of the flap should be cut away to create perpendicular edges for skin closure. Following this debridement, closure is performed in essentially the same manner as for simple laceration.

Small avulsion flaps and gouges, as seen in injuries sustained on newer-model automobile windshields [10] (Fig. 9-3), are best managed by complete excision following normal skin lines whenever possible. Left untreated, or managed solely by a pressure dressing, these tiny avulsion flaps and full-thickness gouges heal with a pebbly skin surface that is difficult to correct later by scar revision [26]. The excision of the small avulsion flap and avulsion injury again converts the injury to a surgical defect that can be sutured with apposing perpendicular edges, thus eliminating the tangential intradermal scarring responsible for the pebbly scar disfigurement.

Pressure dressings play an important part in optimal healing of an avulsion flap and should often be used for several weeks. By minimizing dead space and restricting venous and lymph puddling, they help re-

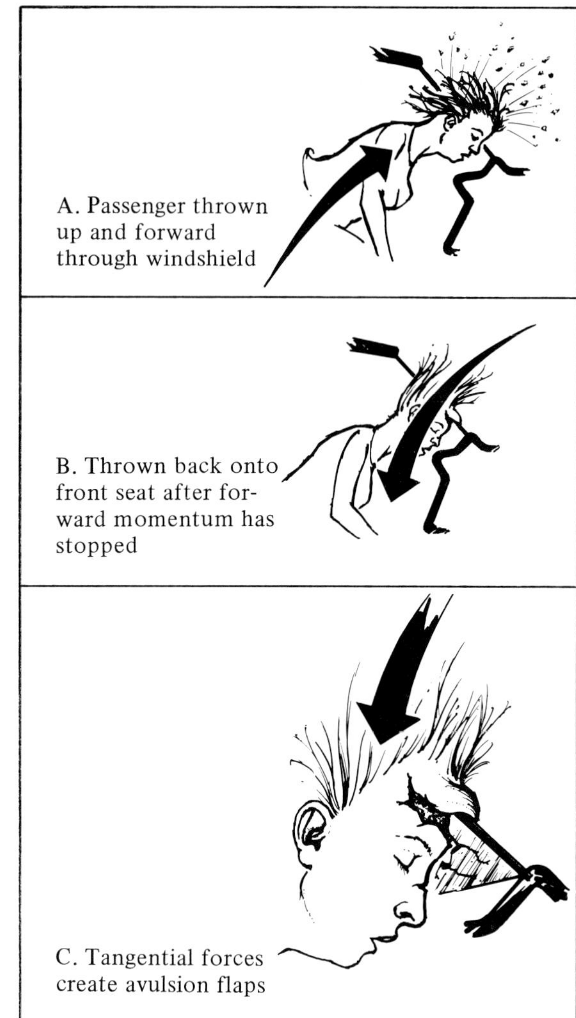

Fig. 9-1. Mechanism of soft tissue injuries from automobile windshields manufactured prior to 1966.

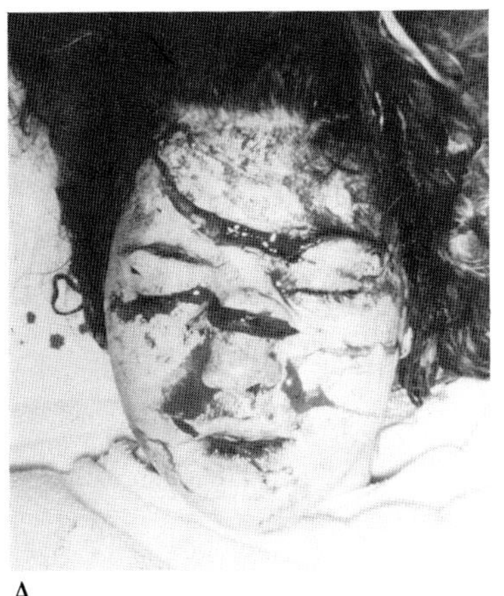

A

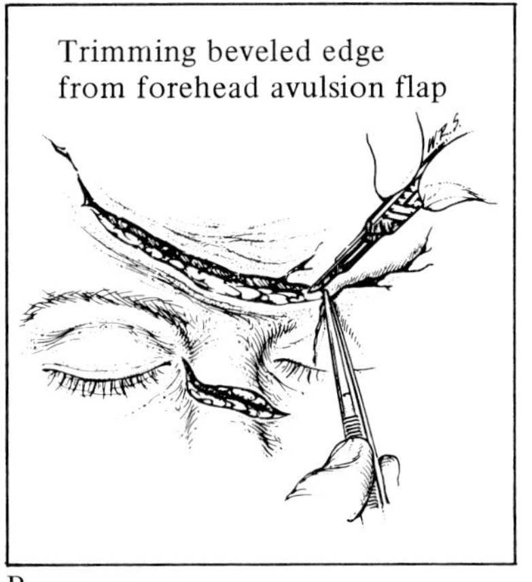

B

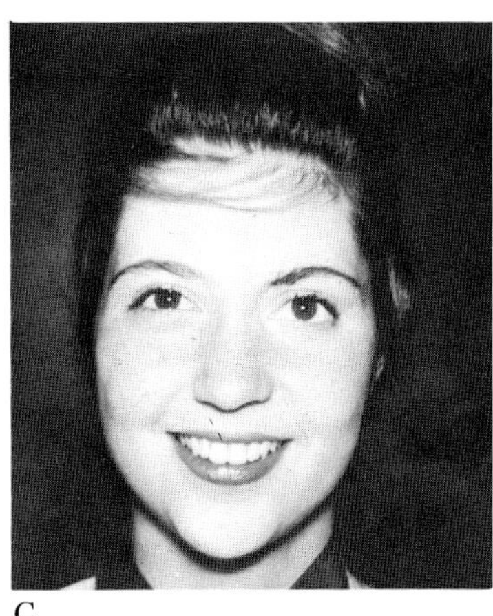

C

Fig. 9-2. Treatment of avulsion flap injuries. A, typical windshield injuries of forehead and nose. B, debridement of thin edge of flap prior to suture. C, healing 18 months following injury.

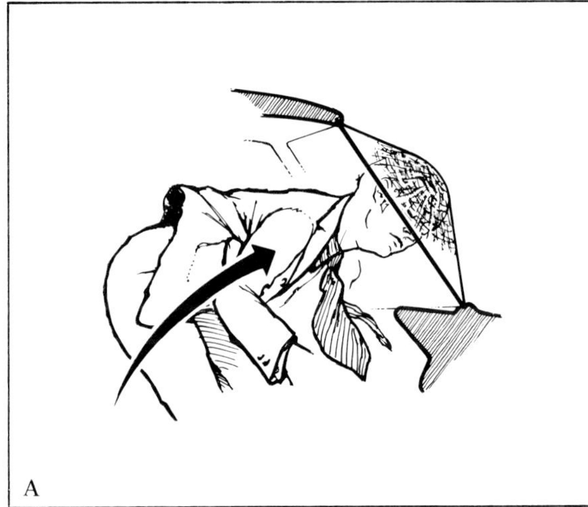

A

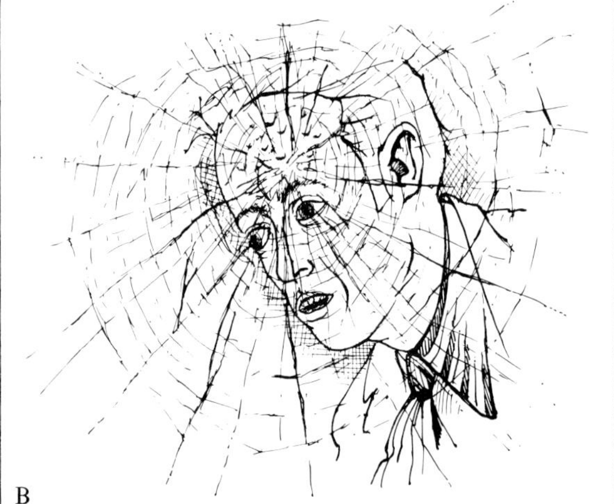

B

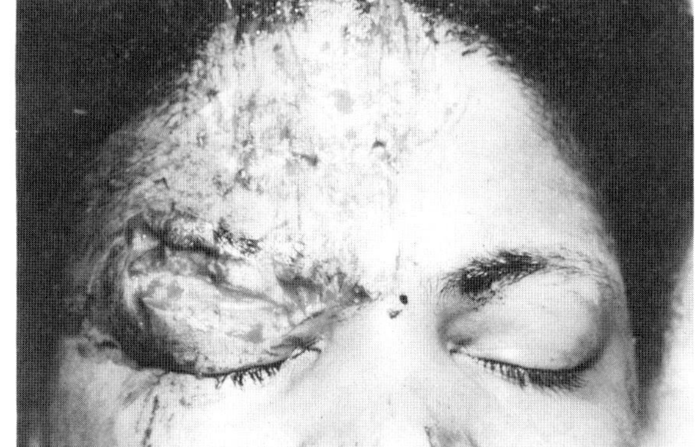

C

Fig. 9-3. Mechanism of soft tissue injury from newer style windshields. A, typical pattern of windshield breakage with ballooning but no penetration. B, mosaic of broken glass imprinted on forehead. C, small avulsion flaps, small lacerations, and superficial avulsion injuries.

duce fibrin deposition and excess scar formation [33].

Ideally, a tissue defect on the face or within the mouth should not be allowed to heal spontaneously by scar [22]. Direct primary closure of adjacent tissue is highly preferable, but if this is not possible, coverage by a skin graft is indicated.

Thick split-thickness skin grafts often provide a definitive repair for large, clean defects. These grafts are usually best taken with a drum-type, hand-operated dermatome. Soft tissue defects should be covered by skin grafts as promptly as the patient's general condition permits, even if the procedure must be performed under local anesthesia. A fresh uncontaminated wound is the best possible bed for accepting a skin graft.

SPECIAL REGIONAL CONSIDERATIONS

Forehead and Brow

The eyebrow is an anatomical feature that should always be preserved as a reference point; it should never be shaved, and must always be repaired with precise attention to its shape and borders.

Muscle division beneath the brow is always repaired to prevent spreading and depression of the scar. Before closure of the brow, however, the surgeon should make sure that there are no fractures of the supraorbital ridge or frontal sinuses, since these fractures are often poorly demonstrated in routine facial x-rays [32].

In planning the repair, the surgeon must keep in mind the fact that forehead scars are the least conspicuous when they occur in or parallel to normal skin lines.

Eyelids

The first consideration in treating patients with injuries to the eyelids is to determine if the globe is injured [9]. The most common error is to miss a foreign body; however, the sudden removal of a foreign body from the globe can be hazardous because of possible further damage. Similarly, removal of blood clots from the globe can be hazardous, because iris tissue may be bound to the clot or confused with it [7]. A wound that penetrates deeply into the orbit through the upper eyelid or globe must be considered a potential intracranial injury since the superior orbital plate is thin and fragile.

Eyelid infection is rare because the blood supply is abundant; nevertheless, eyelid lacerations should be cleaned by irrigation with saline. Avulsed eyelid tissue should be gently cleaned in saline and replaced as an autograft whenever possible [37].

Eyelid lacerations can be divided into two groups: superficial and deep. Superficial lacerations can be further divided into those that parallel the lid margin and those that are perpendicular to it. Superficial lacerations that run parallel require only simple closure of the skin, and smaller ones may not require sutures. Those that are perpendicular to the lid margin cross normal skin lines and tend to gape; they require absorbable sutures in the underlying muscle and subcutaneous tissue prior to skin closure. Many small conjunctival lacerations heal well without suture repair, but when suturing is necessary 6-0 catgut on a swaged ophthalmologic needle is used.

Deep lacerations should be anesthetized and retracted to search for injury to underlying structures. Division of the levator palpebrae or superior rectus muscles should be repaired [5]. Lacerations extending through the lid margin should be repaired promptly. Would gaping and notching of the lid margin result from contracture of the orbicularis muscle fibers that encircle the palpebral fissure. If repair is delayed for 7 to 10 days, these muscle fibers fibrose, the tarsal plate thickens and retracts, and the wound edges can no longer be approximated [33].

Surgeons inexperienced in repairing eyelid lacerations often feel compelled to perform complicated procedures, such as staggered or Z-plasty repairs, in an effort to prevent contracting deformities. The simplest type of anatomically accurate approximation with sutures is generally the best. Greatest care should be taken to approximate the tarsus and ciliary margin accurately. Once these structures have been sutured, the remainder of the eyelid generally falls into place.

Care must also be taken to preserve the integrity of the lacrimal apparatus and the canthal ligaments. A divided and grossly displaced lacrimal system may require cannulation with a fine polyethylene catheter and repair with overlying fine suture. (A 3-0 nylon suture will act as an excellent probe or splint for the lacrimal duct.) However, in instances of incomplete division, the lacrimal system may simply be approximated with expectation of good functional return, often without direct suture [8]. Injury to the upper canaliculus alone rarely results in tearing.

Dacryocystorhinostomy

Despite the apparent logic of performing dacryocystorhinostomy early, it is most often a secondary reconstructive operation performed months after healing of the original naso-orbital injury [33]. It is indicated to relieve epiphora and secondary obstructive dacryocystitis. These symptoms of obstruction in tear flow are caused by a missed or inadequately repaired lacrimal canaliculus, by sac or duct injury, by secondary scarring and stenosis, or by obstruction in the lacrimal collecting system as a result of injury to adjacent bone or medial palbebral ligament [12].

Though many surgical techniques for dacryocystorhinostomy have been described, their shared underlying principle is the reestablishment of unobstructed tear drainage from the conjunctival sac into the nose. In reestablishing the lacrimal collecting system, the medial canthal ligament must frequently be relocated and reattached to adjacent bone of the medial orbital wall. Also, because of bone resorption in the healing of comminuted, telescoped fractures of the nose, secondary bone reconstruction, often with bone grafts, is indicated. Therefore, medial canthoplasty and reconstruction of the nasal pyramid are frequently done in conjunction with a dacryocystorhinostomy. If these procedures are done independently, the later operations become increasingly difficult due to scar formation that results from the previous dissections.

The essence of one operation to reestablish unobstructed lacrimal flow is shown in Figure 9-4. A polyethylene catheter, small red rubber catheter, or Pyrex Jones tube keeps the newly formed drainage system open for 3 to 4 weeks until epithelialization of the constructed lacrimal tract has occurred.

The number of surgical techniques to correct this problem is an indication of persistent problems with all of them. There are numerous instances in which the most logically planned procedure and the most refined surgical technique have had a disappointing outcome. It is most likely that the best way to achieve a high rate of success with this procedure is to perform it within 1 or 2 days following injury [33].

When lower eyelid skin is avulsed or when it is resected because of nonviability, replacement is ideally accomplished either by transposition of skin from the adjacent upper eyelid (Fig. 9-5B) or by a full-thickness skin graft from the opposite upper eyelid or postauricular area. Thin, split-thickness skin grafts fail to provide adequate elasticity, and eyelid contractures result. Similarly, stretching adjacent eyelid skin to cover any but the smallest defect is apt to result in eyelid distortion, especially in the lower lids.

Ears

Primary ear reconstruction is exceedingly important, since secondary repair is not only considerably more difficult but usually much less satisfactory in result [6]. Tissues making up the external ear are unique, and there is no good donor area for their substitution. Therefore, surgical debridement should be conservative and every effort should be made to return tissue to its position of origin. Cutaneous blood supply is abundant, so that narrow, pedicled avulsion flaps and even avulsed or amputated composite tissue segments will often survive if relocated anatomically. If the perichondrial-cutaneous sutures provide sufficient support, sutures in the cartilage may be unnecessary, especially in the conchal region. When sutures are required, nonabsorbable 5-0 monofilament nylon is a good choice, if not tied so tightly as to cut through the cartilage. Absorption of the suture material deep to the perichondrium is exceedingly slow, making the use of catgut sutures in this area somewhat risky.

Information on treatment of amputated portions of the ear and hematoma of the ear is included in Chapter 13.

Nose

With the exception of avulsion or amputation, soft tissue injuries to the nose are generally uncomplicated. Good healing can usually be obtained simply by accurate tissue approximation and refined suture technique. Soft tissues of the nose consist essentially of skin, cartilage, and mucous membrane. The superficial muscle fibers of the nose are sparse and, for the most part, adherent to the skin. Once the bony framework is put right, soft tissues need only be approximated with anatomical accuracy, taking special pains to align the nostril borders accurately.

Septal hematoma can be diagnosed with a nasal speculum. It is evacuated immediately through a small mucosal incision. An untreated septal hematoma will typically resorb and destroy the septal cartilage, especially if infected, leaving a "saddle nose" deformity [4].

For injuries penetrating all soft tissue layers of the nose, it is easiest to repair the mucous membrane lining first, using 4-0 plain catgut suture. Torn septal, upper lateral, alar, and columellar cartilages can usually be reapproximated under direct vision through the wound and held in good position simply by accurate repair of the underlying mucous membrane and the overlying skin [38]. Subcutaneous sutures are usually unnecessary if deep bites are taken through the skin and the sutures tied to achieve a slight eversion of skin edges. Interrupted sutures of 5-0 monofilament nylon are ideal.

Packing of the nose with a petrolatum-impregnated gauze is sometimes done to maintain position of cartilaginous or bony fragments. However, if the supporting structures of the nose are accurately repositioned, packing is usually unnecessary and should be avoided when possible [33]. Not only do such packs interfere with the natural drainage of the nose and the beneficial effects of circulating air, but removal of nasal packs may cause additional bleeding and separation of the repaired mucous membrane.

Skin grafts of the nose are ideally done with full-thickness postauricular grafts, which give the best possible match of color and texture. Thick split-thickness skin grafts can be used, however, and these are best taken from exposed body areas, such as neck or arm, for better color match.

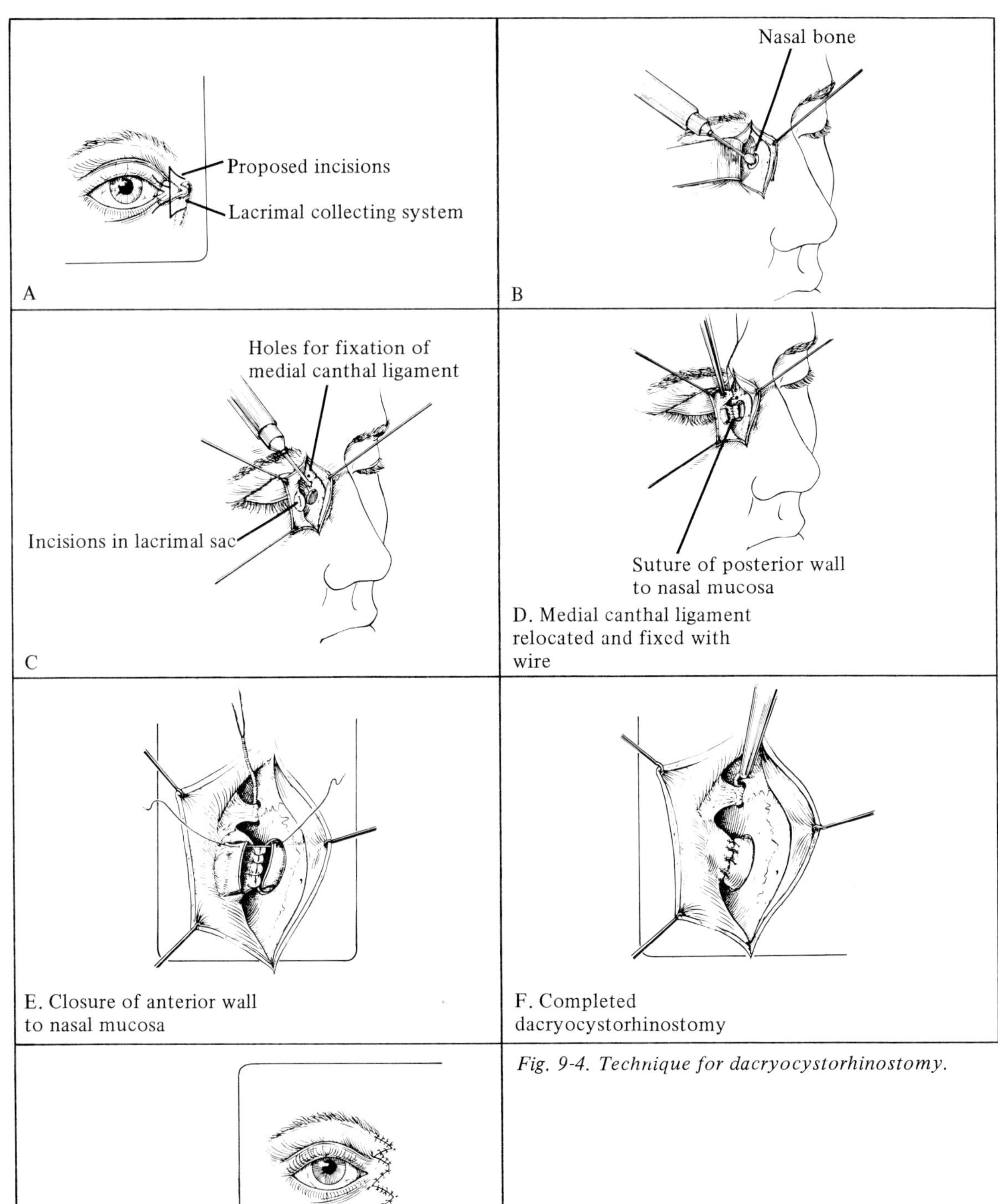

Fig. 9-4. Technique for dacryocystorhinostomy.

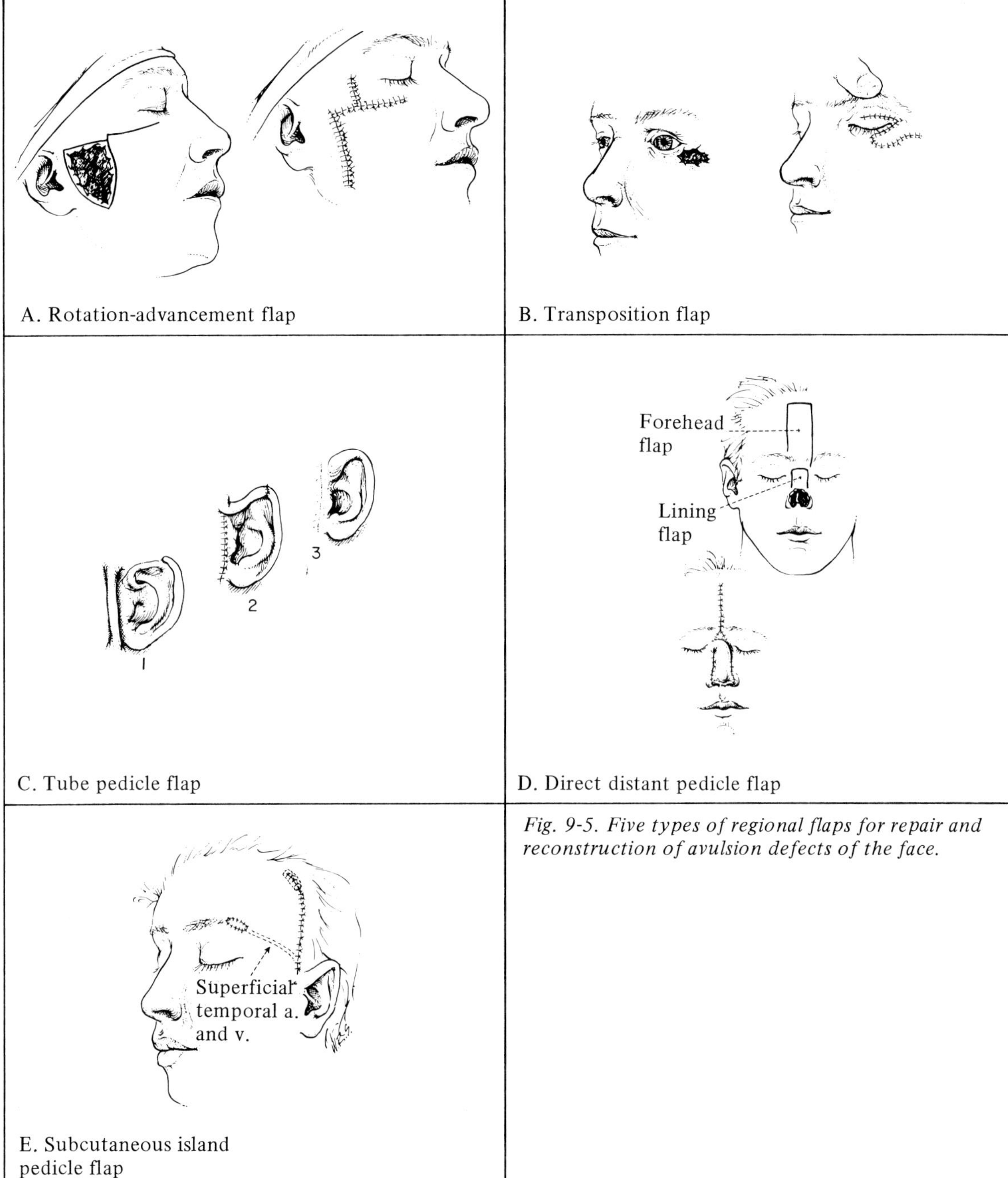

Fig. 9-5. Five types of regional flaps for repair and reconstruction of avulsion defects of the face.

Cheeks and Chin

Laceration of the cheek is the most commonly encountered facial injury. The superficial aspects of this repair are relatively simple, and the outcome should ordinarily be quite satisfactory. However, important structures lying within the cheek deserve special mention. There are (1) branches of the facial nerve, (2) the parotid gland and Stensen's duct, and (3) the muscles of mastication and expression.

BRANCHES OF THE FACIAL NERVE. Soft tissue injuries are of greatest concern when located in the posterior and inferior aspect of the cheek. Within this vital area lie the branches of the facial nerve, the parotid gland and duct, and the masseter muscle.

Major branches of the facial nerve are deep in the cheek, well protected by overlying soft tissue, and are seldom injured by accidental trauma. Exploration is not necessary to determine injury of this nerve; if division has occurred, unmistakable signs of lost muscle function will be present.

The most severe functional deficit of the face from division of a single nerve branch is that of the temporal branch, since this causes paralysis of the eyelid and subsequent exposure of the cornea. The mandibular branch of the facial nerve is sometimes injured with lacerations about the lower jaw. This branch is always deep to the platysma muscle when posterior to the facial artery; it then courses near the lower border of the mandible, sometimes found 1 cm. below it.

Division of nerve branches anterior to the region of the parotid duct (midpupillary line) does not result in permanent loss of muscle function because the superficial facial muscles are innervated in their posterior portions. Repair of these anterior branchings is therefore unnecessary. When there has been a clean division of the posterior portion of the facial nerve branches, as with a razor, the nerve sheaths should be carefully approximated in fascicular units with fine soft suture. When there is greater damage, such as that caused by a blunt, penetrating object, the nerve ends require exploration and debridement prior to repair. This dissection is facilitated by use of a magnifying loupe or operating microscope. If portions of the nerve adjacent to the division have been damaged, the severed ends should be sharply excised prior to anastomosis [1, 15]. A significant amount of nerve regeneration may occur following such a repair, but complete return of function is rare. In general, use of free nerve grafts or crossed anastomosis with other nerves is imprudent at the time of initial care.

PAROTID GLAND AND STENSEN'S DUCT. The parotid gland and duct are more superficial than the branches of the facial nerve and are more exposed to injury. Injury should be suspected when clear fluid is seen leaking from a wound of the posterior cheek. Drooping of half of the upper lip may also be associated with such an injury. The buccal branch of the facial nerve runs parallel to, and sometimes obliquely across, the parotid duct, and they are therefore often divided simultaneously.

The gland itself need not be sutured, but patency of the duct should be determined before the wound is closed. The parotid duct courses along a line from the tragus of the ear to the midportion of the upper lip. A parotid gland fistula will usually close spontaneously within a few days and almost always within 3 or 4 weeks [1, 2]. If the fistula persists for several months, the severed duct can be sutured over a soft tubular splint.

A fine polyethylene catheter, such as an "intracath," may be used to cannulate Stensen's duct. When it is obvious that the duct has been divided and the external wound overlies the point of division, cannulation is most easily done in a retrograde fashion from the point of division. When the point of division is not easily accessible through the external wound, or if division of the duct is uncertain, intubation should be through the ostium opposite the crown of the upper second molar tooth.

Catheterization through the ostium is made easier by retracting the cheek outward, thereby straightening the angulated portion of the cut. The portions of the duct that overlies the masseter muscle are more easily repaired, since the duct is fixed and thicker there. Once catheterized, the divided ends are approximated with fine, soft suture material, such as 6-0 silk, on an atraumatic cutting needle. If the duct has been only partially divided and there is relatively little associated injury in the area, the catheter may safely be removed following repair. If the duct has been completely divided or if there is other local injury, it is best to leave this catheter in place 5 to 7 days, or until most of the edema has resorbed. The catheter is best kept in place by looping it out of the mouth and taping the end low on the cheek or chin to encourage gravitational flow of parotid secretion.

When there is extensive damage to the duct or loss of duct tissue without laceration of the gland, the proximal cut end of the duct can be sutured to a new ostium in the oral mucosa as an alternate procedure to maintain parotid function. The proximal portion of the duct also may be ligated. Following this the parotid gland will atrophy and cease to function.

Fascia, subcutaneous tissue, and skin should be closed over a lacerated parotid gland. If the duct is patent, a subsequent parotid fistula will eventually close spontaneously.

MUSCLES OF MASTICATION AND EXPRESSION. Divided muscles of mastication and facial expression should be repaired routinely. Tissue should be returned to its original location whenever possible. Healing and return of function almost always occur even when these muscles are not repaired, but depression and broad overlying scars can then be anticipated.

Relatively superficial lacerations of the posterior chin may damage the marginal mandibular branch of the facial nerve. This may account for drooping of half of the lip by the loss of innervation of both levator and depressor muscles (mentalis and quadratus labii inferioris) of the lip. Therefore, every effort should be made to discover and repair such a division.

A unique injury can occur at the chin; the soft tissues are avulsed up from the anterior mandible and the oral cavity is penetrated at the base of the lower lip [30]. The wound is tangential and enters the mouth at the level of the lower buccal sulcus. It is important that this perforation into the mouth be recognized and repaired. The intraoral repair requires delicate tissue handling, aided by the use of small atraumatic needles, since the gingival portion of the lower buccal sulcus is vital to proper closure but is easily torn if treated roughly.

Lips

Lip repair is always performed with respect to the vermilion border. "Step-off" or puckering in this area is not only unsightly but often difficult to correct later [17, 20].

Lip musculature should be closed first, using 3-0 or 4-0 catgut. Blood should then be completely cleaned from the vermilion border to make an accurate approximation.

The mucous membrane should be closed next to avoid strain and "seesawing" of sutured skin. The mucous membrane is closed effectively with 3-0 or 4-0 catgut, and these sutures do not require removal. As intraoral mucous membrane is very elastic, this closure should be done with concern for the vermilion border to avoid an excess of tissue on one or the other side.

Intraoral Injuries

Intraoral soft tissue wounds deserve special emphasis, since many reputable medical educators still teach that these may be left to heal spontaneously. This philosophy may have its origin in the observation that intraoral wounds and defects will close rapidly by epithelialization [22]. Unfortunately, such uncon- and imprecise healing results in uncontrolled scarring and imprecise function, just as it does elsewhere in the body.

Intraoral war wounds are managed under different circumstances, and therefore delayed treatment and secondary reconstruction are often necessary [13]. Similar to war wounds are injuries from animal bites and neglected wounds; in general, these wounds are surgically debrided and approximated loosely. This treatment will allow for drainage and will prevent abscess formation while minimizing scarring. A culture for bacteria and sensitivity studies are essential in the management of such injuries. Specific antibiotic therapy and attention to hygiene, such as rinsing with half-strength hydrogen peroxide, promote uncomplicated early healing.

In the mouth as in the skin, nonabsorbable sutures cause less tissue reaction. On the other hand, absorbable sutures (like catgut or synthetics) are easy to work with in the mouth and do not require removal. This convenience is especially appreciated in work with children, in whom suture removal is difficult and trying for both patient and doctor.

Animal Bites

Facial injuries due to dog bites are the commonest in the category of animal bites; they are usually sustained by young children. The injuries are invariably soft tissue wounds of a tearing nature, and tend to follow a rather typical pattern – a crescent-shaped, deep laceration of the cheek, often extending to the oral commissure [35]. There are frequently parallel wounds on the cheek and occasionally a laceration or avulsion defect of the nasal tip. Such wounds of the cheek tend to gape and, at first glance, give the appearance that tissue is missing [17]. Human bites, though not as severe in appearance, have routinely proved to be more virulent from the standpoint of infection.

Animal bite wounds are heavily contaminated with microorganisms from the mouth of the animal; for this reason they are more apt to become infected than are other injuries (with the exception of the human bite wound). Because of this special concern, these wounds are best treated by prompt excision. If the patient is seen more than 6 hours after the injury, a more conservative surgical approach should be followed, anticipating infection. Antibiotics are indicated, but frequently their use does not prevent infection.

Knowledge of the health of the animal is extremely important. When the species and whereabouts of the animal are unknown, the physician is faced with the decision of whether or not to begin rabies vaccination. Persons bitten by rabid dogs are infected in only 10 to 20 percent of instances, the risk varying with wound site and the character of the bite. Bites about the face and neck are the most dangerous. The dog is infectious several days before symptoms appear. The virus is present in the dog's saliva and even an abrasion bathed in saliva may result in rabies infection. In human beings, the incubation period varies between 2 and 8 weeks, whereas in dogs the incubation period is felt to be somewhat shorter. This time differential is the basis for the observation of the confined animal before initiating antirabies treatment of the person who was bitten.

In suburban areas, where most dogs are known and commonly immunized for rabies, the risk of rabies is minimal. The ideal situation for all concerned is to have the animal confined under observation of a veterinarian. In this way, if the animal shows signs of rabies within 10 days, the patient can be treated by rabies vaccination within the incubation period. If the animal is killed, however, it is absolutely essential to have microscopic examination of the brain for Negri bodies or the new fluorescein antibody test to determine if the animal was rabid [33]. When results are positive, rabies vaccination of the patient must begin at once.

ASPECTS OF POSTOPERATIVE CARE

Psychological Aspects

All patients with extensive soft tissue facial injuries are extremely fearful of disfigurement; this is especially true of females. They may even become hysterical in their fear. Firm reassurance by the surgeon, rather than sympathy, is the most effective remedy. However, in this effort to allay fear and reduce anxiety, one must be careful not to promise too much. Implying to the patient that there will be no disfigurement or scars may lead to legal action later. If the patient needs unusual amounts of reassurance, one should give as much comfort as needed, but some responsible member of the family should be realistically informed [33].

The surgeon is commonly asked, "Will I have scars on my face?" Any penetration of the dermis results in scarring, and the patient should not be misinformed in this regard. With the techniques described, scars can often be kept minimal; when the scars are mature, some become unnoticeable.

Infection, Antibiotics, and Immunizations

Infections in facial wounds are uncommon because of the rich vascular supply in this area, but they become far more common following massive bacterial inoculation, as in animal or human bites. It is for this reason that highly contaminated wounds are often excised prior to closure.

Infection of a facial injury is a serious detriment to healing and, subsequently, to function and appearance. Moreover, the infection is particularly dangerous because of ready communication of the organisms through the venous system to the cavernous sinuses. For these reasons, infections of the face deserve prompt attention. Bed rest, warm compresses locally, and specific systemic antibiotics are ordinarily all that is required. When buried foreign material is contributing to the infection, it must be removed.

As in any other wound, the danger of tetanus infection must be considered in facial injuries, especially in puncture wounds. Since tetanus toxoid immunization has become widespread, there is now rarely an indication to use the tetanus antitoxin. When a booster dose of alum precipitated tetanus toxoid seems insufficient to protect against tetanus, human tetanus immune globulin (Hyper-Tet) is much safer to use in the prevention of tetanus infection.

SCARS AND REVISIONAL PROCEDURES

The *nature of facial scars* is often determined more by the character and location of the wound than by the technique of repair. A flat "hairline" scar without distortion of features is the aim of the surgeon.

Scars may heal with bumpy irregularity. This is seen when one side is higher or partially overlaps the other, and following the healing of small avulsion flaps. Such scars can often be improved by surgical abrasion.

Circular or U-shaped scars or those crossing natural skin folds usually benefit by some form of revision involving change in direction, lengthening, or staggering. Revision can be accomplished by Z-plasty, W-plasty, or V-Y techniques [33]. Skin grafting is occasionally necessary when skin has been avulsed or excised, leaving broad areas of contracting scar. However, grafting should be avoided whenever other methods are applicable, since matching facial skin color and texture with a graft is difficult and the results may prove aesthetically disappointing.

Scar Revision

Once scars have matured sufficiently, they may be revised. Red, raised, indurated, ugly scars are the most tempting to revise for the novice. However, these are the very scars that are not ready for revision. The best results are obtained with revision after these scars have softened, faded, and flattened. These signs of maturation indicate control of inflammation and the establishment of capillary and lymphatic flow. The error is not in waiting too long but in beginning too soon.

Most scar revisions of a limited area can be performed under local anesthesia and on an outpatient basis. As is the case for all elective facial operations, these patients should be prepared with a scalp shampoo and oral hygiene; male patients should be clean shaven. The patient should come to the operating room with all cosmetics removed. If the patient has dentures they should be worn, as the appearance and apparent location of scars about the lower face may be changed considerably by the dentures.

First, the scar is outlined with methylene blue or skin marking pen. This is especially helpful when the periphery is irregular. It is much easier to correct mistakes made with the marker than those made with a scalpel.

After the scar is outlined, local anesthetic solution containing epinephrine is slowly injected about its periphery. A relatively bloodless field is available if the surgeon will wait for 7 minutes until the epinephrine takes effect.

Scars are excised as outlined through the full thickness of the skin into the subcutaneous tissue. Most of the subcutaneous portions of the scar should be excised, but compulsive removal of all visible scar tissue is unnecessary and could prove unwise.

When scar excision extends deeply into the subcutaneous tissue or involves fascia and muscle, these deeper layers are best approximated with 4-0 plain catgut suture. For closure of the more superficial layers, a nonabsorbable soft suture, such as white silk or white synthetic material (4-0 or 5-0), can be used. This suture should substantially incorporate the dermis in the closure, with the knot buried beneath the dermis. These sutures not only bring the skin surface into apposition and decrease dependence on the skin sutures but also help prevent subsequent spreading of revised scars. Depending on the location, length, and configuration of the scar, the skin may be approximated with intracuticular, interrupted, or continuous running monofilament nylon suture.

Altering Scar Polarity

Linear scars crossing normal skin folds contract and become hypertrophied. Lengthening and altering the polarity of such a scar by staggering it will relieve the contracture and greatly improve its appearance.

STAGGERING. Simple staggering can be accomplished by putting a deliberate angled limb in the scar, directly in or parallel to the skin fold at the site where the scar crosses it. Such a procedure may suffice, but the classic and more definite correction of linear scar contracture is the Z-plasty.

Z-PLASTY. This procedure not only staggers a linear scar but lengthens it as well by interposing flaps of adjacent tissue. The principle of this simple procedure should be well understood so that it can be modified where necessary to adapt to a particular location on the face.

It is advisable to begin by marking the proposed incisions with methylene blue, since angles and flap lengths may be altered several times before obtaining the pattern desired. Although the classic Z-plasty is described as having equal triangular flaps drawn 60 degrees from the line of contracture, both size and angle may be varied considerably to accommodate a particular feature or facial area. Ideally, Z-plasty flaps should comprise the full length of the contracted scar, but often this is not possible because of adjacent features. In these instances, either the flaps are made somewhat dissimilar for accommodation, or multiple smaller Z's are used.

In a well-planned Z-plasty, the flaps will often transpose themselves, if relocation of tissue in the area is vital. Z-plasties should seldom be tiny, even when in series, since the total area of resulting scar will then retain a linear orientation. Polarity is thus reestablished and contracture reappears.

W-PLASTY. Another procedure designed principally for staggering linear scars is the W-plasty. Since this technique requires the excision of multiple small triangles of normal skin to facilitate closure by interdigitation, little is gained in scar lengthening (Fig. 9-6).

Prior skin marking is important to ensure proper interpositioning of these small triangular flaps. This procedure is probably best for long, depressed linear scars running obliquely across the forehead, cheeks, or chin.

Because of the multiplicity of flaps, angles, and adjacent surfaces, this type of closure may sometimes heal with a pebbly surface. If this occurs, surgical abrasion, using a motorized rotary abrader, may offer additional improvement once the scar has matured.

V-Y PLASTY. Just as the W-plasty is principally used to stagger linear scars, so the V-Y plasty is used principally to lengthen. In practice, converting a V to a Y scar has a minimal lengthening effect unless the scar is lengthened where redundancies form; however, the change in configuration is often beneficial to the surface contour on which the scar lies.

A broad V-shaped scar may become particularly disfiguring due to contracture and edema of the central flap. If the scar is excised, a V-shaped defect results. By closing the bottom of the V in a linear manner, a Y-shaped scar is formed. This also facilitates closure of the long sides to the short sides of the surgical defect. Removal of these "dog ears" will further lengthen the scar.

The procedure is especially useful in revising scars bridging the nasolabial angle at the columella (Fig. 9-7), as well as V-shaped scars at the oral commissures and palpebral canthi.

Avulsion Flaps and U-shaped Scars

Among the most disfiguring scars are those resulting from superiorly based avulsion flaps, particularly from

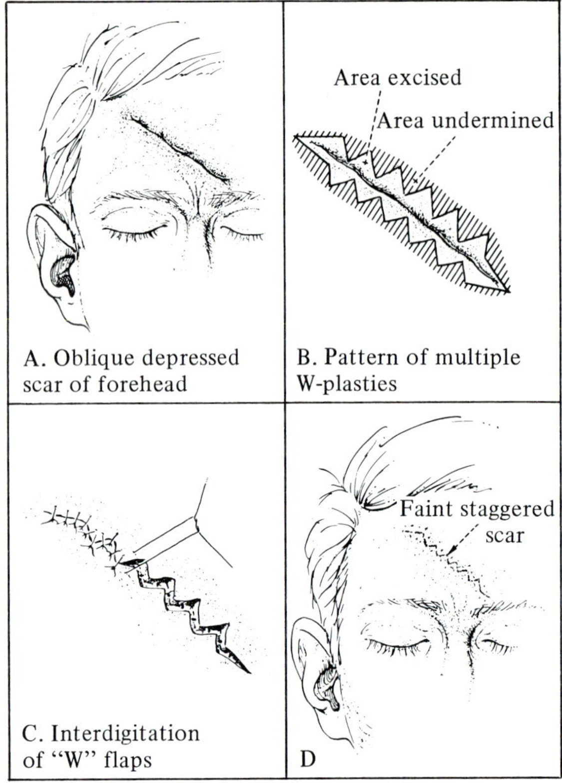

Fig. 9-6. Technique for W-plasty.

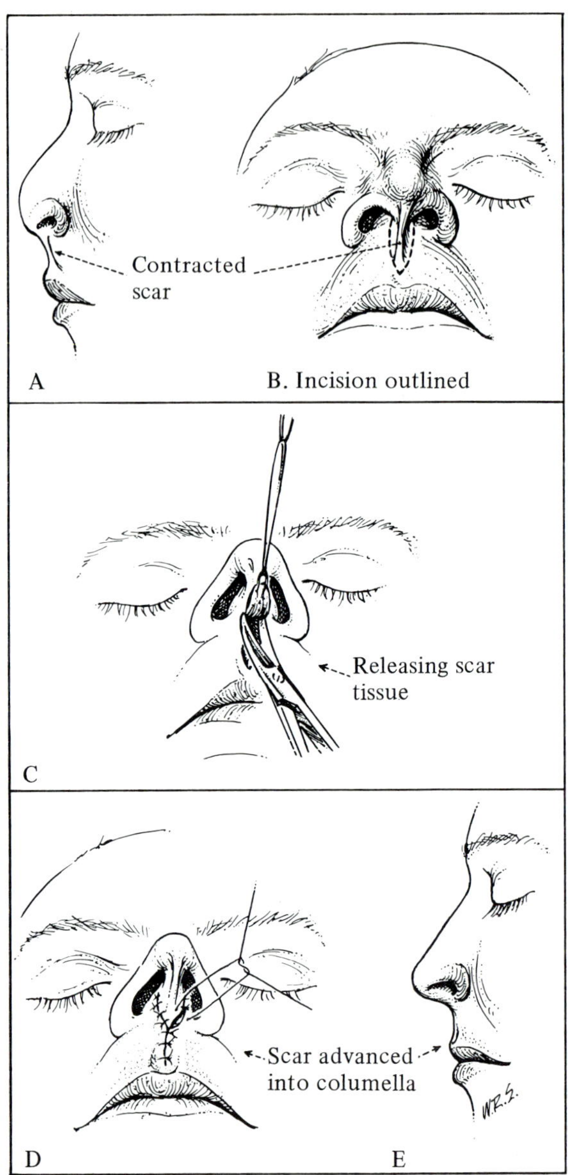

Fig. 9-7. Operative technique for V-Y plasty at nasolabial angle.

windshield injuries. These crescent or U-shaped scars usually are depressed when they heal, with associated edema of the flap. Extensive undermining of the flap and tearing of its borders serve to interpose a broad scar between the flap and its bed.

Softening and maturation of these scars sometimes takes more than a year. Even after several years the appearance is usually disappointing. When avulsion flaps are relatively small and when their location is appropriate, they may be excised with their surrounding scar; if primary closure can be accomplished, the problem is immediately solved. When this is not possible, revision of the peripheral scar with staggering or Z-plasty procedures is indicated. The Z-plasties should be placed at the curved portions of the scars where they cross normal skin lines. In addition to interrupting the constricting nature of the scar in this area, flaps of adjacent tissue interpolated with flaps cut from the avulsion flap bring in undamaged venous and lymphatic channels for improving drainage. Defatting the edematous flap is not corrective and produces still more fibrosis under the flap.

REFERENCES

1. Barton, N. W., Miller, S. H., and Graham, W. P., III. Managing lacerations of the parotid gland, duct, and facial nerve. *Am. Fam. Physician* 13: 130, 1976.
2. Bornstein, L. A., and Simon, B. E. Successful primary repair of severed parotid duct. *Plast. Reconstr. Surg.* 6:217, 1949.

3. Bromberg, B. B. Soft Tissue Injuries of the Face. In Grabb, W. C., and Smith, J. W. (Eds.), *Plastic Surgery*. Boston: Little, Brown, 1975.
4. Clark, G. M. Trauma to the cartilaginous skeleton of the nose. *Eye Ear Nose Throat Mon.* 49:284, 1970.
5. Crawford, J. S. Ptosis as a result of trauma. *Can. J. Ophthalmol.* 9:244, 1974.
6. Dowling, J. A., Foley, F. D., and Moncrief, J. A. Chondritis in the burned ear. *Plast. Reconstr. Surg.* 42:115, 1968.
7. Ellingham, T. R. The immediate care of eye injuries. *Anaesthesia* 31:433, 1976.
8. Flowers, R. S., and Anderson, R. Injury to the lacrimal apparatus during rhinoplasty. *Plast. Reconstr. Surg.* 42:577, 1968.
9. Goldberg, M. F., and Tessler, H. H. Occult intraocular perforations from brow and lid lacerations. *Arch. Ophthalmol.* 86:145, 1971.
10. Huelke, D. F., Grabb, W. C., and Dingman, R. O. Facial injuries due to windshield impacts in automobile accidents. *Plast. Reconstr. Surg.* 37:324, 1966.
11. Iverson, P. C. Surgical removal of traumatic tattoos of the face. *Plast. Reconstr. Surg.* 2:427, 1947.
12. Jabaley, M. E., Lerman, M., and Sanders, H. J. Ocular injuries in orbital fractures. *Plast. Reconstr. Surg.* 56:410, 1975.
13. Kathak, F. F., and Dubrul, E. L. The immediate repair of war wounds of the face. *Plast. Reconstr. Surg.* 2:110, 1947.
14. Kerster, T. E., and McQuarrie, D. G. Surgical management of shotgun injuries of the face. *Surg. Gynecol. Obstet.* 140:517, 1975.
15. McCabe, B. F. Facial nerve grafting. *Plast. Reconstr. Surg.* 45:70, 1970.
16. Mladick, R. A., and Carraway, J. H. Ear reattachment by the modified pocket principle. *Plast. Reconstr. Surg.* 51:584, 1973.
17. Musgrave, R. H., and Garrett, W. S. Dog bite avulsions of the lip. *Plast. Reconstr. Surg.* 49:294, 1972.
18. Ohlsen, L., Skoop, T., and Shon, S. A. The pathogenesis of cauliflower ear. *Scand. J. Plast. Reconstr. Surg.* 9:34, 1975.
19. Pirrucello, F. W. Observation in management of soft tissue injuries of the face: The reconstruction of eyebrows. *Plast. Reconstr. Surg.* 25:548, 1960.
20. Pitts, W., Pickrell, F., and Quinn, G. Electrical burns of lips and mouth in infants and children. *Plast. Reconstr. Surg.* 44:471, 1969.
21. Schultz, R. C. Organized hematoma. *J.A.M.A.* 189:215, 1964.
22. Schultz, R. C. Intraoral sutures. *J.A.M.A.* 195: 400, 1966.
23. Schultz, R. C. Facial injuries from automobile accidents: A study of 400 consecutive cases. *Plast. Reconstr. Surg.* 40:415, 1967.
24. Schultz, R. C. Facial injuries from automobile accidents. *Surg. Gynecol. Obstet.* 127:151, 1968.
25. Schultz, R. C. 760 consecutive cases of facial injury. *Dent. Abstracts* 13:29, 1968.
26. Schultz, R. C. The Changing Pattern and Management of Soft Tissue Windshield Injuries. In Huelke, D. (Ed.), *Proceedings of the 1970 Meeting of the American Association for Automotive Medicine.* Ann Arbor, Mich.: University of Michigan Press, 1970.
27. Schultz, R. C. *Facial Injuries.* Chicago: Year Book, 1970.
28. Schultz, R. C. One thousand cases of major facial injury. *Rev. Surg.* 37:394, 1970.
29. Schultz, R. C. One Thousand Major Facial Injuries from Auto Accidents. In *Proceedings of the International Association for Accident and Traffic Medicine.* Ann Arbor, Mich.: Highway Safety Research Institute, 1971.
30. Schultz, R. C. The changing character and management of soft tissue windshield injuries. *J. Trauma* 12:1, 1972.
31. Schultz, R. C. The nature of facial injury emergencies. *Surg. Clin. North Am.* 52:1, 1972.
32. Schultz, R. C. Facial Injuries. In Condon, R. E., and Nyhus, L. M. (Eds.), *Manual of Surgical Therapeutics* (3rd ed.). Boston: Little, Brown, 1975.
33. Schultz, R. C. *Facial Injuries* (2nd ed.). Chicago: Year Book, 1977.
34. Schultz, R. C., and Baker, S. P. Recurrent problems in emergency room management of maxillofacial injuries. *Clin. Plast. Surg.* 2:65, 1975.
35. Schultz, R. C., and McMaster, W. C. The treatment of dog bite injuries, especially those of the face. *Plast. Reconstr. Surg.* 49:494, 1972.
36. Schultz, R. C., and Oldham, R. J. An overview of facial injuries. *Surg. Clin. North Am.* 57:987, 1977.
37. Shannon, G. M. Treatment of dog bite injuries of eyelids and adnexa. *Ophthalmic Surg.* 6:41, 1975.
38. Tipton, J. B. Dislocation of upper lateral cartilages as a cause for nasal deformities. *Plast. Reconstr. Surg.* 47:459, 1971.

10

Facial Bone Fractures

PAUL NATVIG AND RICHARD K. DORTZBACH

Reduction and immobilization are the two basic principles the surgeon follows in the treatment of fractures of facial bones. Although methods of accomplishing this vary and techniques are multiple, we wish to present methods that are most useful at present. The end result of treatment must offer the patient the best in restoration of function and aesthetics.

Violent accidents may bring about concomitant soft tissue lacerations. It is not unusual, however, to examine a patient who gives a history of a violent force to the face and presents with multiple comminuted fractures of the facial bones with no lacerations save superficial excoriations.

In the United States, the majority of facial fractures result from vehicular accidents. With the increasing number of accidents, automobiles are now being manufactured with more safety devices. Improved seat belts, body harnesses, changes in structural design, and installation of glass that is more shatterproof are some of the improvements. Motorcycles, as they gain in popularity, increase the toll of facial injuries. Proper headgear may lessen the severity of trauma to the face. Nonetheless, these safety devices are only of value if the human elects to use them and to drive the vehicle with equanimity and prudence.

EMERGENCY TREATMENT

An *adequate airway* for the patient with fractures of the facial bones is of prime importance. Following fractures of the facial bones, improper ventilation may result from numerous causes. The facial bones may be so comminuted that there is posterior displacement, with obstruction of the airway by bone fragments and the soft tissues. Hemorrhage into the tissues, causing large hematomas and progressive edema as time passes, are other causes. The examiner should be alert for foreign bodies such as teeth or blood clots, pieces of glass and debris, dislodged and broken dentures, or bits of clothing that may be forced into the oral cavity and the nose.

Profuse hemorrhage requires immediate emergency treatment. The standard methods of hemostasis, with instruments, ligatures, and packing if necessary, are used.

The best time to reduce facial fractures is at the initial operative procedure. This is not to suggest that the plastic surgeon must impetuously rush the patient to the surgical suite soon after admission to the emergency room. The wise surgeon knows that only lifesaving measures require immediate operative intervention in the surgical suite.

The reduction of facial bone fractures can be performed several days after injury. Spinal cord, intracranial, intrathoracic, and intraabdominal injuries, and open fractures to the extremities usually take precedence. It may even be desirable to defer operating on facial fractures to better assess latent signs and symptoms and specialized examinations. One may then correctly identify, for example, epidural or subdural hematomas versus cerebral edema, or a ruptured viscus in the abdomen versus a contusion to the abdominal wall.

It is recommended that a roentgenogram of the cervical spine be completed on all those with severe facial injuries soon after these patients enter the hospital.

CLASSIFICATION OF FRACTURES OF THE FACIAL BONES

Fractures of the facial bones may be classified as *closed* and *open* fractures. Loss of bone may occur in facial fractures. Fractures of the mandible are classified according to anatomic regions (see Fig. 10-4), the zygomatic fractures according to the displacement and rotation of the zygoma (see Fig. 10-9), maxillary fractures according to the three general classifications as described by Le Fort [53] (see Fig. 10-6), and nasal fractures according to the various kinds of fractures (see Fig. 10-7).

DIAGNOSIS OF FACIAL FRACTURES

History

An accurate history of the cause of the injury and a past history of the patient is of high importance and may determine the timing for treatment.

Examination

As soon as a patient has been admitted to the hospital, a thorough physical examination must be completed. All necessary consultations with other surgical or medical specialists should be obtained.

The most common sign of displaced fractures of the facial bones, except for the nose, is *malocclusion of the teeth,* which occurs when a fracture has displaced the mandible or the maxilla, or in fracture of the zygoma when the arch of the zygoma is depressed and the coronoid process of the mandible cannot properly glide behind the arch of the zygoma.

Palpation of the facial bones is a further aid in diagnosis. Palpation of the mandible can be performed by placing the index fingers of both hands on the occlusal or incisal surfaces of the teeth (or, if the patient is edentulous, on the alveolar ridge on either side of the suspected fracture segment) and the thumbs at the inferior border of the mandible, and then demonstrating movement at the fracture site. Stability of the maxillas may be determined by applying the thumb in front of, and the index finger behind, the anterior teeth and then attempting to move the maxillas. Intraoral palpation along the cul-de-sac adjacent to the buccal maxillary mucosa may show irregularities of the maxillas, particularly of the bone anterior and lateral to the maxillary sinuses. The infraorbital margins are palpated with the fingertips to identify displacement of the inferior rim of the orbit, which is part of the maxillas and maxillary process of the zygoma. Palpation over the zygomatic arches may help identify depressed fractures of the arches soon after the injury. However, if hours have elapsed since the injury and there is edema, it may be very difficult to palpate fractures of the zygomatic arches. Palpation on both sides of the nose aids in determining the integrity of the nasal bones and of the frontal processes of the maxillas.

The presence of *edema, hematomas,* and *ecchymosis* of the upper half of the face suggests maxillary, zygomatic, and nasal fractures. These same signs of the lower half of the face suggest fractures of the mandible. Malfunction of the extraocular muscles or *diplopia* suggests fractures of the zygomaticomaxillary bones. *Cerebrospinal rhinorrhea* indicates a fracture through the cribriform plate of the skull.

Roentgenographic Examination

The roentgenogram is a most important adjunct in the diagnosis and treatment of facial fractures. As soon as possible after the injury, radiographs should be obtained.

The single most valuable radiograph for diagnosis is the Waters' projection. This view will show fractures of the maxillas, the maxillary sinuses, the floors and rims of the orbits, the zygomatic bones, the nasal bones, the nasal septum, and the mandible. The visualization of the mandible, however, is not completely satisfactory. A reverse Waters' projection may be useful if the patient cannot be placed in the prone position. Other desirable views of the facial bones include lateral projection of the skull; posteroanterior projection of the mandible; lateral oblique projection of the mandible; lateral projections of the temporomandibular joints; anteroposterior projection of the mandibular condylar processes, including zygomatic arches (modified Towne's projection); inferosuperior projection of the parasymphyseal area and mandible; inferosuperior oblique projection of parasymphyseal area and mandible; superoinferior projection of hard palate; superoinferior oblique projection of hard palate; submental-vertical projection of zygomatic arches; lateral projection of the nasal bones; superoinferior projection of nasal bones; and intraoral dental roentgenograms. Panoramic jaw radiography, where available, may be useful in identifying fractures.

TRACHEOTOMY

Tracheotomy* is the surgical operation of making an artificial opening into the trachea. Tracheotomy is indicated whenever the patient's life is in danger because of obstruction above or in the larynx. The obstruction may be due to lodging of foreign bodies, laryngospasm, edema or hematomas, tumors, or malfunction of muscles of respiration caused by disease or trauma of the central nervous system. Elective tracheotomy is one of the most important adjuncts to the treatment of fractures of the facial bones. It provides an ideal route for the administration of general anesthesia, and the anesthetic equipment is thereby removed from the operative field. Even if one is fortunate enough to have a competent anesthesiologist to convert from nasoendotracheal to oroendotracheal administration during an operative procedure to avoid the use of tracheotomy, there is always edema postoperatively. Nasal packing and dental fixation place the airway in even greater jeopardy. Extensive multiple fractures of facial bones require the presence of a tracheotomy airway in the postoperative period.

If ever there is a reasonable suspicion of a need for tracheotomy, it should be performed.

Tracheotomy may be divided into two types: *superior* and *inferior* tracheotomy (Fig. 10-1.). The superior tracheotomy is also known as the coniotomy and is performed through the cricothyroid (conic) ligament. Coniotomy should be performed only in extreme emergency. When the coniotomy has served its purpose, inferior tracheotomy should be done if it is necessary to maintain the airway. Should the superior tracheotomy be allowed to remain for an extended period of time, laryngeal fibrosis is a likely complication.

The inferior tracheotomy is the desired method. It is usually performed at the level between the third and fourth tracheal rings.

*Tracheotomy is an old, well-founded term. *Tracheostomy* is often used interchangeably with the term *tracheotomy,* but would be better reserved by defining it as the surgical formation of a long-term or permanent opening into the trachea, the edges of the opening being sutured to an opening in the skin of the neck.

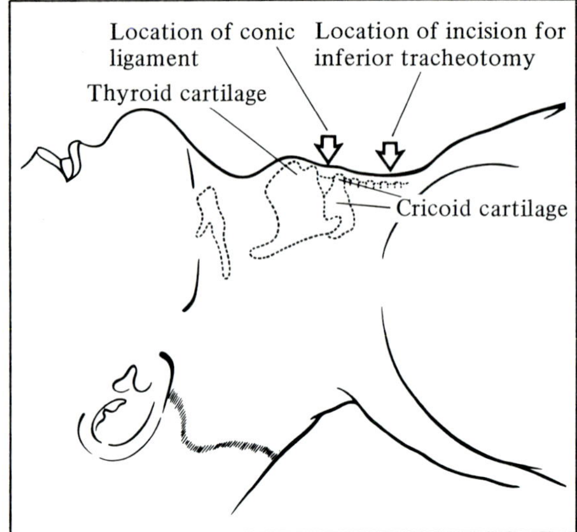

Fig. 10-1. Location for coniotomy and inferior tracheotomy. (Reproduced, by permission, from R. O. Dingman and P. Natvig. Surgery of Facial Fractures. *Philadelphia: Saunders, 1964.)*

THE TEETH AND OCCLUSION

The teeth and their occlusion are the keystone in the treatment of facial bone fractures. Sicher [77] has pointed out that occlusion is dynamic and that positions of occlusion are all those in which contact between some or all maxillary and mandibular teeth occurs. Median occlusion, however, is an intercuspation of the mandibular teeth against the maxillary teeth. Median occlusion may be considered static, or that position where the teeth will be placed in "normal" fixation. Most commonly in anatomical descriptions the terms *medial* and *lateral* or *proximal* and *distal* are in use; however, in dental nomenclature the terms are *mesial* and *distal. If a short imaginary line is drawn in the midsagittal plane between the central incisors, all surfaces of the teeth that face this line are known as the mesial surfaces and all surfaces of the teeth away from this line are known as the distal surfaces.* Hence the distal surface of the right maxillary central incisor approximates the mesial surface of the right maxillary lateral incisor. The mesial or distal surface may also be called the approximal surface. The potential space between teeth is known as the interproximal space.

During one's lifetime, normally two dentitions are present. The deciduous dentition (primary teeth, milk teeth, baby teeth, temporary teeth) consists of 20 teeth: two central incisors, two lateral incisors, two canines, and four molars in each dental arch. The permanent (secondary) dentition is composed of 32 teeth: two central incisors, two lateral incisors, two canines, two first premolars, two second premolars, two first molars, two second molars, and two third molars in each arch. The teeth in both dentitions are divided into anterior and posterior teeth. The anterior teeth are the four central incisors, four lateral incisors, and four canines. *All teeth distal to the canines are known as posterior teeth.* The distal margins of the canines appear to end at the corners of the mouth, and for this reason the surfaces of the anterior teeth that face the lips are the *labial surfaces.* The surfaces of the posterior teeth which face the cheek are the *buccal surfaces.* Collectively, the labial and buccal surfaces are referred to as the *vestibular surfaces.* Inner surfaces of anterior and posterior teeth all approximate the tongue and are the *lingual surfaces* of the teeth. The occluding surfaces of the anterior teeth are the *incisal edges,* and are knifelike. The incisors have simple cutting edges and the canines have a two-armed cutting edge, a mesial arm and a distal arm which join to form an angle. This angulation of the canine gives it a spearlike shape and functions in prehension and tearing of food. The occluding surfaces of the posterior teeth are called the *occlusal surfaces.* The premolars and the molars have an occlusal surface which allows for progressively increased grinding function. The roots of the teeth reflect their function. The incisors and canines have a single root; the root of the canine is the longest, allowing for firm fixation of the tooth for prehension of food. Premolars have one or two roots, and the molars in the mandibular arch have two roots while those in the maxillary arch have three roots. The teeth are seated in the alveolar process of the mandible and maxillas. Each root has its own alveolus or socket. Each tooth is divided into a crown and root or roots. The surface of the crown is covered by enamel and the surface of the root or roots is covered by cementum. The hard inner core of the tooth is composed of dentin (dentine). The center of each tooth has a pulp chamber in its crown and a canal in each root containing nervous and vascular tissues.

An important structure is the periodontal ligament which attaches the tooth to the alveolus.

Approximately between the ages of 6 and 14 years a mixed dentition (i.e., a mixture of deciduous and permanent teeth) is present.

TEETH IN THE FRACTURE LINE

A tooth in the line of fracture need not necessarily be extracted if there is little or no displacement and the tooth is fairly firm in its socket. The old axiom "don't extract yourself out of occlusion" applies. It is desirable to preserve all teeth in treating fractures of the jaws. The teeth aid immeasurably in proper reduction and fixation of the fractures. However, if the tooth has been displaced, is loose, and acts as a wedge or foreign body in the line of fracture, then it should be extracted.

INTERMAXILLARY FIXATION

The Importance of Intermaxillary Fixation

Adapting arch bars to the teeth and ligating the bars with stainless-steel wire to their necks is one of the most important procedures in properly reducing and fixing fractures of the jaws. *"No part of the human body is like the jaws in having appendages that project from bone, appendages that may be realigned for perfect or near-perfect reduction of fractures and locked into position. This surgically convenient feature is peculiar to the mandible and maxilla. Proper intermaxillary fixation is one of the most important factors in treating facial fractures, and the accurate fixation of the teeth is the keystone."** The use of arch bars ligated to the maxillary and mandibular dentition and fixed by intermaxillary traction is the treatment for many fractures of the mandible. However, if there are multiple, oblique, or comminuted fractures, open reduction and interosseous wire fixation are a necessary adjunct. On occasions, intramedullary fixation is used.

Technique of Application of Arch Bars

Dental arch bars may be obtained from several manufacturers; various styles are available. A metallic bar to which small tangs are attached is preferable. The bar is conformed and cut to the length for the maxillary and mandibular arches. The tangs project superiorly from the maxillary arch and inferiorly from the mandibular arch. The bar is ligated with 25 gauge stainless-steel wire firmly hugging the necks of most of the teeth. Ligatures placed first around the premolars aid in initial fixation and simplify ligating the remaining teeth. All of the teeth, with the exception of the incisors, are usually ligated for distribution of force upon the teeth. Incisors are ligated with finer wire in very exceptional cases because ligatures around the incisors may cause evulsion of these teeth. For additional fixation it may be necessary to fix the arch bar with a circumferential wire. Figure 10-2 shows the technique of circumferential wires (see also Fig. 10-21D). Latex bands are attached to the tangs on the maxillary and mandibular arch bars to fix the teeth in occlusion. After the teeth have been held in occlusion for approximately 1 week, fine-gauge wires may be substituted for the rubber bands, removed one by one. This allows the patient to clean his mouth more easily. Supplemental wire ligatures for securing an arch bar are illustrated in Figure 10-3.

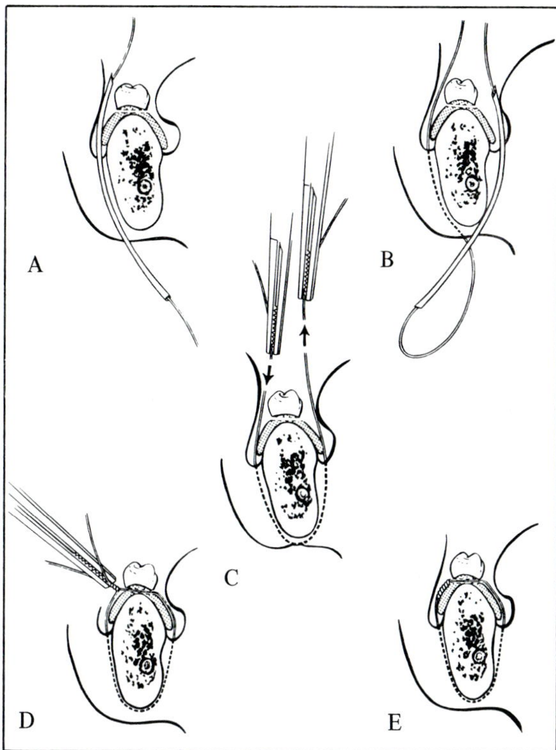

Fig. 10-2. Circumferential wiring of the patient's artificial denture to the mandible. A, a curved passing needle, armed with a wire, punctures the skin at the inferior border of the mandible and passes upward on the lateral surface of the bone into the buccal vestibule; the passing needle is pulled through into the mouth and is slipped off the wire. B, another passing needle, similarly armed with the wire, is inserted through the same puncture wound in the skin and is directed, on the medial surface of the mandible, into the lingual sulcus; the passing needle is slipped off the wire and is removed from the mouth. C, a seesaw motion is applied to the wire to cut through any small fibers of tissue that are trapped in the wire loop; this ensures contact of the wire with the inferior margin of the bone. D, the wire from the lingual side is passed through a bur hole in the artificial denture and twisted securely with the wire from the buccal side. E, the twisted double wire is cut, and its end is pressed firmly against the denture so that the end does not irritate the buccal mucosa.

*Dingman, R. O., and Natvig, P. *Surgery of Facial Fractures.* Philadelphia: Saunders, 1964.

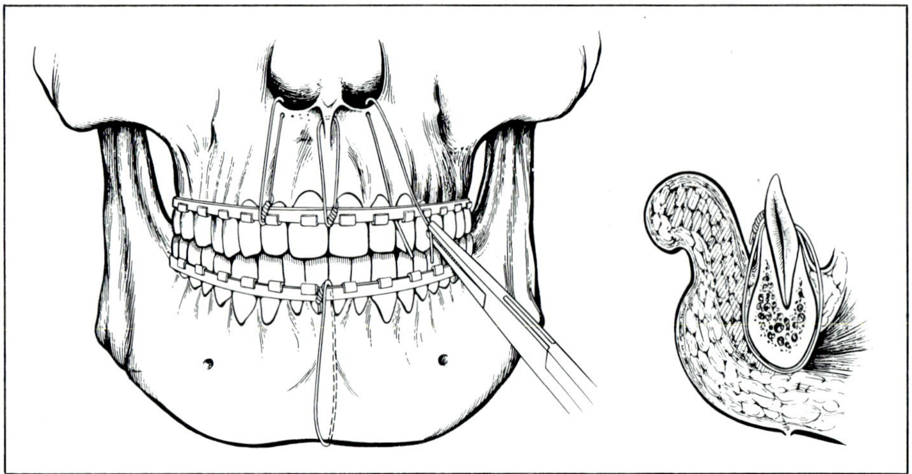

Fig. 10-3. Supplemental wire ligatures for securing an arch bar. Wires are shown through the piriform margins and the nasal spine, along with a circumferential wire around the mandible. The judgment of the surgeon will dictate whether to use one supplemental ligature or a combination of those illustrated. The canines and posterior teeth are also individually ligated but not shown here.

Removal of Intermaxillary Fixation
Arch bars are usually removed 4 to 5 weeks after application. When the latex bands or fine wires have been removed, the stability of the mandible can be determined by palpation. If there is indication that the jaw is not yet fixed firmly, it is advisable to replace the bands and keep the teeth in occlusion for another week or two. Radiographs are of no value in assessing bony healing in the early periods. "Clinical healing" may have occurred, even though radiographic evidence of healing will not be present for several months after the initial trauma.

It is usual for the patient not to be able to open the mouth very wide after removal of the intermaxillary traction. Usually several days must elapse before the jaw will open again to its normal range. For this reason removal of the arch bars might have to be deferred.

FRACTURES OF THE MANDIBLE

About two-thirds of all facial fractures involve the mandible, even though the mandible is the heaviest and strongest of the facial bones. The prominence and position of the mandible expose it to more trauma than the other facial bones.

The causes of mandibular fractures are:

1. External violence – vehicular accidents, fist fights, industrial accidents, falls, kicks, sport accidents, war injuries, gunshot injuries.
2. Local or systemic disease – osteomyelitis, benign and malignant tumors, metastases of malignancy, metabolic dysfunctions, muscular contractions from electroshock therapy.

Fractures of the mandible may be classified according to pathological change of bone and surrounding tissues:

1. Closed fracture – no break in the skin or mucosa.
2. Open fracture – skin or mucosal lacerations.

Any of the above classifications may be further described as oblique, transverse, comminuted, or greenstick. The fractures may be located in the following regions of the mandible [29]: the symphysis, body, angle, ramus, and the condylar, coronoid, and alveolar processes (Fig. 10-4).

The patient usually complains of the following symptoms: pain, malocclusion, excessive salivation, and dysphagia. The most prominent signs noted by the physician are swelling, malocclusion, crepitation, discoloration, deformity, and bad breath.

Muscles That Affect the Movement of the Mandible
Groups of muscles may act in concert to displace fractures at the time of injury. The function of the muscles (Fig. 10-5) may be divided into the following categories:

1. The depressor-retractor group of muscles – the geniohyoid muscles and the digastric muscles.
2. The elevator group of muscles – the masseter muscles, the medial pterygoid muscles, and the temporal muscles.
3. The protrusor muscles – the lateral pterygoid muscles.

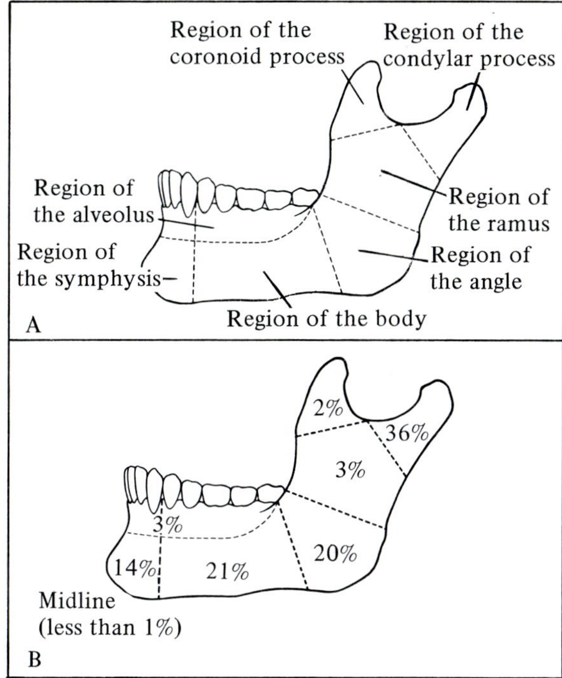

Fig. 10-4. A, the anatomical regions of the mandible. B, the frequency of fractures in those regions.

4. The mylohyoid muscle has practically no influence on the movements of the mandible. The function of the muscle is to elevate the tongue.

Treatment of Mandibular Fractures

As soon after the injury as the patient's general condition allows, reduction and fixation of the fractured mandible should take place. In *nearly all fractures of the mandible it is necessary to place the teeth in occlusion by intermaxillary fixation* (see Fig. 10-20A, D and 10-21B, D). When the fracture is in the region of the *mandibular body and there are teeth on either side of the fracture site, intermaxillary fixation* is the method of choice. Where fractures occur *distal to the teeth,* as in bilateral fractures through the region of the angles, it is most often necessary to perform bilateral *open reduction of the mandible with supplemental intermaxillary fixation* (see Fig. 10-21D). A common injury of the mandible is a fracture in the region of the symphysis along with bilateral subcondylar fractures. This kind of injury is best treated by *open reduction of the fracture in the region of the symphysis along with intermaxillary fixation* (see Fig. 10-19B). *Subcondylar fractures alone are usually treated by wiring the teeth in occlusion.* Fractures of the coronoid process, which are uncommon, are also treated by wiring the teeth in occlusion. Fractures that occur in *edentulous* mandibles are reduced and

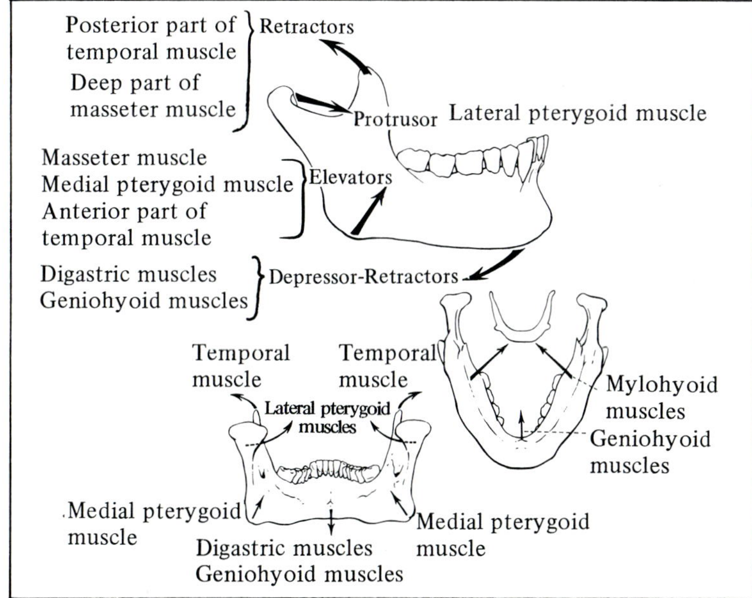

Fig. 10-5. Diagrammatic representation of the main directions of the composite forces of the mandibular muscles.

fixed by *open reduction with the use of the artificial denture fixed with circumferential wires or by intramedullary pin fixation.* The intermaxillary fixation is maintained for 4 to 5 weeks.

CLOSED REDUCTION – WIRING OF ARCH BARS TO TEETH. A commercial dental arch bar is bent to conform to the vestibular surfaces of the teeth. After adapting the bar to the dental arch, 25 gauge stainless-steel wire is placed around the necks of the posterior teeth and the canines, and ligated around the arch bars. The maxillary and mandibular dentitions may then be placed in occlusion, and the small tangs on the arch bars will accept small latex bands, which will hold the teeth in occlusion.

OPEN REDUCTION. Incisions are made below the inferior border of the mandible at the site of the fracture. Sharp dissection is carried up to the fracture and the periosteum dissected away from the bone on either side of the fracture. A small drill hole is made near the margin of the bone on both sides of the fracture and a 25 gauge stainless-steel wire threaded through the small holes. Following reduction of the fracture, the wire is twisted tightly to maintain alignment. The subcutaneous surgical wound is closed in layers with fine catgut. Nylon sutures are used to approximate the skin margins. The adjunct intermaxillary fixation is usually maintained for 4 to 5 weeks.

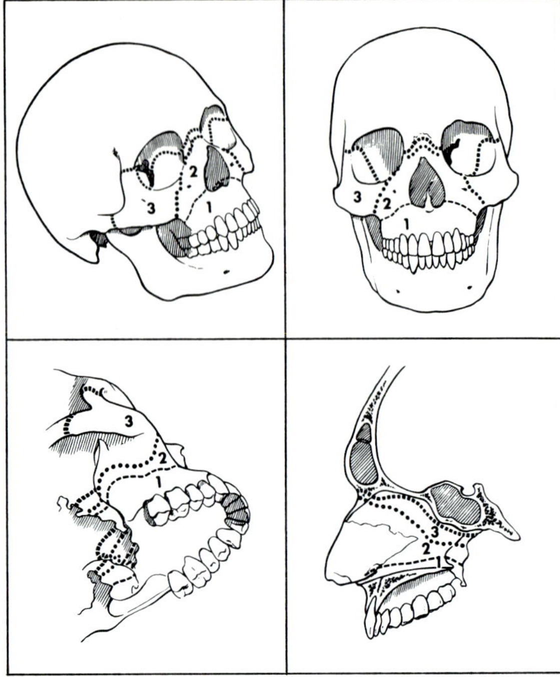

Fig. 10-6. Fractures of the maxillas. 1: Le Fort I (transverse or Guérin) fracture. 2: Le Fort II (pyramidal) fracture. 3: Le Fort III fracture (craniofacial disjunction).

FRACTURES OF THE MAXILLAS

In fractures of the upper jaw it is not uncommon for the two maxillas and palatine bones to be fractured in so-called fractures of the maxillas. Note the classification of fractures of the maxillas and the involvement of approximating bones (Fig. 10-6).

Rowe and Killey [72] and Kazanjian and Converse [49] believe the ratio of fractures of the maxillas to the mandible to be 1 : 4. Recent reports from other centers show, however, that the incidence of fractures of the upper jaw is increasing.

The facial bones, by absorbing violent forces, dissipate these forces in many instances, and this offers protection to the brain and spinal cord.

Fractures of the upper jaw are most commonly the result of transportation accidents. The so-called "guest-passenger" injury occurs when the passenger is thrown against the dashboard or the back of the front seat and smashes the middle third of the face. For this reason, this fracture is sometimes referred to as the "smash injury." Blows by the human fist and industrial accidents are less common causes of fractures of the maxilla.

Classification

Fractures of the maxillas may be classified as follows:

1. Le Fort I, or transverse maxillary or Guérin fracture. This transverse fracture occurs through the maxilla above the level of the teeth. Included in the fracture segment is the alveolar process, portions of the walls of the maxillary sinuses, the palatine bone, and lower portions of the pterygoid processes of the sphenoid bone.
2. Le Fort II, or pyramidal fracture of the maxillas. This pyramidal fracture traverses the nasal bones, frontal processes of the maxillas, lacrimal bones, inferior rims of the orbit, through the floor of the orbit and near or through the zygomaticomaxillary suture. The fracture continues backward along the lateral wall of the maxilla through the pterygoid plates and into the pterygomaxillary fossa.
3. Le Fort III, or craniofacial disjunction. When the traumatic force is so great as to separate the facial bones from their cranial attachments, the fractures usually occur through the zygomaticofrontal, maxillofrontal, and nasofrontal sutures; through the floors of the orbits; and through the ethmoid and sphenoid bones with complete separation of all the structures of the middle facial skeleton.

The symptoms of fracture of the maxillas are pain, malocclusion, excessive salivation, difficulty in swallowing, and epistaxis. The signs are swelling, especially in the periorbital tissues; malocclusion; crepitation; discoloration, especially around the orbit; deformity, elongation of face, donkey-like face except in Le Fort I; bad breath; and cerebrospinal rhinorrhea (Le Fort III).

Treatment of Maxillary Fractures
The important concept in treatment of fractures of the maxillas is stabilization of the fractures to a point superior to the fractures where there is stability of the skeleton.

LE FORT I FRACTURES. This type of fracture is treated by placing arch bars to both dentitions. Utilizing the intact mandible and the intermaxillary fixation, the maxilla is fixed by making small incisions just below the bony margins of the orbit. After drilling small holes through each rim, a 25 gauge stainless-steel wire is threaded through the holes, and with a passing needle the wire and needle are directed into the mouth and secured to the maxillary arch bar.

LE FORT II FRACTURES. An intact mandible is necessary for proper reduction of the pyramidal fracture. In this instance the wire suspension is from the zygomatic process of the frontal bone. A wire is threaded through the hole and the passing needle is directed behind the zygomatic arch into the oral cavity, and the wires are attached to the upper bar (see Fig. 10-21B). Fixation is maintained for 4 weeks. When the mandible is fractured and requires stability, reduction and fixation of the mandible should be performed before reduction of the maxillas.

LE FORT III FRACTURES. Fractures of zygoma and nose are associated with this kind of maxillary fracture. Reduction of the zygomas and nose as described under these headings is performed with the reduction of the maxillas during the same operative procedure. Treatment of the fractured maxillas is the same as described for the Le Fort II (see Fig. 10-20C fracture above.

FRACTURES OF THE NOSE
The nasal bones, frontal processes of the maxillas, nasal cartilages, or nasal septum may be damaged in fractures of the nose. Specific classification of fractures of the nose is difficult to accomplish. Figure 10-7 illustrates different kinds of fractures of the nose.

Symptoms associated with fractures of the nose are pain, swelling, epistaxis, and impairment in breathing. The signs are swelling, intranasal or extranasal lacerations, visible displacement, crepitation or movement, and hemorrhage; late examination may show extensive edema and ecchymosis and preclude diagnosis by palpation.

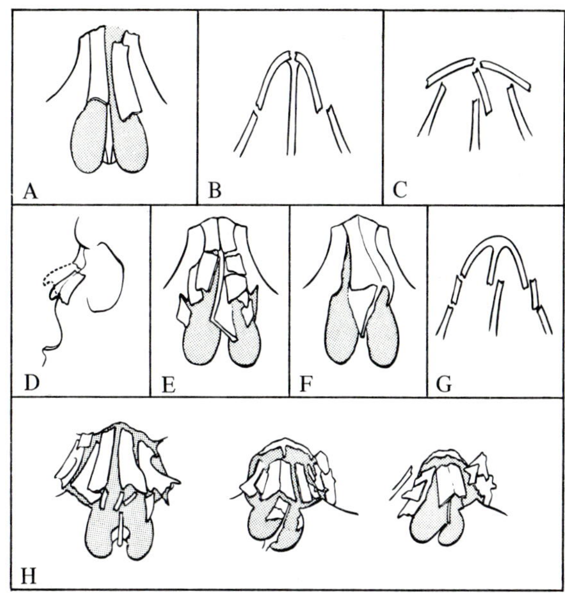

Fig. 10-7. Fractures of the nasal bones. A: Isolation of one nasal bone with inferolateral displacement. B: Diagrammatic horizontal section showing separation of the nasal bones in the midline and from the frontal process of the maxilla; nasal septum intact. C: Fracture of the septum permits a flattening and spreading of the nasal bones; openbook fracture. D: Fracture of the two nasal bones with posteroinferior displacement. E: Comminuted fracture of the nasal bones and the anterior parts of the frontal processes and the nasal septum; displacement mainly down and back. F: Fracture of the nasal septum with separation of the nasal bones from the frontal processes of the maxilla with elevation of the bridge of the nose. G: Cross-sectional diagram of a fracture similar to that in F. H: Three examples of smash fracture of the nose with embarrassment of the interorbital space.

Treatment of Nasal Fractures
Reduction of nasal fractures is accomplished by digital and instrumental manipulation. By placing an Asch forceps (Fig. 10-8) or a large Kelly forceps with rubber tubing over each blade intranasally under the nasal bones, most fractures can be properly reduced along with external digital manipulation. Fractures of the septum that show displacement may likewise be manipulated intranasally. Fractures of the nose that have not resulted in edema and ecchymosis of the surround-

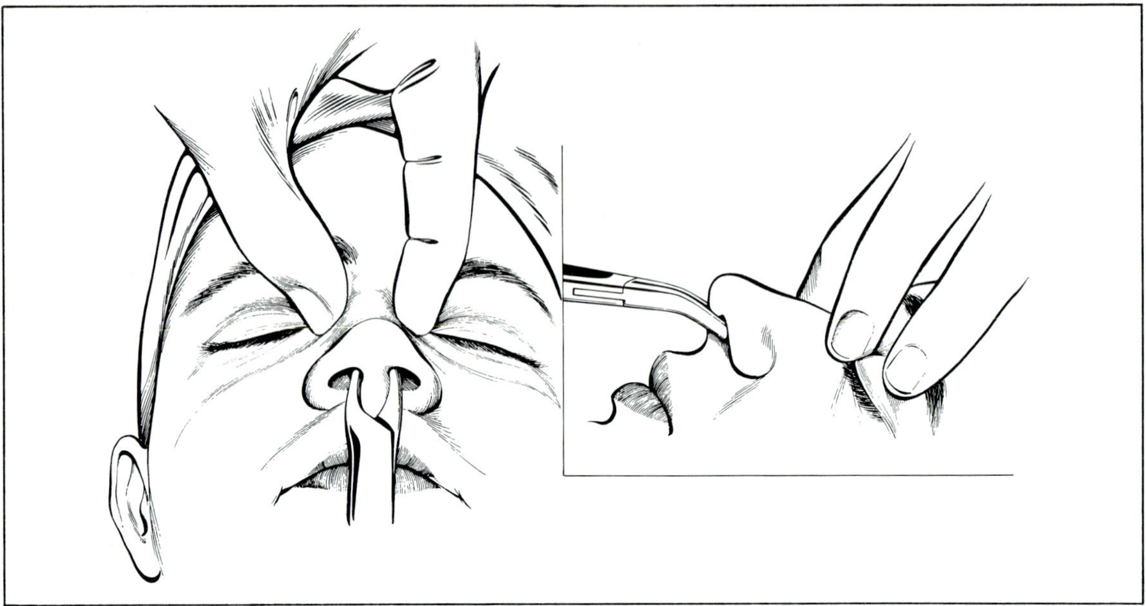

Fig. 10-8. Asch forceps applied intranasally for reduction of a fracture of the nose.

ing tissues may be reduced with moderate ease; after several hours when there is considerable edema and ecchymosis, it is sometimes desirable to wait for the edema to subside in order to allow for more accurate reduction. Nasal fractures that are beyond 1 or 2 weeks old usually require reduction by osteotomy or by modified rhinoplasty procedures. Good light and proper suction equipment are mandatory.

Upon completion of the reduction, intranasal packs impregnated with petrolatum give support to the nasal skeleton. An external splint of a thin metallic material such as copper or aluminum adds additional fixation. Packing is usually allowed to remain in place 4 or 5 days, and the external splint is maintained for about 1 week.

FRACTURES OF THE ZYGOMA

The prominent position of the zygoma and its contour render it very susceptible to fracture. The greater lateral portion of the floor of the orbit is part of the zygomatic bone. The most common fractures of the zygoma (Fig. 10-9) are those in which separation occurs at or near the zygomaticofrontal, zygomaticomaxillary, and zygomaticotemporal suture lines with downward and rotatory displacement, or fracture of the arch only with inward displacement and impingement of the coronoid process of the mandible.

Symptoms in fracture of the zygoma are pain; numbness of the cheek, infraorbital region, and upper teeth on the side affected; swelling of the eyelids with near occlusion of the palpebral fissure; and inability to close the mouth properly if the arch is impinging on the coronoid process of the mandible. Signs in fracture of the zygoma are swelling, edema, and ecchymosis of the periorbital tissues; flatness of the cheek on the affected side, if seen early; irregularity of the infraorbital margin on palpation or depression if the arch is depressed; and irregularity of bone on palpating in the buccal vestibule of the oral cavity.

Treatment of Zygomatic Fractures

Treatment of fractures of the zygoma is by elevating the depressed fracture and maintaining it in the reduced position. Wire sutures ligated through bur holes in the fragments may be necessary for fixation (see Figs. 10-20D and 10-21D). Access to the zygoma is through small incisions in the lateral third of the eyebrow and in the infraorbital region. Through these incisions the zygomaticofrontal suture and zygomaticomaxillary suture may be exposed. It is through these sutures and the zygomaticotemporal suture that fractures most often occur. Through the eyebrow incision a heavy elevator can be placed beneath the arch of the zygoma and the arch reduced and the entire zygoma elevated if required.

Gillies et al. [39] described a method of access to the zygoma through an incision about 2 cm. long in the temporal region, the hair-bearing scalp being shaved. The incision is carried through skin, subcutaneous tissues, and the two layers of the temporal fascia onto the temporal muscle. At this level, a heavy elevator is slipped between the heavy fascia and the

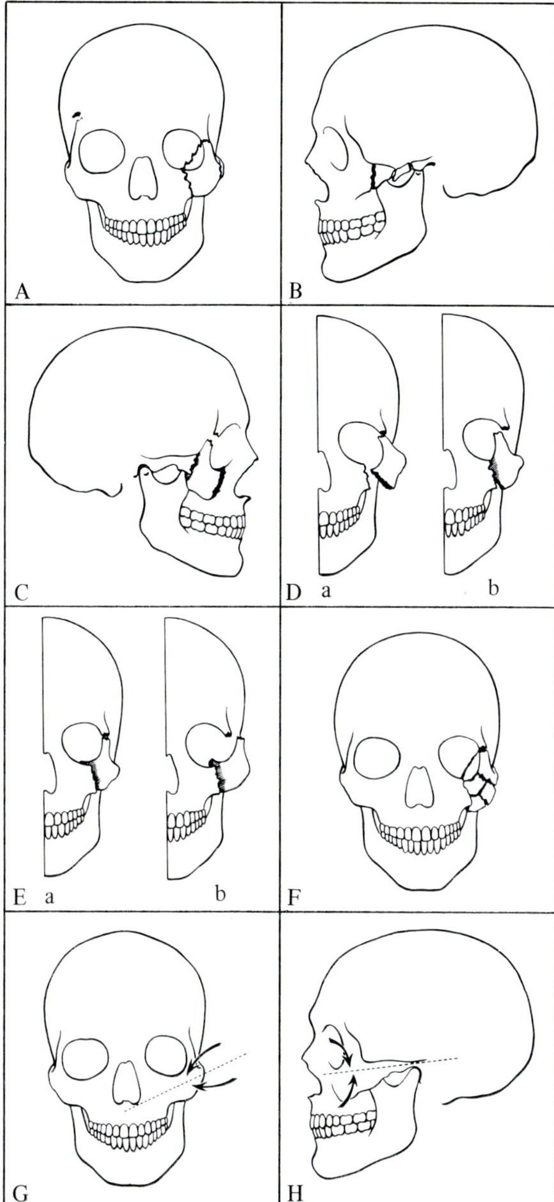

Fig. 10-9. Fractures of the zygoma. A: Group I – no significant displacement. B: Group II – zygomatic arch fractures. C: Group III – unrotated body fractures. D: Group IV – medially rotated body fractures; outward at zygomatic prominence (a) and inward at zygomaticofrontal suture (b). E: Group V – laterally rotated body fractures; upward at infraorbital margin (a) and outward at zygomaticofrontal suture (b). F: Complex fractures. G and H: Directions of force.

muscle to gain access to the undersurface of the zygoma. This method is in use much less today, when an instrument can be placed under the arch more simply through an eyebrow incision (Fig. 10-10).

BLOWOUT FRACTURES

The term *blowout fracture* is reserved for a depressed fracture of the floor of the orbit, usually with some of the contents of the orbit protruding into the maxillary sinus. A true blowout fracture is contained within the area of the orbital floor. Fractures of the orbital rim and adjacent facial bones may be associated with fractures in the orbital floor, but these fractures of the floor are not produced by the "blowout mechanism."

Anatomy of the Orbit

The most common site for a blowout fracture is in the posterior medial part of the orbital floor (Fig. 10-11) of the maxillary bone. In this area the floor is extremely thin, the weakest part of the orbit. Although the ethmoid bones along the medial wall of the orbit are also quite thin, the bony septa in the ethmoid sinuses afford some support.

There are several important inferior orbital structures with which one must be familiar in repairing a blowout fracture of the orbital floor. One should know about the infraorbital groove (Fig. 10-11) through which the infraorbital nerve passes. This groove may be mistaken for the fracture and unnecessary probing in the groove may traumatize the infraorbital nerve. The inferior rectus is the muscle most commonly trapped in a blowout fracture. The inferior oblique muscle may also be involved in the fracture, but in such cases the fracture will extend more toward the anterior part of the floor.

Production of Blowout Fractures

Blowout fractures result from a sudden increase in intraorbital pressure resulting from application of a traumatic force by a nonpenetrating object (larger than the orbital opening) to the soft tissues of the orbital area (Fig. 10-12A, B). The orbital contents are compressed into the smaller volume toward the apex of the orbit, and the orbit has to then "blowout" at its weakest point. This results in a fracture in the posterior medial floor to accommodate the compressed orbital structures. A typical object causing this fracture is a baseball or a fist.

Diagnosis

HISTORY. There will usually be a history of trauma.

DIPLOPIA WITH LIMITATION ON UPGAZE AND DOWNGAZE. The patient may give a history of vertical diplopia, which is exaggerated on upgaze and downgaze. When the extraocular muscle movements are

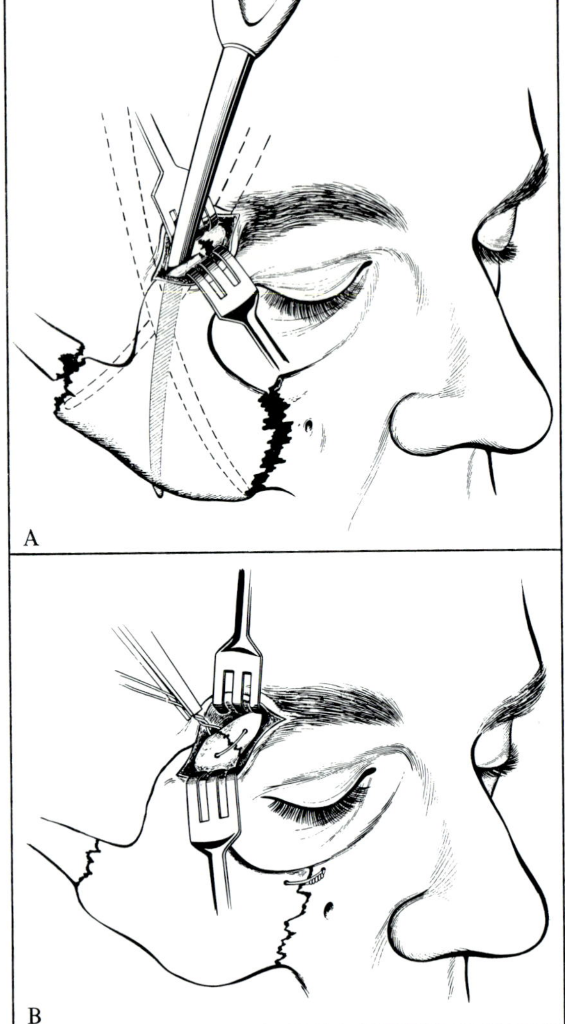

Fig. 10-10. A, tripod fracture of zygoma being elevated through a lateral eyebrow incision. B, wire fixation of fracture at zygomaticofrontal suture line and zygomaticomaxillary suture line.

examined, it is apparent that the movement of the globe is limited and sometimes associated with pain on both upgaze and downgaze. Generally there is no significant limitation on horizontal gaze, either medially or laterally. The red glass test for diplopia and prism measurements in the cardinal fields of gaze can be performed for further evaluation of the degree of diplopia and globe limitation.

Diplopia is caused by entrapment of the inferior rectus muscle, and sometimes the inferior oblique muscle. This can be confirmed by a most important test, the traction test. We have found that the best way to perform this test is to instill a topical anesthetic eyedrop and then to grasp with toothed forceps the conjunctiva and Tenon's capsule near the inferior limbus at the six-o'clock position. An attempt is then made to rotate the globe upward and downward. With a positive traction test, the globe is limited in both upgaze and downgaze, particularly when compared with the uninvolved eye.

Diplopia with entrapment of the inferior extraocular muscles is more likely to occur with smaller blowout fractures. With larger blowout fractures, the muscles are not wedged into the fracture.

ENOPHTHALMOS. If present, this occurs by four mechanisms:

1. A large fracture of the orbital floor may actually allow escape of orbital fat into the maxillary sinus, and this results in inadequate support behind the globe (Fig. 10-13A).
2. At the time of trauma when the orbital contents are compressed toward the posterior orbit and a small blowout fracture occurs, the inferior rectus muscle may be caught in the fracture and hold the globe in a more posterior position in the orbit (Fig. 10-13B).
3. A large fracture of the orbital floor causes sagging of the bone fragments, thus enlarging the orbital cavity (Fig. 10-13C). Because the orbital structures, particularly the orbital fat, expand into a larger orbital volume, there is no longer adequate support for the globe posteriorly and the globe migrates backward.
4. Atrophy of orbital fat may occur following the trauma and result in poor support for the globe posteriorly.

In the first several days following the injury, the enophthalmos may be masked by orbital edema. Enophthalmos should be measured with an exophthalmometer during the initial examination. In instances where orbital edema does mask the enophthalmos, follow-up measurements with the exophthalmometer will disclose the enophthalmos as the orbital edema subsides. Enophthalmos of 3 mm. or less may be within the range of normal. Enophthalmos greater than 4 or 5 mm. is quite noticeable. With significant enophthalmos there is poor support for the upper lid, and a pseudoptosis develops. Measurement of the palpebral fissures on both sides documents pseudoptosis. The superior tarsal fold is also noticeably deepened. In instances where a fracture involves most of the orbital floor, the globe not only drops backward but also downward into the maxillary sinus, causing a ptosis of the globe.

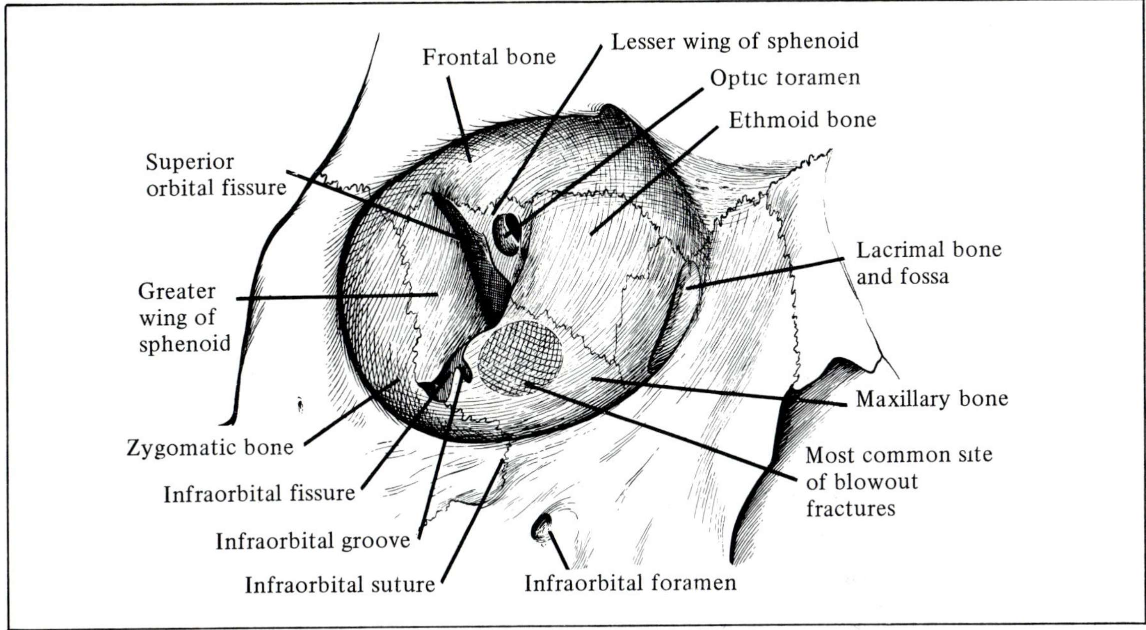

Fig. 10-11. The orbit.

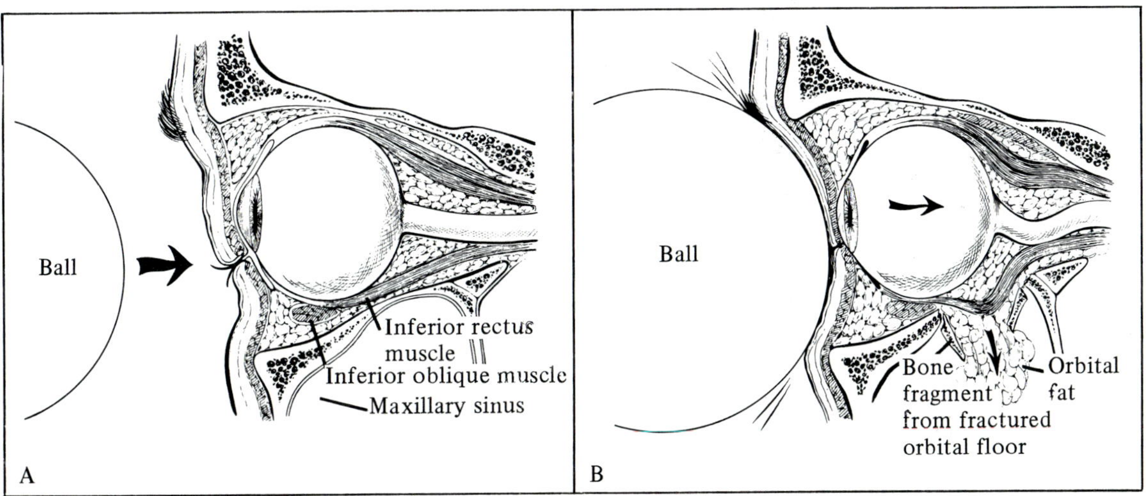

Fig. 10-12. A, orbital structures prior to blowout fracture. B, production of blowout fracture. (Redrawn from B. Smith and W. F. Regan, Jr. Amer. J. Ophthalmol. *44:733, 1957.)*

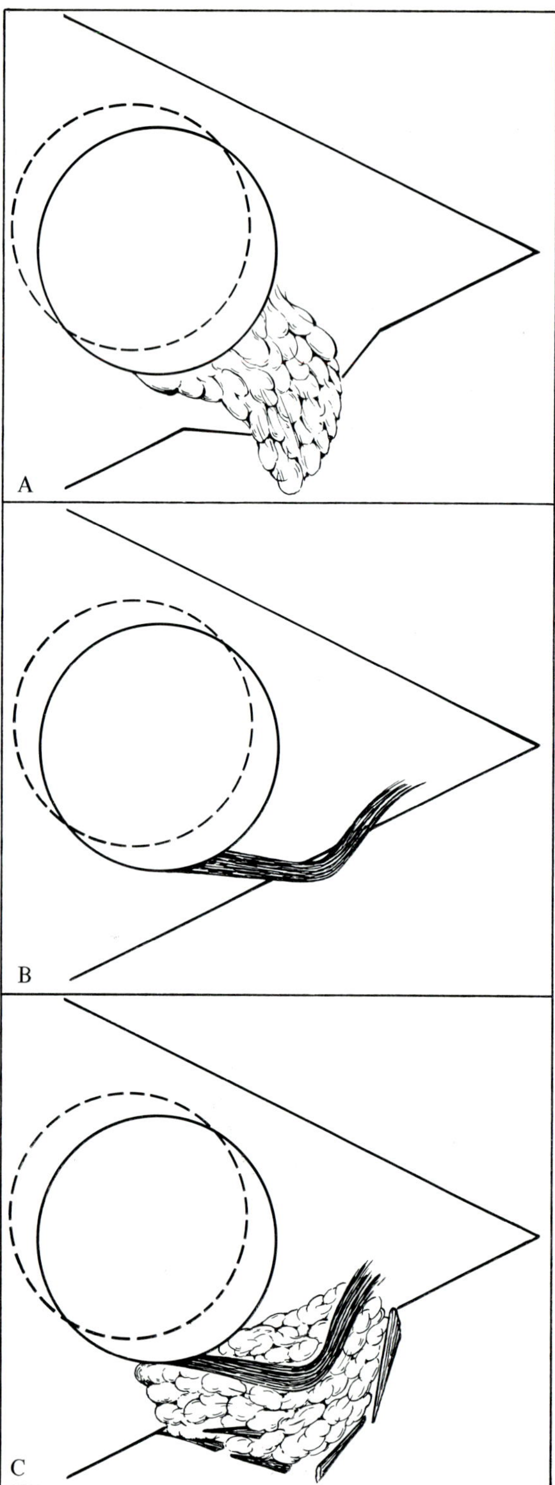

INFRAORBITAL NERVE HYPESTHESIA OR ANESTHESIA. The infraorbital nerve passes through the infraorbital groove and infraorbital canal, and exits through the infraorbital foramen below the inferior orbital rim. The infraorbital nerve carries sensation from the face in the cheek area, extending from the lower lid down to the upper lip and from some of the maxillary teeth. When a blowout fracture extends into the central floor of the orbit, injury may occur to the infraorbital canal. This causes hypesthesia or anesthesia in the area of the face and teeth previously described.

OTHER SIGNS. Additional findings may include periorbital ecchymoses, edema, and emphysema.

RADIOGRAPHS. Stereo Waters' views of the orbital floor and laminograms of the orbital floor are the most helpful in making a diagnosis of a blowout fracture. Radiographs demonstrate fragmentation of the bone of the orbital floor, prolapse of orbital soft tissues into the maxillary sinus, sometimes blood in the maxillary sinus, and sometimes air in the orbit or eyelids due to orbital or periorbital emphysema.

ASSOCIATED INJURIES. There is a high incidence of associated injuries with blowout fractures of the orbital floor. Ocular injuries, such as hyphema and traumatic cataract, are frequent. Avulsion of the medial palpebral ligament and damage to the lacrimal drainage apparatus in the medial canthal area may occur. Damage to the innervation of the levator muscle may result in true ptosis of the upper eyelid. The possibility of associated fractures, particularly of the skull, should be a consideration. Neurological signs and symptoms may be elicited.

Indications for a Surgical Procedure

There are three indications for an operation:

1. Diplopia with limitation on upgaze and downgaze caused by entrapment of the inferior rectus and sometimes the inferior oblique muscle. This can be confirmed with a traction test. If the entrapped muscle is not removed from within the fracture and the fracture repaired, the patient will continue to have diplopia, particularly when the fracture is

Fig. 10-13. A, escape of orbital fat into maxillary sinus. B, globe held back by trapped inferior rectus muscle. C, enlarged orbital cavity with bone fragments sagging down into maxillary sinus. (Redrawn from J. M. Converse. Reconstructive Plastic Surgery, *Vol. 2. Philadelphia: Saunders, 1964.)*

further complicated by ensuing contracture of the muscle.

2. Enophthalmos, which is particularly significant when it is greater than 3 mm. as measured by the exophthalmometer. Enophthalmos is generally associated with radiographic evidence of orbital structures prolapsing through the fracture into the maxillary sinus. If such a fracture is not repaired, the enophthalmos often progresses because of scar formation and contracture of the orbital tissues.
3. Radiographic evidence of a large blowout fracture of the orbital floor. Such large fractures ultimately result in enophthalmos.

Treatment

An operation to repair a blowout fracture should be performed within 7 to 10 days following the injury, before excessive scar tissue develops.

ANTERIOR INFRAORBITAL APPROACH. This is our preferred technique for repair of blowout fractures. Its advantages are that it provides direct observation of a fracture and better exposure of the involved orbital contents (for example, to free bone fragments in or around the inferior rectus muscle) and allows positioning of the prosthesis on the orbital floor.

A slightly curved horizontal incision is made over the inferior orbital rim in the middle of the eyelid in a natural skin crease (Fig. 10-14A). Care should be taken not to extend the incision too far medially where the lacrimal pump will be damaged. If the incision is extended too far laterally and curved upward around the lateral canthus, there is a danger of dividing lymphatic vessels, particularly from the upper eyelid, and causing chronic postoperative lymphedema. The incision is made through the skin and orbicularis oculi muscle down to the periosteum of the inferior orbital rim. The periosteum is incised approximately 3 mm. below the inferior orbital rim. The reason for incising the periosteum below the orbital rim is to provide a better seal when the periosteum is sutured to decrease the chance for extrusion of the implant. A Dingman periosteal elevator is used to raise the periosteum of the floor back to the fracture (Figs. 10-14B and 10-15A). If the inferior rectus muscle is trapped in the fracture, great care should be taken not to pull on the muscle strenuously in an attempt to dislodge it; this may result in additional damage to the muscle. In such instances, we actually enlarge the fracture defect sufficiently to allow the inferior rectus muscle to be lifted gently from the fracture, this minimizing further injury to the muscle.

Various kinds of implants have been used to cover the defect in the orbital floor (Fig. 10-15B). Some materials are Silastic, Teflon, Supramid Extra, Cranioplastic (methyl methacrylate), autogenous and homogenous cartilage, and autogenous bone. No implant is as ideal as the bony floor of the orbit before it has

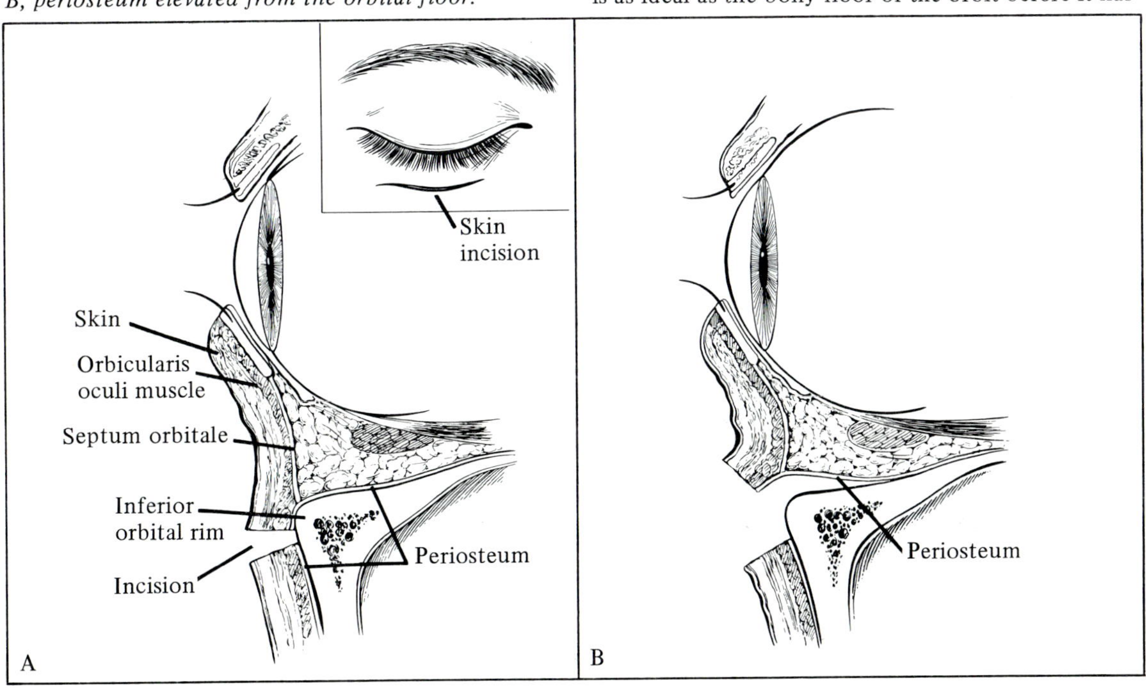

Fig. 10-14. A, incision below the inferior orbital rim. B, periosteum elevated from the orbital floor.

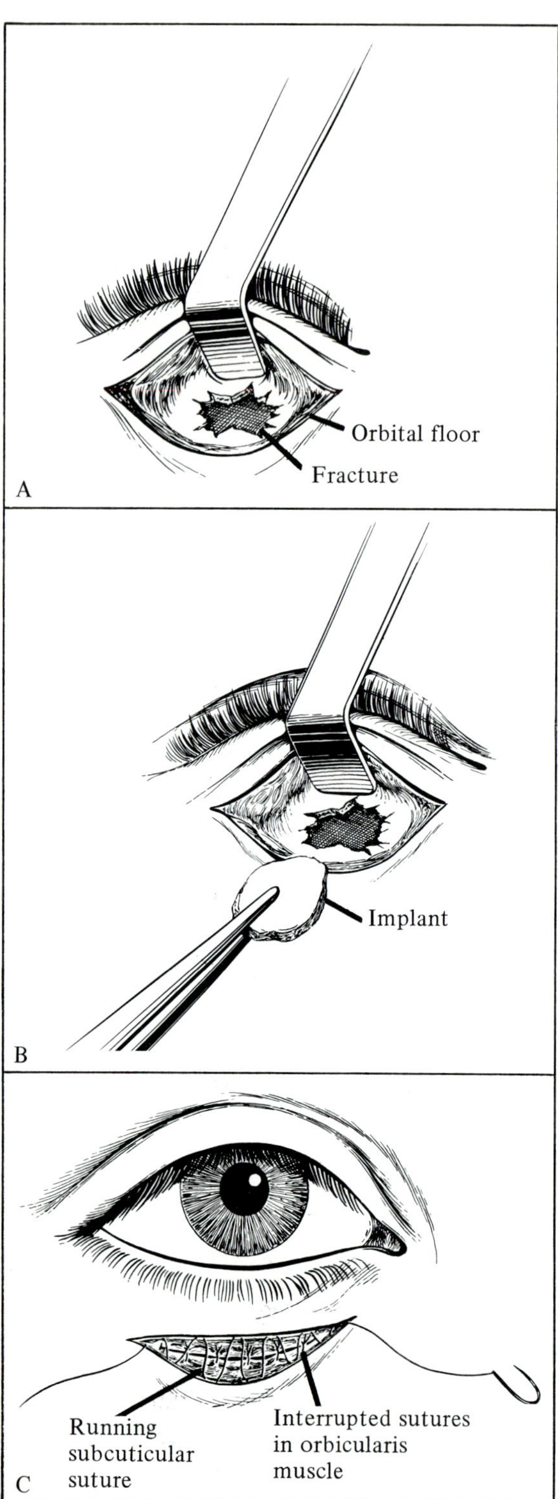

been fractured. We prefer *homogenous cartilage* or a *Silastic* implant to cover small fractures. These are relatively nonreactive and flexible and soft enough to help prevent the globe from future trauma. The main purpose for placing a prosthesis is to cover the fracture and provide a nonadherent surface on the floor. In larger fractures, however, Silastic is too flexible to provide satisfactory support for the orbital contents. In larger defects, we prefer *Teflon,* which is more rigid and supports the orbital tissues better. The Teflon implant, like a Silastic one, has holes cut in the implant through which fibrous tissue can invade and help hold the implant in place. In cases where almost the whole orbital floor is destroyed, even more rigidity is needed in the implant, and we then use *Supramid Extra* (0.8 mm. thickness). In delayed cases of blowout fractures with enophthalmos, much thicker implants are necessary. Carved Silastic up to 4 mm. in thickness may be used. *Autogenous iliac bone grafts* have the advantage that they are the most physiologic and are easily penetrated by systemic antibiotics after vascularization has taken place. However, autogenous grafts have the disadvantage of being more difficult to obtain, and some absorption of the graft may occur, which compromises the correction of the enophthalmos.

After the implant is placed, a traction test should be performed to rotate the globe to be certain that the implant remains in position. If the implant migrates, it can then be wired to the inferior orbital rim. The traction test performed at this time also indicates whether or not a trapped inferior rectus muscle has been released satisfactorily. The periosteum is sutured anteriorly with 4-0 chromic catgut sutures where it had previously been incised just below the inferior orbital rim. The orbicularis oculi muscle is sutured with interrupted sutures of 5-0 plain catgut (Fig. 10-15C). The skin is closed with interrupted 6-0 nylon or silk sutures. It should be pointed out that in the closure of the periosteum, care should be taken not to take "bites" in the orbital septum. If this is done, the septum is shortened, pulling the lower lid downward and causing more sclera to show below the limbus as compared with the other eye (asymmetrical inferior scleral exposure). A light patch and ice packs are applied. No pressure bandage is used because this could contribute to loss of vision if a postoperative hemorrhage should occur, since central retinal artery occlusion may result from the increased intraorbital

Fig. 10-15. A, exposure of fracture. B, placement of implant over fracture site. C, closure of wound. (Redrawn from A. Callahan. Reconstructive Surgery of the Eyelids and Ocular Adnexa. *Birmingham, Ala.: Aesculapius, 1966.)*

pressure [62]. Postoperatively the head of the bed may be elevated 30 to 45 degrees to reduce edema. Antibiotics (local and sometimes systemic) are given during the immediate postoperative period.

CALDWELL-LUC APPROACH. This approach may be used when combined with the anterior infraorbital approach. In general, we feel that it is mainly helpful in very large blowout fractures. The Caldwell-Luc approach has two major disadvantages when used alone to repair blowout fractures: (1) The inferior orbit cannot be visualized well; consequently adhesions between the fracture and the orbital contents cannot always be released. (2) There is danger that bone fragments may be pushed up into orbital structures, such as the optic nerve.

Complications

RESIDUAL DIPLOPIA. It is not uncommon for a trapped inferior rectus muscle to be weak for several weeks following its removal from the fracture. In the majority of these instances the inferior rectus muscle function will return to normal, and the postoperative hypertropia on the involved side clears. If diplopia continues postoperatively, it is our practice to wait at least 6 months or until a constant extraocular muscle deviation is established before performing strabismus surgery. In such cases, we try to achieve fusion in the primary position, and downgaze particularly. Fresnel prisms can also be pressed on the posterior surface of glasses as a nonsurgical method to achieve fusion.

UNDERCORRECTION OF ENOPHTHALMOS. Undercorrection is much more common than overcorrection of enophthalmos, particularly in late cases. The treatment of undercorrection is very difficult because fibrosis of the orbital tissues and atrophy of orbital fat have occurred. Attempts to improve undercorrection are usually made by placing a thicker implant between the periosteum and the bony floor of the orbit. Alloplastics, such as Silastic, have the advantage of a more permanent improvement because they do not absorb. Bone grafts and fascia lata have the disadvantage of absorption.

Another approach to the problem of long-standing residual enophthalmos is not to treat the cause of the enophthalmos directly but to widen the narrowed palpebral fissure, which is secondary to the enophthalmos. A Müller's muscle–conjunctival resection blepharoptosis procedure [68] or a Fassnella-Servat blepharoptosis procedure [7] raises the upper eyelid and thus widens the palpebral fissure enough to make less noticeable the residual enophthalmos that is present.

OVERCORRECTION OF ENOPHTHALMOS. This is an uncommon problem but is observed with the thicker implants. Overcorrection of enophthalmos results in hypertropia and disfigurement. It is not uncommon for overcorrection to be present in the immediate postoperative period, and then for gradual improvement in appearance to be noted over the course of weeks or months.

ASYMMETRICAL INFERIOR SCLERAL EXPOSURE. Asymmetrical inferior scleral exposure refers to more sclera being visible below the inferior limbus on the involved side than on the side of the other eye. This may be due either to mechanical elevation of the globe by the implant, as with overcorrection of enophthalmos, or to vertical shortening of the lower lid. Vertical shortening of the lower lid (lower eyelid retraction) may occur secondary to failure to elevate a depressed bone fragment of the inferior orbital rim or secondary to adhesions of the orbital septum to the inferior orbital rim. These adhesions can occur if one takes "bites" in the septum of the lower lid, rather than through the periosteum, in wound closure at the periosteal level.

Treatment of these problems depends on the cause. Overcorrection of enophthalmos has been discussed and is usually self-correcting. If a depressed fracture of the orbital rim is present, the bone fragments can be reduced and fixed with wire sutures if necessary.

A method for correcting retraction of the lower eyelid has been developed when the cause is shortening or contraction of the orbital septum and/or the lower eyelid retractors [47, 81]. The contracted retractors (the aponeurosis of the capsulopalpebral head of the inferior rectus muscle and the inferior tarsal muscle [Müller's]) and orbital septum require release. After the surgically released area is supple, a homologous scleral graft obtained from an eye bank is placed to fill the defect.

The procedure (Fig. 10-16) is started by incising the palpebral conjunctiva at the base of the tarsus and reflecting it. The lower eyelid retractors and the contracted orbital septum are detached from the base of the tarsus. All restricting scar tissue in the lower eyelid is excised. A donor scleral graft is sutured between the tarsus and the recessed lower eyelid retractors and the orbital septum. The scleral graft should extend across the entire horizontal width of the eyelid and measure twice the vertical height of the amount of eyelid retraction to be corrected, which will allow for postoperative shrinkage of the graft. The palpebral conjunctiva or an autogenous buccal mucous membrane graft is sutured over the scleral graft. Traction sutures from the lower eyelid are taped to the forehead for several days to stretch the lower eyelid tissues and the graft.

While many clinicians are demonstrating good

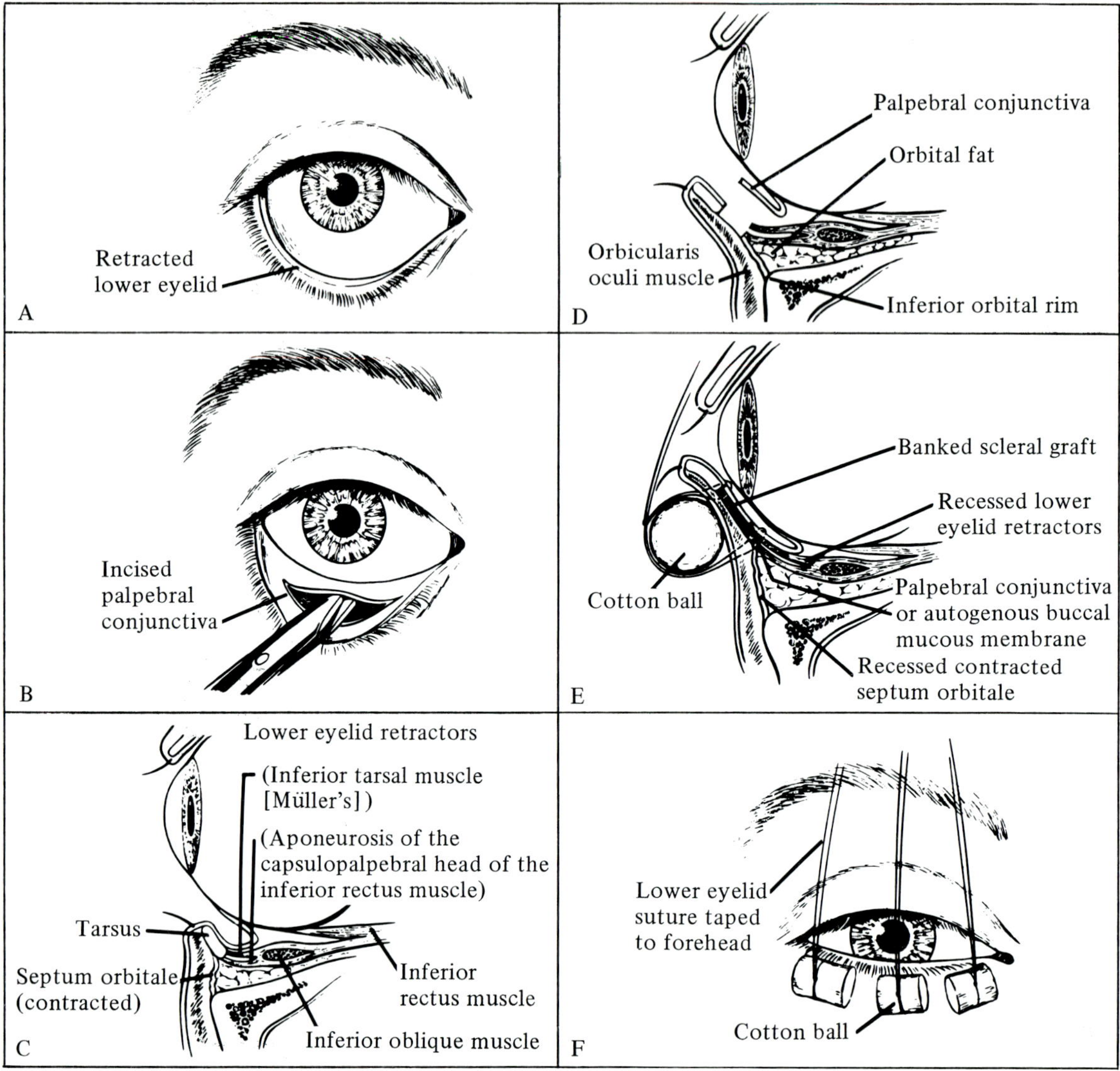

Fig. 10-16. Correction of retraction of the lower eyelid. See text for further details.

results with this technique when there is internal lid contraction, it should be used judiciously. Indeed, there may be only an external restricting scar of the lower eyelid (trauma or postsurgical), in which case excision of the scar and placement of a skin graft taken from either redundant upper eyelid skin or postauricular skin is the better method of correction.

INFECTION. Infection is an uncommon complication following repair of a blowout fracture. Systemic antibiotics are administered; often the orbital floor implant must be removed.

EXTRUSION OF THE IMPLANT. This may be associated with either infection or trauma and is more likely to occur with larger implants. Other causes of extrusion are improper design and carving of the implant and inadequate closure of the periosteum along the inferior orbital rim.

EYELID LYMPHEDEMA. This complication occurs when the incision is curved too far upward and laterally in the lower lid, resulting in division of the lymphatic vessels draining particularly from the upper eyelid. The best treatment for this complication is prevention – more care should be used in making the proper incision. However, lymphedema of the eyelid often resolves slowly over the course of several months.

DAMAGE TO THE LACRIMAL PUMP. Extension of the incision too far into the medial one-third of the lower lid results in damage to the orbicularis oculi muscle and its pumping action on the lacrimal sac. The result is improper drainage of tears and epiphora.

INFRAORBITAL NERVE HYPESTHESIA OR ANESTHESIA. Trauma to the infraorbital nerve by bone fragments or contusion during the operative procedure can effect an alteration in its sensory function. One should take care to avoid damage to the nerve during the operation and remove any bone fragments that may be impinging on the nerve in the infraorbital groove or canal. The area of sensory distribution of the face and teeth supplied by this nerve usually gradually recovers sensation over a period of many months.

FRACTURES OF BONES OF THE FRONTONASOETHMOIDAL REGION

Severe force to the face from below or from the front may cause extensive damage to the frontonasoethmoidal region, causing fractures of the frontal processes of the maxillas; the nasal bones; the bones surrounding the ethmoid sinuses, orbits, and maxillary sinuses; and the base of the skull in the region of the cribriform plate. Sharp spearlike edges from bone in this region may penetrate and lacerate the dura, causing leakage of cerebrospinal fluid. This region of the face includes many specialized structures that require restoration for function and aesthetics. The widening of the interorbital space in facial fractures is referred to as *traumatic interorbital hypertelorism.* The lateral displacement of the medial palpebral ligaments (usually their traumatic avulsion or evulsion) is called *telecanthus.*

By definition *hypertelorism* ([Greek], far + to separate) is abnormal width between two organs or parts. Ocular hypertelorism is a condition resulting from abnormal development of the base of the skull, especially of the sphenoid bone, with an abnormal increase in the space between the eyes (Crouzon's syndrome; hereditary craniofacial dysostosis).

Treatment

The following are considerations in restoration of the interorbital structures:

1. Replace the medial canthus in as normal a position as possible after restoring the position of the medial wall of the orbit (Fig. 10-17).

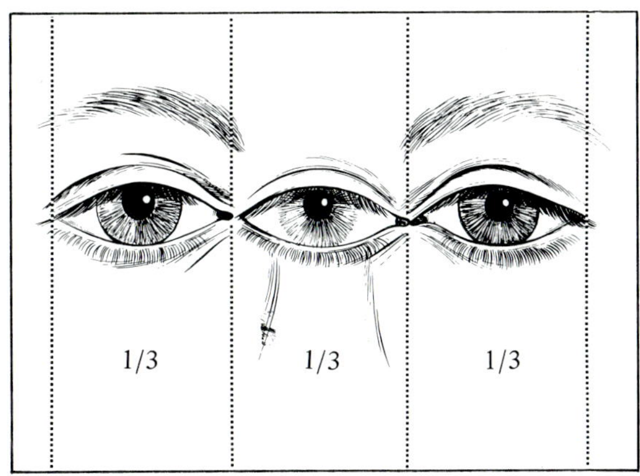

Fig. 10-17. Diagram to express the proper dimensions of the intercanthal space. (After Broadbent and Mathews [7a]).

2. Reestablish continuity or reinsert the medial palpebral ligament.
3. Restore normal function to the nasolacrimal apparatus.
4. Give adequate contour to the bridge of the nose.

Treatment of these fractures should be started as soon as the condition of the patient will permit. Carefully placed incisions in the midfacial region will allow for open reduction and wire fixation of these many fragments. The placing of small incisions and the resultant scars are minimal sequelae compared with the extensive deformity that results when these fractures are not properly reduced (Fig. 10-18). Fractures in this region may cause separation of the strong medial palpebral ligaments arising from the frontal processes of the maxillas and the lacrimal bones embracing the lacrimal sacs. They attach to the tarsi and terminate in the thicker free margins at the medial canthi.

Separation of the medial palpebral ligaments is usually bilateral. The ligaments become separated from their origin because the bone to which they are attached is fractured and the bones and ligaments are displaced. This brings about a greater distance between the medial canthi than is normally present (telecanthus). By threading fine-wire sutures through these ligaments and then drilling a hole from the opposite side of the maxilla or adjacent orbital walls, one can pull the ligaments and bone fragments more medial and into their normal position. There is little danger of overcorrection; undercorrection is the most common complication. The hole into which the ligament is pulled should be superior and posterior to the normal attachment of the ligament (Fig. 10-19A, B).

There is no more deforming or difficult fracture to treat than that of the frontonasoethmoidal area when

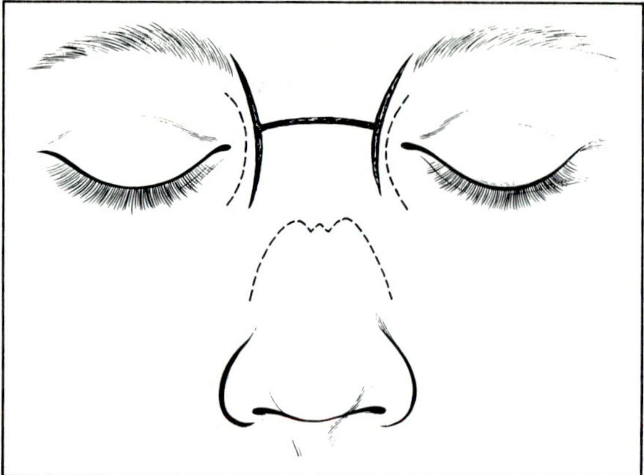

Fig. 10-18. H-type of incision used for exposure of interorbital area.

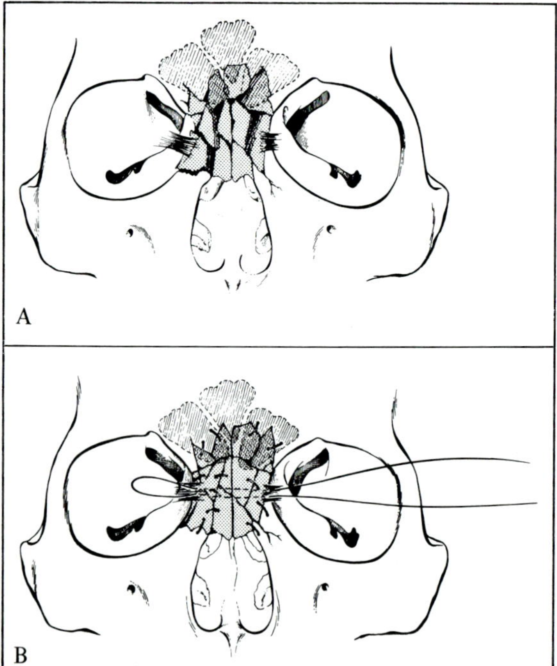

Fig. 10-19. A, extensive interorbital comminuted fractures with traumatic interorbital hypertelorism. B, wire fixation of multiple fractured pieces of bone and wire ligature through medial palpebral ligaments, frontal processes of maxillas, or adjacent orbital bones for restoration of normal intercanthal relationships.

comminution and telescoping are present. The interorbital region is the most challenging to the surgeon in primary and secondary restoration. Converse and Smith [18] have written very extensively on this subject.

Information on reestablishing the nasolacrimal drainage system is included in Chapter 9.

MULTIPLE FACIAL FRACTURES

The treatment of multiple facial fractures requires judgment and skill by the surgeon (Figs. 10-20 and 10-21). The Le Fort III fracture or craniofacial dislocation involves the two maxillas, the two zygomas, the nose, and the frontoethmoidal region in varying degrees. These fractures along with a fracture of the mandible encompass the maximum in facial bone injury. These multiple fractures may reveal loss of bone and soft tissue from a blast or penetrating wounds.

In most cases, multiple fractures require a tracheotomy soon after the injury. Definitive treatment of the fractures begins with the establishment of a stable mandible. In some cases it will be necessary to perform open reduction of the mandibular fractures. After the mandible is stabilized, the remaining facial bones are reduced as described above in the individual sections. The intact mandible is brought into occlusion with the reconstructed upper jaw and the fixation established.

FACIAL FRACTURES IN CHILDREN

Ten percent or less of all facial bone fractures involve children, usually as a result of vehicular accidents; greenstick fractures are the most common. Since bone heals rapidly in children without complications, it is therefore desirable to reduce fractures in children early. Unerupted teeth in the jaws may be deformed if they are in the line of fracture and may erupt abnormally or with deformity.

Treatment of fractures in children follows the same methods employed in adults.

Fractures of the subcondylar region of the mandible may be of concern because of the damage to an important growth center. Most often it is best not to perform open reduction of subcondylar fractures in children. The insult from operative intervention may cause more damage to the growth center than the fracture. If the occlusion is within normal limits, intermaxillary fixation is not even required. If malocclusion is present, however, intermaxillary fixation should be maintained for approximately 3 to 4 weeks.

DISLOCATION AT THE TEMPOROMANDIBULAR JOINT

The acute dislocation of the mandible without fracture occurs anterior to the articular eminence. This is

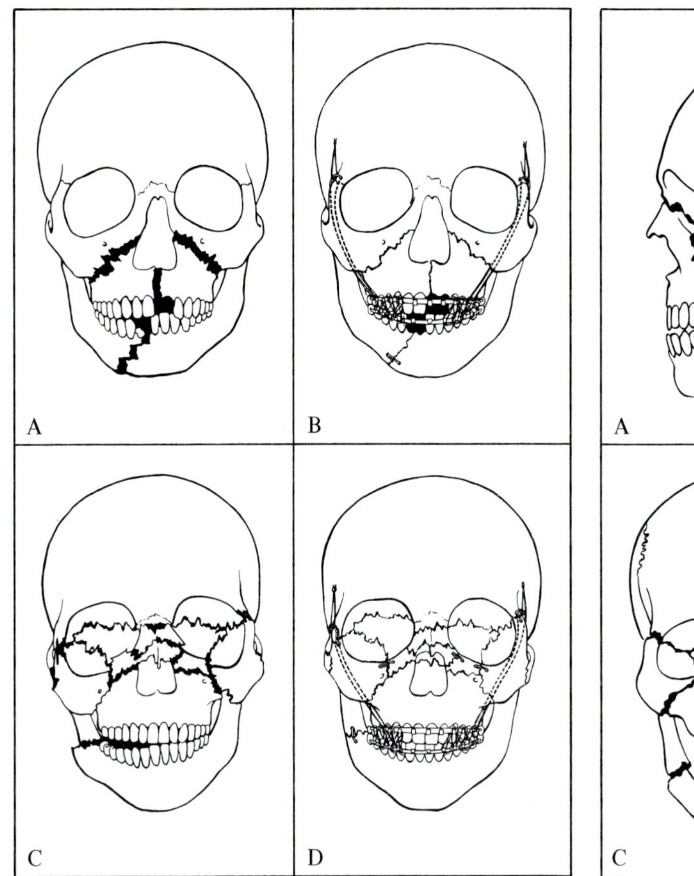

Fig. 10-20. Multiple facial fractures. A, pyramidal maxillary fracture with associated midline fracture of the maxillas and fracture in the region of the symphysis of the mandible. B, treatment by open reduction and interosseous wiring of the mandibular fragments, intermaxillary fixation with arch bars and rubber-band traction, and craniomaxillary fixation with internal suspension wires. C, severe comminuted fractures of the middle third of the face with craniofacial disjunction and fracture of the mandible. D, reconstruction of the mandible with open reduction, intermaxillary fixation, interosseous wiring at the zygomaticofrontal sutures, interosseous wiring of multiple fragments in the infraorbital regions, and craniomaxillary suspension. (Reproduced, by permission, from R. O. Dingman and P. Natvig. Surgery of Facial Fractures. *Philadelphia: Saunders, 1964.)*

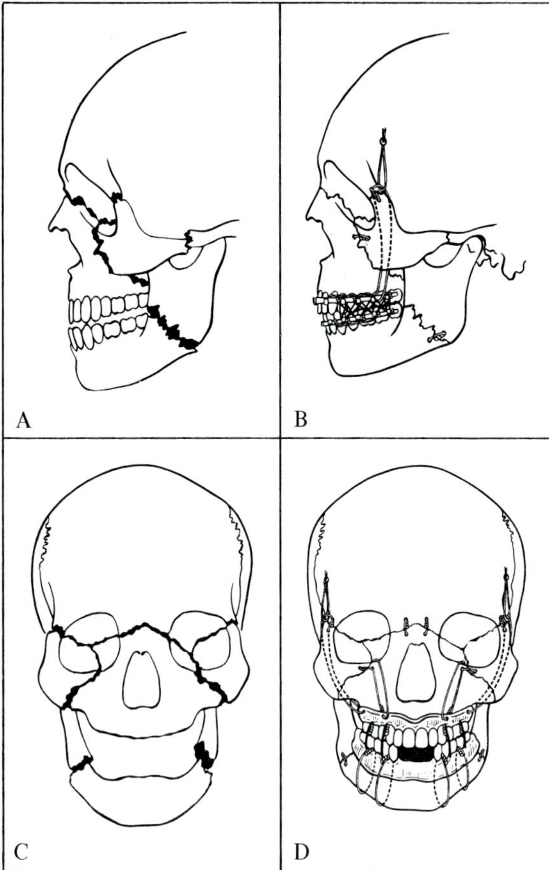

Fig. 10-21. Multiple facial fractures. A, profile view showing fracture of the middle third of the facial bones, open bite deformity, and fracture of the mandible. B, method of fixation following reduction of multiple facial fractures. C, multiple fractures of the middle third of the face, with bilateral mandibular fractures in the edentulous patient. D, the mandibular artificial denture is fixed with circumferential wires to the mandible. The maxillary artificial denture is used to suspend the maxillas and acts as a guide for placement of the maxillary fragments. Open reduction and interosseous wire fixation in conjunction with suspension of the upper denture from the infraorbital rims, and from the zygomatic processes of the frontal bone, provide excellent fixation for extensive fractures in the edentulous patient. (Reproduced, by permission, from R. O. Dingman and P. Natvig. Surgery of Facial Fractures. *Philadelphia: Saunders, 1964.)*

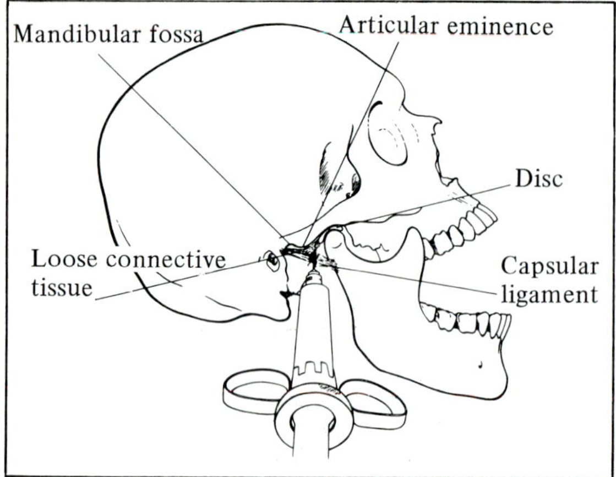

Fig. 10-22. Johnson's method of injection of an anesthetic solution into the nerve-bearing loose connective tissue of the capsule following acute anterior dislocation. Note the attachment of the loose connective tissure to the disc. (Reproduced, by permission, from R. O. Dingman and P. Natvig. Surgery of Facial Fractures. *Philadelphia: Saunders, 1964.)*

almost always bilateral, and the patient is unable to close his mouth.

Reduction is performed by placing the thumbs of both hands on the occlusal surfaces of the molar teeth of the mandible, or alveolar ridge if the mandible is edentulous, and pushing downward and backward. In many instances, severe spasm will prevent reduction without general anesthesia.

Johnson [46] reported a method whereby injection of a local anesthetic solution into the nerve-bearing loose connective tissue of the capsule around the joint diminishes spasm and permits reduction of the dislocation (Fig. 10-22). Injection is performed unilaterally only – even in a bilateral luxation.

Sicher [78] explains this on the basis that in injuries of the capsule neural reflexes maintain spasms of the masticatory muscles. These reflexes stretch over the bilateral group of muscles and can be eliminated by injection on one side only.

POSTOPERATIVE CARE AND COMPLICATIONS OF PATIENTS WITH FACIAL FRACTURES

In the immediate postoperative period the usual high standards of care should be sustained. Electrolyte balance, replacements for proper hydration, and blood volume should be maintained. Medications for pain are administered, and antibiotics if required.

Hygiene of wounds should be attended to daily. Tracheotomy care should be impeccable, and the physician must personally ensure that this is carried out. Proper humidity is mandatory so that the patient who wears a tracheotomy tube is comfortable.

As soon after the operative procedure as possible the patient should be started on an adequate diet. A liquifier or food blender will aid immeasurably in the preparation of the proper foods. Liquid vitamins may be used as supplement.

REFERENCES

1. Adams, W. M. Internal wiring fixation of facial fractures. *Surgery* 12:523, 1942.
2. Adams, W. M., and Adams, L. H. Internal wire fixation of facial fractures; 15-year follow-up report. *Am. J. Surg.* 92:12, 1956.
3. Anderson, R. Ambulatory method of treating fractures of shaft of femur. *Surg. Gynecol. Obstet.* 62:865, 1936.
4. Angle, E. H. Classification of malocclusion. *Dent. Cosmos* 41:248, 1899.
5. Babbitt, D. P. Personal communication, 1967.
6. Barsky, A. J. *Principles and Practice of Plastic Surgery.* Baltimore: Williams & Wilkins, 1950.
7. Beard, C. *Ptosis.* St. Louis: Mosby, 1976, pp. 147–149.

7a. Broadbent, T. R., and Mathews, V. L.: Artistic relationships in surface anatomy of the face: application to reconstructive surgery. *Plast. Reconstr. Surg.* 20:1, 1957.

8. Brown, J. B., Fryer, M. P., and McDowell, F. Internal wire-pin immobilization of jaw fractures. *Plast. Reconstr. Surg.* 4:30, 1949.
9. Brown, J. B., Fryer, M. P., and McDowell, F. Internal wire-pin fixation for fractures of upper jaw, orbit, zygoma and severe facial crushes. *Plast. Reconstr. Surg.* 9:276, 1952.
10. Brown, J. B., and McDowell, F. Internal wire fixation for fractures of jaw: Preliminary report. *Surg. Gynecol. Obstet.* 74:227, 1942.
11. Brown, J. B., and McDowell, F. *Plastic Surgery of the Nose.* St. Louis: Mosby, 1951.
12. Browning, C. W. Alloplastic materials in orbital repair. *Am. J. Ophthalmol.* 63:955, 1962.
13. Cairns, H. Injuries of frontal and ethmoidal sinuses with special reference to cerebrospinal rhinorrhea and aeroceles. *J. Laryngol.* 52:589, 1937.
14. Callahan, A. *Reconstructive Surgery of the Eyelids and Ocular Adnexa.* Birmingham, Ala: Aesculapius, 1966.
15. Campbell, D. A. Discussion. In Glas, W. W., King, O. J., Jr., and Lui, A., Complications of tracheostomy. *Arch. Surg.* 85:62, 1962.
16. Chalmers J. Lyons Club. Fractures involving the mandibular condlye: Posttreatment survey of 120 cases. *J. Oral Surg.* 5:45, 1947.

17. Converse, J. M. *Reconstructive Plastic Surgery* (2d ed.). Philadelphia: Saunders, 1977.
18. Converse, J. M., and Smith, B. Reconstruction of the floor of the orbit by bone grafts. *Arch. Ophthalmol.* 44:1, 1950.
19. Converse, J. M., and Smith, B. Naso-orbital fractures and traumatic deformities of the medial canthus. *Plast. Reconstr. Surg.* 38:147, 1966.
20. Converse, J. M., Smith, B., Obear, M. F., and Wood-Smith, D. Orbital blowout fracture: A ten year survey. *Plast. Reconstr. Surg.* 39:20, 1967.
21. Cornell University Automotive Crash Injury Research. The injury-producing accident: A primer of facts and figures. New York, 1961.
22. DesPrez, J. D., and Kiehn, C. L. Methods of reconstruction following resection of anterior oral cavity and mandible for malignancy. *Plast. Reconstr. Surg.* 24:238, 1959.
23. Dingman, R. O. Use of rubber bands in treatment of fractures of bones of face and jaws. *J. Am. Dent. Assoc.* 26:173, 1939.
24. Dingman, R. O. Symposium: Malunited fractures of zygoma; repair of deformity. *Trans. Am. Acad. Ophthalmol. Otolaryngol.* 57:889, 1953.
25. Dingman, R. O. Local anesthesia for rhinoplasty; and the nasal septum in rhinoplastic surgery. *Plast. Reconstr. Surg.* 28:251, 1961.
26. Dingman, R. O., and Alling, C. C. Open reduction and internal wire fixation of maxillofacial fractures. *J. Oral Surg.* 12:140, 1954.
27. Dingman, R. O., and Grabb, W. C. Surgical anatomy of the mandibular ramus of the facial nerve based on the dissection of 100 facial halves. *Plast. Reconstr. Surg.* 29:266, 1962.
28. Dingman, R. O., and Harding, R. L. The treatment of malunion fractures of the facial bones. *Plast. Reconstr. Surg.* 7:505, 1951.
29. Dingman, R. O., and Natvig, P. *Surgery of Facial Fractures.* Philadelphia: Saunders, 1964.
30. Erich, J. B. Fractures of the facial bones. *Milit. Surg.* 88:637, 1941.
31. Erich, J. B. Treatment of fractures of the upper jaw. *J. Am. Dent. Assoc.* 29:783, 1942.
32. Erich, J. B. Treatment of bilateral fractures of the edentulous mandible. *Plast. Reconstr. Surg.* 9:33, 1952.
33. Erich, J. B., and Austin, L. T. *Traumatic Injuries of the Facial Bones: An Atlas of Treatment.* Philadelphia: Saunders, 1944.
34. Federspiel, M. N. Jaw fractures; the value of orthodontic appliances to immobilize. *Wis. Med. J.* 26:300, 1927.
35. Federspiel, M. N. Maxillo-facial injuries. *Wis. Med. J.* 33:561, 1934.
36. Freeman, B. S. The direct approach to acute fractures of the zygomatic-maxillary complex and immediate prosthetic replacement of the orbital floor. *Plast. Reconstr. Surg.* 29:587, 1962.
37. Gerrie, J. W., and Lindsey, W. K. Fracture of maxillary-zygomatic compound with atypical involvement of orbit. *Plast. Reconstr. Surg.* 11:341, 1953.
38. Gillies, H. D. The Diagnosis and Treatment of Residual Traumatic Deformities of the Facial Skeleton. In Rowe, N. L., and Killey, H. C. (Eds.), *Fractures of the Facial Skeleton.* Baltimore: Williams & Wilkins, 1955.
39. Gillies, H. D. Kilner, T. P., and Stone, D. Fractures of the malar-zygomatic compound, with a description of new x-ray position. *Br. J. Surg.* 14:651, 1927.
40. Glas, W. W., King, O. J., Jr., and Lui, A. Complications of tracheostomy. *Arch. Surg.* 85:56, 1962.
41. Hagan, E. H., and Huelke, D. F. An analysis of 319 case reports of mandibular fractures. *J. Oral Surg.* 19:93, 1961.
42. Hayward, J. R. Treatment methods for jaw fractures. *J. Oral Surg.* 20:273, 1962.
43. Hendrix, J. H., Jr., Sanders, S. G., and Green, B. Open reduction of mandibular condyle. *Plast. Reconstr. Surg.* 23:283, 1959.
44. Holmes, W. N. Personal communication, 1967.
45. Ivy, R. H. Observations of fractures of the mandible. *J.A.M.A.* 79:295, 1922.
46. Johnson, W. B. New method for reduction of acute dislocation of the temporomandibular articulations. *J. Oral Surg.* 16:501, 1958.
47. Jones, L. T., and Wobig, J. L. *Surgery of the Eyelids and Lacrimal System.* Birmingham, Ala.: Aesculapius, 1976, pp. 133–136.
48. Kazanjian, V. H. Treatment of automobile injuries of the face and jaws. *J. Am. Dent. Assoc.* 20:757, 1933.
49. Kazanjian, V. H., and Converse, J. M. *The Surgical Treatment of Facial Injuries* (3d ed.). Baltimore: Williams & Wilkins, 1963.
50. Knight, J. S., and North, J. F. The classification of malar fractures: An analysis of displacement as a guide to treatment. *Br. J. Plast. Surg.* 13:325, 1961.
51. Lang, W. Traumatic enophthalmos with retention of perfect acuity of vision. *Trans. Ophthalmol. Soc. U.K.* 9:41, 1889.
52. Le Fort, R. Fractures de la mâchoire supérieure. *Cong. Int. Med. C. R.* (Paris) 1900, p. 275.
53. Le Fort, R. Etude expérimentale sur les fractures de la mâchoire supérieure. *Rev. Chir.* (Paris) 23: 208, 360, 479, 1901.
54. Lillie, R. H. Personal communication, 1967.
55. Matas, R. Fracture of the zygomatic arch: A simple method of reduction and fixation, with remarks on the prevalence, symptomatology and

treatment of this fracture. *N. Orleans Med. Surg. J.* 49:139, 1896.
56. McCoy, F. J., Chandler, R. A. Magnan, C. G., Jr., Moore, J. R., and Siemsen, G. An analysis of facial fractures and their complications. *Plast. Reconstr. Surg.* 29:381, 1962.
57. Meade, J. W. Tracheotomy – its complications and their management: A study of 212 cases. *N. Engl. J. Med.* 265:519, 1961.
58. Merrill, V. *Atlas of Roentgenographic Positions,* Vol. 2. St. Louis: Mosby, 1949.
59. Meschan, I. *An Atlas of Normal Radiographic Anatomy* (2d ed.). Philadelphia: Saunders, 1959.
60. Mörch, E. T. Tracheostomy and mechanical hyperventilation. *Armamentarium* (Chicago: Mueller) 3:4, 1960.
61. Musselman, M. M. Discussion. In Glas, W. W., King, O. J., Jr., and Lui, A., Complications of tracheostomy. *Arch. Surg.* 85:63, 1962.
62. Nicholson, D. H., and Guzak, S. V. Visual loss complicating repair of orbital floor fractures. *Arch. Ophthalmol.* 86:369, 1971.
63. Panagopoulos, A. P. Management of fractures of the jaws in children. *J. Int. Coll. Surg.* 28:806, 1957.
64. Panagopoulos, A. P., and Dietrich, W. C. Anesthesia in operative procedures on fractures of children's jaws. *Dent. Items Interest* 75:655, 1953.
65. Peacock, E. E., Jr. Management of facial fractures in unconscious patients. *Am. Surg.* 24:639, 1958.
66. Pfeiffer, R. L. Roentgenography of exophthalmos with notes on roentgen ray in ophthalmology. *Am. J. Ophthalmol.* 26:724, 816, 928, 1943.
67. Pfeiffer, R. L. Traumatic enophthalmos. *Arch. Ophthalmol.* 30:718, 1943.
68. Putterman, A. M., and Urist, M. J. Treatment of enophthalmic narrow palpebral fissure after blowout fracture. *Ophthalmic Surg.* 6:45, 1975.
69. Risdon, F. E. Treatment of nonunion of fractures of the mandible by free autogenous bone grafts. *J.A.M.A.* 79:297, 1922.
70. Risdon, F. E. Arthroplasty of the temporomaxillary joint. *J.A.M.A.* 85:2011, 1925.
71. Risdon, F. E. Ankylosis of the temporomaxillary joint. *J. Am. Dent. Assoc.* 21:1933, 1934.
72. Rowe, N. L., and Killey, H. C. *Fractures of the Facial Skeleton.* Baltimore: Williams & Wilkins, 1955.
73. Safian, J. *Corrective Rhinoplastic Surgery.* New York: Hoeber, 1935.
74. Schelble, J. A. Personal communication, 1963.
75. Schneider, R. C., and Thompson, J. M. Chronic and delayed traumatic rhinorrhea as a source of recurrent attacks of meningitis. *Ann. Surg.* 145: 517, 1957.
76. Sicher, H. Structural and functional basis for disorders of the temporomandibular articulation. *J. Oral Surg.* 13:275, 1955.
77. Sicher, H. *Oral Anatomy* (4th ed.). St. Louis: Mosby, 1965.
78. Sicher, H. Personal communication, 1967.
79. Sicher, H., and Tandler, J. *Anatomie für Zahnarzte.* Vienna and Berlin: Springer, 1928.
80. Smith, B., and Regan, W. F., Jr. Blowout fracture of the orbit; mechanism and correction of internal orbital fractures. *Am. J. Ophthalmol.* 44:733, 1957.
81. Soll, D. B. *Management of Complications in Ophthalmic Plastic Surgery.* Birmingham, Ala.: Aesculapius, 1976, pp. 160–163.
82. Stader, O. A preliminary announcement of a new method of treating fractures. *North Am. Vet.* 18:37, 1937.
83. Steffensen, W. H. Reconstruction of the nasal septum. *Plast. Reconstr. Surg.* 2:66, 1947.
84. Straith, C. L. Guest passenger injuries. *J.A.M.A.* 137:348, 1948.
85. Tandler, J. *Topographische Anatomie dringlicher Operationen.* Berlin: Springer, 1916.

Reconstruction of the Scalp, Forehead, and Calvaria

THOMAS D. REES AND RICHARD J. COBURN

ANATOMY AND EMBRYOLOGY

The calvaria is an important coalescence of the several bones that protect the brain. Its vulnerable position makes it subject to injuries. Although this bony capsule is very strong in adult life, it lacks elasticity.

The scalp and forehead are parts of the same structural anatomical unit. The lower border of the forehead is continuous with the anatomy of the face and orbital regions. The scalp and forehead are composed of five layers traditionally remembered by the classic mnemonic word, SCALP: a superficial covering of *S*kin, a rather thick sub*C*utaneous layer, a tough fascial layer the galea *A*poneurosis, and a layer of *L*oose connective tissue overlying the *P*eriosteum.

The thick skin covering the scalp accommodates the hair follicles and sebaceous glands, yet it is firmly attached to the underlying galea. A very rich network of arteries, veins, and lymphatics course through the subcutaneous layer, which is divided into the multiple fat lobules by the interlacing fibrous sheets. These septa limit vessel retraction following injury and are partly responsible for the profuse hemorrhage often associated with scalp lacerations. The galea is continuous with the fascia overlying the frontal and occipital muscles and serves as their origin. The subaponeurotic or subgaleal layer permits free movement of the scalp over the cranium and is the plane where avulsion occurs in scalping injuries. The periosteum or pericranium is adherent at the sutures and thus serves to limit the spread of infection. The calvaria, a membranous bone, consists of an inner table and an outer table that contains the honeycombed diploë.

The sensory nerve supply to the anterior portion of the scalp and forehead arises from the ophthalmic divisions of the fifth cranial nerve. The second cervical nerve, a branch of the greater occipital, supplies the posterior aspect of the scalp. The great auricular nerve extends sensory branches to the region just behind the ear and overlaps with sensory branches of the ophthalmic division of the fifth cranial and greater occipital nerves. The temporal region receives its sensory innervation from the maxillary division of the fifth cranial nerve and the auriculotemporal nerve (Fig. 11-1); there is also considerable overlap here.

The scalp has a particularly rich and abundant source of arterial blood arising from four principal arteries on each side of the head (Fig. 11-1). The occipital, the superficial temporal, and the postauricular arteries (all of which are branches of the external carotid arteries) anastomose with the supraorbital arteries (from the internal carotids). There are abundant communications across the midline. The scalp probably has the richest blood supply of any area of skin. Vessels from this extensive anastomosis penetrate the calvaria and communicate with the intracranial cavity, providing nourishment for the bone and supplementary arterial supply to the meningeal vessels. The veins of this region correspond generally with the arterial supply. Communication between scalp veins, the diploetic veins of the calvaria, the meninges, and the veins of the pterygoid plexus is established whereby facial infections may reach the dural sinuses, producing a meningitis or intracranial abscess.

The lymphatic drainage is unique in that the lymph vessels are not filtered by lymph nodes until the parotid lymph nodes are reached anteriorly. The parotid, preauricular, and postauricular nodes are located on the lateral and anterior aspects of the head. Posterior lymph vessels drain into the occipital, deep jugular, and spinal accessory lymph nodes. Thus, there is no lymph-node filtering system within the scalp itself until these glands are reached.

The scalp also has an overabundance of skin adnexal structures, including sebaceous glands, sweat glands, and hair follicles. These provide a ready source of epithelial growth following injuries such as intermediate-thickness skin burns.

Embryologically, the roof of the skull develops in membranes overlaid by differentiating epidermis and dermis. Growth is appositional with bone deposited on the external surface and resorbed internally to accommodate the rapid cerebral growth. By the third month, primitive follicles begin to develop in the epidermis, and eventually they extend into the dermis. At the seventh month, they appear as surface hair.

CONGENITAL DEFORMITIES

Calvaria

Deformities involving the calvaria include those caused by premature closure of the cranial sutures, the synostoses (Apert's, and Crouzon's syndromes, see Chapter 4), and true congenital abnormalities of the skull shape. Primary correction of synostosis by bony excision and lining is often performed by the neurosurgeon. Correction of the associated facial deformities is discussed in Chapter 5.

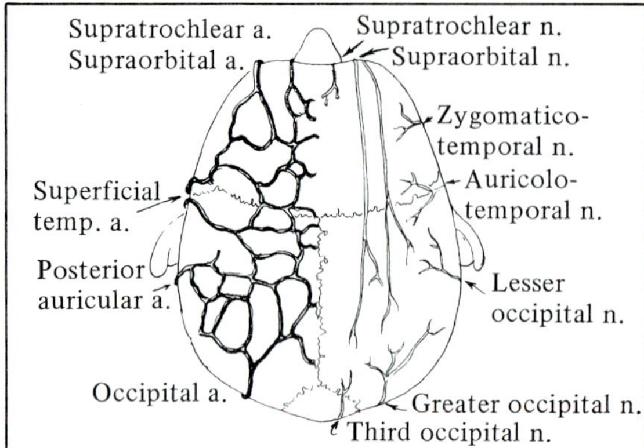

Fig. 11-1. Distribution of vessels and nerves of the scalp.

Defects of Scalp and Calvaria

Congenital defects of both the scalp and calvaria, excluding hemangiomas, are rare. Less than 200 cases have been reported in the European and American literature up to 1970 [1]. Most anomalies affecting the soft tissues of the scalp or the skull (or both) present as protrusions, ulcers, or defects. The vertex, occipital, and postauricular areas are most commonly involved. This deficiency of tissue occurs near or at the midline in 80 percent of the cases. They are usually single, but are multiple in 28 percent of the cases reported. Females are more commonly affected than males, and the first born is usually afflicted [2, 7]. The size of the defect varies from 0.5 to 9.0 cm.

The lesions present at birth most often as a punched-out ulcer, often with dura visible in the base. Usually there is an underlying bone defect corresponding to the size of the scalp deficiency. The small lesions may progress to true ulcer formation with granulating surfaces. Healing usually occurs by epithelialization from the edges, followed by growth of the underlying bone. However, death can occur from hemorrhage from the superior sagittal sinus. The cause is unknown, but hereditary factors, amniotic adhesions, and delayed bony union of the fontanelles have been mentioned [3]. Pap [6] reported the development of a small scalp defect in three successive generations and postulated a dominant inheritance.

Treatment is conservative in the small early lesions. Protective dressings usually prevent infection until epithelialization has occurred. Eventually, this thin non-hair-bearing skin is removed by staged excision. Larger lesions (5–10 cm. in diameter) usually require immediate coverage to prevent infection or hemorrhage. Local flaps or split-thickness skin grafts have been used; with exposure of the superior sagittal sinus, ligation precedes soft tissue coverage [5]. Prior to emergency treatment of the larger defects, a 20 percent perinatal mortality was noted [4]. The bony defect may not close spontaneously in larger lesions, and these require cartilage or bone grafts beneath a scalp flap to provide protection for the brain.

Erydelyi [2] reported an unusual deformity in a 2-year-old girl in whom there was a total absence of hair in the parietal region, as well as in both temporal regions. Reconstruction was accomplished by gradual transfer of a pedunculated hairy flap from the occipital region to the parietal region.

TRAUMATIC DEFORMITIES OF THE SCALP, FOREHEAD, AND CALVARIA

The head is more frequently injured than any other part of the body [13]. The Automotive Crash Research Project of Cornell University showed that injuries of the head occurred in 72.1 percent of 5,959 injury-producing automobile accidents in the United States [14].

Lacerations, contusions, and avulsions are common injuries of the scalp and forehead. Because of the rich vascular anastomoses, healing is exceedingly good, but soft tissue wounds are apt to bleed considerably. Pressure is the best method of controlling hemorrhage in a fresh wound. Lacerations of this region should be carefully closed in layers after thorough cleaning and sharp debridement. Exposed underlying bone should always be carefully examined for fractures. This examination, of course, is confirmed by roentgenograms in most instances.

Lacerations of the Scalp and Forehead

Lacerations, particularly of the forehead, are often due to impact against broken windshields or other sharp objects. In automobile accidents the head is usually flexed abruptly as it strikes the windshield, thus slicing the forehead and creating superiorly based flaps of forehead tissue. These flaps often become trapdoor deformities, with elevated redundant skin partially trapped within the U-shaped scar. It is important to debride the margins of elevated traumatic flaps so that the edges are at a right angle to the skin, rather than beveled. Careful repair and prolonged postoperative pressure dressings help to prevent the formation of chronic edema within the flap. Chronic edema is one of the main causes of fibrosis, which leads to trapdoor deformities.

One of two limbs of these U-shaped flaps can sometimes be repaired by the judicious and immediate use of the Z-plasty principle, when the base of such a flap is sufficiently wide. This also mitigates lymph stasis.

At the time of the initial closure, *small* lacerations of the forehead should be converted to horizontal wounds by elliptical excision in order to follow the lines of facial expression. An exception to this is repair in the region of the glabella where the lines are vertical.

Scalp lacerations require good local care because infection, although uncommon, is the forerunner of subgaleal abscesses, and of greater concern, intradural collections via the diploetic vessels. The wound must be copiously irrigated with saline, contused tissues debrided, foreign material removed, and hemostasis secured prior to the repair. A layered closure is initiated by first approximating the galea with a buried suture to establish a barrier against the spread of a superficial infection. Further information on forehead lacerations is included in Chapter 9.

Contusions of the Scalp and Forehead

Contusions of the scalp heal readily, but one should always watch for signs of subgaleal hematomas, which may become localized with subsequent formation of an encapsulated seroma. The seroma can erode the outer table of the skull to form Pott's puffy tumor.

Any injury causing contusion of the scalp should always make the surgeon wary of an underlying intracranial injury, and the patient should be carefully observed for signs of increased intracranial pressure.

Loss of the Scalp and Forehead

Total avulsion of the scalp is an occupational hazard for women working with rotary machinery; with the current long hair styles, men have also become liable to such injuries [12]. However, more stringent safeguards have virtually eliminated this injury in many industries. The loose areolar layer just beneath the galea facilitates this type of injury. Formerly, many such patients succumbed to chronic infection or intracranial complications, and osteomyelitis, with sequestration, frequently occurred in exposed bone. However, blood transfusions, antibiotics, and surgical therapy have reduced these hazards.

Shock due to extensive blood loss requires immediate whole-blood transfusions. Surgical treatment consists of supplying proper skin coverage to all denuded areas as soon as possible. Usually, the periosteum is intact and lends itself well to the application of intermediate-thickness split-thickness skin grafts. Isolated success has been achieved by replacement of the avulsed tissue [17, 20] or by using the defatted flap as a full-thickness skin graft [24]. However, it is generally agreed that split-thickness skin grafting of the exposed periosteum is the treatment of choice, the graft being taken either from the avulsed scalp itself [24] or from the thigh or buttock [25]. If the graft is taken from the avulsed scalp, it should not be expected to grow hair.

If the outer table of the skull is bared of periosteum, a split graft will not take, and coverage with a skin flap is preferred. Pedicle flap coverage can be achieved by shifting available local tissue or by migration of distant pedicles such as an abdominal jump flap or tubed flap (Fig. 11-2). When local tissue is healthy and sufficient, and the scalp avulsion is not total, it can be shifted by the rotation-flap principle, leaving the pericranium intact on the donor area for coverage with split-thickness skin (Fig. 11-3). This grafting of the flap donor area is essential in order to obviate any tension on the flap. Scalp closures should be layer by layer whenever possible.

Dingman [18] has described the closure of scalp defects with local flaps. A method that helps to extend the scalp tissues, which are limited in elasticity due to the tense galea, is described by Kazanjian and Converse [19], who suggest multiple superficial incisions through the galea on the undersurface of the flap, which permits advancement and extension of tissue (Fig. 11-4). With ingenuity, even large defects can be closed with hair-bearing tissue. Orticochea [23] reported the closure of an 11 X 11 cm. defect, using four local rotation and advancement flaps.

An alternate but less desirable method of covering exposed cranial bone is that of drilling multiple holes through the outer cortical table to facilitate the growth and spread of granulation tissue over the period of a few weeks [16]. Complete removal of the outer table with osteotomes and other bone instruments also can be done, thus exposing the diploë with its rich blood supply and ready disposition to form granulation tissues for the acceptance of subsequent skin grafts (Fig. 11-5). If the calvaria is left exposed and intact, sequestration will occur after many weeks or months.

The most recent and appealing method of reconstruction following scalp evolutions was reported by Miller et al. [22] in 1976. Using the principles of microvascular surgery, the entire scalp was successfully replaced by anastomosing the superficial temporal artery and its paired vein bilaterally. Blood flow was reestablished 4½ hours after injury; at 6 months the hair growth was 8 cm. and frontalis activity had returned.

Primary Treatment of Skull Fractures and Defects

Fractures of the skull, usually the responsibility of the neurosurgeon, are referred to the plastic surgeon when the injury is complicated by soft tissue loss or seventh nerve damage. From 25 to 50 percent of temporal bone fractures have associated nerve injuries. The frequency is lower when the fracture is of the more common longitudinal variety; it is higher with transverse fractures. The longitudinal fractures are treated conservatively, whereas the transverse are best decompressed [21]. Repair of open wounds of the skull, particularly over the frontal bones, may require recon-

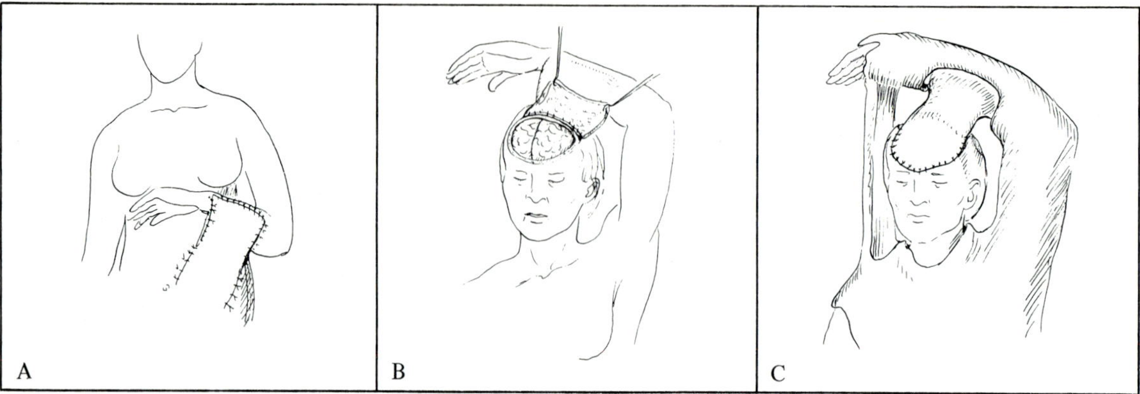

Fig. 11-2. A, B, and C, various stages of transfer of a large open jump flap from the abdomen or thorax carried via the forearm. An interval of 3 weeks or more must separate each of these stages.

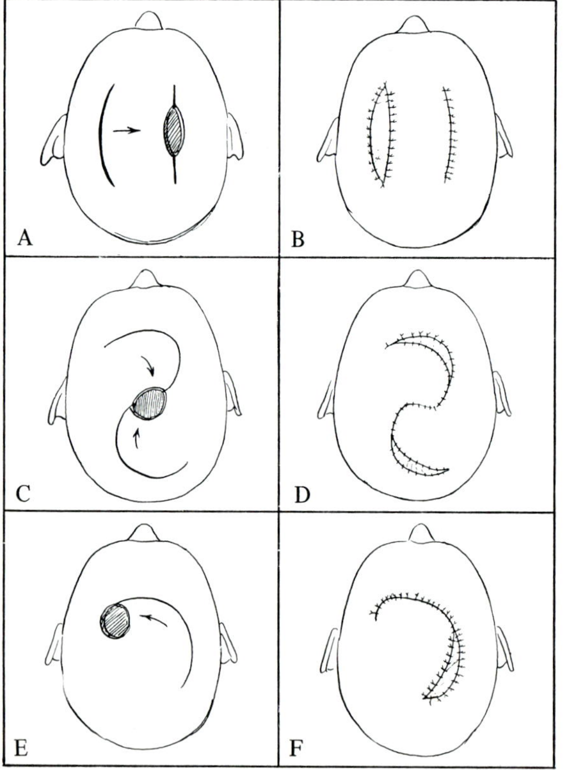

Fig. 11-3. Various methods of closing soft tissue scalp defects with local pedicle flaps. A and B, a bipedicle flap with a split-thickness skin graft to release tension. C and D, the classic double-rotation flap technique; skin grafts are not always necessary, but are usually helpful. E and F, a single pedicle rotation flap.

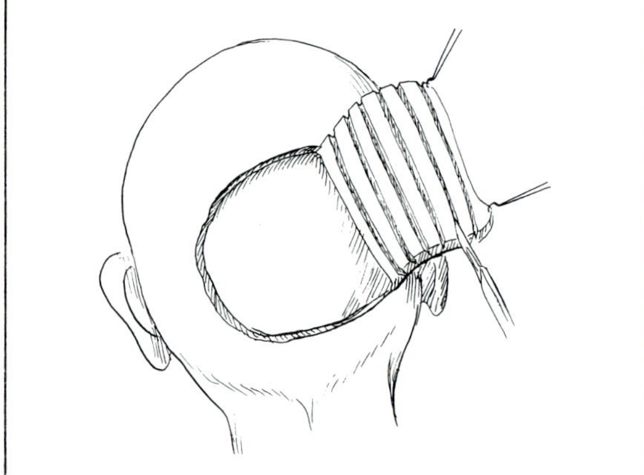

Fig. 11-4. Multiple parallel cuts are made in the galea, which allows the flap to stretch so that further advancement can be achieved much like an accordion.

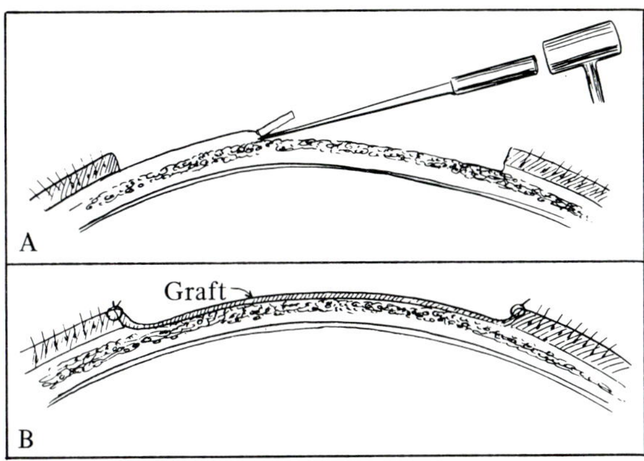

Fig. 11-5. A, decortication of the outer table of the skull, which is necessary when the periosteum is destroyed before a skin graft can be utilized. B, a skin graft in place on the richly vascular diploë beneath. The skin graft is best placed at a second stage after granulations are present.

structive surgery after the neurosurgeon has repaired underlying intracranial structures. Large defects of the meninges can be repaired with fascia lata. Other substitutes, including alloplastic materials, usually have proved unsuccessful on long-term follow-up examination.

Compound fractures of the skull are often comminuted and should not be disturbed except for attention to underlying brain injury, elevation of depressed bone fragments, debridement of all dead tissue, and prompt closure of the soft tissue defect. In large injuries, particularly when there is loss of substance, it may be necessary to do immediate autogenous bone grafting with iliac bone or split-rib grafts for bone restoration. Soft tissue closure may require adjacent scalp flaps, as discussed previously. The surgeon should not hesitate to close the resultant donor wound on the adjacent scalp with a split-thickness skin graft to reduce all tension on the closure.

Reconstruction of Skull Defects Following Loss of Scalp and Calvaria

The loss of soft tissue and bone follows major trauma. Automotive injury and tumor ablation are the two most common causes of these full-thickness defects. Immediate closure following acute injury can be achieved with split-thickness grafts, but definitive reconstruction of the defect usually must be delayed until the patient's general condition has stabilized. A number of biological and nonbiological materials have been used as substitutes for the missing bone: autogenous bone and silicone rubber are currently in favor.

ALLOPLASTIC MATERIALS. Large defects of the cranial vault that require reconstruction are usually seen long after the initial injury or surgical procedure which created them. Various materials have been used for the closure of cranial defects. The most popular alloplastic materials have been Vitallium [27], tantalum [45], stainless steel [41, 42], acrylic resins [44], and silicone polymers [10, 37]. The long-range chance of complications is high when such materials are used. White [46] reported a 10 and 12 percent complication rate with lucite and tantalum cranioplasties. Silastic, a form of silicone rubber, seems to be better tolerated than any substance previously used. Courtemanche and Thompson [26] reported the results in 5 patients with frontal bone defects repaired with silicone rubber prostheses. One implant was extruded secondary to excess tension.

Recently acrylic and polyethylene implants have found renewed favor. Maniscalco [35] describes the fabrication technique using methylmethacrylate. Habal [28] uses a combination polyurethane net in conjunction with cancellous autogenous bone in the frontal area to improve esthetic contouring. Results in 10 patients have been free of complications. (See Chapter 3.)

BONE GRAFTS. There is no substitute for living tissue, and the most satisfactory form of permanent cranioplasty has been achieved with autogenous bone grafts. These grafts have the advantages of being native tissue, and of being molded into position by physical and biological forces with the passage of time. They are usually permanent. Complications, such as infection or extrusion many months following the repair, rarely occur.

Autogenous bone grafts are indicated for defects of the frontal bone near the region of the frontal sinuses where all alloplastic materials act as foreign bodies, and where the long-term complication rate from secondary infection is very high. *Bone is the only suitable substance for reconstruction of the frontal sinus region.*

At the time of frontal cranioplasty, it is important to remove all vestiges of mucous membrane from the frontal sinuses, as any remnants of lining can serve as a focus for infection. The opening of the frontonasal duct should be plugged.

Split-rib grafts [11, 32] *are particularly indicated in children and young adults,* not only because of their rapid regeneration when periosteum is left following removal of the rib, but also because of the possible danger of injury to growth centers when iliac bone is removed and the risk of fracture when osteoperiosteal tibial grafts are used (Fig. 11-6). Growth of the rib grafts is commensurate with the growth of the child.

Longacre and his associates [29, 31, 33, 34] have

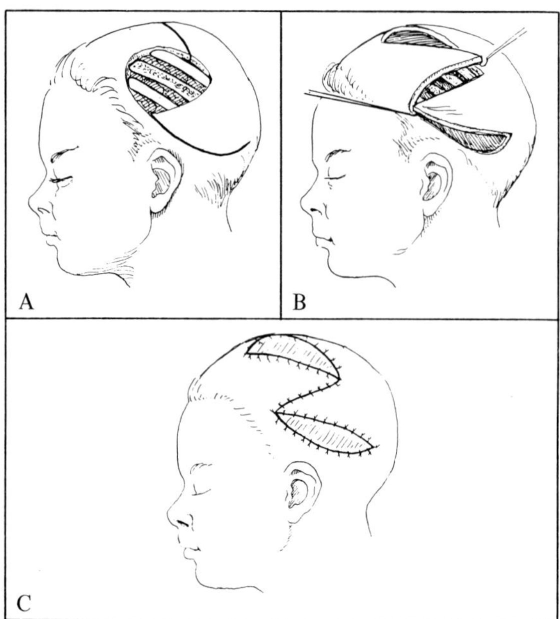

Fig. 11-6. The steps in double-rotation flap closure of a skull defect that has received split-rib grafts. (In actuality the flaps are made much larger than represented here by the artist.) Split-thickness skin grafts are usually necessary in the donor wound to relieve tension.

demonstrated that split-rib grafts can be used to fill in enormous defects of the cranium and that osteogenesis occurs from the edge of the skull to the split-rib grafts, even when the grafts are widely separated. Final and more exacting contour restoration can be obtained by implanting one of the forms of silicone after bony protection has been achieved [37]. Silicone seems an acceptable soft tissue substitute, since the incidence of extrusion is minimal with this material. Silicone is available in several forms of soft or hard rubber as well as sponge. It can be carved to fit any defect. This substance is currently the subject of wide investigation.

The *technique of obtaining rib grafts* requires the use of endotracheal anesthesia. A thoracic incision is made over the seventh rib to expose the rib bed (Fig. 11-7). This may be a short anterior incision or a long posterolateral thoracotomy incision. If necessary, the full length of rib can be resected; however, great care should be taken to strip the periosteum, which is left in situ in the rib bed for regeneration of new bone. *Only alternate ribs are removed.* Suturing the periosteum is not mandatory, but should be done by a running suture when possible. Undue shredding during the stripping procedure should be avoided. If the

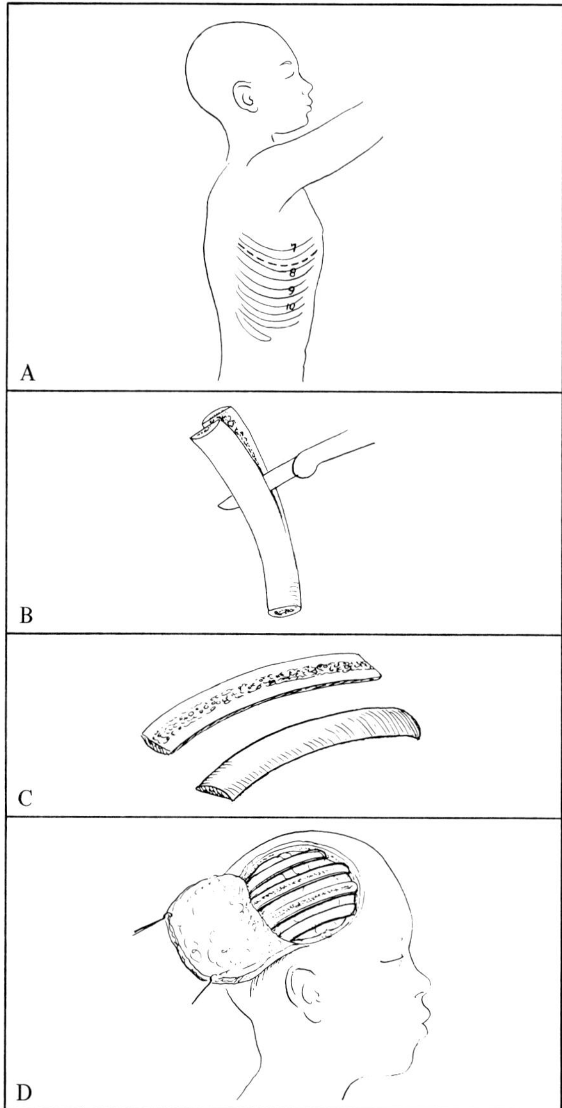

Fig. 11-7. The rib cage of children provides a ready source of bone for cranioplasty. The ribs are soft and easily split with a scalpel as shown. These grafts need not be placed in exact juxtaposition to each other as the gaps in between rapidly heal. A solid bony union results after several months. The adult rib is more ossified, and is generally not as satisfactory as the rib graft in children.

pleura is inadvertently entered, a small suction catheter should be inserted. Following closure of the wound, the lungs can be fully expanded by the anesthetist and the suction catheter removed. An indwelling catheter can be left connected to underwater suction for several days if there is suspicion of air leakage.

Cancellous iliac bone, used as large fitted pieces or as multiple cancellous bone chips, is favored by many for cranioplasty, particularly in the adult [9, 15, 30, 36, 38] (Fig. 11-8). Iliac bone is particularly useful after removal of alloplastic materials [30]. Iliac bone is a highly acceptable donor site for adults, particularly for repair of the frontal region, because of the large bone plates that can be obtained for exacting contour restoration.

When iliac bone is used, the inner table can be exposed through an incision about 8 cm. long which extends posteriorly from the anterior iliac spine (Fig. 11-9). All soft tissues arc divided down to the bone. The periosteum is elevated from the inner table. The full thickness of the iliac wing may be used, or it may be split to use only the inner table. The bone can be removed with the electric saw or by the use of osteotomes and chisels. Care should be taken, particularly when using osteotomes, not to split the bone into the acetabulum. Injury to the bladder or the peritoneum by inadvertent penetration with a sharp osteotome also must be avoided.

The *use of bone* from the *outer table of the iliac crest* was first suggested by Müller [39] in 1890. It was used successfully in 12 patients by Santoni-Rugiu [40] to reconstruct cranial defects. Following exposure of the defect and an adjacent donor area, a series of holes, 5 mm. apart, are drilled through the outer table of the ilium. The bone is then elevated with a large chisel, contoured, seated in the skull defect, and fixed in place. Santoni-Ragiu reported no complications using this technique. X-ray follow-up revealed fully integrated grafts.

Bone dust can also be used in reconstruction of the skull. Shehadi [43] compiled both experimental and clinical evidence supporting the merits of autogenous

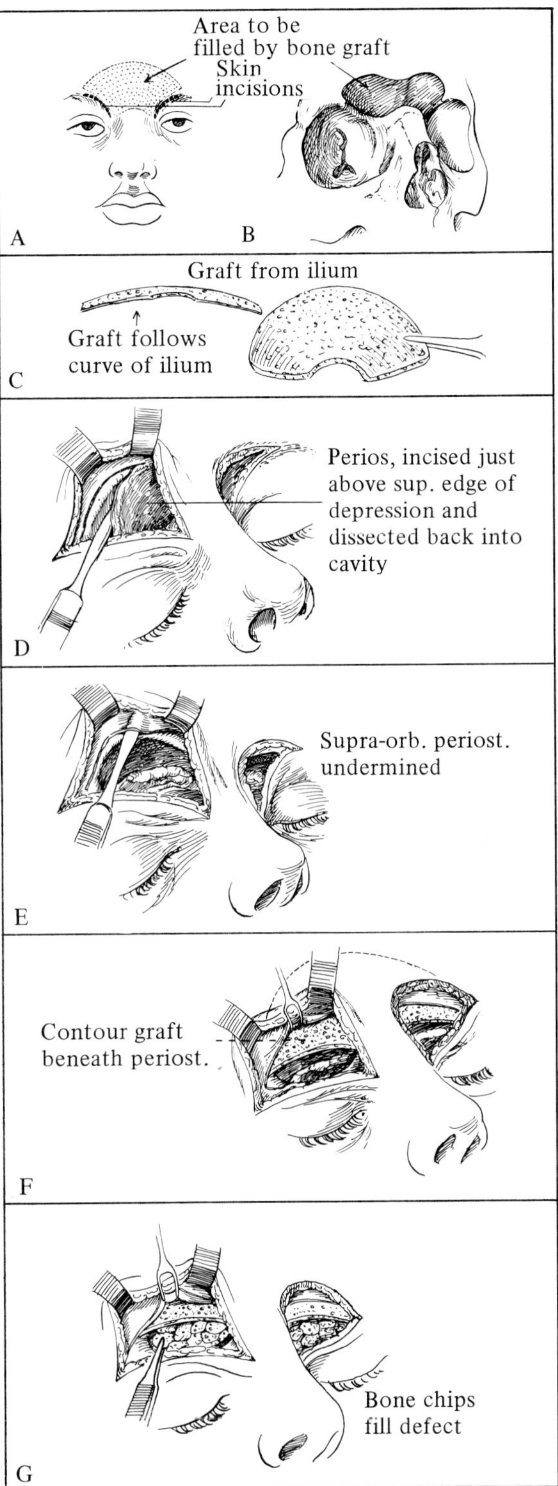

Fig. 11-8. The method advocated by Converse for repair of large frontal defects with a plate of iliac bone. Iliac bone is the graft of choice in the region of the frontal sinus. Foreign bodies are particularly unsuited in this region because of the possibility of infection arising from the frontonasal duct. All mucous membrane should be stripped from the frontal sinus and the duct closed. The plate of ilium is sculptured to fit the defect, and dead spaces are filled with chips. The technique is similar for defects elsewhere in the skull.

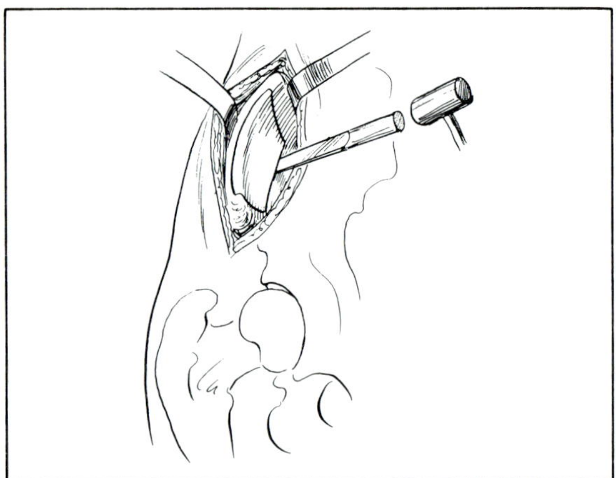

Fig. 11-9. Method for removal of iliac bone graft. The iliac crest is usually split as shown to preserve the rim in order to maintain contour. Cancellous chips are removed at the same time.

bone dust obtained from bur holes for skull reconstruction. The dust-saline paste is spread over the dura at the defect and covered with adjacent scalp. Within 3 months, a defect measuring 5 cm. in diameter was closed; in 1 year, a 12-cm. diameter defect was restored.

SOFT TISSUE CLOSURE. Repair of the soft tissue defect is best accomplished with hair-bearing local flaps prior to grafting. Distant flaps are at best inconvenient but are occasionally necessary. A by-product of microvascular surgery reported by Baudet [8] describes the use of a free thoracodorsal axillary flap in resurfacing large defects of the scalp. The flap artery and vein were anastomosed to the superficial temporal vessels in two patients with 10- and 13-cm. scalp defects.

Reconstruction of Forehead Defects

Small full-thickness skin defects (less than 2 cm. in diameter) can be closed by wide undermining and approximation, preferably in the horizontal plane. Larger defects require either skin grafts or local flaps. Split-thickness grafts to the forehead, though widely used, have two shortcomings: poor color match and the resultant concavity. The Millard crane principle [48] was used by Hamilton and Royster [47] to transport tissue in their two-stage scalp flap procedure for forehead reconstruction. A scalp flap is advanced to the defect and allowed to heal, and subsequently the hair-bearing portion is returned, leaving a bed of galea and subcutaneous fat to which skin is grafted. Worthen [49] reported on four patients in whom local rotation flaps were used to resurface resultant forehead defects following major excisions.

BURNS OF THE SCALP AND FOREHEAD

The scalp and forehead are frequent sites of thermal and occasionally electrical burns. The treatment follows the same general rules as those for burns of other regions. Usually it is preferable to use the exposure technique for the treatment of acute burns of the scalp, forehead, or face.

The presence of many hair follicles on the scalp makes regeneration prompt in burns of intermediate depth. The formation of a dry eschar is encouraged during the initial treatment. When it is clear that the full thickness of skin is affected, early debridement and grafting with split-thickness skin grafts is desirable. Of course, the time of excision and grafting is determined by the general condition of the patient and the response of the local burn.

Deep burns of the scalp may frequently result in exposed areas of cranium. The previously described principles of coverage apply. However, a local skin flap of scalp is rarely available, so decortication of the outer table is usually necessary to encourage rapid granulation. The granulating wound is eventually covered with split-thickness skin grafts. Worthen [52] reported a unique trial wherein the localized segment of devitalized bone following an electrical injury was retained and simply covered with a rotation scalp flap. Biopsy 9 months after injury revealed the bone to be "normal." This suggests that revascularization of the bone proceeded as though a graft had been performed.

After initial coverage of the burned skull or forehead (or both) has been accomplished, further reconstructive procedures can be contemplated. These can include shifting of existing hair-bearing scalp to more esthetically acceptable areas (such as the sideburn or anterior hairline to facilitate the use of hairpieces or wigs). Remnants of hair-bearing scalp should be shifted whenever possible to cover unstable areas of scarred epithelium, which tends to break down.

Cosmetic results are particularly important because of the prominent position of the forehead. When it is heavily scarred by burns or patchy skin grafts, a more harmonious cosmetic result can often be obtained by excising the entire forehead "unit" as a deep split-thickness skin graft and covering the defect with thick split-thickness skin as an overgraft [50, 51]. The epidermis and superficial dermis can be "shaved" with a dermatome or dermabrader, thus leaving the very vascular dermis to provide the best possible bed for the graft. Even when there is heavy scarring, a rich layer of subdermal vessels remains immediately beneath the cicatrix, so that the deep scar layer serves the same purpose as dermis in maintaining a uniform wound size and mitigating subsequent contracture.

Almost all split-thickness overgrafts take because of the available vascularity. The graft is invaded shortly after surgery by capillary buds from the rich blood supply of the underlying dermal bed. The color match of overgrafts is usually superior to that of other split-thickness skin grafts.

RADIATION DEFECTS OF THE SCALP, FOREHEAD, AND CALVARIA

Radiation injury of the skin, subcutaneous tissue, and bone of the forehead is quite common, and the scalp may be affected as well. Fortunately, these lesions are less common now because of the judicious use of ionizing radiation. However, radiation lesions secondary to treatment given many years ago may require resurfacing. The irradiation of hemangiomas or other benign tumors in childhood can result in marked deformity during growth, particularly in the frontal bones. Fortunately, a dose of ionizing radiation large enough to interfere with bone growth or to create skin damage is no longer used for benign lesions. The frequency of epitheliomas after irradiation is another factor against its use.

Treatment of chronic radiation injuries is excision and repair, not only to repair the local defect but also as prophylaxis against future metaplasia. Split-thickness skin grafting of heavily irradiated areas may be disappointing unless all irradiated tissue is excised. Split-thickness skin grafts often do not take on such defects. Robinson and Masters [56] report a loss of about 50 percent of these grafts, an experience similar to that of many others.

When less heavily irradiated lesions have adequate vascularity, split-thickness skin grafts can be used; however, a local rotation or advancement flap of adjacent tissue from the scalp or forehead usually is needed [54, 55]. Split-thickness skin grafting of the flap donor sites should be done to avoid tension on the flap. In some cases, when the injury is not extensive, the irradiated skin can be removed as a thick split-thickness skin graft and repaired by the overgrafting technique.

BENIGN TUMORS OF THE SCALP AND FOREHEAD

The most common benign tumors of the scalp and forehead are sebaceous cysts, hemangiomas, keratoses, and pigmented nevi. Most such tumors are amenable to simple surgery and should be excised.

Hemangiomas

Hemangiomas are excised only when they persist after involution of the capillary elements, or when there is evidence of continuous active growth with or without invasion of the outer table of the skull. Invasion of the skull is exceedingly uncommon, but it can occur, particularly in the region of the brow and orbit. Surgery is rarely justified except in those patients in whom the evidence of growth or invasion is incontrovertibly demonstrated by measurement or roentgenograms.

Flat, extensive hemangiomas are usually of the capillary type known as *port-wine stains.* They are best treated by camouflaging techniques, such as makeup or tattooing [60]. Surgery is occasionally indicated when grapelike papillomatous growths develop, but these are uncommon. Port-wine hemangiomas rarely involve only the forehead; they usually cover one entire side of the face.

In the past, many flat capillary lesions were excised and resurfaced with split-thickness skin grafts. The cosmetic results of this surgery were frequently worse than the original lesion. Deformities secondary to scarring or contracture of these grafts (such as ectropion) were not uncommon.

Some of the persistent *cavernous hemangiomas* can be treated by injection of a suitable sclerosing agent into the lumen of the hemangiomatous system. This method is effective only when the lesion is collapsible so that the intima can be damaged by the injected agent, and adherence of intima-to-intima can occur.

Nevi

Whenever possible, *junctional nevi* should be excised, but this is not always practical. Large nevi of the scalp should be destroyed because they are frequently subjected to minor trauma when the hair is combed, cut, or washed.

The *extensive hairy nevus* is uncommon. When it occurs, it often involves the scalp and forehead. These lesions do not tend to become malignant, and their removal is primarily for cosmetic reasons. Large hairy nevi on the forehead can be treated with resection of the entire skin region as a facial unit, followed by replacement with split-thickness skin grafts. Sometimes it is difficult to define the edges of these lesions, and it is not uncommon to find that a small linear recurrence of the mole is present at the margin of the graft or scar some time after healing. The hairline can be restored by the rotating hair-bearing scalp flaps [61].

If malignancy is suspected, nevi of the scalp or forehead should be excised completely for pathological study. The common compound nevus, typically raised and containing hair, can be electrodesiccated. This can be done with impunity, after "shaving" the elevated lesion for histological examination.

Lymphangiomas

Lymphangiomas of the scalp and forehead are less frequent than hemangiomas. As is the case in capillary or strawberry hemangiomas, these tumors may regress almost completely and gradually be replaced with fibrous tissue. When a significant volume of tumor remains, excision is the treatment of choice.

Wens
Wens or sebaceous cysts of the scalp are very common and frequently multiple. Because they are troublesome and prone to infection, they can and should be excised. The method described by Conway [59] is useful. The wen to be excised is vigorously massaged by the operator immediately before removal. Massage breaks down the fine adhesions between the capsule of the wen and the surrounding areolar scalp tissue. A very small incision is then made in the mouth of the cyst, and the contents are expressed. The emptied sac can then be removed easily, and one suture usually suffices to close the wound.

Aneurysms
Another type of so-called benign tumor is a lesion of blood vessels – *the cirsoid aneurysm.* Technically, it can be considered malignant because of extensive local destruction, high mortality, and difficult surgical control.

These lesions can be small or very extensive. They most frequently involve the parietal region of the scalp with its rich vascular plexus. The entire ear and underlying cranium and occasionally the forehead can be involved. The diagnosis of cirsoid aneurysm is made by palpating a pulsating mass. A bruit is often present.

Operative mortality can be very high indeed, since control of bleeding is difficult. Resection may involve removal of a portion of the ear. Total ablation may leave a large defect that will require a scalp rotation flap from above, or a split-thickness skin graft if the cranium is not exposed.

Neurofibromas
Neurofibromatosis of the scalp is not uncommon, either as isolated lesions or associated with Recklinghausen's disease [63]. The scalp, particularly the parietal areas, can be the site of a very large localized form of neurofibromatosis, in which there is a large, soft tumor. The skin often resembles elephant skin – thus the term *pachydermatocele.* These lesions are highly vascular.

Excision is indicated because approximately 10 percent of these lesions apparently undergo *degeneration into sarcomas,* and because of the severity of the *cosmetic deformity.* Small isolated neurofibromas can be excised without difficulty. When surgical removal of the more extensive lesions is undertaken, several units of whole blood should be available. The surgeon must be prepared to create a large defect which may require (as in the cirsoid aneurysm) rotation of a large scalp flap, or application of a split-thickness skin graft if the base of the excision does not expose the outer table of the cranium.

Turban Tumors
This tumor is very rare and is thought to be of adnexal gland derivation; the exact anlage, whether sweat gland, hair follicle, or sebaceous gland, has not been accurately determined. The tumor, which frequently involves the entire scalp and resembles a turban, has an early onset (usually before 30), is familial, and is more common in women [57]. Chronic irritation of the epidermis from ordinary care of the hair is common, and irritation sometimes leads to ulceration. Malignant dedifferentiation into basal or squamous cell carcinoma has been reported, but this is exceedingly rare [62].

In the differential diagnosis, turban tumors must be distinguished from epithelial or sebaceous cysts, or basal cell carcinoma. However, the typical turban tumor, involving a large area, is difficult to confuse with any other lesion.

The treatment is wide local excision and repair of the resultant defect, either with local rotation flaps or with split-thickness skin grafts. Exposure of the underlying cranium is usually unnecessary; recurrences are unusual.

MALIGNANT TUMORS OF THE SCALP AND FOREHEAD

Malignant tumors of the scalp can be *primary,* the result of *direct extension* from adjacent areas of the head and neck, or *metastatic.*

The most common *primary tumors* are squamous cell carcinoma, basal cell carcinoma, melanoma, and fibrosarcoma. Rare primary tumors are the various types of sarcomas such as rhabdosarcoma and liposarcoma. Primary leukemic infiltrations can also occur on the scalp. Primary malignancies of the scalp are not common when compared with those of other primary sites. According to Conley [64], approximately 2 percent of epithelial tumors of the skin occur on the scalp, with basal cell carcinoma being the most common.

The most common *metastatic tumors* of the scalp are from the breast, stomach, and colon. Other primary sites are the parotid glands, lungs, kidneys, and prostate. Metastases to the scalp or skull may be isolated or multiple. They are usually discovered inadvertently. Histological examination often reveals that these tumors are metastatic. In the histological diagnosis of very undifferentiated tumors, confusion can arise between primary tumors of cutaneous adnexal origin and highly undifferentiated tumors (particularly those originating in the lungs and kidneys). When metastatic disease is suspected, an intensive search for the primary site should be made before treatment of the scalp lesion. Metastasis to the cranium is more common than metastasis to the soft tissue of the scalp. In a large series reported by Conley [64], only three metastatic tumors of the scalp were found, and these were from the parotid gland, breast, and calf (melanoma).

As in malignant tumors elsewhere, the basic cause of malignancies of the scalp is unknown. Exposure to actinic rays, long-standing irritation, ulceration in burn scars, malignant dedifferentiation of benign lesions such as keratoses, and areas of radiation change in the scalp can and do result in malignancies.

Extent of Excision and Method of Repair

When the *excised specimen is larger than 2 cm. in diameter,* repair by direct approximation of the skin edges is virtually impossible on the scalp. Regional pedicle transpositions or free skin grafts must be used.

The subaponeurotic space usually provides sufficient depth for excision of superficial cancers, since this space is a very good barrier to deeper growth. *When larger cancers of the scalp have invaded through the galea, one should include a portion of the outer table of the skull in the excision.* The periosteum or the outer table may not grossly appear to be invaded by malignancy, and *roentgenograms rarely reveal invasion.* However, microscopic foci of invasion can be found in such tumors, particularly in the diploë.

If there is *gross or roentgenographic evidence that the cranial bones are directly involved,* a neurosurgeon should be present during operative excision, so that the full depth of the underlying cranial vault can be removed. In such cases, the preoperative preparation of a large regional flap may be necessary, because a flap is indicated when the underlying dura or brain is surgically exposed. When a flap is not feasible, it should be remembered that split-thickness skin grafts grow without difficulty on the dura. For example, *sarcomas* frequently involve the cranium and require large full-thickness excision. Very large sarcomas may require the preoperative preparation of pedicle grafts or tubed or jump flaps from distant sites (see Fig. 11-2).

Primary Malignant Tumors of the Scalp

Squamous Cell and Basal Cell Carcinoma

These malignancies are fully discussed in Chapter 26.

Adenocarcinoma

Adenocarcinomas, or carcinomas of skin appendages, occur on the forehead and scalp, but they are rare and often difficult to diagnose histologically. Such a lesion should be suspected if an isolated tumor is excised and the histological diagnosis is "undifferentiated carcinoma." *Removal of sweat gland carcinomas should be accompanied by regional dissection of the lymph nodes,* since these tumors are notorious for their metastases to the lymph nodes with resultant high mortality.

Sarcomas

The treatment of sarcoma is radical local excision and repair by an appropriate technique. These tumors are rare. Initial *surgical treatment must be vigorous* indeed if there is to be a chance of cure. *Certain sarcomas may be highly radiosensitive;* when this is so, surgical treatment is often combined with radiotherapy.

Melanomas

Chapter 27 is devoted to this subject.

COSMETIC SURGERY OF THE SCALP

TREATMENT OF BALDNESS. Alopecia, secondary to hereditary causes, disease entities, or trauma, is a condition frequently confronting the plastic surgeon. Male pattern baldness is by far the most common form of baldness. After considering or treating associated disease entities, the plastic surgeon may elect to undertake hair grafting or refer the patient. Regardless of this decision, a working knowledge of the various methods available to restore hair loss is useful.

PATIENT SELECTION. Early male pattern baldness typically involves the temples or the pate. This is the opportune time to begin grafting in order to use the existing hair as camouflage. More extensive loss can be improved but during the immediate treatment period the grafts are obvious. Loss that is nearly complete is best treated nonsurgically with a hairpiece or full wig. Success is predicated on Orentreich's [73] original observation that occipital hair when transplanted anteriorly retains the genetic longevity of the donor site. Thus, patient selection is dependent on adequate parietal and occipital donor sites, a willingness to endure the inconvenience of surgery, and the patience to wait 6 to 8 months before functional hair has regenerated.

Methodology

HAIR PLUGS. The most common method used to restore hair loss is the simple cylindrical composite graft. Typically, a 4.0- or 4.5-mm. skin biopsy punch containing 10 to 15 hair follicles is used to remove the graft from the posterior scalp. A similar or slightly smaller punch is used to prepare a recipient bed from the offending bald area. The composite graft containing skin, fat, and hair follicles is seated in the recipient site with the hair oriented in the direction of existing hair growth (i.e., the frontal hair grows anteriorly). The number of grafts depends on the defect to be covered but as many as 50 to 75 can be done in a

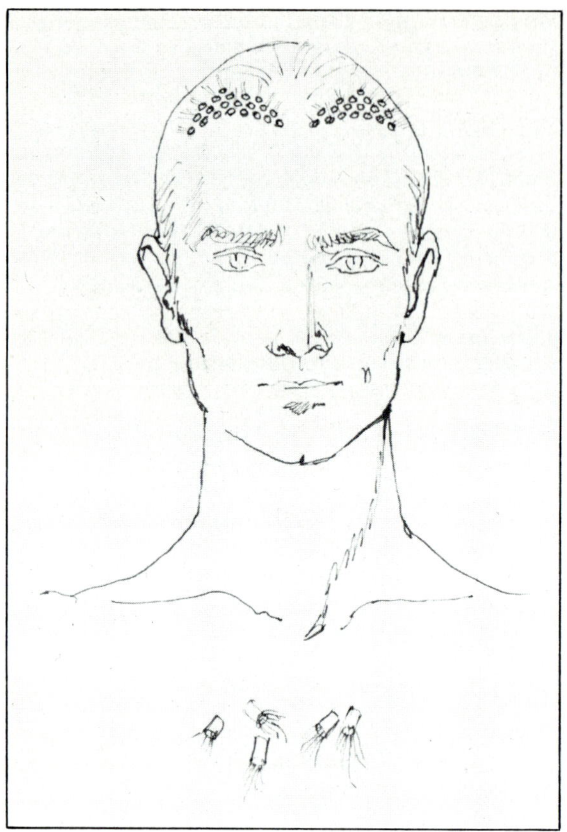

Fig. 11-10. Hair plugs are positioned to resurface the frontal hairline, leaving space for additional grafts at a second session.

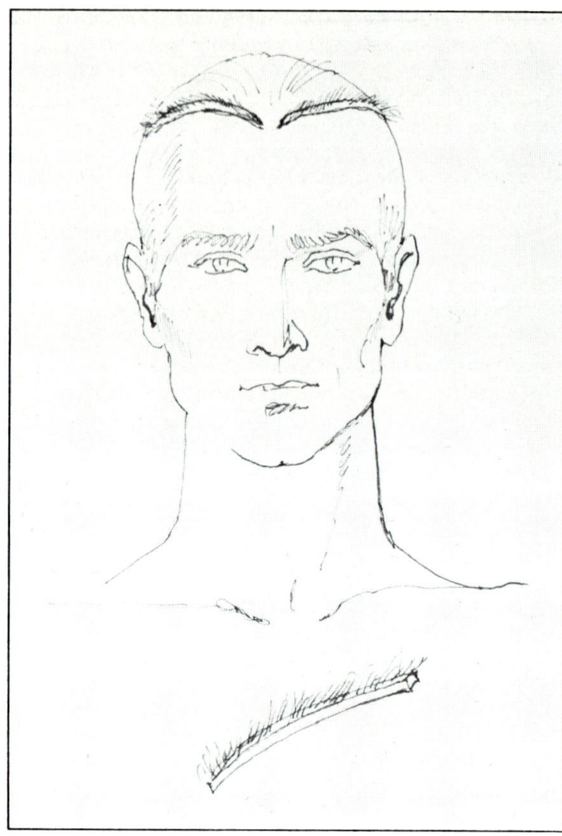

Fig. 11-11. Vallis strip grafts are used to reconstruct a frontal hair line.

session if needed. The grafts are positioned to allow an intervening island which will be removed and planted at the second session (Fig. 11-10). A light bonnet is applied to protect the grafts for 24 hours. A second session can be undertaken within 3 weeks.

STRIP GRAFT. The Vallis [74] strip graft consists of a 6- to 8-mm. wide composite scalp graft of the required length that is cut from the hair-bearing posterior scalp and inserted to reconstruct the frontal hair line. After trimming excess fat from below the follicles, the graft is placed in a simple incision in the recipient area extending through the galea. A running 6-0 nylon suture is used to gain maximum approximation to adjacent tissues. In reconstructing a new frontal hairline, Vallis cautions against trying to restore the original; it is best to settle for a moderate degree of recession. Also the surgeon should be certain to restore the natural curve, avoiding a straight or artificial look (Fig. 11-11). As with hair plugs, the shaft is lost and the transplanted follicle grows a new hair. The principal advantage of the strip is far greater hair density in the recipient site. The disadvantages are that the surgery is more involved and that there is an increased incidence of full or partial graft failure.

SCALP FLAPS. Attempts to restore the hairline by rotating pedicle flaps from the temporal and occipital areas have been successfully accomplished by a number of surgeons. The surgery is much too complicated and massive to undertake routinely for this benign condition. The use of bipedicle and single pedicle flaps for transfering hairy sections of the scalp to bald areas has been reported by Lamont [71], Limburger [72], and Correa-Iturraspe and Arufe [69]. Correa-Iturraspe and Arufe also attempted to reduce the area of baldness by excising full-thickness segments of hairless skin and closing the edges directly – in essence, a multiple-stage technique of advancement of flaps.

Juri [70] has used a delayed parietal flap both unilaterally and bilaterally to recreate the frontal hairline. The result can be spectacular if the patient is sufficiently motivated to undergo the multistaged procedure.

REFERENCES

Congenital Deformities

1. Deeken, J. H., and Caplan, R. M. Aplasia cutis congenita. *Arch. Dermatol.* 102:386, 1970.
2. Erydelyi, R. An unusual malformation of the scalp corrected by plastic surgery. *Plast. Reconstr. Surg.* 35:334, 1965.
3. Hunn, J. M., Huygens, H. J., and Newman, N. M. Hereditary scalp and cranial defects. *Med. J. Aust.* 56:219, 1969.
4. Ingalls, N. W. Congenital defects of the scalp: III. Studies in the pathology of development. *Am. J. Obstet. Gynecol.* 25:861, 1933.
5. Lynch, P. J., and Kahn, E. A. Congenital defects of the scalp: A surgical approach to aplasia cutis congenital. *J. Neurosurg.* 33:198, 1970.
6. Pap, G. S. Congenital defect of scalp and skull in three generations of one family. *Plast. Reconstr. Surg.* 46:194, 1970.
7. Peer, L., and Van Duyn, J. Congenital defects of the scalp. *Plast. Reconstr. Surg.* 3:722, 1948.

Trauma—Soft Tissue Defects

8. Baudet, J., Guimberteau, J. C., and Nascimento, E. Successful clinical transfer of two free thoracodorsal axillary flaps. *Plast. Reconstr. Surg.* 58:680, 1976.
9. Blocker, T. G., and Weiss, L. R. Use of cancellous bone in repair of defects about the jaws. *Ann. Surg.* 123:622, 1946.
10. Brown, J. B., Fryer, M. P., Randall, P., and Lee, M. Silicones in plastic surgery. *Plast. Reconstr. Surg.* 12:374, 1953.
11. Brown, R. C. The repair of skull defects. *Med. J. Aust.* 11:409, 1917.
12. Cantu, R. Complication of long hair. *Lancet* 1:350, 1971.
13. Converse, J. M. Facial disfigurement in automobile accidents. *J.A.M.A.* 185:354, 1963.
14. Cornell University Automotive Crash Injury Research. The injury-producing accident: A primer of facts and figures. New York, August 1961.
15. Crouch, T. H., and Mark, V. H. Repair of cranial defects with anterior iliac bone grafts. *U.S. Armed Forces Med. J.* 9:375, 1958.
16. Davis, J. S. Scalping accidents. *Johns Hopkins Hosp. Rep.* 16:257, 1911.
17. Delak, Z. Successful replacement of the completely avulsed scalp. *Br. J. Plast. Surg.* 8:55, 1955.
18. Dingman, R. O. Surgical treatment of defects of the scalp. *J. Int. Coll. Surg.* 30:148, 1958.
19. Kazanjian, V. H., and Converse, J. M. Reconstruction after radical operation for osteomyelitis of frontal bone. *Arch. Otolaryngol.* (Chicago) 31:94, 1940.
20. Lu, M. M. Successful replacement of avulsed scalp. *Plast. Reconstr. Surg.* 43:231, 1969.
21. McGovern, F. H. Facial nerve injuries in skull fractures, recent advances in management. *Arch. Otolaryngol.* 88:102, 1968.
22. Miller, D. H., Anstee, J. E., and Snell, J. A. Successful replantation of an avulsed scalp by microvascular anastomoses. *Plast. Reconstr. Surg.* 58:133, 1976.
23. Orticochea, M. Application de la technique des quatre lambeaux dans la réconstruction du front et des régions pariétales. *Ann. Chir. Plast.* 2:153, 1969.
24. Osborne, M. P. Complete scalp avulsion. *Ann. Surg.* 132:198, 1950.
25. Robinson, F. Complete avulsion of the scalp. *Br. J. Plast. Surg.* 5:37, 1952.

Bone Defects

26. Courtemanche, A. D., and Thompson, G. B. Silastic cranioplasty following cranio-facial injuries. *Plast. Reconstr. Surg.* 41:165, 1968.
27. Geib, F. W. Vitallium skull plates. *J.A.M.A.* 117:812, 1941.
28. Habal, M. B., Leake, D. L., and Maniscalco, J. E. A new method for reconstruction of major defects in the cranial vault. *Surg. Neurol.* 6:137, 1976.
29. Holmstrand, K., Longacre, J. J., and DeStefano, G. A. Biophysical studies of split-rib grafts in the repair of defects of the cranium: Preliminary results of experimental studies in rhesus monkeys. *Plast. Reconstr. Surg.* 26:286, 1960.
30. Kiehn, C. L., and Grino, A. Iliac bone grafts replacing tantalum plates for gunshot wounds of the skull. *Am. J. Surg.* 85:395, 1953.
31. Longacre, J. J. Surgical Correction of Extensive Defects of Scalp and Cranium with Autogenous Tissues. *Transactions of First International Congress of Plastic Surgeons.* Baltimore: Williams & Wilkins, 1957.
32. Longacre, J. J., and Converse, J. M. Deformities of the Forehead, Scalp, and Cranium. In Converse, J. M. (Ed.), *Reconstructive Plastic Surgery,* 2nd ed. Vol. 2. Philadelphia: Saunders, 1977.
33. Longacre, J. J., and DeStefano, G. A. Further observations of the behavior of autogenous split-rib grafts in reconstruction of extensive defects of the cranium and face. *Plast. Reconstr. Surg.* 20:281, 1957.
34. Longacre, J. J., and DeStefano, G. A. Experi-

mental observations of the repair of extensive defects of the skull with split-rib grafts. *Plast. Reconstr. Surg.* 21:372, 1958.
35. Maniscalco, J. E., and Garcia-Bengochea, F. Cranioplasty. A method of prefabricating alloplastic plates. *Surg. Neurol.* 2:339, 1974.
36. McClintok, N. G., and Dingman, R. O. The repair of cranial defects with iliac bone. *Surgery* 30:955, 1951.
37. Millard, R. Practical variations of cranioplasty. *Am. J. Surg.* 107:802, 1964.
38. Mowlen, R. Cancellous chip bone grafts: Report on 75 cases. *Lancet* 2:746, 1944.
39. Müller, W. Zur Frage der Temporären Schadel Resektion an Stelle der Trepanation. *Zentralbl. Chir.* 17:65, 1890.
40. Santoni-Rugiu, P. Repair of skull defects by outer table osteoperiosteal free grafts. *Plast. Reconstr. Surg.* 43:157, 1969.
41. Scott, M., and Wycis, H. T. Experimental observations of the use of stainless steel for cranioplasty. *J. Neurosurg.* 3:310, 1946.
42. Scott, M., Wycis, H. T., and Murtagh, F. Long term evaluation of stainless steel cranioplasty. *Surg. Gynecol. Obstet.* 115:453, 1962.
43. Shehadi, S. Skull reconstruction with bone dust. *Br. J. Plast. Surg.* 23:227, 1970.
44. Small, J. M., and Graham, M. P. Acrylic resin for the closure of skull defects. *Br. J. Surg.* 33:106, 1945–46.
45. Weiford, B. C., and Gardner, W. J. Tantalum cranioplasty: A review of 106 cases in civilian practice. *J. Neurosurg.* 6:13, 1949.
46. White, J. C. Late complications following cranioplasty with alloplastic plates. *Ann. Surg.* 128:743, 1948.

Forehead Reconstruction
47. Hamilton, R., and Royster, H. P. Reconstruction of extensive forehead defects. *Plast. Reconstr. Surg.* 47:421, 1971.
48. Millard, D. R. The crane principle for the transport of subcutaneous tissue. *Plast. Reconstr. Surg.* 43:451, 1969.
49. Worthen, E. F. Repair of forehead defects by rotation of local flaps. *Plast. Reconstr. Surg.* 57:204, 1976.

Burns of Scalp and Forehead
50. Hynes, W. The treatment of scars by shaving and skin graft. *Br. J. Plast. Surg.* 10:1, 1957.
51. Webster, G. V., Peterson, R. A., and Stein, H. L. Dermal overgrafting of the leg. *J. Bone Joint Surg.* [Am.] 40:796, 1958.
52. Worthen, E. F. Regeneration of the skull following a deep electrical burn. *Plast. Reconstr. Surg.* 48:1, 1971.

Radiation Injury
53. Cannon, B., Randolph, J. C., and Murray, J. G. Malignant irradiation for benign conditions. *N. Engl. J. Med.* 260:196, 1959.
54. Longacre, J. J. The surgical management of local postradiation effects. *Am. J. Surg.* 92:18, 1956.
55. Rees, T. D. Radiation necrosis of the chest wall. *Plast. Reconstr. Surg.* 28:67, 1961.
56. Robinson, D. W., and Masters, F. W. Surgery for radiation injury. *A.M.A. Arch. Surg.* 80:946, 1960.

Benign Tumors
57. Batstone, J. H. F. Turban tumor. *Br. J. Surg.* 54:567, 1967.
58. Braund, R. R., and Pigott, J. D. Surgical treatment of massive scalp lesions. *Cancer* 9:1227, 1956.
59. Conway, H. *Tumors of the Skin.* Springfield, Ill.: Thomas, 1956.
60. Conway, H., and Montroy, R. E. Permanent camouflage of capillary hemangiomas of face by intradermal injection of insoluble pigments (tattooing). *N.Y. State J. Med.* 65:876, 1965.
61. Cronin, T. D. Extensive pigmented nevi in hair-bearing areas. *Plast. Reconstr. Surg.* 11:94, 1953.
62. Davis, C., and Alexander, R. W. Turban tumors of the scalp. *Arch. Surg.* (Chicago) 82:445, 1961.
63. Davis, W. B., Edgerton, M. T., and Hoffmeister, S. F. Neurofibromatosis of the head and neck. *Plast. Reconstr. Surg.* 14:186, 1954.

Malignant Tumors
64. Conley, J. J. Malignant tumors of the scalp: I. Analysis of 92 cases of malignant epithelial and somatic tumors of the scalp. *Plast. Reconstr. Surg.* 33:1, 1964.
65. Conley, J. J. Malignant tumors of the scalp: II. An analysis of 58 cases of melanoma of the scalp. *Plast. Reconstr. Surg.* 33:163, 1964.
66. Masters, F., Georgiade, N., Horton, C., and Pickrell, K. Role of radical surgery in extensive and recurrent malignant lesions of the face and scalp. *A.M.A. Surg.* 68:677, 1954.
67. Mohs, F. *Chemosurgery in Cancer, Gangrene and Infections.* Springfield, Ill.: Thomas, 1956.
68. Ratzer, E. R., and Strong, E. W. Squamous cell carcinoma of the scalp. *Am. J. Surg.* 114:570, 1967.

Cosmetic Surgery
69. Correa-Iturraspe, M., and Arufe, H. N. Plastic surgery of partial alopecia. *Semana Med.* 19:937, 1957.
70. Juri, J. Use of parieto-occipital flaps in the surgical treatment of baldness. *Plast. Reconstr. Surg.* 55:456, 1975.

71. Lamont. G. S. A plastic surgery transformation. *West J. Surg.* 65:164, 1957.
72. Limberger, S. The surgical treatment of hair loss. *Medizinische* 35:1559, 1959.
73. Orentreich, M. Hair transplantation, the punch graft technique. *Surg. Clin. North Am.* 51:511, 1971.
74. Vallis, C. P. Hair transplantation for male pattern baldness. *Surg. Clin. North Am.* 51:519, 1971.

Reconstruction of the Eyelids and Eyebrows and Correction of Ptosis of the Eyelid*

JOHN C. MUSTARDÉ

Reconstruction of the Eyelids and Eyebrows

BASIC PRINCIPLES OF EYELID RECONSTRUCTION

Reconstruction of an eyelid is usually called for when the full thickness of the lid is resected to remove a tumor, but it may be required for congenital lid defects (colobomas) or when the lid has been lost following trauma. When the eye is still present, reconstruction of an eyelid or even a part of it requires a minimum of three elements: an outer layer of skin, an inner layer of mucosa, and a semirigid skeleton interposed between them. Equally as important as provision of these layers is the need to provide a stable margin – one that will neither turn in or out, and will thus prevent possible damage to the cornea from contact with skin, or epiphora.

The upper lid is the most difficult to reconstruct, since it must be movable. There must be some means of opening the reconstructed upper lid in order to see and some mechanism of closing it to protect the globe. If even a small part of the upper lid is lost or distorted, particularly in the center, the cornea may be exposed during sleep, thus incurring the risk of ulceration and even loss of the eye. By contrast, apart from epiphora, loss of the entire lower lid can be tolerated reasonably well. This is one reason why the delicate structures of the active part of the upper lid should not be used in reconstructing the lower lid when any other tissues are available. It is especially unwise to "share" the all-important mobile tarsal portion of the lining of the upper lid in reconstructions of the lower, even though a proportion of cases reconstructed this way can be successful when those cases are of only minor to moderate severity and the procedures are performed by experts. The use of flaps of tarsus and conjunctiva taken from the upper lid to repair the lower may produce undesirable sequelae that affect the function and appearance of both. Only where small amounts of loose orbital skin are needed should the upper lid be considered as a donor site.

*The illustrations in this chapter are reproduced with the permission of Churchill-Livingstone.

The tissues required for reconstructing an upper lid are very specific. To shape the lid to the curvature of the eye it is necessary to have a flexible tarsal skeleton – lined by mucous membrane to prevent keratitis and ulceration of the cornea. In addition there must be a stable margin that will not permit the upper lid skin to roll down and rub against the cornea. Materials good enough to meet these exacting requirements can come from but one place, another eyelid. One possible source is a free graft from the other upper lid, but it is unsuitable as a source for the needed materials. A very satisfactory upper lid, however, can be fashioned from the corresponding lower lid. The whole of the lower lid could, but need not, be donated without hesitation for this purpose, provided the resulting defect can be repaired adequately. This is the first basic principle of sound eyelid reconstruction: *use the lower lid to reconstruct the upper, but use other sources to reconstruct the lower.*

A point of considerable importance to the planning of any reconstruction is that, due to the laxness of the tissues, up to a quarter of an eyelid can be removed and the defect still closed directly. This can often be accomplished without even dividing the lateral canthal ligament. The eyelid tissues of elderly patients may be so relaxed that one-third of the lid can be resected and direct closure of its margins still be accomplished. A second basic principle is that in lid reconstruction, because of the stretch of the tissues, only *three-quarters of either lid need be retained or reconstructed.* (A completely reconstructed lid may not actually stretch to the same length as normal lid tissue, but some lateral shortening will be cosmetically insignificant, and this simplifies the technique of reconstruction.) The basic principles of reconstruction are therefore:

1. Use the lower lid to reconstruct the upper lid, but use other sources to reconstruct the lower lid.
2. Only three-quarters of the width of either lid needs to be reconstructed.

These two fundamental principles allow the planning of either the upper or lower lid reconstruction by a simple scheme based on multiples of a quarter. This reduces the reconstruction to a simple rule which is of greater practical value than providing an illustrated catalogue of cases bearing little relation to the specific problem confronting the surgeon.

Information on dacrocystorhinostomy is included in Chapter 9.

RECONSTRUCTION OF THE LOWER LID

It is quite unnecessary to add a line of lashes in reconstructing a lower lid if the upper lid, with its much stronger and more obvious line of lashes, is present and completely normal. If hairs are transplanted into the margin of the reconstructed lid, they can easily become distorted by scar tissue and rub on the cornea. Furthermore, very few hair-bearing strips inserted at this site ever resemble the normal lash line. Reconstruction of the lower lid must be considered under two headings because *vertical* and *horizontal* (marginal) losses are repaired by different techniques (Fig. 12-1).

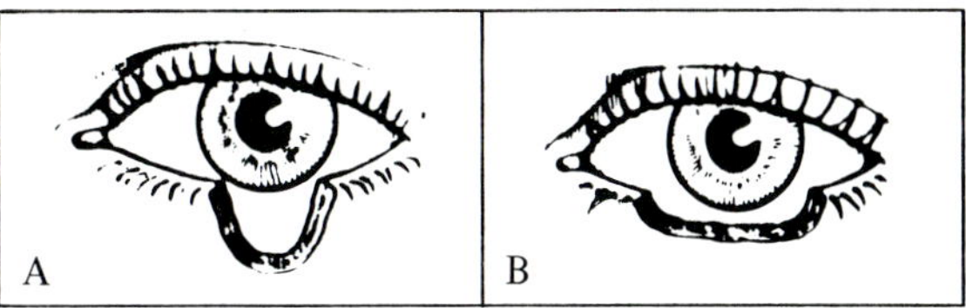

Fig. 12-1. A, vertical loss of lower eyelid. B, horizontal loss of lower eyelid.

Loss in a Vertical Direction

Vertical losses can vary in extent from a minor wedge-shaped U (resection through the margin should always be made vertical to the margin, not obliquely) to complete loss of the lower lid. Since the medial segment of the lid cannot be moved laterally without interfering with the function of the canaliculus, the lateral segment must be moved medially.

In small losses, where three-quarters or slightly less of the original length of the lid remains, the defect can be closed directly (Fig. 12-2A, B), although the lower crus of the lateral canthal ligament may need to be divided. If the loss is greater than this, the limit of stretch usually has been reached. The additional tissue required for the reconstruction is obtained from that part of the eyelid lying beyond the lateral canthus (see Fig. 12-5). Enough must be gained to make the sum of the medial and lateral segments equal to at least three-quarters of the original lid length.

The general plan for reconstruction of the lower lid is to rotate a flap from the cheek and malar region toward the nose, thus carrying the peripheral lid skin, with its lidlike quality, into the defect. If a substitute for inner lining and tarsal plate is needed, it may be secured by using a chondromucosal graft from the nasal septum. A single operation is all that is required, even to reconstruct a complete lower lid.

The surgeon simply designs a large or small flap, depending on the need. Based roughly on multiples of a quarter, the scheme of reconstruction outlined below will enable any surgeon to determine, by reference to the appropriate section, the exact technique to be followed in a particular case.

Loss of Up to a Quarter of the Lower Lid

When three-quarters of the original length of the lid remains, the defect may be closed by direct approximation in three layers (Fig. 12-3). A continuous 6-0 Prolene suture, placed so that it can be removed by the pull-out technique, is used for closing the conjunctiva and tarsus. Interrupted sutures of fine catgut are best for closing the orbicularis oculi muscle, and fine silk is used for the skin. To close the margin accurately a suture is placed in the gray line in the same fashion as when closing a full-thickness vertical laceration of the lid. A "halving" procedure (Fig. 12-4) is neither necessary nor wise because it creates a bigger defect than is actually required and increases the difficulty of closing the gap. If good surgical technique is used, the line of scar will be perfectly satisfactory and notching will not occur. Neither halving nor intramarginal adhesions are required; such techniques cannot serve as a substitute for good surgery. When the defect in the lower lid is only slightly wider than a quarter of the original length, a lateral canthotomy (division of that part of the lateral canthal ligament attached to the lower lid) will allow an increase in the swing of the lateral part of the lid toward the nose to permit the gap to be closed (see Fig. 12-2C, D).

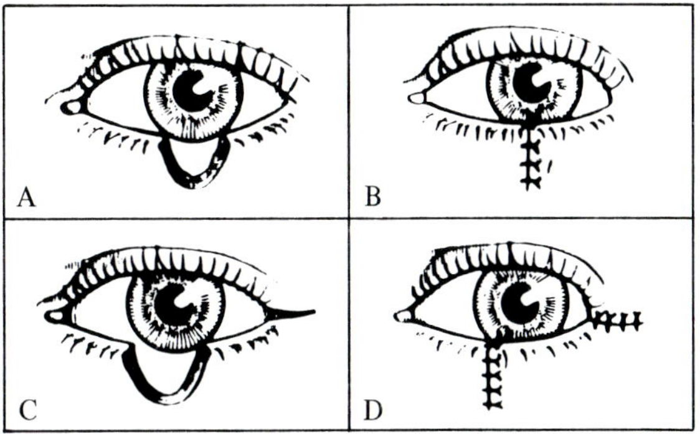

Fig. 12-2. A and B, small vertical losses of the lower lid, where about three-quarters or more of the lid remains, can be closed directly. C and D, slightly larger vertical loss repaired by division of the lateral canthal ligament (lower crus).

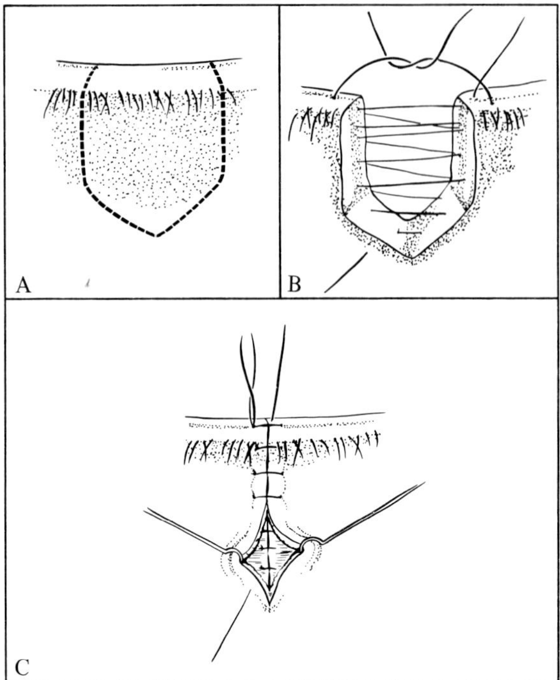

Fig. 12-3. Technique of closing defects of less than a quarter of the lower lid. A, the area to be resected is a pentagon. B, a continuous 6-0, Prolene suture is passed through conjunctiva and tarsus, and finally through skin. This fine suture will not ulcerate the cornea. A single suture unites the gray line at the lid margin. C, fine catgut sutures are used to close the orbicularis muscle and fine silk to close the skin.

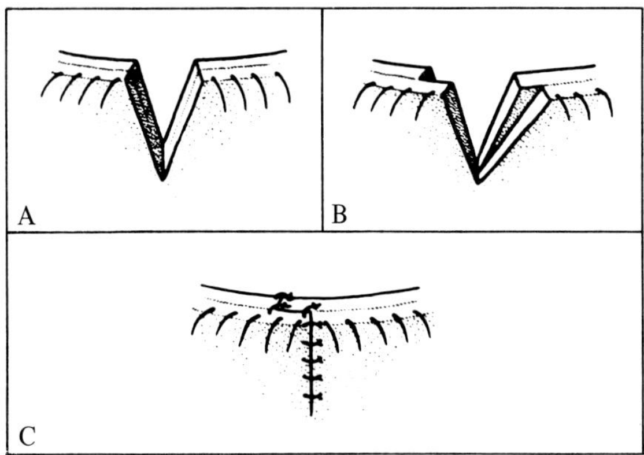

Fig. 12-4. Halving procedure formerly used to close lid defects, but now condemned.

Loss of a Quarter to a Half of the Lower Lid

When a defect in the lid is greater than a quarter but not more than a half of the original length, an additional small amount of lateral lid tissue – up to 8 mm. – must be added to provide a lid of reasonable length. This additional tissue can be obtained from the eyelid skin lateral to the canthus by making a 3- or 4-cm. curving incision upward and outward from the canthus, and by dividing the lateral canthal ligament to the lower lid (Fig. 12-5). The length of the incision is increased until the lid defect can be closed easily. The skin should be undermined over the orbital margin, and the orbital septum – which anchors the lid to the orbital margin – should be freed. The conjunctiva of the lateral fornix can be mobilized for lining the small raw area of the reconstructed lid, or if more lining is required, a graft of nasal septal mucous membrane can be inserted. The margin here will be unstable, but the skin will not rub against the cornea in such a lateral position.

If these lower lid defects do not extend into the lid for any great distance, a triangle of skin and orbicularis, with the base upward (Figure 12-5A), should be excised from beneath the defect. This aids rotation of the cheek flap toward the nose without creating a fold at the point around which it turns.

Loss of More than a Half of the Lower Lid

If more than half of the lid is lost (Fig. 12-6), the curving incision must be carried outward to the preauricular area and down in front of the ear for as far as is needed. This flap is thoroughly undermined. Because the conjunctiva in the lateral fornix will not provide sufficient tissue for lining the new sector of the lid, a graft of mucous membrane will be needed. Buccal mucosa is not satisfactory for this purpose, since it contracts markedly, thus causing a considerable degree of entropion in the unsupported, reconstructed sector, and supporting materials cannot be inserted until 4 to 6 weeks later, when the damage is already done.

Nasal mucosa is undoubtedly the best material for lining the lower lid. A portion of septal cartilage should be left attached to it, on one side. The *graft of nasal mucosa and cartilage* should be removed from the nasal septum in such a way that a strut of cartilage, at least 6 mm. wide, lies in front of and below it to prevent the nasal bridge from collapsing, and mucosa is left on one side. Excellent exposure of the septum is obtained if an incision is made to free the alar soft tissue up to the pyriform opening; the incision is continued on the inside up between the alar cartilages to reach the nasal bridge. Once the composite graft is removed, the resulting septal defect may be packed with Vaseline gauze for a few days, and it epithelializes rapidly. The septal cartilage

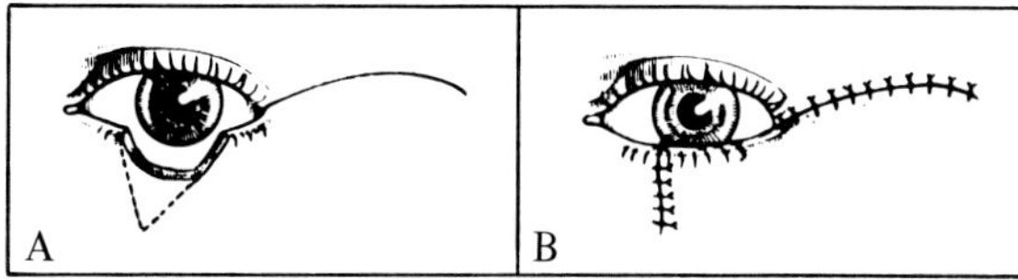

Fig. 12-5. Technique of closing defects of a quarter to a half of the lower lid. A, the pentagonal (or U-shaped) defect is made triangular and a 3- or 4-cm. upward and outward incision is made lateral to the lateral canthus. The lateral canthal ligament is divided, the skin undermined over the orbital margin, and the orbital septum freed. B, appearance of the reconstructed lower lid.

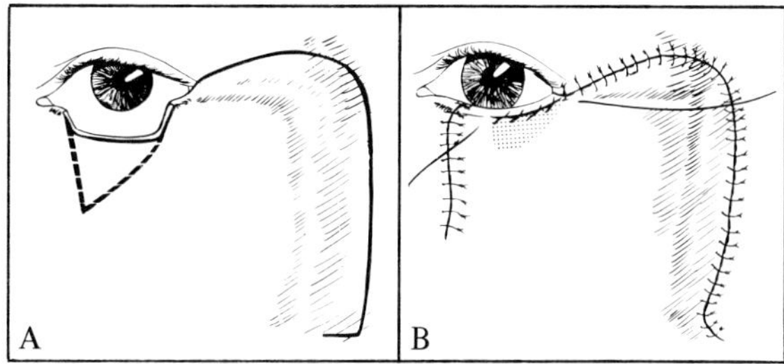

Fig. 12-6. Technique of closing defects of a half to three-quarters of the lower lid. A, the defect of the lower lid is first made triangular, and then a large rotation flap extending to just in front of the ear is moved medially; notice the back cut at the base of this flap. B, a chondromucosal graft from the nasal septum is utilized for lining and support of the reconstructed lid, and to provide a stable margin.

should be thinned and a border of mucosa maintained all around it to ensure quick vascularization; a fringe to lie across the edge of the cartilage should be sutured to the skin flap, which ensures a stable mucosa-covered margin (Fig. 12-7). The cartilage should be of sufficient dimension to rest on the orbital margin.

Total Loss of the Lower Lid

In reconstructing losses of the entire lower lid, the whole cheek must be medially rotated (Fig. 12-8). The incision from the outer canthus of the eye should extend upward and backward, then continue down in front of the ear to a point about 2 cm. below the lobule. At the lower end of the incision a back cut is necessary. When the whole area of the flap has been thoroughly undermined, the back cut will allow additional rotation and yet close easily in a vertical direction. The conjunctival defect is closed by a graft of nasal mucosa and cartilage (sutured into place with a fine Prolene stitch of the pull-out type) and then cov-

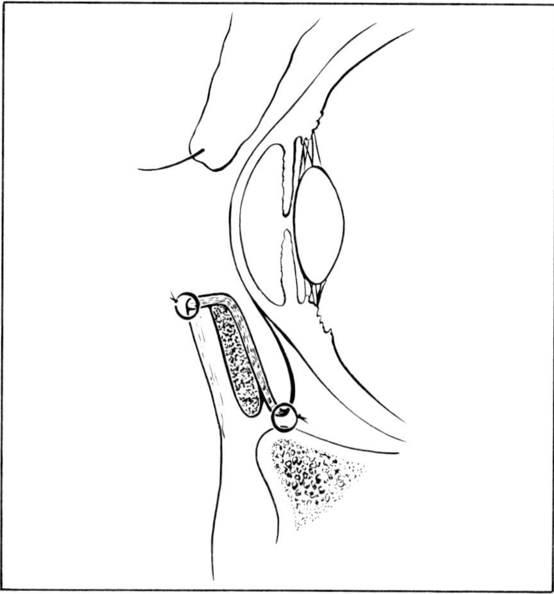

Fig. 12-7. Composite graft of nasal septal cartilage and mucosa; it provides mucus-secreting lining, stiffening skeleton, and mucosa-covered, stable lid margin all at the same time.

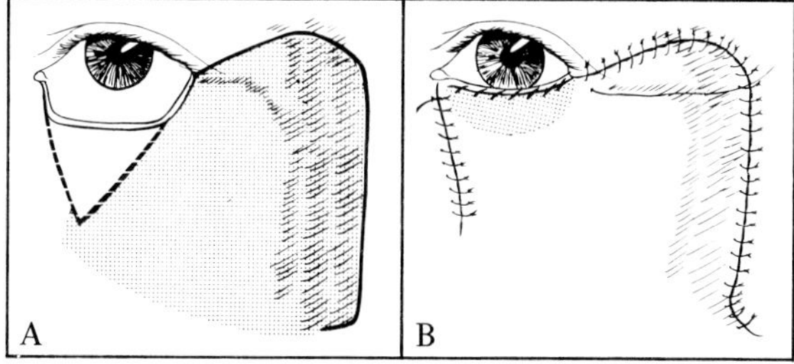

Fig. 12-8. Technique for reconstruction of the entire lower lid. A, large rotation flap of skin including the entire lateral cheek must be used to close the triangulated defect; the stippled area indicates the extent of undermining. B, chondromucosal graft from the septum is necessary for lining and support of lid.

ered by the cheek flap. In total and subtotal losses of the lid, a very deep triangle, based upward, must be removed from below the defect. The *nasal* side of the triangle should be *practically vertical,* so that the flap rises as it advances toward the nose.

Loss in a Horizontal Direction

If the loss from a lower lid is marginal and in a horizontal direction (see Fig. 12-1B), it is not necessary to discard a comparatively large amount of normal tissue from below the defect on the lid to facilitate the rotation of a large cheek flap. Instead, the loose skin of the upper lid can be used for reconstructing the lower lid.

Only the orbital skin (along with underlying orbicularis muscle to preserve the blood supply) of the upper lid (Fig. 12-9) is transferred down from above the supratarsal furrow, where it is abundant, as a bipedicled flap. The conjunctival loss is repaired by using a composite mucosa and cartilage nasal septal graft. Two weeks later the unused parts of the bipedicled flap can be returned to the upper lid. One of the chief difficulties of this operation is a tendency of the rather narrow bipedicled flap to curl on itself. To prevent this, the silk sutures that are inserted into the flap can be left long and tied over a roll of cotton wool or plastic foam (Fig. 12-8C, D).

Bipedicled flap procedures from the upper lid require two stages, but they are technically easy to perform, and the flaps are satisfactory even for wide marginal defects. Defects that are shorter (from side to side), although confined to the margin, can more simply be converted into a V and closed by using a minimal cheek rotation as in vertical loss of lid substance.

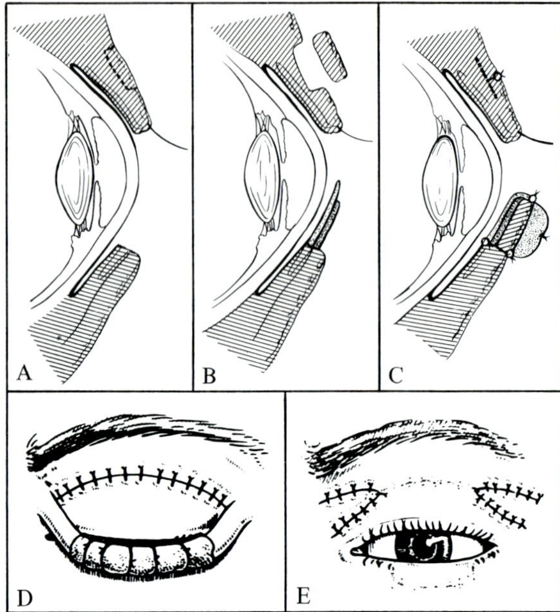

Fig. 12-9. Technique for reconstructing horizontal defects of the lower lid. A and B, composite nasal septal graft of cartilage and mucosa used for support and lining. A bipedicled skin flap is raised from the region of the orbital fold of the upper lid, and a composite nasal septal graft is sutured into the defect to provide skeleton and lining. C and D, the bipedicle flap is brought down and sutured over the composite graft. E, the bases of the flap can be divided in 2 weeks and returned to the upper lid.

Alternative Techniques for Reconstruction of the Lower Lid

For the sake of completeness, other techniques for lid reconstruction must be considered. Almost all of them can be divided into two categories: in the first category, the flap to be used in constructing the new lid supplies the skin cover and subcutaneous tissue, whereas in the second category, it supplies the skeleton and lining of the new eyelid.

Skin Cover and Subcutaneous Tissue Supplied by a Skin Flap

In addition to those already described, many types of skin flaps have been reported, but few are really suitable for eyelid reconstruction. Probably the most commonly illustrated and used flap is the Frické flap. This flap is transposed either from the forehead immediately above the eyebrow (Fig. 12-10) or from the forehead skin immediately below the hairline. When taken above the eyebrow, such flaps create a large secondary defect that tends to elevate the eyebrow, as can be seen by reference to almost any standard textbook of ophthalmic plastic surgery. To avoid this elevation requires a skin graft, and such a patch produces a very obvious defect and an additional facial deformity. A second operation is usually necessary to return the pedicle of the flap or to adjust the fold produced. Such flaps do not provide tissue thin enough for eyelids and are not as suitable as the malar flap. A nasolabial flap can be used, but like a forehead skin

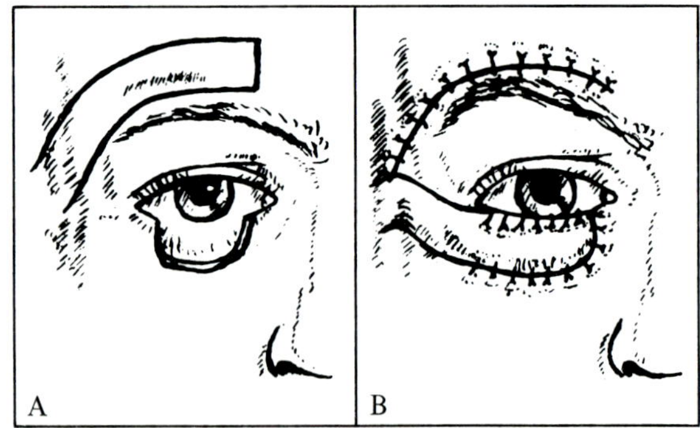

Fig. 12-10. The Frické flap from just above the eyelid to the lower eyelid is an alternative source of skin cover for reconstruction of the lower eyelid.

flap it is much too thick to give a good cosmetic result, although the defect near the nose is readily closed.

Skeleton and Lining Supplied by a Mucosa-Tarsal Flap

In the second category of flaps, skeleton and lining are transferred down from the upper lid. Of the "sharing" techniques, there are two types which utilize the tarsus and conjunctiva of the upper lid: (1) those for reconstructing a partial defect of the lower lid, and (2) those for reconstructing the entire lower lid.

The technique of repairing defects (Fig. 12-11) involves bringing down a flap of conjunctiva from the upper fornix, with several millimeters of tarsal plate attached to the free end, but leaving the margin of the upper lid carrying the lashes still intact. This flap is set into the conjunctival edge of the lower lid defect. Its raw surface is covered, either by a free graft of skin, by a bipedicled skin flap from the upper lid, or by advancing the cheek skin upward. The lids are left closed for 3 months, and then the conjunctival flap is divided.

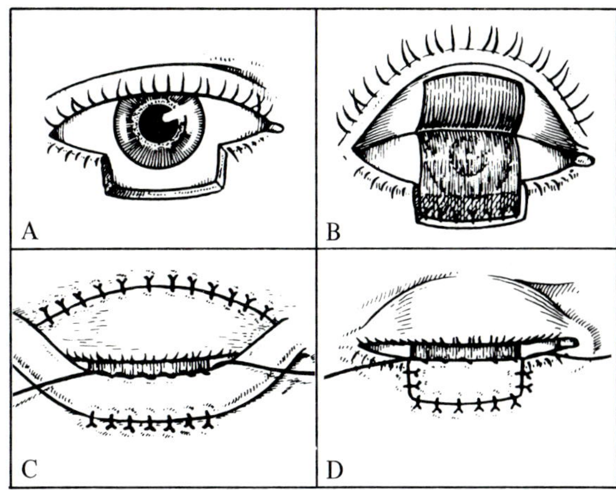

Fig. 12-11. Landolt-Hughes technique. A, horizontal defect of lower eyelid. B, conjunctival flap from upper lid with an attached portion, several millimeters wide, of tarsal plate. C, bipedicled skin flap from upper lid provides skin coverage. D, alternative cover by full-thickness skin graft.

In the Dupuys-Dutemps-Hughes technique of total reconstruction of the lower lid (Fig. 12-12), the upper lid is split into its two laminae through the gray line. The inner lamina, consisting of conjunctiva, tarsus, and levator aponeurosis, is brought downward and sutured to the remnants of the conjunctiva in the lower sulcus. The raw surface of the conjunctiva is covered either by a vertical cheek flap or by a skin graft. The lids are left united for 3 to 4 months; before they are divided a line of lashes is grafted just below the upper lash line.

Both of these above "sharing" operations, but particularly the second, suffer the grave disadvantage that, if the defect in the lower lid is at all deep, there may not be quite enough lining material to supply the two lids adequately. The upper lid may become shortened and may not close fully. There also is a tendency for the lining, when it is short, to pull the lid margins inward and cause entropion. Trichiasis may develop as a result of entropion and scar contracture around the lash follicles. Such deformities may not be found in every case, but the risk of incurring them is always present. Once a complication develops, it is extremely difficult to correct, and each succeeding operation only adds to the difficulty. In addition, and even with the best results, there is no stable margin formed, and in the course of time – even though it may be several years later – the lid will either sink down due to lack of marginal support or, worse, will turn in onto the corner, or turn out to leave much of the conjunctiva exposed. These risks make the "sharing" operations too hazardous to be

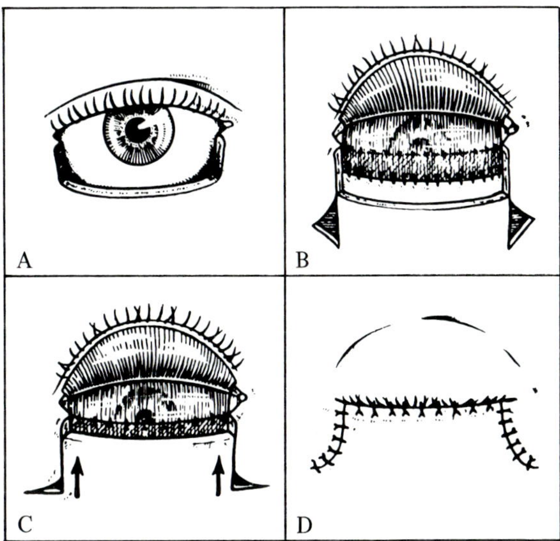

Fig. 12-12. Dupuys-Dutemps-Hughes technique for total reconstruction of lower lid. A, complete loss of lower lid. B, upper lid is split along gray line so that conjunctiva and tarsus can be sutured to conjunctiva of lower lid. C, advancement skin flap used to provide skin coverage. D, the lids are divided in 4 to 6 months.

used, except perhaps in the shallower type of defect. In my opinion it is never justifiable to jeopardize the normal upper lid in any way in order to correct the lower lid, if it is possible to find other satisfactory methods that do not involve the valuable mobile tarsal tissues of the upper lid.

RECONSTRUCTION OF THE UPPER LID

Reconstruction of the upper lid presents a totally different problem from that of the lower lid. Not only is it necessary to fashion a structure that resembles an upper lid while at rest, but it must be capable of moving up and down so that it will rise above the pupil to allow full vision and, at the same time, blink reflexly to assist in lubrication of the cornea. In addition, there must be a stable margin which, while protecting the cornea from rubbing by squamous epithelium, will leave the skin anchored to the deeper tissues in such a way that it cannot slowly roll down and rub on the cornea after the tissues stretch with the advance of the years. It is of such importance that the upper lid be reconstructed as perfectly as possible that there should be no hesitation about using the less valuable lower lid to make up for any deficiency in the upper. The first basic principle here is to *utilize the lower lid to reconstruct the upper and to rebuild the defective lower from other sources.*

Loss in a Vertical Direction

In reconstruction of the upper lid, a wedge of the whole thickness of the lower lid is turned up as a flap on a vascular hinge and fitted into the defect in the upper lid; the lost sector of the lower is repaired by rotating a flap from the cheek as described for lower lid defects.

The problem is considerably simplified when the surgeon applies the second basic principle of lid reconstruction – *it is only necessary to reconstruct a lid three-quarters the length of the original.* As with the lower lid, combining these two simple rules permits the development of a simple scheme, again based on multiples of a quarter, whereby any defect of the upper lid, of whatever degree, may be reconstructed.

As it is only necessary to find enough material to construct a lid three-quarters of the length of the original, the size of the defect may be correspondingly reduced by a quarter of the lid length, and thus the width of the flap of lower lid which must be rotated up need only be *the width of the defect less a quarter of the original lid length.* The chief difficulty is in determining exactly where the hinge of the flap should be placed and in what position the flap should lie, so that it will rotate upward and come to rest accurately in the defect without tension or distortion of the pedicle.

Loss of Up to a Quarter of the Upper Lid

Defects in the upper lid which do not exceed a quarter of its total length may be closed directly in three layers as described for defects of the lower lid. If necessary, the upper portion of the lateral orbital ligament can be divided to relax the lid. In elderly people, losses of up to a third of the lid may be closed in this fashion, but care must be taken to avoid placing too much tension on the reconstructed lid, or a mechanical ptosis may result due to undue tension.

Loss of Between One-Quarter and One-Half of the Upper Lid

If the loss of the upper lid is greater than one-quarter of its total length, it cannot be closed directly without causing a degree of mechanical ptosis, and a wedge-shaped flap of the lower lid tissue must be rotated up to help fill the defect. In theory, the width of the wedge need be equal only to the width of the defect minus the length of a quarter of the original upper lid. However, a flap only a few millimeters wide is technically difficult to rotate and suture into place. The flap should therefore be a *quarter of the lid length* in width, or a few millimeters less if the width of the defect is little more than a quarter. The hinge of the lower lid flap must incorporate the marginal vessels and should lie at the *midpoint* of the defect (Fig. 12-13), with the *flap outlined on either side of the hinge.* The flap, consisting of all layers of the lower lid, is separated from it, except for a hinge 5 mm. wide, which preserves the marginal arcade of vessels. After the defect in the lower lid has been closed directly in three layers, the flap is rotated through 180 degrees and sutured into the defect in the upper lid. A continuous removable suture of 6-0 Prolene closes the conjunctiva, 5-0 catgut sutures approximate the orbicularis, and 6-0 silk sutures close the skin. Two weeks later the hinge is divided and the margins of the lid are carefully reconstructed.

Loss of More than a Half of the Upper Lid

I have recently developed a more up-to-date technique for these larger upper lid reconstructions that is much simpler to carry out and that avoids the risk inherent in using a small vascular pedicle. However, this technique tends, because the upper lid reconstruction takes place in two stages, to produce more transient edema of the upper lid over a longer period. No formula is needed for any particular size of reconstruction and the technique may be summarized as follows:

PARTIAL LOSS OF UPPER LID. Where a part of the upper lid still remains, the pedicle of that part of the lower lid to be brought up should lie *on the same side* as the upper lid remnant. Since the lower lid

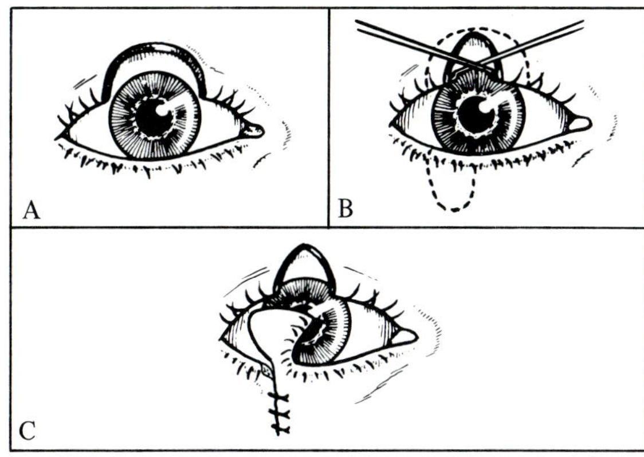

Fig. 12-13. Technique of closing defects of one-quarter to one-half of upper lid. A, vertical defect of one-half of upper lid. B, Abbe-type full-thickness flap of lower eyelid is outlined, based medially on a pedicle 5mm. wide containing marginal arcade of vessels; the width of this flap need only be a quarter of the lid length. C, flap is rotated into upper lid defect. The base of the flap is divided 2 weeks later.

punctum should not be encroached on in any lid reconstruction, the lower lid flap is designed, of adequate size, anywhere on the lateral three-quarters of the lower lid, with its base beneath any existing upper lid remnant, and the pedicle should not be narrower than 7 to 8 mm. (Figs. 12-14 and 12-15). The lower lid defect is closed at the second stage 2 weeks later using the techniques already described.

If the upper lid defect lies in the center of the lid one could bring up a flap based either medially or laterally, but one must always avoid the punctum.

TOTAL LOSS OF UPPER LID. As with a central loss of the upper lid, the pedicle can be placed either medially or laterally, but the lower lid punctum should be preserved (Fig. 12-16). It is probably best to make the base on the lateral side, however, as the primary insertion of the flap will heal with minimal scar tissue and will permit earlier lymphatic drainage from the reconstructed lid. A much larger composite graft will be required to line the new part of the lower lid, or to give it permanent support.

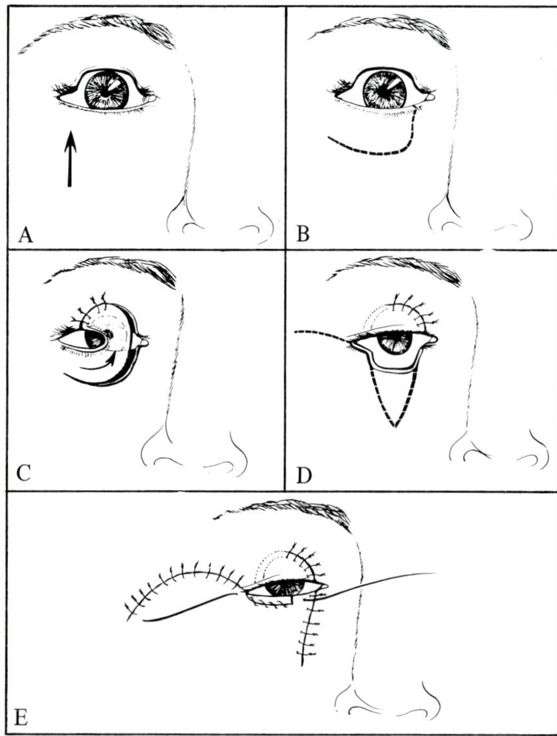

Fig. 12-14. Loss of more than a half of upper lid. A, the largest remnant of upper lid is on the lateral side, therefore the base of the lower lid flap should be on the lateral side. B, lower lid flap outlines: note the avoidance of encroachment on function. C, inset of free end of flap. The levator muscle should be attached to the flap connective tissue as far as possible. The skin is sutured to conjunctiva to close all remaining raw surfaces temporarily. D, the base of the flap is detached and inset in the upper lid. The remaining levator muscle is sutured to the flap tissue, and the lower lid defect is triangulated. E, the lower lid defect is reconstructed by cheek rotation flap, lined by composite graft of nasal septal cartilage and mucosa to provide (1) lining, (2) tarsal stiffening, (3) stable, mucosa-covered lid margin. (Figures 12-14 through 12-16 are taken from J. C. Mustardé, Repair and Reconstruction in the Orbital Region *[2nd ed.]. Edinburgh and London: Churchill-Livingstone (in press), with the permission of the publisher.)*

Loss in a Horizontal Direction

Tumors in the upper lid are much rarer than in the lower, and purely marginal tumors extending horizontally are seldom seen, even in the lower lid. As was the case with horizontal loss of lid substance in the lower lid, defects of the upper lid extending widely from side to side, with only a few millimeters of vertical extension, can be repaired with a bipedicled flap of skin from the lower lid, which must of course be lined either with a flap of tarsus and conjunctiva from the stump of the upper lid or with a free graft of nasal mucosa. The defect in the lower lid must be covered with a full-thickness skin graft and cannot be closed directly for fear of causing ectropion.

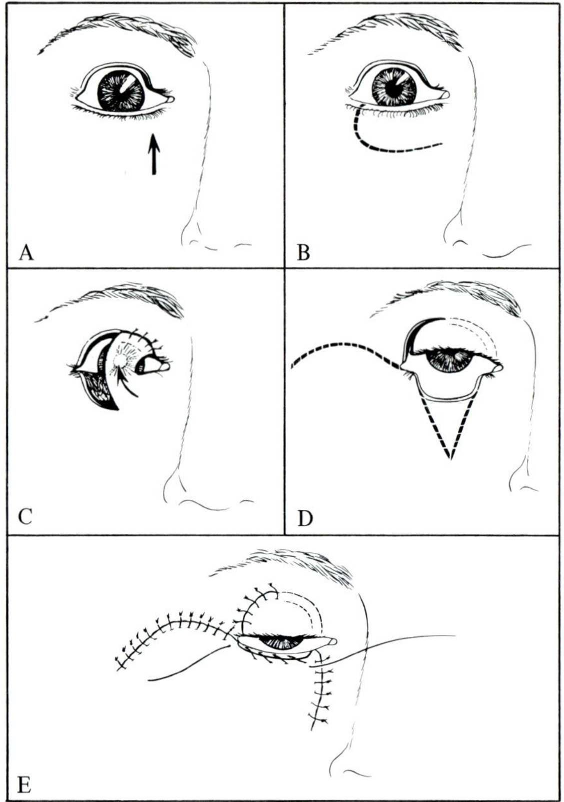

Fig. 12-15. Loss of more than a half of the upper lid. The largest remnant of the upper lid lies on the medial side, hence base of flap must lie on this side. (See Fig. 12-14 for other details.)

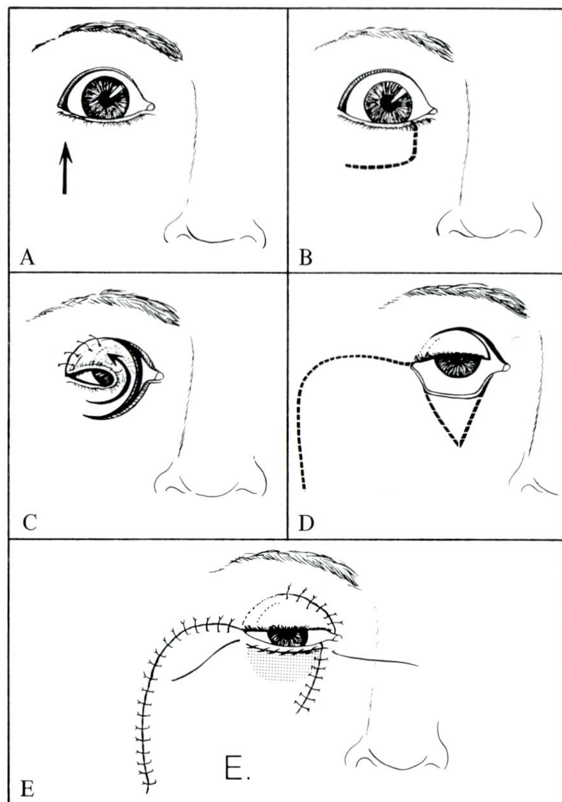

Fig. 12-16. Total loss of the upper lid. *The lower lid flap could be based either on the medial or on the lateral side, but preferably on lateral side, so that primary wound closure can be carried out at lateral side of upper lid reconstruction – thus facilitating lymph drainage and reducing period of edema. (See Fig. 12-14 for further details.)*

An alternative is to bring down a bipedicle flap from the upper part of the upper lid (as shown in Fig. 12-9), and insert a full-thickness skin graft into the higher defect instead of closing it direct. Again, the lining should be a free graft, or a sliding flap of tarsus and conjunctiva from the upper lid – if enough is present.

Such a reconstructed lid margin will have no lashes, and it is wiser to use artificial lashes rather than to resort to inserting a narrow graft of hair-bearing temporal skin, which carries the considerable risk of hair turning in and rubbing on the cornea. These hair-bearing grafts also do not usually look normal.

LOSS OF THE MEDIAL OR LATERAL CANTHUS

Loss of the Lateral Canthus

When the area of the lateral canthus and a part of both lids have been lost, it may be possible to reattach the lids to the canthal ligament if only a small part of each lid is absent. The rest of the defect lateral to this can be covered with a full-thickness skin graft. If, however, the loss from the lids is greater, the defects may be repaired with a flap of skin from other areas – for example, a rotation flap from the cheek or from that portion of the forehead above the eyebrow. It should be lined either with conjunctiva from the lateral fornix or with a free graft of nasal mucosa. No cartilage is required unless the actual reconstruction is greater than 6 to 7 mm., because the actual amount of lid margin which has to be reconstructed (remembering that the first quarter can be ignored) usually is not extensive.

Loss of the Medial Canthus

Minor defects may be dealt with in the same manner

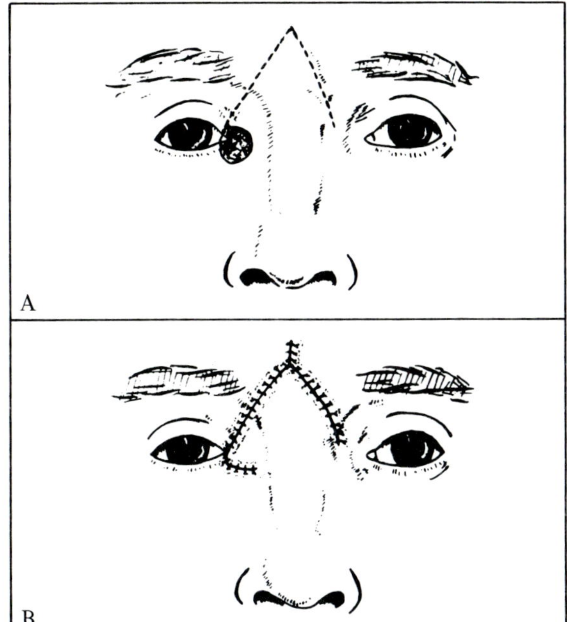

Fig. 12-17. Reconstruction of medial canthus. A rhomboid-shaped glabellar flap can be rotated into the medial canthal defect.

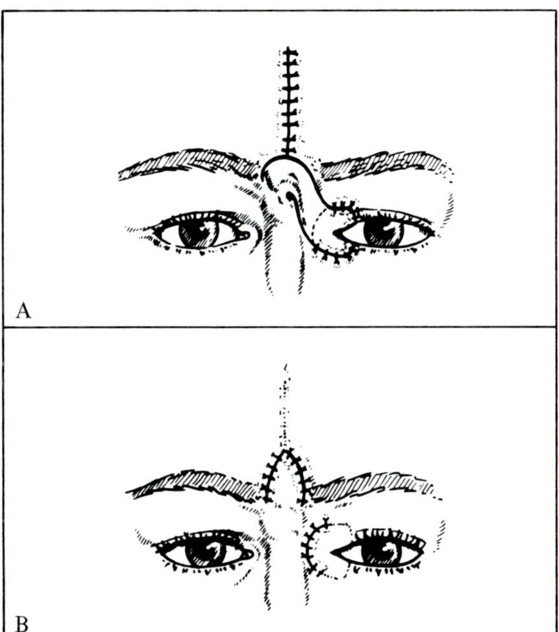

Fig. 12-18. Reconstruction of medial canthus and adjacent eyelids. These larger defects can be closed by a midline forehead flap lined by conjunctiva or nasal mucosa.

as defects involving the lateral canthus. If additional tissue is required for a reconstruction at the medial canthus, a rhomboid-shaped glabellar flap can be rotated downward (Fig. 12-17). The defect above is closed with the use of the V to Y principle. It is best to line the flap with nasal septal mucosa and cartilage when greater amounts of covering tissue such as a midline forehead flap are used in larger losses (Fig. 12-18). A drain for tears may occasionally be reconstructed at the primary operation if there is abundant conjunctiva to spare in the lower fornix. In such cases a flat strip of conjunctiva, 7 or 8 mm. wide, is tunneled medially into the lacrimal sac, or into the cavity of the nose, and allowed to tube itself.

One of the problems of medial canthus reconstruction is to get a good fixation of the canthus to the underlying bone at the site of the medial canthal tendon. A nonabsorbable suture of stainless-steel wire or Prolene may be used, but repeated canthopexy may be required in order to obtain the requisite posterior placing of the new canthus.

LOSS OF BOTH LIDS

Total Loss of Both Lids

Loss of both lids without loss of the underlying eye must be extremely rare, and I have not personally had experience with such a case. In such a circumstance it would be difficult to make lids which would be long enough to function and still protect the cornea. Unless the sight of the other eye is defective, the exposed eye should be protected by covering the cornea with the remnants of the conjunctiva (Fig. 12-19). An opening for drainage should be preserved at the medial canthus. The outer raw surface of the conjunctiva could be covered with a long midline forehead flap, direct closure of the forehead defect being performed. The pedicle of the flap could be returned 2 weeks later. Unless it is imperative to open the lids, the eye should be left permanently covered for protection. In an adult this will not result in amblyopia, and the eye will be "banked" for possible future use. If the lids must be opened, the upper half of the flap could be replaced by a full-thickness skin graft from the postauricular area to provide a thinner lid. When the lids are divided after this has been done, some slight lifting action should be present in this thinner lid. It would be both unnecessary and unsafe to attempt to graft eyelashes onto such an upper lid.

Loss of the Lower Lid and Part of the Upper Lid

Where the lower lid and a part of the upper are lost (Fig. 12-20), the lower lid could be reconstructed by

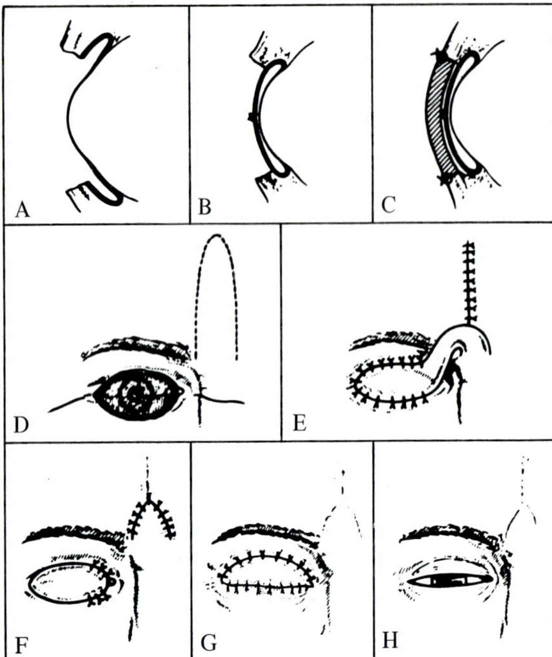

Fig. 12-19. Technique for reconstructing both eyelids. A and B, the remnants of conjunctiva can be used to protect the cornea. C, D, and E, skin coverage is supplied by a midline forehead skin flap. F, the base of the flap is divided 2 weeks later. G, a little more than the upper part of the flap can be replaced in 3 months by a skin graft. H, the lids can then be opened after the skin graft has taken.

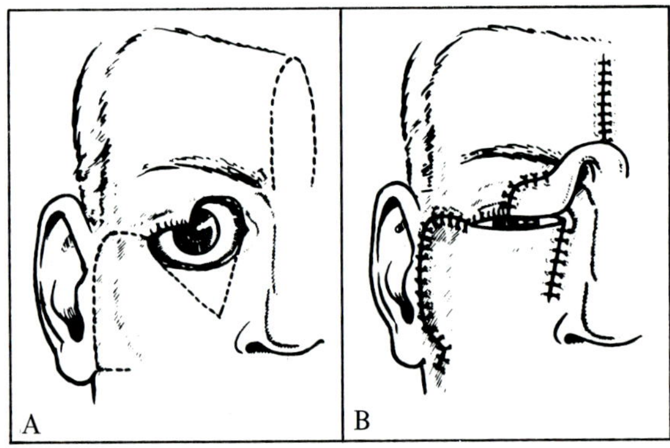

Fig. 12-20. Technique for reconstructing the entire lower lid and part of the upper lid. A and B, the lower lid is reconstructed with a cheek flap lined with nasal mucosa and cartilage. The upper lid is reconstructed with a forehead flap lined by mucosa.

rotating a cheek flap in the usual way, or by a nasolabial flap if the cheek is not suitable, and lining it with nasal mucosa and cartilage, while the defect of the upper lid could be closed using a midline forehead flap lined with mucosa for defects for the medial half, or a Frické flap for defects of the lateral half (see Fig. 12-10). This is one of the few occasions in which a Frické flap is justifiable, as appearance is a secondary consideration in such cases.

Loss of the Upper Lid and Part of the Lower Lid

Loss of the whole of the upper lid and a half of the lower should be dealt with by rotating the remnants of the lower lid upward to make at least part of a satisfactory upper lid; the resultant defective lower lid and the remaining gap in the upper lid are then reconstructed, as already described, using a cheek flap and a flap from the forehead (Fig. 12-21). If the lower lid remnant is on the *lateral* side, the technique is comparatively straightforward, but if it is on the *medial* side, it will require that the flap be doubled over on itself for 2 weeks to obtain a new attachment before being completely set in place, and the rest of the defects are closed (Fig. 12-22). A Buller's glass shield over the whole orbital region, sealed with a strip of tulle gras, may be necessary to protect the cornea during the first stage of this technique.

RECONSTRUCTION OF THE EYELIDS WHERE THE EYE IS ABSENT

When the eye is no longer present, the problem of reconstruction of the eyelids is far simpler than those discussed so far. This is largely because it is no longer necessary to line the new lids with a mucous membrane, but also partly because full movement of the upper lid, though desirable cosmetically, is no longer so essential. Therefore no great effort need be made to obtain such movement or to produce a lid that is supple enough to be capable of motion.

Total Loss of Both Lids

Where both lids are grossly damaged or lost, and especially if the socket is at all contracted, the most practical solution is undoubtedly to provide a good prosthesis on which lids and lashes as well as an eye are incorporated, and attach it to a spectacle frame. This gives a much more natural appearance than any surgical reconstruction of the two lids and the use of an artificial eye.

When this is not possible or acceptable for some reason, or where only one lid is destroyed, a midline forehead flap for reconstruction of the upper lid, or a cheek rotation flap for reconstruction of the lower, can be used, lined in either case with a moderately thick skin graft (one is not here concerned with a

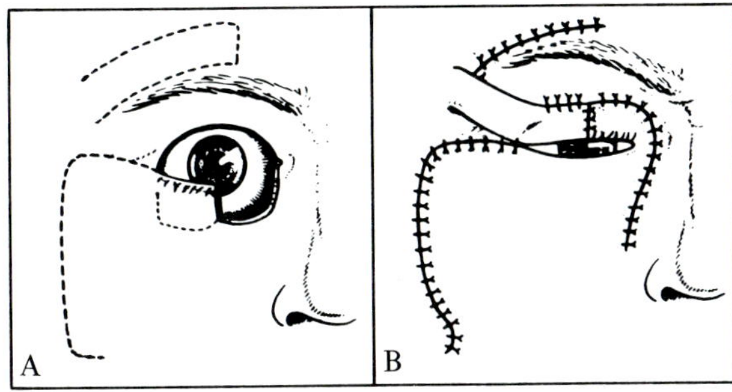

Fig. 12-21. Technique for reconstructing the entire upper lid and part of the lower lid when the remnant is on the lateral side. A and B, the remnant of the lower lid is rotated into upper lid defect, with the lateral cheek flap lined by nasal septal mucosa and cartilage. Remainder of the upper lid is reconstructed by a Frické flap lined with mucosa.

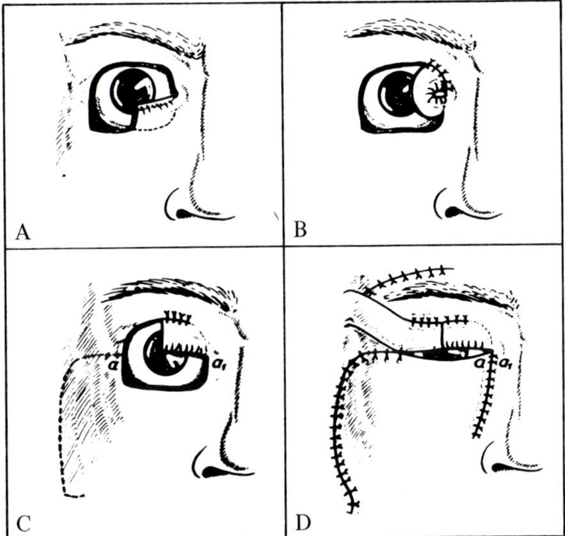

Fig. 12-22. Technique for reconstructing the entire upper lid and part of the lower lid when the remnant is on the medial side. See text for explanation.

stable margin, and a degree of entropion or ectropion is not unacceptable). In some cases the forehead flap will provide skin for both lids.

Partial Loss of Both Lids

Where some of the peritarsal part of a lid remains, the procedure is simplified. The lining of the new lid may be provided by turning over the skin of the remnant of the lid on a base situated where the skin and mu-

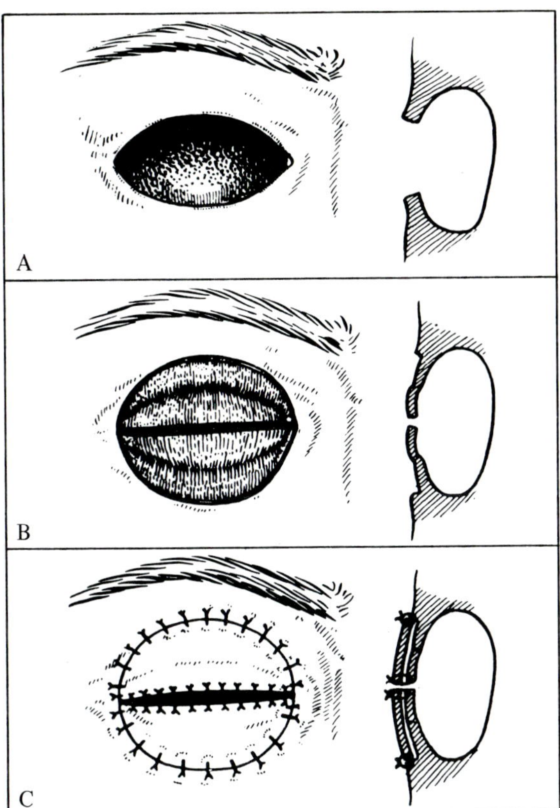

Fig. 12-23. Technique for reconstructing partial horizontal loss of both lids when the eye is absent (A). B, lining is provided by turning in flaps from the lid remnants. C, skin coverage is provided by full-thickness skin grafts.

cosa are fused, a full-thickness skin graft being used for covering (Fig. 12-23).

Smaller defects of either lid may be closed by using the Büdinger-Müller technique (Fig. 12-24), in which a composite skin and cartilage graft is taken from the anterior part of the helix of the ear. Skin is preserved on both sides of the cartilage, and the graft is inserted into the defect after "halving" the area around the latter to give a better blood supply to the graft. Such a three-layer thick composite graft is very likely to be partially or totally lost, however, and this risk must be balanced against the very natural curved lid margin which it produces if it is successful.

A much simpler technique (Fig. 12-25) is to turn in skin flaps from the sides of the defect, or from above, in order to fashion a lining and to cover the whole raw area with a full-thickness skin graft taken from the posterior part of the concha of the ear and

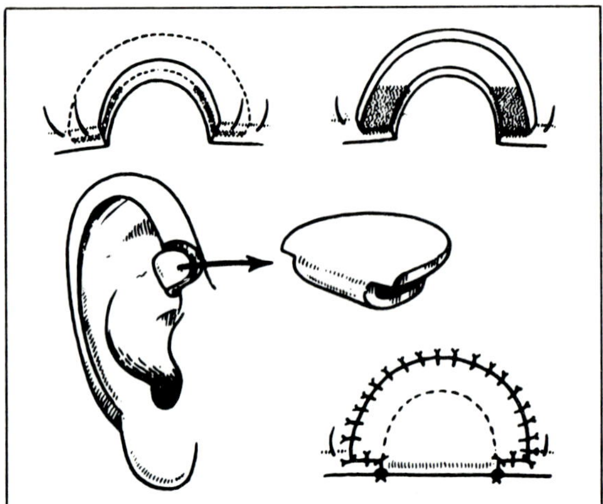

Fig. 12-24. Büdinger-Müller technique for reconstruction of a small vertical loss of the upper eyelid when the eye is absent. A skin-cartilage-skin graft is taken from the helix. A 2- to 4-mm.-wide strip of eyelid skin is removed around the defect and also from the undersurface of the composite graft so as to provide a wider area of blood supply. No point on the composite graft should be more than 1 cm. from the margin of the defect in order to have a reasonable chance for the graft to survive.

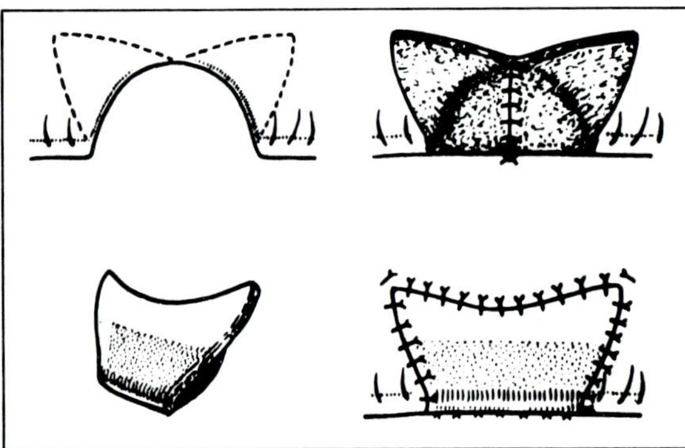

Fig. 12-25. Modified Büdinger-Müller technique, utilizing flaps of lid skin turned in for lining and a composite ear graft for replacing the tarsus and outer cover.

including, if necessary, a strip of the underlying cartilage for stiffening.

RECONSTRUCTION OF THE EYEBROWS

Moderate Loss of the Eyebrow

When all or part of the eyebrow is missing, it can be replaced by using strips of hair-bearing skin from the *opposite eyebrow* or, better still (so as to avoid damaging a normal eyebrow), from the *temporal hair area* or the *occipital region.* Two narrow strips, three follicles wide, should be removed in a direction which will ensure that all the hairs are running along the axis of the graft (Fig. 12-26A). Care must be taken to avoid damaging any follicles; the excess fat may be carefully snipped off to leave the follicles exposed. The site into which the grafts will be inserted is prepared by making two parallel incisions, with an intervening strip of epithelium 2 to 3 mm. in width being left so that both sides of the hair-bearing graft will be exposed to a reasonable blood supply (Fig. 12-26B). The grafts are held in place by sutures passing very superficially through all the structures. A light pressure dressing should be applied for a week and the sutures removed at the end of this time. At first many of the hairs may drop out, but new ones will appear, and after 4 months the intervening bare strip between the grafts may be excised and an additional hair-bearing graft inserted.

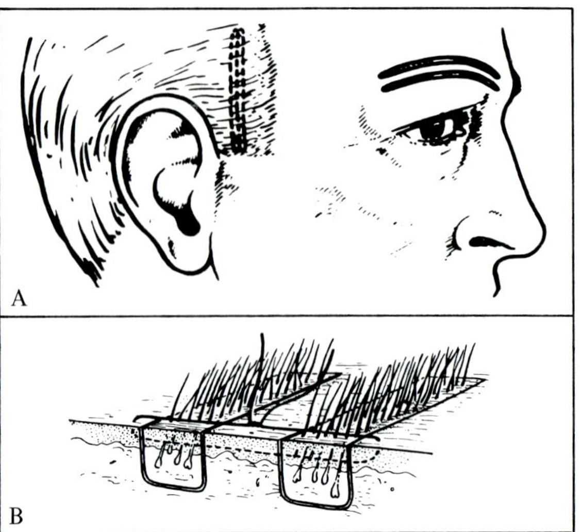

Fig. 12-26. Eyebrow reconstruction by means of hair-bearing scalp grafts that are three follicles wide (A). Two of these hair-bearing grafts can be inserted into two parallel incisions with a 2- or 3-mm. strip of skin between them (B).

Severe Loss of the Eyebrow

When there has been severe deep burning of the eyebrow region, as in unconscious patients, or loss following excision of a neoplasm, it is not sufficient merely to add hair to the area: bulk must also be added to restore the prominence of the eyebrow. This cannot be done adequately by using small grafts of hair-bear-

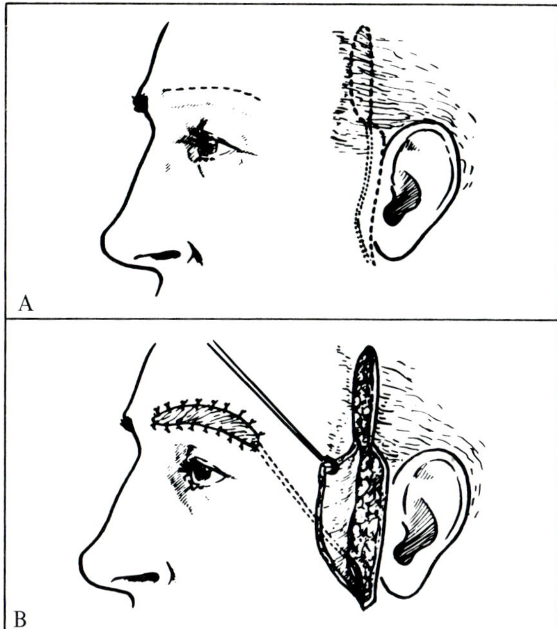

Fig. 12-27. Eyebrow reconstruction with an island flap of temporal scalp based on the superficial temporal artery.

ing skin, especially considering the scarred area into which they may have to be placed. If wider strips are used there is a tendency for areas of follicles and skin to be lost, with a resultant unpleasant, irregular appearance. To overcome this difficulty, a wide strip of hair-bearing skin and fat from the temporal area is raised along with its vascular pedicle, which can easily be visualized once the preauricular skin is reflected (Fig. 12-27). This method is called the "island flap" technique; the hair-bearing flap, after it is raised, is carried through a tunnel in the malar region and set in place in the eyebrow, remaining permanently attached to its artery and vein.

Correction of Ptosis of the Eyelid*

Elevation of the upper lid is carried out by two muscles, the levator muscle and the sympathetically innervated Müller's muscle. In congenital ptosis, whether unilateral or bilateral, the exact cause of the deformity is not clear but failure of development of the affected levator muscle or some obscure myopathic condition has been suggested.

CORRECTION OF PTOSIS OF THE EYELID

Correction of a drooping eyelid has conventionally been carried out by resecting a sufficient amount of the levator complex to raise the lid to a normal height, and this can be done through either an anterior or a posterior route.

Anterior Route (Everbusch)

The levator muscle complex is exposed through the lid skin and orbicularis muscle. Shortening, and eventual closure of the wounds, is effected as shown in Figure 12-28.

Posterior Route (Blascowicz)

The conjunctiva is first dissected away from the overlying Müller's muscle, and the latter, along with the levator aponeurosis anterior to it, is picked up so as to permit resection of the levator muscle itself at a high enough level to lift the lid to the desired position (Fig. 12-29). Double-armed 5-0 silk sutures are passed through the conjunctiva, the cut edge of the levator muscle, and the top edge of the tarsal plate; they are then brought out through the orbicularis muscle and skin and are tied over a small piece of rubber tubing. The sutures are removed in 12 days.

Problems in Ptosis Correction

One of the problems in ptosis correction is that the comparatively thick tarsal plate may act as an antagonist to the defectively acting levator muscle, so that one may have to remove up to 20 mm. of levator complex in order to produce lifting of the lid to a more normal level. The shortened muscle is unable to relax adequately, and in most instances of severe ptosis there is every probability that the lids will remain open (lagophthalmos) to some degree during sleep. If this does occur, a very close watch must be

*Acknowledgment: Apart from the text of the first three paragraphs, the whole of the material for this section is taken from the chapter "The Orbital Region" by J. C. Mustardé in the second edition of *Plastic Surgery in Infancy and Childhood* (edited by J. C. Mustardé), Churchill-Livingstone (1978), with the permission of the publishers.

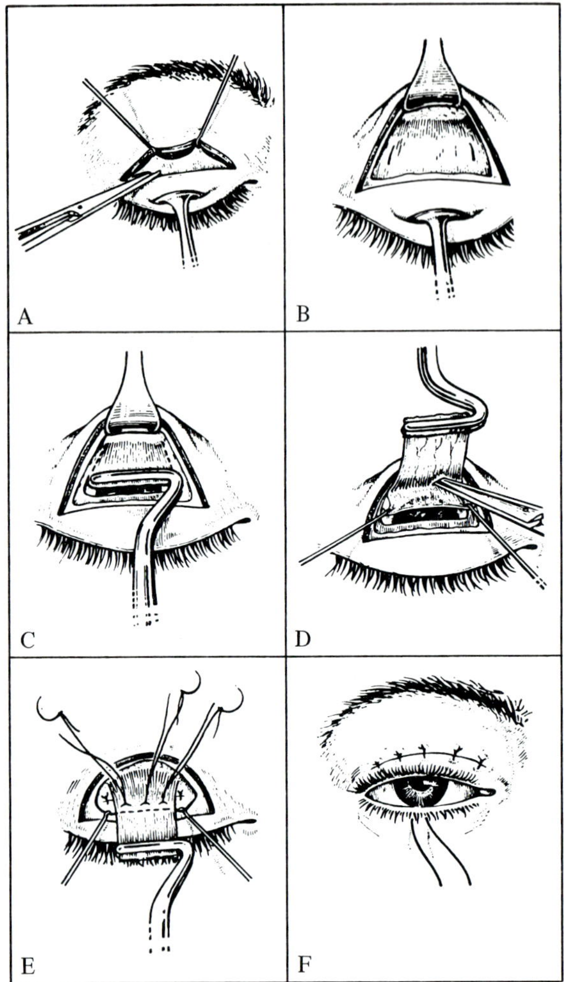

Fig. 12-28. Levator resection for correction of ptosis: anterior approach (Everbusch). A, an incision is made through the skin and orbicularis in the position of desired skin fold. B, the orbital septum is exposed, and incisions are carried through into the upper fornix immediately above the tarsal plate. C, a ptosis clamp is passed through the incisions and the structure is divided distal to the clamp and along the vertical dotted line. D, the orbital septum and conjunctiva are dissected off from the levator flap. E, the conjunctival wound is closed, and the levator flap is brought forward and sutured to the upper edge of the tarsus. The excess levator is excised. F, the skin and orbicularis are closed, and the lower lid is lifted up by a single suture.

kept on the condition of the cornea, and it may be necessary to instill "artificial tears" of methylcellulose or other substances at night.

Apart from the antagonistic bow-string effect of the tarsal plate, the conventional resection of the levator complex necessitates discarding Müller's muscle (which, being sympathetically innervated, contracts independently of the function of the levator muscle). In severe cases of ptosis, Müller's muscle may be the only muscle that is functioning at all; because of this, I have developed an operation that not only preserves the action of Müller's muscle, but also removes about four-fifths of the tarsal plate. Because a wedge of skin and orbicularis muscle is also resected from the drooping lid, the effect is the same as if one had resected a full-thickness wedge of lid tissue 5 to 6 mm. in width, but the resection is carried out at different levels in order to preserve the blood supply to the lid margin.

Split-Level Lid Resection

Where there is good levator function (i.e., 7 mm. or more of movement of the lid attributable to the action of the levator muscle) the operation is carried out as follows:

TECHNIQUE. A wedge of skin about 6 mm. wide is marked out on the skin of the upper lid; the lower line is in the position of the proposed supratarsal sulcus (the lateral end of the incision should not run closer to the lid margin than 7 mm. in order to avoid later edema of the marginal lid skin). The lid is stretched by a temporary suture, and the skin and underlying orbicularis muscle are excised down to the orbital septum (Figs. 12-30A and 31A). The skin and orbicularis muscle inferior to the resection is dissected away from the tarsal plate using thin-bladed, blunt-pointed curved scissors. The dissection is carried almost to the lashes (Figs. 12-30B and 31B).

The lid is then everted over a lid spatula and an incision is made through the conjunctiva and tarsal about 3 mm. from the lid margin. The incision should extend across the entire width of the lid. Following this, the tarsal plate is removed by cutting across immediately above its upper border, thus sectioning it from Müller's muscle, and the levator aponeurosis closely applied to the latter (Fig. 12-31C). Three or four 6-0 catgut sutures are inserted to approximate these structures (along with the attached conjunctiva) to the cut edge of the remaining slip of tarsal plate, burying the knots within the lid tissues. Finally (Fig. 12-31D) the skin wound is closed with five or six 6-0 catgut sutures that pick up the deeper aponeurosis and so create a supratarsal sulcus when the levator contracts as the lid is lifted.

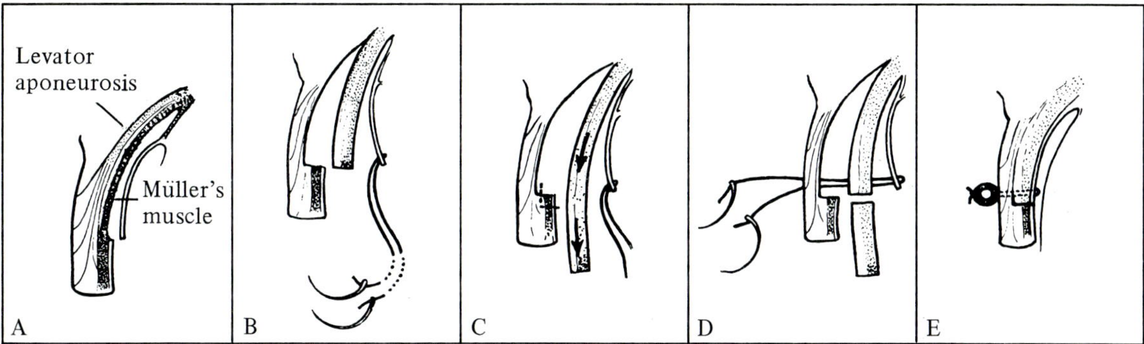

Fig. 12-29. Levator resection for correction of ptosis: posterior approach (Blascovicz). Sagittal section of the upper lid shows the relationship of the double-armed sutures to levator aponeurosis and underlying Müller's muscle. See text for explanation.

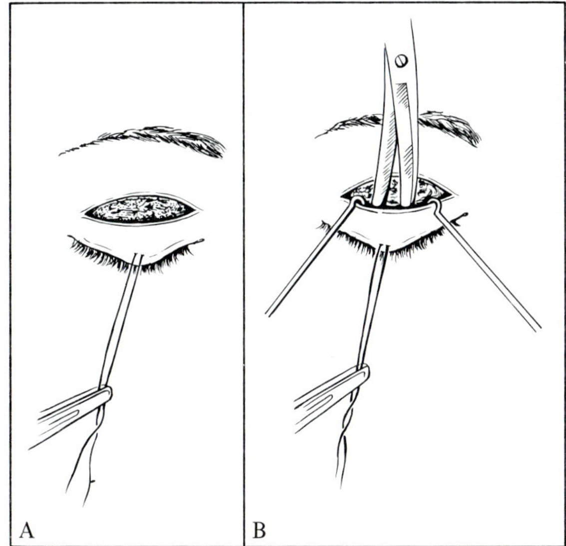

Fig. 12-30. Split-level lid resection. A, the area of skin and orbicularis muscle resected is shown. B, the skin and orbicularis muscle are dissected from the anterior surface of the tarsal plate.

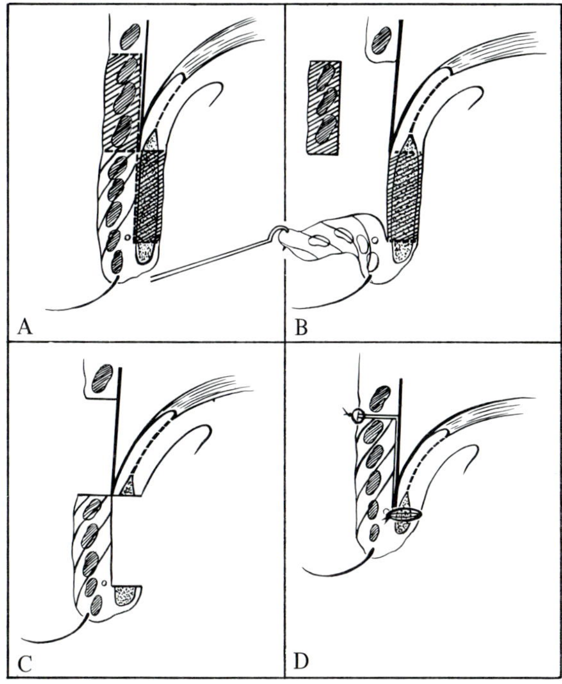

Fig. 12-31. Split-level lid resection. See text for explanation.

Split-Level Lid Resection with Levator Hitch

In patients in whom there is less than 7 mm. of detectable levator function but in whom there is at least 4 mm. of movement present, it is insufficient to carry out a simple split-level lid resection; the levator complex itself must be shortened – but without throwing away any functional tissue. This can be achieved not only by carrying out a split-level lid resection, but in addition turning up the lower half of Müller's muscle and the overlying levator aponeurosis so that it is hitched to itself and can still function despite the shortening.

If there is less than 4 mm. of levator function, but a slight lifting action of the lid margin can definitely be detected, or if there is even only a deepening of the supratarsal fold when the patient looks up, then the whole of Müller's muscle and the levator aponeurosis should be hitched up (i.e., they are turned up for almost 10 mm. from the free edge).

TECHNIQUE. The operation is commenced exactly as for split-level lid resection (Fig. 12-32A, B), but once the anterior surface of the tarsal plate has been exposed, the orbital septum should be incised just above the line where it fuses with the aponeurosis (Fig. 12-32C). This will permit access to the upper part of the aponeurosis and levator muscle and allow them to be drawn downward.

Once the lid has been everted, the conjunctiva is ballooned off from the underlying Müller's muscle and is reflected for about 7 to 8 mm. (Fig. 12-32C). This reflected conjunctiva is excised, and the tarsoconjunctival bloc is resected (Fig. 12-32D).

Once the levator complex (aponeurosis and Müller's muscle) is freed from the tarsal plate, three 6-0 chromic catgut sutures are inserted and knotted on the posterior surface at the level at which it has been decided to turn up the levator complex (Fig. 12-32E). Using these three sutures as holding points, the free edge is then turned up and fixed with three 6-0 chromic catgut sutures to the anterior surface of the levator muscle (Fig. 12-32E). The sutures at the bottom of the loop that has been formed are then passed through the upper free edge of the conjunctiva and the remainder of the tarsal plate (along with its conjunctival cover), burying the knot within the tissue of the lid (Fig. 12-32F). Skin closure is carried out in the same way as is used for split-level lid resection, picking up the levator complex lying immediately deep to the skin wound.

Frontalis Sling Operations

In patients in whom there is no detectable function of the levator, or in those with severe ptosis in whom surgery has failed to make a significant improvement, lifting of the lid may be achieved by attaching the lid

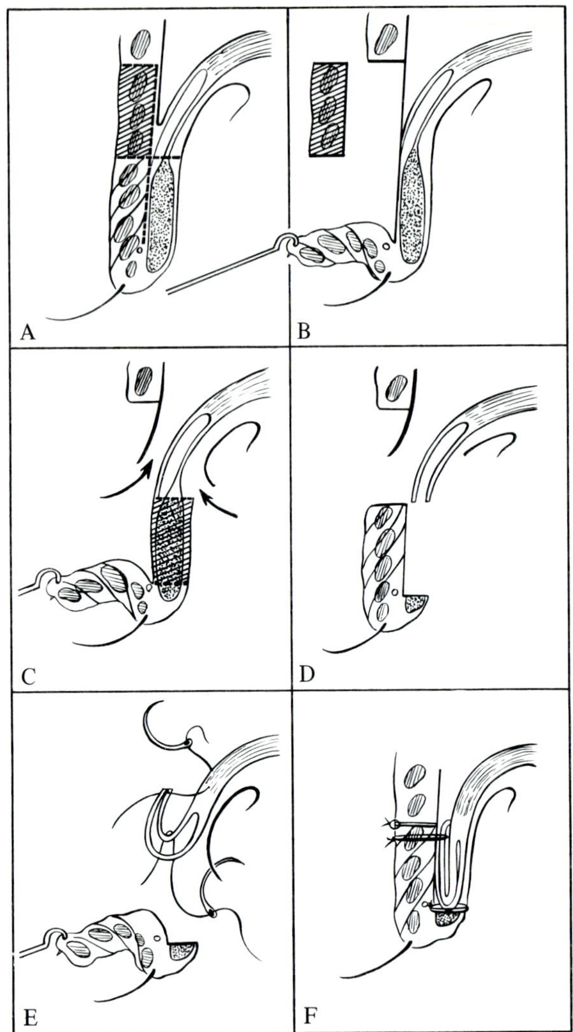

Fig. 12-32. Split-level lid resection with levator hitch. See text for explanation.

to the frontalis muscle by means of a sling. I have in the past used a large number of materials to form this sling, but I have gone back to using autogenous fascia lata because of the greater certainty of its action and the ease of obtaining a strip of fascia lata using a fascial stripper of my own design (Fig. 12-33). A strip of fascia 2 to 3 mm. wide should be fixed to the anterior surface of the tarsal plate by 6-0 Prolene sutures and carried up beneath the orbicularis muscle but in front of the orbital septum, and brought out through the eyebrow in the region of the eyebrow's greatest movement (Fig. 12-34B). A W shape or a rectangular shape of hitch may be used (Fig. 12-34C), but the

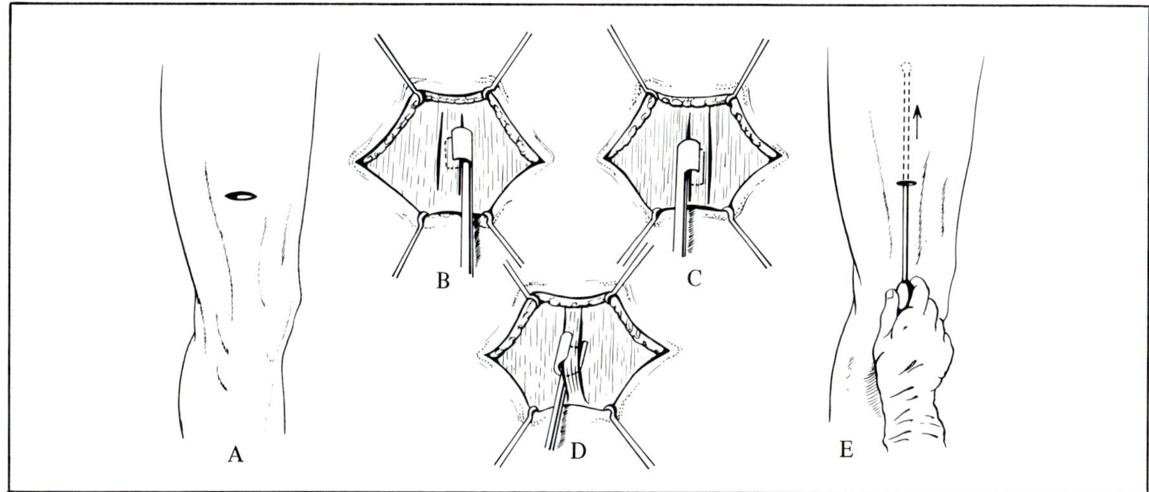

Fig. 12-33. A,B,C, a fascia lata splitter (available from Chas. Thackeray Ltd., Park St., Leeds, England) is used to extend slits made in the fascia just above knee. The instrument is pushed upward to extend each slit; finally, with the isolated strip cradled in the splitter (D), the instrument is again passed up to the full extent of the slitting (E). With counterpressure exerted by a thumb on the thigh immediately above the instrument, an upward thrust of the instrument will enable the sharp upper edge of the splitter to cut through the top end of the fascial strip, which can be withdrawn and resected.

knot in the fascia must be secured with 6-0 Prolene and should be placed deeply just above the periosteum to avoid infection of the whipping stitch from eyebrow hair follicles (Fig. 12-34D).

The height at which the lid is placed should not be so great that there is a marked lagophthalmos, even though good opening is obtained. Because of the problem of judging the optimum height at the time of surgery, a simple adjustable "capstan" may be used; it can be made out of two trouser buttons through which the fascial ends are passed and tied together (Fig. 12-35). Turning the top button tightens the fascia and raises the lid, and if, after fixing the top button with adhesive, the fascia is kept moist with liquid paraffin drops for 24 hours, further adjustment can still be carried out postoperatively if necessary. The fascia sloughs off at skin level after about 2 to 3 weeks.

PTOSIS ASSOCIATED WITH BLEPHAROPHIMOSIS

In patients with blepharophimosis, there is usually a shortage of all the upper lid tissues, including skin; a

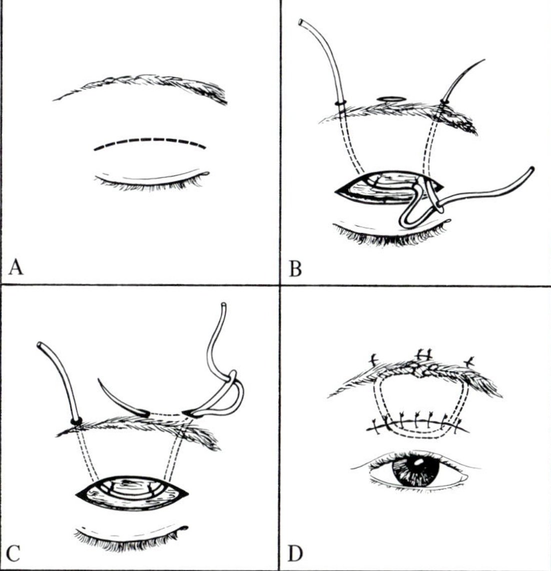

Fig. 12-34. Frontalis hitch. A, an incision is made at the level of the top of the tarsal plate so as to create a supratarsal fold. B, the fascia is sutured to the center of the tarsal plate and exteriorized above the eyebrow. C, the fascia is carried to the deep central wound to permit the placement of a knot in the fascia deep to the follicles in the eyebrow. D, skin closure, totally burying fascia, is shown.

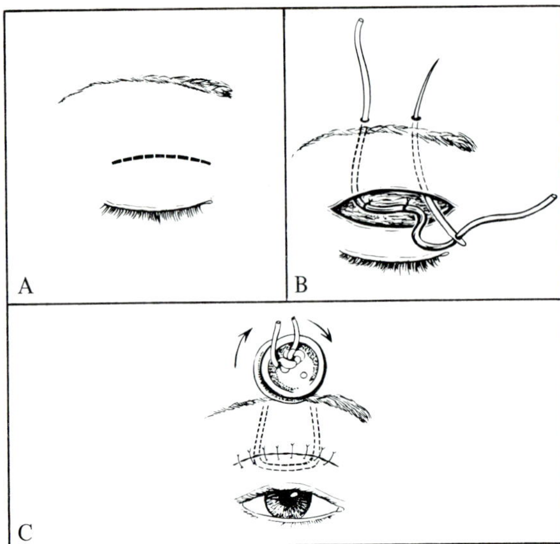

Fig. 12-35. Adjustable fascia lata "capstan" using two trouser buttons. See text for explanation.

split-level lid resection for the ptosis that may be present should *not* be carried out in such patients. If there is obviously reasonable levator muscle function, with a supratarsal sulcus, then a modified split-level and hitch operation is carried out in which no skin or orbicularis is resected and only a half of the tarsal plate is removed. The levator complex is hitched up to itself, making a loop about 5 or 6 mm. deep. Any more radical approach than this will definitely produce lagophthalmos. If a successful result is not achieved, or if the detectable levator action is minimal or nil, then a fascia lata sling should be used. These patients have well-developed frontalis muscle action, and sling operations work better with them than in patients with ordinary unilateral congenital ptosis.

ACQUIRED TRAUMATIC PTOSIS

Acquired traumatic ptosis may result from direct injury to any part of the levator complex. An attempt should always be made to repair such a damaged levator at the time of primary surgery, but if no repair has been carried out and ptosis is present postoperatively, one should wait for 3 or 4 months to determine whether the ptosis is going to resolve spontaneously. If it is apparent that the levator is definitely not attached to the tarsal plate, then an exploratory operation should be carried out and an attempt made to locate and reattach the levator. If it is known that the levator has been reattached but ptosis still results and if there is no improvement after a further 8 or 9 months, a split-level lid resection is likely to prove an effective means of overcoming the drooping of the upper lid by decreasing the factors tending to counteract levator function.

Reconstruction of the Ear*

BURT BRENT

Reconstruction of the auricle is a challenging discipline that prompts innovation and creativity; it also demands strict adherence to the basic principles of plastic surgery and tissue transplantation. The complexity of this surgical enigma has stimulated valuable contributions by a number of interested surgeons. The evolution of a sound method of total ear construction was culminated by the diligent efforts of Tanzer [32–37], who refined the employment of costal cartilage as a supportive framework.

Likewise, Converse [8, 9], Fukuda [16], Brent [2, 3], and others have championed the use of rib cartilage, whereas Cronin [10, 11], Ohmori [24, 25], Edgerton [15], and others [12, 62] have assiduously developed techniques to enhance the employment of alloplastic frameworks.

Since limitations of space prevent the comprehensive inclusion of all techniques, the material for this chapter has been carefully selected to provide the reader with a guideline of practical surgical techniques and sound patient management in auricular surgery.

TOTAL CONSTRUCTION OF THE MICROTIC EAR

Surgical Considerations and Limitations

Total construction of the auricle is one of the greatest challenges that confronts the plastic surgeon. Comprised of a delicately convoluted cartilage frame covered by a fine skin envelope, the ear is a difficult structure to draw or sculpt, let alone to reproduce surgically. Generally, alloplastic frameworks are not well tolerated [7, 12, 23, 63], and contralateral auricular cartilage is inadequate for a total ear framework. At this time, autogenous costal cartilage remains the most reliable tissue for an underlying framework support.

Although costal cartilage can be carved to form a delicate framework [1–3, 6, 32–37], it must be remembered that the volume and detail of the furnished three-dimensional framework are limited by the two-dimensional skin flap under which it is placed. Furthermore, because the retroauricular-mastoid skin that covers the framework is somewhat thicker than the normal delicate anterolateral auricular skin, it blunts the details of a carved framework.

Hence, the plastic surgeon's aim is to achieve accurate representation, which involves the creation of an acceptable facsimile of an ear that is the proper size, in the proper position, and properly oriented to other facial features. Ultimately, the success of the construction is determined by the patient's psychological improvement, and by his willingness to wear a short hairstyle, which displays the constructed ear.

Preoperative Consultation

During the initial consultation, surgical expectations and psychological considerations should be discussed with the patient and his family, emphasizing the earlier stated goals of the reconstruction.

As Tanzer [32–36, 39] has stressed, the age at which to begin the reconstruction is influenced strongly by psychological considerations. Microtia creates significant emotional disturbances in an overwhelming majority of its unfortunate possessors. This deformity, which conceivably might be concealed by long hair, is by no means overlooked by the youngster's peers. It is this factor that prompts surgical consideration at an early age [20].

Since the ear is approximately 85 percent grown by the age of 4 years [14, 16], and since the rib cartilages are of reasonable size to permit fabrication of an adult-sized framework at that age [2], the reconstruction can be initiated before the child is psychologically traumatized by his peers' cruel ridicule and his family's overprotective concern.

Tanzer [33, 34, 36] begins the reconstruction at 6 years, whereas others [1, 29] prefer to wait until the rib cartilages are larger. However, Lindsay [22] performs the cartilage graft at the age of 2, and I prefer to begin their surgery at the age of 5 or 6 years.

General consensus discourages middle ear surgery [32, 39] except in severe bilateral hearing deficits, which are limited almost exclusively to bilateral microtia. In those rare cases, a team approach should be planned with a competent otologist [5].

During the consultation, the previously stated surgical limitations must be fully explained and emphasized to the family. This is best culminated by showing the parents photographs of the surgeon's *average* results, so that they retain realistic expectations. Likewise, accompanying surgical discomforts and inconveniences should be described, including the expected

*Total ear reconstruction requires special artistic skills, in order to obtain the results shown here. Not every surgeon has the artistic training and ability to achieve such good results.

W.C.G.

chest pain, duration of dressings, and protective head gear (as advocated by Converse [39] and Tanzer [32]), to be worn for sleeping during the actual reconstruction and later for contact sports.

Finally, the risks and possible complications of the surgery are discussed thoroughly. These include pneumothorax, cartilage-graft loss secondary to infection, skin-flap necrosis, hematoma, and resorption. It should be stressed that with proper precautions, these risks are comparatively less severe than the emotional trauma created by an absent ear.

Planning and Preparation

The result of a total ear reconstruction depends not only on a surgeon's meticulous surgical technique, but also on careful preoperative planning. It is essential that one practices carving techniques on a volume of human cadaver cartilage prior to any application in live patients. An acrylic or plaster replica of a normal ear serves as an excellent model for practice carvings.

During the patient's second office consultation, preoperative study photographs are obtained, and an x-ray film pattern is traced from the opposite, normal ear (Fig. 13-1). This pattern is reversed, and a framework pattern is designed several millimeters smaller in all dimensions to allow for the extra thickness that occurs when the framework is covered by the retroauricular-mastoid skin flap (Figs. 13-1 and 13-3). After sterilization, these patterns serve as guidelines for framework fabrication at the time of surgery (Fig. 13-3).

The location of the reconstructed ear is predetermined by taping the reversed film pattern to the proposed reconstruction site and then comparing its height from the front view with that of the opposite, normal ear (Fig. 13-2B). From the side, it should be noted that the axis of the ear is roughly parallel to the nasal profile [3, 4, 17, 57] (Fig. 13-2A). Reference marks, as advocated by Tanzer [39], serve as valuable guidelines during surgery.

First Stage of Reconstruction

The actual staging of the individual reconstruction is determined by first assessing the microtic vestiges. If the superior portion of an auricular vestige is substantial and useful for reconstruction, then the vestige is divided and positioned as the first operative stage [39]. Subsequent reconstruction would entail constructing the middle third of the auricle. However, the majority of microtic ears consist of an unfolded, crumpled cartilage nubbin and a relatively normal but displaced earlobe, which is the only tissue worth repositioning. In Tanzer's [32] classic method of a staged total ear reconstruction, he advocates rotation of the lobule to a normal position as the first surgical stage. As his technique has evolved, he has suggested, as an alternative, performing the cartilage graft and lobule rotation simultaneously [36, 37], as is done by Fukuda [16]. I avoid primary lobule rotation, since lobular placement can be more accurately determined when the actual underlying supportive framework is used for reference. Although I occasionally combine lobule rotation with implantation of the cartilage graft, it is generally safer and more accurate to rotate the lobule as a secondary procedure (see Fig. 13-6).

Usually, a first-stage reconstruction entails the implantation of the supportive framework, for which a wide variety of autogenous, homogenous, heterog-

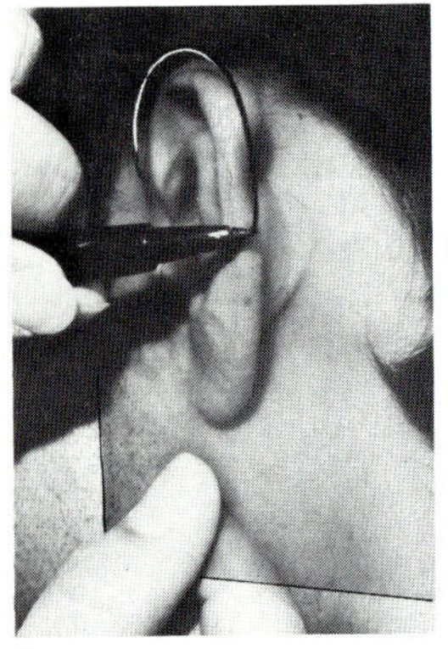

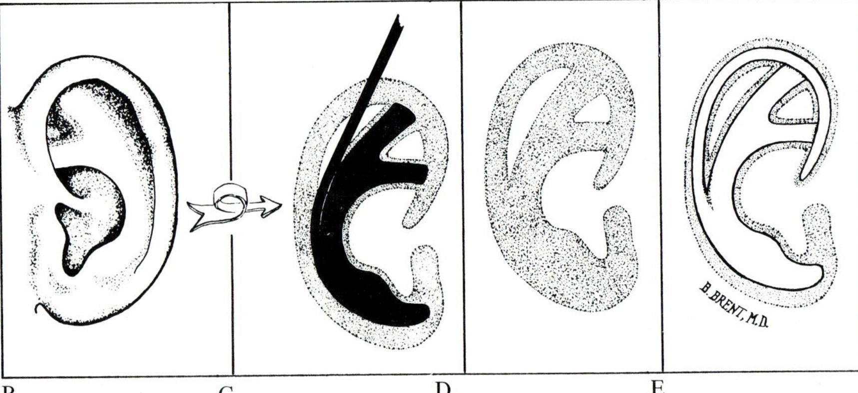

Fig. 13-1. Planning the auricular framework from a reversed film pattern traced from the opposite, normal ear. In this example, an open-spaced pattern has been planned. Note that the framework is designed several millimeters smaller in all dimensions to allow for the extra thickness the skin flap will present. See also Figure 13-3. (From B. Brent, Reconstruction of ear, eyebrow, and sideburn in the burned patient. Plast. Reconstr. Surg. *55:312, 1975.)*

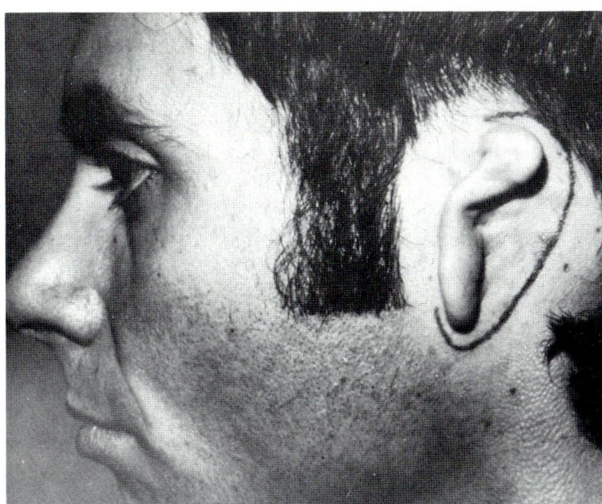

A

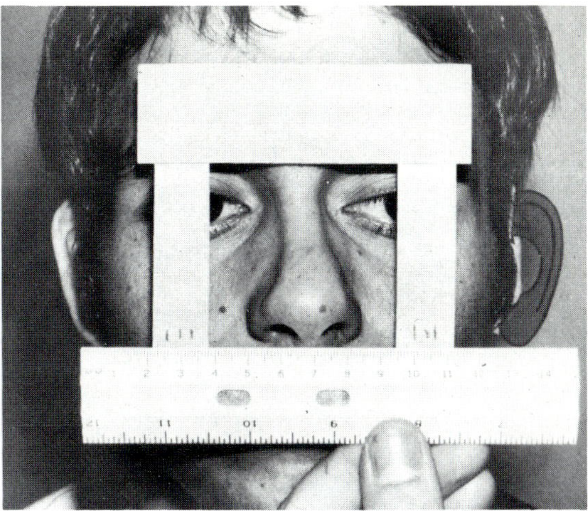

B

Fig. 13-2. Location and orientation of the ear. A, although normal in configuration, the earlobe is often displaced anteriorly and superiorly; note that the axis of the ear should be roughly parallel to the nose. B, the inferior border of the proposed ear is determined by taping the film pattern to the head and comparing its height to the opposite, normal ear.

enous, and alloplastic materials have been used [1–3, 7–13, 15–17, 19, 23, 24–26, 29–40]. Homogenous cartilage undergoes absorption readily [30, 46], and Silastic frameworks suffer a high incidence of extrusion [7, 12, 23]. Cronin [11] minimizes this problem by providing fascia lata for extra autogenous rim coverage, while others provide extra protection over the alloplastic frame with galeal and fascial flaps [15, 25, 40]. To this date, autogenous cartilage has produced the most reliable, lasting result with, comparatively, the least complications [32, 36, 37]. Furthermore, rib cartilage provides the most substantial source for fabricating a total ear framework. Although contralateral conchal cartilage has been used for this purpose [55, 57], it seems best to reserve auricular cartilage for repairing partial ear defects, for which considerably less tissue bulk is needed.

Obtaining the Rib Cartilage

When considering the cartilage configuration in the small child (Fig. 13-3), the rib cartilages are best obtained contralateral to the ear being constructed [35–37]; however, in the adult patient, a suitable supportive structure can be obtained from the ipsilateral side as well [2, 3] (Fig. 13-4). The rib cartilages are removed through a horizontal or slightly oblique incision that is made just above the costal margin (Fig. 13-3A). Following division of the rectus muscle, the film pattern is placed on the exposed cartilages to determine the necessary extent of rib resection.

Likewise, the particular framework design utilized is determined by the individual patient's rib configuration. Tanzer's [32, 61] classic solid-block design provides an excellent supportive framework (Fig. 13-3), whereas an open-spaced framework permits an interesting alternative [2, 3] that is particularly advantageous when skimpy cartilages are encountered. In both of these frameworks, the rim is fashioned separately with cartilage from the first free-floating rib (Figs. 13-3 and 13-4). Excision of this cartilage facilitates access to the synchondrotic region of the sixth and seventh ribs, which supplies a sufficient block to carve the framework body. Extraperichondrial dissection is preferable in order to obtain an unmarred specimen.

In cases where the delicate pleura is entered during this dissection, there is no great reason for concern, as a leak in the lung has not been produced. However, when a pleural tear is discovered, a rubber catheter is inserted well into the chest through the pleural opening; then the chest wound is closed in layers by the assistant, while the surgeon fabricates the framework, thus conserving operative time. When skin closure is complete, the catheter is attached to a suction apparatus, the lung is expanded, and the catheter is rapidly withdrawn. As a final precaution, every patient receives a portable upright chest roentgenogram in the recovery room.

Framework Fabrication

Generally speaking, a novice at ear reconstruction has a tendency to become preoccupied with carving framework details. As experience is gained, it becomes evident that the shortcomings of a reconstruction arise not from a lack of framework detail, but from a

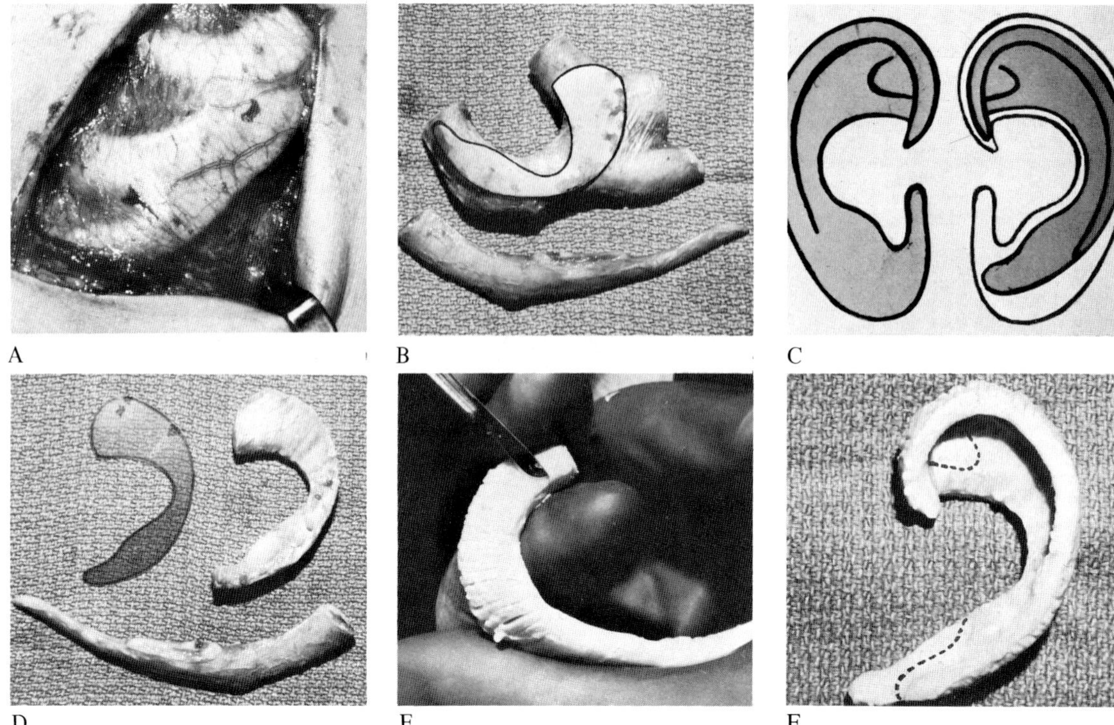

Fig. 13-3. Fabrication of a solid-block cartilage framework (after Tanzer [32]). A, the exposed synchondrosis of the sixth and seventh ribs of the contralateral thorax. B, the excised rib cartilages. C, film patterns; note that the framework pattern is smaller than the ear to be constructed, which allows for the thickness that the skin flap will add. D, the carved basic ear silhouette. E, scoring the rim to facilitate curvature. F, the assembled framework; note that the inferior projection is to be shortened, and the triangular fossa is to be sculpted.

shortage of the skin needed to cover the framework and to permit fine detail.

The surgeon's realistic aim is to fabricate a framework with an exaggerated rim and a distinct posterior conchal wall–inferior crus contour line. This is achieved with scalpel blades and a rounded wood-carving chisel. To minimize possible chondrocytic damage, the use of power tools for sculpting is strictly avoided – one should keep in mind that cartilage-sculpting differs from basic wood carving in that a good long-term result ultimately depends on living tissue.

The basic ear silhouette is carved from the previously obtained cartilage block (Fig. 13-3D). It is necessary to thin very little, if any, of the basic form for a small child's framework, but it is essential for framework fabrication in most older patients. When thinning is necessary, care should be taken to preserve the perichondrium on the lateral, outer aspect of the framework to facilitate its adherence, take, and subsequent nourishment. Because warping must be taken into consideration [45], the surgeon sculpts and thins the cartilage to cause a deliberate warping in a favorable direction.

Finally, the rim is fashioned from the floating rib cartilage, and it is fastened to the framework body with horizontal mattress sutures of stainless steel, with the knots buried on the undersurface of the frame.

Framework Implantation

A cutaneous pocket is created with meticulous technique so as to provide an adequate recipient vascular covering for the framework. Because several hours elapse during the rib removal and framework fabrication, the auricular region is prepared and scrubbed just prior to creating the cutaneous pocket.

Through a small incision anterior to the auricular vestige (Fig. 13-5A), a thin flap is raised by sharp dissection, taking care to preserve the subdermal vascular plexus. Solutions that contain epinephrine are avoided, to enable the surgeon to evaluate the vascular status of the flap and to ensure accurate hemostasis. The surgeon carefully dissects the skin from the gnarled native cartilage remnant, which is then excised and

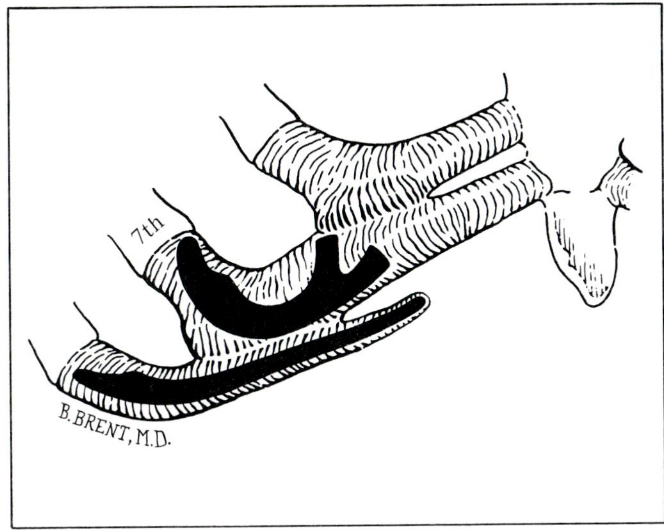

A

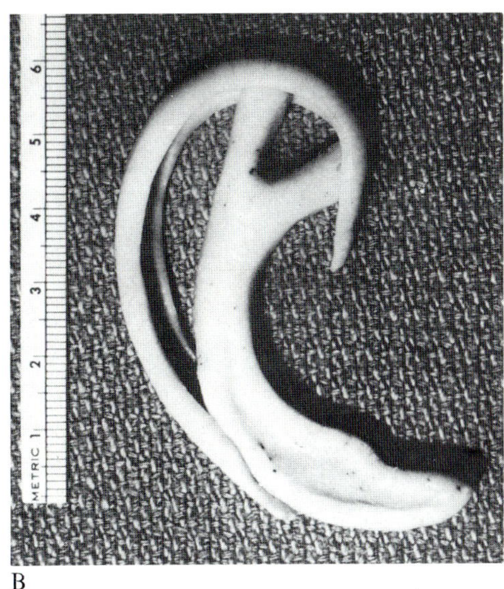

B

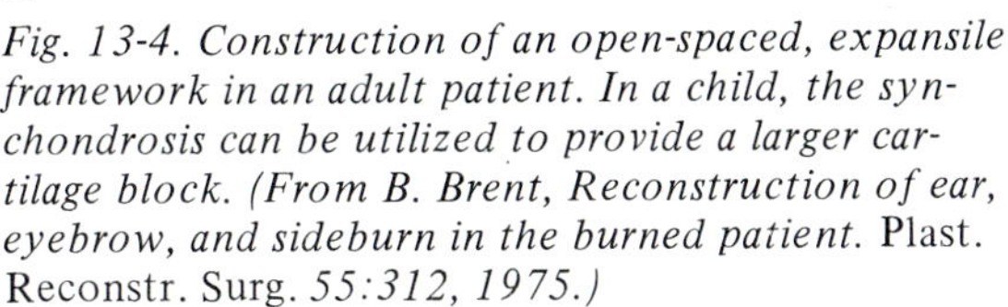

Fig. 13-4. Construction of an open-spaced, expansile framework in an adult patient. In a child, the synchondrosis can be utilized to provide a larger cartilage block. (From B. Brent, Reconstruction of ear, eyebrow, and sideburn in the burned patient. Plast. Reconstr. Surg. *55:312, 1975.)*

discarded. Finally, the pocket is completed by dissecting just peripherally to the projected framework markings (Fig. 13-5A).

Insertion of the framework into the cutaneous pocket takes up the valuable skin slack that was created when the native cartilage remnant was removed. The framework displaces this skin centrifugally in an advantageous posterosuperior direction so as to displace the hairline just behind the rim. This principle of anterior incision and centrifugal skin relaxation, introduced by Tanzer [32], permits advantageous use of the hairless skin in microtia.

The centrifugal skin displacement converts the incision to a conchal defect which can rarely be closed without tension over the cartilage framework. The temptation to close this incision must be resisted, as skin tenting will obliterate form, produce tension, and create dead space – all of which are factors that contribute to the loss of detail and eventual cartilage absorption. Instead, the conchal defect is filled with a full-thickness skin graft, which is usually obtained from the contralateral auriculocephalic sulcus.

Coaption of the skin flap to the underlying framework is attained with either bolster sutures or suction. Tanzer [32–37, 39] advocates the use of mattress sutures tied over gauze bolsters, while Cronin [10] employs suction after implanting his Silastic frameworks. I have employed both methods (Fig. 13-5) but prefer the latter, as it simultaneously prevents fluid collection and minimizes the risk of flap necrosis along the helical margin.

To attain skin coaption with suction, the surgeon fashions a perforated drain from an infusion catheter with the needle inserted into a rubber-topped vacuum tube [18] (Fig. 13-5); the tubes are retained on a rack to observe changes in the quantity and quality of drainage. Although a dressing is applied that accurately conforms to the convolutions of the newly created auricle, firm pressure is unnecessary, as the suction drain provides both hemostasis and skin coaption.

Postoperative Management

Attentive postoperative management is imperative for a successful ear reconstruction that remains unhampered by disastrous complications. The newly constructed auricle is scrutinized frequently and carefully for signs of infection or vascular compromise.

Usually early infection manifests itself, not by auricular pain or fever, but through local erythema, edema, subtle fluctuation, drainage, or a combination of the above. Hence, frequent observations and the immediate institution of aggresive therapy can inhibit an overwhelming infection.

When an infection is suspected, an irrigation drain should immediately be introduced below the flap, and continuous antibiotic drip irrigation should be begun. Appropriate adjustments are made both in the antibiotic drip irrigation and in the systemic therapy when sensitivity studies are available from the initial culture. Cronin [10] has salvaged Silastic-frame reconstructions impressively by this technique, and I have

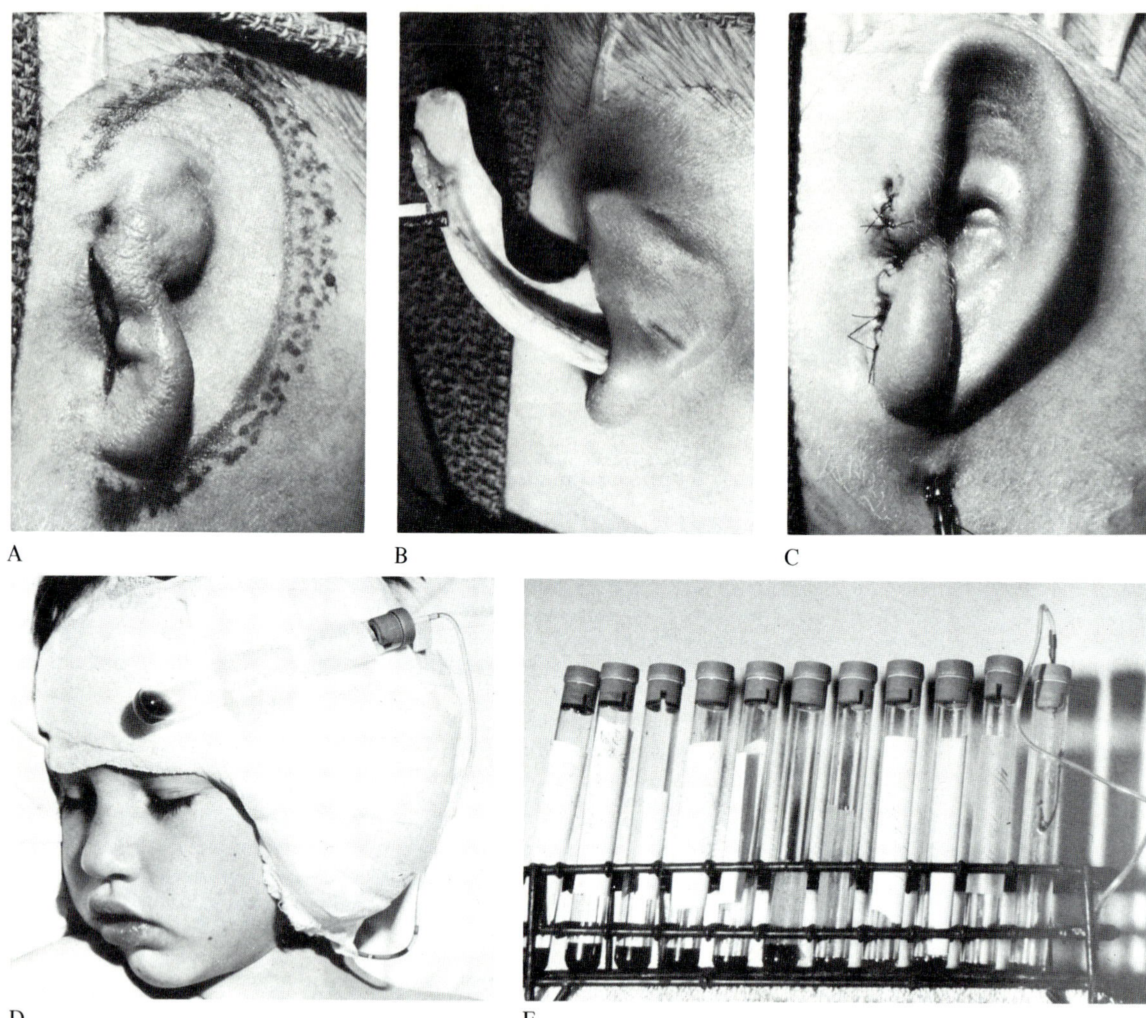

Fig. 13-5. A, the development of a cutaneous pocket via a small anterior incision; the stippled area designates the extent of the dissection peripheral to the proposed implantation site. B, the insertion of the cartilage framework. C, the implanted framework, immediately after the operation; note that the skin coaption has been obtained by a suction-catheter. The lobule will be rotated at the next surgical stage (see Fig. 13-6). D, E, the suction system, consisting of a #19 infusion catheter and a rubber-topped vacuum tube. The display of tubes demonstrates the decreasing quantity of serous fluid, at which time the drain is removed.

had excellent success in managing the occasional infection in cartilage-graft reconstructions.

Skin flap necrosis results from excess tension in an inadequate-sized pocket, tight bolster sutures, or damage to the subdermal vascularity during the flap dissection. This complication is best avoided by meticulous technique; however, once skin necrosis becomes evident, appropriate steps must be taken without delay.

When ischemia is noted below snug bolster sutures, they are removed. Usually, small localized ulcerations heal with good local wound care, although at times a small local flap may be required to cover exposed cartilage. However, major skin flap necrosis merits a more aggressive approach if the framework is to be salvaged. The necrotic skin is excised early, and the framework is covered with an adjacent galeal flap that is surfaced by a skin graft. Although I praise the galeal flap as a salvage procedure, it has been employed as a primary procedure to provide extra tissue protection over Silastic frameworks by Fox and Edgerton [15], Tegtmeier and Gooding [40], and Ohmori [25].

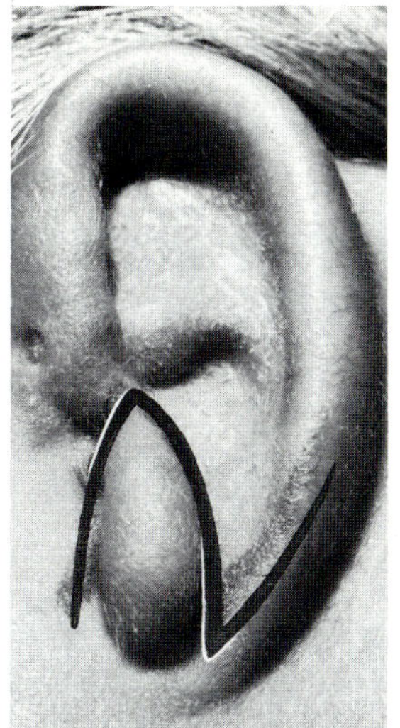

A

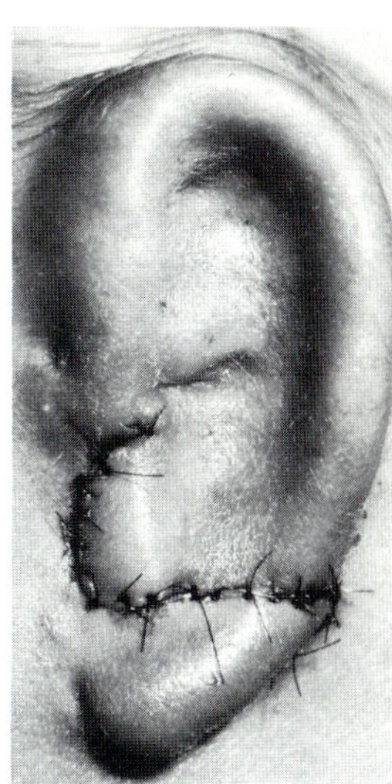

B

Fig. 13-6. Rotation of the lobule; note that the lobular rotation is a Z-plasty transfer and that the accuracy of lobular placement is facilitated by the reference of an underlying framework. The rotation of the lobule is performed as a secondary procedure (in the same patient as in Fig. 13-5). Note that a small cartilage graft has been placed below the anterior flap to simulate a tragal projection.

Other Stages of Auricular Construction

The major stages in auricular construction subsequent to the initial framework implantation are lobule rotation, elevation of the ear, deepening of the concha, and formation of a tragus. These stages can be planned independently or in various combinations, depending on which best achieves the desired end result.

Rotation of the Lobule

The lobule can be rotated in conjunction with framework implantation, as an isolated secondary procedure (Fig. 13-6), or in combination with the elevation and grafting of the lower auricular third segment. Only occasionally do I find it advantageous to reposition the lobule prior to cartilage grafting.

The "rotation" or repositioning of this normal but displaced structure is accomplished essentially by Z-plasty transposition of a narrow, inferiorly-based triangular flap (Fig. 13-6).

Tragal Construction and Conchal Definition

Formation of the tragus, "elevation" of the lower auricular portion, and conchal definition can be achieved separately or in one operation (Fig. 13-7).

The tragus is best formed from a conchal flap, a technique which Tanzer [32–37, 39] advocated and refined during the past three decades. Originally described by Kirkham [19], this method employs an anteriorly based conchal flap (Fig. 13-7A, B). After raising the flap, one attains conchal depth by carefully excising the subcutaneous tissue down to the mastoid periosteum [16, 24, 25]. Finally, the flap is doubled upon itself to simulate a tragus. To ensure lasting detail, I prefer to include a small cartilage graft inside the conchal flap (Fig. 13-7B).

Definition of the lower auricular region is gained by elevation and skin grafting. An incision is made just behind the framework (line *b* in Fig. 13-7A) and the auricle is lifted from its bed by sharp dissection, taking care to avoid exposure of the cartilage itself. The raw area that is created is covered with a skin graft, and the sutures are tied over a gauze bolster.

A "valise-handle" effect may be obtained by continuing the dissection anteriorly until an opening is created in the posterior conchal wall region (Fig. 13-7B). Although Tanzer [32] designed this technique originally to facilitate middle ear surgery, he found that it also served to create the necessary detail in the posterior conchal wall, which is difficult to achieve by any other method.

If one employs the "valise-handle" technique in conjunction with tragal construction, then a full-thickness graft is placed to cover the raw bed from the newly constructed tragus to the posterior incision (Fig. 13-7C). Also, a split-thickness graft serves to cover the inner surface of the "valise-handle." A later closure of the passageway created by the "valise-handle" has been outlined by Tanzer [32, 39] and

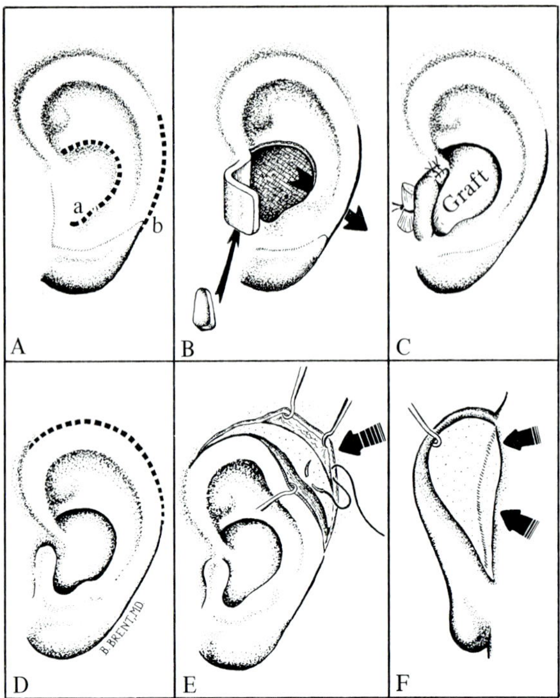

Fig. 13-7. Construction of tragus, by the method of Kirkham (A–C). A, the incision lines are shown: a, *the conchal incision;* b, *the posterior incision to create optional "valise handle." B, the conchal flap is folded upon itself; the inclusion of a small cartilage graft prevents shrinkage. The larger arrow demonstrates the passageway (see text). C, the skin graft is applied to the conchal floor.*

The elevation of the upper auricle (D–F). D, incision. E, dissection of the auricle from the head. E, F, advancement of the scalp toward the auriculocephalic sulcus to decrease the size and visibility of the skin graft.

Converse [9]; however, obliteration of this opening by skin graft contracture at times makes this step unnecessary.

Elevation of the Upper Auricular Region
Elevation of the upper auricular region should not be attempted until the edema has markedly subsided and the auricular details have become well-defined. When this occurs, an incision is made several millimeters behind the rim (Fig. 13-7D), again taking care to preserve a protective layer of connective tissue on the cartilage framework.

I feel that radical elevation should be avoided, since it disturbs the circulation to the cartilage graft and adds nothing to the reconstruction, since ultimately the skin graft will contract and pull the ear close to the head. Instead, projection can be gained later by inserting a cartilage wedge under the framework; this wedge is fashioned from spare cartilage that was banked subcutaneously through the chest wound when the costal cartilage was initially removed.

Touch-up Procedures
Various minor procedures are effective in refining the new auricle so as to achieve the best possible end result. The persistent problem of scalp hair on the reconstructed rim has largely been eliminated in microtia by the anterior incision–centrifugal relaxation principle [32], but the hairline remains a perplexing problem in major acquired auricular deformities.

Although the "scalp roll" and free graft provide a hairless skin cover [21, 39], I prefer to implant the framework first and later eradicate any undesirable hair. Even though depilation by electrolysis has varying degrees of success, I prefer to replace the follicular skin with a full-thickness skin graft.

Rim definition can be enhanced by removing excess fibrous tissue through sulcus incisions [39, 63], or by "eave-flap" procedures as described by Lewin [101] and Cronin [99].

Finally, an otoplasty should be performed concurrently with the final excision of a retroauricular skin graft during the reconstruction, so that the opposite, normal ear is set back to approximate the constructed auricle.

Secondary Reconstruction
In the event of reconstructive failure, any further attempt will be handicapped greatly by the existing scar tissue and by skin shortage. Unstable scars must be excised and the resulting defect resurfaced with a full-thickness graft. Subsequently, a 9 to 12 month waiting period follows, during which the graft matures and becomes soft, pliable, and mobile. After this time, a second reconstructive attempt is begun, but the less favorable skin coverage will limit the results that one can expect to attain.

TOTAL EAR RECONSTRUCTION IN THE ACQUIRED DEFORMITY

Total auricular reconstruction in the acquired deformity presents special problems not encountered in microtia; these problems merit separate consideration. The lack of skin coverage is much more critical than in microtia, since an existing meatus precludes use of the anterior incision, and extra skin, which is usually gained by removing the crumpled microtic cartilage, is not available. This factor compounds the previously mentioned hairline problem. Furthermore, the local tissues are often heavily scarred and must be replaced by skin grafts before the actual reconstruction can begin.

The cutaneous pocket is best developed by incisions above and/or below the proposed auricular site. The somewhat restricted pocket that can be developed in these patients correspondingly restricts the volume of cartilage that can be inserted; thus the surgeon must often be satisfied with a poorly defined rim. Often the only feasible method of attaining rim definition in reconstructing a major acquired deformity is with a delicate supraclavicular tube (see Reconstruction of Acquired Partial Defects).

Auricular Prostheses

The auricular prosthesis should be reserved for patients in whom surgical reconstruction is impractical or contraindicated, or for cases in which an experienced surgeon is unavailable.

For the most part, an auricular prosthesis has no practical value for children, but is worthwhile for older patients who have undergone ablative cancer surgery [41, 43]. Even so, many adults find them undesirable after a short trial experience, since there is always a constant fear that the prosthesis might become dislodged at an embarrassing moment, as well as the psychological discomfort of wearing an "artificial part."

Additional problems that arise are local skin irritation from the adhesive glue that frequently necessitates discontinuance of the prosthesis for a period of time, which in turn causes the patient further embarrassment. Furthermore, an obvious color contrast calls attention to the prosthetic ear in climatic changes, when the prosthetic part remains a constant color while the surrounding skin varies as the patient passes from indoors to outdoors.

When an auricular prosthesis has been decided on for the younger patient, a trial period should ensue, with the realization that surgical reconstruction may be desired later. It is wise to avoid preliminary excision of the microtic lobule or other remnants merely to "gain an improved surface for adherence of the prosthesis," as has been advocated [42]. Should the patient desire surgical reconstruction later, which has often been my experience, then the missing lobule, shortage of skin, and existing scar become a significant handicap.

Acute Auricular Trauma

Because of the delicate nature of the auricle it is exceptionally vulnerable to the various types of trauma for which the plastic surgeon frequently is summoned to the emergency room.

Initially, a good block anesthesia should be administered that will promptly relieve the patient's discomfort and permit proper cleaning, evaluation, and repair of the injury. I prefer 1% lidocaine (Xylocaine) with 1:100,000 epinephrine; the epinephrine is omitted only if there are long thin pedicles of tissue resulting from the injury.

Otohematoma

A common injury in contact sports, otohematoma must be treated aggressively so as to avoid multiple recurrences [69]. While mere needle aspiration is followed almost invariably by recurrent fluid collection, a small incision will permit evacuation of the hematoma under direct vision. Conforming, compressive gauze bolsters are placed on either side of the auricle, and are maintained for 7 to 10 days by horizontal mattress sutures (4-0 nylon) that traverse the bolsters as well as the ear (Fig. 13-8).

The Amputated Ear

A major auricular avulsion presents a complex surgical problem and, until recently, cartilage salvation provided the only measure worthy of effort [73, 75, 76]. Almost invariably, replantation of large composite parts is doomed to failure [65, 68, 70], except when an increased vascular recipient area is prepared first.

Dermabrasion of the amputated part is followed by its reattachment and temporary "pocketing" below a retroauricular flap introduced by Mladick et al. [71, 72] has provided a new and encouraging solution to this difficult problem. The skin flap over the anterior surface of the auricle can be lifted away at 7 to 10 days and the posterior surface separated from the mastoid area at 14 to 17 days.

Removal of the posteromedial skin from the amputated part, followed by "fenestration" of the cartilage (Baudet et al. [64]), provides another excellent method for increasing the recipient vascular surface of the reattached auricle. In this technique, the anterolateral auricular skin is nourished through the cartilage fenestrations by means of direct contact with a vascular bed prepared when a retroauricular flap is raised.

Acute Auricular Burns

The protruding delicate nature of the auricle makes it particularly susceptible to thermal trauma. Often, direct thermal injury may result in a full-thickness loss that is confined to the helical rim. Usually, such an injury heals by autoamputation, a spontaneous separation of the eschar.

A far more dreaded complication of thermal injury is chondritis, which follows infection or external trauma to the burned tissue. The external trauma is usually the result of pillow pressure or friction; it can be prevented by substituting a rolled sheet or doughnut-shaped head support for the offending pillow [78, 83]. Chondritis is characterized by tenderness,

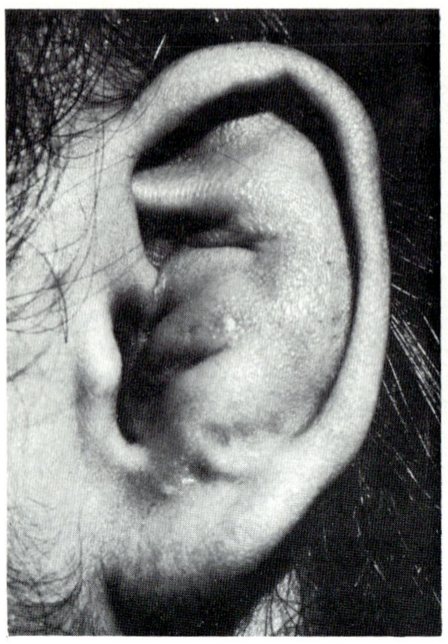
A

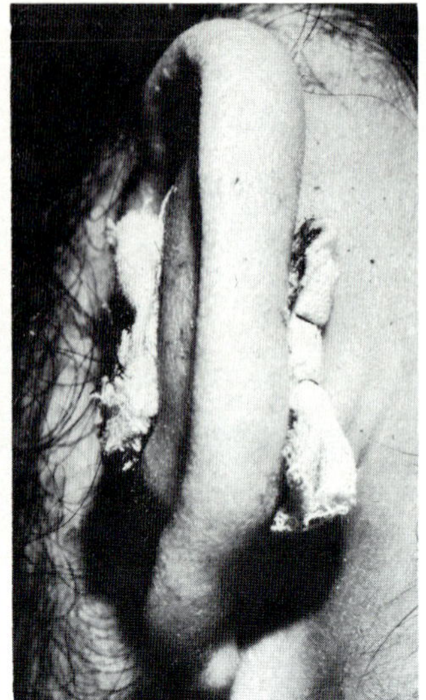
B

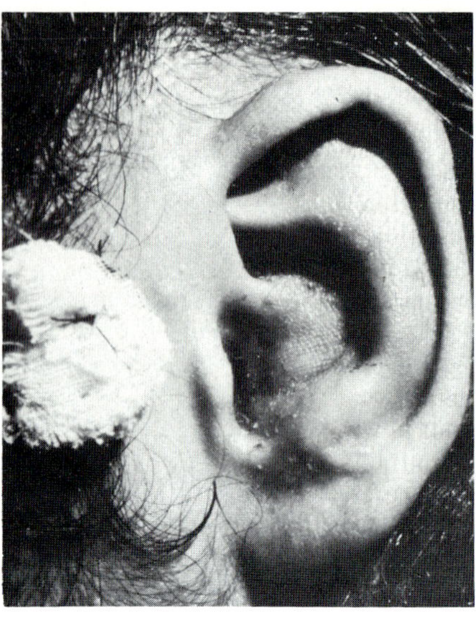
C

Fig. 13-8. Management of acute otohematoma. A, recurrent conchal hematoma, following several aspiration attempts. B, through-and-through bolster sutures, following surgical evacuation of hematoma. C, the auricle, after removal of compression sutures at 10 days.

erythema, warmth, and induration, and it occurs most commonly between the third and fifth week after the burn [80]. This severe complication is largely circumvented by sound wound management, which includes the previously mentioned avoidance of pressure and friction as well as frequent cleaning with soap and water [78] and the liberal use of topical antibiotics [78, 80, 84]. With early tangential excision or dermabrasion of the involved tissue and skin grafting, the incidence of infection is lessened and prompt wound healing is facilitated [83].

However, once chondritis is diagnosed, aggressive steps must be taken to eradicate the infection and prevent subsequent severe deformity. Local instillation of an antibiotic solution and the application of warm compresses have offered a hopeful remedy [77, 79], but if this therapy fails, incision, drainage, and adequate chondrectomy must be performed. When the chondrectomy becomes necessary, the incisions should be planned judiciously to permit later reconstruction, and the helical cartilage should be preserved when feasible.

In burned ears free from chondritis, several salvage procedures are worthy of consideration. A protective retroauricular flap may be employed temporarily to cover a tangentially excised auricular burn or exposed cartilage rim [81, 85], much in the manner of Mladick's "pocket principle" applied to amputated ears [71, 72]. On the other hand, Gorney [82] has amputated the totally burned ear, preserved the cartilage by banking it subcutaneously beneath the skin of the upper arm, and then used it later for the reconstruction.

Frequently, reconstruction of the burned tissue must be preceded by resurfacing, since the healed auricular skin often consists of thin, friable scar tissue. Full-thickness skin grafts are preferable for this purpose; a long waiting period follows the application of the grafts before cartilage implantation is undertaken.

RECONSTRUCTION OF ACQUIRED PARTIAL DEFECTS

Most auricular deformities encountered in everyday practice are acquired partial defects. They present the surgeon with an unlimited variety of unique problems whose reconstructions are influenced by the etiology, location, and nature of each residual deformity.

Utilization of Residual Tissues

In managing acute auricular trauma, initial meticulous reapproximation of tissues and appropriate wound care will greatly facilitate the reconstructive task ahead. Likewise, the innovative utilization of residual local tissues in a post-traumatic deformity will greatly simplify the reconstruction and contribute to a pleasing outcome.

Structural Support

Contralateral Conchal Cartilage

A variety of tissues are available to provide the structural support required for an auricular reconstruction.

Although the quantity of cartilage needed to fabricate a total ear framework necessitates the use of costal cartilage [2, 9, 36, 39], one is rarely compelled to employ this tissue in a partial auricular reconstruction. Because it is almost always possible to utilize an auricular cartilage graft, which is most frequently obtained from the contralateral concha under local anesthesia, the correction of partial losses is less extensive than the procedures to correct total auricular losses.

Auricular cartilage, used as an orthotopic graft in ear reconstruction, is superior to costal cartilage in that it provides a delicate, flexible support covered by perichondrium, and it appears to be more resistant to trauma and the absorptive process than is costal cartilage.

The conchal cartilage graft can be obtained by a posteromedial incision, as described by Adams [53] and Gorney and associates [58], or through an anterolateral approach, which I use more frequently. The anterolateral approach, performed through an incision several millimeters inside the posterior conchal wall–inferior crus contour line, is a simple method of obtaining a precise cartilage graft with direct visual exposure (Fig. 13-9B).

Ipsilateral Conchal Cartilage

In certain partial reconstructions, it is more advantageous to employ an ipsilateral rather than contralateral conchal cartilage graft. However, it is imperative that an intact antihelical strut be present to permit the removal of an ipsilateral conchal cartilage graft without subsequent collapse and further deformity of the ear.

An ipsilateral conchal cartilage graft is particularly advantageous when a retroauricular flap is being raised to repair a major defect in the helical rim (see Fig. 13-10). The elevation of the flap provides the required conchal cartilage exposure without the necessity of an additional incision, and the removal of this cartilage graft subsequently lowers the ear closer to the mastoid region. In effect, this produces a relative gain in length, thus enabling the flap to cover the cartilage graft once it is spliced onto the rim (Fig. 13-10) and eliminating the need for a skin graft in the donor bed of the flap.

Furthermore, the ipsilateral concha may occasionally be used as a composite flap of skin and cartilage (Fig. 13-12G, H). This innovative technique, proposed by Davis [106], is applicable to defects of the upper third of the auricle, and again, should be employed only when the antihelical support remains intact.

Chondrocutaneous Composite Graft

In certain conditions, a composite graft can effectively provide the supportive tissue required for a reconstruction. The success of these grafts is greatly enhanced by removing a portion of the posteromedial skin and cartilage, thus converting part of the wedge to a full-thickness skin graft that is readily vascularized by a recipient advancement flap mobilized from the loose retroauricular skin adjacent to the defect (Fig. 13-13B). A strut of helical cartilage is preserved within the graft to maintain contour and support (Fig. 13-13C).

Free Perichondrial Grafts

An exciting new prospect in ear reconstruction is the use of free perichondrial grafts as a supporting tissue. Inspired by the work of Skoog and associates [50, 51], Ohlsén [49], and Sohn and Ohlsén [52], I have intensely investigated the neochondrogenic potential of the perichondrium in application to auricular and other reconstructive facial surgery. The encouraging results of these laboratory investigations have prompted the use of free perichondrial grafts in varied specific clinical situations [44, 54].

Specific Regional Defects

External Auditory Canal

It is more efficacious to prevent stenosis of the canal than to be faced with treating it once it has occurred. Careful realignment of severed tissues followed by insertion of an acrylic mold will prevent stenosis, provided that the patient retains the obturating device faithfully for at least 3 to 6 months.

Stenosis is best treated by a full-thickness graft carefully applied over an acrylic mold, if a reasonable recipient vascular bed can be prepared [91]. Occasionally, multiple Z-plasties can be utilized to relieve webbing of the orifice [96]; at times, a local flap may be necessary to line the canal and break up the contracture [93, 95].

Helical Rim

Acquired losses of the helical rim may vary from small defects to major portions of the helix. Small defects are usually the result of tumor excisions or minor traumatic injuries, and are best closed by advancing the helix in both directions as described by Antia and Buch [97]. The success of this excellent technique depends on the following factors. (1) The entire helix should be totally freed from the scapha through an incision in the helical sulcus that extends through the cartilage but not through the skin on the back surface of the ear. (2) The posteromedial auricular skin is undermined, dissecting just superficially to the perichondrium until the entire helix is hanging as a chondrocutaneous component of the loosely mobilized skin. (3) Extra length can be gained by a V-Y advancement of the crus helix (Fig. 13-12B), and surprisingly large defects can be closed without tension (Fig. 13-13E, F, G, H).

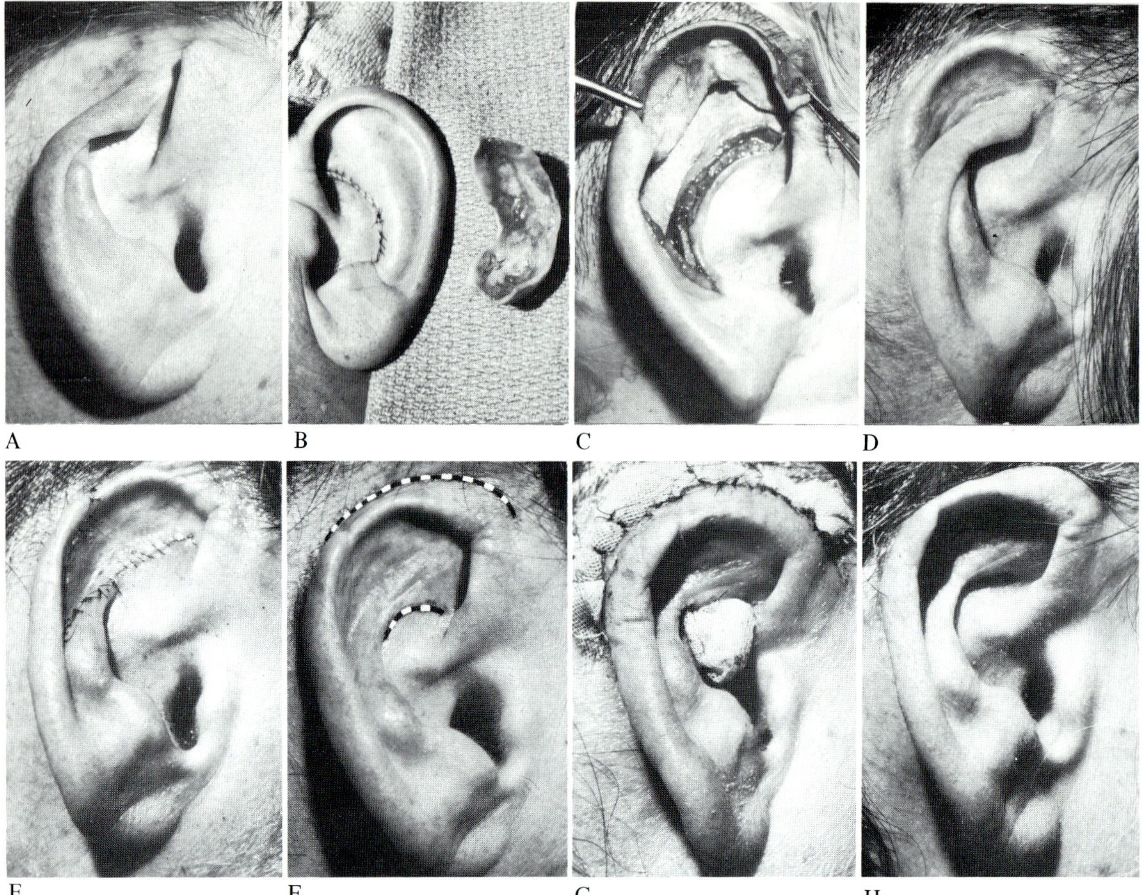

Fig. 13-9. Reconstruction of a major defect of the superior third of the auricle with an auricular cartilage graft. A, the postsurgical deformity. B, the contralateral conchal cartilage graft is removed via an anterolateral approach; note the inconspicuous incision. C, D, the cartilage graft prior to and 6 weeks after implantation. E, the helical component is transposed to a suitable position on the rim. F, G, incisions are planned to create "valise-handle," elevation, skin grafting, and employment of T-shaped tie-over dressing. H, the final result; an excellent definition of inferior crus has resulted from the intentionally created "valise handle." (From B. Brent, The acquired auricular deformity. A systematic approach to its analysis and reconstruction. Plast. Reconstr. Surg. *59:475, 1977.)*

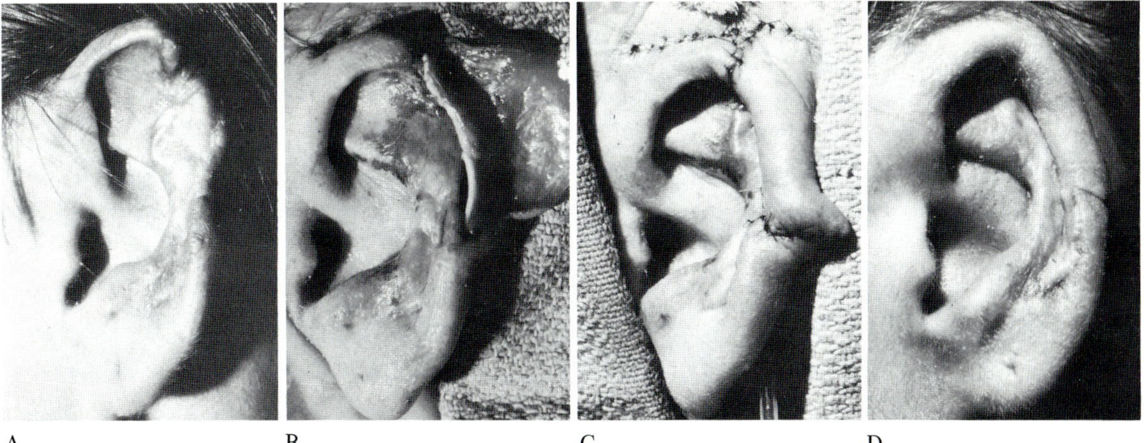

Fig. 13-10. Helical rim reconstruction with an auricular cartilage graft. A, traumatic deformity of helical rim. B, the development of a flap composed of retroauricular and medioauricular skin; an ipsilateral conchal cartilage graft has been spliced onto the rim (see text for further explanation). C, the flap is advanced over the cartilage graft. No attempt has been made to excise the "dog ear," which is removed later when the ear is elevated from the head with a skin graft. D, the final result. (From B. Brent, The acquired auricular deformity. A systematic approach to its analysis and reconstruction. Plast. Reconstr. Surg. *59:475, 1977.)*

Although the technique was originally described for upper-third auricular defects [97] (Fig. 13-12A), I have found that it is even more effective for middle-third defects (Fig. 13-13E, F, G, H), and it is equally applicable in repairing earlobe losses.

Reconstruction of larger helical defects requires a more sophisticated procedure that recreates the absent rim using an auricular cartilage graft covered by an adjacent flap as previously described in the text (Fig. 13-10). Although advancement flaps of local soft tissues have also been employed to provide helical contour [99, 101, 102], I have found that these flaps often suffer a disappointing long-term result unless a strut of cartilage has been incorporated into the repair.

Another sophisticated method of helical reconstruction involves the use of thin-calibered tubes that can successfully create a fine realistic helical rim when meticulous technique is utilized in conjunction with careful case selection (Fig. 13-11). Minor burns often destroy the helical rim and yet leave the auriculocephalic sulcus skin intact, thus providing a superb site for tube construction [104] while minimizing tube migration and the risk of failure and secondary deformity (Fig. 13-11).

If good local skin is unavailable, only then should utilization of a distal tube be considered. Although this method of helical reconstruction should be discreetly reserved for select cases, if one adheres to meticulous technique it is reasonable to consider supraclavicular tubes in males and transverse cervical tubes in elderly patients (Figs. 13-11 and 13-14).

The success of these tiny tubes relies on several important details. One must construct the tube from an 11- to 12-cm. bipedicle flap, which is ideally 13 to 14 mm. wide with a 1.5- to 2-cm. central bridge. In effect, this creates two 5-cm. tubes that are joined 3 to 4 weeks later by tubing the bridge and forming one continuous structure with a caliber that permits the formation of a realistic rim; the excessive length of the structure allows for shrinkage during the transfers. The tube is then allowed to mature sufficiently before subsequent, unhurried migrations are begun.

Upper-Third Auricular Defects

Upper-third defects may be reconstructed by several major methods. Usually, minor losses are confined to the rim and are repaired either by helical advancement, as previously described (Fig. 13-12A), or by a readily accessible preauricular flap (Fig. 13-12C).

Intermediate losses of the upper third are repaired with a banner flap, as described by Crikelair [105]. This flap is based anterosuperiorly in the auriculocephalic sulcus (Fig. 13-12E); it should be used in conjunction with a small cartilage graft to ensure a good long-term result.

Major losses in the superior third are most successfully reconstructed with a contralateral conchal cartilage graft, as classically described in 1955 by Adams [53]. In utilizing this technique, the surgeon must anchor the cartilage graft to the cartilaginous remnant of the helical root by means of a suture placed through a small incision at that point. This prevents the cartilage graft from drifting and ensures helical

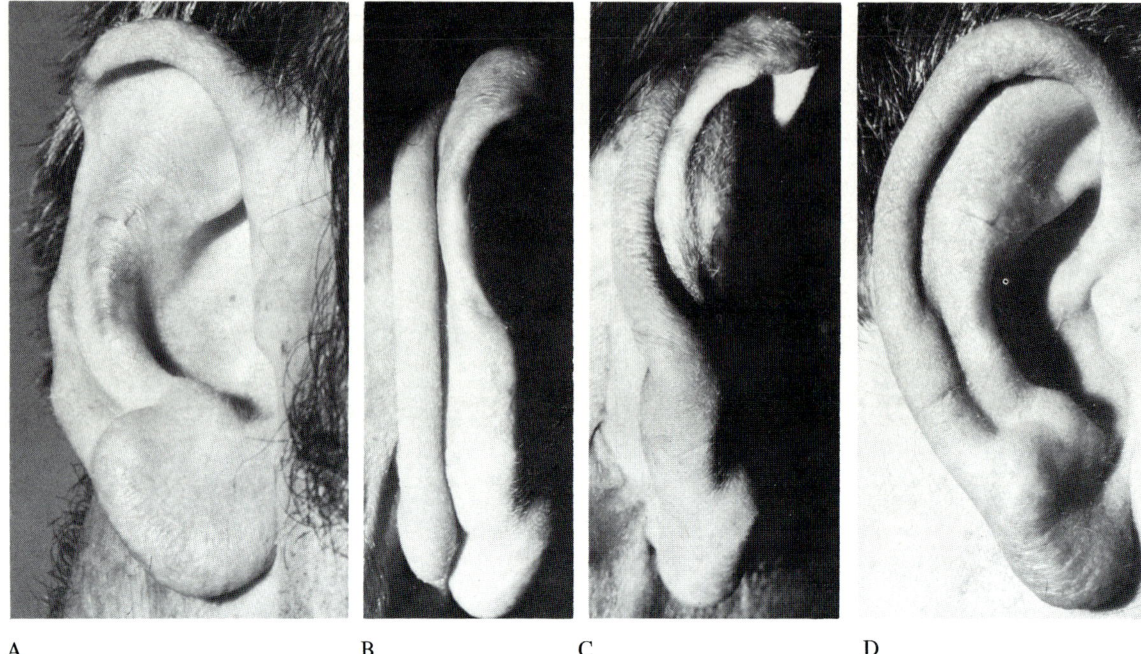

Fig. 13-11. Helical reconstruction with thin-calibered tubes. A, burn deformity of the helix. B, C, the construction and migration of a tube formed in the auriculocephalic sulcus. D, the final result. (From B. Brent, The acquired auricular deformity. A systemic approach to its analysis and reconstruction. Plast. Reconstr. Surg. *59:475, 1977.)*

continuity (Fig. 13-9).

If the existing skin is unfavorable for the above technique, the entire concha may be rotated upward as a chondrocutaneous composite flap on a small anterior pedicle of the crus helix as previously described [106]. This is a demanding procedure technically, and it is restricted to individual instances in which a large concha exists (Fig. 13-12G).

Middle-Third Auricular Defects

Major middle-third auricular defects are usually repaired with a cartilage graft that is either inserted via the Converse tunnel procedure [8], or covered by an adjacent skin flap (Fig. 13-10). Occasionally, conditions may favor a specially prepared composite graft as described previously (Fig. 13-13A, B, C, D).

Middle-third auricular tumors are excised and closed either by a wedge resection with accessory triangles (Fig. 13-13H) or by a helical advancement, as previously described (Fig. 13-13F).

Lower-Third Auricular Defects

Lower-third losses that encompass more than earlobe tissue are an especially complex challenge, and must include a cartilage graft to provide the support necessary to ensure long-term contour.

Although Preaux [114] has described an impressive technique for repairing lower-third defects by means of a superiorly based flap doubled upon itself, I find that contour and support are created and maintained with less risk by primarily inserting a contra-

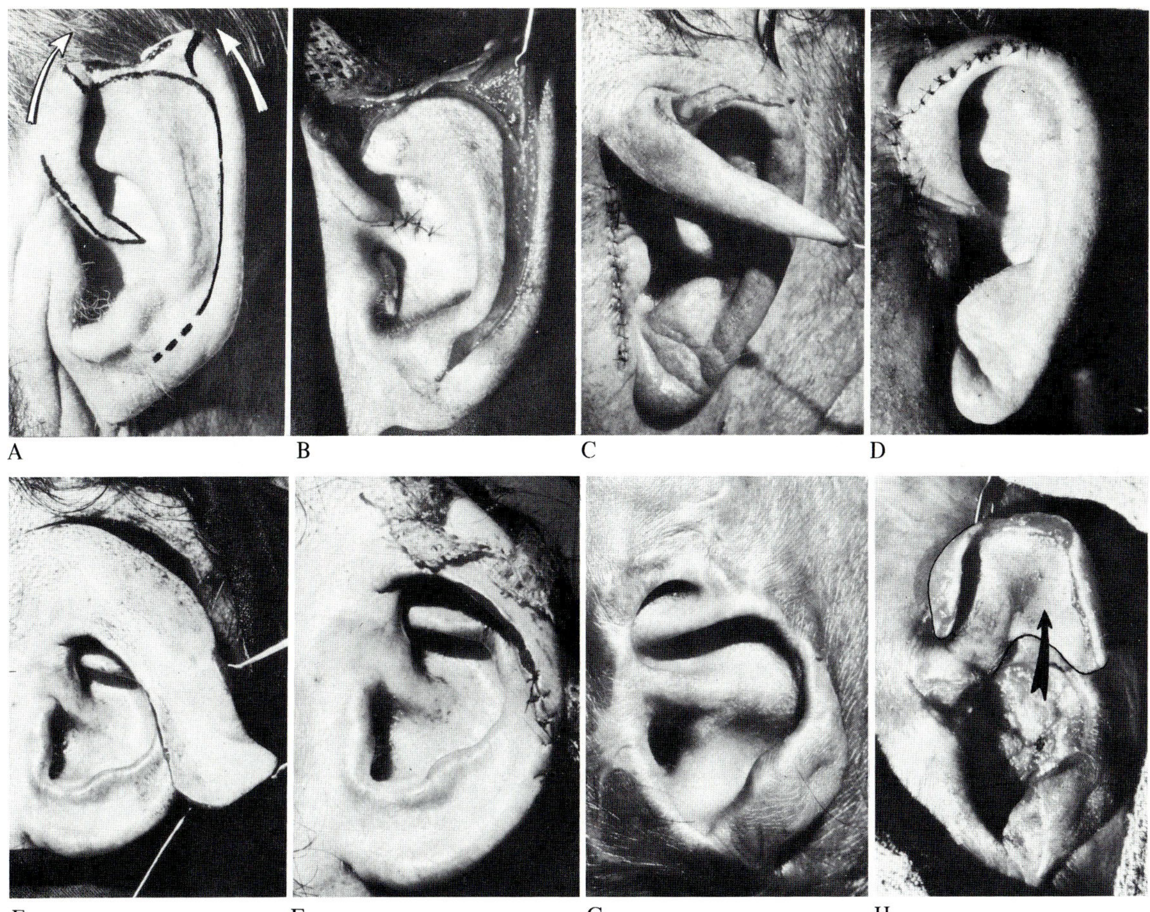

Fig. 13-12. Four different techniques of repairing upper third auricular defects using local flaps. A, B, the advancement of chondrocutaneous helical flaps (after Antia and Buch [97]). Note the extra length gained by V-Y advancement of the crus helix. C, D, the preauricular flap is transposed to repair the minor rim defect. E, F, the banner flap is raised from the auriculocephalic sulcus (after Crikelair [105]). G, H, the upper helicoscaphal thermal loss with a large residual concha favors the transposition of a chondrocutaneous conchal flap to recreate the upper third of the auricle (after Davis [106]). Both the donor bed and the raw surface of the newly created rim are to be grafted. (From B. Brent, The acquired auricular deformity. A systematic approach to its analysis and reconstruction. Plast. Reconstr. Surg. *59:475, 1977.)*

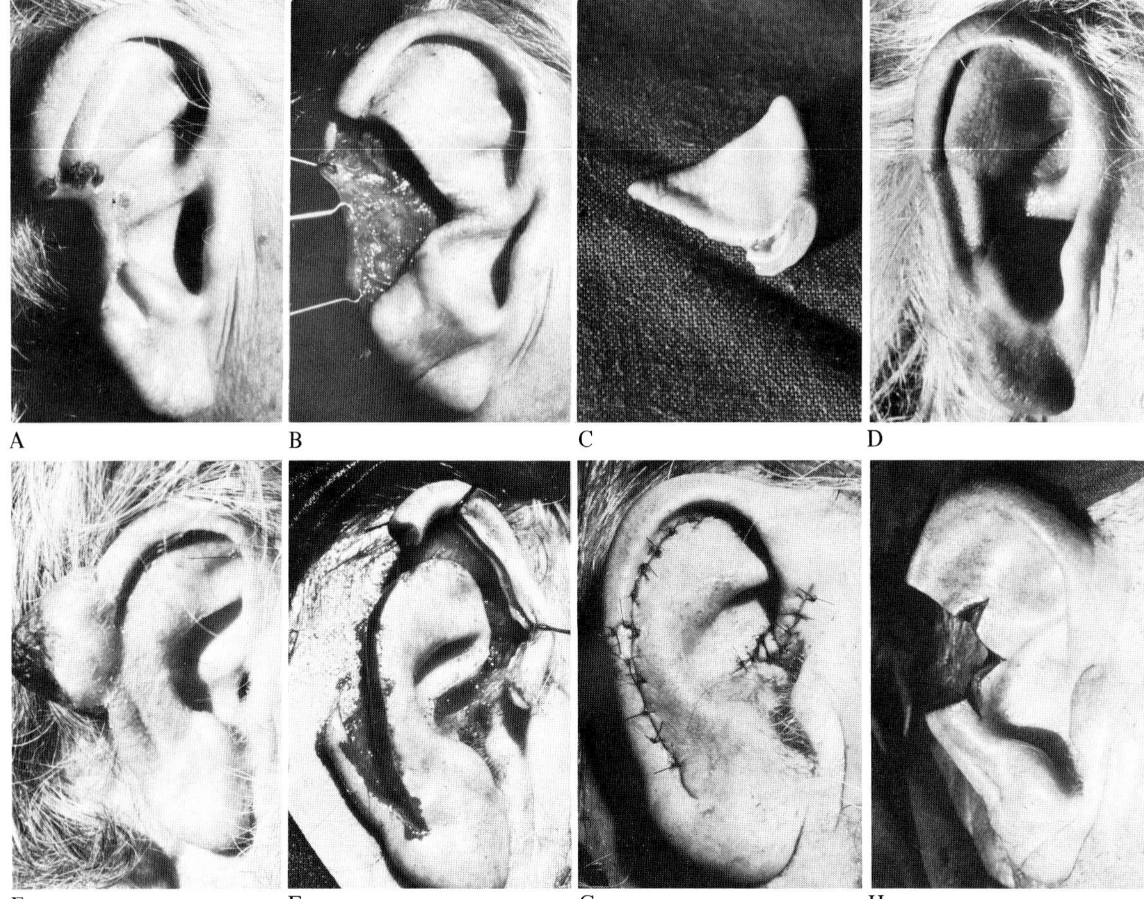

Fig. 13-13. Repair of defects of the middle third of the auricle. A, status after resection of chondrodermatitis in an 83-year-old patient. B, C, the residual diseased tissue is excised and the retroauricular flap is advanced to serve as a recipient bed for the specially prepared composite graft that is illustrated. The survival of the contralateral composite graft has been enhanced by removing the medial auricular skin and cartilage while preserving the cartilage strut in the helical rim for contour and support. (See text for further explanation.) D, the final result. E, large keratoacanthoma. F, G, the excision of the lesion and the preparation and advancement of helical flaps. Note the extent of dissection to mobilize the helix; a small Z-plasty was used to assure a clean splice. H, an alternate method of closure by V wedge. This closure is facilitated by excision of "accessory triangles" as illustrated. (From B. Brent, The acquired auricular deformity. A systematic approach to its analysis and reconstruction. Plast. Reconstr. Surg. *59:475, 1977.)*

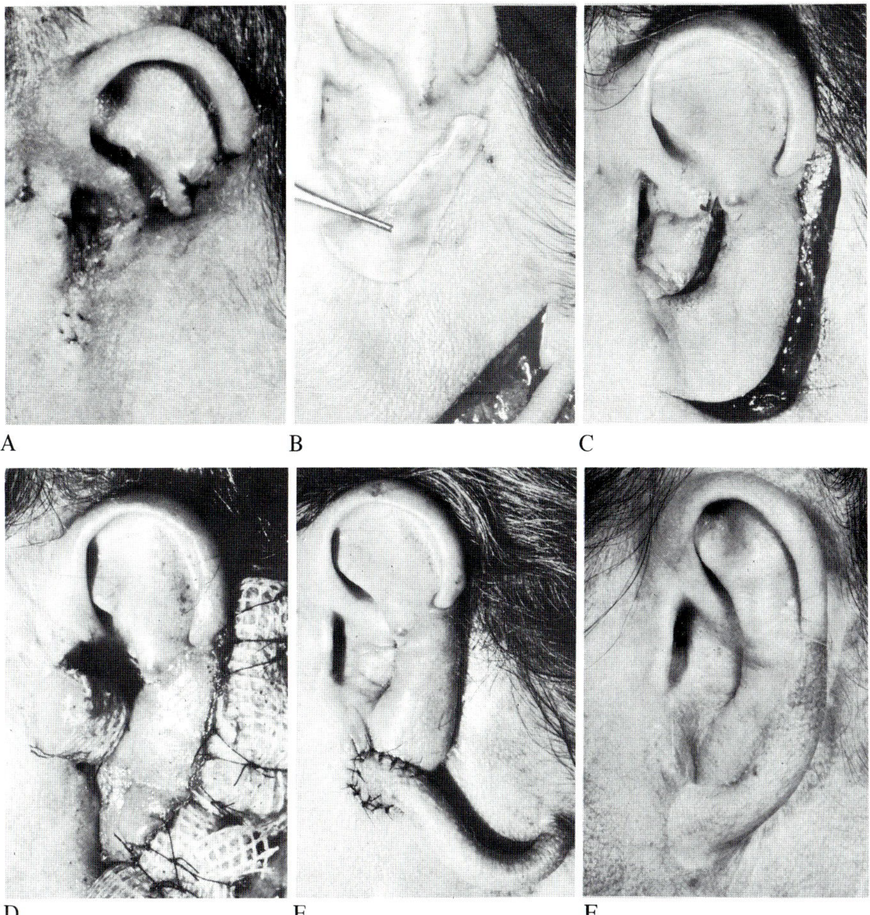

Fig. 13-14. Reconstruction of the lower half of the auricle. A, traumatic loss of the lower auricular region. B, a small cervical tube has been constructed; note that the lower margin of the severed auricle has been previously affixed to the adjacent retroauricular skin to ensure its continuity with the proposed reconstruction. C, D, 6 weeks later, parallel incisions are made adjacent to the previously implanted cartilage, and the composite strap of tissue is elevated and skin grafted; a T-shaped, pull-through, tie-over dressing is inserted. (See text for further explanation.) E, 1 month later, the nearby tube has been migrated to the ear; note the posterior conchal wall definition created by the "valise-handle" procedure. F, the final result, 18 months after insetting the tube. (From B. Brent, The acquired auricular deformity. A systematic approach to its analysis and reconstruction. Plast. Reconstr. Surg. *59:475, 1977.)*

lateral conchal cartilage graft subcutaneously in the proposed site of reconstruction (Fig. 13-14). After 6 weeks or more, the definition of the lower portion of the auricle is obtained by elevation through parallel incisions and creation of a bipedicle, chondrocutaneous composite flap that is backed with a skin graft, thus maintaining a permanent "valise-handle" effect similar to that described previously (see under Total Construction of the Microtic Ear) [32]. This "valise handle" deliberately creates a tunnel, which solves the always difficult task of maintaining definition in the posterior conchal wall region (Fig. 13-14). In addition, the "valise-handle" technique may be employed to simulate the inferior crus contour line (Fig. 13-9).

Acquired Earlobe Deformities

Traumatic clefts and keloids that result from ear piercing are the most common acquired defects of the earlobe. Cleft earlobes, usually occurring from the dramatic extraction of earrings, can be repaired most efficiently by means of Pardue's ingenious adjacent flap [113], which is rolled into the apex of the wedge repair, thus maintaining a tract lined with skin, which permits further use of earrings.

Another common occurrence in everyday practice is the earlobe keloid, which heretofore has been treated, with varying degrees of success, by irradiation and steroid injections [120, 122, 124]. Because there is strong evidence that pressure may play an important role in the future of keloid therapy [123, 125], I have recently developed a constant, light pressure-spring earring device, which suggests a new and effective method of preventing postexcisional recurrence of earlobe keloids [119]. At this time, the results seem encouraging.

Effective techniques for actual reconstruction of the earlobe have been described by Zenteno Alanis [116], Brent [110], and others [111, 112, 115]. Before undertaking any of these more sophisticated techniques, it is advisable to assess the residual local tissues carefully and contemplate the utilization of a simple repair; another option is to employ the helical advancement principle so as to move available tissue downward.

REFERENCES

Total Ear Reconstruction

1. Bǎrinka, L. Congenital malformations of the auricle and their reconstruction by a new method. *Acta Chir. Plast.* (Praha) 8:53, 1966.
2. Brent, B. Ear reconstruction with an expansile framework of autogenous rib cartilage. *Plast. Reconstr. Surg.* 53:619, 1974.
3. Brent, B. Reconstruction of ear, eyebrow, and sideburn in the burned patient. *Plast. Reconstr. Surg.* 55:312, 1975.
4. Broadbent, T. R., and Mathews, V. L. Artistic relationships in surface anatomy of the face: Application to reconstructive surgery. *Plast. Reconstr. Surg.* 20:1, 1957.
5. Broadbent, T. R., and Woolf, R. M. Bilateral Microtia. A Team Approach to the Middle Ear. In Tanzer, R. C., and Edgerton, M. T. (Eds.), *Symposium on Reconstruction of the Auricle.* St. Louis: Mosby, 1974.
6. Brody, G. S. Use of disposable razor band to carve cartilage. *Plast. Reconstr. Surg.* 44:307, 1969.
7. Carroll, D. B. Experiences with Silastic Implants and Autogenous Cartilage in the Treatment of Microtia. In Tanzer, R. C., and Edgerton, M. T. (Eds.), *Symposium on Reconstruction of the Auricle.* St. Louis: Mosby, 1974.
8. Converse, J. M. Reconstruction of the auricle. Parts I and II. *Plast. Reconstr. Surg.* 22:150, 230, 1958.
9. Converse, J. M. Construction of the auricle in congenital microtia. *Plast. Reconstr. Surg.* 32:425, 1963.
10. Cronin, T. D. Use of a Silastic frame for total and subtotal reconstruction of the external ear: Preliminary report. *Plast. Reconstr. Surg.* 37:399, 1966.
11. Cronin, T. D. Use of a Silastic Frame for Construction of the Auricle. In Tanzer, R. C., and Edgerton, M. T. (Eds.), *Symposium on Reconstruction of the Auricle*. St. Louis: Mosby, 1974.
12. Curtin, J. W., and Bader, K. F. Improved techniques for the successful silicone reconstruction of the external ear. *Plast. Reconstr. Surg.* 44:372, 1969.
13. Dupertius, S. M., and Musgrave, R. H. Experiences with the reconstruction of the congenitally deformed ear. *Plast. Reconstr. Surg.* 23:361, 1959.
14. Farkas, L. Growth of Normal and Reconstructed Auricles. In Tanzer, R. C., and Edgerton, M. T. (Eds.), *Symposium on Reconstruction of the Auricle.* St. Louis: Mosby, 1974.
15. Fox, J. W., and Edgerton, M. T. The fan flap: An adjunct to ear reconstruction. *Plast. Reconstr. Surg.* 58:663, 1976.
16. Fukuda, O. The microtic ear: Survey of 180 cases in 10 years. *Plast. Reconstr. Surg.* 53:458, 1974.
17. Gorney, M., Murphy, S., and Falces, E. Spliced autogenous conchal cartilage in secondary ear reconstruction. *Plast. Reconstr. Surg.* 47:432, 1971.
18. Kaye, B. L. "Home-made" suction drain for small areas. *Plast. Reconstr. Surg.* 52:447, 1973.
19. Kirkham, H. L. D. The use of preserved cartilage in ear reconstruction. *Ann. Surg.* 111:896, 1940.
20. Knorr, N. J., Edgerton, M. T., and Barberie, M. Psychologic Factors in Reconstruction of the Ear.

In Tanzer, R. C., and Edgerton, M. T. (Eds.), *Symposium on Reconstruction of the Auricle.* St. Louis: Mosby, 1974.
21. Letterman, G. S., and Harding, R. L. The management of the hairline in ear reconstruction. *Plast. Reconstr. Surg.* 18:199, 1956.
22. Lindsay, W. K. The growth of ear frameworks constructed of autogenous costal cartilage in 2-year-old children. Personal communication, 1976.
23. Lynch, J. B., Pousti, A., Doyle, J. E., and Lewis, S. R. Our experiences with Silastic ear implants. *Plast. Reconstr. Surg.* 49:283, 1972.
24. Ohmori, S., Matsumoto, K., and Nakai, H. Follow-up study on reconstruction of microtia with a silicone framework. *Plast. Reconstr. Surg.* 53:555, 1974.
25. Ohmori, S., and Nakai, H. A refined approach to Silastic ear reconstruction: Preliminary report. Presented at the Annual meeting of the American Society of Plastic and Reconstructive Surgeons. Boston, September 1976.
26. Pierce, G. W. Reconstruction of the external ear. *Surg. Gynecol. Obstet.* 50:601, 1930.
27. Rogers, B. O. Microtic, lop, cup, and protruding ears. *Plast. Reconstr. Surg.* 41:208, 1968.
28. Rogers, B. O. Anatomy, Embryology, and Classification of Auricular Deformities. In Tanzer, R. C., and Edgerton, M. T. (Eds.), *Symposium on Reconstruction of the Auricle.* St. Louis: Mosby, 1974.
29. Spina, V. Kamakura, L., and Psillakis, J. M. Total reconstruction of the ear in congenital microtia. *Plast. Reconstr. Surg.* 48:349, 1971.
30. Steffensen, W. H. Comments on reconstruction of the external ear. *Plast. Reconstr. Surg.* 16:194, 1955.
31. Steffensen, W. H. A method of total ear reconstruction. *Plast. Reconstr. Surg.* 36:97, 1965.
32. Tanzer, R. C. Total reconstruction of the external ear. *Plast. Reconstr. Surg.* 23:1, 1959.
33. Tanzer, R. C. An analysis of ear reconstruction. *Plast. Reconstr. Surg.* 31:16, 1963.
34. Tanzer, R. C. Total reconstruction of the auricle: A 10-year report. *Plast. Reconstr. Surg.* 40:547, 1967.
35. Tanzer, R. C. Secondary reconstruction of microtia. *Plast. Reconstr. Surg.* 43:345, 1969.
36. Tanzer, R. C. Total reconstruction of the auricle. The evolution of a plan of treatment. *Plast. Reconstr. Surg.* 47:523, 1971.
37. Tanzer, R. C. Correction of Microtia with Autogenous Costal Cartilage. In Tanzer, R. C., and Edgerton, M. T. (Eds.), *Symposium on Reconstruction of the Auricle.* St. Louis: Mosby, 1974.
38. Tanzer, R. C., and Chaisson, R. A protective guard for use during reconstruction of the auricle. *Plast. Reconstr. Surg.* 53:236, 1974.
39. Tanzer, R. C., Converse, J. M., and Brent, B. Deformities of the Auricle. In Converse, J. M. (Ed.), *Reconstructive Plastic Surgery* (2nd ed.). Philadelphia: Saunders, 1977.
40. Tegtmeier, R. E., and Gooding, R. A. The use of a fascial flap in ear reconstruction. *Plast. Reconstr. Surg.* 60:406, 1977.

Ear Prostheses

41. Bulbulian, A. H. *Facial Prosthetics.* Springfield, Ill.: Thomas, 1973.
42. Simons, J. N. The Role of the Prosthesis in Correction of Ear Deformities. In Tanzer, R. C., and Edgerton, M. T. (Eds.), *Symposium on Reconstruction of the Auricle.* St. Louis: Mosby, 1974.
43. Snow, R. S. An improved ear prosthesis in silicone rubber incorporating an adhesive surface. *Br. J. Plast. Surg.* 28:289, 1975.

Cartilage and Perichondrial Grafting

44. Brent, B., and Ott, R. Perichondro-cutaneous graft. *Plast. Reconstr. Surg.* 62:1, 1978.
45. Gibson, T., and Davis, W. B. The distortion of autogenous cartilage grafts: Its cause and prevention. *Br. J. Plast. Surg.* 10:257, 1957.
46. Hagerty, R. F., Braid, H. L., Bonner, W. M., Hennigar, G. R., and Lee, W. H. Viable and nonviable human cartilage homografts. *Surg. Gynecol. Obstet.* 125:485, 1967.
47. Hagerty, R. F., Calhoon, T. B., Lee, W. H., and Cuttino, J. T. Characteristics of fresh human cartilage. *Surg. Gynecol. Obstet.* 110:3, 1960.
48. Hagerty, R. F., Calhoon, T. B., Lee, W. H., and Cuttino, J. T. Human cartilage grafts stored in air. *Surg. Gynecol. Obstet.* 110:433, 1960.
49. Ohlsén, L. Cartilage formation from free perichondrial grafts: An experimental study in rabbits. *Brit. J. Plast. Surg.* 29:262, 1976.
50. Skoog, T., and Johansson, S. H. The formation of articular cartilage from free perichondrial grafts. *Plast. Reconstr. Surg.* 57:1, 1976.
51. Skoog, T., Ohlsén, L., and Sohn, S. A. The chondrogenic potential of the perichondrium. *Chir. Plast.* 3:91, 1975.
52. Sohn, S. A., and Ohlsén, L. Growth of cartilage from a free perichondrial graft placed across a defect in a rabbit's trachea. *Plast. Reconstr. Surg.* 53:55, 1974.

Grafts of Conchal Cartilage

53. Adams, W. M. Construction of upper half of auricle utilizing composite concha cartilage graft with perichondrium attached to both sides. *Plast. Reconstr. Surg.* 16:88, 1955.
54. Brent, B. The acquired auricular deformity: A sys-

tematic approach to its analysis and reconstruction. *Plast. Reconstr. Surg.* 59:475, 1977.
55. Davis, J. Repair of Severe Cup Ear Deformities. In Tanzer, R. C., and Edgerton, M. T. (Eds.), *Symposium on Reconstruction of the Auricle.* St. Louis: Mosby, 1974.
56. Falces, E., and Gorney, M. Use of ear cartilage grafts for nasal tip reconstruction. *Plast. Reconstr. Surg.* 50:147, 1972.
57. Gorney, M. The Ear as a Donor Site. In Tanzer, R. C., and Edgerton, M. T. (Eds.), *Symposium on Reconstruction of the Auricle.* St. Louis: Mosby, 1974.
58. Gorney, M., Murphy, S., and Falces, E. Spliced autogenous conchal cartilage in secondary ear reconstruction. *Plast. Reconstr. Surg.* 47:432, 1971.
59. Stark, R. B., and Frileck, S. P. Conchal cartilage grafts in augmentation rhinoplasty and orbital floor fracture. *Plast. Reconstr. Surg.* 43:591, 1969.

Acquired Auricular Deformity

60. Brent, B. The acquired auricular deformity: A systematic approach to its analysis and reconstruction. *Plast. Reconstr. Surg.* 59:475, 1977.
61. Tanzer. R. C. The reconstruction of acquired defects of the ear. *Plast. Reconstr. Surg.* 35:355, 1965.
62. Tanzer, R. C., Converse, J. M., and Brent, B. Deformities of the Auricle. In Converse, J. M. (Ed.), *Reconstructive Plastic Surgery* (2nd ed.). Philadelphia: Saunders, 1977.
63. Tanzer, R. C., and Edgerton, M. T. *Symposium on Reconstruction of the Auricle.* St. Louis: Mosby, 1974.

Acute Auricular Trauma

64. Baudet, J., Tramond, P., and Goumain, A. A propos d'un procédé original de réimplantion d'un pavillon de l'oreille totalement séparé. *Ann. Chir. Plast.* 17:67, 1972.
65. Clemons, J. E., and Connelly, M. V. Reattachment of a totally amputated auricle. *Arch. Otolaryngol.* 97:269, 1973.
66. Edgerton, M. T. Discussion in Tanzer, R. C., and Edgerton, M. T. (Eds.), *Symposium on Reconstruction of the Auricle.* St. Louis: Mosby, 1974.
67. Gorney, M. Discussion of auricular trauma. In Tanzer, R. C., and Edgerton, M. T. (Eds.), *Symposium on Reconstruction of the Auricle.* St. Louis: Mosby, 1974.
68. Grabb, W. C., and Dingman, R. O. The fate of amputated tissues of the head and neck following replacement. *Plast. Reconstr. Surg.* 49:28, 1972.
69. Kellerher, J. C., Sullivan, J. G., Baibak, G. J., and Dean, R. K. The wrestler's ear. *Plast. Reconstr. Surg.* 40:540, 1967.
70. McDowell, F. W. Successful replantation of a severed half ear. *Plast. Reconstr. Surg.* 48:281, 1971.
71. Mladick, R. A., and Carraway, J. H. Ear reattachment by the modified pocket principle. *Plast. Reconstr. Surg.* 51:584, 1973.
72. Mladick, R. A., Horton, C. E., Adamson, J. E., and Cohen, B. I. The pocket principle, a new technique for the reattachment of a severed ear part. *Plast. Reconstr. Surg.* 48:219, 1971.
73. Musgrave, R. H., and Garrett, W. S. Management of avulsion injuries of the external ear. *Plast. Reconstr. Surg.* 40:534, 1967.
74. Ohlsén, L., Skoog, T., and Sohn, S. A. The pathogenesis of cauliflower ear. *Scand. J. Plast. Reconstr. Surg.* 9:34, 1975.
75. Sexton, R. P. Utilization of the amputated ear cartilage. *Plast. Reconstr. Surg.* 15:419, 1955.
76. Spira, M. Early Care of Deformities of the Auricle Resulting from Mechanical Trauma. In Tanzer, R. C., and Edgerton, M. T. (Eds.), *Symposium on Reconstruction of the Auricle.* St. Louis: Mosby, 1974.

Acute Auricular Burns

77. Apfelberg, D. B., Waisbren, B. A., Masters, F. W., and Robinson, D. W. Treatment of chondritis in the burned ear by the local instillation of antibiotics. *Plast. Reconstr. Surg.* 53:179, 1974.
78. Carroll, D. B. Early Treatment of Burned Ears. In Tanzer, R. C., and Edgerton, M. T. (Eds.), *Symposium on Reconstruction of the Auricle.* St. Louis: Mosby, 1974.
79. Collentine, G., Waisbren, B. A., and Mellendor, J. Treatment of burns with intensive antibiotic therapy and exposure. *J.A.M.A.* 200:939, 1967.
80. Dowling, J. A., Foley, F. D., and Moncrief, J. A. Chondritis in the burned ear. *Plast. Reconstr. Surg.* 42:115, 1968.
81. Edgerton, M. T. Discussion of helical exposure. In Tanzer, R. C., and Edgerton, M. T. (Eds.), *Symposium on Reconstruction of the Auricle.* St. Louis: Mosby, 1974.
82. Gorney, M. Discussion of auricular burns. In Tanzer, R. C., and Edgerton, M. T. (Eds.), *Symposium on Reconstruction of the Auricle.* St. Louis: Mosby, 1974.
83. Grant, D. A., Finley, M. L., and Coers, C. R. Early management of the burned ear. *Plast. Reconstr. Surg.* 44:161, 1969.
84. Moyer, C. A., Brentano, L., Gravens, D. L., Margraf, H. W., and Monafo, W. W. Treatment of large human burns with 0.5% silver nitrate solution. *Arch. Surg.* 90:812, 1965.

85. Tolleth, H. Local flap coverage of the burned helico-scaphal complex. Personal communication, 1975.

Composite Grafts

86. Aragamaso, R. V. An ideal donor site for the auricular composite graft. *Br. J. Plast. Surg.* 28:219, 1975.
87. Dufourmentel, C., and LePesteur, J. Les greffes auriculaires composées dans la reconstruction de l'étage inférieur de la pyramide nasale. A propos de 43 greffes. *Ann. Chir. Plast.* 18:199, 1973.
88. Nagel, F. Reconstruction of a partial auricular loss. *Plast. Reconstr. Surg.* 49:340, 1972.
89. Pegram, M., and Peterson, R. Repair of partial defects of the ear. *Plast. Reconstr. Surg.* 18:305, 1956.
90. Symonds, F. C., and Crikelair, G. F. Auricular composite grafts in nasal reconstruction: A report of 36 cases. *Plast. Reconstr. Surg.* 37:433, 1966.

Auditory Canal

91. Conley, J. J. Atresia of the external auditory canal occurring in military service. *Arch Otolaryngol.* 43:613, 1946.
92. Gingrass, R. P., and Pickrell, K. L. Techniques for closure of conchal and external auditory canal defects. *Plast. Reconstr. Surg.* 41:568, 1968.
93. Macomber, W. B., Wang, M. K., and Lueders, H. W. Reconstruction of the traumatically stenosed external auditory canal. *Plast. Reconstr. Surg.* 22:168, 1958.
94. Owens, N. An effective method for closing defects of the external auditory canal. *Plast. Reconstr. Surg.* 23:381, 1959.
95. Pennisi, V. R., Klabunde, E. H., and Pierce, G. W. The preauricular flap. *Plast. Reconstr. Surg.* 35:552, 1965.
96. Steffensen, W. H. A method of correcting atresia of the ear canal. *Plast. Reconstr. Surg.* 1:329, 1946.

Helical Reconstruction

97. Antia, N. H., and Buch, M. S. Chondrocutaneous advancement flap for the marginal defect of the ear. *Plast. Reconstr. Surg.* 39:472, 1967.
98. Argamaso, R. V., and Lewin, M. L. Repair of partial ear loss with local composite flap. *Plast. Reconstr. Surg.* 42:437, 1968.
99. Cronin, T. D. One stage reconstruction of the helix: Two improved methods. *Plast. Reconstr. Surg.* 9:547, 1952.
100. Fan-Hu, K., Hung-Yin, C., and Chu-Jen, H. Experience in the plastic repair of the burned ear. *Chin. Med. J.* 85:47, 1966.
101. Kazanjian, V. H., and Converse, J. M. Traumatic Deformities of the Auricle. In *Surgical Treatment of Facial Injuries* (3rd ed.). Baltimore: Williams & Wilkins, 1974.
102. Lewin, M. L. Formation of the helix with a postauricular flap. *Plast. Reconstr. Surg.* 5:432, 1950.
103. McNichol, J. W. Total helix reconstruction with tubed pedicles following loss by burns. *Plast. Reconstr. Surg.* 6:373, 1950.
104. Steffanoff, D. N. Auriculo-mastoid tube pedicle for otoplasty. *Plast. Reconstr. Surg.* 3:352, 1948.

Upper Auricular Reconstruction

105. Crikelair, G. F. A method of partial ear reconstruction for avulsion of the upper portion of the ear. *Plast. Reconstr. Surg.* 17:438, 1956.
106. Davis, J. Reconstruction of the Upper Third of the Ear with a Chondrocutaneous Composite Flap Based on the Crus Helix. In Tanzer, R. C., and Edgerton, M. T. (Eds.), *Symposium on Reconstruction of the Auricle.* St. Louis: Mosby, 1974.
107. Millard, D. R. The chondrocutaneous flap in partial auricular repair. *Plast. Reconstr. Surg.* 37:53, 1966.
108. Navabi, A. One-stage reconstruction of partial defect of the auricle. *Plast. Reconstr. Surg.* 33:77, 1964.
109. Spina, V. A simpler method of partial reconstruction of the external ear. *Plast. Reconstr. Surg.* 13:488, 1953.

Lower Auricular and Earlobe Reconstruction

110. Brent, B. Earlobe construction with an auriculomastoid flap. *Plast. Reconstr. Surg.* 57:389, 1976.
111. Guerrero-Santos, J. Correction of hypertrophied earlobes in leprosy. *Plast. Reconstr. Surg.* 46:381, 1970.
112. Paletta, F. X. *Trauma. Pediatric Plastic Surgery,* Vol. I. St. Louis: Mosby, 1967.
113. Pardue, A. M. Repair of torn earlobe with preservation of the perforation for an earring. *Plast. Reconstr. Surg.* 51:472, 1973.
114. Preaux, J. Un procédé simple de reconstruction de la partie inférieure du pavillon de l'oreille. *Ann. Chir. Plast.* 16:244, 1971.
115. Subba Rao, Y. V., and Venkaleswara Roa, P. A quick technique for earlobe reconstruction. *Plast. Reconstr. Surg.* 41:13, 1968.
116. Zenteno Alanis, S. A new method for earlobe reconstruction. *Plast. Reconstr. Surg.* 45:254, 1970.

Auricular Tumors and Keloids

117. Arons, M. S., and Savin, R. C. Auricular cancer.

Some surgical and pathologic considerations. *Am. J. Surg.* 122:770, 1971.

118. Blake, G. B., and Wilson, J. S. P. Malignant tumours of the ear and their treatment. *Br. J. Plast. Surg.* 27:67, 1974.
119. Brent, B. The role of pressure therapy in management of earlobe keloids: Preliminary report of a controlled study. *Ann. Plastic Surg.* 1:579, 1978.
120. Converse, J. M., and Stallings, J. O. Eradication of large auricular keloids by excision, skin grafting and intradermal injection of triamcinolone acetonide solution. *Plast. Reconstr. Surg.* 49:461, 1972.
121. Conway, H., and Howell, J. A. Carcinoma of the external ear. Analysis of 100 consecutive cases. *Plast. Reconstr. Surg.* 20:45, 1957.
122. Cosman, B., and Wolff, M. Bilateral earlobe keloids. *Plast. Reconstr. Surg.* 53:540, 1974.
123. Ketchum, L. D., Cohen, I. K., and Masters, F. W. Hypertrophic scars and keloids. *Plast. Reconstr. Surg.* 53:140, 1974.
124. Ramakrishnan, K. M., Thomas, K. P., and Sundararajan, C. R. Study of 1,000 patients with keloids in South India. *Plast. Reconstr. Surg.* 53:276, 1974.
125. Snyder, G. B. Button compression for keloids of the lobule. *Br. J. Plast. Surg.* 27:186, 1974.

14

Reconstruction of the Nose

RONALD R. CAMERON

The nose occupies the most prominent position of the face, a position that makes it vulnerable to distortion by trauma and the most frequent feature involved with skin cancer. It may be ravaged by an infectious process or deformed by congenital abnormality. The reconstructive surgeon may find himself faced with a minor deformity or with the total loss of nasal tissue, either of which may be a major problem to the patient who is unable to disguise this imperfection.

The degree of loss and deformity will usually dictate the type and quantity of tissue required for correction. For the most satisfactory reconstruction the surgeon must consider all of the alternatives to reach the end point with the fewest number of procedures in the most predictable manner and leave the least amount of donor deformity. While few adult noses are attractive in their own right, still they have a definitiveness and at times a delicacy of shape that is demanding in its recreation.

The quality of the skin varies in different areas of the nose itself; the distal skin at times is thickened by sebaceous glands and is entirely unique in its character, while the proximal skin is usually thinner and more like the adjacent forehead or cheek skin. The structure is difficult to segmentalize. Though the domes, alae, columella, dorsum, and side walls have their own characteristics, they flow together to make up a single unit. In rebuilding, a decision must be made about whether to treat the reconstructed areas as a segment in itself or as a part of a larger segment. Hence, while only a portion of the tip may be missing, the best end result may be accomplished by reconstructing the entire tip or the entire nose. One should not discard portions of the nose without regard to the consequences, however. The fine curves of the alae, for instance, cannot be recreated by thick flap tissues with the same delicacy found in undisturbed tissues. The extent of repair may be delineated from the start. The patient may present with a clean, fresh injury or an old, healed one in which the vagaries of scar contracture have reached a mature end point. In such a case the alternatives for repair may be quickly narrowed. Many times this is not the case, however, and the surgeon is faced with a dirty wound perhaps caused by a high velocity missile, a nose that is not yet fully grown, or a neoplasm whose extent cannot be precisely delineated. In these cases all options must be considered until the extent of repair is known. As a generalization, when primary reconstruction can be carried out, the secondary effects of contracting scar on vulnerable cartilagenous tissues and inelastic skin may be considerably limited.

Techniques for utilization of a variety of tissues have been described for nasal reconstruction [6, 10, 18, 34, 55]. The tissues closest to the nose will give the best result, with the most natural appearance, if they are of good quality and satisfactory in quantity. In the adult patient, the surgeon should also consider reduction of the overall nasal size and hence the size of the defect, utilizing the standard techniques of rhinoplasty (particularly shortening the nose and lowering the dorsum). These procedures may also provide some raw materials of help in reconstruction.

The anatomy of the intact nose and its physiological purpose make unique demands for its reconstruction. The nose acts as a duct to filter, moisturize, and moderate the temperature of adequate quantities of air passing to the lungs. Although much of the function of the nose may be compromised when it is necessary to reconstruct the entire structure, as much as possible of the physiology should be preserved with lesser defects. The nose is made up proximally by a rigid bony vault and distally by a cartilagenous superstructure less rigid and hence more able to withstand minor trauma because of its somewhat pliable nature. Both areas are covered by skin externally with a minimum of subcutaneous tissue and by mucosa and skin internally; the internal mucosa and skin are applied directly to the supporting structures. The distal projection is supported not only by the midline septum, but also by thin leaves of cartilage within the outside walls; the cartilage derives strength from its shape and adherence to the lining and cover. Because of this combination, the structural shape is maintained and the airways do not collapse in spite of the strong air currents and repeated minor traumas to which the nose is subjected.

The *precise* surgical duplication of this structure except in relatively minor defects is essentially impossible. The techniques available to us are not well enough refined and the tissues available for rebuilding are too gross or different in character. Our objectives then must be twofold: (1) reconstruct the nose so that the appearance of this most prominent feature will attract a minimum of attention to its imperfection and (2) preserve its remaining physiological purpose. In this chapter a basic assumption will be that there has been loss of tissue and that reconstruction will require its replacement in some degree.

THE NASAL FRAMEWORK

In reconstruction of the tissues of the nose, the replacement of supporting and shaping structures, i.e., bone and cartilage, presents the three basic problems of (1) the determination of need, (2) the selection of the type and source of materials to be utilized, and (3) the timing of this part of the reconstruction.

The determination of need will rest on the residual skeletal framework remaining in place and on whether the soft tissues for cover and lining will require support. This support will serve two functions: projection of the soft tissue to maintain shape, and provision of stiffness in the walls to prevent collapse when the airstream passes through the nose. It is a seeming contradiction that many times a limited reconstruction will require skeletal support, while this need may be minimal in rebuilding of the entire nose. This occurs because the inherent support created by the thicker tissues necessary for complete reconstruction is often not present in the more delicate ones used in segmental replacement. Some degree of secondary contracture can be expected in large flap reconstructions, however, and maintenance of shape and projection will usually require some support in these cases.

The selection of the type and source of materials to be utilized is based on several variables. The material must be readily available, must provide the functions it is expected to perform, and must be likely to remain in place without creating secondary problems. As in most reconstruction, autogenous materials rate first consideration. Both bone and cartilage are usually available in adequate amounts. Bone provides greater predictability in maintenance of shape; however it is rigid and hence more subject to fracture with minor trauma when utilized as tip support.

Though limited in quantity, the septum may provide cartilage of good quality in thin strips or a broad sheet useful for building up the dorsum, providing side wall stiffness, or giving projection and definition to the tip. Millard has demonstrated the advancement of a chondromucosal L-shaped flap from residual septal structures to give projection and support to the nasal tip [56].

Cartilage may also be obtained from the helical or conchal areas of the ear or from the ribs. Ear cartilage is thin, and its strength is imparted to some degree by its shape. If it is possible to precisely pattern the cartilage removed and utilize it in its natural configuration, this strength will be maintained to some degree in the transfer. However, the resiliency of this material does tend to decrease with age. Care should be taken to minimize the donor ear deformity. Rib cartilage may have a tendency to warp in the healing process, though this tendency can be minimized by appropriate procurement of the graft [26]. Gibson and Davis [31] described excision of the cartilage graft in a "balanced cross section" that eliminates the distorting forces.

Bone may be procured from the septum in small pieces which have a delicacy not found elsewhere. These may be ideal for small areas of loss on the side walls or minor defects in the dorsum. When somewhat larger pieces are necessary, particularly for dorsal struts of the cantilever type, the clavicle and proximal ulna are satisfactory sites of procurement. Utilizing fine sharp osteotomes, a precise graft can be removed; the graft will be quite straight if the donor area is properly chosen. The ribs are also available and utilized principally in reconstruction in children. The major source for large grafts of bone is the iliac crest. This is mostly cancellous bone and may be difficult to sculpt finely, but it can be chiseled from the bed in a precise size; utilizing the anterior superior spine, an L-shaped configuration can be removed. In all cases the surgeon will benefit from creating the graft in the desired size and shape as much as possible directly in the bed from which it is removed. Whether cartilage or bone is being used, the graft should be refined to the least degree of bulk that will give satisfactory support and withstand the stresses of scar contracture and the degree of external trauma to which the nose will be subjected under normal circumstances.

TRANSFER AND FIXATION

There is considerable discussion as to the proper timing for placement of structural support in nasal reconstruction. This is because the variables here are unique to the feature. Delicate flaps and/or grafts will contract in healing if not properly supported; however, unless coverage of bone or cartilage is secure, exposure will result in their loss. These problems in general are best handled along the following guidelines:

1. Soft tissue replacements should be done in units so that the lines of scar contracture will least distort the structure when not supported.
2. Adequate or even slightly excessive amounts of soft tissue should be utilized to allow for some shrinkage.
3. Grafts of bone, cartilage, or other materials should not be transferred to the bed until their secure coverage has been assured. This certainly means that it should not be done in a wound that might be contaminated, and it should not be done until there is complete soft tissue healing with the return of softness and mobility to the tissues. This is not likely to occur for at least a month after soft tissue repair and usually not for several months.

Fixation of the supporting structures is usually indicated. Though cartilage does not need to be in intimate contact with other cartilage or bone to survive, both cartilage and bone must be secure in their position to prevent shifting and hence distortion of the reconstructed feature. This means anchoring the graft to an intact portion of the facial skeleton. Except in rare instances, a significant part of the nasal bony pyramid will be present. This can be grooved to accept the graft, which is then held with one or two wire sutures placed through drill holes in the bone [18]. A simple strut of bone so fixed will suffice in most cases and is called a *cantilever graft* (Fig. 14-1). Should there not be enough residual nasal bone to serve as a base, the graft will have to provide its own distal or tip support. This is done by fashioning the graft in an L shape and fixing its contacts with the facial skeleton by whatever method is available. Millard has described the placement of a proximal bone block as a base for supporting a cantilever bone graft in complete nasal loss [52].

There may be instances where the skeletal loss is segmental, with proximal and distal support, and where the simple provision of a pocket for the graft will be adequate. The surgeon is cautioned, however, to provide additional fixation in most cases, particularly if the graft is providing primary support and not simple augmentation of contour.

ALLOGRAFTS AND ALLOPLASTIC IMPLANTS

At this time the use of allografts and alloplastic implants in the primary reconstruction of the nose should be greatly limited. Although one is tempted by the availability of these materials, there are several reasons that make their use in nasal reconstruction undesirable.

Allograft tissues either fresh or preserved have the disadvantage of a higher degree of latent resorption than occurs with autografts [30]. The synthetic materials such as silicone will frequently become exposed if there is the slightest amount of stress on the tissues covering them. Once exposed, loss of the implant will usually occur. In either case, use is recommended only when autogenous tissue is not available (a rare instance) or when temporizing procedures are being carried out, as in children. Soft tissue coverage must be absolutely secure and stress on the implant absolutely minimal if long-term success is to be anticipated.

FREE SOFT TISSUE GRAFTS

A number of free soft tissue grafts have a significant place in nasal reconstruction not only when skin loss alone is present, but in conjunction with other types of repair. The proper utilization of these tissues can enhance the reconstruction, but the converse is also quite true. It is important to remember that free grafts depend on the ingrowth of blood vessels from the recipient bed for their survival. Bone or cartilage stripped of soft tissue coverage, dense scar, and irradiated tissues may not have the ability to produce these vessels in adequate supply, and grafting in these situations is contraindicated.

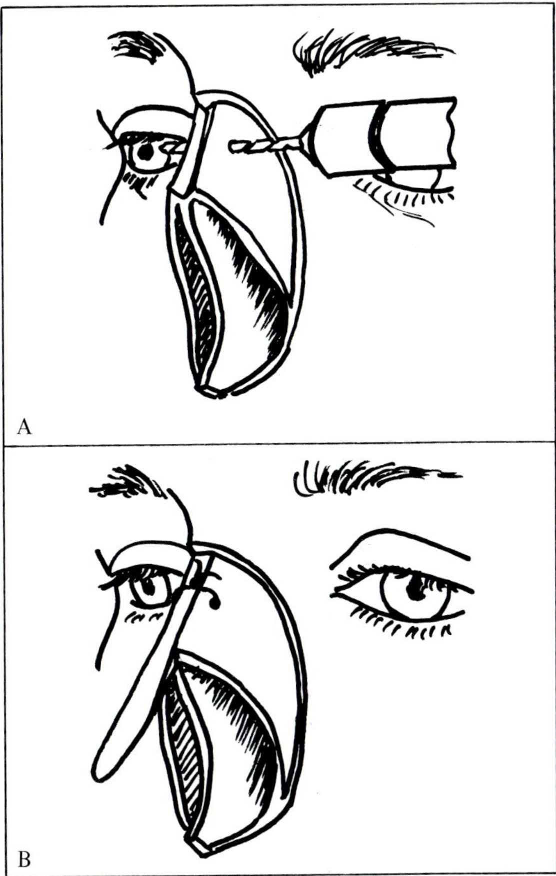

Fig. 14-1. Fixation of "cantilever" bone graft. A, the bone of dorsum is grooved with sharp chisel or bur. One or two holes are drilled through the intact bone. B, the bone graft is precisely fashioned to fit the groove and provide distal support; it is secured with a wire suture as indicated to maintain position. (After Converse [18] and others.)

Split-Thickness Skin Grafts

Split-thickness skin has a limited usefulness in this type of repair. Large areas of skin loss are usually accompanied by subcutaneous tissue loss of some degree, and thicker tissue is needed for replacement. The contracture of split skin is also a disadvantage on the nose. There are cases, however, in which the split graft may be used for cover; in these cases the best donor areas are the neck, infraclavicular, lateral chest, and inframammary areas, in that order of preference for color match [24]. Utilization of the neck and inframammary areas is often associated with secondary donor site changes that must be considered because of the difficulty in covering these areas, particularly in women. Grafts from other areas are usually of poor color and texture, and they should be avoided except to provide lining.

Full-Thickness Skin Grafts

When the defect requiring coverage needs only skin, the full-thickness graft is the one of choice in most instances. With a satisfactory take of the graft, there is little contraction and texture is more nearly normal if the donor site is carefully chosen. Postauricular skin is the most popular for facial resurfacing, and in many instances it produces a satisfactory result on the nose. Nasolabial, upper eyelid, and supraclavicular skin can also be utilized [4]. Bennett and Thurston [5] describe the use of preauricular skin for good match of color and texture with minimal donor deformity. They also suggest that angular defects as opposed to oval or round ones will heal with less residual deformity when grafted. I would agree that this technique – or even more radical segmentalization of the defect – will frequently disguise the deformity to the patient's benefit. In all cases the surgeon should analyze the particular color and texture characteristics of the patient at hand and utilize donor skin that will most closely match that to be replaced. In general the skin about the root of the nose will be lighter in color, thinner, and smoother in texture than that at the tip.

Composite Grafts

Composite grafts are those that concurrently utilize more than one type of tissue. The ear, by virtue of its dense vascularity and unique structure of skin closely apposed to cartilage (in most areas on two sides), is an excellent source for such grafts in small defects of the nose [8, 9, 33, 44]. Grafts of full-thickness skin from the postauricular crease with a small amount of subjacent fat still attached are helpful in depressed defects about the nasal tip. The border of the ear lobe with skin and fat may be used to fill a small columellar deficit (Fig. 14-2A).

Appropriate portions of the ear with its skin and cartilage may be selected to reconstruct the alae, tip, columella, and nasal side walls. Since the usual composite graft should not be larger than 2 cm. in greatest dimension (or 1 cm. from the recipient area blood supply), there are definite limits to such reconstruction. The posterosuperior portion of the helical rim is most often used; if the graft is small enough and removes as a wedge, the donor area may be closed primarily with minimal defect. Larger portions removed may leave deformities that must be repaired with sliding flaps or other methods. Cartilage grafts from the conchal area with the postauricular skin and/or conchal skin attached are sometimes appropriate to fill side wall nasal defects (Fig. 14-2D).

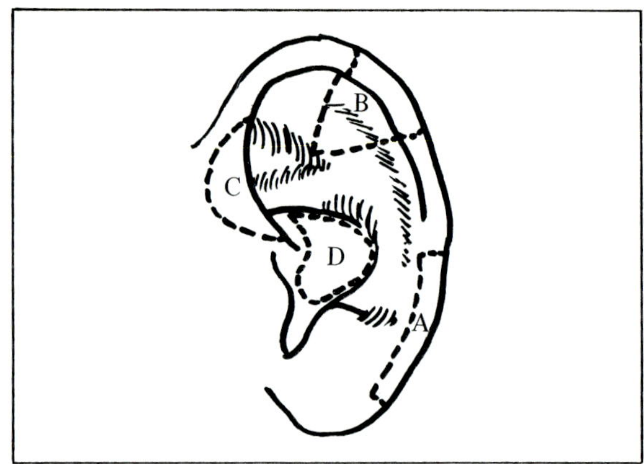

Fig. 14-2. Common areas for securing composite grafts from the ear. A, *skin and fat for columellar replacement.* B *and* C, *cartilage with skin on the anterior and posterior surfaces for the alar rim.* D, *conchal floor for side wall, dome, and upper lateral cartilage replacement.*

When utilizing composite grafts, the recipient area should be developed to enable the base to bear maximum circulation. For instance, if tissue adjacent to an alar defect can be turned down to form the lining and a viable bed for an overlying cartilage-skin composite graft, the chances of successful take will be enhanced (Fig. 14-3). Should this not be possible, meticulous technique in the excision of the scar about the periphery of the defect, careful hemostasis, accurate tailoring of the graft to the defect, support from within with light packing, and postoperative iced compresses for 48 to 72 hours will favor survival of the graft [16, 60]. It is routine for these grafts to appear quite tenuous for several days; however, with careful attention to the details of transfer, success usually follows.

SKIN FLAPS

For most significant defects of nasal structure, flap tissue will prove the best reconstructive material. Myriad flaps have been described for these purposes derived from local, regional, or distant sources. The history of plastic surgery is intertwined with the use of flap tissue for nasal reconstruction. As early as 600 B.C., the ancient Hindus utilized first cheek and later forehead flaps to rebuild noses that had been cut off as punishment for theft, adultery, and other crimes

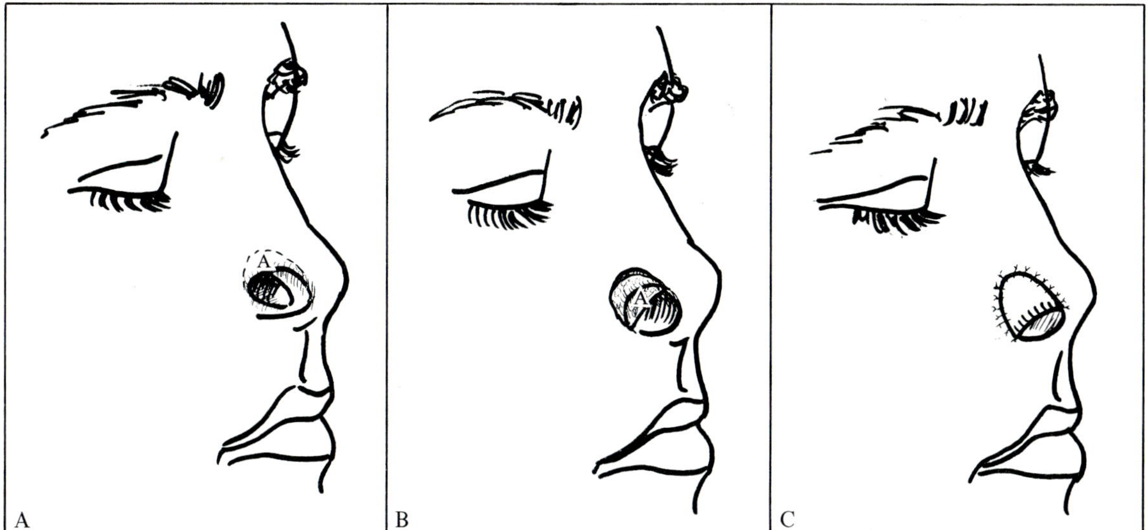

Fig. 14-3. Composite graft of skin and cartilage to rebuild ala. A, loss of ala. B, the superior margin flap has been elevated and turned down as a hinge to provide lining and broaden the vascular base. C, the composite graft from the helical rim is sutured in place.

[13, 47, 51]. In the fifteenth and sixteenth centuries, the Brancas and Tagliocozzi carried out nasal reconstruction with arm flaps in a manner that is now classic [35, 66]. In the nineteenth century, European surgeons used these flaps; Dieffenbach described many variations in the mid 1800s [22, 23]. Further variations of these techniques closely paralleled the development of plastic surgery itself through the first and second world wars until the present time. There have been well over a thousand references in the surgical literature of the world on nasal reconstruction, most of them describing techniques for the use of flaps.

Flap tissue fulfills most of the requirements of nasal reconstruction. It is usually available in quantity that is adequate for rebuilding any part of the nose, or the entire nose, and in quality that matches the normal skin in acceptable color and consistency. Flaps can usually be prepared thin enough that their shape can be modeled and yet with enough resiliency to maintain contour, at least temporarily. When used as lining and cover, flap tissue presents a cleavage plane that will accept supporting bone or cartilage and provide it with intact cover. The tissue may be available from the nose itself, from the adjacent cheeks or forehead, or from other areas of the head and neck or other parts of the body. The choice of tissue source will depend on the requirements of the case.

Local Flaps

When the defect to be covered is small, local tissue for repair has the obvious advantages of similar color and consistency. The use of thicker flap tissue also obviates the depression that sometimes results when a graft is utilized for such a defect. Even though there is little redundancy of skin in the normal nose, some shifting is possible, utilizing various techniques. A simple rotational or "banner"-type flap often may be used when the defect is within or adjacent to the more mobile skin of the proximal two-thirds of the nose [25]. The flap is usually raised along the superior border of the defect with its base toward the cheek. Generally, the flap width should be equal to or greater than that of the defect, and it should be slightly longer than the defect. Rotation is made possible by undermining about the base. The donor area is closed primarily and the flap set into the defect. If there is difficulty in closure of the donor area, a second, smaller flap can be raised around the axis of rotation and utilized to fill the donor defect. This creates a bilobed flap; this type of flap is defined as one consisting of two lobes separated by an angle of approximately 90 degrees and based on a common pedicle [21, 71]. The angle between the flaps should be designed to take advantage of the skin laxity of the area in question.

Limberg [48] and Lister and Gibson [50] have thoroughly studied the physical properties of skin in regard to extensibility and the geometry of its transfer based on these limitations. These properties are important on the nasal surface, where there is minimal mobility over a convex surface. The Limberg flap is designed to close a rhomboid defect that has acute angles of 60 degrees and equal sides (Fig. 14-4). A

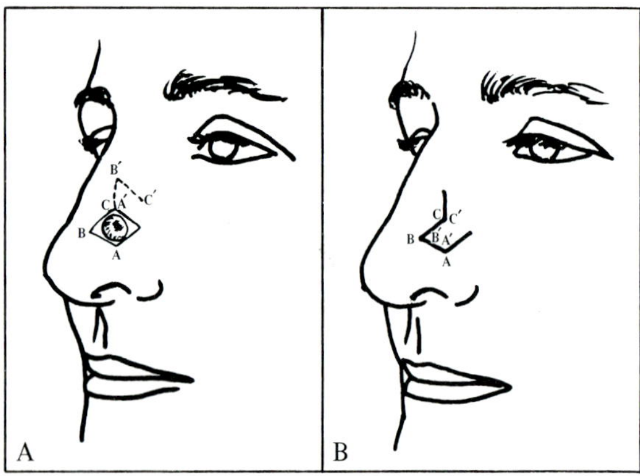

Fig. 14-4. Limberg flap. A, the lesion of the nasal wall is outlined for excision in rhomboid configuration. The Limberg-type flap is represented by a dotted line. B, the flap is rotated into position as indicated.

quadrangular flap is developed by extending the short axis of the defect a distance equal to one side of the defect and then cutting back at a 60-degree angle a similar distance [39, 48, 50]. This flap, like the simple rotational and bilobed flaps, should be designed to rotate about the axis of greatest mobility and skin extensibility, which minimizes the tension on closure of the donor area.

When a small local flap cannot be satisfactorily developed to cover a small defect, particularly about the nasal tip, the skin of the entire nose may be elevated and advanced or rotated to close such a deficit. Incisions are made at the juncture of the nose with the surrounding structures and adjacent to the defect, with a base maintained on the appropriate side. The tissue can then be advanced across the nose for defects on the opposite side [49] or rotated and advanced toward the tip [62]. These flaps have been satisfactory for coverage of defects up to 2 cm. wide in older individuals, but their use in younger persons should be limited [5].

Nasolabial Cheek Flaps

The tissue of both cheeks, particularly that outpouching directly lateral and superior to the juncture of the cheek and upper lip, has most of the qualities necessary for good nasal reconstruction (Fig. 14-5). It has the advantages of location, color match, excellent blood supply, minimal donor deformity, absence of hair, and ease of transfer (usually under local anesthesia) [12]. The most significant limitation to the use of this tissue is its quantity, though in appropriate patients with proper planning of the flaps almost the entire nasal dorsum can be resurfaced from this source [27] (Figs. 14-6, 14-7, and 14-8).

Under optimum circumstances nasolabial flaps up to 3 cm. in width and 10 cm. in length can be developed with relative safety. The only width limitation is that which prohibits primary donor site closure, and even this limitation can be overcome by utilizing the bilobed flap principle or rotation-advancement of cheek flaps. Delay is usually not necessary except when the flap is exceptionally long or narrow. These flaps may be based superiorly (when used to reconstruct the alae, nasal dorsum, etc.) or inferiorly (for the nasal floor, adjacent upper lip, septum, etc.). The flaps should be thin, consisting only of the skin and the immediately subdermal fat. This will generally not adversely affect circulation and it allows the doubling of the flap on itself to provide whatever lining and cover are required for alar reconstruction; however, it results in tissue which is not overly bulky [11].

Nasolabial flaps may be tubed to allow transfer across intact skin; these are transferred on subcutaneous pedicles and passed through incisions in the ala or side wall to reach the columella or septum [29]. These flaps may be used in combination with flaps from the other side and with grafts of skin and/or cartilage and bone. The versatility of this tissue (and that of the forehead) is dependent primarily on the ingenuity of the surgeon, and success is directly related to the care in planning and the technique.

Subcutaneous Pedicle and Island Flaps

When the need is for a limited quantity of skin and subcutaneous tissue for nasal reconstruction, the shifting of this tissue on subcutaneous or arterial pedicles may have some advantages. Principal among these are (1) the possibility of maintaining intact skin between donor and recipient areas, (2) the potential for minimizing "dog ears" and other deformities created by the rotation and advancement of tissues, and (3) the ability to bring flap tissue from a distance without intermediate steps (Fig. 14-9).

The arterial flap differs from the subcutaneous pedicle only in that a known artery is included within the pedicle [36, 41]. This allows for a longer pedicle, but otherwise the technique for transfer is quite similar. The pedicle in both of these flaps is developed in two planes, one subdermal and the other just superficial to the deep fascia (Fig. 14-9B). The pedicle should be somewhat longer than the distance from its base (point of rotation) to the recipient area. When a known artery is not included, the subcutaneous pedicle should be as wide as is convenient [2, 3].

Island flaps developed from the nasolabial folds may be adapted to defects of the nasal tip, dorsum, or side wall. They should be based laterally or inferiorly for the most dependable blood supply [37]. Those from the midforehead can be conveniently based on supratrochlear vessels [19] and those from the lateral forehead on the temporal vessels [36, 41].

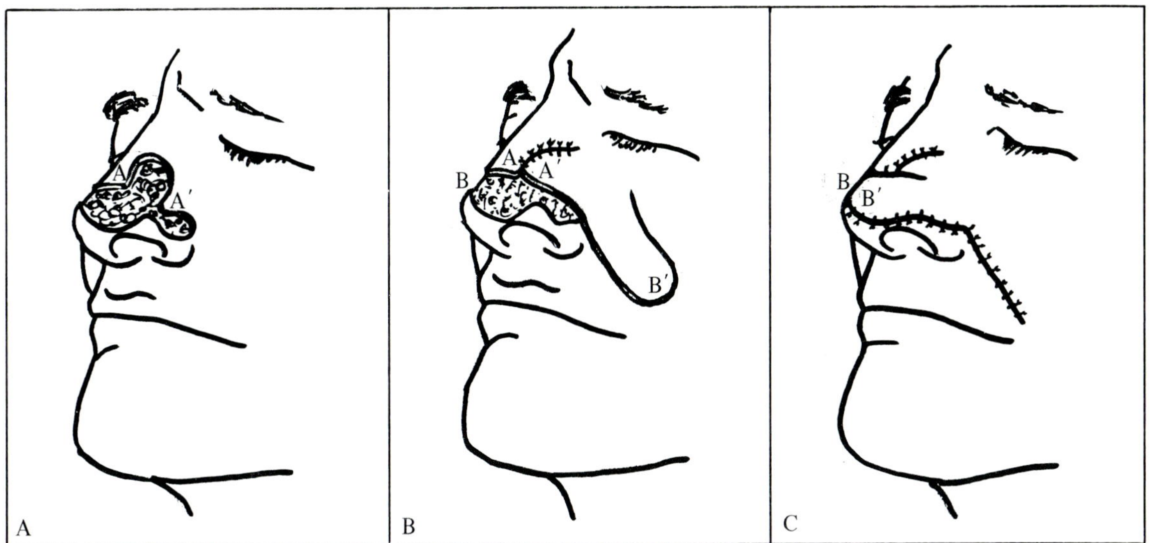

Fig. 14-5. A local rotational flap is used in conjunction with a nasolabial flap. A, the defect left by excision of three small, adjacent basal cell carcinomas is shown. B, the local flap A′ *is rotated and advanced to close the most superior portion of the defect. C, the nasolabial flap* B′ *is developed on the common pedicle with the local flap and rotated to cover the remaining defect.*

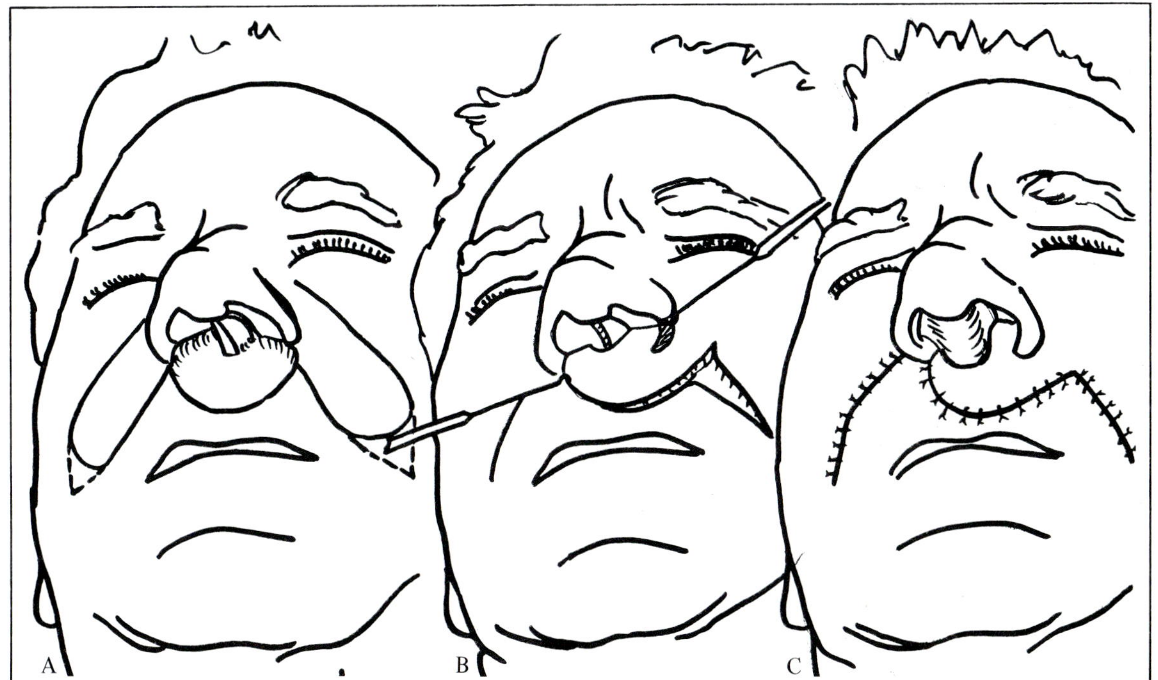

Fig. 14-6. Bilateral nasolabial flaps are utilized to reconstruct columellar and nasal floor defects. A, the defect from excision of large basal cell carcinoma and bilateral nasolabial flaps are outlined. B, the left nasolabial flap is rotated to cover the defect of the nasal floor and upper lip. C, the right nasolabial flap is passed through the incision in the alar fold to cover the columellar defect. (After Georgiade et al. [29].)

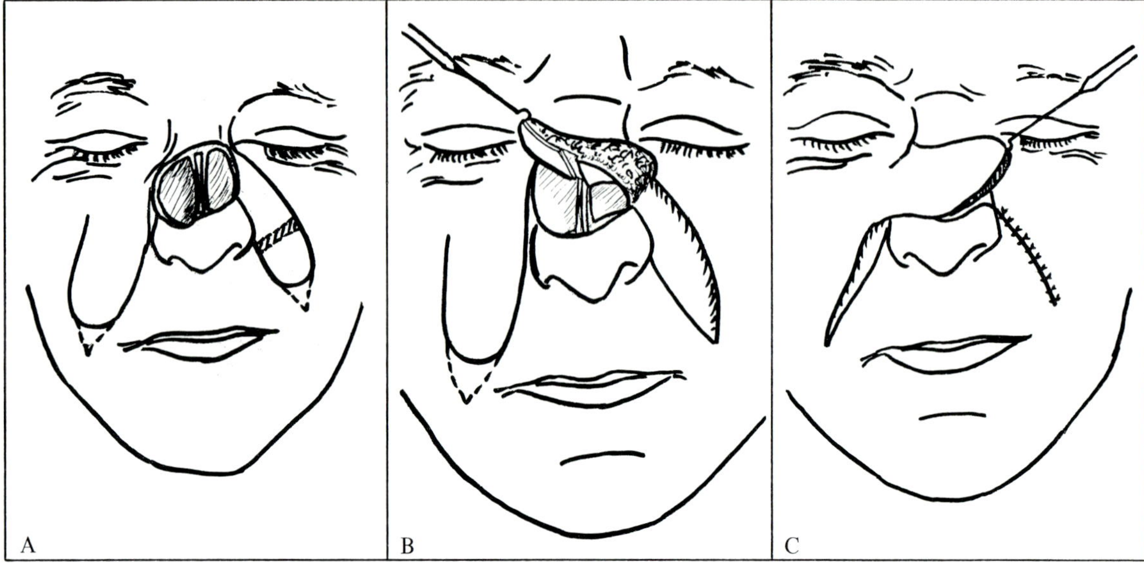

Fig. 14-7. Bilateral nasolabial flaps for lining and coverage of the midnasal defect. A, extensive full-thickness defect of nasal walls from wide excision of recurrent basal cell carcinoma. The bilateral naso-labial flaps are outlined. B, the left nasolabial flap is turned over with the pedicle at the base of the defect to provide lining. The epithelial strip is removed in the area of the septum. C, the right flap is brought across the nose for skin cover.

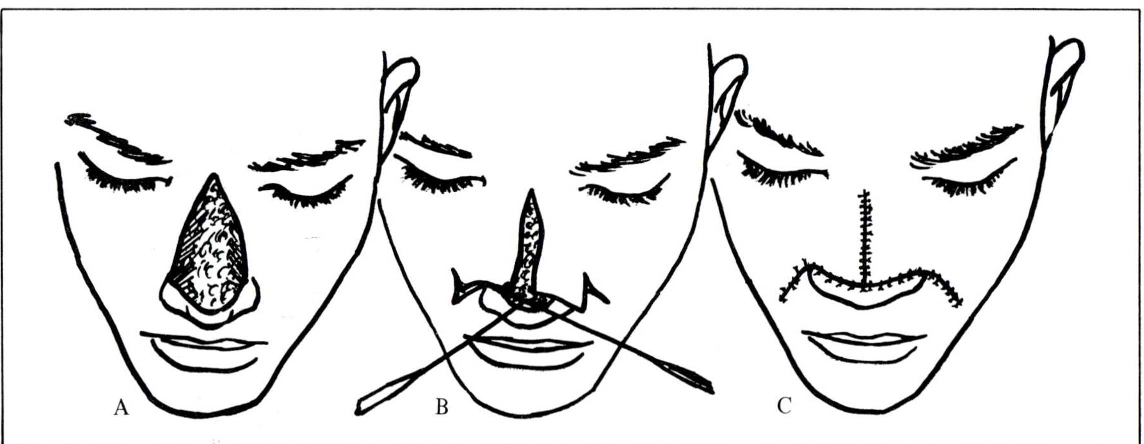

Fig. 14-8. Resurfacing of the nasal dorsum with bi-lateral cheek flaps. A, excision of nasal skin. B, the bilateral cheek flaps are elevated and advanced. C, the flaps are sutured in place; the deficit was diminished by rhinoplastic shortening of the nose.

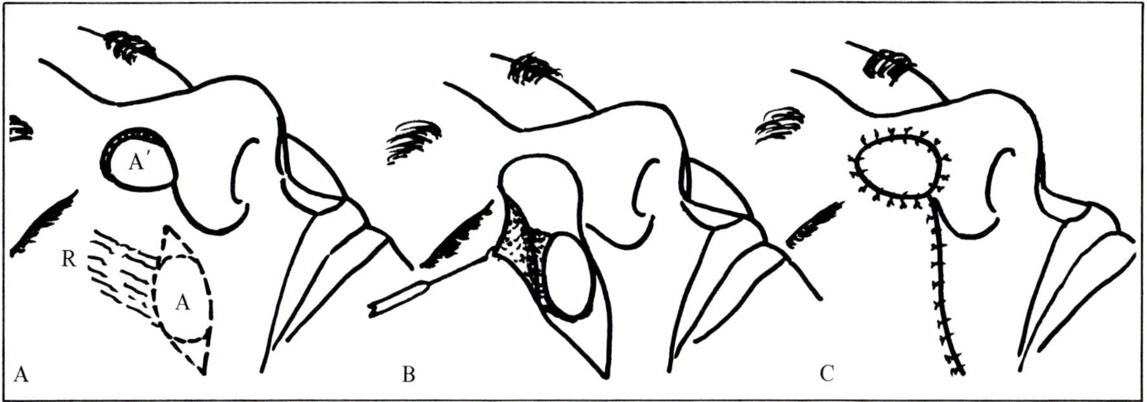

Fig. 14-9. Nasolabial subcutaneous pedicle flap. A, defect of nasal side wall A′ *and outline of nasolabial flap. Wavy lines represent subcutaneous pedicle.* R *is the point of rotation; the distance* R–A *should be slightly longer than* R–A′. *B, the pedicle is developed by dissecting immediately subdermally and on a plane beneath the subdermal plexus. C, the flap is sutured in place and the donor area is closed primarily.*

Forehead Flaps

The skin of the forehead has the same advantages in general as that of the nasolabial fold and cheek in nasal reconstruction. In addition there is usually more than adequate quantity available. There is a consistent, predictable vascular supply that allows transfer usually without delay unless long, narrow, or complex flaps are utilized [54, 56]. For these reasons this is the most widely used tissue for major nasal reconstruction, though the donor site deformity may be significant.

For purposes of simplification, forehead flaps may be divided into three classifications: (1) midline flaps with donor sites that can be closed primarily (Figs. 14-10 and 14-11), (2) vertically oriented flaps (including "up and down" flaps), and (3) horizontally oriented flaps. The last group, based primarily on the superficial temporal arteries, find their most frequent utilization in other areas than the nose [38] and, hence, will not be dealt with in detail here. They are basically sound flaps, however, and in particular circumstances their use in nasal reconstruction should be evaluated [52].

The midline forehead flap was the basis for the ancient Hindu nasal reconstruction. These artisans apparently left the donor area to heal secondarily but nonetheless obtained remarkable results for the state of the art [20, 47]. Kazanjian [40] refined this flap and described primary closure of the donor site. This technique will provide tissue up to 3 cm. in width [14], with adequate length to reach the nasal tip and with residual tissue to fold under for lining. Length may be gained by extending the flap obliquely away from the midline, deviating to one side at the hairline [63], or extending superiorly to include the hair-bearing scalp (later replaced by a graft) [61]. Extension of the vertical portion may be made bilaterally to reconstruct the alae in gull wing fashion as described by Millard [54, 56]. These extensions will require delay. The width can be increased but this will require grafting of the donor area with secondary deformity.

The basic technique requires parallel incisions to the periosteum from the hairline to the glabella. These incisions are connected at the hairline and the flap is elevated. The skin incisions only are extended inferiorly to the area of the nasion; gentle blunt dissection is used, and care is taken to mobilize the pedicle through which the supratrochlear vessels supply the flap. The flap may then be turned 180 degrees for use on the nose and the midline defect is sutured. The redundancy about the pedicle can be relieved in about 3 weeks by sectioning and rerotation of the base [18].

Gillies [32] extended the use of the midforehead flap by carrying his incisions cephalad into the hair-bearing scalp, then inferiorly parallel to the initial flap. He called this an "up and down" flap, and its increased length made it more versatile. The scalping flap technique of Converse [17] further expanded this technique, which is probably the most widely accepted method of supplying skin cover for total and subtotal nasal reconstruction (Fig. 14-12). This flap is based on the supratrochlear, supraorbital, and superficial temporal vasculature of one side of the forehead and brings down tissue from the opposite side in an "up and down" fashion. The actual tissue that is utilized for reconstruction originates from the temporal forehead and is made up of skin and immediate subcutaneous tissue only. The temporalis muscle is left in its bed in this area and grafted with post-auricular or supraclavicular skin if possible. These measures soften the degree of donor deformity. Most

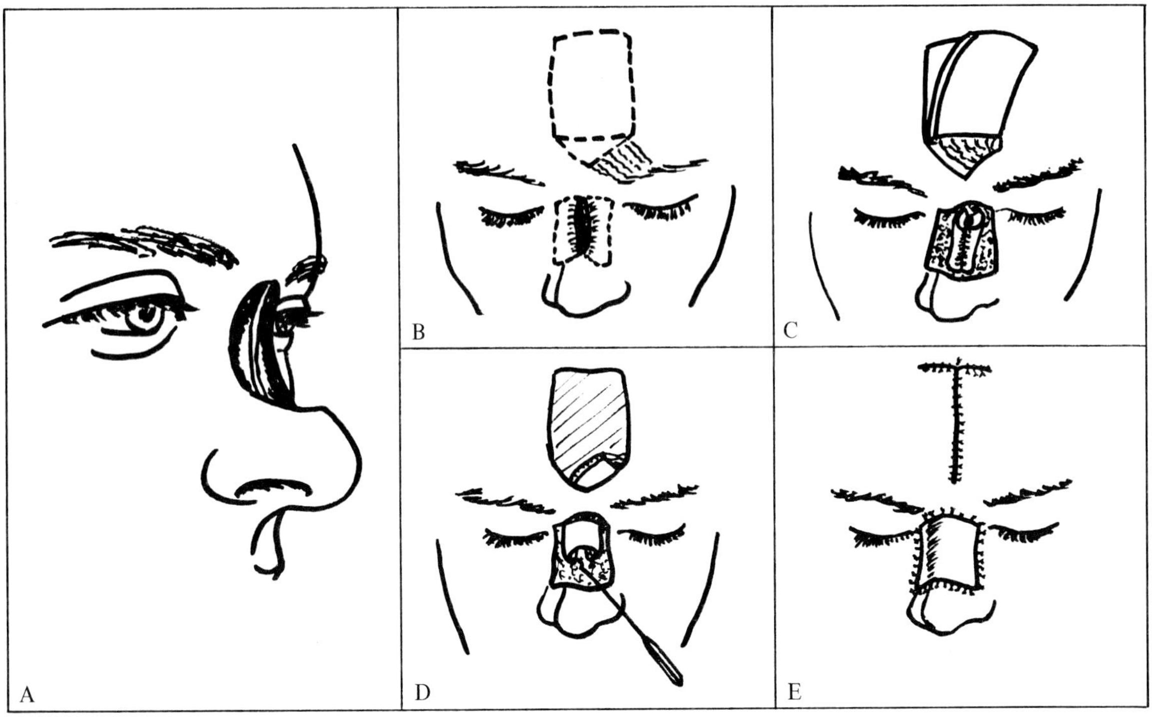

Fig. 14-10. Forehead island flap. A, proximal nasal defect. B, the raw surfaces are allowed to heal and the edges to mature. The midforehead and local flaps are outlined. The local flaps should be based on their medial borders. C, the midforehead flap is elevated and a subcutaneous pedicle containing supratrochlear vessels is preserved. The local flaps are developed from their lateral borders and turned upward toward each other; the edges are inverted and sutured together to form the nasal lining. D, the forehead flap is rotated and passed through a tunnel to the defect. E, the flap is sutured in place for cover and the donor site is closed primarily.

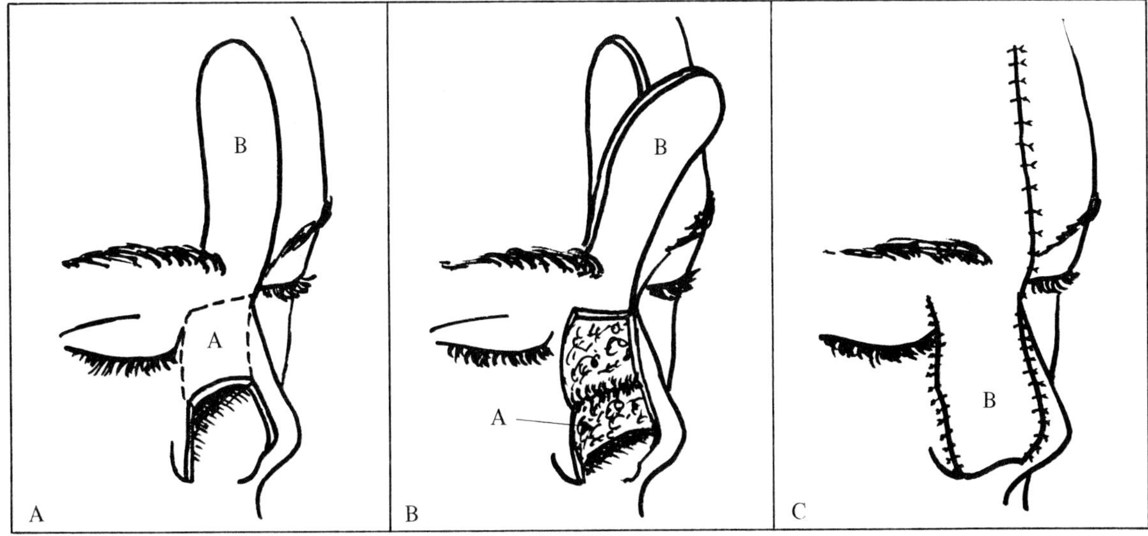

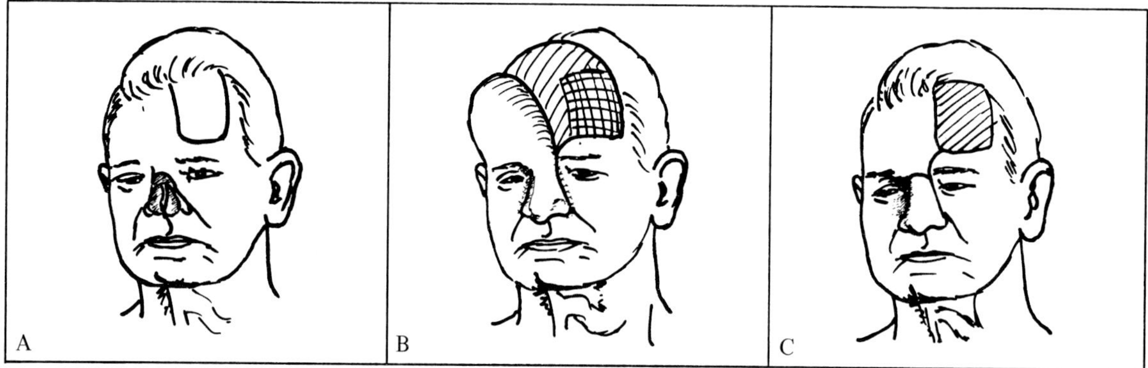

Fig. 14-12. Forehead scalping flap for subtotal nasal reconstruction. A, subtotal nasal loss is shown, with the area of tissue on left forehead to be used for reconstruction outlined. B, the flap for nasal reconstruction is elevated, leaving the frontalis muscle in place. The remaining forehead and anterior scalp are elevated to the depth of the galea and are folded and brought downward; the nasal tip is shaped and the flap is sutured in place. The raw surface may be dressed or grafted with split-thickness skin graft. C, after 18 to 21 days, the flap is transected at the base of the nose, unfolded, and returned to its original position. The donor area is grafted with postauricular or cervical skin if possible to lessen the deformity.

of the remaining incisions are placed within the hair-bearing scalp; the body of the flap incorporates the frontalis muscle. Extending cephalad to the area of the coronal suture line, the incision over the top of the head ends several centimeters above the ear. The large flap thus created is folded on itself with the distal end brought down to the nasal defect. By suturing the lateral corners of the distal edge to one another and then invaginating this, a columella and alar wings are developed. These are sutured in place as indicated. The raw surface over the calvaria is temporarily covered with a split-thickness skin graft or dressed. After 18 to 21 days, the folded portion of the flap is detached at the root of the nose, unfolded, and reapplied in its original position.

Other Flaps (Regional and Distant)

There are times when the circumstances of a case dictate the utilization of soft tissues for reconstruction other than from the forehead, cheeks, or nose itself. The postauricular, cervical, and clavicular areas have been successfully utilized for such tissue transfers, which provide tissue matches that may be quite satisfactory.

The postauricular area has some limitations as to the quantity and quality of skin for nasal reconstruction; however, it may match up quite well and the donor area is obscure. Washio [69] has demonstrated that the superficial temporal and retroauricular arteries connect in an anastomosis 8 to 10 cm. cephalad to the anterior end of the helix. Utilizing this anastomosis, he has designed a flap based anterior to the ear; this flap will carry postauricular skin to the midfacial region. Fujino, Harashina, and Nakajima [28], utilizing the techniques of microvascular anastomosis, have transferred postauricular skin to the nose as a free flap in sufficient quantity for complete nasal coverage.

The cervical and clavicular areas have long been sources of flap material for nasal reconstruction [32] (Fig. 14-13). These flaps may be based at either mastoid area and tubed with a distal "pancake" of skin and subcutaneous tissue for the reconstruction. While several preliminary delays are necessary, the actual transfer can be done with a minimal amount of inconvenience to the patient [7, 14, 70]. It would be possible to transfer a strut of clavicle as an integral part of one of these flaps, utilizing the technique described by Snyder et al. [65].

Though many techniques for the transfer of tissues below the clavicle to the nose have been described, the inadequacies of the tissue increase with the distance from the nose. Acromiothoracic [32] and deltopectoral [1] tissues can be transferred directly, as can arm tissues. Abdominal tissue can be transferred, utilizing the forearm as an intermediate carrier [42, 43,

---

Fig. 14-11. Midforehead flap to cover half of the nose (hemirhinoplasty after Millard [53]). A, the distal nasal wall defect is shown, with the superior nasal flap A *and the midforehead flap* B *outlined. B, flap* A *is turned down, hinged at the superior border of the defect, to form the nasal lining. Should additional lining be required, a nasolabial flap can also be utilized. C, midforehead flap is rotated 180 degrees to cover the raw surface, with the distal end folded on itself to create the alar border.*

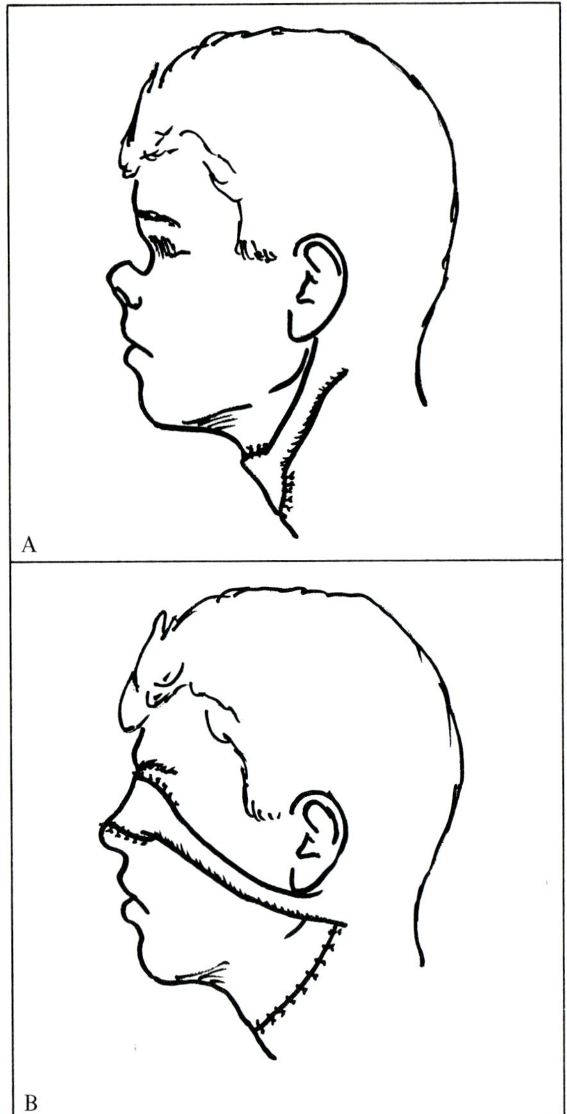

Fig. 14-13. Cervical flap for nasal reconstruction. A, nasal defect and adjacent cheek and eyelid loss are shown. Tubed pedicle with a delayed distal "pancake" is ready for transfer. B, the flap is transferred to nose and adjacent areas for reconstruction. The donor site is closed primarily. The pedicle may usually be transected in three weeks or less.

45]. In each case, however, the quality of the skin will differ in color and texture from normal facial skin and the thickness of the skin and subcutaneous tissue will limit the refinement of the finished product. In addition to these drawbacks, the complexity of the transfer and the immobilization of the patient are definite deterrents, particularly in elderly patients.

THE PLAN FOR RECONSTRUCTION

The raw materials are available for nasal reconstruction with an acceptable result. The surgeon must supply the judgment, ingenuity, and technical acumen to do the job. Thorough study of the problem at hand and determination of a basic detailed operative plan with alternatives should precede any surgery. The quality of the result will more directly reflect sound planning than spectacular surgical gymnastics.

The provisional plan should be developed through several stages:

1. Determination of the precise size and character of the defect: The eventual tissue deficit may differ from whatever situation the surgeon first encounters. The nose torn by fresh trauma may be further distorted by scar contracture. The seemingly well-localized basal cell lesion may have unexpected extensions noted on pathological section.
2. Determination of available local tissues that will enhance and simplify the reconstruction. Portions of residual tissue that the inexperienced surgeon might be tempted to discard may be quite valuable in reconstruction. Skin adjacent to the defect may be turned over to serve as lining or rotated or advanced to create an alar border if the margins of the defect are mature and scar will not interfere with vascular supply.
3. Study of the nasal remnants to determine if rhinoplasty techniques will lessen the size of the defect or simplify reconstruction. Nasal shortening and/or hump removal may often be valuable steps in this regard.
4. Determination of timing of the repair. This may be affected by contamination of the wound, uncertainty as to neoplastic residuum, age of the patient, availability of tissues for repair, and other factors.
5. Determination of sources of tissue for transfer. The most desirable tissues may be impaired by concurrent or previous injury, neoplasia, radiation injury, or other problems that limit their use.
6. Preparation of alternative plans. Should intervening infection, flap necrosis, secondary injury, spread of neoplasm beyond expected limits, or any one of many other problems arise, the surgeon must be prepared to alter his course.

As a general statement, the best nasal reconstruction will result from the simplest, most direct combination of available raw materials that in the end present this feature as a single unit. Techniques that result in a piecemeal accumulation of "crazy quilt" design will do a disservice to the patient.

NASAL PROSTHETICS

It is not unusual to encounter circumstances in which a prosthetic device will benefit the patient as either a temporary or permanent solution to a nasal defect. This may amount simply to a Band-Aid over a sidewall defect or a cover molded from an aluminum nasal splint or sheet of malleable plastic. Temporary appliances such as this will be helpful in the patient awaiting surgery when the initial healing is incomplete following trauma or when the margins of a basal cell lesion are uncertain. The patient who is not a candidate for reconstruction because of age, general condition, or personal preference will require a more permanent solution.

The construction of prosthetic maxillofacial appliances requires an artistic bent, a knowledge of the technique, and the availability of the raw materials and necessary equipment. Ideally, the materials utilized are easily processed and should accept pigments incorporated in them or applied to their surface, resemble the texture of the tissues they are to simulate, and retain their form and detail. They should not cause irritation, toxicity, or allergic response on prolonged contact with the skin, yet should be light but strong, durable, and stain resistant. The need to adhere to the skin during facial movements particularly along inconspicuous edges demands a degree of flexibility. Though the list of qualifications is demanding, recent years have produced the development of silicone, polyvinyl, polyurethane, and methylmethacrylate, which are available in varied forms; alone or in combination they pass most of the tests [15, 46, 59, 64].

A certain amount of basic knowledge in working with these materials using a limited number of tools would allow the reconstructive surgeon to make molds and fabricate acceptable prostheses for temporary use. Patients who are likely to wear such appliances permanently are generally best served by consultation with a professional prosthetist.

REFERENCES

1. Bakamjian, V. Y. The Deltopectoral Flap. In Grabb, W. C., and Myers, M. B. (Eds.), *Skin Flaps.* Boston: Little, Brown, 1975.
2. Barron, J. N. Subcutaneous Pedicle Flaps. In Grabb, W. C., and Myers, M. B. (Eds.), *Skin Flaps.* Boston: Little, Brown, 1975.
3. Barron, J. N., and Emmett, A. J. J. Subcutaneous pedicle flaps. *Br. J. Plast. Surg.* 18:51, 1965.
4. Beare, R. L. B., and Bennett, J. P. The nasolabial full thickness graft. *Br. J. Plast. Surg.* 25:315, 1972.
5. Bennett, J. E., and Thurston, J. B. Cancer of the nose: Ablation and repair. *Clin. Plast. Surg.* 3:461, 1976.
6. Blair, V. P., and Byars, L. Hits, strikes and outs in the use of pedicle flaps for nasal restoration. *Surg. Gynecol. Obstet.* 82:367, 1946.
7. Bromberg, B. E., Oakley, R. S., and Wickstrom, O. W. Total reconstruction of the nose. *Plast. Reconstr. Surg.* 14:298, 1954.
8. Brown, J. B., and Cannon, B. Composite free grafts of skin and cartilage from the ear. *Surg. Gynecol. Obstet.* 82:253, 1946.
9. Brown, J. B., Cannon, B., Lischer, C. E., Moore, A., and Murray, J. Further reports on the use of composite free grafts of skin and cartilage from the ear. *Plast. Reconstr. Surg.* 1:130, 1946.
10. Brown, J. B., and McDowell, F. *Plastic Surgery of the Nose.* Springfield, Ill.: Thomas, 1965.
11. Cameron, R. R. Nasal Reconstruction with Nasolabial Cheek Flaps. In Grabb, W. C., and Myers, M. B. (Eds.), *Skin Flaps.* Boston: Little, Brown, 1975.
12. Cameron, R. R., Latham, W. D., and Dowling, J. A. Reconstruction of the nose and upper lip with nasolabial flaps. *Plast. Reconstr. Surg.* 52:145, 1973.
13. Carpue, J. C. An account of two successful operations for restoring the nose from the integuments of the forehead. London: Longman, 1816. Reprinted (in part) in *Plast. Reconstr. Surg.* 44:174, 1969.
14. Carson, W. E., Cameron, R. R., and Latham, W. D. Naso-orbital reconstruction in war casualties. *Plast. Reconstr. Surg.* 45:536, 1970.
15. Chalian, V. A., Drane, J. B., and Standish, S. M. *Maxillofacial Prosthetics.* Baltimore: Williams & Wilkins, 1971.
16. Conley, J. J., and Vonfraenkel, P. H. The principle of cooling as applied to the composite graft in the nose. *Plast. Reconstr. Surg.* 17:444, 1956.
17. Converse, J. M. Reconstruction of the nose by the scalping flap technique. *Surg. Clin. North Am.* 39:335, 1959.
18. Converse, J. M. *Reconstructive Plastic Surgery.* Philadelphia: Saunders, 1964.
19. Converse, J. M., and Wood-Smith, D. Experiences with the forehead island flap with a subcutaneous pedicle. *Plast. Reconstr. Surg.* 31:521, 1963.
20. Daver, B. M., and Antia, N. H. Large indian forehead rhinoplasty. *Plast. Reconstr. Surg.* 55:360, 1975.

21. Dean, R. K., Kelleher, J. C., Sullivan, J. G., and Baibak, G. J. Bilobed Flaps. In Grabb, W. C., and Myers, M. B. (Eds.), *Skin Flaps.* Boston: Little, Brown, 1975.
22. Dieffenbach, J. F. Surgical observations of the restoration of the nose. *Operative Chirurgie* 1:359, 1833.
23. Dieffenbach, J. F. *Die operative Chirurgie.* Leipzig: Brockhaus, 1845.
24. Edgerton, M. T., and Hansen, F. C. Matching facial color with split-thickness skin grafts from adjacent areas. *Plast. Reconstr. Surg.* 25:455, 1960.
25. Elliott, R. A., Jr. Rotation flaps of the nose. *Plast. Reconstr. Surg.* 44:147, 1969.
26. Fry, H. Cartilage and cartilage grafts: The basic properties of the tissue and the components responsible for them. *Plast. Reconstr. Surg.* 40:426, 1967.
27. Fryer, M. P. Subtotal nose reconstruction with a cheek flap. *Plast. Reconstr. Surg.* 53:436, 1974.
28. Fujino, T., Harashina, T., and Nakajima, T. Free skin flap from the retroauricular region to the nose. *Plast. Reconstr. Surg.* 57:338, 1976.
29. Georgiade, N. G., Mladick, R. A., and Thorne, F. L. The nasolabial tunnel flap. *Plast. Reconstr. Surg.* 43:463, 1969.
30. Gibson, T., Curran, R. C., and Davis, W. B. The survival of living homograft cartilage in man. *Transplant. Bull.* 4:105, 1957.
31. Gibson, T., and Davis, W. B. The distortion of autogenous cartilage grafts: Its cause and prevention. *Br. J. Plast. Surg.* 10:257, 1958.
32. Gillies, H. D. Experiences with tubed pedicle flaps. *Surg. Gynecol. and Obstet.* 60:291, 1935.
33. Gillies, H. D. A new free graft applied to the reconstruction of the nostril. *Br. J. Surg.* 30:305, 1943.
34. Gillies, H. D., and Millard, D. R. *The Principles and Art of Plastic Surgery.* Boston: Little, Brown, 1957.
35. Gnudi, M. T., and Webster, J. P. *The Life and Times of Gaspare Tagliacozzi, Surgeon of Bologna,* 1545–1599. New York: Reichner, 1950.
36. Heanley, C. The subcutaneous tissue pedicle in columella and other nasal reconstruction. *Br. J. Plast. Surg.* 8:60, 1955.
37. Herbert, D. C., and Harrison, R. G. Nasolabial subcutaneous pedicle flaps. *Br. J. Plast. Surg.* 28:85, 1975.
38. Hoopes, J. E. Forehead Flaps. In Grabb, W. C., and Myers, M. B. (Eds.), *Skin Flaps.* Boston: Little, Brown, 1975.
39. Jervis, W., Salyer, K. E., Vargas Busquets, M. A., and Atkins, R. W. Further applications of the Limberg and Dufourmentel flaps. *Plast. Reconstr. Surg.* 54:335, 1974.
40. Kazajian, V. H. The repair of nasal defects with the median forehead flap: Primary closure of the forehead wound. *Surg. Gynecol. Obstet.* 83:37, 83:37, 1946.
41. Kernahan, D. A., and Littlewood, A. H. M. Experience in the use of arterial flaps about the face. *Plast. Reconstr. Surg.* 28:207, 1961.
42. Kilner, T. D. Plastic Surgery. In Maingot, R. (Ed.), *Postgraduate Surgery,* Vol. 3. New York: Appleton-Century-Crofts, 1937.
43. Kivrakirov, V. On the problem of total rhinoplasty with a Filatov's flap stripped of fat. *Acta Chir. Plast.* 3:241, 1961.
44. Koenig, F. Ueber Nasenplastik. *Beitr. Klin. Chir.* 94:515, 1914.
45. Krauss, M. Reconstruction of subtotal defects of the nose by abdominal tube flap. *Br. J. Plast. Surg.* 17:70, 1964.
46. Lepley, J. B. Current practices in maxillofacial prosthetics. *Surg. Clin. North Am.* 54:787, 1974.
47. Letter to the Editor, Gentlemen's Magazine, London, October, 1794. Reprinted in *Plast. Reconstr. Surg.* 44:67, 1969.
48. Limberg, A. A. Design of Local Flaps. In Gibson, T. (Ed.), *Modern Trends in Plastic Surgery.* London: Butterworth, 1966.
49. Lipshutz, H., and Penrod, D. S. Use of complete transverse nasal flap in repair of small defects of the nose. *Plast. Reconstr. Surg.* 49:629, 1972.
50. Lister, G. D., and Gibson, T. Closure of rhomboid skin defects: The flaps of Limberg and Dufourmentel. *Br. J. Plast. Surg.* 25:300, 1972.
51. McDowell, F., Valone, J. A., and Brown, J. B. Bibliography and historical note on plastic surgery of the nose. *Plast. Reconstr. Surg.* 10:149, 1952.
52. Millard, D. R. Total reconstructive rhinoplasty and a missing link. *Plast. Reconstr. Surg.* 37:167, 1966.
53. Millard, D. R. Hemirhinoplasty. *Plast. Reconstr. Surg.* 40:440, 1967.
54. Millard, D. R. Reconstructive rhinoplasty for the lower half of a nose. *Plast. Reconstr. Surg.* 53:133, 1974.
55. Millard, D. R. Total and Subtotal Reconstructive Rhinoplasty. In *Transactions of the Sixth International Congress of Plastic and Reconstructive Surgery.* Paris: Masson, 1976.
56. Millard, D. R. Reconstructive rhinoplasty for the lower two thirds of the nose. *Plast. Reconstr. Surg.* 57:722, 1976.
57. New, G. B. Sickle flap for nasal reconstruction. *Surg. Gynecol. Obstet.* 80:497, 1945.

58. Orticochea, M. A new method for total reconstruction of the nose: The ears as donor area. *Br. J. Plast. Surg.* 24:228, 1971.
59. Rahn, A. O., and Boucher, L. J. *Maxillofacial Prosthetics: Principles and Concepts.* Philadelphia: Saunders, 1970.
60. Rees, T. D., Wood-Smith, D., Converse, J. M., and Guy, C. L. Composite grafts. Presented at the Third International Congress of Plastic Surgery, Washington, D.C., 1963.
61. Richardson, G. S., Hanna, D. C., and Gaisford, J. C. Midline forehead flap nasal reconstructions in patients with low browlines. *Plast. Reconstr. Surg.* 49:130, 1972.
62. Rieger, R. A. A local flap for repair of the nasal tip. *Plast. Reconstr. Surg.* 40:147, 1967.
63. Sawhney, C. P. A longer angular midline forehead flap for the reconstruction of nasal defects. *Plast. Reconstr. Surg.* 58:721, 1976.
64. Smith, W. In Gibson, T. (Ed.), *Modern Trends in Plastic Surgery,* Vol. 1. Washington, D.C.: Butterworth, 1964.
65. Snyder, C. C., Bateman, J. M., Davies, C. W., and Wardim, G. D. Mandibulo-facial restoration with live osteocutaneous flaps. *Plast. Reconstr. Surg.* 45:14, 1970.
66. Tagliacozzi, G. *De Curtorum Chirurgia per Institionem.* Venice: G. Bindonus, 1597.
67. Taylor, G. I., and Daniel, R. K. Free Flap Transfers by Microvascular Anastomosis. In Grabb, W. C., and Myers, M. B. (Eds.), *Skin Flaps.* Boston: Little, Brown, 1975.
68. Taylor, G. I., and Daniel, R. K. The anatomy of several free flap donor sites. *Plast. Reconstr. Surg.* 56:243, 1975.
69. Washio, H. The Retroauricular Temporal Flap. In Grabb, W. C., and Myers, M. B. (Eds.), *Skin Flaps.* Boston: Little, Brown, 1975.
70. Young, F. The surgical repair of nasal deformities. *Plast. Reconstr. Surg.* 4:59, 1949.
71. Zimany, A. The bilobed flap. *Plast. Reconstr. Surg.* 11:424, 1953.

15

Reconstruction of the Facial Muscles, Lips, and Cheeks

BARD COSMAN AND JORGE NIKLISON

FACIAL MUSCULATURE

Anatomy of Facial Musculature

The facial musculature can be separated into two groups: the *muscles of expression* and the *muscles of mastication.* The muscles of expression are often referred to as the facial muscles.

Muscles of Expression

Divided into *superficial* and *deep* groups, the muscles of expression arise as second branchial arch derivatives and are innervated on their deep, lateral, and posterior portions by the facial nerve (Fig. 15-1). These muscles are unique in the body in that they move the soft tissues of the face rather than acting to move the underlying bones. The clinically significant muscles are listed below:

A. *Superficial group of muscles*
   1. *Frontalis muscle* arises from the epicranial aponeurosis, inserts into the skin of the eyebrow, providing for elevation of the eyebrows and causing the transverse forehead lines.
   2. *Orbicularis oculi muscle* arises from the medial palpebral ligament, nasal process of frontal bone, lacrimal crest of maxilla, and inferior orbital rim. On contraction of this muscle, the eyelids close forcibly. A milking action on the lacrimal gland and lacrimal sac, facilitating the flow of tears and their collection by the nasolacrimal apparatus, is produced by alternate contraction and relaxation.
   3. *Quadratus labii superioris muscle* arises in three parts:
      a. Zygomatic, from the zygomatic bone inserting into the skin and muscle of the upper lip angle, producing elevation and lateral pull of the commissure.
      b. Infraorbital, from the infraorbital margin inserting into skin and muscle of the lateral half of the upper lip, producing elevation of lip.
      c. Angular, from the frontal process of the maxilla inserting into the alar cartilage of the nose and the orbicularis oris muscle of lip, producing retraction of the lip and alar elevation.
   4. *Zygomaticus muscle* arises from the zygomatic bone, inserts into the angle of mouth, and produces lip retraction.
   5. *Quadratus labii inferioris muscle* arises from an oblique line on the mandible, inserts into the skin of the lower lip and orbicularis oris, and draws the lower lip down and laterally.
   6. *Orbicularis oris muscle,* a complex, interwoven, generally circular sphincter, is continuous with the surrounding musculature. It compresses, everts, and inverts the lips.

B. *Deep group of muscles*
   1. *Corrugator muscle* arises from the frontal bone beneath the frontalis and orbicularis oculi muscles, inserts into the skin of the eyebrow, and pulls the eyebrows medially, giving rise to vertical glabellar frown lines.
   2. *Buccinator muscle* arises from alveolar processes of the mandible and maxilla, and the pterygomandibular raphe; it inserts into the orbicularis oris muscle, compressing the cheeks and maintaining tone.

Muscles of Mastication

The muscles of mastication can be divided into those *superficial* (masseter and temporalis) and those *deep* (internal and external pterygoid) to the mandible. All of them are innervated by branches of the trigeminal nerve.

The *temporalis muscle* arises from the temporal fossa, passes deep to the zygomatic arch, and inserts on the coronoid process and anterior border of the mandibular ramus. It acts to close the jaws and retract the mandible. The anterior and posterior temporal nerves innervate this muscle, entering on its deep surface.

The *masseter muscle* arises from the zygomatic arch and the maxilla and inserts into the angle and lower one-half of the mandibular ramus. It acts to close the jaws and receives its innervation on the deep surface from the masseter nerve. The parotid duct is superficial to this muscle, running 1.5 cm. below the zygomatic arch, and passing through the buccinator muscle into the mouth at the anterior border of the masseter. The buccal branch of the facial nerve runs transversely across the midportion of the muscle. The mandibular branch of the facial nerve courses forward just above the angle of the mandible in most persons, though in about 20 percent of patients it passes in an arc just below (1 cm. or less) the angle of the mandible, finally crossing the inferior mandibular border anteriorly at the level of the facial artery.

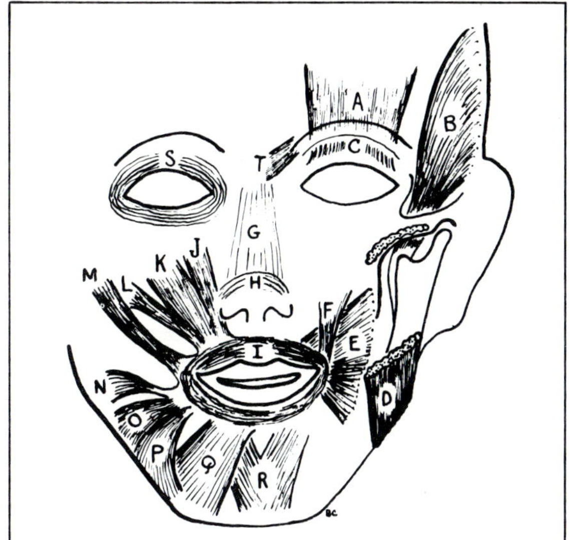

Fig. 15-1. Muscles of expression and mastication. A, frontalis; B, temporalis; C, levator palpebrae; D, masseter, with segment removed to show mandibular ramus; E, buccinator; F, caninus (levator anguli oris); G, procerus; H, nasalis; I, orbicularis oris; J, angular head of quadratus labii superioris; K. infraorbital head of quadratus labii superioris; L, zygomatic head of quadratus labii superioris; M, zygomaticus; N, risorius; O, platysma; P, triangularis; Q, quadratus labii inferioris; R, mentalis, S, orbicularis oculi; T, corrugator.

The *internal pterygoid muscle* arises from the medial and lateral pterygoid plate of the sphenoid bone, the maxillary tuberosity, and the pyramidal process of the palatine bone. The muscle passes downward, backward, and laterally to insert on the medial surface of the ascending ramus of the mandible. The *external pterygoid muscle* consists of two fasciculi. The superior fasciculus arises from the pterygoid crest and great wing of the sphenoid and inserts on both the capsular ligament in front of the articular disc and the upper third of the condylar neck. The inferior fasciculus arises from the lateral surface of the lateral pterygoid plate and inserts on the condylar neck. Motor nerve supply to the pterygoid muscles is from a branch of the trigeminal nerve. The internal pterygoid acts to close and medially displace the mandible while the external pterygoid protrudes and medially displaces the mandible.

Facial Palsy

Facial muscle paralysis of seventh cranial nerve origin is the most significant condition affecting the facial muscles.

Etiology

Facial palsy may be congenital or acquired. The *congenital* type may be an isolated nuclear paralysis, or it may be associated with other cranial nerve palsies, as in the Möbius syndrome. Four forms of interruption of facial nerve function are responsible for *acquired palsy.* (1) Central nervous system damage as in strokes, meningitis, or infantile paralysis may affect the intracerebral nucleus of the facial nerve. (2) Intracranial damage to the nerve may be caused by acoustic neuromas or the surgery for their removal. (3) Intratemporal bone canal damage may occur accidentally in middle ear surgery; it may also occur when inflammatory swelling compresses the nerve in the bony canal, as in Bell's palsy. (4) Peripheral nerve damage may occur in facial lacerations or in the planned or accidental excision of the nerve in parotid gland surgery. A large portion of acquired paralyses are idiopathic, apparently related to acute swelling of the nerve in its unyielding intratemporal canal, and are called Bell's palsy.

Characteristic Defect of Facial Palsy

Subtotal unilateral paralysis is the most common palsy encountered. The patient presents a characteristic appearance with component abnormalities that involve the nonparalyzed side as well as the paralyzed side of the face (see Fig. 15-4A). The forehead wrinkles are absent over the paralyzed frontalis muscle, and the eyebrow droops; the unbalanced frontalis action on the nonparalyzed side accentuates this difference by wrinkling the forehead excessively and lifting the eyebrow.

On the abnormal side the palpebral fissure is widened, and it remains this way as facial expressions narrow the palpebral fissure on the nonparalyzed side. The lagophthalmos on the paralyzed side is due to the action of the levator palpebral muscle of the upper lid, which is unopposed by the paralyzed orbicularis oculi, and to the descent of the lower lid, whose muscle is deprived of its tone. The lower lid tends to fall away from the globe, with tears collecting in and spilling over from a central lake, rather than being directed to the medial canthus and the lower lid punctum. With this paralytic ectropion, the inferior punctum tends to turn out and often stenoses because of exposure. Epiphora is exaggerated further by this and by the constant minor and occasional major degree of exposure keratitis of the cornea, which further stimulates lacrimal secretion. The exposed caruncle hypertrophies. The affected lids can often close to a considerable degree, but closure is not completed, the pupil turns up (Bell's sign), and white scleral conjunctiva remains unpleasantly exposed.

The paralyzed cheek sags and its nasolabial fold is erased. Plosives are garbled in speech as air pressure is lost because of blowing out on the paralyzed side, which is without its buccinator function. The cheek on the nonparalyzed side, however, shows hyperactivity; there is no doubt that the grimaces originating in the imbalance of the nonparalyzed side musculature are more objectionable aesthetically then the inexpressive facies on the paralyzed side.

The nose and philtrum are deviated to the nonparalyzed side by this excessive muscle activity. The lip angle sags on the affected side. Drooling may occur. Articulation of labial sounds is often impaired. On the nonparalyzed side the lip angle is pulled up, out, or down, or is puckered by varying combinations of the hyperactive quadratii, the zygomaticus, and the orbicularis oris muscle.

Patients with partial facial palsies can show varying degrees of the complete defect. On the nonparalytic side, hyperactivity is usually less of a problem. Congenital unilateral palsies are often not complete, show more muscle tone on the paralyzed side, and exhibit less marked weakness of the oribcularis oculi.

Bilateral complete palsy is rare. Drooling may be a problem. However, the bilateral inexpressivity of the face is less objectionable cosmetically than the facial appearance with the unilateral condition.

Indications for Reconstructive Procedures

There is no question that *early repair* of any part of the facial nerve or *replacement* of a resected segment by a nerve graft is desirable and is at least partially successful [12, 15]. There is also no question that *the great majority of patients with Bell's palsy* can be expected to show a degree of recovery that precludes the need for reconstructive procedures. When early facial nerve repair is not feasible but peripheral facial nerve branches are present, *nerve crosses* employing hypoglossal, spinal accessory, or phrenic nerves may be used; however, these procedures are less desirable than nerve repair because of the mass movements produced and the additional deformities created by sacrificing the "donor nerves" [11, 24, 34]. To preserve the unique facial nerve function, contralateral facial nerve branches have been joined to the persisting branches on the paralyzed side using microsurgical technique and free nerve grafts to bridge across the face [2, 20, 39, 40] (see Fig. 15-4). *If more than a year has elapsed* after the onset of palsy, motor endplate degeneration makes successful nerve crosses unlikely, although good results have been claimed for direct nerve implants into the facial musculature [14]. If the continuity of the facial nerve has been definitely interrupted or if repair and replacement are not feasible, reconstructive procedures can be begun before a year has elapsed. The phenomenon of *facial nerve regeneration* in the absence of an intact facial nerve probably occurs in 15 percent of cases, probably involves pathways other than the facial nerve, cannot be depended on, and yet is not prejudiced by the performance of the reconstruction [13, 25].

Reconstructive Procedures

The correction of deformities due to facial paralysis is not simple, and *no single measure* will correct the several variable components of the defect. In each case the forehead, eyebrows, eyelids, eyes, cheeks, and lips on *both the affected and the normal side* must be considered separately from the standpoint of the functional and aesthetic deformities involved. From such consideration the corrections needed and the procedures to follow should emerge.

The techniques that have evolved may be divided into several general categories:

A. *Static*
   1. Insertion suspension – use of fascia lata, tendon, or alloplastic materials to suspend eyelids, cheeks, or lips from fixed points such as zygomatic arch, infraorbital rim, or temporalis fascia [4, 8, 15].
   2. Intrinsic suspension – use of local structures as in medial and lateral canthoplasty to suspend the lower eyelid, plication of paretic muscles to suspend the lips, or use of dermal pedicle slings for the nasolabial region and lips [9, 21, 28].
   3. Excision suspension – removal of local tissue as in supraorbital excision to raise the eyebrow, rhytidectomy to lift the face, or nasolabial fold excision to suspend the lips [7, 9, 35].

B. *Dynamic*
   1. *On paralyzed side*
      a. Muscle transfer – use of the temporalis, masseter, anterior belly of digastric, or sternocleidomastoid to move the forehead, eyelids, cheeks, and lips [1, 3, 16, 17, 27, 29, 36].
      b. Muscle division – transection of the levator palpebrae in the affected eyelid to reduce lagophthalmos [33].
      c. Muscle transplant – use of previously denervated autogenous muscles with their motor nerves anastomosed to a neural supply from the normal side [20, 23, 44].
      d. Nerve transfer – use of normal facial nerve branch or another motor nerve for direct insertion into the paralyzed muscle or for anastomosis to peripheral facial nerve branches on the paralyzed side [2, 14, 39, 40].
      e. Nerve transplant – use of the sural nerve or other nerve graft to bring the facial nerve or other motor nerve supply to muscle or peripheral facial nerve branches on the paralyzed side [2, 39, 40].

2. *On normal side*
   a. Muscle transplant – use of previously denervated autogenous muscle grafts with muscle bellies on the normal side for neurotization and tendons arranged on the paralyzed side to move the forehead, eyelids, cheeks, or lips [18, 20, 22, 41–44].
   b. Muscle division – excision of blocks of facial muscle, especially around the lips, to reduce grimacing on the normal side [32, 33, 37].
   c. Nerve division – transection of the facial nerve branches to reduce normal side hyperactivity in the forehead and lips [10, 32, 33].

C. *Dissimulative*
Surgical creation of wrinkles in forehead and nasolabial fold [9, 19].

D. *Mechanical*
Alloplastic devices for suspension of the eyelids, eyebrows, cheeks, and lips, and for depression of the upper eyelids [5, 6, 30, 31, 38].

Treatment of Facial Palsy
The treatment of facial palsy may be divided into two areas: (1) *frontal-palpebral* or *upper facial paralysis,* and (2) *buccal-labial* or *lower facial paralysis.*

UPPER FACIAL MUSCLE PARALYSIS IN THE FRONTAL AREA. A method for restoring symmetry to the forehead is neurectomy of the frontal branch of the facial nerve on the nonparalyzed side together with supraorbital skin excision on the paralyzed side [33]. Neurectomy of the frontal branch can be done under general or local anesthesia. With the former, accurate location of the nerve by faradic stimulation is possible. Local anesthesia interferes with nerve conduction, thus preventing location of the nerve by faradic stimulation. However, the exact localization of the nerve is not vital. The nerve pathway can be identified by tracing two divergent lines extending from a point just in front of the ear lobe to the uppermost and lowermost forehead wrinkles. Within these limits and approximately one fingerbreadth above the zygomatic arch, the local anesthetic is injected. The frontalis muscle should become motionless in a few minutes. The needle is left in situ for subsequent guidance. A temporal hairline incision is made and the selected portion of the epicranial layer is resected, removing the desired nerve rami. An objectionable consequence of this procedure is the drooping of the eyebrow that may ensue.

On the paralyzed side, the eyebrow can be raised by the closure of a wide lozenge-shaped skin resection just above the eyebrow [7]. An initial overcorrection on the paralyzed side is necessary. An insufficient degree of lift is obtained with the excision of skin only at the hairline of the forehead. Additional lift and further simulation of normality can be achieved by creation of surgical wrinkles through the excision of narrow transverse ellipses using a figure-of-eight suture to compress the tissue and anchor it to the deep fascia [19].

UPPER FACIAL MUSCLE PARALYSIS IN THE PALPEBRAL AREA. For mild degrees of palpebral fissure widening, where sagging of the lower lid plays a part, *lateral canthoplasty* (tarsorrhaphy) is a useful method of suspension. Preservation of the upper lid eyelashes is important cosmetically in maintaining the oval shape of a normal fissure (Fig. 15-2).

With more advanced degrees of sagging of the lower lid and punctum dysfunction, where epiphora is significant and where ectropion is occurring, medial and lateral canthoplasty and a canalicular opening

Fig. 15-2. Technique of medial and lateral canthoplasty with canalicular opening. A, incision for medial canthoplasty in the eye with widened palpebral fissure; note the hypertrophied caruncle and the lower lid ectropion with outward turning of the punctum. B, further skin excision medially to accommodate for direct advancement of triangular flap; lateral canthoplasty begun with excision of the conjunctiva and tarsus in the upper lid, preserving the eyelashes and excising the skin and lashes in the lower lid. C, enlargement of the punctum and laying open of the canaliculus by the indicated incisions (three-snip procedure). D, turned in lid margins cover the caruncle medially; raw areas laterally are coapted with mattress retention sutures. E, completed canthoplasties and canalicular opening; note preservation of the eyelashes laterally.

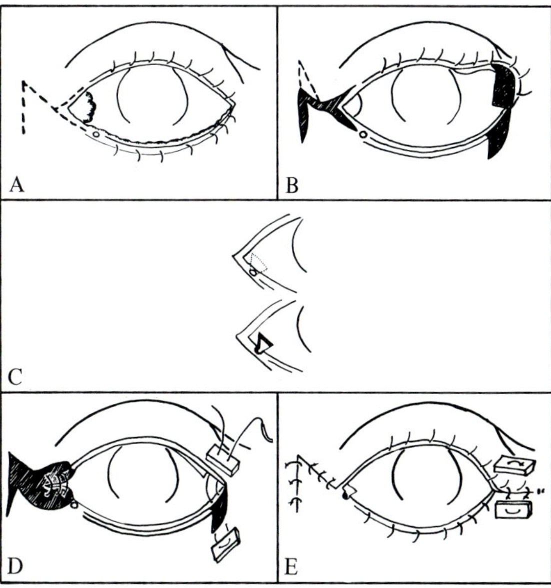

have given good esthetic and functional results [28] (Fig. 15-2). Extreme flaccidity of the lower lid requires additional shortening by the Kuhnt-Szymanowski method (see Chapter 4). The insertion of wire devices for mechanical support of eyelids and eyebrows has been widely practiced in Europe [30, 31]. In mild cases of lagophthalmos insertion of a weight into the upper lid has been of use [6, 38].

The *transfer of temporalis muscle and fascia* to paralyzed eyelids, as modified from Gillies's original technique, has been used widely in treating the lagophthalmos of leprosy [27, 29]. The temporalis fascia is exposed through an incision in the temporal region. Parallel vertical incisions permit the freeing of a ribbon of fascia, which is then detached from the zygoma and reflected off the underlying muscle, preserving the muscle-fascial attachment superiorly. The muscle-fascial junction is incised horizontally above the upper edge of the temporalis muscle, and a segment of muscle, slightly wider than its attached fascial strip, is freed from the skull. The muscle is reflected downward to the level of the lateral canthus, its nerve and vessel supply being preserved. Excising wedges of fascia adjacent to the base of the muscle strip will aid in rotating the muscle-fascia unit toward the eye. It is passed through a subcutaneous tunnel to exit in a small incision at the lateral canthus. Tunnels are created beneath the skin along each lid margin, and half of the fascial slip is passed to the medial canthus on each side. Making a small incision through the skin at the midportion of each lid greatly facilitates threading the fascia to the medial canthus. The fascial strips are crisscrossed beneath the medial canthal ligament and sutured to it and to each other under tension sufficient to overlap the upper lid on the lower. Practice with chewing motions is begun in 2 to 3 weeks. Adaptation of such motion to eye closure is said to be rapid [29].

The *use of free muscle grafts* neurotized on the normal side to achieve eye closure was initiated by Thompson [41–44] (see Fig. 15-3). Two or three stages are required, with the patient under general anesthesia. Denervation of the muscle to be transplanted and formation of a transnasal tunnel constitute the first procedure. The second stage involves transplanting the muscles onto the orbicularis on the normal side and the passage of the tendons to the paralyzed side. In nearly all cases tenolysis of the tendons in the tunnel has been necessary 3 to 6 months later [22]. The recommended muscle is the extensor digitorum brevis of the foot, since at least two of its four muscle bellies correspond in size to the recipient areas of the orbicularis oculi on the normal side. The complexity of this procedure and its several stages is apparent. More experience will be needed before the effective spontaneity of the motion achieved can be evaluated.

LOWER FACIAL MUSCLE PARALYSIS. Complete treatment requires attention to both the paralyzed and the nonparalyzed side.

1. *Paralyzed side correction.* The insertion of *autogenous fascia lata* to suspend the paralyzed cheek and lips was one of the earliest and remains one of the most widely practiced procedures in paralysis of the lower facial muscles (Fig. 15-4) [4, 8, 15]. Autogenous fascia is obtained via a small transverse incision in the thigh approximately three fingerbreadths above the lateral condyle in the midaxial line. The decussating fascia lata fibers are exposed, and a strip of fascia with its base proximal is raised until the vertical fibers are encountered. The fascia is threaded into the Masson fascia stripper and removed.

A perioral loop of fascia is threaded from just beyond the midline of the upper lip around the angle of the mouth to just beyond the midline of the lower lip (Fig. 15-4), a Blair fascia passer or a large autopsy needle being used. The procedure can be accomplished through small intraoral incisions and a nasolabial skin incision. The ends of the loop are sutured into the facial musculature just beneath the dermis. The angle of the loop should include orbicularis musculature.

At a second stage, 2 to 4 months later, when the perioral loop has healed in place, an additional strip or strips of fascia lata are obtained and passed via a preauricular rhytidectomy incision to the angle of the mouth, looped around the previously inserted fascia, and carried back to the temporalis fascia where, after pulling up and overcorrecting the lips, the fascial strips are interwoven with the temporalis fascia and sutured in place with nonabsorbable sutures (Fig. 15-4). The two-stage procedure ameliorates the problem of the anchoring sutures of the initial fascial loop pulling away. The rhytidectomy incision offers the opportunity of adding a modified face lift dissection and skin excision and suspension to the fascia insertion procedure. Other anchors for the fascia strips have been of use, including the zygomatic arch, the infraorbital rim, and the angle of the mandible. A *single-stage fascia insertion* is possible using as the distal anchor a dermal-fat flap at the nasolabial crease [9]. Care must be taken not to include hair follicles in the dermal flap, which is pulled up by the fascia and fixed beneath the cheek.

Masseter and temporalis muscle transfers are the major muscle transfers for reanimation of the paralyzed side [1, 16, 36]. Popularized by McLaughlin [28], the temporalis transfer requires a tendon or fascia extension. Transfer of the anterior two-thirds of the masseter to the angle of the mouth is generally considered to be easier and equally effective. The degree of animation achieved is quite variable. The suspensory function may be somewhat inferior to that achieved with the insertion of fascia lata. Various

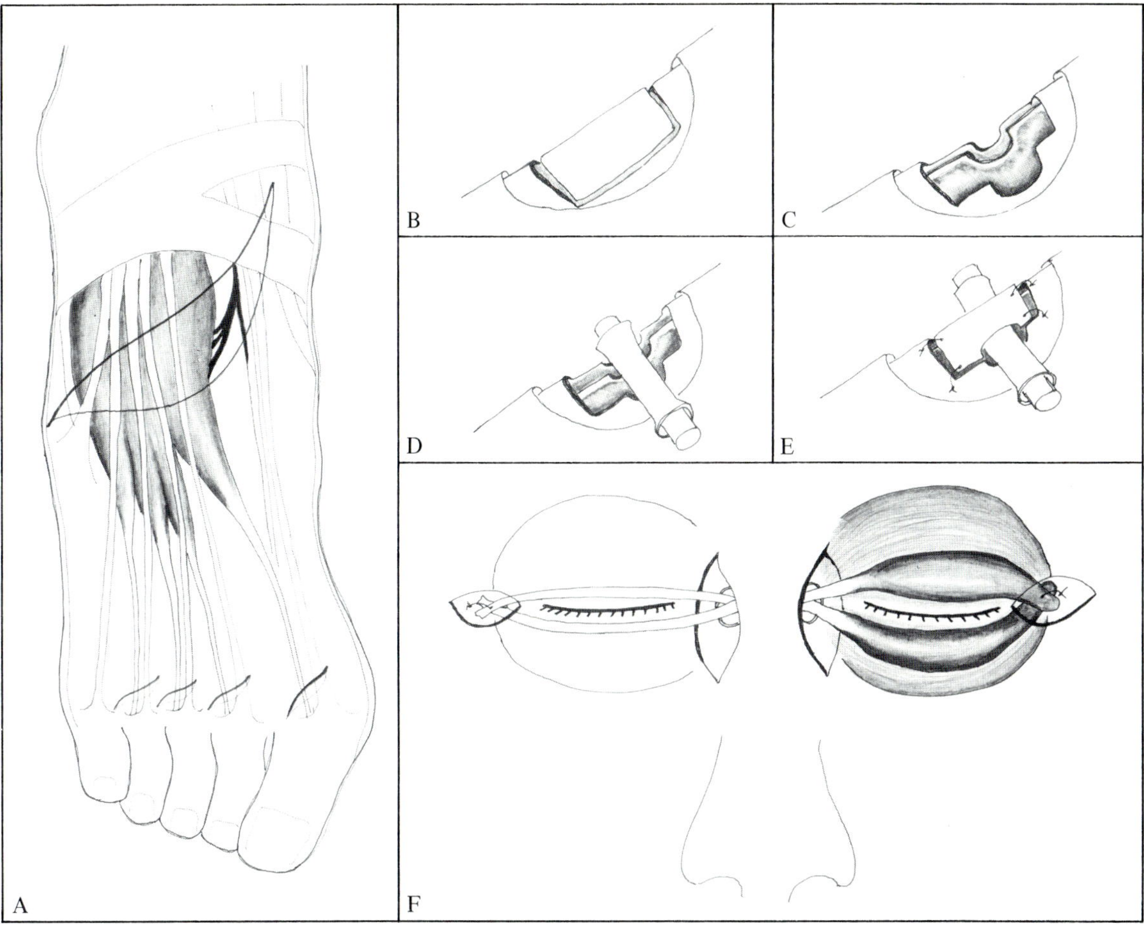

Fig. 15-3. Technique of free muscle graft for lid closure. A, drawing of the extensor digitorum brevis muscle with its nerve supply from the deep peroneal nerve emerging beneath the lower border of the inferior extensor retinaculum and just lateral to the dorsalis pedis artery exposed via the dorsal incision. All branches of the nerve are divided at the first stage as it disappears under the first muscle belly of the extensor, since the sensory component supplies only a small area of the first and second toes. A saphenous vein graft is obtained from the leg. B, through a dorsal nasal incision, a block of bone is removed at the level of the medial canthal ligaments, preserving the underlying nasal mucosa. C, a further slot is cut in the bone and septum. D, the vein graft is passed over the silicone rod and placed in the slot. E, the bone block is slotted and replaced, and the wound is closed, leaving the vein and silicone rod ends subcutaneously.

At the second stage 2 to 3 weeks later, the extensor muscle is resected through the old dorsal wound and separate interdigital incisions. F, two muscle bellies are chosen, divested of fascia, and tunneled through the medial and lateral canthal incisions on normal side (right) so that they lie against the orbicularis. The tendon ends are crossed, pulled through the tunnel as the rod is removed, tunneled through the lids, and sutured to each other and the lateral palpebral ligament on the paralyzed side (left).

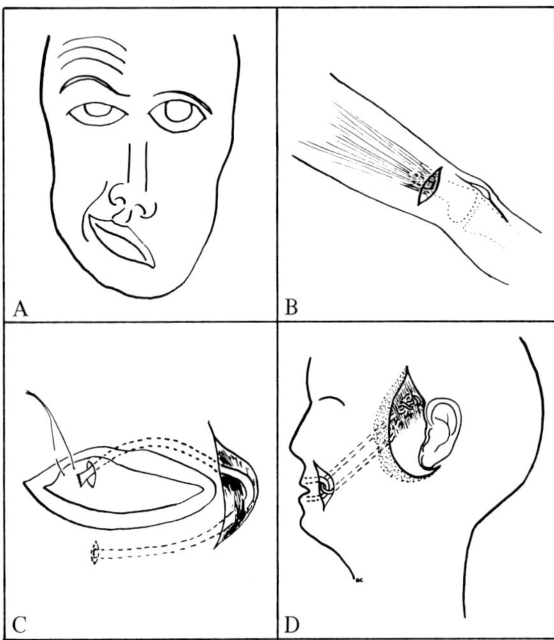

Fig. 15-4. Facial suspension with autogenous fascia lata in complete unilateral facial palsy. A, distorted features of complete left facial palsy (see text for details). B, strip of incised fascia lata in the lateral thigh prior to introducing the Masson fascia stripper; note the decussating fibers whose inclusion in the resected strip makes possible splitting of the band obtained with the decussation reinforcing the loop. C, insertion of fascia strip periorally through labial mucosal incisions and a nasolabial fold skin incision; note interweaving with the orbicularis oris muscle. D, suspension of the previously inserted perioral loop by the fascia strip inserted through a face lift incision. The ends of the fascia are woven through the temporalis fascia and sutured to it and to each other. The stippled area indicates the extent of skin excision that adds skin suspension to the procedure. A standard rhytidectomy incision can be used.

combinations of suspensions with fascia lata along with attached masseter, temporalis, and digastric muscle transfers have been reported.

Free muscle grafts are the most recent attempts to achieve dynamic action. These procedures involve one stage for denervation of the muscle to be grafted and at least one stage for the transplant. *Three types of application* have been described: (1) all of the muscle graft is in contact with normal innervated muscle; (2) only a part of the graft is in such contact; (3) the graft is in contact with partially denervated muscle (see Fig. 15-5). In addition to the extensor digitorum brevis, the palmaris longus muscle is a useful graft. Its motor nerve branches from the median nerve just above the elbow; at the initial denervation it is identified by stimulation. Its use as the first type of graft in the cross zygomaticus procedure is complicated by the extra stage involved and the mechanical inefficiency of the arrangement required to redirect its muscle action (Fig. 15-5A, B). Used as the second type of graft, the split palmaris offers a firm suspension in addition to whatever dynamic activity it acquires through its neurotization from the functioning side of the orbicularis oris (Fig. 15-5C). Use of extensor digitorum brevis muscle onlays (the third type of graft) to strengthen weak action in congenital palsies has been favorably reported [22] (see Fig. 15-5D). The elaborate procedures of cross facial nerve graft and free muscle graft with direct neurotization as well as neurovascular-muscle pedicle transfer have recently been added to this group of procedures (Fig. 15-5F) [20, 23, 44].

2. *Nonparalyzed side correction.* Hyperactivity of musculature on the normal side is generally due to the actions of four muscles: the orbicularis oris puckers the lips toward the normal side; the quadratus labii superioris elevates the upper lip; the zygomaticus retracts the angle of the mouth; and the quadratus labii inferioris pulls the lower lip and corner of the mouth downward [32, 33] (see Fig. 15-1). Usually the function of only two or three of these muscles needs to be eliminated.

The elimination of *specific muscle function* may be accomplished by *neurectomy, myomectomy, or both.* The operative approach may be by a *skin incision* or an *intraoral mucosal incision.* The latter has the advantage of direct access and lack of visible scarring, and it is the incision generally preferred. Marking the skin provides a helpful guide showing the position of the muscles, after which two sutures are passed intraorally through the whole thickness of the lip at the muscle borders. Traction on these sutures facilitates appropriate eversion of the lip and its exposure, and it marks the limits of the muscle fibers to be dissected.

The *actual operative techniques* are as follows:

1. *Zygomaticus.* This muscle is well defined and the easiest to find and cut. An incision 2 cm. from the corner of the lips permits dissection and resection of approximately 1 cm. of muscle at the point where its fibers intermingle with those of the orbicularis oris (Fig. 15-6A).
2. *Quadratus labii superioris.* This muscle is ill-defined, with its fibers adherent to the skin. A 3-cm. incision is made parallel to the lip margin where the abnormal pulling takes place (Fig. 15-6B). Muscle fibers are cut through until the undersurface of the

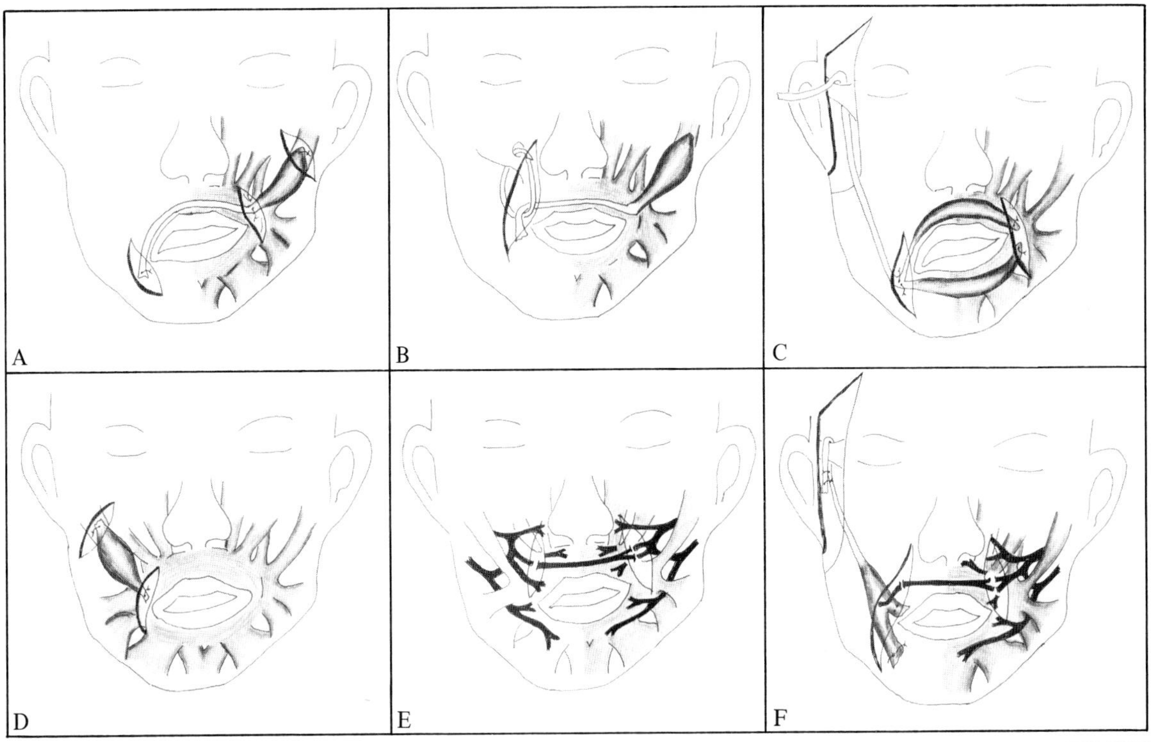

Fig. 15-5. Varieties of autogenous free muscle, nerve, and nerve-muscle grafts in inferior facial paralysis. A, cross zygomaticus graft procedure involves two stages after denervation of palmaris longus. A, initial placement of muscle graft over the fully innervated zygomaticus is followed 2 to 3 weeks later by elevation of the paralyzed angle of the mouth by a tendon pulley passed through a hole drilled in the lower edge of the malar eminence (B). C, the split palmaris muscle is passed around the mouth so that about one-half of each belly is in contact with the innervated orbicularis. The tendon is passed around the zygomatic arch and then pulled up to elevate the corner of the mouth on the paralyzed side. D, the muscle belly of the extensor digitorum brevis is placed over the partially denervated zygomaticus in a case of congenital palsy in order to strengthen function. E, several small branches of the functioning facial nerve on the normal side are joined by microsurgical technique to a sural nerve graft that, in turn, is anastomosed to the persisting facial nerve branches on the paralyzed side, thus accomplishing a cross face facial nerve graft. F, a similar cross face facial nerve graft is used to bring an immediate neural supply to a free, partially split palmaris graft. The palmaris tendon is passed around the zygomatic arch and the corner of the mouth of the paralyzed side is pulled up before the nerve graft is joined to the palmaris muscle motor nerve.

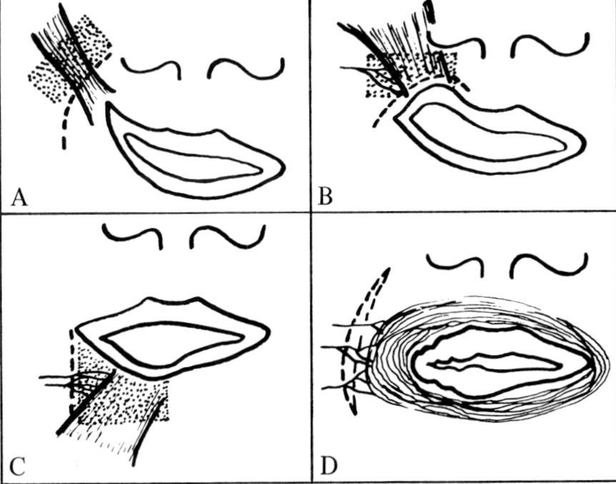

Fig. 15-6. Major muscles involved in distortion of the nonparalyzed side in patients with unilateral facial palsy. Dash line indicates incision; stippling indicates area of excision. A, zygomaticus distortion treated by intraoral incision 2 cm. from lip angle and myomectomy. B, quadratus labii superioris distortion treated by nerve and muscle resection via an intraoral incision parallel to the lip margin. C, quadratus labii inferioris distortion treated by neurectomy and myomectomy by intraoral approach. D, orbicularis oris distortion treated by selective neurectomy via nasolabial skin fold incision.

labial skin is exposed. This layer is then cut away from the vermilion border by scissor dissection. Nerve fibers reaching the lateral aspect of the muscle are eliminated at the same time.

3. *Quadratus labii inferioris.* This muscle is also ill-defined and adherent to the skin. A vertical incision is made extending down from the level of the labial commissure (Fig. 15-6C). The muscle fibers are found toward the midline. Dissection is carried out as in the quadratus labii superioris. Nerve fibers reaching the muscle transversely lie on the lateral external aspect and should be resected after proper identification.
4. *Orbicularis oris.* This is the most difficult muscle to regulate, since only a partial paralysis is usually required. Neurectomy is carried out through a skin incision in the nasolabial fold and after faradic stimulation to identify the branches that are responsible for the localized pull or partial deformation of the orbicular ring (Fig. 15-6D).

Evaluation of Results of Facial Palsy Treatment

While improvement may be expected no procedure or combination of procedures will restore normality to the paralyzed face. Suspension procedures may need to be repeated or the slings tightened over the years. Successful muscle transfer operations may produce unpleasant mass movements. The degree of long-term function of such muscle transfers has been questioned. The development of spontaneous appropriate action in free muscle grafts has sometimes been difficult to demonstrate. Many have also considered that the effect of myomectomy and neurectomy on the normal side is only transient, although good long-term results have been obtained. As a final note of caution, it must be pointed out that no significant series of cases exists in which patients matched for etiology of paralysis have had different procedures performed with comparisons being made after long periods. These deficiencies in clinical studies preclude the universal endorsement or condemnation of any of the multiple approaches to the problem of facial paralysis and leave the field open to further research and practice.

Hypertrophy of Facial Muscles

Benign masseteric hypertrophy is the most significant hyperplasia of the facial musculature [26]. Its cause is essentially *unknown* but may be related to grinding of the teeth. It is characterized by a soft, nontender, ill-defined *contractile mass* that becomes firm when the teeth are clenched. A spur of cortical bone may be found at the angle of the mandible where the hypertrophied muscle inserts.

Treatment of Benign Masseteric Hypertrophy

The prime indication for surgical treatment is cosmetic. In the external operative approach, an incision is made beneath the angle of the mandible, the tail of the parotid gland is retracted, and the mandibular and buccal branches of the facial nerve are identified and protected. The central two-thirds of the insertion of the masseter muscle is freed from the inferior border of the mandible, and resection of the hypertrophied muscle is carried out on the medial surface of the masseter. The underlying bony spur is also removed. The remaining muscle belly is sutured back to the free margin of the mandible. An intraoral approach is equally possible and avoids the danger of injury to the parotid duct or facial nerve, since these structures are located lateral to the muscle.

LIPS

Reconstruction of the lip has challenged the ingenuity of generations of surgeons. Repair of congenital defects of the lip is described in Chapter 7. Techniques for ameliorating the residua of trauma, burns, infections, and tumor excisions are considered here.

Anatomy of the Lips

The lips are the *anterior sphincter* of the oral cavity. The skin on their external surface meets the highly colored epithelium of the vermilion at the *red line.* Just superior to this junction is a surface prominence of paler skin which forms the *white line.* Infringement of this border is often the most noticeable part of any irregularity of the vermilion margin. Superficial landmarks specific to the upper lip are the *philtrum* hollow, its eminences, and the associated curving of the white and red lines into the *Cupid's bow.*

The vermilion blends into the oral mucosa. The inner and outer epithelial surfaces of the lips enclose the *orbicularis oris muscle* and the labial glands located between the muscle and the oral mucosa. The orbicularis oris muscle accomplishes the *sphincter function* of the lip, the *damming of saliva,* and the *formation of labial sounds.* Its innervation is by branches of the buccal and mandibular divisions of the facial nerve; the former supplies the upper lip and the latter the lower lip, primarily. Lip sensation is mediated by the infraorbital and mental branches of the trigeminal nerve. The labial arteries of the upper and lower lips are branches of the facial artery. They form an anastomosing coronary system and are located just beneath the mucosa on the inner surface of the lip just below its free border.

Reconstructive Procedures

Ideally, the reconstruction of lip defects would be by innervated, muscle-containing flaps, with inner and outer epithelial linings, and with the free edge covered by vermilion. Thus the emphasis is on *local flaps* in lip repair.

Defects involve the upper or lower lip and may be classified as being primarily of the skin surface, mucosal surface, full thickness of the lip, the commissure, or the vermilion.

Upper Lip Reconstruction

SKIN SURFACE DEFECTS. *Scars* are the major superficial defects and can be treated by excision or dermabrasion or both. *Replacement* of an area of scar can also be accomplished by a local flap from an area such as the nasolabial fold. Larger areas of scar, such as in burn scar *ectropion* of the lip, can be replaced by free skin grafts within the margins of the *esthetic unit* outlined by the nasolabial folds. The hair-bearing skin of the upper lip can be replaced imperfectly by a skin flap transferred from the scalp or by tattooing the skin in the reconstructed lip with India ink. The loss of local anatomical landmarks in all surface replacements of the lips is to be avoided whenever possible.

MUCOSAL SURFACE DEFECTS. Scarring between the lip and the alveolus, with or without *entropion,* can be released by transposing *a flap of local mucosa* if the involved area is small. *Free mucosal grafts* can be used for somewhat broader areas, and *skin grafts* are required for the still larger defects. Grafts may be placed on the labial surface alone, allowing the alveolar surface to reepithelialize spontaneously [51]. Non-hair-bearing skin should be used for intraoral grafts when possible.

FULL-THICKNESS LIP DEFECTS. The loss of the upper lip may be partial in the median or lateral regions, or the complete lip may be lost. In the case of *median loss,* small defects can be treated simply by extending the defect as a triangular *wedge resection,* closing it as a straight line, and using a small step at the vermilion margin to prevent a scar contracture. *Free composite grafting* of the full thickness of the lip from the lower to the upper lip has been reported but is hazardous [55, 57]. Relatively large median losses can be compensated for by advancing *lateral lip* segments toward the midline. Advancements are facilitated by the excising of a Bürow's triangle from each nasolabial area or by *perialar crescentic excisions* [71]. The *fan flap* is a useful flap of the lateral advancement-rotation type [59] (Fig. 15-7). The oral aperture narrowed by any significant flap advancement requires secondary revision. Loss of the philtrum landmark also occurs. This may be avoided by combining an Abbe flap with the advancement of lateral flaps. The Abbe flap alone is the procedure of

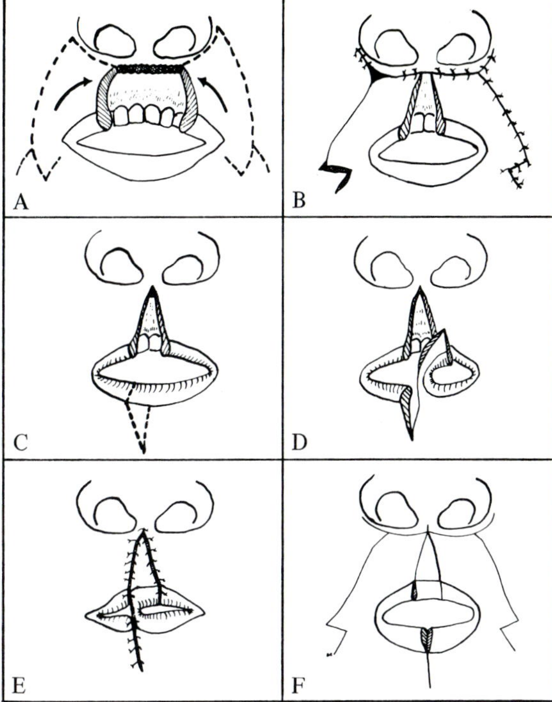

Fig. 15-7. Median loss of the upper lip treated by fan flap rotation and Abbe flap transposition. A, fan flaps outlined and their rotation-advancement indicated by arrows. Z-plasty flaps at the base help to both close the donor defect and support the advancement. B, closure of incisions with the central defect still remaining. C, Abbe flap outlined, the labial artery in the vermilion-mucosal base on one side being preserved though the vermilion in this base can be carefully incised on its surface (dotted line) to facilitate wound closure. The flap is made approximately one-half the width of the defect to be filled so that the upper and lower lip share in the width reduction. The base of the flap must be placed so that after closure of the donor defect it will lie approximately opposite the upper lip defect. The apex of the defect has been excised for better simulation of the philtrum. D, Abbe flap incised and rotated. E, suturing of the Abbe flap closes the lips together. F, flap divided 10 to 14 days later and revision of donor and recipient incisions accomplished. The Abbe flap simulates the philtrum.

choice in moderate-sized median defects, since the scars of the flap insertion simulate the philtrum margins and the lip commissures are not altered (Fig. 15-7). Variations in design of the Abbe flap permit the transfer of more vermilion than lip substance if the reconstructive needs require this [56, 65]. Occasionally, tumor excisions in the upper lip may leave intact vermilion but full-thickness loss above. The Abbe flap procedure may be modified, filling the defect by passing beneath the vermilion bridge with later excision of the vermilion of the Abbe flap itself [50].

The most useful procedure for small to moderate *lateral loss* of the upper lip is the *Estlander flap.* Like the Abbe flap, it is a triangular flap rotated on a vascular pedicle. In losses of the upper lip it is rotated from the lateral lower lip into the upper lip, with the donor site closed by direct approximation. The rounding at the angle of the lip requires revision, although modification in design can reduce this requirement [74]. Larger defects justify cheek flaps of varying shape. Simultaneous mucosal flaps must be developed to supply vermilion.

For *complete loss* of the upper lip, the treatment of choice *combines local cheek and lip flaps* advanced by perialar or Bürow triangular excisions *with an Abbe flap centrally* (Fig. 15-7). Forehead flaps lined by local turned over nasolabial tissue or by a skin graft placed prior to transferring the flap are feasible but distinctly less desirable techniques.

Lower Lip Reconstruction

Counteracting the *pull of gravity* by supplying either supporting tissue or suspensory function is a necessity in reconstruction of the lower lip. Creating a *labio-alveolar sulcus* of sufficient dimension to collect saliva and prevent drooling is also a major consideration. Preserving sensory and motor innervation is an important aid in achieving this functional result.

SKIN SURFACE DEFECTS. The procedures just discussed for the upper lip are applicable to the lower lip. In addition, the neck is a potential site for obtaining large *bipedicle* or *unipedicle* flaps for transfer as well as for creating *direct advancement* flaps which may be freed in a second stage.

MUCOSAL SURFACE DEFECTS. *Entropion* is more common in the lower lip than in the upper because the former usually suffers the major insult from an electrical or chemical burn. Methods of repair are similar to those used for reconstruction of the upper lip.

FULL-THICKNESS DEFECTS. Small to moderate losses lend themselves to repair by triangular wedge excision and closure or by the Hagedorn rectangular flap technique [45]. A variety of other procedures have been described for median losses [47]. A "step" bilateral rectangular flap advancement utilizes the line of the lip-chin crease to mask the scars [61]. In the case of *large median loss,* the defect is adequately reconstructed by a procedure in which one border of the defect is mobilized as a *rectangular flap* that is based inferiorly and slid in a medial direction, the resulting lateral defect being filled with an *Estlander flap* from the upper lip (Fig. 15-8). The Stein procedure, an Abbe flap from the central upper lip, removes the philtrum of the lip and is therefore undesirable. Still larger defects can be handled by fan flaps based superiorly or by the *Bernard operation* [58]. The latter uses the excision of Bürow's triangles of partial thickness from the nasolabial folds and employs the unresected mucosa to restore the vermilion on the lateral portions of the advanced quadrilateral cheek flaps.

In larger *lateral loss* of the lower lip, the Estlander-type procedure is the best method of reconstruction (Fig. 15-8). Nasolabial and lateral rotation flaps are also feasible.

TOTAL LOSS OF LOWER LIP. Total loss of the lower lip is more frequent than loss of the upper lip since squamous cell carcinoma involves it more often. Such defects can be reconstructed by the modified *Dieffenbach procedure,* in which large bilateral cheek flaps based on the anterior facial vessels and neck are elevated from the mandible and advanced medially. The donor defect is closed externally by the V-Y technique. The deficiency of internal mucosa and the absence of vermilion are made up by mucosal flap advancements [64]. The reconstituted lip is without innervation and, while better than that afforded by distant flaps, leaves much to be desired. Nevertheless, local tissue is to be preferred to distant lined flaps, pedicles, or muscle-skin composite transfers [66]. The preservation of innervated muscle, combined with the extension of the Bürow triangular excision principle above and below the flaps, in the procedure designed by Webster is an important principle [72] (Fig. 15-9). The formation of *neurovascular local cheek-lip flaps* under direct vision has been demonstrated by Karapandzic [63]. In this technique, myocutaneous flaps of orbicularis oris are separated from the surrounding facial musculature with minimal mucosal separation; these flaps have been proved effective in achieving innervated lower lip reconstruction in nearly total loss [60].

Commissure Reconstruction

Restoration of the commissure is required following tumor excisions or reconstructive procedures that narrow the oral stoma as well as after chemical or electrical burns of the lips that produce the same result. *Electrical burns of the mouth* are most frequent in children who chew, suck, or salivate on loose electrical outlet connections and suffer a typical low voltage, high temperature, arc type full-thickness burn of the lips and corner of the mouth [53, 68]. Early care involves tetanus immunization, clear fluids by mouth (rarely tube or intravenous routes are needed),

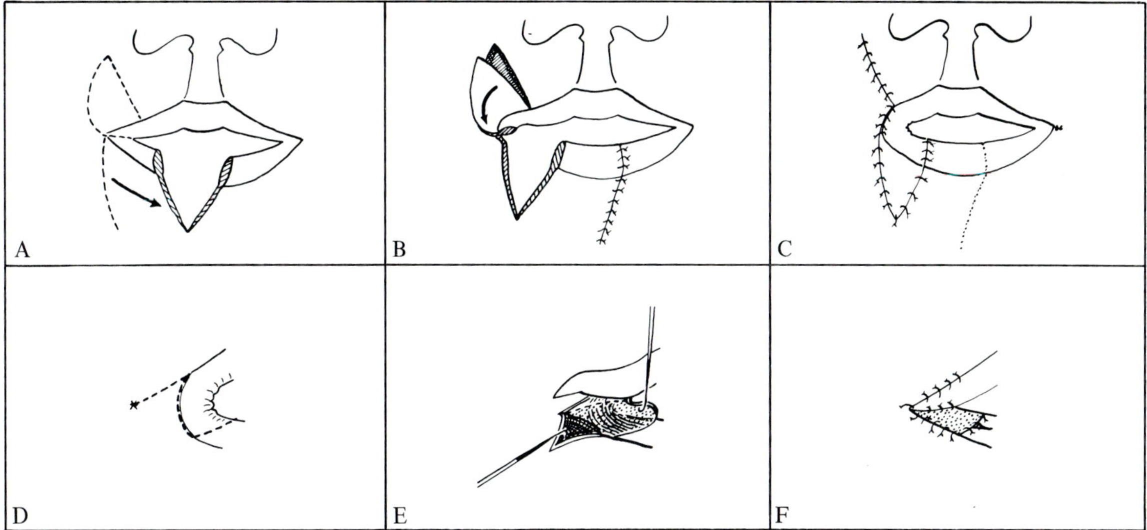

Fig. 15-8. A–C, medial lower lip loss treated by sliding medially a local rectangular flap, using an Estlander flap from the upper lip for the lateral defect. A, flaps outlined, with the Estlander flap having the labial artery preserved in the vermilion of the pedicle. B, rectangular flap shifted medially; Estlander flap incised and ready for rotation. C, closure of the donor site and the flap incisions causes a shortened, rounded commissure that requires secondary revision. D–F, commissure extension [59]. D, angle of the new commissure is to be at the site of the star. Incisions through the skin, red line, and vermilion are made as indicated by the dash line. E, vermilion flap is elevated, leaving orbicularis muscle fibers and mucosa (stippled) behind. Cross-hatched skin flap (lower left) is excised and the mucosa and muscle flap are incised along the dash line and rotated outward to form the lower lip vermilion. F, adjustment of the adjacent lower lip vermilion after the vermilion and mucosal flaps are sutured. It might be thought that the vermilion flap should be used to reconstruct the lower rather than the upper lip; however, this leads to a distinctly inferior result.

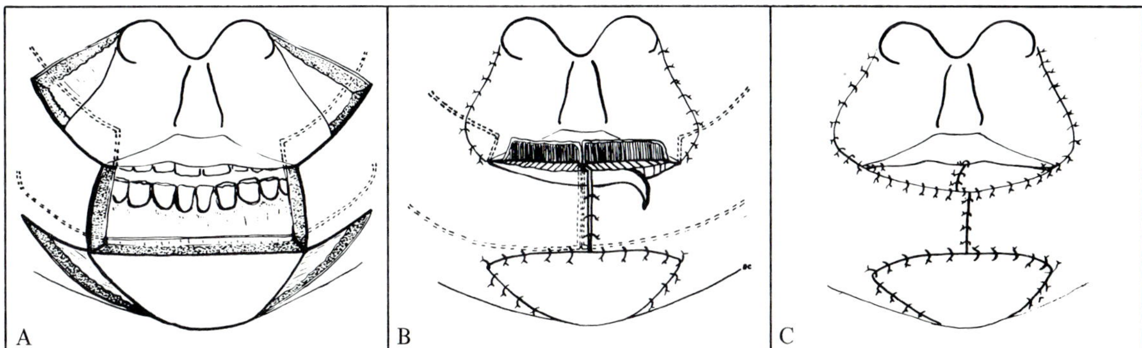

Fig. 15-9. Reconstruction of total loss of the lower lip [72]. A, rectangular cheek advancement flaps created by excising Bürow's triangles from the nasolabial region and the perimentum, preserving the oral mucosa. Mucosal incisions (double-dash lines) are placed at the level of the skin incisions inferiorly but at a higher level superiorly. B, cheek flaps advanced medially and sutured. The superior border of the cheek flaps is denuded of epithelium along the site of the future free margin of the lower lip (wide bare surface). The mucosal flaps (narrow bare surface) are incised, then folded forward over the cheek flaps to form the vermilion. C, closure of wounds after the nasolabial and perimentum tissue advancements; offset of vermilion-mucosal and cheek flap closure lines.

and brief observation to ensure the absence of any more significant form of electrical damage. Subsequent therapy is controversial. Immediate excision and reconstruction require emergency anesthesia, with its hazards, as well as involving the technical difficulties of operating in an acutely inflamed area. Delay for the approximately 3 weeks required for spontaneous separation of slough is more usual. Labial artery bleeding may occur and is controlled by finger pressure and suture ligation. Insertion of dental splints with commissure extensions at this time has been advocated [48]; they are used for 4 to 12 months to ameliorate contracture. Reconstruction by tongue flaps at this 2- to 3-week period has also been presented as a means of avoiding commissure contracture [73]. The conservative approach allowing complete spontaneous healing and scar resolution for 6 or more months prior to reconstruction is based on the fact that these injuries are often much less extensive than they initially appear and their residual deformities are usually amenable to limited reconstructive measures.

Lateral splitting of a scarred and shortened commissure with *direct advancement* of vermilion flaps is successful only in minor degrees of deformity. Splitting of the superficial tissue, excising excess skin and fat along the lines of the new opening, and replacement of vermilion by *two mucosal flaps* or a single *bilobed* one is better, but there is a tendency for the new commissure to shorten and round up. The addition of a *third small mucosal flap* at the angle itself, together with sutures to cinch up the orbicularis muscle fibers, is a more permanent solution. A well-tested and efficacious method is the combination of *vermilion and mucosal flaps* [59] (see Fig. 15-8D, E, F). More extensive losses may be treated by variants of the Estlander procedure in reverse [49].

Vermilion Reconstruction

Defects of the vermilion may be divided into those of line, of contour, and of combinations thereof. Among the *linear defects,* irregularities of the red line can be corrected by Z-plasty. The suggestion of a *Cupid's bow* can be simulated by skin excisions and direct vermilion flap advancement [59]. This procedure, however, destroys the white line and gives an artificial effect. No good method is yet available for reconstructing the white line.

Among the *contour defects,* small notch deformities can be removed by *wedge excision* and closed with step or Z-plasty technique. Broader notches, including the whistle deformity of some repaired cleft lips, can be improved by V-Y advancement of *mucosal flaps* based on the vermilion margin or by shifting *vermilion and muscle flaps* from the lip segments lateral to the defect [54, 62, 70]. Thin, cryptic vermilion can be expanded by broad *mucosal "roll"* advancement flaps, or by insertion of *dermal fat grafts,* fascia, or tendon beneath the epithelial surface [67].

Vermilion Abbe flaps or *mucosal "apron flaps"* are satisfactory for *local* vermilion replacement [56, 59]. More extensive replacement can be achieved by direct mucosal advancement as in the vermilionectomy procedure, by a tubed pedicle of mucous membrane, or by a bipedicle mucosal flap from the upper lip [69]. Young children cannot be expected to cooperate in maintaining their lips together postoperatively, and, for them, joining the two lips together is hazardous. A unilateral mucosal tube, using coronary artery and mucosa of the upper lip, transferred at once to the lower lip is possible in these cases [52]. Where no mucosa is available, as in some total reconstructions of the upper and lower lips, vermilion reconstruction can also be accomplished by use of flaps and tubes from the *tongue* [46].

CHEEKS

Defects of the cheeks requiring repair can be classified as those of the *skin surface, mucosal surface, full thickness,* and *general contour* of the cheek.

Anatomy

The cheeks are the watertight muscular side walls of the oral cavity. Their epithelial and mucosal surfaces enclose a fat pad in which the facial muscles, in particular the buccinator, are found. The cheek tissue is both redundant and extensible, permitting unrestricted jaw opening. The *prime requirement* in cheek reconstruction is *tissue ample enough* to permit mandibular movement and provided with an *inner and outer lining.*

Reconstructive Procedures of the Cheek

Skin Surface Defects

Small defects should be closed along lines that parallel the axis of the skin lines. When possible, larger defects should be replaced by *local flaps rather than free skin grafts* for the best appearance. Where grafts are needed, and the size of the defect permits, full-thickness preauricular and postauricular, cervical, and supraclavicular skin offers the best color and texture match.

Transposition flaps from the *neck* and the *preauricular and postauricular region,* with the donor sites closed by the V-Y technique, are useful in cheek coverage [78, 79]. There are limits to this method, however, and the massive replacements of giant nevi or burn scars of the cheeks and face by local flap advancements in multiple stages are rarely as successful as their diagrammatic representations. Distant tissue in the form of skin tubes or flaps, when required, can be carried to the face on a forearm attachment. Such tissue placed over broad facial areas does not allow the facial expression to show and produces an unpleasant masklike effect. Such broad areas of superficial surface defect are better treated by free skin grafts.

Mucosal Surface Defects

The redundancy of the cheek lining makes the *direct approximation* and closure of even moderate-sized defects possible. *Mucosal flap* rotations and transpositions are well tolerated. The rapidity of epithelialization of the buccal mucosa permits considerable liberty in leaving open the donor sites of such local flaps. Where the excision of a tumor or the effect of a chemical burn results in larger intraoral losses, *skin graft replacement* is necessary. Applied with a bolus dressing, these grafts are usually successful in spite of the motion and moistness of the recipient site [98]. A *contracture of about 33 percent* in size must be planned for in the initial grafting. Following extirpative procedures in the oropharynx, in which either the primary repair was tight or closure with a tongue flap was carried out, it may become necessary to release the tongue and add more lining material to the oral surface. Proper planning can often eliminate the latter disadvantage [75, 80]. *Inlay skin grafts* for the release may be suitable in many cases, but when a nearly full-thickness loss exists, flap tissue may be needed. *Cervical and temporal skin flaps* as well as *tubed pedicles,* let into the mouth through cheek or inframandibular incisions, are superior to using the oral aperture and will prove more comfortable [77].

Full-Thickness Cheek Defects

Severe trauma such as gunshot injuries, through-and-through excisions for carcinoma, radiation damage with associated osteoradionecrosis, and gangrenous stomatitis (noma) are common causes of full-thickness cheek losses [75, 82, 88]. Repair requires an *inner,* preferably non-hair-bearing, lining as well as *external* coverage. The internal lining can be supplied by an extensive *mobilization of mucosal flaps* from the margins of the defect or by *local turnover flaps* where suitable [89]. External nasolabial flaps may be turned in for lining [81]. When there is insufficient mucosa or when local skin is damaged or hair-bearing, *distant flaps* may be *lined* by skin grafts prior to transfer or so constructed that the end of the flap can be folded on itself for lining [90, 92]. Either of these methods can be carried out with a forehead flap based on the superficial temporal vessels [76, 77, 90]. The flap base can be modified so as to be useful even in cases in which the external carotid has been ligated [86]. Deltopectoral flaps may be combined with temporal flaps, and cervical and pectoral flaps can also be employed [91, 97]. A compound cervical flap, skin lined and including the sternocleidomastoid muscle, can be used for large defects [94]. The need for inner lining also can be met by inserting a tube pedicle into the defect in "doughnut" fashion and then closing the hole in the middle. When the lip commissure has been lost in continuity with the cheek defect, it is advisable whenever possible to *reconstruct the lip angle first,* transforming the defect into one of the cheek alone [85]. Simultaneous repair of both is possible, however. Recent advances in microvascular technique have led to the successful use of large free flaps for oral and pharyngeal cavity reconstruction [83, 84, 87, 95].

Contour Defects

Local areas of depression may occur in the cheek secondary to trauma or infection, which presumably initiate a local resorption of fat. Dermal fat grafts inserted intraorally offer a convenient means of repair; but they will undergo some resorption and tend to become fibrotic.

Massive contour defects of the cheeks occur in facial hemiatrophy (Romberg's disease). The treatment of choice is the insertion of large abdominal tubes or flaps, denuded of epithelium and secondary skin appendages. They can be introduced into the defect through a temporal hairline incision, and placed with their own dermis beneath the dermis of the facial skin [93]. Direct injection of Silastic remains an experimental technique at the present. Some other forms of contour defects may be ameliorated by the implantation of preformed Silastic or acrylic prostheses [96]. (For additional information on implantation materials see Chapter 3.)

FACIAL PROSTHETIC DEVICES

Both patients and plastic surgeons generally share the desire to use autogenous tissue for permanent facial reconstruction. The apparent ease of prosthetic replacement as well as the force of special circumstances, however, may lead to the choice of this approach.

Rationale for Facial Prostheses

Temporary prostheses may be of use in *camouflaging* the defects from facial resections when there is uncertainty as to whether the malignancy has been totally eradicated. Such a circumstance might preclude immediate surgical reconstruction, but at the same time the defect could be large enough to compromise the patient's function. Temporary *supporting* function may be of value in holding both bone and soft tissue in place during the healing of either surgical or traumatic defects prior to their definitive repair [99, 100, 105].

Permanent prostheses may be considered when extreme age or medical conditions preclude further operations. The technical difficulty of surgical repair is occasionally a factor. Permanent cosmetic prostheses may also be substituted to avoid creating secondary defects of autogenous tissue donor sites.

Types of Facial Prostheses

Some of the types of facial prostheses are as follows:

1. *Orbit.* An artificial eye is a common prosthetic device. Use of graduated globes for expansion of microphthalmic orbits is a form of functional prosthetic inlay. The difficulty of complete surgical orbital reconstruction following loss of both the eye and the eyelids is such that a total prosthetic external onlay retained by glasses is a common method of treatment [100].
2. *Nose.* Total replacement of the external nose with a prosthesis can be effective. A nasal cavity acrylic inlay prosthesis is a vital support for the skin flap in cases having undergone the Gillies type of treatment for congenital syphilitic nose.
3. *Ear.* Total external ear prosthetic devices of silicone or acrylic have had limited acceptance by patients and physicians [102].
4. *Lips.* Plumping devices of acrylic attached to upper dentures are of definite use in rehabilitation after cleft lip repair.
5. *Maxilla and palate.* Obturators for closing palate fistulas have long been successful. Both the immediate and the permanent support given to the cheek and the obturator effect on the palate may make the immediate prosthetic replacement of maxillary resections a useful technique. A permanent inlay prosthesis that is inserted after healing is the present standard approach to correcting the resulting defect [101, 107].

REFERENCES

Facial Muscles

1. Adams, W. The use of the masseter, temporalis and frontalis muscles in the correction of facial paralysis. *Plast. Reconstr. Surg.* 1:216, 1947.
2. Anderl, H. Reconstruction of the face through cross-face-nerve transplantation in facial paralysis. *Chir. Plast.* 2:19, 1973.
3. Antia, N. H. The scope of plastic surgery in leprosy: A ten year progress report. *Clin. Plast. Surg.* 1:69, 1974.
4. Ashley, F. L., Grazer, F. M., Machida, R. C., McConnell, D. V., and Morgan, S. C. A modified operation for the correction of facial paralysis. *Plast. Reconstr. Surg.* 41:58, 1968.
5. Banuelos, A. Combined operation for facial palsy. *Arch. Ophthalmol.* 89:329, 1973.
6. Barclay, T. L., and Roberts, A. C. Restoration of movement to the upper eyelid in facial palsy. *Br. J. Plast. Surg.* 22:257, 1969.
7. Beard, C. Canthoplasty and brow elevation for facial palsy. *Arch. Ophthalmol.* 71:386, 1964.
8. Brown, J. B., McDowell, F., and Fryer, M. P. Facial paralysis supported with autogenous fascia lata. *Ann. Surg.* 127:858, 1948.
9. Clodius, L. Reconstruction of the nasolabial fold. *Plast. Reconstr. Surg.* 50:467, 1972.
10. Clodius, L. Selective neurectomies to achieve symmetry in partial and complete facial paralysis. *Br. J. Plast. Surg.* 29:43, 1976.
11. Colman, C. C., and Walker, J. C. Technic of anastomosis of the branches of the facial nerve with the spinal accessory for facial paralysis. *Ann. Surg.* 131:960, 1950.
12. Conley, J. Facial rehabilitation following radical parotid gland surgery. *Arch. Otolaryngol.* (Chicago) 66:58, 1957.
13. Conley, J. Accessory neuromotor pathways to the face. *Trans. Am. Acad. Ophthalmol. Otolaryngol.* 68:1064, 1964.
14. Conley, J. The treatment of long-standing facial paralysis – a new concept. *Trans. Am. Acad. Ophthalmol. Otolaryngol.* 78:386, 1974.
15. Converse, J. M. (Ed.). *Reconstructive Plastic Surgery* (2nd ed.). Philadelphia: Saunders, 1976.
16. Conway, H. Muscle plastic operations for facial paralysis. *Ann. Surg.* 147:541, 1958.
17. Correia, P. C., and Zani, R. Masseter muscle rotation in the treatment of inferior facial paralysis: Anatomical and clinical observations. 52:370, 1973.
18. Dessapt, B., Morin, A., Janvier, H., and Masson, Ch. L. Les greffes musculaires: Etude anatomique et technique de prélèvements des muscles pédiux et petit palmaire. *Ann. Chir. Plast.* 19:235, 1974.
19. Frackelton, W. H. Surgical creation of wrinkles. *Plast. Reconstr. Surg.* 9:565, 1952.
20. Freilinger, G. A new technique to correct facial paralysis. *Plast. Reconstr. Surg.* 56:44, 1975.
21. Guerrero-Santos, J., Ramirez, M., and Espaillat, L. Treatment of facial paralysis of static suspension with dermal flaps. *Plast. Reconstr. Surg.* 48:325, 1971.
22. Hakelius, L. Transplantation of free autogenous muscle in the treatment of facial paralysis. A clinical study. *Scand. J. Plast. Reconstr. Surg.* 8:220, 1974.
23. Harii, K., Ohmori, K., and Tarii, S. Free gracilis muscle transplantation with microneurovascular anastomosis for the treatment of facial paralysis: A preliminary report. *Plast. Reconstr. Surg.* 57:133, 1976.
24. Kessler, L. A., Moldaver, J., and Pool, J. L. Hypoglossal facial anastomosis for treatment of facial paralysis. *Neurology* 9:118, 1959.

25. Martin, H., and Helsper, J. T. Spontaneous return of function following surgical section or excision of the seventh cranial nerve in the surgery of parotid tumors. *Ann. Surg.* 146:715, 1957.
26. Masters, F., Georgiade, N., and Pickrell, K. The surgical treatment of benign masseteric hypertrophy. *Plast. Reconstr. Surg.* 15:215, 1955.
27. Masters, F. W., Robinson, D. W., and Simons, J. N. Temporalis transfer for lagophthalmos due to seventh nerve palsy. *Am. J. Surg.* 110:607, 1965.
28. McLaughlin, C. R. Permanent facial paralysis. *Lancet* 2:647, 1952.
29. Mitler, S. H., and Wood, A. M. Surgical treatment of facial nerve involvement caused by leprosy. *Am. J. Trop. Med. Hyg.* 25:445, 1976.
30. Morel-Fatio, D., and Lalardrie, J-P. Palliative surgical treatment of facial paralysis: The palpebral spring. *Plast. Reconstr. Surg.* 33:446, 1964.
31. Morgan, R. L., and Rich, A. M. Four years' experience with the Morel-Fatio palpebral spring. *Plast. Reconstr. Surg.* 53:404, 1974.
32. Niklison, J. Contribution to the subject of facial paralysis. *Plast. Reconstr. Surg.* 17:276, 1956.
33. Niklison, J. Facial paralysis: Moderation of nonparalyzed muscles. *Br. J. Plast. Surg.* 18:397, 1965.
34. Perret, G. Results of phrenicofacial nerve anastomosis for facial paralysis. *Arch. Surg.* 94:505, 1967.
35. Puckett, C. L., Neale, H. W., and Pickrell, K. L. Dynamic correction of unilateral paralysis of the lower lip. *Plast. Reconstr. Surg.* 55:397, 1975.
36. Rubin, L. R., Bromberg, B. E., and Walden, R. H. Congenital Bilateral Facial Paralysis, Moebius Syndrome, Surgical Animation of the Face. *Transactions of the Fourth International Congress of Plastic and Reconstructive Surgery* (1969). Amsterdam: Excerpta Medica, 1969.
37. Rubin, L. R. The anatomy of a smile: Its importance in the treatment of facial paralysis. *Plast. Reconstr. Surg.* 53:384, 1974.
38. Smellie, G. D. Restoration of the blinking reflex in facial palsy by a simple lid-load operation. *Br. J. Plast. Surg.* 19:279, 1966.
39. Smith, J. A New Technique of Facial Animation. *Transactions of the Fifth International Congress of Plastic and Reconstructive Surgery* (1971). Melbourne, Australia: Butterworth, 1971.
40. Smith, J. W. Advances in facial nerve repair. *Surg. Clin. North Am.* 52:1287, 1972.
41. Thompson, N. Treatment of Facial Paralysis by Free Muscle Grafts. *Transactions of the Fifth International Congress of Plastic and Reconstructive Surgery* (1971). Melbourne, Australia: Butterworth, 1971.
42. Thompson, N. Autogenous free grafts of skeletal muscle. *Plast. Reconstr. Surg.* 48:11, 1971.
43. Thompson, N. A review of autogenous skeletal muscle grafts and their clinical applications. *Clin. Plast. Surg.* 1:349, 1974.
44. Thompson, N., and Gustavson, E. H. The use of neuromuscular free autografts with microneural anastomoses to restore elevation to the paralysed angle of the mouth in cases of unilateral facial paralysis: With an analysis of late results of muscle grafts in the treatment of 103 cases of facial hemiparesis. *Chir. Plast.* 3:165, 1976.

Lips

45. Andrews, E. B. Repair of lower lip defects by the Hagedorn rectangular flap method. *Plast. Reconstr. Surg.* 34:27, 1964.
46. Bakamjian, V. Use of tongue flaps in lower lip reconstruction. *Br. J. Plast. Surg.* 17:76, 1964.
47. Bretteville-Jensen, G. Reconstruction of the lower lip after central excisions. *Br. J. Plast. Surg.* 26:247, 1973.
48. Colcleugh, R. G., and Ryan, J. E. Splinting electrical burns of the mouth in children. *Plast. Reconstr. Surg.* 58:239, 1976.
49. Converse, J. M. The "over and out" flap for restoration of the corner of the mouth: Case report. *Plast. Reconstr. Surg.* 56:575, 1975.
50. Converse, J. M. The bridge flap for reconstruction of a full-thickness defect of the upper lip. *Plast. Reconstr. Surg.* 57:442, 1976.
51. Cosman, B., and Crikelair, G. F. Release of the prolabium in the bilateral cleft lip. *Cleft Palate J.* 3:122, 1966.
52. Cosman, B., Gong, K., and Crikelair, G. F. Horizontal cross-lip flap with pedicle at commissure: Case report. *Plast. Reconstr. Surg.* 41:273, 1968.
53. Crikelair, G. F., and Dhaliwal, A. S. The cause and prevention of electrical burns of the mouth in children: A protective cuff. *Plast. Reconstr. Surg.* 58:206, 1976.
54. Crikelair, G. F., and Hickey, M. J. Correction of the "whistle deformity." *Surg. Gynecol. Obstet.* 104:759, 1957.
55. Dufourmentel, C., Mouly, R., Preaux, J., and Marchac, D. The free composite graft from lip to lip. *Ann. Chir. Plast.* 12:119, 1967.
56. Fischl, R. A. Hemifacial atrophy: Unusual cross-lip flap. *N.Y. State J. Med.* 73:313, 1973.
57. Flanagin, W. S. Free composite grafts from lower to upper lip. *Plast. Reconstr. Surg.* 17:376, 1956.
58. Fries, R. Advantages of a basic concept in lip reconstruction after tumour resection. *J. Maxillofac. Surg.* 1:13, 1973.
59. Gillies, H. D., and Millard, D. R., Jr. *Principles and Art of Plastic Surgery.* Boston: Little, Brown, 1957.

60. Jabaley, M. E., Orcutt, T. W., and Clement, R. L. Applications of the Karapandzic principle of lip reconstruction after excision of lip cancer. *Am. J. Surg.* 132:529, 1976.
61. Johanson, B., Aspelund, E., Breine, U., and Holmström, H. Surgical treatment of non-traumatic lower lip lesions with special reference to the step technique: A follow up on 149 patients. *Scand. J. Plast. Reconstr. Surg.* 8:252, 1974.
62. Kapetansky, D. I. Double pendulum flaps for whistling deformities in bilateral cleft lips. *Plast. Reconstr. Surg.* 47:321, 1971.
63. Karapandzic, M. Reconstruction of lip defects by local arterial flaps. *Br. J. Plast. Surg.* 27:93, 1974.
64. May, H. One stage operation for closure of large defects of lower lip and chin. *Surg. Gynecol. Obstet.* 73:236, 1941.
65. Millard, D. R., Jr. A lip fleur-de-lis flap. *Plast. Reconstr. Surg.* 34:34, 1964.
66. O'Brien, B. A muscle-skin pedicle for total reconstruction of the lower lip. *Plast. Reconstr. Surg.* 45:395, 1970.
67. Pickrell, K., Masters, F., Georgiade, N., and Horton, C. Restoration of lip contour using fascia, tendon, and dermal grafts. *Plast. Reconstr. Surg.* 14:126, 1954.
68. Pits, W., Pickrell, K., Quinn, G., and Massengill, R. Electrical burns of lips and mouth in infants and children. *Plast. Reconstr. Surg.* 44:471, 1969.
69. Spira, M., and Hardy, S. B. Vermilionectomy: Review of cases with variations in technique. *Plast. Reconstr. Surg.* 33:39, 1964.
70. Watson, A. C. H. An innervated neuro-muscular flap for the correction of defects of the vermilion border of the lip. *Br. J. Plast. Surg.* 26:355, 1973.
71. Webster, J. P. Crescentic peri-alar cheek excision for upper lip flap advancement with a short history of upper lip repair. *Plast. Reconstr. Surg.* 16:434, 1955.
72. Webster, R. C., Coffey, R. J., and Kelleher, R. E. Total and partial reconstruction of the lower lip with innervated muscle-bearing flaps. *Plast. Reconstr. Surg.* 25:360, 1960.
73. Zarem, H. A., and Grier, D. M., Jr. Tongue flap for reconstruction of the lips after electrical burns. *Plast. Reconstr. Surg.* 53:310, 1974.
74. Zisser, G. A contribution to the primary reconstruction of the upper lip and labial commissure following tumour excision. *J. Maxillofac. Surg.* 3:211, 1975.

Cheeks

75. Bakamjian, V. Y. The surgical management of cancer of the cheek. *J. Surg. Oncol.* 6:255, 1974.
76. Campion, R. Closure of full-thickness cheek loss by forehead flap. *Br. J. Plast. Surg.* 13:76, 1960–61.
77. Conway, H., Stark, R. B., and Kavanaugh, J. D. Variations of the temporal flap. *Plast. Reconstr. Surg.* 9:410, 1952.
78. Crow, M. L., and Crow, F. J. Resurfacing large cheek defects with rotation flaps from the neck. *Plast. Reconstr. Surg.* 58:196, 1976.
79. De Cholnoky, T. The repair of extensive soft tissue losses of the cheek: The use of sliding skin flaps from the preauricular and parotid region. *Plast. Reconstr. Surg.* 16:288, 1955.
80. Edgerton, M. T., and Des Prez, J. D. Reconstruction of the oral cavity in the treatment of cancer. *Plast. Reconstr. Surg.* 19:89, 1957.
81. Elliott, R. A., Jr. Use of nasolabial skin flap to cover intraoral defects. *Plast. Reconstr. Surg.* 58:201, 1976.
82. Farina, R., Neto, D. S., Santos, P. S., and Castro, O. Surgical treatment of sequelae of gangrenous stomatitis (noma). *Plast. Reconstr. Surg.* 16:47, 1955.
83. Finseth, F., Kavarana, N., and Antia, N. Complications of free flap transfers to the mouth region. *Plast. Reconstr. Surg.* 56:652, 1975.
84. Fujino, T., and Saito, S. Repair of pharyngoesophageal fistula by microvascular transfer of a free skin flap. *Plast. Reconstr. Surg.* 56:549, 1975.
85. Gillies, H. D., and Millard, D. R., Jr. *Principles and Art of Plastic Surgery.* Boston: Little, Brown, 1957.
86. Hamaker, R. C., and Conley, J. Modified nondelayed forehead flap. *Arch. Otolaryngol.* 101: 189, 1975.
87. Harashima, T., Fujino, T., and Aojagi, F. Reconstruction of the oral cavity with a free flap. *Plast. Reconstr. Surg.* 58:412, 1976.
88. Ivy, R. H. The repair of full-thickness cheek defects following irradiation necrosis. *Plast. Reconstr. Surg.* 4:188, 1949.
89. Kaplan, I., and Plaschkes, J. Closure of fistulae of head and neck by combined inverted and rotation flaps. *Br. J. Plast. Surg.* 14:334, 1961.
90. Kavarana, N. M. Use of a folded forehead flap for reconstruction after a large excision of the full thickness of the cheek. *Plast. Reconstr. Surg.* 56:629, 1975.
91. McGregor, I. A., and Reid, W. H. Simultaneous temporal and deltopectoral flap for full thickness defects of the cheek. *Plast. Reconstr. Surg.* 45: 326, 1970.
92. Naryanan, M. Immediate reconstruction with bipolar scalp flap after excision of huge cheek cancers. *Plast. Reconstr. Surg.* 46:548, 1970.
93. Neumann, C. G. The use of large buried pedicled flaps of dermis and fat; clinical and pathological evaluation in the treatment of progressive facial hemiatrophy. *Plast. Reconstr. Surg.* 11:315, 1953.

94. Owens, N. A compound neck pedicle designed for the repair of massive facial defects: Formation, development and application. *Plast. Reconstr. Surg.* 15:369, 1955.
95. Panje, W. R., Bardach, J., and Krause, C. J. Reconstruction of the oral cavity with a free flap. *Plast. Reconstr. Surg.* 58:415, 1976.
96. Rhodes, R. D., III. Restoration of facial defects with individually prefabricated silicone prostheses. *Plast. Reconstr. Surg.* 43:201, 1969.
97. Shons, A. R., and McQuarrie, D. G. Cervical-pectoral flaps in the treatment of advanced oral cancer. *J. Surg. Oncol.* 7:213, 1975.
98. Slanetz, C. A., Jr., and Rankow, R. M. The intraoral use of split thickness skin grafts in head and neck surgery. *Am. J. Surg.* 104:721, 1962.

Facial Prosthetic Devices

99. Bulbulian, A. H. Maxillofacial prosthetics: Its origin and present status. *Mayo Clin. Proc.* 39:3, 1965.
100. Bulbulian, A. H. *Facial Prosthetics.* Springfield, Ill.: Thomas, 1973.
101. Corso, P. E., and Schachter, A. Making a folded denture or intraoral prosthesis for insertion into a small mouth. *Plast. Reconstr. Surg.* 52:94, 1973.
102. Fromm, B. E., Knutson, P-O., and Stenström, S. J. Prosthetic ears – two methods of fixing to a reconstructed auditory meatus. *Plast. Reconstr. Surg.* 34:252, 1964.
103. Masson, J. K. Relationship of surgery to prosthetic reconstruction of maxillofacial areas. *Mayo Clin. Proc.* 39:20, 1964.
104. McConnell, D. V., and Nixon, M. A simplified method for the construction of facial prostheses. *Plast. Reconstr. Surg.* 33:278, 1964.
105. Salyer, K. E., Rinkle, R. D., Hahn, G. W., and Layton, J. G. Interrelated role of maxillofacial prosthetics and reconstructive surgery. *Am. J. Surg.* 126:496, 1973.
106. Schaaf, N. G. Color characterizing silicone rubber facial prostheses. *J. Prosthet. Dent.* 24:198, 1970.
107. Schaaf, N. G., and Carl, W. Prosthetic rehabilitation of the head and neck cancer patient. *J. Surg. Oncol.* 6:311, 1974.

Primary Intraoral Tumors

DWIGHT C. HANNA

TUMORS OF THE TONGUE

Since Billroth [3] first made the statement, "Without inflammation, cancer does not exist," many authors have studied and written about various types of irritation to the tongue in their search for the cause of cancer. The irritating role of tobacco, either chewed or smoked, has received great emphasis in recent years. Most authors who have studied the incidence of multiple intraoral cancers agree that a patient with an intraoral cancer has a greater potential of developing another tumor [22, 29, 37, 48]. Moore [35] has tried to show that patients who continue to smoke after the development of a primary intraoral cancer incur a far greater possibility of developing a second cancer than those who stop smoking. Kuehn et al. [25] have also shown that smoking probably has a role in the development of oral, laryngeal, esophageal, and bladder cancer, and if patients live long enough for a second or third malignancy to develop, all of these organ systems may be affected.

History

Down through the ages the tongue has been amputated as a punitive measure, but nothing was recorded in literature about the treatment of lingual cancer until 1635, when Alexander Read [39] first described cancer of the tongue. In 1664, deMarchetti [5] published the first report of a surgical excision of the tongue. From then until the early 1900s various surgeons excised cancers of the tongue and individual metastatic lymph nodes of the neck. In 1906, however, Crile et al. [13] gave us the first clear understanding of the importance of removing all of the cervical lymphatics. He presented a carefully planned procedure designed to remove the regional lymphatics along with the primary lesion. This plan included primary lesions of the tongue and floor of the mouth in continuity with a dissection of the neck. With minor modifications, the neck dissection that he described is the standard procedure used today.

However, modern techniques of anesthesia, current understanding of fluid balance, and miracle antibiotic drugs were not available then, so infection, fistulas, and high morbidity and mortality figures forced surgeons to give way to radiation treatment. In 1902 Dickson employed x-ray and Dominici introduced radium as a means of treatment [30]. The description of interstitial implantation by Stevenson [44], in 1914, laid the groundwork for therapy techniques employed by modern radiologists. Martin et al. [31, 32] and many others, with the use of endotracheal anesthesia, antibiotics, and the administration of blood transfusions, brought the treatment of intraoral cancers back into the field of surgery, and a significant improvement in morbidity, mortality, complication, and survival figures began to appear. Now the pendulum has swung again toward the combined use of radiation [49], chemotherapy [15], and surgery. Perhaps from these modalities of treatment will eventually arise the best means of treating cancer of the tongue.

Incidence

Over 95 percent of tongue cancers are of the squamous cell variety, with most of the cancers occurring on the lateral border of the middle one-third of the tongue [42]. The next most common area is the posterior third of the tongue, then the anterior third, and last the undersurface of the tip. Tumors of the tongue make up about 1 to 3 percent of all cancers of the body and about 24 percent of all intraoral lesions. In a recent study from Memorial Hospital in New York of 758 patients with cancer of the oral cavity, in 9 percent of the cases the original lesion was in the buccal cavity, 20 percent in the floor of the mouth, 25 percent in the anterior two-thirds of the tongue, and 15 percent in the posterior one-third of the tongue [41]. Our experience is that tongue cancers make up 40 percent of intraoral cancers seen in our clinic [20].

A definite increase in the number of women affected by cancer of the tongue has been noted over the years. In 1940 Martin et al. [31] reported that out of 556 patients with cancer of the tongue, 13 percent were women, whereas in 1956 Berridge and James [2] reported that 27.4 percent of 102 cases were women. More recently Botstein and his colleagues [4] reported a 38.5 percent incidence and Mendelson, Woods, and Beahrs [33] a 42 percent incidence. Norway, Sweden, Finland, and Russia report much higher incidences in women, but this is thought to be due to the Plummer-Vinson syndrome [36].

Classification and Staging

Anyone treating cancer of the tongue should be thoroughly familiar with the TNM system (T denotes primary lesion and its extent, N indicates the status of the regional lymph nodes from 0 to 3, and M the presence of distant metastasis from 0 to 1) for classification and staging of cancer developed by the American Joint Committee for Cancer Staging and End-Results Reporting [9] (Tables 16-1, 16-2). By being familiar with this system one will be better able to choose proper treatment and better understand the eventual result and prognosis following treatment. The TNM system is a clinical staging system that is carried out before any definitive therapy is given; it is not changed to account for any subsequent finding of regional or distant metastasis.

Table 16-1. Definition of T Categories of the Oral Cavity

Category	Definition
T_{is}	Carcinoma in situ
T_1	Tumor 2 cm. or less in greatest diameter
T_2	Tumor greater than 2 cm. but not greater than 4 cm. in greatest diameter
T_3	Tumor greater than 4 cm. in greatest diameter
T_4	Massive tumor greater than 4 cm. in diameter with deep invasion involving antrum, pterygoid muscles, root of tongue, or skin of neck

Table 16-2. Cervical Lymph Node Classification

Category	Definition
N_0	No clinically positive node
N_1	Single clinically positive homolateral node less than 3 cm. in diameter
N_2	Single clinically positive homolateral node 3 to 6 cm. in diameter or multiple clinically positive homolateral nodes, none greater than 6 cm. in diameter
N_{2a}	Single clinically positive homolateral node 3 to 6 cm. in diameter
N_{2b}	Multiple clinically positive homolateral nodes, none greater than 6 cm. in diameter
N_3	Massive homolateral node(s), bilateral nodes, or contralateral node(s)
N_{3a}	Clinically positive homolateral node(s), one greater than 6 cm. in diameter
N_{3b}	Bilateral clinically positive nodes (in this situation each side of the neck should be staged separately; that is, N_{3b} – right N_{2a}, left N_1)
N_{3c}	Contralateral clinically positive node(s) only

Pathology

For the most part cancers involving the *anterior two-thirds* of the tongue are highly differentiated squamous cell carcinomas (Grades I and II), whereas 80 percent of the cancers in the base or *posterior third* of the tongue are nonkeratonizing carcinomas [31]. The epithelium of the base of the tongue arises from the primitive foregut, entodermal in origin, and thus responds to radiation in a manner similar to that of tumors of the hypopharynx. The undifferentiated and transitional cell carcinomas of the tongue are fast growing and spread early to lymph nodes. Spindle cell epidermoid carcinomas and adenocystic carcinomas occur in the tongue but are very uncommon and thus are not discussed in detail.

The *incidence of metastasis to the lymph nodes* in the neck varies with the experience of different authors. One of the lowest percentages of metastatic involvement, 40 percent, was reported by Berridge and James [2] in 1956, and incidences to as high as 68.8 percent were reported by Gibb et al. [21] in 1949. My own experience has shown cervical metastases to be present in 65 percent of the cases when the patient was first seen [20]. There appears to be a definite correlation between the size of the primary tumor and the incidence of metastasis. Southwick [42] states that in all lesions over 2 cm. in diameter (T_2, T_3, and T_4) there is a yield of over 50 percent positive nodes.

Many textbooks have described the lymphatic spread in patients with cancer of the tongue. Ward and Hendrick [47] described the drainage from the anterior one-third of the tongue to the submental, submaxillary, and internal jugular chain. Larson et al. [26] confirmed this, except that they found no drainage into the submental nodes. They further demonstrated that no crossover of lymphatics to the opposite side exists until the cancer causes lymphatic obstruction. When obstruction occurs, the valves are destroyed and retrograde flow is possible, resulting in lymph node involvement high in the neck and also, perhaps, flow to the contralateral side.

Benign Lesions of the Tongue

Cancer of the tongue must be differentiated from a variety of benign or premalignant conditions involving the tongue.

Benign Changes in the Tongue

In each of these conditions reassurance is all the care that the patient needs.

1. *Hairy tongue* caused by elongated papillae that become stained by food or tobacco (Fig. 16-1); a toothbrush and hydrogen perioxide can improve the appearance.

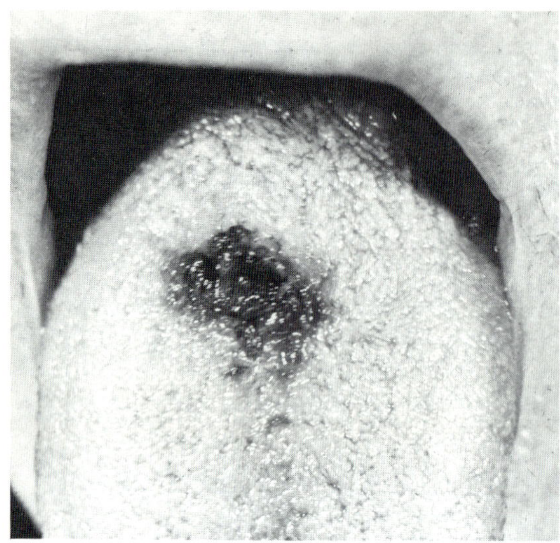

Fig. 16-1. Hairy tongue. The darkened area in the center of the tongue is made up of elongated papillae that become stained by food or tobacco.

2. *Congenital fissured tongue.* There is no break in the mucosa and no real fissure, but rather long papillae falling apart in rows; it is easily cared for by good oral hygiene.
3. *Geographic tongue.* Red desquamated patches are surrounded by white borders of thickened papillae.
4. *Stomal ulcers.* These are extremely painful, sudden in onset, surrounded by a red halo, and they disappear spontaneously in 2 or 3 weeks (Fig. 16-2).

Benign Tongue Tumors Not Requiring Excision

1. *Glossitis rhomboidica medians.* This condition is found in the center of the tongue at the junction of the middle and posterior third of the tongue; its cause is unknown (Fig. 16-3).
2. *Small areas of leukoplakia* that are not ulcerated and that frequently disappear when smoking ceases or dentures are adjusted.
3. *Mucoceles,* which are usually found on the underside of the tongue.
4. *Hemangiomas or lymphangiomas* that remain small and cause few symptoms (Fig. 16-4).
5. *Lingual tonsils,* which are generally found on the lateral aspect of the posterior one-third of the tongue without ulceration and without change in size over a prolonged period of observation.

Benign Tongue Tumors Requiring Excision

1. *Papillomas,* both small and large; they represent squamous epithelial proliferations developing into folds or finger-like projections and require com-

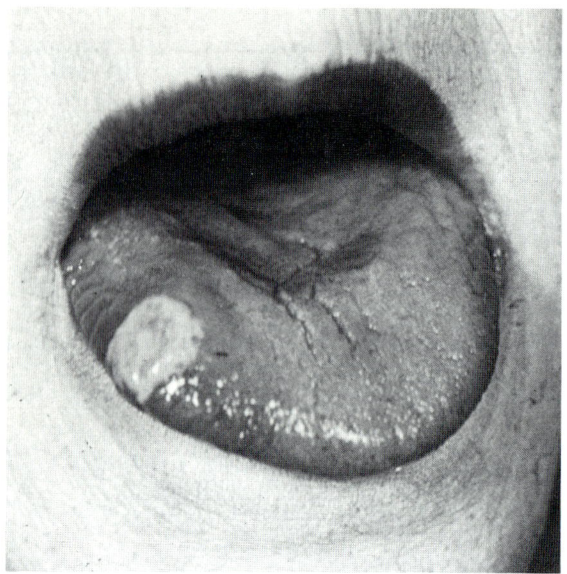

Fig. 16-2. Benign ulcer of tongue. This stomal ulcer has a rapid onset, is very painful, and disappears spontaneously in 2 or 3 weeks.

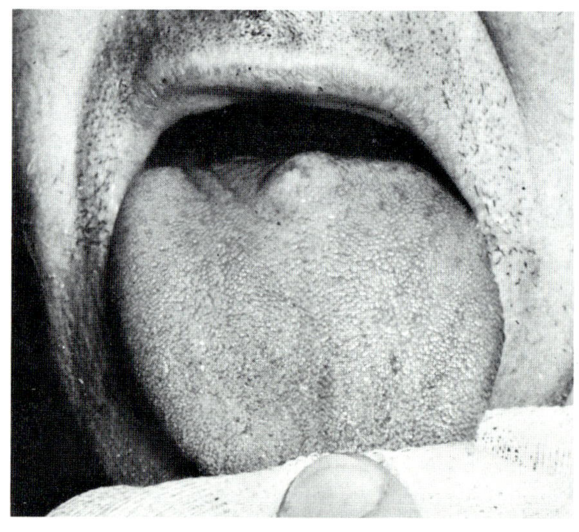

Fig. 16-3. Glossitis rhomboidica medians appears as a painless, slightly firm, elevated lesion in the midline of the tongue at the junction of the middle and posterior third. No treatment is required.

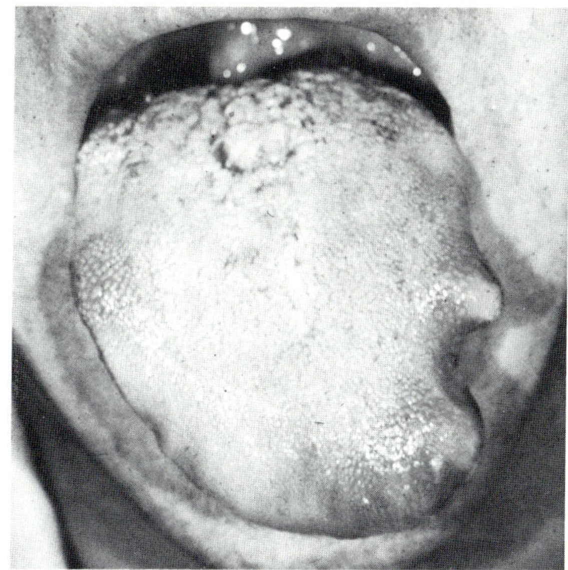

Fig. 16-4. Hemangioma of tongue. The purplish-red compressible lesion is evident along the margins of the tongue in this patient.

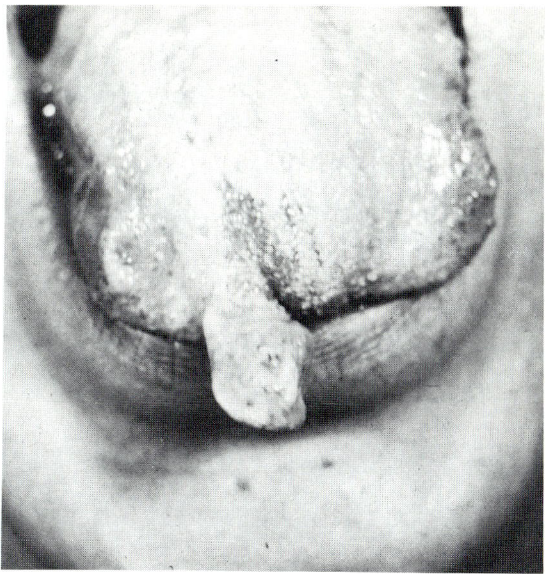

Fig. 16-5. Papilloma of tongue. Growth may occur from a narrow base. Though usually epithelial in origin, they may be fibromas or neurofibromas.

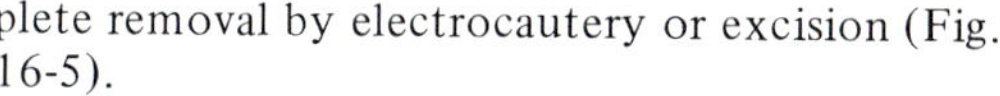

plete removal by electrocautery or excision (Fig. 16-5).

2. *Condylomas,* which are large confluent papillomas of the tongue and are best removed by electrosurgery.
3. *Granular cell myoblastomas,* which usually occur as submucosal swellings in the middle third of the dorsum or lateral border of the tongue, without ulceration, and appear as a firm, discrete, yellowish or grayish-white tumor on transection; they are frequently confused with an epidermoid cancer but respond well to wedge excision.
4. *Large patches of leukoplakia* that show some thickening but do not completely disappear when smoking ceases.
5. *Pregnancy tumor of the tongue* occurs as a granuloma that is usually very vascular and difficult to differentiate histologically from an infected hemangioma; it can be excised if troublesome, although it will often disappear following pregnancy (Fig. 16-6).
6. *Ulcers caused by syphilis and tuberculosis,* which can be diagnosed by biopsy and treated medically (Fig. 16-7).

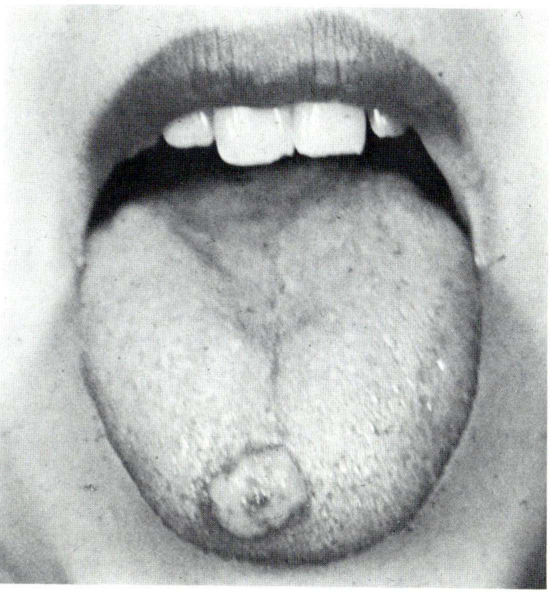

Fig. 16-6. Pregnancy tumor of tongue. This granuloma usually disappears spontaneously following pregnancy.

Diagnosis of Cancer of the Tongue

Very few cancers of the tongue will be found on a routine examination. Usually the patient presents himself at the doctor's or dentist's office because of

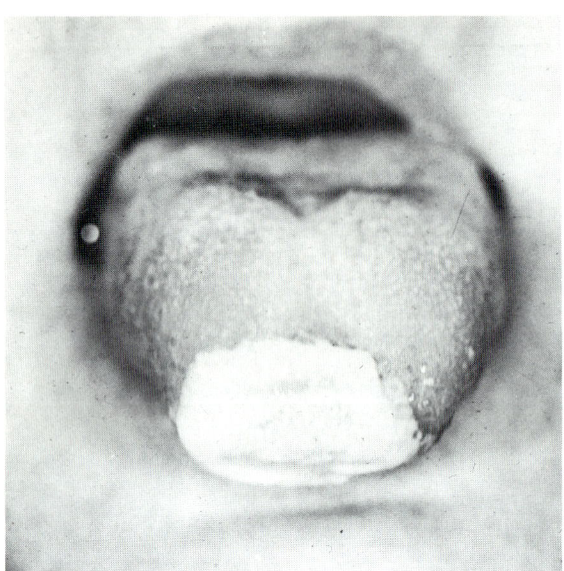

Fig. 16-7. Syphilitic chancre of tongue. White patches such as this are often scattered over the surface of the tongue; ulcerations may also occur.

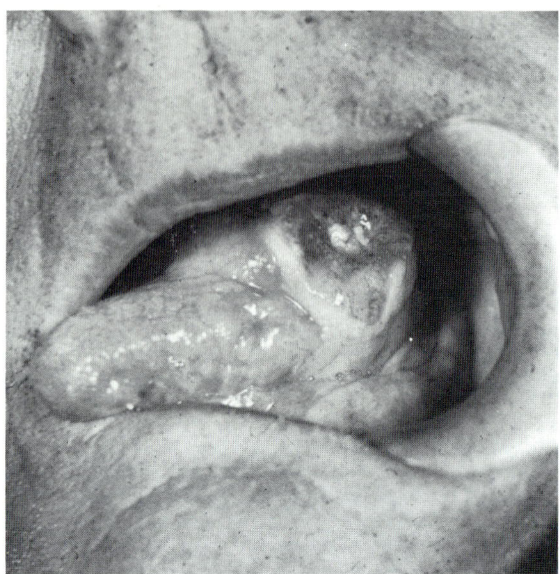

Fig. 16-8. Cancer of tongue. The typical lesion is round or slightly irregular, raised on the lateral edge of the tongue with firm rolled edges and a central ulcer with a fine granular base.

a painful ulcer of the tongue. The diagnosis at this time should not be difficult if the doctor or dentist considers the possibility of cancer. Therefore, any swelling, ulcer, or bleeding that does not disappear promptly within 2 weeks should be examined carefully and usually *biopsied.* Too often the patient is adequately concerned, but either the dentist or physician chooses to pass the condition off as unimportant or he loses valuable time by treating the lesion with antibiotics and mouth washes or by extracting teeth without obtaining a biopsy. This is particularly true when ulcerations appear on the tongue of a patient under 30 years of age. Although rare, such tumors do occur, often without the history of smoking, bad oral hygiene, or alcoholism as a causative agent [7].

The diagnosis of a typical cancer of the tongue is not difficult. The lesion most commonly presents on the lateral surface of the tongue and has firm rolled edges, is round or irregular, and has a central ulcer crater with a finely granular base (Fig. 16-8). These cancers are often not painful when small, but as they increase in size and the ulcer becomes more prominent, they become tender and painful.

Lesions that vary from the typical often are difficult to diagnose even when seen by an experienced observer. One of these variations presents as a soft villous-type squamous epithelioma that is clinically slow growing, shows little or no ulceration, and can persist for long periods without evidence of metastases. Microscopically, it is reported as showing borderline changes or being a very low-grade cancer. It often accompanies badly fitting dentures or sharp carious teeth. Another variation is the adenocarcinoma of the posterior third of the tongue. It is difficult to diagnose because it is not easily seen except by a laryngeal mirror and may ulcerate late, thus producing few symptoms for some time. Then the patient usually complains of a sore throat, which again is first treated with antibiotics without the real nature of the disease being suspected.

The differential diagnosis of cancer of the tongue is important, for all the benign tumors of the tongue previously noted must be ruled out. Cancer must then be differentiated from leukoplakia of long standing; chancre, which is now quite rare; tuberculosis ulcer, which usually has accompanying pulmonary involvement and neighboring inflammation; and herpes, which is painful but will spontaneously disappear in a short time.

Treatment of Cancer of the Tongue

Cure rates for epidermoid carcinoma originating in the oral cavity have improved slightly over the last few years primarily because of earlier diagnosis and not because of the constantly changing treatment modalities. However, as experience continues to accumulate, certain guidelines have developed in the treatment of cancer of the tongue. The surgeon who assumes the responsibility of caring for these patients must be adequately trained in general surgery and reconstructive procedures such as skin grafts, skin flaps, and bone grafts; he must have a working knowledge of radiation therapy – its advantages and disadvantages; and he must be interested not only in active treatment but also in the follow-up care, as is well pointed out by Gaisford [18]. One of the most important considerations in the follow-up care is insistence that the patient treated for cancer absolutely refrain from smoking. It has been shown with little doubt that the incidence of a second and frequently fatal cancer is much higher in the patient who continues to smoke than in the patient who stops smoking after treatment of the original cancer [35].

Treatment of cancer of the tongue is divided among radiologists and surgeons, depending in a large degree upon the availability of adequate facilities and the skill, training, and interest of the physician treating the patient. Where good facilities are available in both radiation therapy and surgery, preference depends upon the anatomical location of the primary tumor, the size and extent of involved adjacent tissues, and whether or not metastases have occurred. For instance, most radiologists agree that a *small cancer on the tip of the tongue* can best be treated by primary surgical excision [10]. This form of treatment produces minimal disability and is quickly and easily done, whereas the treatment by external radiation is either prolonged or rendered difficult by technical problems in retaining radiation needles easily.

Radiologists believe that cancer involving the *middle third of the tongue* is best treated by radiation, and surgeons believe that it is best treated by surgery. Proponents of both modalities of treatment report equal survival rates when treatment is carried out by competent physicians. However, when clinically positive nodes exist at the time of the initial diagnosis (N_1 or N_2), most physicians in this field would favor surgery with the radical neck and tongue excision done en bloc. If the nodes are histologically positive, postoperative irradiation is given to the original site and to the ipsilateral neck. Million [34] claims that survival rates are significantly improved by elective irradiation to the neck. In our own clinic, surgery of the neck combined with surgery of the primary lesion has been preferred in *T_2, T_3, and T_4 lesions* because of the high incidence (65 percent) of clinically positive lymph nodes (N_1 or N_2) [20]. In addition, our experience parallels that of Mendelson, Woods, and Beahrs [33], who found in studying neck specimens that 25 percent of the lymph nodes thought to be negative clinically showed tumor microscopically. However, we will select patients with tumors *measuring less than 2 cm.* ($T_1 N_0$) for radiation therapy or partial glossectomy. Cure rates drop significantly when the tumor exceeds 2 cm. and nodes in the neck are positive [43].

Lesions of the tongue that most radiologists agree are best treated by surgery are [10]:

1. Small tumors close to the tip of the tongue.
2. Small tumors on the dorsum of the tongue.
3. Lesions in conjunction with a positive Kahn test, even without a syphilitic glossitis.
4. Tumors in very old patients.
5. Multiple primary tumors.
6. Lesions extending into the mandible.
7. Lesions in alcoholics and heavy smokers.

Lesions that most surgeons would agree should be treated by irradiation are:

1. Sarcomas and poorly differentiated epidermoid tumors of the tongue (usually the posterior third), tonsil, and hypopharynx.
2. Tumors of the anterior two-thirds of the tongue in patients with simultaneous medical conditions such as active tuberculosis that would preclude a safe anesthetic administration or constitute a danger to the personnel in the operating room.
3. Tumors considered inoperable and thus incurable but where the symptoms need palliation.
4. Curable tumors when the patient absolutely refuses surgery but will consider having irradiation.

Extending the scope of surgery in recent years has given a comfortable life with minimal or moderate deformity to a group of patients formerly destined to a horrible death of pain and partial starvation. These patients have extensive tumors involving most of the tongue but have cervical metastases that can be regarded as resectable. Total glossectomy with a simultaneous bilateral neck dissection can salvage such patients in many instances. This is made feasible by various reconstructive techniques using skin grafts to line the raw surfaces inside the mouth and interdigitating skin flaps to build up the chin. Such a procedure has been described by Bakamjian and Cramer [1], who show conclusively that patients with this extended surgery can live a useful and comfortable life. (Details of these surgical procedures are contained in Chapter 17.)

Prognosis of Cancer of the Tongue

Both the surgical treatment and the radiation therapy have undergone considerable improvement in recent years. *Preoperative irradiation* to a level of 2,000 R in 4 days has been shown to reduce local recurrence but has not altered the 5-year cure rate [41]. However, combined therapy as suggested before has now shown the following *average 5-year survival rates* (Table 16-3).

Table 16-3. Average 5-year Survival Rate According to TNM Category of Patients with Cancer of the Tongue

Category	Survival Rate
T_1N_0	80–95%
T_2N_0	80–90%
T_3N_1	60–70%
T_4N_2	20–30%

Mortality and morbidity rates vary considerably with each clinic. In a carefully supervised clinic with adequate facilities, both rates can be kept at a minimum. Our experience is that we have a 3.5 percent overall mortality related to the surgical treatment of cancer of the tongue and a 17 percent morbidity or complication rate [20]. Morbidity and mortality can never be completely eradicated if every patient is going to be offered a chance for cure. Realistically then, surgery will occasionally be attempted on poor-risk patients with the hope that a cure might be obtained, even though the odds are very much against such an outcome.

TUMORS OF THE JAW

Though tumors arising in the upper and lower jaws are very uncommon, their management becomes very important because of the resulting deformities. This is significant, for the jaw is necessary for proper eating and talking, and alterations of its shape produce external changes in the patient's appearance that are difficult to hide. The surgeon must therefore use all his talents and imagination, first to produce a cure and, second, to reconstruct the deformity so as to minimize the loss as much as possible.

Tumors of the upper and lower jaw are so similar that they are discussed together. However, the treatment involves different techniques, which are emphasized under the heading, Treatment of Jaw Tumors.

Incidence

Cancers of the jaw are very rare, comprising less than 0.5 percent of all cancers in the body. They occur about three times more often in men than in women. Benign growths of the jaw are seen and are sometimes treated by the dentist or the oral surgeon. The jaw is most commonly involved by cancers that originate in the tongue, floor of the mouth, and alveolus and secondarily invade the jaw. Metastatic tumors to the jaw are rare: they come from the breast, thyroid gland, adrenal glands, stomach, prostate, melanomas, and neuroblastomas.

Primary malignant tumors of the mandible or maxilla are still more uncommon, making up only about 5 percent of jaw tumors [14]. Most of these are osteogenic sarcomas, which constitute 4 to 6 percent of all osteogenic sarcomas in the body (usually in the long bones). Coley [11], Schwartz and Alpert [40], and Kragh et al. [24] found the greatest incidence of mandibular osteogenic sarcoma in the second and third decades, with the incidence in males twice that in females. Triedman [46] recently reported 2 cases and Looser and Kuehn [28] reported 11 more cases. Our experience in a very small series of cases is that mandibular osteogenic sarcomas offer a good prognosis because of an apparently low grade of malignancy. Dahlin and Coventry [14], however, in reviewing 600 cases of osteogenic sarcomas of the body, found that 40 percent of jaw sarcomas were of a high grade of malignancy.

Pathology

A knowledge of the embryology of the area is necessary to understand the variety of tumors that may involve the jaw. At the fourth week of gestation the stomodeum ruptures, establishing continuity between the endoderm of the pharynx and the ectoderm of the first branchial arch. The mandibular process of the first branchial arch gradually develops into the lower lip, jaw, tongue, dental enamel, lower face, and oral covering. A thickening of the ectoderm covering over the mesodermal mass forms localized protrusions into the ectodermal covering. The bone of the mandible forms from mesoderm, enamel of the teeth from ectoderm, dentin of the teeth from mesoderm, and the alveolus from ectoderm.

Tumors, therefore, can originate (1) from the ectoderm of the alveolus, floor of the mouth, or tongue by invading the jaw, or (2) as metastatic tumors from elsewhere carried in by the blood vessels, or (3) from the jaw bone itself. The rather complex embryological formation of the jaw and teeth allows many varieties of benign tumors and cysts to develop; these often are treated by the oral surgeon. Only when these tumors become very large or are malignant do the head and neck surgeons see them for treatment.

Diagnosis

Treatment must be guided by the proper diagnosis. Most tumors of the jaw, except those beginning in the alveolus, floor of the mouth, or tongue, will present as a swelling that is usually painless. X-ray examination will confirm osteolytic or osteoblastic activity and its extent, but it will not indicate what pathological process is going on. This can only be determined by careful examination of the patient to rule out other primary tumors and subsequently by biopsying the tumor.

A classification of the various jaw tumors and their treatment suggested by Conley [12] is as follows:

I. Benign lesions of the alveolus
   A. *Gingival hyperplasia* – flange of denture cutting into gum – remove dentures.
   B. *Papillomas* – simple excision.
   C. *Pregnancy tumors* – granulomas that frequently disappear spontaneously at end of pregnancy (Fig. 16-6).
   D. *Epulis* – peripheral giant cell tumor that needs local excision with the removal of some bone.
   E. *Leukoplakia* – excision or electrocautery if it does not spontaneously disappear on removing the irritant (e.g., cigarette smoking).
   F. *Hemangiomas* – frequently no treatment needed.
   G. *Mixed tumors* – usually benign, and most commonly seen on the hard palate.

II. Malignant tumors of the alveolus
   A. *Epidermoid cancer* – usually occurs in conjunction with leukoplakia and may involve both upper and lower jaw. (For additional information refer to Chapter 17.)
   B. *Adenocarcinoma* – grows rapidly, forming a bulky tumor that invades bone early and involves both upper and lower jaw.
   C. *Fibrosarcoma* – prone to frequent local recurrences and difficult to differentiate from scar in recurrent cases.
   D. *Melanoma* – a very poor prognosis because of rapid spread through the lymphatics and constant massage of the tumor by eating and talking.
   E. *Malignant salivary tissue tumors* – such as malignant mixed tumors and mucoepidermoid cancers, which have a fairly good prognosis because of slow growth.
   F. *Rare malignant tumors* – such as liposarcomas, reticulum cell sarcomas, lymphosarcomas, and neurosarcomas.

III. Benign tumors of the jaw
   A. *Cysts* – such as dentigerous, radicular, periodontal, and congenital, some of which become very large.
   B. *Osseous tumors:*
      1. *Exostosis* – such as the torus mandibularis or palatinus, which may need removal when dentures are worn.
      2. *Osteomas* – respond well to simple excision.
      3. *Giant cell tumors* – frequently look malignant clinically but respond well to excision.
      4. *Ameloblastomas* (adamantinomas) – require large excisions but immediate reconstruction by a bone graft is usually possible.
   C. *Connective tissue tumors* – such as fibromas, angiomas, and fibrous dysplasia presenting soft tissue problems that occasionally defy correction.

IV. Malignant tumors of jaw
   A. *Osteogenic sarcoma* – differs from osteogenic sarcoma elsewhere in the body (see under Treatment of Jaw Tumors).
   B. *Malignant giant cell tumor* – quite rare.
   C. *Neurogenic sarcoma* – apparently begins in the alveolar nerve – requires radical treatment surgically; usually radioresistant.
   D. *Other rare tumors* – such as Ewing's tumor, angiosarcoma, chondrosarcomas.

V. Metastatic malignant tumors of the jaw
   A. *Carcinomas* from breast, prostate, kidney, and melanomas.
   B. *Sarcomas* – such as myelosarcomas and lymphosarcomas.

Other classifications have been suggested, such as one by Byars and Sarnat [6] that uses the x-ray findings as the basis for differentiation. However, the method described above with various alterations seems best.

Treatment of Jaw Tumors

Benign Tumors

Benign cysts or tumors of the jaw can be treated by simple excision or curettage through an intraoral approach. Because of this and because so many are related to the dentition, the oral surgeons more commonly see and treat these lesions. However, when a cyst becomes large enough to involve the whole horizontal ramus of the jaw, an external approach becomes necessary. In these cases, the lingual plate of the jaw containing the teeth and alveolar nerve with the branches can be saved, giving a foundation for new bone formation that will restore the jaw to a more normal shape and size. The major exceptions to this are in the treatment of the ameloblastomas (adamantinomas) and hemangiomas that require through-and-through resections in good bone on either side of the tumor. The high incidence of recurrence in *ameloblastomas* treated by the conservative intraoral route indicates the need for resection of the tumor through an external approach in order to completely eradicate it. This in turn requires more extensive reconstructive procedures (see Chapter 17). *Hemangiomas,* on the other hand, carry a considerable risk when a conservative intraoral approach has been used. Massive hemorrhage can occur from the extraction of a tooth or a biopsy in a jaw containing hemangioma, and even deaths have been reported when such intraoral surgery was attempted [45]. Treatment through an extraoral incision, with adequate blood available for replacement and with the use of hypothermia or hypotensive anesthesia, is preferred. Fortunately, immediate bone grafting with iliac crest or rib yields excellent results, because sufficient soft tissue remains to provide adequate cover for the graft.

Fibrous dysplasia of the craniofacial bones is a distinctive benign fibroosseous change that occurs in skeletal bones first described by Lichtenstein [27] in 1938. The ratio of fibrous to osseous elements varies considerably from one patient to another but all elements appear to stop growing. Therefore, conservative therapy is the treatment of choice with bone contouring an acceptable method of treatment [38].

Malignant Tumors

Malignant tumors of the alveolus that are relatively small (under 2 cm.) and show no clinical evidence of metastasis to the cervical lymph nodes may be treated by local intraoral excision. This involves removal of a border of normal soft tissue around the tumor as well as the adjacent bone. A through-and-through excision of the bone is seldom necessary, and sufficient soft tissue remains to allow an easy primary closure. Larger malignant tumors of the alveolus of longer duration usually require the combined procedure of radical neck dissection in continuity with resection of the jaw. (The operative technique is discussed in Chapter 17.) Frequently, bone replacement is not necessary following a hemimandibulectomy, but even when bone grafting is desirable, it may not be possible to perform the surgery because of insufficient soft tissue to cover the graft adequately. If bone is used, however, we have found that autogenous bone is superior to homogenous bone or implantation materials.

Metastatic malignant jaw tumors seldom become surgical problems because the primary disease usually has not been adequately controlled, or the metastasis to the jaw represents only one of many metastases, making cure improbable.

Primary malignant tumors of the jaw consist mostly of osteogenic sarcomas, which are rare, highly malignant bone tumors in which surgery is the treatment of choice. Local recurrence is the usual reason for treatment failure (60 percent reported by Caron, Hajdu, and Strong [8]), so that aggressive surgery with or without irradiation should be used. This usually means that a delay in bone replacement is preferred, to ensure adequate tumor control. Radical neck dissection is seldom needed, since there is little tendency for these tumors to spread to lymph nodes.

Primary malignant tumors of the palate when under 2 cm. can be excised locally in most cases. When larger excisions prove necessary, a Weber-Fergusson incision through the midline of the upper lip, around the base of the nose, up along the side of the nose, and across beneath the lower eyelid just 0.5 cm. below the lid margin gives adequate exposure. An electrical cautery knife can be used to dissect the soft tissues on the palate, and the underlying bone is widely resected well beyond the visible tumor with an osteotome and mallet. After bleeding is controlled, a split-thickness skin graft is used to line the raw surface of the cheek pedicle. After healing has occurred, an upper dental prosthesis can be made with an obturator that fits into the skin-graft-lined operative defect and supports the cheek.

Prognosis

The prognosis of all *benign jaw tumors* including ameloblastomas is good, provided that an adequate excision has been carried out. Inadequate excisions in ameloblastomas have led to recurrences that eventually may prove to be malignant. Metastatic spread from malignant ameloblastomas has been reported, probably of the acanthoma variety in which epithelial pearl formation is not uncommon. Hemangiomas may involve surrounding soft tissue, making adequate excision improbable or impossible without destroying vital structures. Patients with hemangiomas can live comfortably for many years without treatment.

The prognosis of *malignant tumors of the alveolus* depends on: the size of tumor, duration of tumor, presence or absence of metastasis, and histological classification of the tumor.

When primary epidermoid cancer of the alveolus is less than 2 cm. without neck metastasis, an 80 percent 5-year cure rate has been reported. However, this rate falls rapidly when larger tumors are included, and Martin reports an overall 30.6 percent 5-year survival. Our own experience is an overall survival rate of 42 percent [19]. Our prognosis for palate lesions is similar to that for the alveolus. However, when the lesion begins in the antrum, the prognosis is extremely poor. Patients with these antral lesions are usually best treated by irradiation or the combination of irradiation and surgery. The prognosis of *osteogenic sarcomas of the mandible* ranged between 25 and 36 percent [46], in spite of the fact that few metastasize to the lung. This is much better prognosis than that for osteogenic sarcoma of the long bones.

TUMORS OF THE FLOOR OF THE MOUTH

Benign Tumors

The most common benign lesion is a *ranula.* This cyst, which results from obstruction of the sublingual salivary glands, is best treated by marsupialization. Some of these cysts become so large that they interfere with speech and mastication (Fig. 16-9). When repeated conservative management fails to eradicate them, only

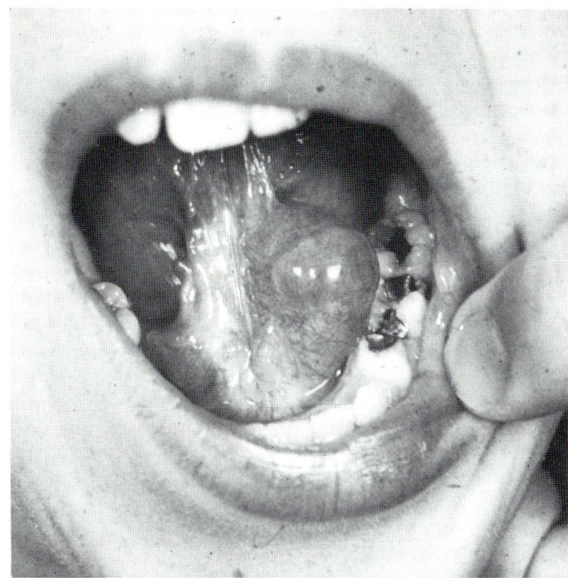

Fig. 16-9. Ranula of floor of mouth. This cyst of the sublingual gland can be treated by marsupialization, if it is symptomatic.

surgical removal of the submaxillary and sublingual glands can provide relief.

Malignant Tumors

Squamous cell carcinomas are the most common malignant tumors seen in the floor of the mouth and are primarily found in older patients. Because surgery and irradiation offer the same prognosis for T_1 and T_2N_0 lesions, irradiation is the preferred treatment [23], since resection of this area, particularly the anterior floor of the mouth, produces a considerable deformity requiring extensive reconstructive procedures. However, in the presence of clinically positive nodes in the neck or in T_3 and T_4 lesions, surgery followed by irradiation is the treatment of choice. Marginal resection of the jaw is usually possible, reducing the amount of deformity and reducing the amount of reconstruction necessary. A cervical flap provides an excellent method for reconstruction of the soft tissue in this area [23].

Mucoepidermoid carcinomas arising in the sublingual gland are extremely rare and usually respond poorly to irradiation. Surgery, therefore, is the treatment of choice. *Adenoid cystic carcinomas* are also seen in the anterior floor of the mouth, are usually slow growing, and respond to both surgery and irradiation. *Melanomas* also are seen but are very rare and very lethal.

REFERENCES

1. Bakamjian, V., and Cramer, L. Surgical management of advanced cancer of the tongue. *Ann. Surg.* 152:1058, 1960.
2. Berridge, F. E., and James, H. G. Management of lingual cancer. *Surg. Gynecol. Obstet.* 102:595, 1956.
3. Billroth, T. Über die Exstirpation ausgedehntner Zungencarcinome von der Regio suprahyoidea *Arch. Klin. Chir.* 16:1, 1874.
4. Botstein, C., Silver, C., and Ariaratnaum, L. Treatment of carcinoma of the oral tongue by radium needles implantation. *Am. J. Surg.* 132:523, 1976.
5. Butlin, H. T., and Spencer, W. G. *Diseases of the Tongue* (2nd ed.). London: Cassell, 1900. Quoting from deMarchetti, P., *Obstet. Med. Chir. Rar. Sylloge Patavini,* 1664, obs. 33, p. 62.
6. Byars, L. T., and Sarnat, B. G. Mandibular tumors. *Surg. Gynecol. Obstet.* 83:355, 1946.
7. Byers, R. M. Squamous cell carcinoma of the oral tongue in patients less than thirty years of age. *Am. J. Surg.* 130:475, 1975.
8. Caron, A. S., Hajdu, S. I., and Strong, E. W. Osteogenic sarcoma of the facial and cranial bones. *Am. J. Surg.* 122:719, 1971.
9. Chandler, J. R., Guillamondegui, O. M., Sisson, G. A., Strong, E. W., and Baker, H. W. Clinical staging of cancer of the head and neck: A new "New" system. *Am. J. Surg.* 132:525, 1976.
10. Chu, A., and Fletcher, G. H. Incidence and causes of failure to control by irradiation the primary lesions in squamous cell carcinomas of the anterior two thirds of the tongue and floor of mouth. *Am. J. Roentgenol. Radium Ther. Nucl. Med.* 117:502, 1973.
11. Coley, B. L. *Neoplasms of Bones* (2nd ed.). New York: Hoeber, 1960. P. 270.
12. Conley, J. J. Treatment of the tumors of the inferior alveolus and the mandible. *Ann. Otol.* 61:62, 1952.
13. Crile, G. W. Excision of cancer of the head and neck with special references to the plan of dissection based on one hundred and thirty-two operations. *J.A.M.A.* 47:1780, 1906.
14. Dahlin, D. C., and Coventry, M.D. Osteogenic sarcoma. A study of six hundred cases. *J. Bone Joint Surg. [Am.]* 49:101, 1967.
15. DesPrez, J. D., Kiehn, C. L., Benson, J. W., and Damm, H. Combination of surgery and chemotherapy in the treatment of oral cancer. *Am. J. Surg.* 108:583, 1964.
16. Farr, H. W., and Arthur, K. Epidermoid carcinoma of the mouth and pharynx, 1960–1964. *J. Laryngol. Otol.* 86:243, 1972.
17. Flynn, M. B., and Moore, C. Marginal resection of the mandible in the management of squamous can-

cer of the floor of the mouth. *Am. J. Surg.* 128: 490, 1974.
18. Gaisford, J. C. Tumors of the head and neck—The who, when and how of treatment. *Plast. Reconstr. Surg.* 36:447, 1965.
19. Gaisford, J. C., Hanna, D. C., Atwell, R. B., and Terry, J. L. Evaluation of radical neck dissections and jaw resections. *Plast. Reconstr. Surg.* 25:39, 1960.
20. Gaisford, J. C., Hanna, D. C., Richardson, G. S., and Walker, G. R. Surgical pathology and its relationship to the management of head and neck tumors. *Plast. Reconstr. Surg.* 36:185, 1966.
21. Gibbel, M. I., Cross, J. H., and Ariel, I. M. Cancer of the tongue. *Cancer* 2:411, 1949.
22. Goodner, J. T., and Watson, W. L. Cancer of the esophagus: Its association with other primary cancers. *Cancer* 9:1248, 1956.
23. Hanna, D. C. Cancer of the floor of the mouth. *Symposium on Malignancies of the Head and Neck.* St. Louis: Mosby, 1969. Vol. 11, Chap. 17, pp. 110–116.
24. Kragh, L. V., Dahlin, D. C., and Erich, J. B. Osteogenic sarcoma of the jaws and facial bones. *Am. J. Surg.* 96:496, 1958.
25. Kuehn, P. G., Beckett, R., and Reed, J. F. Tissue specificity in multiple primary malignancies. *Am. J. Surg.* 111:164, 1966.
26. Larson, D. L., Lewis, S. R., Rapparport, A. S., Coers, C. R., and Blocker, T. G. Lymphatics of the mouth and neck. *Am. J. Surg.* 110:625, 1965.
27. Lichtenstein, L. Polystotic fibrous dysplasia. *Arch. Surg.* 36:874, 1938.
28. Looser, K. G., and Kuehn, P. G. Primary tumors of the mandible. *Am. J. Surg.* 132:608, 1976.
29. Marchetta, F. C., Sako, K., and Camp, F. Multiple malignancies in patients with head and neck cancer. *Am. J. Surg.* 110:537, 1965.
30. Martin, H. E. The history of lingual cancer. *Am. J. Surg.* 48:703, 1940.
31. Martin, H. E., Del Valle, B., Ehrlich, H., and Cahan, W. G. Neck dissection. *Cancer* 4:441, 1951.
32. Martin, H. E., Munster, H., and Sugarbaker, E. L. Cancer of the tongue. *Arch. Surg.* (Chicago) 41: 888, 1940.
33. Mendelson, B. C., Woods, J. E., and Beahrs, O. H. Neck dissection in the treatment of carcinoma of the anterior two thirds of the tongue. *Surg. Gynecol. Obstet.* 143:75, 1976.
34. Million, R. R. Elective neck irradiation for TxNO squamous carcinoma of the oral tongue and floor of mouth. *Cancer* 34:149, 1974.
35. Moore, C. Smoking and mouth-throat cancer. *Am. J. Surg.* 108:565, 1964.
36. Pack, G. T., and Ariel, I. M. *Treatment of Cancer and Allied Diseases* (2nd ed.). Vol. 8, *Tumors of the Head and Neck,* New York: Hoeber, 1959.
37. Rae, M. V. Multiple malignancy. *Med. Serv. J. Canada* 14:193, 1958.
38. Ramsey, H. E., Strong, E. W., and Frazell, E. L. Fibrous dysplasia of the craniofacial bones. *Am. J. Surg.* 116:542, 1968.
39. Read, A. The Cherurge Call Lectures of Tumors and Ulcers. Treat. 2, Lect. 26, p. 313. London, 1635.
40. Schwartz, E. T., and Alpert, M. The clinical course of mandibular osteogenic sarcoma. *Oral Surg.* 16:769, 1963.
41. Shah, J. P., Cendon, R. A., Farr, H. W., and Strong, E. W. Carcinoma of the oral cavity. *Am. J. Surg.* 132:504, 1976.
42. Southwick, H. W. Cancer of the tongue: Symposium on head and neck surgery. *Surg. Clin. North Am.,* 53:147, 1973.
43. Spiro, R. H., and Strong, E. W. Discontinuous partial glossectomy and radical neck dissection in selected patients with epidermoid carcinoma of the mobile tongue. *Am. J. Surg.* 126:544, 1973.
44. Stevenson, W. C. Preliminary clinical report on a new and economical method of radium therapy by means of emanation needles. *Br. Med. J.* 2:9, 1914.
45. Taylor, B. G. Hemangiomas of the mandible and maxilla presenting as surgical emergencies. *Am. J. Surg.* 108:574, 1964.
46. Triedman, L. J. Osteogenic sarcoma of the mandible. *Am. J. Surg.* 110:580, 1965.
47. Ward, G. E., and Hendrick, J. W. *Tumors of the Head and Neck.* Baltimore: Williams & Wilkins, 1950.
48. Warren, S., and Gates, O. Multiple primary malignant tumors: A survey of the literature and a statistical study. *Am. J. Cancer* 16:1358, 1932.
49. Watson, T. A. Irradiation in the management of tumors of the head and neck. *Am. J. Surg.* 110: 542, 1965.

Radical Neck Dissection for Oral Cancer

LESTER M. CRAMER AND NORRIS K. CULF, JR.

Radical neck dissection is one of the best operations available for the treatment of cancer because the en bloc principle can be applied so readily. It is well to emphasize that there are many varieties of radical neck dissection and that the specific type should be determined by the location of the primary lesion and by histological studies. Common to all varieties is the basic tenet that the entire system of lymphatic drainage for a tumor must be removed. To accomplish this, one must excise the anterior portion of the carotid sheath; the internal jugular vein; the sternocleidomastoid, omohyoid, stylohyoid, and digastric muscles; the spinal accessory and ansa hypoglossi nerves; and the contents of the submaxillary triangle. In addition, including the platysma muscle with the removed specimen ensures a wider field and more adequate resection, within which the tumor, the intervening lymphatics, and the lymph nodes are treated as an untouchable entity. The monoblock technique, best accomplished by wide exposure and wide excision to ensure adequate margins, appears radical; actually, this radical treatment is the conservative approach to this disease. An understanding of the basis for this philosophy helps the conservative surgeon make the conservative decision for radical surgery.

As has been described in the previous chapters nearly all primary lesions of the head and neck can be demonstrated by looking and seeing, by feeling and thinking. Good light, comfortable and optimal positioning, and the use of mirrors and endoscopes facilitate finding the primary lesion so that a tissue diagnosis can be made by biopsy. Ten percent of patients with such lesions will eventually show a second primary lesion in the head and neck region. When there is a primary lesion available for biopsy, palpable cervical lymph nodes should never be biopsied, as dissection of the neck without prior biopsy will give an increased cure rate. More than 90 percent of the time, cervical lymph nodes will be positive for tumor if an experienced clinician feels that they are clinically positive. More than 70 percent of the time, the neck with a palpable positive lymph node will have other positive nodes [1]. Clinically negative necks will have microscopic nodes 25 to 50 percent of the time [27].

TNM CLASSIFICATION

One should be familiar with the coding classification which conforms with the TNM classification for oral tumors for the American Joint Committee for Cancer Staging and End-Results Reporting, and the TNM Committee of the International Union against Cancer (1967).

TNM System of Clinical Staging

T = Primary tumor
- T_1 – less than 2 cm.
- T_2 – 2 cm. to less than 4 cm.
- T_3 – 4 cm. or greater

N = Regional node metastasis
- N_0 – none
- N_1 – hemilateral
- N_2 – bilateral or contralateral
- N_3 – fixed

D = Distant metastasis
- M_0 – none
- M_1 – present

Stage 1 – T_1N_0
Stage 2 – T_2N_0
Stage 3 – T_3N_0, and T_1, T_2, or T_3 with N_1
Stage 4 – T_1, T_2, or T_3, with N_2, N_3, or M_1

This classification system has been a very useful adjunct in the coding and the evaluation of significant statistical data since its development; it allows for reasonably accurate clinical description of head and neck lesions, so that different institutions can compare the results of similar lesions in assessing effective treatment programs.

TREATMENT PROGRAM

The decision to do a radical dissection is arrived at by evaluating the following factors. The determination of what proper modality of treatment should be used (surgery, radiation, chemotherapy, or combinations of these) remains one of the most difficult decisions in treating patients with carcinoma of the oral cavity. Our policy, the rationale for which will be outlined subsequently, assumes equal expertise in all participating specialties, i.e., surgery, radiation, and chemotherapy.

Important General Principles

1. The survival rates of Stages 2, 3, and 4 in head and neck cancer are too low when single modality

therapy is used [9]. Half of the failures are usually due to persistent or recurrent disease at the primary site and half are due to tumor involvement of the regional nodes [14]. The overall therapeutic effect of radiation therapy is about the same (within 5 to 10 percent) as that of surgery.

2. Attempts to salvage patients with recurrent disease at the primary site or in the neck after initial treatment has been rendered are very disappointing (less than 33 percent) [14]; therefore, the initial therapeutic attack should be vigorous with an aim for cure. This involves utilization of multimodality therapy for Stages 2, 3, and 4 lesions both at the primary and regional nodal sites.

3. Low-dose radiation (2,000 to 4,000 rads) followed by radical surgery does not significantly alter the survival rate, although a slight increase in local disease control does occur. It falls far short of an acceptable survival rate.

4. Two paramount points should be made: (A) Combined-modality therapy, especially radiation and surgery, gives significantly higher survival rates and control of local disease (at times twice as good as does single-type therapy) [7, 9, 17, 21, 24]. (B) Contrary to popular belief, radical surgery and therapeutic radiation can be used consecutively in a preplanned combination without significantly increasing the morbidity and mortality rates. The mortality should be no greater than 14 percent and morbidity no greater than 5 percent if the management program is properly executed [19]. This presumes close liaison between radiation therapist, surgeon, and chemotherapist, as well as expertise in all areas of care including preoperative work-up, dental care, anesthesiologists, operating room technicians, nurses, intensive care units, and rehabilitative facilities. In particular, the surgeon not only should be expert in extirpative surgery, but also should utilize properly designed incisions, afford adequate coverage of the carotid artery (preferably with local muscle flaps), and when necessary be able to supply adequate tissue replacement by the use of local or regional flaps or grafts to secure water-tight suture lines with viable tissue.

5. Therapeutic radiation therapy administered 3 to 6 weeks following radical surgery also significantly increases local and regional control and survival rates [21]. If one is concerned about mortality and morbidity from preoperative radiation, then it can be given postoperatively with just as good results. The important factor is that the pretreatment plan (including port sizes and areas, time dosage schedules, etc.) is not changed and follows in an orderly fashion (within 6 weeks) unless the patient's condition precludes this. Lindberg [21] could find no difference in local recurrences or distant metastasis between 5,000 rads given preoperatively and 6,000 rads given postoperatively.

6. Both radiation and chemotherapy fail when there are residual foci of tumor, usually centrally located; surgery fails because of field recurrence, usually at the periphery of the lesion or area. Therefore, surgery is complementary to both radiation and chemotherapy. Radiation and chemotherapy are not complementary to each other because they both fail for similar reasons. Chemotherapy, however, does not have the detrimental effect on normal adjacent tissue that radiation has, but it has a systemic toxicity especially with hematopoietic and mucosal tissue, and also with the kidney and liver.

7. Timing of combined-modality therapy is important to afford optimal accomplishment of the mission. Usually chemotherapeutic and radiation treatments are carried out concomitantly unless intraarterial regional infusion is utilized (in this situation, the patient is admitted 2 weeks preoperatively for the chemotherapy). When preoperative radiation is used, radical surgery should not be scheduled until 6 to 8 weeks after termination of radiation. If the patient is operated upon sooner, there is poor definition of surgical planes, edema and wound healing problems. If later, the main problems are related to delayed wound healing secondary to the obliterative endarteritis of the smaller vessels with the inevitable decrease in local blood supply, especially to the overlying skin. Postoperative radiation should begin 3 to 6 weeks after the operation (assuming healing has been by primary intention) and consists of 6,000 rads over 6 weeks to the primary site and the entire neck [17].

8. Discontinuous surgery, whether done as separate operative procedures or at the same surgical sitting, adversely affects the survival rate (i.e., in continuity en bloc surgery is preferable) [28, 39].

9. When surgery and radiation are combined or used as single entities together (i.e., radiation to the primary site and surgery to the neck), it must be carefully planned so that overlapping coverage at the borders of adjacent treatment fields is afforded.

10. In combined therapy, careful team planning is necessary. Treatment fields, ports, margins of the lesion, and margins of the proposed resection must be determined and should not be modified once outlined initially, regardless of the response the disease undergoes as a result of initial therapy. An accurate description, a diagram, and possibly a photograph or tattooing of the margins are helpful adjuncts in keeping to the original plan. Even though a tumor has shown a good response with significant regression to chemotherapy or radiation, as substantiated by negative biopsies, one should hold fast since a tumor is frequently found around these negative biopsy sites at a later time. As experience is gained in multimodality therapy, it may be possible, once proper guidelines

are established, to modify the surgical margins if good tumor regression has occurred with chemotherapy and/or radiation therapy [24].

11. Surgery for radiation failures is often more effective than radiation for surgical failures. Factors that worsen prognosis are: size and location of the primary lesion; the degree of anaplasia as well as the incidence of nodal metastasis; location in the pharynx and hypopharynx as opposed to the anterior oral cavity; infiltration of the tumor; extracapsular extension of disease in cervical nodes; involvement of soft tissue, or multiple nodes at multiple levels; bilateral nodes; and nodes lower in the neck.

Specific Treatment Program

In T_1N_0 (Stage 1) lesions, usually no neck treatment is necessary. The primary lesion may be treated by a single modality (wide surgical excision or therapeutic radiation). It is probably not necessary to add chemotherapy to this regimen, although it certainly might be considered if the circumstances suggest an aggressive lesion (rapid growth or infiltrating nature).

Because of the aggressive behavior of intraoral malignancies, the neck needs some type of treatment in most oral cancers if the primary lesion is T_2N_0 (Stage 2) or greater. Even if the neck is clinically negative, microscopic metastases are present in 25 to 60 percent of cases [27]. A further argument for treating the clinically negative neck is exemplified by carcinoma of the tongue. Cervical metastases develop in 30 percent of Stage 1 and 43 percent of Stage 2 lesions [26, 28]. The strongest argument against single-modality therapy in Stage 2 is the poor survival rate. Therefore, we favor combined therapy to the primary lesion and the neck in all cases of Stage 2 and above except in the noninvasive, exophytic, well-localized Stage 2 lesion, where the choice might be radiation therapy or surgery to the primary lesion, combined with radiation or surgery to the neck. In the clinically negative neck, especially in T_2N_0, one option may be to treat it only with radiation. Lindberg [21] has shown that 4,000 to 5,000 rads will sterilize 90 percent of the occult disease.

Most lesions in Stage 3 (T_3N_0, T_1N_1, T_2N_1, T_3N_1) as well as in Stage 4, with the exception of those with distant metastasis, should have the benefit of combined-modality therapy to the primary lesion and the neck. It is worthwhile in all of these cases to add chemotherapy to the program. Also to be considered are the preradiation sensitizers, such as hydroxyurea [9].

Recommendations on treatment regimens are included in Table 17-1.

On the Horizon

Very little further variation or modification of the surgical attack appears possible. However, as surgery becomes more sophisticated with the use of such techniques as the carbon dioxide laser [18], transplantation of composite tissue from a distance using microsurgical techniques [25] for small vessel anastomosis, and large vessel replacement, more patients may fall into the operable category.

Chemotherapy, depending as it does on arrest of cellular mitoses, is well established as a valuable adjunct in head and neck cancer. The most commonly used and thus far the most effective of these agents has been methotrexate [34]. This drug may be given as a local arterial infusion which leads to the highest percentage of tumor regression but also to a significant number of complications [11]. It may also be administered in high doses parenterally using the citrovorum factor (folinic acid) rescue technique. Another alternative is to use low doses (45 to 60 mg. per square meter) administered intravenously every 7 to 10 days [34].

Many drugs are now undergoing studies in terms of their use both alone and in combination with other drugs, with radiation, and with surgery. These drugs include bleomycin, cytarabine, doxorubicin, and imidazole carboxamide. A basic tenet with all these agents is that the best results are obtained when they are incorporated into the initial multimodality treatment program before recurrent or distant metastatic disease develops. Continued investigation will lead to new drugs or improved combinations of drugs to add to our armamentarium.

Table 17-1. Summary of Treatment Recommendations

	Treatment	
TNM Stage	Primary Site	Regional Nodes (neck)
T_1N_0 (Stage 1)	Radiation or surgery	Careful observation
T_2N_0 (Stage 2)	Radiation and surgery with or without chemotherapy	Radiation before or after surgery, or either radiation or surgery alone
T_3N_0, T_1N_1, T_2N_1 (Stage 3)	Radiation with surgery and chemotherapy (radiation is given before or after surgery)	Radiation and surgery (radiation is given before or after surgery)
Stage 4	Same as for Stage 3	Same as for Stage 3

Radiotherapy shows some exciting and potentially helpful developments in this area. Improvement of cure rates with conventional supervoltage radiation has not been as effective as one would hope for in comparison to those treated with orthovoltage radiation. However, with the advent of the betatron and cyclotron, and with the use of particulate radiation therapy to replace electromagnetic radiation, new modalities are available and currently under study with moderately encouraging results [6, 8, 21, 32]. Neutron beams and negative pions are two entities that appear to be effective against both hypoxic and oxygenated tumor cells. These rays produce a higher number of ionization events within the cell, due to a higher linear energy transfer, which causes cell death faster than previously used modalities. The expense of this type of equipment will prolong the investigatory program; however, theoretically it seems that they should be helpful.

The use of hydroxyurea and 5-fluorouracil, which have in common a tumorcidal effect as well as an ability to presensitize the tumor cells to radiation (thereby making radiation therapy more effective in tumor ablation), continues under study [9, 20, 24].

Immunological Frontier

Immunocompetence can be tested by administration of antigens intradermally or by the demonstration of delayed hypersensitivity to contact antigens such as dinitrochlorobenzene [22]. The degree of skin reaction (flare) is an indication of immune competence or of systemic cellular immune function. This has been found to be decreased in patients with head and neck cancer and somewhat parallels the course of the disease (i.e., generally the worse the disease becomes, the lower the immune response). Immunoglobulin A in serum and saliva has been shown to be increased in these patients [12]. Usually, there is a return to the normal level if the patient is cured and an increase if recurrence develops. Radiation does affect the immune response by depressing it, but this is short lasting (2 months) and probably not clinically significant [31].

Immunotherapy, as such, has not proved helpful in head and neck tumors thus far. The use of BCG vaccine as an immune-response stimulant has met with varied results. It is open to speculation as to whether or not specific vaccines or a more intense manipulation of the immune response may be developed.

RADICAL NECK DISSECTION

General Aspects

The factors to be evaluated to help make the decision of inoperability of the neck are invasion of the base of the skull, blockage of the skin lymphatics, and possibly fixation to deeper structures, although this is rarely a deterrent by itself. The patient with an operable primary lesion may have any one of the following neck situations: (1) neck nodes negative, (2) neck nodes positive with anatomical discontinuity, (3) neck nodes positive with anatomical continuity, or (4) neck nodes positive with anatomical and pathological continuity. The situation also may occur in which (1) the neck nodes are positive but no primary lesion is found, or (2) the neck nodes are positive but the primary lesion is not obvious. The treatment modality may vary if anatomical discontinuity exists, i.e., irradiation for the primary lesion and surgery for the neck nodes, or vice versa. Exceptions to neck dissection in these lesions include cases in which the primary lesion is in the lip or maxilla, or on one laryngeal cord; intraoral lesions of less than 1 cm. in diameter; and patients with low-grade-type malignancies in whom the neck is clinically negative. Radical neck dissection may then be deferred.

Both the operative and postoperative morbidity are much less if radical neck dissection is done alone, rather than in combination with resection of the primary lesion. However, the cure rate with this plan is significantly less than with the monoblock technique. The average radical dissection has a strikingly low operative and postoperative morbidity. The procedure should rarely exceed 3 hours, and frequently it requires no blood transfusion or tracheotomy. The period of hospitalization is usually less than 10 days. The patient can be ambulated the evening of the operation, has minimal pain, may drink liquids by the first postoperative day, and is on a full liquid diet within 2 weeks. The symptoms secondary to the neck dissection include hollowing of the neck; an inconspicuous scar; decreased sensation from excision of the cervical plexus, which in most cases will return; and the typical shoulder deformity with a drooping and winging of the scapula secondary to division of the spinal accessory nerve. Some patients, particularly those who are elderly or who have had radiation therapy, may need a tracheotomy to help during the immediate postoperative phase. This same group, especially if one glossopharyngeal or superior laryngeal nerve is taken on the operative side, may have problems with swallowing, but these problems gradually improve. A small percentage of patients will also develop a Frei-type syndrome or Horner's syndrome.

It must be realized that performing a composite resection (primary lesion and a radical neck dissection in continuity) adds considerably to the morbidity. Attempts to decrease this morbidity have been directed to either immediate reconstruction or radiation therapy. A thorough knowledge of the use and management of skin grafts and local rotation skin flaps is a prerequisite to adequate reconstruction in these patients. If the radiation therapist can anticipate a high rate of cure for certain primary lesions, such as those on the lateral border of the tongue or tonsillar pillar, it is most tempting to treat them with radiation therapy. By extending the lower border of the radiation port to the level of the hyoid bone, the subsequent neck dissection will remove the lower end of a completely treated field, thus completing the monoblock treatment. Careful selection of the combination treatment of radiation for the primary lesion and surgery to the neck can render this treatment program very effective. One must not allow the wish to decrease deformity to interfere with the cure rate. In the majority of instances, even after radical extirpative therapy, immediate and carefully planned reconstruction can produce quite satisfactory results from both a functional and cosmetic point of view.

When the primary lesion is one for which the radiation therapist cannot expect a high cure rate or if the lesion encroaches on the mandible, the initial approach must be a surgical excision of the primary lesion, combined with radical neck dissection. This usually is done within a few days after the diagnosis is established, though it may be postponed from 3 to 10 weeks to allow for preoperative radiation, preoperative chemotherapy, or a combination of both. Occasionally the neck dissection must be postponed while skin flaps are delayed in preparation for reconstruction of the defects.

Technique of Radical Neck Dissection

The essential anatomy of the neck as it relates to the technique of radical neck dissection [13] is outlined in Figure 17-1. The veins, arteries, and nerves of the neck, as well as the nodal drainage, are illustrated.

The patient is placed on the operating table in a supine position with a head tilt of approximately 25 degrees. The cautery plate is placed beneath the patient, and an intravenous drip is begun in an arm vein. The neck is extended and maintained in the position by support under the shoulders, and the ipsilateral shoulder is depressed toward the waist. The chin is turned toward the opposite side and elevated about 10 degrees. An endotracheal tube can be inserted through either the mouth or the nose unless a tracheotomy has been planned. One indication for a tracheotomy is in patients who may have pulmonary problems, especially if the mandible is removed. A tracheotomy will also be needed if the tumor is located in such a position that oral or nasal intubation will traumatize the tumor. In these circumstances, it is best to do the tracheotomy first, under local anesthesia, and then to proceed with the patient under general anesthesia, inserting an endotracheal tube within the tracheotomy. Draping the patient should permit access to the whole neck, the lower face, and the second intercostal space on the same side. This should be done in a way by which the head can be independently turned or moved during the procedure without disturbing the neck or chest drapes. If only the radical neck dissection is being done, no antibiotics are used. In a combined resection, it is advisable to give the patient antibiotics, which can be started by intravenous drip at the beginning of the operative procedure.

Incision

The upper incision, drawn with the chin in neutral position, at the level of the hyoid bone, should be transversely placed in a prominent neck crease but curved upward gently at either end (Fig. 17-2A). Posteriorly, this curved part of the incision will lie over the mastoid process; anteriorly, it extends to the mandible just below the mandibular symphysis. The remainder of the incision can be varied greatly. Keeping the design of an incision simple will ensure survival of the skin flap. If a vertical incision is used (Fig. 17-2B), it should be placed 2.5 cm. anterior or posterior to the carotid vessels, so that its superior portion joins the transverse incision at a right angle. The inferior limb should be curved reciprocally in an S shape down over the clavicle. The safest flap for a radical neck dissection requires two transverse incisions (Fig. 17-2A). The lower incision is placed 2.5 cm. above the clavicle and extends 1 cm. from the midline of the neck laterally to the anterior border of the trapezius muscle. (The other superior incision at the level of the hyoid bone has been described above.) This approach is especially recommended when operating on a previously irradiated neck; however, it is a utilitarian and safe flap that can be recommended for all neck dissections. Our policy is to utilize this McFee-type incision in all cases except in the patient with a short neck. In this case, an S-shape vertical type (Fig. 17-2B) described earlier is utilized. This essentially ensures primary wound healing, which is essential if carotid blowouts are to be avoided.

Flap Elevation

The skin flaps are raised by dissecting along the superficial plane of the platysma perimysium (Fig. 17-3A, B). Superior traction on the skin at right angles and countertraction of both the muscle and the skin of the wound inferiorly facilitate bloodless, rapid, and atraumatic elevation of the flaps (Fig. 17-3C). There has been some controversy whether the platysma should be left with the skin flaps or included with the specimen. Those favoring leaving platysma with the skin flaps believe that it protects the flaps and thus decreases the incidence of flap necrosis. This reasoning can be true only if the surgeon injures the skin flaps when raising them from the platysma. No actual protection of a flap can be provided by a denervated and devascularized muscle. Good incision design, gentle tissue handling, correct flap design, correct flap elevation, and avoidance of tension on suture lines eliminate flap necrosis. By dissection of the skin flaps along the deep side of the fascial plane overlying the platysma, directly on the perimysium of the platysma, one avoids trauma to the skin flaps. In our experience, we have had no flap loss in the nonirradiated neck and none in the irradiated neck since we began using the double transverse incisions. Taking the platysma with the specimen helps protect the monoblock principle, keeps the dissection at a greater distance from the specimen, and may decrease local recurrence. The only advantage in leaving the platysma attached to the skin flaps is the time saved, since it is much quicker to dissect deep to this muscle than superficial to it. However, the few operative minutes saved are rarely a major gain.

Upper Dissection

The contents of the neck must be separated from the face and jaw unless there is a combined resection being done for an intraoral or oropharyngeal primary lesion. The platysma is transected at the level of the lower border of the mandible. The ramus mandibularis of the seventh nerve does not actually run directly beneath the platysma, but is separated from its deep surface by the superficial layer of the cervical fascia. This fascia is transected with the exposure of the nerve that transgresses the limits of the submaxillary triangle. This appears to be clinically significant only when the primary tumor is in the lip or when there is a high incidence of metastatic disease in the submaxillary triangle. In these instances, the nerve should be sacrificed and taken with the specimen, without entering the submaxillary triangle. The nerve is located 2 cm. anterior to the angle of the mandible, superficial to the adventitia of the anterior facial vein and artery (Fig. 17-3D). It is isolated here, protected by a rubber drain, which is used for gentle traction, and followed both proximally and distally. It is important to dissect out the nerve distally along the body of the mandible and proximally through the substance of the tail of the parotid so that subsequent dissection in this area and removal of the neck contents do not allow inadvertent injury to the nerve (Fig. 17-3E). The anterior facial vein and external maxillary artery can be divided just below the level where they are crossed by the ramus mandibularis; the distal end of the artery is sutured to the skin flap superiorly, making a sling to protect the nerve (Fig. 17-3F). Posteriorly, the parotid gland is transected on a line of the angle of the mandible to the tip of the mastoid process. During this section of the parotid gland, the facial nerve will not be injured because of

Fig. 17-1. A, triangles of the neck. Anterior triangle: *medial border = anterior midline of neck, lateral border = sternocleidomastoid muscle, superior border = lower border of mandible. Subdivisions of anterior triangle are (1) submaxillary triangle: between the anterior and posterior bellies of the digastric muscle and the lower border of the mandible; (2) submental triangle: medial border = anterior midline of the neck beneath chin, lateral border = anterior belly of the digastric muscles, inferior border = hyoid bone; (3) superior carotid triangle: anterior and inferior borders = superior belly of the omohyoid muscle, superior border = posterior belly of the digastric muscle, posterior border = sternocleidomastoid muscle; and (4) inferior carotid triangle: medial border = anterior midline of the neck, superior border = superior belly of the omohyoid muscle, posterior border = sternocleidomastoid muscle.* Posterior triangle: *medial border = sternocleidomastoid muscle, posterior border = trapezius muscle, inferior border = clavicle. Subdivisions of the posterior triangle are (1) occipital triangle: anterior border = sternocleidomastoid muscle, posterior border = trapezius muscle, inferior border = posterior belly of the omohyoid muscle; and (2) subclavian triangle: anterior border = sternocleidomastoid muscle, superior border = posterior belly of the omohyoid, inferior border = clavicle.*

B, lymphatics of the neck, showing the progression of lymph node drainage from the head and neck region. In general this proceeds in an orderly fashion, cephalad to caudad. However, multiple cross-overs both from ipsilateral to contralateral as well as skip areas are possible, depending on the potency of the lymphatics (i.e., blockage by metastatic disease or radiation treatment).

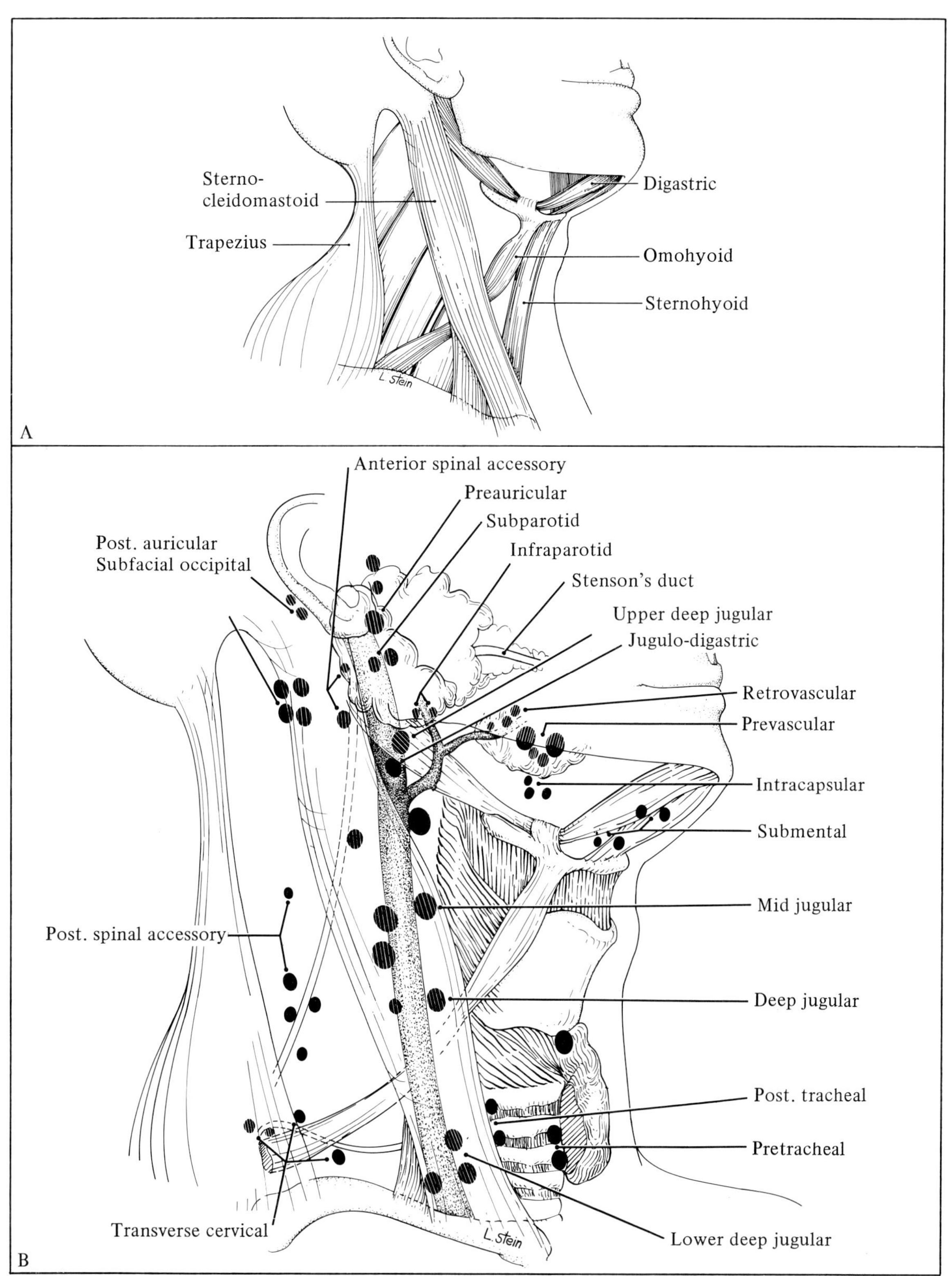
Sterno-
cleidomastoid
Trapezius
Digastric
Omohyoid
Sternohyoid
A
Anterior spinal accessory
Preauricular
Subparotid
Post. auricular
Subfacial occipital
Infraparotid
Stenson's duct
Upper deep jugular
Jugulo-digastric
Retrovascular
Prevascular
Intracapsular
Submental
Mid jugular
Post. spinal accessory
Deep jugular
Post. tracheal
Pretracheal
Transverse cervical
Lower deep jugular
B

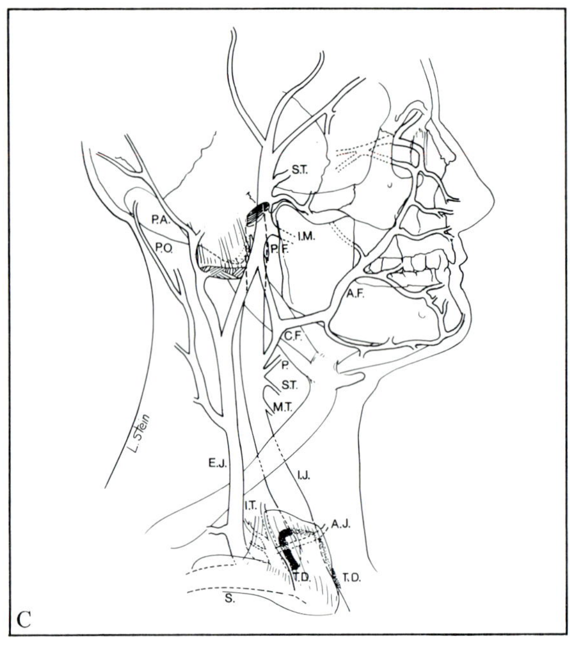

Fig. 17-1 (Continued). C, veins of the neck. S. = *sub-clavian;* A.J. = *anterior jugular;* E.J. = *external jugular;* M.T. = *middle thyroid;* P. = *pharyngeal;* A.F. = *anterior facial;* I.M. = *internal maxillary;* P.O. = *posterior occipital;* T.D. = *thoracic duct;* I.T. = *inferior thyroid;* I.J. = *internal jugular;* S.T. = *superior thyroid;* C.F. = *common facial;* P.F. = *posterior facial;* S.T. = *superficial temporal;* P.A. = *posterior auricular.*

D, the arteries of the neck are outlined. Of note is the relationship of the transverse cervical and suprascapular arteries, which are branches of the costocervical trunk coming from the subclavian artery. They are initially superficial to the prevertebral fascia, as is the thoracic duct. During their lateral course, they may perforate the fascia and become deep to it. S. = *subclavian;* T.C. = *thyrocervical trunk;* S′. = *suprascapular;* I.F. = *inferior thyroid;* S.T. = *superior thyroid;* E.C. = *external carotid;* A.F. = *anterior facial;* I.M. = *internal maxillary;* P.A. = *posterior auricular;* I.Mm. = *internal mammary;* V. = *vertebral;* T. = *transverse cervical;* C.C. = *common carotid;* A.P. = *ascending pharyngeal;* I.C. = *internal carotid;* M. = *mental;* S.T′ = *superficial temporal;* P.O. = *posterior occipital.*

E, superficial nerves of the neck encountered during a neck dissection. All of the nerves depicted, except the ramus mandibularis and cervical facial branch of the facial nerve to the platysma, are cervical sensory nerves. A.N. *represents the eleventh motor nerve to the sternocleidomastoid and trapezius muscles.* M.S. = *medial supraclavicular;* L.O. = *lesser occipital;* C.F. = *cervical facial branch of seventh nerve to the platysma;* L.S. = *lateral supraclavicular;* A.C. = *anterior cervical;* G.A. = *greater auricular;* R.M. = *ramus mandibularis of seventh nerve to the lower lip.*

F, deep nerves of the neck. These are in general the major nerves encountered during a neck dissection, excluding the nerves visualized, such as the branches of the vagus and the glossopharyngeal and cervical sympathetic nerves. It should be recalled that the hypoglossal nerve crosses superficial to both the internal and external carotid arteries and just deep to the inferior border of the midposterior belly of the digastric muscle. P. = *phrenic from C2, 3, and 4 of the cervical plexus;* D.C. = *descendens cervicalis;* V. = *vagus (tenth);* M.H. = *mylohyoid branch from the inferior dental nerve division of the fifth cranial nerve;* J.F. = *jugular foramen;* A. = *ansa hypoglossus;* D.H. = *descendens hypoglossi;* H. = *hypoglossal (twelfth);* L. = *lingual nerve (a branch from the third division of the fifth cranial nerve);* S.A. = *spinal accessory nerve (eleventh).*

G, common areas of nodal metastasis from known primaries. A = *anterior floor of the mouth, lower middle third of the lower lip;* B′ = *anterior floor of mouth and tongue, buccal mucosa, submaxillary gland, sublingual glands, mandibular tumors;* D = *hypopharynx, intrinsic and extrinsic larynx;* F = *posterior triangle metastases, which are usually noted late in head and neck tumors (the most notable exception to this is with primaries in the nasopharynx, with metastasis high in the posterior triangle);* H = *skin of the temporal scalp;* B = *lower lip, buccal mucosa;* C = *oral and hypopharynx, parotid, nasopharynx, posterior two-thirds of tongue, lateral pharyngeal wall, soft palate, tonsillar fossa;* E = *thyroid, larynx, cervical esophagus;* G = *thyroid, lung, stomach;* I = *external and middle ear and occipital scalp.*

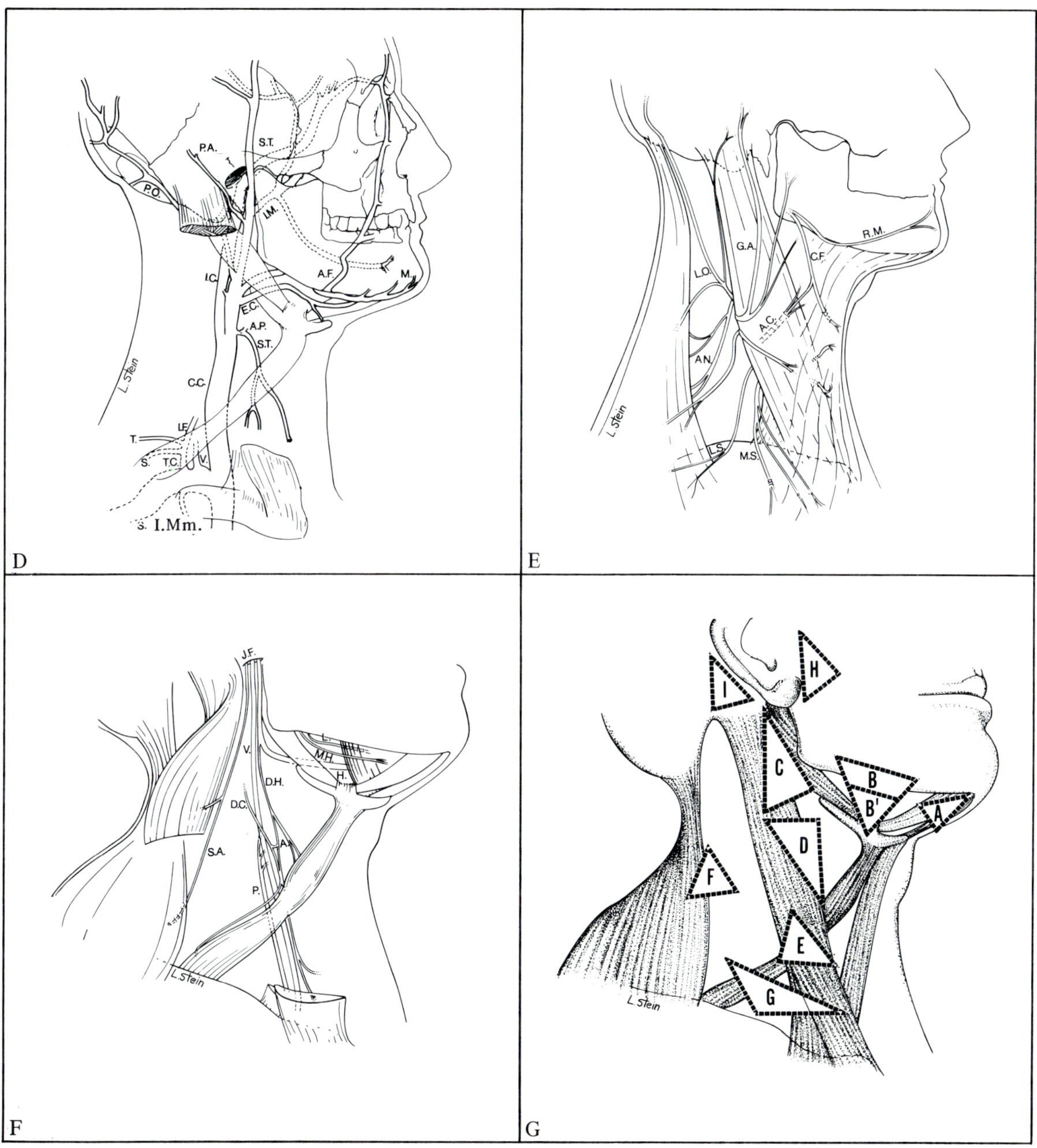
P.A.
S.T.
T.
P.O.
I.M.
A.F.
M.
I.C.
E.C.
A.P.
S.T.
C.C.
L.F.
T.
S.
T.C.
V.
S. I.Mm.
L. Stein
D
G.A.
R.M.
L.O.
C.F.
A.C.
A.N.
L.S.
M.S.
L. Stein
E
J.F.
L.
M.H.
H.
V.
D.H.
D.C.
S.A.
A.
P.
L. Stein
F
H
I
C
B
B'
A
D
F
E
G
L. Stein
G

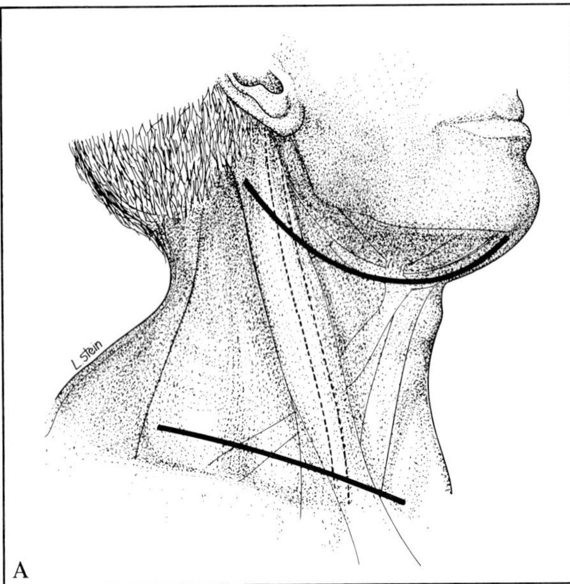

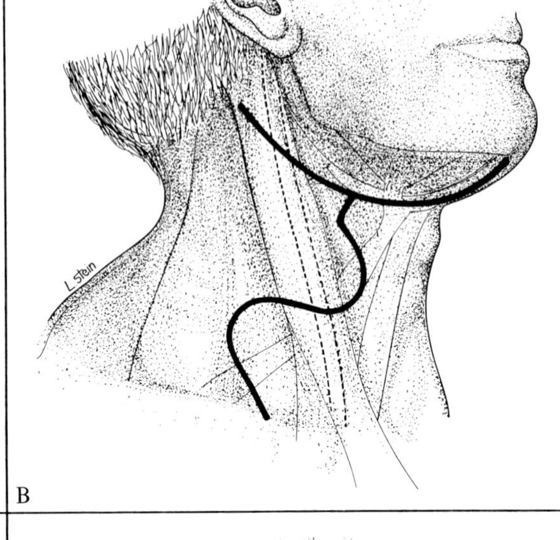

Fig. 17-2. A, biparallel neck incisions (McFee). The carotid system is outlined deep to the sternocleidomastoid muscle. The upper incision is approximately 4 cm. below the lower border of the mandible in a prominent skin crease and crosses from the submental region posteriorly to the tip of the mastoid. The lower incision is approximately 2.5 cm above and parallel to the clavicle, coming close to the midline anteriorly and to the leading edge of the trapezius muscle posteriorly. This is a utilitarian type of incision, considered most safe for primary wound healing in the neck both in patients who had previously received radiation and in other patients. (See text for further description.)

B, this S type of reciprocal vertical limb incision is preferred in patients who have a short thick neck. The upper incision is similar to that in the biparallel incisions. Of note is the fact that the perpendicular portion from the upper neck incision comes off approximately 2.5 cm. anterior or posterior to the palbable underlining carotid system, which will keep end corners in the suture line away from this critical area. The remainder of the incision is a reciprocating type in an S type fashion down to the clavicle. This has the advantage of preventing linear vertical contraction because of the contour of the final scar, as well as good blood supply to its component flaps, with no suture lines of significance lying directly over the carotid artery.

C, the Bakamjian deltopectoral flap is outlined. As this has been described it is based on the perforating internal mammaries, vessels that can be seen on the contralateral side of the parasternal region, giving anatomical arterial supply and venous drainage to this versatile flap. It is shown in conjunction with the lower McFee-type incision to demonstrate the ease with which this flap can be passed deep in the neck to the bipedicle neck incision for use in the reconstruction of the oral cavity or cervical esophagus. The ideal patient for this has a broad shoulder width with a short neck, allowing maximal length of the flap.

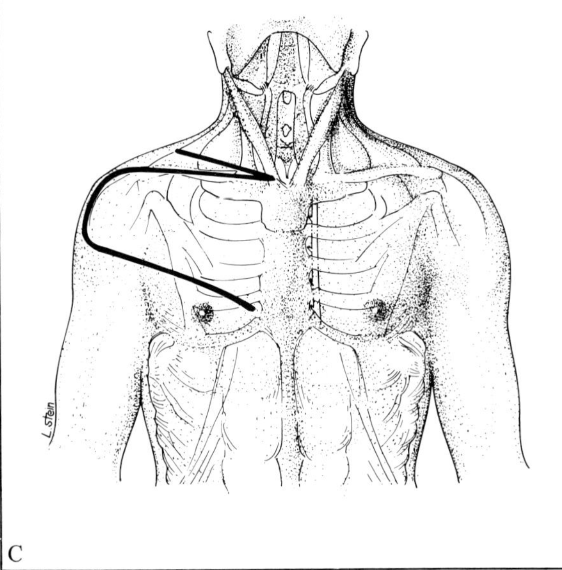

the previous isolation of the ramus mandibularis. The posterior facial vein lying within the tail of the parotid gland is also ligated. The nerve will pass superficial to this structure in most instances, usually well above the lower border of the mandible. The sternocleidomastoid muscle is separated from its tendinous insertion into the mastoid, thus exposing the posterior belly of the digastric muscle and the stylohyoid muscle, which may be transected at this time, exposing the external surface of the splenius capitis muscle. It is important to remember that the sternocleidomastoid muscle has actual dermal insertions, and sharp dissection is necessary to separate them from the posterior neck skin.

Attention is then directed anteriorly where the insertion of the anterior belly of the digastric muscle is detached from the mandible (Fig. 17-3G). The submental triangle from the contralateral anterior digastric over the floor of the mylohoid is cleared, keeping it in continuity with the specimen. The posterior margin of the mylohyoid is identified and retracted anteriorly, exposing the contents of the submaxillary triangle. Outward and downward traction on the specimen with anterior retraction of the mylohoid and hypoglossus would then expose the floor of the submaxillary triangle and allow removal of the lymph nodes and glandular elements of the submental and submaxillary triangles. Protection of the lingual and hypoglossal nerves is accomplished by this direct vision. The submaxillary duct lies between the lingual nerve superiorly and the hypoglossal nerve inferiorly. Wharton's duct is divided between nonabsorbable sutures to complete this phase of the operation. The superior skin flap is then turned back on the wound and covered with a moist pad, which prevents acute angulation of the vessels supplying the base of this flap. Some surgeons may prefer to leave the submaxillary dissection portion of the procedure until later on in the operation.

Lower Dissection

The remaining skin flaps are then elevated and rubber drains placed around the bipedicle neck flap for traction purposes (Fig. 17-3H). Leaving the clavicular periosteum intact, the platysma and superficial cervical fascia are divided along the upper border of the clavicle from the sternal notch to the anterior border of the trapezius muscle. Anterosuperior traction places the tissues on the necessary stretch. The sternocleidomastoid muscle is divided 1.3 cm. superior to its sternal and clavicular attachments. The anterior border of the dissection is easy to identify at the lateral border of the strap muscle (at the junction of these muscles and the leading edge of the sternocleidomastoid muscle). At the posterior border of the clavicular origin of the sternocleidomastoid muscle lies the external jugular vein, which is ligated, care being taken to avoid the transverse scapular and transverse cervical arteries, which are located deep to the prevertebral fascia. The lower and posterior angle of the dissection is defined by locating and dividing the posterior belly of the omohyoid muscle, clearing away the fat and lymph nodes above the prevertebral fascia overlying the brachial plexus (Fig. 17-3I). The anterior part of the inferior region is not completed until the posterior and deep surfaces of the internal jugular vein have been dissected relatively free, deferring ligation of the internal jugular vein until later, which helps to decrease the amount of bleeding encountered until a later stage.

Posterior and Deep Dissection

When the McFee incision only is used, the lower half of the neck dissection is done through the lower incision. The specimen is separated from the anterior border of the trapezius muscle from the clavicle to the midneck. A common error is to miss the presenting edge of the trapezius muscle by going too deep in the neck initially. This is easily avoided if the operator remembers that the trapezius muscle is immediately below the skin and is readily identified by its surface landmarks. During this phase of the procedure, the spinal accessory nerve must be severed. Retracting the trapezius muscle posteriorly and, at the same time, lifting the neck contents anteriorly aid in the identification of the deep cervical fascia on the floor of the neck. This elevation separates it from the prevertebral fascia, defining the plane between them for safe incision and dissection. More medial dissection is continued along the deep cervical floor, just superficial to the vessels supplying the muscles of the floor (scalenus anticus, scalenus posticus, levator scapulae, and splenius capitis), and avoiding these vessels, the phrenic and accessory phrenic nerves, and brachial plexus. If one stays above the prevertebral fascia, which admittedly is somewhat thin and attenuated in certain portions of the neck, injuries to these structures will be avoided. In reality, the prevertebral fascia is usually taken with the specimen. The sensory branches of the cervical plexus are placed on stretch to delineate it from the phrenic nerve. Stretching these nerve branches prior to cutting may allow the proximal ends to retract into the muscular floor and prevent painful neuromas. The carotid sheath is now approached at its posterolateral border in the low neck. Wide visualization of the vagus nerve, the thoracic and cervical ducts, and the internal jugular vein is now possible. The carotid sheath is opened anteriorly, and the internal jugular vein is quadruply ligated and then divided. The vagus nerve and carotid artery are identified prior to clamping the vein. The jugular vein is initially isolated 2.5 cm. above the clavicle.

(Text continues on p. 382)

Fig. 17-3. A, McFee incisions have been outlined. Dotted lines represent the lower border of the mandible and the leading edge of the trapezius muscle. The perpendicular hash mark represents the area where the anterior facial artery crosses the lower mandibular border. The mastoid process and angle of the mandible are also marked. This represents the level of transection of the tail of the parotid. The ramus mandibularis is identified 2 cm. anterior to the angle of the mandible, superficial to the anterior facial artery and vein, 1 cm. below the lower mandibular border. Note that at strategic points the drapes are sutured to the skin to ensure maintenance of a sterile field. They are not sutured in the supraclavicular area; this allows easy access to the anterior chest, which has also been prepped, to control an inadvertent pneumothorax on bleeding from the jugular vein at the root of the neck.

B, traction on the upper neck incision for elevation of the superior flap, superficial to the platysma muscle. Injury to the ramus mandibularis nerve will not occur if one stays superficial to the platysma muscle during this flap elevation. Also note that the traction and countertraction principle is followed with sponge traction inferiorly and skin hook traction to the upper flap.

C, the dissection of the upper skin flap has been completed. The platysma muscle can be seen lying in situ. Posteriorly, the anterior border of the sternocleidomastoid has come into view. The dissection is carried to the upper border of the body of the mandible. If the neck dissection is being done for a lip carcinoma, then this dissection must be considerably higher than the region of the anterior facial artery and vein, as is described in the text.

D, the anterior facial artery and vein are isolated approximately 1 cm. below the inferior margin of the mandible, transected and doubly ligated. The right hemostat in this photograph is underneath these vessels. The left hemostat is under the nerve that crosses superficial to these vessels. Crossing just beneath the superficial cervical fascia, deep to the transected platysma muscle, can be seen the faint proximal outline of the ramus mandibularis (arrow). This is gently isolated and dissected free from the area, with care taken not to go deep into the confines of the submaxillary triangle.

E, the hemostat to the left is under the mobilized ramus mandibularis, which has been freed both anteriorly and posteriorly so that it will not be injured later on in the dissection. The nerve will now be displaced cephalad by suturing the ligated distal ends of the facial artery to the undersurface of the upper skin flap.

F, the nerve (arrow) is now well isolated from the operative field, being held in that position by the previously described technique of suturing the transected anterior facial artery and vein to the upper skin flap. The posterior isolation of the nerve has continued through a portion of the parotid substance, and the tail of the parotid has been transected with ligation of the posterior facial vein at this time. Thereby, under direct vision there is no chance of injuring the proximal portion of the ramus mandibularis when the tail of the parotid is being transected.

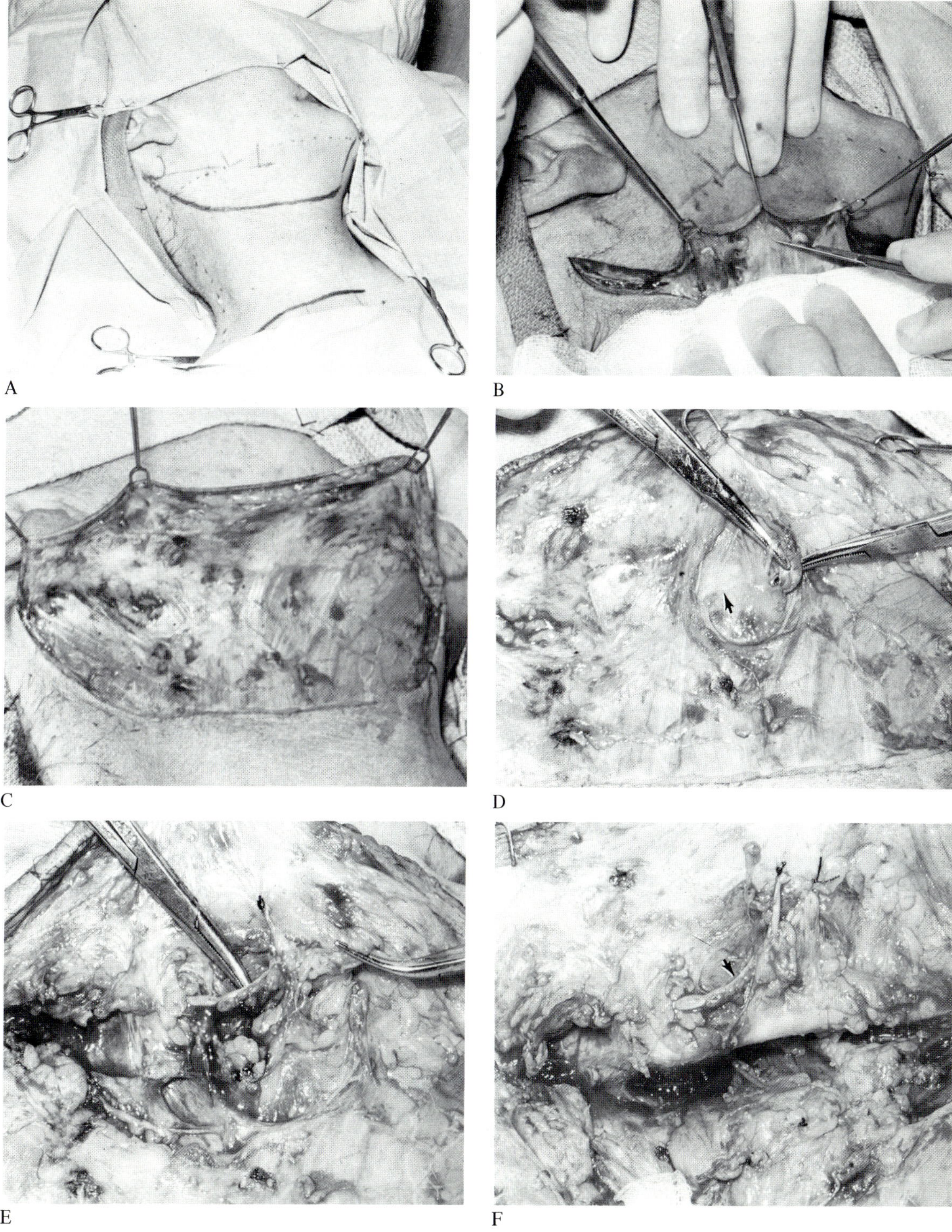
A
B
C
D
E
F

Fig. 17-3 (Continued). G, anteriorly, the anterior digastric muscle is detached from the mandible to be included with the specimen. In this particular situation the periosteum over the external and lingual aspects of the mandible has been included with the specimen. The masseter muscle is seen at its insertion into the midposterior body of the mandible. At the same time, the contralateral submental triangle is identified and cleaned out over the mylohyoid muscles. Anterior traction on the posterior border of the mylohyoid muscle allows easy entrance into the submaxillary triangle, and its contents can be easily removed. The base of this triangle is the hyoglossus muscle.

H, the bipedicle neck flap between the two parallel incisions is elevated, staying superficial to the platysma muscle. Soft rubber drains are placed anteriorly and posteriorly around this flap so that gentle traction can be used to afford adequate exposure. Note that the upper skin flap has been returned to its anatomical position, with a sponge in the depths of the upper neck wound so that blood supply to this flap will not be compromised during the remainder of the operative procedure.

I, depicted in this cross-sectional schematic drawing at C6 level are several points to be noted. The prevertebral fascia is overlying the scalenus muscles, the phrenic nerves, and the brachial plexus. The prevertebral fascia extends well laterally into the posterior triangle of the neck, deep to the overlying trapezius muscle, forming a portion of the floor of the posterior triangle. The cervical sympathetics lie just anterior to the prevertebral fascia but posteromedial to the common carotid artery. The investing layer of cervical fascia splits to embrace both the sternocleidomastoid and trapezius muscles. The carotid sheath embraces the carotid artery and vagus nerve, with only a very filmy sheath actually being present around the internal jugular vein. If one keeps this diagram in mind while carrying out a neck dissection, it will be much easier to maintain the proper planes for a more satisfactory procedure with less loss of blood.

J, lower neck dissection. The clavicular and sternal origins of the sternocleidomastoid muscle have been transected. The omohyoid muscle has been transected well laterally and can be seen held in the clamp at the upper left. The anterior border of the trapezius has been identified and dissected to the midneck level. The contents of the posterior triangle, including some of the prevertebral fascia, have been removed from the floor of the posterior triangle. Gentle traction on the omohyoid muscle is useful in delineating the anterior limit of the dissection up to the hyoid bone. The lower hemostat is under the internal jugular vein, which has been isolated approximately 2.5 cm. above the clavicle before being transected and doubly transected. Prior to ligation of the internal jugular vein, the common carotid artery, vagus nerve, and phrenic nerve are positively identified. The thoracic duct and its ramifications are also transected and ligated at this time.

K, the carotid sheath has been opened, with exposure of the vagus nerve and the common carotid artery. The lateral border of the strap muscles and the omohyoid serve as a guide line as dissection is continued cephalad. One must be cautious not to injure the phrenic nerve; the dissection should not be deep enough to expose the lower cervical sympathetic ganglia, which are deep to the common carotid artery. Again the principle of traction and countertraction makes this procedure quite easy. In patients who have had previous irradiation, however, there may be a significant amount of stickiness, difficulty in obtaining satisfactory tissue cleavage planes, and bothersome bleeding because the vessels do not contract.

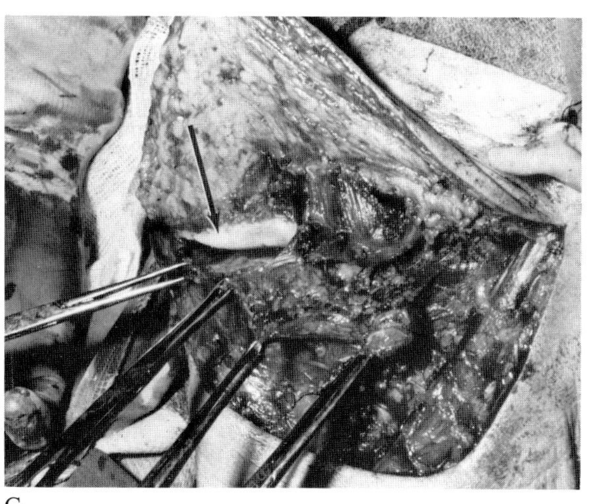

G

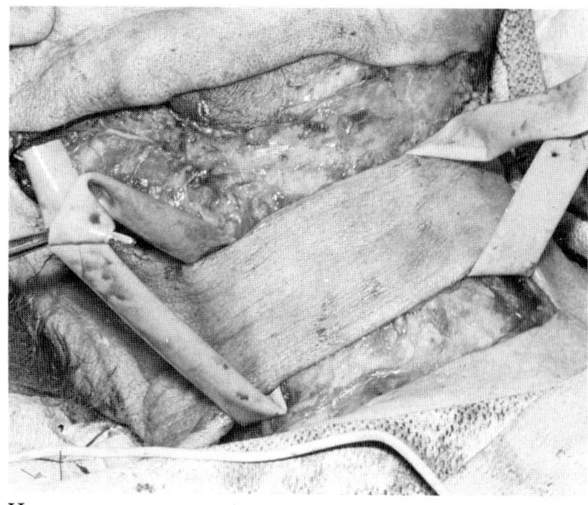

H

Ligamentum nuchae
Semispinalis cervicis
Semispinalis capitis
Posterior primary ramus of C6
Scalenus medius
Prevertebral fascia
Cervical sympathetic
Roof of post. triangle
Carotid sheath and vagus nerve
Pretracheal fascia
Thyroid gland
Investing layer
Pretracheal fascia
Cricoid
Sternocleidomastoid
Platysma
Infrahyoid muscles
External jugular vein
Internal jugular vein
Retropharyngeal space
Scalenus anterior and phrenic nerve
Longissimus capitis
Levator scapulae
Splenius cervicis
Multifidus
Trapezius
C6

I

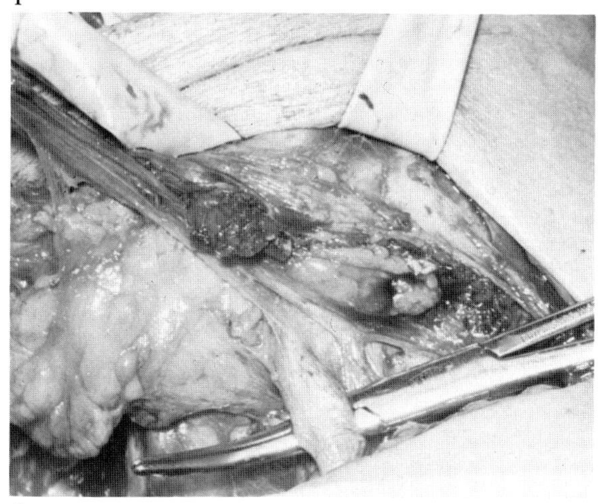

J

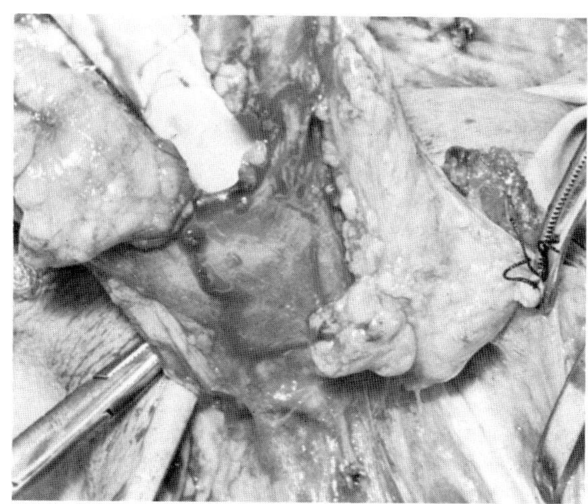

K

Fig. 17-3 (Continued). L, the dissection continues on the muscular floor of the neck to the midneck level, usually just above the superior thyroid cartilage. The cervical sensory nerves are best transected after one has followed and positively identified the take-off point of the phrenic nerve from the cervical plexus. The sensory nerve should be transected close to the bifurcation to reduce the possibility of neuroma formation in a long unprotected stump. The lower neck portion of the dissection is shown here. The next maneuver entails passing the specimen underneath the bipedicle flap and retracting the cephalad incision for completion of the neck dissection.

M, the specimen has been passed through to the upper neck. Dissection is continued up the leading edge of the trapezius muscle, as well as the carotid artery and vagus nerve, until it joins the previous dissection. This occurs at the submental and submaxillary areas anteriorly, posteriorly at the tail of the parotid, and where the insertion of the sternocleidomastoid muscle has been transected. Bifurcation of the carotid artery can be injected with 1% procaine into the adventitia, if necessary, to prevent hypotension. The hypoglossal nerve, which passes superficial to both the internal carotid and external carotid systems, is usually spared. However, metastatic disease frequently occurs in the area around the jugular digastric nodes. If there is significant disease in this area, the hypoglossal nerve should be included with the anatomical specimen for a true in-continuity type resection.

N, the completed neck. The external carotid artery is usually taken just a bit distal to the superior thyroid take-off. However, in this particular case, it remains in place and the specimen is removed. Prior to wound closure, copious irrigation with sterile saline is carried out. Approximately 2 L. is used, and a search for any bleeding points is done and cared for.

O, the closed wound is depicted. Prior to closure, two plastic catheters are inserted and brought out at the posterior inferior base of the posterior triangle and attached to suction. The suction apparatus is instituted prior to closing the wound and kept working throughout the closure so that clots will not form, and the flaps will remain well seated against the underlying neck tissue. The catheters are so arranged that one goes up the anterior and the other the posterior neck without significant pressure on the carotid vessels. The wound is then closed with inverting dermal type sutures. The skin is closed with subcuticular 5-0 nylon continuous-type pull-out sutures or a combination of vertical mattress and simple interrupted sutures. A pressure dressing is required over the supraclavicular fossa so that skin in this area will not tent across the trapezius to the clavicle and allow fluid to collect.

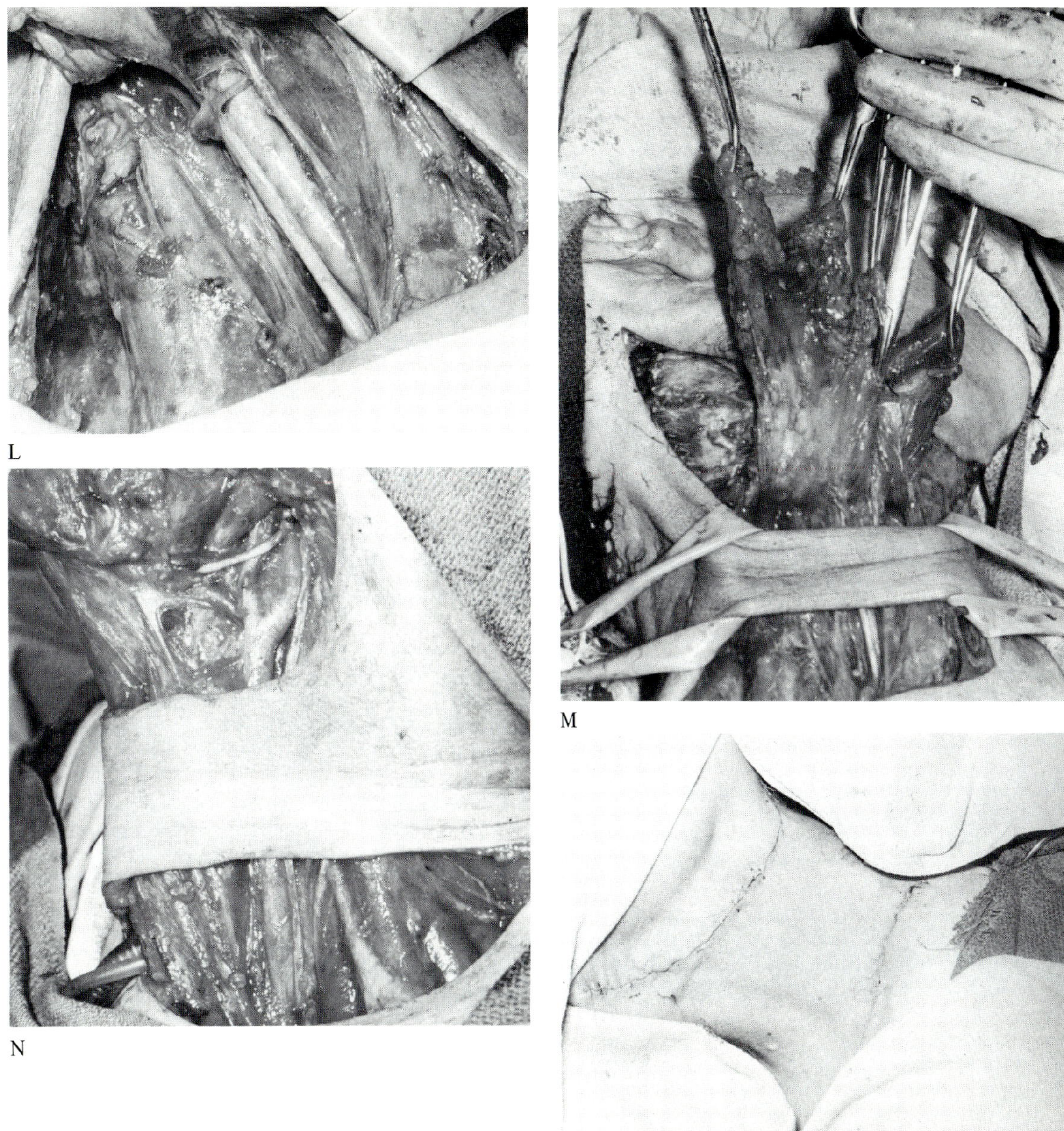

L

M

N

O

It is mobilized and then ligated at the root of the neck. This allows for better control of the proximal stump if troublesome bleeding is encountered. Serial clamping and ligation are done at the lateral border of the vein at the root of the neck to ensure that all lymphatics in this area have been adequately controlled. The anterior half of the carotid sheath is removed with the vein progressing upward to the carotid bifurcation (Fig. 17-3J, K).

It is advantageous at this point to define the medial border. This is facilitated by downward and posterior traction on the omohyoid muscle. The anterior border of this muscle is then followed to the hyoid bone. At this time, the specimen is passed beneath the skin of the neck and brought through the upper incision (Fig. 17-3L, M).

At the bifurcation of the carotid artery, the adventitia is infiltrated with anesthetic solution to abolish the sinus reflex. Distal to the superior thyroid artery, the external carotid artery is ligated and divided between the ties. The distal segment of the external carotid artery is passed beneath the hypoglossal nerve, which lies superficial to it. With the hypoglossal nerve thus preserved, the external carotid artery with its branches ligated and transected distally is now taken with the specimen. The cleaning of the internal carotid artery up to the base of the skull can be done quickly and with little blood loss. Care must be taken at this point to avoid damage to the superior cervical ganglion, which lies just behind the vagus nerve and the posterior carotid sheath. The submaxillary triangle is then resected as described earlier, if this has not already been done. The dissection at the anterior border of the trapezius is now completed from the midneck to the mastoid, where it joins the previous dissection at the lateral surface of the splenius capitis muscle. The posterior digastric belly, as well as the stylohyoid muscle, is transected and removed with the specimen, if this has not been done previously. The spinal accessory nerve is divided, the vagus and hypoglossal nerves are protected, and the specimen is delivered after ligation of the internal jugular vein (Fig. 17-3N).

Copious irrigation is performed, 2 L. of normal saline being used. Plastic drainage tubes are placed, one medial and one lateral to the carotid artery. Each is drawn through a separate dependent stab wound in the infraclavicular area or the lateral neck skin and attached to suction through a Y connector before the flaps are replaced and sutured (Fig. 17-3O). This prevents clogging of tubing and pulling of clots within the depths of the wound while closure is being carried out. The only dressing used is a compression dressing over the supraclavicular fossa. Continuous suction by a wall or motorized pump is carried out for 48 hours, after which the standard portable suction unit is used. The drainage tubes are left in place for 5 to 6 days, or until the 24-hour drainage is less than 25 ml.

Modifications of Radical Neck Dissection

The points of difference in the dissection for each primary anatomical site are discussed below.

PRIMARY LESION IN THE LIP. The upper border of the neck dissection should not lie on the lower border of the mandible but rather 2 cm. above it, especially in the anterior two-thirds of the dissection. The ramus mandibularis of the seventh nerve cannot be preserved because of the high incidence of involved nodes in the region where the anterior facial vein crosses the mandible. In order to clean the submental and submaxillary triangle in a more radical fashion, the periosteum of the lateral inferior and medial portions of the body of the mandible is included with the specimen (Fig. 17-4).

INTRAORAL PRIMARY LESION. The definition of the upper border of the radical neck dissection is not done, i.e., the mandibular periosteum and musculature are not incised. This tissue will remain attached to the mandible, since a portion of the mandible will

Fig. 17-4. This depicts the drainage from carcinomas of the lower lip, the majority of which drain primarily to the prevascular components of the submaxillary group of nodes. These nodes are located adjacent to the anterior facial artery and vein superficial to the mandible. The submental nodes may also be involved, although somewhat less frequently. The importance here lies in the fact that if a supraomohyoid or radical neck dissection is done, it must be modified so that the dissection carries well above the upper border of the mandible including the periosteum of the mandible in that area, as well as the anterior facial artery and vein. (See text for further discussion.)

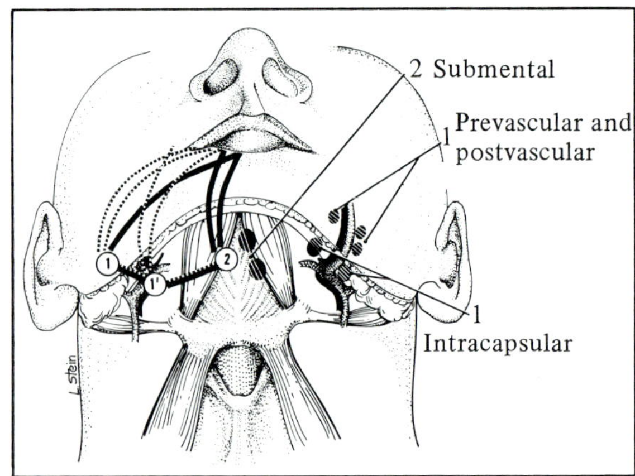

be resected in continuity with the lesion. Likewise, as soon as the carotid bifurcation has been cleaned and the external carotid artery ligated, a decision is made concerning the hypoglossal nerve. If hemiglossectomy is contemplated, the hypoglossal nerve stays with the specimen. If the tongue is to be preserved, after protection of the hypoglossal nerve, the dissection does not progress superiorly toward the submaxillary triangle, to avoid entering the upper neck triangles. Rather, at this point, the lip is split, the lip-cheek flap elevated, and the anterior section of the mandible done. Traction on the bone and on the neck contents as a unit, with retraction of the lip-cheek flap, facilitates exposure of the oral lesion and allows for adequate mucosal and muscular excision. As the primary lesion is freed, the posterior site of the mandibular resection at the base of the ascending ramus is done and internal pterygoid muscles are divided 1 cm. distal to the level of the bone section. After the bone is removed, the proximal fragment of the ascending ramus is covered by suturing the masseter to the internal pterygoid, providing a muscle cradle to prevent erosion of the mucosa by the bony fragment.

PRIMARY LESION IN THE OROPHARYNX. There are three major modifications when operating on oropharyngeal lesions. (1) Avoid entrance into the submaxillary triangle when there is a possibility that metastatic nodes may be located there; therefore, the ramus mandibularis is resected. (2) Maintain an adequate bulk of tissue in composite resection attached to the mandible between the primary and the neck nodes; this effectively prevents inadvertent surgical encroachment on the intervening lymphatics. (3) With a posteriorly located lesion, dissection must include the retropharyngeal lymph nodes. This is ensured by incising the prevertebral fascia just lateral and posterior to the carotid sheath, great care being taken not to injure the vagus nerve, the superior sympathetic ganglion, and the sympathetic trunk, which lie superficial to the prevertebral fascia (Fig. 17-31). Medial dissection to the midline behind the oropharynx can be done in this prevertebral plane in a quick, bloodless fashion.

PRIMARY LESION IN THE HYPOPHARYNX. There are four major modifications of the radical neck dissection technique – three to widen the field of dissection for inclusion of the lymphatics draining inferiorly through the thyroid capsule, and one to lessen the dissection superiorly. Ipsilateral thyroidectomy and removal of all strap muscles on the involved side are mandatory. In order to complete the partial pharyngectomy (occasionally total pharyngectomy) or laryngectomy (or both), the opposite side of the neck must be entered, and, while preserving the thyroid lobe and the superior thyroid artery, the strap muscles are removed with the specimen. As with the oropharyngeal lesions, it is necessary to modify the standard radical neck procedure by dissecting the retropharyngeal lymph nodes and including these with the monoblock resection. The superior border does not have to be a wide resection because metastases to the submaxillary and submental triangles are infrequent.

Radical Neck Dissection after Radiation Treatment

The best time to perform an elective radical neck dissection is within 6 to 8 weeks after the radiation treatment, when the acute radiation reaction has subsided, when the patient is eating and has stopped losing weight, and before the inexorable blood vessel damage begins to be a significant factor for avascularity. When considerable time has elapsed between the radiation therapy and the opportunity to perform the neck dissection, the possibilities of wound complications are greatly enhanced. In this event, two factors have improved the results and decreased the risk of complications: (1) the use of two transverse skin incisions, so that the skin flaps are safer, and (2) the use of flaps designed from the muscles of the floor of the posterior triangle to serve as protection for the blood vessels. The most common and utilitarian of these muscle flaps is a local rotation or turnover flap of the levator scapulae muscle (Fig. 17-5), based anterosuperiorly [10]. Should this be unavailable, a lateral turnover flap of the splenius capitis muscle or a portion of the scaleneus muscle, the trapezius muscle, or the strap muscles can be used. Each of these latter flaps is based medially. Muscle flaps are used in preference to free dermal grafts [15, 30].

THE SUPRAOMOHYOID NECK DISSECTION

There are times when a procedure less extensive than a radical neck dissection is indicated for control of the cervical lymph glands. When circumstances call for less than a radical neck dissection, supraomohyoid dissection must be done. The specific indication to do less than a radical dissection must be clearly understood. The wide dissection of the upper neck is not a substitute for the radical dissection, but rather a supplement to it. The adverse notoriety gained by the supraomohyoid dissection stems from poor selection for its use, lack of understanding of the extent of removal, and technical difficulty. Knowledge of its use and attention to technical details can make the supraomohyoid dissection a valuable tool in increasing the cure rate in malignancies of the lip, floor of the mouth, and alveolar ridge, as well as in some lingual malignancies.

The major indication for the use of supraomo-

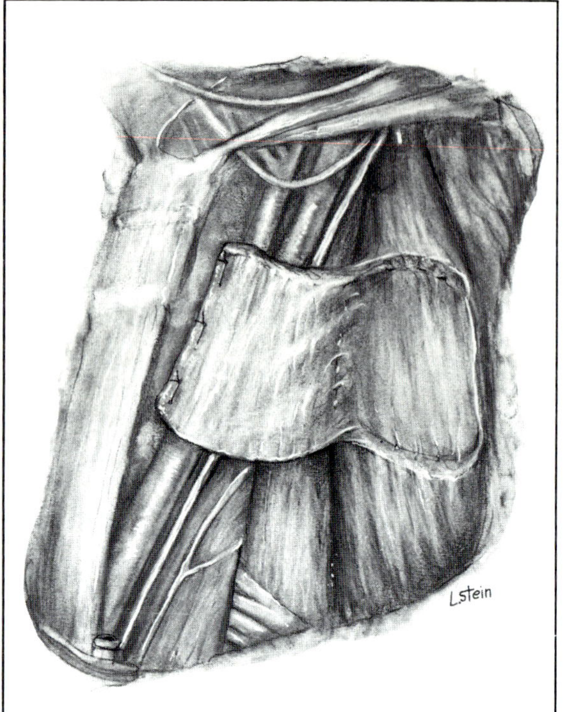

A

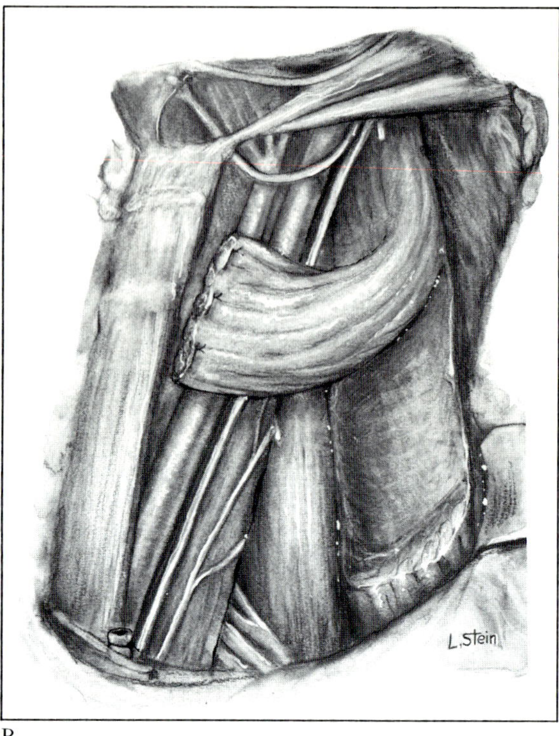

B

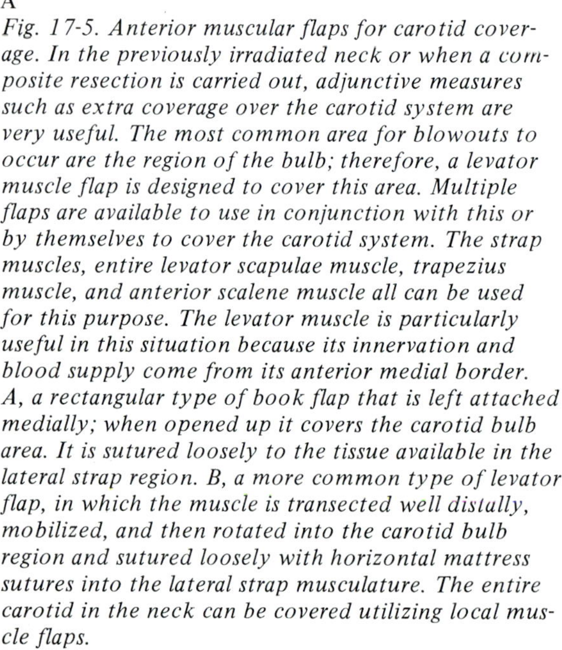

Fig. 17-5. Anterior muscular flaps for carotid coverage. In the previously irradiated neck or when a composite resection is carried out, adjunctive measures such as extra coverage over the carotid system are very useful. The most common area for blowouts to occur are the region of the bulb; therefore, a levator muscle flap is designed to cover this area. Multiple flaps are available to use in conjunction with this or by themselves to cover the carotid system. The strap muscles, entire levator scapulae muscle, trapezius muscle, and anterior scalene muscle all can be used for this purpose. The levator muscle is particularly useful in this situation because its innervation and blood supply come from its anterior medial border. A, a rectangular type of book flap that is left attached medially; when opened up it covers the carotid bulb area. It is sutured loosely to the tissue available in the lateral strap region. B, a more common type of levator flap, in which the muscle is transected well distally, mobilized, and then rotated into the carotid bulb region and sutured loosely with horizontal mattress sutures into the lateral strap musculature. The entire carotid in the neck can be covered utilizing local muscle flaps.

hyoid dissection is part of the monoblock dissection for a unilateral lesion in the floor of the mouth that approaches or crosses the midline. Radical neck dissection is done on the side of the lesion, and supraomohyoid dissection is done contralaterally in continuity if there are no palpable lymph nodes on the contralateral side. Use of supraomohyoid dissection on the ipsilateral side should be limited to situations in which there is no palpable adenopathy and the primary tumor is a small, well-differentiated lesion of the alveolus or lip. Bilateral supraomohyoid dissection may be done for central lower lip carcinoma with high palpable nodes or a small central lesion in the anterior floor of the mouth.

Technique of Supraomohyoid Neck Dissection

The upper portion of the dissection is accomplished in the same manner as that in the radical technique. As the parotid tail is transected and the mastoid approached, the superior end of the sternocleidomastoid is not transected. Rather the fascia along the outer border of the sternocleidomastoid is opened, cleaning this border inferiorly until the omohyoid tendon is reached. Strong posterior retraction of the muscle and anterior lifting of the fascia expose the floor of the muscular triangles and the carotid sheath.

Anteriorly, the dissection proceeds downward from the insertion of the anterior belly of the digas-

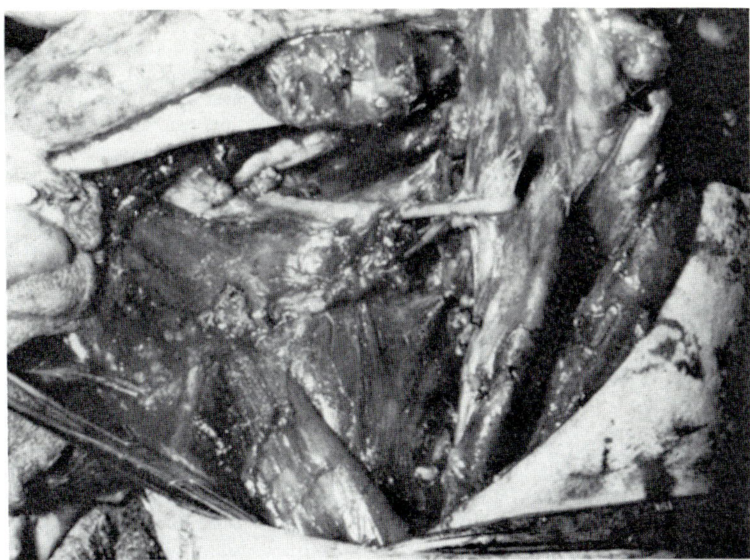

Fig. 17-6. Completed left supraomohyoid dissection. As described in text, the superior limits are the mandible, including, if necessary, the region well above the upper border of the mandible: the anterior limits are the contralateral submental triangle, the lateral border of the strap muscles down to the point where the sternocleidomastoid muscle approaches the strap muscles, which is in the lower third of the neck. The posterior margin is the retracted anterior border of the sternocleidomastoid muscle, which allows cleaning of the internal jugular vein nodes up to the jugular foramen.

tric, which is transected, in the midline to the hyoid bone. The contents of the contralateral and the ipsilateral submental triangles are removed with the specimen, the depth of the dissection being the presenting surface of the mylohyoid muscle. The fascia overlying the anterior belly of the omohyoid is incised to meet the posterior and inferior dissection.

The carotid sheath incision is begun at this low level, and the stripping of the internal jugular vein and carotid artery on the floor of the neck proceeds upward until the upper dissection is joined. This maneuver is facilitated on the floor of the neck by retracting the posterior belly of the digastric cephalad and following the internal jugular vein as far as possible toward the base of the skull, then transecting the fascia close to the jugular foramen (Fig. 17-6).

RADICAL NECK DISSECTION OF THE OTHER SIDE OF THE NECK

Radical neck dissection on the side of the neck contralateral to the lesion increases morbidity greatly, so that a bilateral procedure must be reserved for a few specific situations. In order to make the correct decision, all of the various situations that may occur should be considered. Only in some of the following situations will bilateral radical neck dissection be indicated:

A. Primary Lesion
   1. Unilateral
   2. Unilateral encroaching on the midline
   3. Unilateral crossing the midline
   4. Midline
B. Cervical Lymph Nodes
   1. Ipsilateral negative, contralateral negative
   2. Ipsilateral positive, contralateral negative
   3. Ipsilateral negative, contralateral positive
   4. Ipsilateral positive, contralateral positive

The unilateral lesion will have bilateral cervical metastases in less than 10 percent of the cases. If the ipsilateral lymph nodes are negative, rarely will the contralateral nodes be positive.

When a unilateral primary lesion encroaches on the midline, there may be invasion of the lymph drainage on the opposite side. If the contralateral nodes are clinically negative, a supraomohyoid neck dissection should be performed on the contralateral side in continuity with the resection of the primary lesion and the ipsilateral radical neck dissection. If the unilateral lesion has actually crossed the midline, it must be considered in the same category as the midline lesion and a bilateral radical neck dissection carried out. If the lymph nodes are clinically negative on both sides, the decision rests between doing a bilateral radical dissection on the one hand and an ipsilateral radical procedure with supraomohyoid dissection on the lesser involved side. Usually the bilateral simultaneous radical dissection is reserved for patients with midline lesions and palpable adenopathy on both sides of the neck or for those with lesions in which it would be necessary to cut across the tumor if only a unilateral neck dissection were done.

Because the performance of the second neck dissection can give such an increased morbidity, biopsy of the palpable cervical lymph nodes may be recommended, contrary to the recommendation prior to an initial procedure. The method of performing this cervical biopsy is critical. This should not be done under local anesthesia or through a small incision; neither should a needle biopsy be performed. The procedure of choice consists of preparing the patient for a radical neck dissection by administering a general endotracheal anesthesia, by outlining the flaps for the contemplated dissection, and by elevating widely only the flap necessary to expose the area of the node. Tissue for the frozen section can then be obtained, great care being taken to prevent contamination of the tumor field. If the node is negative for tumor, all that has been lost is the risk of a short general anesthesia and a slightly longer scar. If the biopsy is positive for tumor, the region can be readily included in the resected specimen to minimize local recurrence.

RESECTION OF THE MANDIBLE

The overlying mandibular body and ramus should be generally included in the resection when primary lesions are located in the tongue, the lateral floor of the mouth, or the tonsillar region. This permits both wider exposure and wider resection, allowing the operator to stay well away from the tumor and still visualize it clearly. Encroachment on the intervening lymphatics between the primary lesion and the deep anterior cervical chain is less likely. There is no doubt that many experienced surgeons can perform either the mandibular swing or the pull-through operation for selected lesions, but these procedures are not recommended for the usual lesion in this region.

There does not seem to be any good reason for replacing the lateral mandible when less than a hemimandibulectomy has been performed. The resultant flattening of the face is not a severe cosmetic deformity. The function of swallowing is not disturbed, although there may be some disturbance of chewing. Most patients secondarily decline a bone graft replacement, believing that it is not necessary on either cosmetic or functional grounds. This is particularly true when control of the distal mandibular fragment is maintained by some means. We favor the use of intraoral appliances that are applied preoperatively or at the time of the operation; these appliances help maintain the normal occlusal relationship of the mandible to the maxilla. One of these appliances consists of a lateral guide bar on the mandibular denture that glides on a vertical guide plane on the maxillary teeth or denture. It is placed on the unoperated side and worn approximately 3 or 4 months postoperatively, which helps to prevent wound contraction with deviation of the chin toward the affected side and allows reeducation through proprioceptive fibers within the masticatory muscles on the unoperated side to compensate and maintain the mandible in a more optimal position (Fig. 17-7).

However, major resection of the anterior oral cavity for lesions of the anterior alveolus or floor of the mouth which encroach on the mandible creates cosmetic and functional defects that are uniquely different from those resulting from the lateral resections. Addition of lining material when large defects have been created can be done primarily when it does not unduly increase the risk, when it is absolutely necessary to provide tissue to accomplish wound closure, or when the nonreconstructed deformity is incompatible with satisfactory patient management. However, the dorsal mucosa of the tongue can close surprisingly large defects adeptly and acceptably in this area. Primarily or secondarily, the addition of anterior oral lining can be accomplished by skin grafts, local rotation mucosal flaps, bipedicle (Visor) lingual flaps, nasolabial skin insertion flaps, cervical skin flaps, or forehead flaps.

Immediate restoration of the mandibular arch accomplishes support of the pharynx, chin, and lip; creates chin protrusion and the submental-cervical angle; facilitates early removal of the tracheotomy; and diminishes the drooling secondary to the temporary labiolingual synechia.

The use of a thin Kirschner wire covered with a silicone rod provides the most direct, quickest, and safest mandibular arch restoration. This rod can be threaded or not. This wire should be curved to simulate the contour of the mandibular arch, stabilized by countersinking it into cortical bone, covered adequately by well-vascularized soft tissue, and securely immobilized. Suspension of the larynx to prevent aspiration can be accomplished by passing a wire through the upper border of the thyroid cartilage and attaching it to the Kirschner wire. This is necessary when the suprahyoid musculature is removed bilaterally. A tracheotomy protects the wire from trauma during postoperative pulmonary toilet. These details ensure long-term survival of the wire, which may be left in situ indefinitely. If the wire is removed and no replacement is contemplated, it may be easily done under local anesthesia on an outpatient basis. Soft tissue scar of the chin alone may support function and appearance; however, a bone graft will give

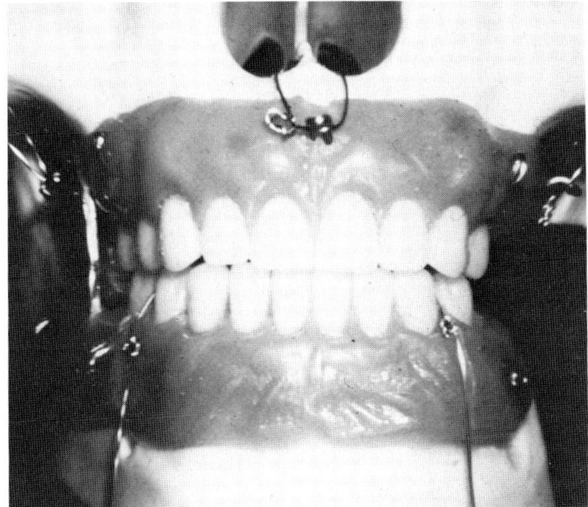

A

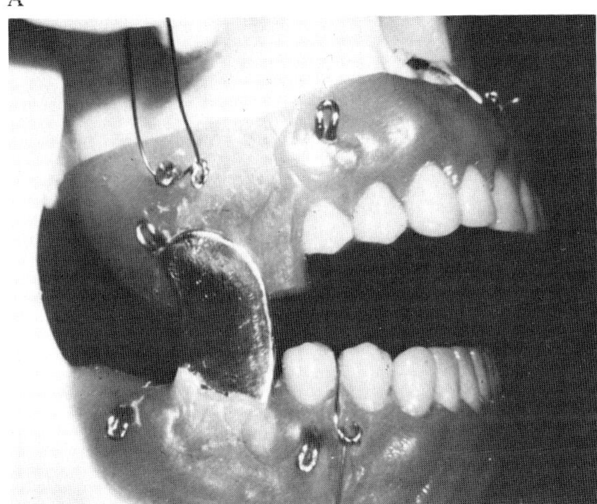

B

Fig. 17-7. Control of the remaining mandibular fragment following mandibular resections can prevent chin shifting to the operative side as well as improve appearance and masticatory function. Several means are available for obtaining this. One such technique is demonstrated in A and B, which show a buccal type vertical guide bar that is attached to the mandibular denture. A, the denture is wired to the remaining mandible with circummandibular wires incorporating the denture in the wire (i.e., on the unoperated side). This vertical guide bar then glides on an acrylic guide plane that is attached to the maxillary denture or teeth. B, when the mouth opens and closes, the guide bar glides up and down the guide plane, thus preventing shift of the mandible toward the operated side. After 2 to 3 months, the majority of the patients will not need this, and their mandible will stay in a relatively good occlusive position without wearing this appliance. This is apparently due to reeducation of, and compensation by, proprioceptor units within muscle fibers on the normal side.

even more improvement in the appearance and allow for more satisfactory mastication, since dentures can then be used.

A different approach, the use of a pull-through technique, with marginal resection, attempts to preserve contour and support by preserving part of the anterior mandible. This approach should be used only when there is considerable space between the lesion and the bone. It is accomplished by removing all of the mandible contiguous to the floor of the mouth, a strip of the lower border and outer cortex of mandibular bone being preserved (this strip of mandible is susceptible to fracture). The technique involves the use of a mechanized saw or drill to cut the bone at its lateral ends vertically to within 5 mm. of the lower mandibular border. Connecting these two cuts by an on-the-bias cut, which maintains the 5 mm. strip of outer cortex while removing the inner cortex, does not encroach on the tumor block.

WHAT TO DO WITH THE UNKNOWN PRIMARY LESION WITH A LUMP IN THE NECK?

In somewhere between 5 and 12 percent of patients who present with a metastatic mass in the neck, the primary lesion has not been located. Barrie et al. [5] describe 123 patients; in this group, 71 biopsies were performed, 61 by the needle aspiration technique and the remaining 10 by open biopsy. The search for the primary lesion was quite extensive, including careful direct and indirect laryngoscopy and nasopharyngoscopy, and many patients had blind biopsies of the nasopharynx and base of the tongue. Other examinations, such as routine chest x-rays and skeletal surveys, were done. Specialized procedures, such as bronchoscopy with washings and cytological examinations, esophagrams, and sinus x-rays, were carried out as indicated. The important thing to remember is that the site of the primary lesion remained unknown in 70 percent of these patients. In 85 percent of the patients, the metastatic lesion represented epidermoid carcinoma.

In the 30 percent of the patients in whom the primary lesion was eventually located, the lesions falling under the epidermoid classification arose from the supraglottic larynx, the nasopharynx, the base of the tongue, and the tonsillar fossa; other lesions included adenocarcinoma and melanoma. The absolute 5-year survival rate following treatment by a radical neck dissection was approximately 25 percent.

Since a relatively high percentage of these patients show a primary lesion in the nasopharynx, thought

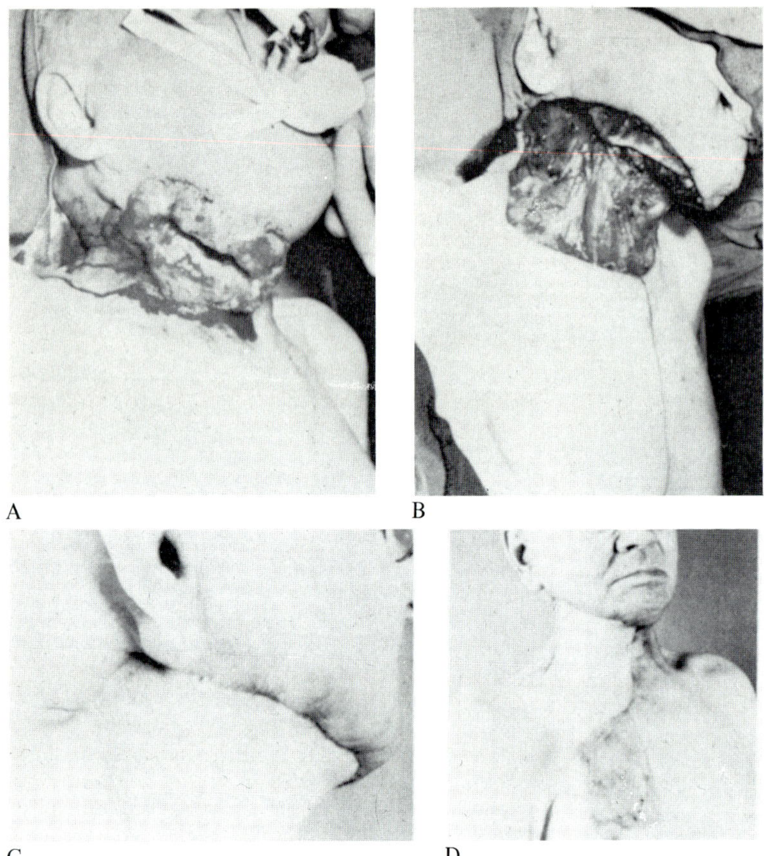

Fig. 17-8. Surgical and radiation treatment elsewhere did not control squamous metastasis. A, the patient entered the hospital emitting a foul smell; he was anemic despite repeated transfusions and was in extreme pain. B, radical neck dissection was done, although cure was not the aim; the dissection necessitated removal of all cervical skin, and a large laterally based deltopectoral flap was needed for wound closure. C, several months later, palliation has succeeded; the patient is living at home free from pain and odor, and without need for transfusions. There is persistent disease. D, close view of the thoracoacromial laterally based deltopectoral flap on the neck.

should be given to initial treatment with radiation therapy that would include the suspected area of the primary lesion, as well as the neck, or a combined approach, using both irradiation and surgery. Marchetta et al. [23] and Bagshaw and Thompson [2] have shown higher survival rates over shorter periods of time when radiation treatment was used in this group of patients. This again appears to be a group who would experience a better cure rate with a joint treatment approach, using a combination of irradiation and surgery.

PALLIATIVE NECK DISSECTIONS

Usually the surgeon sends patients with inoperable or recurrent cancer to the radiotherapist or to a chemotherapist for palpation. Occasionally this situation must be reversed, since there are several situations when the surgeon can palliate recurrences after either irradiation or chemotherapy. Subtotal excision of necrotic tumor masses covered by imaginative flaps of skin and muscle can relieve pain, heal infected wounds, and improve appearances for unexpectedly long periods (Fig. 17-8).

Other adjunctive measures have been described previously. In particular, irradiation and surgery show 5-year survival rates that in general vary 5 to 10 percent from each other, but both are low. However, when these methods are used conjointly as a purposeful program for an initial therapeutic plan, the survival rate may be very significantly improved. Unfortunately, the good survival rates occur in similar regions with both modali-

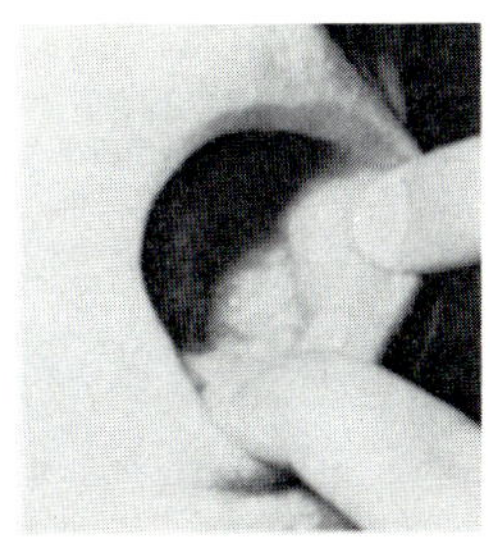
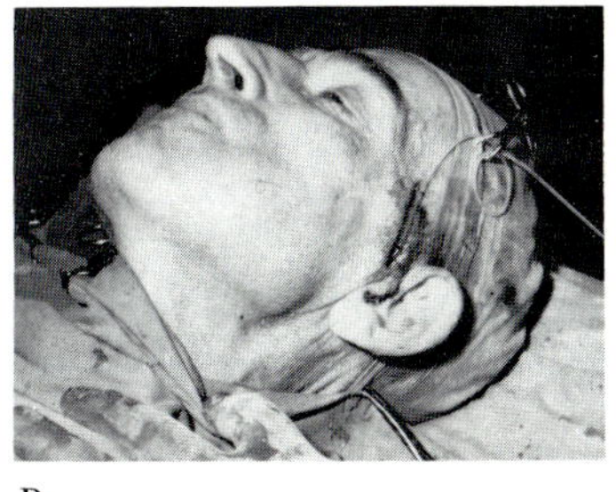
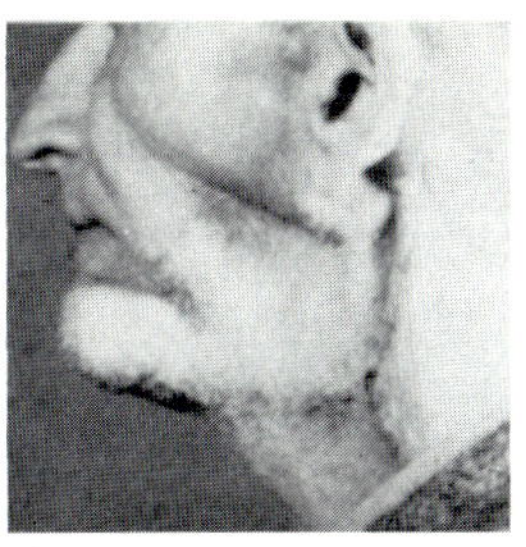

A B C

Fig. 17-9. The place for preoperative and intraoperative chemotherapy by infusion or perfusion is not yet completely determined. This patient represents the combined approach of the surgeon and the chemotherapist. A, the massive intraoral squamous lesion invaded the buccal mucosa and obstructed the lymphatics of the buccal skin. B, preoperative methotrexate infusions were delivered to the lesion and to the cheek via retrograde cannulation of the external carotid artery. The primary lesion regressed to 50 percent of its pretreatment size, and the tumor obstruction of the cheek skin disappeared, so that several weeks later combined resection was performed. The buccal skin was preserved, eliminating a through-and-through cheek defect. C, one year later, there has been no recurrence.

ties. However, there is a theoretical advantage when they are used together. The area in which surgery is the weakest is in the periphery when small foci of cells are not readily recognizable, and this is the area in which radiation therapy is most effective. In contrast to this, with the decreased oxygenation on the central tumor area, radiation therapy is less effective, whereas surgery is much more reliable. Hydroxyurea capsules, 80 mg./kg. orally once every third day, given concomitantly with irradiation seem to potentiate the effect of radiation therapy on the tumor cells [20, 24]. Unfortunately, preoperative radiation therapy with subminimal dosage (2,000 to 3,000 rads) of cobalt 60 in 5 days does not significantly increase the 5-year survival rate.

Methotrexate used as an infusion-type drug can be very impressive, leading to significant regression of the lesion, as well as relief from pain. Unfortunately perfusion techniques with this drug are not practical. Oral and intravenous administrations of the drug appear to be less effective than the infusional route (Fig. 17-9). Cryotherapy can also be used in palliating nonresectable lesions that are secondarily infected, causing pain, discomfort, and bad odor.

REFERENCES

1. Ackerman, L. V., and del Regato, J. A. *Cancer: Diagnosis, Treatment, Therapy* (3rd ed.). St. Louis: Mosby, 1966.
2. Bagshaw, M. A., and Thompson, R. W. Elective irradiation of the neck in patients with primary carcinoma of the head and neck. *J.A.M.A.* 217: 456, 1971.
3. Bakamjian, V. Y. Reconstruction of the Pharynx and Cervical Esophagus. In Gaisford, J. C. (Ed.), *Cancer of the Head and Neck: Total Treatment and Reconstructive Rehabilitation.* St. Louis: Mosby, 1969.
4. Bakamjian, V. Y., Culf, N. K., and Bales, G. W. Versatility of the Medially Based Delto-pectoral Skin Flap in Primary Reconstruction in Head and Neck Surgery. In *Transactions of the Fourth International Congress of Plastic Surgery,* 1967. Amsterdam: Excerpta Medica, 1969.
5. Barrie, J. R., Knapper, W. H., and Strong, E. W. Cervical node metastases of unknown origin. *Am. J. Surg.* 120:466, 1970.
6. Berry, H. C., Parker, R. G., and Gerdes, A. J. Preliminary results of fast neutron teletherapy of metastatic cervical adenopathy. *Cancer* 37:2613, 1976.
7. Carifi, V. G., Ohanion, M. L., David, A. B., Greenlaw, R., and Rush, B. F., Jr. Results of high dose radiation and surgery in the treatment of advanced carcinoma of the head and neck. *Am. J. Surg.* 128:580, 1974.
8. Catteral, M., Sutherland, I., and Bewley, D. K. First results of a randomized clinical trial of fast neutrons compared with x or gamma rays in treatment of advanced tumors of the head and neck. *Br. Med. J.* 2:653, 1975.
9. Chambers, R. G. Combined Therapy in the Treatment of Intraoral Cancer. In Anderson, R., and Hoopes, J. E. (Eds.), *Symposium on Malignancies of the Head and Neck.* St. Louis: Mosby, 1975.
10. Cramer, L. M., and Culf, N. K. Use of Pedicle Flap Tissues in Conjunction with a Neck Dissection. In Gaisford, J. C. (Ed.), *Cancer of the Head and Neck: Total Treatment and Reconstructive Rehabilitation.* St. Louis: Mosby, 1969.
11. Desprez, J., Kiehn, C., Sciotto, C., and Ramirez-Gonzales, M. Response of oral carcinoma to pre-

operative methotrexate infusion therapy. *Am. J. Surg.* 120:461, 1970.
12. Eilber, F. R., Morton, D. L., and Ketcham, A. S. Immunologic abnormalities in head and neck cancer. *Am. J. Surg.* 128:534, 1974.
13. Elliot, R. A., Jr. Technique of Radical Neck Dissection. In Gaisford, J. C. (Ed.), *Cancer of the Head and Neck: Total Treatment and Reconstructive Rehabilitation.* St. Louis: Mosby, 1969.
14. Farr, H. W., and Arthur, K. Epidermoid carcinoma of the mouth and pharynx. *Mem. Sloan-Kettering Cancer Center Clin. Bull.* 1:130, 1971.
15. Jacques, D. A., Harvey, L. M., and Chambers, R. G. Carotid artery protection by means of a trapezius muscle flap. *Am. J. Surg.* 122:744, 1971.
16. Jesse, R. H., Barkley, H. T., Jr., Lindberg, R. D., and Fletcher, G. H. Cancer of the oral cavity. *Am. J. Surg.* 120:505, 1970.
17. Jesse, R. H., and Lindberg, R. D. The efficacy of combined radiation therapy with a surgical procedure in patients with cervical metastasis from squamous cell carcinoma of the oropharynx and hypopharynx. *Cancer* 35:1163, 1975.
18. Kaplan, I., and Aronoff, B. L. The CO_2 Surgical Laser in Surgery for Cancer of the Head and Neck. In Chambers, R. G. (Ed.), *Cancer of the Head and Neck.* Amsterdam: Excerpta Medica, 1975.
19. Ketcham, A. S. Complications and Sequelae of Surgery for Cancer of the Head and Neck. In Anderson, R., and Hoopes, J. E. (Eds.), *Symposium on Malignancies of the Head and Neck.* St. Louis: Mosby, 1975.
20. Lerner, H. J., Beckloff, G. I., and Godwin, M. C. Concomitant hydroxyurea and radiotherapy in the management of 60 patients with head and neck cancer. *Am. J. Surg.* 35:525, 1969.
21. Lindberg, R. D. Present Day Role of Radiation Therapy in Treatment of Head and Neck Cancer. In Chambers, R. G. (Ed.), *Cancer of the Head and Neck.* Amsterdam: Excerpta Medica, 1975.
22. Mandell, M. A. Skin testing for prognosis or therapy formulation in cancer patients. *Plast. Reconstr. Surg.* 57:621, 1976.
23. Marchetta, F. L., Murphy, W. T., and Rovarie, J. J. Carcinoma of the neck. *Am. J. Surg.* 106:976, 1963.
24. Richards, G. J., and Chambers, R. G. Combined Therapy in Treatment of Carcinomas of the Head and Neck. In Chambers, R. G. (Ed.), *Cancer of the Head and Neck.* Amsterdam: Excerpta Medica, 1975.
25. Serafin, D., Georgiade, N. G., and Peters, C. R. Microsurgical composite tissue transplantation; a method of immediate reconstruction of the head and neck. *Clin. Plast. Surg.* 3:447, 1976.
26. Shear, M., Hawkins, D. M., and Farr, H. W. The prediction of lymph node metastasis from oral squamous carcinoma. *Cancer* 37:1901, 1976.
27. Southwick, H. W. Elective neck dissection for intraoral cancer. *J.A.M.A.* 217:454, 1971.
28. Spiro, R., and Strong, E. Epidermoid carcinoma of the mobile tongue. Treatment by partial glossectomy alone. *Am. J. Surg.* 122:707, 1971.
29. Spiro, R. H., and Strong, E. W. Epidermoid carcinoma of the oral cavity and oropharynx. Elective vs. therapeutic radical neck dissection as treatment. *Arch. Surg.* 107:382, 1973.
30. Staley, D. J. A muscle cover for the carotid artery after radical neck dissection. *Am. J. Surg.* 102:815, 1961.
31. Stefano, S., Kerman, R., and Abbate, J. Serial studies of immunocompetence in head and neck cancer patients undergoing radiation therapy. *Am. J. Roentgenol. Radium Ther. Nucl. Med.* 126:880, 1976.
32. Tobin, D. A., Hall, W., and Scott, R. M. Electron beam therapy in head and neck tumors. *Am. J. Roentgenol. Radium Ther. Nucl. Med.* 126:1251, 1976.
33. Wilson, J. S. P. Major Flaps in Reconstruction of Defects of the Head and Neck. In Chambers, R. G. (Ed.), *Cancer of the Head and Neck.* Amsterdam: Excerpta Medica, 1975.
34. Woods, J. E. Current status of chemotherapy in the treatment of head and neck cancer. *Arch. Surg.* 111:1055, 1976.

Primary Tumors of the Salivary Glands and Neck

JOHN E. HOOPES

PAROTID GLAND TUMORS

The parotid gland is subject to a variety of inflammatory processes, benign tumors, and malignant neoplasms, which may either originate in the gland or involve the parotid by direct or lymphatic extension. Increased awareness of the natural history of benign mixed tumors and improved surgical training have resulted in increased success in the management of parotid pathology in recent years.

Incidence

Tumors of the major salivary glands are rare [1]. In the states of New York and Connecticut, they constitute only 0.4 percent of all malignant tumors diagnosed. In the 1947 United States survey, the age-adjusted incidence per 100,000 population was 2.1 and 2.0 for male and female whites and 2.5 and 2.6 for male and female nonwhites, respectively. One in four salivary gland tumors occurred in patients under 40 years of age. Benign tumors are approximately twice as common in females as in males. The average age at time of diagnosis is 42 years for benign tumors and 53 years for malignant tumors.

Pathology

This discussion is limited to malignant disease and the benign tumors peculiar to salivary gland tissue. Lymphoepithelial tumors and the myriad of benign soft tissue tumors that may be found in the salivary glands are excluded [3]. Tumors are more common than inflammatory conditions.

Benign Tumors

Approximately 80 percent of all benign tumors of salivary gland origin arise within the parotid, 80 percent of all primary parotid tumors are benign, and 80 percent of all benign parotid tumors are mixed tumors. *Benign mixed salivary gland tumors* have no true capsule. Local extension may be widespread, and the incidence of recurrence is excessive if adherence to basic principles is neglected. Considerable evidence supports the thesis that malignant transformation of benign mixed tumors occurs and is enhanced following inadequate excision.

Warthin's tumor (papillary cystadenoma lymphomatosum) occurs primarily in males beyond the age of 50 years. The tumor has no malignant implications; recurrence is unusual following adequate excision. *Benign adenoma* is encountered infrequently; it has no malignant potential, and recurrence is uncommon.

Major salivary gland tumors may occur in more than one gland and as multiple foci in a single gland. Warthin's tumor is the most common multiple tumor [10].

Malignant Tumors

Seventy-five percent of malignant tumors of salivary gland origin are primary in the parotid. The tumors are classified histologically in order of frequency as follows [2]:

Undifferentiated carcinoma	27.7%
Mucoepidermoid carcinoma (includes malignant mixed tumor)	24.4%
Cylindroma	16.0%
Acinic cell carcinoma	14.8%
Adenocarcinoma	12.9%
Squamous cell carcinoma	5.0%

They are classified further on the basis of their clinical course:

A. *Low-grade malignancy*
   1. Mucoepidermoid carcinoma
   2. Cylindroma
   3. Acinic cell carcinoma

B. *High-grade malignancy*
   1. Squamous cell carcinoma
   2. Undifferentiated carcinoma
   3. Adenocarcinoma
   4. Malignant mixed tumor

Parotid gland carcinoma is highly invasive locally but metastasizes to the cervical lymph nodes infrequently and late in the course of the disease. Squamous cell and undifferentiated carcinoma involve the cervical nodes earlier and more frequently than other histological types [6, 8].

The efferent lymphatics of the upper face and scalp course through the superficial lobe of the parotid gland. Involvement of the parotid by squamous cell carcinoma and melanoma is not uncommon. Malignancies primary in the oral cavity and paranasal sinuses involve the parotid gland by contiguous spread.

Diagnosis

Benign neoplasms are asymptomatic almost uniformly. The patient has usually been aware of the presence of a mass for a considerable period before seeking medical attention. The most common location of the mass is immediately inferior to the lobule of the ear

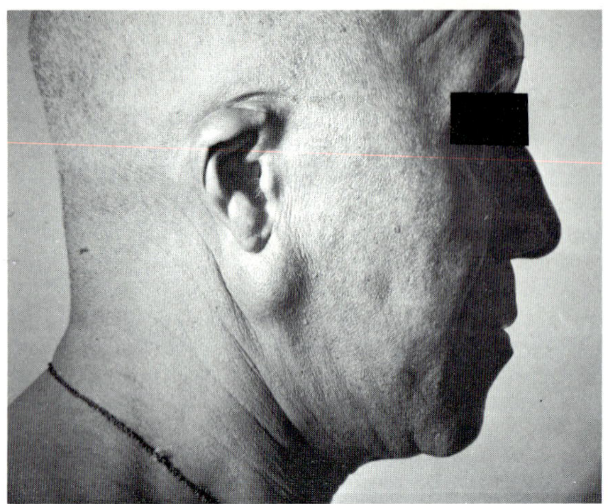

Fig. 18-1. The typical location and appearance of a benign mixed tumor of the parotid gland.

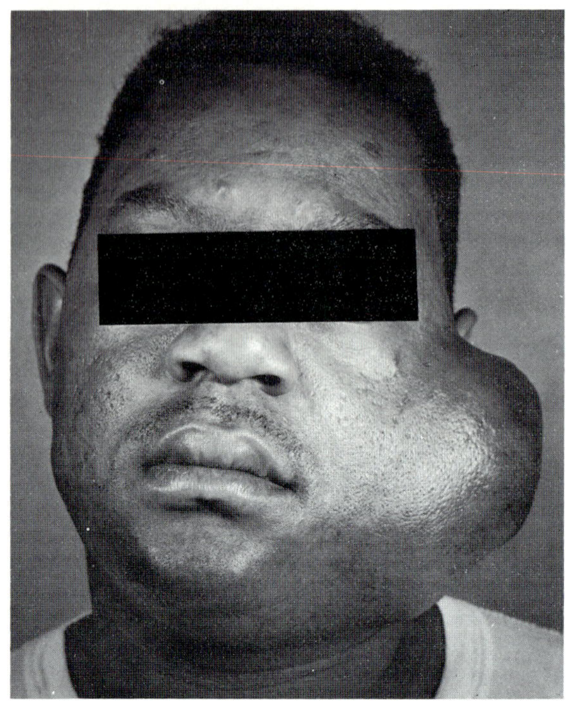

Fig. 18-2. Benign parotid tumor of considerable size without associated symptoms. Note the absence of facial palsy.

(Fig. 18-1). Regardless of the size and local extent of the tumor, pain or impairment of function is minimal, and facial nerve palsy is seen rarely (Fig. 18-2).

Malignant tumors rapidly invade the complex anatomy of the parotid region. Pain and trismus are common presenting complaints. Examination frequently reveals skin fixation or ulceration, invasion of the external auditory canal, and facial nerve palsy. Extensive radiological evaluation is essential to accurate tumor delineation.

Needle aspiration biopsy is used with reservation in tumors suspected of being malignant, and subsequent resection should incorporate the entire needle tract. Sialography has not proved of consistent value as a diagnostic adjunct.

Treatment

Parotid gland surgery should be undertaken only by a well-trained surgeon thoroughly versed in the pathology of salivary gland tumors, the complex anatomy of the parotid region, and basic reconstructive techniques. The advent of this understanding in recent years has resulted in a decreased incidence of recurrence and increased survival figures.

A brief anatomical review is pertinent at this point. The parotid gland extends from the zygomatic arch to 3 cm. inferior to the angle of the mandible, and from the mastoid to the anterior margin of the masseter muscle. It is covered externally by the dense parotid fascia; its medial surface is intimately related to the pterygoid fossa and the lateral aspect of the pharynx. The gland is divided into superficial and deep components by the facial nerve. The superficial lobe is larger than the deep lobe and is closely applied to the masseter muscle and ramus of the mandible. The facial nerve exits from the skull via the stylomastoid foramen, passes anteriorly lateral to the styloid process, and enters the parotid 1 cm. inferior to the bony margin of the external auditory canal. Upon entering the parotid, the nerve divides into temporofacial and cervicofacial branches.

In the usual case of a mass limited to the parotid gland, superficial parotidectomy should be the minimal biopsy procedure [6]. Immediate frozen-section diagnosis is obtained. Superficial parotidectomy is adequate treatment for benign mixed tumors in this part of the gland (Fig. 18-3). The parotidectomy is completed if a diagnosis of malignancy is returned. Deliberate violation of the tumor cannot be condemned too strongly.

Utilization of this precise anatomical approach has reduced the incidence of recurrence of benign mixed tumor from 25 to 30 percent to less than 10 percent. Successful management of benign mixed tumor rests almost entirely with the initial resection. The recurrence rate following secondary procedures approximates 30 percent [8]. A recurrent "benign" mixed tumor may be more difficult to eradicate than a

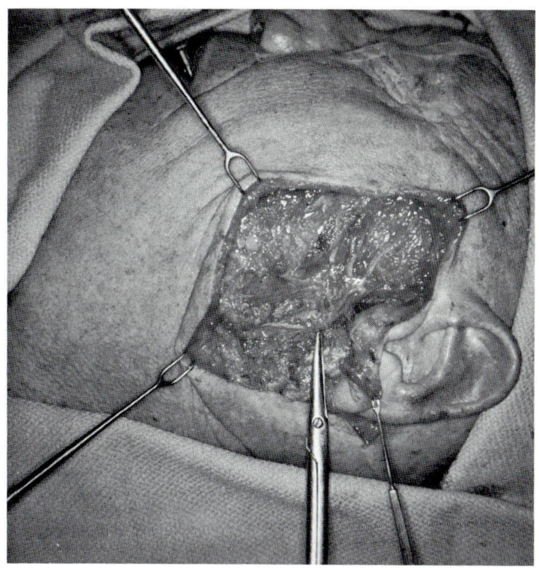

Fig. 18-3. Superficial parotidectomy with meticulous dissection and preservation of the facial nerve.

malignancy. Application of the principle of en bloc resection with adequate margins is mandatory in the management of parotid tumors, whether they are benign or malignant.

The complex anatomy of the parotid region allows involvement of multiple structures by contiguous spread of malignant tumors. Sacrifice of the overlying skin frequently is required and demands coverage by a pedicle flap. Resection of the mandible is indicated if invasion of the masseter is present. The mastoid, zygoma, and temporal bones may be involved by direct extension. Medial extension requires resection of the lateral aspect of the pharynx.

Sacrifice of the facial nerve is not determined by the histological composition of the parotid tumor, but rather by the nearness or involvement of the nerve by cancer [8]. Immediate reconstitution of resected branches is performed with a great auricular or cervical plexus nerve graft. A lateral tarsorrhaphy is performed routinely if the continuity of the facial nerve is interrupted. Dynamic muscle transfers are reserved for secondary, elective reconstruction. Temporalis transfer to the upper and lower eyelids and coronoid transfer to the oral commissure yield entirely satisfactory results. The preferred, single-stage reconstructive procedure consists of the contralateral front neurectomy and intraoral partial myomectomy together with ipsilateral creation of a nasolabial fold.

Radical neck dissection is not indicated routinely in the management of parotid malignancy. An in-continuity neck dissection is performed in the presence of clinically suspicious lymph nodes. In the case of squamous cell and undifferentiated carcinoma, the superior jugular nodes are included with the parotid specimen and a neck dissection is performed if metastases are demonstrated in the neck [11].

Approximately 10 percent of parotid malignancies are radiosensitive. Radiotherapy is indicated postoperatively in the management of anaplastic tumors in which the resection margins are questionable and in the management of inoperable recurrences [5].

Melanoma and adequate resection of squamous cell carcinoma of the scalp that has metastasized to the cervical lymph nodes requires in-continuity superficial parotidectomy if the lesions are so situated that the efferent lymphatics drain through the parotid region.

Prognosis

A 5-year follow-up period is not adequate for benign mixed tumors. Recurrence has been noted 10 to 20 years after initial therapy. The incidence of recurrence should be less than 5 percent in primary cases and approaches 30 percent following second procedures.

The overall 5-year survival rate for parotid malignancy approximates 65 percent [4]. Low-grade mucoepidermoid carcinoma has the most favorable prognosis, with a 5-year survival rate in exesss of 90 percent [9]. The tumors classified as high-grade malignancy yield 5-year survival figures of 33 percent (Table 18-1). The local recurrence rate for adenoid cystic carcinoma approximates 70 percent [7]. Squamous cell and undifferentiated carcinoma have the most unfavorable prognosis.

SUBMAXILLARY GLAND TUMORS

The submaxillary gland is involved more commonly by inflammatory conditions than by neoplasms. Tumors of the submaxillary gland have a greater incidence of malignancy than those of the parotid gland.

Incidence

Neoplasia is more frequent in females than in males. The average age at the time of diagnosis is 37 years for benign tumors and 45 years for malignant tumors.

Pathology

Fifteen percent of benign, and 10 to 15 percent of malignant, salivary gland tumors occur in the submaxillary gland. Sixty percent of submaxillary gland tumors are benign, and 95 percent of the benign tumors are benign mixed tumors. An occasional Warthin's tumor is encountered. Malignant tumors are of the same histological type as those found in the parotid gland but with somewhat different frequency. Cylindroma comprises 40 to 50 percent and

Table 18-1. Parotid Tumors; 5-Year End Results (1930–1959) [4]

Type of Tumor	No. Cases Observed	No. Cases Determinate	Percent[a] Survivals	Percent[a] Cures
Benign Tumors				
Benign mixed	908	741	99	97.5
Warthin's tumor	94	59	98	97
Oncocytoma	9	3	100	100
Benign lymphoepithelial lesion	9	7	100	100
Malignant Tumors				
Malignant mixed	111	98	55	45
Mucoepidermoid – low grade	126	104	96	96
Mucoepidermoid – high grade	66	63	14	11
Squamous cancer	38	33	36	33
Adenocarcinoma:				
Adenoid-cystic	34	30	40	30
Acinic cell	33	28	82	82
Adenocarcinoma not otherwise specified	91	80	48	43
Cystic papillary lesion	6	4	100	100
Malignant tumor unclassified	24	17	24	24

[a]Based on determinate cases.
From E. L. Frazell. Observations on management of salivary gland tumors. *Cancer* 18:235, 1968.

mucoepidermoid carcinoma 20 to 25 percent of malignant tumors of the submaxillary gland [12]. Distant metastases are encountered twice as frequently as with malignant tumors of parotid gland origin.

Diagnosis

As with parotid gland tumors, benign tumors present as asymptomatic enlargement of the submaxillary gland. The lesions are slow growing and may reach considerable proportions without producing significant symptoms.

Malignant disease is highly invasive locally, and metastasis occurs relatively early. Pain is a prominent symptom. Examination frequently reveals skin fixation, extension to the mandible and the floor of the mouth, and involvement of the hypoglossal and lingual nerves.

Soft tissue radiography and sialography may be helpful in demonstrating calculi. Sialography is of no value in tumor diagnosis and evaluation. Radiological evaluation of the mandible is essential to preoperative planning if malignancy is suspected.

Treatment

The submaxillary gland lends itself to straightforward anatomical dissection and total removal without functional or cosmetic deformity. Needle aspiration biopsy and incisional biopsy are to be avoided. If the clinical diagnosis is uncertain, resection of the submaxillary gland and frozen-section diagnosis provide the necessary information. A diagnosis of malignancy frequently is obvious clinically, and management consists of adequate resection of the local extent of the tumor in continuity with a radical neck dissection. Sacrifice of the overlying skin and soft tissue, the mandible, and the floor of the mouth frequently is required. Provision must be made for stabilization of the mandible and replacement of oral mucosal lining.

Reconstitution of the soft tissue defect is best accomplished by the use of a cervical pedicle flap. Loss of the marginal mandibular branch of the facial nerve is compensated for by anchoring the orbicularis muscle at the commissure with fascia lata to the inferior margin of the mandible. Mandibular stabilization is accomplished with a bone plate or Kirschner wires (see Chapter 17). Replacement of the oral mucosal lining is achieved primarily with either an ipsilateral forehead flap based on the temporal vessels and turned into the mouth of a large nasolabial flap turned into the floor of the mouth through the nasolabial crease.

Radiation therapy is palliative and is reserved for the management of inoperable recurrence.

Prognosis

The incidence of recurrence of benign tumors is less than 5 percent. Malignancy of the submaxillary gland has a less favorable prognosis than primary parotid tumors [4] (Table 18-2).

Table 18-2. Submaxillary Tumors; 5-Year End Results (1930–1959)

Type of Tumor	No. Cases Observed	No. Cases Determinate	Percent[a] Survivals	Percent[a] Cures
Benign Tumors				
Bengin mixed	90	64	100	100
Oncocytoma	3	1	100	100
Malignant Tumors				
Malignant mixed	15	15	33	20
Mucoepidermoid – low grade	12	10	100	100
Mucoepidermoid – high grade	8	8	25	25
Squamous cancer	13	12	25	25
Adenocarcinoma:				
Adenoid-cystic	36	34	38	24
Adenocarcinoma not otherwise specified	19	17	12	6
Malignant tumor unclassified	2	1	–	–

[a]Based on determinate cases.

SUBLINGUAL AND ACCESSORY SALIVARY GLAND TUMORS

Although neoplastic disease of the minor salivary glands is not strictly included among the primary tumors of the neck, a brief resumé of minor salivary gland pathology is warranted to complete and place in proper perspective the discussion of salivary gland tumors (Table 18-3).

Neoplastic disease of the minor salivary glands is more frequent in females than in males. Of all benign tumors of salivary gland origin, 5 to 10 percent occur in the minor salivary glands; of all malignant tumors of salivary gland origin, 10 to 15 percent occur in the minor salivary glands. Forty percent of tumors originating in the minor salivary glands are benign; essentially, all of the benign tumors are benign mixed tumors. An occasional Warthin's tumor is encountered.

The histology of minor salivary gland malignancies is the same as that of the parotid and submaxillary glands. Of the malignant tumors, approximately 40 percent are adenoid cystic carcinoma and 40 percent are mucoepidermoid carcinoma [13].

Malignant tumors exhibit extreme local invasiveness. Cervical lymph node metastasis occurs early in the course of the disease.

Benign neoplasms present as asymptomatic submucosal masses. The hard palate is the most common location, and the lesion is usually asymmetrical, in contradistinction to torus palatinus. The mucosa is intact and freely movable over the underlying tumor.

Widespread extension at the time of diagnosis is the rule with malignant tumors. Pain is a prominent feature. Mucosal ulceration is confined to the central portion of the tumor mass and is limited in extent as compared with that found with squamous cell carcinoma. Thorough radiological evaluation is essential to accurate delineation of malignant tumor extension and is helpful in differential diagnosis. Needle or incisional biopsy is not recommended, since tumor spillage should be avoided.

Resection of benign mixed tumors requires adequate mucosal and bony margins. For the usual tumor located on the hard palate, the underlying hard palate is resected with preservation of the nasal mucosa. Immediate reconstruction is accomplished either with local buccal or palatal flaps or with a skin graft. Resection of the maxilla to a greater or lesser degree frequently is indicated. Surgical management of the oroantral fistula is far superior to obturation with dental prostheses.

Adequate treatment of minor salivary gland cancer requires en bloc resection of the local extent of the tumor without regard for anatomical boundaries and in-continuity radical neck dissection. Considerable sacrifice of oral mucosal lining is the rule. Immediate reconstruction is accomplished with a variety of pedicle flaps.

Adequate resection of benign tumors is curative. The incidence of recurrence does not exceed 5 percent. The prognosis for malignant tumors of minor salivary gland origin is guarded. Five-year survival figures approximate 25 percent.

THYROID TUMORS

Perhaps no area of oncology is debated more exhaustively than the management of thyroid cancer. "Carcinoma of the thyroid" is not a single entity.

Table 18-3. Salivary Gland Tumors

Gland	Sex Predominance		Average Age (yr.)		Distribution (%)		Pathology		Histology		5-Year Survival with Malignant Tumor (%)
	Benign	Malignant	Benign	Malignant	Benign	Malignant	Benign	Malignant	Benign	Malignant	
Parotid	Female (2:1)	Equal	42	53	76	74	80	20	80[a]	68.1[b]	65
Submaxillary	Female	Female	37	45	15	13	60	40	95[a]	70.5[c]	50
Minor	Female	Female	—	—	9	13	40	60	95[a]	65.0[d]	25

[a] Benign mixed tumor.
[b] Undifferentiated, 27.7%, mucoepidermoid, 24.4%, cylindroma, 16.0%.
[c] Cylindroma, 47.0%, mucoepidermoid, 23.5%.
[d] Adenocarcinoma.

Confusion has resulted from inadequate definition of the problem, from the fact that similar results are obtainable by a variety of surgical approaches, and from impressions based on inadequate duration of follow-up studies. Proper evaluation of data demands critical appraisal of the age and sex of the patients, the histological classification of the tumors, and the duration of follow-up study.

Incidence

Thyroid cancer is not a common neoplasm. The sex-age-adjusted incidence for malignant tumors of the thyroid gland in the 1947 United States survey was 1.0 and 3.4 per 100,000 for males and females, respectively [1]. The incidence is highest in the ages between 40 and 70 years, with an average age of 42 years at the time of diagnosis of papillary carcinoma. In males past 55 years of age and in females past the age of 65 years, the rates are more than double the average rates and gradually increase, by three to five times the average rates, in patients past 80 years of age. Papillary carcinoma occurs relatively frequently in children under the age of 17 years, and a history of radiation therapy to the cervical region can be elicited in 70 percent of these cases. Tumors demonstrating a highly malignant potential occur infrequently before the age of 40 years.

Pathology

Malignant tumors of the thyroid gland are classified histologically into four groups: papillary, follicular, solid (including Hürthle cell), and anaplastic (including spindle and giant cell types). Any given tumor commonly exhibits a mixed histological pattern. Papillary carcinoma comprises 50 to 60 percent and follicular carcinoma 20 to 25 percent of thyroid cancer; less than 10 percent of tumors are anaplastic. The incidence of anaplastic carcinoma is directly proportional to age and occurs rarely in children.

Thyroid carcinoma metastasizes via the lymphatics to the pericapsular and jugular nodes and via the blood stream to lung and bones. All except the anaplastic tumors exhibit a clinical course compatible with low-grade malignancy. Papillary carcinoma is usually slow growing in the neck but may metastasize widely early in the course of the disease, particularly in children. The incidence of blood-borne metastases is slightly higher with follicular than with papillary carcinoma. Anaplastic carcinoma is highly invasive locally and metastasizes early.

Multicentric origin or intraglandular dissemination (or both) of thyroid cancer is undeniable. An incidence of multicentricity ranging from 20 to 58 percent, and averaging approximately 35 percent, is reported [14–16, 24, 25]. Meticulous total gland studies have revealed intraglandular dissemination or involvement of the contralateral pericapsular nodes in 88 percent of specimens. The same studies indicated 46.3 percent residual disease on the basis of total thyroidectomy performed after a preceding "definitive" excision [16].

The incidence of cervical node involvement is appreciable. Neck dissections performed in the absence of clinically suspicious nodes reveal microscopic metastases in 25 to 61 percent of patients [19, 24]. When neck dissection is performed routinely regardless of clinical findings, the incidence of metastasis is reported to be 80 percent [24]. Studies in children reveal that in 40 percent of patients positive nodes will develop bilaterally at some time during the course of the disease [21].

The precise clinical significance of intraglandular dissemination and involvement of the cervical lymph nodes is not readily apparent. The incidence of recurrence in a retained lobe is reported as 0 to 5 percent [18, 24]. The incidence of development of clinical metastasis in patients with clinically negative nodes in whom no neck dissection was performed is reported as 4 to 15 percent [18, 25]. The capricious nature of thyroid cancer has been well documented. Many patients with widespread metastasis have been followed for considerable periods. The observed discrepancy between pathological and clinical findings is possibly attributable to inadequate duration of follow-up study. The average interval from primary surgery to recurrence is 5 years.

Diagnosis

Thorough statistical analyses relating thyroid cancer to various types of goiter are readily available. Cancer is found in 15 to 20 percent of solitary nodules, in 5 percent of multinodular goiters, and uncommonly in diffuse goiter. Benign thyroid nodularity increases with age. Hyperthyroidism and cancer are not mutually exclusive.

The majority of patients present with an asymptomatic, asymmetrical mass in the thyroid gland detected either by themselves or by their physician. Enlarged cervical nodes are the first indication of disease in a significant percentage of patients with papillary carcinoma. The term *lateral aberrant thyroid* refers to metastatic papillary carcinoma. Fifty percent of thyroid nodules in children are malignant [21].

Pain, hoarseness, and dysphagia appear late in the course of the disease and indicate extraglandular extension. On examination, the thyroid gland is fixed to adjacent structures.

All patients being subjected to thryoid exploration for suspicion of malignancy should be evaluated by means of preoperative radioisotope studies. A 40 percent incidence of malignancy has been demonstrated in nonfunctioning nodules which fail to respond to thyroid-stimulating hormone [20]. Thyroid and total-body scanning serves not only as an aid to diagnosis but also as a guide to future therapy.

Treatment

The capricious nature of thyroid cancer and the similar results obtainable with a variety of surgical approaches have been emphasized. Advocates can be found for surgical management ranging from lobectomy and "node-picking" to radical en bloc resection of the thyroid gland, adjacent structures, and bilateral pathways of lymphatic drainage. The occurrence of papillary carcinoma in children and young women introduces an emotional factor which influences judgment.

Operative management consists of *total lobectomy as the minimal biopsy procedure,* with immediate frozen-section diagnosis. Malignant thyroid neoplasms are never truly encapsulated, and the danger of spillage attendant upon incisional biopsy or "shelling out" procedures is excessive. Reliable histological diagnoses are made readily on the basis of a frozen section by a trained pathologist.

Surgical management of carcinoma of the thyroid consists of ipsilateral total lobectomy and isthmusectomy and contralateral subtotal lobectomy; in-continuity resection of the lymphatic drainage pathways is performed only in the presence of clinically positive nodes [17, 23].

Long-term survival with residual papillary carcinoma is well documented. A surgical procedure in which tumor is knowingly excluded from the resection violates the basic tenets of cancer management. If esthetic considerations are a major factor, a thorough radical neck dissection may be performed, with preservation of the sternocleidomastoid muscle. A modified node dissection without sacrifice of major structures imposes neither significant morbidity nor deformity.

An attitude of extreme pessimism exists relative to anaplastic thyroid carcinoma [19, 26]. Surgical extirpation followed by radiation therapy is the most effective form of management presently available and should be applied to its technical limits. This implies *radical en bloc resection of the entire local extent of the tumor with formal bilateral radical neck dissection; sacrifice of the larynx and cervical esophagus is performed, if indicated.*

The *complications* of total thyroidectomy include hypothyroidism, hypoparathyroidism, and damage to the recurrent laryngeal nerves. Hypothyroidism presents no problems. The recurrent laryngeal nerves are sacrificed only if indicated by tumor extension. Hypoparathyroidism occurs in 30 percent of cases, but proves to be permanent in only a third of those exhibiting tetany [16, 24].

The more well-differentiated thyroid malignancies are to some extent hormone dependent. Postoperatively, all patients are placed permanently on suppression therapy with either desiccated thyroid or one of the synthetic l-triiodothyronine substitutes.

Metastatic disease is best managed with radioactive iodine if it can be demonstrated that the metastases are functional. Total-body scanning before and after stimulation with thyroid-stimulating hormone will elucidate this point. Preoperative thyroid scanning and submission of the specimen for autoradiography provides valuable information. Follicular carcinoma is more susceptible to iodine ablation than papillary carcinoma. Total removal of functioning thyroid tissue in the cervical region must precede treatment of metastasis with radioactive iodine. Many patients have apparently been cured of metastatic disease by radioactive iodine therapy.

Radiation therapy is palliative and is indicated in the management of inoperable recurrence.

Prognosis

The importance of inadequate duration of follow-up study cannot be emphasized too strongly: meaningful data must be based on observation periods of over 10, 15, or 20 years. Surgical management of thyroid tumors classified as low-grade malignancy will yield 5-year and 10-year survival figures of 90 percent and 75 percent, respectively. The majority of patients with anaplastic thyroid cancer will be dead within 18 months of diagnosis.

LARYNGEAL CARCINOMA

The management of laryngeal carcinoma is undergoing continuous evolution. Precise classification of these tumors on the basis of site of origin and degree of extension is essential to obtaining meaningful data [30].

Incidence

In the 1947 cancer survey in the United States, the age-adjusted incidence of cancer of the larynx was found to be 7.6 and 0.6, respectively, for male and female whites and 5.7 and 0.6, respectively, for male and female nonwhites per 100,000 population. For men 35 to 39 years of age, the incidence is only 0.7, but it rises rapidly thereafter to over 50.0 per 100,000 in those over 79 years of age. In recent years, there has been a reduction in the male-female ratio.

Pathology

Essentially all malignant tumors of the larynx are squamous cell carcinoma. The tumors are classified on the basis of anatomical location as being either intrinsic or extrinsic. *Intrinsic carcinoma* is defined as malignant disease confined to the true vocal cords or ventricular bands, with no extension superior or inferior to these limits. Tumors involving the aryepiglottic folds, epiglottis, base of the tongue, and pyriform sinuses are defined as *extrinsic*.

Metastatic involvement of the cervical lymph nodes (Table 18-4) occurs frequently and early in the course of the disease with both intrinsic and extrinsic lesions [27]. Microscopic metastases in clinically negative nodes are demonstrated in 25 percent of patients undergoing routine radical neck dissection in the management of laryngeal cancer. The incidence of nodal involvement increases in direct proportion to the degree of extension of the tumor. Intrinsic lesions with cord fixation exhibit twice the incidence of metastasis as intrinsic lesions without fixation. Involvement of contralateral cervical nodes occurs in 15 to 20 percent of all patients with extrinsic tumors. Distant metastasis occurs infrequently and late in the course of the disease.

Table 18-4. Incidence of Early Cervical Metastasis in Intrinsic and Extrinsic Laryngeal Carcinoma

Involvement of Cervical Node	Intrinsic	Extrinsic
At time of diagnosis	7.3%	37%
At some time during the course of the disease	19.1%	57%

Diagnosis

Hoarseness is the outstanding symptom of patients with intrinsic carcinoma of the larynx. Pain is an unusual complaint, although "sore throat" is relatively common. Dysphagia is a late manifestation and indicates tumor extension. Hemoptysis occurs rarely. It cannot be emphasized too strongly that a complaint of hoarseness demands thorough investigation.

Patients with extrinsic laryngeal carcinoma present with symptoms referable to the location and extent of the disease. Pain is the most common complaint. Hoarseness, sore throat, dysphagia, and hemoptysis are seen frequently. A significant percentage of patients note an asymmetrical mass in the neck as the first sign of disease.

Adequate evaluation of laryngeal pathology demands direct laryngoscopy, with precise tumor delineation by multiple biopsies. Early lesions may escape detection at initial examination; patients with significant symptoms but with negative findings must be scheduled for reexamination, under general anesthesia if necessary, within a reasonably brief time. Biopsies obtained following a course of radiation therapy are notoriously misleading.

Treatment

Intrinsic Lesions

Early intrinsic carcinoma of the larynx may be cured by a variety of therapeutic modalities [31]. The 5-year survival rate for lesions that are limited to the true cord without cord fixation and that are treated either by radiation or by surgical excision is approximately 92 percent. The usual patient undergoing laryngofissure is discharged from the hospital 1 week postoperatively and is allowed to return to work after an additional week of convalescence. The resection includes the involved cord, the anterior commissure, and the anterior one-fourth of the normal cord. Hoarseness is a constant sequela of operation and is exceedingly variable in degree; the voice is uniformly serviceable.

Radiation therapy entails a 4- to 6-week period of disability, and mucositis of a significant degree is a common problem. Increasing data tend to indicate that radiation therapy is the treatment of choice for intrinsic lesions and for superficial or exophytic lesions of the epiglottis [29]. A substantial percentage of radiation failures can be cured by subsequent resection.

More extensive intrinsic lesions are not candidates for radiation therapy as the definitive treatment of choice [29]. Planned preoperative radiation therapy followed by resection offers considerable promise but has received insufficient evaluation to justify advocation as a routine approach.

Conservation surgery, in terms of frontolateral partial laryngectomy and horizontal partial laryngectomy, has received intensive investigation in recent years [30]. Strict criteria have been established for the performance of these modified procedures and must be observed rigorously. Misguided efforts to preserve the voice by compromising the resection court inevitable recurrence. An in-continuity formal radical neck dissection is performed on the side of the lesion; the contralateral node-bearing tissues, limited by the carotid sheath laterally, the anterior belly of the digastric superiorly, and the sternoclavicular joint inferiorly, are included with the specimen.

Extrinsic Lesions

Management of extrinsic carcinoma of the larynx demands precise preoperative evaluation and planning [28]. Treatment consists of en bloc resection of the larynx (or a conservation procedure, if indicated) and bilateral radical neck dissection. A formal radical neck dissection is performed on the side of predominant disease; on the contralateral side, the dissection is of similar extent, but the jugular vein and spinal accessory nerve are preserved.

Sacrifice of the base of the tongue or the pyriform sinus and lateral aspect of the pharynx is frequently required to obtain an adequate tumor margin when dealing with extrinsic carcinoma. Preoperative preparation must include careful planning with regard to reconstitution of the mucosal defect. The usual surgical approach utilizes a large cervical apron flap extending from mastoid to mastoid and crossing the midline at the level of the proposed tracheotomy. Reconstruction of the hypopharynx and cervical esophagus is best accomplished with the deltopectoral flap [32]. The time-honored Wookey procedure may be utilized if chest flap tissue is unavailable. Immediate reconstruction of lateral pharyngeal defects is accomplished with an ipsilateral forehead flap. Primary closure of the hypopharynx is preferable to any method of reconstruction. This is performed whenever sufficient mucosa remains to allow closure about a #16 Fr. catheter.

The most common complication of laryngectomy, which occurs in approximately 10 to 15 percent of patients, is a pharyngocutaneous fistula. The incidence of this complication is increased markedly if previous radiation therapy has been given. Small fistulas will close spontaneously; larger fistulas require operative management with the introduction of healthy tissue.

Radiation therapy has little to offer as the primary treatment of extrinsic carcinoma of the larynx. The 3-year and 5-year survival figures are considerably inferior to those obtainable with surgical management. Severe mucositis, permanent dryness of the mucous membranes, chronic hypopharyngeal fibrosis, a 10 percent incidence of cartilaginous necrosis, fistula formation, and an excessive local recurrence rate constitute strong arguments against this modality of treatment. Radiation therapy serves to obscure tumor margins, impose additional tissue damage, increase rather than decrease the magnitude of the resection, increase the incidence of postoperative wound problems, and complicate reconstruction by negating the use of local tissue.

The value of planned preoperative radiation has not been clearly established. Available evidence tends to indicate that improved results may be obtained with this regimen. In general, radiation therapy is reserved for the palliative management of unresectable recurrence.

Cancer of the larynx is a local disease. Failure to control the disease in the neck is responsible for mortality.

Prognosis

Carcinoma in situ and tumor localized to the true cords yield 5-year survival figures in excess of 90 percent with adequate management. *Intrinsic carcinoma* of the larynx carries a relatively good prognosis, with overall 5-year survival figures of approximately 75 to 80 percent. The overall 3-year survival rate of 35 percent for *extrinsic carcinoma* of the larynx indicates the inadequacy of present management. The 3-year survival approximates 10 to 15 percent in those patients who present with clinically involved nodes.

HYPOPHARYNX AND CERVICAL ESOPHAGUS TUMORS

Cancer of the hypopharynx and cervical esophagus is a lethal disease demanding the utmost in diagnostic, resective, and reconstructive skills if a successful outcome is to be anticipated. Inadequate treatment courts disaster in the form of inevitable, uncontrollable recurrence or impairment of function to the extent of precluding useful existence.

Incidence

Malignant disease of the hypopharynx and cervical esophagus occurs predominantly in males. An outstanding exception is postcricoid carcinoma, the majority of which occurs in females. The peak age incidence is 40 to 60 years. A history of significant alcoholism is obtained almost uniformly.

Pathology

Essentially all malignant tumors originating in this anatomical area are squamous cell carcinoma.

A majority of the female patients with postcricoid cancer will exhibit Plummer-Vinson's syndrome – that is, anemia, achlorhydria, and mucosal atrophy. The precise relationship between this degenerative disorder and cancer is not clearly defined.

Cancer of the hypopharynx and cervical esophagus rapidly involves the structures of the neck by contiguous spread. Accurate assessment of the degree of lateral spread is virtually impossible following intensive radiation therapy.

Metastatic involvement of the cervical lymph nodes is present in the majority of patients seeking consultation. Microscopically demonstrable metastases are present in two-thirds of patients undergoing a staged contralateral neck dissection.

Diagnosis

Pain and dysphagia are the outstanding symptoms referable to hypopharyngeal lesions. Cough, hoarseness, "sore throat," and hemoptysis are common. A significant number of patients note cervical lymphadenopathy as the first sign of disease.

Adequate preoperative evaluation of the local extent of the tumor is of paramount importance and is usually accomplished satisfactorily only under general anesthesia. Meticulous direct laryngoscopy and esophagoscopy, with biopsy of all suspicious areas, is mandatory. Delineation of the distalmost extent of the tumor requires careful examination and is essential to preoperative planning.

Treatment

Many patients with hypopharyngeal lesions present for evaluation following previous inadequate treatment, usually in the form of radiation therapy. The problems associated with all aspects of management are magnified tremendously in such patients. Tumor invasion is exceedingly difficult to outline, thereby necessitating extensive sacrifice of soft tissue. Impoverishment of local blood supply greatly complicates reconstruction.

Adequate treatment of cancer of the hypopharynx and cervical esophagus requires *en bloc resection of the local extent of the tumor and bilateral radical neck dissection* [35]. The neck dissection contralateral to the side of predominant disease is modified to preserve the internal jugular vein. The functional disability imposed by such a resection is tremendous, and thorough application of the principle of in-continuity resection has awaited the development of satisfactory methods of reconstruction.

Total glossectomy is usually necessitated by sacrifice of the blood supply to both sides of the tongue.

It is the unusual case in which the larynx can be preserved. Inclusion of the larynx in the resected specimen may be required on the basis of tumor involvement or on the basis of functional considerations. Repeated, uncontrollable aspiration pneumonia results from interruption of the sensory or motor innervation of the larynx or from sacrifice of its muscular and ligamentous support. Injudicious preservation of the larynx invites recurrence and may subject the patient to intolerable functional impairment. Secondary laryngectomy to prevent pulmonary complications is common.

Lateral extension of the primary tumor poses the threat of carotid artery involvement. This is particularly true when dealing with recurrence in heavily irradiated patients. There is no reliable clinical guide as to which patients will tolerate loss of the carotid artery. Demonstration of adequate cross-filling via a patent anterior communicating artery is the most valuable index. Rarely will the characteristics of the wound allow carotid artery grafting.

Restoration of satisfactory function is of prime importance in the management of this disease. Reconstruction at the time of resection is achieved whenever possible. If immediate reconstruction is not feasible, preparations for reconstruction are begun as soon as the patient's general condition and the wound permit. Flap preparation prior to resection is advantageous in those patients who have received intensive radiation therapy, since wound complications can be expected. Three basic methods of reconstruction are available: primary closure of the hypopharynx, local and distant pedicle flaps, and transplanted bowel.

Resection of the entire circumference of the hypopharynx and cervical esophagus is usually required. Primary closure can be accomplished if 2 cm. of mucosa remain – that is, sufficient mucosa to allow tension-free closure around a #16 Fr. catheter. Function is entirely satisfactory.

Immediate reconstruction with the deltopectoral flap at the time of resection is the method of choice [32, 34, 36]. The major disadvantages of the Wookey method of repair are the meticulous nursing care required, multiple stages, and prolonged periods of hospitalization [37].

Reconstruction of the cervical esophagus with intestine, either as a free graft or as a transposition pedicled on the mesenteric vessels, has been attempted with variable success [33]. The magnitude of the procedure is prohibitive, and the incidence of complications in the form of necrosis and fistula formation is excessive.

Complete rehabilitation of these patients requires instruction in esophageal speech. Perfectly acceptable esophageal speech is attainable following the methods of reconstruction described above.

Prognosis

The management of cancer of the hypopharynx and cervical esophagus with radiation therapy yields 5-year survival figures not exceeding 10 percent. Adequate surgical treatment of this type of cancer consistently yields 5-year survival figures of 30 to 40 percent.

MISCELLANEOUS TUMORS OF THE NECK

Obscure Primary Tumor

The most common cause of an asymmetrical mass in the neck of an adult is cancer. A number of patients seek medical evaluation regarding the appearance of a cervical mass without associated symptoms. If thorough examination of the head and neck is negative, repeat examination under general anesthesia, particularly of the nasopharynx, together with a biopsy of the cervical mass is indicated. The biopsy incision is planned as a portion of a radical neck dissection. Occasionally, the histology of the metastasis will suggest the site of the primary lesion. More commonly, the pathology report is metastatic squamous cell carcinoma. Meticulous search for the primary malignancy must include chest x-ray, paranasal sinus films, bronchoscopy, and esophagoscopy. Should thorough evaluation fail to disclose the site of origin, a radical neck dissection is indicated, with the anticipation of 5-year survival in the range of 20 to 25 percent [38].

Primary Branchiogenic Carcinoma

Squamous cell carcinoma arising in a congenital branchial cleft cyst occurs rarely, if ever [39]. The patients present with an asymmetrical cervical mass, thorough evaluation is negative, and biopsy reveals squamous cell carcinoma. Radical neck dissection is curative. This lesion possibly explains some of the patients who do not exhibit further evidence of disease following a radical neck dissection in the absence of a demonstrable primary tumor.

Carotid Body Tumor

The carotid body is situated within the carotid artery bifurcation and represents the largest collection of chemoreceptor cells in the body. Tumors of the carotid body are infrequent; evidence suggests a significant familial tendency.

Considerable controversy surrounds the pathology and treatment of carotid body tumors. The consensus is that these neoplasms are benign; nevertheless, extensive invasion of adjacent structures and distant metastasis have been reported. Long-term survival in the presence of metastatic disease is well known. It is most probable that true malignant invasion occurs infrequently, and metastasis is rare.

The usual patient gives a history of a slowly enlarging cervical mass over a long period. The mass may produce minimal discomfort, but significant symptoms are absent. On examination, the tumor is located immediately inferior to the angle of the mandible, it is firm and rubbery in consistency, and it is freely movable in an anteroposterior direction but fixed in the vertical direction. The tumor may reach considerable proportions before the patient seeks medical attention.

The morbidity associated with surgical management of carotid body tumors need not be excessive [40, 43]. In the usual case, the tumor can be dissected from the carotid artery without injury to, or occlusion of, the vessel. The dissection must be meticulous and must be undertaken only by a well-trained surgeon. Local recurrence is inevitable following inadequate resection.

Sarcoma

Sarcoma of the head and neck, excluding lymphosarcoma, is seen infrequently. The tumors may arise from any of the mesenchymal tissues of the head and neck; they commonly arise in sites not usually the origin of primary tumors, and they are usually somewhat bulky and slow growing. Radiation-induced osteogenic sarcoma following treatment of head and neck lesions has become a recognized entity.

Fibrosarcoma is the most common histological type. Rhabdomyosarcoma, osteogenic sarcoma, chondrosarcoma, liposarcoma, lethal midline granuloma, and sarcomas of neurogenic origin are seen infrequently [41, 42].

Treatment is surgical and consists of adequate local resection of the tumor. Radical neck dissection is performed only in the presence of clinically suspicious lymph nodes [44].

Fibrosarcoma and liposarcoma offer the best prognosis. Cure is unlikely when dealing with other histological types. Administration of a necrotizing dosage of radiation therapy to osteogenic sarcoma before resection enhances survival.

REFERENCES

Parotid Gland

1. Ackerman, L. V., and Del Regato, J. A. *Cancer: Diagnosis, Treatment, and Prognosis* (4th ed.). St. Louis: Mosby, 1970.
2. Beahrs, O. H., Woolner, L. B., Carveth, S. W., and Devine, K. D. Surgical management of parotid lesions. *A.M.A. Arch. Surg.* 80:890, 1960.
3. Foote, F. W., and Frazell, E. L. Tumors of the Major Salivary Glands. *Atlas of Tumor Pathology,* Sect. IV, fasc. 11. Washington, D.C.: Armed Forces Institute of Pathology, 1954.
4. Frazell, E. L. Observations on management of salivary gland tumors. *Cancer* 18:235, 1968.
5. Guillamondegui, D. M., Byers, R. M., Luna, M. A., Chiminazzo, H., Jesse, R. H., and Fletcher, G. H. Aggressive surgery in treatment for parotid cancer: Role of adjunctive postoperative radiotherapy. *Am. J. Roentgenol. Radium Ther. Nucl. Med.* 123:49, 1975.
6. Richardson, G. S., Dickason, W. L., Gaisford, J. C., and Hanna, D. C. Tumors of the salivary glands: An analysis of 752 cases. *Plast. Reconstr. Surg.* 55:131, 1975.
7. Spiro, R. H., Huvos, A. G., and Strong, E. W. Adenoid cystic carcinoma of salivary origin: A clinicopathologic study of 242 cases. *Am. J. Surg.* 128:512, 1974.
8. Spiro, R. H., Huvos, A. G., and Strong, E. W. Cancer of the parotid gland: A clinicopathologic study of 288 primary cases. *Am. J. Surg.* 130:452, 1975.
9. Thorvaldsson, S. E., Beahrs, O. H., Woolner, L. B., and Simons, J. N. Mucoepidermoid tumors of the major salivary glands. *Am. J. Surg.* 120:432, 1970.
10. Turnbull, A. D., and Frazell, E. L. Multiple tumors of the major salivary glands. *Am. J. Surg.* 118:787, 1969.
11. Woods, J. E., Chong, G. C., and Beahrs, O. H. Experience with 1,360 primary parotid tumors. *Am. J. Surg.* 130:460, 1975.

Submaxillary Gland

12. Simons, J. N., Beahrs, O. H., and Woolner, L. B. Tumors of the submaxillary gland. *Am. J. Surg.* 108:485, 1964.

Sublingual and Accessory Salivary Gland Tumors

13. Rankow, R. M., and Mignogna, F. Cancer of the sublingual salivary gland. *Am. J. Surg.* 118:790, 1969.

Thyroid Gland

14. Black, B. M., Kirk, T. A., Jr., and Woolner, L. B. Multicentricity of papillary adenocarcinoma of the thyroid: Influence on treatment. *J. Clin. Endocrinol.* 20:130, 1960.
15. Buckwalter, J. A., Soper, R. T., Madaras, J. S., Jr., and Mason, E. E. The effectivensss of treatment of well differentiated thyroid carcinoma. *Surg. Gynecol. Obstet.* 113:427, 1961.
16. Clark, R. L., White, E. C., and Russell, W. O. Total thyroidectomy for cancer of the thyroid: Significance of intraglandular dissemination. *Ann. Surg.* 149:858, 1959.
17. Crile, G., Jr., and Hawk, W. A. Carcinomas of the thyroid. In Anderson, R., and Hoopes, J. E. (Eds.), *Symposium on Malignancies of the Head and Neck.* St. Louis: Mosby, 1975.
18. Crile, G., Jr., McNamara, J. M., and Hazard, J. B. Results of treatment of papillary carcinoma of the thyroid. *Surg. Gynecol. Obstet.* 109:315, 1959.
19. Frazell, E., and Foote, F. Papillary thyroid carcinoma: Pathological findings in cases with and without clinical evidence of cervical node involvement. *Cancer* 8:1164, 1955.
20. Gibbs, J. C., Jr., Halligan, E. J., Grieco, R. V., and McKeown, J. E. Scintiscanning the thyroid nodule. *A.M.A. Arch. Surg.* 90:323, 1965.
21. Hayles, A. B., Johnson, L. M., Beahrs, O. H., and Woolner, L. B. Carcinoma of the thyroid in children. *Am. J. Surg.* 106:735, 1963.
22. Marchetta, F. C., Sako, K., and Matsuura, H. Modified neck dissection for carcinoma of the thyroid gland. *Am. J. Surg.* 120:452, 1970.
23. Strong, E. W. The Treatment of Thyroid Cancer – A Summary. In Chambers, R. G., de Limpens, A. M. P. J., Jaques, D. A., and Routledge, R. T. (Eds.), *Cancer of the Head and Neck.* Amsterdam: Excerpta Medica, 1975.
24. Tollefsen, H. R., and DeCosse, J. J. Papillary carcinoma of the thyroid. Recurrence in the thyroid gland after initial surgical treatment. *Am. J. Surg.* 106:728, 1963.
25. Tollefsen, H. R., and DeCosse, J. J. Papillary carcinoma of the thyroid. *Am. J. Surg.* 108:547, 1964.
26. Wychulis, A. R., Beahrs, O. H., and Woolner, L. B. Papillary carcinoma with associated anaplastic

carcinoma in the thyroid gland. *Surg. Gynecol. Obstet.* 120:28, 1965.

Larynx

27. Baker, R. R., and Cherry, J. Carcinoma of the larynx. *A.M.A. Arch. Surg.* 90:449, 1965.
28. Loré, J. M. Radical Surgery of the Larynx and Laryngopharynx. In Chambers, R. G., de Limpens, A. M. P. J., Jaques, D. A., and Routledge, R. T. (Eds.), *Cancer of the Head and Neck.* Amsterdam: Excerpta Medica, 1975.
29. Marchetta, F. C., Sako, K., and Mattick, W. L. Squamous cell carcinoma of larynx. *Am. J. Surg.* 116:491, 1968.
30. Ogura, J. H., and Sessions, D. G. Cancer of the Larynx and Hypopharynx. In Anderson, R., and Hoopes, J. E. (Eds.), *Symposium on Malignancies of the Head and Neck.* St. Louis: Mosby, 1975.
31. Petti, G. Management of anterior commissure carcinoma of the larynx. *Bull. N.Y. Acad. Med.* 49:915, 1973.

Cervical Esophagus

32. Bakamijian, V. Y. Total reconstruction of pharynx with medially based deltopectoral skin flap. *N.Y. J. Med.* 68:2771, 1968.
33. Ballantyne, A. J. Methods of repair after surgery for cancer of the pharyngeal wall, postcricoid area, and cervical esophagus. *Am. J. Surg.* 122: 482, 1971.
34. Fujino, T., and Saito, S. Repair of pharyngoesophageal fistula by microvascular transfer of free skin flap. *Plast. Reconstr. Surg.* 56:549, 1975.
35. Loré, J. M. Carcinoma of the Hypopharynx and Cervical Esophagus. In Anderson, R., and Hoopes, J. E. (Eds.), *Symposium on Malignancies of the Head and Neck.* St. Louis: Mosby, 1975.
36. Petty, C. T., Theogaraj, S. D., and Cohen, I. K. Secondary reconstruction of the cervical esophagus. *Plast. Reconstr. Surg.* 56:70, 1975.

Primary Branchiogenic Carcinoma

37. Wookey, H. The surgical treatment of carcinoma of the pharynx and upper esophagus. *Surg. Gynecol. Obstet.* 75:499, 1942.

Obscure Primary Tumor

38. Barrie, J. F., Knapper, W. H., and Strong, E. W. Cervical nodal metastasis of unknown origin. *Am. J. Surg.* 120:466, 1970.
39. Batsakis, J. G. *Tumors of the Head and Neck.* Baltimore: Williams & Wilkins, 1974.

Carotid Body Tumors

40. Anderson, R., and Bevin, E. G. Carotid Body Tumors. In Anderson, R., and Hoopes, J. E. (Eds.), *Symposium on Malignancies of the Head and Neck.* St. Louis: Mosby, 1975.
41. Batsakis, J. G. Soft Tissue Tumors of the Head and Neck: Unusual Forms. In *Tumors of the Head and Neck.* Baltimore: Williams & Wilkins, 1974.
42. Batsakis, J. G. Fibrous Lesions of the Head and Neck: Benign, Malignant, and Indeterminate. In *Tumors of the Head and Neck.* Baltimore: Williams & Wilkins, 1974.
43. Chambers, R. G., and Mahoney, W. D. Carotid body tumors. *Am. J. Surg.* 116:554, 1968.

Sarcoma

44. Gaisford, J. C., and Hanna, D. C. Sarcomas of the head and neck. *Plast. Reconstr. Surg.* 29:250, 1962.

Surgery of the Eyelids*

SALVADOR CASTAÑARES

In my experience the correction of protrusion (herniation) of intraorbital fat, producing the "baggy eyelid" deformity, is one of the most gratifying aesthetic plastic surgical operations. Apart from the purely cosmetic factors involved, there are some important physiological ones related to this deformity [2].

The intraorbital fat, protruding through the weakened tarsoorbital fascia and orbicularis muscle, produces the characteristic baggy bulging of the lower eyelids, and very frequently of the upper lids as well. For the sake of brevity, it will suffice here to say that there are two definite and distinct compartments of fat in the upper eyelid and three in the lower. Frequently, protrusion or herniation of intraorbital fat coexists with blepharochalasis, a condition characterized by atony and redundancy of the skin of the eyelids [6].

The conditions of blepharochalasis and dermochalasis (or ptosis adiposa of Sichel) involve only the skin of the lids, primarily the upper lids. Because the treatment of both conditions is simple – consisting of a proper resection of the excessive redundant skin and a plastic surgical closure – no further mention will be made of them here [6]. This presentation deals exclusively with protrusion (herniation) of intraorbital fat, which is by far the major cause of the baggy eyelid deformity. This deformity appears in both sexes, and is not related to a general obese constitution of the patient. The etiology is not known, but there is a definite hereditary predisposing factor in its development.

The term *herniation* (of intraorbital fat) is often used because it is convenient for descriptive purposes, although in the true sense of the word there is no hernia comparable, for example, to an inguinal or ventral hernia, in which there is a definite break or rent of the fascia and musculature.

SURGICAL TECHNIQUE

Anesthesia

The operation may be done under local or general anesthesia. I prefer local infiltration anesthesia with lidocaine 1% and epinephrine 1:100,000, almost without exception.

Incisions and Excisions of Skin

The lines of incision (Figs. 19-1 through 19-4) for both lids may be marked with brilliant green before the surgical preparation and before the anesthetic agent is injected. (The brilliant green will remain even after the routine preparation is performed.) The lines follow the classic pattern with slight modification. The preliminary markings all are made with the patient in the sitting position, and are completed while the patient is in the recumbent position.

The upper lid skin resection is made in S fashion, curving and placing the incision line in the recess of the orbitopalpebral fold, except laterally, where it slants outward and upward. The amount of skin resected depends on the severity of the deformity and the age of the patient. The upper part of Figure 19-1 shows the shape of the elliptical skin resection in a relatively young patient (see Fig. 19-6). Normally more redundant skin is found at the lateral region; the resection in that area must be made according to the calculations (and marking) made while the patient was in the sitting position. The lower incision of the elliptical wedge must be 8 to 9 mm. from the palpebral margin at the center, so that the final incision line rests at the orbitopalpebral sulcus.

It is surprising how much skin may be resected safely from the upper lid, but this is not the case with the lower lid. In the lower lid (Fig. 19-1, bottom), a wedge of no more than 4 to 5 mm. of skin should be resected in the younger patient. The maximum wedge resection at the center in an older patient, in whom there is excessive skin, should be 8 to 9 mm. (or more in very rare cases). The correction of the excessive and wrinkled lower lid skin is actually performed through a lid rhytidectomy – that is, by gently stretching it and pulling it laterally and upward (Fig. 19-4B), rather than by excising skin. The resulting lateral triangle of excessive skin is trimmed off in the usual manner (Fig. 19-4C). This maneuver ensures against ectropion or buckling of the lower lid.

Approach to the Protruding Intraorbital Fat

I prefer to start with the upper eyelid, leaving the incisions open after the fat removal, and keeping a moist saline sponge over it while operating on the lower lid. After finishing the fat removal of the lower lid, a moist saline sponge is placed over the open lower eyelid while the upper is sutured.

This order of procedure allows observation of possible late bleeding, which thus may be easily con-

*This presentation complements a previous one (Blepharoplasty for Herniated Intraorbital Fat: Anatomical Basis for a New Approach, published in *Plastic and Reconstructive Surgery* [1]) and others that followed [3–5].

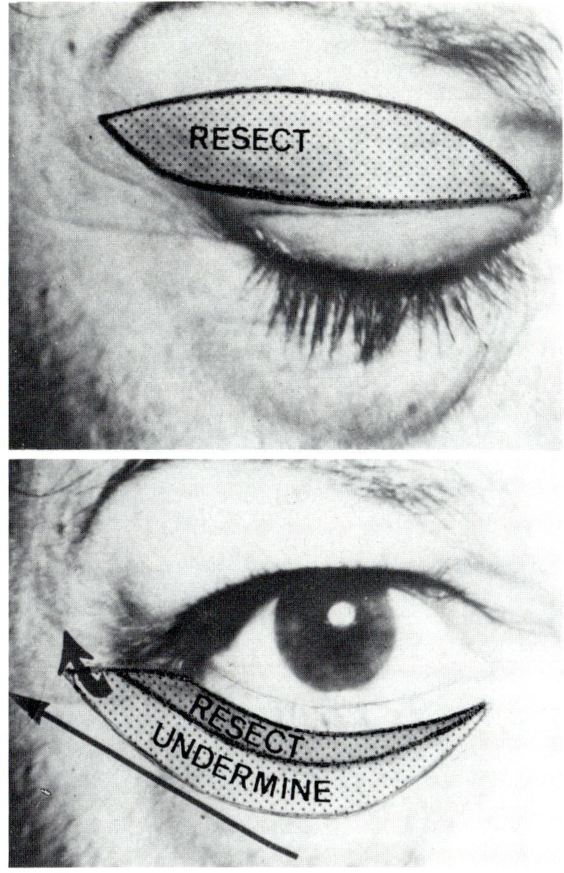

Fig. 19-1. Design for resection of the skin of the upper and lower lids. Only the lower lid is undermined in the area indicated. The undermining extends to midway between the palpebral border and the infraorbital bone rim. The skin attached to the lower part of the weak orbicularis will permit the desired lateral and upward tensioning of skin and muscle, as indicated by the arrows.

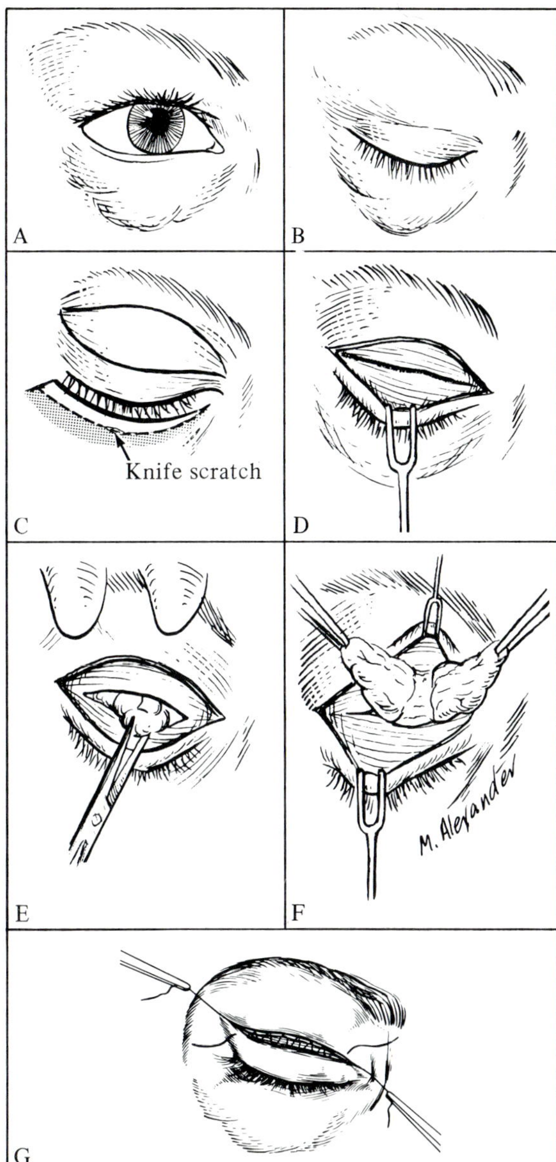

Fig. 19-2. A, B, a typical case of herniation of intraorbital fat in a relatively young patient (for example, the patient shown in Fig. 19-6). C, markings are made with brilliant green. Note the large amount of upper lid skin resection and the narrow wedge of lower lid removal, 4 or 5 mm. wide at the center. Stippling of the lower lid indicates the extent of undermining. Note the knife scratch made underneath after infiltration of the anesthetic at the center of the inferior border of the wedge of skin to be resected later. D, the line of incision of the orbicularis oculi muscle at the vault of the bulge. E, cutting the orbicularis oculi muscle; the fat protrudes readily. F, the two definite compartments of fat of the upper lid are shown; these are transected at their base with fine straight hemostats and resected. G, closure of the upper lid with a 5-0 Dermalon subcuticular suture. (From S. Castañares. Correction of the Baggy Eyelid Deformity Produced by Herniation of Orbital Fat. In Smith, B., and Converse, J. M. (Cochairmen), Proceedings of the Second International Symposium on Plastic and Reconstructive Surgery of the Eye and Adnexa. *St. Louis: Mosby, 1967.)*

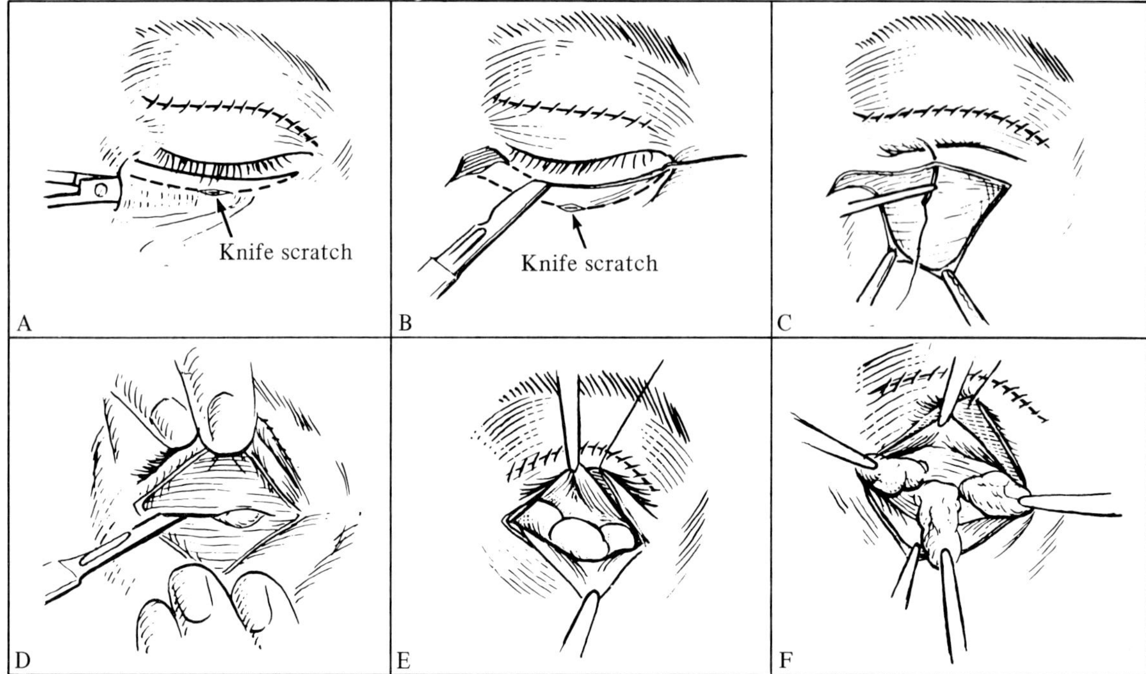

Fig. 19-3. A, undermining of the lower lid through the lateral incision with fine blunt scissors (the lateral incision prolongation is usually horizontal, not vertical as it appears in the drawing). B, using the knife to cut cleanly at the mark 2 mm. below the lid margin. The wedge of skin will be resected at the end of the lower lid operation before suturing at the level of the knife scratch. C, the tension suture to be held with a hemostat over the head of the patient protects the eye and gives good exposure. D, cutting the orbicularis oculi muscle, as in the upper lid. E, the three compartments of fat of the lower lid often appear well defined. F, each compartment is isolated and its capsule nicked. The fat is then delivered, transected at its base, and resected.

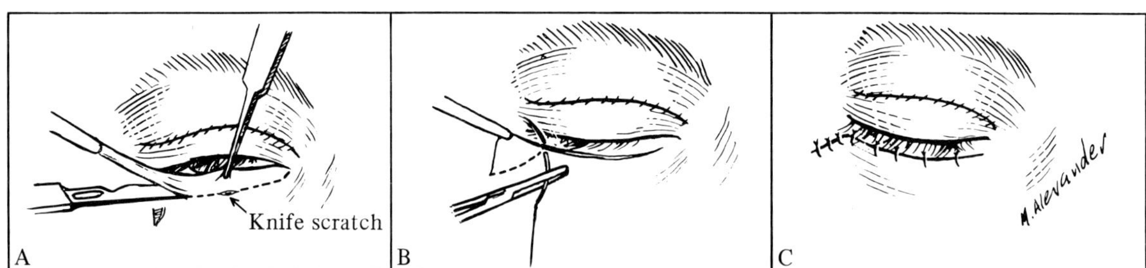

Fig. 19-4. A, cutting the calculated wedge of skin of the lower lid, while tensing the skin laterally and upward. The wedge resection measures 4 to 8 mm. only at the center (see text). B, the wedge has been resected as a final step before the suturing. A deep key suture is applied to the tensed and elevated skin. C, the appearance at completion, after resection of the triangle of excessive skin. In actual practice the upper lid skin is closed by a subcuticular suture (Fig. 19-2G), not a continuous one as shown here for purposes of simplicity. Three or four interrupted fine silk or Dacron sutures for the central portion of the lower lid incision are all that is necessary. More sutures are required for the lateral incision extension, which has the most tension.

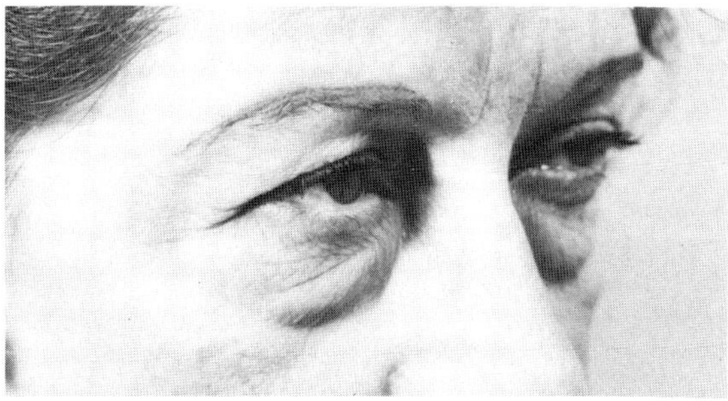

A

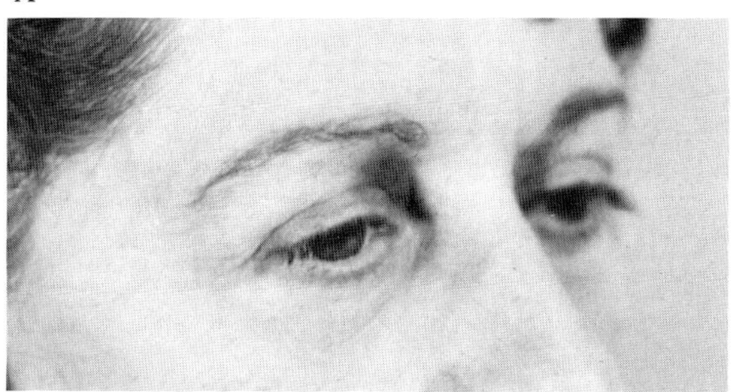

B

Fig. 19-5. A, preoperative photographs are helpful in determining which compartments are predominant. B, the same patient 1 year after the blepharoplasty.

trolled before the final skin suturing. The same is done with the other eye (Figs. 19-2 through 19-4).

When the orbicularis muscle is exposed, gentle digital pressure over the eyeball causes the muscle to bulge, due to the protruding orbital fat underneath (Fig. 19-2D). The apex or vault of the bulging muscle is cut, preferably with the #15 blade, almost from canthus to canthus (Fig. 19-3D). This affords a clear view of the fat compartments and greatly facilitates the fat resection (Fig. 19-3E). Upon cutting the orbicularis, the compartments of encapsulated fat promptly protrude through the incision, but the fat cannot be delivered properly until each individual capsule is nicked with sharp pointed scissors or with the knife (Fig. 19-2E). Gentle digital pressure over the closed eye is continued to make the herniated fat bulge out.

The two compartments of fat of the upper lid, and later the three compartments of the lower lid, are carefully identified (Figs. 19-2F and 19-3E). The amount of excess fat to be removed is calculated by grasping the apex of the individual protruding fat compartment with a small hemostat, and by gently pulling it while maintaining gentle digital pressure over the eyeball (Figs. 19-2F and 19-3F). Clinical judgment is easily gained with a little experience to determine the amount of fat to be removed. In general the amount that is easily and gently pulled out is the amount to be removed. Another way to determine the amount to be removed in the lower lid is to observe the amount that presents itself above the level of the infraorbital ridge after gentle pulling. The bony structure may readily be identified by palpation and by its glistening appearance.

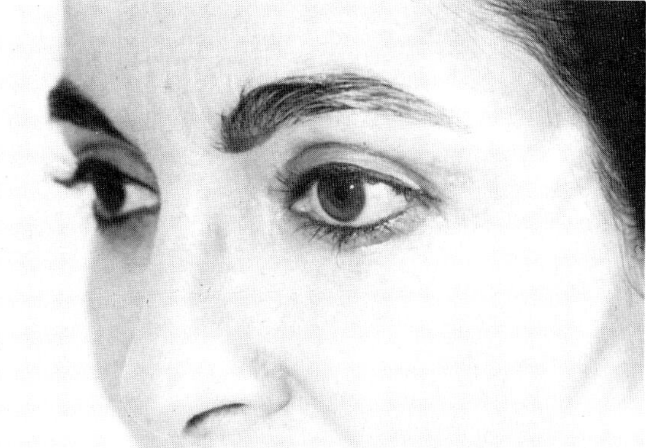

A

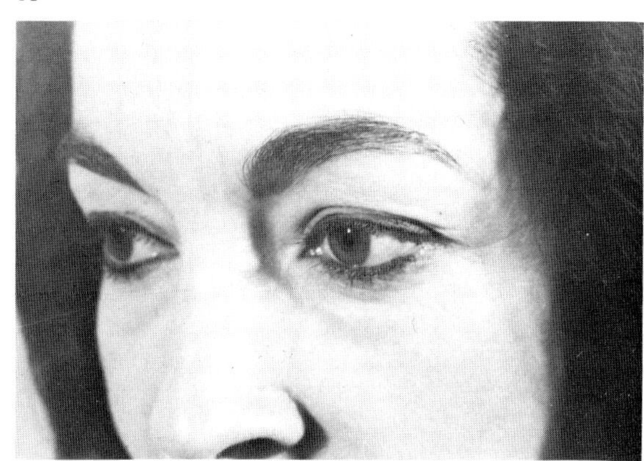

B

Fig. 19-6. A relatively young patient with early baggy eyelid deformity. A, the patient is shown before the procedure. B, 3 weeks postoperatively.

Enough fat must be removed from each one of the three fat compartments, or the operation may be only partially successful. Preoperative photographs are very helpful in determining which of the fat compartments are more prominent; particular attention should be directed to those compartments (Figs. 19-5 through 19-8). On the other hand, care must be exercised not to remove too much fat of the lower lid, since this would result in a slightly sunken or hollow appearance. (This is a very rare complication. I have seen only three such cases in consultation in my many years of practice.)

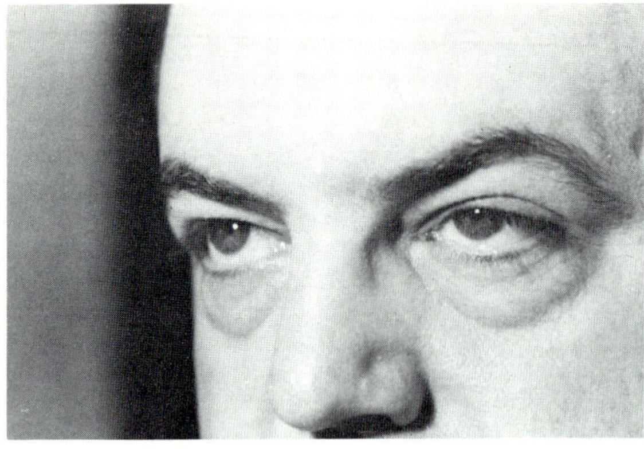

A

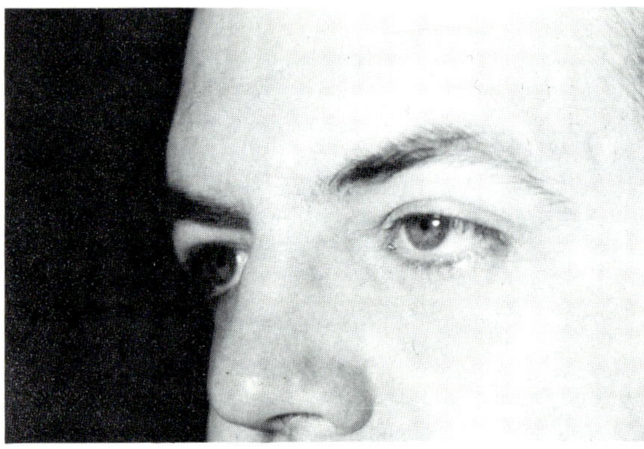

B

Fig. 19-7. A, a relatively young patient with typical protrusion of the intraorbital fat of the upper and lower lids. B, 6 months after surgery.

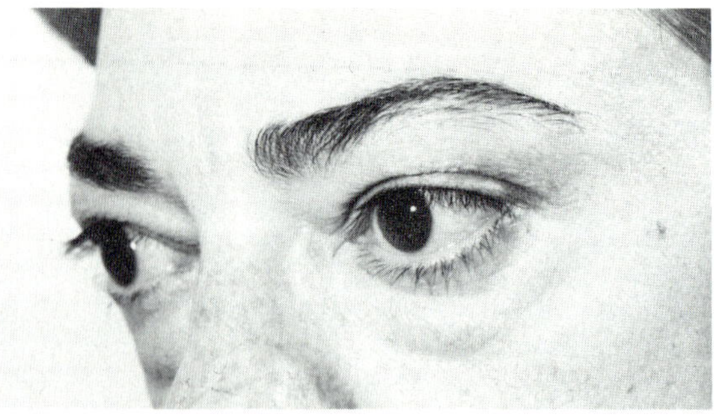

A

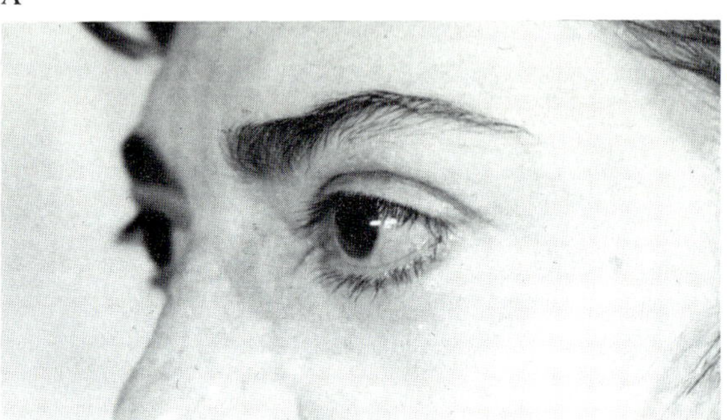

B

Fig. 19-8. A, exophthalmos with herniation of intraorbital fat, showing the condition of the eyes after the ablation of the thyroid. B, 1 year after blepharoplasty; concomitant anterior decompression of the orbit has been done through the blepharoplasty.

No attempt is made to repair the defective and tenuous orbital septum; it falls in line under the orbicularis muscle in the upper and lower lids. No sutures should be applied to the edges of the split orbicularis. Not only is this unnecessary, but experience has shown that suturing the muscle edges in the lower lid may result in temporary ectropion when the lower part of the split orbicularis is tensed laterally with the skin, dragging the upper part of the split orbicularis and causing the slight ectropion.

The skin of the upper lid incision is closed with a fine suture (5-0 Dermalon or similar material), which is removed in 5 to 7 days postoperatively (Fig. 19-2G). The subcuticular suture normally results in a fine inconspicuous scar, and minimizes the formation of milia.

The lower lid incision is closed in two sections: the central or palpebral part requires only three or four interrupted fine silk or Dacron sutures, while the lateral extension (from the canthal area toward the temple) requires more sutures, either continuous or interrupted, since it is here where the greatest tension is located (Fig. 19-4B, C).

An occlusive dressing (not a pressure dressing) may be applied for 12 to 24 hours, primarily for complete rest of the eyes to minimize edema and ecchymosis. All dressings are removed at the end of 24 hours and are replaced with small covering dressings, or dressings may be omitted, in which case the patient should wear dark glasses for psychological reasons.

All skin sutures may be removed on the third or fourth postoperative day, except for the subcuticular sutures, which may remain for 5 to 7 days after the surgery.

A small Micropore adhesive tape support is applied to the external lower canthal incision (the lid-cheek incision line) for 4 or 5 more days.

Rapid uneventful recovery is the general rule.

REFERENCES

1. Castañares, S. Blepharoplasty for herniated intraorbital fat. Anatomical basis for a new approach. *Plast. Reconstr. Surg.* 8:46, 1951.

2. Castañares, S. Baggy Eyelids. Physiological Considerations and Surgical Technique. In *Transactions of the Third International Congress of Plastic Surgery,* 1963. Amsterdam: Excerpta Medica, 1964.
3. Castañares, S. Correction of the Baggy Eyelids Deformity Produced by Herniation of Orbital Fat. In Smith, B., and Converse, J. M. (Cochairmen), *Proceedings of the Second International Symposium on Plastic and Reconstructive Surgery of the Eye and Adnexa.* St. Louis: Mosby, 1967.
4. Castañares, S. Cosmetic Eyelid Plasty: Correction of Baggy Eyelid Deformity Produced by Herniation of Intraorbital Fat. In Masters, F., and Lewis, J. R., Jr. (Coeditors), *Symposium on Aesthetic Surgery of the Face, Eyelid and Breast.* St. Louis: Mosby, 1972.
5. Castañares, S. Blepharoplasty in the Aging Face; Surgical Technique. In Tessier, P., Callahan, A., Mustardé, J., and Salyer, K. (Eds.), *Symposium on Plastic Surgery in the Orbital Region.* St. Louis: Mosby, 1976.
6. Castañares, S. Classification of baggy eyelids deformity. *Plast. Reconstr. Surg.* 59:622, 1977.
7. Converse, J. M., Johnson, J. B., and Hadley, R. L. The Aging Face. In Converse, J. M. (Ed.), *Reconstructive Plastic Surgery,* Vol. 3. Philadelphia: Saunders, 1964.
8. Fox, S. A. *Ophthalmic Plastic Surgery.* New York: Grune & Stratton, 1952.
9. Fuchs, E. *Textbook of Ophthalmology* (8th ed.). Translated by A. Duane. Philadelphia: Lippincott, 1924.
10. González-Ulloa, M., and Stevens, E. The treatment of palpebral bags. *Plast. Reconstr. Surg.* 27:381, 1961.
11. Hadley, H. G. Dermatolysis palpebrarum (blepharochalasis). *Rocky Mt. Med. J.* 37:517, 1940.
12. Hotz, F. C. Uber das Wesen und die Operation der Sogenannten Ptosis Atonica. *Arch. Augenh.* 9:95, 1880.
13. Lewis, J. R., Jr. (Ed.). *Atlas of Aesthetic Surgery.* Boston: Little, Brown, 1973.
14. Rees, T. D., and Guy, C. L. Patient selection and techniques in blepharoplasty and rhytidoplasty. *Surg. Clin. North Am.* 51:22, 1971.

Cosmetic Surgery of the Aging Face

JAMES W. SMITH

SIGNS OF AGING IN THE FACIAL SKIN

Upper Face

Telltale signs of aging are evident not only in the general texture of the skin but also in such local alterations as those that occur on the forehead, where transverse lines deepen and become more evident than they were during youth. Especially unattractive and distressing are the vertical frown lines that lie at the inner aspect of the eyebrow and extend from the margin of the superior orbital rim upward to the area of the transverse frown lines [16, 17]. These lines are accentuated by the action of the corrugator muscles.

Ptosis of the eyebrows downward from their normal position along the superior orbital rim is sometimes a more subtle mark of aging. The relaxed brow may fall well below the orbital rim to produce or accentuate redundancy of the eyelid skin. In the lateral portion of the brow, this downward displacement often produces a hooded effect. To correct it may require excision of redundant skin from the eyelid or removal of skin from above the lateral portion of the eyebrow in order to elevate it.

A third area of aging can be seen at the base of the nose. Transverse wrinkle lines accompany the downward sag of the eyebrow and the stretching of eyelid skin. The presence of transverse folds at the glabella suggests the need to inspect the location of the eyebrow.

The so-called "crow's-feet," a number of lines radiating outward from the eyelid, lateral to the outer canthus of each eye, become especially apparent with smiling. These lines are accentuated as the facial skin loses its elasticity. The fact that a number of muscles of expression insert into the skin along these lines helps each facial gesture to accentuate them.

Cheeks and Mouth

In the cheeks may be found such additional signs of aging as the prominence of the nasolabial folds, especially in the area adjacent to the upper lip and corners of the mouth. Often the accentuated folds, rather than stopping at this point, continue downward in an almost C-shaped fashion onto the submandibular region. This change in combination with the downward displacement of tissues from the cheek produces jowls and a square-looking face in contrast to the heart-shaped line of youth (see Fig. 20-1). The jowl and the squared lower part of the face are usually accompanied and accentuated by flattening of the malar prominence. This loss of "high cheekbones," due to a downward displacement of the subcutaneous tissue from this region, adds significantly to the impression of aging. To restore the youthful look, it is necessary that this prominence of the malar region be restored.

As one ages, the corners of the mouth are commonly marked with deep creases that join those of the nasolabial folds and may be accompanied by fissuring. In addition, there are vertical lines on the upper and lower lips; these lines, of course, lie at right angles to the underlying orbicularis oris muscle, and they seem to deepen with age and perhaps with a loss of subcutaneous tissue.

Neck

The neck is a common site for telltale signs of aging [1]. Deep transverse lines often ring it as in trees, to mark out the years. There is also a loosening of skin, so that vertical lines or folds are created that extend from the margin of the mandible down onto the neck. The third and perhaps most common finding is the presence of a "double chin," which seems to be due to an accumulation of fat between the mandible and the hyoid bone and stretching of the skin in this area. Because there is less fat over the hyoid bone and the skin is more firmly attached in this area, the double chin tends to fall over it. This change can make it difficult for women to wear necklaces or turtleneck sweaters, whereas for men it may cause constant soiling of the shirt or tie. Many patients with double chins or vertical folds seem to use their platysma and sternocleidomastoid muscles a great deal in making facial gestures and in movements. It is entirely possible that repeated contraction of these muscles accentuates the aging process.

ETIOLOGY

Much of the aging process has been attributed to the fact that skin merely stretches with age and loses its elastic fibers. This may not be entirely true [20, 30, 32]. If the tissues that constitute a jowl or double chin are rolled between the thumb and index finger, it becomes apparent that a second major component of this aging tissue is subcutaneous tissue. Flattening of the malar prominence and a hollowing in the preauricular area support the suggestion that the difficulty may indeed be a relaxing of skin and superficial subcutaneous tissue on the deep fascia and that it prolapses downward as its vascular pedicles stretch out.

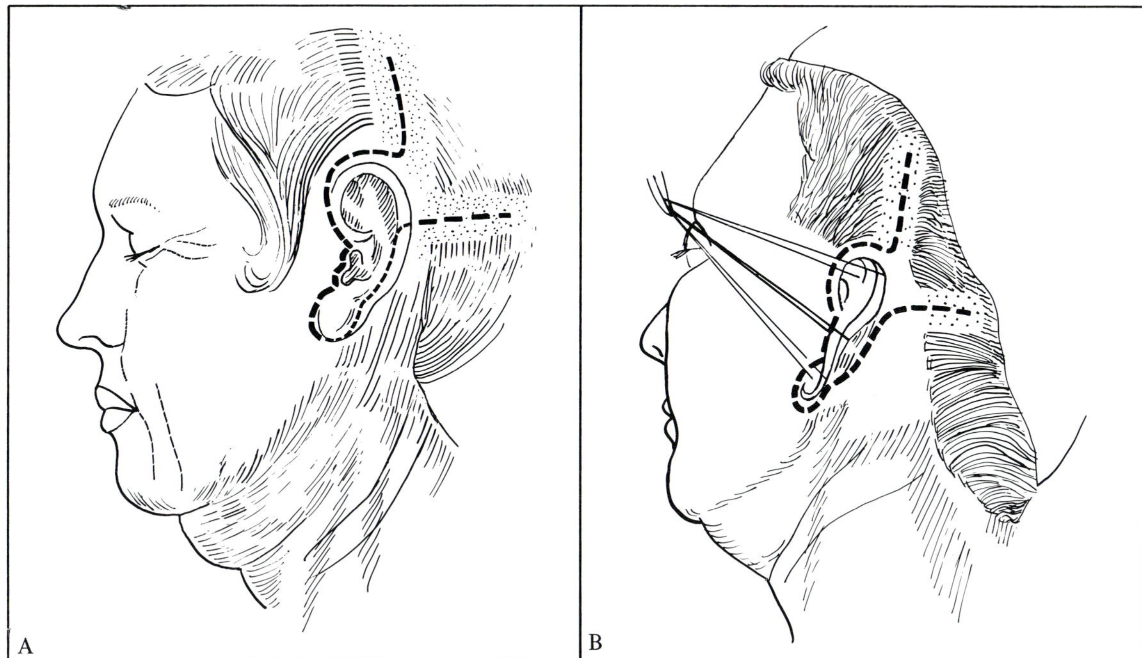

Fig. 20-1. The incision for rhytidectomy. A, the incision is placed well back in the hair-bearing scalp so that it remains hidden. In the preauricular area it follows the skin folds normally found just anterior to the ear. Stretch the skin of the cheek forward when marking this part of the incision; otherwise the final scar may not lie as close to the ear complex and be as well hidden. B, the lower margin of the incision is curved in a V-shaped fashion on the flat skin adjacent to the ear lobule and not in the groove. Posteriorly it curves back into the hairline at a 90-degree angle, eliminating a sharp angle; this minimizes the chance of skin necrosis and removes the scar from an area that might prevent the patient from wearing her hair "up" on the top of her head.

No matter how the process occurs, the fact that the jowl and double chin contain skin and fat makes the treatment of both skin and fat a necessity [10, 11].

Not only does the excess skin need to be removed, but also the excess fat must be removed or repositioned in order to restore the contour of youth [36, 38]. In addition, treatment must be considered for the fine vertical wrinkles located in such areas as the upper and lower lips [39]. Something must be done to even out the hills and valleys created by the aging process.

The discussion that follows deals mainly with the techniques of treatment as they apply to the female patient. Facial surgery in the male patient is discussed on page 418.

PREOPERATIVE PREPARATION

The role each of the above factors plays in the aging process needs careful evaluation. The surgeon must decide, for example, whether a redundancy in the lower eyelid is primarily related to the lid itself or associated with and perhaps more completely a part of an inward and downward ptosis of the adjacent cheek. Each area must be analyzed to determine which change is primary and which is secondary. If the redundant skin of an eyelid is removed when the major portion of the redundancy was due to a ptosis of the eyebrow, the result will be disappointing unless the eyebrow is also elevated at the time of the eyelid surgery [9]. In such a circumstance, both factors must be corrected.

The use of photographs is important in the preoperative planning. By a careful study of the eyes, face, and neck, one may pinpoint the signs of aging.

Preoperative evaluation should include a search for the presence of hypertension or any bleeding or clotting disorder. In patients with a history of excessive menstrual bleeding, easy bruisability, or excessive bleeding from minor injuries, a sufficient hematological work-up must be undertaken to make certain that there is no underlying disorder of the bleeding or clotting mechanisms. If none is found, the administration of vitamin C 250 mg. and vitamin K 10 mg., twice a day for 5 to 7 days before surgery, may be of benefit.

Scars on the body should be carefully studied to determine whether the patient has any tendency to form keloids or hypertrophic scars. If either of these abnormalities of healing is found, it may be advisable to use a minimum of buried sutures and nonreactive suture materials for skin closure. It is advisable to have the patient wash her face and hair with a surgical soap several days before admission to the hospital. When the patients have an unusual degree of apprehension about hospitalization or surgery, it may be useful to give a sedative (for example, phenobarbital 30 mg. three or four times a day) or a tranquilizer such as diazepam (Valium) 5 to 10 mg. three or four times a day, in preparation for surgery.

I prefer to extend the preauricular and postauricular incisions into the hair-bearing scalp rather than to locate them at the juncture of facial and hair-bearing skin. Consequently, a small channel about 1.5 cm. in width is shaved preoperatively (see Fig. 20-1). The hair on either side of it is pulled out of the way with rubber bands and fixed with povidone-iodine (Betadine) soap (this is the thick soap that surgeons use in the scrub room). If applied 10 to 15 minutes prior to surgery and allowed to dry, it forms a thick matted coagulum. Postoperatively it washes out easily when the patient is placed in the shower.

The surgery should be planned so that, from the preauricular region, the anterior line of incision follows the normal curve of the ear up to the highest point of the superior pole, then extends in a C-shaped fashion up into the hair along a line approximately 3.5 to 5 cm. back in the hair-bearing scalp, to the level of the widow's peak (see Fig. 20-1). Posteriorly the line of incision is extended backward from a point level with the antitragus and continued slightly downward into the hair-bearing scalp for approximately 5 cm. After the area has been shaved, the Betadine soap and rubber bands can be applied to hold the hair out of the way.

ANESTHESIA

Anesthesia may be either general or local. The disadvantage of general anesthesia is that an endotracheal tube makes it necessary to work around the tube at the time of the neck surgery.

When the patient is cooperative, local anesthesia is probably more desirable from the surgeon's point of view. A proper level of sedation can be achieved by giving the patient some combination of medications such as that listed below:

1. Pentobarbital (Nembutal) 100 mg. and diazepam 5-10 mg. at bedtime the night before surgery.
2. Nembutal 100 mg. 90 minutes before surgery.
3. Morphine 10 mg., Nembutal 100 mg., and prochlorperazine (Compazine) 10 mg. 30 minutes before surgery.

If the combination listed above does not produce the desired degree of narcosis, we prefer to use intravenous diazepam (Valium) in the operating room to gain the desired level of narcosis; 5 to 20 mg. is injected slowly during the surgery, usually in 2.5-mg. doses, as it is needed. It is best to give it through an intravenous drip of dextrose and water so that the Valium will be diluted when it enters the vein. This lessens any discomfort to the patient and makes it easier to flush out the vein after administration to lessen the chance of a chemical phlebitis.

SURGICAL TECHNIQUES

Surgery on the face may be done either alone or in combination with eyelid surgery.

Preoperative Marking

I find it advantageous to mark topographical lines on the face prior to surgery. This allows better symmetry and aids in ascertaining that the same amount of elevation and rotation is accomplished on each side of the face.

With the patient in the supine position and the back slightly elevated, the patient is asked to smile, exposing the teeth. This helps to identify the nasolabial folds on either side so that they can be marked; the midline mark is continued down onto the neck to the level of the mandibular notch. Then, with the head slightly flexed, the transverse crease lines in the neck are identified and marked. Only two or three of the most prominent of these need be marked. Attention is given to determining which one will specifically represent the point of creasing between the underside of the chin and the neck, and where the vertical bands, if any, are located.

Once this has been accomplished, the patient is asked to sit up with her feet over the side of the operating table. The "shadow line" is marked along the lower face to represent the junction between the lower border of the mandible and the neck. This line is carried backward and upward until it reaches the point where the jawline attaches to the earlobe. Then the juncture between the skin of the lower lid and the cheek should be marked. The skin texture of the lower lid usually is easy to identify and separate from that of the cheek. With age this margin often has a sag to it and looks like a hammock that hangs too low. At surgery an attempt is made to raise this to a position closer to its normal level.

The line marking the most inferior portion of the lid usually comes to lie just at the height of the malar prominence. If a finger is placed here and laid flat against the cheek, an additional line can be marked that runs essentially from a finger breadth below this high point backward to the level of the tragus. The forward position or location where the finger is placed establishes the location on the face where an upward and backward pull achieves the greater reduction of the heaviness of the nasolabial folds. It is along this line that a plication of soft tissue is made to try to eliminate some of the sagging of the cheek and to restore an appearance of high cheekbones. If forehead surgery is also contemplated, any deep transverse forehead lines are also marked. Scowl lines are also noted if the patient wants them treated. The patient is returned to the reclining position and the lines are reinforced with methylene blue or brilliant green in order to make the lines more permanent for the operation.

One might ask why it is necessary to do all of this preoperative marking. In return for a few minutes of preparation, one gains a greater assurance of symmetry, and one can ascertain that the lines of pull and tension are essentially the same on both sides of the face. Prior to institution of this plan, patients frequently complained that one earlobe was higher than the other or that there were other asymmetries relating to the surgery on the two sides of the face. Now, this is seldom a problem, which saves a great deal of time postoperatively.

Technique of Incision

The patient's head is placed on a rubber-padded neurosurgical headrest; this type of headpiece facilitates the operation. The head is usually turned to the side, with the patient supine in a partially sitting position. To minimize bleeding it is important to have the head elevated above the level of the heart. If local anesthesia is to be used, a solution of 0.5% lidocaine with epinephrine 1:200,000 will prove helpful and yet not exceed the maximal allowable dose of this solution for any given period.

The skin is prepared with an anesthetic and sterile drapes are applied. We find it is best to cover all the hair initially; then, once the remainder of the drapes are in place, we suture the head towels to the forehead, just above and just behind the area where the forehead joins the scalp in the midline. The towels can then be pulled back on either side so that the ears and the posterior margins of the upper and lower channels in the hair-bearing scalp are identified. Small wheals of 0.5% lidocaine with adrenalin are infiltrated to anesthetize the area before the towels are sutured into place. All sutures are placed within the hairline to prevent any possible marks on the forehead skin.

The incision for rhytidectomy begins about 3 cm. behind the widow's peak on the forehead. It extends in a C-shaped fashion downward along the narrow channel from which the hair has been clipped or removed to the point where the upper posterior part of the ear would touch the head. From here the incision continues forward and then downward immediately in front of the ear within the small groove that is normally present there.

After making a small V in the crus of the helix, the incision is carried down along the margin of the tragus to the narrow shallow groove that lies between the tragus and antitragus. From here it again comes forward and downward, passing around the earlobe. The incision continues upward and backward in the groove created first by the earlobe and the flat surface of the neck and then by the concha and the neck. At a point about two-thirds of the way up, it turns backward and slightly downward into the hair-bearing scalp at an angle of about 90 degrees. At the lower pole of the ear, do not place the incision in the groove; rather, the incision is placed just on the flat surface of the facial skin adjacent to the earlobe. In this way the normal curvature formed by the earlobe and its junction with the skin of the face is not disturbed. The repair looks more natural because of the greater accuracy gained in approximating the two cut, but flat, surfaces.

Dissection

Initial undermining is carried out in the superficial subcutaneous tissue. I think it is helpful to begin posteriorly, incising and elevating the skin of the posterior scalp. If the right plane is found, a great portion can be done with the fingers in a "scalping" fashion. The mastoid fascia and the sternocleidomastoid muscle can be seen, with the greater auricular nerve crossing superficially over the sternocleidomastoid muscle as it heads in the general direction of the earlobe. As dissection continues anteriorly, it is important to stay superficial to the more lateral fibers of the platysma muscle. Sometimes it is helpful to switch to preauricular incision after elevating some of the skin in this area and to connect the anterior area of undermining with the posterior one so that the proper plane can be maintained. In the neck the dissection is maintained at a level superficial to the platysma and carried down across the midline when fat needs to be removed and prominent bands of platysma muscle must be divided (Fig. 20-2). I now use a small submandibular incision to remove any excess fat and to approximate the edges of the platysma muscles from either side in the midline. Then below the plication I divide the cordlike vertical folds that span across the neck to the underside of the chin. Dividing larger sections of the platysma and trying to tack them backward under tension or not mobilizing them at all after division seem to cause a great deal of induration in the neck. When the skin is stretched so that it is under the tension seen in the young neck, a great deal more irregularity of contour and a less smooth appearance of the skin seem to result.

In dividing any section of the platysma muscle,

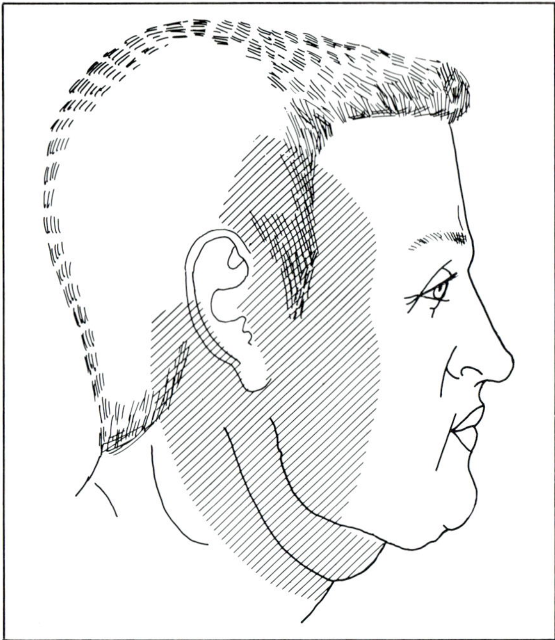

Fig. 20-2. Area of skin to be undermined in a rhytidectomy. The amount, of course, varies with each case. In hair-bearing areas, the dissection should be carried out deep to the level of the hair follicles.

one should be careful not to damage or divide the mandibular branch of the facial nerve [18, 19, 31, 33, 35]. The course of this nerve has been described by Dingman and Grabb [14]. It is always deep to the platysma muscle but in about 20 percent of patients it will lie as much as 1 or 1½ cm. below the mandible between the angle of the jaw and the mandibular notch. In the remaining 80 percent, the mandibular branch of the facial nerve lies on the mandible throughout its whole course.

Over the cheek area the skin is usually dissected from the parotid-masseteric fascia anteriorly to about the anterior border of the masseter muscle [35]. Once this is completed, it is best to make the superior scalp incision and free the temple and forehead skin down to meet the lower dissection. Undermining should be deep to the galea aponeurotica in the hair-bearing areas to preserve the follicles and to prevent hair loss. Thus, the dissection in the hair-bearing area of the temple should be beneath the fascia until the hairline is reached. At the hairline the dissection becomes superficial again to connect with the undermining in the preauricular area. In the region of the zygomatic arch, the superficial layer of temporal fascia has deep attachments onto the arch. When the temporal skin flap is separated from the arch, the line of fascial detachment should be kept superficial. It may be necessary to divide the frontal branch of the temporal artery and its accompanying veins with this maneuver, but this should not cause concern. Once the flaps are freed and elevated, hemostasis is easily controlled.

Plication and Closure

In spite of all the arguments to the contrary, I find it advantageous to plicate the superficial component parts of the superficial musculoaponeurotic system [30, 40]. The parotid fascia is plicated transversely if there is a prominent nasolabial fold or heavy jowl (Fig. 20-3). It is also plicated vertically if the whole cheek appears to have dropped or sagged. In the transverse plication, I run a continuous over and over suture such as 4-0 Vicryl just inferior and parallel to the zygomatic arch. A second plication suture is run from the area of the earlobe attachment up to the zygomatic arch (Fig. 20-4). A third row of sutures is located along the posterior border of the platysma muscle. This tightens the anterior portion of the platysma muscle upward and stretches out the skin in an upward and backward fashion as imbrication of the platysma muscle proceeds. I use sutures of either 3-0 white silk or white cotton and mobilize the posterior edge of the platysma back over the sternocleidomastoid and suture it under moderate tension. Nylon does not appear to be as satisfactory for this maneuver because it does not produce the inflammatory reaction necessary to help fix the plicated tissues together. Several times in the past, nylon sutures have popped when one of my patients turned her head suddenly; this was followed by an immediate return of the sag that had been present before the surgery.

When the plication has been completed, the posterior skin flap is pulled up and backward, and one suture is inserted at the angle of the posterior flap of the ear. The second suture is placed at the point where the incision angles upward from the upper pole of the ear (Fig. 20-5). These sutures serve as key points for further suturing. Before additional sutures are inserted, a narrow Penrose drain is placed as a vent in the neck along the line paralleling the mandible. It is brought out along the posterior portion of the hair-bearing scalp incision (Fig. 20-6). The second Penrose drain is placed over the masseter muscle and extends upward to exit through the superior incision in the hair-bearing portion of the scalp. It emerges along the flat part of the incision so that the skin margins will fall together once the drain is removed. Once the two sutures are in place, it is then possible to close the nearly S-shaped incision by using a number of almost linear closures.

If the redundant skin lying just in front of the ear is pulled up over it, the excess or redundant skin over

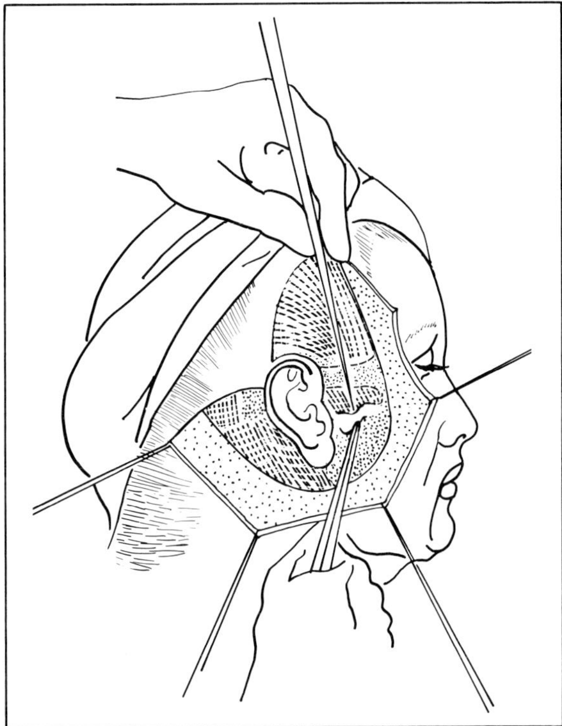

Fig. 20-3. With the flaps elevated and hemostasis achieved, the sternocleidomastoid muscle covered by its fascia is visible posteriorly as it extends down into the neck from the mastoid process. Care must be taken not to injure the greater auricular nerve, which crosses this muscle and continues in the direction of the lobule. On the temple it is important to keep all dissection superficial anterior to the hair-bearing skin. Above the point where the parotid fascia attaches along the zygomatic arch, branches of the facial nerve to the forehead lie in the superficial tissues forward of the hair-bearing scalp. All plicating sutures should be placed below the level of the zygomatic arch, except those that will lie behind the origin of junction between hair-bearing and non-hair-bearing skin on the forehead. These sutures should be directed to pull the subcutaneous tissue upward and back in a direction which somewhat parallels that of the lower border of the mandible.

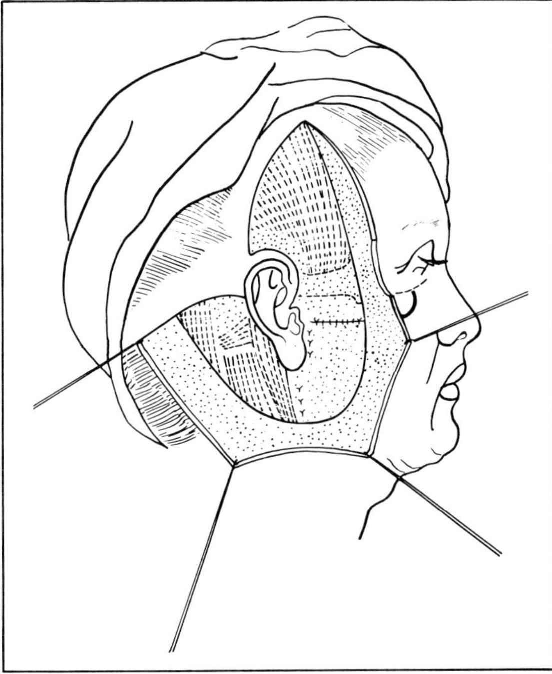

Fig. 20-4. Lines of plication at their completion. If the plication is confined to the areas shown, it is difficult to damage branches of the facial nerve because they lie either deep within the parotid gland or in front of the hair-bearing skin on the scalp. Plications around the lobule are placed so that they tighten the fascia without affecting the position of the lobule itself.

the two points located just above and just below the tragus can be determined by incising in from the skin margin. These are fairly fixed points. The topographical line previously drawn with methylene blue to the midpoint of the tragus with the plication usually ends up near the V identation at the top of the tragus or just above as a result of the underlying plication. If this same point is attached to the V of the tragus on either side, it gives the same comparative degree of elevation. The methylene blue line that was drawn on the skin along the lower margin of the jaw preoperatively will usually remain in a similar relationship to the lobe of the ear as the excess skin is advanced up and excised.

After the two points are identified on either side of the tragus, temporary tacking sutures of 3-0 black silk are placed there to hold the two sides of the incision together. Then the corresponding curve of the incision from the tragus to the top key suture can be duplicated upon the redundant overlying skin and the excess skin removed. The excess skin can also be easily identified in front of the tragus and removed.

The closure can now be carried out in the region of the mastoid after the redundant skin is excised. A sharp pointed scissor or curved clamp should be used to identify the point at which the redundant skin overlaps the posterior incision at the top of the lobe and its junction with the concha. Then the straight or slightly curved incision on the redundant

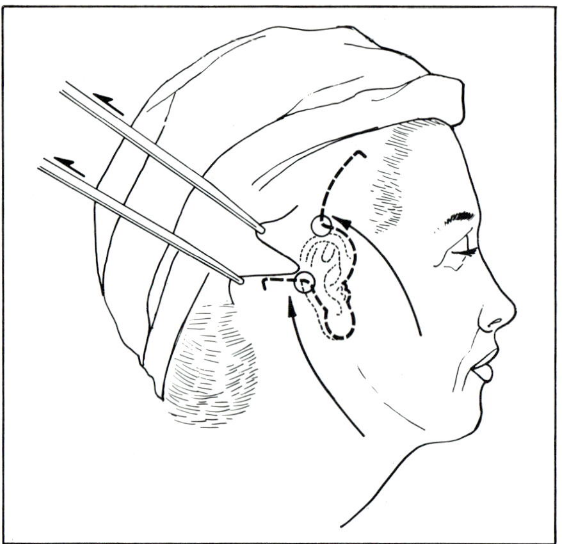

Fig. 20-5. The key to excision of excess skin and closure lies in drawing the skin flaps upward and back (direction shown by arrows) over the ear and placing key sutures (circles) at the two angles as shown here. (The dotted line corresponds to eventual suture line.) These angle sutures should be tied down, even if only temporarily, because they aid in fixing these points for the rest of the closure. Keep both sutures in place while trimming of the overlapping skin is being carried out, for this helps to prevent errors in outlining the flaps. Note the cut backs at the ends of the original incision to allow greater rotation and easier closure. Once the posterior excision has been performed, begin the suturing posteriorly and continue up to the postauricular angle. The temporal region is closed next by this technique. Finally the postauricular and preauricular areas are closed. Dividing the wound up in this fashion transforms an S-shaped incision into a number of straighter suture lines and decreases the chances of making errors.

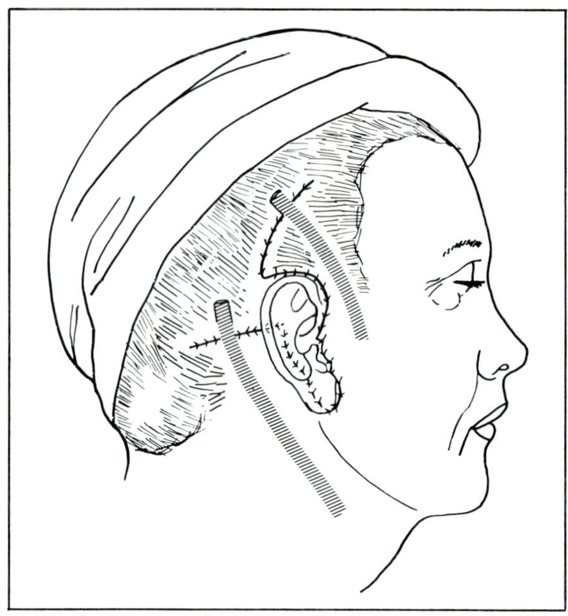

Fig. 20-6. Small Penrose drains serving as vents are placed in the temporal and cervical areas. These vents exit along a linear portion of the closure so that once they are removed the margins flatten. A small safety pin with a wire attached to it is fixed to each of these drains and the ends of the wires are passed into the upper part of the dressing so that it is possible to remove the drain in 24 hours without changing the dressing. This maintains constant skin compression and prevents the accumulation of fluid along the tracts where the drains were located. The head dressing is removed at 48 hours.

skin behind the ear down to the lobe should be marked and the excess skin excised. A fixing suture is placed between this flap and the skin margin at the posteroinferior border of the concha. Once this is done it becomes a comparatively easy maneuver to incise a V in the excess skin overlying the earlobe and remove it so that the lobe will fit in a natural way into the V and not pull, tug, or distort it. If the lower margin of the wound appears to be longer than the upper in this portion of the closure, the lower skin flap can be drawn up posteriorly a little more or advanced up a little more in front until the earlobe fits properly into the V-shaped cut that has been made through the redundant skin overlying it. It is important not to exert any tension on the skin of the ear lobe, since a downward pull eliminates the natural curved appearance of the lobe and replaces it with a less natural look that years ago was called "the drawing room giveaway."

An excision of the excess skin can now be carried out in the superior hairline and the wound closed from the most superior part down to the point located at the junction at the upper part of the ear with the head.

The last part of the closure can be carried out after the redundant skin in the mastoid region is excised (Fig. 20-6). Suturing here should begin posteriorly and continue upward to the postauricular angle to ensure keeping the margin of the hairline intact behind the ear.

Dressing and Postoperative Care

After the head has been turned on the opposite side and a similar procedure performed, the dressing can be applied. Safety pins with #28 or #30 wires attached are placed through the Penrose drains to permit their removal without necessitating a removal of the dressing. This not only saves time but also prevents any serum from accumulating along the drain tracts after the drains are removed 24 hours following surgery. A firm dressing is placed over the face with cotton around the ears to minimize discomfort here. The bandage usually consists of a Kling or Kerlex roll and Ace bandages placed to give a slight pressure over the operative areas. The ends of the wires are brought out through the dressing posteriorly and tagged with a piece of tape, which makes it easy to identify the drain wires for removal. At 24 hours gradual traction is placed on the ends of the wires with a clamp and the drains are removed. At 48 hours the large dressing is removed and the patient allowed to shower.

Preauricular sutures are usually removed in 3 to 5 days, whereas the postauricular incisions and those lying in the hair-bearing areas should be removed in 8 to 14 days.

REGIONAL SURGERY

Submental Lipectomy and Excision of Excess Skin

In spite of the improvement in neck contour gained in the face lift operation, submental fat or a double chin frequently persists [27, 28, 29]. If this remains it is usually for one of two reasons. (1) There is often an excess of fat in the midline that is difficult to identify and reach from the lateral incision. (2) Some patients have a transverse deep indentation or crease between the chin line and the normal neck crease. Between these lines lies a second pocketing of fat, which is accentuated by the fibrous septum that extends from the skin in the surface to the fascia overlying the platysma. Splitting this fascia to release its deep attachment and remove some of the fat often does a great deal to help correct this latter problem. However, the area is usually approached through the submandibular incision, which can tremendously increase the technical difficulties. These difficulties include: difficulty in resecting just the right amount of fat to prevent having a recurrence of the fullness; removing too much fat centrally and leaving lateral bulges (which tends to make the patient feel that the surgery was incomplete); having the skin become adherent in the midline (which indents it and again accentuates the suggestion of a lateral fullness); and creates irregularities in skin smoothness (which makes the result look less crisp and exacting and leaves the patient displeased). Anesthesia is obtained with a local infiltration of 1% lidocaine with epinephrine. If one studies the patient preoperatively, it is easy to see and mark the inferior border of the mandible; just inferior to that is a submental skin crease, which usually separates the neck fat into a smaller anterior accumulation and a greater portion posteriorly. The incision is made just inferior to the submental skin crease and deepened down to the level of the muscular layer. From this point undermining continues inferiorly, above the fascia, down to the crease line that would be between the transverse and vertical portions of the neck if it were well developed. Once the undermining has been completed, it is also important to undermine in a reverse direction, anteriorly, to the anterior edge of the mandible – just above the muscular layer. The submental fat pad is excised from the posterior flap, but at the same time sufficient fat should be left on the flap to prevent it from adhering to the deep tissues over the mandible and creating an unsightly depression between the skin and the submental area. Hemostasis is achieved and the posterior fat sutured to the fat anteriorly or to the periosteum of the mandible so as to keep it from falling posteriorly. It is also important to consider advancing toward the midline the fat deposits of the remaining fat that lies laterally, in order to lessen the lateral fullness that can result from central removal and lateral fat and subcutaneous tissue retraction. If this is not done, a bulge sometimes results on either side of the central neck area.

If skin had to be removed, either a triangle can be removed and the closure completed or a vertical triangle can be made by removing the skin from either side of the midline and having a short T scar. To do this, one takes the lateral skin and advances it past the margin of the midline; the overlapped portion is resected. This is also done on the opposite side, and then the two flaps are approximated anteriorly as well as to one another in the midline area.

For this dissection in the neck as well as for undermining the flaps, either a fiber-optic retractor or a fiber-optic headlight, such as the Malis headlight* (sold by Designs for Vision), is truly helpful for increasing the ease of surgery. The fiber-optic headlight assures the surgeon a well lighted view of the operating area at all times, because its beam is directed from a midpoint between the eyes and therefore follows the same course as the eyes.

Correction of Eyebrow Ptosis

Ptosis in the eyebrow occurs in certain individuals; it is usually greater in the lateral portion of the brow than the medial part. As a matter of fact this deformity often accentuates the downward creasing of the eyelid. Castañares [9] has described various skin excisions that can be made above the eyebrow in order to raise it and lessen the sag. We do not favor this approach when the problem is minimal, and prefer to

*Designs for Vision, Inc., 120 E 23rd St., New York, N.Y. 10010.

make the excisions through the eyelid incision itself at the time of upper lid blepharoplasty. At the most lateral portion of the eyelid incision, one can identify the point where the dissection lies nearest to the bony orbital rim laterally. It is here that the brow can be positioned at a higher level, by identifying the superior margin of the orbicularis oculi muscle and anchoring it at a slightly higher level to the underlying periosteum.

Removal of Deep Forehead Wrinkles

Skoog [37] and Kaye [23] have discussed the steps necessary to remove the deep furrows and transverse folds that develop on the forehead due to overactivity of the frontalis muscle. Another problem that frequently accompanies deep forehead wrinkle lines is the sagging of the brow. Both problems can be improved by the forehead lift [41, 42].

The surgical exposure is gained through a crescentic scalp flap located about 5 cm. above the hairline. (This procedure is less popular in the men because of the frequency of male pattern baldness.) Dissection is carried down between the paracranium and the galea aponeurotica above and the frontalis muscles below. The scalp flap is raised to a point just above the supraorbital rim, preserving the sensory innervation to the area. Small strips of frontalis muscle are excised in a transverse fashion from the deep surface of the flaps to diminish the activity of the forehead and lessen the conspicuousness of the deep lines.

The glabellar frown lines, which are produced by the contraction of the two corrugator supercilii muscles, are treated by either removing a portion of the corrugator muscles or lessening their effectiveness. This can be done when the scalp flap used to treat the deep transverse forehead wrinkle lines is turned down, or the operation can be performed more locally.

Another way to eradicate these glabellar wrinkle lines is with chemosurgery, which is discussed under the heading, Chemical Face Peel (Chemosurgery).

Upper Face Lift – The "Temple Tuck"

A great number of patients first become dissatisfied with their appearance when they note deepening nasolabial folds and see beginning jowls, usually without sagging of the neck. In such cases if surgery is selected, it can be confined to the temple and cheek areas. A combined temple and preauricular incision is made. The fullness in the jowl area can be lessened by longitudinal plication just beneath the zygomatic arch. This plication also improves the nasolabial lines.

After the plication is complete the face lift flaps are rotated in a superoposterior direction to further enhance the lift. If the initial anterior dissection is carried down to the level of the earlobe and no further, once the elevation has been completed the excess skin in the preauricular region and just beneath the earlobe can be more easily excised. By comparison, it seems that freeing the skin around the earlobe initially makes it more difficult to evaluate the excess of skin and to get the same degree of lift.

After the excess skin has been excised, positioning or fixing sutures are placed between the fresh edges of the skin flap and the notches above and below the tragus for flap fixation. I place an absorbable suture such as Vicryl or Dexon from the posterior surface of the notch that is located between the tragus and antitragus through the cartilage, into the dermis of the flap, and back out; this suture can serve as a tension or stay suture. It can be left in for a long period of time if it is not tied too tightly and will serve to take the tension off of the skin surface for better healing along the margin.

Incisions are closed in the same manner as with the standard facial operation, and a small Penrose drain or vent is brought out along the superior portion of the closure in the hair-bearing area.

Penrose drains still are used rather than others, such as the Jackson-Pratt suction drains, because the Penrose drains seem to clog less frequently and have greater simplicity of drainage and ease of removal. Furthermore a great deal of additional attention is required when suction tubes are attached to the ends of a drain. It becomes necessary to see that they remain firmly attached and working, and that they are emptied at regular intervals.

Since the only place of dissection and suturing lies adjacent to the ear, in front of the ear, and over the cheek area, a modified facial dressing can be used. This consists of an Owen's nylon dressing and several layers of gauze that can be slit down the center and slipped over the ear to pad it; at the same time it provides some compression over the area of the surgery. Then some cotton can be placed over the ears for additional contouring and comfort with the remainder of the dressing being made up of a Kling roller dressing and Ace bandages. The bandages are removed at 48 hours when the patient washes her hair. Preauricular sutures are removed at 3 to 5 days and those sutures lying in the hairline at from 7 to 10 days.

FACE LIFTING IN THE MALE PATIENT

There seems to be an increasing demand for facial surgery in the male patient [4]. However, it seems to me that it is more difficult to give men as satisfactory a result as is possible for women [15]. Furthermore, because of hair length, hair style, and beard, compromises are necessary. It is more important to attempt to minimize the scar in the male face lift, because the scar is truly a problem that must be contended with. Another problem is the difficulty that arises if there is too marked a narrowing of the sideburn.

There has been a great deal of discussion about the placement of the incisions away from the creases and folds posteriorly, but this has not been a cause for complaint on the part of my patients. The dissection is done very much in the same manner as in the female, except that the extent of the surgery is not quite as great, and frequently in the male the face lift must be done in conjunction with a midline excision [13].

COMPLICATIONS

The most common complications of the face lift operation are hematoma, hair loss, skin loss, and nerve injury [3, 6, 12, 25].

Hematomas

Hematomas are probably the most frequent complication (occurring in about 2 percent of cases); they are caused by small bleeding points that temporarily stop but start again after closure and after the local anesthesia has worn off. Hematomas are no doubt sometimes caused by rebound hyperemia; they may also result from a rise in the patient's blood pressure after the local anesthesia has worn off. Occasionally a hematoma may be due to coughing or vomiting immediately following surgery, but it is often difficult to pinpoint the cause of a hematoma in the average case. Probably the most important point that can be made about hematomas is the clue that alerts one to their presence – an increasing asymmetry can be seen in the swelling of the face at some point between 1 and 36 hours following surgery. The patient with a hematoma appears especially to develop swelling of one eye or one side of the mouth, and the conjunctiva of the eye usually has an ecchymotic appearance. This patient sometimes complains of pain in association with the swelling because as the hematoma expands the dressing tightens. When the problem is in the upper face, the eye on the involved side is usually closed. It is important to remove the dressing and examine the face if there is any suspicion of this problem.

If the hematoma is large enough to cause these symptoms, then it should be evacuated, usually in the operating room. Sutures should be removed, the clots evacuated, and the bleeding point found. Usually the procedure can be done under sedation and local anesthesia, thus avoiding the problem of intubation of the trachea. With the hematoma removed, there is less difficulty in healing, a decreased likelihood of excessive scar tissue formation, and a reduced chance of flap necrosis, which certainly can follow the delay in revascularization of the flap.

Hair Loss

Hair loss can also be a major problem, which usually results from direct injury to the hair follicles or from excess tension along the suture line. It is important to dissect beneath the fascia to avoid damaging hair follicles.

Skin Sloughs

Skin sloughs are probably seen most frequently behind the ears. It is often possible for sloughing of the skin to follow swelling and/or hematoma and increased flap tension. It also may accompany excess pressure from the dressing, or it may result from the damage to the blood supply of the skin that occurs when too superficial a dissection is made, with damage to the subdermal plexus.

When a suture is tight and a line of ischemia or ecchymosis appears from the point of the suture down into the flap (indicating a compromise of blood supply), the suture should be released temporarily to let the margin separate slightly. Secondary healing occurs rapidly and does not produce as bad a scar as one might suspect.

Nerve Loss

A partial facial paralysis is a serious complication following facial surgery [34]. If the paralysis is noted immediately after surgery and a subsurface plication has been performed, immediate reexploration and removal of the plication sutures should be done, because muscle weakness or paralysis can be the result of compression of the nerve by a suture.

The most common types of facial paralysis following face lifting are paralysis of the frontal, buccal, and submandibular branches. Most authors report a 1 to 2 percent incidence of facial palsy from facial surgery [36].

SPECIAL ANCILLARY TECHNIQUES

Dermabrasion

Dermabrasion (or sanding of the skin) is a technique that is used to smooth scars and reduce surface irregularities such as result from acne vulgaris or chickenpox [22, 24]. It is also helpful in removing foreign body tattoos, especially during the emergency phase of treatment [21] (see Chapter 9). Professional tattoos, however, are more difficult to eradicate by this technique because so many of the particles of pigment are located in the lower layers of the dermis or in the subcutaneous tissue. Total removal of such pigment usually also destroys all the skin in the area and produces excessive scarring.

Irregular scars often can be improved by sanding, equalizing the margins, and eliminating any elevations [8, 36]. Fine wrinkling, such as the wrinkling that appears around the mouth with aging, can also be improved by abrasion, even if only temporarily. An easy way to firm the lips for this treatment is to have the patient open his mouth, a maneuver that puts the skin on a stretch. If the surgeon then places the fingers of one hand under the lip and stretches it out, the other hand can be used to manipulate the abrader over the surface with excellent control. Abrasion, however, seems to give less of a lasting result than the use of a skin peeling technique on the lip.

Most often dermabrasion or planing is carried out with the Stryker unit, a motor-driven instrument that revolves at a high speed (24,000 r.p.m.) and is controlled by varying the pressure on a foot pedal. To it is attached a cylinder of sandpaper or a wire brush. The wire brushes have a cutting width that varies from about 2 to 12 mm. The cylinders of sandpaper are available in three sizes; the larger cylinders are used for sanding broad flat surfaces, while the smaller ones are helpful in abrading narrower sites and complex surfaces such as those around the nose. The Dremel unit is a less painful sander that was developed for model makers; it can be purchased in toy stores and model shops. This unit is inexpensive and smaller, and it has the advantages of slower speeds and less power. It seems capable of doing as good a job as the Stryker unit, and the middle-sized sanding disc will fit it.

Local anesthesia for the sanding can be achieved by freezing the skin with an ethyl chloride or Freon spray. This method has the advantage of temporarily hardening or fixing the skin and yet preserving its usual surface contour. Because the anesthetic effect is so short with either of these agents, the abrasion is usually planned so that one area 5 to 7 cm. square is frozen and abraded before proceeding to the next.

Many surgeons prefer to use sedation and to infiltrate the area with a local anesthetic containing epinephrine so that oozing from the raw surface during treatment is diminished. This prevents blood from obscuring the surface and saves a great deal of time. Infiltration anesthesia, however, does have the disadvantage of altering existing surface configurations; thus it is advisable to mark the bottom of pits or depressions with methylene blue so that they can be identified.

The goal in treating irregular surfaces is to sand down the high points or elevations so that the low ones appear less deep. Improvement is achieved because once the dermis has been thinned by this technique, it never regains its original thickness. As the wound heals after abrasion, a new layer of epidermis forms over the raw dermal surface. The rate and success of healing depend on the outgrowth of epithelial cells from the portions of hair follicles and sweat glands remaining in the area following treatment. This healing process is similar to that of a skin graft donor site.

Because the speed of healing is related to the adnexal structures present, the face and scalp respond better, and with less reaction, to sanding than any other place on the body. The backs of hands do moderately well, whereas the chest and the upper and lower arms, especially on their inner or flexor surfaces, do poorly. The lower legs and feet are also slow to heal and may scar excessively. Because such lesions as burn scars, keloids, hypertrophic scars, and radiodermatitis all lack the number of adnexal skin structures needed for reepithelialization, they usually do not respond well to this type of treatment. People with dark skin do poorly because the treated areas often become darker than the normal adjacent skin.

After the area has been cleaned and anesthetized, the skin is placed on the stretch using gloved hands alone; gauze sponges must be kept at a distance to prevent them from catching in the machine. The abrading drum should remain parallel to the surface of the skin as the sanding proceeds with a light brushing stroke at right angles to the plane of rotation of the instrument. As the epidermis comes away, the dermal papillae will be noted as tiny sites of bleeding. A little deeper, the layers of the dermis appear as parallel ridges of collagenous tissue. These fibers begin to fray if the depth of abrasion is increased, and eventually break up into short, white interrupted threads, giving the area a shredded appearance. Any sanding deep to this layer should be done cautiously because minute holes soon begin to appear in the dermis, with yellow fat from the subcutaneous tissues herniating through the holes.

Any surface being abraded should be irrigated copiously with saline solution during and following the treatment to remove any blood and all remnants that have accumulated. Abraded areas can be treated postoperatively by exposure, but a thick uncomfortable coagulum forms, which later cracks and falls away. Probably a more comfortable technique for dressing the wound is to apply a layer of Owens gauze* (saponified cellulose acetate) to the raw surface and on top of this a layer of gauze sponges moistened with saline solution. Finally, a layer of dry fluffed gauze, a Kling or Kerlex roll, and an Ace bandage, if desired, complete the dressing. This method encourages any excess blood to filter through the Owens gauze and be absorbed into the moistened sponges rather than to coagulate on the surface. The outer dressing can be removed after 24 hours when the oozing has stopped, leaving the Owens gauze attached to the abraded skin until it separates after 3 to 5 days. The coagulum between the Owens gauze and the healing surface is so thin that any sense of confinement or immobilization is minimized by this

*Davis and Geck, American Cyanamid Co., 1 Casper St., Danbury, Conn. 06810.

technique. After 3 days the patient can shower, and the Owens gauze easily comes away, leaving the thin coagulum behind, beneath which the process of reepithelialization continues undisturbed. Cocoa butter, mineral oil, or cold cream is applied to the scar or coagulum to aid in removing it as well as in lubricating the surface beneath, which tends to be dry. If there was a surface infection at the time of treatment, as in a subacute case of acne, it may be desirable to apply saline soaks or Furacin ointment to the outer surface of the Owens gauze after 24 hours if odor or drainage suggests surface infection.

Powder and makeup can be applied after the abraded surface has healed, but patients should be told of the importance of washing the area well each day and lubricating it if necessary.

Erythema can persist for several months or even longer following abrasion, and patients should be advised to avoid direct or indirect sunlight during this time because it may produce areas of hypopigmentation or hyperpigmentation. Sun-screening agents are an aid in avoiding these complications. If such complications do occur, these areas can cause a "splotchy" appearance that may persist for a long time.

Milia frequently appear postoperatively and are due to a temporary blockage of ductal orifices during the reepithelialization process. If patients with this problem use a wash cloth for cleaning the area, its mildly abrasive effect usually removes these pinpoint areas of white cebum and leaves the duct orifice open.

Chemical Face Peel (Chemosurgery)

The chemical face peel has been termed "facial rejuvenation" by Litton [26] because it restores to the skin a somewhat healthier, younger appearance. However, it has only limited usefulness in treating problems of aging tissue because it tightens loose skin only slightly. Its major advantage is that it helps to eliminate fine wrinkles and such skin blemishes as keratoses. The peel is sometimes used as an isolated procedure when there is fine wrinkling with little or no associated prolapse of the facial tissues. When the problems of both ptosis and wrinkling are present, it serves best as an adjunct to the surgical face lift. Women with fair skin, fine wrinkling, and a minimum of gross sag are ideal candidates. Those with a more olive complexion are less satisfied because the treated areas are so much lighter in color than the adjacent untreated areas.

The most satisfactory results from this technique are obtained on the forehead, eyelids, and lips when the problem is primarily multiple creases or fine wrinkles. It seems especially unsatisfactory on the neck because it can result in hypertrophic scarring. Considerable nursing care is required for these patients since there is often marked edema of the eyelids, which makes it difficult to see [2, 5, 7]. When the lower face has been treated, the patient must not talk or move about and is given a slate and chalk to use for communication; fluids are administered orally through a straw.

The dangers of this treatment are its potential systemic toxicity and the scarring and blotchy discoloration of the skin that can result if the treatment is unskillfully performed.

When it is to be employed, peeling of a limited area such as the upper lip may be done at the same time as a surgical face lift. A surgical face lift and extensive chemical peel are never done at the same time. If both are to be used in treating the patient's problem, the face peel is scheduled approximately 4 to 6 weeks after the rhytidectomy. The chemical face peel can be used to treat the entire face in one procedure.

The solution used for this procedure contains 3 ml. of phenol (U.S.P.), 2 ml. of distilled water, 3 drops of croton oil, and 8 drops of liquid soap. A fresh solution is mixed for each application and administered with ordinary cotton applicators. Care must be taken to apply the solution only to the areas where it is desired and to use particular caution in working around the eyes, to prevent any of it from accidentally coming into contact with the conjunctiva. By using almost dry cotton swabs, any chance of the solution splashing on these other areas can be minimized.

It is necessary to give patients some sedation before treatment to minimize their discomfort, because immediately after the solution is applied the patient will experience a burning sensation. This will rapidly subside as the local anesthetic properties of phenol take effect. The treated area develops a white, frosty appearance, which lasts several minutes, and then a dark red hue appears. Two or three layers of ordinary waterproof adhesive tape are applied to meticulously cover the area that is being peeled. This mask is left in place for 24 to 48 hours and then carefully removed. A narcotic is usually required for this step in the procedure. Thymol iodide (U.S.P.) powder is immediately dusted onto the chemically treated surfaces in liberal quantities after the tape is removed; the powder is reapplied several times during the following 24 hours until a thick crust forms. The crust should be kept dry and intact for 3 to 5 days. Talking and chewing should be kept to a minimum because they frequently will cause the crusts to crack. This in turn may result in a delay of healing, cause a localized infection, or deepen the peel at this site.

After 3 to 5 days or when the crust becomes really uncomfortable, a mild ointment such as boric acid ointment (5%) can be applied to the crust. This softens the crust as does washing the area with soap and water. After washing, pat the skin dry gently with a towel, and leave it open to the air for a few minutes; then apply the ointment again. After this treatment has been used for several days, the crusts will usually lift away, leaving behind a pink-colored skin. This pink color lasts from 6 to 12 weeks. The severity of the redness can be lessened by having the patient apply triamcinolone cream to the area two times a day.

After the crusts have separated from the face, the skin is gently cleaned and a mild facial cream is applied to the skin if it is dry. Prolonged exposure to sunlight is to be avoided for 3 to 4 months [2]. If the patient has complaints of itching, this can sometimes be diminished by the application of a vegetable oil (for example, Crisco) or the triamcinolone cream.

REFERENCES

1. Adamson, J. E., Horton, C. E., and Crawford, H. H. The surgical correction of "turkey gobbler" deformity. *Plast. Reconstr. Surg.* 34:598, 1964.
2. Baker, T. J. Chemical face peeling and rhytidectomy. *Plast. Reconstr. Surg.* 29:199, 1962.
3. Baker, T. J., and Gordon, H. L. Complications of rhytidectomy. *Plast. Reconstr. Surg.* 40:31, 1967.
4. Baker, T. J., and Gordon, H. L. Rhytidectomy in males. *Plast. Reconstr. Surg.* 44:219, 1969.
5. Baker, T. J., Jr., and Gordon, H. L. Chemical Face Peeling. In Goldwyn, R. M. (Ed.), *The Unfavorable Result in Plastic Surgery: Avoidance and Treatment.* Boston: Little, Brown, 1972.
6. Baker, T. J., Gordon, H. L., and Mosienko, P. Rhytidectomy, a statistical analysis. *Plast. Reconstr. Surg.* 59:24, 1977.
7. Baker, T. J., Gordon, H. L., and Seckinger, D. L. A second look at chemical face peeling. *Plast. Reconstr. Surg.* 37:487, 1966.
8. Campbell, R. M. Surgical and chemical planing of the skin. *Plast. Reconstr. Surg.* 1:187, 1964.
9. Castañares, S. Forehead wrinkles, glabellar frown and ptosis of the eyebrows. *Plast. Reconstr. Surg.* 34:406, 1964.
10. Connell, B. F. Lipectomies combined with platysma muscle flaps for severe neck contour problems. Presented at the Tenth Annual Meeting of the American Society of Aesthetic Plastic Surgery. Los Angeles, Calif., March 1977.
11. Connell, B. F., and Peterson, R. Rhytidectomy with special emphasis on the lower face and neck. Presented at the Tenth Annual Meeting of the American Society of Aesthetic Plastic Surgery. Los Angeles, Calif., March 1977.
12. Conway, H. The surgical face lift – rhytidectomy. *Plast. Reconstr. Surg.* 45:124, 1970.
13. Cronin, T. D., and Biggs, T. M. The T-Z plasty for the male turkey gobbler neck. *Plast. Reconstr. Surg.* 47:534, 1971.
14. Dingman, R., and Grabb, W. C. Surgical anatomy of the mandibular ramus of the facial nerve based on the dissection of 100 facial halves. *Plast. Reconstr. Surg.* 20:266, 1962.
15. Edgerton, M.T., Webb, W. L., Slaughter, R., and Meyer, E. Surgical results and psychosocial changes following rhytidectomy. *Plast. Reconstr. Surg.* 33:503, 1964.
16. Gonzalez-Ulloa, M. Facial wrinkles. *Plast. Reconstr. Surg.* 29:658, 1962.
17. Gonzalez-Ulloa, M., and Stevens, E. F. Senility of the face. Basic study to understand its causes and effects. *Plast. Reconstr. Surg.* 36:239, 1965.
18. Guerrero-Santos, J., Espaillat, L., and Morales, F. Muscular lift in cervical rhytidoplasty. *Plast. Reconstr. Surg.* 54:127, 1974.
19. Guy, C. L., Converse, J. M., and Morello, D. C. The Aging Face. In Converse, J. M., and McCarthy, J. G., (Eds.), *Reconstructive Plastic Surgery.* Philadelphia: Saunders, 1977.
20. Hollander, M. M. Rhytidectomy: Anatomical, physiological, and surgical considerations. *Plast. Reconstr. Surg.* 20:218, 1957.
21. Iverson, P. C. Surgical removal of traumatic tattoos. *Plast. Reconstr. Surg.* 2:427, 1947.
22. Iverson, P. C. Further developments in the treatment of skin lesions by surgical abrasion. *Plast. Reconstr. Surg.* 12:27, 1953.
23. Kaye, B. L. The forehead lift. *Plast. Reconstr. Surg.* 60:101, 1977.
24. Kurtin, A. Corrective surgical planing of skin; new technique for treatment of acne scars and other skin defects. *A.M.A. Arch. Dermatol. Syph.* 68:389, 1963.
25. Leist, F. D., Masson, J. K., and Evich, J. B. A review of 324 rhytidectomies, emphasizing complications and patient dissatisfaction. *Plast. Reconstr. Surg.* 59:525, 1977.
26. Litton, C. Chemical face lifting. *Plast. Reconstr. Surg.* 29:371, 1962.
27. Marino, H., Galeano, E. J., and Gandolfo, E. A. Plastic correction of double chin. *Plast. Reconstr. Surg.* 31:45, 1963.
28. Millard, D. R., Jr., Garse, W. P., Beck, R. L., and Thompson, I. D. Submental and submandibular lipectomy in conjunction with a face lift, in the male or female. *Plast. Reconstr. Surg.* 49:385, 1972.
29. Millard, D. R., Jr., Pigott, R. W., and Hedo, A. Submandibular lipectomy. *Plast. Reconstr. Surg.* 41:513, 1968.
30. Mitz, V., and Peyronie, M. The superficial musculo-aponeurotic system (SMAS) in the parotid and cheek area. *Plast. Reconstr. Surg.* 58:80, 1976.
31. Owsley, J. Q. Platysma-facial rhytidectomy. *Plast. Reconstr. Surg.* 60:843, 1977.
32. Pangman, J. Cosmetic surgery of the face and

neck. *Plast. Reconstr. Surg.* 27:544, 1961.
33. Peterson, R. Rhytidoplasty with emphasis on SMAS. Presented at the Forty-Sixth Annual Convention of the American Society of Plastic and Reconstructive Surgeons. San Francisco, Calif., November 1977.
34. Pitanguy, I., and Ramos, A. S. The frontal branch of the facial nerve: The importance of its variations in face lifting. *Plast. Reconstr. Surg.* 38:352, 1966.
35. Rees, T. D., and Aston, S. J. A clinical evaluation of the results of submusculo-aponeurotic dissection and fixation in face lifts. *Plast. Reconstr. Surg.* 60:851, 1977.
36. Rees, T. D., and Wood-Smith, D. *Cosmetic Facial Surgery*. Philadelphia: Saunders, 1973.
37. Skoog, T. *Plastic Surgery*. Philadelphia: Saunders, 1975.
38. Spira, M., Gerow, F. J., and Hardy, S. B. Cervicofacial rhytidectomy. *Plast. Reconstr. Surg.* 40:551, 1967.
39. Stark, R. B. A rhytidectomy series. *Plast. Reconstr. Surg.* 59:373, 1977.
40. Tipton, J. B. Should the subcutaneous tissue be plicated in a face lift? *Plast. Reconstr. Surg.* 54:1, 1974.
41. Uchida, J. I. A method of frontal rhytidectomy. *Plast. Reconstr. Surg.* 35:218, 1965.
42. Vinas, J. C., Cariglia, C., and Cortinas, J. L. Forehead rhytidoplasty and brow lifting. *Plast. Reconstr. Surg.* 57:445, 1976.

21

Aesthetic Rhinoplasty

GEORGE C. PECK

Aesthetic rhinoplasty was first recorded in medical history by the Branca brothers in Sicily in the 15th Century. However, it was Jacque Joseph [5] who gave us the first manual of rhinoplasty technique, which became the basis for today's rhinoplasty. Later, it was masters like Aufricht [1, 2] and Safian [16] who refined the techniques. By the early 1960s, rhinoplasties had become a commonplace operation. However, the results were not always predictable, and patients frequently were left with tell-tale rhinoplastic signs. The techniques described in this chapter have been developed over the past 20 years; they are predictable and produce a nose that is anatomically normal – the two most important criteria of a satisfactory technique.

PREOPERATIVE EVALUATION

Aesthetic reduction rhinoplasty begins in the office with the initial consultation. The patient must want the aesthetic improvement; the goals, which must be realistic, should be discussed. The nose is examined and palpated. It must be determined whether the skin is thin or thick and how much bone and cartilage are in the hump. Most important is a thorough examination of the nasal tip. Certain important questions must be answered. Is the alar cartilage strong and resilient, or is it thin and weak? What is the nasal tip projection – is it too high, about right, or too low? Is the nose too long from the glabella to the nasal tip? Is there a drooping tip or hanging columella in profile? What is the angle of the glabella in profile? What is the nasolabial angle? Is the upper lip crowded by the nasal spine? Are the alar rims wide? Is the bridge wide? Is the chin receding or weak? Is there difficulty with breathing?

With these questions answered and noted on the chart, a preliminary plan is evolved for the aesthetic refinement, and that plan is discussed with the patient. Photographs (3 in. × 5 in.) are taken of the patient (Figs. 21-1 and 21-2), including front view, profiles, and a "worm's eye view," with serious and smiling expressions. The pictures and the preliminary plan are used in the evolution of a final plan for the patient. Not to be forgotten is a good medical history, with such important points as allergies to drugs, hypertension, diabetes, and bleeding tendency.

Prior to surgery, the patient must have a laboratory profile, with studies including a complete blood count, bleeding tendency profile, prothrombin and partial thromboplastin time, blood smear for platelets, urinalysis, blood urea, and blood sugar.

PREOPERATIVE MEDICATION AND PREPARATION

One hour before surgery the patient is given preoperative medication, which may vary considerably; a typical combination might involve a narcotic such as opium alkaloids (Pantopon) 15 mg. administered with pentobarbital (Nembutal) 90 mg. and dimenhydrinate (Dramamine) 100 mg. In the operating room intravenous diazepam (Valium) is given until the patient has slurring of speech. At that time, the patient is ready for local anesthesia.

The nose is again thoroughly examined. The alar cartilages are palpated, and the caudal border of the alar cartilage is drawn on the skin (Fig. 21-3). Depending upon the height of the nasal tip – that is, the nasal tip projection – the sculpturing or intracartilaginous line is outlined on the external skin. This line represents the sculpturing incision that will be made in the vestibular skin (Fig. 21-4). If the nasal tip projection is high, maximum reduction in tip height is sought, and consequently a narrow rim (3 to 5 mm.) of alar cartilage is left in continuity in the alar rim (Fig. 21-5). If the tip projection is acceptable prior to surgery, the goal is to preserve as much alar cartilage as possible. The intracartilaginous incision is made high, leaving 5 to 10 mm. or more; the intent is primarily to produce the desired sculpturing line (Fig. 21-6).

LOCAL ANESTHESIA

The nose is now anesthetized with 1% lidocaine and adrenalin, using a mixture of 50 ml. of 1% lidocaine with 0.6 ml. of 1:1,000 adrenalin. With a #27 needle and a 5 ml. syringe (no larger), a regional block is performed. It is important to avoid injecting into the nasal bridge and tip, since this will distort the nasal bridge and tip. Surgeons performing this procedure should consider themselves as sculptors, and as such it is to their benefit to see the results of their work immediately, which would not be possible if the tissues were distorted with local anesthetic. The vestibular skin and septum are injected intranasally; this usually takes 10 to 15 ml. of the local anesthetic. Care must be taken not to inject too much at the nasal spine, since this will produce a false elevation of the nasal tip. It is better to radiate the needle around the nasal

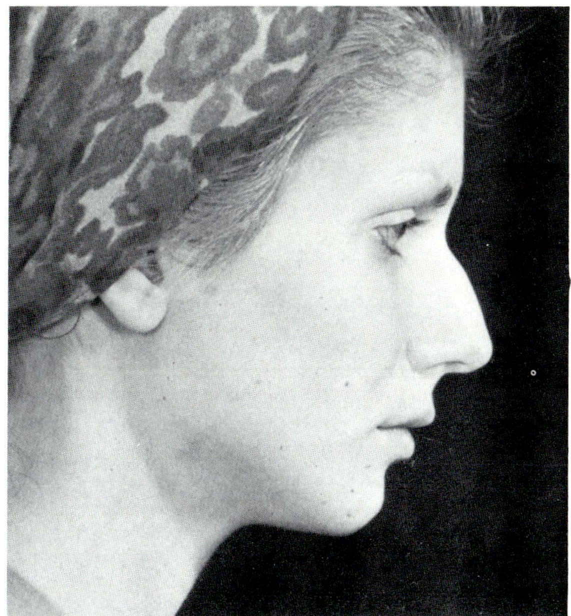

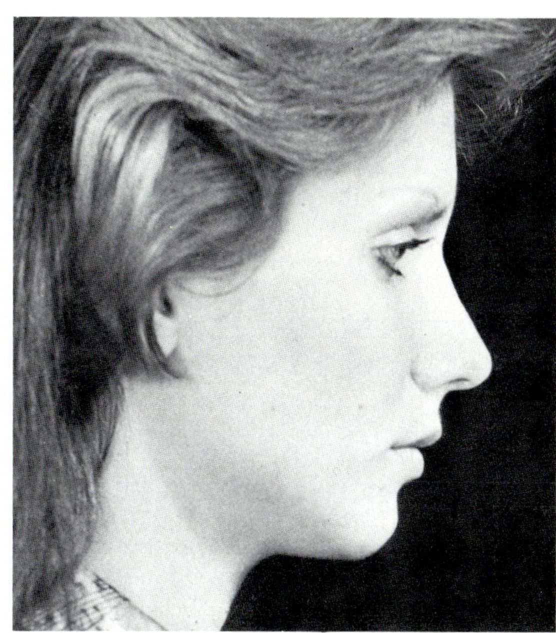

Fig. 21-1. Photographs before and after rhinoplasty of a 20-year-old woman with minor deformities of nasal lines, which required subtle refinements. Note the preservation of normal anatomical lines.

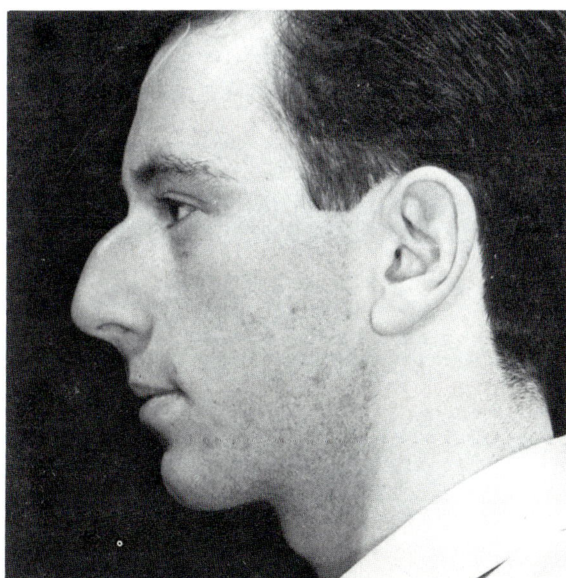

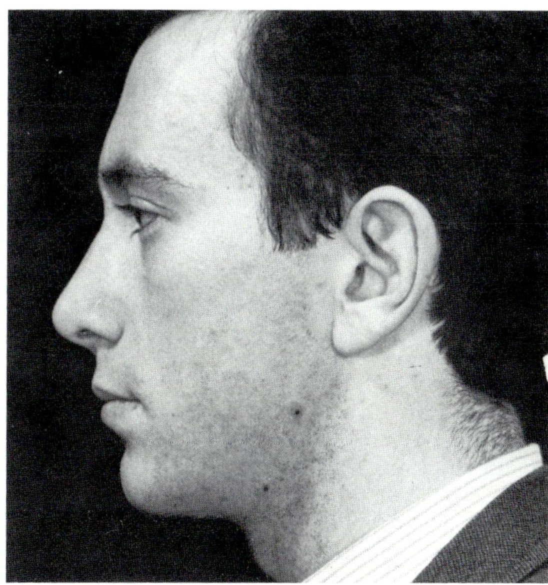

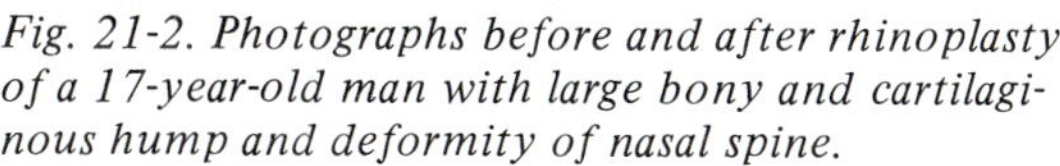

Fig. 21-2. Photographs before and after rhinoplasty of a 17-year-old man with large bony and cartilaginous hump and deformity of nasal spine.

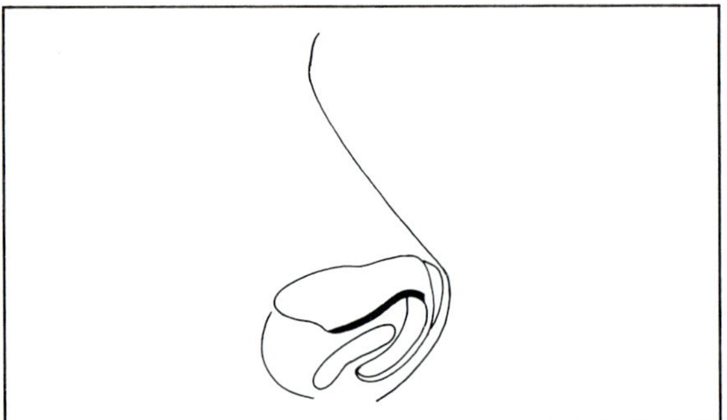

Fig. 21-3. The caudal end of the alar cartilage is marked on the external skin.

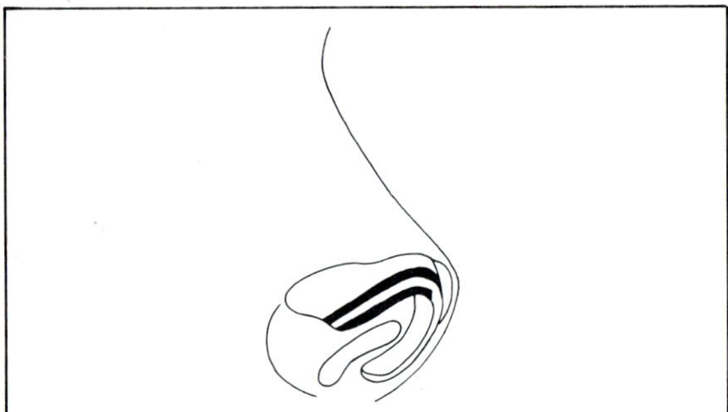

Fig. 21-4. The external skin is marked, showing the position of the intracartilaginous incision.

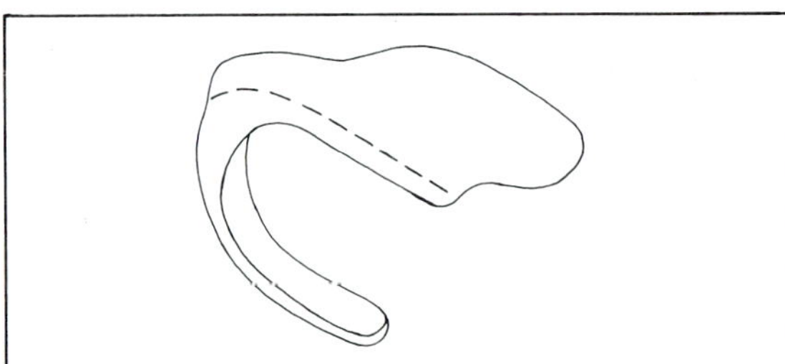

Fig. 21-5. In the high projecting tip, a narrow rim (3 to 5 mm.) of alar cartilage is left in continuity.

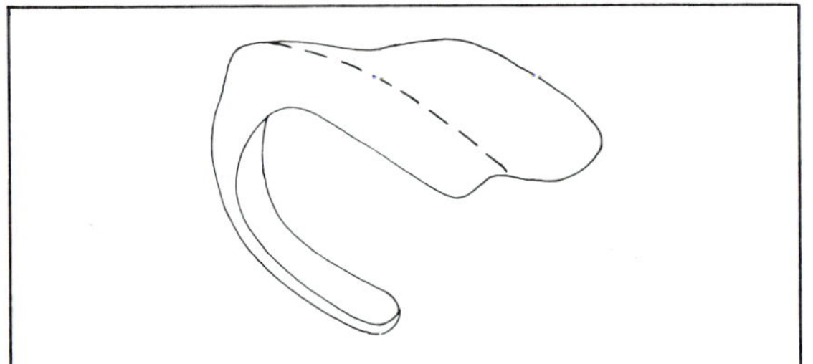

Fig. 21-6. In the low or good projecting tip, as much alar cartilage is preserved as possible.

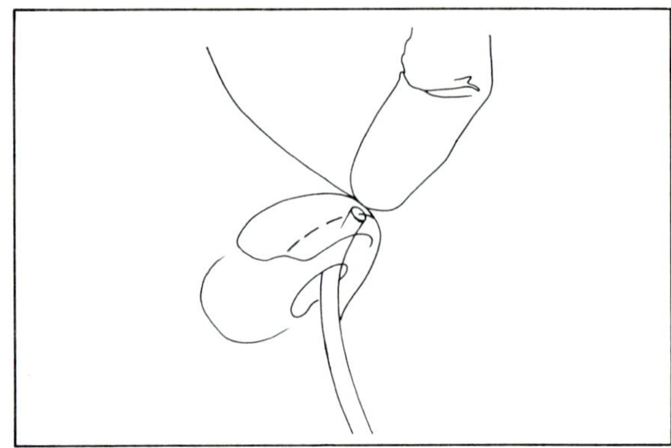

Fig. 21-7. The suction tip is used as a guide to mark the position of the intracartilaginous incision.

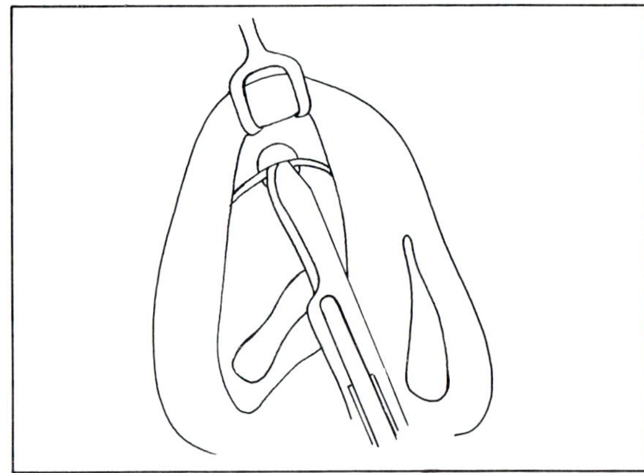

Fig. 21-8. The intracartilaginous incision begins at the imprint made by the suction tip.

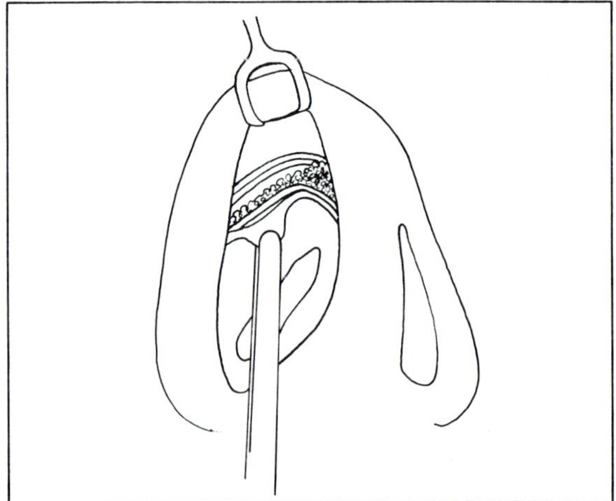

Fig. 21-9. The vestibular skin is grasped with a hemostat.

tip, injecting minute amounts upon withdrawal of the needle. Three cotton applicators, dampened with 10% cocaine solution, are then placed intranasally, one along the nasal floor, one under the inferior turbinate, and one under the nasal roof. With the injections completed, it is necessary to wait a minimum of 10 minutes for the anesthesia and adrenalin to take effect (this can be easily seen by the blanching of the entire nasal skin). While waiting, the nasal vibrissae can be trimmed and, if it is necessary, the chin augmentation performed.

OPERATIVE TECHNIQUE

Surgery of the Nasal Tip

Surgery begins with the intracartilaginous incision [10, 11]. In order to locate the exact position of the incision, the suction tip is utilized. It is placed intranasally, directly under the intracartilaginous line that has been drawn on the skin. By pressing with the index finger of the opposite hand, an imprint is made in the vestibular skin, which is now our guide (Fig. 21-7). With a #15 blade, the sculpturing incision is made (Fig. 21-8). Care is taken not to injure the dermis of the skin, since this will show up postoperatively.

If the nasal tip is to be elevated, or if the columella is hanging, we must continue our intracartilaginous incision into the transfixion incision, that is, the separation from the septal angle to the nasal spine of the membranous columella from the caudal end of the septal cartilage. With the septal cartilage exposed, the entire line can now be elevated as necessary according to the preoperative plan. Most important is the resulting angle that is created, which must be an obtuse angle and never a straight line. This is true because the columella must always hang in profile below the alar rim. The position of the obtuse angle gives an excellent safety factor, since the anterior one-third of the line is only being elevated from the nasal spine to the nasal tip. The retruse columella, or piglike look, is consequently prevented. Since the alar nasal openings are situated in the posterior two-thirds of this line, one is only elevating the fleshy nasal tip; consequently, the front-view open nostril appearance is prevented.

At this time, if the lip is crowded, the nasal spine and contiguous cartilage are removed, in order to shorten the overall length of the nose and increase the vertical length of the upper lip.

The attention now returns to the sculpturing of the alar cartilages. The vestibular skin on the cephalad side of the incision is grasped with a straight hemostat (Fig. 21-9), and the skin is undermined from the alar cartilage and contiguous fibrofatty tissue with a blunt curved Joseph scissor (Fig. 21-10). With a straight sharp-pointed scissor, the vestibular skin is separated from the intranasal side of the alar cartilage (Fig. 21-11). The alar cartilage is grasped with a curved hemostat (Fig. 21-12); utilizing the tip of the sharp scissors, one can peel the vestibular skin from the alar cartilage medially and laterally. The alar cartilage is amputated laterally (Fig. 21-13), together with the fibrofatty tissue. Note the preservation of the tail of the lateral crus. Most individuals have an external depression in this area; its removal will accentuate the depression, producing a pinched effect. Therefore, only in individuals with fullness in this area must the tail be excised.

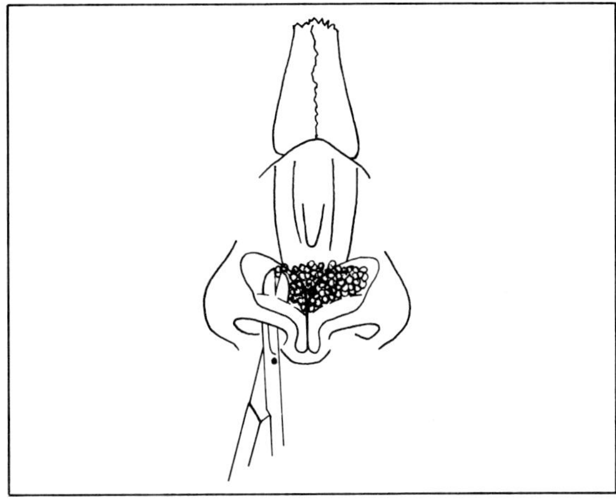

Fig. 21-10. With a blunt-tip scissor, the external skin is undermined from the fibrofatty tissue beneath.

With the cephalad alar cartilage removed bilaterally, the sculpturing of the nasal tip has been completed. These lines are now readily visible. A level discrepancy has been produced at the intracartilaginous incision. In the area between the incision and the upper lateral cartilage, there is nothing but external skin and internal vestibular skin. Below the incision, in cross section, there is full thickness of skin, fibrofatty tissue, alar cartilage, and vestibular skin. The level discrepancy will produce a light shadow on the external skin, much the same as it would on a scar with one side higher than the other. Therefore, if the intracartilaginous incision is properly placed, the proper aesthetic lines will be sculptured into the nasal tip. Until an operator has attained experienced skill in judgment, it is wise to leave a *wider margin* of alar cartilage in the alar rim [14].

It is important to understand what happens to the nasal tip pyramid when the alar cartilage has been refined, as described. If a large volume of alar cartilage is removed, the total volume of the nasal pyramid is always reduced; that is, both the height and the width of the nasal tip are reduced. If the tip is too wide or too high after completing the sculpturing,

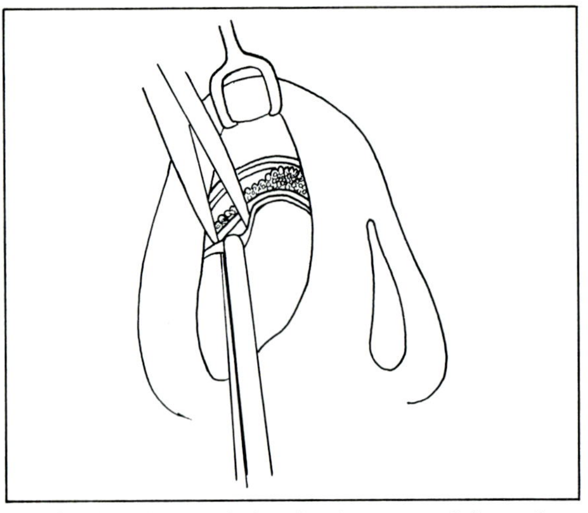

Fig. 21-11. The vestibular skin is separated from the alar cartilage with a sharp-pointed scissor.

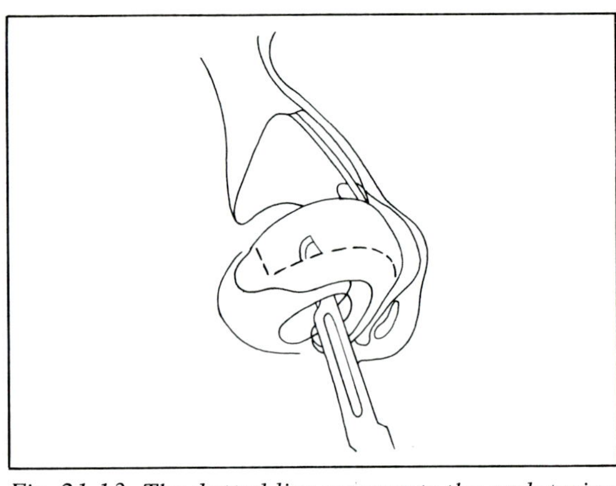

Fig. 21-13. The dotted line represents the sculpturing incision. Note the preservation of the tail of the lateral crus.

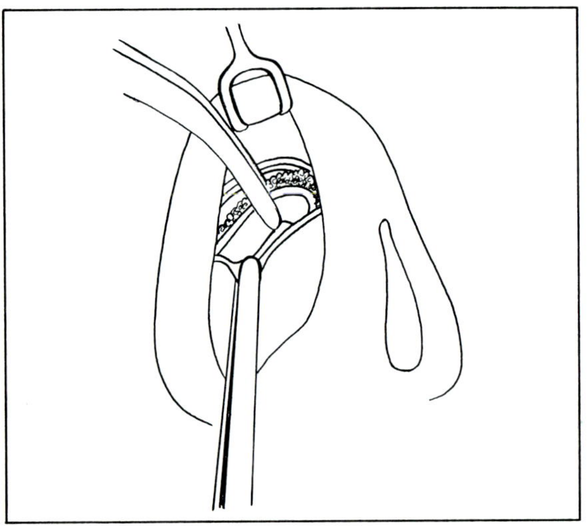

Fig. 21-12. The cephalad portion of the alar cartilage and contiguous fat are fully exposed prior to removal.

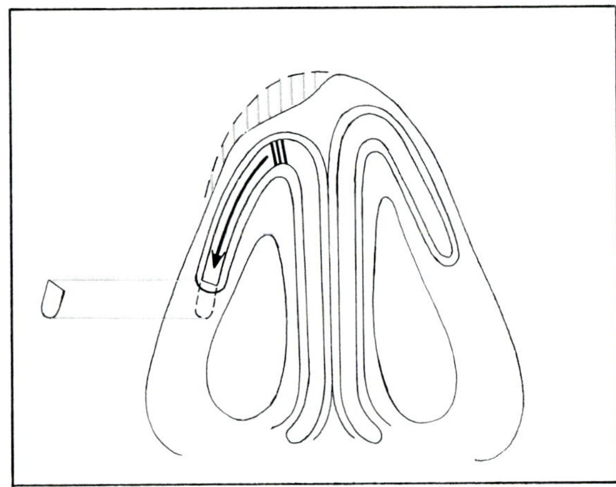

Fig. 21-14. In the high projecting tip, the technique of lateral rotation is used.

lateral rotation of the alar cartilage (Figs. 21-14, 21-15, and 21-16) is done [4, 12]. However, unless there is an extreme deformity in width or height, it is better to leave the tip alone, since healing and contracture will usually achieve a satisfactory result. One must remember that later correction is always possible, and a minor secondary revision, with good control, is often the wisest course. In the bifid tip, a midline columellar incision with suturing of the medial crural cartilages at the dome is a necessary primary procedure.

The most important concern has been to preserve the continuity of the alar cartilages and normal anatomical lines; this prevents the pinched, irregular boxy tip [15, 20]. However, in a slightly wide tip there is no objection to crosscutting the dome in order to break the resiliency, so long as the crosscutting does not go completely through the cartilage [8]. If the tip projection is short, a high sculpturing incision is planned, with very little alar cartilage being removed; then the nasal tip is augmented with an autogenous septal cartilage graft, a process that is well described by Sheen [17–19]. This graft is placed in a pocket between the caudal end of the medial crura and the nasal tip skin, occupying the outer one-

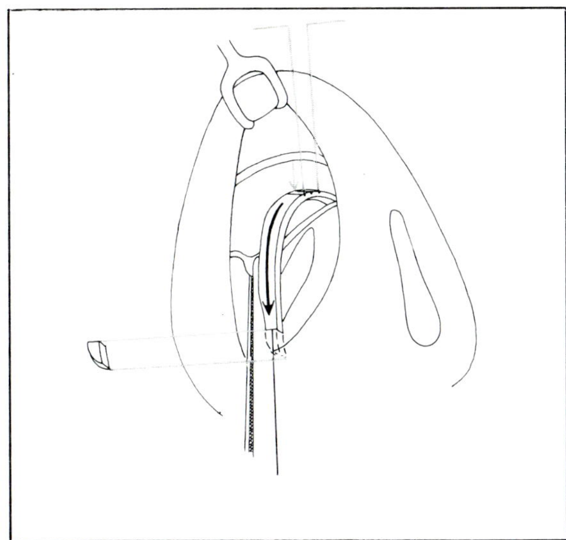

Fig. 21-15. The position of crosscuts at the dome is shown, with the cartilage excised laterally.

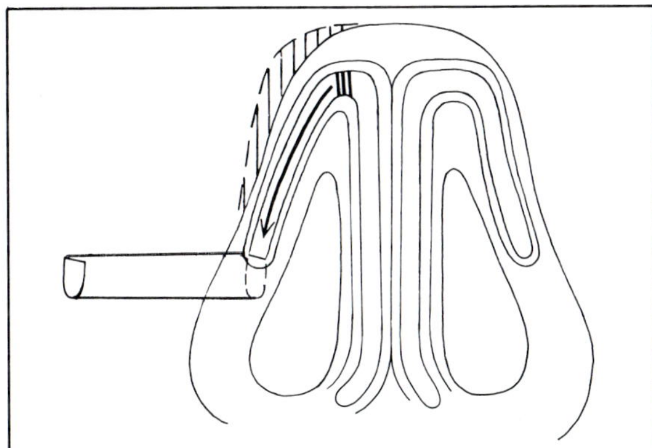

Fig. 21-16. In the broad tip, the lateral crus is delivered from its pocket and shortened, and the dome is crosscut.

third of the line between the nasal tip and the nasal spine.

Nasal Bridge

With the tip completed, one now proceeds to the nasal bridge. The nasal tip is almost always completed before the nasal hump, since reduction of the hump is an adjustment of that line to the new nasal tip height. If a tip appears almost perfect preoperatively, the hump may be done primarily through a high intracartilaginous incision.

Surgery of the hump begins with undermining the skin from the hump through the intracartilaginous incision. The bony portion of the hump is usually a very small component, and it has not been found necessary to elevate the periosteum. The skin undermining should extend laterally over the hump, but should *not* separate the skin from the lateral nasal bones. The sharp pull-rasp is inserted into the pocket and the bony component of the hump is lowered (Fig. 21-17).

With a #15 blade (Fig. 21-18) placed over the lowered dorsal bone, the cartilaginous portion of the hump is removed by cutting caudally with the scalpel. The cartilaginous hump incision is consequently an extension of the rasped dorsal bone line. By adjustment with a little rasping of bone and trimming of the hump cartilage, one finally reaches a point where the nasal tip projects from the line of the nasal bridge. By pressing on the nasal tip, it is possible to make an immediate check of the dorsal line, which must be perfectly straight. Palpation and direct visualization will reveal any minute irregularities (Fig. 21-19). The removal of the cartilaginous portion of the hump included the hump portion of the upper lateral cartilages and the septal cartilage. After removing the cartilaginous hump, inspection of the area will often reveal a continuity of the mucosa extending from the remaining upper lateral cartilages to the septum (Fig. 21-20). It is important to preserve this continuity of mucosa when it exists, since it has been found to give a smooth appearance to the dorsum of the central third of the nasal bridge. In the patients with an extremely large hump, the mucosa is obviously amputated with removal of the hump. In these patients the surgeon will frequently see the edges of the bone and upper lateral cartilages showing through the dorsal skin, especially if the skin is thin. A definitive answer cannot be given at this time to this problem, but the submucosal dissection and preservation of the mucosa, as described by Jost [6], may be an answer.

Nasal Bone Fracture

The lateral osteotomy is the next step and is performed by placing a 4-mm. chisel at the pyriform fossa and piercing the vestibular skin. The chisel is turned at a 45-degree angle, and in a steplike manner, the lateral osteotomy is carried up to an imaginary horizontal line through the medial canthi. In performing the lateral osteotomy, a subperiosteal pocket is not necessary.

At this point, thumb pressure on the nasal bone will infracture the bone, unless it is too thick. If the bone does not infracture, the horizontal fracture is made by placing a 4-mm. chisel under the dorsal skin; usually two taps will produce the fracture (Fig. 21-21). It is important to note that it is rarely necessary to make the horizontal fracture line above the

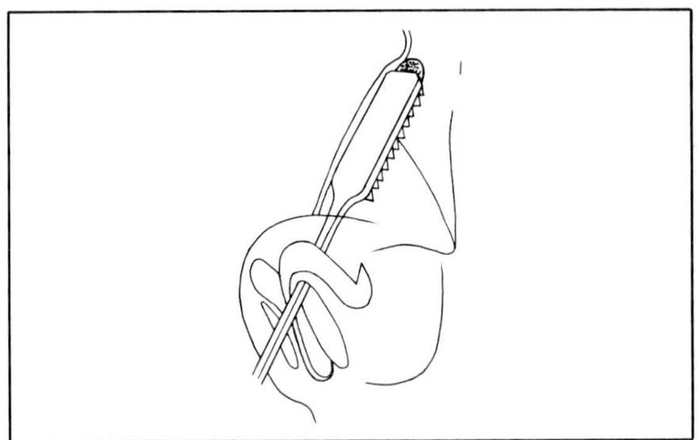

Fig. 21-17. The bridge is rasped with a pull-rasp (the secret to rasping is a sharp rasp).

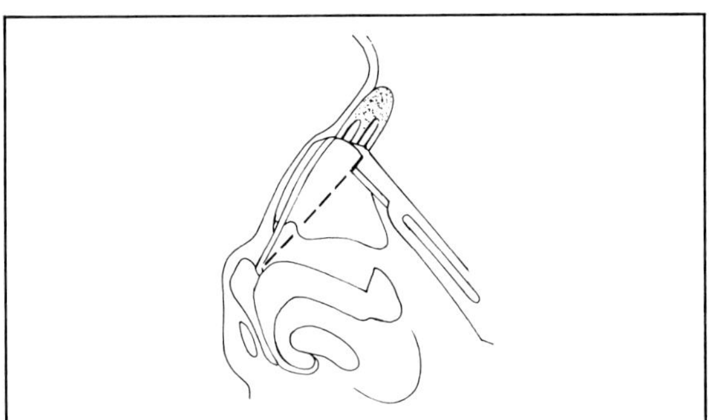

Fig. 21-18. The cartilaginous component of the hump is trimmed with the scalpel.

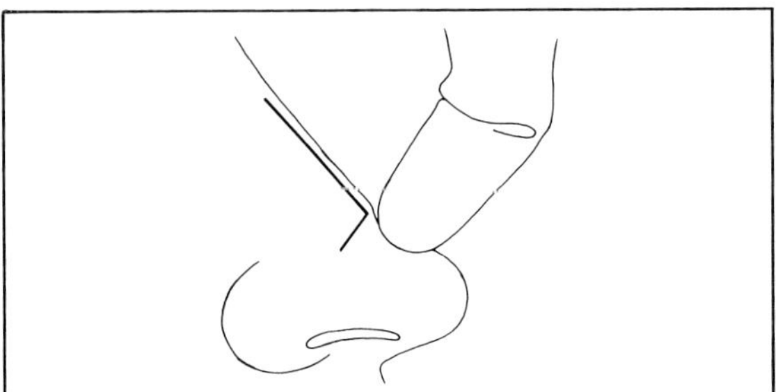

Fig. 21-19. By pressing on the nasal tip, the straight dorsal line can be seen, and any irregularities can be evaluated.

imaginary line through the medial canthi. The aim is to produce a narrowing of the nose between the glabella and the nasal tip. An attempt to produce a fracture line too high in the glabella is difficult and can prove disastrous, because of the thickness of the glabella in that area. It has been found that the fracture of the thin nasal bony plate at the point where

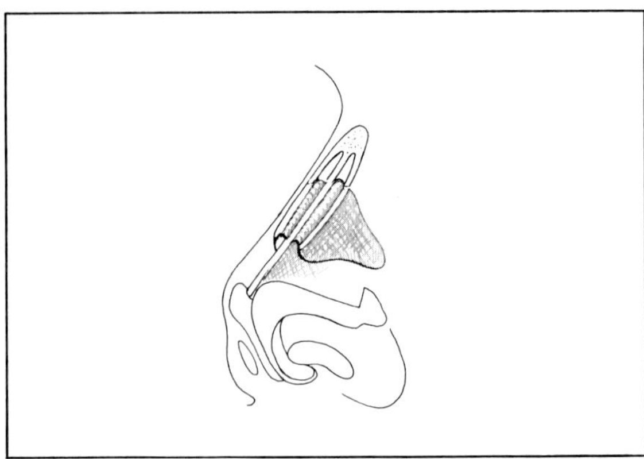

Fig. 21-20 If the mucosa between the septum and upper lateral cartilages is intact, it is preserved.

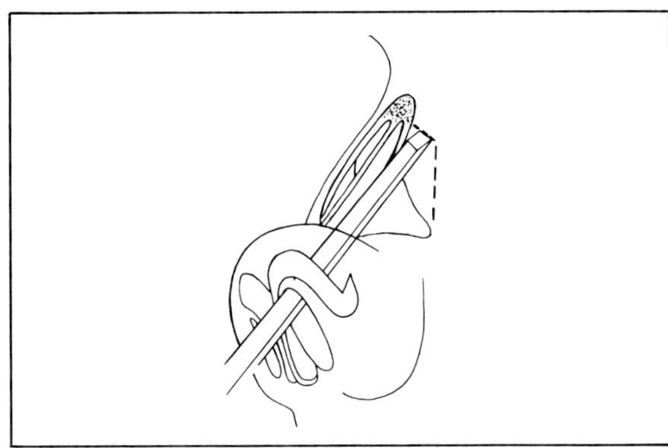

Fig. 21-21. The 4-mm. chisel can also be used to perform the horizontal osteotomy.

it meets the thick glabella is relatively safe and will produce an excellent aesthetic line (Fig. 21-22). With the hump reduced and the nasal bones infractured, it is necessary to make a final check of the dorsal bridge line. Sometimes slight irregularities that were not discernible will now become obvious; they are easily trimmed or rasped. At this time a thorough visual inspection of the hump area is made, looking for any irregularity or soft tissue excess. The nasal pocket is thoroughly cleaned out with a rongeur.

Upper Lateral Cartilages

The upper lateral cartilages are inspected. If the nasal tip has been appreciably elevated, the upper lateral cartilages may project caudally downward and will have to be trimmed (Fig. 21-23). However, the amount of trimming is usually minimal. Excess trimming of the caudal end of the upper lateral cartilages can produce an objectionable pinching in the middle

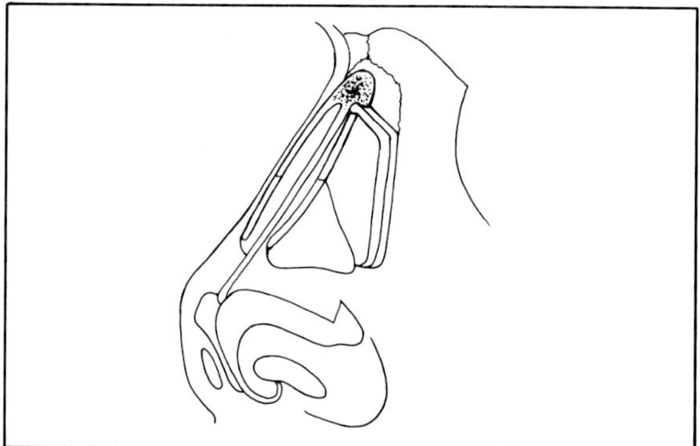

Fig. 21-22. The nasal bones are infractured. Note the level of the horizontal osteotomy and the glabella.

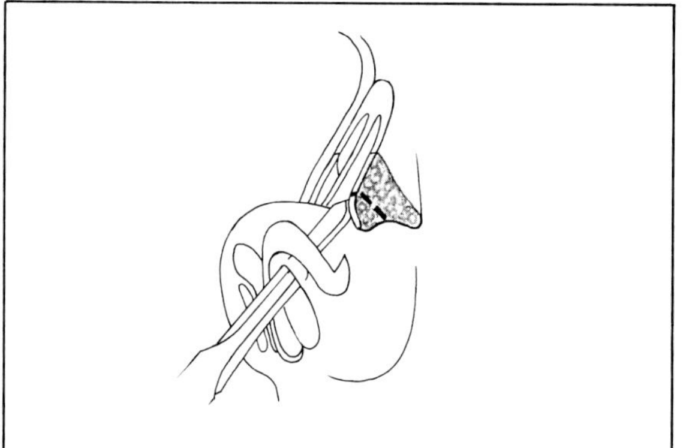

Fig. 21-23. The caudal ends of the upper lateral cartilages are trimmed if the nose has been shortened.

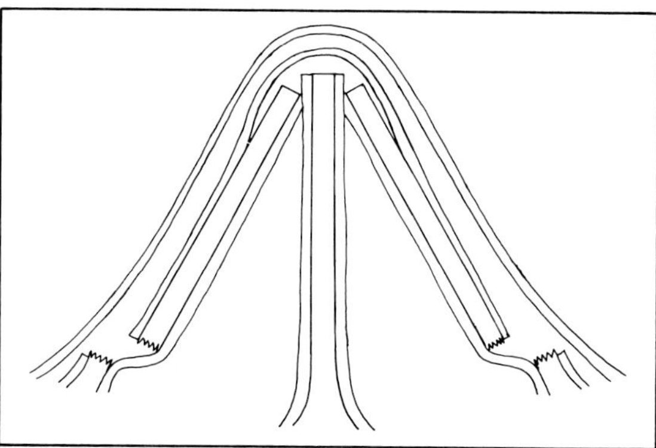

Fig. 21-24. At the lateral osteotomy, the nasal bones rarely, if ever, rest on the maxillary ledge. Note the preservation of periosteal attachment to the nasal bones.

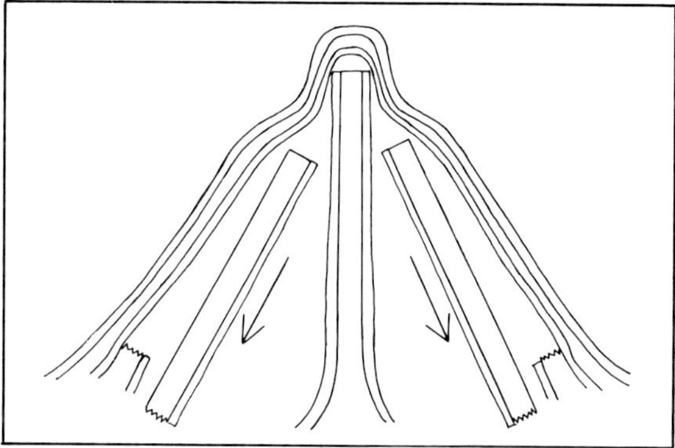

Fig. 21-25. The nasal bones can collapse into the nasal vault if all soft-tissue attachments are lost.

third of the nose. On the other hand, if a patient has a very wide central third of the nose, there are two adjunctive procedures to use. The fibrofatty tissue lying on the upper lateral cartilages between the skin and the cartilage is removed by sharp dissection. The mucosal attachment, if it exists, may also be separated between the upper lateral cartilages and the septum. This latter step skeletonizes the middle third of the nose; it should not be performed unless necessary in the nose with a wide bridge or thick skin.

It had been believed that infracture of the nasal bones would cause the nasal bones to be moved medially, to rest on the medial edge of the maxilla. This is not true, which has been confirmed by x-rays (modified Waters view). These x-rays showed a definite space between the maxillary ledge and the fractured nasal bone (Fig. 21-24). Therefore, it is important to remember that the nasal bones will be suspended by the soft tissue attachment to the bone. Elevation of the periosteal attachment can cause the nasal bones to fall into the nasal vault (Fig. 21-25). Thus, the periosteal and soft tissue attachment to the nasal bones must always be preserved.

The membranous columella and septum are now sutured with two transfixion sutures of 1-0 chromic catgut (Fig. 21-26). The nasal tip must not be distorted during this suturing. An attempt to raise the tip with the suture will not be successful. All redundant mucosa on the columellar septum must be trimmed.

Alar Rims

The alar rims are approached next. In 90 percent of patients it has been found that an alar base wedge resection is necessary to improve the flaring that exists in the alar rims. One can think of the tip projection as a tent pole. If the height of the tent pole

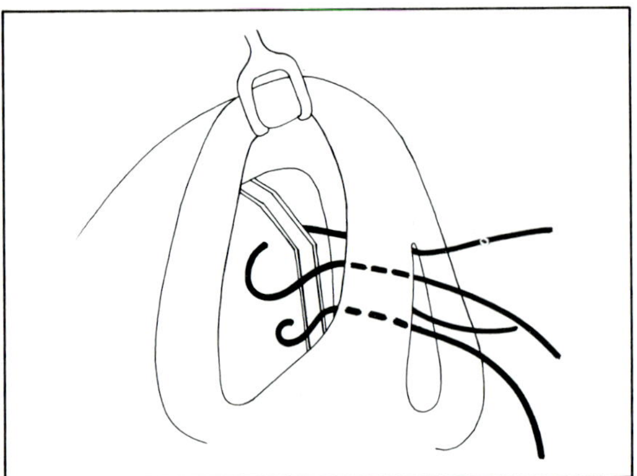

Fig. 21-26. The transfixion sutures close the septocolumellar incision. Attempts to raise or lower the tip with these sutures are fruitless.

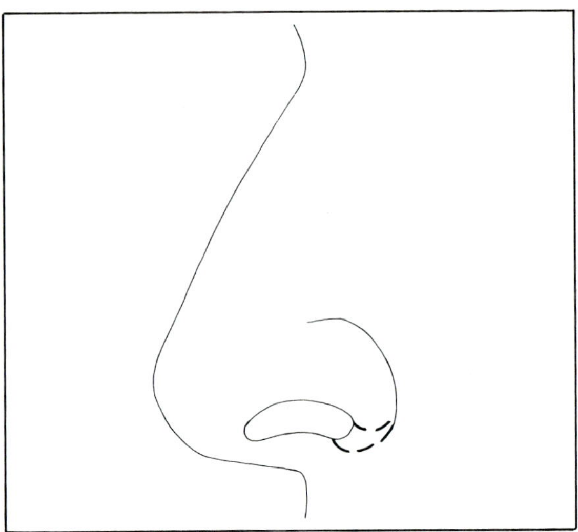

Fig. 21-27. The alar crease wedge excision. The dashed line is in the alar crease.

is lowered, a baggy tent results and it is necessary to reef in the tent sides at the base. The same is true in the nasal pyramid. In the "worm's eye view," the extent of flaring can be ascertained; it is corrected by excising a wedge from the nostril floor (Fig. 21-27). The incision begins in the alar floor and estends posteriorly in the alar crease. It is practically never essential to carry this incision in the crease more than 5 mm. The second incision removes the desired amount, making a pie-shaped excision of alar base. It might appear that the incision would go through-and-through into the vestibular floor in order to prevent a dog ear. However, this produces notching of the alar rim, which can be prevented by cutting horizontally across the alar rim (Fig. 21-28). The rim is sutured with 5-0 nylon; two or three sutures suffice, with either none in the crease, or a buried chromic catgut.

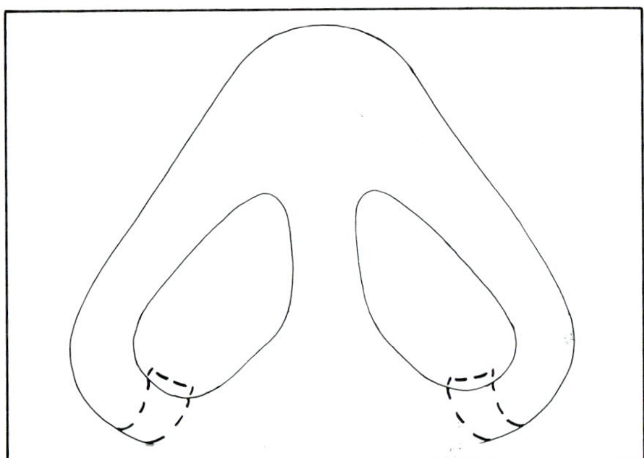

Fig. 21-28. The horizontal vestibular incision preserves vestibular skin and prevents alar rim notching.

Packing and Dressing

Before packing the intranasal passages, the dorsal pocket is suctioned of any blood clot. The packing consists of Oxycel cotton and Adaptic gauze or carbazine (½-in. wide). The nasal speculum is inserted into the nasal passageway, holding the dorsal vestibular skin in position as the packing is inserted. No suture of vestibular skin is necessary. The packing should occlude the passageway without distorting the nose or tip.

The nasal bridge is covered by ½-in. Steri-Strips, beginning from the supratip area and extending to the glabella. At this point one can see the newly created dorsal profile line and the tip setting out gracefully from the straight dorsal bridge line. The nasal bridge is tape-splinted and a dental stent (black compound) is applied over the bridge and forehead.

Crushed ice is placed in two surgical gloves, which are tied together and positioned over the eyes and against the dental stent.

Chin Implant

In order to achieve good profile symmetry, the balance between the forehead, nose, and chin is most important [3, 7]. An examination of the profile pictures will immediately determine the chin position. A simple criterion involves the examination of the position of the upper lip and chin. If the chin recedes behind the upper lip when a vertical line is dropped from the glabella through the upper lip, an augmentation of the chin will produce a better balance of the profile. The chin implant is Silastic, which can be carved to the desired shape; it may be placed in a pocket over the mental prominence. The approach may be either internal or external. In making the incision into the pocket, the portal to the pocket must always be smaller than the pocket so that the implant will not work back to the incision. After suturing the incision, the chin should be tape-splinted for occlusive pressure. It is not necessary to use sutures to hold the implant in the pocket, since the pocket should be made only as large as the implant. In this manner, migration of the implant is almost always prevented [9].

RHINOPLASTY IN THE ADOLESCENT

The techniques that have been described have been utilized in adolescents between the ages of 13 and 15 years with no signs of further growth of the nose or of any adverse changes of nasal physiology. The indications for surgery are a matured, large nose with a high projecting nasal tip. If the nasal tip projection is short, surgery should not be done until growth has ceased. Of primary concern in the nasal tip surgery is the preservation of the continuity of the alar cartilage.

RHINOPLASTY IN THE ELDERLY

The techniques as described have been used in patients up to the age of 65 years. Age is not a contraindication to rhinoplasty, and fear of redundant skin is unwarranted. Peterson [13] described an open-flap rhinoplasty utilizing an inconspicuous external excision at the glabella. Rhinoplasty in the elderly can be an important adjunct to face lifting. If the surgeon makes a face look younger with a face lift when the nose is old looking, the purpose of the procedure is defeated.

REFERENCES

1. Aufricht, G. Joseph's rhinoplasty with some modifications. *Surg. Clin. North Am.* 51:299, 1971.
2. Aufricht, G. Total Concept of Rhinoplasty. In Millard, D. R. (Ed.), *Symposium on Corrective Rhinoplasty.* St. Louis: Mosby, 1976.
3. González-Ulloa, M. Quantitative principles in cosmetic surgery of the face (profileplasty). *Plast. Reconstr. Surg.* 29:186, 1962.
4. Gordon, H., and Baker, T. Primary cosmetic rhinoplasty. *Clin. Plast. Surg.* 4:9, 1977.
5. Joseph, J. *Nasenplastik und sonstige Gesichtsplastik nebst Mammoplastik.* Oxford, England: Meeuws, 1931.
6. Jost, G. Defaut de projection de la pointe du nez. *Ann. Chir. Plast.* 17:245, 1972.
7. Lewis, J. The Nasal Profile. In Millard, D. R. (Ed.), *Symposium on Corrective Rhinoplasty.* St. Louis: Mosby, 1976.
8. Lipsett, E. A new approach to surgery of the lower cartilaginous vault. *Arch. Otolaryngol.* 70:42, 1959.
9. Millard, D. Adjuncts in augmentation mentoplasty and corrective rhinoplasty. *Plast. Reconstr. Surg.* 36:48, 1965.
10. Peck, G. C. Surgery of the Nasal Tip. In Millard, D. R. (Ed.), *Symposium on Aesthetic Surgery of the Nose, Ears and Chin.* St. Louis: Mosby, 1976.
11. Peck, G. C. Sculpturing the Nasal Tip. In Millard, D. R. (Ed.), *Symposium on Corrective Rhinoplasty.* St. Louis: Mosby, 1976.
12. Peck, G. C. The difficult nasal tip. *Clin. Plast. Surg.* 4:103, 1977.
13. Peterson, R. Open-flap Rhinoplasty. In Millard, D. R. (Ed.), *Symposium on Corrective Rhinoplasty.* St. Louis: Mosby, 1976.
14. Rees, T., and Wood-Smith, D. *Cosmetic Facial Surgery.* Philadelphia: Saunders, 1973.
15. Rogers, B. O. Rhinoplasty. In Goldwyn, R. (Ed.), *The Unfavorable Result in Plastic Surgery: Avoidance and Treatment.* Boston: Little, Brown, 1972.
16. Safian, J. Fact and fallacy in rhinoplastic surgery. *Br. J. Surg.* 11:45, 1958.
17. Sheen, J. Achieving more nasal tip projection by the use of a small autogenous bone or cartilage graft. *Plast. Reconstr. Surg.* 56:35, 1975.
18. Sheen, J. Secondary rhinoplasty. *Plast. Reconstr. Surg.* 57:137, 1975.
19. Sheen, J. Finesse in Rhinoplasty. In Millard, D. R. (Ed.). *Symposium on Corrective Rhinoplasty.* St. Louis: Mosby, 1976.
20. Williams, J. Pinched nasal tip. *Clin. Plast. Surg.* 4:41, 1977.

22

Secondary Rhinoplasty

JACK H. SHEEN

It is better to consider secondary rhinoplasty in terms of rehabilitation rather than of revision. Unsatisfactory primary rhinoplasty frequently causes functional and aesthetic impairment due to tissue deficit and damage. To say surgical revision or "redoing it" does not fully acknowledge the need to deal with a new set of problems, not just to find new or better ways to deal with the original problems.

Usually the major goals of a secondary procedure are to restore nasal function and to restore nasal contour to a near-normal condition, that is, to rehabilitate the nose. Scarring, tissue deficit, and decreased vascularity are factors that, if the surgeon fails to recognize their significance, may foil attempts at secondary correction.

Since secondary rhinoplasty requires the recognition and skillful treatment of special problems which worsen with each subsequent procedure (often causing irreversible tissue damage), it may be a disservice to patients to refer them back to their original surgeons who performed two or more unsuccessful operations. Patients must be spared the devastating effects of a series of untoward rhinoplasties.

GROUND RULES FOR SECONDARY RHINOPLASTY

Because of the singularity and complexity of the problems in secondary rhinoplasty, there cannot be a standardized technique. However, there are ground rules that should be followed for a successful result:

1. Defer surgery until there is final resolution of tissues.
2. Limit the surgical dissection.
3. Use only autogenous graft material.
4. Have a well-defined aesthetic goal.

Defer Surgery

Minor surgical revision can be performed in six months; however, major reconstruction should be deferred for at least one year. In some cases, two or more years are required for final resolution of tissues. The number and extent of prior procedures and the extent of the planned reconstruction are determinants for the timing of secondary rhinoplasty.

Limit the Surgical Dissection

The surgeon should dissect only those areas that require surgical correction. A major difference between virgin and operated tissues is the decreased vascularity present in the latter. Injudicious undermining or incisions can further compromise vascularity, thereby sabotaging what might otherwise have been a good result.

Use Only Autogenous Graft Material

The use of alloplastic material in secondary rhinoplasty is detrimental to the patient because of its poor long-term acceptance in the operated nose. The use of synthetic material is responsible for a high percentage of irreparably deformed noses since the tissues respond to infection and extrusion of the implants by disfiguring scarring (Fig. 22-1).

Autographs of septal tissues, ear cartilage, rib bone, or cartilage and iliac bone are readily obtainable and provide the best chance for a permanent result.

Have A Well-Defined Aesthetic Goal

A well-defined aesthetic goal is not a vague generalization, but rather a clearly defined set of relationships that harmoniously integrate all of the anatomical parts of the nose.

With the above ground rules in mind, I will discuss the obtainment of graft material and its application to the most common problems in secondary rhinoplasty.

SEPTAL CARTILAGE

Whereas proficiency in the techniques of septal surgery is helpful for the plastic surgeon performing primary rhinoplasty, it is absolutely essential for the surgeon attempting to do secondary rhinoplasty because: (1) The patient requesting a secondary procedure usually has nasal airway impairment and (2) septal cartilage is the best material for nasal reconstruction. Improving the appearance of the nose using material removed to improve function is a winning combination. The surgeon's ability to extract the necessary material without jeopardizing the structure or function of the nose can make the difference between success and failure.

To harvest septal cartilage one must use an instrument that will provide as much cartilage as possible in continuity with ethmoid to obtain optimum length of the graft. For this reason the use of a Ballenger knife is discouraged. In addition, the Ballenger knife cannot cross the osseochondral junction and is therefore useless for the correction of functional problems involving the ethmoid or vomer. The Jackson nasal scissors is ideally suited to obtain excellent strips of donor

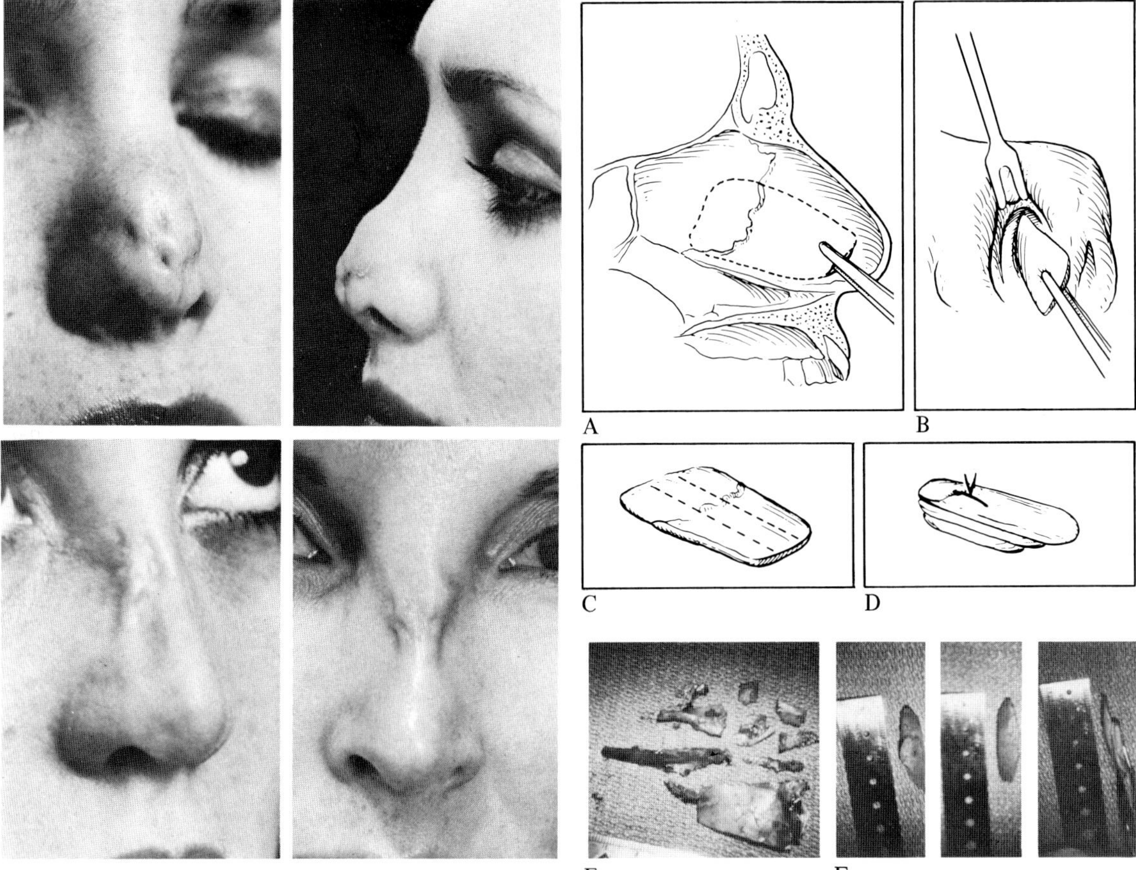

Fig. 22-1. Patients following extrusion of alloplastic material with subsequent disfigurement.

Fig. 22-2. A–D, available donor area and planned dorsal graft. E, F, septal material obtained and dorsal graft ready for insertion.

cartilage with ethmoid attached and can easily transect irregular or distorted ethmoid and occasionally can be used to sever parts of the vomer.

Figure 22-2A illustrates the available donor area of the septum. Beveled septal cartilage can nicely reduplicate the dorsum and has the effect of realigning the nasal contour by providing a straight, central framework for the soft tissues. The planning and preparation of a three-tiered graft for dorsal augmentation are shown in Figure 22-2C and D. E and F are photographs of the material obtained and the prepared graft ready for insertion.

The patient on whom this graft was used is 23 years old, shown ten years following a primary rhinoplasty (Fig. 22-3A). In Figure 22-3B the patient is shown following insertion of the above graft. Revision of the irregular tip cartilages and chin augmentation were also done.

EAR CARTILAGE

Ear cartilage provides an abundant and readily available source of reconstructive material. The natural convolution of ear cartilage can make a superb dorsal graft. In obtaining ear cartilage, the anterior approach, as described by Burt Brent [1], is the simplest and the least deforming technique. It also produces the maximum amount of cartilage. Ear cartilage cannot be crushed or trimmed as satisfactorily as septal cartilage. However, it is more elastic and can be rolled into a usable graft and secured by nonabsorbable circumferential sutures.

Figure 22-4 illustrates a specimen obtained from the concha of an ear using the anterior approach. This maximal amount should be resected only if it is needed. Since structure of the ear is better if the concha cavum remains, just that amount necessary for a dorsal graft is removed.

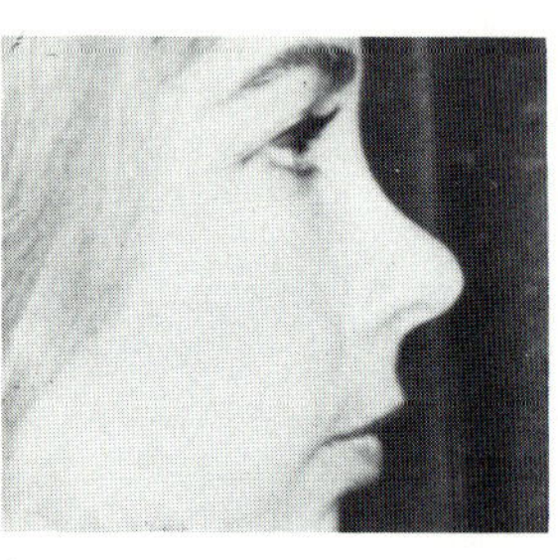
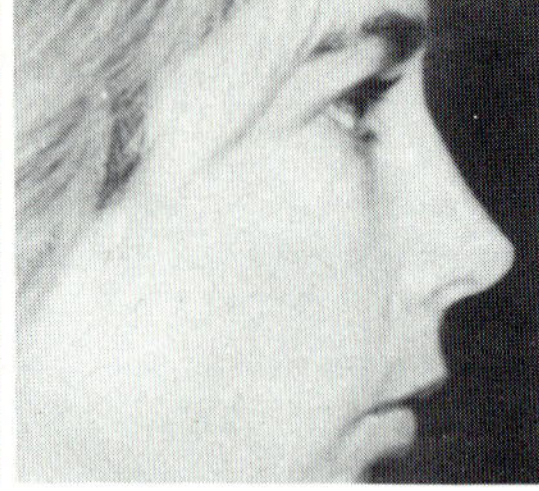

A B

Fig. 22-3. A, patient prior to insertion of graft (Fig. 22-2F). B, following insertion of graft and chin augmentation.

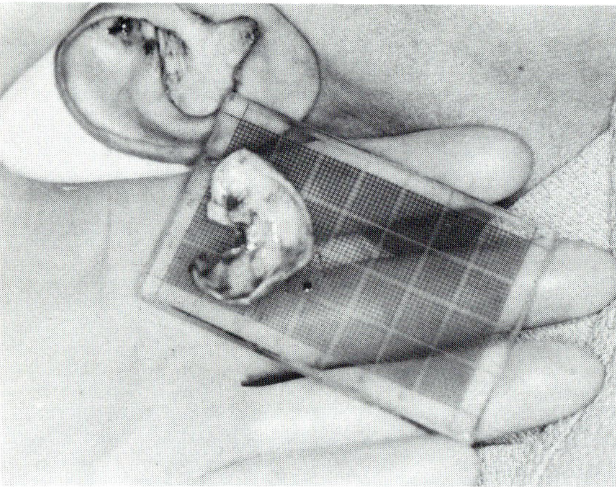

Fig. 22-4. Conchal cartilage graft following removal from ear using Brent anterior approach.

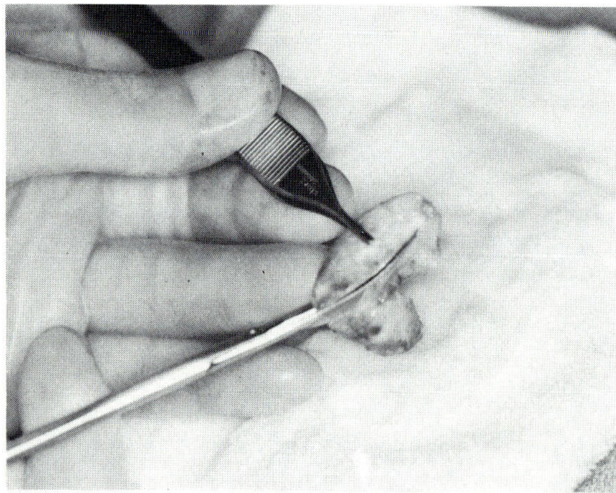

Fig. 22-5. Careful planning ensures the largest usable contour of the graft.

The graft should be designed so that the longest, most uniform part is obtained (Fig. 22-5). Most often the concha cavum is not used.

The completed graft (Fig. 22-6A, B), shown on dorsal and ventral views, demonstrates the use of circumferential nonabsorbable sutures to maintain form. The height and the width of the graft can be controlled using this technique.

The patient shown in Figure 22-7A, C had undergone five prior surgeries, which included removal of most of the bony and cartilaginous septum. There was a 1½-cm. perforation at the angle of the septum. An alloplastic implant had been inserted through the tip, followed by infection and rejection, leaving a central scar and more distortion. The specimen shown in Figure 22-6A was used in the reconstruction of the dorsum. The effect of straightening the nose is apparent (Fig. 22-7B, D) with the new straight dorsal framework. In addition, the patient had bilateral flap rotations from the posterior membranous septum to close the septal perforation, a tip graft, lateral wall augmentation, and ethmoid bone grafts to the alar rims.

THE FLAT TIP

A flattened, round, and nonprojecting tip is a hallmark of the secondary rhinoplasty patient. A loss of tip definition usually is the result of surgical overtreatment of the lower lateral cartilages during primary rhinoplasty.

The use of supportive tip grafts of septal cartilage [2, 3] has proved to be a suitable method for achieving more projection of the nasal tip. Septal cartilage is the material of choice and has no equal. Ear cartilage may be used successfully, but too often lacks the necessary rigidity. Vomer has the necessary rigidity; however, it may be absorbed.

The patient in Figure 22-8A, B illustrates the dramatic effect of tip elevation on a secondary rhinoplasty patient whose flattened nasal tip was the primary cause of the unsatisfactory appearance of her nose.

THE CROOKED NOSE

Crookedness is frequently the result of asymmetry of lateral contour rather than deviation of the central skeleton. Septal cartilage, intact or crushed, can be used to fill out lateral concavities to create the appearance of straightness.

The 44-year-old patient shown in Figure 22-9A had a crooked nose that was a consequence of asymmetrical medial movement of nasal bones following osteotomy. The left nasal bone moved in too far because of the concavity of the septum on that side – the right nasal bone was held out laterally by the septal convexity on the right. Following correction of the septal impac-

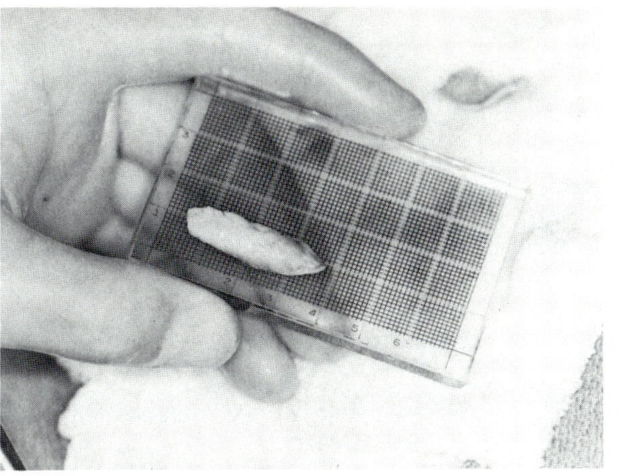

A

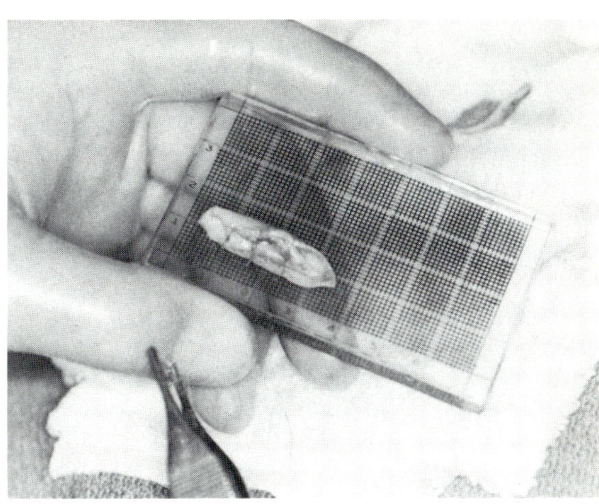

B

Fig. 22-6. A, dorsal view of prepared graft prior to insertion. B, ventral view of graft.

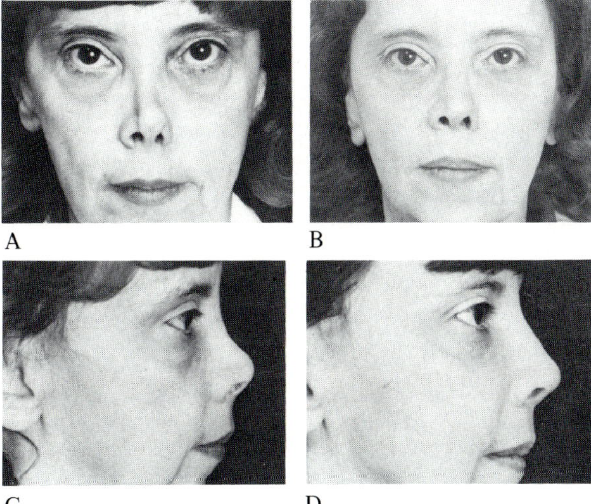

A B C D

Fig. 22-7. A, C, patient following five procedures with no septal cartilage or bone available. B, D, following sixth procedure using ear cartilage graft for reconstruction.

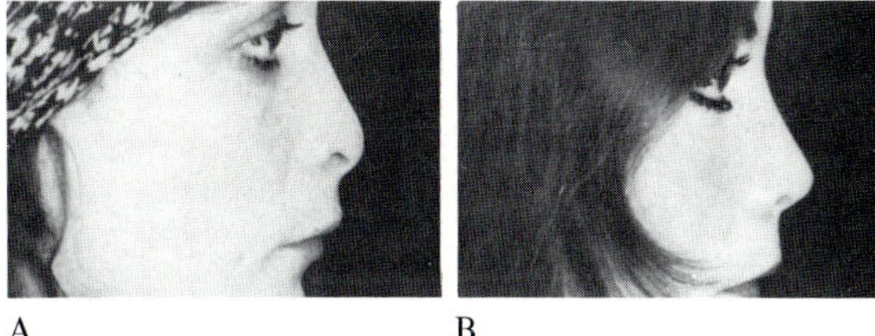

A B

Fig. 22-8. A, patient with flattened nasal tip following primary rhinoplasty. B, following secondary rhinoplasty which included use of septal cartilage tip graft.

tion against the right nasal bone, crushed cartilage was used to reform the contour of the nose providing the illusion of straightness (Fig. 22-9B). No fractures of nasal bones were done.

Occasionally, a single dorsal graft can provide the illusion of straightness by creating a straight and uniform dorsal support. Often this must be combined with lateral grafts, especially in patients who have very thin tissues; otherwise the edges of dorsal graft become visible as lateral walls sink.

The patient in Figure 22-10A had a low dorsum and a crooked-appearing nose following two previous rhinoplasties. A dorsal graft of ear cartilage provided a more symmetrical nasal contour that showed less evidence of surgery.

SUPRATIP DEFORMITY

The terms *supratip deformity, ram's head deformity,* and *parrot's beak* or *poly beak deformity* are used synonomously to describe a postsurgical fullness or convexity of the dorsal line, cephalad to the nasal tip. This is not the transient supratip swelling which frequently occurs in the immediate postoperative period, but it is a supratip fullness which is definite and persistent.

This unattractive hump of tissue is one of the most frequently found complications following primary rhinoplasty and though it has been recognized and

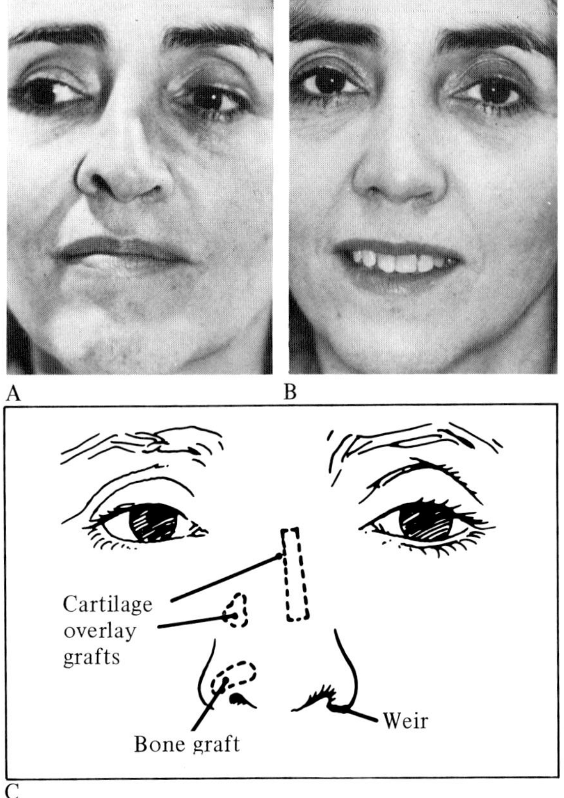

Fig. 22-9. A, B, frequently patients can have crooked appearing noses straightened by lateral onlay grafts of cartilage which provide the illusion of straightness as illustrated by this patient. C, schematic drawing of graft placement.

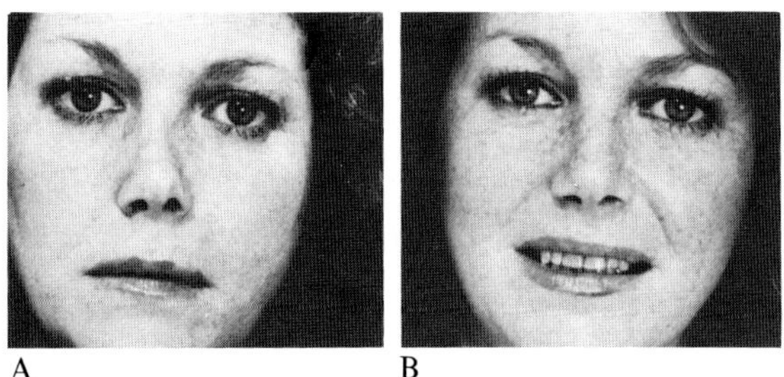

Fig. 22-10. Straightening nasal contour using ear cartilage graft which provided a straight dorsal edge on tissues to drape over. Lateral grafts were also used.

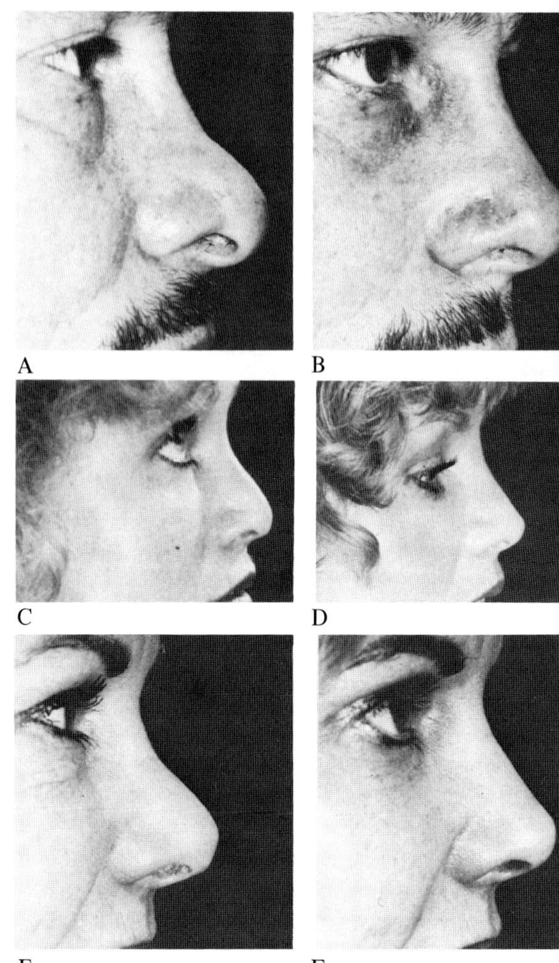

Fig. 22-11. Patients with supratip deformity treated by augmentation. No dorsal tissues were resected from any of patients shown.

described, I think that the problem and treatment have not been clearly understood.

In my opinion, the most frequent cause of supratip deformity is the reduction of dorsal skeleton to the point where the overlying soft tissue cannot drape over it. The thin tissue overlying the upper third of the nose tends to contract easily to the reduced dorsum, whereas the tissue overlying the caudal part of the nose does not. If this theory is correct, augmentation of the dorsal skeleton would correct the problem. And in my experience, this has proved to be true.

One hundred consecutive secondary rhinoplasty patients on whom I operated during 1978 were analyzed as follows:

Males	23
Females	77
Average age	28.9 (youngest 16/oldest 67)
Average number of procedures	1.7 (greatest number 8)

The treatments employed were:

Dorsal augmentation	82 (with or without tip graft)
Tip augmentation only	8
Reduction of dorsum	8
External excision	7 (5 with dorsal augmentation)
Supratip thinning	0

It is of significance that 82 percent of the patients in this series were treated by augmentation. Resection of scar tissue was not done in any of the cases.

The series of patients shown in Figure 22-11A-F all have varying degrees of supratip fullness. Each of these patients was treated with dorsal augmentation without resection of any tissues to achieve the results presented.

REFERENCES

1. Brent, B. Personal communication, 1977.
2. Brown, J. B. Secondary Nasal Operations. In *Plastic Surgery of the Nose* (2d ed.). Springfield, Ill.: Thomas, 1965.
3. Converse, J. M., et al. Rhinoplasty. In J. M. Converse (Ed.), *Reconstructive Plastic Surgery*. Philadelphia: Saunders, 1964.
4. Goldwyn, R. M. *The Unfavorable Result in Plastic Surgery*. Boston: Little, Brown, 1972.
5. Millard, D. R. Secondary corrective rhinoplasty. *Plast. Reconstr. Surg.* 15:404, 1955.
6. Peer, L. A. Fate of Autogenous septal cartilage after transplantation in human tissue. *Arch Otolaryng.* 34:697, 1941.
7. Rees, T. D., Krupp, S., and Wood-Smith, D. Secondary rhinoplasty. *Plast. Reconstr. Surg.* 46:332, 1970.
8. Rogers, B. O. The importance of delay in timing secondary and tertiary corrections of post-rhinoplastic deformities. In *Trans. Fourth Internat. Cong. Plast. Reconstr. Surg.* Amsterdam: Excerpta Medica, 1967.
9. Sheen, J. H. Achieving more nasal tip projection by the use of a small autogenous bone or cartilage graft. *Plast. Reconstr. Surg.* 56:35, 1975.
10. Sheen, J. H. *Aesthetic Rhinoplasty*. St. Louis: Mosby, 1978.
11. Sheen, J. H. Secondary rhinoplasty. *Plast. Reconstr. Surg.* 56:135, 1975.

Deformities of the Ears

STEN J. STENSTRÖM

This chapter is primarily devoted to the subject of *prominent ears, lop ears, invaginated ears, shell ears,* and *satyr ears.*

ANATOMY

The external ear is formed embryonically from the mandibular and hyoid portions of the branchial arches. The former contributes to the tragus, crus helicis, and conchal floor and the latter to the remaining portions, which amount to approximately 85 percent of the adult auricle (Fig. 23-1) [35].

The *framework* of the auricle consists of a single piece of yellow fibrocartilage with a complicated relief on the anterior, concave side and a fairly smooth configuration on the posterior, convex side. The covering skin is thin and firmly adherent on the anterior surface but movable on the posterior surface. The Darwinian tubercle, which is present in some people, lies in the descending part of the helix and corresponds to the true ear tip of the long-eared mammals [30]. The lobule merely contains subcutaneous tissue.

The profuse *blood supply* of the auricle is derived from the superficial temporal and posterior auricular arteries. Venous drainage is by way of the external jugular and the superficial temporal veins. Lymphatic drainage goes into the lymph nodes near the mastoid tip.

The normal auricle is said to be attached to the head at an angle of about 30 degrees. More exact specifications indicate an *average angle between the auricular and median planes* of 25 to 26 degrees in boys and 17 to 18 degrees in girls, between the ages of 8 and 16 years. It is considered that the right ear often protrudes from the head about 1 degree more than the left [19].

There are two angles in the postauricular space, one between the skull and the concha (cephalochonchal angle) and another between the concha and the scapha (scaphoconchal angle). The *cephaloconchal angle* is, broadly speaking, the same in all ears and averages about 90 degrees. The size of the *scaphoconchal angle,* on the other hand, varies considerably; in the normal ear this angle is about 90 degrees, but it may be as much as 120 degrees [21].

The ear may also vary in its vertical position. Normally the opening of the external auditory meatus is located at the level of the upper margin of the ala nasi [18].

According to several authors, the ear is almost fully grown at the age of 7 or 8. It has been shown recently on the basis of a large series that in the average child at 3 years of age, 85 percent of ear development has been achieved. Growth in the height of the ear continues until into adulthood. The width and the distance of the ear from the scalp change little after 10 years of age. The average adult sizes are described as 6.5 cm. in length and 3.5 cm. in width. The two ears of the same individual often vary in size and shape [28].

A striking difference in the size of the ears has been observed among different races [2]. The longest and widest ears are found among Asiatics (Alaskan Eskimos). Negroes have the shortest ears, while Caucasians have ears of medium length but similar to the Negroes' ears in width. A racial characteristic of the Japanese is the direct connection between the lobule and the skin of the upper neck [3].

PROMINENT EARS

Ears appear especially prominent when there is an increased scaphoconchal angle, an increased height of the posterior conchal wall, or a combination of the two. This prominence may be unilateral or bilateral. In the bilateral cases, there is often a difference between the two sides as to the degree of protrusion. Two centimeters appears to be the upper limit of normal in measuring between superior helical rim and the scalp.

Whether or not an ear appears to be prominent may depend on its size [13]. A small ear may appear quite normal even if the scaphoconchal angle is very wide, whereas a large ear with a similarly obtuse antihelical fold can seem prominent. Children's ears, because of early maturation, are comparatively large in relation to the size of their heads. One may judge a child's ears to be prominent, only to find later that the deformity becomes less noticeable or disappears altogether as the head grows.

These ear deformities have been given many names, but as yet none has gained general acceptance. Though the term *lop ear* is often used, it must be considered to be grammatically incorrect. McEvitt [21] maintains quite appropriately that "lop means to hang limply, and the protruding ear certainly does not hang and is anything but limp." Other terms include *protruding ears, outstanding ears, bat ears, flaring ears, obtrusive ears, unfolded ears,* and *obtusely*

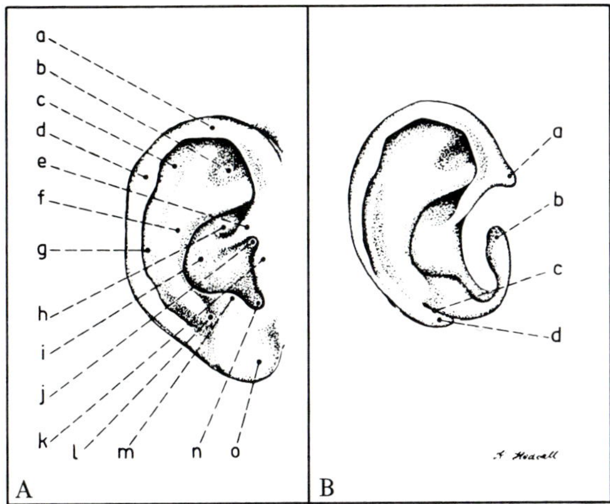

Fig. 23-1. Diagram of the normal ear. A, front view of the auricular prominences and depressions. a, helix with ascending (in front), horizontal, and descending parts; b, fossa triangularis; c, fossa helicis; d, Darwin's tubercle; e, crus helicis; f, antihelix with anterior crus (plica principalis) and posterior crus; g, scapha; h, cymba conchae; i, cavum conchae; j. incisura anterior; k, tragus; l, sulcus auriculae posterior; m, antitragus; n, incisura intertragica; o, lobulus. B, front view of the cartilaginous framework. a, spina helicis; b, lamina tragi; c, fissura antitragico-helicina; d, cauda helicis (tail of the helix).

angulated ears. As Tucker [42] pointed out, a number of these appellations are inaccurate. He suggested instead the term *prominauris,* made up of Latin roots, and meaning projecting ear. I prefer the term *prominent ears.*

Indications and Timing for Correction of Prominent Ears

The primary reason for operating on prominent ears is to eliminate the psychological effect that the ear deformitv produces. Ju [14] has discussed this deformity in relation to its psychological effect. Many children have become emotionally disturbed as they are reminded again and again of their deformity. I recall a 6-year-old boy with prominent ears who had suffered from the misunderstanding and cruelty of those around him. When he was warned that he would feel a little pain from the anesthetic needle, he declared, "I don't care a jot how much it hurts as long as I'm made well and they don't call me Mickey Mouse any more."

Women can conceal a moderate degree of ear deformity with their hair. If the ears are very prominent, practically no hair style can hide them.

The ideal time for the correction of prominent ears is considered to be during the year or two before a child starts school. In the preschool age group the deformity is often unnoticed by playmates and so the psychic trauma is minimized. Once school begins, however, the situation changes.

Principal Methods of Correcting Prominent Ears

In 1845 Dieffenbach [9] suggested the removal of a wedge of skin from the postauricular sulcus. This procedure can be considered in the first group of otoplasty techniques. Now reduction of the cephaloconchal angle and an abnormal conchal depth is performed by conchal-mastoid sutures [10] or excision of conchal cartilage [29, 32, 33].

The most important cause of an ear's prominence is that the antihelical fold is not sufficiently pronounced, and hence the scaphoconchal angle is abnormally large. Luckett [20] was the first person to clearly describe this flattening of the antihelical fold. He described an operation to excise a strip of skin and cartilage on the posterior auricular surface along the future antihelical line and to evert the cut edges of the cartilage with Lembert sutures, thus forming an antihelical ridge on the anterior surface. Luckett's method and the many variations of it, representing the second otoplasty group, thus entail *cutting through the full thickness of the cartilage, which unfortunately tends to create a sharp antihelical fold.* This is not so, however, in the case of "tubing" of the antihelix and posterior crus [7, 40, 41].

A third group of operational techniques provides a more smoothly rounded contour of the antihelix by leaving the anterior surface of the ear intact when *the cartilage is thinned out in various ways on the posterior surface* along the line of the desired fold. Pierce and colleagues [27] seem to have been the first advocates of this treatment. They recommended the use of 8 to 10 parallel incisions along the future antihelical sulcus. I used their method for a time but later slightly modified it, scratching the cartilage with 15 to 20 razor blades bound together in a holder. In this way the scratching was very superficial and the risk of the knife slipping through the cartilage was eliminated.

A fourth otoplasty technique, described by Mustardé, produces folding of the antihelix by means of permanent matress sutures inserted at the base of the fold from behind the ear after removing an ellipse of postauricular skin [6, 22–24].

A fifth otoplasty technique involves the *morsalization of a 6-mm. width of auricular cartilage along the line of the proposed antihelical fold.* After excising postauricular skin and undermining the anterior auricular skin as described by the author below, a curved double-bladed morsalizing instrument is inserted near the tail of the helix. The multitoothed opposing blades of the morsalizer break up the architecture of the cartilage, releasing its spring. Morsalization is carried over into the upper posterior conchal wall and along the entire antihelical fold to produce a wide smooth fold that can be maintained with permanent Mustardé-type sutures in the cartilage [11a].

A sixth otoplasty group is composed of those techniques that wholly or partially *exploit the tendency of the cartilage to curl away from the side where it is scratched or thinned* [5, 15, 25, 37, 44]. In these cases, too, the antihelical fold acquires a smoothly rounded contour. I described a technique of this kind in 1961 [36, 39].

Why the Scratched Ear Bends Toward the Side of the Skull

Bergman and Stenström [4] have shown that there is good reason to believe that, contrary to current opinion, *it is the perichondrium that causes the ear cartilage, and also other types of cartilage, to curl.* When the cartilage is split up into fine sections parallel to the surface, this curling tendency may still be there to some degree, even after one has observed macroscopically that the perichondrium level has been passed. However, microscopic examination discloses remains of the perichondrium in the diffuse transitional area before the pure cartilage tissue is reached. In the pure cartilage, no curling occurs whatsoever. This finding would seem to indicate that, using my scratching method, reduction of the perichondrium on the anterior side of the ear cartilage leads to contraction of the intact perichondrium on the posterior side. Thus a curling of the ear back toward the skull takes place. The strongest evidence for the importance of the perichondrium would seem to be the fact that where there is no perichondrium the cartilage lacks the capacity to curl.

Author's Method of Correcting Prominent Ears

After the operative field has been thoroughly cleaned, it is draped by rolling a length of stockinette over the head and neck, a procedure recommended by Gelb and described by Stark [34]. The stockinette material is kept in sterilized packs, having previously been cut to a suitable length, rolled up to form a ring, and knotted at one end. After the stockinette has been applied, it is tied around the neck by making a cut up each side and knotting the resultant corners together. The ears are exposed through very small apertures. If the patient has long hair, it is fastened above and behind the ears with rubber bands or tape before draping to prevent it from contaminating the operative field. If the ears are to be made symmetrical, it is absolutely essential that the position of both ears be compared during the operation.

Either local or general anesthesia can be used for this operation. Young children usually require general anesthesia, and patients over 10 years of age usually do well under local anesthesia, if properly sedated. Local anesthesia is obtained by infiltrating the local anesthetic agent, with a vasoconstrictor, circumferentially around the base of the auricle and also around the external auditory canal orifice.

The first step in the operation is to fold the ear back in order to produce the new antihelical and posterior crural folds, which are then outlined with dye. When the posterior conchal wall is high, it is important to mark the new antihelical fold part way down the posterior wall. A traction suture is inserted through the middle of the descending helix to hold the ear forward. A plug of gauze is placed in the auditory canal to prevent blood from collecting there.

EXPOSING THE EAR CARTILAGE. The preliminary planned skin excision on the posterior side of the ear is drawn with parallel sides and pointed ends, with the course of the new antihelical fold and posterior crus serving as the axis (Fig. 23-2A). The proximal side is marked particularly clearly, for it must be visible even during the closing stages of the operation. Five diagonal lines mark the corresponding points on both sides. They are useful when the ears are sutured at the end of the operation.

First an incision is made along the distal side and a flap is undermined and based along the proximal side (Fig. 23-2B). The tail of the helix is exposed together with a large part of the descending helix, thereby affording good access to the anterior surface of the cartilage. Undermining is then performed over the entire anterior area except the conchal bottom.

SCRATCHING. This should be performed over the entire anterior cartilage surface, but with more intensity along the antihelix, anterior and posterior crura, and posterior conchal wall (Fig. 23-2C). The effect of the scratching instrument* on the cartilage surface can easily be checked visually. Special attention must be given to those parts that are particularly resistant. This is almost always the case with the lower part of the descending helix. If the posterior conchal wall is too high, it is lowered by a deepening of the cleft between the tail of the helix and the concha and by extra scratching of the upper part of the conchal wall. The deepening incision should gently slant 10 to 15 mm. in direction toward the conchal bottom.

As far as is possible all scratching should be performed with one finger on the posterior side of the ear, pushing the cartilage forward to convexity (Fig.

*Available from Stille-Depuy Inc., Warsaw, Indiana 46580, or Stille-Werner, P.O. Box 4051, S-10261 Stockholm 4, Sweden.

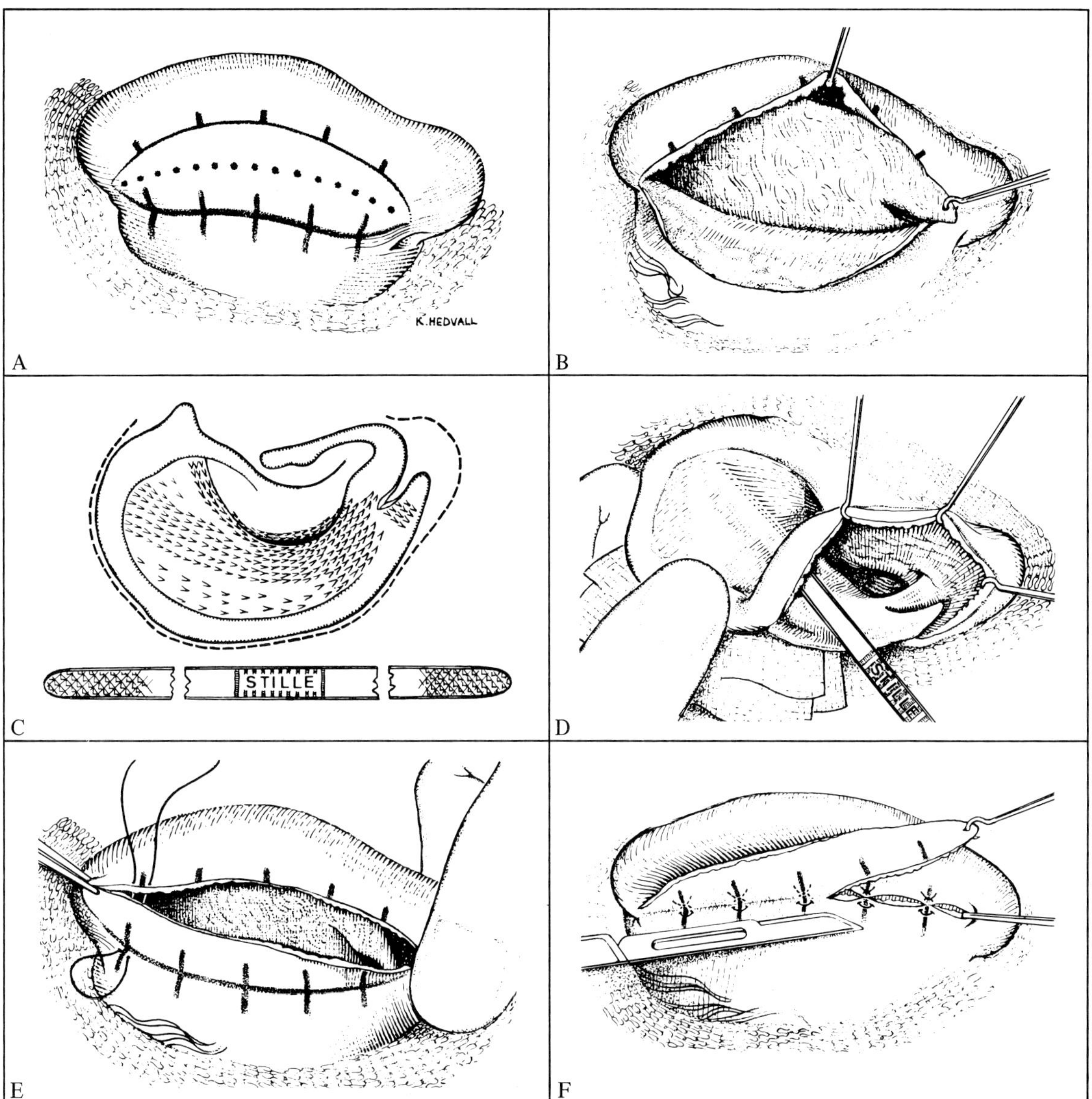

Fig. 23-2. Otoplasty for prominent ear. A, diagram showing the approximate dimensions of the later skin excision of the posterior auricular surface. The dotted line corresponds to the course of the new antihelix. B, the circumscribed area is raised as a flap based along the proximal line. The tail of the helix and a large part of the descending helix are exposed, with good access to the anterior surface of the cartilage. C, extent and intensity of scratching on the cartilage surface of the ear of average prominence. Our present scratching instrument consists of a rasp that has differing degrees of fineness at each end. D, the scratching has greater effect if the cartilage surface is bent forward convexly by a finger held behind the ear. The use of a compress gives a firmer grip. E, the first cranial mattress suture is inserted. The base line of the flap serves only as a guide line for the suture grips. The tension required in each case to place the ear in the correct position determines if the grips should be at line level or proximally or distally to it. F, sutures inserted through the diagonal lines. Overlapping skin is cut away.

23-2D). By doing this it is possible to feel how the anterior cartilage surface yields and stretches out at almost every stroke of the scratching instrument. In order to get a firm grip on the ear, a gauze sponge should be held at the back of it. The undermining and scratching of the left ear is easier if the surgeon stands on the opposite side.

SKIN EXCISION. It is not at all necessary to scratch the ear cartilage so much that the ear is thereby bent toward the side of the skull. It is sufficient if one can bring about a marked reduction of the cartilage spring. This can be tested by light pressure with the fingertips over the descending helix. Once the reduction of spring has been achieved, the ear is brought into the desired position by means of suturing of an adequate excision on the posterior side of the ear. The first tightening sutures are inserted before the skin is cut away. Mattress sutures are used, beginning at the cranial end of the wound and at first only through the five diagonal lines (Fig. 23-2E). Should the position not be satisfying when closely checked from the front, some or all of the mattress sutures are removed and new ones inserted, gripping proximally or distally to the base line according to the tension required to get a correct position. Occasionally it may be useful to introduce the rasp between the sutures into the undermined area where resistant parts of the cartilage can be treated further. With the mattress sutures through the diagonal markings definitely inserted, the overlapping skin is excised, after which suturing is completed with interrupted stitches (Fig. 23-2F). Naturally the shape of the skin excised when using this technique varies from case to case. This shows with all desirable clarity that no one can say in advance what the correct shape of the excision should be.

PERSISTENT PROMINENCE OF THE LOBULE. Special measures are occasionally necessary. In most cases the prominence can be corrected if the excision on the posterior side of the ear is widened and continued still further down the lobule. If this does not help, the crosswise scratching on the anterior surface of the helical tail is repeated until the tail no longer protrudes. Furthermore, when the antitragus is pronounced it is sometimes necessary to level it off.

PROTRUSION OF THE UPPER POLE OF THE EAR. If a critical examination of the shape of the ear is made at the end of the operation, it is not unusual to find that the superior portion of the ear is overhanging a bit more than is consistent with an absolutely perfect result. This is a problem that arises whatever operational techniques are used. Sometimes the ear falls outward in a very disturbing way, especially when

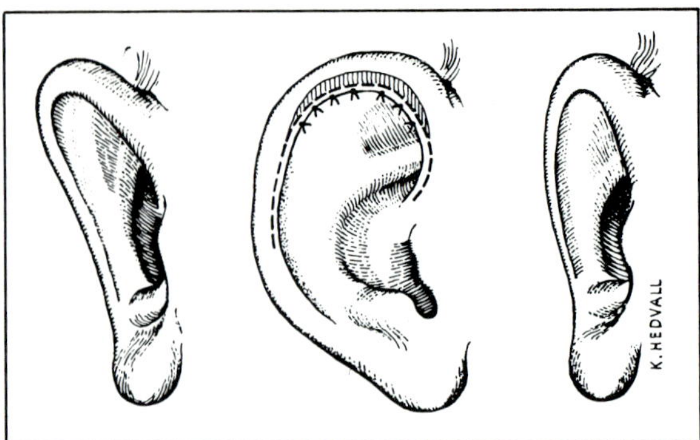

Fig. 23-3. Correction of overhanging upper pole of the ear. If the upper portion of the ear is overhanging, excision of a marginal piece of the horizontal helical cartilage will make the ear perfectly erect.

the horizontal helix is wide. Neither more skin excisions nor scratching helps very much in this situation. An immediate full effect is achieved if one exposes the horizontal helical cartilage from an incision along the lower edge and a marginal piece of cartilage is excised (Fig. 23-3). No reduction of the skin of the helix should be made. If the suturing is done with care, no trace remains. In some slight cases of prominent ears, such marginal excision from the horizontal helix plus adequate scratching from this upper approach are the only measures required.

Webster [43] considers "the tail of the helix as a key to otoplasty." I agree that it is a very important part of the auricle, but I think it is also time that the horizontal helix was given proper attention in the treatment of prominent ears.

DRESSING. Any simple type of dressing may be used, since no special care need be taken to consolidate or preserve the shape and position of the ears that have been achieved by the operation. If the result achieved is good, it will remain so. There is no need to be concerned about a recurrence of protruding ears. I use dressings moistened with 3% boric acid. A layer of crepe kraft paper [38], bent over double, is placed on top of the wet gauze sponges and is fixed in place with a strip of adhesive tape. An elastic bandage forms the outer layers of the dressing (see Fig. 23-5D). The kraft paper covering is pressed into the shape of a fairly firm cup by the elastic bandage and provides perfect support around each ear.

The dressing is changed on the second postoperative day. The "paper cups" are then opened by cutting through the adhesive tape anteriorly. When new wet gauze sponges have been laid around and over the ear, the "paper cups" are put back into place and refastened by a small piece of adhesive tape. Such dressings are generally used for a week after the operation, but sometimes they can be discarded 2 or 3 days earlier. *No protective cap is required at night following removal of the dressings.* The sutures are removed 2 weeks after the operation.

It is a common fallacy that the correction of prominent ears is easy. On the contrary, it is difficult to obtain a perfect result. To obtain consistently good results in correcting this deformity, both experience and technical ability are required.

Results of the Author's Method of Correcting Prominent Ears

One hundred and sixty-seven patients who were operated on by 20 different surgeons during the period 1965 to 1976 at the Department of Plastic Surgery, Umeå University Hospital, Umeå, Sweden, returned for an evaluation 1 to 12 years after operation. The patients at the time of operation were 5 to 25 years of age.

PATIENTS' ASSESSMENTS. Of the 167 patients examined, 40 percent were very satisfied, 49 percent were satisfied, and 4 percent fairly satisfied. Only 1 patient was dissatisfied because of overcorrection; 74 percent of the patients would recommend the operation to others with the same deformity.

ASSESSMENTS BY MY ASSOCIATE, DR. JADWIGA HEFTER. In 82 percent of the patients, the overall result was considered good. Symmetry and setting were noted as good in 71 percent of the cases. No patient had ptosis of the upper portion of the ear. There was negligible incomplete correction in 4 percent, slight overcorrection in 19 percent, and marked overcorrection in 6 percent. An antihelix with a round and natural appearance was noted in 81 percent of the patients, a sharp antihelix in 14 percent, and the occurrence of isolated small nodules in 5 percent. A superior crus with a round and natural shape was seen in 83 percent of the patients; 7 percent had a sharp superior crus. It was only in the considerably overcorrected cases that there was a cartilage deformity in the form of a sharp antihelix and/or superior crus. Overcorrection was mainly related to the surgeon, since some surgeons had a large number of overcorrections, while others had none at all.

ABNORMAL CONCHAL DEPTH WITH NORMAL ANTIHELICAL FOLD

In the ear with abnormal conchal depth and normal antihelical fold, a less common type of protruding ear, correction can be obtained by conchal-mastoid sutures, often in combination with scratching the anterior surface of the superior crus.

Furnas [10] describes the excision of an ellipse of posterior auricular skin to expose the posterior surface of the conchal cartilage (Fig. 23-4). The fibers of

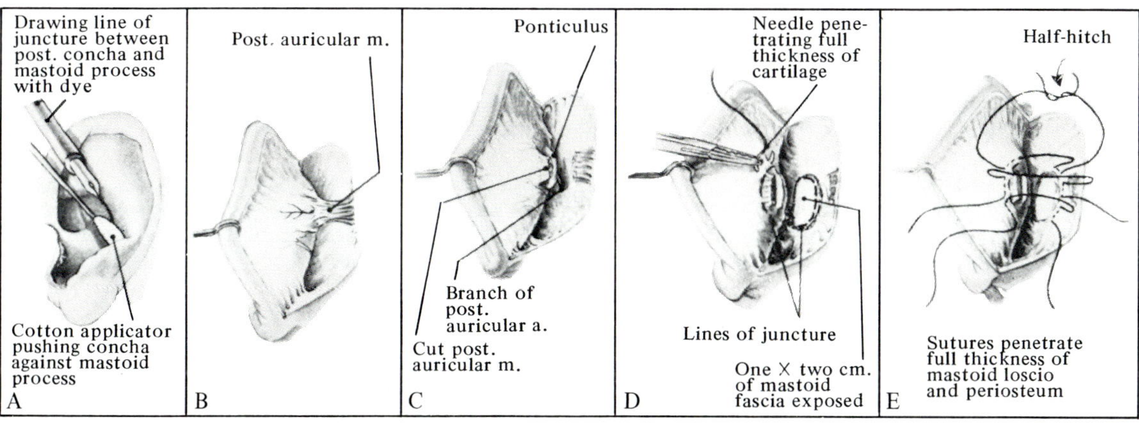

Fig. 23-4. Technique of the conchal-mastoid suture. A, a cotton-tipped applicator is used to push the concha back against the mastoid and a line is drawn at the junction between the posterior concha and the mastoid process. B, the posterior auricular muscle is exposed. C, the small branches of the greater auricular nerve in this area should be preserved; once the posterior auricular muscle is divided the ponticulus will be noted at the point of insertion of this muscle on the cartilage. D, the horizontal mattress suture of 4-0 clear nylon being passed through the conchal cartilage posterior to the ponticulus, avoiding the skin of the anterior surface. The dye mark on the anterior surface of the concha serves as a guide. E, the suture is tightened with a single half hitch so the operator can note how the ear is affected. If distortion occurs, the suture is removed and a slightly different site is tried. (From D. W. Furnas. Correction of prominent ears by conchal-mastoid sutures. Plast. Reconstr. Surg. *42:189, 1968.)*

the posterior auricular muscle are divided and a 1 × 2 cm. area of mastoid fascia is exposed. Three or more conchal-mastoid sutures of 4-0 clear nylon are passed through the conchal cartilage and then through the solid mastoid periosteum, following which the sutures are tied down. Care should be taken that the sutures do not pull the concha forward and reduce the diameter of the external auditory canal. Often the superior crus of the auricular cartilage is still flat, so that scratching of the anterior surface of the cartilage as described below will be necessary.

LOP EARS

The lop ear deformity derives its name from the fact that the upper posterior portion of the ear hangs downward. At the beginning of the third month of pregnancy, the posterior edge of the ear folds forward like a flap so that the forward pointing edge comes into contact with the crus helicis and covers the antihelix [12]. Over the next few weeks the flap opens again, and the edge of the ear returns to its original position. If this process does not take place, or if it occurs only partially, the folding of the ear will persist.

The lop ear is usually prominent too, with an indistinct antihelix and crura. The length of the helix is shortened. Sometimes it is better described as a *cupped ear* [16] or a *cat's ear.* It always looks small, and the term *microtia* may sometimes mistakenly be applied. However, once the deformity has been corrected there is little or no difference in size when compared with the normal ear (Fig. 23-5A, B).

Author's Method of Correcting Lop Ears

Since the helix of the lop ear is too short to permit the ear to be raised up to the normal position it must inevitably be lengthened. The procedure I use in order to lengthen the helix is as follows: *I cut the helical crus and the ascending helix free as far as is necessary* along the bottom of the fold of the drooping part of the ear (Fig. 23-6B). The ear can then be fully erected and usually assumes an amazingly normal appearance immediately. So that this shape may be retained, the drooping tendency must be counteracted. One takes advantage of the good access one already has to the anterior side of the ear and undermines and scratches all parts (especially the drooping fold) that prevent the ear from becoming properly erect and from losing its prominence. The ascending helix is then adjusted into its new erect position, with great care being taken to keep it vertical. It has a marked tendency to assume a forward-inclined position, which can detract considerably from the cosmetic result. The skin defect in the area of the helical crus is closed by mobilization of the skin in front of the ear. The final stage in the operation entails increasing the antihelical fold and posterior crus in order to stabilize the new shape of the ear and to correct protrusion. This is achieved by making a skin excision on the posterior side of the ear similar to the one described for prominent ears.

If the deformity is unilateral, the position of the normal ear should be adjusted until it is symmetrical with the corrected one. This is easier than the other way round. If there is a noticeable difference in the size of the ears, both of them should be set closer to the skull so that the difference is less noticeable.

INVAGINATED EARS

"Congenital invagination of the external ear" is the terminology coined by Gosserez and Piers [11] to describe a deformity in which the upper portion of the ear is more or less embedded beneath the scalp (Fig. 23-7A). Cowan [8] reported on the postulated causes of the deformity. According to one of the theories [11], a genetic defect of the scapha causes a secondary invagination of the superior helix beneath the temporal skin. The terms *cryptotia* and *pocket ear* have also been suggested for this condition. In pronounced cases, the patients are unable to wear glasses because the postauricular sulcus is absent.

The shape of the ear varies in other cases. In 1 of the 2 patients operated on by me, the upper part of the ear was pointed because of a helical fold within the area of the fossa helicis. This helical fold, together with underdevelopment of the scapha, seems to be a characteristic feature. In the patient just mentioned, the upper half of the ear was almost an exact mirror image of the lower half. In both patients the lower half of the ear was prominent because the posterior lower conchal wall was relatively high.

The operative treatment is aimed at releasing the upper part of the ear and creating a better postauricular sulcus. To cover the defect that follows this step, Kubo [17] applied a triangular flap of skin from the supraauricular area to the denuded part of the ear. Gosserez and Piers [11] covered the posterior surface of the ear with a free skin graft and closed the skull side of the defect by use of the Z-plasty technique.

I have had satisfactory results using a procedure described by Šercer [31] (Fig. 23-7). In this operation the skin deficiency in the upper part of the postauricular sulcus is corrected by advancing a flap of skin from the lower part of the sulcus as a Y-V advancement. The lower part of the sulcus is tightened at the same time, which helps to prevent the repositioned ear cartilage from sliding back to its original location. In both patients mentioned above, a simultaneous correction of the prominent ears was performed. Lowering of the posterior conchal wall lifts the upper part of the ear away from the skull very nicely. By scratching the abnormal folding inside the

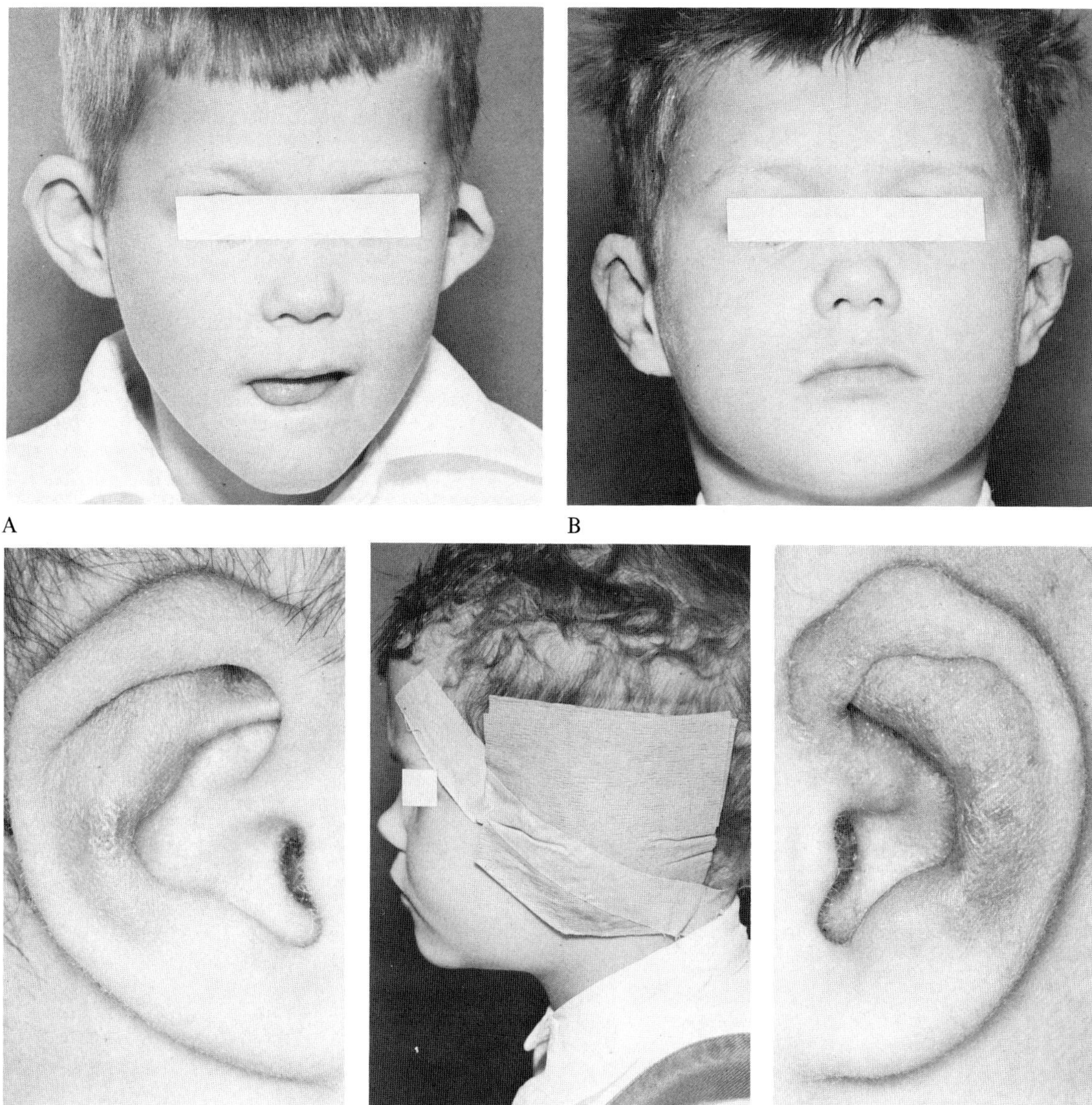

Fig. 23-5. Five-year-old boy with a prominent ear on the right and a lop ear on the left. A, preoperative view. B, postoperative view. C, close-up postoperative view of the right ear. D, dressing consists of wet gauze sponges, covered with a double layer of crepe kraft paper fixed by adhesive tape; an elastic bandage then goes around the head. E, close-up postoperative view of the left ear.

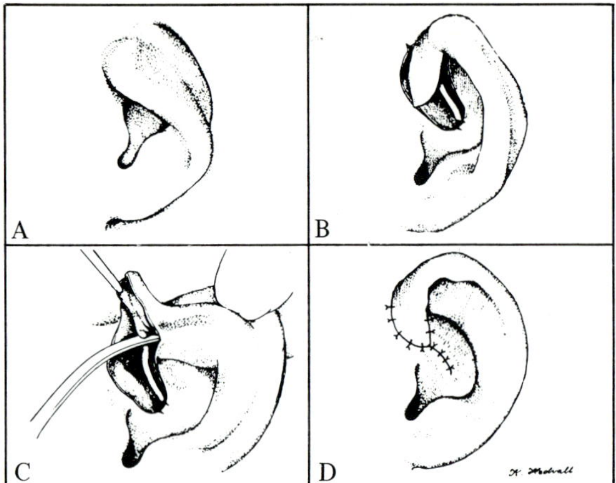

Fig. 23-6. Otoplasty for lop ear. A, lateral preoperative view. B, the helical crus and the ascending part of the helix are cut free so that the ear can be unfurled. C, the ear is bent backward. Undermining is executed as for a prominent ear. Scratching is done in the drooping fold and in all other parts of the cartilage surface that are resistant to folding along the antihelix and posterior crus. D, the ear is folded back by means of a skin excision on the posterior side of the ear.

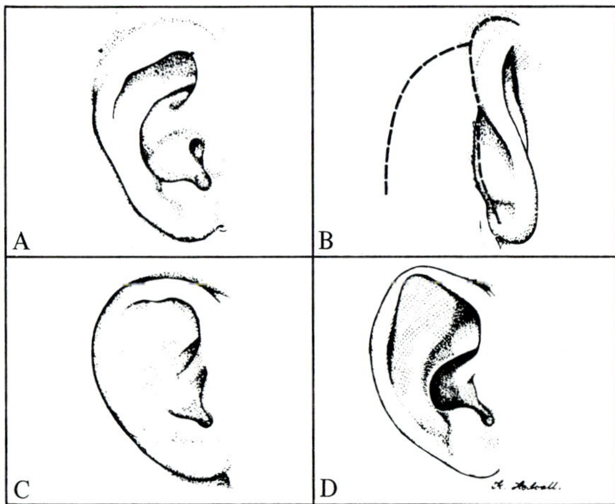

Fig. 23-7. Invaginated ear. A, the upper edge of the auricular cartilage can be seen under the scalp. B, flap cut for correction of the deformity by Y-V advancement; flap should be continued far down toward the lobule, since this makes it more mobile. C, shell ear; the concha and scapha merge into each other directly without a break, and the helix is largely uncurled. D, satyr ear; the auricle's satyr tip is very noticeable due to incomplete curling of the helix at this point.

fossa helicis, this part can be unfolded to give the ear a more normal contour.

SHELL EARS

When the shell ear deformity is pronounced, it can be described as a prominent ear with little or no curling of the helix and with an absence of the antihelix and crura so that the concha and scapha merge directly into each other (Fig. 23-7C).

Padgett and Stephenson [26] suggested that the deformity should be corrected by creating a normal antihelix and increasing the prominence of the helix by excising several V-shaped pieces with their base at the rim of the auricle. When the defects are sutured, the external rim of the ear is shortened, thus producing marked curvature of the helix.

I prefer to begin the operation as for prominent ears, but then to bring about an increase in the curling of the helix by scratching along its posterior edge. This is achieved by undermining over a 1-cm.-wide zone of cartilage from below, rather than exposing the posterior margin of the helix by means of a skin excision. When outlining the antihelix and crura, careful attention must be paid to trace their course. Sometimes the line is faint, but it will appear more obvious when the ear is drawn back toward the skull. The scratching must have a subtle gradation to it in order to more or less sculpt out the details. On each occasion that I have formed the helix curl by scratching, a narrow strip of skin along the anterior side of the helix has been excised.

SATYR EARS

Characteristic of the satyr ear deformity is a pointed contour and incomplete curling at some point along the horizontal portion of the helix, and a deformity of the posterior crus (Fig. 23-7D).

According to Schwalbe [30], the free edge of the ear curls during the last months of gestation. Before that time, the highest point of the helical margin looks like the vertex of an angle – a satyr tip. Darwin's tubercle can be seen lower down along the posterior edge of the ear. The satyr tip corresponds to the anterior upper edge of an animal's ear, while Darwin's tubercle corresponds to the tip of an animal's ear.

To correct the satyr ear, Becker [3] makes an incision in the cartilage parallel to the rim and folds it on itself. A flap of skin is then raised on the posterior surface of the auricle and rolled over on itself to help to form the helix. In addition, a new posterior crus is created.

REFERENCES

1. Adamson, J. E., Horton, C. E., and Crawford, H. H. The growth pattern of the external ear. *Plast. Reconstr. Surg.* 36:466, 1965.

2. Bean, R. B. Some characteristics of the external ear of American whites, American Indians, American Negroes, Alaskan Eskimos and Filipinos. *Am. J. Anat.* 18:201, 1915.
3. Becker, O. J. Correction of the protruding deformed ear. *Br. J. Plast. Surg.* 5:187, 1952.
4. Bergman, F. O., and Stenström, S. J. Curling Tendency of Various Types of Distortionable Cartilages. *Transactions of the Fifth International Congress of Plastic and Reconstructive Surgery.* Melbourne, Australia: Butterworth, 1971.
5. Bowen, J. A method for correction of prominent ears. *Br. J. Plast. Surg.* 27:92, 1974.
6. Bruck, H. G. Correction of prominent ears. *Arch. Otolaryngol.* 98:10, 1973.
7. Converse, J. M., Nigro, A., Wilson, F. A., and Johnson, N. A technique for surgical correction of lop ears. *Plast. Reconstr. Surg.* 15:411, 1955.
8. Cowan, R. J. Cryptotia. *Plast. Reconstr. Surg.* 27:209, 1961.
9. Dieffenbach, J. F. *Die Operative Chirurgie.* Leipzig: Brockhaus, 1845.
10. Furnas, D. W. Correction of prominent ears by concha-mastoid sutures. *Plast. Reconstr. Surg.* 42:189, 1968.
11. Gosserez, M., and Piers, J. H. Invagination congénitale du pavillon de l'oreille. *Ann. Chir. Plast.* 4:143, 1959.
11a. Grabb, W. C. Personal communication, 1977.
12. Henke, F., and Lubarsch, O. *Handbuch der speziellen pathologischen Anatomie and Histologie.* Zwölfter Band. Berlin: Springer, 1926.
13. Jayes, P. H., and Dale, R. H. The treatment of prominent ears. *Br. J. Plast. Surg.* 4:193, 1951.
14. Ju, D. M. C. The psychological effect of protruding ears. *Plast. Reconstr. Surg.* 31:424, 1963.
15. Kaye, B. L. A simplified method for correcting the prominent ear. *Plast. Reconstr. Surg.* 52:184, 1973.
16. Kislov, R. Surgical correction of the cupped ear. *Plast. Reconstr. Surg.* 48:121, 1971.
17. Kubo, I. Über das "taschenohr" (Kubo) und die plastische Operation dieser Missbildung. *Otologia* 6:105, 1933.
18. Langer, C. Über die Form- und Lageverhältnisse des Ohres. *Mitt. Anthropol. Ges.* (Wien) 2:115, 1882.
19. Linder, L. The angle of the external ear to the median plane of the skull in children. *Acta Genet.* (Basel) 1:92, 1948.
20. Luckett, W. H. A new operation for prominent ears based on the anatomical deformity. *Surg. Gynecol. Obstet.* 10:635, 1910.
21. McEvitt, W. G. The problem of the protruding ear. *Plast. Reconstr. Surg.* 2:481, 1947.
22. Mustardé, J. C. The correction of prominent ears using simple mattress sutures. *Brit. J. Plast. Surg.* 16:170, 1963.
23. Mustardé, J. C. The Correction of Prominent Ears with Buried Mattress Sutures. In Gibson, Th. (Ed.), *Modern Trends in Plastic Surgery.* London: Butterworth, 1964.
24. Mustardé, J. C. Problems in the Correction of Prominent Ears for Television Demonstration. *Transactions of the Fifth International Congress of Plastic and Reconstructive Surgery.* Melbourne, Australia: Butterworth, 1971.
25. Neuner, O. A simple method for the correction of prominent ears. *Plast. Reconstr. Surg.* 47:111, 1971.
26. Padgett, E. C., and Stephenson, K. L. *Plastic and Reconstructive Surgery* (1st ed.). Springfield, Ill.: Thomas, 1949.
27. Pierce, G. W., Klabunde, E. H., and Bergeron, V. L. Useful procedures in plastic surgery. *Plast. Reconstr. Surg.* 2:358, 1947.
28. Rubin, L. R., Bromberg, B. E., Walden, R. H., and Adams, A. An anatomic approach to the obtrusive ear. *Plast. Reconstr. Surg.* 29:360, 1962.
29. Schneider, K., and Clodius, L. Conchal hypertrophy and the correction of protruding ears. *Br. J. Plast. Surg.* 26:115, 1973.
30. Schwalbe, G. Das Darwinsche Spitzohr beim menschlichen Embryo. *Anat. Anz.* 4:176, 1889.
31. Šercer, A. Beitrage zur Kenntnis der Formanomalien des äusseren Ohres. *Acta Otolaryngol.* (Stockh.) 20:59, 1934.
32. Small, A. Prevention of meatal stenosis in conchal setback otoplasty. *Laryngoscope* 85:1782, 1975.
33. Smith, R., and Teachey, W. S. Medial conchal excision in otoplasty. *Laryngoscope* 85:738, 1975.
34. Stark, R. B. *Plastic Surgery.* New York: Harper & Row, 1962.
35. Stark, R. B., and Saunders, D. E. The first branchial syndrome. *Plast. Reconstr. Surg.* 29:229, 1962.
36. Stenström, S. J. Utstående öron. *Nord. Med.* 69:222, 1963. (Paper read in Umeå Medical Society, October 13, 1961.)
37. Stenström, S. J. A "natural" technique for correction of congenitally prominent ears. *Plast. Reconstr. Surg.* 32:509, 1963.
38. Stenström, S. J. Kraft paper in wet dressings. *Plast. Reconstr. Surg.* 34:307, 1964.
39. Stenström, S. J. A simple operation for prominent ears. *Acta Otolaryngol.* [Suppl.] 224:393, 1967.
40. Tanzer, R. C. The correction of prominent ears. *Plast. Reconstr. Surg.* 30:236, 1962.
41. Tanzer, R. C. Correction of Prominent Ears. *Transactions of the Fifth International Congress of Plastic and Reconstructive Surgery.* Melbourne,

Australia: Butterworth, 1971.
42. Tucker, A. L. Prominauris. *Plast. Reconstr. Surg.* 30:685, 1962.
43. Webster, G. V. The tail of the helix as a key to otoplasty. *Plast. Reconstr. Surg.* 44:455, 1969.
44. Wieland, H. Die einfache Ohrmuschelkorrektur. *Laryngol. Rhinol.* 53:556, 1974.

III

Skin and Adnexa

Thermal Burns

J. B. LYNCH

About two million burns occur annually in the United States. Of these, one-half are limited or require only first aid treatment for the relief of pain. Approximately 250,000 are more severe and require bed rest or home treatment. Approximately 70,000 burn patients are hospitalized annually in the United States, with 12,000 deaths. Although extensive burns continue to carry a high mortality, the National Safety Council Bulletin indicates that the mortality per 100,000 from burns has dropped from 9 to 4 since 1910.

With improved understanding of the mechanism and treatment of shock, attention within recent years has been directed toward the altered pathophysiology of burns, which includes protein disequilibrium, anemia, endocrine and metabolic abnormalities, local and systemic infection, and full-thickness skin loss that necessitates tissue transplantation. Surgical excision of the burn wound, either in one or in multiple stages, has been evaluated in many burn centers. Although useful in limited burns, it has done little to decrease the overall mortality or morbidity in major burns.

Regardless of the method of treatment, a third-degree burn represents a very serious injury. Under optimum conditions, the initial period of hospitalization will vary from 3 to 12 weeks, and the period of convalescence and reconstruction may consume many additional months or even years. The financial impact of such an unexpected disaster and the necessity of prolonged treatment are difficult to comprehend and impossible for the average family to manage despite the increasing insurance coverage of the American public. When the tragedy involves the head of the household, the problem is compounded by loss of wages during the period of treatment and convalescence.

The current trends in burn management have been toward standardization and simplification of care for the average burn patient and improved recognition and management of complications occurring during the course of the burn.

HISTORICAL ASPECTS

An excellent summary of the ancient history of the treatment of burns has been presented by Blocker [7]. Beginning with Hippocrates (460 to 377 B.C.), the observations and writings of Selsus (about A.D. 100), Galen (129–199), Albucasis (936–1013), Hispanus (1220–1277), Fallopius, Fabricius, and others were traced to the end of the eighteenth century. In 1797, Edward Kentish [20] published one of the most important early discussions of burns in the English language, a monograph entitled *An Essay on Burns Which Happen to Workmen in Mines.* This essay advocated exposure therapy in the early stages but the later use of occlusive dressings. James Earl, about the same time, published a series of discussions about burn treatment, including the use of ice for initial pain, in 1799. Few changes were made in therapy throughout the nineteenth century, and articles in textbooks by the end of the nineteenth century indicate little or no emphasis on burn physiology and supportive therapy. These textbooks do advocate a wide variety of local agents for burn treatment, including carbolic acid, bichloride of mercury, carron oil, lead carbonate, zinc oxide, lard, colodian, silver nitrate, castor oil, and a wide variety of other medications. A classic paper published by Sneve [41] in 1905, entitled "The Treatment of Burns and Skin Grafting," advocated early exposure therapy. In 1906, Oppenheimer [36a] advocated picric acid therapy, which was used intermittently for many years following this publication. By 1919, numerous reports on the exposure therapy of burns had appeared. The use of paraffin wax or Ambrine was popularized by Barthe de Sandfort [4], and it became widely used.

Davidson [11] published a paper on "Tannic Acid in the Treatment of Burns" in 1925 and inaugurated the era of chemical escharotic agents, which lasted for several years. Other agents in wide use at that time included silver nitrate, saline packs, and gential violet. With the introduction of sulfanilamide in the early 1940s, the era of topical antibiotic agents began. However, it was not until 1964, with the reports of Moyer and co-workers [32], that topical bacteriostatic agents with ability to penetrate the eschar became available.

In 1943, the National Research Council manual [35] abandoned tannic acid and other types of chemical escharotic agents, and the publication of Allen and Koch [1] emphasized the use of pressure dressings.

With the report of A. B. Wallace [42] in 1949, exposure treatment of burns was revived in the literature as an acceptable procedure. Blocker [6] and Pulaski [40] were primarily responsible for reintroducing exposure therapy to the United States at that time.

In the past 25 years, there has developed better understanding of the metabolic, nutritional, hematologic, fluid, and electrolyte problems; methods of combating shock have improved; and a large number of papers have appeared on all aspects of burn care from around the world. In recent years, specialized institutions for the treatment of burns have been developed in many countries, and a large number of national and international burn meetings are regularly held.

ETIOLOGY OF BURNS

A statistical analysis of 1,000 burn patients was presented by Blocker and his co-workers [9]; it showed that the overwhelming majority of burns in their area were due to direct contact with flash or flame (78.3 percent), following by scalds (12 percent), with direct contact with burning agents, chemical burns, and electrical burns making up the remainder. The frequency of burns from various sources will vary somewhat depending on the geographical part of the country, and the patient population in hospitals will vary, depending on the population that they serve. National statistics for the incidence of burns are compiled annually by the National Burn Information Exchange. It is tragic to note that approximately half of the burns annually occur in the home and, of these, approximately two-thirds could be prevented. In recent years, there have been stringent federal and state laws related to flame retardant treatment of clothing and modification of building codes to help minimize the possibility of accidental burns, but the need for further preventive measures is apparent.

AGE DISTRIBUTION OF BURN PATIENTS

Although the age of the patient admitted to the hospital with a burn varies widely according to the area and type of hospital service, the frequency of accidental burns in children deserves special consideration. An analysis of the age distribution of burn patients reveals that 50 percent occur in individuals under the age of 20. A major burn during a child's formative years may leave him with a functional or cosmetic impairment requiring physical as well as emotional adjustment. In addition, children must be kept under close observation to correct any secondary deformities that may develop during their growing years.

PHYSIOLOGICAL DERANGEMENT OF BURN PATIENTS

Acute Phase

Circulatory Derangement

In the immediate postburn period, the primary physiological alterations are related to the circulatory system. Capillary permeability is altered, allowing loss of fluid rich in protein and electrolytes, particularly sodium, into the burn wound. This produces the obligatory burn edema which is clinically most evident in the head and neck region, where tissues are more relaxed. The resulting hypovolemia leads to decreased renal blood flow, decreased glomerular filtration, and oliguria. Decreased venous return to the heart and decreased cardiac output then occur. Compensatory peripheral vasoconstriction results in a transient rise in blood pressure followed by a gradual decline, although not as severe as that seen in hemorrhagic shock. As plasma volume reduction continues, hemoconcentration develops, followed by blood cell agglutination and abnormalities of blood flow in the microcirculation.

Anemia

There is a variable amount of red blood cell destruction in the burn area as a result of the injury. In addition, there is loss of effective circulating red cells from agglutination in capillary beds and inactivation by the sludge phenomenon. The absolute amount of red cell destruction averages approximately 15 percent, but it can vary from 5 to 40 percent of the total red blood cell mass, depending on the extent and depth of the burn [34]. In addition to the relative and absolute decrease in circulating red cells, there is an accelerated rate of hemolysis from increased red cell fragility, which reduces the half-life of the red blood cells.

Metabolic Response

Following a burn, a number of physiological and chemical changes occur, involving protein, carbohydrate, fat, fluid and electrolytes, vitamins, and endocrines; at one time or another, almost any organ system of the body may be involved. Metabolic response to injury may include: increased heat production, weight loss, negative nitrogen balance, negative potassium and phosphorus balances, disturbed carbohydrate utilization, fat mobilization, retention of sodium chloride and water, and alteration in the metabolism of certain vitamins. In general, the severity of the changes parallels the extent of the injury, and the responses are most accentuated in previously healthy patients.

Subacute Phase

As the shock phase subsides and diuresis occurs, mobilization of sodium occurs and urinary output increases. As the edema fluid in the burn wound accumulates, there is an increased lymph flow from the burn area. Though this suggests an attempt to reestablish equilibrium, studies indicate that the equilibrium is incomplete, particularly as far as the protein is concerned [25, 30]. As the clinical edema subsides, anemia becomes manifest, and a negative nitrogen balance usually persists until the burn wounds are virtually healed. In addition to the protein disequilibrium, the patient has disordered fat metabolism, evidence of impairment of hepatic function, various endocrine disturbances, and bone and joint changes. More detailed discussion of the multiple facets of burn pathophysiology can be found in reports such as those by Levenson [22], Artz and Moncrief [2], and Dolocek [12]. Wilmore [43–46] has contributed a number of excellent reports in recent years on various metabolic aspects in the burn patient.

MORBIDITY AND MORTALITY OF BURN PATIENTS

The patient and his family usually ask almost immediately about the chances for survival; they also ask for an estimate of the length of hospitalization, the number of surgical procedures required during initial treatment, and the probability of subsequent scarring and deformity. Obviously, the time required for healing depends on the extent and depth of the wound, the location of the burns, the patient's general condition, and whether or not local and systemic complications develop.

In general, *second-degree burns* will heal in 7 to 21 days, depending on their depth. In some very deep second-degree burns, sufficient hair follicles, sebaceous glands, and sweat glands remain in the dermis so that reepithelialization will take place even though healing requires many weeks. Since the resulting scar following spontaneous healing after several weeks of very deep second-degree burns is frequently thin, brittle, and vulnerable to trauma, this type of wound is often best managed by early application of skin grafts, particularly in the hand and over flexion areas. Some preparation of the burn surface, such as dermabrasion, may be helpful in removing residual debris in preparation for grafting of these deep second-degree burns.

Unless they are extremely small in area, *third-degree burns* will require skin transplants. The time required to obtain healing in third-degree burns depends on the number of skin grafting procedures necessary and on the development of local and systemic complications. Studies have shown that even small areas of 5 to 10 percent full-thickness skin loss require nearly twice as long a treatment period as extensive (30 to 40 percent) second-degree burns. Early excision and skin grafting, when feasible, is the procedure of choice in treating small, localized third-degree burns. However, excision and grafting should be limited to burns that involve 15 percent of the body surface or less and lesions that are clearly third degree, such as would occur in the laundry worker who catches her hand in the laundry press. In the more extensive third-degree burns, about 3 weeks of hospitalization are required before the first skin grafting procedure. Patients with injuries involving *20 percent or less* of the body surface will usually need only one or two grafting operations and can be discharged about *6 weeks* after injury. In burn injuries involving *20 to 50 percent* of the body surface, an average of *10 weeks* of hospitalization is required; if over *50 percent* of the body surface is affected, a minimum of *14 weeks* will elapse before the patients are ready for discharge.

Although the mortality rates reported in various studies in the literature show wide variation, a number of factors are important in estimating the mortality due to burns. It is interesting to note that in recent years the pattern of deaths in extensive burns has changed. The National Research Council manual *Burn, Shock, Wound Healing and Vascular Injuries* in 1943 reported that between 50 and 75 percent of burn deaths were the result of shock [35]. At the present time, it is unusual for the patient even with the most extensive burn to succumb in the initial shock phase when any of the currently available methods of intravenous fluid replacement therapy are properly administered. After the first 2 or 3 days, the patient's circulatory system and general condition usually stabilize for a few days, so that the majority of deaths now occur after the first week and are most commonly related to the development of infectious complications. The mortality for hospitalized burn patients is currently in the range of 20 to 25 percent and is related to magnitude of the injury and the general condition of the patient (Table 24-1).

It must be remembered that patients at the extremes of life tolerate burning poorly, the mortality being high even in burns involving small body-surface areas in those under the age of 1 year and past the age of 60. In patients with third-degree burns of up to 30 percent of the body surface and who are under the age of 50, the mortality is low. If the extent of body-surface involvement increases beyond 30 percent, the mortality rises in all age groups. As the age of the patient increases beyond 50, the risk grows, even in burns of less than 30 percent. The *age of the patient* and the *extent of body-surface involvement* are the two most important factors in estimating the magnitude of the injury in third-degree lesions.

Although the age of the patient, the extent of body-surface area involved, and the depth of the burn are the most important factors contributing to mortality or prolonged morbidity, there are other factors: the anatomical location of the lesion, obesity, alcoholism, any preexisting disease state such as cardiac or renal disease, concomitant metabolic disease such as diabetes or arthritis, and any associated fractures or soft tissue injuries. Cardiac complications probably contribute to mortality and morbidity more often

Table 24-1. Predicted Mortality in Males (%)*

Age (yr.)	Percent of Body Surface Burned 10	20	30	40	50	60	70	80	90	100
2	0	5	17	40	63	80	92	98	100	100
4	0	5	16	39	63	79	92	98		
8	0	4	14	37	60	78	91	97		
12	0	4	13	36	59	77	91	97		
16	0	3	13	35	59	77	90	97		
20	0	3	13	35	59	77	90	97		
24	0	4	14	37	60	78	91	97		
28	0	4	15	38	62	78	92	97		
32	0	5	17	40	63	80	92	98		
36	1	6	19	44	66	81	94	98		
40	1	7	22	47	69	84	94	98		
44	2	9	27	52	71	87	95	99		
48	3	11	32	56	75	89	96	99		
52	4	15	39	62	79	92	97	100		
56	6	20	45	67	83	94	98			
60	9	27	53	72	87	96	99			
64	13	36	59	77	91	97	100			
68	19	45	67	83	94	98				
72	29	54	73	88	96	99				
76	40	63	80	92	98	100				
80	51	71	86	95	99					
84	61	78	92	97	100					
88	71	86	95	99						
90	75	89	97	99						

Modified from J. A. McCoy et al., *J.A.M.A.* 203:644, 1968.
*The mortality in females at each age bracket is generally the same or increased by only one percentage point.

than is realized. Stress diabetes, which may occur as a transient stage following a burn, or latent diabetes of the hereditary type, may become manifest after thermal injury. Emergency therapy of associated injuries should take precedence over local management of the burn wound. The possibility of respiratory-tract injury must be kept in mind in any burn involving the face or neck or in patients who may have inhaled smoke or noxious fumes.

EVALUATION OF THE MAGNITUDE OF THE INJURY

At the time of initial examination, it is important to determine the extent of the burned area and the depth of the burn for treatment purposes and to determine whether inpatient or outpatient care is required, the necessity for intravenous fluid therapy, and the prognosis for survival and length of hospital stay.

A number of factors must be taken into consideration in making this assessment; the more important factors include:

1. Extent of body surface involved.
2. Burn depth.
3. Age.
4. Causative agent (chemical, electrical, flame, etc.).
5. Fractures or other associated injuries.
6. Concomitant disease, such as preexisting renal or cardiopulmonary disease; metabolic diseases, such as diabetes, obesity, alcoholism, epilepsy.
7. Burns complicated by inhalation of smoke or carbon monoxide.

Estimation of Burn Area

In estimating the burned area, the common practice is to employ the tables which have been devised by Berkow or to modify the Rule of Nines (Fig. 24-1). The Rule of Nines* is sufficiently accurate to enable

*The Rule of Nines used to approximate surface area allows 9% for the head and neck, 9% for each upper extremity, 18% for each lower extremity, 18% for the anterior thorax and abdomen, and 18% for the back and buttocks.

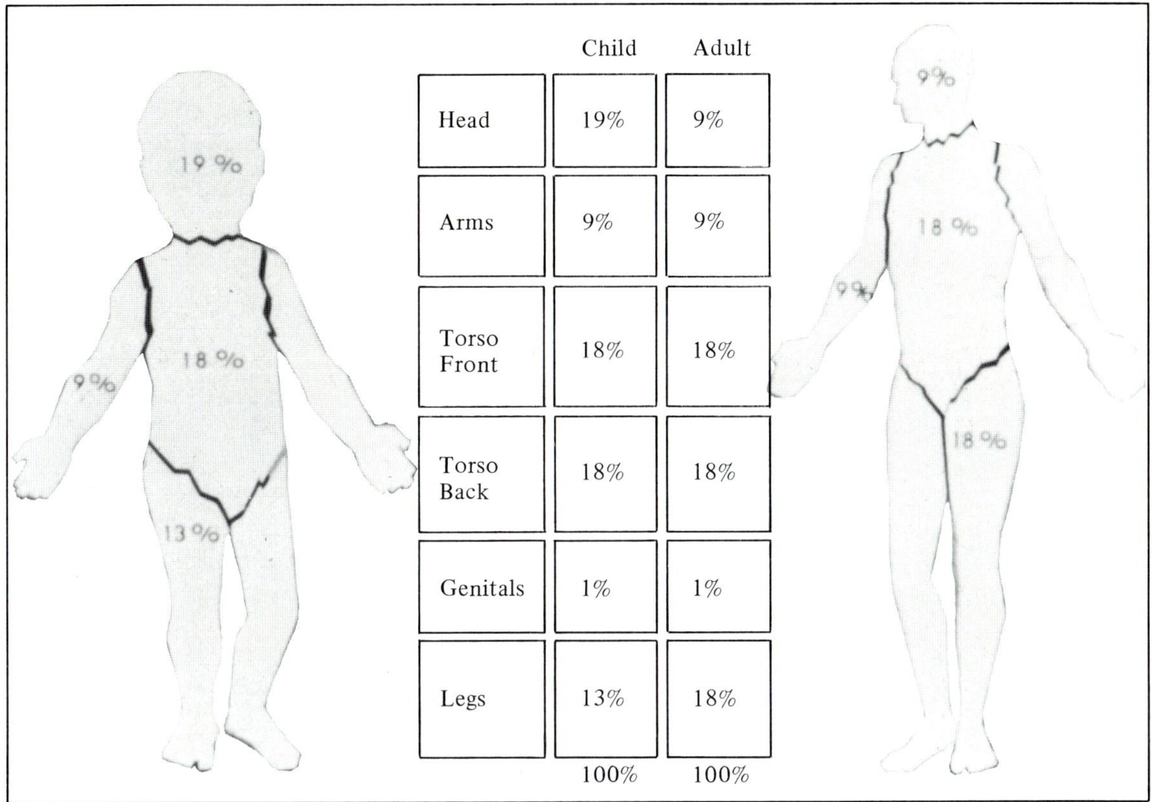

	Child	Adult
Head	19%	9%
Arms	9%	9%
Torso Front	18%	18%
Torso Back	18%	18%
Genitals	1%	1%
Legs	13%	18%
	100%	100%

Fig. 24-1. The Rule of Nines is useful for immediate estimation of the extent of body-surface involvement.

the examining physician to make an initial estimate of the approximate body-surface area involved. For more accurate records it is essential that the detailed surface areas be plotted, utilizing the charts derived from Berkow as illustrated in Figure 24-2.

Estimation of Depth of Burn

In general, the depth of burn is dependent on the temperature of the burning agent and the duration of contact. Burns are classified as first, second, and third degree depending on the amount of tissue destroyed (Fig. 24-3). A *first-degree burn* is characterized by erythema and edema of the skin and involves only the epidermis. This superficial burn usually requires no therapy except for relief of pain. *Second-degree burns,* ordinarily characterized by blister formation and weeping, destroy the epidermis and a portion of the dermis. These burns heal with minimum scarring if infection can be avoided, although pigment changes may persist for some months. *Third-degree burns* destroy the full thickness of the skin and often involve the underlying tissue as well; unless these areas are very small, they must be skin grafted. The term *fourth-degree burn* is sometimes utilized to indicate the involvement of underlying structures such as muscle or bone. It is frequently difficult to differentiate a second-degree from a third-degree burn, and in the early stages it may sometimes be impossible. Helpful diagnostic points related to the depth of the burn include:

1. Type of burning agent.
2. Appearance of lesion.
3. Presence or absence of sensation.
4. Dye and other tests.
5. Course of healing process.

TYPE OF BURNING AGENT. Since different burning agents often produce characteristic injuries, the most reliable early guide to the depth of the burn may be the knowledge of the causative agent. Electrical burns sustained from high-tension wires are, as a rule, the most severe. These lesions, and those due to chemical agents, tend to be much deeper than indicated on initial examination and frequently involve underlying muscles, tendons, nerves, and bone. Next in order of severity are flame burns and burns from liquids at

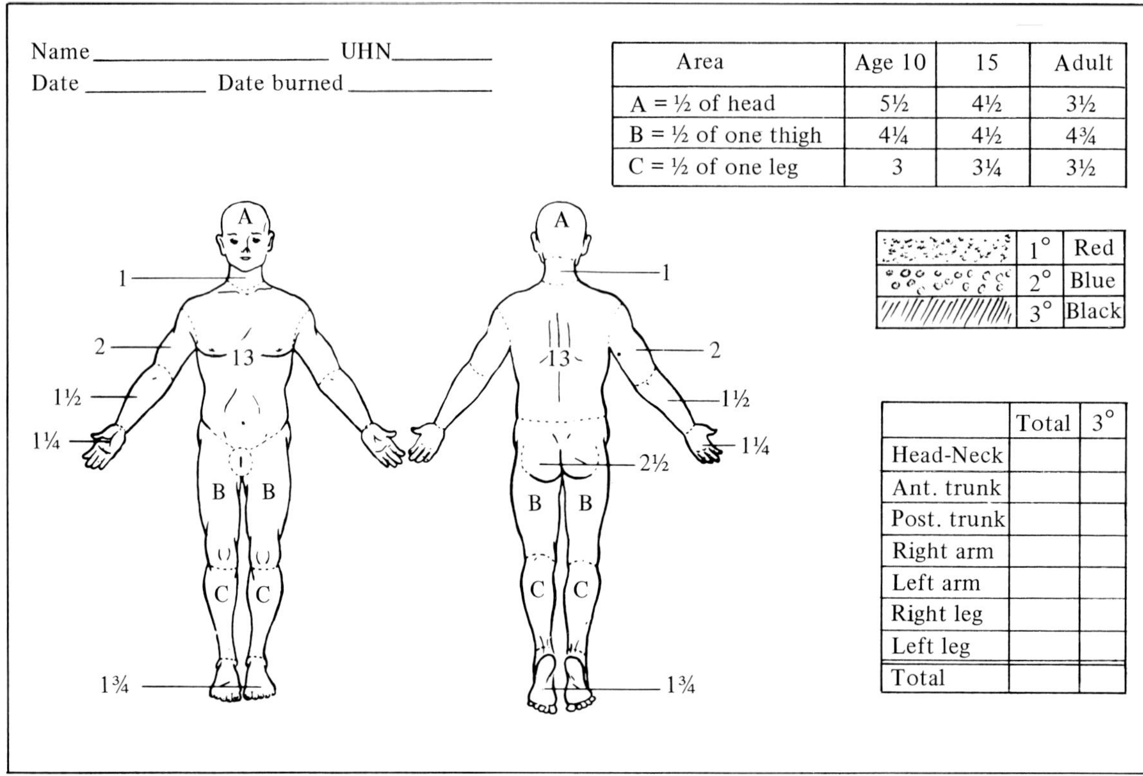

Area	Age 10	15	Adult
A = ½ of head	5½	4½	3½
B = ½ of one thigh	4¼	4½	4¾
C = ½ of one leg	3	3¼	3½

	1°	Red
	2°	Blue
	3°	Black

	Total	3°
Head-Neck		
Ant. trunk		
Post. trunk		
Right arm		
Left arm		
Right leg		
Left leg		
Total		

Fig. 24-2. Diagrams used to calculate the percentage of the skin area that has been burned.

extremely high temperatures, which are almost invariably third-degree injuries. Immersion in hot water, which produces damage from conduction of heat to the deeper tissues, is much more serious than simple scalds. Exposure to a flash explosion without direct flame contact results in second-degree burns largely confined to the exposed area, such as the face and hands.

APPEARANCE OF LESION. Second-degree burns are characterized by the formation of blisters. The burned area is edematous and may be elevated in relation to the surrounding normal skin; if the blisters are denuded, the surface is frequently red in color, with a profuse exudate. In third-degree burns the lesion may be pale, white, brown, or even frankly charred. The wound surface is frequently depressed in relation to the surrounding unburned skin and the wound is usually dry if the burn results from direct contact with flame. The appearance of coagulated vessels in waxy-appearing skin is diagnostic of third-degree injury.

PRESENCE OR ABSENCE OF SENSATION. Since third-degree burns destroy the sensory endings in the skin, sensation to pinprick is usually absent. This sensation may be retained in second-degree burns but may be obliterated as edema progresses. Although determination of the presence or absence of sensation is helpful in distinguishing second-degree from third-degree burns, this test is not infallible.

DYE AND OTHER TESTS. Various techniques of staining tissue with dyes such as fluorescein, patent blue, and others to delineate second-degree from third-degree wounds have been developed. Thermography and radioisotope techniques have been reported as helpful diagnostic aids for evaluating the depth of the burn. Although these methods may be helpful in individual cases, they are subject to considerable technical difficulty and error and are not routinely used in most burn centers.

COURSE OF HEALING PROCESS. The most experienced observer may be unable to determine whether a given area of burn is second degree or third degree in the early stages. In such cases, it is frequently necessary to make the diagnosis in retrospect after waiting to determine whether spontaneous healing

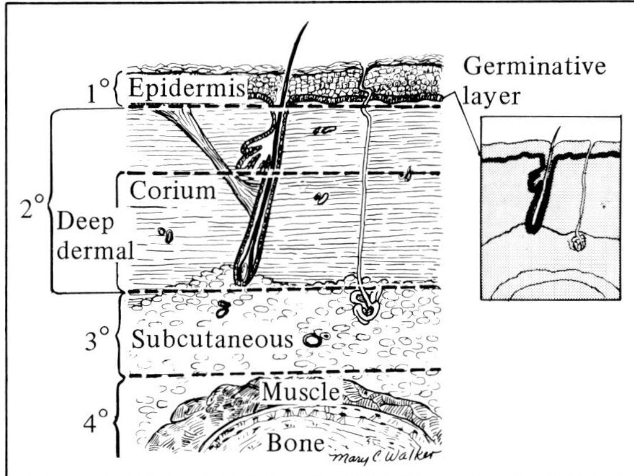

Fig. 24-3. Cross section of skin indicating the degree of burns. The inset depicts the way second-degree burns heal from the epithelium of the skin appendages.

occurs or whether separation of the burn eschar results in a granulating wound. This is particularly true in burns caused by both flash and flame, which often have a patchy distribution of mixed second- and third-degree areas.

CLASSIFICATION OF BURN INJURIES

Since burn injuries may vary from a very minor lesion (limited sunburn or a small superficial flash burn of the finger sustained while lighting an oven) to injuries that may be judged on initial examination to have a fatal outcome, a basic classification of burns according to their severity is useful for disposition and treatment purposes. Burn casualties may be classified into three categories for disposition and treatment:

1. *Critical or major burns* (hospitalization required with full therapeutic approach as outlined later in this chapter).
   a. Second-degree burns exceeding 30 percent of the body surface.
   b. Third-degree burns exceeding 10 percent of the body surface.
   c. Burns complicated by respiratory-tract injury, major soft tissue injury, and fractures.
   d. Electrical burns.
   e. Third-degree burns involving critical areas, e.g., the hands, face, and feet.
2. *Moderate burns* (hospitalization recommended for observation, but therapeutic requirements are usually less than for critical burns).
   a. Superficial second-degree burns of more than 15 percent of the body surface.
   b. Deep second-degree burns of 15 to 30 percent.
   c. Third-degree burns of less than 10 percent – excluding the hands, face, and feet.
3. *Minor burns* (can usually be managed on an outpatient basis in the absence of complications).
   a. First-degree burns.
   b. Second-degree burns of less than 15 percent of the body surface.
   c. Third-degree burns of less than 2 percent of the body surface.

FIRST AID AND TRANSPORTATION

First Aid

The majority of burns occur in the home, at the place of employment, or in recreational areas. Usually some type of topical first-aid medication will be applied before the patient seeks professional assistance. Home remedies vary widely and include such materials as butter, petroleum jelly, topical local anesthetic or antibiotic creams or sprays, and ice water. In general, first-aid measures for an acute burn should be aimed at avoiding undue contamination of the wound and at positioning the patient for comfort; topical medications that are not water soluble should be avoided, since they may be difficult to remove later. The following specific suggestions are useful first-aid measures:

1. *First-degree burns.* No medication required. A dry, clean dressing may be useful to avoid further wound trauma.
2. *Small second-degree burns.* Oral medication for pain may be helpful (type and amount should be noted for the information of subsequent medical personnel). The wound may be cleaned gently with bland soap and water, blotted dry, and covered with a clean, dry dressing. Do not use absorbent cotton on the wound as it may become adherent and difficult to remove. Blisters should *not* be broken. The application of ice packs to localized burn areas is helpful in minimizing initial pain and edema. The ice should be sealed in a plastic bag for application to the burned surface. A burned extremity should not be immersed in ice water, and addition of salt to ice water solutions can produce tissue damage.
3. *Severe burns* (10 percent in a child and 15 percent in an adult). Do not attempt to clean wounds or break blisters. Cover wounds with clean, dry dressings if possible. If the hands are involved, they should be elevated. If the legs are involved, the patient should not walk. Elevate the head of the patient if the face is burned. Applying cold water to the burned surface is not recommended for extensive burns, but localized cold packs (as for the face) may be helpful. If transportation is to be

delayed for more than 30 minutes, allow only salt solution (no ice water) orally. A number of electrolyte solutions have been developed commercially that are preferable to the ingestion of plain water. The amount of oral liquids should be restricted to only a few sips to allay the intense thirst the patients have. If allowed unlimited access to oral fluids, patients can ingest surprising quantities, with resulting acute gastric dilatation. In addition, burn patients often spontaneously develop an ileus, which can result in nausea and vomiting. Therefore, most patients with major burns should be permitted no oral intake if transfer to an appropriate medical institution can be accomplished in a reasonable period of time. Alcoholic beverages should not be allowed.

Transportation

Under ordinary circumstances, a patient can be transported to a treatment facility within an hour, in which case transportation is usually not a great problem. Most communities are now served by an emergency medical service with transportation vehicles that are well-equipped for instituting limited initial medical treatment. The staffing of such units with well-trained emergency medical technicians has contributed greatly to the transportation of critically ill patients, such as those with burns. If an individual with a major burn is to be moved from a community hospital to a major medical center, the time of transportation must be considered. Patients with large burns usually tolerate transfer well for the first 24 hours, provided that the initial resuscitative measures have been adequate and that provisions are made for trained personnel to continue therapy during travel. After 24 hours, edema is usually maximal, and it is wise to defer transfer until 4 or 5 days after the burn, when the patient's general condition will usually be stabilized.

OUTPATIENT TREATMENT OF MINOR BURNS

Wound Cleaning

After initial pain control, the wound should be thoroughly cleaned, using a bland soap and water; the use of antiseptics, alcohol, or hexachlorophene should be avoided. The washing should be gentle and primarily of the irrigation type unless there is imbedded foreign material or other bits of debris. Blisters that rupture easily should be cleaned, but blisters do not necessarily need to be broken initially if there is no other foreign material present.

In general, all burns treated on an outpatient basis do better if dressings are utilized. An exception is a second-degree burn of the face, which is best managed by repeated applications of moist compresses for 15 minutes three or four times per day, followed by the application of a triple antibiotic ointment. Essentially, all other burn wounds treated on an outpatient basis will benefit from a dressing for wound protection.

A dressing should cover the entire wound and be substantial enough to result in some even compression with splinting of the involved part. The dressings on outpatients should be changed at 2- to 3-day intervals or at any time that the patient complains of pain or exhibits a rise in temperature, and when the dressing shows signs of significant exudation through the dressing material. At the time of dressing change, the outer portions of the bandage material can be removed; soaking the inner layers of the dressing with saline solution will soften the bandage material and make its removal easier and less painful.

Antibiotics and Tetanus Prophylaxis

If burns are sufficiently minor that outpatient treatment is elected, it is usually unwise to administer broad-spectrum antibiotics. If the wound involves 10 percent of the body surface or more, administration of penicillin for the first 4 or 5 days is permissible, but no other antibiotics are required. Although wounds may appear to be only second degree, the administration of a tetanus toxoid booster is wise as a precautionary measure.

During the course of outpatient treatment, if the wound becomes suppurative or clinically shows signs of erythema or infection, a culture should be taken and the patient placed on appropriate systemic antibiotic therapy. The bandages utilized for outpatient treatment tend to promote a warm, moist environment that facilitates proliferation of bacteria. Obviously, if significant infection develops or if the superficial infection involves significant areas of the body surface (as much as 10 percent), immediate hospitalization and appropriate treatment should be instituted.

Minor Grafting

After the burn victim has been treated for a few days as an outpatient, it will become readily apparent if the wounds are second degree or third degree; if third-degree areas develop, evaluation for grafting is required. In general, small, patchy, third-degree areas in second-degree wounds may reepithelialize quite satisfactorily with outpatient treatment. On the other hand, if it is apparent after several days that there are third-degree areas that exceed 2 cm. in diameter, the morbidity will be lessened and rehabilitation enhanced by covering these areas with skin grafts. If the areas are small and limited in number, grafting can often be accomplished under local anesthesia without hospitalizing the patient. If wounds that initially appeared to be second degree turn out to show significant areas of third-degree involvement, it is usually wise to hospitalize the patient for appropriate skin grafting in the operating room.

After the first few days, when the wounds have stabilized and are sealed with stable second-degree crusts or reepithelialization, dressings should be discontinued and the patient encouraged to soak and appropriately exercise the involved area, which hastens maximum functional recovery.

TREATMENT IN THE HOSPITAL

The immediate treatment for an extensive burn should be rendered efficiently and in an orderly manner to avoid unnecessary handling and moving of the patient. Adequate assistance should be obtained, and all personnel in immediate contact with the patient should wear gloves. The establishment of a definite program of management will ensure that the more urgent needs of the patient are met before the treatment of less important aspects. The following plan is suggested as a workable guide:

1. Evaluation of the patient's general condition and classification of burns and other injuries.
2. Establishment and maintenance of an adequate airway, with oxygen if required.
3. Emergency sedation if required.
4. Appropriate fluid replacement therapy.
5. Insertion of an indwelling catheter.
6. Monitoring of central venous pressure
7. Prophylaxis against tetanus.
8. Initial antibiotic therapy.
9. Program of oral fluids and nutritional requirements.
10. Provision of other supportive measures as indicated.
11. Management of local burn wound.

Included later in this chapter (p. 475) is a list summarizing the treatment program.

Evaluation of the Patient's General Condition and Classification of Burns and Other Injuries

A pertinent history should be obtained relative to the cause of the burn and the time elapsed since burning, together with any previous treatment administered. Basic information of immediate importance includes the patient's age, any known allergies to drugs, status of tetanus immunization, and whether the patient is currently receiving any medication, particularly insulin, digitalis, phenytoin (Dilantin), cortisone, or other major drugs.

The patient's clothing should be completely removed for examination of the burn area. A rapid physical examination should be performed immediately to detect any major injury or disease state that might influence subsequent therapy (Fig. 24-4). Important aspects of the initial physical examination include recording the temperature, pulse, and respiration, and evaluating the mental status of the patient as far as degree of alertness, presence of confusion, coma, and ability to cooperate are concerned. Note should be made of the skin temperature and turgor, and examination of the nose and mouth should include observation for singed nasal hairs or the appearance of soot, erythema, or ulcers of the pharynx, which may herald later respiratory difficulty. Examination of the chest should be made for breath sounds and for the presence of rhonchi or rales. Examination of the abdomen should be made for distention and for the presence or absence of bowel sounds. Following accidents or explosions, skeletal examination for associated fractures or other injuries is imperative. The initial history and physical examination consume only a few moments and can ordinarily be performed while the patient is being transferred from the stretcher to a hospital bed and while intravenous solutions, catheter trays, and other equipment are being made ready. While supplies and personnel are being assembled, early photographs should be taken; it should be remembered that these constitute an invaluable part of the record for subsequent reference and for medicolegal purposes.

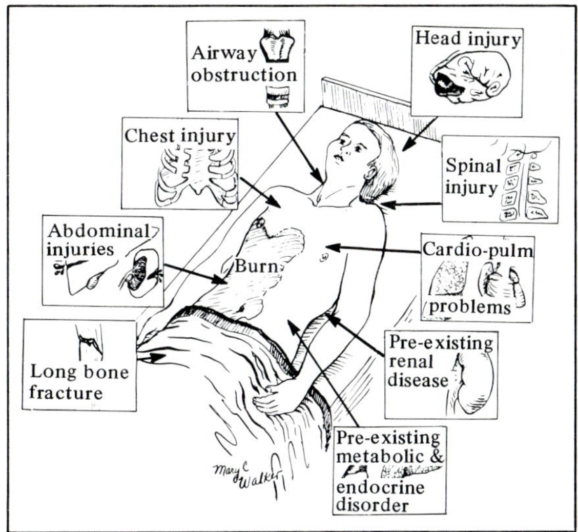

Fig. 24-4. An evaluation of the burn patient may reveal a variety of preexisting abnormalities or associated injuries.

This rapid preliminary overall evaluation should be performed to assess the magnitude of injury and to establish priority for treatment. Treatment should be instituted prior to a meticulous recording of a detailed history and performance of a physical examination, which are, of course, essential.

Establishment and Maintenance of an Adequate Airway, with Oxygen if Required
An adequate airway is essential. If there is associated head and neck trauma or facial fractures, a careful inspection and removal of necrotic material and stabilization of the fractures may be required. A nasopharyngeal airway may be helpful. In the absence of associated trauma, the oral mucous membranes should be inspected for evidence of direct burn injury. Although prophylactic tracheotomy was once considered indicated in patients with extensive head and neck burns, or in patients showing evidence of inhalation of smoke or fumes, this procedure is not recommended at the present time. The institution of a tracheotomy considerably increases the nursing requirements of the patient; in addition, the cannula can be a source of mechanical trauma as well as infection. For these reasons, prophylactic tracheotomy should not be performed. If early postburn edema produces some mechanical upper airway obstruction, temporary endotracheal intubation utilizing a soft endotracheal tube is preferable. These are usually tolerated quite well by patients for a period of 5 to 7 days. At the present time, tracheotomy should be reserved for the occasional patient who develops later pulmonary complications requiring ventilatory assistance.

Nasotracheal intubation with a soft, cuffed tube may also be required for patients suffering smoke inhalation in addition to their burns. This permits ventilatory assistance and is monitored by blood gases and pH. An occasional patient is seen with compromised pulmonary exchange due to constricting third-degree eschar of the chest wall; multiple escharotomies of the thorax can improve ventilation.

In patients with burns involving the head and neck, elevation of the head of the bed makes the patient more comfortable and is helpful in minimizing head and neck edema. Most patients benefit from the administration of oxygen during the acute burn phase. The use of a humidified atmosphere is also helpful (Fig. 24-5). *Undue restlessness in a patient during the immediate postburn period is often a manifestation of hypoxia.*

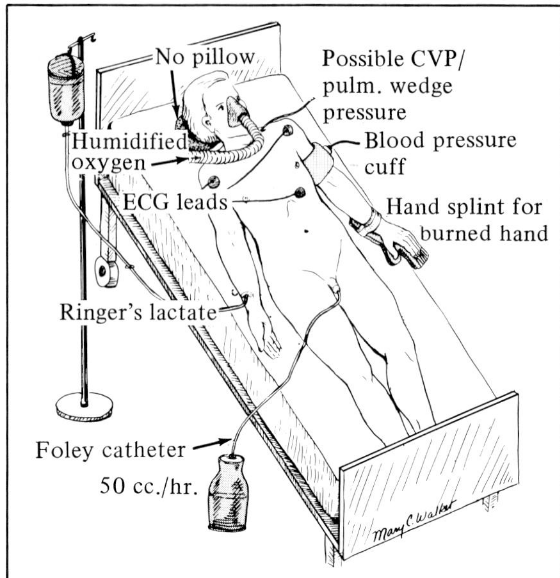

Fig. 24-5. This diagram illustrates the minimum requirements for care of the patient with an acute burn. For those with face and ear burns, a soft pillow can produce additional trauma and should be avoided.

Emergency Sedation if Required
A narcotic for sedation is usually the first medication administered by a patient's family physician or by the emergency room personnel. If sedation is required, a full therapeutic dose of morphine sulfate (10 mg. for adults and 1 mg. per year of age in children) is recommended and should be administered intravenously to ensure absorption. It must be kept in mind that patients with third-degree burns are often free from severe pain except during dressing procedures or position changes. Much of the patient's initial reaction may reflect fear, excitement, and apprehension, as well as true physical pain. For this reason, a calm, reassuring approach by the surgeon may be as valuable as any medication. In any event, the temptation to order narcotics every 4 hours should be resisted, and after 24 to 48 hours oral analgesics can usually be substituted, except when preoperative or postoperative medication is required. The regular use of small amounts of barbiturates may be helpful in unusally apprehensive patients. Although small amounts of tranquilizing agents may be helpful in occasional adult patients, one should not use them as a routine measure; it is important to keep in mind that some of these drugs (such as diazepam) can produce an undesirable degree of mental confusion in burn patients. The use of phenothiazine prior to tubbing or dressing is particularly helpful in children.

Appropriate Fluid Replacement Therapy
In general, intravenous fluid replacement therapy is required for burns of 20 percent or more in adults and 15 percent or more in children. Because the maintenance of an intravenous pathway is critical, insertion of a plastic catheter must be performed instead of simple insertion of a needle in the vein. An initial venipuncture should be performed to obtain blood for cross-matching, hemoglobin, hematocrit,

blood count, serum electrolytes, and blood urea nitrogen tests. In addition, if there is any indication from the history and physical examination, additional blood determinations, such as glucose, cholesterol, and liver function tests, and others, may be performed as indicated.

Estimation of Fluid Requirements

The reason for the burn shock with the resultant necessity for fluid replacement is threefold:

1. The internal fluid and electrolyte shift from the intravascular to the extracellular space (outlined under Physiological Derangement of Burn Patients, earlier in this chapter). The magnitude of this fluid shift is very extensive, and several thousand milliliters of fluid can accumulate in the burn wounds of the trunk without producing clinically obvious evidence of edema. A burn of the lower extremity that results in an increase in ankle circumference of 2.5 cm. and increase of thigh circumference of only 8 cm. requires 2.4 L. of edema fluid in an adult. Clinically apparent edema is usually most obvious in burns involving the head and neck and burns of the upper extremity.
2. Evaporative water loss from the surface of the burn wound. The amount of evaporative water lost through the burn wound surface is greater than generally appreciated. Various studies available in the literature show that on the average 4,000 ml. of fluid per square meter of burns are lost per day. The requirement for replacement of this volume of fluid is evident. The metabolic demands that this evaporative water loss places on the patient is of importance, since each 1,000 ml. of evaporative fluid loss is attended by a loss of 576 kilocalories.
3. The combined moisture excretion through the lungs, kidneys, and gastrointestinal tract. The loss of fluid from the lungs may be increased somewhat, but the lung, kidney, and gastrointestinal fluid loss are usually in the physiological range of 1,500 to 3,000 ml. per day.

Prior to 1940, programs for the treatment of burn shock by the replacement of fluids were developed largely on the basis of trial and error. After the first blood transfusion was administered to a burn patient in 1925, increasing emphasis was placed on whole-blood transfusions as an important part of the initial management. This policy was climaxed in the late 1940s by replacement programs where 4 or 5 L. of blood would be administered to the patient with an acute burn during the first 24 hours. Doubtless, the lifesaving value of massive transfusions to war casualties contributed to this policy. By such a regimen, however, many patients were overtransfused, with resulting elevation of hematocrit and, in some instances, thrombosis. In 1950 Evans and colleagues [15] presented a formula based on experience for estimating the fluid replacement therapy in acute burns. Their initial formula allowed 1.0 ml. of colloid per kilogram of body weight for each 1 percent of body-surface area burned, with an equal amount of electrolyte solution. The mainstay of the colloid regimen was whole blood. Since this original formula was presented, many formulas and calculations have been developed based on body weight, elevation of hematocrit, or modifications of the original Evans formula (Table 24-2).

Since some patients, particularly those with partial-thickness wounds, are overtransfused with the Evans formula, the *Brooke Army formula* [3] has been widely publicized in recent years.

The Brooke formula recommends the same total volume as the Evans formula but reduces the amount of colloid by 50 percent. The Brooke formula also relies on plasminate for the colloid component instead of whole blood, as originally advocated by Evans. Colloid administered during the first few hours post-burn tends to be lost from the vascular compartment. Colloid is lost over a period of time and exerts a transient osmotic effect, so that the judicious use of small amounts of colloid, particularly in the very elderly patients or the very young patients, may be beneficial in decreasing the total volume of intravenous fluids required. In most healthy patients, however, perfectly

Table 24-2. Examples of Replacement Fluid Formulas

Formulas	Colloid	Electrolyte Solution	H_2O
Evans	1 ml./kg./% burn	1 ml./kg./% burn	2,000 ml./day
Brooke	0.5 ml./kg./% burn	1.5 mg./kg./% burn	2,000 ml./day
Moore's budget	10% body wt./48 hr. (colloid solution in isotonic electrolytes)	1,500 ml.	1,000 ml./day
Parkland regimen		4 ml./kg./% burn	

adequate resuscitation for the first 24 hours can be accomplished with the use of electrolyte solutions alone. The use of colloids can, therefore, be deferred until the second 24 hours in the majority of patients. There has been some evidence presented to suggest that colloid administered during the first few hours postburn may be lost from the circulatory system and, in part, accumulate in the lungs and interfere in pulmonary exchange.

From time to time, other plasma expanders, such as serum albumin, dextran, hypertonic saline, and others, have been evaluated, but these are not now in widespread use.

Our current understanding of the initial fluid requirements for burn patients may be summarized as follows:

1. In the absence of preexisting anemia, fractures, or other associated injuries, the magnitude of red blood cell destruction at the time of the burn (average 15 percent) is not great enough to impair the oxygen-carrying capacity of the blood. Therefore, red blood cells are not required during the first 24 to 48 hours of resuscitation.
2. Colloid administered during the first few hours after the burn exerts a very transient effect and is lost from the vascular compartment where it may produce secondary difficulties. In most healthy patients, perfectly adequate resuscitation for the first 24 hours can be accomplished without the inclusion of colloid solutions in the treatment regimen.
3. The sodium ion is the key to fluid resuscitation in the burn patient. The use of a buffered electrolyte solution is satisfactory for initial resuscitation in the majority of patients.

Recommended Fluid Replacement

Initial fluid resuscitation in the average burn patient should consist of lactated Ringer's solution. The initial estimate of the amount required can be based on 4 ml. per kilogram for each percent of body-surface area burned (Parkland regimen). It must be emphasized that this formula is useful as an initial estimation only and should not be rigidly followed. A urinary output of 50 to 75 ml. per hour is the best guide to adequacy of fluid replacement therapy. The volume of fluid administered to the burn patient during the first several hours after the injury is frequently large, and the possibility of pulmonary congestion or edema is always present. The necessity for rapid intravenous digitalization must be kept in mind. Since the myocardium of burn patients is more sensitive to digitalis than is that of normal patients, necessary digitalization should be carried out intravenously, using multiple small doses at repeated intervals to minimize the possibility of arrhythmia. If digitalization is required it should be performed in an ICU setting with a cardiac monitor attached to the patient.

It must be kept in mind that following the burn there is normally an elevation of the serum potassium as a result of cellular destruction and electrolyte redistribution. Since the serum elevation of potassium occurs at a time when urinary output may be compromised, the administration of exogenous potassium must be limited. The 4 mEq. of potassium per liter contained in lactated Ringer's solution is acceptable for intravenous infusion except in infants or patients with inadequate urinary output; in these cases potassium administration should be strictly avoided until satisfactory renal function is established.

The serum sodium level is usually in the low-normal range (or below) immediately after the burning, since sodium selectively enters the edema fluid in the burn wound. *As a result, the chief requirement of electrolyte therapy is to supply sodium.* Despite the fact that the Brooke and Evans formulas point out the necessity to replace insensible fluid loss, the administration of sodium-free water as 5% glucose solution should be avoided in the immediate postburn period. Free water should be administered only after the hypovolemia has been partially corrected with electrolytes and colloids and a good urinary output has been established and maintained for some time. One of the common errors that inexperienced personnel make in the fluid therapy of burns is to order 5% glucose in water as one of the initial measures. This tends to further dilute the serum sodium and can produce symptomatic hyponatremia.

The average patient with full-thickness skin burns of major extent requires repeated *whole-blood* transfusions for replacement of red cell losses due to increased hemolysis and bleeding during dressing and grafting procedures. The total blood required usually averages 1 ml. for each 1 percent of body-surface area involved multiplied by the number of days of hospitalization following the resuscitation period. A patient with a 30 percent burn hospitalized for 10 weeks will hence require about 2,000 ml. of blood, with the administration concentrated during the pregrafting phase and immediately after surgery. Whole blood is preferable to packed cells for maintenance of hemoglobin and hematocrit levels, because the proteins in the former are partially effective in combating the negative nitrogen balance and hypoproteinemia that accompany extensive burns. During the first several days following the burn, there is a gradual decline in serum protein levels and particularly in the serum albumin component. Adequate data are available to demonstrate that in the burn patient, it is important to maintain the serum albumin level at a minimum of 3 gm. per 100 ml.

The hazard of serum hepatitis from multiple blood transfusions must be kept in mind. The incidence of hepatitis associated with blood transfusions varies among available reports but probably averages about 1 case in 300 transfusions. In large burn centers where multiple transfusions are administered to many patients over a prolonged period, the incidence appears to be considerably lower. It has been theoretically postulated that this is due to the fact that the multiple transfusions are not administered in a short period of time, as occurs in acute trauma, but are spread out as repeated transfusions over many days or weeks. The gamma globulin from the multiple spaced transfusions may exert a protective effect against serum hepatitis in the burn patient.

Schedule Rate of Fluid Administration

Since the internal fluid shifts are maximal in the immediate postburn period and transudation proceeds thereafter at a progressively slower rate, fluid therapy should be intensified for the first few hours after injury. As a general rule, about *one-half of the first 24-hour fluid requirements should be administered in the first 8 hours, one-quarter in the second 8 hours,* and the *final one-quarter in the third 8 hours.* It should be remembered that this schedule is related to the time the burn occurred and not to the time of admission to the hospital.

About *one-half of the fluids given in the first 24 hours will be sufficient during the second 24-hour period,* and fluids are administered orally and intravenously as indicated thereafter. In general, the earlier the patient with an extensive burn is admitted and fluid therapy started, the smaller the problem of maintaining adequate hydration and urinary output. When initiation of therapy has been delayed for some hours, the fluid requirements for the first 24 hours are often considerably greater. Again, it must be emphasized that these rules are statistical averages and must be individualized for each patient. In fact, there is considerable evidence that the majority of the internal fluid shift has occurred by the end of the first 18 hours, which reemphasizes the necessity for concentrating the fluid therapy during the first few hours following the burn.

Diuretics

The use of osmotic diuretics may be helpful in an occasional patient exhibiting hemoglobinuria or myoglobinuria or in whom resuscitation has been delayed, resulting in a period of oliguria. Urinary output can be increased by the use of osmotic diuretics, which minimize the precipitation of protein or hemoglobin casts in the renal tubules with mechanical plugging. Since the excretion of these agents requires excretion of water, mobilization of fluids from the unburned portion of the body can result in dehydration if excessive amounts of the diuretic are administered. For this reason, the use of diuretics should be judicious and *must be preceded by prior restoration of circulatory blood volume to more normal levels.*

Over the years, agents such as 4% urea, mannitol, and dextran have been utilized as osmotic diuretic agents. These are not widely utilized at the present time.

However, furosemide is a very potent and widely used agent that is very useful in occasional patients, but it can produce a profound diuresis with water and electrolyte depletion in underperfused patients. The occurrence of decreasing urinary output during the initial phase of burn treatment is usually an indication for intensifying the fluid replacement, perhaps supplemented with osmotic diuretics, but the osmotic diuretics alone are not proper treatment if the underlying mechanism is inadequate fluid replacement. There is evidence that the judicious use of osmotic diuretics combined with adequate fluid resuscitation has beneficial effects on the microcirculation as well as the kidney.

Insertion of an Indwelling Catheter

During the shock phase of therapy, the blood pressure and pulse are unreliable guides to the adequacy of hydration, as significant fluid deficits can exist when these parameters are relatively normal. The insertion of a Foley catheter is essential for monitoring urinary output during the acute phase. *The maintenance of urinary output between 50 and 75 ml. per hour is the best guide to the adequacy of fluid replacement therapy,* although not an infallible one. In infants and small children, the rate should be maintained according to the child's age, in accordance with the figures listed in Table 24-3. If the urinary output falls below these desired levels, the rate of fluid administration should be intensified. If the urinary output consistently runs above these levels, the patient should be reevaluated, since the extent of burn may have been overestimated, and fluid administration should be cautiously decreased.

Maintenance of satisfactory urinary output does not guarantee, of course, that the patient's prognosis is favorable. In the converse situation, where urinary output is low, the possibility of *acute renal insuffi-*

Table 24-3. Adequate Urinary Output According to Age

Age	Urinary Output
0 to 1 year	8 to 20 ml./hr.
1 to 4 years	20 to 25 ml./hr.
4 to 10 years	25 to 30 ml./hr.
10 years plus	30 to 50 ml./hr.

ciency must be kept in mind. Fortunately, acute renal insufficiency rarely occurs early, except in overwhelming burns; in most cases, a decreased urinary output signifies a need for increased fluid administration.

An occasional patient is encountered in whom there is scanty urinary output during the initial period of fluid administration or in whom the urinary output decreases during the course of treatment. The possibility of acute tubular necrosis is always raised and must be differentiated from inadequate fluid replacement therapy. As a general rule, acute tubular necrosis is uncommon during the first 24 to 48 hours of burn treatment if the patient has been admitted early and if initial fluid resuscitative measures have been adequate. In the majority of patients in whom urinary output is, or becomes, inadequate, the lowered output is related to insufficient fluid replacement therapy. Nonetheless, the differentiation of these two conditions is essential since the management is diametrically opposed. To differentiate between acute tubular necrosis and inadequate fluid therapy, the following points are helpful:

1. Urinary output tends to be scanty or almost absent in true renal failure, while there is usually a small urinary output when inadequate fluid replacement is the problem.
2. In early renal failure, the specific gravity of the urine will tend to be in the range of 1.015 to 1.020, and will usually exceed 1.025 when inadequate fluid therapy exists.
3. The differential between urinary and serum osmolarity and urinary sodium excretion studies is helpful in differentiating the two conditions.
4. It is usually essential to make an early test of the response to a fluid test load (i.e., bolus of fluid).

When decreased urinary output is present or appears during the course of treatment, the simple bedside test of *urinary specific gravity* and the patient's response to a *bolus of fluid* are the most important diagnostic aids. As a general rule, no patient should be considered to have acute tubular necrosis until the patient has demonstrated failure to respond to a fluid test load. It is important to remember that a plugged catheter or other mechanical problems can block external urinary excretion and *total absence of urinary output is almost always related to mechanical obstruction of the drainage system,* rather than to acute tubular necrosis or inadequate fluid replacement.

The administration of 1,000 ml. of lactated Ringer's solution over a 30- to 45-minute period is suggested as a fluid test load. During this infusion, a slight, transient, or absent response will be noted in acute tubular necrosis, while some evidence of increased urinary output usually occurs in the patient with inadequate fluid therapy unless his fluid deficiency is very large. If there is increased urine output suggesting inadequate fluid replacement, the fluid administration should be intensified; after urinary volume increases, the judicious use of an osmotic diuretic may be helpful in maintaining adequate glomerular filtration and minimizing renal tubular precipitates. If the patient is in acute tubular necrosis, the infusion of 1,000 ml. of fluid at this stage will ordinarily not unduly complicate his fluid load and the information gained by his failure to respond is very helpful in subsequent fluid restriction and other treatment.

Monitoring of Central Venous Pressure

Monitoring central venous pressure is not required for the vast majority of burn patients. The average patient with a 30 to 50 percent burn who had been in good health prior to injury, who was admitted within a reasonable time after the burn, and in whom adequate initial fluid resuscitation is instituted can ordinarily be followed adequately for clinical purposes without central venous pressure determinations. On the other hand, in patients who have failed to respond adequately to appropriate immediate treatment or in whom pulmonary or cardiac abnormalities exist, the monitoring of central venous pressure can be a very important adjunct. For monitoring central venous pressure, a plastic catheter is placed in the external jugular or subclavian vein and passed into the intrathoracic vena cava; one should attempt to estimate the length of tubing required to place the tip of the catheter at or near the right atrium. The antecubital, basilic, or cephalic veins may also be utilized, but the increased length makes estimation of the tip location more difficult. The catheter is then connected through a three-way stopcock to a manometer, which is positioned at the same height as the right atrium. The positioning of the catheter, the subsequent positioning of the manometer, and the respiration of the patient at the time the reading is made all contribute to technical errors in the reading.

A central venous pressure reading of 7 cm. of water or less indicates inadequate venous return and suggests that fluid therapy is inadequate. If this is corroborated by decreased urinary output and other clinical signs of hypovolemia, fluid therapy should be intensified. If the central venous pressure reading is from 7 to 15 cm. of water, and if that finding is corroborated by adequate urinary output and satisfactory clinical signs, the intravenous therapy should be continued at the same rate. When the central venous pressure rises above 15, great caution should be exercised, since the possibility of pulmonary edema exists and the need for rapid digitalization may occur.

Although the recording of central venous pressure

Anemia and Hypoproteinemia in the Chronic Burn Patient
In addition to periodic transfusions and caloric and protein intake as outlined, therapeutic administration of plasminate at intervals may be necessary in chronic burn patients referred late with emaciation and hypoproteinemia. Intravenous administration of albumin exerts such a transient effect that it is not helpful except in an occasional patient in whom the serum albumin may fall below 3 gm. per 100 ml. Total parenteral alimentation may be necessary in some patients with gastrointestinal or other complications and in occasional patients as nutritional support. Gamma globulin has been suggested as an adjunct to massive antibiotic therapy in the treatment of overwhelming septicemia, and it may have some very limited value. There has also been evidence presented to suggest that adrenal insufficiency may develop late in the course of some burn patients with extensive injuries, but the early administration of steroid preparations or ACTH as a routine measure appears to be of no value and should be avoided.

Position Patient Carefully and Institute Physiotherapy
Although burn contractures cannot be totally prevented, an attempt to minimize deformities should include positioning of extremities and other joint surfaces in extension when feasible. The patient should be made as comfortable as possible, and the head of the bed should be elevated initially for burns of the upper portion of the body to facilitate breathing and minimize edema. Bed patients should be encouraged to exercise various muscle groups actively; in fact, physiotherapy should be started shortly after admission to the hospital in order to preserve muscle tone and strength. Foot drop may be prevented by the use of foot boards to avoid plantar flexion; double mattresses may be employed in those patients who are confined in the prone position so that their feet may extend over the end of the mattress.

For patients with severe burns who are unable to cooperate during the first few days of treatment and those who develop complications during the course of treatment that make their cooperation with physical therapy difficult, consideration should be given to functional splinting of joints. Custom splints can be readily constructed to maintain elbows, knees, ankles, or hands in functional positions to minimize the possibility of soft tissue contractures developing. These are most helpful for the hands and are regularly used as night splints during the initial treatment of patients with deep hand burns. Prolonged splinting and immobility are to be avoided when possible, and continuous active range-of-motion exercises are preferable. For patients unable to cooperate, for those in whom severe complications develop, and to minimize contractures occurring during sleep, the use of splinting as a temporary or intermittent measure to minimize the development of contractures can be very helpful.

Management of Local Burn Wound

Initial Phase
The majority of flash-and-flame burns require no cleaning, and blisters may be left intact initially. Adherent clothing, dirt, or other foreign material may be cleaned by general rinsing with bland soap and warm water. Chemical burns should be treated with copious irrigations of water. Total body cleaning utilizing *hexachlorophene*-containing compounds should be avoided since significant amounts of hexachlorophene can be absorbed from open burn wounds, with resulting central nervous system symptoms. Circumferential burns of the extremities must be inspected carefully for evidence of circulatory impairment, and decompression incisions made as indicated (Fig. 24-6B and 24-7).

After initial evaluation of the patient and his burn wounds and inspection for tourniquet effect, the patient is positioned in bed. Patients who have sustained burns of the head and neck are usually more comfortable if the head of the bed is elevated. If there are circumferential burns of the lower extremity, slight elevation on pillows is used. Patients who have sustained burns of the hands should have their hands elevated for the first 2 or 3 days to minimize edema. Active and passive exercises are essential at regular intervals during the day. The use of a splint to maintain the wrist in dorsiflexion and the thumb in abduction and opposition with the metacarpophalangeal joints flexed is helpful for positioning the hands at night and in patients who are unable to cooperate with their exercise program for the first few days. The use of Stryker frames or Circa beds to permit turning and alternative exposure of opposite surfaces of the body is desirable in patients with circumferential trunk burns.

Formerly, dressings utilized for the care of the burn wound were impregnated with nitrofurazone, petrolatum, glycerin, or a variety of other compounds. Conventional antibiotics lack the ability to penetrate the eschar to exert any effect on the bacterial proliferation in the depths of the eschar. Similarly, systemically administered antibiotics could not reach this subeschar space since the circulation to this area is not intact. In recent years, several compounds have been developed that exert a bacteriostatic effect on the burn wound by virtue of their ability to penetrate the eschar. The use of these compounds minimizes bacterial proliferation in the tissue, prevents conver-

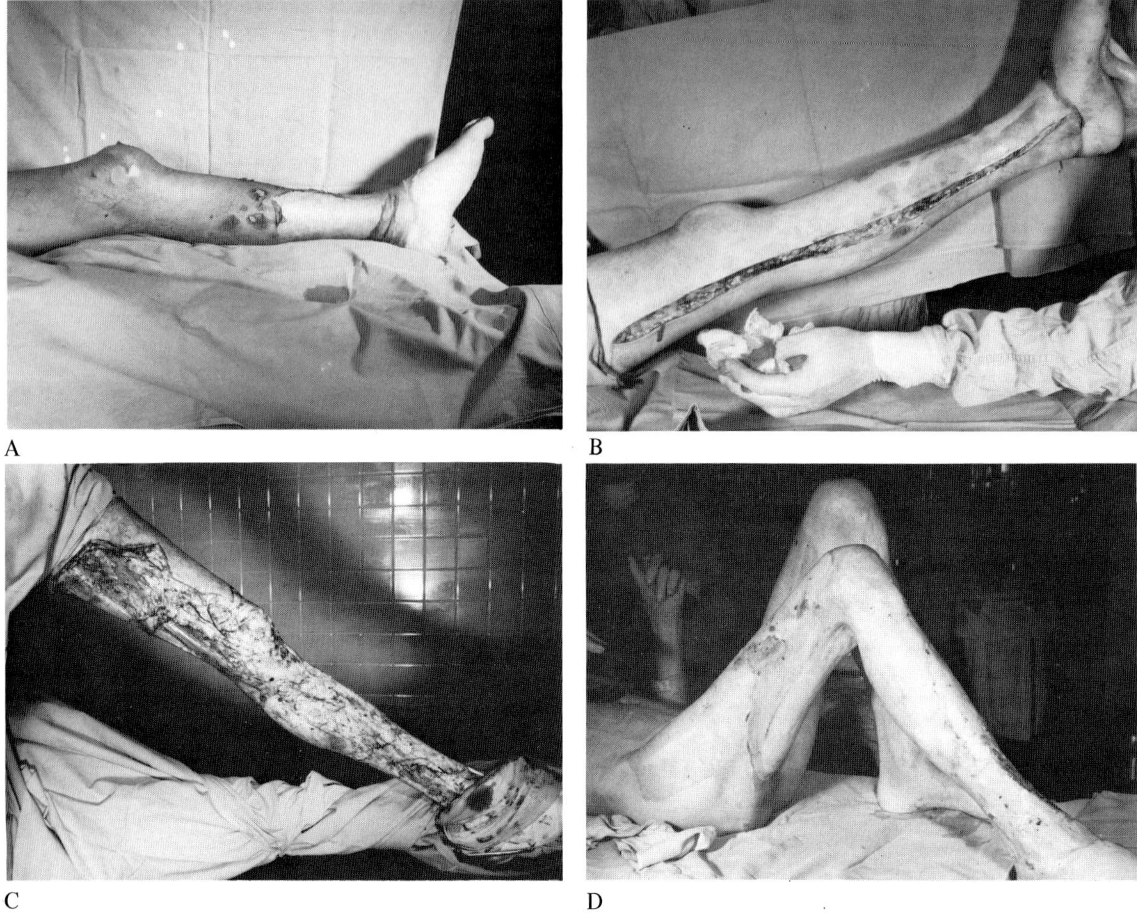

Fig. 24-6. A, circumferential third-degree burn extending from the ankle to above the knee. B, cleaning of wound and relaxing incision at the time of admission. C, surgical excision of the burn wound on the fifth postburn day; compression dressings were applied for 48 hours to obtain hemostasis, and then skin grafts were applied. D, appearance 2 weeks after application of grafts.

sion of deep second-degree burns into third-degree wounds, and has decreased the frequency of secondary septic complications. The first effective topical agent was 0.5% silver nitrate soaks, as reported by Moyer and colleagues [32]. This was followed shortly by Lindberg and associates' [24] report on Sulfamylon. More recently, Fox [17] has introduced silver sulfadiazine, and other agents continue to be evaluated.

Silver nitrate, Sulfamylon, and silver sulfadiazine possess the following advantages:

1. Good bacteriostatic properties.
2. Ability to permeate and penetrate the eschar.
3. Ease of use.
4. Decrease in the frequency of septic complications.
5. Elimination of the putrid odor formerly associated with burn wards.
6. Less conversion of second-degree to third-degree wounds by secondary infection.

The main disadvantages of 0.5% silver nitrate include some delay in eschar separation by inhibition of bacterial autolysis in the burn wound; electrolyte abnormalities (consisting primarily of dilutional hyponatremia and hypokalemia); intense black discoloration of the wound, dressings, bed linens, personnel,

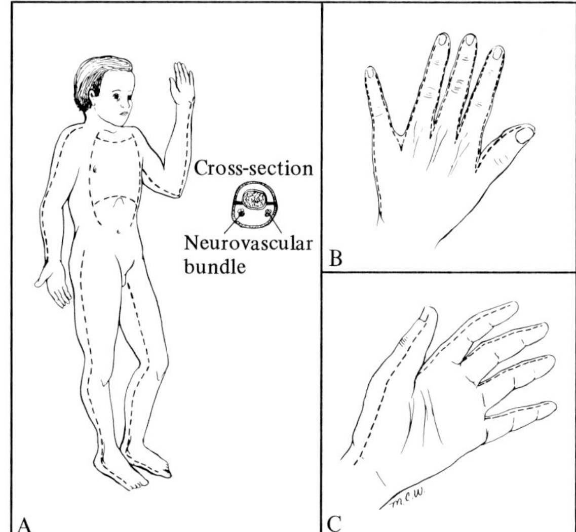

Fig. 24-7. Suggested incisions for escharotomies. The doppler is useful for evaluating circulation in the digits and finger escharotomies can be beneficial.

etc.; and the time-consuming necessity of changing the bulky dressings every 12 hours. The main disadvantages of Sulfamylon are that it is frequently painful on application; produces sensitivity skin rashes in 10 to 15 percent of the patients; delays eschar separation; and, as a potent carbonic anhydrase inhibitor, tends to produce acidosis.

Silver sulfadiazine appears to possess all of the advantages of silver nitrate and Sulfamylon with minimum disadvantages. Silver sulfadiazine is easy to apply, is better tolerated by the patients than Sulfamylon, possesses good bacteriostatic properties, and does not contribute to electrolyte abnormalities; sensitivity reactions, if they occur at all, are quite rare. A transient leukopenia has been reported in many patients treated with silver sulfadiazine, although the exact mechanism is not clear. Because silver sulfadiazine possesses all of the advantages of silver nitrate and Sulfamylon with minimal side effects, it is now the most widely used topical chemotherapeutic agent in the treatment of burns.

REMOVAL OF NECROTIC TISSUE. After the initial wound evaluation and institution of topical therapy, the burn wound requires no specific therapy for the first few days. Management of burn shock and general supportive measures take precedence over local wound management at this time.

Between 7 and 10 days after the burn injury, the intact eschar begins to show autolysis and liquefaction so that the conservative removal of necrotic material is necessary. This is best accomplished by daily tubbing in the Hubbard tank, which can be started on the third to fifth day postburn. Daily immersion in the Hubbard tank is an effective method of removing the topical agent in order to allow inspection and evaluation of the burn wounds. This serves as an excellent time also for the physical therapist to conduct intensive range-of-motion exercises, which may be more comfortable to the patient while he is immersed in the tub. After removal from the Hubbard tank, any gentle cleaning and debridement required can be easily accomplished prior to reapplication of the topical agent being utilized.

When the Hubbard tank cleaning method is utilized on a daily basis, the wounds can be followed until there is healing of the second-degree burns or until the third-degree burns are ready for grafting. An occasional patient will benefit from an operating room debridement procedure after 2 or 3 weeks to complete the removal of the adherent eschar and facilitate earlier grafting than would be possible if complete spontaneous separation of all eschar is allowed. When a suitably large area is ready for grafting, coverage should be accomplished even if some remaining eschar is present over the remainder of the burn wounds.

Experimental studies have indicated that there is a tendency for some retardation of epithelialization of experimental wounds using any of these topical agents. For that reason it is sometimes wise in second-degree burns after a period of 10 days to 2 weeks when the crusts have been removed and a clean wound base is present to discontinue the topical medication in order to facilitate more rapid wound epithelialization.

Excision and grafting of the burn wound can be effective in certain patients. In patients with limited burns, surgical excision of the burn tissue followed by skin grafting, either at the same sitting or after 24 to 48 hours to obtain hemostasis, is a satisfactory method of therapy (Fig. 24-6C). This method is particularly applicable to burns over the dorsum of the hand, where early wound coverage and functional restoration are important. Hand burns, which initially appear to be third degree by clinical criteria, often reepithelialize spontaneously, probably due to prevention of bacterial destruction of viable remnants of skin appendages in the deep dermis by the currently used topical agents. Healing of these deep dermal burns often results in excessive hypertrophic scarring, which can be incapacitating on the hands. Hand rehabilitation is so important that, if hand burns have not healed spontaneously in 3 weeks, it is assumed that the depth of the burn is sufficient to increase the possibility of severe hypertrophic scarring. Instead of allowing additional time to see if healing will occur, patients with hand burns are taken to the operating room before 3 weeks postburn, and the wounds are prepared for grafting by excision, abrasion, scraping, or any appropriate method of eliminating residual crusts and eschar with application of grafts, either immediately or after 24 to 48 hours (Fig. 24-8).

Although conventional excision, either in one stage or repeated stages, has been evaluated over the years in many burn centers, it has accomplished little in reducing the overall mortality and morbidity in large burns. Burke and associates [10] have recently reported encouraging results using a highly sophisticated experimental method of surgical excision combined with allograft coverage and immunosuppression. For the average hospital, however, excision therapy should still be limited to burns involving 15 percent or less of the body surface area and wounds that are clearly third degree in depth.

TANGENTIAL EXCISION. Because all of the effective topical chemotherapeutic agents retard bacterial autolysis of the eschar and tend to delay the time for initial grafting, other methods have been evaluated for hastening eschar removal. One method is that of tangential excision [19]. This technique is performed 2 to 5 days after the burn, utilizing a dermatome or skin graft knife to remove repeated superficial slices of the burn eschar until a bleeding surface is obtained, with immediate application of skin grafts. Jackson and Stone [18] have reported earlier wound closure by this method without increased mortality. The application of grafts is essential following tangential excision, since the excision alone appears to have no advantage. This method appears to be most useful in very deep dermal burns mixed with patchy third-degree areas in which some dermal base persists for application of the grafts. When burns extend into the subcutaneous fat, tangential excision results in a wound bed that is not satisfactory for uniform take of skin grafts.

Experimental evaluation of the carbon dioxide laser as a technique for removal of the eschar indicates that this may have little, if any, beneficial effect in the majority of patients.

ENZYMATIC DEBRIDEMENT. Despite disappointment with earlier attempts at enzymatic debridement of the eschar, there is continued interest in this area, because early chemical removal of the eschar to facilitate early grafting would be very beneficial for the burn patient. Since the report of McCann and coworkers [29] on a neutral proteinase of high specific activity obtained from bacillus subtilis, considerable clinical interest in this compound has resulted and many different authors have reported beneficial effects from the use of this enzyme. The use of this enzyme has been reported to be helpful in accomplishing early debridement of the necrotic eschar [21, 37]. Application of this agent requires that it be kept continuously moist and that it be applied to a limited area of the body not to exceed 10 percent of the body surface at one time. It must be instituted within 2 or 3 days after the burn when the patient's general condition is stabilized, and it becomes progressively less effective late in the course of the burn when the stable leathery eschar has existed for several days. In addition to being inactivated by drying, this enzyme is also inactivated by heavy metals.

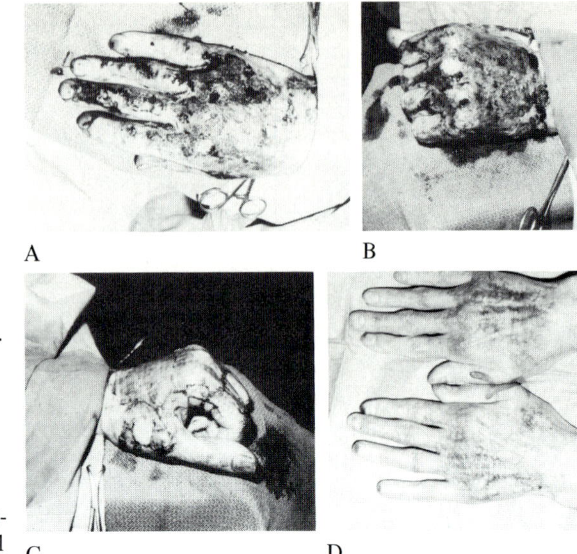

Fig. 24-8. A, at 2 weeks after the burn, both hands show mixed deep second- and third-degree burns. B, the wounds have been freshened to provide a uniform surface by superficial abrasion in preparation for grafting. C, a sheet of skin has been applied over the dorsum with the metacarpophalangeal joints flexed. D, final appearance with a full functional range of motion.

Grafting Phase

It is not necessary to wait until all burned areas are ready for grafting before applying the initial skin coverage. No specific preparation of the burn wound is required in the majority of patients, although continuous wet dressings for 24 hours may be helpful in locally infected wounds.

Donor sites, in order of preference, are the back, abdomen, upper thighs, chest, upper arms, buttocks, legs, and dorsum of the feet. The lower thighs, legs, and feet are to be avoided if early ambulation is anticipated. The patient's age and sex, and the extent and distribution of the burn, may alter the usual order of preference. In some patients, the extent of the burn may be so great that donor sites are extremely limited. Under these circumstances, any available skin should be utilized, including such areas as soles of the feet and the scalp. The scalp skin can be easily harvested and heals rapidly for early recropping if required. The electrical dermatome or the air-powered dermatomes are useful for rapidly removing large amounts of skin in sheets.

Skin thickness of 0.008 to 0.010 of an inch is satisfactory in children and 0.012 to 0.015 of an inch in adults. If repeated crops of autografts from the same donor areas are anticipated in extensive burns, the skin grafts are proportionately thinner. The donor site may be covered with a single layer of fine mesh gauze. A moist pad is applied in the operating room to promote hemostasis, but it should be removed at the conclusion of surgery, leaving the gauze with incorporated blood and serum to form a crust as it dries within 48 to 72 hours. By this time pain in the donor site is usually minimal and the gauze may be left undisturbed until spontaneous separation occurs as healing takes place. (See Chapter 1 for further information on skin grafting.)

When *applying the skin grafts,* an effort should be made to use large pieces of skin as opposed to postage-stamp size or thin strips. The grafts are spread out on the granulating surface and trimmed to fit the defect. If the wound can be positioned for exposure, no sutures or dressings are required, as the skin grafts rapidly become adherent to the underlying wound (Fig. 24-9B).

In occasional patients the extent of the burn wound may be so great that the available donor sites are grossly inadequate for coverage. Under these circumstances, the use of the mesh graft or a similar technique for expansion of a limited amount of skin to obtain a larger area of coverage is worthwhile. These expanded grafts are most useful over the broad surface areas of the trunk, back, and buttocks; efforts should be made to minimize their use over joint spaces, where potential contractures can develop. It must be kept in mind that the "cobblestone" appearance of these grafts is permanent, and the cosmetic result is inferior to that obtained with broad sheets of skin grafts.

In dependent areas or circumferential wounds of the extremities, the skin grafts may be held in place with bulky occlusive dressings. As an alternative to such dressings, particularly in difficult areas where exposed grafts are subjected to mechanical dislodgement and dressings are difficult to apply, skeletal traction is helpful (Fig. 24-10). This is not required routinely, but in a problem patient with a difficult burn of the axilla or lower extremity, it represents the most feasible method of protecting skin grafts until they have taken. Complications from the use of Steinmann pins are rare even when they are placed immediately adjacent to burn wounds. The use of skeletal traction can be particularly helpful in exposing burns of the hand for grafting while maintaining the hand in a functional position. The use of skeletal traction is also very useful to position extremities in extension to minimize the possibility of subsequent contracture; in fact, gentle prolonged traction over a few days is an effective method of reducing contractures prior to the application of skin grafts.

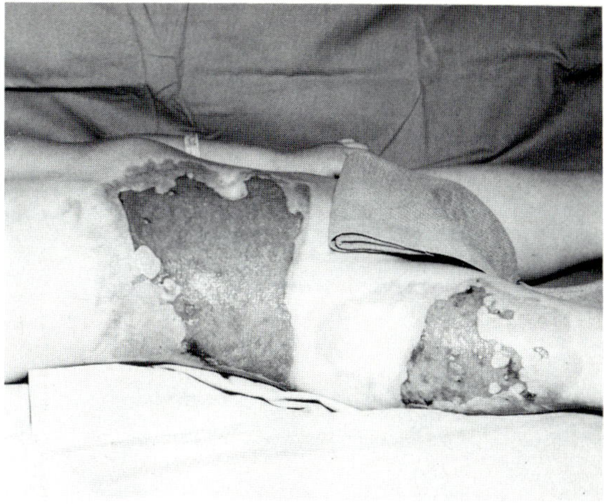

A

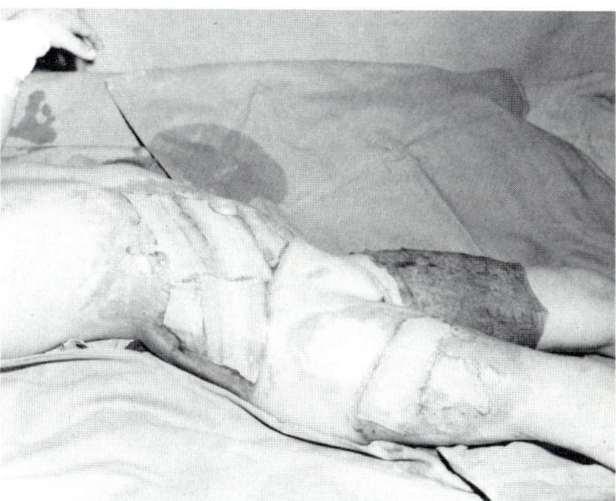

B

Fig. 24-9. A, wound prepared for grafting without removal of granulations. B, skin grafts are applied to the wounds without the use of sutures or bandages.

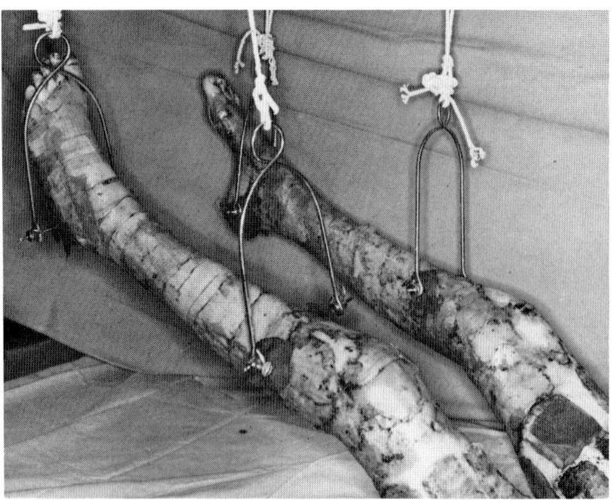

Fig. 24-10. In some patients, the use of skeletal support may facilitate the application of skin grafts.

ALLOGRAFTS. At times, the use of *allograft skin* may be lifesaving. In some burn centers, the use of allografts is prevalent, and they have been advocated as biological dressings in wounds not quite ready to risk the take of autogenous skin grafts. Since procurement is not always easy, and since the useful life of allografts is limited, they are most valuable in patients with extensive burns and large granulating wounds where adequate donor sites are not available for autogenous skin. Since many patients with massive burns do not survive long enough for granulating areas to exceed available donor sites, their use is somewhat restricted. In addition, many massive burns will have some areas ready for grafting before other portions of the wound have formed adequate granulation tissue. In these instances, repeated crops of available autogenous skin may be preferable to the application of allografts. Since the rejection of allografts is usually associated with considerable exudation and shredding of tissue, it is preferable to remove the allografts after several days and replace them with autografts whenever feasible. If adequate fresh cadaver allografts are available, their quality and survival period are comparable to those removed from members of the patient's family and have the additional advantage of avoiding the hospitalization and morbidity associated with utilization of live donors. Permanent survival of allografts of skin will probably not be a reality in the immediate future, and their useful life at the present time is about 2 weeks or less in the majority of cases, despite occasional reports of prolonged survival in burn patients. Only in identical twins can permanent survival be expected.

XENOGRAFTS. With the limited availability of allografts, certain xenografts, particularly pigskin, have been extensively evaluated in recent years and are currently used as an alternative to human allografts in many centers. The pig xenografts may be derived from animals maintained near the burn facility or can be purchased commercially. In general, the xenografts can be used as biological dressings to facilitate the microdebridement and preparation of a wound for autografting, with the grafts being changed at 24- to 72-hour intervals, or they may be applied over second-degree burns and donor areas, with some clinical suggestion that they enhance the rapidity with which second-degree wounds and donor areas become reepithelialized.

Postgrafting Phase

Following the application of skin grafts, patients should be positioned in bed for exposure of the skin grafts and donor sites if feasible. The use of a gooseneck lamp for short intervals during the first 1 or 2 days may hasten the drying of donor sites and avoid complicating infections. In small children, where exposed skin grafts are used without suturing, restraints may be necessary for the first 3 to 5 days. Within 48 hours after grafting, the discomfort in the donor site has usually subsided, and the patients are reasonably comfortable. During this time, any small collections of serum or pus can be evacuated from the skin grafts on the ward. Our routine postgrafting management provides that nursing personnel "roll" grafts with cotton-tipped applicators at hourly intervals for the first 24 to 48 hours postgrafting. With the use of the cotton-tipped applicator, any small accumulations of serum, blood, or purulent material beneath the grafts can be rapidly expressed, resulting in a greatly improved graft take. As the grafts mature, the frequency of this "rolling" maneuver is decreased. Although sutures are not required for stability of the grafts, Steri-strip is used generously to maintain the grafts in their desired position for the short period of time until adherence to the wound surface occurs.

The grafts are usually sufficiently stable and mature in 7 to 10 days for the patients to resume daily bathing in the Hubbard tank. It is usually possible to remove any Steinmann pins placed for skeletal traction at about this same time, although they have been left for a few weeks without undue complications. When the wounds have been virtually covered with skin grafts, with only multiple small granulating areas remaining, daily tubbing in detergent solution in the Hubbard tank for cleanliness and exercise is useful. Following soaking and exercising in the tank, the small raw surfaces are blotted dry.

After the acute phase of the burn, ambulation is encouraged in most patients. In patients with burns of the lower limbs, dependency requires the use of elastic supports during ambulation. Elastic supports are worn until circulatory equilibrium has been completely restored; in some cases, these are worn permanently.

TREATMENT SUMMARY AND ADMISSION ORDERS FOR THE ACUTE BURN

With the above information in mind, the evaluation and treatment (with suggestions for admission orders) for the patient with an acute burn may include any or all of the following:

A. General evaluation.
  1. History.
    a. Patient's age.
    b. Type of burn and circumstances.
    c. Time since burn.
    d. Any prior burn treatment, including sedation, intravenous therapy, and the use of other medications.
    e. Status of tetanus immunization.
    f. Known allergies to medication.
    g. Current medications (digitalis, steroids, etc.).
    h. History of peptic ulcer or cardiopulmonary, renal, or metabolic disease.
    i. Symptoms since burn, including mental status, vomiting, and voiding.
  2. Physical Examination.
    a. Evaluate mental status (e.g., alert, confused, comatosed).
    b. Evaluate state of hydration.
    c. Estimate extent of burn (Rule of Nines).
    d. Estimate depth of burn.
    e. Check for constricting circumferential wounds and perform decompressing incisions as needed.
    f. Check temperature, pulse, respiration, and blood pressure (if unburned areas are available).
    g. Check nasal and oral mucous membranes for soot, singed hair, or other evidence of direct injury.
    h. Chest: check for rales or rhonchi.
    i. Abdomen: check for distention: check for bowel sounds.
    j. Skeletal: check for fractures or other injuries.
    k. Weight is taken on admission and daily.

B. Maintain adequate airway.
  1. Check for unstable facial fractures.
  2. Remove any foreign material from the oropharynx.
  3. Evaluate the need for oral airway or endotracheal intubation.
  4. Elevate the head of the bed for burns of the upper half of body.
  5. Use humidified oxygen initially for burns of the upper body.
  6. Reserve tracheostomy for later complications.
  7. Undue restlessness is often due to hypoxia.

C. Immediate sedation.
  1. Morphine sulfate 10 mg. or meperidine (Demerol) 75 mg. in adults; in children, morphine 1 mg./year of age.
  2. Give slowly intravenously – not intramuscularly or subcutaneously.
  3. Reassure the patient and use a calm, confident attitude.
  4. Try to restrict narcotics to the first 48 hours except for preoperative and postoperative medication.
  5. Use oral analgesics when possible.
  6. Small regular doses of barbiturates may be helpful.
  7. Tranquilizers should be limited but may be helpful in occasional patients.

D. Institute fluid therapy (full therapeutic intravenous regimen for burns of 20 percent or more in adults and 15 percent in children).
  1. Insert a plastic catheter into a large vein.
    a. This provides an adequate intravenous line for the majority of burns in healthy patients with less than 50 percent body surface involvement.
    b. For patients with burns over 50 percent, in elderly patients, and in those with burns complicated by cardiopulmonary or renal problems, insert central venous pressure lines through the external jugular or subclavian vein.
    c. Maintain central venous pressure between 7 and 15 cm. water.
    d. Following subclavian puncture, obtain portable chest x-ray to rule out pneumothorax.
    e. Remove all intravenous catheters as soon as possible after the general condition stabilizes (4 to 7 days).
    f. If the intravenous line must be maintained longer, change the intravenous site after 5 to 7 days.
  2. Estimate the initial fluid requirements at 4 ml. × body weight (kg.) × percent body-surface area burned.
    a. This estimate is only a guide and fluid administration must be adjusted to maintain urinary output (see 2g.).
    b. Begin fluid therapy with lactated Ringer's solution.
    c. Do not give glucose solutions in free water for the first 24 hours.
    d. In elderly patients or patients with cardiopulmonary or renal complications, consider the judicious use of small amounts of plasminate after some initial infusion of Ringer's solution to decrease volume of resuscitation fluid required.

e. In most patients, infusion of colloids can be deferred until the second 24 hours.
f. Concentrate fluid therapy in first few hours after the burn.
g. Quantitate type and rate of fluid administration to maintain 50 to 75 ml. urinary output per hour in adults.
h. Blood pressure and pulse are *not* reliable guides to the adequacy of fluid therapy.
i. Be aware of possible need for intravenous digitalization if pulmonary congestion develops.

3. Draw the following baseline blood studies:
   a. Complete blood count, hemoglobin, and hematocrit.
   b. Blood urea nitrogen and serum electrolytes.
   c. SMA 6 or 12 as available.
   d. Additional blood studies as indicated.
   e. Arterial blood gases if complications are present.
   f. Repeat hematocrit or hemoglobin in 12 hours.
   g. Repeat other blood studies as needed.
   h. Serum protein determinations at least weekly; serum albumin should be maintained above 3 gm. per 100 ml.

E. Insert a Foley catheter.
   1. Record initial quantity and character of bladder urine (presence of hemoglobin, etc.).
   2. Record output hourly (the specific gravity determined at the bedside may occasionally be helpful).
   3. Maintain output at 50 to 75 ml. per hour in adults.
   4. Send initial specimen for urinalysis, culture, and sensitivity.
   5. Remove catheter as soon as possible (in 3 to 7 days).

F. Tetanus toxoid 0.5 ml. is administered if the patient was previously immunized. If not, 250 ml. immune globulin is given on admission and every 2 weeks until the wounds close.

G. One million units of aqueous penicillin is added to the intravenous fluids daily (if the patient is not sensitive) for 5 days. Thereafter, antibiotics are given as indicated clinically, guided by culture and sensitivity reports. No initial broad-spectrum antibiotics are given in the absence of pulmonary injury or when the patient has concurrent injuries (compound fractures) or associated infections.
   1. Obtain swabs for culture and sensitivity of representative areas of the burn wound initially.
   2. Repeat wound cultures are obtained as needed (at least weekly).
   3. Anticipate a temperature of about 38°C. in most patients with large burns. When the temperature is above 39°C., the following steps should be taken:
      a. Ensure respiratory toilet by encouraging the patient to turn, cough, and breathe deeply.
      b. Obtain a chest x-ray.
      c. Antipyretic medications are used for patients with a temperature greater than 39.4°C.
      d. Draw blood cultures for those with a temperature greater than 39.4°C.
      e. Urine culture should be performed, along with a search for other infections.
      f. Make a careful reevaluation of burn wound for abscesses, etc. Quantitative bacterial cultures may be helpful.
      g. Start potent antibiotics if clinical signs of sepsis are present; do not wait for culture report.

H. Nothing is given by mouth to patients with major burns initially. Nasogastric suction is used for all patients with burns over 40 percent and any burn patient with distention, hypoperistalsis, or nausea. After 12 to 24 hours, if there is no distention and peristalsis is present, start oral fluids. Avoid citrus juices for the first 3 or 4 days. Milk, 100 to 250 ml. per hour, is an excellent starting fluid. On the second and third days, a soft diet is given; on the fourth through seventh days, a high-calorie high-protein diet is administered. Supplementary tube feedings are required in most major burns. Total parenteral alimentation can be lifesaving in patients with gastrointestinal complications. A multiple-vitamin preparation and ascorbic acid, 1,000 mg., are given daily.

I. Chest x-ray is made on admission; a portable technique is frequently required. Repeat x-ray is done for patients with an unexpected temperature elevation, and chest x-ray is done following subclavian puncture. A baseline electrocardiogram is recorded on all patients over 50, in all those with electrical burns, and as indicated in patients with cardiac complications. Early photographs should be obtained.

J. Wound care involves the following:
   1. Position the patient appropriately.
   2. Use Circa beds for circumferential trunk wounds.
   3. Place the patient on clean sheets with the wounds exposed and cradles over the bed.
   4. For burns of the upper half of the body, elevate the head of the bed.
   5. If the legs are burned, elevate them on pillows initially.
   6. If the hands are burned, splint them when they are not actively exercising.
   7. The burn wound may be gently cleaned by rinsing, although blisters need not necessarily

be broken for the first 24 to 48 hours.

8. Copious prolonged irrigation is needed for chemical burns.
9. Make decompression incisions if required for circumferential wounds.
10. Cover burn wounds with silver sulfadiazine.

K. General.

1. Record a detailed history with results of the physical examination and burn diagrams.
2. Patients with burns in excess of 25 percent should be placed on the critical list initially.
3. Consultations are obtained as required.
4. Physical therapy for joint motion and maintenance of muscle tone should be started on the day of admission.
5. Analgesics and sedatives are used as required.
6. Antacids and antispasmodics are administered for epigastric pain or distress.
7. Laxatives are given as needed.
8. Steroids are not required.
9. Begin daily cleaning in Hubbard tank after 2 or 3 days, when the patient's general condition has stabilized.
10. Heat lamps and/or small doses of chlorpromazine (Thorazine) are given for excessive shivering after Hubbard tank therapy.
11. Whenever possible, ambulate patients after 2 or 3 days, when the general condition has stabilized.
12. Other appropriate therapeutic measures are employed as required by the individual patient.

COMPLICATIONS OF BURNS

Respiratory Tract Injury

During the immediate postburn period, the status of the respiratory tract must be continually evaluated. Phillips and Cope [38] have emphasized the importance of respiratory tract injury as a cause of death in burn patients. Patients sustaining burns about the face and those who are burned in closed areas with inhalation of smoke and fumes are particularly likely to sustain such injury.

In general, respiratory tract problems of *two types* may be encountered. The *first* is the early postburn problem associated with edema of the head and neck and mechanical airway obstruction, which is usually encountered 24 to 48 hours after the burn. These patients are best managed by the use of humidified oxygen and the use of a temporary endotracheal tube for the first 3 to 5 days until the edema subsides. Tracheotomy ordinarily should be avoided at this period. The transient edema with mechanical airway obstruction usually resolves spontaneously by the fourth to fifth day, and in almost all patients the endotracheal tube can be removed by the seventh day.

The *second* type of respiratory complication that occurs is the *"burn-lung syndrome."* This is more insidious at onset and usually does not become clinically manifest until 2 to 5 days after the burn injury. The first clinical symptom may be nothing more than an *increased respiratory rate,* which is followed progressively by gradual difficulty in breathing. At this stage the blood gas determinations and blood pH may begin to show some desaturation of the arterial oxygen, although the chest x-ray film may be clear. As the condition progresses, patchy infiltrates appear on the chest x-ray film, associated with some audible rales and ronchi and clinical evidence of increasing respiratory difficulty associated with progressive arterial oxygen desaturation. The course can progress rapidly over 24 to 72 hours to result in progressively greater respiratory distress, confluent pneumonia on the chest x-ray film, severe arterial oxygen desaturation, and death of the patient. There is suggestive evidence that the use of Sulfamylon in the immediate postburn period may, in some way, be implicated in the pathogenesis of this particular pulmonary problem; since silver sulfadiazine has largely supplanted Sulfamylon, the frequency of this problem appears to have diminished. The exact mechanism producing this sequence of events is unclear, but is probably not specific for the burn injury, since a similar condition known as the "shock-lung syndrome" is seen following other types of trauma. Common features include loss of pulmonary compliance with interstitial edema (followed by decreased perfusion across the alveolar membrane) and arterial oxygen desaturation, secondary infection, pneumonia, and death. One predisposing cause is *overhydration,* which should be avoided, particularly in elderly burn patients or in burn patients with a history of having sustained their injury in a closed space. Treatment consists of prophylactic broad-spectrum antibiotics, use of a high-oxygen atmosphere, tracheotomy with mechanical ventilatory assistance if required, and other supportive measures. The use of a pharmacological dose of steroids is sometimes helpful in the early stages of this condition to minimize the edema and inflammatory component. If required, the steroids should be administered at pharmacological doses and if necessary may be repeated in 4 to 6 hours for an additional dose or two. Bronchodilators and aminophylline are of limited value, but may be of some benefit in occasional patients.

The onset of burn lung syndrome after a latent period of 2, 3, or 4 days represents an extremely ominous complication. The mortality with this complication remains extremely high.

Shock

The other major complications occurring during the

immediate postburn period are those related to the circulatory system and shock. It is uncommon for acute renal failure to develop in patients who have been adequately treated, and acute tubular necrosis requiring medical management or dialysis is a rare complication in burn centers. An occasional elderly patient with massive, deep burns is still seen in whom there is no clinical response to treatment for shock and in whom death occurs in a matter of a few hours, apparently as a result of the overwhelming injury.

Infection

The major group of complications occurring in burn patients are in the infectious category. The respiratory tract injury and subsequent bronchopneumonia have previously been mentioned.

Urinary Tract Infections

Urinary tract infections can develop with the prolonged use of indwelling catheters. In general, the catheter should be removed as soon as it is no longer required for evaluation of intravenous replacement therapy during the shock phase, or when it is not required to facilitate nursing care in children or elderly patients, particularly during the grafting phase. While the catheter is in place, the use of a urinary antibiotic such as sulfisoxazole (Gantrisin) (1.0 gm. initially followed by 0.5 gm. four times a day), methenamine mandelate (Mandelamine), or nitrofurantoin (Furadantin) will minimize urinary tract infections. If urinary catheters are left in for an indefinite period, urethral strictures or fistulas may develop.

Septicemia

By far the most important complicating infection developing in the burn patient is septicemia. The usual portal of entry still appears to be the burn wound, although considerable discussion and much research effort have been devoted to this subject. The wound is continuously colonized by various bacteria from the time of injury until healing has occurred. Studies have demonstrated that as the bacteria proliferate in the interface between the normal tissue and burn eschar tissue, invasion becomes manifest at a tissue concentration of about 10^5 organisms per 1 gm. of tissue. With tissue invasion, local arteritis with thrombosis occurs, producing the characteristic satellite lesions around the burn wound. Septic emboli also enter the blood stream, producing multiple liver, lung, kidney, and brain abscesses. The advent of the currently available topical antibacterial burn wound agents has been helpful in minimizing the frequency with which this complication occurs.

Septicemia may be caused by either gram-positive or gram-negative organisms. Formerly, the incidence of gram-positive and gram-negative septicemia was approximately equal. In recent years, there has been an increasing incidence of gram-negative septicemia, with the *Pseudomonas* organism being particularly troublesome. Patients who develop gram-positive septicemia can frequently be salvaged by massive doses of appropriate antibiotics combined with blood transfusions and other supportive measures.

Drugs that are useful for the treatment of gram-positive staphylococcal septicemia include: methicillin, utilizing intramuscular doses in adults of 1 gm. every 4 to 6 hours, or intravenously, giving 1 gm. every 6 hours; lincomycin, utilizing adult doses of 600 mg. intramuscularly every 12 to 24 hours, or 600 mg. every 8 to 12 hours intravenously; oxacillin in adult doses of 500 mg. every 4 to 6 hours intramuscularly or intravenously; and erythromycin, 2 to 4 mg. per kilogram of body weight repeated at 8- to 12-hour intervals. Other effective antibiotics include the cephalosporins, nafcillin, and the tetracyclines.

The occurrence of gram-negative septicemia represents a grave therapeutic situation. The onset is frequently detected by the development of hypothermia and a leukopenia in the presence of a clear sensorium. These clinical findings are quite different from the high spiking temperature, marked leukocytosis, and toxic delirium that clinically characterize septicemia due to gram-positive organisms and other severe infections. The hypothermia and leukopenia of a gram-negative septicemia may be followed by anuria and death before the laboratory reports the growth of gram-negative bacteria from the blood cultures.

The most common gram-negative organism recovered from the blood stream of burn patients is *Pseudomonas aeruginosa.* Culture and sensitivity studies are desirable for appropriate treatment of this organism. The most effective agents available at the present time for most strains of *Pseudomonas* include gentamicin intramuscularly in three or four doses of 2 to 3 mg. per kilogram of body weight per 24 hours and carbenicillin, which can be administered intravenously at levels of 4 to 5 gm. every 6 hours. Other drugs that may be helpful for gram-negative organisms include colistin sulfate, polymixin B, and amikacin.

The sensitivity of the various organisms producing septicemia varies from one medical center to another and from time to time within the same medical center. In addition, new antibacterial agents are continually being evaluated; thus these specific drug recommendations should be adapted for the local circumstances in any specific hospital.

With the improved prognosis in recent years in the management of burn wound sepsis and gram-negative septicemia, there is emerging, with increasing frequency, colonization of the burn wound with yeast type organisms. Reports of patients undergoing burn therapy, utilizing topical antibacterial agents, who develop septicemia with yeast organisms (most commonly *Candida albicans*) are emerging with increasing frequency.

Curling's Ulcer

The development of acute gastrointestinal bleeding during the course of a burn represents a serious complication. The onset is usually 7 to 10 days after injury; it is quite unusual for bleeding to develop during the first week of therapy. Although less common in children than in adults, this complication may occur in patients of any age. The premonitory symptoms of epigastric pain, discomfort, or tenderness frequently herald the onset of bleeding, and immediate therapy consisting of sedation, antispasmodics, and antacids should be started. In the presence of massive bleeding, conservative therapy consisting of transfusions as indicated and nasogastric suction is necessary to keep the stomach empty should be instituted. The exact mechanism of acute gastroduodenal bleeding is unclear despite numerous studies aimed at delineating such problems as the role of histamine and the involvement of the adrenal cortex [27, 36, 39].

Bone and Joint Abnormalities

The most frequent abnormality occurring in the burn patient is flexion contractures developing over joint surfaces during the postburn period as a result of scarring. During the course of the acute burn, malpositioning of the joints by allowing them to remain in flexion can result in joint contractures, which may be very difficult to overcome secondarily. This tendency for contracture deformity can be minimized by basic splinting and pressure during the acute phase of the burn.

During the course of burn treatment, it is not uncommon for areas of bone to become exposed. This happens most frequently over the anterior tibia, where the skin and subcutaneous covering are relatively thin; over the scalp, often a result of electrical injuries; and over the distal phalanges and interphalangeal joints of the hand. In the absence of underlying fractures or other abnormalities, exposure of small amounts of bone, such as over the tibia, can be anticipated to result in healthy granulation tissue that will accept skin grafts after a period of time. The development of granulation tissue in this manner is related to gradual absorption of the superficial cortex of the bone, which allows granulation tissue to develop. If the exposed areas of bone are larger, the length of time required for development of granulation tissue is unacceptable. Under these circumstances, the best treatment is to remove the outer portion of the bone. This can also be accomplished with chisel or burs if care is exercised to prevent the bone from being overheated. The technique frequently described in the past of drilling multiple small holes in the bone to allow granulation tissue to develop all too often results in the development of multiple buds of granulation with persistent areas of exposed bone between the islands of granulation tissue. This method can require an inordinately long time for the development of a surface that will accept skin grafts; the use of the Hall drill or a hammer and chisel for removal of the uniform portion of the outer part of the bone is more effective. After removal of this superficial exposed bone, it is important to prevent the base of the wound from drying, either by continuous applications of moisture for 24 to 48 hours or by immediate placement of skin grafts. Skin grafts can be expected to take on exposed bleeding bony surfaces, and exposed bone does not necessarily require pedicle flap coverage.

In addition to joint contracture and exposure of bone during the treatment of acute burns, a wide variety of musculoskeletal abnormalities have been described by Evans [13, 14]. Evans' classification of bone and joint abnormalities is as follows:

1. Alterations limited to bone.
   a. Osteoporosis.
   b. Periosteal new bone formation.
   c. Irregular ossification.
   d. Diaphyseal exostoses.
   e. Acromutilation of fingers.
   f. Pathological fractures.
   g. Osteomyelitis.
   h. Necrosis and tangential sequestration.
2. Alterations involving pericapsular structures.
   a. Pericapsular calcification.
   b. Heterotopic paraarticular ossification.
   c. Osteophytes.
3. Alterations involving the joint proper.
   a. Septic arthritis.
   b. Spontaneous dissolution.
   c. Ankylosis.
   d. Dislocation.
4. Alterations secondary to soft tissue contracture.
   a. Muscle contracture.
   b. Malposition of joints.
   c. Scoliosis.
5. Abnormalities of growth.
6. Nonviability of extremity, leading to amputation.

According to Evans, each of these complications occurs in approximately 1 to 2 percent of hospitalized patients.

One of the most frequent complications is septic arthritis resulting from exposure of the joint or from hematogenous spread during septic episodes. The joints most likely to be exposed during the course of burn treatment are the interphalangeal joints of the fingers, ankle joints, wrist joints, and elbow joints. If the area of joint exposure is small, the joint should be irrigated by frequent flushing with normal saline solution containing antibiotics and positioned to promote drainage and prevent accumulation or pocketing of purulent material. If the joint opening is small, if it can be kept clean, and if early coverage can be obtained, the joint can frequently be salvaged, especially in children. If the exposure is extensive, ankylosis should be anticipated, and the joint should be positioned for functional efficiency.

Metabolic Considerations and Complications in the Burn Patient

Following any severe trauma, and particularly in the burn, there is a complicated series of metabolic reactions that normally occur, including a variety of chemical and physiological changes related to protein metabolism, carbohydrate metabolism, fat metabolism, water and electrolyte shifts, vitamin metabolism, and certain endocrine changes. These complex metabolic changes may be summarized in an oversimplified fashion as follows: increased heat production, negative nitrogen balance with weight loss, disturbed carbohydrate metabolism, fat mobilization, retention of sodium, chloride, and water, and alteration in the metabolism of certain water soluble vitamins. These changes are usually accompanied by leukocytosis, adrenal cortical hypertrophy with an increase in secretion of certain adrenal hormones, increased excretion of antidiuretic hormone, and lymphoid involution with changes in the reticuloendothelial system. Extensive studies related to thyroid function, pituitary function, and liver function have produced inconsistent results.

Protein Metabolism

Protein metabolism has been the most extensively studied of all the metabolic changes occurring in the burn patients. Under normal circumstances, the average individual takes in each day about 100 gm. of protein, containing 10 to 15 gm. of nitrogen. A small amount of nitrogen (1 to 2 gm.) is excreted from the gastrointestinal tract each day and 10 to 15 gm. in the urine. This maintains the individual normally in nitrogen equilibrium. Following a major burn, the urinary nitrogen begins to increase to levels of two to three times normal urinary excretion and the patient remains in negative nitrogen balance, which continues until the wounds are essentially closed. Since the main source of this nitrogen appears to be from skeletal muscle, extreme degrees of muscle wasting can be seen if vigorous attempts to maintain adequate protein and nitrogen intake are not accomplished. The marked increase in metabolism with negative nitrogen balance is associated with increased anabolic capacity, and provision of adequate protein and calories can minimize the negative nitrogen balance. There are also changes in plasma protein concentration because of fluid shifts and water loss, together with loss of water, electrolytes, and protein through the burn wound. The greatest decrease in serum proteins is usually in the albumin fraction, and in severe injuries there may be a decrease in prothrombin and fibrinogen concentrations. These anticipated metabolic alterations are best managed clinically by providing the largest intake of calories and protein that the patient can tolerate; the most severely burned patients will require supplementary tube feedings and, in some instances (if complications develop), the use of intravenous alimentation as well. These protein metabolic abnormalities usually persist until the burn wounds are healed, at which time the excessive nitrogen excretion decreases and protein intake is utilized for rebuilding body stores.

Carbohydrate Metabolism

Hyperglycemia and acidosis may occur during the course of burn treatment and may persist over a period of time. There is often some decrease in glucose tolerance and some increased resistance to insulin, which may also last for several days. This condition has been referred to in the literature as the stress "pseudodiabetes" of the burn patient. Although the exact mechanism is not clear, the hyperglycemia seems to result from increased liver glycogenolysis secondary to epinephrine release. It may also be caused in part by increased adrenal glucocorticoid secretion resulting in an increase in gluconeogenesis and in peripheral carbohydrate breakdown. Altered secretions of growth hormone, insulin, and glucagon have been studied, but their role in this abnormality is uncertain.

Fat and Vitamin Metabolism

Changes in fat metabolism in burns are poorly understood, although clinically there is a rapid loss of body fat during the postburn period. Various studies related to vitamin metabolism have also revealed some changes following burns, with the most notable for clinical purposes being a decrease in the plasma concentration and urinary excretion of ascorbic acid. For clinical purposes, routine supplements of the B complex vitamins should be administered, with 1,000 mg. of ascorbic acid daily. An ideal goal to strive for in burn patients is to achieve an intake of 2 to 4 gm. of protein per kilogram of body weight per day and 50 to 80 calories per kilogram of body weight per day. Obviously, such an intake is very difficult to achieve; however, from the available studies, the more closely this level of intake can be approached, the more the negative nitrogen balance and severe wasting and emaciation can be minimized.

Toxic Psychosis

The development of a toxic psychosis is occasionally seen during the first few days of burn therapy. The most frequent cause for an acute toxic psychosis is withdrawal from excessive alcohol intake or habitual use of drugs. In many patients, the burn in itself may have been the result of smoking in bed while the patient was drinking; under suggestive circumstances of this type, the possibility of withdrawal symptoms should be anticipated. The use of drugs is now particularly widespread in our society, and severe withdrawal may precipitate spectacular symptoms in some patients. An immediate and thorough inquiry should be made from friends and members of the family about excessive alcohol intake or habitual use of sedatives or other drugs. Treatment consists of adequate intravenous hydration, infusion of adequate amounts of vitamins, and sedation as required to control convulsions or undue restlessness during a period of severe withdrawal. Although the use of intravenous alcohol has been advocated from time to time for the treatment of patients undergoing acute withdrawal symptoms, this is not recommended for the burn patient, and infusion of alcohol may only serve to delay the withdrawal symptoms and complicate the recovery.

The development of acute toxic symptoms after the first week of burn treatment is most commonly due to the development of sepsis.

Miscellaneous Complications

In addition to the complications previously mentioned, a wide variety of others (e.g., electrolyte abnormalities, metastatic abscesses, congestive heart failure, thrombophlebitis, and pulmonary embolism) may occur. Many others may develop during the course of therapy. One very common problem encountered in patients with burns of the ears is the associated chondritis. When this occurs, wide incision of the ear with removal of the involved cartilage is required. Localized incision and drainage result in a chronic chondritis that persists until all the involved cartilage has been removed. Time and morbidity can be saved if the initial incision and removal of cartilage are adequate.

REHABILITATION

Following discharge from the hospital, the patient is encouraged to be ambulatory and to participate in active exercise programs within the tolerance of his strength and taking into account the location of the wounds. In many instances, supervised physical and occupational therapy may be helpful. At this time, the patients usually undergo a rapid weight gain and regain their sense of well-being.

As a rule, the healed burn scars become hypertrophic. These scars are often thick, red, and inelastic, and they may itch intensely. This is a normal phase of postburn healing and does not necessarily represent keloid formation. The use of lanolin or other bland ointment three or four times daily, with a few minutes of gentle massage, facilitates scar maturation and improves patient comfort. The use of antipruritic medication may be helpful in selected patients for a time. In some patients, the itching and stinging symptoms can often be minimized by injection of steroid preparations (e.g., triamcinolone acetonide) directly into the scar if the burn scars are relatively localized. The application of pressure in the form of custom-fitted compression bandages is probably the most helpful single measure in hastening the resolution of the scar hypertrophy. With the passage of weeks or months, the scars fade in color and become softer and more supple, and the itching and discomfort subside. Unless the deformity is severe, needed reconstruction should be delayed until the scar tissue has completed this normal process of maturation. This may require a period of 12 to 18 months.

Children may develop contractures due to growth and must be kept under periodic observation throughout their adolescent period. If there is significant deformity or disability, as from hand burns or a major amputation, vocational counseling, and, in some instances, vocational retraining may be necessary. It is always wise to correct functional disability before attempting cosmetic improvement of existing scars. In general, the more severe the initial injury, the greater will be the residual deformity and disability, and the more realistic should be the reconstructive effort.

REFERENCES

1. Allen, H. S., and Koch, S. L. The treatment of patients with severe burns. *Surg. Gynecol. Obstet.* 74:914, 1942.
2. Artz, C. P., and Moncrief, J. A. *The Treatment of Burns* (2nd ed.). Philadelphia: Saunders, 1969.
3. Artz, C. P., and Reiss, E. *The Treatment of Burns.* Philadelphia: Saunders, 1957.
4. Barthe de Sandfort, E. De la keritherapie. Nouvelle application thermale des paraffines. *Bull. Acad. Med. Paris* 26:249, 1914.
5. Baxter, C. R. Response to Initial Fluid and Electrolyte Therapy of Burn Shock. In Lynch, J. B., and Lewis, S. R. (Eds.), *Symposium on the Treatment of Burns.* St. Louis: Mosby, 1973.
6. Blocker, T. G., Jr. An Introduction to Disaster Problems. *Symposium on Burns.* (National

Research Council.) Washington, D.C.: National Academy of Sciences, 1950.

7. Blocker, T. G., Jr. History of the Treatment of Burns. In Lynch, J. B., and Lewis, S. R. (Eds.), *Symposium on the Treatment of Burns.* St. Louis: Mosby, 1973.
8. Blocker, T. G., Jr., and Blocker, V. *Report on Visit to Peru.* Annual Report, U.S. Army Contract DA-49-007-MD-447, 1964.
9. Blocker, T. G., Jr., Washburn, W. W., Lewis, S. R., and Blocker, V. A statistical study of 1000 burn patients admitted to the plastic surgery service at the University of Texas Medical Branch, 1950–59. *J. Trauma* 1:409, 1961.
10. Burke, J. F., May, J. W., Albright, N., Quinby, W. C., and Russell, P. S. Temporary skin transplantation and immunosuppression for extensive burns. *N. Engl. J. Med.* 290:269, 1974.
11. Davidson, E. C. Tannic acid in the treatment of burns. *Surg. Gynecol. Obstet.* 41:202, 1925.
12. Dolecek, R. *Metabolic Response of the Burned Organism.* Springfield, Ill.: Thomas, 1969.
13. Evans, E. B. Orthopaedic measures in the treatment of severe burns. *J. Bone Joint Surg.* [Am.] 48:643, 1966.
14. Evans, E. B. Bone and Joint Changes Secondary to Burns. In Lynch, J. B., and Lewis, S. R. (Eds.), *Symposium on the Treatment of Burns.* St. Louis: Mosby, 1973.
15. Evans, E. I., Purnell, O. J., Robinett, P. W., Batchelor, A., and Martin, M. Fluid and electrolyte requirements in severe burns. *Ann. Surg.* 135:804, 1952.
16. Foley, F. D. Early Recognition of the Infected Burn Wound. In Lynch, J. B., and Lewis, S. R. (Eds.), *Symposium on the Treatment of Burns.* St. Louis: Mosby, 1973.
17. Fox, C. L., Jr. Use of Silver Sulfadiazine in Burned Patients. In Lynch, J. B., and Lewis, S. R. (Eds.), *Symposium on the Treatment of Burns.* St. Louis: Mosby, 1973.
18. Jackson, D. M., and Stone, P. A. Tangential excision and grafting of burns. The method and a report of 50 consecutive cases. *Br. J. Plast. Surg.* 25:416, 1972.
19. Janzekovic, A. A new concept in the early excision and immediate grafting of burns. *J. Trauma* 10:1103, 1970.
20. Kentish, J. *An Essay of Burns Which Happen to Workmen in Mines.* Edinburgh: Robinson, 1797.
21. Krisek, T. J., and Robson, M. C. Clinical experience with Travase ® for enzymatic debridement in the burned patient. Presented at the Annual Meeting of the American Society of Plastic and Reconstructive Surgeons. Houston, Texas, October 1974.
22. Levenson, S. M. Pathophysiology of Burns—An Overview of Some Aspects of the Metabolic and Nutritional Response to Burns. In Lynch, J. B., and Lewis, S. R. (Eds.) *Symposium on the Treatment of Burns.* St. Louis: Mosby, 1973.
23. Lewis, S. R., Lynch, J. B., Wolf, C. W., Goolishian, H., and Blocker, T. J., Jr. Psychological studies in burn patients. *Plast. Reconstr. Surg.* 31:323, 1963.
24. Lindberg, R. B., Moncrief, J. A., Switzer, W. E., Order, S. E., and Mills, W. The successful control of burn wound sepsis. *J. Trauma* 5:601, 1965.
25. Lynch, J. B., Bray, J. P., Lewis, S. R., and Blocker, T. G., Jr. Studies with radioisotope labeled albumin in experimental burn wounds. *J. Surg. Res.* 4:226, 1964.
26. Malm, O. J., and Slawikowski, G. J. M. An Evaluation of the Burn Toxin-Antitoxin Theory, with Emphasis on Experimental Methods. (Monograph, Office of the Surgeon General.) Washington, D.C.: U.S. Government Printing Office, 1961.
27. Mason, A. D., Jr., and Pruitt, B. A., Jr. Curling's Ulcer. In Lynch, J. B., and Lewis, S. R. (Eds.), *Symposium on the Treatment of Burns.* St. Louis: Mosby, 1973.
28. Matter, P., Chambler, K., Bailey, B., Lewis, S. R., Blocker, T. G., Jr., and Blocker, V. Experimental studies with reference to antigen-antibody phenomena following severe extensive burns. *Ann. Surg.* 157:725, 1963.
29. McCann, J. D., Tsuru, D., and Yasonubu, K. T. *Bacillus subtilis* neutral proteinase: A zinc enzyme of high specific activity. *J. Biol. Chem.* 239:3706, 1964.
30. Millican, R. C. S^{35} plasma and erythrocyte distribution in tourniquet-shocked mice. *Am. J. Physiol.* 179:513, 1954.
31. Monasterio, F., Rebeil, A. S., Barrera, G., Araico, J., Bosque, R. G., Escobosa, J. E., and Barreto, F. R. Comparative Study on the Treatment of Extensive Burns With and Without Antibiotics. In Artz, C. P. (Ed.), *Research in Burns.* Washington, D.C.: American Institute of Biological Sciences, Pub. 9, 1962.
32. Moyer, C. A., Brentano, L., Gravens, D. L., Margraf, H. W., and Monafo, W. W. Treatment of large human burns with 0.5% silver nitrate solution. *A.M.A. Arch. Surg.* 90:812, 1965.
33. Moyer, C. A., and Butcher, H. R. *Burns, Shock and Plasma Volume Regulation.* St. Louis: Mosby, 1967.
34. Muir, I. F. Red cell destruction in burns, with particular reference to the shock period. *Br. J. Plast. Surg.* 14:273, 1961.
35. National Research Council, Committee on Surgery. *Burn, Shock, Wound Healing and Vascular Injuries.* Philadelphia: Saunders, 1943.
36. O'Neill, J. A., Jr. The influence of thermal burns

on gastric acid secretion. *Surgery* 67:267, 1970.

36a. Oppenheimer, L. S. The treatment of burns. *N.Y. Med. J.* 84:646, 1906.

37. Pennisi, V. R., Capozzi, A., and Friedman, G. Travase ®, an effective enzyme for burn debridement. *Plast. Reconstr. Surg.* 51:371, 1973.

38. Phillips, A. W., and Cope, O. Burn therapy: II. The revelation of respiratory tract damage as a principal killer of the burned patient. *Ann. Surg.* 155:1, 1962.

39. Pruitt, B. A., Jr., Foley, F. D., and Moncrief, J. A. Curling's ulcer: A clinical pathology study of 323 cases. *Ann. Surg.* 172:523, 1970.

40. Pulaski, E. J. Exposure Method. *Symposium on Burns.* (National Research Council.) Washington, D.C.: National Academy of Sciences, 1950.

41. Sneve, H. The treatment of burns and skin grafting. *J.A.M.A.* 45:1, 1905.

42. Wallace, A. B. Treatment of burns; a return to basic principles. *Br. J. Plast. Surg.* 2:232, 1949.

43. Wilmore, D. W., Mason, A. D., Johnson, D. W., and Pruitt, B. A. Effect of ambient temperature on heat production and heat loss in burn patients. *J. Appl. Physiol.* 38:593, 1975.

44. Wilmore, D. W., Mason, A. D., and Pruitt, B. A. Impaired glucose flow in burned patients with gram-negative sepsis. *Surg. Gynecol. Obstet.* 143:720, 1976.

45. Wilmore, D. W., Mason, A. D., and Pruitt, B. A. Insulin response to glucose in hypermetabolic burn patients. *Ann. Surg.* 183:314, 1976.

46. Wilmore, D. W., Orcutt, T. W., Mason, A. D., and Pruitt, B. A. Alterations in hypothalamic function following thermal injury. *J. Trauma* 15:697, 1975.

25

Radiation Injury and Electrical Burns

Radiation Injury

SHATTUCK W. HARTWELL, JR.

PATHOGENESIS AND EPIDEMIOLOGY

Pathogenesis

Living tissue can be injured by *ionizing radiation* from a variety of sources. This ionizing radiation includes: particulate radiation, and that portion of the electromagnetic spectrum in which the rays carry enough energy to produce ionization in materials that absorb them.

The state of ionization is estimated to last 10^{-8} seconds. The precise mechanism of injury following radiation is not clear, but there are several theories: the formation of ion pairs within a cell may inactivate or damage enzyme systems; toxic breakdown products as a consequence of ionization diffuse throughout the cell; and genetic or metabolic patterns may be injured by the ionization of key molecules within the molecular anatomy of the cell. Recent studies demonstrate sensitivity of deoxyribonucleic acid (DNA) to ionizing radiation. Both structural and functional damage can be assessed in vitro. Protection from radiation to DNA has been provided in vitro by bis-(2-guanidoethyl)disulphide, and it is postulated that molecular bonding on the surface of DNA is responsible for protection. Clinical use of these important discoveries is not imminent. Although patients with xeroderma pigmentosum are well known to develop skin malignancy because of their sensitivity to ultraviolet light, it has only recently been discovered that these patients lack normal fibroblasts in the skin. In normal skin, fibroblasts are able to repair damage to DNA in the skin after exposure to ultraviolet light. Here, at least, may exist a clue to pinpointing the abnormalities that ultimately appear in patients as postirradiation cancer.

Particulate radiation is the product of the decay of radioactive or fissionable material. Examples of particulate radiation are the alpha particle, which is the nucleus of the helium atom; the neutron, which is a component of the nuclear structure; and the beta particle, or electron, which is a much smaller subatomic particle that is capable of ionizing the molecules within the cells of living tissue. There are many subatomic particles, but not all of them are importantly related to biological disorders. These particles, traveling at various speeds and with variable energy, are capable of causing radiation injury due to the ionization of molecules within the cells of living tissue by the displacement of electrons from the molecular structure. The electron, or beta particle, will ordinarily ionize tissue to a depth of only a few millimeters in the skin unless it is part of a high-energy electron beam that is capable of delivering ionizing beta radiation to tissues deep beneath the surface. Such high-energy electron beams, as produced by the betatron with its many millions of electron volts, are also capable of generating from appropriate targets the second classification of ionizing radiation – namely, the *extremely short rays in the electromagnetic spectrum,* x-rays and gamma rays.

The *electromagnetic spectrum* includes, in decreasing order of wavelength, radio waves, visible light, ultraviolet light, grenz rays, x-rays, and gamma rays. All electromagnetic radiations have an equal speed of propagation (3×10^{10} cm. per second). The capacity of these radiations to penetrate living tissues depends on their frequency and wavelength. Only the shortest rays in the electromagnetic spectrum (x-rays and gamma rays) are capable of significantly penetrating and ionizing molecules within living cells. The shorter the wavelength, the greater the energy and penetrating power of the rays.

The ionizing effect is *cumulative* over the lifetime of the individual, which explains the inherent danger in repeated exposure. "Soft" x-rays are of longer wavelength and are used in treating dermatological disorders such as acne and superficial mycoses. The additive effect from these longer x-rays may be particularly harmful to skin. The "hard" x-rays are of shorter wavelength and are therefore more penetrating. Lower voltage x-ray machines always emanate a mixture of soft and hard radiation. Thin metal plates are used as filters in the radiation beam when it is desirable to filter out the longer x-rays. This allows the shorter x-rays to ionize at deeper levels without the otherwise damaging absorption at skin levels. Diagnostic machines operate at 30 to 80 kilovolts, giving selective absorption in tissues of varying depth and density for the best quality films. Most of the radiation is soft and is therefore capable of damaging the skin at dosage levels that would be harmless with hard x-rays.

Epidemiology

The acute response to radiation is most commonly seen in the skin and tissues of patients undergoing treatment for malignant disease. New supervoltage sources of radiation with proper filtration can spare the injury to the skin that has been such a problem in the past. The acute changes of radiation injury, anticipated in the planning of radiation therapy, are only temporary.

Prolonged exposure during fluoroscopy while searching for foreign bodies or in attempting to reduce fractures has been the cause of many cases of acute radiation injury. Deep injuries are also reported from the careless handling of radioactive materials in conjunction with the development of atomic energy.

Physicians, dentists, veterinarians, and technical personnel using roentgenographic equipment or radioactive materials are easily injured. Not only acute but chronic radiodermatitis results from exposure to ionizing radiation. Particularly notable are those patients who had been irradiated for the removal of unwanted hair; the skin has been pitifully injured in many of these individuals. Unskilled practitioners who had a poor understanding of radiation and who were unconcerned about careful calibration of dosage have inflicted dreadful acute and chronic radiation injuries in the treatment of both malignant and benign disease.

Chronic radiodermatitis may occur insidiously over a period of many years, during which time the patient or unwary practitioner is repeatedly exposed to radiation. There may be no history of an acute episode, the resulting injury being expressed 5 to 20 years after exposure; chronic radiodermatitis may also occur after an episode of acute radiodermatitis distinctly related to one exposure or a series of closely spaced exposures 5 years or more earlier.

CLINICAL AND HISTOPATHOLOGICAL SEQUELAE

Acute Radiation Injury – Signs and Symptoms

No part of the body skin is immune to the changes induced by radiation. Unlike the thermal burn, which produces an immediate subjective awareness of acute injury, the effects of a radiation injury are not immediately felt, except for a tingling sensation in some cases. The shorter the wavelength of radiation, the longer the *latent period* before signs and symptoms develop. Following infrared radiation injury, the pain and swelling of a burn are prompt; burns from ultraviolet radiation have a latent period of from 2 to 12 hours; manifest injury from x-rays may take as long as 14 days to appear. There is no known explanation for the intracellular course of events constituting the latent period. From several hours to several days must elapse before the signs and symptoms become well developed. Just as for the thermal burn, the quantity of the exposure determines the extent of the injury. At one extreme there may be only a slight erythema and an increase in pigmentation that develop within a few days of exposure to radiation, and these changes soon fade. At the other extreme, the acute radiation injury may cause an extensive necrosis of the skin to develop within 7 to 10 days. This may be preceded by erythema, swelling, extreme tenderness, and vesication of the skin.

Acute radiation injuries sustained by technical personnel handling radioactive materials have been documented most carefully. In such cases, the ionization of the molecules within the cells causes immediate irreparable damage to cellular metabolism and mitosis; biological death of the damaged cells ensues, with the necrosis of an entire digit, hand, or extremity.

The acute phase of radiation injury to the skin may result in *moist desquamation,* or incomplete destruction of the epithelium, a condition less frequently seen now than in the past when the modern supervoltage radiation machines were not available and the skin suffered as a result of an intense radiation dosage delivered to a deep tumor. In time, the moist desquamation heals, leaving dermal and epidermal changes recognized as a radiation scar. Subsequently, there may be hyperpigmentation or depigmentation of the skin. The epithelium may even be completely destroyed and an ulcer may develop. The more penetrating radiation now achieved with supervoltage and appropriate filtration spares the skin from these cumulative effects caused by the longer wavelengths of ionizing radiation.

Chronic Radiation Injury – Signs and Symptoms

Chronic radiodermatitis is characterized by gross atrophy of the skin and its appendages (Fig. 25-1). The skin becomes scaly, brittle, and scarred, and it has a tendency to appear eczematoid. Cracks and fissures in the skin appear. Telangiectases are common. Fibrosis occurs in the deeper tissues Injuries in the epidermis allow the ready access of bacteria, and the ensuing ulceration and infection are frequent clinical problems. The impairment of vascularity and reparative processes hinders the normal regional response to this insult.

Chronic radiodermatitis expresses itself in a wide range, extending from slight hyperkeratosis and atrophy of the epidermis to extensive changes in the skin, subcutaneous tissue, and deeper tissues. Some of the more extensive changes are ulceration, osteoradionecrosis, and malignancy. In carefully administered therapeutic radiation, there is no relationship between the severity of the early initial skin reaction and late changes. The early and late changes are independently variable, and this is true in patients of all complexions and skin colors. The reason is unknown.

When *acute ulceration* is the initial response to radiation, healing may be followed many years later

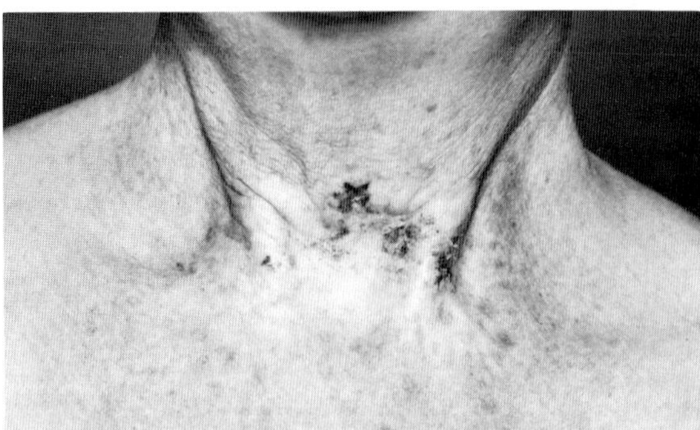

Fig. 25–1. Overlying skin damaged after x-ray treatment to the thyroid gland. Note loss of pigmentation, atrophy of the skin, with disappearance of wrinkles, thinning of the skin, hyperkeratosis, and crusting.

by skin breakdown and *secondary ulceration.* This is often the final expression of a chronic course of radiodermatitis. As the reparative processes are impaired, such ulceration is frequently initiated by repeated wear and tear to the injured region or by ultraviolet radiation from the sun, or it may be the result of a chronic infection that has become established in the defective skin. If the dermis and the subcutaneous tissues are severely scarred and their blood supply is impoverished, the ulcer will be deep. Though painstaking bandaging and topical care may bring about healing of these ulcers, they are sure to recur in this poor quality tissue.

Osteoradionecrosis is commonly seen in the maxillofacial region where large doses of radiation have been given to control primary or metastatic carcinoma about the mouth and upper neck. Radiated bone, which is secondarily infected, presents a distressing problem. All of the features of a chronic osteomyelitis are present, so that along with the impaired reparative processes in the bone and adjacent tissues, an exposed, infected, and chronically draining bone invariably results. Osteoradionecrosis of the jaws, an occational complication of radiotherapy in excess of 6,000 rads for definitive treatment of squamous cell carcinoma of the oral cavity and nasopharynx, is minimized by hygienic dental conservation or, if extractions of teeth are necessary, by allowing complete healing of extraction sites prior to commencing radiotherapy. Osteoradionecrosis that is not septic is not a difficult problem unless growth is impaired. Irradiation in children must always be calculated in consideration of underlying bone and its growth potential.

Malignant change is the ultimate expression of radiation injury. Successive generations of cells, initially altered by the ionizing property of radiation, may become frankly malignant. In the skin the most common malignancy is squamous cell carcinoma. Basal cell epitheliomas, as well as areas of sarcomatous change, may also be found. Although fibrosis may be dense around foci of squamous cell carcinoma, these tumors are not always entrapped and can metastasize to regional lymph nodes. Any area of ulceration, unusual keratinizing proliferation, or other change in an area of radiodermatitis should be biopsied. Such malignant changes generally develop at least 5 years after the time of injury, with many instances of malignant change occurring as late as 20 to 30 years after a period of radiation exposure. In a series of 361 patients treated for radiation-induced malignancy of the head and neck, 10 percent died of their cancer.

Histopathological Changes

Histopathological examination of radiated skin will show atrophy of the dermal appendages (Fig. 25-2). There is a loss of the normal interface between the dermis and the epidermis, with hyalinized collagenous stroma beneath the intact epidermis. The epidermis itself may show hyperkeratosis, parakeratosis, extreme thinning, and atrophy. These changes reflect the chronicity of the disease and the amount of the radiation injury.

In the dermis itself, telangiectasia and a thickening of the intima of small arterioles may occur. Perivascular edema and fibrillation of collagen may be seen. Thrombosis of the vessels may occur, and there may be considerable evidence of chronic inflammation with round cell infiltration in various areas of the dermis. Chronic inflammation in the dermis often reflects the degree of change that has occurred in the overlying epidermis. The dermal appendages may be unchanged, atrophic, or destroyed.

An analysis of the histopathological changes that take place as a result of radiation injury is easily related to the clinical problem. The ionizing effect on the genetic material within the cells necessarily affects the succeeding generations of cells in subtle ways that may not be initially apparent after radiation insult. Bizarre dysplastic fibrocytes are often found in the collagen, sometimes simulating sarcoma. The cellular patterns of metabolism are also impaired, and the cumulative effects of these changes are passed down to succeeding generations of cells. Reparative ability in response to injury is notably damaged.

TREATMENT OF RADIATION INJURY

General Principles

The management of *acute radiodermatitis* depends on the extent of the injury. With incomplete epidermal loss, the use of bland ointments and protective dressings on exposed, tender, or easily injured areas

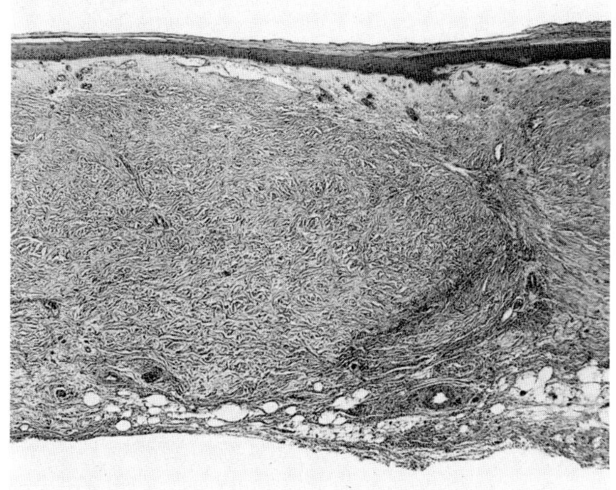

Fig. 25–2. Chronic radiation dermatitis, showing loss of the normal pattern between dermis and epidermis, with a densely hyalinized collagenous stroma in the dermis. There is atrophy of the epidermis with some hyperkeratosis. Note the telangiectases close to the dermal-epidermal junction (X 10).

may be required for many weeks. When the hands and fingers have been acutely injured, active and passive exercises and dynamic splinting help to maintain motion and reduce pain. Agonizing pain and necrosis induced by enormous doses (as much as 250,000 rads has been reported) of accidental radiation to the hands must be treated by excision and resurfacing using either skin grafts or flaps.

Basic to all considerations in the care of *chronic radiodermatitis* is the realization that this is an *irreversible process.* Furthermore, the smaller the extent of the lesion, the easier it is to treat. Medical treatment must include an ointment to keep the skin soft and well lubricated in areas of chronic radiodermatitis. Even so, recurring patches of hyperkeratosis and small ulcerations will relentlessly appear. Areas of hyperkeratosis may be pared or sanded. Markedly proliferative patches should be excised. Sunlight, unnecessary trauma, and additional radiation should be avoided. Solar protective agents should be used on exposed surfaces of radiodermatitis. When the hands are affected, gloves or small ready-made bandages should be worn for even the most inconsequential tasks in order to protect areas of radiodermatitis from injury or exposure. A vigil must be kept for many years by physicians caring for patients with radiogenic changes in the skin.

General principles for the management of open areas of ulceration are similar to those for the management of ulcers due to other causes. Cleanliness, debridement, careful bandaging, and sometimes antibacterial therapy are indicated. Resurfacing procedures may be necessary.

Excision and Resurfacing of Radiation Injuries

Operative excision of areas of chronic radiodermatitis or of one of the undesirable sequelae, such as chronic ulceration or a malignant lesion, is quite effective. Local advancement of the wound edges into a defect created by simple excision may be followed by postoperative complications, such as infection, hemorrhage, or poor wound healing. Wound closures with a split-thickness skin graft or skin flap are the methods of choice.

Procedures to resurface cutaneous areas of *chronic radiation change* involve the use of *split-thickness skin grafts and skin flaps.* The split-thickness skin graft is most often used for resurfacing these areas and is the most generally successful method of treatment. As there is poor vascularity of the recipient bed, there are almost always scattered spots where the graft does not take. These gradually epithelialize from the margins. Because of the changes in the blood vessel walls of this radiated tissue, the vessels do not contract easily and absolute hemostasis may be difficult to obtain. For this reason, delay of grafting for 24 to 48 hours is often necessary.

A skin flap must be used for coverage when there is bone, cartilage, tendon, or intense scarring in the base of the wound. Only nonirradiated tissue should be used in such a flap. A skin flap will fail if the tissue within the flap is injured by radiation. This is the hazard of flaps created in tissue adjacent to the areas to be resurfaced. Pedicled flaps, tubed and transposed from a distance, are necessary when adjacent tissue is involved or affected by the radiation injury. Radionecrosis of the chest wall and axilla may occur either before or after mastectomy for cancer. Resurfacing the defects following treatment may require large flaps, or skin grafts may be placed on an arterialized flap of greater omentum transposed to fill the defect.

Septic osteoradionecrosis in bone is managed by excision of all necrotic bone. The osteotome, rongeur, and high-speed bur are very useful in excising necrotic bone of the mandible and other facial bones. Subsequent replacement with bone grafts or other material is rarely successful because of the fibrosis and secondary radiogenic changes in the adjacent soft tissue that must support or invest the substituted graft or prosthesis. Stainless-steel Steinmann pins may be useful as mandibular substitutes to maintain the position of the chin after mandibulectomy in densely irradiated tissue. Most of these will ultimately be removed, however, leaving the chin in a relatively central position. Mandibulectomy may not always be necessary in instances of chronic exposed osteoradionecrotic mandible. Coverage of segments of such exposed and debrided mandible by forehead island flaps or delto-pectoral flaps may permit salvage of an intact and functional mandibular arch.

Malignant change increases the seriousness of chronic radiodermatitis. Squamous cell carcinoma, basal cell epitheliomas, basosquamous cell carcinoma, fibrosarcoma, and undifferentiated malignant neoplasms of the epithelium and dermis may arise in chronic radiodermatitis. Treatment of the primary foci of these cancers is resection of the involved skin; occasionally, amputation may be required. Again, the split-thickness skin graft is the most commonly used method of resurfacing after resection where primary wound closure is not feasible. Flaps may be necessary.

Squamous cell carcinomas can become metastatic in regional lymph nodes, but radical resections of clinically negative regional lymph nodes at a distance from the primary tumor should not be done as a "prophylactic" measure. The reason for this is that much of the squamous cell carcinoma will be incidental, small, hyperkeratotic, and multifocal in resected specimens of chronic radiodermatitis. The regional lymph nodes will be clinically negative. Perhaps the dermal fibrosis investing these kinds of foci is an effective barricade against tumor metastasis.

There are cases of ulcerative radionecrosis of skin, chronic eczematoid dermatitis, and bulky ulcerative squamous cell carcinomas. Regional lymphadenopathy will always be present in such cases, and lymphadenectomy should then be done. The lymph node resection may be conveniently delayed 3 or 4 weeks after the resection of the primary tumor. Chronic ulceration and eczematoid dermatitis by themselves will cause hyperplastic or even granulomatous lymphadenitis; but with the additional diagnosis of squamous cell carcinoma, only a lymph node resection can assure the patient of adequate cancer treatment. Preoperative lymphangiography may be helpful, but is not always reliable; chronic granulomatous lymphadenitis can simulate neoplastic replacement radiographically, and the question of metastatic disease will still remain unanswered without a surgical specimen.

Too often surgical treatment is tardy. Operations are fraught with the problems of infection and languid healing. Poor blood supply and indolent reparative processes in these areas impair chances of an uneventful postoperative course. It cannot be overly stressed that reconstructive procedures in irradiated tissue are bound to have a significantly higher percentage of surgical difficulties. This should be made clear to the patients preoperatively. To obviate the difficulties of far-advanced radiation-induced changes in the skin and subcutaneous tissue, it is better to proceed with operation in the earlier stages of radiodermatitis, affording reconstructive procedures and replacement of tissue before the occurrence of ulceration or malignant degeneration. The complications of reconstructive procedures are fewer if this course of action is followed.

Electrical Burns

REX A. PETERSON AND JOHN GIBNEY

An estimated 1,100 fatalities due to electrical trauma occur annually in the United States, with an overall incidence of 6 per million population. Approximately 7 percent of all patients admitted to hospitals for burn treatment incurred thermal injury secondary to electrical trauma. Electrical burns parallel in all parameters the devastating effects on human life seen in the most extensive thermal burns.

For many years an aura of mystery and confusion has surrounded the electrical injury. A seemingly insignificant electrically induced wound may be followed by loss of limb or life. The perplexing nature of the damage is further enhanced by the lack of knowledge of all the exact mechanisms by which electrical current causes tissue destruction.

PATHOGENESIS

Electrical thermal injury produces tissue destruction that is extended in depth and plane, as opposed to the surface damage seen in purely thermal burns. The electrical current enters the body at the point of contact with a conducting source, traverses the body through the pathway of least resistance, and finally exits at the site of grounding. The significance of the injury at the "entrance" and "exit" sites is one of high-temperature thermal injury, while the more devastating effects of the passage of the current through the body are less obvious in the immediate period after contact; however, these effects are of equally as great importance as the damaging effects caused by the trauma. The passage of electrical current may damage any body tissue, including subcutaneous tissue, muscles, tendons, bones, joints, arteries and nerves, and distant organs.

Electrical burns vary from localizing punctate lesions of less than 1 cm. in diameter to extensive, deep charring and remote vascular and organ damage. The severity of the electrical burn injury is determined by (1) the voltage of the current, (2) the intensity or amperage, (3) the resistance at the point of contact, (4) the resistance at the point of grounding (if grounding occurs), (5) the duration of the contact, (6) the pathways of the current through the body, (7) the type of current, (8) the surface area of contact, and (9) the victim's individual susceptibility to electrical current. There can be a great number of combinations of these factors, so a myriad of forms of electrical burn injuries may occur in one patient. Each electrical burn victim presents unique problems, depending on the extent and types of electrical burns he sustains. Voltage and duration of contact are the principal factors that determine the extent, depth, and multiplicity of the electrical burn damage.

In order to adequately treat electrical injury, an understanding of the basic variables involved is necessary.

Voltage

Voltage may be defined as the tension or potential of the electrical current. The thermal damage sustained by the victim of electrical contact is directly proportional to the voltage. Extensive thermal injury occurring after high-tension electrical accidents is caused by arcing of the current. This electrical arcing produces extremely high temperatures, which may exceed 2,500° to 4,000°C. in such high-voltage injuries. Under normal atmospheric conditions, the ionized air particles will arc approximately 3 cm. for each 10,000 volts; once a high-voltage arc has been established, it may extend for 3 m. before interruption of the circuit will occur.

Amperage

The real potential threat to life is directly related to the amperage. Ohm's equation indicates that the amperage or intensity is equal to the voltage divided by the resistance; hence, it is difficult to ascertain the true intensity of the current at the time of contact, since the resistance is unknown. Likewise, the heat generated at the point of contact and exit is in direct proportion to the amperage and the resistance. As seen in the Joule effect, heat in centigrade is equal to (0.24) amperage^2 $\times$ resistance.

Resistance

Upon coming in contact with an electrical source, the body becomes an integral part of the current circuit, presenting a number of resistors to the transmission of the current. The resistance offered by each tissue varies. Bone offers the greatest resistance to the transmission of electrical current, followed in descending order by fat, tendon, skin, muscle, nerves, and blood vessels. The fluid medium of blood vessels offers the least resistance and provides the most accessible pathway for transmission. At the point of entrance of the current, the skin reveals the greatest variance to resisting the current. Dry skin may present a skin resistance in the order of one megaohm (1 million ohms), while sweaty skin has a resistance of approximately 35,000 ohms, thoroughly wet skin 10,000 ohms, and the body immersed in water a mere 1,000 ohms. Hence, it may then be understood how a relatively low voltage may cause electrical fatality when coming in contact with a body immersed in water, whereas the same voltage causes minimal damage coming in contact with dry skin. Since the heat developed by passage of the current through the tissues is in direct proportion to the resistance offered, the extreme temperature of high-voltage transmission causes severe local and adjacent damage and may coagulate blood in vessels for some distance from the contact or grounding points. If the principal veins and arteries of an extremity are so damaged, gangrene of the digits or a major portion of the extremity occurs. In those cases in which gangrene develops, circulatory impairment is obvious at the time of injury. This vascular impairment may be localized and adjacent only to the burn, or it may be extensive. The necrosis that results from electrical vascular damage is no different from that caused by crush injuries or other vascular trauma or insufficiency.

Type of Current

Alternating current is considered more dangerous than direct current. The tetanizing effect alternating current produces on muscles prevents the contact with the electrical circuit from being easily interrupted, thereby causing increased duration of contact, as well as more severe damage. At high voltages, direct current becomes as destructive as alternating current. It has been shown that at 1 to 2 milliamps of an alternating current, a tingling sensation in the skin will occur. Twenty milliamps has been defined as the "let go" current; 90 milliamps will lead to respiratory center depression as well as respiratory arrest, and at 100 milliamps, ventricular fibrillation will result.

If the electrical burn is permitted to demarcate and slough, bacterial invasion of adjacent tissue of depressed vitality results in necrosis that is apparently in excess of the original burn. This enigma of "progressive necrosis" has led to the belief that electrical burns should not be excised because they are always worse than they appear. This is a fallacy; within the first 24 to 72 hours after an electrical burn, one can recognize and excise those tissues completely destroyed and those tissues that have a significant degree of partial burn necrosis. Histological examination of tissues at the margin of the "red zone" reveals spotty areas of coagulation necrosis and vascular damage. Larger vessels usually remain patent and demonstrate damage to the intima and media, as well as surface thrombi. This may explain the phenomena of delayed hemorrhage or complete thrombosis. Smaller vessels show injury to the vessel wall, as well as complete thrombosis, accounting for muscle necrosis and injury to areas some distance from the path of current. Additional histological studies on both permanent and frozen sections of muscle damaged along the pathway of electrical current revealed clumping of the nuclear chromatin and coagulation of myofibrillar proteins, as well as disruption of the myofilament bundles, indicating myonecrosis.

Every electrical burn has a central charred point of contact or grounding. This point is surrounded by a gray-white, inwardly contracted, dry zone, about which is a peripheral areola of blood-red coagulation necrosis of the skin. *All these areas involve full-thickness skin burns.* The damage to the deep tissues is most severe directly under the blackened central portion and diminishes peripherally (Figs. 25-3 and 25-4A).

As a guide to clinical practice, electrical burns may be classified as follows:

A. Low-voltage injuries (less than 1,000 volts).
   1. Flash.
   2. Contact.
B. High-voltage injuries (more than 1,000 volts).
   1. Flash.
   2. Arc or contact.
      a. Punctate, small and large.
      b. Extensive.
      c. Extensive with vascular impairment.
C. Associated thermal burn – ignition of clothing or surrounding materials.

TREATMENT

General Principles

If the victim of an electrical burn survives the contact and is brought to the hospital for treatment, physical and laboratory evaluation of the patient's condition are of primary importance. The physician must be aware of the patient's age, general physical condition, and health before injury. He should also determine the mode of injury, the voltage and duration of contact, and any history of a forceful fall (including whether unconsciousness occurred or there had been a need for artificial resuscitation).

The patient should be examined for associated injuries, such as skull fracture or other broken bones, cardiovascular abnormalities, intraabdominal injuries, and thermal burns. The location of burns should be charted, so that a plan of treatment can be determined.

Shock and electrolyte imbalance are rare, but may be severe in patients with multiple extensive high-voltage burns. When these disorders are present, there are usually associated injuries, distant organ or vascular damage, or thermal burns. The laboratory evaluation should be adapted to the severity of the injuries. In extensive multiple high-voltage burns, an electrocardiogram, skull x-rays, complete blood count, urinalysis, urine myoglobin and hemoglobin, and blood chemistry studies are advisable. If major thermal burns are present, all the laboratory examinations normally required for adequate continuing evaluation are indicated. Myoglobinuria and hemoglobinuria foretell the possibility of renal tubular obstruction

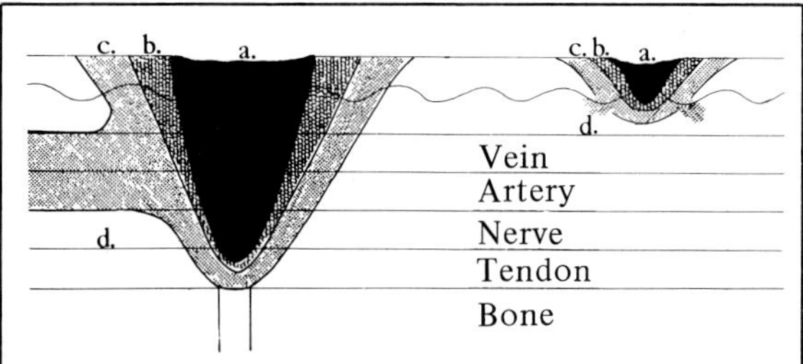

Fig. 25–3. Schematic representation of two electrical burns of different degree, but having the same characteristics. On the left, a high-voltage extensive burn with vascular impairment. On the right, a low-voltage burn or a high-voltage punctate burn. a, central charred zone of complete necrosis; tissues obliterated. b, surrounding gray-white zone of necrosis; tissues intact. c, peripheral partial coagulation necrosis (the "red zone"); as the heat is dissipated, less damage results. d, coagulation of vessels from heat produced as current is transmitted along vascular channels.

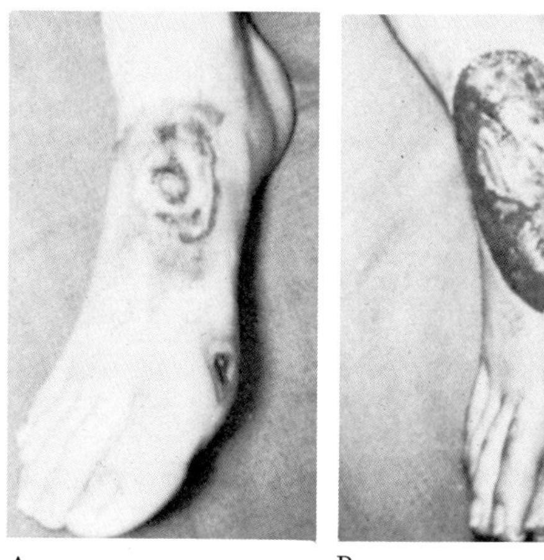

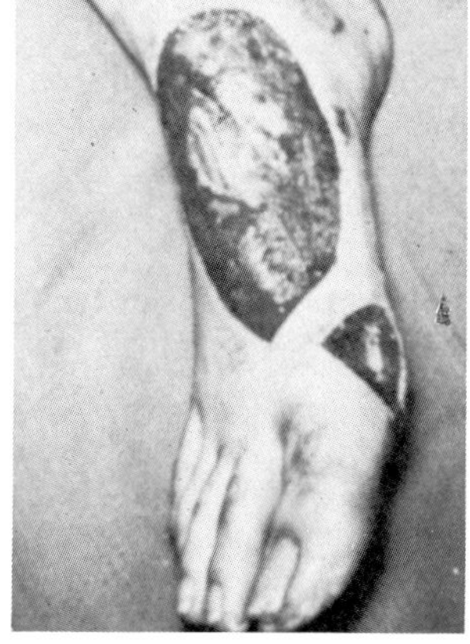

A B

Fig. 25–4. A, high-voltage electrical burns of the foot, extensive *over the dorsum and* punctate *over the metatarsophalangeal joint. In each, note the central charred zones, the surrounding gray-white zone, and the peripheral red zone. B, 4 days after the excision, both wounds are granulating well except under the central charred area. There is no "progressive necrosis," and coverage with a split-thickness skin graft was successful.*

with subsequent failure. Repeat blood counts are advisable as bone marrow depression may occur in certain cases. When internal organ damage is suspected, liver function studies should be obtained.

Appropriate resuscitative measures should be instituted. Intravenous fluid therapy is difficult to calculate according to any preset formula. Urine output should be monitored closely as a guide to fluid therapy. The hourly urine output should be kept between 50 and 75 ml. (or higher if myoglobinuria or hemoglobinuria becomes apparent). Mannitol or other diuretics may be useful adjuvants to fluid resuscitation. Anticlostridial prophylaxis is especially indicated in all patients with high-voltage injuries because of the deep tissue necrosis. In addition to antitetanus measures (with tetanus toxoid, tetanus hyperimmune human globulin, or tetanus antitoxin), prophylactic antibiotics are indicated.

Early and adequate excision of the burned tissues should also be carried out. If the patient's general condition permits and if he does not have extensive thermal burns, excision of the electrical burn within the first 24 to 72 hours is preferable; however, if the burns remain dry and intact, complete early excision of the necrosing tissue may be accomplished satisfactorily within a few days after injury.

In excision of burns of the extremities, the bloodless field obtained by the use of the pneumatic tourniquet assists in determining the extent of deep tissue necrosis. Frozen sections for histological examination at the time of the debridement may also assist in determining the adequacy of the removal of nonviable tissues. Damaged tendon, muscle, nerve, and joint capsule are easily identified. In the most severe injuries, structures may be charred or obliterated. It is equally important to remove those that are necrosed, but not so obviously damaged. Necrosed tendons, areolar tissue, and fascia lose their glistening appearance and appear dry and slightly more brownish or tan in color. Necrotic fat is more opaque and pinkish gray compared to normal yellow. Necrosed nerves may be swollen, soft, friable and grayish tan in color, or may be firm and fibrotic, thin, and tapered. Coagulated muscle has a light brown color similar to milk chocolate. Coagulated skin has the blood-red color often seen in third-degree thermal burns. Adequate excision of these necrosed tissues is essential to a successful repair.

If the surgeon doubts the adequacy of his early excision, repair can be delayed for several days for a "second look," at which time additional tissue may be removed if the primary excision has been incomplete or additional progressive necrosis has occurred. In a patient who has had multiple electrical burns and thermal burns, staged systematic excision and repair of the burn wounds at intervals of 3 to 5 days provides the earliest complete closure of the burn and facilitates rehabilitation. This regimen is readily combined with the presently accepted methods of treating thermal burns utilizing topical antibacterial dressings.

Operative Technique

Low-Voltage Injuries

Low-voltage electrical flash burns are thermal injuries of the skin caused by the heat of the nearby electrical flash. The epidermis is blackened, giving the appearance that the injured part is charred. Cleaning usually reveals that the discoloration is superficial and that the injury involves only a partial thickness of skin. Voltages of 24 volts or less are generally considered safe under all conditions. Flash injuries are treated by cleaning the burned surface with a surgical detergent and sterile saline solution or water, debridement as indicated, and sterile dressings with petrolatum gauze, multiple-ply coarse-mesh plain gauze without cotton filling, bias stockinette wrap, or other similar dressing material. Antibiotic ointments such as neomycin, bacitracin, or polymyxin B may be of benefit for topical application. Daily dressing changes under sterile conditions should be performed thereafter until the wound is completely healed. Daily hydrotherapy in balanced Locke's solution is employed to assist in the debridement and maintenance of function of the injured extremities.

Low-voltage contact burns are usually localized because the heat produced is not as intense as in high-voltage injuries. The skin lesion has a characteristic central blackened area, the surrounding grayish white zone, and the peripheral halo of blood-red coagulation necrosis. All of these areas are full-thickness skin burns and should be excised. Necrotic subjacent tissues should also be removed at the initial excision and repair effected by split-thickness skin graft if bones, joints, and tendons are not exposed, or by a local rotation skin flap or a flap from a distance if they are exposed.

A common low-voltage injury in small children is the full-thickness skin burn of the mouth and lips sustained when an infant chews on an electric lamp cord or socket. Controversy exists as to whether these burns should be treated by early complete excision or by a conservative approach of delaying surgery until the eschar separates and the scar softens. Adhering to the philosophy of early excision, the burn wound is removed to the point where healthy tissue begins within the first 24 to 72 hours. Frequently, the excision amounts to no more than a wedge resection of the commissure of the upper or lower lip, and a direct repair provides excellent results. If later reconstructive surgery is necessary, early excision affords prompt healing without an infection or undue cicatrization, and it provides the best surgical field for reconstruction of the residual defect. When early excision has not been carried out, it is best to allow the necrotic tissue to slough spontaneously. At least 6 months should pass before beginning reconstructive procedures. (Techniques of lip reconstruction are included in Chapter 15.)

High-Voltage Punctate Lesions

High-voltage punctate lesions vary from a few millimeters to several centimeters in diameter. They are usually charred or blackened and have little or no grayish white and hyperemic peripheral zones. Early excision is not indicated if they are small, because they may be treated conservatively and will gradually demarcate and extrude without significant deformity. They may be excised and repaired by split-thickness skin graft if more than 1 or 2 cm. in diameter in size and if located on the fingertips, over interphalangeal joints, over weight-bearing areas of the foot, or about the scalp or face. If tendons, nerves, or joints are exposed, a local skin flap is preferred for wound closure.

High-Voltage Electrical Flash Burns

High-voltage electrical flash burns are more apt to be full-thickness and more extensive than low-voltage flash burns because the heat generated by the high-voltage flash is greater. They should be treated by initial cleaning, debridement, and application of sterile dressings, with subsequent sterile dressing changes daily until their depth is known. If they are extensive or of deep partial-thickness or full-thickness involvement, they may be treated by any of the currently accepted modes of topical therapy (e.g., topical antibacterial dressings or biological dressings of homograft or xenograft), frequent daily dressing changes, and hydrotherapy in balanced Locke's solution. Systematic, staged surgical debridement and repair are indicated as for any thermal burn.

Extensive High-Voltage Injuries

Extensive high-voltage injuries are caused by sufficient contact with a high-voltage current to char the tissues and produce thermal damage to the adjacent superficial and deep structures. These lesions are larger and deeper than low-voltage or high-voltage punctate burns. If the patient's condition permits, they should be treated by early excision of all necrosed tissue. It is frequently best to delay the repair for a few days after the excision to determine if the necrosing tissue has been completely excised. Further excision is necessary in areas in which granulation tissue fails to form. After excision of any residual necrosis at this "second look" operation, repair can usually be completed. If the surgeon still doubts the adequacy of excision, the burn wound may be dressed to await a "third look" a few days later.

Early excision and repair are superior for electrical burns of the hands, because a lingering, open, infected wound of the hand contributes to stiffness and loss of function. Mobilization of the structures of the hand can be obtained only by early closure of the burn wounds.

In excision of the electrical burn of the hand, after all the damaged skin and subcutaneous tissue are excised, the deep fascia over the tendons and nerves should be carefully examined for burn damage and removed only if there is deeper necrosis. If they are obliterated or necrosed, the tendons should be removed; however, they should be spared at the initial operation unless they are obviously necrotic. Nerves should be spared unless they have lost continuity, since they have a remarkable power of recovery, even if exposed in granulation tissue. The release of the tourniquet will reveal the adequacy of the excision because viable tissue will bleed readily. At the first operation, conservation of the important deep structures is indicated, even if they are of doubtful viability. Should it be necessary to expose tendons, nerves, bones, or joints, a repair with a skin flap is advisable; otherwise, coverage with a split-thickness skin graft is sufficient. Coverage with a skin flap is essential for later major reconstructive procedures of tendon, nerve, bone, and joints.

When an extensive high-voltage burn involves the scalp and skull, the devitalized scalp should be excised and repaired by split-thickness grafts if there is a viable recipient area. However, if the dry outer table of the skull is bared, the surgeon may leave it exposed until the other wounds are closed before removing the nonviable bone by multiple shallow bur holes and delicate tangential osteotomies with a curved-gouge osteotome (the osteotomy depth is to bleeding bone). An interval of several days permits formation of granulations for repair by split-thickness skin graft. If it is necessary to remove the full thickness of skull, a split-thickness skin graft may be applied directly to the dura. If dura is not intact, the dural defect may be reconstructed by a free graft of pericranium and covered by an adjacent scalp flap. It is necessary to reconstruct the full-thickness skin and subcutaneous tissue with a local or distant skin flap before consideration of cranioplastic procedures. (For additional information, see Chapter 11.)

Extensive High-Voltage Injuries with Vascular Impairment

The most severe form of electrical injury is the extensive high-voltage burn with vascular impairment. These injuries are caused by prolonged high-voltage contact, which produces extreme heat and extensive damage to the skin, subcutaneous tissue, muscles, tendons, nerves, bones, joints, and major blood vessels. They frequently occur on the palm of the hand or the plantar surface of the foot. During the prolonged contact, the electrical current is transmitted proximally along the blood vessels and muscle planes, and the vascular damage may extend for great distances and lead to gangrene of the extremity. In these cases there are usually signs of circulatory impairment of the parts involved. Cold, mottled, and pulseless extremities are indicative of impending gangrene. Damaged arteries may secondarily rupture and produce late, massive hemorrhage. Immediate escharotomy and fasciotomy are indicated under such circumstances.

The high-voltage current transversing the body may actually penetrate the surface at flexion creases of the wrist, elbow, axilla, and groin, causing additional severe electrical injuries at these points. The reduced resistance of the generally moist skin at a flexion crease, the thinness of the skin, and the relatively superficial course of the underlying blood vessels and nerves all play a part in allowing penetration to occur.

When there is a tourniquet-like contracture of the burn eschar about the wrist or foot, early surgical decompression by excision of the eschar may improve the circulation and salvage the extremity. If all the major vessels supplying the extremity are thrombosed, amputation will be required; it is desirable to amputate early because these wounds are susceptible to bacterial invasion with coagulase-positive *Staphylococcus aureus, Pseudomonas,* and *Clostridium perfringens.* If clostridial contamination occurs, daily doses of antigas serum and increased doses of penicillin or other antibiotics should be given until excision of the burn necrosis is completed or the extremity amputated. Early excision for decompression is only the first step in treatment. Repair should follow subsequent surgical dressing changes and staged excision of the burn areas. Wound closure is obtained by split-thickness skin grafts, skin flaps, or by amputation of the gangrenous or useless parts as soon as feasible.

ASSOCIATED INJURIES

Additional extensive thermal burns may occur in combination with electrical thermal injuries when ignition of clothing or other combustible materials has occurred. (Treatment for thermal burns is outlined in Chapter 24.)

The incidence of renal failure is somewhat higher in electrical burns than seen in purely thermal burns. This higher incidence may result from the initial shock, a direct electrical injury to the kidneys or renal vessels, renal toxic breakdown products, or hemoglobinuria or myoglobinuria. Adequate fluid therapy as well as excision of devitalized tissue has been shown to reduce the incidence of renal failure.

Intraabdominal organ injury is rare. When it does occur, it usually consists of mural necrosis of hollow viscera, such as the gall bladder or intestine. Appropriate surgical exploration and intervention are necessary under such circumstances.

Electrical injuries about the face or head may cause cataracts to develop. These may occur as an acute or as a delayed (6 to 8 months) response after the accident has occurred. The patient should be informed of these possibilities, and appropriate ophthalmological consultation should be employed.

REFERENCES

Radiation Injury – Epidemiology

1. Abrahams, A., Harris, S. J., Paul, I., and Paul, G. W. Radiological hazards due to exposure to low-energy radiation in veterinarians; environmental study. *A.M.A. Arch. Ind. Health* 14:521, 1956.
2. Bedwinek, J. M., Shukovsky, L. J., Fletcher, G. H., and Daley, T. E. Osteonecrosis in patients treated with definitive radiotherapy for squamous cell carcinomas of the oral cavity and naso- and oropharynx. *Radiology* 119:665, 1976.
3. Brown, J. B., McDowell, F., and Fryer, M. P. Radiation burns, including vocational and atomic exposures: Treatment, and surgical prevention of chronic lesions. *Ann. Surg.* 130:593, 1949.
4. Cannon, F., Randolph, J. G., and Murray, J. E. Malignant irradiation for benign conditions. *N. Engl. J. Med.* 260:197, 1959.
5. Cole, H. N. Acute and chronic radiodermatitis as seen in physicist, physician and dentist. *Postgrad. Med.* 13:133, 1953.
6. Crikelair, G. F., Beasley, R. W., and Cosman, B. Irradiation dermatitis and the Tricho institute. *N.Y. J. Med.* 64:1193, 1964.
7. Leddy, E. T., and Rigos, F. J. Radiodermatitis among physicians. *Am. J. Roentgenol.* 45:696, 1941.
8. Mohs, F. E. Roentgen ray cancer of the hands in dentists. *J. Am. Dent. Assoc.* 45:160, 1952.
9. Robinson, D. W., and Masters, F. W. Surgery for radiation injury. *A.M.A. Arch. Surg.* 89:946, 1960.
10. Smith, S. M. Subjective experiences during a 32-year period after resurfacing of hands for severe and acute radiation burns. *Plast. Reconstr. Surg.* 51:23, 1973.
11. Warren, S. The pathological effects of small doses of radiation. The Fifth Annual Ross Golden Lecture of the New York Roentgen Society. *Bull. N.Y. Acad. Med.* 34:633, 1958.

Radiation Injury – Pathogenesis

12. Cleaver, J. E. Defective repair replication of DNA in xeroderma pigmentosum. *Nature* (London) 218:652, 1968.
13. Dunlap, C. E. Effects of Radiation. In Anderson, W. A. D. (Ed.), *Pathology* (5th ed.). St. Louis: Mosby, 1966.
14. Epstein, E. *Radiodermatitis.* Springfield, Ill.: Thomas, 1962.
15. Fox, B. W., and Lajtha, L. G. Radiation damage and repair phenomena. *Br. Med. Bull.* 29:16, 1973.
16. Glasser, O., Quimby, E. H., Taylor, L. S., Weatherwax, J. L., and Morgan, R. E. *Physical Foundations of Radiology* (3rd ed.). New York: Hoeber, 1961.
17. Hempelmann, L. H. Acute radiation injuries in man. *Surg. Gynecol. Obstet.* 93:385, 1951.
18. Knowlton, N. P., Jr., Leifer, E., Hogness, J. R., Hempelmann, L. H., Blaney, L. F., Gill, D. C., Ochs, W. R., and Slafev, C. L. Beta ray burns of human skin. *J.A.M.A.* 141:239, 1949.
19. Kollman, G., Castel, N., and Shapiro, B. Further studies on protection of DNA against ionizing radiation. *Int. J. Radiat. Biol.* 18:587, 1970.
20. Moss, W. T. *Therapeutic Radiology; Rationale, Technique, Results.* St. Louis: Mosby, 1959.
21. Teloh, H. A., Mason, M. L., and Wheelock, M. C. A histopathologic study of radiation injuries of the skin. *Surg. Gynecol. Obstet.* 90:335, 1950.
22. Wolbach, S. B. A summary of the effects of repeated roentgen-ray exposures upon the human skin, antecedent to the formation of carcinoma. *Am. J. Roentgenol.* 13:139, 1925.

Radiation Injury – Sequelae

23. Arcangeli, G., Friedman, M., and Paoluzi, R. A quantitative study of late radiation effect on normal skin and subcutaneous tissues in human beings. *Br. J. Radiol.* 47:44, 1974.
24. Brown, J. B., and Fryer, M. P. High energy electron injury from accelerator machines (cathode rays): Radiation burns of chest wall and neck – 17-year follow up of atomic burns. *Ann. Surg.* 162:426, 1965.
25. Chu, F. C., Glicksman, A. S., and Nickson, J. J. Late consequences of early skin reactions. *Radiology* 94:669, 1970.
26. Cronin, T. D., and Brauer, R. O. Radiodermatitis and necrosis. *Surgery* 26:665, 1949.
27. Daland, E. M. Symposium on cancer: Radiation damage to tissue and its repair. *Surg. Gynecol. Obstet.* 72:372, 1941.
28. Malbec, E. F., and Quaife, J. V. Plastic surgery in radiation burns. *Plast. Reconstr. Surg.* 20:232, 1957.

29. Malbec, E. F., Quaife, J. V., and Vieyra Urquiza, H. A. Carcinomatous complication in radiodermatitis. *Plast. Reconstr. Surg.* 32:447, 1963.
30. Robinson, D. W. The hazards of surgery in irradiated tissue. *A.M.A. Arch. Surg.* 71:410, 1955.
31. Robinson, D. W., and Boley, J. O. Irradiation fibromatosis and fibrosarcoma. *Am. Surg.* 22:33, 1956.
32. Sutton, R. L., Jr. Transverse band pigmentation of fingernails after x-ray therapy. *J.A.M.A.* 150:210, 1952.

Radiation Injury – Treatment

33. Barnes, W. E., Hoffman, G. W., and Pickrell, K. Surgical treatment of irradiation injuries of the perineum. *Surg. Gynecol. Obstet.* 118:1067, 1964.
34. Brown, J. B., McDowell, F., and Fryer, M. P. Surgical treatment of radiation burns. *Surg. Gynecol. Obstet.* 88:609, 1949.
35. Converse, J. M., Campbell, R. M., and Watson, W. L. Repair of large radiation ulcers situated over heart and brain. *Ann. Surg.* 133:95, 1951.
36. Conway, H. The surgical management of post-radiation scars and ulcers. *Surgery* 10:64, 1941.
37. Conway, H., and Hugo, N. E. Radiation dermatitis and malignancy. *Plast. Reconstr. Surg.* 38:255, 1966.
38. Conway, H., Hugo, N., and Tulenko, J. *Surgery of Tumors of the Skin.* Springfield, Ill.: Thomas, 1966.
39. Gaskins, J. A., Ertugrul, G., and Rush, B. F., Jr. Tolerance to stainless prostheses in patients after postradiation hemimandibulectomy. *Am. J. Surg.* 117:375, 1969.
40. Glover, D. M. Surgical treatment of irradiation dermatitis and carcinoma. *Am. J. Surg.* 74:735, 1947.
41. Greeley, P. W. Reconstruction following irradiation injuries. *Arch. Surg.* (Chicago) 56:741, 1948.
42. Gue, S. Omental transfer for the treatment of radionecrosis of the chest wall. *Aust. N.Z. J. Surg.* 45:390, 1975.
43. Hartwell, S. W., Jr., Huger, W., Jr., and Pickrell, K. Radiation dermatitis and radiogenic neoplasms of the hands. *Ann. Surg.* 160:828, 1964.
44. Hultberg, S. Local enzymatic treatment of radiation necroses of the skin. *Acta Radiol.* 39:343, 1953.
45. Krizek, T. J., and Ariyan, S. Severe acute radiation injuries of the hands. *Plast. Reconstr. Surg.* 51:14, 1973.
46. Martin, H., Strong, E., and Spiro, R. H. Radiation-induced skin cancer of the head and neck. *Cancer* 25:61, 1970.
47. Masters, F. W., and Robinson, D. W. Early operation, a conservative approach to the treatment of chronic irradiation injury. *J. Trauma* 1:583, 1961.
48. Matton, G., and D'Hooghe, P. Reconstructive plastic surgery in radionecrosis of the breast and thoracic wall. *Acta Chir. Belg.* 73:301, 1974.
49. Nickell, W. B., Vasconez, L. O., Jurkiewicz, M. J., and Salyer, K. E. One stage surgical repair of mandibular osteoradionecrosis with jaw preservation. *Am. J. Surg.* 126:502, 1973.
50. Pathak, M. A., Fitzpatrick, T. B., and Frenk. E. Evaluation of topical agents that prevent sunburn – superiority of para-aminobenzoic acid and its ester in ethyl alcohol. *N. Engl. J. Med.* 280:1459, 1969.
51. Robinson, D. W. Surgical problems in the excision and repair of radiated tissue. *Plast. Reconstr. Surg.* 55:41, 1975.

Electrical Burns

52. Artz, C. P., and Reiss, E. *The Treatment of Burns* (2nd ed.). Philadelphia: Saunders, 1969.
53. Baldridge, R. R. Electric burns: Report of a case. *N. Engl. J. Med.* 250:4649, 1954.
54. Bowe, J. J. Primary excision in third degree burns. *Plast. Reconstr. Surg.* 25:240, 1960.
55. Brown, J. B., and Fryer, M. P. Repair of industrial electrical burns. *Plast. Reconstr. Surg.* 18:177, 1956.
56. Burke, J. F., et al. Patterns of high tension injury in children and adolescents and their management. *Am. J. Surg.* 133:492, 1977.
57. Dale, R. H. Electrical accidents: A discussion with illustrated cases. *Br. J. Plast. Surg.* 7:44, 1954.
58. Davies, R. M. Burns caused by electricity. *Br. J. Plast. Surg.* 11:288, 1959.
59. Fleury, A. F. Electrical burns of the lips: A modified plan of treatment. *Am. Surg.* 25:328, 1959.
60. Frank, G. Primary and accelerated early plastic surgery for burns. *Plast. Reconstr. Surg.* 23:313, 1959.
61. Gatewood, J. W., and McCarthy, H. H. The treatment of electric burns of the skull. *Am. J. Surg.* 93:525, 1957.
62. Goulian, D. Early differentiation between necrotic and viable tissue in burns. *Plast. Reconstr. Surg.* 27:359, 1961.
63. Hyslop, V. B. Treatment of electric burns of the lips. *Plast. Reconstr. Surg.* 20:315, 1957.
64. Hyslop, V. B., and Miller, E. W. Treatment of electric burns. *J. Int. Coll. Surg.* 23:481, 1955.
65. Kragh, L. V., and Erich, J. B. Treatment of severe electric injuries. *Am. J. Surg.* 101:419, 1961.
66. Lewis, G. K. Burns from electricity. *Ann. Surg.* 131:80, 1950.

67. Lewis, G. K. Electric burns of the upper extremities. *J. Bone Joint Surg.* [Am.] 40:27, 1958.
68. Maisel, D. O., and Saad, M. N. Early surgery in the treatment of burns. *Br. J. Surg.* 56:466, 1969.
69. Mann, R. J., et al. Early decompression fasciotomy in the treatment of high-voltage electrical burns of the extremities. *South. Med. J.* 68:1103, 1975.
70. McLaughlin, C. W., Jr., and Coe, J. D. Management of electrical burns. *Arch. Surg.* (Chicago) 68:531, 1954.
71. Moyer, C. A., Brentano, L., Gravens, D. L., Margraf, H. W., and Monafo, W. R. Treatment of large human burns with 0.5% silver nitrate solution. *A.M.A. Arch. Surg.* 90:812, 1965.
72. Muir, I. F. K. The treatment of electrical burns. *Br. J. Plast. Surg.* 10:292, 1957–58.
73. Oeconomopoulos, C. T. Electrical burns in infancy and early childhood. *Am. J. Dis. Child.* 103:35, 1962.
74. Peterson, R. A. Electrical burns of the hand – Treatment by early excision. *J. Bone Joint Surg.* [Am.] 48:407, 1966.
75. Poate, W. J., and MacAfee, A. L. Gas gangrene following electrical burns. *Br. J. Plast. Surg.* 15:17, 1962.
76. Poticha, C. P., Bell, J. L., and Mehn, W. H. Electrical injuries with special reference to the hand. *A.M.A. Arch. Surg.* 85:852, 1962.
77. Rank, B. K., and Wakefield, A. R. *Surgery of Repair as Applied to Hand Injuries.* Baltimore: Williams & Wilkins, 1960.
78. Robins, R. H. C. *Injuries and Infections of the Hand.* Baltimore: Williams & Wilkins, 1961.
79. Skoog, T. The surgical treatment of burns. *Acta Chir. Scand. [Suppl.]* 305:86, 1963.
80. Snyder, C. C. The Hand Injured by Electricity. *Transactions of the International Society of Plastic Surgeons* (Second Congress). Edinburgh: Livingstone, 1960.
81. Wells, D. B. Treatment of electrical burns by immediate resection and skin graft. *Ann. Surg.* 90:1069, 1929.

Basal Cell and Squamous Cell Carcinoma of the Skin

EDWARD W. GIBSON AND JORGE LOPEZ-GARCIA

This chapter will be confined to the treatment of the two most common malignant tumors of the skin – basal cell carcinoma and squamous cell carcinoma. Brief reference will be made to keratoacanthoma; although it is a benign lesion, it can cause dangerous confusion with squamous carcinoma.

AIMS AND MODES OF TREATMENT

The aims of the treatment of skin cancer can be simply stated as follows: to eliminate the disease – both the primary site and the site of metastatic spread, if applicable – and to secure the best functional and cosmetic result.

The main accepted modes of treatment are surgery, radiotherapy, Mohs' chemosurgery, and perfusion or local application of cytotoxic drugs. All these modalities of treatment have their place. Surgery can probably make the greatest contribution to the treatment of skin malignancy at present, but in many countries radiotherapy is used most often to treat this condition.

Surgery

Surgical treatment offers:

1. A high cure rate – better than 98 percent for basal cell carcinoma.
2. The opportunity to treat the patient by one operation, often during a single short hospital stay.
3. Good cosmetic and functional results; happily, in the age group in which most of these lesions occur, healing results in excellent scars with very little trouble from scar hypertrophy or keloid.
4. The opportunity to confirm the diagnosis and adequacy of excision by histological examination.
5. The opportunity for in-continuity lymph node dissection when this is applicable.

Radiotherapy

Radiotherapy offers a good cure rate in competent hands and an acceptable cosmetic result in most cases, but it exposes the patient to the hazards of radiation (and in particular radionecrosis), especially if a course of treatment is repeated for a recurrent lesion or a closely adjacent new lesion. Furthermore, unless a separate biopsy procedure is carried out beforehand, the diagnosis cannot be established with certainty by histological examination.

Similarly, the adequacy of treatment – particularly in depth – is dependent on the skill of the radiotherapist in assessing the depth of the lesion, and choosing the appropriate type of radiation and dosage to meet the requirements.

In spite of these obvious difficulties and limitations, one must concede that the skilled radiotherapist or dermatologist treats a large number of patients with skin malignancy successfully, when measured by the yardsticks of cure rate and cosmetic standards.

Some patients choose a regimen of radiotherapy even if it means many visits to the radiotherapist over the long time that fractional doses may require. In spite of the demands on the patient's time and convenience, they prefer this to what they imagine is the mutilation associated with surgery. Radiotherapy became firmly established in the treatment of skin cancer in many countries at a time when surgical treatment was in the hands of general surgeons not equipped with the refinements of modern reconstructive techniques. Surgeons see the failures of radiotherapy and therefore are prone to get a distorted and unfair impression of the value of this mode of treatment. However, the following recommendations are made in regard to the use of radiotherapy in the treatment of skin malignancy:

1. Radiotherapy should be *avoided* in the treatment of lesions of the inner canthus, eyelids, tip of the nose and alar region, base of the ala nasi, preauricular region, external ear, and auditory canal.
2. Surgery should be offered as a *preferred alternative* in the treatment of lesions of the backs of the hands, front of the lower legs, and lips.
3. Radiotherapy should not be used to treat lesions recurrent after previous radiotherapy.

No doubt many radiotherapists will contest these recommendations and cite successes with radiotherapy when used to treat lesions in these problem areas. However, it is undeniable that the chances of radionecrosis together with all its unhappy consequences are much greater in those regions where cartilage or tendon lies close beneath the skin.

It is not our intention to discuss the techniques of radiotherapy and the reader is referred to standard textbooks for this information [1–3].

Radiation-damaged tissue is itself prone to malignant degeneration. Texier and Preaux [4] reported on 456 patients with radiodermatitis; of those patients, 20 percent developed malignant change, with basal cell carcinoma predominating in the face and trunk and squamous carcinoma in the hand and extremities.

Mohs' Chemosurgery
Mohs' chemosurgery is a form of treatment that has not found much support, although the early reports were encouraging [5, 6]. We are sure the whole conception of the treatment does not appeal to the surgical mind, since en bloc removal of cancer, when possible, is one of the first tenets of the surgical creed. The essential approach of the cancer surgeon is to outflank his enemy and attack him from the rear and all sides so that he is removed in one piece all at the same time.

However, at some surgical centers, this technique is used for treatment of extensive carcinoma about the nose and orbit and for basal cell carcinoma recurrent after irradiation. Satisfactory results are claimed, but it is a tedious procedure requiring special skills in preparing and interpreting the histological sections.

Topical Cytotoxic Therapy
The use of cytotoxic drugs in an ointment base has found some supporters in recent years. Belisario [8], who has written extensively on the subject, favors a 5% concentration of 5-fluorouracil, but he has not yet presented a completely documented and controlled series of cases. Ryan and colleagues [12] have also reported favorably on the use of 5-fluorouracil cream to define suitable donor areas for reconstructive procedures. They claim that nonvisible basal cell carcinomas are often hidden under normal-appearing surface epithelium. The application of 5-fluorouracil cream can cause these hidden lesions to become apparent in 10 days or so. He recommends that areas of skin which are to be used as flaps for reconstruction following excision of a skin cancer should be treated with 5-fluorouracil cream to reveal the presence of occult basal cell carcinomas. We feel that this is an unnecessary precaution in the vast majority of cases. Careful inspection of potential donor area by naked eye or 2 to 2½ times magnification will usually reveal the presence of any active lesions.

Litwin and colleagues [10] and Ryan and coworkers [12] also report on the use of 5-fluorouracil cream in the treatment of skin lesions. The former report favorable results in lesions of the head and neck [10], but appear to use a higher concentration of 5-fluorouracil (up to 20%) than most other workers. Litwin and Ryan and their associates [11] describe the use of 5-fluorouracil cream in the treatment of advanced cutaneous malignancy with encouraging results.

Anderson and associates [7] report a study on 46 cases of skin malignancy treated with 5-fluorouracil cream. Short-term cures were achieved in only 7 out of 22 basal cell carcinomas, 5 out of 10 solar keratoses, 7 out of 10 Bowen's disease, and 1 out of 1 case of keratoacanthoma.

Everall [9] reported unfavorably on the results of the treatment of basal cell carcinoma with topical cytotoxic ointment. He reported a relapse rate of 33 percent over 3 years, in comparison with a 12 percent relapse rate for radiotherapy and 5 percent for surgery (including incision, diathermy, and curettage).

Dermabrasion
The use of dermabrasion in the treatment of patients with a high susceptibility to skin carcinoma has been reported by Burke and co-workers [33]. These authors reported on their experience based on 5 years' observation of 15 half-face planings. They claim the degree of improvement based on the opinion of seven inspectors was 85 percent cosmetically and 92 percent therapeutically.

The exact way in which skin planing benefits these patients (if in fact it does) has not been determined. Histological studies after skin planing demonstrate a zone of new fibrous tissue between the area of solar degeneration and the epidermis that contains elastic fibers. Perhaps this new zone of fibrous and elastic tissue rejuvenates the epithelium and isolates it from the area of solar degeneration, thereby lessening its susceptibility to premalignant and malignant changes. Alternatively, it might be that elimination of the old epidermis and its replacement by a new secondary epithelium that has grown from remaining dermal elements may offer the explanation. It is unlikely that dermabrasion can offer a safe and effective treatment for skin degeneration that has progressed beyond solar degeneration and hyperkeratosis. We must also admit the possibility of dissemination or stimulation of unrecognized squamous carcinoma, should this be present.

THE GENERAL PLAN OF SURGICAL TREATMENT

The plan of surgical treatment must be carefully worked out before actually embarking on treatment. This may be a very simple matter in a small localized lesion or may be a vastly complicated exercise.

Diagnosis

The diagnosis of the lesion should be established by clinical examination, with the aid of a biopsy and microscopic examination of the histological sections if necessary. Many small lesions can be so readily excised and repaired that even if doubt exists about diagnosis, preliminary biopsy is not necessary.

Assessment of Extent of Involvement

In superficial, mobile lesions the extent of involvement can usually be established quite easily. In deep lesions, however, especially those involving bone or cartilage or recurrent lesions (especially recurrent after previous radiotherapy), assessment of extent can be very difficult.

Duration of the lesion gives an indication of probable extent of spread. Malignant melanoma, if present long enough, will almost certainly spread by lymphatic paths or the blood stream. Squamous cell carcinoma commonly will spread through the lymphatics, and basal cell carcinoma will practically never spread to a distant site.

Clinical examination helps this assessment. *Size* of the lesion is the next consideration. In general, the larger the lesion, the deeper the spread and the more the chance of distant spread in a metastasizing lesion. *Mobility* of the lesion is a most valuable index of spread. Fixation to deep fascia, cartilage, or bone is strongly suggestive that the malignancy has spread to these tissues. *Internal examination* of the relative cavities, notably nose and mouth, should be made to detect spread to the lining of these cavities. *X-ray examination* may be helpful if bony involvement is suspected.

Plan the Limits of Excision

Having assessed the limits of involvement, the surgeon then proceeds to plan the limits of excision, which must include a margin of normal tissue beyond the estimated extent of involvement.

It is difficult to define precise limits for the margin of normal tissue to be included in the excision in various tumors. The experienced surgeon develops a judgment in this decision based on his knowledge of the pathology of the particular tumor and his previous experience in such excisions when his assessment of a safe margin has been confirmed or proved wrong by the pathologist's report or by local recurrence. In addition, the limits for this margin of normal tissue are influenced by the anatomical site – it is apparent that one can include the upper limits where ample tissue is available, but one may need to stay within the lower limits where more radical excision would sacrifice vital structures and impose serious disability or disfigurement. However, as a general guide the following margins are recommended for the three most common malignant tumors: for basal cell carcinoma 5 to 10 mm.; for squamous carcinoma 10 to 15 mm.; and for malignant melanoma 4 to 6 cm.

Burg and colleagues [13] attempted to give more precise guidelines for the limits of excision in basal cell carcinomas. They attempted to measure the spread of basal cell carcinoma beyond the visible margins in different situations. In this study, the authors measured the visible limits of the lesion and then removed the lesion completely (or as completely as possible) by Mohs' chemosurgery and measured the defect. The difference they called the subclinical extension. The average subclinical extension for the whole series was 7.6 ± 4.5 mm. As would be expected, this subclinical extension was greater in the recurrent than in primary lesions, being 8.9 mm. in comparison with 5.5 mm. It was also greater in morphea-like lesions than solid lesions, being 9.3 mm. as opposed to 6.5 mm. When we look at the great variation in behavior of these lesions, it is difficult to accept such precise quantification as this. Although this paper provides interesting information on the spread of basal cell carcinoma, the recommendation of a 2-mm. margin of excision beyond the visible edge in the normal case and a 5- to 10-mm. margin in high-risk areas is far too conservative in our opinion.

It seems that carcinoma will at first usually take the line of least resistance and spread laterally rather than penetrate certain natural tissue barriers such as bone, cartilage, and deep fascia. Accordingly, when it is suspected that the tumor is closely approaching such tissue barriers, an excision should be planned to include such barriers, thereby safely confining the tumor within the limits of the tissue excised.

The Resection of the Tumor

Having determined the limits of excision, the surgeon then proceeds with the actual excision. The surgeon should ensure that he has the most favorable conditions for this exercise, especially in extensive resections. This means that bleeding should be minimized by some or all of the following aids:

1. Local anesthesia or general anesthesia perhaps combined with induced hypotension.
2. Appropriate posture of the patient whereby the operative field is elevated – giving the operating table a foot-down tilt can reduce bleeding substantially from an operative field in the head and neck.
3. Local infiltration of peripheral tissues or packing of cavities with vasoconstrictor agents.

The resection then proceeds in a logical and systematic manner, the surgeon ever on the watch for unexpected extension of the tumor across the limits of the planned excision. In soft tissues *the surgeon's finger* is often a helpful guide to a safe margin of uninvolved tissue in depth between the plane of excision and the tumor – the indurated tumor can be felt through the soft yielding normal tissue and the finger indicates, like the depth sounder on a ship, the safe course for the surgical navigation.

Doubts about adequacy of excision may be confirmed or dispelled by *frozen section* or *cytodiagnosis.* No doubt the reader is familiar with the former technique. In the latter, a small portion of suspect tissue is spread on a microscope slide and stained with hemotoxylin and eosin. The experienced cytologist can usually give an accurate opinion as to whether tumor cells are present.

Later, when the specimen has been removed, its correct orientation should be clearly marked by sutures or other means. The histologist can then carry out a careful systematic histological examination by paraffin section to determine as accurately as possible whether in fact the tumor has been completely removed. Coating the undersurface of the excised specimen with india ink may assist the pathologist in determining adequacy of excision. Distortion and shrinkage of normal tissue beyond the tumor may sometimes mislead the pathologist in the assessment of adequacy of excision.

The Repair

Having extirpated the tumor, the surgeon is then faced with the problem of repair. This may mean no more than a few well-placed sutures, or he may be presented with a disfiguring and devastating defect that taxes to the utmost the resources of the skilled and experienced reconstructive surgeon.

Simple defects can be repaired at the time of excision, usually with minimal disfigurement or disability. However, when faced with *large and complicated defects,* the surgeon is presented with the dilemma of whether to carry out an immediate definitive repair or to settle for a temporary repair that achieves healing and prepares the way for a later definitive repair or the fitting of a prosthesis.

Timing of Repair

The considerations discussed in this section relate to the question of timing of repair after major resection for skin cancer, and apply particularly to the head and neck region. The traditional and more conservative approach to this subject, especially in dealing with recurrent lesions, was to effect a temporary repair only, at the time of the resection, sufficient to achieve healing and minimize disability. At a later time, after a period to permit careful observation for recurrence, the definitive repair was carried out. This method of management has been described by one of us (E. W. G.) previously [17].

In recent years there has been a changed attitude to this problem. We consider that the fear of recurrence has occupied our minds too much and that it is in the patient's interest to carry out more repairs at the time of the ablative surgery or soon afterward. This more ambitious approach to the problem has been discussed by Edgerton [15] and ourselves [18] in regard to head and neck surgery, and also by Millard [20] in regard to reconstruction of the lower jaw.

In regard to the timing of repair after cancer resection, the patients belong to one of three groups:

1. Patients in whom immediate repair is *mandatory.*
2. Patients in whom immediate repair is *contraindicated.*
3. Patients in whom immediate repair is *desirable.*

The first and second groups are mentioned briefly, with most consideration being given to the more difficult third group.

IMMEDIATE REPAIR MANDATORY. Immediate repair is demanded when vital structures are exposed and life would be threatened by their continued exposure or when local necrosis would proceed if these structures were left exposed. Such vital structures are the dura mater or brain, bone and cartilage, and major vessels or nerves.

The repair is carried out by use of local tissue if available – we usually use scalp, neck, cheek, or forehead flaps. If, due to the cosmetic considerations, a suitable local flap cannot be found, one must then seek tissue from afar. This usually means an abdominal or chest flap or tube must be fabricated in advance, ready to transfer to the defect at the time of the ablative operation. Island flaps based on specific vascular pedicles (temporal, supraorbital, etc.) or dermal or subdermal pedicles can make a most useful contribution to the mucosal lining component in the immediate repair of compound defects, as described by Davies [14].

IMMEDIATE REPAIR CONTRAINDICATED. When serious doubt exists about the adequacy of excision or when the technical difficulties of immediate repair are too great, immediate repair should not be done. This usually means that the defect is covered by a split-thickness skin graft, or skin and mucosa are united at the margins of the defect. One must *always* attempt to achieve primary healing even if one does not attempt primary repair.

IMMEDIATE REPAIR DESIRABLE. When one is reasonably sure of completeness of excision, and especially if severe deformity or functional disturbance will follow, an attempt should be made to carry out an immediate repair. While it would be obvious folly to repair a defect when recurrence is reasonably likely, there are a number of issues to evaluate.

The greatest chance of cure of extensive lesions is the first major surgical attack. If this first attack is unsuccessful, the chance of cure after second or third operations for recurrence is fairly remote. Therefore, why deny the patient the benefit of an immediate or early repair solely to enable one to recognize a possible recurrence that probably means a fatal outcome for the patient in any case?

Many of the patients undergoing this surgery are in an older age group. It is unkind to inflict on them gross disfigurement or the discomfort of dribbling saliva or inadequate mastication for long periods, when this does not *very significantly* increase their chances of ultimate cure. It is an axiom of cancer surgery that the best chance of cure is at the first operation. A corollary to this is that this first operation must be carefully planned and radical enough to remove the entire tumor. Since one is contemplating a primary repair, one may tend toward a wider and safer excision than would be done if a temporary repair only were being planned.

A decision on the wisdom of primary repair could be made following an assessment of the following factors:

1. The *age and life expectancy* of the patient. If the patient is elderly and his life expectancy short, one would incline toward primary repair to make the concluding period of life as comfortable as possible and to minimize the burden imposed on the family or those responsible for the patient's care.
2. The same considerations apply to patients whose life expectancy is seriously reduced by *other diseases.* It is a kindness to spare them the anguish of disfigurement if it is to be added to the burden of their other conditions.
3. The *natural history of the neoplasm.* Many of these carcinomas (especially basal cell carcinomas in old people) progress very slowly indeed. Some have taken 10 years or more to reach troublesome proportions. Lesions of this sort can often be excised and repaired at once with the knowledge that a failing heart or senility will kill the patient before any signs of recurrence develop.
4. The *degree of disfigurement and disability* from temporary repair. This may range from a small disfigurement that can be left exposed or covered by a small dressing, to a large defect in the mouth, lower lip, and jaw, which can make a patient's life a misery and bring him close to suicide. The constant dribbling of saliva from mouth defects or external buccal or pharyngeal fistulas is one of the most distressing discomforts a patient can be called on to endure. Patients of advanced years may be denied one of the few pleasures left to them – eating a good meal. Mandibular defects and an incompetent oral sphincter may make eating and drinking extremely difficult, and meals become an unsatisfying and frustrating ordeal. If repair is deferred to permit observation for recurrence, one must measure a year's misery of this sort against the possible opportunity to detect a recurrence earlier and permit an earlier *second* attempt to eradicate the tumor.
5. The *physical fitness* of the patient to stand extensive surgery for the excision and what might be *equally* extensive surgery for the repair if done at the same time. This, of course, can be decided only at the time of operation for the particular patient. However, with proper preoperative preparation and competent anesthesia, patients can tolerate long extensive operations with little risk to life.
6. The *psychological fitness* of the patient and the possibilities of postoperative psychological complications. Surgeons are often shamefully unaware of the subtler changes in their patients' psychological state, and the influence for the worse which major surgery can produce in the state of their minds. This subject has been discussed in a most thoughtful and valuable paper by Maddison [19], who reports that as many as a third of older patients undergoing major operations showed serious postoperative mental changes.
7. The *extreme technical difficulties* of a primary repair. Certain deep defects, especially those communicating with the nasal or buccal cavity or paranasal sinuses, may provide an unsurmountable challenge to the surgeon aiming at primary repair. These must wait for a secondary repair or prosthesis.
8. The *ability of patients to cope* with the deformity. While in general advocating primary or early repair, we must be fully aware of how well patients can cope with what appear to be major deformities, and the natural enthusiasm to restore patients to normal must not blind one to this fact. For example the loss of half the mandible may not produce the disfigurement and disability that is commonly supposed, provided that the patient has a competent oral sphincter. This has been emphasized by Gaisfor and Hanna [16].

While trying to avoid the folly and disappointment of seeing recurrence develop in the repair, one should realize that often the proper and humane course may lie in taking a calculated risk to permit patients to live out their remaining years in greater comfort and happiness.

THE RESECTION AND THE REPAIR: ONE SURGEON OR TWO?

It has been suggested by some – including even the illustrious Halsted – that in the surgery of skin cancer, especially advanced disease of the head and neck, one surgeon (or surgical team) should do the resection and another the repair. The inference is that the extirpating surgeon could be inhibited in resecting the lesion adequately by a knowledge of the difficulties of the repair that lie ahead. This seems to us a denial of the intellectual integrity of the surgeon who is charged with, and must accept, the full personal responsibility for the welfare of his patient. Surely none would suggest that one surgeon resect the bowel and another perform the anastomosis. We find this division of responsibility unacceptable for the following reasons:

1. The trained reconstructive surgeon has the technique of repair immediately available and, strengthened by this knowledge, can often take a bolder line in his excision, with better hope of cure, than the surgeon not so equipped.
2. The surgeon not trained in reconstructive work may well sacrifice tissue valuable for the repair, which does not in any way contribute to the chances of cure.
3. Surgeons involved in treating malignancy of the skin and head and neck generally are constantly meeting the challenge of assessing the extent of spread of malignancy, often with only superficial access to the tumor (see under the heading, Planning the Surgical Treatment). The correctness or otherwise of their assessment is then subject to the searching eye of the histologist's microscope.

It must be admitted that many of these operations are long and laborious, making heavy demands on the physical and nervous resources of the surgeon. We feel that this situation would be met best by two expert reconstructive surgeons, each with his own assistant, perhaps working simultaneously, one mainly concerned with the resection while the other is preparing the repair tissues. The final reconstructive phase can then probably be done jointly.

SPECIAL CONSIDERATIONS IN LOCAL EXCISION OF SKIN MALIGNANCIES

Excision of Carcinoma of External Auditory Canal

When carcinoma of the ear involves the *external auditory canal,* special problems arise. The following points in management have emerged from a considerable experience with this condition [29].

1. If the dissection is likely to proceed in the vicinity of the facial nerve, this nerve should be formally exposed beforehand, even if resection of the parotid gland is not contemplated.
2. Carcinoma confined to the external auditory canal can usually be resected as a sleeve of tissue (with the adequacy checked by frozen section) and the defect repaired by an inlay free graft. Stenosis of the canal is not a problem in this type of case.
3. When the carcinoma involves bone, a skin flap repair is usually indicated, and stenosis becomes a serious problem if an attempt is made to preserve the external auditory canal. Removal of both the lining of the canal and the ear drum, before applying the flap, resolves this problem. It seems that secondary middle ear epithelium seals off the middle ear deep to the flap. Impairment of hearing on one side seems to cause little concern to the patient.
4. In extensive resections, temporary occlusion of the external carotid artery facilitates the dissection. However, permanent ligation is not recommended because this could jeopardize the blood supply to the scalp flap, which could well be needed for the repair. In addition, if an inoperable recurrence should develop, previous ligation of the external carotid artery might preclude the effective use of regional perfusion.

Contrary to our experience, Pless [30] reports a predominance of squamous carcinoma of the external ear over basal cell carcinoma (67 percent squamous cell carcinoma, as opposed to 30 percent basal cell carcinoma). Blake and Wilson [28] report on a high recurrence in carcinoma of the auricle; they report a 16 percent recurrence after surgery and 47 percent recurrence after radiotherapy. Wilson and associates [32] give a sound comprehensive report on carcinoma extending into the auditory canal and also into the temporal bone.

MULTIPLE CARCINOMAS OF THE SKIN

One of the most challenging problems facing the surgeon charged with treating basal cell and squamous cell carcinoma is the management of the patient with multiple carcinomas of the skin. These patients present repeatedly with successive crops of skin carcinomas, endure half a lifetime of treatment, and often succumb in the end to the persistent attacks of their malignancy. We advocate a radical attack on this problem in very carefully selected cases [34].

Rationale of the Treatment

It seems that skin usually takes many years of conditioning by exposure to solar rays before carcinoma develops. We see many patients in their fifties or sixties in whom multiple skin cancers suddenly develop. It is unusual for new lesions to develop in skin grafts removed from unexposed areas. We often see a free graft on such a patient as an island of sound skin in a sea of carcinoma. It is therefore suggested that susceptible patients who show numerous widespread cancerous and precancerous lesions should have the whole of the affected skin removed and replaced by skin taken from an unexposed part of the body.

The Technique of Massive Skin Replacement

In planning the actual skin excision, the involved skin

should be removed in units that permit the location of graft margins in inconspicuous hairlines or natural skin folds. This approach has been emphasized by González-Ulloa [35] in his writings on aesthetic units in skin replacement on the face. Such units are the total forehead, each cheek, total nose, upper lip, lower lip, and chin.

Certain areas permit massive skin replacement with very satisfactory cosmetic and functional results. These areas are the forehead, nose, eyelids, hands, and forearms. Difficulties exist in areas such as the cheeks, lips, and ears, because free grafts tend to contract and become corrugated over the mobile tissues of the lip and cheek, and in addition contour irregularities in the fullness of the cheek are conspicuous. Massive skin replacement over the ear is difficult because excision of even early lesions is liable to expose bare cartilage – a poor base for a free graft.

Such surgery carried out in a single stage would be very time consuming, so that we usually carry out the procedure in two stages.

At the *first stage* the area to be excised is removed under local anesthetic and the raw area dressed with a nonadherent dressing. Several days later at the *second stage,* a healthy, fresh granulating surface presents itself that is readily covered by a thick dermatome graft. It is, of course, apparent to the reader that a free graft will take as readily on a fresh surgically prepared bed as on a clean granulating surface, provided that perfect hemostasis is achieved. However, in these large areas, in a region of rich blood supply, complete hemostasis may be difficult to achieve in spite of all the aids, such as locally applied epinephrine (Adrenalin) and topical thrombin. It is for this reason that a two-stage operation is sometimes used. It has been found that replacement of one forehead, the nose, or two cheek units is all that can reasonably be done at one operation.

Malignant Potential

It seems that the malignant potential of the skin of patients with multiple carcinomas increases as time goes by. A number of patients, after suffering many low-grade lesions over the years, acquire highly malignant anaplastic cancers. We have on our records a patient who, after suffering numerous basal cell carcinomas and squamous cell carcinomas, acquired in turn a sarcoma, an anaplastic squamous carcinoma, and a malignant melanoma. Awareness of this increasing malignant potential offers further justification for massive skin replacement in patients highly susceptible to cancer who have multiple lesions.

The Terebrating (Boring) Basal Cell Carcinoma

Some basal cell carcinomas display a sinister characteristic of burrowing under the skin – sometimes deeply – far beyond obvious visible limits. This characteristic is also sometimes seen in squamous cell carcinomas and sweat gland carcinomas.

How is the surgeon alerted to the fact that he is dealing with a potentially troublesome burrowing type of lesion? The biopsy report, recurrence after previous x-ray therapy, or recurrence after previous surgery may sound a warning. Clinical examination may indicate to the examining finger induration deep to skin and well beyond the visible superficial limits of the tumor. This is probably the most significant and ominous sign. Biopsy of such a suspicious area before surgical treatment may confirm this suspicion.

PLANNING THE SURGICAL TREATMENT. We believe that, except in exceptional circumstances, the treatment of the burrowing lesion should be surgical. When faced with a lesion of terebrating proclivities, one should plan carefully a sufficiently radical approach to encompass the lesion completely with a margin of normal tissue beyond.

The excision should be planned to include a natural tissue barrier, fascia, bone, or cartilage, which we can assume has not been penetrated by the lesion. Sacrifice of such tissue may not significantly complicate the repair but may ensure a complete removal of the tumor. Frozen section of tissue on the edge of the specimen or on the margin of residual tissue may be helpful in determining the adequacy of excision.

The use of a special knife with double parallel blades 2 mm. apart, as designed by McCoy, is recommended by Moore [37]; this knife permits the excision of a 2-mm. strip at the margin of the planned line of excision. This strip is then examined by frozen section after careful orientation. Any residual tumor can be identified and appropriate reexcision carried out.

In more advanced lesions where real concern about the adequacy of excision exists, it could be advisable to repair the defect by an inlay graft. *This permits inspection of the actual plane of excision over the next few months to observe any recurrence.* It can also provide tissue that may be utilized in the late definitive repair.

It is our view that surgical treatment is indicated in almost all of these cases, although some would propose that Mohs' chemosurgery has a place for some cases.

The behavior of the burrowing basal cell carcinoma is well illustrated in the inner canthus region, where the basal cell carcinoma will tend to spread backward along the nasal bone to the ethmoid region. This is particularly liable to happen if the lesion has been inadequately treated by x-ray therapy. Residual surviving cells in the depth of the lesion can be separated from the surface of the skin by a barrier of scar tissue.

The tumor will then take the line of least resistance and spread backward to the ethmoid region. The extent of this posterior spread may be not at all apparent from superficial examination. Bostwick [36] refers to frequent extension into the soft tissues of the orbit in this type of lesion, but in our experience this is unusual. We consider that the modern air drill is a better instrument for bone resection in this region than the osteotome, which is advocated by Bostwick.

Another area in which this burrowing characteristic can give trouble is the alar base. Here a lesion that was inadequately treated by either surgery or x-ray therapy can spread through the adjacent lip to become attached to the maxilla and create a major surgical problem.

In aggressive and extensive basal cell carcinomas, a large deep tissue defect may be left after excision. Such a defect may be suitable for repair by a free flap transfer (Poole [38]). For this technique to be used, two criteria must be met – first the surgeon must be certain that the lesion has been completely excised, and second, there must be a suitable recipient blood vessel in the vicinity to anastomose to the vessels of the free flap.

THE COMMON MALIGNANT TUMORS

Since *basal cell carcinomas* practically never metastasize, the surgeon is required only to ensure adequate local removal – although even this can be a difficult task. On the other hand, in the case of *squamous carcinoma* and *malignant melanoma,* he is charged with the responsibility of encompassing established or potential distant spread. The question of prophylactic lymph node dissection is discussed later in this chapter.

Basal Cell Carcinoma

When we consider the high incidence of basal cell carcinoma, it is interesting to recall that its identity was only clearly established by Jonathan Hutchinson and Carl Thiersch barely a century ago. As Bennett [39] pointed out, from the middle ages until the nineteenth century the lesions we call basal cell carcinoma were known as *noli me tangere* ("touch me not"); these were not distinguished from squamous carcinomas, syphilitic ulceration, and lupus vulgaris.

The essential treatment of basal cell carcinoma is to ensure adequate local removal. This requirement can be met by excision and repair in accordance with the methods described earlier in this chapter.

Sound comment on the management of these lesions, especially in regard to the respective roles of surgery and radiotherapy, is provided in papers by Rank and Wakefield [46, 47]. They also offer wise advice on the treatment of advanced lesions and assessment of operability. The reader is referred to an earlier section of this chapter for comment on the treatment of advanced and recurrent lesions.

Basal cell carcinoma is a very common lesion and without doubt the most common malignancy in countries whose population is exposed to a high dosage of ultraviolet irradiation from the sun. In persons of northern European origin with fair or sandy coloring whose skin is exposed for long periods to direct sunlight, solar degeneration and hyperkeratosis will certainly develop and a great many of these lesions will continue on to frank carcinoma [41]. Harris [43] writes of one patient in northern Australia who, commencing at 27 years of age, had 150 lesions excised in 4 years. He states that in northern Queensland 13 percent of all males between 20 and 80 years of age will develop skin cancer.

Regional and Sex Incidence

Table 26-1 shows the high incidence of this tumor in the head and neck. In 4,123 histologically proved tumors examined at Royal Prince Alfred Hospital, Sydney, between 1950 and 1964, 3,069 occurred in this region. It will also be noted that the incidence in males is almost twice that in females.

Clinical Types

Enthusiastic dermatologists have classified these lesions into a large number of clinical types. However, for the practicing surgeon a classification into the following five types will enable him to determine treatment and general management:

1. *The papulo-pearly type.* This is the most common variety and presents itself as a nodule or ulcer with a rolled pearly edge. This pearly edge is made more apparent by stretching the skin over it with the finger.
2. *The cystic type.* This is a circumscribed lesion raised above the surface in which the round cysts may be apparent to the naked eye or may be revealed under the microscope.

Table 26-1. Site and Sex Incidence of Basal Cell Carcinoma – Royal Prince Alfred Hospital, Sydney, 1950 to 1964

Site	Males	Females	Total
Head and neck	1,918	1,151	3,069
Trunk	235	94	329
Upper limb	224	73	297
Lower limb	166	59	225
Not stated	131	72	203
Total	2,674	1,449	4,123

3. *The sclerosing and morpheic types.* These types are separately identified by some dermatologists but for practical purposes may be grouped together. They present as slow-growing ill-defined indurated lesions that may show little surface growth and in fact even give a depressed scarlike appearance.
4. *The cicatricial type.* This variety shows itself as a very slow-growing, peripherally spreading invasion of the skin tissues by basal cell carcinoma. As the lesion spreads peripherally, the skin left behind has the appearance of thin papery scar and usually comprises scar tissue with little or no active carcinoma. The behavior of this variety has been likened to a slowly burning forest fire that spreads peripherally and leaves behind the scarred and burned-out remnants.
5. *The pigmented type.* This may appear as a pearly nodule varying in color from light brown to black. Its special importance is that it may be extremely difficult to distinguish it from a malignant melanoma and each should be considered in the differential diagnosis of the other.

The histological appearance of these lesions may be inferred from the clinical appearance. The papulopearly and cystic types are clearly localized clinically and well defined histologically. Masses of basal cells are scattered through the connective tissue, but the limits of spread are clearly demarcated. The peripheral layer of basal cells in these masses typically shows a palisade arrangement of their nuclei. In the cystic type, some of the masses of cells are expanded into cysts. The sclerosing and morpheic types are as ill-defined histologically as they are clinically. Cords of basal cells extend widely through tissues from the main focus.

Certain practical considerations emerge from the above review of the clinical and pathological varieties of basal cell carcinoma. The well-circumscribed lesions can be readily excised completely by including a small margin of normal tissue (4 or 5 mm.) beyond the visible limits. The infiltrating lesions need much wider excision in lateral extent and depth, possibly 1 to 1.5 cm., beyond the visible limits; very careful histological scrutiny of the specimen; and regular and careful follow-up examination of the patient.

Furthermore, the infiltrating sclerosing types are less sensitive to irradiation, and many dermatologists advise surgical treatment for this condition.

Special Considerations in Recurrent Lesions

It has been clearly demonstrated that many basal cell carcinomas are multifocal in origin. This fact should not be seized upon, however, to explain recurrences in surgical scars of previous excisions or recurrences at the site of previous irradiation. Lesions that appear at these sites should be regarded as recurrences both for statistical purposes and for the desirable chastening influence on the surgeon.

The chance of further recurrence following secondary treatment for a basal cell carcinoma recurrent after previous surgery or irradiation is much higher than the expected recurrence rate following the primary surgical treatment. Rank and Wakefield [47] quote a 15 percent recurrence rate for the former and a recurrence rate of less than 1 percent for the latter. In a more recent paper Binns and Sherriff [40] report a recurrence rate of 0.5 percent in patients with basal cell carcinomas treated by surgery without having had previous irradiation.

When excising lesions recurrent after previous irradiation, the excised tissue should include, if possible, all adjacent radioatrophic tissue for two reasons: (1) radioatrophic tissue is itself especially prone to malignant change [4], and (2) healing may be delayed when radioatrophic tissues are sutured or grafted, and actual radionecrosis may develop subsequently in the atrophic tissue.

Basal Cell Carcinoma of the Eyelids

The eyelid is a common site for basal cell carcinoma, which presents special problems for the following reasons:

1. The eyelid has a complex structure consisting of skin, conjunctiva, muscle, tarsal plate, and eyelashes. A good reconstruction should provide all five elements.
2. The eyelids are required to cover and protect the eye – they provide cover during sleep and they protect the eye from trauma and desiccation during waking hours. The reconstructed lid must serve these functions.
3. The eyelid is close to other important structures, particularly the tear-draining mechanism.

Holmström and co-workers [44] report an ingenious technique for repair of the upper lid whereby a skin island from the lower lid on a conjunctival pedicle is transferred beneath the lower lid margin to the defect in the upper. In some patients this could present a risk of lower lid ectropion. (See Chapter 12 for additional information.)

Multiple Nevoid Basal Cell Carcinoma and Congenital Anomalies

Reference must be made to a rare but interesting syndrome in which multiple basal cell carcinomas of a nevoid type occur in association with a number of congenital abnormalities. Gorlin and Goltz [42] described the association of multiple basal cell carcinomas with jaw cysts and bifid ribs. Rayner and associates [48] later assembled from their own experience and the literature a remarkable array of associated abnormalities; the list includes calcification of the falx cerebri, palmar and plantar pits, scoliosis, hypertelorism, mandibular prognathism, high palate, high scapulae, diabetes, ovarian tumors, mesenteric cysts, cataract, glaucoma, mental retardation, cerebral tumor, and undescended testes! Rayner recommends that the bone cysts be treated by enucleation and curettage of the bone by a bur.

X-ray examination of the mandible should be performed in young people with multiple basal cell carcinomas. Families showing a history of this condition should be under surveillance and those at risk identified. Members of such families should also be offered genetic counseling.

Murphy [45] reports metastatic basal cell carcinoma with squamous appearance in a patient with Gorlin's syndrome.

Squamous Cell Carcinoma

As compared with basal cell carcinoma, we find, in general, that squamous cell carcinoma has a more rapid and wider local spread. In addition, the squamous lesion has the capacity for distant spread by blood stream and lymphatics.

Regional and Sex Incidence

Again the high incidence of this tumor on the exposed skin of the head and neck is illustrated by the figures from Royal Prince Alfred Hospital, Sydney (Table 26-2). Over the period of 1950 to 1964, of 2,479 patients with histologically proved squamous carcinomas, 1,578 had lesions situated on the head and neck region. The very high relative incidence in males compared with females can be noted – over five times as many lesions in the head and neck and nearly four times as many overall.

Clinical Considerations

The base of the lesion usually shows induration and proliferation and an opaque appearance, compared with the pearly edge of the basal cell carcinoma. If untreated, the lesion usually ulcerates. As ulceration proceeds, the lesion may be covered by a keratin layer (like a keratoacanthoma) or by a serous crust, or the lesion may merely present a raw granular surface that bleeds readily. In general these lesions pursue one of two clinical courses – either they develop as an exuberant cauliflower-like growth or they progress as an invasive tumor with infiltration of adjacent tissues; the former tends to be more differentiated with less tendency to metastasize, the latter less differentiated with more tendency to metastasize.

Table 26-2. Site and Sex Incidence of Squamous Cell Carcinoma – Royal Prince Alfred Hospital, Sydney, 1950 to 1964

Site	Males	Females	Total
Head and neck	1,326	252	1,578
Trunk	32	16	48
Upper limb	448	186	634
Lower limb	87	31	118
Not stated	70	31	101
Total	1,963	516	2,479

Treatment

LOCAL TREATMENT. Local excision is carried out along the lines described above under the heading of Special Considerations in Local Excision of Skin Malignancies. In general a wider excision will be carried out than in basal cell carcinoma, the surgeon aiming to leave a margin of apparently normal tissue about 1 to 1.5 cm. beyond the obvious edge of the lesion. This recommendation in regard to margin of normal tissue is intended only as a general guide. The actual margin of normal tissue which should be included is influenced by:

1. *The degree of malignancy of the tumor,* as indicated by gross appearance (fungating or infiltrating); histological differentiation; clinical history in regard to size, duration, and rate of growth; and the age of the patient.
2. *The anatomical site* – for example, some areas permit a liberal margin of normal tissue in lateral extent, whereas others with vital underlying structures may tax the surgeon's judgment in determining a safe plane of excision.

In addition, the question of lymph node involvement must be considered. On occasion it will be necessary to carry out immediate or delayed lymph node dissection.

Local excision of areas of leukoplakia and squamous carcinoma in the mouth requiring grafting can present technical problems because of persistent bleeding and movement. McGregor [52] suggests a "quilting" technique whereby multiple quilting sutures are passed through the bed holding the graft in contact. The graft is then perforated by multiple stab wounds between the quilting sutures. The grafts take well even in the presence of free bleeding.

LYMPH NODE DISSECTION. The following principles probably represent the usual current practice in this matter:

1. The vast majority of squamous carcinomas may be excised locally and careful follow-up observation maintained to detect any local recurrence or involvement of draining lymph nodes. Should lymph node involvement occur, appropriate surgery should be carried out unless contraindicated by such factors as advanced age, the general condition of the patient, or widespread dissemination of the carcinoma. In such circumstances radiotherapy might be considered.
2. If lymph nodes are clinically involved at the time of initial treatment of the *primary* lesion, then simultaneous (and in-continuity if possible) lymph node dissection should be carried out, provided that there is a reasonable chance of controlling the primary. However, the same contraindications as mentioned in paragraph 1 might apply.
3. If lesions are *recurrent* (especially after previous surgery), *large* (more than 2 cm. across), of *anaplastic* histology, and in the *younger age group* (under 55 years), serious consideration should be given to prophylactic lymph node dissection (either simultaneous or delayed), provided that their anatomical location makes such lymph node removal a practical proposition.
4. Early squamous cell carcinoma of the lip can probably be safely excised locally; assuming that regular follow-up examinations can be maintained, lymph node dissection can be delayed until clinical evidence of spread to this site is apparent.

Harris [51] finds, at least in Queensland, that squamous carcinomas usually run a more benign course than we had generally believed in the past. In 219 patients with squamous carcinoma, 2 percent had involved nodes when first seen, and only 5.3 percent developed them later. In regard to histological differentiation, he found 76 percent well differentiated, 31 percent moderately differentiated, and 8 percent poorly differentiated.

Some authorities [41] advocate routine prophylactic lymph node dissection in all cases of squamous carcinoma of the lip. They support this stand by quoting the high incidence of positive lymph node involvement (up to 25 percent) when such nodes are very minutely examined. However, since this high incidence of positive nodes comes from a clinic that attracts a large number of patients from distant places – many of whom had had previous treatment – this figure may not represent a true incidence of lymph node involvement. When all early lesions are included in a series, and in a country where all practitioners, and even the public, are alerted to the potential hazards of persistent cracks, sores, or nodules of the lip, and therefore seek early treatment, the incidence of lymph node involvement is lower.

The excision of advanced lesions of the lower lip should be accompanied by lymph node dissection, simultaneous and en bloc if possible.

A new and interesting development in the immunological field in relation to squamous carcinoma is reported by Ariyan and associates [49]. Squamous carcinoma cells grown in tissue culture (some from other patients) were exposed to lymphocytes from patients with squamous carcinoma in cytotoxicity studies. Lymphocytes from such patients killed from 40 to 60 percent of the tumor cells during 48 hours of incubation. The same lymphocytes did not show any killing potential against cultured melanoma cells or cultured fibroblasts. This demonstrates an immune response that is specific to tumor antigen. There was no evidence of any serum-blocking factor, because the killing potential of these lymphocytes was not significantly altered by the addition of the patients' sera.

Bowen's Disease

Bowen's disease is a low-grade, slow-growing variant of the squamous carcinoma in which the growth of the tumor is essentially intraepidermal. Its development and progress are similar to those of the other intraepidermal carcinomas – Paget's disease of the nipple, erythroplasia of Queyrat, and Borst-Jodassohn intraepidermal carcinoma.

The incidence of Bowen's disease seems to show great regional variation. Conway and co-workers [54] report 31 cases from an examination of 1,764 malignant skin tumors at the New York Hospital over a 30-year period. At the Royal Prince Alfred Hospital, Sydney, over a 15-year period 419 histologically proved tumors were reported, of which 233 were in males and 186 in females.

Several authors have found a common association of other malignancies with Bowen's disease. McGovern [55] found an incidence of 7 percent of serious internal cancer (bladder, bronchus, esophagus, breast, reticulum cell) and an incidence of 54 percent of other forms of skin cancer including 2 cases of malignant melanoma in 100 successive unselected cases of patients with Bowen's disease. Although the explanation for this association has not been provided, the association is common enough to warrant a careful search for other malignancies in a patient who presents with Bowen's disease.

Clinical Features

The lesion shows itself as a fairly circumscribed, slightly raised pink or brown patch covered by gray scales. The lesions are often multiple, and show a special predilection for the trunk and lower legs, but can also occur on the hands and face, including the conjunctiva.

The clinical course of the lesion is usually one of slow-spreading growth extending over many months or years. Sometimes the lesions will develop into frank invasive squamous carcinoma and even metastasize. The development of squamous carcinoma is shown by the appearance of a raised nodule, which will often be covered by a keratinous crust.

Treatment

Since the lesion commonly presents on the trunk and extremities, surgical excision and repair usually present no problems. Since the lesion is noninvasive and its activity strictly localized, it can be excised with a narrow margin of normal tissue. Either direct closure or free skin graft will deal with the defect. If the lesion involves the face or eyelids, greater demands will be made on the surgeon's repertoire of repair techniques. If invasive squamous carcinoma develops, the management will be on the same general lines as indicated in the section on squamous carcinoma.

Keratoacanthoma

It is only in recent years that the frequency of keratoacanthoma has been recognized, and its differentiation from squamous carcinoma delineated [56].

Hueston [57] rather aptly refers to it as a sheep in wolf's clothing. However, on some occasions one cannot be sure of the nature of the animal that lurks within, as the wolf will in fact masquerade in the sheep's clothing. Although a benign lesion, the keratoacanthoma is included briefly because confusion with squamous carcinoma can operate both ways. We have personal knowledge and experience with a number of cases assumed to be typical keratoacanthoma (even after preliminary biopsy) subject to the very limited treatment required by keratoacanthoma. Subsequently they recurred as squamous carcinomas.

Clinical Features

On clinical grounds one's suspicions of keratoacanthoma are aroused by a history of rapid growth, often over a period of 3 to 6 weeks. The typical keratoacanthoma is a raised lesion 1 to 3 cm. in diameter with pale ballooned margins and a central keratin plug. If the keratin plug is removed, an underlying papillary appearance is revealed. The base of the tumor shows no true induration and no evidence of deeper fixation than the dermis.

It seems probable that trauma can be an initiating cause of this condition. We have on record a patient in whom a keratoacanthoma arose exactly on the site of a recently healed laceration. The origin of the lesion at the site of the scar could be clearly seen in the histological section.

Treatment

We consider that the correct treatment is limited but complete local excision, followed, of course, by histological examination. One cannot recommend any of the very limited local treatments (such as slicing off at skin level), except in areas where significant disfigurement would follow even limited local excision or where considerable reconstructive problems would present themselves. If the last-mentioned difficulties do arise, very limited local treatment or a period of waiting for resolution might be justified after biopsy has supported the diagnosis of keratoacanthoma.

REFERENCES

Radiotherapy

1. Carling, R., Windeyer, B. W., and Smithers, D. W. *British Practice in Radiotherapy*. London: Butterworth, 1955.
2. Murphy, W. T. *Radiation Therapy*. Philadelphia: Saunders, 1955.
3. Paterson, R. *Treatment of Malignant Disease by Radium and X-rays*. London: Arnold, 1963.
4. Texier, M., and Preaux, J. Skin Cancer in Radiodermatitis. *Transactions of the Sixth International Congress of Plastic and Reconstructive Surgery*. Paris: Masson, 1976.

Mohs' Chemosurgery

5. Mohs, F. E. Chemosurgery, microscopically-controlled method of cancer excision. *Arch. Surg.* (Chicago) 42:279, 1941.
6. Mohs, F. E. Chemosurgical treatment of cancer of the lip. *Arch. Surg.* (Chicago) 48:478, 1944.

Topical Cytotoxic Therapy

7. Anderson, F. E., et al. Preliminary studies in the use of 5-fluorouracil cream in the treatment of skin tumours. *Med. J. Aust.* 2:385, 1969.
8. Belisario, J. C. The Treatment of Skin Cancer and Pre-cancer with Topical Cytotoxic Ointments. *Proceedings of the Thirteenth International Congress of Dermatology*, Munich. 1:99, 1967.
9. Everall, J. Comparison of Therapeutic Results in Basal Cell Carcinomas. In *Melanoma and Skin Cancer. Proceedings of the International Cancer Conference*, Sydney, 1972.
10. Litwin, M. S., et al. Topical chemotherapy of cutaneous malignancy of the head and neck. *South. Med. J.* 62:556, 1969.
11. Litwin, M. S., Ryan, R. F., Reed, R. J., and Remetil, E. T. Topical chemotherapy of advanced cutaneous malignancy with 4-fluorouracil cream. *J. Surg. Oncol.* 3:351, 1971.
12. Ryan, F. R., Litwin, M. S., Reed, R. S., and Pollock, W. J. The use of 5-fluorouracil cream to define suitable areas. *Plast. Reconstr. Surg.* 46:433, 1970.

Planning the Limits of Excision

13. Burg, G., Hirsch, R. D., Konz, B., and Braun-Falco, O. Histographic surgery: Accuracy of visual assessment of the margins of basal cell epithelioma. *J. Dermatol. Surg.* 1:21, 1975.

The Timing of Repair

14. Davies, D. Immediate Local Flap Repair of Lining Defects of the Oral Cavity. *Transactions of the Third International Congress of Plastic Surgeons* (1963). Amsterdam: Excerpta Medica, 1964.
15. Edgerton, M. T. Timing of head and neck reconstruction in cancer patients. *Trans. South. Surg. Assoc.* 73:429, 1962.
16. Gaisford, J. C., and Hanna, D. C. Mandibular resection. Personal communication, 1965.
17. Gibson, E. W. Some Aspects of the Management of Recurrent Basal Cell Carcinoma. In Wallace, A. B. (Ed.), *Transactions of the International Society of Plastic Surgeons (Second Congress,* 1959). Baltimore: Williams & Wilkins, 1960.
18. Gibson, E. W. Timing of repair following surgery for malignancy of the head and neck. Read at Annual Scientific Meeting, Royal Australasian College of Surgeons, 1962.
19. Maddison, D. C. Psychological aspects of surgical practice. *Aust. N.Z. J. Surg.* 30:9, 1960.
20. Millard, D. R. Immediate reconstruction of the lower jaw. *Plast. Reconstr. Surg.* 35:60, 1965.

Island Flaps

21. Barron, J. N., and Emmet, J. J. Subcutaneous pedicle flaps. *Br. J. Plast. Surg.* 18:51, 1969.
22. Converse, J. M., and Wood-Smith, D. Experiences with the forehead island flap with a subcutaneous pedicle. *Plast. Reconstr. Surg.* 31:521, 1963.
23. Gibson, E. W. Some variations of the island flap. Read at Annual Scientific Meeting, Royal Australasian College of Surgeons, 1965.
24. Kernahan, D. A., and Littlewood, A. H. M. Experience in the use of arterial flaps about the face. *Plast. Reconstr. Surg.* 28:207, 1961.
25. Littler, J. W. The neurovascular pedicle method of digital transposition for reconstruction of the thumb. *Plast. Reconstr. Surg.* 12:303, 1953.
26. Littler, J. W. Neurovascular Skin Island Transfer in Reconstructive Hand Surgery. In Wallace, A. B. (Ed.), *Transactions of the International Society of Plastic Surgeons (Second Congress,* 1959). Baltimore: Williams & Wilkins, 1960.
27. Millard, D. R. The island flap in cleft palate surgery. *Surg. Gynecol. Obstet.* 116:297, 1963.

Ear Repair

28. Blake, G. B., and Wilson, J. S. P. Malignant tumours of the ear and their treatment: I. Tumours of the auricle. *Br. J. Plast. Surg.* 27:67, 1974.
29. Gibson, E. W. Carcinoma involving the external auditory canal. Read at Annual Scientific Meeting, Royal Australasian College of Surgeons, 1963.
30. Pless, J. Carcinoma of the external ear. *Scand. J. Plast. Reconstr. Surg.* 10:147, 1976.
31. Tanzer, R. C. The reconstruction of acquired defects of the ear. *Plast. Reconstr. Surg.* 35:355, 1965.
32. Wilson, J. S. P., Blake, G. B., Richardson, A. E., and Westbury, G. Malignant tumours of the ear and their treatment: II. Tumours of the external auditory meatus, middle ear, cleft and temporal bone. *Br. J. Plast. Surg.* 27:77, 1974.

Massive Skin Replacement

33. Burke, J. W., Marascalco, J., and Clark, W. H., Jr. Half-face planing of precancerous skin after five years: An evaluation. *Arch. Dermatol.* (Chicago) 88:572, 1963.
34. Gibson, E. W. Massive Skin Replacement in Cancer-Susceptible Subjects. *Transactions of the Third International Congress of Plastic Surgeons* (1963). Amsterdam: Excerpta Medica, 1964.
35. González-Ulloa, M. Restoration of the face covering by means of selected skin in regional aesthetic units. *Br. J. Plast. Surg.* 9:212, 1956.

Terebrating Basal Cell Carcinoma

36. Bostwick, J., Vasconez, L. O., and Jurkiewicz, M. J. Basal cell carcinoma of the medial canthal area. *Plast. Reconstr. Surg.* 55:667, 1975.
37. Moore, J. R. Treatment of cicatrising basal cell carcinomas. *Plast. Reconstr. Surg.* 47:371, 1971.
38. Poole, M. D., Cochrane, T. D., and Bowen, J. Aggressive non-irradiated basal cell carcinoma of forehead treated by free flap transfer. *Br. J. Plast. Surg.* 28:142, 1975.

Basal Cell Carcinoma

39. Bennett, J. P. From noli-me-tangere to rodent ulcer: The recognition of the basal cell carcinoma. *Br. J. Plast. Surg.* 28:144, 1974.
40. Binns, J. H., and Sherriff, H. M. Low incidence of recurrence in excised but non-irradiated basal cell carcinomas. *Br. J. Plast. Surg.* 28:133, 1975.
41. Douglas, G., Silverstone, H., and Smithurst, B. A. The Epidemiology of Skin Cancer in Australia. In *Melanoma and Skin Cancer. Proceedings of the International Cancer Conference.* Sydney, 1972. P. 23.
42. Gorlin, R. J., and Goltz, R. W. Multiple nevoid basal cell epithelioma, jaw cysts and bifid ribs. *N. Engl. J. Med.* 262:908, 1960.
43. Harris, T. J. Skin cancer in sunny Queensland. *Br. J. Plast. Surg.* 29:61, 1976.

44. Holmström, H., Bartholdson, L., and Johanson, B. Surgical treatment of eyelid cancer with special reference to tarsoconjunctival flaps. *Scand. J. Plast. Reconstr. Surg.* 9:109, 1975.
45. Murphy, K. J. Metastatic basal cell carcinoma with squamous appearance in the naevoid basal cell carcinoma syndrome. *Br. J. Plast. Surg.* 28:331, 1975.
46. Rank, B. K. Surgery and Skin Cancer. *Melanoma and Skin Cancer. Proceedings of the International Cancer Conference,* Sydney, 1972. P. 323.
47. Rank, B. K., and Wakefield, A. R. Surgery of basal cell carcinoma. *Br. J. Plast. Surg.* 45:531, 1958. See also reference [17].
48. Rayner, C. R. W., Towers, J. F., and Wilson, J. S. P. What is Gorlin's syndrome? The diagnosis and management of the basal cell naevus syndrome, based on a study of thirty-seven patients. *Br. J. Plast. Surg.* 30:62, 1977.

Squamous Carcinoma

49. Ariyan, S., Krizek, T. J., and Mitchell, M. S. Identification of squamous cell carcinoma of the head and neck by tissue culture and immunological testing. *Plast. Reconstr. Surg.* 59:386, 1977.
50. Brown, J. B., and McDowell, F. *Neck Dissections.* Springfield, Ill.: Thomas, 1954.
51. Harris, T. J. Squamous carcinoma in Queensland: A relatively benign lesion. *Br. J. Plast. Surg.* 29:68, 1976.
52. McGregor, I. A. Quilted skin grafting in the mouth. *Br. J. Plast. Surg.* 28:100, 1975.

Bowen's Disease

53. Conway, H. *Tumors of the Skin.* Springfield, Ill.: Thomas, 1956.
54. Conway, H., Hugo, N. E., and Tulenko, J. F. *Surgery of Tumors of the Skin.* Springfield, Ill.: Thomas, 1966.
55. McGovern, V. J. Personal communication, 1965.

Keratoacanthoma

56. Bruner, J. M. Keratoacanthoma. *Plast. Reconstr. Surg.* 31:281, 1963.
57. Hueston, J. T. Molluscum sebaceum. *Aust. N.Z. J. Surg.* 26:25, 1956.

Malignant Melanoma*

FREDERICK R. EILBER, E. CARMACK HOLMES, AND DONALD L. MORTON

INCIDENCE AND EPIDEMIOLOGY

The incidence of malignant melanoma is increasing in the United States [17, 33]. The American Cancer Society estimated that there would be approximately 13,600 new cases (13 per 100,000 population) of malignant melanoma in the year 1979 [1]. This increase would make melanoma more common than Hodgkin's disease or primary brain tumor. Therefore, it seems appropriate to reappraise the therapeutic recommendations for patients with melanoma.

Although the etiology of this tumor is unknown, certain of its demographic factors warrant discussion. An increase in both the incidence of and death rate from malignant melanoma is noted – with decreased latitude, the exposure to the sun is greater, and the incidence is higher [3, 18, 27, 29]. For example, the incidence of melanoma in Queensland, Australia, is the highest in the world and is twice (16 per 100,000 population) the incidence in New South Wales or the United States [13].

Another interesting fact concerns the relationship of the overall increase in incidence of melanoma to particular anatomical sites – on the legs of females and on the trunk in males [33]. There has been no increase on head and neck areas or on areas of the extremities that are constantly exposed to the sun. Genetic factors, too, may have a relationship to the occurrence of melanoma, specifically in the peoples of Celtic origin – the Welsh and Irish appear to incur this type of cancer more often than Latins or Blacks [45]. To date, no relationship between exposure to air-borne or work-related carcinogens and incidence of malignant melanoma has been clearly established [2, 36].

RECOGNITION OF MALIGNANT MELANOMA

Since melanoma is a disease of skin, it has the potential for early diagnosis. Color changes of nevi that lead to a suspicion of malignancy are a blue mixed with brown or black. Borders or boundaries of such transforming lesions are usually irregular [13, 34, 35].

Descriptions of malignant melanoma have been divided into three basic categories [8, 34]: lentigo maligna, superficial spreading malignant melanoma, and nodular malignant melanoma.

Lentigo Maligna

Lentigo maligna, or the melanotic freckle of Hutchinson, is usually located on the sun-exposed surfaces such as the head and neck, hands, and legs, and occurs mostly in older age groups (median age, 70 years). This lesion has no sex predilection. Lesions may be present for 5 to 15 years, and the size is rather large (median, 3 to 4 cm.).

Superficial Spreading Malignant Melanoma

Superficial spreading malignant melanoma can occur on all body surfaces and in younger age groups (median age, 56 years). There is some sex predilection, since this tumor occurs more frequently on the lower extremities of females. The usual duration of growth before invasion is 1 to 5 years. The margin of the lesion is indistinct and irregular.

Nodular Malignant Melanoma

Nodular malignant melanoma can occur on all body surfaces (median age, 49 years). There is no sex predilection and its history of duration is much shorter – a few months to 2 years. This lesion is distinctly raised and nodular and may be amelanotic in appearance.

Results of Treatment

Results of therapy based on these gross descriptions of the different types of melanoma have varied from the patients with probable cure and extended survival to those with some early benefit, but eventual recurrence and ultimate death. Specifically, the superficial spreading melanoma and lentigo melanoma appeared to respond to treatment more favorably than the nodular melanomas, which are renowned for extreme virulence [9, 51].

HISTOLOGICAL EVALUATION OF MALIGNANT MELANOMA

Histopathology

One of the most significant improvements for the evaluation of patients with malignant melanoma was provided by the excellent histopathological classification systems introduced by Clark and co-workers [8], Breslow [5, 6], and others, who developed the microstaging techniques for primary malignant mela-

*Supported by U.S. Public Health Service grants CA 12582, CA 09010; National Institute of Health contract CB 64076-TQ (awarded by the National Cancer Institute, Department of Health, Education, and Welfare); and the Medical Research Service of the Veterans Administration.

noma. Clark's findings were based on the retrospective observation that with increasing depth of invasion, there was an increasing mortality. Clark defined Level I melanoma, or melanocytic hyperplasia, as a clinically benign lesion that does not penetrate the basement membrane; Level II extends into the papillary dermis; Level III passes through the papillary dermis to the junction of the reticular interface; Level IV invades the reticular dermis; Level V penetrates the subcutaneous fat [8] (Fig. 27-1). Breslow [5, 6] devised a similar system, in which depth of invasion could be quantitated by an ocular micrometer and measurement from the basal layer. In the retrospective and now in prospective studies, it appears that lesions measuring greater than 1.7 mm. in thickness have a very high metastatic potential. Lesions that are 0.7 to 1.5 mm. have a lesser potential, whereas the thinner lesions have a very low incidence of spread and a high survival rate for the patient.

Thus, the clinician who now is called upon to treat the patient with malignant melanoma can base prognosis on depth of invasion as well as on the gross appearance of the lesion before making the decisions for treatment.

Biopsy

The biopsy must be the first topic for discussion. Accurate histopathology is absolutely essential if the clinician is to make a reasonable therapeutic decision for the treatment of malignant melanoma. It is our feeling that all pigmented lesions brought to the attention of the physician warrant biopsy. Although certain gross characteristics may be highly suspicious for malignant melanoma, it is impossible to make an absolute determination of malignancy without a biopsy. Because microstaging and depth of invasion are so important, an incisional biopsy must include all layers of the epidermis and dermis. Therefore, for the majority of malignant melanoma lesions of 2 cm. or less, excisional biopsy is appropriate. This biopsy method complete removes the lesion and allows the pathologist adequate tissue for determining the depth of invasion. For lesions larger than 2 cm. and for those situated on the face, we suggest an incisional biopsy at the portion of the lesion that appears most nodular or irregular or in which recent change has been observed, including a portion of adjacent normal skin. Shave biopsies are mentioned only to be condemned, since they do not permit accurate microstaging.

Clinical Staging

Once the diagnosis of malignant melanoma has been established, a thorough evaluation must be done to determine the clinical extent of the disease. Of all the human malignancies, melanoma is the least predictable with a propensity for spread to any organ in the body, including the heart and spleen.

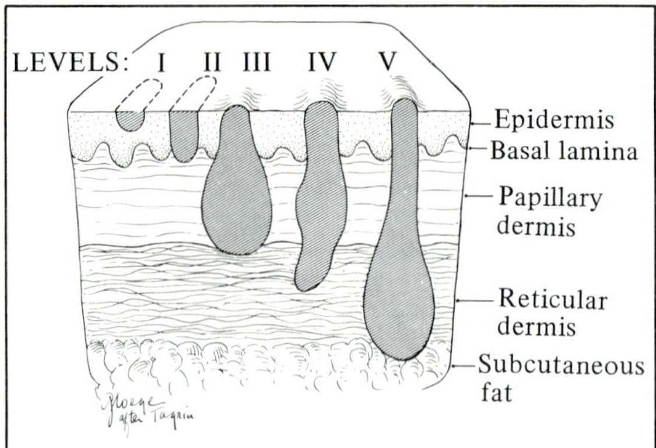

Fig. 27-1. Clark's levels of invasion (see text for explanation).

The extent of disease spread determines the preoperative clinical stage:

Stage I: disease confined to the primary site.
Stage II: metastases from the primary site to the regional lymph nodes.
Stage III: metastases beyond the regional lymph nodes.

The evaluation required for staging includes a complete history and physical examination. Laboratory examination includes complete blood count, SMA-12*, urinalysis, and chest x-ray studies. Patients with Stage I disease who are asymptomatic and have a normal physical exam and normal laboratory values do not require any additional diagnostic procedures [42]. Patients with palpable regional nodes or abnormal test results, and those who are symptomatic, require liver, brain, and bone scans. Additional tests for those patients who have abdominal symptoms should include an intravenous pyelogram and an upper gastrointestinal x-ray series, with small bowel follow-through.

TREATMENT OF PRIMARY MELANOMA

If after biopsy the diagnosis is malignant melanoma at Level II, III, IV, or V, or if there is greater than 0.75 mm. of invasion at any level, appropriate treatment of the primary lesion becomes paramount. The justification for a more extensive surgical excision is based on the original work of Sampson-Handley [43], which showed that a 5-cm. margin

*Battery of 12 blood chemistry tests.

of normal tissue must surround the primary lesions [12, 13, 47]. (This measurement is done with a ruler during the definitive surgical procedure.) Closure of the resultant circumferential defect on an extremity usually requires a skin graft, whereas on the trunk, such a defect may be accomplished by primary closure or rotational flaps. It has been shown that lesser excisions than the recommended 5-cm. margin had a high incidence of local recurrence. Furthermore, Cochran [9] demonstrated antigenic changes, and Wang [55] has shown melanocyte activation up to 4 cm. away from the primary tumor in areas of skin that appear grossly normal.

Clearly, in the head and neck area a 5-cm. margin is not possible. Most investigators and experienced clinicians reason that *a 2.5-cm. margin is the absolute minimum margin.* The incidence of local recurrence with this measurement has been very small indeed [13].

Depth of excision is equally important. Since the goal of the primary therapy is complete excision of the tumor, a dissection down to and including the underlying fascia must be accomplished. The excellent work of Olson [37, 38] indicated that although the lymphatics do not penetrate the underlying fascia, melanomas can certainly extend to this depth. Therefore, we recommend that the underlying fascia be removed for all deeply penetrating lesions (Levels IV and V), although this procedure may not be required for the more superficial lesions of Level III. By the same token, the less invasive lesions of Levels I and II may only necessitate operative margins of 2 to 3 cm. [7].

Since subcutaneous tissue and fascia are nonexistent in the subungual areas, appropriate treatment for melanoma in these locations involves amputation at a level of the distal interphalangeal joint.

The question of the acceptability of less extensive surgery or a smaller margin is constantly put forth, but, because there are few reliable studies in the literature, no one can answer with certainty. However, it seems unlikely that a smaller margin could improve the therapeutic results. When dealing with a very malignant tumor, the clinician must consider its complete eradication as his mandatory goal.

CONSIDERATION FOR REGIONAL LYMPHADENECTOMY

There is very little disagreement regarding adequate surgical treatment for patients presenting with palpable regional nodes [12, 20, 31]. These patients must undergo a regional lymphadenectomy at the time of operation for their primary lesion. The incidence of false positive regional lymphadenopathy (enlarged lymph nodes without micrometastases) is less than 5 percent; in this instance, no biopsy is required [22, 25]. It is doubtful that biopsy before lymphadenectomy is harmful, although there may be a higher incidence of local recurrence with a preoperative biopsy.

There is a major controversy in the literature over whether an elective node dissection in patients with nonpalpable regional nodes should be performed at the time of the diagnosis of the primary melanoma [12, 31, 41]. Although this controversy has been debated for the past 40 years, unfortunately, no one has been able to give a definitive answer. However, several randomized prospective studies from the Mayo Clinic [52] and from the Eastern Cooperative Group [14] suggest that there is no difference in the overall survival in patients who were found to have pathologically involved lymph nodes whether the lymph node dissection was performed electively or when the nodes became palpable.

Although it is probable that the patients who have occult regional node metastases and elective lymph node dissection may not enjoy an improved survival over those who have palpable disease, it is clear that a regional lymphadenectomy is the only available staging procedure. Patients with primary melanoma without regional lymph node metastases enjoy an 80 to 90 percent survival rate, whereas at least 50 percent of patients with metastases to the lymph nodes have recurrent disease within 3 years of their surgical procedure [11, 13]. Therefore, therapeutic advantage or disadvantage becomes a moot point because lymphadenectomy is the only method for achieving adequate pathological staging. The clinician cannot inform the patient of his or her general prognosis nor can he identify those patients at high risk (those with positive nodes) for recurrence in order to include them in possibly beneficial postoperative adjuvant therapy trials.

Recent reports of prospective trials by Wanebo and colleagues [54], Holmes and associates [25, 26], and others [21] showed how the microstaging techniques of Clark and Breslow were used to determine those patients that would most benefit from regional lymphadenectomies for purposes of adequate staging. It was clear that as the melanoma increased its depth of penetration, there was an increased incidence of lymph node metastases (Table 27-1). Thus, it would appear that the consideration of regional lymphadenectomy for staging must be based upon some method for ascertaining those who are at high risk for developing lymph node involvement. We suggest that patients with melanoma invasive to 0.75 mm. or deeper, or Clark's Levels III to V, should be considered for regional lymphadenectomy [26].

Furthermore, it is evident that if this procedure is done for staging, the entire chain of nodes in the region must be dissected. Although Sappey [44] showed that the lymphatic system of the forehead,

Table 27-1. Depth of Invasion and Incidence of Regional Lymph Node Metastases

		Palpable Adenopathy		Nonpalpable		
Level of Primary	No. of Patients	Clinically Positive	Pathologically Positive	Clinically Positive	Pathologically Positive	Total Pathologically Positive
III	112	17	15(88%)	95	17(18%)	32(29%)
IV	78	19	17(90%)	59	16(27%)	33(42%)
V	12	6	5(83%)	6	2(33%)	7(58%)
TOTAL	202	42	37(87%)	160	35(26%)	72(43%)

cheek, and anterior ear drained first to the parotid lymph nodes many years ago, this fact seems to have escaped common clinical recognition (Fig. 27-2). These parotid nodes are within the capsule of the parotid gland; when a melanoma of the head or neck is located in this area, a regional lymphadenectomy must, of necessity, include a superficial parotidectomy [50].

A second area of controversy concerns the lymphatic areas of the trunk from which lymph shed is equivocal. Again, Sappey [44] defined a line that is 2 cm. wide and encircles the trunk just above the umbilicus (Fig. 27-3). In general, lesions above this line drain to the axillary nodes and those below it drain to the inguinal nodes [32, 50]. However, there are a number of patients who have midline lesions that could drain to all four node areas, particularly when the primary lesion is in the umbilical area or midline back; although this group of patients is in a minority, they present a very difficult and perplexing problem. However, a recent report by Fee and Robinson and their co-workers [19] described a new technique using injectable colloidal gold and subsequent scanning to demonstrate the lymph shed from these marginal areas. This method shows great clinical promise and appears to be useful in these difficult situations.

One of the major reasons why regional lymphadenectomies have been controversial is their attendant morbidity. Although the morbidity from an axillary lymph node dissection seems to be minimal (but with some rare lymphedema), that from the inguinal node dissection can be as high as 40 to 60 percent [39, 41]. A recent report by Holmes and associates [26] described a modified technique for inguinal lymph node dissection that appeared to markedly reduce morbidity associated with inguinal lymphadenectomy to less than 10 percent. Furthermore, several studies of cervical lymph node dissections have shown that a modified neck dissection, one that preserves the sternocleidomastoid muscle, is possible in patients with nonpalpable metastases to the neck.

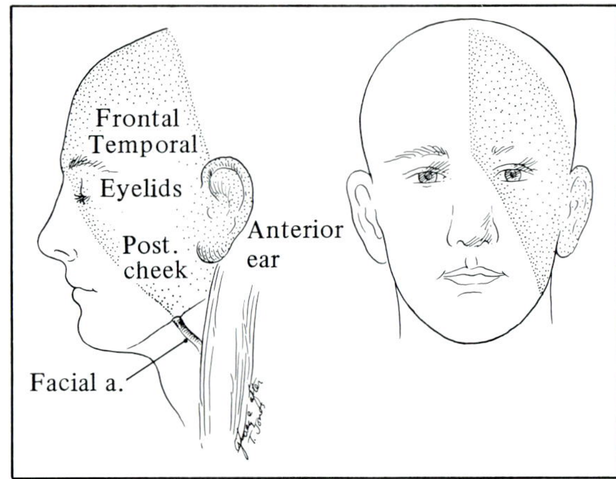

Fig. 27-2. Lymphatic drainage system of the forehead, cheek, and anterior ear to the parotid lymph nodes according to Sappey [44].

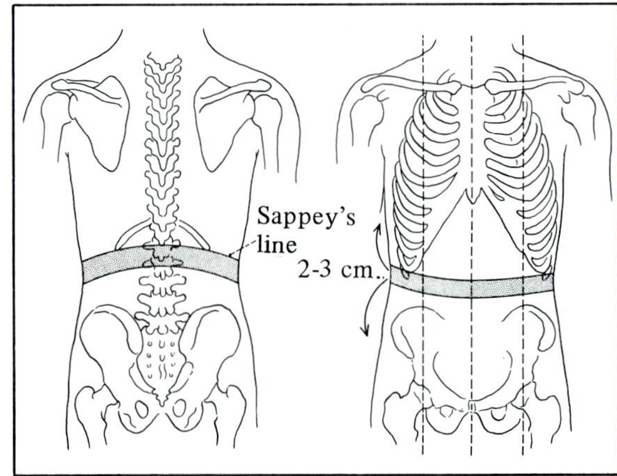

Fig. 27-3. Sappey's line defining lymph drainage. The area above the line drains to the axillary nodes, while the area below the line drains to inguinal nodes.

REGIONAL PERFUSION

In clinical practice, the exact role of chemotherapy when used in isolated limb perfusion has not yet been defined. The results of Stehlin [49] and McBride [30] obtained with melphalan and hyperthermia indicate benefit from this technique for controlling locally recurrent or in-transit melanoma (i.e., between sites of primary and regional nodes) to avoid amputation. However, perfusion for patients with primary nonrecurrent disease on the extremity is controversial simply because the results from wide excision and regional lymphadenectomy seem to be comparable [51]. Stehlin also reported encouraging results using chemotherapy with dimethyltriazeno imidazole carboximide (DTIC) by infusion for patients with locally recurrent disease [50].

CLINICAL RESULTS

Historically, the overall survival statistics for malignant melanoma have not been encouraging. However, as more is known about this disease, it becomes increasingly apparent that multiple important prognostic variables must be considered before any determination of the ultimate survival can be made [53]. Clearly, the depth of invasion plays an essential role, but it is equally important to have a clinical estimate of the regional nodes involved and their absolute number, in addition to the sex and age of the patient and the location of the primary lesion. It is impossible to make an overall statement concerning prognosis for all patients who have malignant melanoma. However, recent reports [11] indicate that the 5-year survival of patients with pathologically uninvolved regional nodes is from 80 to 90 percent, whereas that for pathologically involved nodes is 35 to 50 percent (Table 27-2). Therefore, it seems that elective or therapeutic regional lymphadenectomy is not only an effective staging procedure, but in fact is therapeutic in a large number of patients with positive nodes.

Prognosis for patients with melanoma metastatic to lungs, liver, or a distant subcutaneous or nodal site is much less encouraging, since the majority die of their disseminated disease within 12 months of diagnosis regardless of the type of chemotherapy or surgical procedure.

POSTOPERATIVE ADJUVANT STUDIES OF MALIGNANT MELANOMA

Patients with metastases to the regional nodes appear to be at high risk for systemic disease recurrence. In an effort to benefit these patients, postoperative adjuvant therapy trials have been underway in the United States and throughout the world for the past 4 or 5 years. The first of these employed the chemotherapeutic agent DTIC, which has a 20 percent response rate, with a median duration response of from 3 to 4 months [28]. In an adjuvant setting following surgical resection of regional lymph nodes, this agent has not improved the overall survival rate for patients with disseminated malignant melanoma [24]. Thus, at the present time, there is no known adjuvant chemotherapy regimen to benefit patients with regional lymph node metastases.

The current results of immunotherapy trials for malignant melanoma are preliminary [48] and it is not possible to determine whether immunotherapy with BCG has any definite role in the treatment schedule. Eilber and co-workers [15, 16] and Gutterman, Mavligit, and Hersh [23] have shown an apparent reduction of disease recurrence for patients treated with BCG immunotherapy. Trials reported from the World Health Organization have shown similar improved benefits [4]. However, Pinsky and colleagues [40] showed no apparent improvement from BCG treatment. Therefore, although there are some encouraging results from adjuvant immunotherapy, it is impossible to state that BCG immunotherapy benefits all patients with regional lymph node metastases. However, we hope that in the near future it will be possible to determine if there is a subset of patients with certain prognostic factors who would benefit from adjuvant BCG immunotherapy.

Table 27-2. Level of Invasion and Pathological Evaluation of Regional Nodes and Incidence of Recurrence[a]

	Regional Lymph Nodes			
	Histologically Positive (79)		Histologically Negative (130)	
Clark Level	NED[b]	Recurred	NED[b]	Recurred
III	23/36	13/36(36%)	82/83	1/83(1%)
IV	24/37	13/37(35%)	38/41	3/41(7%)
V	1/6	5/6 (83%)	5/6	1/6(17%)

[a]Median follow-up, 18.5 months.
[b]NED = no evidence of disease during follow-up period.

REFERENCES

1. American Cancer Society. Estimated New Cancer Cases and Deaths for All Sites, 1979. In *Cancer Facts and Figures.* New York: American Cancer Society, 1978. P. 10.
2. Bahn, A. K., Rosenwaike, I., Herrmann, N., Grover, P., Stellman, J., and O'Leary, K. Melanoma after exposure to PCB's. *N. Engl. J. Med.* 295:450, 1976.

3. Beardmore, G. L. The Epidemiology of Malignant Melanoma in Australia. In McCarthy, W. H. (Ed.), *Melanoma and Skin Cancer.* New South Wales: Sidney Government Print, 1972.
4. Beretta, G. Controlled Study for Prolonged Chemotherapy, Immunotherapy, and Chemoimmunotherapy as an Adjuvant to Surgery. In Terry, W. D., and Windhorst, D. (Eds.), *Immunotherapy of Cancer: Present Status of Trials in Man.* New York: Raven Press, 1978.
5. Breslow, A. Thickness, cross sectional areas and depth of invasion in the prognosis of cutaneous melanoma. *Ann. Surg.* 172:902, 1970.
6. Breslow, A. Tumor thickness, level of invasion and node dissection in Stage I cutaneous melanoma. *Ann. Surg.* 182:572, 1975.
7. Breslow, A. Personal communication, 1977.
8. Clark, W. H., From, L., Bernardino, E. A., and Mihm, M. C. The histogenesis and biologic behavior of primary human malignant melanomas of the skin. *Cancer Res.* 29:705, 1969.
9. Cochran, A. Malignant melanoma: A review of 10 years experience in Glasgow, Scotland, *Cancer* 23:1190, 1969.
10. Creech, O., and Krementz, E. T. Regional perfusion in melanoma of limbs, *J.A.M.A.* 188:131, 1964.
11. Das Gupta, T. Results of treatment of 269 patients with primary cutaneous melanoma: a five-year prospectives study. *Ann. Surg.* 186:209, 1977.
12. Das Gupta, T., and McNeer, G. The incidence of metastasis to accessible lymph nodes from melanoma of the trunk and extremities – its therapeutic significance. *Cancer* 17:897, 1964.
13. Davis, N. C., McLeod, R. G., Beardmore, G. L., Little, J. H., Quinn, R., and Holt, J. Primary cutaneous melanoma: A report from the Queensland melanoma project. *CA* 26:80, 1976.
14. Eastern Cooperative Group. Personal communication, 1977.
15. Eilber, F. R., Holmes, E. C., Ramming, K. P., Sparks, F. C., and Morton, D. L. Adjuvant immunotherapy of stage II malignant melanoma. *N. Engl. J. Med.* 294:237, 1976.
16. Eilber, F. R., Townsend, C. M., Jr., and Morton, D. L. Results of BCG adjuvant immunotherapy for melanoma of the head and neck. *Am. J. Surg.* 132:476, 1976.
17. Elwood, J. M., and Lee, J. A. H. Recent data in the epidemiology of malignant melanoma. *Sem. Oncol.* 2:149, 1975.
18. Elwood, J. M., Lee, J. A. H., and Walter, S. D. Relationship of melanoma and other skin cancer mortality to latitude and ultraviolet radiation in the U.S. and Canada. *Int. J. Epidemiol.* 3:325, 1974
19. Fee, H. J., Robinson, D. S., Sample, W. F., Graham, L. S., Holmes, E. C., and Morton, D. L. The determination of lymph shed by colloidal gold scanning in patients with malignant melanoma: A preliminary study. *Surgery.* 84:626, 1978.
20. Fortner, J. G., Booker, R. J., and Pack, G. T. Results of groin dissection for malignant melanoma in 220 patients. *Surgery* 55:485, 1964.
21. Goldman, L. I., Clark, W. H., Bernardino, E. A., and Ainsworth, A. M. The accuracy of predicting lymph node metastases in malignant melanoma by clinical examination and microstaging. *Ann. Surg.* 184:537, 1977.
22. Goldsmith, H. S., Shah, T. T., and Kim, D. H. Prognostic significance of lymph node dissection in the treatment of malignant melanoma. *Cancer* 26:606, 1970.
23. Gutterman, J. U., Mavligit, G. M., Hersh, E. M. Postoperative BCG Immunotherapy for Malignant Melanoma with Regional Lymph Node Metastases. In Terry, W. D., and Windhorst, D. (Eds.), *Immunotherapy of Cancer: Present Status of Trials in Man.* New York: Raven Press, 1978.
24. Hill, G. J., Metter, G. E., Moss, S., Krementz, E. T., Fletcher, W., Minton, J., and Golomb, F. DTIC therapy for melanoma. *Proc. Am. Soc. Clin. Oncol.* 17:244, 1976.
25. Holmes, E. C., Clark, W., Morton, D. L., Eilber, F. R., and Bochow, A. Regional lymph node metastases and the level of invasion of primary melanoma. *Cancer* 37:199, 1976.
26. Holmes, E. C., Mosley, H. S., Morton, D. L., Clark, W., Robinson, D. S., and Urist, M. M. A rational approach to the surgical management of melanoma. *Ann. Surg.* 186:481, 1977.
27. Lancaster, H. O., and Nelson, J. Sunlight as a cause of melanoma: A clinical survey. *Med. J. Aust.* 1:452, 1957.
28. Luce, J. K. Chemotherapy of melanoma. *Sem. Oncol.* 2:179, 1975.
29. Masen, T. J., and McKay, F. W. U.S. cancer mortality by country: 1950–1969. Department of Health, Education and Welfare Publication (NIH) 74-615. Washington, D.C.: U.S. Government Printing Office, 1974.
30. McBride, C. M. Advanced melanoma of the extremities. *Arch. Surg.* 101:122, 1970.
31. McCarthy, J. A., Haagensen, C. D., and Herter, F. P. The role of groin dissection in the management of melanoma of the lower extremity. *Ann. Surg.* 179:156, 1974.
32. McNeer, G., and Das Gupta, T. Routes of Lymphatic Spread of Malignant Melanoma. In *Malignant Melanoma.* New York: American Cancer Society, 1965.
33. Melanoma Clinical Cooperative Group. Unpublished observations, 1978.

34. Mihm, M. C., Clark, W. H., and From, L. The clinical diagnosis, classification, and histogenic concepts of the early stages of cutaneous malignant melanoma. *N. Engl. J. Med.* 284:1078, 1971.
35. Mihm, M. C., Clark, W. H., and Reed, R. The clinical diagnosis of malignant melanoma. *Semin. Oncol.* 2:105, 1975.
36. National Academy of Science Report. Halocarbons: Environmental effects of chlorfluoromethane release. Washington, D.C., 1976.
37. Olsen, G. *Malignant Melanoma of the Skin.* Copenhagen: Finsen Institute and Radium Centre, 1966.
38. Olsen, G. The malignant melanoma of the skin: New theories based on the study of 500 cases. *Acta Clin. Scand.* 365(SI):1, 1966.
39. Papachristow, D., and Fortner, J. G. Comparison of lymphedema following incontinuity and discontinuity groin dissection. *Ann. Surg.* 185:13, 1977.
40. Pinsky, C. M., Hirshaut, Y., Wanebo, H. J., Fortner, J., Mike, V., Shottenfeld, D., and Oettgen, H. F. Surgical Adjuvant Immunotherapy in Patients with Malignant Melanoma: A Prospective Randomized Trial. In Terry, W. D., and Windhorst, D. (Eds.), *Immunotherapy of Cancer: Present Status of Trials in Man.* New York: Raven, 1978.
41. Polk, H., Cohn, J. D., and Clarksen, J. C. An Appraisal of Elective Regional Lymphadenectomy for Melanoma. In Zuidema, G. D., and Skinner, D. B. (Eds.), *Current Topics in Surgical Research.* New York: Academic Press, 1969.
42. Roth, J. A., Eilber, F. R., Bennett, L. A., and Morton, D. L. Role of radionucleide scanning in malignant melanoma. *Arch. Surg.* 110:1211, 1975.
43. Sampson-Handley, W. The pathology of melanotic growths in relation to their operative treatment. *Lancet* 1:966, 1907.
44. Sappey, M. P. C. Traite d'Anatomie Descriptive. In *Anatomie, Physiologie, Pathologie des Vaisseauz Lymphatiques Consideres Chez l'Homme et les Vertebres* (4th ed.). Paris: Delahaye and Lecrosnier, 1888.
45. Shah, J. P., and Goldsmith, H. S. Malignant melanoma in the North American Negro. *Surg. Gynecol. Obstet.* 133:437, 1971.
46. Sim, F. H., Ivins, J. C., Taylor, W. P., Pritchard, D. J., and Soule, E. H. A preoperative randomized study of the efficacy of routine prophylactic lymphadenectomy in the management of malignant melanoma: Preliminary results. *Cancer.* In press.
47. Southwick, H. W. How much surgery? *Minn. Med.* 47:1233, 1964.
48. Spitler, L. E., Sagebiel, R., Wong, P., Malm, T., Chase, R., and Gonzalez, R. A Randomized Double Blind Trial of Adjuvant Therapy with Levamisole in Patients with Malignant Melanoma. In Terry, W. D., and Windhorst, D., (Eds.), *Immunotherapy of Cancer: Present Status of Trials in Man.* New York: Raven, 1978.
49. Stehlin, J. S. Hyperthermic perfusion with chemotherapy for cancers of the extremity. *Surg. Gynecol. Obstet.* 129:305, 1969.
50. Storm, F. K., Eilber, F. R., Sparks, F. C., and Morton, D. L. A prospective study of parotid metastasis. *Am. J. Surg.* 134:115, 1977.
51. Sugarbaker, E. V., and McBride, C. M. Survival and regional disease control after isolated-perfusion for invasive Stage I melanoma of the extremities. *Cancer* 37:188, 1976.
52. Sugarbaker, E. V., and McBride, C. M. Melanoma of the trunk: The results of surgical excision and anatomic guidelines for predicting nodal metastases. *Surgery* 80:22, 1976.
53. Valenzulea, L. A., Pickren, J. L., and Moore, R. H. A clinicopathological study of prognostic factors in cutaneous malignant melanoma. *Surg. Gynecol. Obstet.* 144:32, 1977.
54. Wanebo, H. J., Fortner, J. G., Woodruff, J., MacLean, B. S., and Binkowski, E. Selection of the optimum surgical treatment of Stage I melanoma by depth of microinvasion. *Ann. Surg.* 182:302, 1975.
55. Wang, C. K. The study of melanocytes in normal skin surrounding malignant melanoma. *Dermatologica* 141:215, 1970.

Hemangioma, Lymphangioma, and Arteriovenous Fistula

HUGH G. THOMSON

In a pediatric plastic surgery practice, the most common cutaneous tumor is the congenital endothelial hamartoma. Each congenital lesion of endothelial origin has a slightly different clinical course and, therefore, prognosis [9, 12, 16, 57, 86–88, 102, 107, 128]. Basic research has been limited to the rat, and clinical applications of this research have been negligible [59, 60].

It is extremely important for the patient, the parents, and the physician to appreciate the natural history of each tumor in order to prepare the family unit for a specific treatment overview. In this regard, the most pivotal issue is the classification of a confusing nomenclature that can be of either a clinical or pathological nature. It is important that we all talk about the same lesion and not an admixture of different terms; otherwise, there is confusion on confusion. A simple (but not totally inclusive) clinical classification is outlined in Table 28-1.

CAPILLARY HEMANGIOMA (SUPERFICIAL)

The capillary hemangioma is the most common group seen in a pediatric practice. It represents an accumulation of embryonic mesodermal rests of superficial vasoformative tissue. The subepidermal and deep dermal layers are primarily involved.

Port-Wine Stain (Nevus Flammeus)

The port-wine stain presents in the neonate and is located primarily on the face in areas supplied by the sensory branches of the fifth cranial nerve. It can also occur on an extremity alone or in combination with a lesion on the face. There is no tendency for spontaneous regression of this particular lesion; rather, it becomes darker and may develop verrucous eruptions in adulthood. The true nevus flammeus in the periorbital and glabellar regions of the neonate must be differentiated from the pale nevus flammeus neonatorum, which is self-limiting, usually over a period of 2 to 6 months.

There are two worrisome problems associated with the facial port-wine stain: (1) Sturge-Weber syndrome, which is an intracranial involvement of the choroid and pia mater with hemangioma (Fig. 28-1). The hemangioma is usually located in the frontotemporal lobes with early clinical manifestation. Less frequently, it will remain quiescent for long periods in the occipital lobes. Characteristically, the patient with this syndrome presents with involvement of the opthalmic and maxillary divisions of the trigeminal nerve (VI and V2) and a history of epileptic seizures, sometimes intractable. They may require hemispherectomy if seen in infancy and should have relatively little residual physical defect. This syndrome must not be confused with other hemangioma syndromes of Osler-Weber-Rendu, von Hippel Lindau, blue rubber bleb nevus, and Maffucci. (2) The patient with glaucoma (or one in whom glaucoma is suspected) has involvement of the ipsilateral eye; this is assumed in 50 percent of patients who have a combination of a trigeminal VI and V2 distribution [117, 118]. Conjunctival injection or apparent spread by itself does not indicate glaucoma. If glaucoma is anticipated and diagnosed in the first 6 months of life, it can be medically treated, which should preclude blindness. This requires an awareness on the part of the plastic surgeon and early referral to an ophthalmologist for sophisticated anterior chamber examination, such as slit lamp analysis and tonometry.

Table 28-1. Hemangiomas and Lymphangiomas, a Simplified Clinical Classification (excluding syndromes and malignancies)

- Capillary hemangioma
  - Port-wine stain
  - Strawberry
    - Wild-fire
    - Ulcerated
    - Spontaneous regression
  - Salmon patch
  - Campbell de Morgan
  - Telangiectasia
  - Pyogenic granuloma
- Capillary-cavernous hemangioma
- Cavernous hemangioma
- Other hemangiomas
  - Verrucous
  - Keratotic
  - Venous
- Lymphangioma
  - Circumscripta
  - Simplex
  - Cavernous
  - Cystic hygroma
- Lymphangiohemangioma and hemangiolymphangioma
- Arteriovenous malformation
- Vascular gigantism

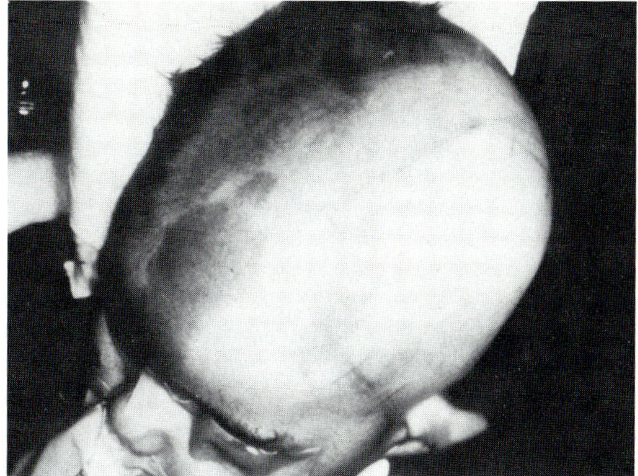

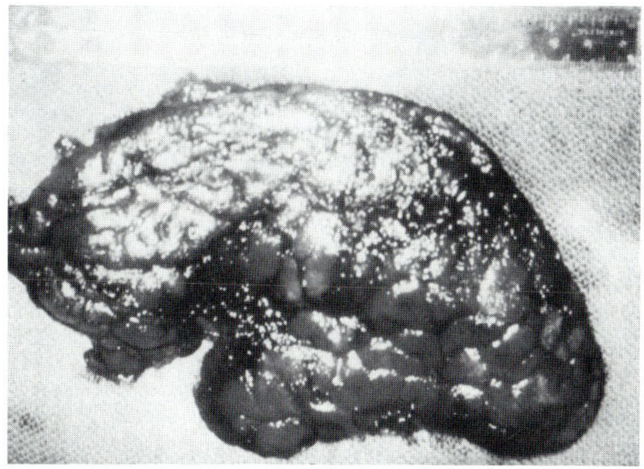

Fig. 28–1. The Sturge-Weber syndrome. Top, the distribution of the ophthalmic and maxillary divisions of the trigeminal nerve (V1 and V2) bilaterally with intractable seizures. Bottom, hemisphere resected.

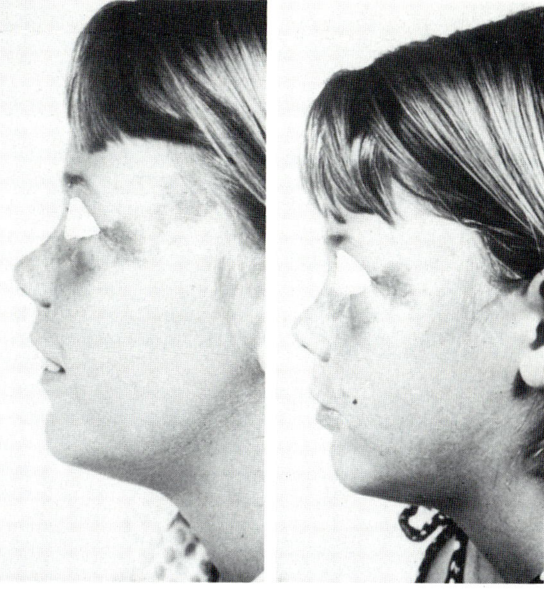

Fig. 28–2. Port-wine stain in the lateral distribution of the maxillary division of the trigeminal nerve (V2), with posterior segment demonstrating the result after electrocoagulation.

Satisfactory treatment of the patient with a port-wine stain has escaped all investigators [2, 3, 15, 20, 22–25, 50, 51, 63, 114, 115, 123, 124, 126]. Treatment with thorium X radiation, cryotherapy, laser beam, excision and skin graft or flap replacement, surgical tattooing, and even electrocoagulation has not totally provided for the patients' needs (Fig. 28-2). Cosmetics (for example, Covermark or Cover Girl) still remain as sound back-up support for these patients. Surgical tattooing does make it possible for females to use lighter cosmetic coverage and therefore appear less clownlike than with heavy cosmetics. The leaching out or fading of the inserted pigment after a few years is the major drawback with tattooing. The amount of leaching appears to be much less in adult patients.

Strawberry Hemangioma

The strawberry hemangioma is bright red and raised; it grows rapidly and is present either at birth or within the first 2 weeks. It grows much faster than the child and does so until the age of 6 to 8 months, when it appears to reach a growth plateau; subsequently, it parallels the growth of the patients. These lesions may be single or multiple and are frequently found in the head and neck region. They may be small and innocent or large and ulcerated. The Kasabach-Merritt syndrome (platelet trapping or disseminated intravascular coagulopathy) can occur in association with this type of lesion [4, 10, 11, 31, 48, 55, 61, 62, 64, 66, 70, 71, 78, 90, 100, 112, 116, 119, 132].

Most patients with a strawberry hemangioma do not require local treatment; actually, the therapy is reserved for the parents. This is done by frequent, reassuring office visits every 2 weeks, then monthly, and at intervals as needed later. Assurance of spontaneous regression, which will occur in 95 percent of all patients by the age of 6 years, is the pivotal statement (Fig. 28-3A, B). The first sign of regression is

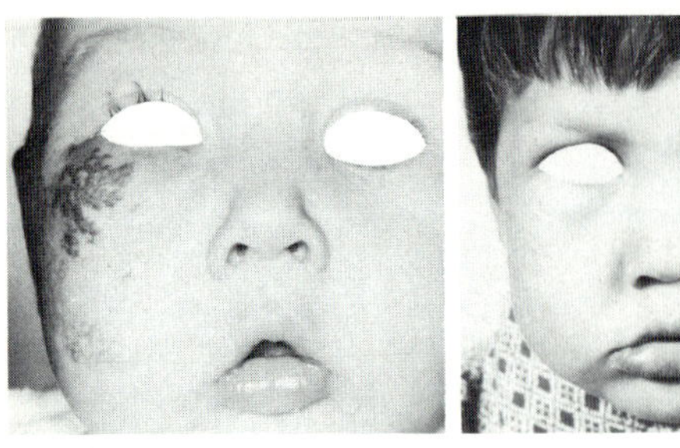

A B

Fig. 28–3. A, an infant with capillary (strawberry) hemangioma of the right malar prominence with some associated telangiectasia. B, spontaneous regression without treatment after 3 years.

evidenced by central gray spots; these spots gradually coalesce and reduce the zone of raised red hemangioma, which by this time has reduced its angry red hue to a quieter purplish-red.

In case of sharp or blunt trauma, the parents must be instructed to apply direct pressure for 5 minutes.

If the lesion develops a small ulceration or, indeed, develops the wild-fire, pseudomalignant destructive ulceration, the specific lesion requires topical cleaning, the use of an antibiotic, and, in some patients, excision and skin graft coverage (Fig. 28-4). These are the two instances in which the patient might bleed and/or develop a disseminated intravascular coagulopathy. They are the exceptions to the rule and may require a surgical approach. Indeed, in massive hemangiomas of this type, disseminated intravascular coagulopathy may develop in the postoperative period, particularly if only part of the hemangioma is removed.

If the lesion is massive (regardless of location) and particularly if the patient demonstrates disseminated intravascular coagulopathy, consideration should be given to a treatment program combining prednisone (20 to 30 mg. per day for 1 month), very selective low dosage radiation, and, when possible, compression bandaging [17, 33, 37, 43, 65, 79, 85, 92, 94, 99, 137]. Various surgical techniques may have to supersede this program in certain instances – for example, when deprivation or astigmatic amblyopia is a real risk (Fig. 28-5A, B) [118a].

Pyogenic Granuloma

Pyogenic granuloma is a capillary hemangioma that has an intrinsic inflammatory cell infiltrate; it could be labeled the "Band-Aid" disease. In the child 2 to 10 years old, there is a short onset of 1 to 2 months with the development of a bright red, smooth or warty excrescence that is initially sessile and then semipedunculated. This demonstrates, by history and

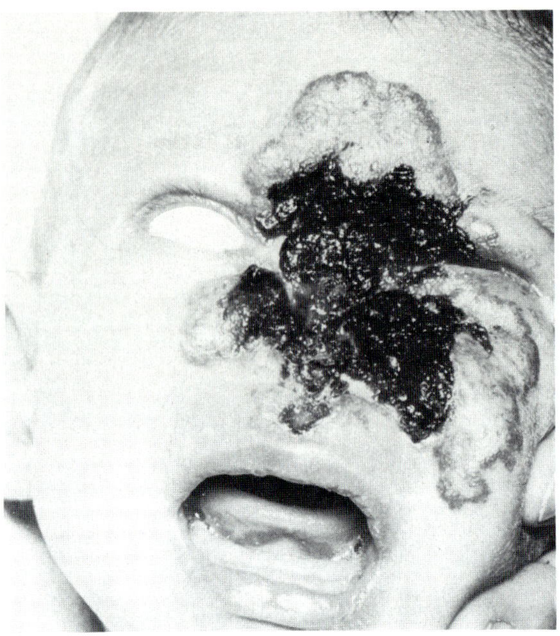

Fig. 28–4. Pseudomalignant or wild-fire strawberry hemangioma with nasal infarction.

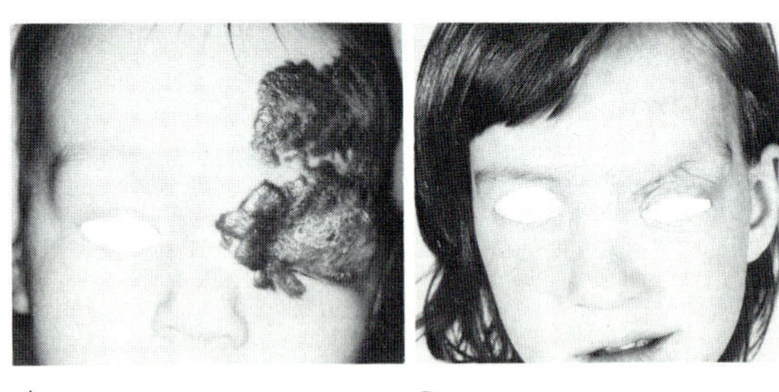

A B

Fig. 28–5. A, strawberry (capillary) lesion obtunding the left upper lid during neonatal and infant period. B, even with delayed surgical intervention, the deprivation amblyopia was complete.

appearance, a friability that precipitates profuse and disturbing bleeding to both the patient and the parents (Fig. 28-6). The patients usually present in the office covered with a blood-tinged Band-Aid.

Topical sclerosants are usually unsuccessful, and excision is too radical. These lesions respond nicely to shaving flush with the skin and electrocoagulation of the bleeding arterioles. This technique also permits a pathology specimen to rule out malignant hemangioendothelioma.

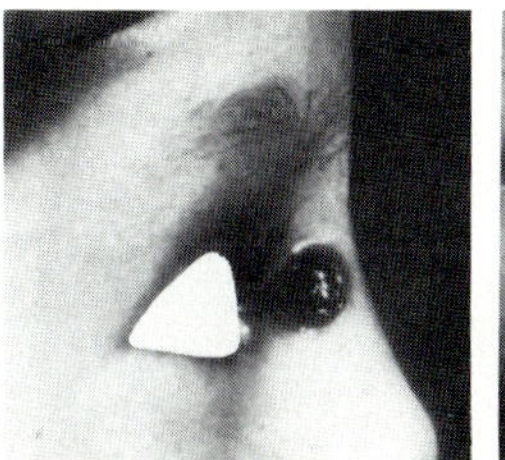
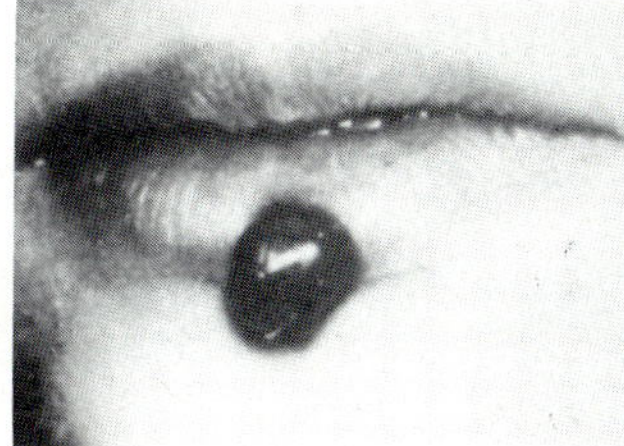

Fig. 28–6. Pyogenic granuloma of the nose and lower lip.

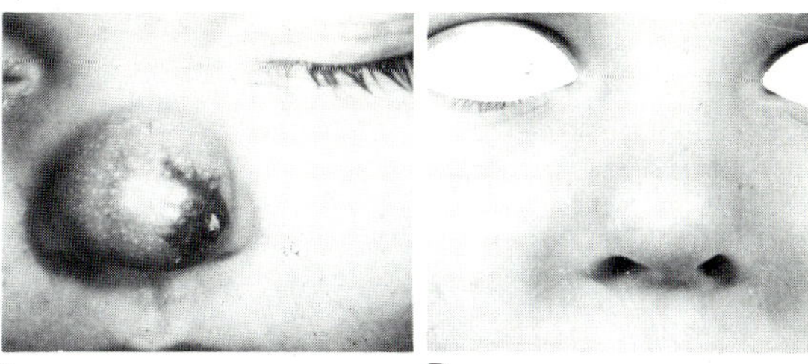

A B

Fig. 28–7. A, cavernous hemangioma of the nose with a small capillary component during infancy. B, 8 years later, almost total spontaneous resolution has occurred without surgical intervention.

CAVERNOUS HEMANGIOMA (DEEP)

The cavernous hemangioma has a similar congenital onset but is more subtle in nature; therefore, the developmental time is not always exact. It involves a more mature endothelial cell organization and presents as a deep, blue, diffuse swelling, frequently in the head and neck, with an apparent gigantism if it involves a specialized part, such as the eyelid. In this particular site, whether small or large, this tumor has the potential to cause anisometropic (astigmatic) and/or deprivation amblyopia during the sensitive first 6 months of life if the eyelid partially obtunds the pupil [28]. This particular issue should push the surgeon to a more aggressive treatment plan rather than a wait-and-see attitude.

The surgeon must always be aware of the differential diagnoses in the neonate and infant, which would include rhabdosarcoma and fibrosarcoma. If there is any doubt in subsequent visits, a biopsy is certainly justified.

There is at least a 60 to 70 percent chance of total regression of all these lesions by the age of 8 years if the parents will permit this approach [89, 129, 134]. However, there are always exceptions to this rule, and the lesion in the lower lip is a good example, It does tend to regress, but rarely totally, due to the blood supply from the labial artery. Surgery is frequently needed in this situation when the associated gigantism makes peer criticism a problem. If the lesion has bony involvement (most commonly in the mandible), great care must be taken at surgery. The bleeding is excessive, as occurs in the case of an aneurysmal bone cyst; it may even cause operative death [1, 5, 18, 27, 32, 35, 38, 39, 44, 53, 68, 69, 72, 73, 80, 83, 91, 93, 103, 106, 111, 113, 122, 127, 131, 133, 135].

A cavernous hemangioma of the nose with or without a capillary component presents as a situation involving parental pressure. The nasal tip is usually the involved site, creating a "Cyrano" nose.

Continued support of the parents is the hallmark of the management program and, indeed, can act as a protection for the child, since this eliminates the very significant scarring that might otherwise be created by various surgical techniques. I have found that of 22 patients with cavernous hemangiomas, the long-term results were vastly superior with conservative as opposed to operative treatment (Fig. 28-7A, B) [125].

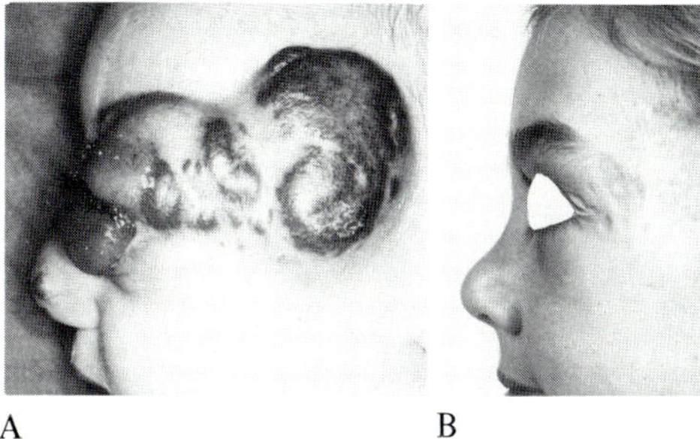

A B

Fig. 28–8. A, extensive capillary-cavernous hemangioma in the temporal-orbital-nasal region. B, after 9 years, almost complete spontaneous resolution has occurred.

If surgery is necessary because of extreme parental pressure, it should remain well localized and confined to the nasal tip itself. For this type of localized cavernous hemangioma and other cavernous hemangiomas, wide excisional and replacement techniques are all ill-advised, since they create otherwise unnecessary scarring and increase morbidity [136].

The parents usually accept the physician's frequent support with conservatism in mind. However, in some areas, after resolution undesirable skin redundancy remains; it can be readily treated without being destructive, since the lesion itself has almost completely regressed.

CAPILLARY-CAVERNOUS HEMANGIOMA (SUPERFICIAL AND DEEP)

The capillary-cavernous hemangioma contains deep cavernous and superficial capillary components (Fig. 28-8A, B). The response to maturation, incidence

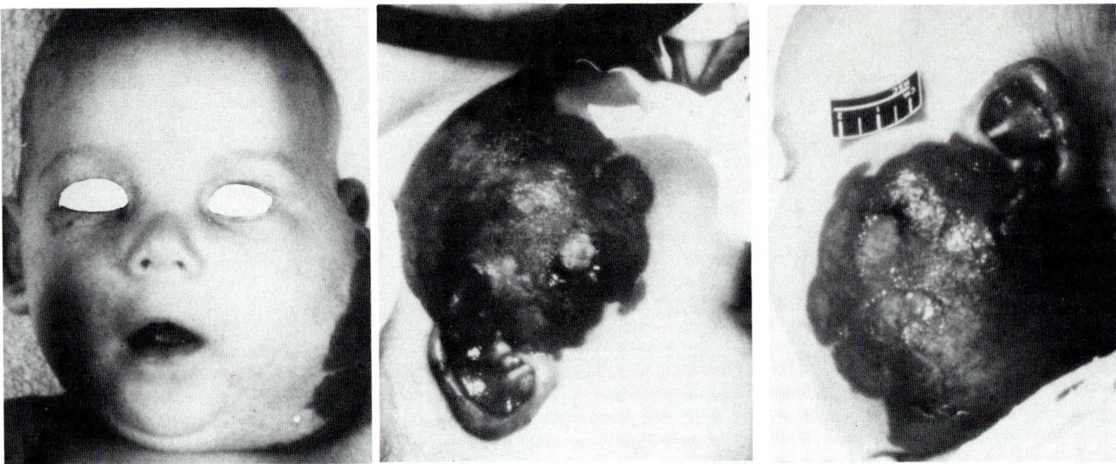

Fig. 28–9. Extensive capillary-cavernous hemangioma with a microarteriovenous shunt demonstrating immediate postembolization appearance.

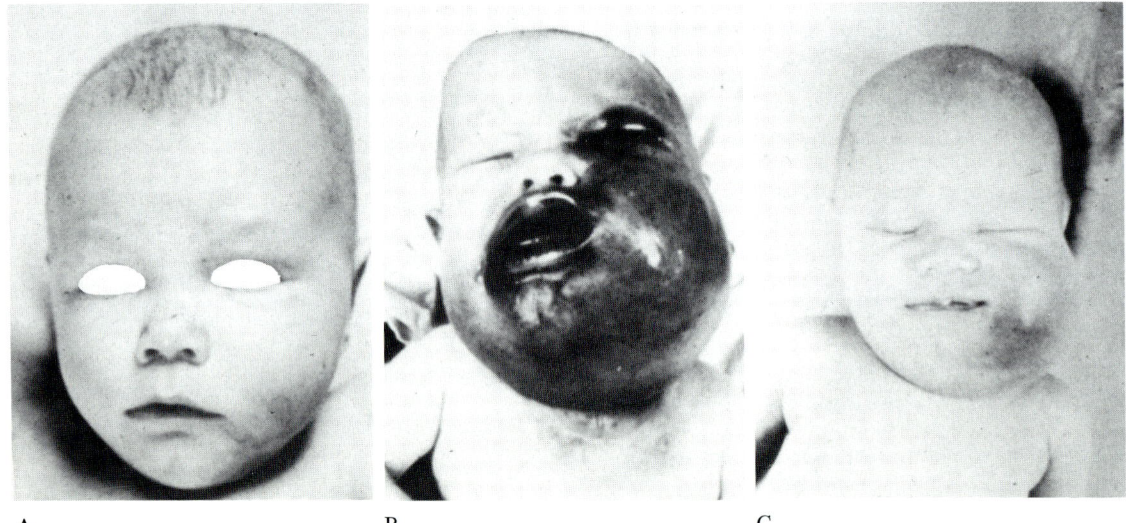

A B C

Fig. 28–10.A, capillary-cavernous hemangioma of the left cheek. B, demonstrating subsequent massive enlargement and firmness with associated Kasabach-Merritt syndrome treated with radiation and prednisone. C, considerable improvement occurred after 6 weeks of therapy.

of complications, and other characteristics are the same as for each component as described previously.

The occasional overwhelming lesion that has microarteriovenous fistulas demonstrates no regression, continues to grow and expand, is hot to touch, and may be threatening to the patient with such problems as Kasabach-Merritt syndrome, amblyopia, and tracheal obstruction.

Microembolization with microspheres, muscle, or Gelfoam can be considered as a reasonable form of treatment, coupled with prednisone and/or radiation (Figs. 28-9 and 28-10) [6, 30, 36, 74, 75, 81, 82, 97, 105, 108].

VERRUCOUS OR KERATOTIC HEMANGIOMA

The verrucous or keratotic hemangiomas occur less frequently than the preceding groups. It is consistent in appearance and is characterized by purplish-red, warty, irregular patches that appear very superficially in the dermis and may be isolated or diffuse. There

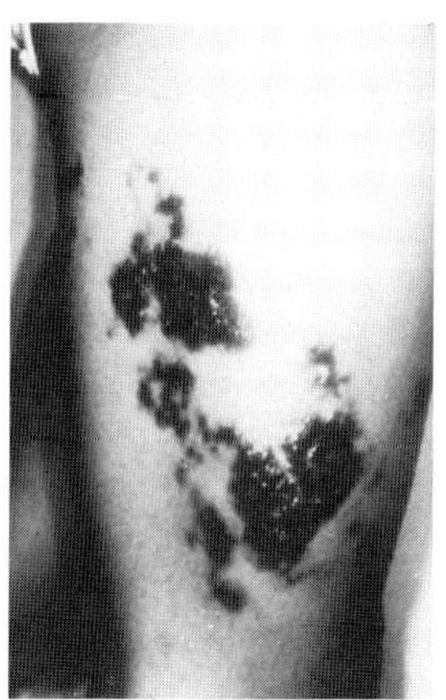

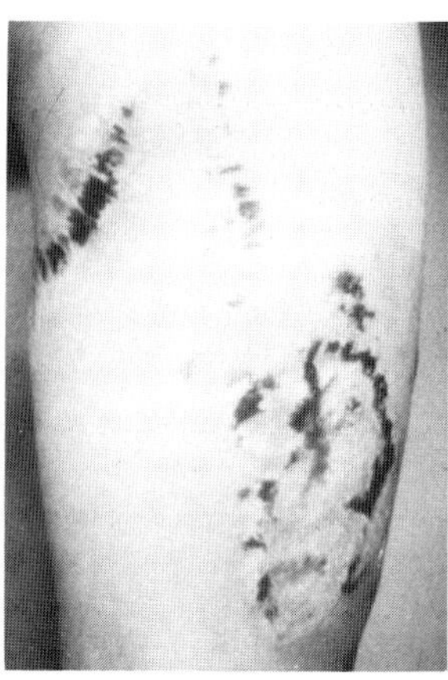

A B

Fig. 28–11. A, verrucous hemangioma with purple raised areas giving rise to occasional episodes of bleeding. B, after simple excision and closure with a skin graft, some persistent hemangioma remained.

are silvery keratotic flakes covering the purple lesions; these are usually associated with frequent small hemorrhages. Occasionally, there is an element of regional gigantism because the lesions are, indeed, not superficial, but tend to involve deep dermal and subcutaneous fat and even muscle. This is important from an excisional viewpoint as the lesion tends to reappear along the scar margin, or it may infiltrate the graft itself (Fig. 28-11).

LYMPHANGIOMA

The lymphangioma is a relatively avascular congenital lesion that continues to confuse surgeons by its response to maturation and surgery [7, 14, 19, 41, 42, 46, 84, 104, 109]. The group can be divided into simplex, cavernous, and hygromatous.

The *simplex form* is a rare, very superficial, cutaneous lesion composed of capillary-sized lymphatic channels; it poses no specific clinical problem.

The *cavernous lesion* involves deeper structures and is characterized by superficial and deep endothelial-lined lymphatic vessels with small cystic spaces; it has a spongy yet firm consistency. If the cutaneous portion ulcerates and becomes infected with an associated lymphangitic response, the resulting fungoid appearance is suggestive of carcinoma.

The *cystic hygroma* involves the head and neck; like the cavernous lesion, it has cellular and cystic components. It can be unilocular or multilocular. The latter is the most common, with many grapelike clusters of various sized cysts filled with straw-colored fluid. It is usually present at birth, but can develop thereafter; it is usually slow-growing, unless there is

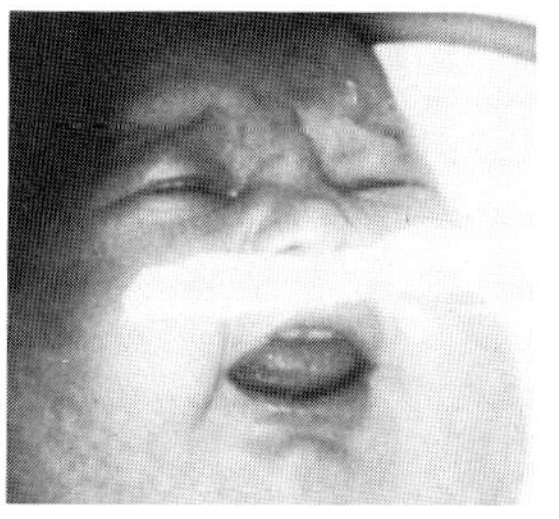

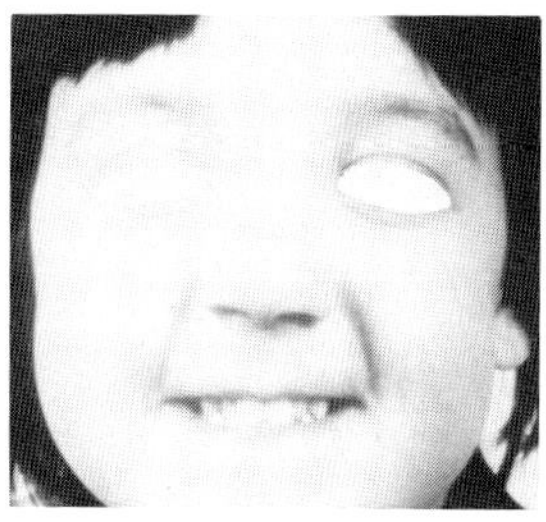

A B

Fig. 28–12. A, bilateral cystic hygroma causing respiratory distress, treated by marsupialization, electrocoagulation, and tracheotomy. B, the patient's appearance 6 years later.

an associated internal venous hemorrhage or lymphangitis due to infection. The infection usually responds rapidly to penicillin, but the acute fullness tends to regress slowly.

The initial major concern is upper airway obstruction, which is particularly true if the cystic hygroma crosses the midline in the postpharyngeal area and presents as a bilateral lesion (Fig. 28-12).

It is occasionally a diagnostic challenge to rule out similar lesions, such as lymphangiohemangioma or hemangiolymphangioma. This differentiation can be accomplished using technetium isotope flow studies, which reveal the cystic hygroma to be singularly cold as compared to the other two. This finding is also important from a prognostic viewpoint.

Along with other observers, I believe that all pure cystic hygromas *tend to involute unless there is a hemangiomatous component* and that cystic hygromas are not present in adults. There are others who feel that there is no regression and, therefore, that active surgical intervention is important. The lesion has an apparent disregard for anatomical planes and involves all tissues extensively, which makes it impossible to excise totally. In an attempt to do so, there is an increased morbidity due to transection of peripheral cranial nerves and other complications.

Respiratory distress is certainly a surgical emergency, and the patient who presents with opisthotonos due to the hygromatous bulk requires some form of decompression and/or tracheotomy. This can be achieved by the insertion of multiple Hemovac tubes; by marsupialization of the cysts with or without wound closure, with or without sclerosing with iodine or electrocautery (Fig. 28-13); or by wide extensive excision. If the lesion primarily involves a few large cysts, Hemovac decompression is promising, but if there are a myriad of smaller cysts, decompression is impossible.

The rarer combined cellular hemangiolymphangioma has a high blood volume flow (as demonstrated

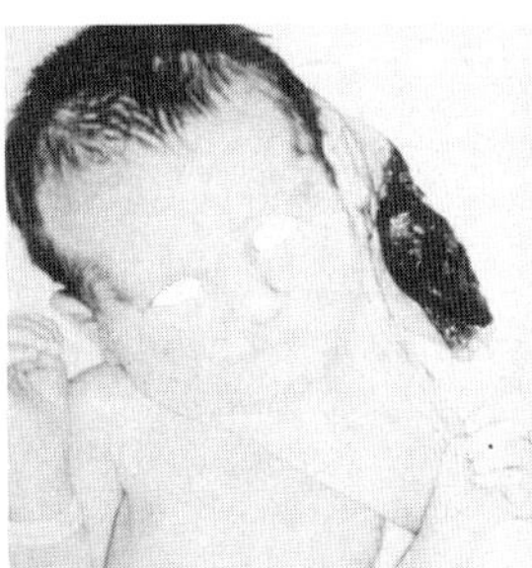
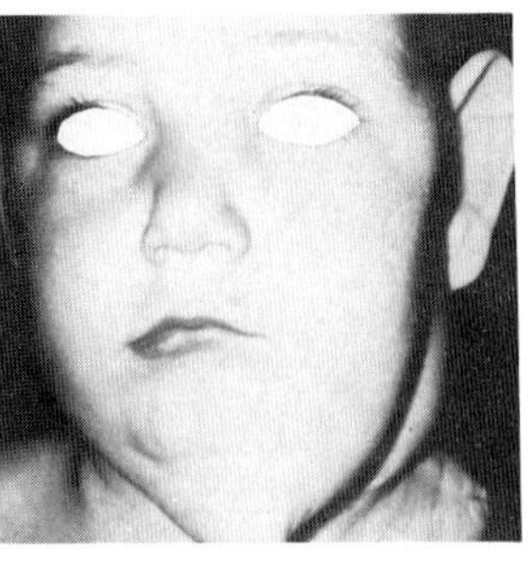

A B

Fig. 28–13. A, cystic hygroma of the left side after drainage decompression. B, the same patient 4 years later, after skin trimming, had some residual cystic hygroma.

clinically and by technetium isotope flow studies) and may be associated with Kasabach-Merritt syndrome. The lesion may respond to radiation and cortisone, but it has a poor long-term prognosis because there are repeated bouts of lymphangitis and extension into the tongue and sublingual area. Attempts at surgical treatment are exercises in absolute frustration. It is important to differentiate these lesions, from both a therapeutic and a prognostic point of view.

ARTERIOVENOUS MALFORMATION

The patient with true macroshunting congenital arteriovenous fistula has a potentially lethal surgical problem for which there has been very little promising therapy until recently [8, 21, 26, 29, 34, 40, 45, 47, 49, 52, 56, 76, 77, 95, 98, 101, 110, 120, 121, 130].

Over 50 percent of these lesions involve the head and neck region. These lesions should be differentiated from the hot, microshunting type of fistulization found in the arteriovenous aneurysm and found in the capillary-cavernous lesions and the lesions that are only cavernous. In either clinical condition, left ventricular strain or, indeed, failure can develop. A bruit and/or thrill is a constant physical finding in the macroshunting lesion.

There is clinical evidence to support the need for wide resection under hypotensive anesthesia if any resection is to be done at all. Clinical experience has shown that single or multiple ligations of vessels simply worsen the condition because a more extensive collateral circulation develops, presumably secondary to opening up of vestigial rests. This radical concept becomes a serious aesthetic decision when the lesion involves the face. In some instances, embolization has made it possible for delayed excision, with encouraging results [97] (Fig. 28-14A, B).

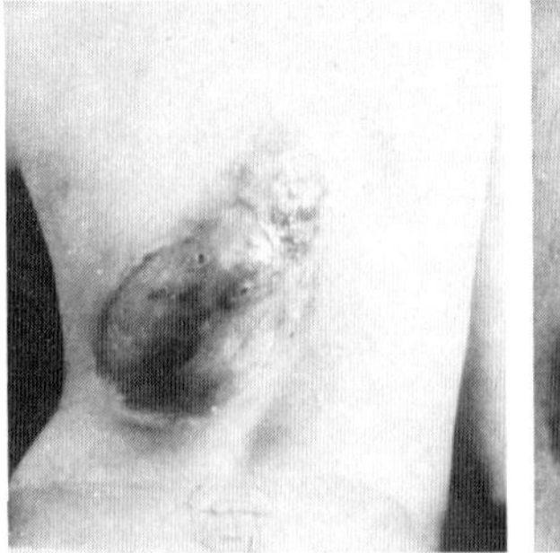
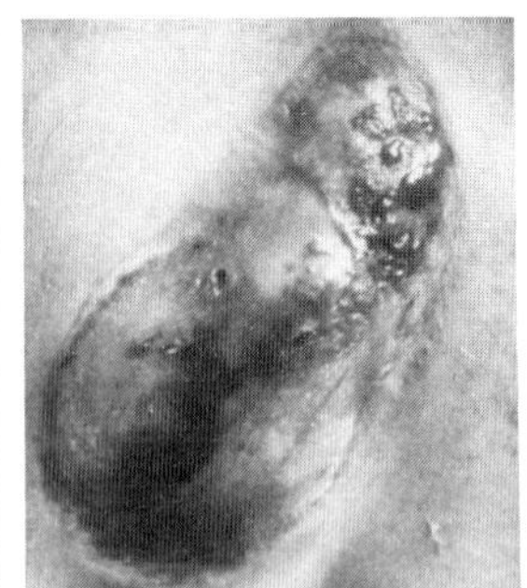

A

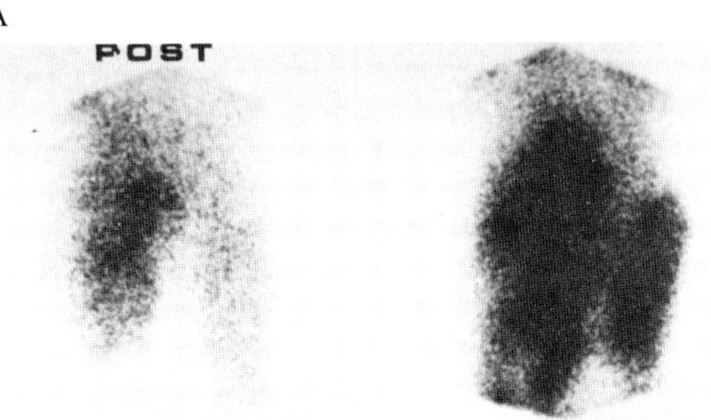

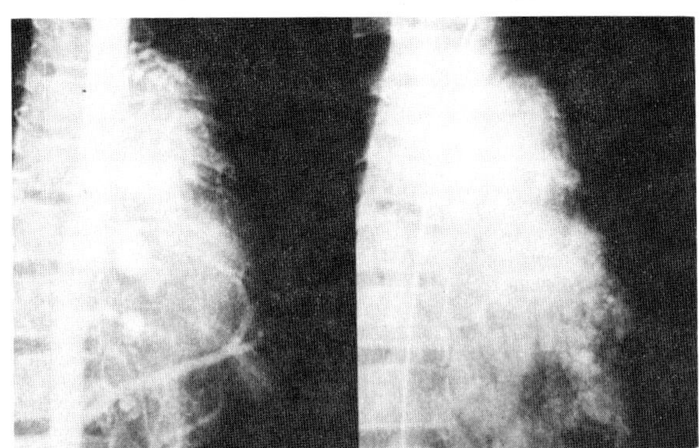

B

Fig. 28–14. A, macrocongenital arteriovenous fistula of the back with bruit and thrill. B, the technetium and arteriogram x-ray studies demonstrated vascularity.

VASCULAR GIGANTISM (KLIPPEL-TRENAUNAY-WEBER SYNDROME)

Enlargement of an extremity due to vascular involvement can be localized or diffuse, superficial or deep, venous or arteriovenous, and with microshunting or macroshunting (Fig. 28-15A, B). It is not infrequent to have diffuse tissue overgrowth including bone [13, 54, 58, 67, 96]. However, hypoplasia can occasionally occur. This type of gigantism must be differentiated from that associated with plexiform

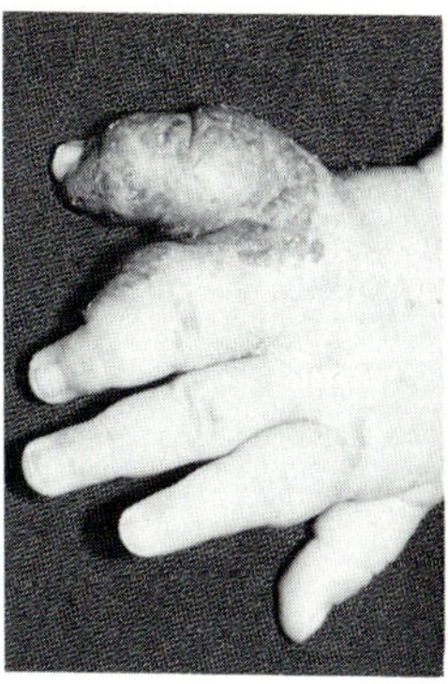
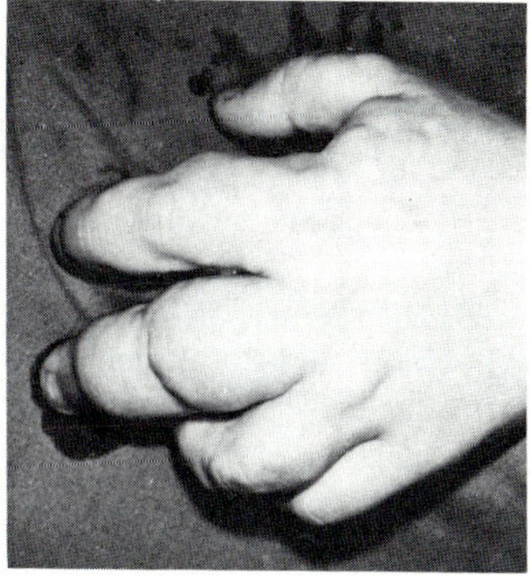

A B

Fig. 28–15. Hemangiomatous gigantism of the hand (Klippel-Trenaunay) in two patients demonstrating two different types of vascular lesions. A, capillary-cavernous microshunting. B, venous engorgement with dilated veins and soft and bony tissue overgrowth.

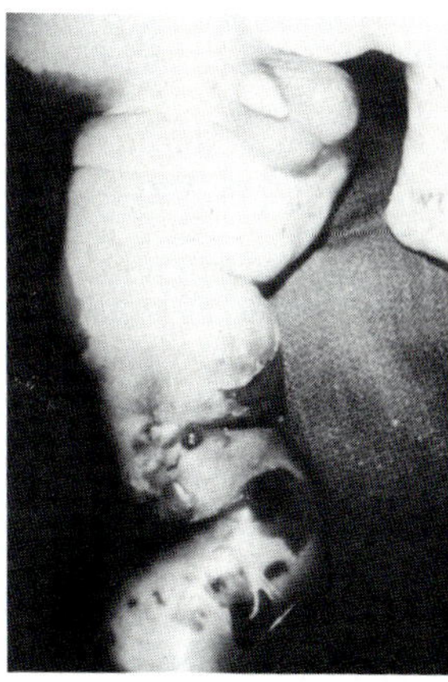
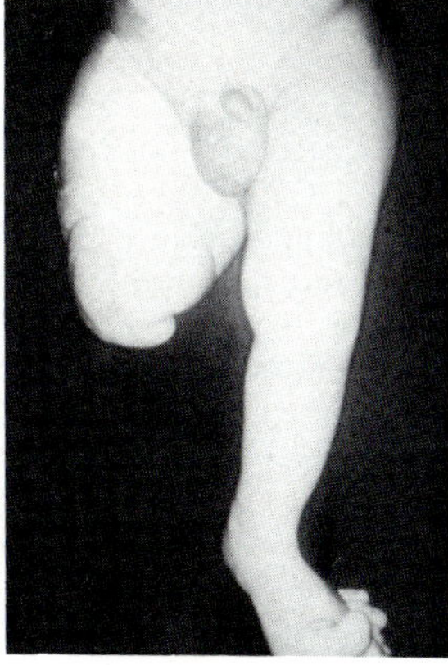

Fig. 28–16. Extensive lymphangiohemangiomatous lesion of the right leg associated with diffuse intravascular coagulopathy. Amputation was necessary.

neurofibromatosis and fibrolipoma and other hamartomatous enlargements.

If the zone of involvement is large and the lesion feels hot, microshunting should be anticipated; in the infant, this may cause left ventricular hypertrophy or failure and necessitate digitalis therapy. A compression elastic bandage or a Jobst stocking may be helpful in controlling the problem; in some instances, it will result in some degree of spontaneous regression.

Occasionally, the gigantism is associated with ipsilateral organomegaly; it may be so diffuse and severe in the extremities that it causes a multiplicity of problems as suggested above, along with ulceration and superinfection, disuse due to sheer weight, and diffuse intravascular coagulation. Amputation may therefore be necessary (Fig. 28-16).

For the more localized and quiescent-looking forms of digital and hand vascular gigantism, the surgeon may consider some form of soft tissue reduction such as a filletting procedure, osteotomy, or epiphysiodesis. However, treatment should be tempered by the fact that wound healing is usually delayed and skin infarction is common. The surgeon should proceed with great care in such cases.

REFERENCES

1. Abramson, B. S. Central hemangioma of the mandible: Report of a case. *J. Oral Surg.* 23:66, 1965.
2. Andrews, G. C., cited by Conway, H. Evolution of treatment of capillary hemangiomas of the face with further observation on the value of camouflage by permanent pigment injection (tattooing). *Surgery* 23:389, 1948.
3. Apfelberg, D. B. Argon laser management of cutaneous vascular deformities – A preliminary report. *West. J. Med.* 124:99, 1976.
4. Atkins, H. L., Wolf, J. A., and Sitarz, A. A giant hemangioma with secondary thrombocytopenia purpura. *Am. J. Roentgenol.* 89:1062, 1963.
5. Battersby, T. G. Cavernous angioma of mandible. *Br. Dent. J.* 103:347, 1957.
6. Bennett, J. E., and Zook, E. G. Treatment of arteriovenous fistulae in cavernous hemangiomas of face by muscle embolization. *Plast. Reconstr. Surg.* 50:84, 1972.
7. Bill, A. H., Jr., and Sumner, D. S. A unified concept of lymphangioma and cystic hygroma. *Surg. Gynecol. Obstet.* 120:79, 1965.
8. Bingham, H. G., and Lichti, E. L. Use of ultrasound transducer (Doppler) to localize peripheral arteriovenous fistulae. *Plast. Reconstr. Surg.* 46:151, 1970.
9. Bivings, L. Spontaneous regression of angiomas in children. *J. Pediatr.* 45:643, 1954.
10. Blix, S., and Aas, K. Giant hemangioma, thrombocytopenia, fibrinogenopenia and fibrinolytic activity. *Acta Med. Scand.* 159:63, 1961.
11. Bogin, M., and Thurmond, J. Hemangioma with purpura, thrombocytopenia and erythrocytopenia. *Am. J. Dis. Child.* 81:675, 1951.
12. Bowers, R. E., Graham, E. A., and Tomlinson, K. M. The natural history of the strawberry nevus. *Arch. Dermatol.* 82:667, 1960.
13. Brihaye, J., Milaire, J., Dustin, P., and Pietif, J. Local gigantism of the hand associated with a plexiform

neurofibroma of the ulnar nerve. *J. Neurosurg. Sci.* 18:271, 1974.
14. Broomhead, I. W. Cystic hygroma of the neck. *Br. J. Plast. Surg.* 17:225, 1964.
15. Brown, J. B., and Byars, L. T. Interstitial radiation treatment of hemangiomata. *Am. J. Surg.* 39:452, 1938.
16. Brown, J. B., and Fryer, M. P. Treatment of hemangiomas. *Arch. Surg.* 65:417, 1952.
17. Brown, S. H., Neerhout, R. C., and Fonkalrud, E. W. Prednisone therapy in the management of large hemangiomas in infants and children. *Surgery* 71:168, 1972.
18. Castleman, B. Case records of the Massachusetts General Hospital, weekly clinicopathological exercises. Case 42021: Haemangioma of the mandible. *N. Engl. J. Med.* 254:70, 1956.
19. Chait, D., Yonkers, J, Beddoe, G. M., and Yarington, C. T. Management of cystic hygromas. *Surg. Gynecol. Obstet.* 139:55, 1974.
20. Clodius, L. Excision and grafting of extensive facial hemangiomas. *Br. J. Plast. Surg.* 30:185, 1977.
21. Coleman, C. C., Jr., and Hoopes, J. E. Congenital arteriovenous anomalies of the head and neck. *Plast. Reconstr. Surg.* 47:354, 1971.
22. Conway, H. The permanent camouflage of port wine stains of the face by intradermal injection of insoluble pigments (tattooing). *N. Y. J. Med.* 48:2040, 1948.
23. Conway, H., and Docktor, J. P. Neutralization of color in capillary hemangiomas of the face by intradermal injection (tattooing) of permanent pigments. *Surg. Gynecol. Obstet.* 84:866, 1947.
24. Conway, H., McKinney, P., and Climo, M. Permanent camouflage of vascular nevi of the face by intradermal injection of insoluble pigments (tattooing): Experience through twenty years with 1,022 cases. *Plast. Reconstr. Surg.* 40:457, 1967.
25. Conway, H., and Montroy, R. E. Permanent camouflage of capillary hemangiomas of the face by intradermal injection of insoluble pigments (tattooing): Indications for surgery. *N. Y. J. Med.* 65:876, 1965.
26. Coursley, G., Ivins, J. C., and Barker, N. W. Congenital A-V fistulae in the extremities: An analysis of 69 cases. *Angiology* 7:201, 1956.
27. Cran, J. A. Cavernous hemangioma in the mandible. *Br. J. Oral Surg.* 3:32, 1965.
28. Not used.
29. Cross, F. S., Glover, D. M., Simeone, F. A., and Oldenburg, F. A. Congenital arteriovenous aneurysms. *Ann. Surg.* 148:649, 1958.
30. Cunningham, D. S., and Paletta, F. X. Control of arteriovenous fistulae in massive facial hemangioma by muscle emboli. *Plast. Reconstr. Surg.* 46:305, 1970.
31. Dargeon, H. W., Amparo, C. D., and Pack, G. T. Hemangioma with thrombocytopenia. *Pediatrics* 54:285, 1959.
32. Davies, D. Cavernous hemangioma of the mandible. *Plast. Reconstr. Surg.* 33:457, 1964.
33. Degreef, H., Flour, M., Eggermont, E., et al. Treatment of hemangiomas with corticosteroids. *Arch. Belg. Dermatol.* 30:195, 1974.
34. Devine, K. D., Beahrs, O. H., Lovestedt, S. A., and Erich, J. B. Congenital arteriovenous fistulae of the face and neck. *Plast. Reconstr. Surg.* 23:273, 1959.
35. Dibble, P. A., and Whelan, T. J. Cavernous haemangioma of the mandible. *Arch. Otolaryngol.* 75:114, 1962.
36. Djindjian, R. Embolization of angiomas of the spinal cord. *Surg. Neurol.* 4:411, 1975.
37. Edgerton, M. T. The treatment of hemangiomas: With special reference to the role of steroid therapy. *Ann. Surg.* 183:517, 1976.
38. Erich, J. Central hemangioma of the mandible: Report of a case. *Am. J. Orthod.* 33:611, 1947.
39. Figi, F. A. Haemangiomas of the mouth. *Ann. Otol.* 56:853, 1947.
40. Fisher, H. C., and Johnson, M. E. Congenital arteriovenous communications. *Am. Surg.* 23:112, 1957.
41. Fonkalsrud, E. W. Lymphangiomas in infancy and childhood. *Pediatr. Dig.* 11:29, 1969.
42. Fonkalsrud, E. W. Surgical management of congenital malformations of the lymphatic system. *Am. J. Surg.* 128:152, 1974.
43. Fost, N. C., and Esterly, N. B. Successful treatment of juvenile hemangiomas with prednisone. *J. Pediatr.* 72:351, 1968.
44. Geschickter, C. F., and Maseritz, I. H. Primary haemangioma involving bones of the extremities. *J. Bone Joint Surg. [Br.]* 20:888, 1938.
45. Girard, C., Graham, J. H., and Johnson, W. C. Arteriovenous hemangioma (arteriovenous shunt): A clinicopathological and histochemical study. *J. Cutan. Pathol.* 1:73, 1974.
46. Goetsch, E. Hygroma colli cysticum and hygroma axillere: Pathologic and clinical study and report of twelve cases. *Arch. Surg.* 36:394, 1938.
47. Gomes, M. M., and Bernatz, P. E. Arteriovenous fistulae: A review and 10-year experience at the Mayo Clinic. *Proc. Staff Meet. Mayo Clin.* 45:81, 1970.
48. Good, T. A., Carnazzo, S. F., and Good, R. A. Thrombocytopenia and giant hemangioma in infants. *Am. J. Dis. Child.* 90:260, 1955.
49. Habal, M. B., and Murray, J. E. The natural history of a benign locally-invasive hemangioma

of the orbital region. *Plast. Reconstr. Surg.* 49:209, 1972.
50. Hall, R. R., Beach, A. D., Baker, E., and Morrison, P. Incision of tissue by carbon dioxide laser. *Nature* 232:131, 1971.
51. Hall, R. R., Hill, D. W., and Beach, A. D. A carbon dioxide surgical laser. *Ann. R. Coll. Surg. Engl.* 48:181, 1971.
52. Halsted, W. S. Congenital arteriovenous and lymphaticovenous fistulae. *Trans. Am. Surg. Assoc.* 37:262, 1919.
53. Hartley, J. H., Jr., and Schatten, W. R. Cavernous hemangioma of the mandible: Case report. *Plast. Reconstr. Surg.* 50:287, 1972.
54. Herrington, J. L. Congenital angiomatous malformation involving the entire lower extremity: Report of hemipelvectomy in a 25-day-old infant. *Surgery* 34:759, 1953.
55. Hill, G. J., and Longino, L. A. Giant hemangioma with thrombocytopenia. *Surg. Gynecol. Obstet.* 114:304, 1962.
56. Holman, E. Clinical and experimental observations on arteriovenous fistulae. *Ann. Surg.* 142:840, 1940.
57. Hopkins, J. G. Vascular nevus with spontaneous involution. *Arch. Dermatol. Syph.* 43:1033, 1941.
58. Horton, B. T. Hemihypertrophy of the extremities with arteriovenous fistulae. *J.A.M.A.* 98:373, 1932.
59. Howell, J. S. Skin tumours in the rat produced by 9,10-dimethyl-1-2-benzanthracene and methylcholanthrene. *Br. J. Cancer* 16:101, 1962.
60. Howell, J. S. The experimental production of vascular tumours in the rat. *Br. J. Cancer* 17:653, 1963.
61. Inglefield, J. T., Jr., Tisdale, P. D., and Fairchild, J. P. A case of hemangioma with thrombocytopenia in the newborn infant treated by total excision. *J. Pediatr.* 59:238, 1961.
62. James, D. H., Jr., and Tuttle, A. H. Congenital hemangioma with thrombocytopenia. *J. Pediatr.* 59:234, 1961.
63. Jarzab, G. Clinical experience in the cryosurgery of hemangioma. *J. Maxillofac. Surg.* 3:146, 1975.
64. Johnson, H. A. Expanding hemangioma with associated thrombocytopenia. *Br. J. Plast. Surg.* 12:69, 1959.
65. Kasabach, H. H., and Merritt, K. K. Capillary hemangioma with extensive purpura. *Am. J. Dis. Child.* 59:1063, 1940.
66. Katz, H. P. Thrombocytopenia Associated with Hemangiomata: Critical Analysis of Steroid Therapy. Eleventh International Congress of Pediatrics, Tokyo, 1965.
67. Khaw, J. H., and Datuk, O. b. D. Localized gigantism of the extremities. *Med. J. Malaysia* 27:292, 1973.
68. Kiehn, C. L., Des Prez, J. D., and Kaufman, B. Cavernous hemangiomas of the head and neck. Indications for arteriography and surgical treatment. *Plast. Reconstr. Surg.* 33:338, 1964.
69. Kilgour, C. S. Hemangioma of the mandible. *Br. J. Plast. Surg.* 10:60, 1957.
70. Knox, W. C., Stanley-Brown, E. G., and Dargeon, H. W. Surgical management of extensive hemangioma associated with severe hemorrhage in an infant: A case report. *Surgery* 49:406, 1961.
71. Kontras, J. B., Green, O. A., King, L., and Duran, R. J. Giant thrombocytopenia. *Am. J. Dis. Child.* 105:188, 1963.
72. Kroh, F. Fatal haemorrhage after extraction of tooth (abstract). *J.A.M.A.* 86:236, 1926.
73. Laborde, S. Cavernous hemangioma of the jaws: Treatment in infants. *Dent. Abstr.* 4:25, 1959.
74. Lang, E. R., and Bucy, P. C. Treatment of carotid-cavernous fistula by muscle embolization alone. The Brooks method. *J. Neurosurg.* 22:387, 1965.
75. Larson, S. J., and Worman, L. W. Internal carotid artery flow rate during craniotomy and muscle embolization for carotid cavernous fistula. *J. Neurosurg.* 29:60, 1968.
76. Lawton, R. L., Tidrick, R. T., and Brintnall, E. S. A clinicopathological study of multiple congenital A-V fistulae of the lower extremities. *Angiology* 8:161, 1957.
77. Leonard, F. C., and Vassos, G. A. Congenital A-V fistulae of the lower limb: Report of a case successfully treated by total excision. *N. Engl. J. Med.* 245:885, 1951.
78. Levine, R., Holcomb, T. M., and Lutzner, M. A. Hemangioma associated with thrombocytopenia. *Arch. Dermatol.* 82:94, 1960.
79. Li, F. P., Cassady, J. R., and Barnett, E. Cancer mortality following irradiation in infancy for hemangiomas. *Radiology* 113:177, 1974.
80. Lichtenstein, L. Aneurysmal bone cyst. *Cancer* 3:279, 1950.
81. Longacre, J. J., Benton, C., and Unterthiner, R. A. Treatment of facial hemangioma by intravascular embolization with silicone spheres: Case report. *Plast. Reconstr. Surg.* 50:618, 1972.
82. Luessenhop, A. J., Kachmann, R., Jr., Shevlin, W., and Ferrero, A. A. Clinical evaluation of artificial embolization in the management of large cerebral arteriovenous malformations. *J. Neurosurg.* 23:400, 1965.
83. Lund, B. A., and Dahlin, D. C. Hemangioma of the mandible and maxilla. *J. Oral Surg. Anesth. Hosp. Dent. Serv.* 22:234, 1964.
84. Lynn, H. B. Cystic hygroma. *Surg. Clin. North Am.* 43:1157, 1963.

85. Mangus, D. J. Continuous compression treatment of hemangiomata: Evaluation in two cases. *Plast. Reconstr. Surg.* 49:490, 1972.
86. Margileth, A. M., and Museles, M. Current concepts in diagnosis and management of congenital cutaneous hemangiomas. *Pediatrics* 36:410, 1965.
87. Margileth, A. M., and Museles, M. Cutaneous hemangiomas in children. *J.A.M.A.* 194:523, 1965.
88. Martin, L. W. Angiomas in infants and children. *Am. J. Surg.* 107:511, 1964.
89. Matthews, D. N. Hemangiomata. *Plast. Reconstr. Surg.* 41:528, 1968.
90. Meeks, E. A., Jay, J. B., and Heaton, L. D. Thrombocytopenia purpura occurring with large hemangioma. *Am. J. Dis. Child.* 90:349, 1955.
91. Meyer, I. Comments. On Abramson, B. S., Central hemangioma of the mandible: Report of a case. *J. Oral Surg.* 23:68, 1965.
92. Miller, S., Smith, R., and Shochat, S. Compression treatment of hemangiomas. *Plast. Reconstr. Surg.* 58:573, 1976.
93. Mohnac, A. M. Central hemangioma of the mandible: Report of a case. *J. Oral Surg.* 25:445, 1967.
94. Moore, A. M. Pressure in the treatment of giant hemangioma with purpura. *Plast. Reconstr. Surg.* 34:606, 1964.
95. Nisbett, N. W. Congenital arteriovenous fistula in the extremities. *Br. J. Surg.* 41:658, 1954.
96. Noh, E., and Steckenmesser, R. Der angeborene Riesenwuchs Klinische und arteriographische Befunde an Hand und Arm beim Klippel-Trenaunay-Syndrom. (Congenital gigantism – clinical and radiographic findings in hand and arm.) *Z. Orthop.* 112:243, 1974.
97. Olcott, C., Newton, T. H., Stoney, R. J., and Ehrenfeld, W. K. Intra-arterial embolization in the management of arteriovenous malformations. *Surgery* 79:3, 1976.
98. Orbach, S. Congenital arteriovenous malformations of the face. *Oral Surg.* 42:2, 1976.
99. Overcash, K. E., and Putney, F. Subglottic hemangioma of the larynx treated with steroid therapy. *Laryngoscope* 83:679, 1973.
100. Paletta, F. X., and Walker, J. Hemangioma-thrombocytopenia syndrome. *Plast. Reconstr. Surg.* 23:615, 1959.
101. Pemberton, J. D., Jr., and Saint, J. H. Congenital arteriovenous communications. *Surg. Gynecol. Obstet.* 46:470, 1928.
102. Phelan, J. T., and Grace, J. T. Conservative management of cutaneous capillary hemangioma. *J.A.M.A.* 185:246, 1963.
103. Pizer, M. E. Cavernous hemangioma occurring in the body of the mandible. *Oral Surg.* 7:1201, 1954.
104. Ravitch, M. M. Cystic Hygroma. In Mustard, W. T., Ravitch, M. M., Snyder, W. H., Jr., Welch, K. J., and Benson, C. D. (Eds.), *Pediatric Surgery* (2nd ed.). Chicago: Year Book, 1969.
105. Robles, C., and Carrasco-Zanin, J. Treatment of cerebral arteriovenous malformations by muscle embolization. *J. Neurosurg.* 29:603, 1968.
106. Rohan, R. F. Hemangioma of the mandible presenting as epistaxis. *J. Laryngol. Otol.* 74:178, 1960.
107. Ronchese, F. Spontaneous involution of cutaneous vascular tumors. *Am. J. Surg.* 86:376, 1953.
108. Rush, B. F., Jr. Treatment of a giant cutaneous hemangioma by intra-arterial injection of nitrogen mustard. *Ann. Surg.* 164:921, 1966.
109. Saijo, M., Munro, I. R., and Mancer, K. Lymphangioma: A long-term follow-up study. *Plast. Reconstr. Surg.* 56:513, 1975.
110. Sako, Y., and Varco, R. Arteriovenous fistula: Results of management of congenital and acquired forms, blood flow measurements and observations on proximal artery degeneration. *Surgery* 67:40, 1970.
111. Shira, R. B. Central cavernous hemangioma of the mandible: Report of a case. *J. Oral Surg.* 23:636, 1965.
112. Silver, H. K., Aggeler, P. M., and Crane, J. T. Hemangioma (capillary and cavernous) with thrombopenia purpura. *Am. J. Dis. Child.* 76:513, 1948.
113. Smith, H. W. Haemangioma of the jaw. *Arch. Otolaryngol.* 70:579, 1959.
114. Snyderman, R. K., and Wynn, W. D. Complete replacement of port wine stains. *N.Y. J. Med.* 66:1910, 1966.
115. Solomon, H., Goldman, L., Henderson, B., Richfield, D., and Franzen, M. Histopathology of the laser treatment of port wine lesions. *J. Invest. Dermatol.* 50:141, 1968.
116. Southard, S. G., De Sanctis, H. C., and Waldron, R. J. Hemangioma associated with thrombocytopenia purpura. *J. Pediatr.* 38:732, 1951.
117. Stevenson, R. F., and Morin, J. D. Ocular findings in naevus flammeus. *Can. J. Ophthalmol.* 10:136, 1975.
118. Stevenson, R. F., Thomson, H. G., and Morin, J. D. Unrecognized ocular problems associated with "port wine" stain of the face in children. *Can. Med. Assoc. J.* 111:9, 953, 1974.
118a. Stigmar, G., Crawford, J. S., Ward, C. M., and Thomson, H. G. Ophthalmic sequelae of infantile hemangiomas of the eyelids and orbit. *Am. J. Ophthalmol.* 85:806, 1978.
119. Sutherland, D. H., and Clark, H. Hemangioma associated with thrombocytopenia: Report of a case and review of the literature. *Am. J. Med.* 33:150, 1962.

120. Szilagyi, D. E., Elliott, J. P., De Russo, F. J., and Smith, R. F. Peripheral congenital arteriovenous fistulae. *Surgery* 57:61, 1965.
121. Szilagyi, D. E., Smith, R. F., Elliott, J. P., et al. Congenital arteriovenous anomalies of the limbs. *Arch. Surg.* 111:423, 1976.
122. Taylor, B. G., and Etheridge, S. N. Hemangioma of the mandible and maxilla presenting as surgical emergencies. *Am. J. Surg.* 108:574, 1964.
123. Thomson, H. G., Birdsell, D. C., and Freiberg, A. Surgical tattooing: An experimental study. *Plast. Reconstr. Surg.* 37:536, 1966.
124. Thomson, H. G., Douglas, L., and Munro, I. R. Surgical tattooing: An experimental study (Part II). *Plast. Reconstr. Surg.* 39:291, 1967.
125. Thomson, H. G., and Lanigan, M. The Cyrano nose – a clinical review of hemangioma of the nasal tip. *Plast. Reconstr. Surg.* 63:155, 1979.
125b. Thomson, H.G., Ward, C., Crawford, J. S., and Stigma, R. G. Hemangiomas of the eyelid: Visual complications and prophylactic concepts. *Plast. Reconstr. Surg.* 63:641, 1979.
126. Thomson, H. G., and Wright, A. Surgical tattooing of the port wine stain. Operative technique, results and critique. *Plast. Reconstr. Surg.* 48:113, 1970.
127. Villa, V. G., and Limchayseng, F. Central hemangioma of the mandible (central angioma): Report of a case. *Oral Surg.* 8:1254, 1955.
128. Wallerstein, R. O. Spontaneous involution of giant hemangioma. *Am. J. Dis. Child.* 102:233, 1961.
129. Walter, J. On the treatment of cavernous hemangioma with special reference to spontaneous regression. *J. Fac. Radiol.* 5:134, 1953–1954.
130. Warren, J. V., Nikerman, J. L., and Elkin, D. C. The cardiac output in patients with arteriovenous fistulae. *J. Clin. Invest.* 30:210, 1951.
131. Weinstein, I., Yamanaka, H., and Fuchihata, H. Resection and reconstruction of the mandible for removal of central hemangioma. *Oral Surg.* 16:2, 1963.
132. Weissman, J., and Tagnon, H. J. Syndrome of hemangioma and thrombocytopenia purpura in infants. *Arch. Intern. Med.* 92:523, 1953.
133. Wilde, N. J. Hemangioma of the mandible: Report of a case. *J. Oral Surg.* 24:549, 1966.
134. Williams, H. B. Hemangiomas of the parotid gland in children. *Plast. Reconstr. Surg.* 56:29, 1975.
135. Williams, W. J., and Gilbert, R. K. Hemangioma of the mandible. *Br. Dent. J.* 98:445, 1955.
136. Wynn, S. K. Aesthetic reduction of "Pinocchio" nose hemangioma. *Arch. Otolaryngol.* 102:416, 1976.
137. Zarem, H. A., and Edgerton, M. T. Induced resolution of cavernous hemangiomas following prednisone therapy. *Plast. Reconstr. Surg.* 39:76, 1967.

29

Benign Growths and Generalized Skin Disorders

HARVEY A. ZAREM AND ALLAN L. LORINCZ

BENIGN GROWTHS

Pigmented lesions present the physician with the dilemma of which are potentially malignant or frankly malignant and which are lesions that may be treated as benign. Clinically, the distinction between benign and malignant skin lesions is usually clear, but the physician must be cautious to remove those lesions that arouse suspicion of malignancy or that create anxiety to the patient. The characteristics of malignant melanoma have been defined in numerous articles, and most physicians are fully aware of the need to remove pigmented lesions that are enlarging, crusting, or bleeding, or that show such activity as deepening pigmentation with surrounding inflammation. The real challenge is to understand the nature of the lesions that do not have obvious signs of malignancy but may possibly create trouble in the future. Pathologists now agree that malignant melanoma may arise from a preexisting pigmented lesion or that it may arise de novo. The majority of malignant melanomas that arise from preexisting pigmented lesions do so from a melanotic freckle of Hutchinson [52]. Much less commonly, junctional or compound nevus cell nevi, in particular those large nevus cell nevi that are present since birth, can be the site of malignant melanoma. The ordinary nevus cell nevus – junctional, compound, or intradermal – is rarely complicated by the evolution of malignant melanoma [49, 50].

The *junctional nevus* clinically is a smooth, flat, irregularly pigmented lesion. It may occur at any site on the body, but pigmented nevi on palmar or plantar skin or on transitional epithelium (such as vermilion border of lip, glans penis, or vulva) are usually junctional nevi and remain so. Junctional nevi may appear at any age, but particularly in childhood, adolescence, and young adult life. The junctional nevus seen in childhood is less common in adults, presumably from the transformation of the junctional nevus to an intradermal compound nevus in adulthood.

Although it is uncommon for malignant melanoma to arise from an *intradermal* or a *compound* nevus, it still may occur. However, it is generally agreed that unless such a lesion exhibits a notable change in size, crusting, surrounding inflammation, or increasing pigmentation, it need not be excised for fear of malignant degeneration.

The *melanotic freckle of Hutchinson* (Fig. 29-1) early in its course resembles the junctional nevus, but is characterized by continuing slow growth to form a patch of irregular, polycyclic, and variegated pigmentation usually larger than 1 cm. Although it characteristically occurs on the face, the melanotic freckle of Hutchinson may be seen on the neck, back, or anywhere else on the body. This lesion frequently precedes a superficial malignant melanoma, and its recognition is critical so that removal may be carried out before frank invasive melanoma develops. The excision of the melanotic freckle of Hutchinson need not be radical, but the entire lesion must be removed.

Benign juvenile melanoma has been clearly discussed in a comprehensive review article by Kopf and Andrade [26]. This lesion, despite some histological characteristics that in the past led to confusion with malignant melanoma, is a variant of the nevus cell nevus and does not behave as a malignant lesion. These frequently nonpigmented pale red papular lesions usually occur before puberty and may even be present at birth. In 15 percent of cases, they are observed initially in adolescence or adulthood. The benign juvenile melanoma occurs most frequently on the face; only occasionally is it melanized. Although true malignant melanomas may occur rarely in infants and children, it is important to recognize the more common benign juvenile melanoma to avoid unnecessary radical operative procedures necessary for the treatment of a malignant melanoma.

The *giant pigmented nevus* (Fig. 29-2) is a congenital lesion that sometimes demonstrates a tendency to occur in the distribution of dermatomes, or it may occur in bathing trunk, vest, sleeve, or stocking pattern. It most commonly occurs on the head or pelvic area, appearing as a large, pigmented, hairy, soft verrucose lesion. The reported incidence of malignant melanoma arising in the giant pigmented nevus is quite variable – from less than 1 percent to as high as 10 to 25 percent [41]. The issue of the malignant potential of congenital nevi is an important but confusing one. The "true incidence" of malignant degeneration in giant pigmented nevi is likely to be in the range of 1 to 2 percent, which was found in a 40-year follow-up in 110 defined cases of giant pigmented nevi; in that study, 2 cases of melanoma developed at the ages of 28 years and 40 years, as cited by Dellon [10] and by Kaplan [22]. Kaplan reviewed the literature of 59 cases of malignant melanoma developing in giant pigmented nevi, adding 7 other cases from their own institution, and demonstrated

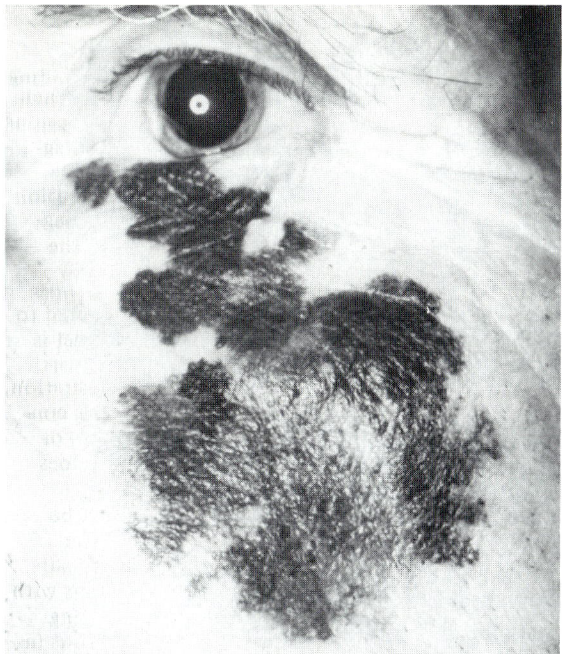

Fig. 29-1. Melanotic freckle of Hutchinson showing irregular borders and variegated pigmentation. This should be excised since there is a high incidence of progression to malignant melanoma.

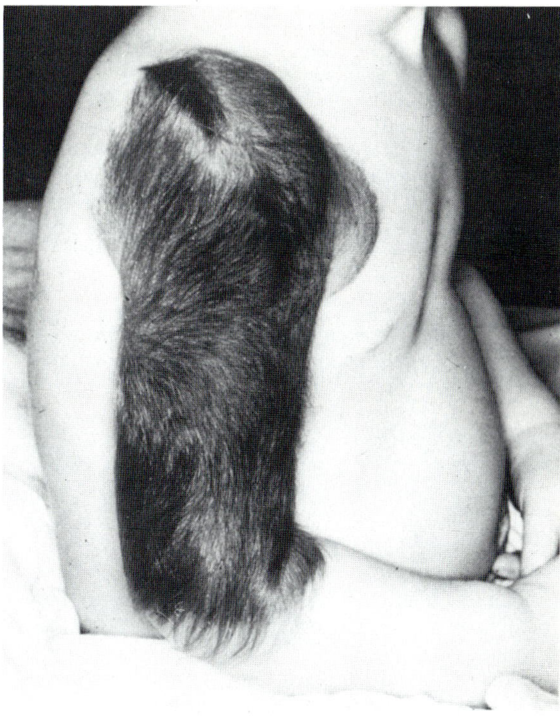

Fig. 29-2. Giant hairy pigmented nevus.

a peak incidence of malignant melanoma arising in congenital giant pigmented nevi during the first 5 years of life.

It appears that those lesions which exhibit verrucose characteristics with deep pigmentation and thick skin are more likely to be complicated by malignant change and warrant operative removal. Most children or parents will seek removal of these lesions because of aesthetic disfigurement. The giant pigmented nevus creates a surgical challenge, especially about the face. Today, it is generally agreed that such lesions on the face are best removed and the face reconstructed with local skin flaps. Lesions on the trunk may be excised in stages with ultimate total removal. The extremity lesions are generally removed and resurfaced with free skin grafts. The melanocyte proliferative activity is frequently more extensive than is apparent from the margins of clinical pigmentation, so that the appearance of pigmented cells in the scars or adjacent to the scars of previous excisions is not uncommon. For this reason *it is important to remove some margin of seemingly normal skin* beyond that indicated by the presence or absence of pigment.

Lentigo senilis is not a nevus cell lesion, but consists of a smooth, dark brown patch measuring up to 1.5 cm. in diameter in which there are increased numbers of normal melanocytes. Lentigo senilis is frequently multiple in middle-aged or older people and appears especially in areas exposed to actinic rays, such as the dorsum of the hands, face, neck, and arms. Although lentigo senilis is on occasion difficult to differentiate clinically from freckles, junctional nevi, incipient seborrheic keratosis, and Hutchinson's melanotic freckle, lentigo senilis is rarely confused with malignant lesions. When the diagnosis of lentigo senilis is established, removal may be accomplished by operative excision when feasible or by proper cryotherapy.

A *freckle* (ephelis) represents a pigmented lesion with a normal number of melanocytes that produce an abnormally large amount of melanin granules. The melanocytes in the freckle show no proliferative activity and as such do not exhibit any malignant potential.

The *blue nevus* is a firm, well-defined small intradermal nodule composed of dermal melanocytes. Although malignant degeneration in blue nevi is a rarity, malignancy can occur in the lesions that clinically resemble a blue nevus. Occasionally the differential diagnosis is difficult between blue nevus, metastasis of a malignant melanoma, and Kaposi's sarcoma. A venous lake or other hemangioma may also present diagnostic confusion with the blue nevus, but usually compression of the lesion that is a hemangioma will illustrate some sponginess and blanching, which are not characteristic of the blue nevus.

The *nevus of Ota* is a blue-gray discoloration of the face in a pattern following the first and second branches of the fifth cranial nerve. The nevus of Ota most commonly involves the eye and the periorbital regions [57], and 60 percent are present at birth or within the first decade of life; 80 percent of the nevus of Ota lesions are seen in females. The lesion must be distinguished from a malignant melanoma, which it can closely resemble clinically.

Epidermal Lesions

Nevus verrucosus is a papillomatous yellowish-tan keratotic plaque that appears at birth or during childhood. The lesion may be patchy or linear and often has the deceptive appearance of being limited to the superficial epidermis clinically. Superficial abrasion or electrodesiccation rarely removes the lesion permanently because there is an underlying dermal disturbance that induces the epidermal changes. Those lesions that create a significant diagnostic problem or cause a noticeable deformity can be excised with a full-thickness of skin in order to ensure that they will not recur.

Keratosis follicularis (Darier's disease) is a hereditary disorder of keratinization resulting in greasy, crusted warty masses on the face, neck, chest, axilla, and inguinal areas. The unpleasant, malodorous masses have not responded to conservative treatments, and irradiation has been recommended in some dermatological literature. A recent article has reported the successful treatment of these lesions by partial thickness removal with split-thickness shaving or dermabrasion [9].

Tylosis (keratosis palmaris et plantaris) is a hereditary thickening of the palms and soles, which become painful. Patients who are sufficiently symptomatic from the painful fissures may be treated with excision of the involved skin and resurfacing with split-thickness skin grafting [25].

Seborrheic keratosis is a common lesion often seen in large numbers, especially on the trunk, face, and arms of middle-aged and older individuals. The seborrheic keratosis is a sharply circumscribed, cauliflower-like, waxy papillomatous lesion with a friable hyperkeratotic surface. Most descriptively it has a "stuck-on appearance." Pigmentation of seborrheic keratoses is quite variable, from mild to deep black. The experienced physician can readily recognize the seborrheic keratosis by its appearance and by its characteristic superficiality, which allows the lesion to be readily scraped off level with surrounding skin, revealing a raw surface. Nevertheless, seborrheic keratoses are the most commonly encountered lesions in surgical pathology laboratories erroneously diagnosed by the clinician as malignant melanoma. Because many of these lesions are broad based, excision is limited to those lesions where there may be diagnostic uncertainty. Superficial examination of the histological pattern of a seborrheic keratosis may create confusion with squamous carcinoma in those inflamed lesions that have recently been subjected to trauma or irritation. The experienced pathologist is usually able to distinguish the seborrheic keratosis from the squamous cell carcinoma without hesitation. Adequate treatment of the seborrheic keratosis consists of curettage, superficial electrodesiccation, or freezing with liquid nitrogen, since this lesion does not undergo malignant degeneration.

The *actinic keratosis* (senile keratosis) must be distinguished from the seborrheic keratosis. The actinic keratosis is found primarily on exposed surfaces as discrete, flat, or slightly elevated lesions with hard, dry adherent hyperkeratosis and underlying erythema. Since these lesions are often numerous in elderly people with weather-beaten skin, it may be impractical to excise all of them. The physician must select for excision those senile keratoses that occur in relatively young people, those lesions that have become thickened or verrucose, and those that exhibit surrounding inflammation or crusting. Many dermatologists feel secure in removing lesions that do not have a suspicious characteristic by nonsurgical means such as liquid nitrogen or topical 5-fluorouracil. Histologically, the actinic keratosis may be similar to Bowen's disease. Except for the very early superficial actinic keratotic lesions that are removed nonsurgically by the dermatologist, those lesions exhibiting the symptoms of activity with thickening skin, inflammation, and crusting must be adequately removed operatively and thoroughly examined histologically, since one may be dealing with a presquamous cancer lesion.

Bowen's disease (Fig. 29-3) presents as a persistent red, rough, scaly patch that tends to spread slowly. When these lesions occur on the penis, they are referred to as *erythroplasia of Queyrat.* Bowen's disease is an intraepidermal squamous cell carcinoma or a squamous cell carcinoma in situ, which can deteriorate to an invasive squamous cell carcinoma if untreated. One-third of the Bowen's lesions occur secondary to chronic arsenic poisoning (such as from Fowler's solution), and they are associated with arsenical keratoses, leukomelanoderma, and a high incidence of visceral carcinoma, especially squamous cell carcinoma of the respiratory epithelium. The patient with multiple Bowen's lesions of the skin

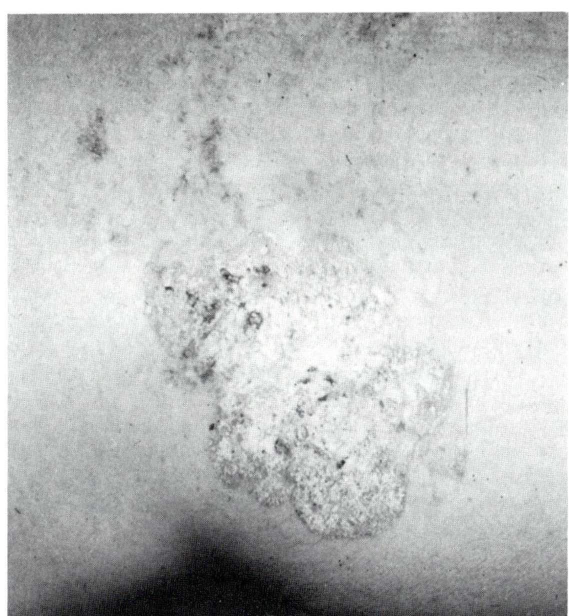

Fig. 29-3. Bowen's disease on leg, showing rough, scaly patch with polycyclic borders.

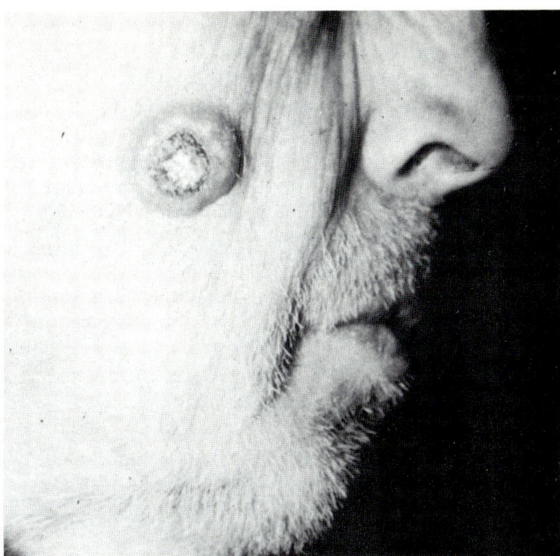

Fig. 29-4. Keratoacanthoma on the check with massive central keratotic core.

consistent with the arsenical-ingestion pattern deserves a visceral work-up, with repeated examinations [18].

Keratoacanthoma (Fig. 29-4) is a lesion that has been the subject of much discussion because of its unique qualities [8]. It is a rapidly growing papule that enlarges to 1 to 2 cm. within a period of several weeks. It then undergoes spontaneous resolution within 6 months of its onset. The round, smooth, pink nodule encircles a massive keratinous plug. Histologically, the keratoacanthoma may be difficult to distinguish from a squamous cell carcinoma, and frequently the diagnosis depends on the gross architecture of the lesion. Since the most critical diagnostic criterion of a keratoacanthoma may be spontaneous resolution, diagnosis with absolute certainty is often difficult. If the lesion does not show tendency to regress after several months, the physician should deal with the lesion as a squamous cell carcinoma. Rather than allow the lesion to declare itself as a benign keratoacanthoma, it is usually our preference to remove the tumor as if treating an early squamous cell carcinoma.

Adnexal Tumors

In adnexal tumors the relationships between epithelial and stromal components are maintained, even though distorted to varying degrees. Differentiation in the direction of hair follicles, sebaceous glands, apocrine or eccrine sweat glands, or various combinations of these cutaneous appendages occurs. Such tumors are classified according to their level of differentiation, as well as their direction of differentiation, and a continuous spectrum ranging over all combinations of both parameters exists. Some general synonyms for adnexal tumors as a whole are organoid tumors, appendageal tumors, nevoid tumors, and hamartomas.

Where there is simply a localized excess of well-differentiated, fully mature cutaneous appendageal structures with normal surrounding stroma, the lesions are called nevi of such appendages. The term *adenoma* is used when maturation of benign tumors is incomplete and their organization is distorted, whereas *epithelioma* tends to be applied to poorly organized and immature tumors.

Tumors Showing Hair Follicular Differentiation

Hair follicle nevus (trichofolliculoma) presents on the face or scalp as a single, small, skin-colored papule, often with a highly characteristic central pore from which a wisp of white cottony hairs protrudes. Simple excisional biopsy suffices for diagnosis and treatment.

Multiple trichoepithelioma (epithelioma adenoides cysticum) is frequently a dominantly inherited disorder in which smooth, shiny, slightly translucent, firm, pale papules appear in increasing numbers during puberty or early adult life in somewhat symmetrical distribution chiefly on the face, especially about the eyes, but also on the scalp. Lesions may begin in early childhood, and they tend to be encountered more frequently in women. The lesions are benign and are best treated by electrodesiccation. Histologically, their differentiation from keratotic basal cell epithelioma may be difficult, whereas clinically they often resemble syringoma or the facial angiofibromas that characterize the tuberous sclerosis syndrome. So-called solitary trichoepithelioma is perhaps best included in the most highly differentiated end of the spectrum of keratotic basal cell epitheliomas.

Pilomatricoma (calcifying epithelioma of Malherbe) occurs as a single, hard, deeply seated, firm nodule covered by normal skin, usually from 0.5 to 3.0 cm. in size. It is found most commonly in children and young adults, especially on the face and arms. Clinically, it can be confused with calcified epithelial cyst or even at times with carcinoma when cutting into it because of its solid hard consistency. The lesion is benign and consists of an encapsulated mass of epidermoid cells with areas of small basophilic cells gradually merging into zones of pale eosinophilic "shadow" cells, among which there is usually calcium deposition. It is properly treated by simple excision.

Tricholemmoma shows downward proliferating buds of large, light-staining, glycogen-rich, follicular sheath–type epithelial cells extending from the surface into the corium. The tumor buds are surrounded by a row of cells showing nuclear palisading to resemble the outer root sheath of hair follicles. This benign tumor usually occurs on the scalp and is amenable to simple excision.

Tumors Showing Eccrine Differentiation

Syringomas present occasionally as single, but more often as multiple, flesh-colored, pinkish or yellowish-tan papules, usually 2 to 3 mm. in diameter. They are often confused with trichoepithelioma, nevus, xanthelasma, or basal cell epithelioma. These lesions occur most often in adult women and usually involve the lower eyelids and upper cheeks, although they may also be found on the trunk, neck, and extremities. Removal for cosmetic purposes is best accomplished by electrodesiccation or cryotherapy with liquid nitrogen.

Eccrine hidrocystoma may resemble syringoma in distribution, but the lesions are translucent and appear as tense, slightly bluish, deep vesicles. These lesions are seen especially on the face of older women exposed to heat, which stimulates profuse perspiration. They subside in a cool environment and represent passively dilated, obstructed sweat ducts. Avoidance of heat and simple puncturing of the lesions suffice for treatment.

Eccrine poroma usually occurs on plantar or palmar skin as a firm, sessile, reddish, papular or nodular tumor in a shallow cup-shaped depression surrounded by a narrow hyperkeratotic ridge. Clinically, it is easily confused with granuloma pyogenicum, amelanotic melanoma, or even Kaposi's sarcoma. The lesions are benign and can be removed by simple excision biopsy or by punch biopsy for diagnosis followed by curettage and electrodesiccation.

Eccrine spiradenoma in 90 percent of cases is either painful, tender, or both. Paroxysms of severe pain triggered by manipulation may lead to clinical confusion with glomus tumor. The lesions are usually solitary, deep dermal or subcutaneous tumors about 1 cm. in diameter and occur most often in young adults, frequently on the upper ventral body.

Eccrine acrospiroma (clear cell hidradenoma) may occur anywhere on the body, usually as a single, solid or cystic nodular, sometimes lobulated lesion, flesh colored or reddish, and most often 1 to 2 cm. in diameter. A few are tender on pressure, and a few will show drainage or ulceration. *Nodular hidradenoma* is another term sometimes applied to this lesion as well as to other histological variants of nodular benign solid sweat gland tumors. All are easily treated by simple excision. Very rarely, *malignant clear cell hidradenoma* and even *malignant eccrine poroma* have been noted, and these can be usually grouped under the general category of sweat gland carcinomas, which altogether are very rare.

Cylindroma (turban tumor) (Fig. 29-5) occurs predominantly on the scalp or forehead as either solitary or multiple, firm, pink, smooth nodules, ranging in size up to several centimeters. They usually begin in adult life and are slow to grow. A dominantly inherited form, sometimes associated with multiple facial trichoepitheliomas, may form extensive grape-

Fig. 29-5. Cylindroma (turban tumor) of scalp and forehead.

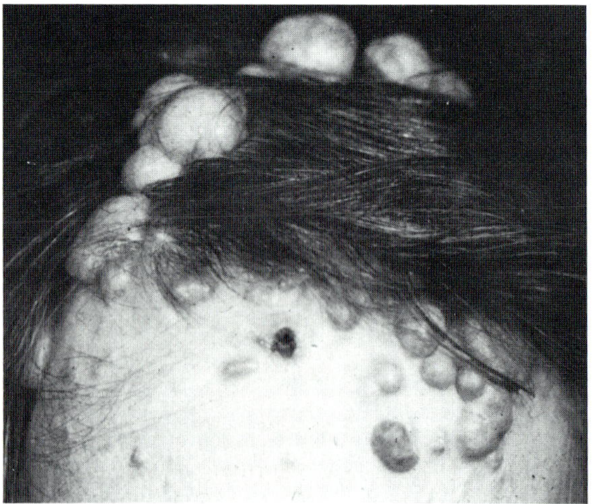

like clusters covering the entire scalp like a turban. Simple excision suffices for treatment. In extensive cases, surgical removal of the most conspicuous tumors may be the most practical approach [17].

Tumors Showing Apocrine Differentiation
Apocrine cystadenoma is a small, benign, nevoid, dome-shaped, often translucent nodule, usually appearing on the face. It is frequently pigmented and on incision may contain brownish fluid. It may be clinically confused with pigmented or blue nevi and even with melanoma or pigmented basal cell epithelioma.

Syringocystadenoma papilliferum is usually a verrucose lesion that occurs most commonly on or near the scalp. It is a hamartomatous growth that frequently develops within an associated organoid nevus of the nevus sebaceous type. These lesions often begin to develop in childhood and vary in size and appearance. They may be bulbous and exude fluid. Small lesions may be umbilicated and resemble molluscum contagiosum. Foci of basal cell epithelioma occur in about 10 percent of the lesions. Treatment consists of full-thickness excision of the lesion, as well as any surrounding sebaceous nevus.

Chondroid syringoma (mixed tumor of skin, salivary gland type), like other mixed tumors, has both epithelial and mesenchymal tissue components, in this case sweat gland elements (syringoma) and cartilage-like chondroid. The lesions are stable, firm, asymptomatic, cutaneous nodules easily separated from the surrounding tissue and usually not connected to the normal overlying epidermis. These lesions are benign, and simple excision is needed only for cosmetic and diagnostic purposes.

Tumors Showing Sebaceous Differentiation
Nevus sebaceous (Jadassohn), also called *organoid nevus,* is a well-circumscribed verrucose or finely nodular, orange-colored, raised, irregular, hairless plaque occurring most frequently on the scalp and less often on the face and neck. It is present at birth and persists throughout life, being quiescent during childhood and tending to become verrucose and nodular during puberty. Clinically, it may resembel nevus verrucosus. In later stages of development, other tumors tend to arise in these lesions, with *basal cell epithelioma arising in 15 to 20 percent.* Syringocystadenoma papilliferum and other adenomatous appendageal tumors may also develop in them as well as keratoacanthoma. Very rarely, even squamous cell carcinoma has been observed in the overlying epidermis. Because of the potential risk of aggressive tumor development in these lesions, their removal by simple excision during childhood or when first recognized is advisable.

Senile sebaceous hyperplasia occurs commonly on the face of middle-aged or older persons, especially males with seborrheic complexions. The lesions usually present as multiple, soft, elevated 2- to 3-mm. papules, with central umbilication and edges composed of confluent pinhead-sized yellowish-white subunits. Fine superficial telangiectatic vessels may course over the edges of the papules. They often are easily mistaken for small basal cell epitheliomas. Treatment is usually not indicated, except for cosmetic purposes; they can be removed by simple electrodesiccation. *Sebaceous adenomas* are rare and benign; they are solitary, smooth, firm tumors on the face or scalp, usually less than 1 cm. in diameter.

Sebaceous epithelioma essentially looks and behaves clinically like basal cell epithelioma, except that their color is sometimes yellowish and there is a notable histological tendency for their component cells to show sebaceous differentiation. These lesions are radiosensitive, but are best treated by either excision or electrocoagulation and curettage, depending on size and location. It may be necessary to differentiate this lesion from rare malignant sebaceous carcinoma, which usually develops in the tarsal region of the eyelids and may metastasize.

Smooth Muscle Tumors
Benign cutaneous tumors consisting of smooth muscle proliferation are called *leiomyomas.* Multiple cutaneous leiomyomas occur in widely varying numbers, sometimes diffusely scattered on the trunk, face, or extremities. They tend to gradually increase in number and are usually firm, pale, reddish-brown, intradermal nodules less than 1 cm. in size. Frequently, they harden and become painful on pressure or application of cold. These multiple lesions are believed to arise from arrectores pilorum muscles. *Solitary angioleiomyomas* are usually small encapsulated subcutaneous nodules less than 2 cm. in size and are seen mainly on the legs. They may be sensitive to pressure and cold and are believed to arise from venular smooth muscle. A third variety is the *solitary genital leiomyoma* located in the subcutis on either the scrotum, labia majora, or nipple area. They may reach larger sizes of up to several centimeters. Solitary tender leiomyomas need to be differentiated at times from glomus tumor and eccrine spiradenoma. Excision is the only suitable treatment for symptomatic leiomyomas. There is a fairly high tendency for recurrences.

Epithelial Cysts
Squamous epithelium-lined cysts of several types that contain lipid and keratinous material in the past have been encompassed under the general designation of sebaceous cysts. They are specifically classified as follows:

Epidermoid cysts are tense, somewhat fluctuant, smooth swellings attached to the dermis but freely movable over underlying tissues. They vary in size up to several centimeters in diameter and commonly occur on the face, neck, and trunk. Tending to enlarge very slowly, they contain cheesy lipid-rich material composed mainly of a lamellated horny substance. Their squamous epithelial lining shows orderly keratinizing differentiation through a well-developed granular layer. At times a central comedo-like point is present. These cysts may become infected, after which they are difficult to enucleate with the entire cyst wall because of adherence to surrounding tissues. There are no sebaceous glandular structures in the linings of these keratin cysts. Simple excision is the most suitable treatment for noninfected lesions. Small cyst linings can at times be teased out entirely through a small incision, which can heal with scarcely perceptible scarring. It is important to remove the lining sac completely, or recurrence is likely. Mildly infected cysts with redness and tenderness can be treated with an oral antibiotic such as tetracycline for a few days until inflammation subsides, before excision is undertaken. Severely infected cysts may require incision, drainage, and curettage of the lining, followed by packing with iodoform gauze to allow healing from within.

Pilar cysts (also called *wens* or *trichilemmal cysts*) clinically resemble epidermoid cysts, except that they occur in 90 percent of cases on the scalp. They contain nonlamellous keratinous material that is not as cheesy as occurs in epidermoid cysts, and their lining shows pilar-type keratinization, with plump luminal cells without keratohyalin granules. They are managed similarly to epidermoid cysts. The dominant familial occurrence of large numbers of wens or epidermoid cysts should alert the clinician to look for the possible presence of Gardner's syndrome, with multiple polyposis of the colon and rectum. The extremely high risk of early death from colon cancer in such patients makes early diagnosis and treatment by total colectomy imperative.

Milia or *whiteheads* are tiny 1- to 2-mm. superficially situated epidermal inclusion cysts that are miniature epidermoid cysts. They tend to occur most frequently about the eyes, where they are occasionally mistaken for xanthelasma, syringoma, or trichoepithelioma. They also tend to develop at healing blister sites in some bullous diseases, such as epidermolysis bullosa, prophyria cutanea tarda, and pemphigus. They may also develop at dermabrasion sites. Treatment by simple needle teasing is effective, and the use of abrasive cleaners may also be helpful.

Steatocystoma multiplex is an autosomal dominantly inherited disorder in which numerous small (no larger than 1 cm.) cystic intradermal nodules are found most commonly on the skin of the upper anterior midtrunk, axillae, scrotum, arms, and thighs. These small cysts contain an olive oil–like fluid, and sebaceous glandular elements are found in their thin squamous epithelial linings of 2 or 3 cell layers. Small lanugo hairs are also present in these cysts. Because of the large numbers of these harmless small lesions, their removal by excision is frequently impractical.

Dermoid cysts are congenital hamartomas, probably deriving from anomalous developmental inclusion of embryonic epidermis along embryonic cleft closure lines. Their most common sites are the lateral ends of the eyebrows and along the midline in the nasal root, sublingual, neck, sternal, perineal, scrotal, and sacral areas. They are of variable size, at times as large as 10 cm. They are subcutaneous in location, resemble steatocystomas or epidermoid cysts, and usually have sebaceous glandular, rudimentary hair follicle and sweat gland elements attached to their epithelial linings. At times, even cartilage and bone may be present. Dermoid cysts should be completely excised.

Fibrous Tumors

Cutaneous tags and *papillomas* occur in a variety of sizes and are soft and frequently pedunculated. They have been variously called cutaneous papilloma, fibroepithelial polyp, fibroma pendulum, acrochordon, soft fibroma (fibroma molle), and fibroma molluscum. They have a papillomatous loose, finely fibrillar dermal core and often show epidermal changes resembling those in seborrheic keratoses. Occasionally, lesions on thin stalks become twisted, inflamed, and infarcted. The lesions are easily removed by clipping the stalks and lightly electrodesiccating the bases, or by simple excision of the broad-based sessile lesions.

Dermatofibroma, histiocytoma, nodular subepidermal fibrosis, fibroma simplex, sclerosing hemangioma, noduli cutanei, and fibroma durum are various terms that have been applied to a very common benign nonencapsulated, reactive, lenticular intradermal nodular lesion composed of proliferating fibrocytes, irregularly arranged bundles of fine collagen fibers, capillary blood vessels, histiocytes, and mononuclear inflammatory cells in varying proportions. At times, the histiocytes in the lesions accumulate hemosiderin or become somewhat xanthomatized. The lesions are firm and range in color from pale skin hues through various shades of red, brown, and yellow. They occur most often on the lower extremities but also are seen on the arms and trunk in adults. They rarely exceed 1 or 2 cm. in size. It is believed that some of these lesions develop at sites of minor trauma such as mosquito bites. No treatment is usually needed unless excision becomes warranted for cosmetic or symptomatic reasons. Excision for histological establishment of the diagnosis may be necessary. Incomplete removal tends to be followed by recurrence.

Acquired digital fibrokeratoma is a smooth, pinkish, hyperkeratotic, well-demarcated, partly fleshy, hornlike projection emerging from a collarette of elevated skin on a finger. It may closely resemble a rudimentary supernumerary digit or small cutaneous horn. The core of the lesion contains thick collagen bundles. Excision at skin level with electrodesiccation of the base suitably removes this benign growth.

Pseudosarcomatous lesions are of interest because several clinically benign localized fibromatous proliferative lesions may show cellular changes and numerous mitoses that easily lead to mistaken diagnosis of fibrosarcoma. Among such pseudosarcomatous lesions are the following: (1) Nodular pseudosarcomatous fasciitis (subcutaneous pseudosarcomatous fibromatosis), which occurs most often on the upper extremities as a rapidly developing slightly painful nodule, 1 to 3 cm. in size, attached to deep fascia. (2) Infantile digital fibromatosis, which is a rare pseudosarcomatosis characterized by asymptomatic, firm, red, smooth nodules up to 1 cm. in size on the dorsal and lateral aspects of the distal phalanges of the toes and fingers in infancy and childhood. Surgical excision is the recommended treatment, but recurrences are reported to be frequent. (3) Atypical fibroxanthoma is a more common psuedosarcomatous lesion, which appears on chronically sun-exposed parts of the head and neck, particularly in the preauricular area in older persons. The tumor is a small, firm nodule which may show some crusting and can resemble basal cell epithelioma. The bizarre, highly atypical spindle or histiocytoid cells and giant cells of the tumor, with abundant mitoses, are separated from the epidermis by a thin zone of collagen. Treatment is by simple excision.

Dermatofibrosarcoma protuberans usually presents as a slowly growing, hard, nodular protuberant mass arising in the dermis, mostly on the trunk and thighs. It may be erythematous or slightly dusky in color and covered by smooth shiny epithelium, which gives a keloidal appearance. There may be complicating ulceration, infection, and scarring. As this local disorder becomes extensive, it may cause severe pain, contractures, and invalidism. Histologically, there is a characteristic "cartwheel" pattern of the hypercellular fibrous bundles in these nonencapsulated tumors which extend finger-like processes into adjacent subcutis and fascia. Mitotic figures may be numerous. Wide excision, including the deep fascia, is necessary to prevent recurrence. Long-standing, inadequately excised lesions have been known to metastasize [31].

Angiofibroma (Fig. 29-6) occurs on the lower central portions of the face and nose as firm, pale, sometimes telangiectatic fibrous or slightly erythematous papules, 1 to 3 mm. in size. Solitary lesions are inconsequential and can be removed for histological diagnosis and cosmetic purposes by superficial biopsy and electrodesiccation. When multiple, these lesions had in times past been called adenoma sebaceum (Pringle type) and are associated with the tuberous sclerosis complex (Bourneville's disease). The fibrous papules of tuberous sclerosis that occur on the forehead, cheeks, chin, and nasolabial folds can be distressing to the patient. Dermabrasion and limited excision offer some improvement [34]. Characteristic periungual and subungual protruding digitate fibromas (Koenen's periungual tumors) also are often present in this syndrome.

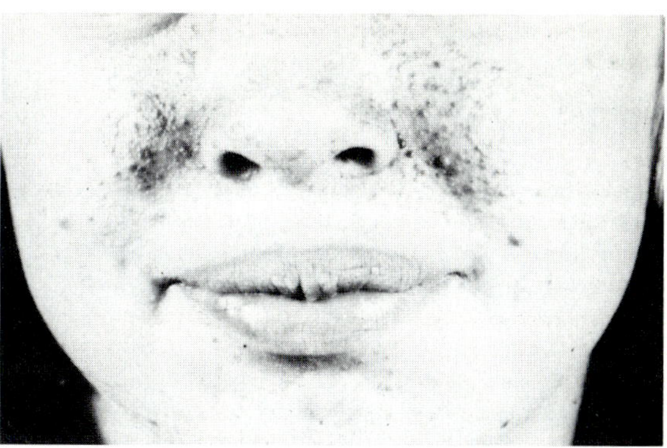

Fig. 29-6. Multiple angiofibromas (adenoma sebaceum, Pringle type) associated with tuberous sclerosis.

Myxoid cysts, less appropriately called synovial cysts in the past, occur particularly on the dorsa of the distal phalanges of the fingers, just proximal to the nails. They are smooth translucent nodules, usually less than 1 cm. in size, which are filled with a crystal-clear mucin or jelly-like fluid. They are not truly cysts because they are not encapsulated by any lining. Their myxoid contents simply compress the adjacent superficial dermis. Removal can be achieved by excision or electrodesiccation and curettage.

True myxomas are rare tumors, resembling embryonal mesenchyme, which show infiltrating growth and have uniform cellularity in contrast to the nonuniformity in mucinous cysts and mucinous degeneration. These tumors usually originate from deep fascia but in the skin may occur subungually. They require wide excision because of their high tendency to recur.

Miscellaneous Skin Tumors

Xanthomas represent a variety of skin lesions characterized by focal accumulations of lipid-laden histiocytes and giant cells with foamy cytoplasm. Often these lesions are associated with a variety of hyperlipoproteinemias, and at times the morphological type of xanthoma provides a clinical clue to the specific underlying lipidosis.

Xanthelasma palpebrarum, the most common kind of xanthoma, occurs on the eyelids, usually near the inner canthi. It presents in the form of soft, thin, yellowish, slightly raised, elongated plaques, often symmetrically distributed. In a little over half of individuals presenting with these lesions there is associated hyperlipoproteinemia, a high risk of early atherosclerosis, and the accompanying cardiovascular complications. In many cases, there is no apparent associated general disturbance of lipid metabolism, and xanthelasma is simply a local cosmetic problem. Extensive xanthelasma may also occur in biliary cirrhosis, with associated xanthomatosis, and in histiocytic disorders, such as reticulohistiocytoma cutis, Hand-Schüller-Christian disease, and xanthoma disseminatum. Treatment of the cosmetic problem is relatively easy as the lesions can be simply excised superficially, lightly electrodesiccated, or even treated topically with trichloracetic acid carefully applied with a flat toothpick applicator. A 20-year retrospective study on xanthelasma palpebrarum reviewed 68 patients; 34 percent of these patients had an increased serum cholesterol, but only 5 percent had a documented hyperlipemia [32]. Recurrence of the xanthelasma was noted in 40 percent of the patients who underwent excision of the xanthelasma; of the patients who had already had a recurrence of the xanthelasma after excision, a tertiary excision resulted in a recurrence of the xanthelasma in 60 percent of the patients.

Xanthoma planum resembles xanthelasma, but may involve extensive areas beyond the eyelids, especially palmar creases, axillae, flexor areas of the extremities, the neck, inner thighs, trunk, and shoulders.

Glomus tumor (glomangioma) is a benign vascular hamartomatous derivative of the glomus body, a normal intradermal arteriovenous anastomosis that arises from the normal neuromyoarterial glomus and presents as a skin-colored or bluish firm nodule a few millimeters to 1 to 2 cm. in diameter. It is usually exceedingly sensitive, and paroxysms of severe radiating pain are often triggered by the slightest manipulation of the lesion. Nonpainful glomus tumors, however, can also occur. The lesions may be single or multiple, and they most characteristically occur on the hands and feet, especially subungually. Glomus tumors have also been reported on the face [6]. Treatment of symptomatic lesions requires complete excision, which dramatically relieves the severe episodes of pain. Subungual highly sensitive lesions may be small and difficult to locate visibly. *Hemangiopericytoma* may resemble a painless glomus tumor, is quite rare and solitary, and may grow up to 10 cm. in size. Very rarely hemangiopericytoma may be malignant. Diagnosis requires histological examination.

Chondrodermatitis nodularis chronica helicis is a fairly common chronic inflammatory, painful, papular lesion on the upper rim of the ear, occurring with overwhelming preponderance in males. The lesions are very tender and firmly attached to the cartilage, which histologically shows focal degenerative change and surrounding perichondritis. Overlying hyperkeratosis and acanthosis are present. Clinical differentiation from solar keratosis or incipient carcinoma may be difficult. Simple excision with removal of the focus of underlying degenerated cartilage suffices for treatment.

Granular cell myoblastoma (Abrikossoff) or granular cell schwannoma is a usually solitary, but occasionally multiple, very hard, smooth, brownish-red to flesh-colored intracutaneous nodular tumor, ranging up to 3 cm. in size. Occasionally ulceration may occur, in which case it may clinically resemble squamous cell carcinoma. A third of the lesions occur on the tongue. Some may occur in internal organs, and rarely some behave in malignant fashion and metastasize. The lesions grow slowly and show characteristic, nonlipid-containing cells that resemble xanthoma cells, except that they have granular rather than foamy cytoplasm. Current opinion favors a relationship of these cells to Schwann rather than muscle cells. The lesions are best removed by simple complete excision. Recurrence is likely if excision is incomplete.

GENERALIZED DISORDERS

DISCOID LUPUS ERYTHEMATOSUS. This is a chronic dermatitis (Fig. 29-7) that results in extensive atrophic scarring. The lesions of chronic lupus erythematosus may occur on the scalp, face, lips, and extensor surface of the arms, and less often on the trunk. Although satisfactory treatment has been accomplished with topical steroid therapy and with antimalarial drugs such as chloroquine, there are many patients in whom discoid lupus erythematosis has caused persistent scarring and deformity of the nose and face that require the attention of the surgeon. The lesions are usually discrete, and surgical removal of the involved tissue permits successful reconstruction with the use of either free skin grafts or adjacent pedicle flaps after the activity of the lesion has been suppressed with the proper medical therapy. Past treatment of discoid lupus erythematosus with irradiation resulted in a significant incidence of squamous cell carcinoma over long periods of time. Mladick and colleagues [33] reported a case of squamous cell carcinoma developing on the face of a patient with discoid lupus erythematosus who had had no pre-

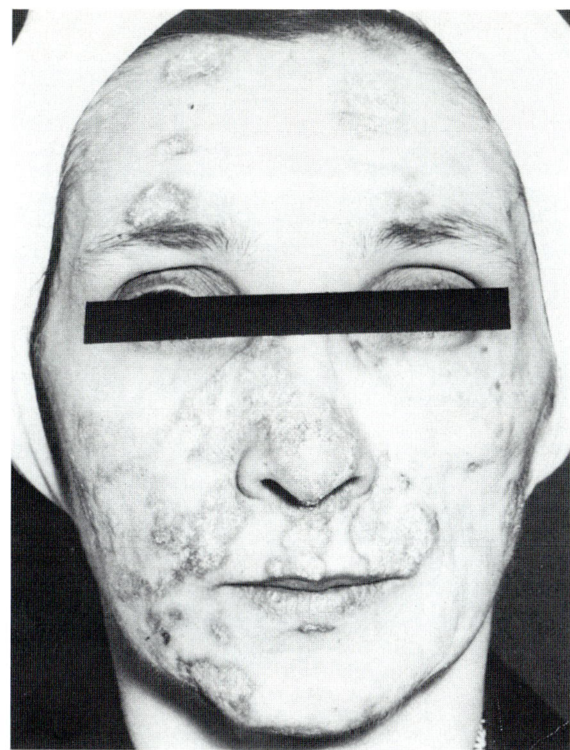

Fig. 29-7. Chronic discoid lupus erythematosus.

vious radiation therapy. Chronically active discoid lupus erythematosus lesions that result in severe atrophic scars complicated by secondary erosion and ulceration should be excised after conservative measures have controlled the activity in the lesions, because it is these long-standing chronically ulcerated scarred lesions that particularly have the risk of carcinoma.

SYSTEMIC LUPUS ERYTHEMATOSUS. This disease can vary from a mild to a severe and fatal disease. The activity of lupus erythematosus is often reflected by leukopenia, anemia, increased erythrocyte sedimentation rate, positive antinuclear factor tests and lupus erythematosus preparations, and positive cutaneous immunofluorescence tests. Low serum complement levels are also present with active vasculitis. After the systemic disease has been properly evaluated and controlled with appropriate therapy, the operative management of associated lesions has been safe. The use of skin grafts and of flaps in reconstructive surgery in the patient with systemic lupus erythematosus has been successful in the presence of steroid therapy. It is clear that the benefits of steroid therapy in suppressing the vasculitis far exceed the drawbacks of delayed wound healing when undertaking an operative procedure in patients with this disease. *Sjögren's syndrome* [5], consisting of xerostomia, keratoconjunctivitis sicca, and rheumatoid arthritis, has been associated in some instances with systemic lupus erythematosus. A patient with Sjögren's syndrome may occasionally appear with a parotid mass secondary to parotitis, which may be asymmetrical or unilateral. Awareness of this entity should avoid a disastrous set of events from the erroneous diagnosis of a parotid tumor without appreciation of systemic implications.

SYSTEMIC SCLERODERMA. This disease is seen most frequently in the acrosclerotic form, especially in women between the ages of 20 and 50 years. Since the initial process often begins in the distal extremities, with such vasospastic changes as Raynaud's phenomenon and sclerodactylia, the surgeon is often consulted initially. Sclerodactylia designates the characteristic hand changes consisting of hide-bound atrophic skin of the fingers held in partial flexion with limitation of motion in both flexion and extension. The cutaneous changes that lead to hide-bound atrophy and inelasticity of the skin, flexion deformities of the fingers, and ulcerations over joint and finger-tip surfaces demand extreme conservatism in treatment. In the early stages of the disease, medical sympathetic block has been of some value in many people's minds. Alpha-methyldopa and guanethidine have been used as sympatholytic agents with some success in early scleroderma. Systemic steroid therapy has not helped the course in this type of disease. Operative intervention in scleroderma requires careful judgment since the wound-healing characteristics of the tissues are quite tenuous. In the face of ulceration and gangrenous changes, the wound must be treated similarly to an ischemic ulcer, with careful debridement of the wound and resurfacing with split-thickness skin grafts when vascularity permits. Although operative procedures, such as skin flaps and skin grafting, have been successful in some patients [30], aggressive resection of tissue has been discouraging, since there may be progression of the necrosis following operative intervention. Although in the common acrosclerotic form of scleroderma steroid therapy has not been effective, there have been reports of cases of so-called mixed connective tissue disease which often present scleroderma-like features and do respond to steroid therapy [48].

SCLERODERMA CIRCUMSCRIPTUM. Morphea and bandlike lesions characterize this disease and often follow a dermatome pattern on the trunk or an extremity or appear in the paramedian region of the forehead, a condition referred to as scleroderma *en coup de sabre.* This latter lesion has been associated with progressive hemifacial atrophy in children. Severely deforming atrophy of skin, subcutaneous tissues, muscle, and bone may result from scleroderma. The eventual extent of the disease is unpredictable in its early stages, and spontaneous resolution may occur in some cases. The treatment must be conservative as long as there is active disease. When activity has ceased, the evidence suggests that subsequent operative intervention and correction of the deformity is safe and effective.

VON RECKLINGHAUSEN'S NEUROFIBROMATOSIS. Known also as multiple neurofibromatosis (Fig. 29-8), von Recklinghausen's neurofibromatosis is a hereditary disorder manifested by numerous cutaneous neurofibromas, café-au-lait pigmentation, and neurofibromas, producing bone lesions and intracranial and gastrointestinal symptoms, and is occasionally associated with mental retardation. The diagnosis is made on the basis of multiple neurofibromas, café-au-lait spots, and axillary freckling. Although the skin pigmentation may have been present since birth or early childhood, tumor formation is generally most aggressive at the time of puberty. The course of the disease is unpredictable. There is a rough correlation between the age of onset of the neurofibromas and the probable severity of the disease. Patients seen in youth with disfiguring masses may go on to progressive difficulties, including palsies and pituitary hypofunction. To the surgeon, the most common presenting form of neurofibromatosis in the young patient is facial deformity with neurofibromatous masses, which are soft, flaccid subcutaneous tumors. The treatment consists solely of excising the symptomatic lesions. Operative correction of these lesions is often only partial, since total excision of a large lesion in the facial area may create extensive deformity. The vascular pattern with large thin-walled veins obscures the anatomy and makes hemostasis difficult. In the face, bony involvement results in facial deformity and asymmetry, in addition to the soft tissue masses and thick unsightly gingiva. Although malignant degeneration in multiple neurofibromatosis has been reported, it is not feasible to excise all of the lesions in anticipation of malignant changes.

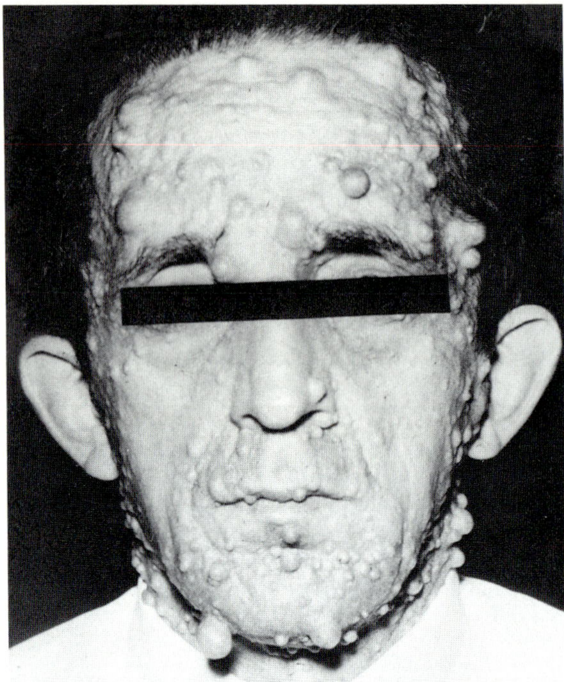

Fig. 29-8. Von Recklinghausen's neurofibromatosis.

XERODERMA PIGMENTOSUM. This is an inherited disorder characterized by unusual sensitivity to actinic rays. Normally, there are special cellular enzyme systems which can remove and replace ultraviolet damaged segments of DNA in which thymidine dimers have formed. In many cases of xeroderma pigmentosum, this DNA repair mechanism has been found deficient [7]. Theoretically, if the patient could be completely screened from actinic rays, the skin would be protected and no lesions would occur. The patient develops keratoses and spotty pigmentation which ultimately involve all of the exposed surfaces of the body. Basal cell carcinomas, squamous cell carcinomas, and malignant melanomas occur. Patients with xeroderma pigmentosum may develop all of the cutaneous malignant neoplasms known. Most of these patients succumb to this disease by early adulthood, but in the past decade careful protection from actinic rays, aggressive treatment with topical chemotherapeutic agents such as 5-fluorouracil, extensive dermabrasion, excision of malignant and premalignant lesions, and resurfacing with skin grafts have significantly improved the outlook of these patients.

DYSTROPHIC EPIDERMOLYSIS BULLOSA. This is a hereditary disease of the skin and mucosa characterized by the formation of bullae after minor trauma, which heal with scarring (Fig. 29-9). Excessive epidermal collagenase activity has been found in this disorder [15, 37]. This enzyme is believed to attack the most superficially situated papillary dermal collagen fibers at a level where blister formation often begins. Although the entire skin and mucosa of the hypopharynx and esophagus are subject to this break-

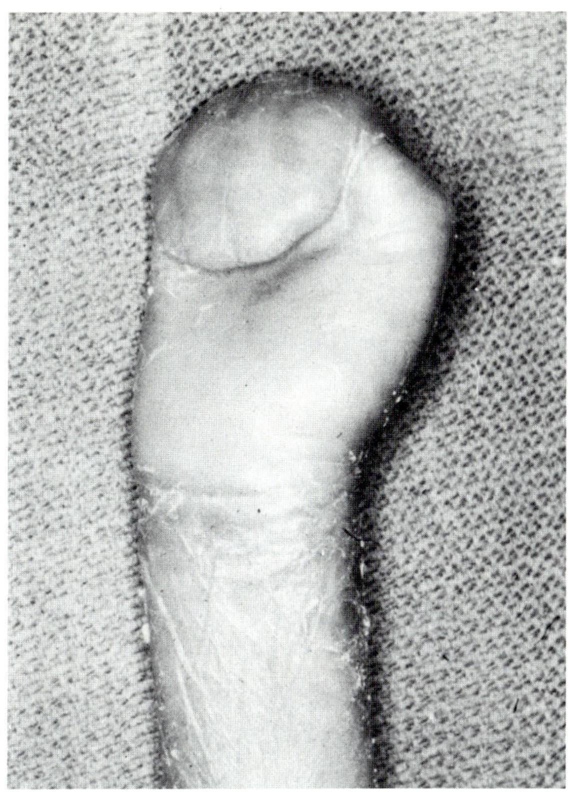

Fig. 29-9. Dystrophic epidermolysis bullosa in 6-year-old girl, showing entrapment of digits in scar cocoon.

down, scarring secondary to the recurrent minor trauma is most obvious on exposed surfaces. The typical deformity is progressive encasement of the digits in a cocoon of atrophic scar. Subsequent loss of the use of fingers and thumbs results. There are varying degrees of clinical expression of this entity; some patients have a relatively normal life, but most patients suffer greatly and require careful attention on the part of the family and treating physician and surgeon. To date, there is no basic therapy to remedy the defect that results in the formation of bullae. In some patients the vigorous use of topical steroid therapy has seemed to help reduce blistering and scar formation. Efforts to correct the severe hand deformities have been frustrating [21, 44]. Although the fingers are surprisingly mobile after being encased in a skin cocoon for many years, retention of the corrected position of the fingers after resection of the cocoon and resurfacing with skin grafts or flaps has been limited. Patients and the patients' families have been enthused over the operative correction of the finger and thumb deformities, but objectively there is loss of much of the correction with rescarring of the fingers. Our own experience with a modest number of patients has led us to correct the finger deformities repeatedly at intervals of several years, because the patients feel that it has improved their personal lives [58]. However, the patients must be realistically informed that the corrections are usually temporary.

CUTIS LAXA. This entity is a rare skin disorder in which the skin hangs in loose folds due to inadequacy of elastic fibers throughout the body, especially in the skin, lungs, and aorta [12, 42]. The defective elastic fibers in part account for the tendency to develop cardiorespiratory difficulties, which make the patient a significant operative risk. The systemic involvement in some patients contraindicates operative procedures. The primary presenting symptom is the extreme laxity of the skin, which causes the skin to hang in loose folds. The patient usually complains of appearing prematurely aged. Beighton, Bull, and Edgerton point out that the skin is not unduly fragile, wound healing is normal, and excessive bleeding is not a problem in these patients [3]. In the absence of cardiorespiratory difficulties, operative correction of the prematurely aged skin, excision of redundant tissues, and application of the standard rhytidectomy concepts have been gratifying.

PSEUDOXANTHOMA ELASTICUM. This condition is a heritable disorder in which the mechanically stressed skin (especially base and sides of neck and axillae) takes on the texture of plucked chicken skin [23, 28]. The loose, inelastic skin has a yellowish, pebbled thickening. Widespread severe arteriosclerosis commonly develops as early as the third decade of life.

CUTIS HYPERELASTICA. Known also as Ehlers-Danlos syndrome, this is a heritable disorder that should not be confused with cutis laxa [29]. Cutis hyperelastica is characterized by skin that is hyperextensible in a patient with extremely lax joints. These patients have a distinct fragility of the skin and blood vessels, and the patients report that their skin damages easily with frequent bruising and hematoma formation. In addition, these patients heal poorly, with gaping wounds that retract. The skin has a low tensile strength and does not hold suture material. The surgeon must clearly distinguish the patient with cutis hyperelastica from the patient with cutis laxa, since elective operative procedures are fraught with disaster.

VASCULITIS. Many disease processes have been termed some form of vasculitis, with the common denominator being an inflammation of blood vessels with subsequent thrombosis, ischemia, and necrosis of tissues. For clinical purposes, these diverse entities of necrotizing vasculitis can be classified according to the size of vessels and organ systems involved [54]. Pulmonary, renal, and gastrointestinal involvement may present severe problems in some forms. Large vessels are involved in periarteritis nodosa and temporal arteritis. Small vessel involvement occurs in such entities as Henoch-Schönlein's purpura and the Waterhouse-Friderichsen syndrome (where it is leukocytoclastic) and in granulomatous forms of angiitis such as Wegener's syndrome. The necrotic ulcers in various forms of necrotizing angiitis are ischemic lesions that are slow to debride and to granulate. Recognition of the particular disease entity as a systemic necrotizing vasculitis and the initiation of systemic treatment, often with steroid or immunosuppressive agents, are of primary concern [11]. If the systemic disease can be brought under control, careful debridement and operative management require attention similar to that required for ischemic tissues [20]. Withdrawal of steroid therapy and activation of the vasculitis are a serious threat to the successful management of necrotic lesions secondary to vasculitis.

Skin necrosis has occurred in many entities that result in increased coagulability or sludging of the blood. The Waterhouse-Friderichsen syndrome secondary to meningococcemia [47] and leg ulcers secondary to sicklemia are well known entities to surgeons [55]. Cases of skin necrosis secondary to cryoglobulinemia and other paraproteinemias have been reported [46]. The presence of cryoglobulin in the blood has been associated with multiple myeloma, various collagen diseases, and malignant lymphomas, as well as occurring idiopathically. Recent reports have documented the occurrence of skin necrosis following anticoagulant therapy, associated primarily with coumarin congeners [35, 39].

NECROBIOSIS LIPOIDICA. This condition is commonly associated with diabetes mellitus [4] (Fig. 29-10). Necrobiosis lipoidica may occur in patients without diabetes, and it may precede the clinical onset of diabetes mellitus. The lesion begins as a dusky red plaque that slowly progresses to atrophy of the skin; it may ulcerate in the center, secondary to minimal trauma. There is a distinct yellowish cast in the atrophic telangiectatic center of the lesion, which is characteristic. There seems to be a predilection for the pretibial area. The lesion is progressive, and control of diabetes and other medical modalities of treatment have not been effective. Some young women with necrobiosis lipoidica will present with the primary complaint of disfigurement of the anterior lower legs. Although not widely recommended, operative resection of the involved area and resurfacing with split-thickness skin grafts have been successful [13].

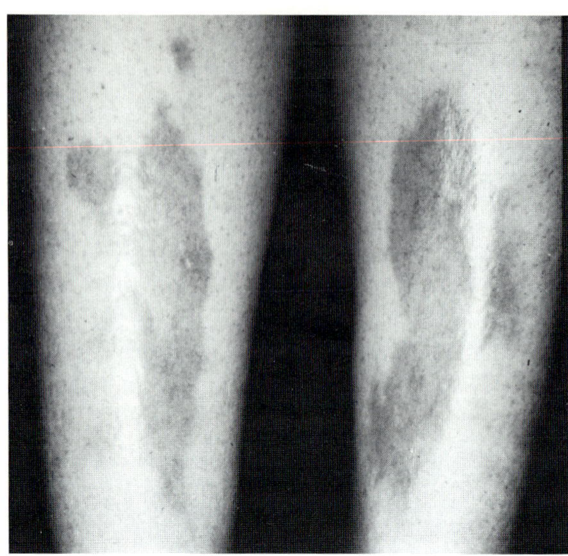

Fig. 29-10. Necrobiosis lipoidica on shins of 32-year-old female diabetic.

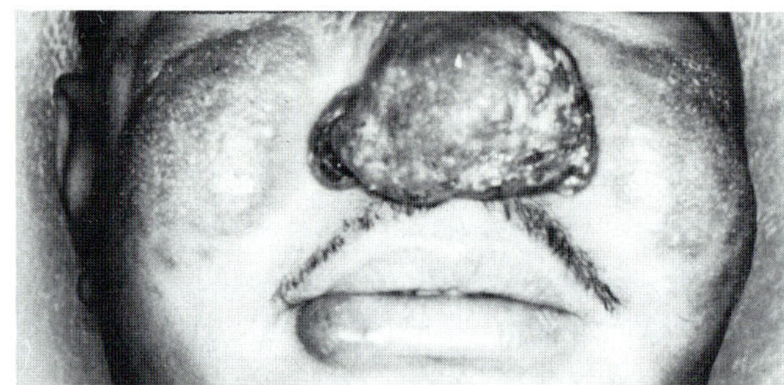

Fig. 29-11. Sarcoidosis with large nodular masses on cheeks and nose.

SARCOIDOSIS. The cutaneous manifestations of sarcoidosis (Fig. 29-11) may present initially either as erythema nodosum, reddish-tan translucent smooth papules on the eyelid and nasal margins, or as a variety of deeper indurated plaques and nodules. When the disease requires steroid therapy for control of systemic manifestations, the cutaneous lesions often respond in due time. Large disfiguring nodular masses may be excised after an adequate trial of medical therapy has failed to resolve the lesions [36].

MYCOSIS FUNGOIDES. This condition is a cutaneous form of lymphoma that presents with pruritic erythematous scaly patches, infiltrated plaques, and irregular skin nodules and ulcers (Fig. 29-12). The diagnosis is established by histological examination. The usually extensive skin involvement precludes any definitive

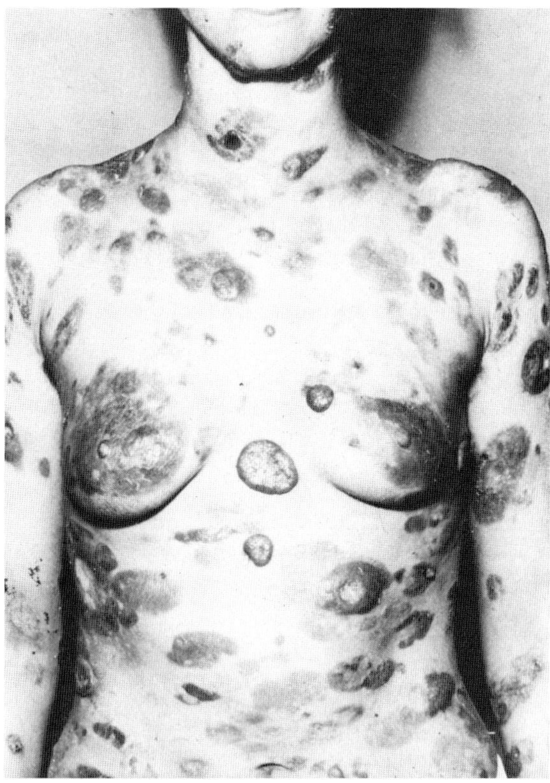

Fig. 29-12. Extensive mycosis fungoides in 20-year-old woman.

operative treatment except for purposes of diagnosis and for the management of ulcerations. Topical nitrogen mustard and electron beam therapy have achieved remissions, but ulcerations in the treated areas are frequent. In the presence of induration and skin breakdown, the therapeutic approach depends on the underlying pathology. Ulcerations may occur in the areas of lymphomatous involvement, in which case these lesions will respond to topical nitrogen mustard or electron beam therapy. If the ulceration is secondary to irradiation, then the lesion must be managed conservatively or with appropriate debridement and resurfacing with split-thickness skin grafts or adjacent pedicle flaps when feasible. In most instances when irradiation ulcerations have occurred, the extent of the disease and the extent of the previous electron beam therapy preclude the availability of adjacent tissues for pedicle flaps. Although mycosis fungoides is eventually a fatal disease, in some cases the course may be prolonged, and extensive debridement and resurfacing of ulcerated areas with skin grafts or pedicle flaps are appropriate when the lesions create sufficient discomfort.

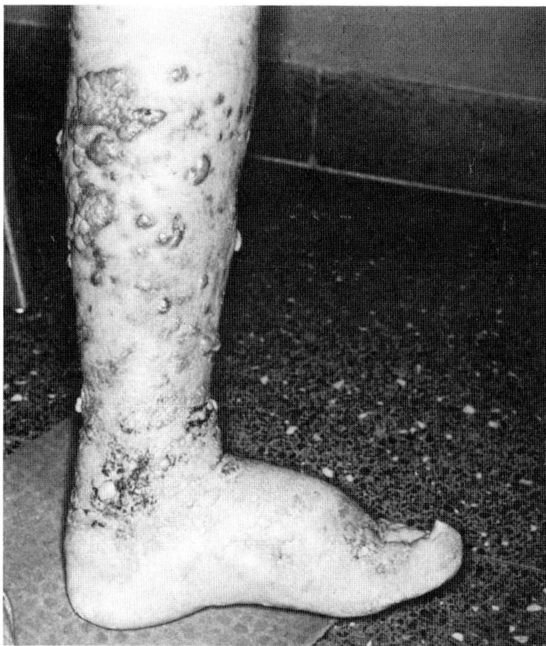

Fig. 29-13. Kaposi's sarcoma of 12-years' duration.

KAPOSI'S SARCOMA. This is a multicentric proliferative disorder of vasoformative tissue which ultimately follows a malignant neoplastic course (Fig. 29-13). The disease usually affects males, middle-aged or older, and has a predilection for people of Mediterranean racial origin, including Jews, Italians, Greeks, and Ugandans. The course of the disease is slow, and it is common to see survivals of more than 10 years after the onset of the disease. In the early stages, lesions present as purplish pigmented patches of purpura, with hemosiderosis most often on the feet and lower legs. Later indurated plaques and firm vascular polypoid excrescences appear. Chronic lymphedema also develops in affected areas. Radiotherapy has been the treatment of choice. The surgeon is often asked to manage ulceration secondary to radiotherapy. The tissue diagnosis of the ulceration to distinguish irradiation necrosis from active tumor is mandatory to determine whether further x-ray treatment or operative intervention is indicated. Surgical excision of the primary lesion in Kaposi's sarcoma is futile, since the disease is multicentric. In the early stages of the disease, the surgeon must have awareness of this entity and its features so that the mistaken diagnosis of localized sarcoma and inappropriate radical operative excision will not be undertaken.

ACNE VULGARIS. This is a common skin disorder seen in adolescents and young adults, consisting of seborrhea, small comedones, and inflammatory papulopustules or cysts. In some instances the disease can be severe, with deep cysts and burrowing sinus tracts resulting in extensive scarring of the face, back, and anterior chest. The most severe form of cystic acne (acne conglobata) can be disabling, with undermining of the skin of the forehead, temporal regions, cheeks, and chin, and with extensive pockets of a sanguinopurulent exudate. The usual pathogenic organisms are not found in these lesions. Incision of the cystic lesions with a fine pointed blade or electric needle will drain the cysts and reduce the inflammation which produces the scarring. Dietary control, which in the past was an unpleasant ritual for patients with acne, is not thought to be important today. Topical medications with preparations containing sulfur, benzoyl peroxide, or vitamin A acid, and careful skin hygiene, combined with long-term administration of systemic antibiotics such as tetracycline, have been helpful in controlling the disease. Ultraviolet rays are also beneficial. Although superficial x-ray therapy had been effective in controlling acne, the consequent atrophy of the skin and the increased risk of skin carcinomas have rendered this mode of therapy obsolete.

After the patient with acne has been under an optimal dermatological regimen, dermabrasion in selected cases has been an effective tool in reducing the unsightliness of the acne scarring. Activity of the disease is not a contraindication to dermabrasion, and in some instances the dermabrasion seems to alleviate active pustules. Although frequently the objective improvement in the quality of the skin is not dramatic (perhaps 60 percent improvement), in most instances the results have yielded sufficient improvement in the appearance of the skin to gratify the patient. Shallow, sharply demarcated pits appear to benefit the most from dermabrasion. The dermabrasion essentially reduces the depth of the acne scar, and the resultant skin contracture further decreases the depth of the scar. Shadows are thereby minimized, and the patients are able to effectively disguise the scarred acne skin with appropriate cosmetics. Patients with olive or darker complexions are subject to depigmentation or hyperpigmentation after healing of the dermabrasion, so that the coloring of the skin may be blotchy. If the patient and the surgeon agree that the blotchy appearance will present less of a problem than the degree of pitting and scarring, dermabrasion may be undertaken so that the judicious use of cosmetics will yield a pleasant skin texture. Females are willing to use cosmetic make-up to disguise the blotchiness sooner than males, who consider make-up inappropriate; this must be taken into consideration in selecting the appropriate patients for dermabrasion. When the limitations of dermabrasion and the potential hazards of disturbed pigmentation are taken into consideration by the surgeon and patient, dermabrasion is a major means of alleviating the suffering of patients with acne vulgaris scarring.

Patients with severe cystic acne may develop extensive areas of undermining with epithelium-lined tunnels which harbor a sanguinopurulent material. These lesions do not heal and are a continuous source of purulent discharge that is unpleasant and embarrassing for the patient. Unroofing of the epithelium-lined tunnels helps to control the lesions and improves the gross appearance of the skin to the satisfaction of the patient.

ACNE ROSACEA AND RHINOPHYMA. Acne rosacea occurs primarily in middle-aged individuals in the flush areas of the face. The nose, the medial aspects of the cheeks adjacent to the nose, and the chin exhibit patulous, dilated follicular openings, with a lobulated dermal fibrosis that takes on a purplish hue with superficial large telangiectasis. This disease has been associated with alcoholics because alcohol and spicy foods enhance the vasodilatation of the central face in those patients predisposed to acne rosacea.

Rhinophyma (Fig. 29-14), severe acne rosacea of the nose, carries the stigma of alcoholism as popularized in literature. It is frequently the rhonophyma that is the source of embarrassment for patients with acne rosacea, causing them to seek medical help. Understanding of the disease and control of the underlying process with an optimal dermatological regimen are critical. Once rhinophyma is established, operative treatment with dermabrasion, surgical shaving of the thickened skin combined with dermabrasion, and total excision of the skin of the nose and

Fig. 29-14. Rhinophyma.

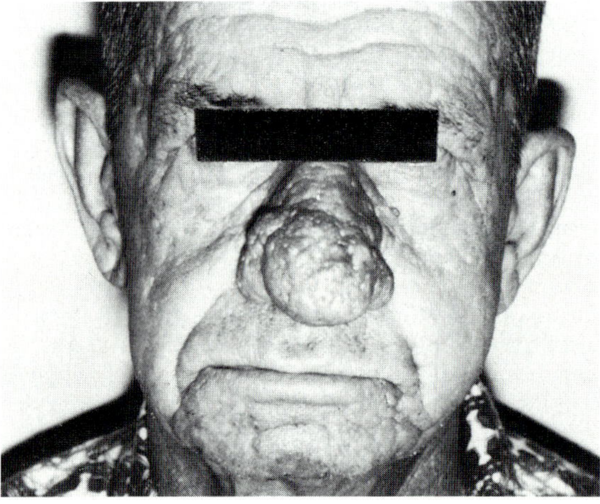

resurfacing with skin grafts are each effective treatments for this disease entity.

Although some surgeons have advocated excision of the diseased skin on the nose, our preference remains to shave the rhinophyma in most cases. The deep pores allow shaving of the thickened skin to a depth that leaves sufficient appendages for epithelialization. We have been unable to describe this level definitively, but in the thickened skin shaving may be carried to a depth beyond that which one would ordinarily estimate without experience with this disease entity. Shaving is usually supplemented with dermabrasion to smooth the chiseled surface and to reduce the thickened skin on the medial cheeks adjacent to the nose.

After shaving and dermabrasion, hemostasis is aided by the application of a gauze saturated with epinephrine in saline 1:200,000. Recently we have applied a porcine graft dressing to the denuded nose rather than an antibiotic ointment and a greased gauze. Early experience suggests that the epithelialization under the porcine graft is comfortable and clean. After the healing of the shaved nose, contracture of the newly epithelialized surface further enhances the reduction of the bulbous nose.

When the surgeon chooses to excise the rhinophymatous skin, care should be taken to preserve the underlying perichondrium of the lateral cartilages for vascular support of a skin graft and to preserve the cartilage, which gives the natural contour of the nose. The alar rim should be incised external to the nares in order to preserve the normal alar contour. Occasionally, excisions of the alar base are helpful in reducing the elongated nose. Resurfacing of the rhinophymatous nose after excision is best done with a full-thickness skin graft or thick split-thickness graft from a blush area when feasible. In some instances it might be necessary to obtain a skin graft from a nonblush area, which is our primary objection to grafting in preference to shaving. The texture and color match of skin from the arm or trunk are rarely satisfactory compared with the natural blushed texture of the face, which is exaggerated in these patients.

ALOPECIA. The most common form of alopecia is early male pattern baldness. Although surgeons have been correcting hair defects on the scalp for many years for patients with congenital absence of hair-bearing skin, burn scars, or traumatic scalp loss, recent popularity of hair follicle transplants to correct male pattern baldness has brought a rash of patients to the dermatologist and plastic surgeon seeking correction of baldness.

Prior to undertaking any procedure, the differential diagnosis of alopecia must be considered. *Alopecia areata* consists of circumscribed patches of total baldness with otherwise normal scalp skin. Hair at the edges of active bald patches is easily extracted, and the root ends can be seen to taper to a point. Alopecia areata in children tends to be more extensive, and the return of hair is less likely. After puberty it is usually a self-limited disease, and the regrowth of hair in bald areas commonly occurs. The disease is not entirely predictable and may progress to permanent hair loss. Hair transplants in a patient with active alopecia areata would be injudicious. *Cicatricial alopecias* present bald patches associated with areas of atrophy scarring. They occur after various disorders, including fungal and other infections and in chronic discoid lupus erythematosus. After cicatricial alopecia has become inactive, it is appropriate in selected cases to undertake either excision of the scarred area or hair transplants if the vascularity of the tissue appears adequate to support such transplants.

Three operative procedures are available – insertion of plugs of scalp containing hair follicles, transplantation of strips of scalp hair, or transferring local scalp flaps from the hair-bearing parietal region to the anterior scalp. The effectiveness of these procedures in satisfactorily correcting male pattern baldness is an unanswered question in our minds. We have had sufficient experience to raise our skepticism over the ultimate success of these procedures. The plug technique consists of removing cylinders of hairless scalp with a sharp 4-mm. round punch. Hemostasis is enhanced by cutting the cylinder with the punch and placing a cotton swab dipped in an epinephrine solution 1:200,000 into the defect while obtaining the hair-containing plugs. The plugs containing follicles are then obtained with a 5-mm. punch from the lateral and posterior hair-bearing scalp. Instruments are available which facilitate taking plugs at an angle parallel to the hair follicle. On placing the plugs, the shafts of hair should be oriented away from the direction in which the hair will lie in order to camouflage the scalp scar. Planning the area of implantation, including the hair styling, allows some camouflage of the plugs with the existing hair. Strips of hair no wider than 1 cm. can also be implanted in the hairless scalp to give a thick hairline. In the totally hairless area of the apex of the skull, it has been our experience that placement of plugs and strips has not given a natural appearance, and we have seen a significant number of patients who are dissatisfied. We have also not been able to offer these patients anything beyond further hair transplants to attempt to thicken the hair or to cover up the spottiness of the transplants. Enthusiasm for this procedure on the part of other plastic surgeons and dermatologists implies that their experience has been more favorable than our own. We feel obligated to offer a word of caution that many males who have had hair follicle transplants by plugs and by strips have been dissatisfied and have been dismayed to learn that there is no significant way of improving their situation once the procedures have been carried out. Our own position in this regard is one of extreme caution.

HYPERHIDROSIS. Some individuals are prone to hyperhidrosis, excessive sweating on the palms of the hands, the soles of the feet, and the axillae. Although these patients actually perspire more all over the body than the average person, these areas usually represent the focus of their complaint. Continued wetness of the hands, feet, and axillae is a source of great discomfort and extreme social embarrassment to the patient. Although these patients are somewhat improved in cool dry climates, even under these conditions the perspiration is excessive, and there is literally a dripping of perspiration from the axillae. The condition may be improved with the usual antiperspirants, but the improvement is often insignificant. With excessive hyperhidrosis of the feet and hands, medical sympathetic block or surgical sympathectomy has been effective in carefully selected patients. Axillary hyperhidrosis has been treated effectively by wide elliptical excision of the apex of the axilla, which includes most of the eccrine sweat glands, which are concentrated in the axillary vault [45, 51].

The sweat glands extend in some areas below the dermis into the subcutaneous tissues, and for this reason some surgeons have advocated removing the subcutaneous tissues as well. It is more likely that any benefit from removing the subcutaneous tissue is derived from denervation of the remaining eccrine glands. On this basis we have chosen simply to do as wide an elliptical excision as feasible to permit primary closure and to undermine the adjacent tissues just below the dermis to adequately denervate the remaining eccrine glands and to facilitate skin closure.

EXCESSIVE HAIRINESS. In young women this condition is of particular concern when present on the face, especially the upper lip or chin. The patient may require a medical work-up to rule out endocrine abnormalities, if this seems warranted. If there is no systemic basis for hirsutism, diathermy or electrolysis is a permanent means of hair removal, but these procedures do require the skill of an experienced operator to avoid scarring. Temporary removal of the hair is accomplished with the use of depilatories or an epilating wax, which is acceptable in minor cases. Bleaching is also a means for reducing the conspicuousness of unwanted hair about the face. Shaving is an effective approach, despite the inaccurate belief that repeated shaving causes thickening of the hair.

SKIN INFECTIONS

HIDRADENITIS SUPPURATIVA. This inflammatory disease of the apocrine glands presents most frequently as deep recurrent abscesses in the axillae, which may result in scarred deep sinus tracts, fluctuant draining abscesses, and excruciating pain with limitation of abduction of the shoulder. Although seen most commonly in young females in the axillae, it also occurs in the groin and perineum and in the areolae. Early acute cases may be treated with local therapy, such as incision and drainage of the abscess, followed by control with long-term antibiotic therapy. However, once the disease entity is established with deep scarring and sinus tracts, the only appropriate therapy is surgical excision of the involved area. These patients are too frequently not offered the alternative of operative management of this disease until an unpleasant and rather prolonged course of conservative treatment for abscesses and pain has elapsed. Rarely must patients be convinced of the need for operative intervention, since they have usually suffered extensively with the discomforts and unpleasantness of this disease. Culture of the purulent discharge and appropriate antibiotic therapy for a period of at least 10 days prior to operative intervention are important.

Excision of all of the involved tissue is the ultimate goal of the operative procedure. Primary closure can be accomplished with large defects as pointed out by Pollock, Virnelli, and Ryan [40], but if necessary the surgeon must not compromise the excision in order to accomplish primary closure. Large areas of involvement (8 × 15 cm.) can be excised and closed primarily if the wound is closed with heavy retention sutures to approximate the axillary fascia and subcutaneous tissues and if a careful subcuticular skin closure is accomplished (Fig. 29-15). When primary closure is not feasible, split-thickness skin grafts and immobilization of the arm with Velpeau dressings would be the next choice. We have not found it necessary to use any type of skin flap to accomplish skin coverage in the axillary vault after excision of hidradenitis suppurativa.

When the disease has extended beyond the axilla onto the chest wall or onto the upper arm, it is preferable to excise the involved areas entirely and apply split-thickness skin grafts. It has been our practice to undertake the excision and grafting on one axilla at a time so that the patient will not be totally disabled during the healing period. When the surgeon can clearly excise and close the wounds primarily, it is feasible to undertake the correction of the disease in both axillae in one operative procedure. Good healing and lack of wound infection are usual when all of the diseased tissue is properly excised. If the scarred sinuses or involved glands are not completely excised, then delayed wound healing and infection are common.

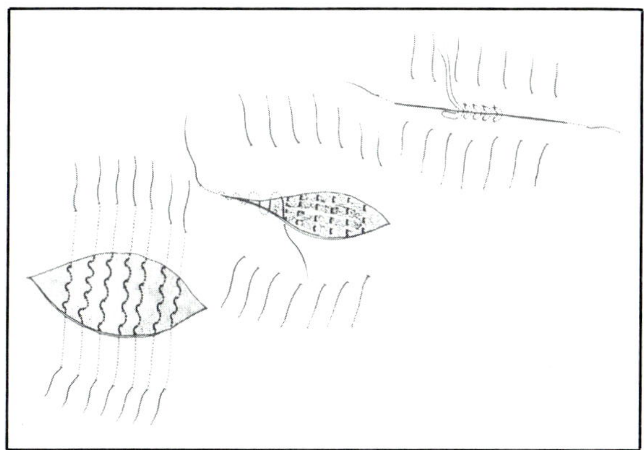

Fig. 29-15. Excision and primary closure of axillary skin up to 8 × 15 cm. (measured in contracted state) can be excised. Retention sutures of #1 nylon are placed about 4 cm. from the wound edges, picking up the axillary fascia or two or three points (left). A 2-0 nylon subcuticular suture is then inserted (center), followed by interrupted 4-0 nylon vertical mattress sutures (right). (Reproduced, with permission, from W. J. Pollock, et al. Plast. Reconstr. Surg. *49:22, 1972.)*

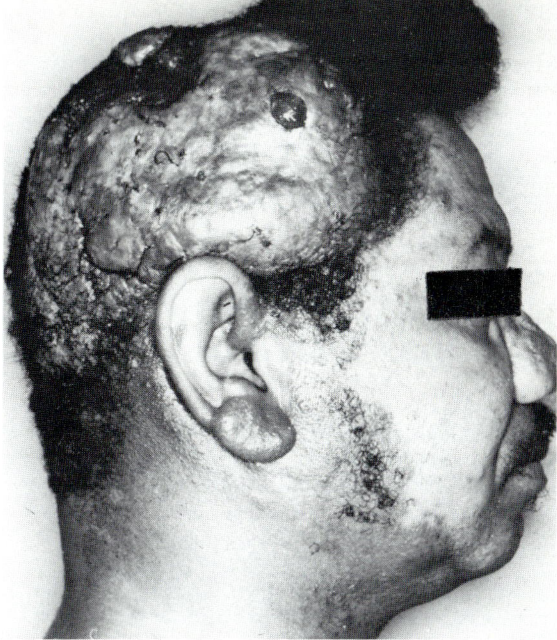

Fig. 29-16. Dissecting cellulitis of scalp.

Since these patients have had limited abduction of the shoulder for long periods prior to the operative intervention, exercises to abduct the arm must be stressed, and the patients should be followed until full abduction is accomplished.

DISSECTING CELLULITIS OF THE SCALP. Known also as perifolliculitis chronica abscedens et suffodiens, this disease (Fig. 29-16) occurs most often in black men and is a disease entity of the scalp similar to hidradenitis suppurativa. The scalp is involved with a perifolliculitis resulting in burrowing, encysted epithelium-lined tracts, with associated chronic infection and granulation tissue. The conservative management of this extensive folliculitis has been discouraging. The only effective treatment, once this disease entity is established, is excision of the scarred, infected areas and resurfacing with split-thickness skin grafts or skin flaps from the adjacent scalp if the disease is limited.

PYODERMA GANGRENOSUM. Multiple skin abscesses with necrosis and undermining ulcerations occur in this necrotizing lesion of the skin often associated with ulcerative colitis (50 percent of patients). It has been reported to occur in association with other gastrointestinal disorders (diverticulosis, regional enteritis, peptic ulcer disease, hepatitis, and carcinoid tumor) as well as rheumatoid arthritis, pulmonary diseases, and hematological disorders. In 20 percent of the cases of pyoderma gangrenosum, no systemic disease is evident [24, 38, 56]. No specific organism or combination of organisms has been identified with this disease entity, although frequently *Proteus* and other gram-negative organisms and beta-hemolytic streptococci have been cultured from these wounds. Systemic and topical antibiotic therapy has been of some use in controlling the active disease process. It appears today that the basic lesion is not a primary infection but is a necrotizing cutaneous equivalent of ulcerative colitis, with rapidly developing hemorrhagic liquefying tissue necrosis of the skin. It is characterized by ulceration surrounded by bluish hemorrhagic cribriform edges. The course is protracted and in some instances fulminant. Careful control of pathogenic bacteria with culture and sensitivity tests preceding antibiotic therapy, associated with conservative debridement of the necrotic tissues, has been successful in many instances. It appears important to debride only the grossly necrotic tissue and not to incise the adjacent intact tissues to avoid extension of the disease beyond the operative debridement. Local and systemic steroid therapy and systemic sulfones with their antiinflammatory effects have been helpful in this disease entity as in ulcerative colitis.

LUPUS VULGARIS. Although once common, this disease (Fig. 29-17) is now a rare form of cutaneous tuberculosis; it can produce slowly progressive destruction of soft tissues followed by atrophic scarring. Active areas of the disease are studded with superficial intradermal small reddish-tan lupus nodules. Lupus vulgaris is a specific form of cutaneous tuberculosis to be distinguished from scrofuloderma (cold abscess), either primary in the skin or extending to it secondarily from tuberculosis of bone or lymph nodes. Lupus vulgaris is controlled with appropriate antituberculosis chemotherapy (long-term isoniazid administration). If resultant scarring is a problem, excision of the lesion, with prior antituberculous therapy, is effective and safe [2]. Treatment of lupus vulgaris with irradiation is now obsolete. It is now appreciated that irradiation for treatment of lupus vulgaris contributed to the development of squamous cell carcinomas in these areas. Seventy-four percent of the patients seen by Griffith in 1957 [19] with a carcinoma in the area of a lupus vulgaris lesion had previous radiotherapy. In a group of patients with healed lupus vulgaris without previous radiotherapy, there was a 2 percent incidence of carcinoma. Rees [43] has demonstrated that there is an incidence of carcinoma in the unhealed lupus vulgaris lesion, even in the absence of irradiation.

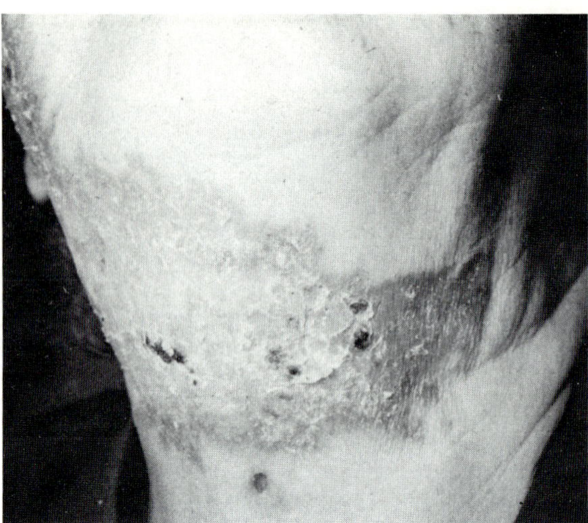

Fig. 29-17. Lupus vulgaris of 20-years' duration, with atrophic scarring and active lupus nodules at edges.

LEPROSY. This disease affects primarily the skin and peripheral nerves to produce deformities that are of particular interest to the plastic surgeon. The classic picture of lepromatous leprosy incorporates the lepra facies, which has become a repulsive concept in our culture. Enna and Delgado [16] indicate three prerequisites before undertaking facial reconstruction in leprosy – (1) disease inactivity, (2) intact healthy skin, and (3) a stabilized deformity. The authors point out the common deformities that are typical of the face in leprosy: (1) megalolobule of the external ear, (2) loss of eyebrows, (3) nasal deformity, (4) sagging and wrinkled redundant facial skin, and (5) lagophthalmos. Correction of the nasal deformity associated with leprosy has been described in an experience with 86 patients, utilizing skin grafts to restore the nasal lining [1]. The problems encountered in leprosy subsequent to peripheral neuropathy have resulted in extensive literature on the management of hand deformities. The most commonly presenting dysfunction of the hand in the leprosy patient is ulnar nerve palsy, with inability to fully extend the fingers for grasp, and median nerve palsy, with the inability of the thumb to oppose.

NOMA. Cancrum oris (noma) is a destructive infection of the face in African or Asian children under 5 years of age; this condition results in extensive unilateral loss of the lips, oral commissure, nose, cheek, and occasionally lower eyelid. The bones of the maxilla, nose, zygoma, and mandible may be eroded, and the masticatory muscle involvement often causes trismus [14].

FINGERNAIL INFECTIONS. Disturbances of the nail are frequent sources of concern for patients. Trauma, fungal infections, and psoriasis are the most common causes of nail deformities that lead patients to seek medical advice. Treatment of an *acute paronychia* consists of adequate drainage. The *chronic paronychia* presents a different problem. The surgeon should first look for a subungual abscess associated with a chronic paronychia. The small area of pus under the nail adjacent to the paronychia can be subtle and can result in a recurrent paronychia, requiring repeated operative drainage and a search for an exotic causative organism. When the subungual abscess is recognized, unroofing the nail bed results in a certain solution to the problem. In the true chronic paronychia without a subungual component, *candidiasis* is the usual offender. The diabetic and patients whose hands are constantly wet – housewives, waitresses, bartenders, or dentists – are susceptible to chronic paronychia associated with candidiasis. The treatment of chronic paronychia associated with candidiasis is to remedy the wetness of the hands, local application of nystatin, and flushing the crevices and pockets under the nail with acetone to eliminate moisture. Congenital paronychia (Jadassohn-Lewandowski syndrome) may require excision of the nail bed and nail plate, which can be resurfaced with split-thickness grafts [53].

WART VIRUS INFECTION. This results in well-circumscribed hyperkeratotic verrucose papules, nodules, spicules, or spiny clusters on the skin. On pressure-bearing plantar surfaces, large thick overlying callus accumulations can cause tenderness and pain on walking. In intertriginous and genital areas, such infections yield vegetating, gray or pinkish cauliflower-like papillomatous soft excrescences and confluent masses called "condylomata acuminata." These lesions are at times macerated and secondarily infected and inflamed with malodorous purulent secretions developing in their crevices. Giant condyloma acuminata (Buschke-Löwenstein tumor) show pseudoepitheliomatous hyperplasia and may be clinically and histologically difficult to differentiate from epidermoid carcinoma. Plantar warts can be difficult to differentiate from corns and calluses. Black specks of degenerating hemorrhage and honeycomb patterning in the overlying hyperkeratosis are clinical signs that favor the diagnosis of wart. *Tuberculosis verrucosa cutis* (prosector's wart) may mimic the common wart but usually has some inflammatory reaction at its base and may show some exudation as well. Common warts and especially plantar warts are not suitably treated by excision and suturing, for aggravated recurrences along the suture line from inoculated virus are common. Small lesions are best managed dermatologically with either curettage and electrodesiccation or liquid nitrogen. A host of other dermatological approaches with such agents as caustics, vesicants, and formalin are available for the management of warts in addition to temporizing and suggestion that may result in suitable clearing. The surgeon is best advised to avoid futile attempts at clean excision. Massive condylomata acuminata at times may require some surgical excision as part of the management program.

MOLLUSCUM CONTAGIOSUM. This is a pox virus infection of the epidermis which results in the formation of translucent, umbilicated, smooth, pale semiglobular papules 1 to 3 mm. in size. Rarely such lesions may become large (1 to 2 cm.) and develop an inflammatory base, hyperkeratosis, and secondary infection; the lesions then resemble carcinoma or other skin tumors. Lesions in adults occur especially about the genital area and may be venereally transmitted. There is a characteristic histological picture in which infected cells develop huge cytoplasmic basophilic inclusions which compress the cell nucleus to a peripheral crescent. The lesions are best treated by curettage or light electrodesiccation and not by surgical excision.

REFERENCES

1. Antia, N. H., and Pandya, N. J. Surgical treatment of the nasal deformities of leprosy. *Plast. Reconstr. Surg.* 60:768, 1977.
2. Barker, L. P. Lupus vulgaris occurring in a skin graft. *Arch. Dermatol. Syph.* 54:758, 1946.
3. Beighton, P., Bull, J. C., and Edgerton, M. T. Plastic surgery in cutis laxa. *Br. J. Plast. Surg.* 23:285, 1970.
4. Binkley, G. W. Dermopathy in the diabetic syndrome. *Arch. Dermatol.* 92:625, 1965.
5. Block, K. J., Buchanan, W. W., Wohl, M. J., and Bunim, J. J. Sjögren's syndrome: Clinical, pathological, and serological study of 62 cases. *Medicine* 44:187, 1965.
6. Charles, N. Multiple glomus tumors of the face and eyelid. *Arch. Ophthalmol.* 94:1283, 1976.
7. Cleaver, J. E. DNA damage and repair in light sensitive human skin disease. *J. Invest. Dermatol.* 54:181, 1970.
8. Cohen, N., Plaschkes, Y., Pevzner, S., and Loewenthal, M. Review of 57 cases of keratoacanthoma. *Plast. Reconstr. Surg.* 49:138, 1972.
9. Dellon, A. L., Chretien, P. B., and Peck, G. L. Successful treatment of Darier's disease by partial thickness removal of skin. *Plast. Reconstr. Surg.* 59:823, 1977.
10. Dellon, A. L., Edelson, R. L., and Chretien, P. B. Defining the malignant potential of the giant pigmented nevus. *Plast. Reconstr. Surg.* 57:611, 1976.
11. DePalma, R. G., Moskowitz, R. W., and Holden, W. D. Peripheral ischemia and collagen disease: Clinical manifestations, diagnosis, and treatment. *Arch. Surg.* 105:313, 1972.
12. Dingman, R. O., Grabb, W. C., and Oneal, R. M. Cutis laxa congenita – generalized elastosis. *Plast. Reconstr. Surg.* 44:431, 1969.
13. Dubin, B. J., and Kaplan, E. N. Surgical treatment of necrobiosis lipoidica, diabetocorum. *Plast. Reconstr. Surg.* 60:421, 1977.
14. Durrani, K. M. Surgical repair of defects from noma (cancrum oris). *Plast. Reconstr. Surg.* 52:629, 1973.
15. Eisen, A. Z. Human skin collagenase: Relationship to the pathogenesis of epidermolysis bullosa dystrophica. *J. Invest. Dermatol.* 52:449, 1969.
16. Enna, C. D., and Delgado, D. Surgical correction of common facial deformities due to leprosy. *Plast. Reconstr. Surg.* 42:422, 1968.
17. Given, K., Pickrell, K., and Smith, D. Dermal cylindroma (turban tumor). *Plast. Reconstr. Surg.* 59:582, 1977.
18. Graham, J. H., and Helwig, E. B. Bowen's disease and its relationship to systemic cancer. *Arch. Dermatol.* 80:133, 1959.
19. Griffith, B. H. The surgical treatment of lupus vulgaris and lupus carcinoma. *Plast. Reconstr. Surg.* 20:155, 1957.

20. Hill, E. J. Skin grafting in periarteritis nodosa. *Plast. Reconstr. Surg.* 15:186, 1955.
21. Horner, R. L., Wiedel, J. D., and Bralliar, F. Involvement of the hand in epidermolysis bullosa. *J. Bone Joint Surg. [Am.]* 53:1347, 1971.
22. Kaplan, E. N. The risk of malignancy in large congenital nevi. *Plast. Reconstr. Surg.* 53:421, 1974.
23. Kaplan, E. N., and Henjyoji, E. Y. Pseudoxanthoma elasticum: A dermal elastosis with surgical implications. *Plast. Reconstr. Surg.* 58:595, 1976.
24. Kelley, M. L. Skin lesions associated with chronic ulcerative colitis. *Am. J. Dig. Dis.* 7:255, 1962.
25. Kisner, W. H., and Hendrix, J. H., Jr. Keratosis palmaris et plantaris. *Plast. Reconstr. Surg.* 51:424, 1973.
26. Kopf, A. W., and Andrade, R. Benign Juvenile Melanoma. In the *Year Book of Dermatology* (1965–1966 Series). Chicago: Year Book, 1966.
27. Lanier, V. C., Jr., Pickrell, K. L., and Georgiade, N. G. Congenital giant nevi: Clinical and pathological considerations. *Plast. Reconstr. Surg.* 58:48, 1976.
28. Lorincz, A. L. Pseudoxanthoma Elasticum. In Demis, D. J., Crounse, R. G., McGuire, J., and Dobson, R. L. (Eds.), *Clinical Dermatology.* Hagerstown: Harper & Row, 1972. 1:Section 4, Unit 2.
29. Lorincz, A. L. Ehlers-Danlos Syndrome (Cutis Hyperelastica). In Demis, D. J., Crounse, R. G., McGuire, J., and Dobson, R. L. (Eds.), *Clinical Dermatology.* Hagerstown: Harper & Row, 1972. 1:Section 4, Unit 3.
30. Losken, H. W., Davies, D., and Gordon, W. Coverage of scalp and skull defect in a patient with the systemic form of scleroderma. *Plast. Reconstr. Surg.* 51:212, 1973.
31. McPeak, C. J., Cruz, T., and Nicastri, A. D. Dermatofibrosarcoma protuberans: An analysis of 86 cases – five with metastasis. *Ann. Surg.* 166:803, 1967.
32. Mendelson, B. C., and Masson, J. Xanthelasma: Follow-up on results after surgical excision. *Plast. Reconstr. Surg.* 58:535, 1976.
33. Mladick, R. A., Pickrell, K. L., Thorne, F. L., and Hall, J. H. Squamous cell cancer in discoid lupus erythematosus. *Plast. Reconstr. Surg.* 42:497, 1968.
34. Morgan, J. E., and Mulliken, J. B. Dermabrasion and limited excision of the fibrous papules of tuberous sclerosis. *Plast. Reconstr. Surg.* 59:124, 1977.
35. Nalbandian, R. M. Skin necrosis induced by coumarin congeners. *Excerpta Medica* 2:58, 1971.
36. O'Brien, P. Sarcoidosis of the nose. *Br. J. Plast. Surg.* 23:242, 1970.
37. Pearson, R. W. Mechano-Bullous Diseases (Epidermolysis Bullosa). In Fitzpatrick, T. B., Arndt, K. A., Clark, W. H., Eisen, A. Z., Van Scott, E. J., and Vaughan, J. H. (Eds.), *Dermatology in General Medicine.* New York: McGraw-Hill, 1971.
38. Perry, H. O., and Brunsting, L. A. Pyoderma gangrenosum: Clinical study of 19 cases. *Arch. Dermatol.* 75:380, 1957.
39. Pierre, M., Jouglard, J. P., and Tramier, H. A case of skin necrosis following anticoagulant therapy. *Excerpta Medica* 2:109, 1971.
40. Pollock, W. J., Virnelli, F. R., and Ryan, R. F. Axillary hidradenitis suppurativa: A simple and effective surgical technique. *Plast. Reconstr. Surg.* 49:22, 1972.
41. Reed, W. B., Becker, S. W., Sr., Becker, S. W., Jr., and Nickel, W. R. Giant pigmented nevi, melanoma, and leptomeningeal melanocytosis. *Arch. Dermatol.* 91:100, 1965.
42. Reed, W. B., Horowitz, R. E., and Beighton, P. Acquired cutis laxa. *Arch. Dermatol.* 103:661, 1971.
43. Rees, T. D. Surgical repair of lupus vulgaris. *Plast. Reconstr. Surg.* 20:147, 1957.
44. Rees, T. D., and Swinyard, C. A. Rehabilitative digital surgery in epidermolysis bullosa. *Plast. Reconstr. Surg.* 40:169, 1967.
45. Rigg, B. M. Axillary hyperhidrosis. *Plast. Reconstr. Surg.* 59:334, 1977.
46. Riu, R., Ruth, L. D., and Snyder, C. C. Skin necrosis secondary to cryoglobulinemia: Case report. *Plast. Reconstr. Surg.* 46:510, 1970.
47. Schultz, R. C. Skin sloughs in Waterhouse-Friderichsen syndrome. *Plast. Reconstr. Surg.* 42:598, 1968.
48. Sharp, G. C., Irvin, W. S., Tan, E. M., Gould, R. G., and Holman, H. R. Mixed connective tissue disease – an apparently distinct rheumatic disease syndrome associated with a specific antibody to an extractable nuclear antigen (ENA). *Am. J. Med.* 52:148. 1972.
49. Stegmaier, O. C. Natural regression of the melanotic nevus. *J. Invest. Dermatol.* 32:413, 1959.
50. Stegmaier, O. C., and Montgomery, H. Histopathologic studies of pigmented nevi in children. *J. Invest. Dermatol.* 20:51, 1953.
51. Tipton, J. B. Axillary hyperhidrosis and its surgical treatment. *Plast. Reconstr. Surg.* 42:137, 1968.
52. Wayte, S. M., and Helwig, E. B. Melanotic freckle of Hutchinson. *Cancer* 21:893, 1968.
53. White, R. R., and Noone, R. B. Paronychia congenita (Jadassohn-Lewandowski syndrome). *Plast. Reconstr. Surg.* 59:855, 1977.
54. Winkelmann, R. K., and Ditto, W. B. Cutaneous

and visceral syndromes of necrotizing or "allergic" angiitis: A study of 38 cases. *Medicine* 43:59, 1964.

55. Wolfort, F. G., and Krizek, T. J. Skin ulceration in sickle cell anemia. *Plast. Reconstr. Surg.* 43:71, 1969.
56. Wustrack, K., and Zarem, H. A. Pyoderma gangrenosum: Recognition and management. *Plast. Reconstr. Surg.* Submitted for publication.
57. Yeschua, R., Wexler, M. R., and Neuman, Z. The nevus of Ota. *Plast. Reconstr. Surg.* 55:229, 1975.
58. Zarem, H. A., Pearson, R. W., and Leaf, N. Surgical management of hand deformities in recessive dystrophic epidermolysis bullosa. *Br. J. Plast. Surg.* 27:176, 1974.

GENERAL REFERENCES

59. Braverman, I. M. *Skin Signs of Systemic Disease.* Philadelphia: Saunders, 1970.
60. Demis, D. J., Crounse, R. G., McGuire, J., and Dobson, R. L. (Eds.). *Clinical Dermatology.* Hagerstown: Harper & Row, 1972.
61. Domonkos, A. N. *Andrews' Diseases of the Skin* (6th ed.). Philadelphia: Saunders, 1971.
62. Fitzpatrick, T. B., Arndt, K. A., Clark, W. H., Eisen, A. Z., Van Scott, E. J., and Vaughan, J. H. (Eds.). *Dermatology in General Medicine.* New York: McGraw-Hill, 1971.
63. Rook, A., Wilkinson, D. S., and Ebling, F. J. G. *Textbook of Dermatology.* Oxford and Edinburgh: Blackwell, 1968.

Hypertrophic Scars and Keloids

LYNN D. KETCHUM

In the last 20 years, significant strides have been made in the understanding and treatment of hypertrophic scars and keloids. In both areas, much is still left to be learned. However, the majority of lesions are now rendered manageable.

DIAGNOSIS AND ETIOLOGY

Hypertrophic scars and keloids are variations of a normal wound healing process. It is difficult to define precisely the term *normal wound healing,* since the fine line scar is a rarity in dark-skinned races. However, to establish a starting point, one may arbitrarily say that in the normal wound healing process, an equilibrium occurs between the anabolic and catabolic phases of wound healing at about 3 to 4 weeks after the injury. At this time the strength of the wound is approximately 30 to 40 percent that of normal skin; as maturation occurs with progressive cross-linking of the collagen fibers across the wound, the tensile strength will continue to improve without appreciable increase in the collagen content of the wound. At this time, the scar is somewhat hyperemic, as evidenced by its pink color, and may still have evidence of a healing ridge, which is involuting (Fig. 30-1). Over the next 3 to 4 months, hyperemia will subside, and the scar will be flat and pliable although 2 to 3 mm. wide.

In the abnormal scar, an equilibrium does not occur between the anabolic phase and the catabolic phase at 3 to 4 weeks; instead, there is a continued increase in the production of collagen above that which is degraded. The wound expands in all directions; it is elevated above the skin and is also deeper and wider than normal. Although it is a stronger scar, this does not benefit the patient; a "normal" scar, which has a tensile strength weaker than that of normal skin, nevertheless is sufficiently strong to withstand without disruption the forces imposed on the scar in normal living activities.

There are two types of abnormal scars – hypertrophic scars and keloids. Hypertrophic scars are more common; they are wide, red, elevated scars, as seen in Figure 30-2. Keloids likewise are wide, raised, and deep scars, but in addition, they continue to grow beyond the point at which hypertrophic scars plateau (Fig. 30-3). They exceed the original dimensions of the wound and grow mounds upon mounds of collagen in a pseudotumor fashion. There is a gray zone between the two lesions; however, in the extreme cases, it is clinically not difficult to recognize a keloid when it becomes distorted. A hypertrophic scar never becomes distorted but is uniformly raised and wide. Histologically the two lesions cannot be differentiated by either light or electron microscopy. Tissue culture studies of the two lesions are inconclusive at this time. The work by Conway and colleagues [3] 20 years ago has never been reproduced, though several attempts have been made to do so. Recently, however, Hoehn [6] has described a new cell of neural origin that heretofore has not been described in tissue culture work dealing with keloids; this work is still in progress.

Since the clinical differentiation between keloids and hypertrophic scars is a subjective one, the only true objective differentiation between the two lesions is biochemical. Cohen and associates [2], in 1971, found that although the collagenase level in hypertrophic scars was similar to that in normal scars, the rate of collagen production was increased in hypertrophic scars, resulting in an abnormally large scar. However, in keloids, both the anabolic and catabolic phases of collagen metabolism were increased, with the production of collagen proceeding at a greater rate than that of degradation.

Etiology

At this time the etiology of keloid formation is unknown; however, this is not true for hypertrophic scars. In the same area of the same patient can be found hypertrophic scars and "normal" scars in close proximity. This biological experiment has been repeated many times fortuitously with the aid of surgical incisions and traumatic wounds. Even within the same scar, a segment of it may become hypertrophic while an adjacent segment remains soft and flat. Since the causes of hypertrophic scars, which will be mentioned subsequently, are largely preventable, therefore much in the way of treatment of hypertrophic scars can be accomplished by proper planning before an incision is made and by excellent intraoperative and postoperative care.

One factor in the etiology of hypertrophic scars is infection, as seen in Figure 30-4. In this example, the inferior aspect of the wound became infected, whereas the superior aspect healed uneventfully, resulting in a widened but soft and flat scar. The inferior aspect of the wound enkindled a much greater inflammatory response than did the superior part of the wound,

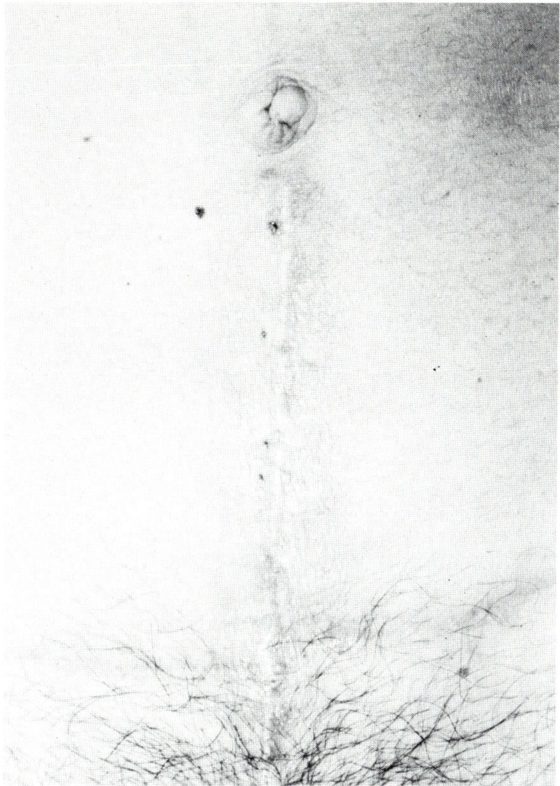

Fig. 30-1. The healing ridge in this normal scar will begin to fade 3 or 4 weeks after repair.

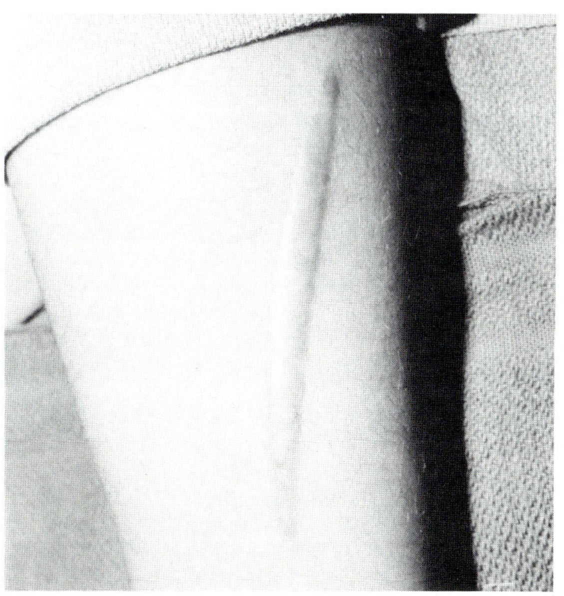

Fig. 30-2. A hypertrophic scar is shown that is fairly uniformly thick. In addition to being wide, this scar is at least as deep as it is elevated.

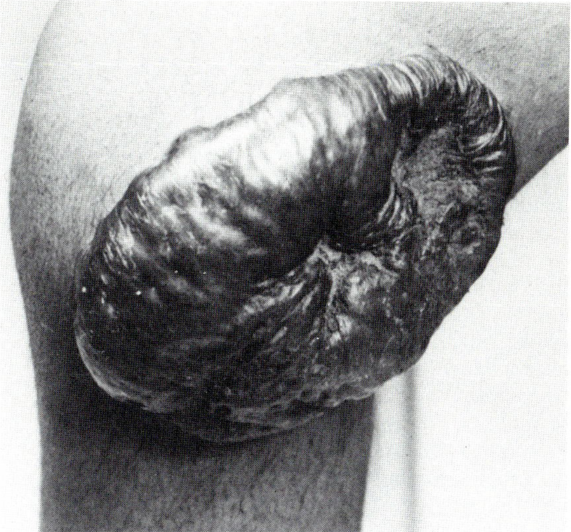

Fig. 30-3. This true keloid located on the knee has escaped the boundaries of the original wound. It is not uniformly thick but has mounds and mounds of collagen heaped up above the level of the skin.

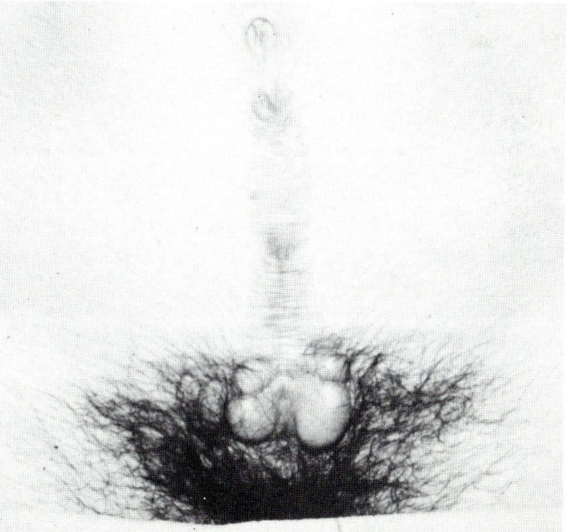

Fig. 30-4. An infection or other factors may increase the stimulus for inflammation during wound healing. In this patient, there was an increased stimulus in the inferior aspect of the wound, and thus there has been an increased amount of collagen formed.

which also produced an inflammatory response, one that is necessary for normal wound healing. One of the principles of wound healing is that inflammation is necessary for wound healing, particularly these three components of the inflammatory process – oxygen, macrophages, and fibroblasts. Without oxygen, fibroblasts cannot manufacture collagen and macrophages cannot opsonize bacteria. Without macrophages, fibroblasts do not multiply. Through an unknown mechanism, macrophages send a message to the fibroblasts that stimulates them to multiply and secrete collagen. As a corollary, with a greater stimulus for inflammation, there will be more macrophages and more fibroblasts and more collagen secreted. Therefore scar formation is directly dependent on the amount of the inflammatory response. It follows that one of the methods of modifying wound healing surgically is to eliminate any factor that would increase the inflammatory response. Obviously a gross infection must not be allowed to develop. There should be a minimum amount of foreign material, including suture material – even so-called nonreactive monofilament suture materials should be minimized, since the area where a suture is knotted will result in a small area of ischemia and necrotic tissue. Dead spaces are to be eschewed, since they will be filled with fibrous tissue. Modifying the inflammatory response can also be augmented chemically (see the section on triamcinolone).

The next etiological factor that produces hypertrophic scars is tension, as seen in Figure 30-5. Here within a 4-cm.-square area, in the same individual, can be seen a flat, narrow scar crossed perpendicularly by a wide, raised scar; thus, the same individual is capable of producing both normal scars and hypertrophic scars, in the same area of the body. Why is one hypertrophic and the other one not? There are definite directions of tension on the skin everywhere on the body produced by both the underlying musculature and skeletal system. Although the musculature is not always contracting, the skeleton is always imposing tension in a definite direction in different areas of the body, just as tent poles produce tension on canvas. Without a skeleton, the skin would be a spherical or cylindrical bag, depending on the area of the body. There are areas of the body where tension is greater than others and within a particular area the tension flows in a given direction [1].

On the shoulder, for example, one of the areas of increased tension, the lines of relaxed skin tension imposed by the underlying skeleton flow in a transverse direction, not longitudinally down the limb. The collagen fibers in the skin also flow in the same direction as the lines of relaxed skin tension. If an incision is made parallel to the lines of skin tension, two forces develop: (1) the distracting force of the wound, which is in a longitudinal direction, and (2) the force imposed by the lines of skin tension, which is in a transverse direction. This results in a haphazard arrangement of collagen fibers going across the wound, which in turn results in a smaller and weaker scar than one in which the wound crosses perpendicular to the lines of skin tension (Fig. 30-6). In such a scar, Sussman [14] has shown that both forces, the distracting force and the force of skin tension, are traveling in the same direction. Somehow this increase in force is translated into a stimulus for increased inflammatory reaction; a much greater quantity of collagen is produced with the fibers all running in the same direction, producing a stronger scar that is also wider and thicker. The lesson to be learned from this is that in areas of inherently greater tension on the healing wound (such as the shoulder, upper back, and presternal area) there would be a tendency to thicker scars than in areas with decreased tension. When

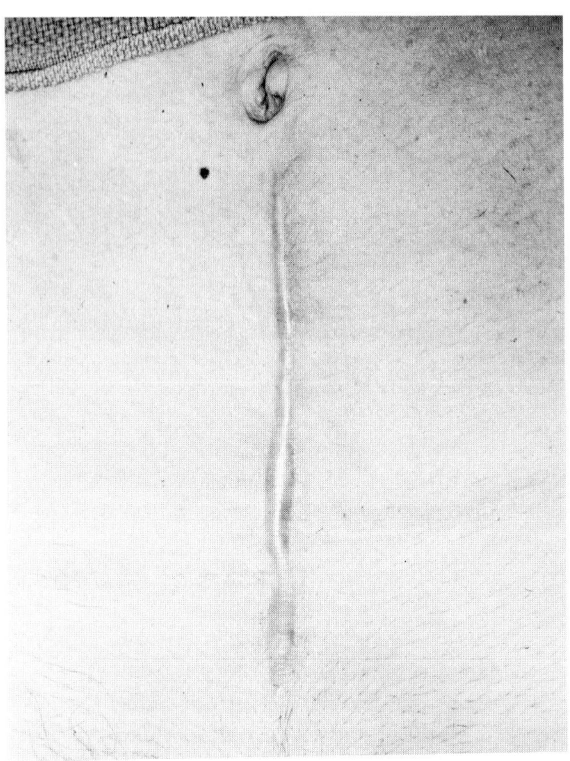

Fig. 30-5. The transverse scar in the suprapubic area is barely discernible, whereas the midline scar that crosses it is hypertrophic. Here in this very small area, the patient is capable of forming either a fine line scar or a hypertrophic scar. The reason for this is the difference in tension on the wound edges imposed by the direction of the scar.

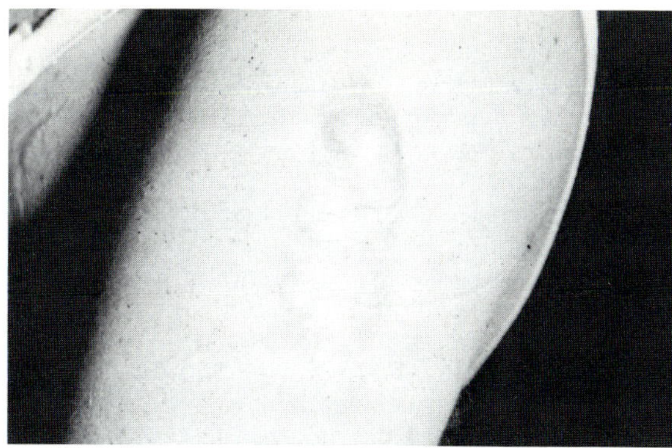

Fig. 30-6. The deltoid, presternal, and upper back regions are areas of increased tension on the skin. In addition, the lines of relaxed skin tension run transversely in this area of the upper arm. This hypertrophic scar runs perpendicular to the lines of relaxed skin tension.

possible, the direction of the scar should be changed, either by election in planning a surgical incision or by redirecting the scar with the use of a Z-plasty, and if tension on the wound edges exists because of an absolute loss of tissue through an avulsion or ablation, it can be reduced by shifting in tissue from an area of decreased tension or by applying a skin graft.

Another etiological factor is thought to be age. No one will argue that the metabolic rates in children are greater than those in adults, and no one will argue that there is a high incidence of hypertrophic scars in children. However, adults into the sixth and seventh decades are also capable of forming hypertrophic scars with a relatively high frequency when incisions are made perpendicular to the lines of resting skin tension. To prove this, one has only to visit the office of a cardiovascular surgeon who uses the routine midline presternal incision for coronary bypasses.

Race and Abnormal Scarring

It is a well-established fact that there is an increase in the incidence of thicker scars in dark-skinned races. The reason for this is unknown at this time but Koonin [9] suggests that there is a relationship between pigment cells and hypertrophic scars, especially keloids. He points out that keloids are rarely, if ever, found on the palms and the soles of the feet, where melanocytes are sparse. He also mentions that hydrocortisone is an inhibitor of melanocyte-stimulating hormone, and hydrocortisone is also an inhibitor of inflammation, which reduces scar formation. The most potent analogue of hydrocortisone is triamcinolone (9-alpha-fluoro-hydrocortisone). When this agent is injected into a keloid, it frequently will atrophy; as the atrophy occurs, the keloid blanches in color or becomes less hyperpigmented. If injected by accident into normal skin, this agent will produce atrophy of normal skin and depigmentation.

Although the work of Hoehn [6] in finding a new cell of neural origin in the tissue culture of keloids is yet uncompleted, it should be noted that melanocytes are also of neural origin.

TREATMENT

At present there are five modalities that can be used in treating the abnormal scar. The role of surgery has already been alluded to earlier in this chapter. The use of sound surgical principles and atraumatic technique is absolutely essential in the prevention and treatment of abnormal scars. In addition, surgery is also helpful in reducing the size of an established keloid, rendering it more amenable to treatment by pressure, steroids, or irradiation. The only occasion in which surgery alone would be indicated in the treatment of hypertrophic scarring is in reorienting the direction of the scar if the direction is perpendicular to the lines of relaxed skin tension, or if the scar is the result of an infection; in these cases the scar can then be revised, taking care to prevent a recurrence of the initial causes of the infection. Otherwise the excision of an abnormal scar converts it into a fresh wound in which the inflammatory process inherent to normal wound healing is subject to modification by pressure, steroids, or irradiation. Irradiation and steroids, when begun immediately upon the onset of wound healing, reduce the inflammatory phase of wound healing and thus the subsequent multiplication of fibroblasts and production of collagen.

Radiation

Immature dividing fibroblasts are particularly vulnerable to the ionizing effects of radiation and are either killed or sterilized, preventing further multiplication of the treated cells. This effect is both permanent and additive, so that if subsequent irradiation for malignancy is required in the treated area, it will be limited by the amount of irradiation given for the benign scar. Furthermore, irradiation is not indicated in the treatment of scars in children or in any growing tissue. Irradiation, furthermore, is inconvenient and is an added expense to the surgical procedure. Irradiation is only effective in newly forming scars, not established scars, and requires multiple visits to the radiotherapist. I feel that the only indication for the use of irradiation is in an individual who has a diathesis to keloid formation and who has a rather large keloid that cannot be managed with the use of steroids and pressure alone. If irradiation is to be used in combination with other modalities, there is no advantage to giving preoperative irradiation; however, it should be started soon after surgery. Moss and Brand [12] recommend giving three or four daily treatments of 300 to 400 gm. each to the surface at 100 kv with 2-mm. AL filters, beginning on the third postoperative day.

Pressure

One of the two significant advances in the treatment of hypertrophic scars and keloids in the last decade has been the use of pressure. First demonstrated by Fujimori, Hiramoto, and Ofufi [4] in 1967, in the last several years, Larson and co-workers [10] have expanded the use of pressure in the treatment of hypertrophic burn scars and the use of traction in overcoming burn scar contractures (Fig. 30-7).

The great advantage in the use of pressure in the treatment of abnormal scarring is that large areas can be treated with this modality – for example, severe burn scars. Although total body irradiation has been used for rare malignant conditions, irradiation of a large segment of the body is not recommended. Similarly, triamcinolone is limited by dosage to approximately 40 sq. cm. at any one given time, so that if a patient had hypertrophic scars over 20 to 25 percent or greater body surface, it would require a long period of time for effective treatment with triamcinolone. In contrast, the entire area can be managed with pressure simultaneously.

Larson and colleagues [10] and Kischer and associates [8] have shown that pressure reorients collagen bundles parallel to the surface of the skin and converts them from a ropelike weave to individual filaments that are thicker and more mature than those seen in bulky hypertrophic scars. Pressure also has some effect on the level of chondroitin sulfate associated with hypertrophic scars, decreasing it while at the same time increasing levels of hyaluronic acid to those of normal skin. The mechanism of action of pressure is unknown, but it is thought that hypoxia may play a causative role in these effects.

There are definite disadvantages to the use of pressure, however: it must be maintained continuously for a minimum of 9 months, and premature release is frequently followed by recurrence of the lesion. If pressure is reapplied once the lesion has recurred, it will regress again, but if pressure is then left on for an adequate period of time, the lesion will not recur once the pressure is released. This may mean wearing an elastic face mask for 9 months to a year. Although such an elastic reduces the size of the lesion, which is the goal of the treatment, it visually isolates the patient, with obvious psychological disadvantages (although the scars themselves have at least an equal psychological disadvantage). In addition, in warm weather, the use of such compression bandages is uncomfortable.

The pressure must be discontinued if ulceration or tissue breakdown occurs, and this may allow recurrence of the lesion. The pressure must be resumed as soon as reepithelialization occurs. The simplest way of applying pressure is to place a piece of foam rubber directly over the exact dimensions of the scar and then compress it with an elastic bandage, or the patient may be measured for a custom-fitted elastic garment that fits snugly over the contour of the area involved. Although the skin must be cleaned from time to time, pressure should not be relieved for more than 30 minutes at a time.

Triamcinolone

Triamcinolone, which has been used clinically for the last 17 years, is the first agent that produces atrophy in an established keloid. This effect was first reported by Maguire [11] in 1965 and by Griffith [5] and Ketchum and co-workers [7] in 1966 (Fig. 30-8). In 1963, Murray [13] showed that the injection of steroids into the wound edges following excision of a

Fig. 30-7. The effect of compression on a hypertrophic scar. A, this patient had sustained hypertrophic burn scars of the hand and forearm following a thermal burn. B, with the application of a Jobst glove, the scar was flattened to the level of normal skin.

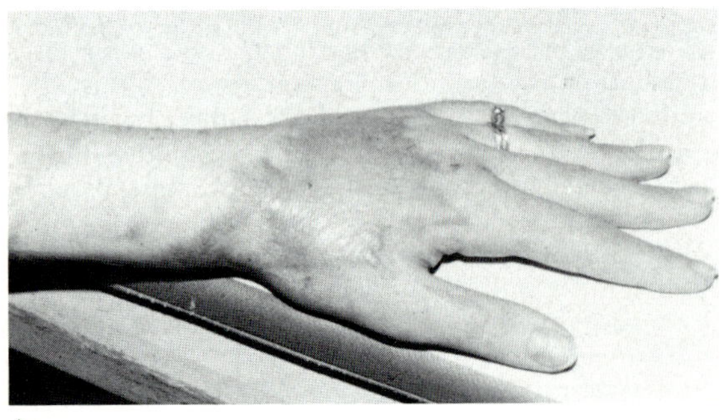

A

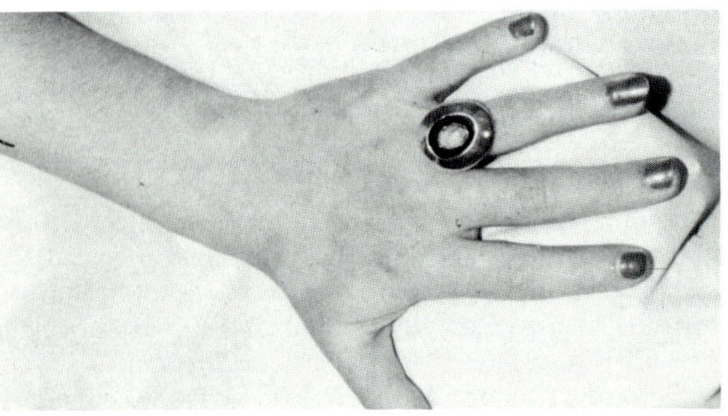

B

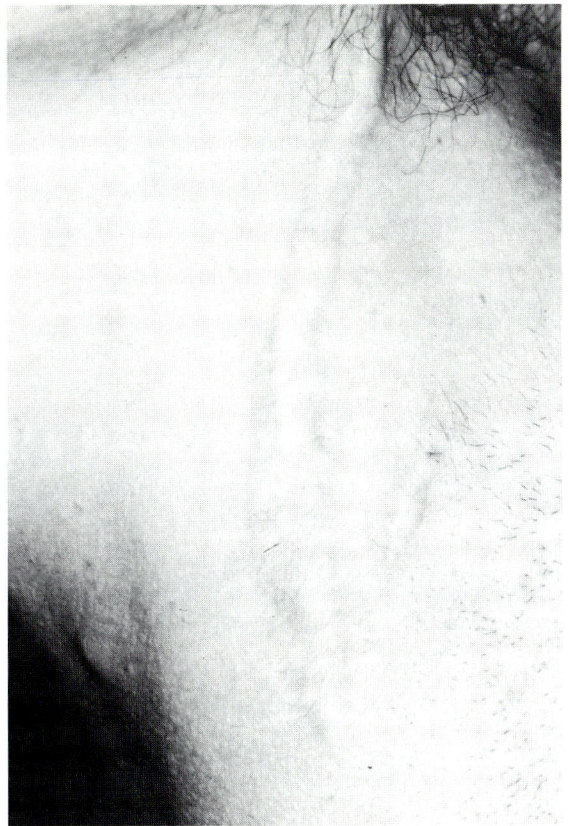

Fig. 30-8. An intralesional injection of triamcinolone was made into the lower aspect of a hypertrophic scar, whereas the upper half served as a control; the lower half flattened and softened, whereas the upper half remained unchanged.

hypertrophic scar would prevent its recurrence.

Triamcinolone is a powerful antiinflammatory agent that exerts several effects. When injected into the edges of a newly made wound, it modifies the inflammatory response. There will be fewer macrophages and subsequently fewer fibroblasts and less collagen secreted, so that the scar will be a smaller scar. However, when injected into an established hypertrophic scar, its mechanism of action is different, since it activates endogenous collagenase to degrade the mature collagen to more soluble forms, which are extracted from the wound. Once it is extracted, the hypertrophic scar does not reform.

I have had extensive experience with the use of this agent, having injected more than 600 lesions, and I am still amazed at the way that a hypertrophic scar will melt away after a course of injections. Because these scars may be extremely dense, it is often not possible to instill much fluid into the scar at all at the time of the first injection; thus a priming dose is required, whereby the material is injected directly under the scar. In a month the scar can be reinjected; at that time the scar does not appear to be smaller but the material can now be instilled in a greater quantity into the scar. In approximately 3 weeks, the scar will begin to respond by becoming softer and somewhat smaller, depending on the size of the scar. A series of injections over a period of months may be required to achieve a soft, flat scar. At the end point, the scar will remain wide but it is soft, flat, and nonpruritic. All of the complications with the use of triamcinolone are caused by overdosage or instillation of the drug into normal tissue.

Complications consist of excessive atrophy of normal tissue around and under the scar, telangiectasia, and depigmentation. All of these complications can be avoided by injecting triamcinolone into the scar; as the final result is approaching, one should observe the scar an extra month to ensure that further resolution of the scar will not occur without the injection, and then titrate the dose to avoid atrophy. Atrophy is not a permanent complication; the tissue will thicken though it may take 6 to 12 months to do so. In this regard, this atrophy is similar to the effects of pressure, as seen in a paraplegic patient who sits on one ischial tuberosity while allowing an ulcer on the contralateral side to heal. The skin will atrophy from the pressure but if the pressure is then relieved, the skin will thicken and return to its normal thickness.

A dosage schedule for triamcinolone is seen in Table 30-1. A maximum dose of 120 mg. should not be exceeded in any 1-month period, but it may be repeated at monthly intervals; the dosage is tailored appropriately for children.

Table 30-1. Dosage Schedule for Triamcinolone

Age of Patient and Size of Lesion	Dosage
1 to 5 years	40 mg. (maximum dose)
6 to 10 years	80 mg. (maximum dose)
ADULTS	
1- to 2-sq.-cm. lesion	20 to 40 mg.
2- to 6-sq.-cm. lesion	40 to 80 mg.
6- to 10-sq.-cm. lesion or larger	80 to 120 mg. (maximum dose is 120 mg.; may be repeated once a month for 4 to 6 months)

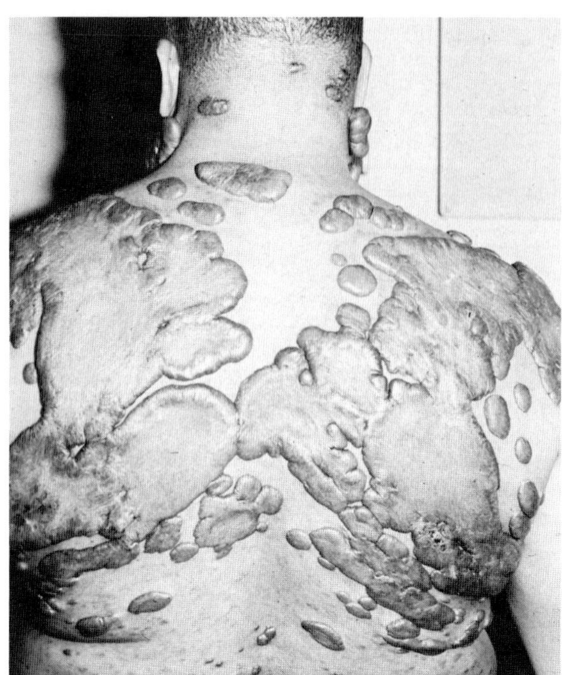

Fig. 30-9. This individual has morbid fibrosis in which keloids developed from furuncles on the back. Nodules of collagen were then formed that coalesced in a pseudotumor fashion.

Combination Therapy

The only indication for a combination of all of the modalities mentioned above is in the patient subject to keloid formation plus morbid fibrosis – a tendency to form true keloids in a significant area of the body (Fig. 30-9). In such an individual, it may be necessary to reduce the bulk of the keloid by a surgical excision, eliminate tension on the wound by appropriate means, inject the wound edges with triamcinolone, irradiate the wound, and apply pressure. This combination should only be used as a last resort in individuals with lesions, in whom pressure and the combination of pressure and steroids are not effective.

REFERENCES

1. Borges, A. F., and Alexander, J. E. Relaxed skin tension lines, Z-plasties on scars, and fusiform excisions of lesions. *Br. J. Plast. Surg.* 15:242, 1962.
2. Cohen, I. K., Keiser, H. R., and Sjoerdsma, A. Collagen synthesis in human keloid and hypertrophic scar. *Surg. Forum* 22:488, 1971.
3. Conway, H., Gillette, R. W., Smith, J. W., and Tindley, A. Differential diagnosis of keloids and hypertrophic scars by tissue culture technique with notes on therapy of keloids by surgical excision and decadron. *Plast. Reconstr. Surg.* 25:117, 1960.
4. Fujimori, R., Hiramoto, M., and Ofufi, S. Sponge fixation method for treatment of early scars. *Plast. Reconstr. Surg.* 42:322, 1968.
5. Griffith, B. H. Treatment of keloids with triamcinolone acetonide. *Plast. Reconstr. Surg.* 38:202, 1966.
6. Hoehn, R. Personal communication, 1976.
7. Ketchum, L. D., Smith, J., Robinson, D. W., and Masters, F. W. Treatment of hypertrophic scars, keloids, and scar contracture by triamcinolone acetonide. *Plast. Reconstr. Surg.* 38:209, 1966.
8. Kischer, C. W., Shettar, M. R., and Shettar, C. L. Alteration of hypertrophic scars induced by mechanical pressure. *Arch. Dermatol.* 3:60, 1975.
9. Koonin, A. J. The aetiology of keloids; a review of the literature and a new hypothesis. *S. Afr. Med. J.* 38:913, 1964.
10. Larson, D. L., Abston, S., Evans, E. B., et al. Techniques for decreasing scar formation and contractures in the burned patient. *J. Trauma* 11:807, 1971.
11. Maguire, H. C. Treatment of keloids with triamcinolone acetonide injected intralesionally. *J.A.M.A.* 192:325, 1965.
12. Moss, W. R., and Brand, W. N. *Therapeutic Radiology* (3rd ed.). St. Louis: Mosby, 1967.
13. Murray, R. D. Kenalog and the treatment of hypertrophied scars and keloids in Negroes and whites. *Plast. Reconstr. Surg.* 31:275, 1963.
14. Sussman, M. Effect of increased tissue fraction on tensile strength of cutaneous incisions in rats. *Proc. Soc. Exp. Biol. Med.* 123:38, 1966.

Tattoos

JOSEPH AGRIS

There are three principal categories of tattoos: *adventitious, medical,* and *decorative.*

ADVENTITIOUS (TRAUMATIC) TATTOOS

Adventitious tattooing may be defined as the accidental deposition of pigmented particles within the dermis. Carbon, in the form of road blacktop, is the most common material found in such tattoos, and it leaves black to blue color blemishes, depending on the depth of embedment. Other than the fact that it results from trauma (abrasive or explosive forces), the final result is not much different from commercially placed tattoos, except that the designs are nonrepresentational splotches and are cosmetically objectionable. Once the particles are embedded, removal without scarring becomes difficult. This can be obviated by treatment immediately following injury [1].

The *abrasive* form of adventitious tattooing is very common; it results from damage to the skin by friction, scraping, or scratching, with concurrent impregnation of pigmented particles. Blacktop surfaces, macadam roads, and cinder tracks are the usual sources of foreign particles. The sites of deposition of pigment (in descending order of frequency) are face, forehead, chin, hands, knees, lateral aspect of thighs, shoulders, breasts, forearms, and back.

The *explosive* form of adventitious tattooing, which is less common, usually involves the face, neck, and hands. Gunpowder (in the form of firearms, firecrackers, homemade bombs, and dynamite), gasoline, and household gas are the usual chemical causes. Granules permeate all layers of the skin, characteristically producing a dense central focus and decreasing to a finite circumferential and more superficial peripheral deposition of particles. Because of the depth of the deposition of granules, especially in the central focus of the explosion, the granules are difficult to remove, often requiring multiple excisions [2].

Treatment of Adventitious Tattoos

For the *abrasive* form of adventitious tattooing, treatment involves gently washing the involved areas with surgical soaps and rinsing with saline. The pigmented area is outlined with methylene blue. If the patient will not require a general anesthetic for the treatment of associated injuries, 0.5% lidocaine with 1:200,000 epinephrine is infiltrated locally into and around the involved area in a fanning out motion. The deposition of local anesthetic is facilitated by using a 25-gauge, 3-inch spinal needle and a 10-cc. syringe. After anesthesia is achieved, the area is cleaned with a sterile, hard, natural-bristle toothbrush or surgical scrub brush, utilizing a solution of physiological saline and surgical soap (Fig. 31-1). The area should be kept moist with the soap solution. Repeated rinsing and blotting with a wet 4 X 4 inch sponge will keep the area clear and help ensure that all embedded pigment is removed. Larger particles may be removed manually with a #11 blade and a fine pair of jeweler's forceps. Gentle pressure will provide the necessary hemostasis [3]. After being cleaned, the abrasive wounds are left open. The patient is instructed to wash the involved areas four times daily and to apply a topical antibiotic preparation. Healing proceeds in the course of 2 to 3 weeks (Fig. 31-2). Protection against exposure to sunlight is advised for 1 year to minimize the danger of excessive melanization.

The *explosive* form of adventitious tattooing is initially managed as described above; however, because of the larger number of particles and the greater depth of penetration, further treatment is needed [5, 6]. Abrasive therapy utilizing a revolving sandpaper disc or wire brush is often necessary [13, 14]. Dermaplaning may even be required. Individual,

Fig. 31-1. The particles are removed utilizing a toothbrush or an operating room scrub brush with a circular motion, keeping the surface moist with a sterile saline solution. (Figs. 31-1 and 31-3 are from J. Trauma *16:798, 1976. Copyright © 1976 by The Williams & Wilkins Co., Baltimore.)*

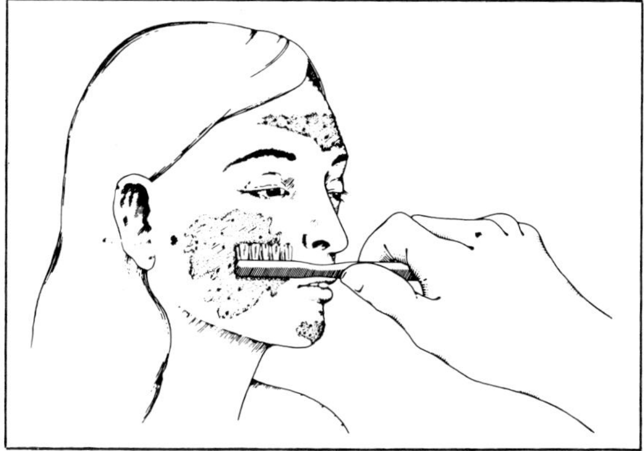

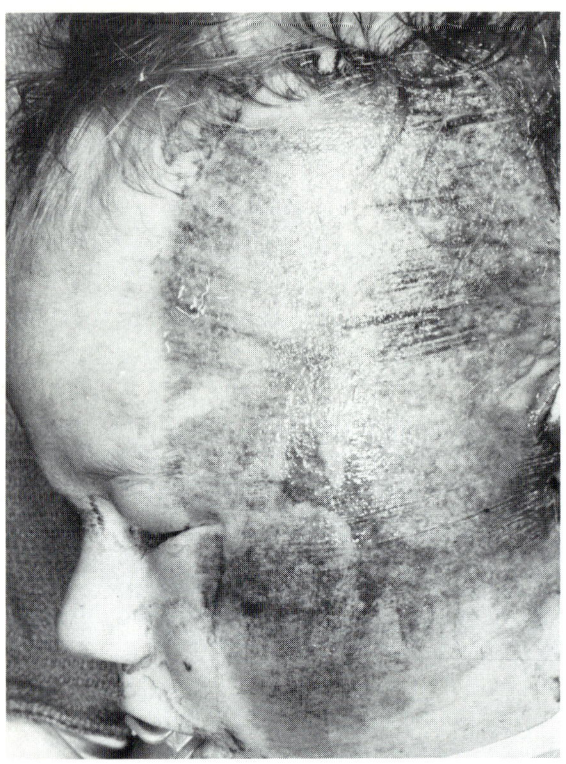

A

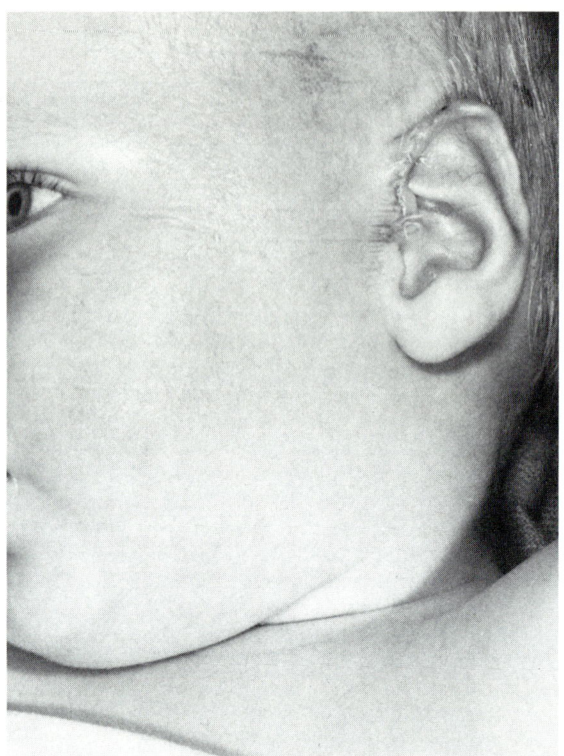

B

Fig. 31-2. A, pedestrian–motor vehicle accident, in which blacktop is embedded over the left side of the face. B, after immediate removal of debris with coarse abrasive brush, the wound is left open to the air and a topical antibiotic is used.

deeply impregnated granules can be removed with a 1- or 2-cm. dermal punch (Fig. 31-3).

Recently, microsurgical methods have been used with good results in patients with explosive adventitious tattooing. An operating microscope with two ocular heads is utilized, allowing two surgeons to work simultaneously, thus minimizing the length of anesthesia time. Utilizing a #2 Bonnie forceps or a #3C jeweler's forceps, each small wound is incised. Any particulate matter is scraped from the wound with a #67 Beaver blade. An assistant provides continuous irrigation over the area with a saline solution. If this technique fails, the wound edges are grasped with the Bonnie forceps, the pigmented area of the skin is trimmed away with a #65 blade, and the defect is then closed with an 8-0 monofilament nylon suture. If an appreciable amount of pigment is involved, the procedure can be carried out utilizing alternating teams of surgeons, or it can be repeated the following morning [10].

MEDICAL TATTOOS

Medical tattooing involves the insertion of colored pigments into the skin utilizing sterile techniques with multiple minute punctures, in order to conceal, replace, or recreate a state that appears more anatomically normal. Surgical tattooing was first pioneered by Hance and co-workers [12] in 1944. Since that time medical tattooing has been utilized on the cornea (chiefly to conceal leukomatous spots), in the recreation of the breast areola (due to loss from burns or from trauma), and to cover skin blemishes, particularly port-wine stains *(nevus flammeus)*. (The use of medical tattooing for port-wine hemangioma is discussed in detail in Chapter 28.)

DECORATIVE TATTOOS

Decorative tattoos consist of planned impregnation of fine particulate material into the skin to create an artistic design or pattern. Decorative tattoos can be divided into two categories: professional and nonprofessional (amateur) tattoos. Professional tattoos are those placed by an artist trained in the art of tattooing and having a degree of artistic skill. Professional tattoos usually have a regular, thin, well-demarcated outline, with fine details. The central portion of the design is usually multicolored. Pigment is evenly dis-

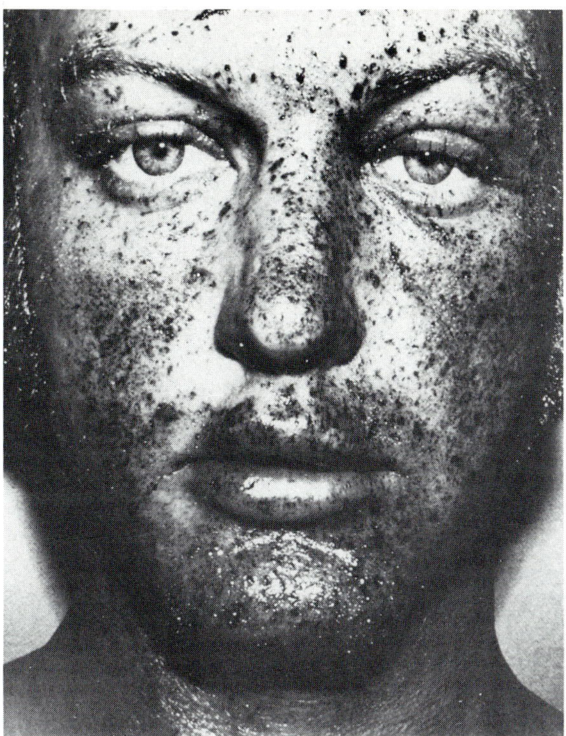

A

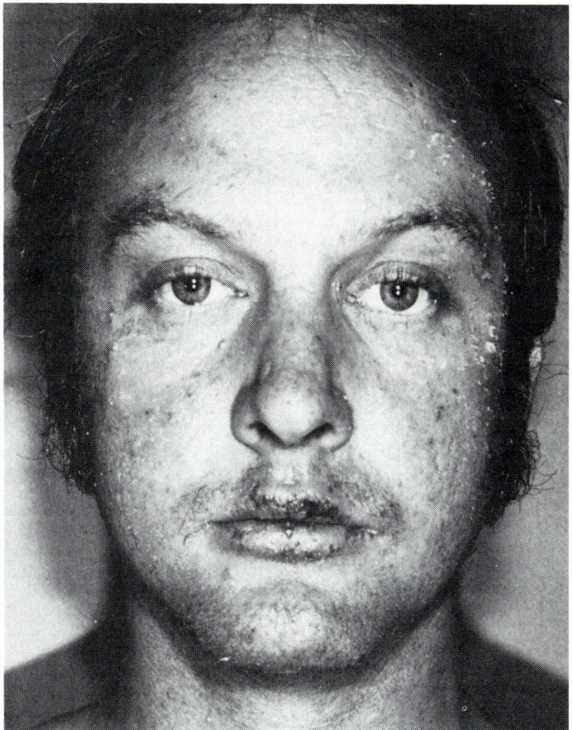

B

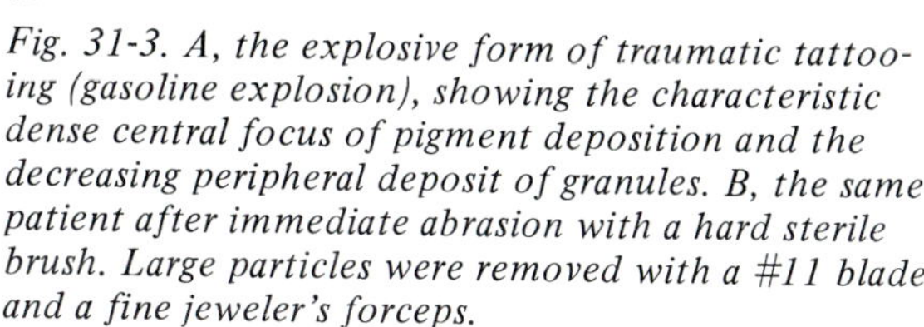

Fig. 31-3. A, the explosive form of traumatic tattooing (gasoline explosion), showing the characteristic dense central focus of pigment deposition and the decreasing peripheral deposit of granules. B, the same patient after immediate abrasion with a hard sterile brush. Large particles were removed with a #11 blade and a fine jeweler's forceps.

tributed. The design is homogeneous, and colors blend well.

Nonprofessional tattoos tend to have outline form only. The outline is often irregular and thick, containing pigmentation variations and omissions. Designs are rather simple and they are usually placed on the distal portion of the extremity for convenience. Since 40 to 50 percent are self-inflicted and most people are right-handed, the majority of such tattoos occur on the left arm or the left leg. There are almost never any colors seen in the nonprofessional tattoos, because the materials utilized by the nonprofessional tattooist are those items conveniently available (india ink, mascara, boot black, pencil lead). The outlines tend to be elevated and often have a granular consistency when palpated (Table 31-1). Until recently, most tattoos found on women were nonprofessional, since most women would not visit a tattoo parlor. In a series of 332 tattooed women reported in 1957, only 5 of the tattoos were done in a tattoo parlor; however, this has changed in the past several years. Women today receive 40 to 50 percent of all professional tattoos in this country. In males, there are as many professional as nonprofessional tattoos seen. In the male, the tattoos tend to be more extensive, and more consideration is given to the anatomical location for these complex, multicolored, and expensive tattoos.

The majority of tattoos are placed when the subject is between 12 and 24 years of age, a time when there is great personal instability, and the need for identification with peer groups is very strong. Often the first tattoos are done under the pressure of one's peer group and the need to "belong." Quite often these tattoos combine letters, numbers, dots, and interposed lines in a symbolic manner intended to be understood only by those in the "group" [4].

It is usually in the mid to late twenties that the individual finds the decorative tattoo a liability. It is at this point that social pressure and stigmata relative to the tattoo become apparent to the individual, and the removal of the tattoo is sought. Often such individuals have attempted to remove a portion of the tattoo themselves by burning the area with a hot object or abrading the area with salt or sandpaper,

Table 31-1. Relationship of Tattoos to Subject and Materials Used in Tattooing in Women

Person Who Applied the Tattoo	Percent	Materials Used in Tattooing	Percent
Self	45	Inks (ball point, india, etc.)	75
Friend	40	Pencil lead	14
Boyfriend or husband	7	Cosmetics (eyeliner, mascara, etc.)	10
Brother or sister	5	Paint	4
Parent	2	Shoe polish	4
Professional	1		

only to find it painful and the scarring that results as objectionable as the tattoo (Fig. 31-4).

Removal of Decorative Tattoos

A wide variety of techniques have been described for the obliteration of decorative tattoos [4, 16, 17, 19–21]. No one technique is completely satisfactory, and each case must be individualized. One must be sure it is the patient who wants it removed – not a parent, spouse, or close friend. The physician must be sure the patient understands what the residual will be following removal. However, in a survey of some 2,200 tattoo removals, most patients felt that the residual scarring was much more acceptable than the tattoo and could be explained more easily [4].

The history and physical examination are most important in determining the method of choice for a particular tattoo removal. One must first elicit whether the tattoo is professional or nonprofessional. Professional tattoos placed with an electrical needle tend to be between 0.4 and 0.8 mm. from the skin surface; their fine outlines and multiple colors lend themselves to dermabrasion or superficial dermaplaning. In contrast, pigments used in the nonprofessional tattoos will vary from just under the skin surface to the subcutaneous layers. The outlines are rather thick and the designs are often filled in with the same material, thus requiring excision, multiple excisions, or excision with skin graft to achieve complete removal.

One of the pitfalls in examining a tattoo is the tendency to focus on the tattoo itself. An important consideration is whether the tattoo was used to cover up track marks of narcotic injections, old previous scarring, or perhaps a previously placed tattoo that was objectionable (this technique is known as *overtattooing*). In any of the aforementioned instances, the only way to remove the pigment is to excise full-thickness skin and often subcutaneous tissue in order to remove the deeper lesion as well as the pigments. Depending on the size of the lesion, it may be possible to close it primarily; otherwise, the application of a skin graft would be needed. In any case, the presence of a tattoo is not in itself a reason for removal.

Various techniques – surgical, mechanical, chemical, electrical, overtattooing, retattooing, or a combination of these methods – have all been utilized in tattoo removal. In small lesions, excision followed by primary closure is the method of choice. In the smallest of lesions, a biopsy punch can be utilized to remove dots, dashes, small figures, and letters. The biopsy punch is particularly applicable to small areas on the face and the dorsum of the hand and fingers.

Tattoos are removed by the following methods:

Fig. 31-4. Examples of some primitive attempts at removal of tattoos. A, burning the skin with cigarettes and heated knife blade. B, salt abrasion. C, commercial sandpaper abrasion.

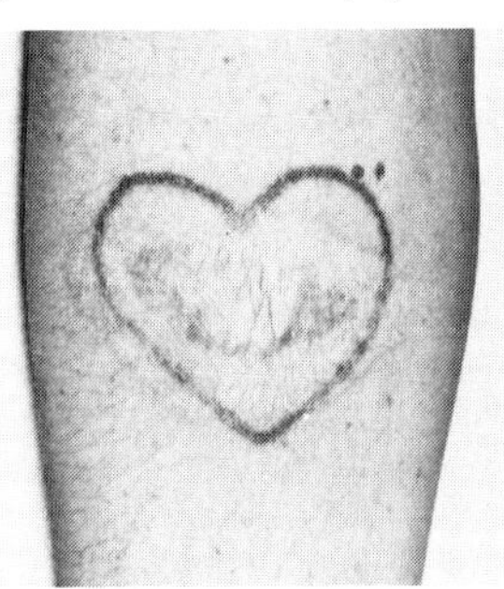

A

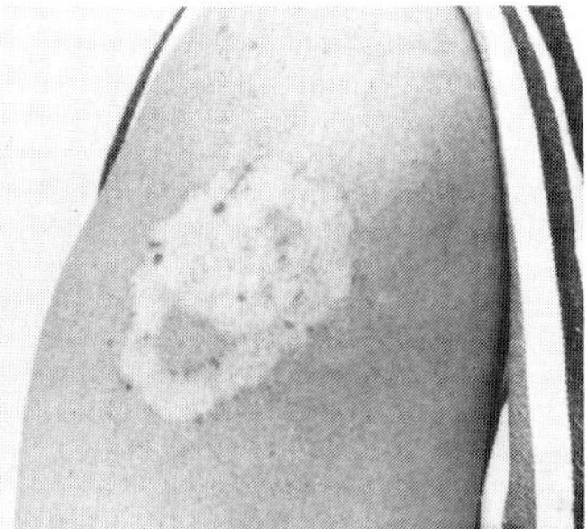

B

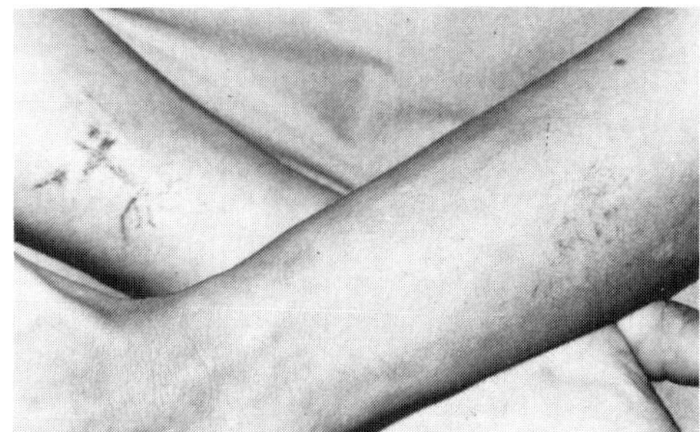

C

1. Surgical removal.
   a. Biopsy, punch method.
   b. Direct incision.
   c. Multiple excisions.
   d. Excision and flap transfer.
   e. Excision and grafting.
2. Mechanical removal.
   a. Pure dermabrasion (full thickness).
   b. Superficial dermabrasion.
3. Chemical removal.
4. Combination methods.
   a. Mechanical and chemical removal.
   b. Surgical and chemical removal.
5. Overtattooing or retattooing.
6. Electrical removal.
   a. Cautery.
   b. Laser beam.
   c. Combination with chemical.
   d. Combination with mechanical.

Surgical Excision

For lesions not exceeding 4 cm., excision and primary closure produce a very satisfying result, and that method is particularly applicable for small to moderate-sized lesions of the extremity (Fig. 31-5). Lesions exceeding 4 cm. in diameter on the extremity and the torso can be removed with multiple excision and primary closure. Multiple excisions should be spaced 6 to 12 months apart. An adequate area of undermining is necessary in order to achieve the desired result. Excision and closure with a local flap (utilizing a bilobed configuration) are particularly applicable to intermediate-sized lesions on the lateral and dorsal aspect of the foot and upper thigh and portions of the upper extremity. Extremely large lesions (those that exceed 8 cm. in diameter) of the extremity and torso can be removed completely by excision and application of a skin graft to the defect.

Dermabrasion and Sialabrasion

Intermediate (4 to 8 cm.) and large (8 to 15 cm.) multicolored professional tattoos can be removed by dermabrasion or sialabrasion with any of the standard motor-driven sanding devices. I have found that multicolored professional tattoos do well with two to four superficial dermabrasions, producing minimal scarring and a very acceptable result (Fig. 31-6).

The intermediate-sized tattoo can be dermabraded in its entirety, while larger tattoos can be subdivided and completed in two or three stages. The areas are first cleaned with surgical soap solution and injected with local anesthetic. Ethyl chloride can also be utilized; it has the advantage of providing a firm skin surface against which the abrasion is more easily performed. The majority of tattoos can be removed in the office or as an outpatient procedure utilizing this very fast, simple, yet effective method. With the skin now anesthetized, the rotary sanding disc or diamond fraise is gently directed over the surface of the tattoo in an even and symmetrical progression. It is of the utmost importance to continue moving the rotary instrument over the entire tattoo and not to concentrate on a particular area of dark pigment or on the outline. The depth of the abrasion should be uniform; otherwise, areas of uneven topography (gauging) and third-degree burns with full-thickness loss will result. As the dermis is removed, *a brightening and a glistening of the tattoo pigment occurs, followed by the appearance of pigment particles in the abraded material.* This is the end point of the procedure. It should be remembered that in superficial dermabrasion the purpose is not to remove the pigment with the dermabrader, but to allow the pigment to migrate to the skin surface.

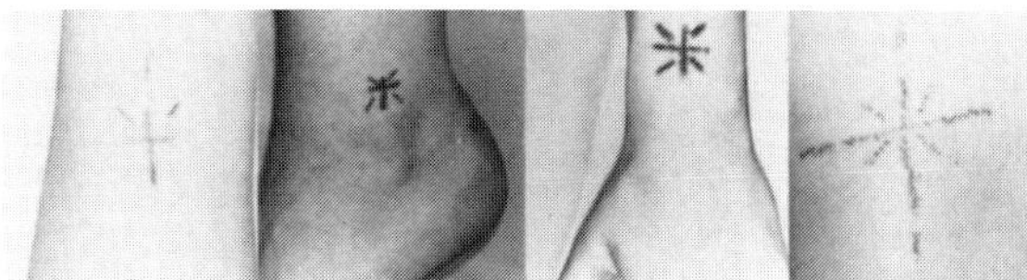

Fig. 31-5. The pachuco mark – a "tough guy" symbol that originated in Sicily and is now used by street gangs in the United States. The central portion can be removed with an elliptical incision and primary closure. The remaining portions of the tattoo are removed at the same time with a punch biopsy or smaller individual excisions. Sutures are left in place for 10 days to 2 weeks on the extremities.

Dermabrasion in combination with vital dye (2% aqueous gentian violet) has been said to help cause the pigment to migrate to the surface. However, I have found that covering the dermabraded area with a saline solution dressing which is dampened every four hours will produce the same result. The dressing is changed again in 48 to 72 hours. At this dressing change, it will be noted that the migrated pigmented particles will be deposited on the bandage. The amount of pigment on the bandage is variable, but will often give a mirror image of the tattoo that has been dermabraded. The patient is instructed to wash the area with soap and water and change the dressing once in the morning and once in the evening. Continued removal of pigment may be observed during the ensuing dressing changes. In about 15 days, the wound is healed and the patient is advised to lubricate the area and to prevent exposure of the area to sunlight for 1 year. As is the case with sialabrasion, 60 to 70 percent of pigment is removed with the first dermabrasion; subsequent superficial dermabrasion or spot abrading is carried out 3 to 6 months later, if needed.

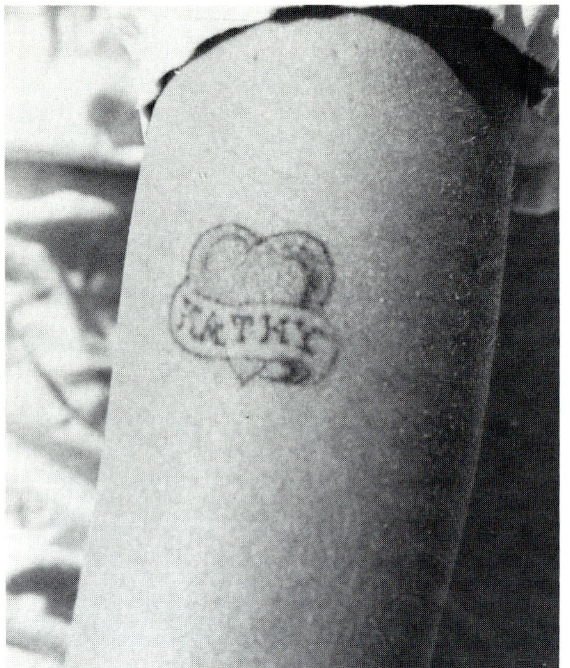

A

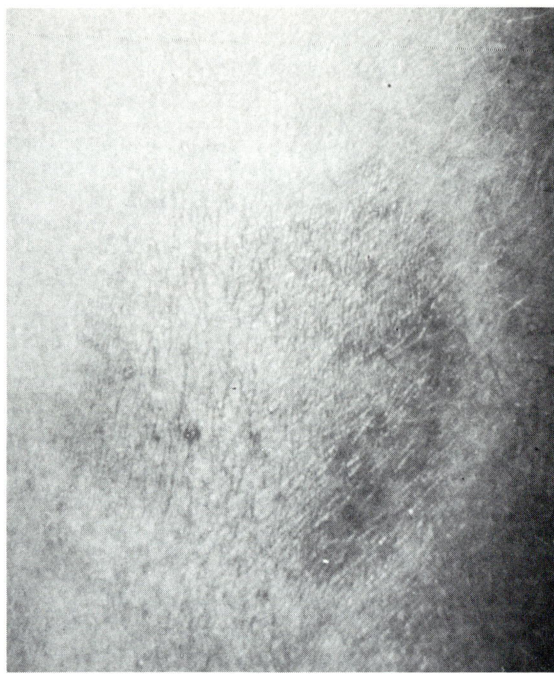

B

Fig. 31-6. A, this multicolored professional tattoo was removed by two superficial dermabrasions under local anesthesia. Superficial dermabrasion can be accomplished quickly, safely, easily, and inexpensively, leaving an excellent cosmetic result. B, postoperative view.

Superficial dermabrasion lends itself to the professional multicolored tattoo. Nonprofessional tattoos utilizing india ink, lamp black, and pencil lead do not lend themselves to optimal results because of the variation in the depth of pigment deposition.

The use of salt for superficial abrasion of the skin is not new. Aëtius, a Greek physician, was the first to describe the use of salt for tattoo removal in A.D. 543. Cittenden demonstrated the usefulness of table salt for this purpose and named the process *sialabrasion.*

The area to be treated is first washed with a soap solution and then thoroughly rinsed. After this, the skin is infiltrated with local anesthetic, or the application of ethyl chloride is sufficient. A rotating sanding disc is then used to remove the overlying keratin layer. Any commercially available electrical or air driven rotary device can be utilized. When this is completed, there will be some local erythema and minimal bleeding. A sterile medicine glass containing ordinary table salt (sodium chloride) is then moistened with enough sterile saline to allow the crystals to adhere. The salt paste is applied over the dekeratinized area with gentle rotary motion, using a sterile toothbrush. The rotary motion with the toothbrush is continued for approximately 5 minutes, during which time the area is irrigated periodically with saline to determine the depth of the abrasion. Additional salt paste is added as needed. The area should develop the appearance of a donor site after removal of a thin split-thickness skin graft. At the conclusion, the abraded area is again irrigated, and a topical antibiotic and sterile dressing are applied. The patient is instructed to wash the area and change the dressing once in the morning and once in the evening over the following 5 to 7 days. In about a week, the edema and erythema have disappeared and a thin brown eschar appears. Between the tenth and fifteenth day, the eschar will begin to separate from the underlying dermis; with the eschar, approximately 60 to 70 percent of the tattoo pigments will be removed. At this point, a gauze dressing containing a petroleum base is applied daily until the wound is completely healed. It will now require an additional 3 to 4 weeks before complete healing has occurred.

Patients are informed prior to the procedure that not all pigments will be removed with a single sialabrasion and that the remaining pastel pigments will fade and blend with the surrounding tissue in time. However, the blue-black color of the outline may require an additional treatment. The patients are also instructed to keep the area covered in order to avoid sunlight (ultraviolet radiation) to the area. It is suggested that the area be covered with a dressing, clothing, or the application of sunscreen lotion for at least 1 year following treatment. I also advise my patients to keep a pressure dressing on the area for 1 year to minimize any untoward scarring. This can easily be accomplished on the extremities by the use of an Ace elastic wrap.

If a second or third treatment is required, there is a 3- to 6-month wait before repeating the sialabrasion. If small scattered areas of outline pigment remain, these areas are removed with minimal scarring utilizing a disposable dermatological biopsy punch of 2 or 3 mm.

Untoward results of superficial dermabrasion and sialabrasion include hyperpigmentation, hypopigmentation, atrophy of the overlying skin, and hypertrophic scar formation. Hyperpigmentation is the most commonly seen; it is transitory and usually fades, though not completely, over a period of several months, and it does not constitute a significant cosmetic problem. In contrast, hypertrophic scar formation is an infrequent untoward result, but the most cosmetically displeasing. There is an increased incidence of hypertrophic scar formation in individuals with dark pigmented skin. There is also an increased incidence when the scar is located over the chest, shoulder, or upper back. Hypertrophic scarring can also be the result of abrading too deeply or the conversion of the wound to a full-thickness loss as a result of secondary infection.

The result of superficial dermabrasion or sialabrasion is considered good to excellent by 70 to 80 percent of patients, while 10 to 15 percent are happy that the tattoos have been removed but had hoped for a more cosmetic appearance. The remaining 5 percent consider the result poor, but still better than the tattoo.

Chemical Agents

Chemical agents have been used for many years, both professionally and by the public. Most contain various quantities of phenol and result in a second-degree burn which causes the skin to slough and the pigment to surface. Often the burn is deeper than anticipated and results in full-thickness loss as well as infection, leaving a prolonged painful course and an undesirable scar. This technique is only mentioned to be condemned.

Laser

Electrical devices have also been used, including the standard operating cautery and more recently the laser beam [11, 15, 25]. Those tattoos that I have seen treated by a Q-switch ruby laser resulted in a complete removal of the pigment; however, the scarring leaves much to be desired. It is not yet known exactly what happens to the pigment. Some feel that the pigment is actually volatilized and the gas passes through the skin. Laser treatment for tattoos is relatively new; the long-term effects of treating large skin areas with a laser beam are yet unknown.

Overtattooing

Overtattooing or retattooing should not be forgotten. Many patients find their present tattoo socially objectionable, but would be willing to have it overtattooed if a pleasing and more sociably acceptable design could be obtained. This approach is often overlooked; I think it is only fair that this be presented as one of the possible methods for correcting the problem, particularly if it is not the presence of a tattoo that bothers the patient, but the content of the design itself.

REFERENCES

1. Agris, J. Adventitious tattooing. *J. Dermatol. Surg.* 2:72, 1976.
2. Agris, J. Traumatic tattooing. *J. Trauma* 16:798, 1976.
3. Agris, J. Traumatic tattooing, suggestion for management. *J. Mod. Med.* March 15, 1977. P. 100.
4. Agris, J. Tattoos in women. *Plast. Reconstr. Surg.* 60:22, 1977.
5. Bunke, J. J., and Conway, H. S. Surgery of decorative and traumatic tattoos. *Plast. Reconstr. Surg.* 20:67, 1957.
6. Campbell, R. M. Surgical and Chemical Planing of the Skin. In Converse, J. M. (Ed.), *Reconstructive Plastic Surgery* 2nd ed. Philadelphia: Saunders, 1977.
7. Conway, H., Hug, N. E., and Tubensko, J. F. *Tumors of the Skin* (2nd ed.). Springfield, Ill.: Thomas, 1966. P. 105.
8. Conway, H., McKinney, P., and Climo, M. Permanent camouflage of vascular nevi of the face by intradermal injection of insoluble pigments (tattooing). *Plast. Reconstr. Surg.* 40:467, 1967.
9. Conway, H., and Montroy, R. E. Permanent camouflage capillary hemangiomas of the face by intradermal injection of insoluble pigments (tattooing). Indications for surgery. *N.Y. J. Med.* 65:876, 1965.
10. Furnas, D. W., and Somers, G. Microsurgery and prevention of traumatic tattoos. *Plast. Reconstr. Surg.* 58:631, 1976.
11. Goldman, L., Rockwell, R. J., Meyer, R., Otten, R., Wilson, R. G., and Kitzminer, K. W. Laser treatment of tattoos. *J.A.M.A.* 201:841, 1967.
12. Hance, G., Brown, J. B., Byars, L. T., and McDowell, F. Color matching of skin grafts and flaps with permanent pigment injection. *Surg.*

Gynecol. and Obstet. 70:624, 1944.
13. Iverson, P. C. Further developments in the treatment of skin lesion by surgical abrasion. *Plast. Reconstr. Surg.* 12:27, 1953.
14. Iverson, P. C. Surgical removal of traumatic tattoos. *Plast. Reconstr. Surg.* 2:427, 1947.
15. Laub, D. R., Yuler, R., Arras, M., Murray, D. E., Crawley, L., and Chase, R. Ruby lessar radiation on dermal tattoos in man. *J. Surg. Res.* 8:220, 1968.
16. Manchester, G. H. Tattoo removal, a new simple technique. *Calif. Med.* 18:10, 1973.
17. McDowell, A. J., Brown, J. B., and Cannon, B. Permanent pigment injection of capillary hemangioma, *Plast. Reconstr. Surg.* 1:106, 1946.
18. McDowell, F. Tattoo erasing (Editorial). *Plast. Reconstr. Surg.* 53:580, 1974.
19. Shie, M. J. The study of tattooing, a method of its removal. *J.A.M.A.* 90:94, 1928.
20. Soussaline, M. Trial of a new technique in the surgical treatment of tattoos (Part I). *Ann. Chir. Plast.* 19:193, 1974; Part II. 19:251, 1974.
21. Tattoos, sialabrasion (Editorial). *Med. J. Aust.* 2:352, 1973.
22. Thomson, H. G., Birdsell, D. C., and Freidberg, A. Surgical tattooing: An experimental study. *Plast. Reconstr. Surg.* 37:536, 1966.
23. Thomson, H. G., Douglas, L., and Monroe, I. Surgical tattooing. An experimental study: II. *Plast. Reconstr. Surg.* 39:291, 1967.
24. Thomson, H. G., and Wright, A. M. Surgical tattooing of the port wine stain. *Plast. Reconstr. Surg.* 48:113, 1971.
25. Yules, R. B., Laub, D. R., Honey, R., Vassiliadis, A., and Crowley, L. Effect of Q-switched ruby lessar radiation on dermal tattoo pigment in man. *Arch. Surg.* 95:179, 1967.

IV

Hand and Upper Extremity

Fingertip Injuries, Amputations, and Infections of the Hand and Upper Extremity

JOHN M. MARKLEY, JR.

The fingertips are the focal point of the complex, coordinated neural, cutaneous, musculotendinous, skeletal, and circulatory components of the upper extremity. The apexes of stable balanced strength and mobility, they project the body into the world with force and precision, speed and delicacy, in an infinite variety of gestures, grips, pinches, percussions, strokes. Their motion encompasses a range of surfaces from the infinitely small to the infinitely large. They are complex sensory receptors of exquisite sensibility. Their movement and touch may convey nuances of motion unequalled by language. Their repair is not to be taken lightly. When the fingertips are injured, the attendant loss of structure and function may result in significant temporary or lifelong personal and socioeconomic disabilities. Several million injuries of fingertips [88] (from 15 to 20 percent of all bodily injuries [72]) occur each year. In the United States, 30 to 40 percent of the total annual industrial compensation payments result from all types of injuries to the hand; injuries of the fingertip contribute to a large proportion of those injuries.

The repair of injured fingertips should be performed with a skill and delicacy commensurate with the precision demanded of the fingertips. Success, as in all surgery of the hand, depends upon sound knowledge of functional anatomy, atraumatic technique, and reliable judgment.

Anatomy of the Fingertip

In this chapter, the term *fingertip* will be defined as the skin, soft tissues, bone, and nail of the digit distal to the insertion of the extensor and flexor tendons at the base of the distal phalanx.

Skin

The volar skin of the fingertip is of the unique palmar and plantar type with deep parallel papillary ridges, numerous eccrine sweat glands, and a thick cornified layer, which responds to increased demands on durability with increased cornification. The dorsal skin is smooth and less cornified; at midphalanx it becomes specialized into the nail structures.

Soft Tissue

The pulp and fascial structure of the fingertip have been described in detail by Shrewsbury and Johnson [82]. The digital pulp is thickest in the ungual fossa. The distal ungual pulp is more fibrous, less fatty, and less mobile than the proximal pulp, from which it is divided by a fibrous barrier at the level of the ungual spines. The proximal pulp and the distal ungual pulp are bounded dorsolaterally by the strong lateral interosseous ligaments (Fig. 32-1). While the distal ungual pulp is firmly attached to the ungual tuberosity by strong fibrous elements, compartmentalization into multiple discrete pockets within the distal pulp is apparently incomplete [49].

Nerves and Vessels

The volar digital nerves enter the terminal segment at the distal joint crease level volar to their accompanying digital arteries and divide into terminal branches to the pulp and nail bed. At the level of the distal joint crease, the nerves are still 1 to 1.5 mm. in diameter and contain 60 percent of the approximately 5,000 endoneural tubes that enter each finger [96]. In the thumb, the volar nerve supplies only the nail bed dorsally, while the dorsal skin is usually supplied by branches of the radial nerve. In the fingers, the innervation of dorsal skin is shared variably by the dorsal nerves and dorsal branches of the volar digital nerves. The branches of nerve and vessel to the nail bed pass through the rima ungualum.

Nail

The nail is composed of the nail plate, matrix (or germinal matrix), nail bed (or sterile matrix), lunula, hyponychium, eponychium (proximal fold), and lateral nail folds. The relationships are illustrated in Figure 32-2. The nail plate is formed by nongranular keratinization of the cells of the germinal matrix [100]. The nail bed contributes a very few cells to the process. The lunula is the most distal edge of the germinal matrix, always present but often hidden beneath the eponychial fold. The shape of the distal nail plate edge is dictated by the contour of the lunula [51]. The nail bed has no subcutaneous tissue; its dermis is directly adherent to the dorsal phalangeal periosteum. The hyponychium is the skin beneath the free edge of the nail plate and, like the nail bed, is rich in glomus bodies. The eponychial fold with its cuticle is a double layer of skin, dermis to dermis, with a thin areolar layer intervening, which is the site of paronychia.

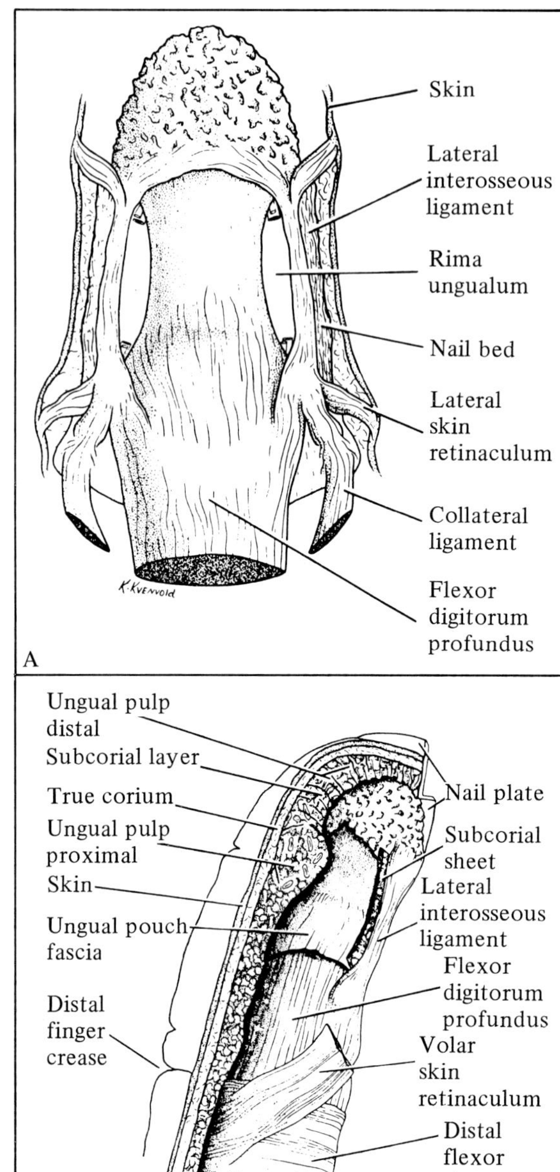

Fig. 32-1. A, a volar view of the deep dissection of the distal phalanx with the various fibrous attachments to the lateral tubercles at its base. Note the presence of the lateral interosseous ligaments with their proximal and distal fibrous continuations. B, a composite lateral view of a partial sagittal section of the digital pulp on the volar surface of the distal phalanx. (From M. Shrewsbury and R. K. Johnson, The fascia of the distal phalanx. J. Bone Joint Surg. *[Am.] 57:784, 1975.)*

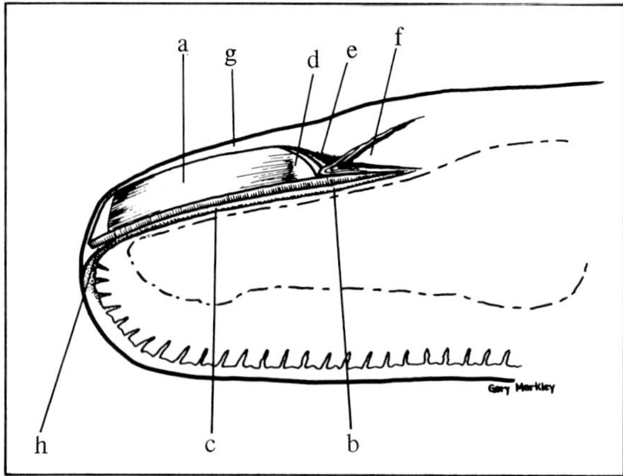

Fig. 32-2. Fingernail anatomy, a, *nail plate;* b, *germinal matrix;* c, *nail bed;* d, *lunula;* e, *eponychial fold;* f, *site of paronychia;* g, *lateral nail fold;* h, *hyponychium. (Redrawn from M. Shrewsbury and R. K. Johnson,* J. Bone Joint Surg. *57:784, 1975.)*

Type of Injury

Fingertip wounds can be subdivided in two ways: (1) a simple laceration as compared with more complicated ones from which there has been a loss of substance of skin, soft tissue, and deeper structures; and (2) sharp, "tidy" wounds as compared with complex, crushed, contaminated, "untidy" wounds.

Important observations in fingertip injuries are: the level of injury and the amount, if any, of the exposed phalanx; the obliquity of injury and the proportion of volar pad involved relative to remaining length; and the degree of involvement of the nail structures.

Hand dominance, occupation, avocation, the specific digit or combination of digits involved, age, and any special needs of the patient require careful individual consideration and may modify the application of the guidelines for treatment.

Goals of Treatment

It is desirable to restore the injured digits to fullest possible function after the shortest possible period of disability. The goal is to provide stable, durable, corniferous skin, protected from underlying bone by pliable soft tissue, with functional and pain-free sensibility. The contour should approach normal. Nail deformity and unnecessary loss of nail should be avoided when possible. Preservation of length is important, particularly in the thumb and index finger as well as in multiple losses, but has sometimes been overemphasized. A tender, painful, cold-sensitive finger resulting from direct closure or flap coverage under excessive tension or free graft in direct contact with bone is far more disabling than a nonpainful, stable, sensible digit of lesser length. The worst that can result from the latter is exclusion of the digit; the worst result from the former involves exclusion of the hand. It is of greater importance to preserve stable length in the thumb and index tips distal to the functional nail matrix than in the proximal one-half of the distal segment in order to preserve the precise, fine pick-up function of the nail [66, 74]. Reconstructive donor area deficits should be functionally insignificant and cosmetically minimal.

Application of Specific Techniques

The available methods of treatment, with or without shortening of bone, are: dressing with repair by epithelialization and wound contraction, direct suturing of the skin, free autogenous split-thickness and full-thickness skin grafts, local flaps, distant flaps from adjacent portions of the same hand, distant flaps from elsewhere in the body, and replantation.

Reports comparing results of several graft and flap techniques fail to show any uniformity. The following section presents the more common variants of fingertip injuries and recommendations for management.

Initial Considerations

In every case, careful preparation of the hand and cleaning of the wound are necessary. Exposure of the wound to direct contact with antiseptic is deplored, since some degree of additional cellular damage will result. The injured skin should be carefully prepared, preferably with an organic iodine compound, and the wound itself is meticulously cleaned with large volumes of sterile balanced saline solution. A pulsatile irrigating jet may be of some help.

The choice between emergency room, clinic, or major operating room as the site for operation is individual to the proposed procedure and to the facility in which the patient is cared for; the choice is based on the ready availability of proper lighting, instruments, assistants, sterile technique, bloodless field, and suitable anesthesia. In this regard, excess is preferable to insufficiency.

Regional anesthesia is well suited to these cases. Techniques of regional block are well described by Chase [17]. Of particular importance is the placement of local anesthetic in the loose space between the metacarpal heads for regional anesthesia of individual digits, rather than placing it within the digit itself distal to the web.

Repair by Wound Contraction

The method of repair by wound contraction, attributed to Fisk by Bossley [9], has recently received increasing attention [16, 35, 37]. It is particularly applicable to children but may be useful in adults as well.

The skin is prepared and the wound is irrigated and freed of nonvital tissue. In children the bone is not trimmed, since some restoration of length covering exposed bone that is not rongeured appears to occur, suggesting some regeneration. In adults the phalanx should be rongeured 1 to 2 mm. proximal to the soft tissue level. A layer of nonadherent gauze followed by a compact soft dressing is applied. The dressing is changed weekly until epithelialization is complete. The patient (or the parents) is cautioned at the time of treatment that the digit will appear inflamed or unpleasant at the first dressing change. Four to ten weeks are necessary for completed wound closure.

In my opinion this is the method of choice for treatment of fingertip injuries of children. The upper age limit is not established. In adults it is well suited for small areas of slicing skin loss, but in most adults I prefer to use a very thin split skin graft, as described in the following section.

Repair of Injuries When the Bone Is Not Exposed

Transverse or Slightly Oblique Loss of Skin and Pulp

In these cases (Fig. 32-3), the normal process of wound contraction will, with time, resurface the defect by advancement of the normal, sensible, cornified adjacent volar and lateral skin over the wound. Since the skin is relatively elastic and the nail bed–periosteum at the tip is relatively nonelastic, the final scar lies just below the nail edge. This result may be achieved either by the previously described wound contraction method or, as is my preference, by the application of a *very thin* (less than 0.25 mm. or less than 0.010 inches) split-thickness skin graft. (The statement is often encountered that the thinner the skin graft is, the more it will contract. This is incorrect; contraction takes place at the wound interface with the graft and is usually inhibited to a lesser extent by thin than by thick grafts.) The important

Fig. 32-3. Transverse or slightly oblique loss of skin and pulp without bone exposure.

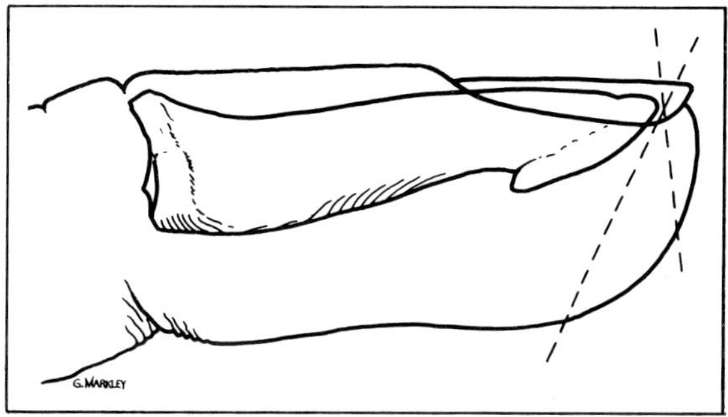

concept in the skin-graft technique is that the graft is not intended as the final cover but rather as an early epithelial barrier producing a healed protected wound in 4 to 7 days without inhibiting wound contraction appreciably. Many patients are able to return to work with a small finger dressing in place within 7 to 10 days with less tenderness and less danger of infection than occurred with the dressing technique.

PROCEDURE. The digit is properly prepared. Hemostasis, which is essential, is gained by careful compression, occasionally with precise pinpoint electrocoagulation. The thinnest possible graft is cut, free hand or with the use of a small dermatome such as the Silver knife* or the Goulian knife†. The graft may be secured either by fine sutures with a tie-over bolster dressing or by crisscrossed sterile adhesive strips. A gentle compressive bolus of cotton wool or a piece of sponge from a disposable skin prep kit is applied over a single layer of nonadherent flexible gauze; an external dressing of tubular gauze is applied, with the proximal interphalangeal joint left mobile. The initial dressing is removed in 5 to 7 days, and it may be replaced by a light dressing or Band-Aids thereafter. Delay in application of the graft for 48 hours is advisable in injuries with severe crushing, since the microvasculature may undergo thrombosis not evident at the time of injury.

A variety of donor sites are available, none of which are ideal. Volar lateral hypothenar skin is useful for medium-thickness split-thickness grafts [68] or full-thickness grafts [52], but its thick cornified layer is a disadvantage for very thin grafts. Volar forearm and upper inner arm skin is excellent; however, a mild cosmetic deformity may result. The upper lateral thigh is of lesser cosmetic importance, but grafts from this area tend to hyperpigment significantly. Selection is individual.

Tangential Loss of the Volar Surface

Tangential loss of the volar surface commonly results from an accident with a sharp knife or meat slicing machine. If the loss is of skin only and less than 5 to 7 mm. transversely, the wound may be sutured or allowed to heal spontaneously. Greater involvement requires resurfacing in a manner designed to prevent wound contraction (Fig. 32-4). When all pulp has been lost with resultant exposure of phalanx and flexor insertion, the use of flap coverage (such as cross finger flap or volar advancement flap) is advised (as discussed under the heading Repair of Skin and Pulp Loss with Bone Exposed). Commonly 50 percent or more of the pulp thickness will remain; in these cases a thick split-thickness or full-thickness hypothenar skin graft provides excellent results [52]. Full-thickness groin skin may also be used. A lenticular-shaped piece of full-thickness skin equal in width to that of the full volar surface of the middle finger may be removed from the volar lateral aspect of the hypothenar pad. Linear closure of the donor defect is readily accomplished, especially if aided by a 5-mm. mobilization of the margins. Initially a mild depression at the donor site results but in my experience this remodels nicely; such donor scars have been without troublesome sequelae. The graft is immobilized with a gently compressive dressing, which remains in place for 10 to 12 days.

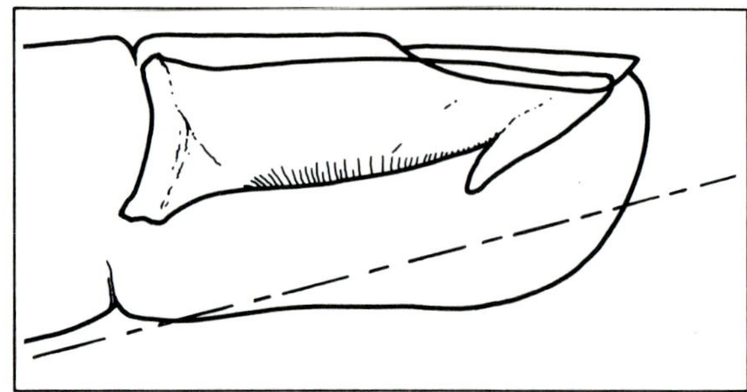

Fig. 32-4. Tangential loss of the volar surface.

If the injury involves only the radial volar aspect and the distribution of the ulnar digital nerve is intact at the tip, the ulnar volar skin may be transferred to the defect, without tension, as a local neurovascular flap; the new ulnar defect is then surfaced with a free graft, as described by Littler [54].

Repair of Skin and Pulp Loss with Bone Exposed

The critical factors of sensibility, durability, length, and freedom from pain are most at risk when the bone has been exposed. Preservation of length of the index finger and thumb is most important in the zone from the tip of the bony phalanx to the level of the lunula in order to provide phalangeal support of the nail, which is essential to fine pick-up and helpful in support of the terminal pulp [66].

Transverse or Oblique Injury with Greater Preservation of Volar Skin at or Distal to the Eponychial Fold

This type of injury is illustrated in Figure 32-5.

THUMB. The volar advancement flap is recommended [66, 86]. Other satisfactory choices are index cross finger flap with radial nerve innervation [1, 9], the flag flap [38, 95], the rotation advancement flap of Argamaso [2], or the index cross finger flap [40, 62].

*Storz Instrument Co., 3365 Tree Court Industrial Blvd., St. Louis, Mo. 63122.

†Edward Weck & Co., Inc., 49-33 31st Place, Long Island City, N.Y. 11101.

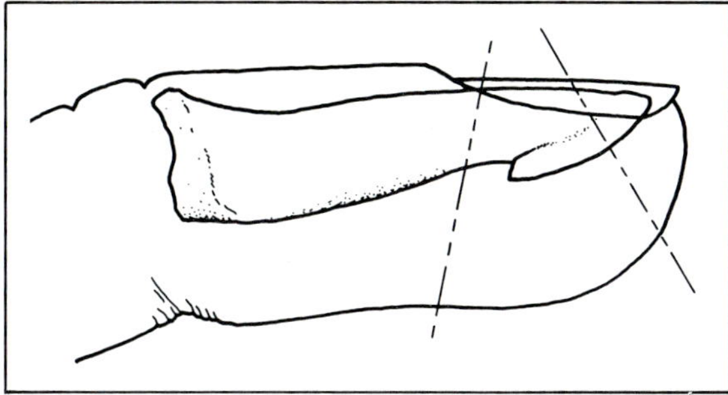

Fig. 32-5. *Transverse or oblique injury with greater preservation of volar skin at or distal to the eponychial fold.*

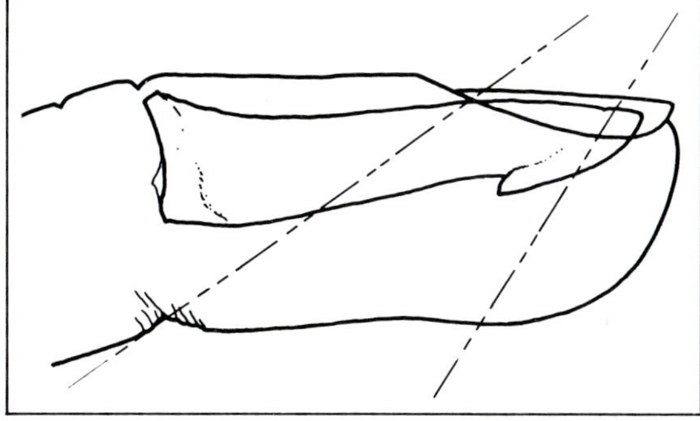

Fig. 32-6. *Oblique injury with volar loss extending proximally, at or distal to the eponychial fold.*

INDEX FINGER. The volar V-Y advancement (Kleinert flap) [3] is recommended. If the injury is oblique greater preservation of the volar tissues, the volar neurovascular advancement flap is satisfactory but is more difficult to mobilize adequately than in the thumb. Both of these flaps offer the greatest chance for normal sensibility. Other satisfactory choices are the laterally based dorsal transposition flap [62], a cross finger flap from the middle finger, or the Hueston volar transposition flap [36].

MIDDLE, RING, AND SMALL FINGERS. The volar V-Y advancement or bone shortening with direct closure is recommended.

Oblique Injury with Volar Loss Extending Proximally, at or Distal to the Eponychial Fold

This injury is illustrated in Figure 32-6.

THUMB. Either the volar neurovascular advancement flap with mobilization of neurovascular bundles and proximal skin graft [54] or radial innervated index cross finger flap is recommended. An index cross finger flap without nerve transfer is also acceptable.

In an untidy wound situation, it may at times be wise to attain initial healing with a thin split-thickness skin graft and proceed with definitive repair 1 to 3 weeks later, lessening the chance of complications (but losing the advantage of one-stage repair).

INDEX FINGER. The cross finger flap from the middle finger is recommended. The volar transposition flap of Hueston may also be suitable.

MIDDLE, RING, AND SMALL FINGERS. Bone shortening with dorsal flap closure is recommended.

Injury Proximal to the Eponychial Fold

This injury is illustrated in Figure 32-7.

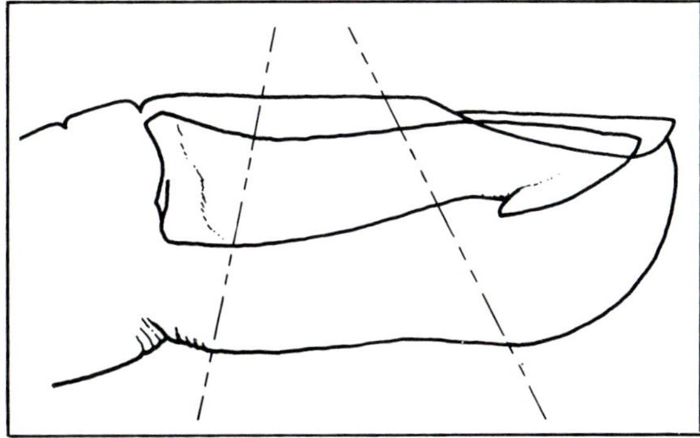

Fig. 32-7. *Injury proximal to the eponychial fold.*

THUMB. Depending upon individual assessment of the need for length, the Littler volar advancement flap with proximal graft or the index cross finger flap may be used, or the bone may be shortened to allow direct tension-free closure.

INDEX, MIDDLE, RING, AND SMALL FINGER. If tension-free direct closure can be attained by disarticulation at the distal joint, this procedure is recommended since it will result in the greatest number of functional repairs with the most rapid healing time. Care must be taken with removal of nail matrix remnants. If direct closure is not possible, the cross finger flap is recommended. The volar V-Y advancement flap may give less good results [97].

Degloving of Distal Phalanx with Distal Interphalangeal Joint Function Intact

THUMB. This injury may be an indication for immediate neurovascular island flap transfer from another digit, but this procedure should be undertaken only by surgeons experienced in elective neurovascular island transfers. Otherwise, distant pedicle resurfacing from the chest, opposite arm or forearm, or groin flap, with secondary neurovascular island or index radial innervated cross finger flap coverage, is preferable if the distal phalanx is to be preserved. Several reports describing only a poor return of sensibility have made the value of the neurovascular island flap controversial. It is probable that these poor results are in part due to technical difficulties that can be overcome [58].

For distal phalangeal degloving of digits other than thumb, distal phalangeal amputation is advised [13].

Flap Techniques

Attention to details of technique and anatomy is necessary to success; accordingly it is recommended that the reader become acquainted with the articles referred to in the text.

Bone Shortening and Direct Flap Closure

See under the heading Amputation of Digits.

Cross Finger Flap

This flap [40, 62] may be laterally or proximally based. The distal base is hazardous, since perfusion is diminished. The skin of the dorsum of the proximal and middle phalanges may be used, but the skin over the proximal interphalangeal joint should be spared if possible. The flap may extend from one midaxial line to the space along the opposite midaxial line. It is raised in the loose plane over the extensor tendon, leaving areolar tissue on the tendon. Clelland's ligaments are cut at the base as necessary for mobility. The margins of the recipient defect should be altered to conform to lines of elective incision if necessary. The flap is designed to place the digits in a position of least possible interphalangeal flexion. The donor defect is covered with a thick split-thickness or full-thickness skin graft dressed with a tie-over bolus. Care is taken not to kink or twist the pedicle. The digits are dressed and immobilized in a plaster splint or shell cast. A transarticular Kirschner wire may be useful in some cases. The flap base is divided and inset in 2 to 2½ weeks, and mobilization of the digits is begun. Insetting of the flap should be delayed for several days if the flap is congested and edematous after division of its pedicle.

Innervated Cross Finger Flap

This flap [1, 29] is based proximally at the index metacarpophalangeal joint level. It is elevated in the same plane as the standard cross finger flap and is sutured to the thumb defect without tension; the donor site is resurfaced with a free graft. In 2 to 3 weeks the flap base is divided, but care is taken to preserve the branches of the radial nerve to the flap. The nerve is mobilized through a zig-zag incision from the base of the flap to the dorsum of the first web. The incision is then continued distally along the midaxis of the thumb to meet the base of the inset flap when the nerve is moved into the thumb incision completing the transfer. The flap also may be based along its volar lateral edge and the nerve transferred at the first stage, leaving only the division of the pedicle for the second stage [1].

A similar two-stage technique for transfer from middle finger to index finger, utilizing a dorsal branch of the digital nerve, is described by Joshi [42].

Sensory distribution of the intended donor nerves should be mapped preoperatively with local anesthetic nerve blocks when using these techniques.

Flag Flap

The flag flap of Iselin uses middle or proximal phalangeal skin (the flag) on a narrow proximal pedicle (the flag pole) for a one- or two-stage transfer to dorsal or volar defects of the same or adjacent digit. Branches of the radial nerve may be transferred with the flap. Its blood supply is said to be from the dermovascular plexus. The reader is referred to the papers by Iselin [38] and Villain and Dupuis [95], since I have not used this flap myself.

Dorsal Transposition Flap

The base of this flap [52, 83] is along one midaxial line, the tip is at or near the other, the distal margin is the level of amputation injury, and the proximal margin is parallel to the distal interphalangeal extension crease. The flap is elevated in the extensor plane and transposed over the exposed end of the digit. It may be used as a bipedicle, but the mobility of the flap is thus limited. The donor site is resurfaced with a free split-thickness graft.

Volar Triangular V-Y Advancement Flap

This triangular flap [3] has a proximal subcutaneous pedicle bearing the terminal digital nerve and vessel filaments. The triangle is designed with the distal cut edge of skin as base and is of width slightly greater than the nail; a V incision of skin only, with its apex near the distal joint crease, completes the triangle. The flap is immobilized by division of the fibrous strands along the phalanx and fibrous sheath, followed by careful division of the fibrous strands along the V incision, especially at the apex, until the flap moves distally. Dissection at this point must not be deep, to avoid dividing the neurovascular supply. The distal edge of the flap is sutured to the edge of nail and matrix. The V defect is closed as a Y, but if the closure is under tension, a very thin split-thickness graft may be applied to the V defect instead. Atraumatic handling of this flap is essential. Similar flaps based laterally as described by Kutler may also be fashioned. Freiberg and Manktelow [27] have reported 19 cases of Kutler flaps with little or no residual symptoms; however, these findings are contradicted in the 31 cases of Weston and Wallace [97].

Volar Advancement Flap
In the volar advancement flap (Snow [86]), midaxial incisions are made from the defect to a point 2 cm. proximal to the interphalangeal joint level in the thumb or 1 cm. proximal to the proximal interphalangeal joint in the finger. Clelland's ligaments are divided and the entire volar skin and soft tissue with neurovascular bundles intact are freed by sharp dissection from the fibrous flexor sheath. Care must be taken to avoid damaging the volar plates or injuring the dorsal branches of the digital nerves near the proximal interphalangeal joint. The tip of the flap may be made to fit the tip of the amputation by suturing the preserved lateral triangles at the end of the flap if desired. The flap is advanced to the tip and the midaxial incisions are sutured. Considerable interphalangeal joint flexion may be required for closure in the finger but less is needed with the thumb. Mobilization is begun after 2 weeks.

Volar Advancement Flap with Proximal Skin Graft
In the volar advancement flap with proximal skin graft (Littler [54]), the volar skin is mobilized as for the volar advancement flap. The skin and subcutaneous tissue are divided transversely near the metacarpophalangeal crease (thumb), avoiding injury of the neurovascular bundles, which are gently mobilized. The flap is then drawn distally as much as 1.5 cm. and sutured in the defect. The proximal bare area is covered with a full-thickness skin graft. Mild flexion of the interphalangeal joint may be required. The thumb is dressed and immobilized; remobilization is begun in 12 to 14 days.

Hueston Volar Transposition Flap
This flap is based on one entire neurovascular bundle; it is transposed obliquely distally, leaving a proximal triangular donor defect to be covered by a free skin graft. The reader is referred to the paper by Hueston [36] for technical details and report of 1 case.

Neurovascular Island Flap
A thorough discussion of this flap is beyond the scope of this chapter. The technique should be used only by experienced hand surgeons. For review of the pertinent literature and technical aspects, see the article by Markley [58].

Thenar and Palmar Flaps
I prefer to avoid the use of these flaps and agree with the observation of Rank, Wakefield, and Hueston [72] that it is unwise to create a secondary defect in the sensory region of the palm against which the injured tip will oppose. In addition, the marked flexion of the proximal interphalangeal joint required for thenar flaps can cause severe joint stiffness in adults. However, there are reports of satisfactory results of thenar and palmar flaps [63, 88].

Replantation
Replantation and revascularization of severed fingertips by microvascular anastomoses are discussed in Chapter 43.

Nail Bed Reconstruction
At times it may be desirable to attempt reconstruction of the nail primarily for cosmetic reasons. The folded skin-graft nail-pouch technique with insertion of a modified commercial plastic artificial nail [12] or a custom-made acrylic nail [6] can be used in these cases. McCash [59, 60] has reported 10 cases of free nail transplantation from the toes, with results varying from excellent appearance and function to brittle and fragmented nails.

FINGERNAIL AVULSION. In crush injury of the fingertip, the base of the nail plate is often avulsed from the cul-de-sac, with or without fracture of the phalanx. Replacement of the nail seems logical but is undesirable, since subacute paronychia or subungual infection may result. Also, if the phalanx is fractured, a torn edge or fold of the nail bed may be trapped in the fracture line and will be hidden by the overlying replaced nail, resulting in nonunion or epidermal cyst formation [54, 80]. It is preferable to excise the proximal one-third to one-half of the nail plate and repair the soft tissues only. If it is felt absolutely necessary to replace the nail base, the drainage hole and traction suture technique of Schiller should be used [81].

AMPUTATION OF DIGITS

Functional loss resulting from amputation of a portion of one or more digits, whether by accident or election, may be lessened by careful selection of the level and technique of repair. As with fingertip injuries, the single most important feature of successful repair is the provision of stable, sensible, pain-free, well-padded skin. Preservation of length at the expense of quality of cover is inadvisable [18, 66, 73]. There are several situations in which the use of local or distant flap techniques to preserve length with good cover (rather than direct closure with bone shortening) is indicated. These situations are: loss in the thumb distal to the eponychial fold and losses greater than the proximal 1 cm. of the proximal phalanx; loss in the index finger distal to the midshaft of the middle phalanx; and multiple digital losses in which any remaining length may be of value. In these cases the salvage of portions of one digit for use in reconstruction of another should be considered and the use of free grafts and any viable local flaps to gain cover is advised [17, 69, 89].

The Thumb

The most significant functional loss with amputation of the thumb distal to the proximal centimeter of the proximal phalanx is the inability to pick up fine objects due to loss of thumbnail. All the other prehensile functions (e.g., key pinch and power grip) are preserved at normal or near normal levels, provided that the stump is stable and pain free, as demonstrated by Ratliff [74] and discussed by Murray [66]. Thus, direct closure with normal volar skin and with shortening of bone as required is indicated when the final healed level falls between the proximal and distal centimeter of the thumb. However, when the amputated part is replantable, this may be the procedure of choice because it restores the thumbnail (see Chapter 43). The proximal centimeter may be preserved through the use of local volar and/or dorsal skin flaps, flag flaps, cross finger flaps, or forearm flaps when necessary.

When total amputation of the thumb with no opportunity for replantation occurs, a healed and stable wound should be attained in the most rapid and uncomplicated manner available by the use of free grafts and/or local flaps. Subsequently the thumb may be reconstructed by index finger transposition, osteoplastic thumb reconstruction with transfer of island neurovascular flap, toe to hand transfer, or the use of a prosthetic pinch post. Recently an immediate groin flap containing an iliac bone graft was used in the reconstruction of a thumb amputation; this procedure may be of help in selected cases [23].

Index Finger

When shortened proximal to the midshaft of the middle phalanx, the index finger will usually be excluded from hand function and held in the hyperextended posture of "index habitus" to allow its functional replacement by the adjacent middle finger. Thus, index amputations at this level should be resurfaced without further shortening. The volar triangular flap or cross finger flap is recommended in this circumstance. When the amputation is more proximal, consideration may be given to primary index amputation at the proximal one-quarter of the metacarpal. In most cases it may be wise, however, to close the amputation at a nonfunctional level and allow the patient to anticipate for himself, with the surgeon's guidance, the potential value of removal of the nonfunctional index stump.

Middle and Ring Fingers

Amputation at any level distal to the proximal interphalangeal joint may be shortened and closed. When the level of amputation is proximal to the proximal interphalangeal joint, the resulting gap between the adjacent fingers often results in loss of ability to contain small objects in the cupped hand. This may be corrected and the appearance strikingly improved by metacarpal amputation and transfer of the index to the middle metacarpal or small to ring metacarpal (see under the heading Digital Ray [Metacarpal] Amputation).

Small Finger

Amputation distal to the proximal interphalangeal joint is closed primarily. Proximal to this level, resection obliquely just distal to the metacarpal base is usually indicated.

Multiple Digital Loss and Proximal Amputations

When several digits are amputated, all possible length should be preserved. Consideration should be given to possible replantation. (Discussion of management of transmetacarpal, transcarpal, and wrist disarticulation amputations with the use of static and dynamic prostheses is beyond the scope of this chapter. The reader is referred to the articles by Tooms [94], Mansfield and Knight [57], and Swanson [89].)

Technical Aspects of Digital Amputation

Flaps

The volar flap is preferred when possible. When designing these flaps, the lateral incisions should be somewhat volar to the midaxial line (Fig. 32-8), which will minimize dog ears and provide a smooth contour [92]. In oblique traumatic amputations with relative loss of volar skin, dorsal or lateral flaps may be designed to make maximum use of available tissue. Hemostasis and closure should be meticulous. Fine monofilament nonabsorbable suture is preferred. When suturing is completed, the skin should be neither under tension nor patulous.

Treatment of the Bone End

When a digital amputation is to be at the level of a joint, the articular coverage of the remaining phalangeal head should not be removed, although such removal is often recommended [92]. Whitaker and

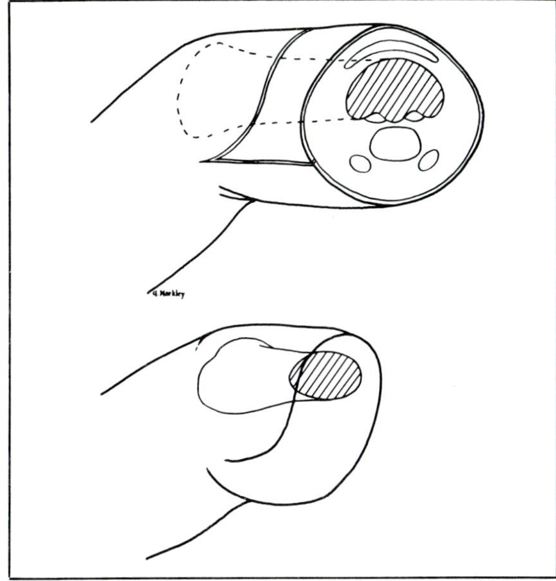

Fig. 32-8. Design of volar flap for digital amputation.

colleagues [99] have shown that preservation of the articular cartilage results in less inflammation and better mobility, resilience, and comfort of the stump. The condylar flare may be trimmed for better contour. When the amputation is not at a joint, the medullary cavity may be closed, with results similar to preservation of articular cartilage with an osteoperiosteal flap [50].

Tendon

The tendons are withdrawn, severed cleanly, and allowed to retract. In no case should the tendon ends be sutured across the bone end for padding, since this will result in tenodesis with imbalance of the intrinsic and extrinsic systems and derangement of function of the stump and of the remaining digits.

Nerves and Neuromas

The digital nerves should be dissected gently 2 to 3 mm. proximal to the level of amputation and divided cleanly with a fresh blade. Traction on the nerve and ligation of the nerve are undesirable, since either action may result in increased scar adherence of the neuroma. A painful neuroma is one of the primary sources of disability following digital amputation. Formation of the terminal neuroma is a natural result of healing of the severed peripheral nerve. Why some neuromas should be tender while others, formed under apparently identical circumstances, are not is unclear. Methods to eliminate painful neuromas are numerous and of variable effectiveness. In my experience, the technique described by Herndon, Eaton, and Littler [34] is the most reliable; in this technique, the neuroma is left intact with the nerve and is gently dissected from the surrounding scar and soft tissue. The nerve is mobilized proximally by sharp dissection until the neuroma can be transposed proximally into a protected, soft position *without tension on the nerve.* Insertion of the nerve into bone, or silicone capping if done meticulously and precisely, may also be effective [90].

Fingernail

In amputations near the base of the distal phalanx, careful attention to ablation of the nail matrix is important.

Digital Ray (Metacarpal) Amputation

When the level of finger amputation is through the proximal phalanx or at the metacarpophalangeal joint, the resulting stump may be excluded from (or interfere with) coordinated hand function, may result in loss of small-object containment by cupping of the hand, and is often of unpleasant appearance. With loss of the restraint of the intervolar plate ligament, malrotation and divergence of adjacent fingers may result. All of these problems may be relieved by resection of the remaining portion of the ray near the metacarpal base and, in the case of the central digits, transfer of the adjacent marginal digit to the more central position. The resulting three-finger hand will suffer some reduction in grip strength [14, 67] and the decrease in width at the level of the metacarpal heads may somewhat diminish torsional force of the hand, but this is generally overshadowed by the increase in dexterity and coordinated function. Cold intolerance and hyperesthesia of the new first web may present difficulty postoperatively [67]. Caution is advised in subjecting the chronically painful hand to ray amputation, because pain will often persist despite a technically perfect procedure.

Technical details of index and small finger ray resection, middle finger resection with metacarpal shift of index, and ring finger resection with metacarpal shift of small finger may be found in several articles [17, 62, 69, 89]. Several important features warrant emphasis (Fig. 32-9):

1. Skin incisions should be planned to transfer a full web rather than allowing the final scar to run through a web.
2. Positive identification of digital nerves and vessels to adjacent fingers must be made prior to division of those to the digit being removed to avoid error due to anomalous neurovascular patterns.
3. Metacarpal resection should be subperiosteal.
4. Metacarpal stumps of border digits should be

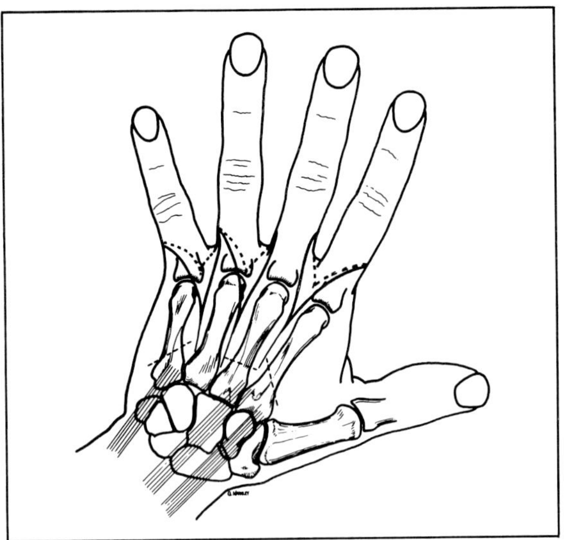

Fig. 32-9. Composite of skin incisions and osteotomy sites for index, ring, and small fingers. Skin incisions for middle finger amputation with index transfer, not illustrated, are similar to those for index ray amputation. Note the insertions of wrist extensors. Solid incision lines are dorsal, broken lines are volar.

beveled for smooth contour.

5. In index ray amputation, the extensor indicis proprius may be sutured to the extensor digitorum communis of the middle finger to improve independent function. Care must be taken to avoid excessive tension in this transfer.
6. The first dorsal interosseous tendon may be transferred to the middle finger following index ray amputation to provide greater abduction force; this tendon may be inserted either into the phalangeal base or into the radial intrinsic tendon. If the latter insertion is used, great care must be taken to prevent undue tension, which would result in intrinsic deformity. The same is true of abductor digiti minimi transfer to the ring finger for small finger amputation.
7. Digital nerve stumps should be kept long and transferred without tension into a soft portion of the interosseous muscle mass.
8. Bases of index, middle, and small finger metacarpals should not be resected, since these are the sites of insertion of the wrist extensor tendons.
9. The small finger metacarpal may be transferred in two ways: (a) the ring finger metacarpal may be disarticulated at the carpometacarpal joint [14], or (b) transverse osteotomy at the proximal one-third with fusion of the metacarpals may be done [69]. If the ring metacarpal is disarticulated, the fifth metacarpal base will shift radially. This eliminates the possible complications of nonunion and changes in extrinsic/intrinsic tendon balance. However, osteotomy with fusion has the advantage of allowing modest advancement of length of the transferred small finger to closer balance with the index and middle fingers. Usually this is limited to 5 mm., or undue tension will be placed on the extrinsic tendons, resulting in imbalance.
10. Careful attention must be paid to proper rotational position of the metacarpal to avoid finger crossing.
11. The intermetacarpal ligament must be preserved and reconstituted to prevent splaying of the fingers.
12. Use of an intramedullary bone peg cut from the resected metacarpal may be used to aid fusion of the metacarpals.

Problems Related to Fingernail Remnants

When the eponychial fold and lunula are preserved in fingertip loss, I believe that the residual nail should be allowed to prove its value or lack thereof. Often even a short, downward-curved nail remnant may provide useful function. At times, however, the residual nail may snag objects, cause local irritation or pain, and be cosmetically unsatisfactory. In such cases, it should be secondarily ablated. When the tip loss has been proximal to the eponychial fold, the residual matrix should be completely removed initially, since the regrowth of a nail remnant in this situation is nearly always disabling. Successful complete removal of the germinal matrix requires excision from midaxial to midaxial line and from the lunula and eponychial cul-de-sac proximally along the dorsum of the phalanx until the extensor insertion is reached.

Nail Splitting

Scarring of the germinal matrix may result in split nail deformity. Removal of the nail, excision of the scar, and bipedicle mobilization together with meticulous repair of the matrix (as described by Johnson [39]) may result in significant improvement.

INFECTIONS OF THE HAND

Infection in the hand, if unchecked, can partially or totally destroy the hand's function. In 1907 Kanavel [43] set forth principles of anatomy and technique that remain pertinent. However, the advent of antibiotics and an increased awareness of the significance of hand infection have resulted in a change in patterns of infection and a general decrease in occurrence of severe complications and sequelae [8].

The goal of treatment (as for any hand affliction) is to overcome the infection with minimum tissue damage (due to either the pathological process or the treatment) and with maximum restoration of function. Before treatment can begin, a correct diagnosis must be made. (Features of anatomical diagnosis are covered in the following sections on specific types of infection.) Bacteriological diagnosis depends first on a presumptive diagnosis based on statistical data for hand infections, supplanted when possible by specific diagnoses attained with smear, gram stain, and anaerobic and aerobic cultures with determination of antibiotic sensitivity.

Any infection is an interaction between three variables (Fig. 32-10). Proper treatment is predicated on decreasing organism dose and virulence and increasing host resistance.

Organism dose can be reduced by adequate drainage of pus, by dilution with irrigation, and by serial dressing changes ("dilution is the solution to pollution"). Organism dose and, in part, virulence may be reduced by appropriate antibiotic therapy provided that the drug has ingress to the organism by means of an intact circulation. Host resistance may be improved by:

1. Rest, with immobilization of the hand in the balanced functional position. The wrist, key to the posture of the hand, should be included in the immobilization. A light, nonconstrictive plaster shell over a gently conforming gauze dressing is effective and, when properly applied, less hazardous than a splint wrapped with elastic bandages [44].
2. Elevation of the hand, improving venous return and decreasing edema, thus improving microcirculation and in addition decreasing long-term stiffness.
3. Careful elimination of clearly nonvital tissue.
4. Diagnosis and control insofar as possible of resistance-depressing factors, such as diabetes mellitus, antimetabolic drugs, and chronic lymphedema.

A variety of bacteriological studies of hand infection over the past 10 years suggests that gram-positive organisms account for 75 to 85 percent of all organisms in hand infections and that *Staphylococcus aureus* is the dominant organism (Bell [8] 61 percent; Stone [87] 59 percent; Eaton [20] 47 percent). At the present time, most staphylococci will be penicillin resistant (Bell 67 percent; Eaton 64 percent; Stone 56 percent; Freiberg [28] 88 percent). These studies suggest that methicillin, oxacillin, cephalothin, and erythromycin are the empirical choices pending specific culture and sensitivity results in all hand infections, including those due to human bites [56]. If large numbers of gram-negative organisms are present on gram strain, the initial use of either cephalothin

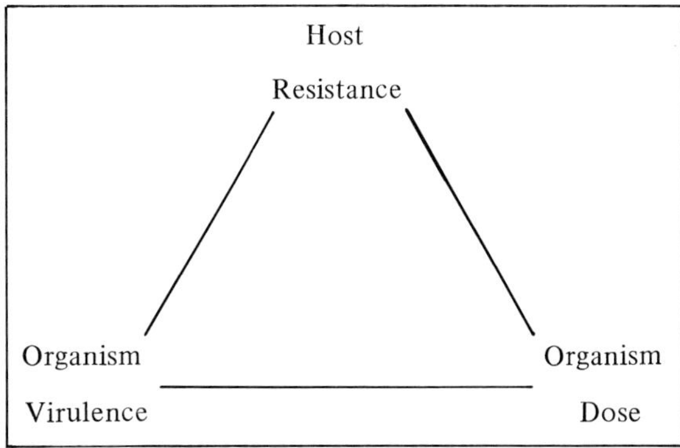

Fig. 32-10. The triangle of infection.

or a combination of semisynthetic penicillin and kanamycin may be indicated, depending on the severity of infection. However, Fitzgerald and co-workers' [26] study of mutilating hand injuries due to farm implements indicates that in this specific entity the flora is predominately of mixed gram-negative organisms. They are often resistant to kanamycin, cephalothin, and ampicillin. In such cases, these authors recommend delaying the use of any antibiotic until wound culture data are available; they stress meticulous wound care and delayed closure.

It is emphasized that the use of antibiotics is an aid to, not a replacement for, proper surgical management with drainage, meticulous wound care, and immobilization of the infected hand.

Type of Infection

Description of types of invasive hand infection according to anatomical locus has been the conventional method and is useful. It is important to recognize that unchecked infection may breach the boundaries of the various compartments, obscuring anatomical landmarks and increasing the severity of damage.

Subcutaneous Infection

Subcutaneous infection more commonly involves the dorsal aspect of the digits and hand. It is usually localized; upon careful examination, it does not present the signs of deep infection. The initial stage of cellulitis should be treated by elevation, rest, and antibiotics, without incision. Drainage in this stage serves no purpose and should be avoided unless a localized abscess has occurred. Infections of the subcutaneous space of the dorsum of the hand superficial to the extensor tendons may be particularly misleading, since the loose areolar layer permits accumulation of so much edema that abscess may be mimicked by diffuse cellulitis, precipitating fruitless attempts at drainage.

Collar-Button Abscess
Subcutaneous abscess of the palmar aspect, characteristically in the web space, may penetrate the space between metacarpal heads more easily than the tough palmar corniferous skin and present dorsally, forming a vertically oriented dumbbell or collar-button configuration. Penetration of the lumbrical canal may occur, with potentially devastating effect. Drainage is by dorsal and palmar incisions between the metacarpal heads, sparing the web; curved or angled incisions are made if the distal palmar crease is crossed.

Felon
Pyogenic infection of the ungual pulp is termed *felon,* a name of obscure origin. As noted previously in this chapter, the proximal boundary of the ungual pulp is a fibrous sheet at the distal flexion crease. Fibrous strands connect phalanx and dermis but do not form a system of closed compartments as is sometimes inferred [49]. The distal segment is red, tense, painful, and exquisitely tender, but cutaneous pointing of the abscess may not be evident. If not drained, felon may result in distal phalangeal osteomyelitis or penetration into the flexor sheath or both. If the abscess is pointing distally or anteriorly, drainage by a longitudinal midline incision as described by Kilgore is recommended (Fig. 32-11A). If the abscess is deep and/or proximal, my preference is to make an incision 1 mm. below the distal edge of the nail, continued along one lateral margin well above the midaxial line, skimming the volar surface of the phalanx (Fig. 32-11B). Incisions placed between those incisions just described should be avoided, even though they are often seen illustrated, because painful scars and pulp instability will usually result from their use. Care must be taken not to open the intact flexor sheath during drainage. A small piece of a thin rubber drain should remain in the wound, loosely, for 48 hours; the digit should be immobilized in the balanced position.

Paronychia
Insufficient attention has been given to differentiating three distinct entities often lumped together as *paronychia;* these are acute subungual abscess, acute paronychia, and chronic paronychia.

Acute subungual abscess is an abscess occurring between the nail plate and the nail bed. It is treated by removal of the proximal portion of the nail plate, including that beneath the eponychial fold. No skin or soft tissue incision is necessary.

Acute and chronic paronychia appear in the same anatomical site but differ in etiology. The thin subcutaneous layer sandwiched between the skin of the eponychial fold and the germinal layer of the eponychial cul-de-sac is the locus of infection. In acute paronychia, the introduction of pyogenic bacteria,

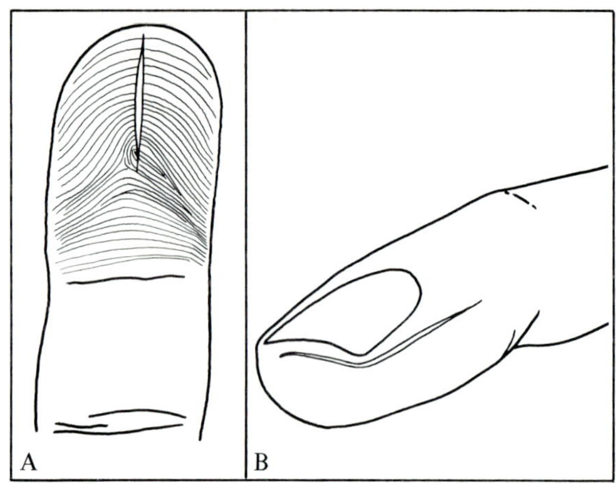

Fig. 32-11. Incisions for felon. (See text for further details.)

usually *Staphylococcus aureus,* by minor trauma results in acute inflammation and abscess formation in part or all of this space. If undrained, the abscess may extend deep to the nail or into the pulp space secondarily. Various incisions for drainage have been described that involve cutting through the margin of the eponychial fold at one or more points [62, 75]; this can result in somewhat deforming scars with notching of the cuticular margin. I believe acute paronychia can be best drained with lesser deformity by the same marsupialization technique as advocated for chronic paronychia by Keyser and Eaton [48].

Chronic paronychia is characterized by chronic inflammation with thickening of the eponychial fold, loss of cuticle, and grooving of the nail plate, which most commonly occurs in women with frequently macerated hands. The responsible organism is *Candida albicans,* sometimes with an associated mixed bacterial flora. The technique of eponychial marsupialization is effective for both chronic and acute paronychia. A crescentic piece of skin and subcutaneous tissue is excised. The piece of tissue is 5- to 6-mm. wide, its distal edge parallels the nail fold 1 to 2 mm. away, and its tips extend to both lateral nail margins (Fig. 32-12). The underlying matrix of the cul-de-sac is thus exposed but not injured. The wound is dressed daily after the first 48 to 72 hours and reepithelializes in approximately 2 weeks. In acute paronychia if extension into the pulp space by way of the rima ungualum has occurred, counterdrainage as for felon may be indicated.

Flexor Sheath Infection
Acute infection in the flexor sheath is now uncommon, contributing from 0.5 to 1.5 percent of the hand

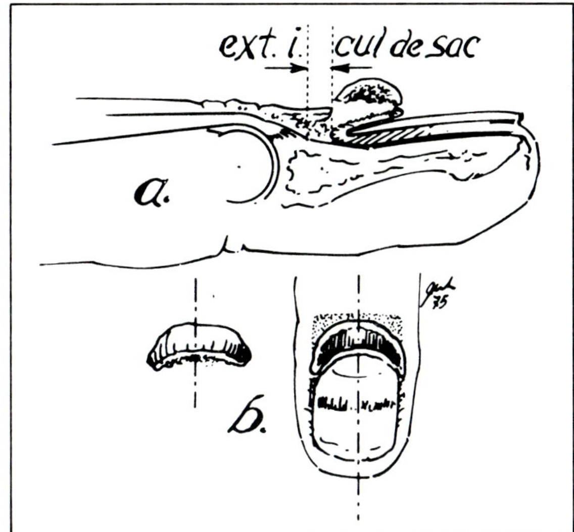

Fig. 32-12. Eponychial marsupialization. (From J. J. Keyser and R. J. Eaton, Surgical cure of chronic paronychia by eponychial marsupialization. Plast. Reconstr. Surg. *58:67, 1976.)*

infections in several recently reported series [70, 75]. However, familiarity with diagnosis and treatment of this infection is important because of its destructive potential. If the infection is controlled in the early, exudative phase, nearly full function may be regained; however, with progression of infection, extensive flexor adherence, necrosis, and spread to the deep planes of the hand may occur with disastrous results.

Usually there is a history of a digital injury, often a minor one, but at times no precipitating event can be found. The characteristic signs are: a semiflexed and motionless finger, diffuse swelling of the entire digit, tenderness along the course of the fibrous flexor sheath, and severe pain with passive motion [43]. When testing for pain on passive motion gently hold the distal segment along the lateral margins to avoid causing localized pain due to pressure on a tender volar aspect. In cases where diagnostic signs are obscured by other antecedent or coincident disease processes, very careful needle aspiration may be of help in diagnosis [77].

Surgical drainage is nearly always required except in the rare case seen extremely early (less than 12 hours from onset of symptoms); in the early case, the process may be reversed within 12 hours by using systemic antibiotics and immobilization. Drainage should be done under tourniquet ischemia with regional or general anesthesia. As with all hand infections, when establishing the bloodless field the hand should be exsanguinated by elevation prior to inflating the tourniquet to avoid the spread of infection by rubber bandage compression. An oblique incision passing distally from the distal palmar crease or a transverse incision at the distal palmar crease is made, the proximal end of the flexor tendon sheath is exposed and opened, and the exudate or pus is taken for culture and smear. If there is a digital wound or skin necrosis, this is excised; an incision may be extended along the midaxial line for exposure and opening of the flexor sheath. If there is no wound, the sheath is opened through a midaxial incision along the middle phalanx. Carter recommends a transverse digital incision rather than the axial incision when a catheter is used [15]. If there is tendon necrosis, the entire sheath should be opened and all necrotic material removed. A small plastic catheter is placed in the sheath through the palmar incision, and 2 to 4 ml. of semisynthetic penicillin solution is instilled every 4 hours for approximately 48 hours [15, 70]. Immobilization is maintained until the infection is controlled, and then remobilization is rapidly begun. Systemic antibiotics are used in addition to the irrigations.

The flexor sheath of index, middle, and ring fingers usually ends at the level of the metacarpophalangeal joints. That of the thumb extends proximally into the distal wrist, where it is termed the radial bursa. The sheath of the small finger extends at the ulnar bursa to the wrist as well and usually extends to envelop the middle and ring finger flexors in the proximal palm and wrist, separate from the digital flexor sheaths. The radial and ulnar bursae may communicate in the wrist; with the rupture of either, infection may spread into the subcutaneous space of Parona.

Deep Fascial Space Infection

The thenar and midpalmar spaces are potential planes of easy dissection lying between the deep interosseous and adductor fascia and the fascia deep to the flexor and lumbrical compartments. A plane of fascia from index flexor sheath to the third metacarpal separates the thenar from the palmar space. The detailed anatomy has been well described [4, 24, 43]. Deep fascial space infection has become quite rare. Diagnosis is based on deep swelling, palmar pain and tenderness, and loss of motion of the index finger and thumb (thenar) or the middle and ring (midpalmar) fingers. The midpalmar abscess is drained by any incision following lines of election for access to the ring finger flexors; the thenar space is exposed by either a first web space or a palmar thenar crease approach to the adductor pollicis [53, 62].

Special Problems

Opportunistic Infections

Since the report of Kelly and associates [47] in 1963, atypical mycobacterial infection of the hand has been recognized with increasing frequency [33, 46]. *Mycobacterium marinum, M. kansasii, M. intracellularis,* and *M. avium* have all been reported in hand infections. The typical clinical presentation is of a chronic, indolent, tender digital synovitis, often accompanied by carpal tunnel syndrome, in a middle-aged, otherwise healthy person. History of a preceding injury, particularly in association with marine fauna in the case of *M. marinum,* may be elicited, but this is not always the case. The patient is usually afebrile. If the infection is untreated, severe damage will result.

Diagnosis depends upon suspicion followed by synovial biopsy, acid-fast smear, and culture. Presence of granulomas histologically is of prime significance. Treatment is indicated for the combination of characteristic clinical findings, granulomatous synovitis histologically, and positive smear, and it should precede culture results. Treatment consists of thorough synovectomy surgically and chemotherapy with ethambutol, rifampin, and isoniazid. Cultures should be done at both 37 and 31°C. to include all varieties of atypical mycobacteria.

Fungi, particularly *Nocardia,* may also cause chronic synovial infection but more characteristically present as abscess or pyarthrosis. Treatment is by surgical drainage plus systemic sulfonamides and trimethoprim [85].

Diabetes Mellitus

Increased severity of hand infection and dire prognosis are associated with diabetes mellitus. Small vessel disease, peripheral neuropathy, and inhibition of leukocytic phagocytosis all play a role in this problem. In one series of 20 diabetic patients with hand infection, 50 percent required amputation at some level to control the disease or improve function [56]. In this series, aerobic gram-negative organisms predominated. A high suspicion is necessary in severe hand infections to identify patients not previously known to have diabetes mellitus. Recommended treatment according to Mann and Peacock includes aggressive repeated debridement, antibiotics aimed at gram-negative organisms (until culture results are known), early motion, and proper insulin management.

Drug Addiction

In the last decade, injection of various narcotic and psychedelic drugs (often "cut" with nonpharmacological agents) into the vessels and soft tissues of the upper extremity has increased markedly. With chronic use of such agents, vascular sclerosis and extravasation often result in subcutaneous fibrosis and lymphedema, producing a so-called puffy hand. Infection is frequently a sequel, expressed as inflamed seropurulent nodules, cellulitis, chronic ulceration, abscess, and pyarthrosis (particularly of the proximal interphalangeal joint as it accompanies a boutonnière injury) [20, 78]. The chronic lymphedema may mimic deep space infection when none is present. A conservative approach with splinting, moist dressing, elevation, and intramuscular or oral antibiotics has been recommended in joint infections [98]. However, a localized soft tissue abscess may be masked by the chronic edema; in such cases, as well as in those of drug-induced slough of tissue, prompt definitive and aggressive treatment is indicated [20, 61].

REFERENCES

1. Adamson, J. E., Horton, C. R., and Crawford, H. H. Sensory rehabilitation of the injured thumb. *Plast. Reconstr. Surg.* 40:53, 1967.
2. Argamaso, R. V. Rotation transposition method for soft tissue replacement of the distal segment of the thumb. *Plast. Reconstr. Surg.* 54:366, 1974.
3. Atasoy, E., Ioakimidis, E., Kasdan, M. L., Kutz, J. E., and Kleinert, H. E. Reconstruction of the amputated fingertip with a triangular volar flap. *J. Bone Joint Surg.* [Am.] 52:921, 1970.
4. Bailey, D. H. *The Infected Hand.* London: H. K. Lewis, 1963.
5. Barclay, C. L. The late results of fingertip injuries. *Br. J. Plast. Surg.* 8:38, 1955.
6. Bautista, B. N., and Nery, S. B. Replacement of a malformed fingernail with acrylic resin material. *Plast. Reconstr. Surg.* 55:234, 1975.
7. Beasley, R. W. Reconstruction of amputated fingertips. *Plast. Reconstr. Surg.* 44:349, 1969.
8. Bell, M. S. The changing pattern of pyogenic infections of the hand. *Hand* 8:298, 1976.
9. Bossley, C. J. Terminal digit amputations. *J. Bone Joint Surg.* [Br.] 57:254, 1975.
10. Brody, G. S., Cloutier, A. McL., and Woolhouse, F. M. The fingertip injury—an assessment of management. *Plast. Reconstr. Surg.* 26:80, 1960.
11. Buncke, H. J., Jr., and Gonzalez, R. J. Fingernail reconstruction. *Plast. Reconstr. Surg.* 30:452, 1962.
12. Burton, R. I., and Littler, J. W. Non-traumatic Soft Tissue Afflictions of the Hand. In *Current Problems in Surgery*. Chicago: Year Book, 1975.
13. Carroll, R. E. Ring injuries in the hand. *Clin. Orthop.* 104:175, 1974.
14. Carter, S. J., and Mersheimer, W. L. Use of Catheters in Treatment of Infections of the Hand. In Littler, J. W., Cramer, L. M., and Smith, J. W.

(Eds.), *Symposium on Reconstructive Hand Surgery,* Vol. 9. St. Louis: Mosby, 1974.
15. Chase, R. A. *Atlas of Hand Surgery.* Philadelphia: Saunders, 1973.
16. Conolly, W. B. Spontaneous healing of hand wounds. *Aust. N.Z. J. Surg.* 44:393, 1974.
17. Conolly, W. B., and Goulston, E. Problems of digital amputations: A clinical review of 260 patients and 301 amputations. *Aust. N.Z. J. Surg.* 43:118, 1973.
18. Crawford, J., Horton, C. E., and Oakley, R. S. Skin avulsions of fingers. *Plast. Reconstr. Surg.* 10:46, 1952.
19. Eaton, R. G. Hand Complications of Drug Addiction. In Littler, J. W., Cramer, L. M., and Smith, J. W. (Eds.), *Symposium on Reconstructive Hand Surgery,* Vol. 9. St. Louis: Mosby, 1974.
20. Eaton, R. G., and Butsch, D. P. Antibiotic guidelines for hand infections. *Surg. Gynecol. Obstet.* 130:119, 1970.
21. Edwards, D. H. The spectrum of hand injuries. *Hand* 7:46, 1975.
22. Entin, M. A. Infections of the hand. *Surg. Clin. North Am.* 44:981, 1964.
23. Finseth, F., May, J. W., Jr., and Smith, R. J. Composite groin flap with iliac bone flap for primary thumb reconstruction. *J. Bone Joint Surg.* [Am.] 58:130, 1977.
24. Fisher, R. H. The Kutler method of repair of fingertip amputations. *J. Bone Joint Surg.* [Am.] 49:317, 1967.
25. Fitzgerald, R. H., Jr., Cooney, W. P., III, Washington, J. A., II, Van Scoy, R. E., Linscheid, R. L., and Dobyns, J. H. Bacterial colonization of mutilating hand injuries and its treatment. *J. Hand Surg.* 2:85, 1977.
26. Flatt, A. E. *The Care of Minor Hand Injuries* (3rd ed.). St. Louis: Mosby, 1972.
27. Freiberg, A., and Manktelow, R. The Kutler repair for fingertip amputations. *Plast. Reconstr. Surg.* 50:371, 1972.
28. Freiberg, A., and Waddington, J. P. Selection of antibiotics in hand infections. *J. Bone Joint Surg.* [Am.] 54:896, 1972.
29. Gaul, J. S. Radial-innervated cross finger flap from index to provide sensory pulp to injured thumb. *J. Bone Joint Surg.* [Am.] 51:1257, 1969.
30. Gruneberg, R., and Spence, A. J. Finger amputations and ability to work. *Hand* 6:236, 1974.
31. Guba, A. M., Jr., Mulliken, J. B., and Hoopes, J. E. The selection of antibiotics for human bites of the hand. *Plast. Reconstr. Surg.* 56:538, 1975.
32. Gunther, S. F., and Elliott, R. C. *Mycobacterium kansasii* infection in the deep structures of the hand. *J. Bone Joint Surg.* [Am.] 58:140, 1976.
33. Gunther, S. F., Elliot, R. C., Brand, R. L., and Adams, J. P. Experience with atypical mycobacterial infection in the deep structures of the hand. *J. Hand Surg.* 2:90, 1977.
34. Herndon, J. H., Eaton, R. J., and Littler, J. W. Management of painful neuromas in the hand. *J. Bone Joint Surg.* 58:369, 1976.
35. Holm, A., and Zachariae, L. Fingertip lesions: An evaluation of conservative treatment vs free skin grafting. *Acta Orthop. Scand.* 45:382, 1974.
36. Hueston, J. T. Local flap repair of fingertip injuries. *Plast. Reconstr. Surg.* 37:349, 1966.
37. Illingworth, C. M. Trapped fingers and amputated fingers in children. *J. Pediatr. Surg.* 9:853, 1974.
38. Iselin, F. The flag flap. *Plast. Reconstr. Surg.* 53:374, 1973.
39. Johnson, R. K. Nail plasty. *Plast. Reconstr. Surg.* 47:275, 1971.
40. Johnson, R. K., and Iverson, R. E. Cross finger pedicle flaps in the hand. *J. Bone Joint Surg.* [Am.] 53:913, 1971.
41. Joshi, D. B. One stage repair for distal amputation of thumb. *Plast. Reconstr. Surg.* 45:613, 1970.
42. Joshi, D. B. A sensory cross finger flap for use on the index finger. *Plast. Reconstr. Surg.* 58:210, 1976.
43. Kanavel, A. B. *Infections of the Hand* (6th ed.). Philadelphia: Lea & Febiger, 1933.
44. Kelleher, J. C., Sullivan, J. G., Baibak, G. J., and Dean, R. K. The distant pedicle flap in surgery of the hand. *Orthop. Clin. North Am.* 1:227, 1970.
45. Kelleher, J. C., Sullivan, J. G., Baibak, G. J., and Dean, R. K. "On-top plasty" for amputated fingers. *Plast. Reconstr. Surg.* 42:242, 1968.
46. Kelly, P. J., Karlson, A. G., Weed, L. A., and Lipscomb, P. R. Infection of synovial tissues by mycobacteria other than *Mycobacterium tuberculosis. J. Bone Joint Surg.* [Am.] 49:1521, 1967.
47. Kelly, P. J., Weed, L. A., and Lipscomb, P. R. Infection of tendon sheaths, bursae, joints, and soft tissues by acid-fast bacilli other than tubercle bacilli. *J. Bone Joint Surg.* [Am.] 45:327, 1963.
48. Keyser, J. J., and Eaton, R. J. Surgical cure of chronic paronychia by eponychial marsupialization. *Plast. Reconstr. Surg.* 58:66, 1976.
49. Kilgore, E. S., Jr., Brown, L. G., Newmeyer, W. L., Graham, W. P., III, and Davis, T. S. Treatment of felons. *Am. J. Surg.* 130:194, 1975.
50. Larsen, R. D., and Oneal, R. M. Use of osteoperiosteal flaps in amputation in the hand. *Plast. Reconstr. Surg.* 38:529, 1966.
51. LeGros Clark, W. E., and Buxton, L. H. D.

Studies in nail growth. *Br. J. Dermatol. Syph.* 50:221, 1938.
52. Lie, K. K., Magargle, R. K., and Posch, J. L. Free full-thickness skin grafts from the palm to cover defects of the fingers. *J. Bone Joint Surg.* [Am.] 52:559, 1970.
53. Littler, J. W. Hand, Wrist and Forearm Incisions. In Littler, J. W., Cramer, L. M., and Smith, J. W. (Eds.), *Symposium on Reconstructive Hand Surgery,* Vol. 9. St. Louis: Mosby, 1974.
54. Littler, J. W. Principles of Reconstructive Surgery in the Hand. In Converse, J. M. (Ed.), *Reconstructive Plastic Surgery,* Vol. 4 (2nd Ed.). Philadelphia: Saunders, 1977.
55. Mann, R. J., Hoffeld, T. A., and Farmer, C. V. Human bites of the hand: 20 years of experience. *J. Hand Surg.* 2:97, 1977.
56. Mann, R. J., and Peacock, J. M. Hand Infections in Patients with Diabetes Mellitus. Presented at the thirty-first annual meeting of The American Society for Surgery of the Hand, January, 1976.
57. Mansfield, O. T., and Knight, J. S. Treatment of congenital amputations through the forearm. *Br. J. Plast. Surg.* 16:23, 1963.
58. Markley, J. M., Jr. The preservation of close two-point discrimination in the interdigital transfer of neurovascular island flaps. *Plast. Reconstr. Surg.* 59:812, 1977.
59. McCash, C. R. Free nail grafting. *Br. J. Plast. Surg.* 8:19, 1955.
60. McCash, C. R. Toe pulp free grafts in fingertip repair. *Br. J. Plast. Surg.* 11:322, 1958.
61. McKay, D., Pascarelli, E. F., and Eaton, R. G. Infections and sloughs of the hands in drug addicts. *J. Bone Joint Surg.* [Am.] 55:741, 1973.
62. Milford, L. *The Hand.* St. Louis: Mosby, 1971.
63. Miller, A. J. Single fingertip injuries treated by thenar flap. *Hand* 6:311, 1974.
64. Miller, S. H., and Rusenas, I. Changes in primate pacinian corpuscles following volar pad excision and skin grafting. *Plast. Reconstr. Surg.* 57:627, 1976.
65. Mosher, J. F. Split thickness hypothenar grafts for skin defects of the hand. *Hand* 9:45, 1977.
66. Murray, J. F. The Missing Thumb. In Littler, J. W., Cramer, L. M., and Smith, J. W. (Eds.), *Symposium of Reconstructive Hand Surgery,* Vol. 9. St. Louis: Mosby, 1974.
67. Murray, J. F., Carman, W., and MacKenzie, J. K. Complications and Hand Strength Following Transmetacarpal Amputation of the Index Finger. Presented at the thirty-second annual meeting of The American Society for Surgery of the Hand, February, 1977.
68. Patton, H. S. Split skin grafts from hypothenar area for fingertip avulsion. *Plast. Reconstr. Surg.* 43:426, 1969.
69. Peacock, E. E., Jr. Metacarpal transfer following amputation of a central digit. *Plast. Reconstr. Surg.* 29:345, 1962.
70. Pollen, A. G. Acute infection of the tendon sheath. *Hand* 6:21, 1974.
71. Porter, R. W. Functional assessment of transplanted skin in volar defects of the digits. *J. Bone Joint Surg.* [Am.] 50:955, 1968.
72. Rank, B. K., Wakefield, A. R., and Hueston, J. T. *Surgery of Repair as Applied to Hand Injuries* (4th ed.). Edinburgh and London: Churchill-Livingston, 1973.
73. Ratliff, A. H. C. Amputation of the finger and thumb. *Hand* 1:137, 1969.
74. Ratliff, A. H. C. Amputations of the distal part of the thumb. *Hand* 4:190, 1972.
75. Robins, H. C. Infections of the hand. *J. Bone Joint Surg.* [Br.] 34:567, 1952.
76. Robins, H. C. Fingertip injuries. *Hand* 2:119, 1970.
77. Ryan, J. J., and Hoopes, J. E. Needle aspiration of the flexor digitorum sheath as an aid in diagnosing tenosynovitis. *Plast. Reconstr. Surg.* 56:152, 1975.
78. Ryan, J. J., Hoopes, J. E., and Jabaley, M. E. Drug injection injuries of the hands and forearms in addicts. *Plast. Reconstr. Surg.* 53:445, 1974.
79. Salaman, J. R. Partial thickness skin grafting of fingertip injuries. *Lancet* 1:705, 1967.
80. Sandzen, S. C., and Oakey, R. S. Crushing injury of the fingertip. *Hand* 4:253, 1972.
81. Schiller, C. Nail replacement in fingertip injuries. *Plast. Reconstr. Surg.* 19:521, 1957.
82. Shrewsbury, M., and Johnson, R. K. The fascia of the distal phalanx. *J. Bone Joint Surg.* [Am.] 57:784, 1975.
83. Slocum, D. B. Amputation of the fingers and the hand. *Clin. Orthop.* 15:35, 1959.
84. Smith, J., and Bom, A. F. Evaluation of the fingertip reconstruction by cross finger and palmar pedicle flap. *Plast. Reconstr. Surg.* 35:409, 1965.
85. Smith, J., and Ruby, L. Nocardia asteroides thenar space infection: A case report. *J. Hand Surg.* 2:109, 1977.
86. Snow, J. W. Use of a volar flap for repair of fingertip amputations. *Plast. Reconstr. Surg.* 60:163, 1967.
87. Stone, N. H., Hursch, H., Humphrey, C. R., and Boswick, J. A. Empirical selection of antibiotics for hand infections. *J. Bone Joint Surg.* [Am.] 51:899, 1969.
88. Sturman, M. J., and Duran, R. J. Late results of fingertip injuries. *J. Bone Joint Surg.* [Am.] 45:289, 1963.
89. Swanson, A. B. Levels of amputation of fingers and hand – considerations for treatment. *Surg. Clin. North Am.* 44:1115, 1964.

90. Swanson, A. B., Boeve, N. R., and Lumsden, R. M. The prevention and treatment of amputation neuromata by silicone capping. *J. Hand Surg.* 2:70, 1977.
91. Tempest, M. N. Cross finger flaps in the treatment of injuries to the fingertips. *Plast. Reconstr. Surg.* 9:205, 1952.
92. Thompson, R. V. Essential details in the technique of fingertip amputation. *Med. J. Aust.* 2:14, 1963.
93. Thomson, H. G., and Sorokolet, W. T. The cross finger flap in children: A follow-up study. *Plast. Reconstr. Surg.* 39:482, 1967.
94. Tooms, R. E. Amputation injury in the upper extremity. *Orthop. Clin. North Am.* 3:383, 1972.
95. Villain, R. and Dupuis, J. F. Use of the flag flap for coverage of a small area on a finger or the palm. *Plast. Reconstr. Surg.* 51:397, 1973.
96. Wallace, W. A., and Coupland, R. E. Variations in the nerves of the thumb and index finger. *J. Bone Joint Surg.* [Br.] 57:491, 1975.
97. Weston, T. A. M., and Wallace, W. A. The use of locally based triangular skin flaps for the repair of fingertip injuries. *Hand* 8:54, 1976.
98. Whitaker, L. A., and Graham, W. P., III. Management of hand infections in the narcotic addict. *Plast. Reconstr. Surg.* 52:384, 1973.
99. Whitaker, L. A., Graham, W. P., III. Riser, W. H., and Kilgore, E. Retaining the articular cartilage in fingertip amputations. *Plast. Reconstr. Surg.* 49:542, 1972.
100. Zaias, N., and Baden, H. R. Disorders of Nails. In Fitzpatrick, T. B., Arndt, K. A., Clark, W. H., Jr., Eisen, A. Z., Van Scott, E. J., and Vaughan, J. H. (Eds.), *Dermatology in General Medicine.* New York: McGraw-Hill, 1971.

33

Fractures and Joint Injuries of the Hand

RICHARD G. EATON AND RICHARD A. SPERLING

Treatment of fractures in the hand involves the same principles as treatment of fractures elsewhere, although they must be applied with greater expertise [11]. Reduction must be as anatomical as possible and with a minimum of trauma. Edema induces scar formation, and a crude reduction, without regard for the soft tissue structures surrounding the fracture, may produce an aligned fracture at the price of a fibrosed stiff digit.

The surgeon charged with the primary care of a hand fracture should perform a thorough examination to locate possible associated injury to nerve, tendon, or blood vessels. In phalangeal fractures, *true posteroanterior* (PA) *and lateral radiographs of the finger,* in addition to the hand, are required for accurate assessment of the fracture and the areas surrounding the injury. Remember that the responsibility for *accepting* an imperfect radiograph lies with the physician rather than the technician who took the film. Fractures that will be clearly visible on the true lateral film may not be noticed in a film with just a few degrees of obliquity. The patient must be questioned in detail as to the mechanism of injury, since this may lead the examiner to check for an associated injury. A knowledge of the anatomy and biomechanical forces responsible for the deformity seen on the radiograph is essential, for it is precisely these forces that must be overcome in obtaining and maintaining reduction. An awareness of deforming forces will make apparent a method of reduction applicable to many variations and will obviate the need for a cookbook approach.

A regional anesthetic such as the wrist block is ideal for fracture reduction in fingers, although digital blocks may be sufficient for the more distal fractures. The patient's hand frequently must be placed in an uncomfortable position for reduction, so the more proximal block makes the procedure more tolerable.

Internal fixation with a Kirschner wire, is not in itself adequate immobilization for a fracture. It is, in effect, an internal suture, which will maintain a reduction only if external immobilization is provided. Neither is a splint by itself usually adequate for maintaining a significantly displaced fracture in the reduced position. Fractures of the metacarpals, proximal phalanges, and frequently the middle phalanges should be immobilized in a circumferential carefully padded plaster dressing to provide uniform gentle compression. The cast should begin at the distal forearm and extend to immobilize the joint distal to the fracture, as well as the adjacent finger in most cases. Immobilization for fractures, and for dislocations, must always be for at least the minimum time necessary to achieve healing. Immobilization for 3 weeks is usually sufficient, while 4 weeks is the maximum period for any metacarpal or phalangeal fracture.

Metacarpal Fractures

Fractures of the metacarpals are relatively common and may follow a direct blow, torque, or axial compression. A direct blow commonly results in a transverse fracture, usually midshaft. Although these fractures are often easily reducible and stable, angulation is not uncommon. Rotational deformities are common for fractures of the second and fifth metacarpals. This is because they have only unilateral support from the intervolar plate ligament. Rotational deformities are also found when metacarpal fractures are multiple. Torque applied to the proximal phalanx may cause a spiral fracture of the metacarpal shaft. Malrotation is frequent. Both spiral and transverse fractures are reduced by placing traction on the proximal phalanx and then flexing the metacarpophalangeal (MP) joint to 90 degrees. Malrotation is corrected by the fist position maneuver, using adjacent uninjured digits as guides. In the normal fist, the middle finger points to the tubercle of the scaphoid while the other fingers assume a position parallel to the middle one. Malrotation should become immediately apparent in this flexed position, and it can be corrected by simply rotating the injured finger until it lines up in proper position relative to its neighbors. Reduction is best maintained by immobilization on a splint with the MP joint flexed 60 degrees.

If the reduction appears unstable or if redisplacement occurs at any time, percutaneous internal fixation with Kirschner wires will be necessary. Usually one wire, inserted from the metacarpal head and passed longitudinally down the shaft, is sufficient. Once the pin is through the skin, the extensor tendon is swept aside and penetration avoided. Multiple fractures may also require transverse pins through the metacarpal heads, in addition to the longitudinal wires, for control of rotation.

Axial compression results in the frequently seen "boxer's fracture," a fracture of the metacarpal neck with variable degrees of volar angulation. Usually the fourth or fifth metacarpals are involved. Up to

45 degrees of angulation is acceptable and requires no reduction. With greater angulation, reduction is necessary and may be achieved by applying vertical compression to the flexed proximal interphalangeal (PIP) joint with the MP joint maximally flexed. Counterpressure is simultaneously applied to the metacarpal neck dorsally just proximal to the fracture. Neck fractures with angulation greater than 55 degrees are unstable; these require the use of a longitudinal Kirschner wire, as described previously. Immobilization for all types of metacarpal fractures is secured with plaster from the midforearm to the distal one-third of the proximal phalanx, with the injured and an adjacent digit included. *It is essential to leave the PIP joints free.* The MP joints are kept at 60-degree flexion. It is desirable to extend the padding and plaster just beyond the metacarpal heads of the digits not included with the injured ray as an aid in controlling edema. The cast and pins are removed at 3 weeks and active motion is begun with the injured finger taped to its neighbor. Passive stretching may be added the following week if necessary.

Occasionally a metacarpal fracture will prove irreducible and open reduction will be necessary. Exposure is through a curved longitudinal dorsal incision. Internal fixation is usually necessary; Kirschner wires may be placed as described previously, or they may be passed out the metacarpal head through the distal fragment and then passed retrograde across the fracture site after reduction. Intraarticular fractures of the metacarpal head require precise restoration of joint contours, an objective that may be impossible with closed reduction. Operative exposure may be through a longitudinal dorsal incision, dividing the ulnar shroud fibers and retracting the extensor mechanism radially. Internal fixation is necessary using the smallest available pins. Despite considerable comminution, one major articular fragment is usually present and can be securely transfixed. Immobilization in 60 to 70 degrees of MP flexion is important to keep the collateral ligaments at maximum length. Immobilization for 4 weeks is required.

Complications of metacarpal fractures include malrotation, impaired flexor or extensor tendon gliding, and joint stiffness. If fractures are the result of a crush injury, interosseus fibrosis may develop. Nonunion is rare in the absence of infection.

Fractures of the Thumb Metacarpal

Fractures of the thumb metacarpal are usually caused by a direct blow or axial compression applied to the clenched fist while striking a blow. A transverse fracture of the shaft or base follows. As might be expected, fracture deformities of the first metacarpal may be worse than those of the other metacarpals because of the lack of the stabilizing influence of an adjacent metacarpal or intervolar plate ligament.

Fractures of the shaft are usually flexed at the distal fragment due to the combined pull of the thenar intrinsic muscles, while the proximal fragment is extended and abducted proximally by the abductor pollicis longus. Reduction is by traction, slight carpometacarpal joint flexion, and pronation applied to the thumb. Displaced fractures are notoriously unstable because of these forces; they may require pinning with a longitudinal and occasionally an oblique wire to control rotation. Immobilization is for 3 weeks, with plaster extending to the interphalangeal (IP) joint with the thumb in the fist projection. (Intraarticular fractures of the metacarpal base are discussed under the heading of Joint Injuries.)

Proximal Phalangeal Fractures

Fractures of the proximal phalanx may result from hyperextension of the MP or PIP joints, a direct blow, or a torque applied to the proximal phalanx. These fractures, particularly those of spiral-oblique configuration, are difficult to treat because of the intimate relationship of the bone to the delicate gliding structures. In the proximal phalanx the tendons of the flexor and extensor mechanism are separated from a fracture site by only a thin layer of periosteum. So they can easily become entrapped in a fracture callus and have movement of the more distal joints more limited as a result. Gentle anatomical reduction and precise immobilization are more crucial in this region than anywhere else in the hand. The chances for acquiring a normally functioning finger are directly related to the degree of fibrosis and external callus fixation of contiguous gliding structures.

In most proximal phalangeal fractures, the forces responsible for the deformity are the same regardless of the configuration of the fracture. The proximal fragment is flexed by the intrinsic muscles and the distal fragment is extended by the extrinsic extensor tendon. Telescoping or shortening occurs by the combined actions of the extrinsic flexors and extensors. The shortening forces acting through the configuration of the fracture (especially in fractures with a spiral component) tend to maintain malrotation in much the same way that vertical compression applied to the handle of an automatic screwdriver will produce rotation. Reduction is accomplished by applying traction to the middle phalanx while flexing the MP joint to 90 degrees and the PIP joint to 45 degrees. This relaxes the deforming forces and allows molding and realignment of the fragments within their periosteal sleeve. Malrotation is corrected by assumption of the fist position.

Transverse fractures at the base of the proximal phalanx result from hyperextension and are usually stable when reduced and held in flexion. Midshaft transverse fractures usually result from a direct blow and are often unstable. Reduction may be maintained with a longitudinal Kirschner wire passed from the metacarpal head down through the proximal phalanx (Fig. 33-1) with the MP joint flexed 60 degrees. It is neither necessary nor desirable to cross the PIP joint with the wire. Immobilization is for 3 weeks, with plaster extending just proximal to the PIP joint unless the fracture is adjacent to that joint, in which case it is extended to the distal interphalangeal (DIP) joint.

A torque force applied to the flexed PIP joint results in a spiral fracture. These fractures are unstable and require internal fixation. Even if an x-ray shows minimal displacement, such fractures should be pinned, because they usually slip during the period of immobilization. We prefer to perform reduction and internal fixation in the operating room, with the aid of the image intensifier. A fracture clamp (Fig. 33-2) is invaluable here in holding and often improving the reduction achieved by the traction-flexion maneuver, as well as serving as a marker to help guide accurate placement of the pins. The clamp should be tightened just enough to bring the fragments together. If it is too tight, especially in fractures with an intercondylar component, overriding may result. Transverse pins of the smallest caliber are now passed across the fracture site using the power drill. Accurate placement of these pins is of key importance. Transverse pins have approximately seven to ten times greater resistance to the compression stress of an oblique fracture than obliquely placed pins [1]. At least two pins are required, and these should be placed parallel and as far apart as possible for maximum stability. Placement of the pins along the midaxial line will allow active motion without producing tension on the skin. The hand is placed in a cast with the plaster extending to the DIP joint over the involved and adjacent fingers, keeping the MP joint flexed at 60 degrees and the PIP joint at 20 degrees. After 7 to 14 days, depending on the estimated stability of the reduction, the volar portion of the cast is trimmed to permit active PIP flexion; this reduces the tendency to fixation of contiguous gliding structures. The dorsal portion of the cast remains as an extension restraint. Pins and cast are usually removed at 3 weeks and full active motion is begun. If significant swelling or stiffness of the PIP joint remains for more than a week after plaster removal, it is our practice to give a 5-day course of prednisone, starting at 40 mg. per day, and reducing the amount each day.

Closed reduction is not always successful, and open reduction may be required. This is particularly true when soft tissue interposition has occurred or when displacement has persisted longer than 5 to 6 days. Since articular fractures demand as nearly perfect

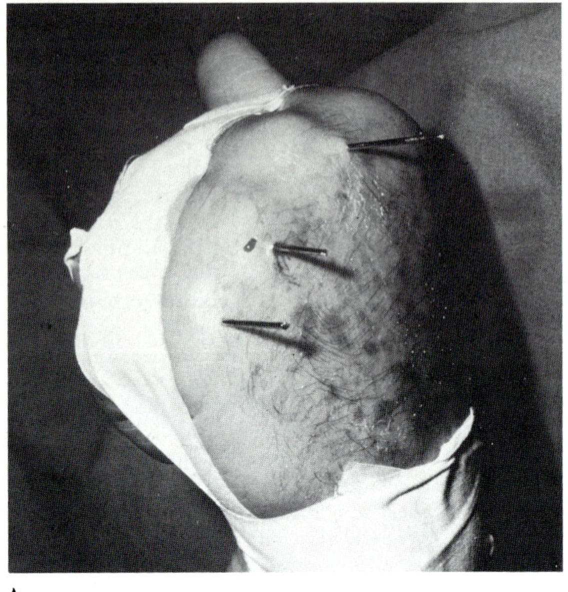

A

B

Fig. 33-1. A, for immobilizing fractures of the proximal phalanges, Kirschner wires are passed through the metacarpal head in line with the medullary canal of the proximal phalanx. Note that the proximal interphalangeal joint is not pinned, permitting early motion in most patients. B, this x-ray shows the alignment and fixation of transverse fractures with these longitudinal pins. Early proximal interphalangeal motion produces compression at the fracture site.

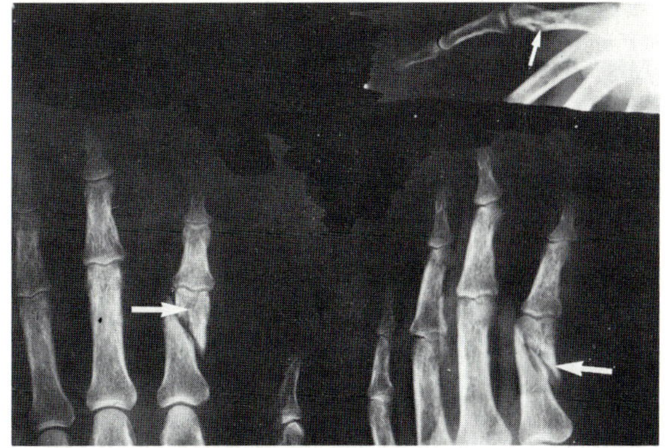

A

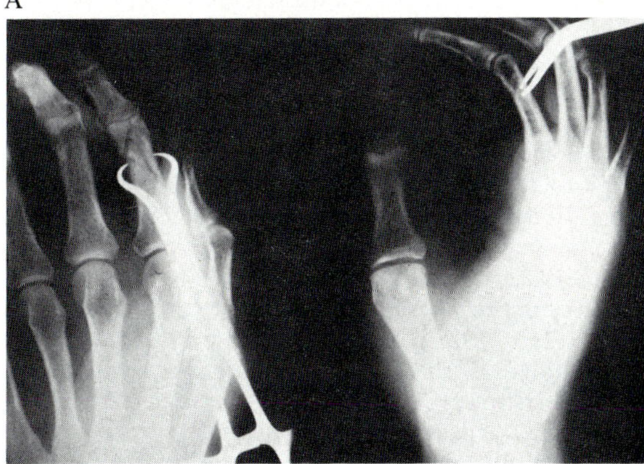

B

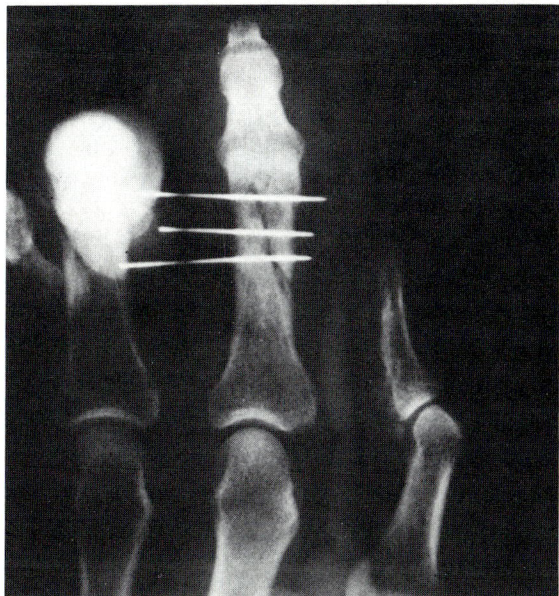

C

reduction as possible, open reduction is the rule.

Exposure of the fracture is obtained through a midaxial or dorsolateral incision. *The lateral band overlying the fracture site is excised,* eliminating one potentially fixed gliding surface. The undamaged opposite lateral band and central tendon provide adequate extensor power. Stripping of periosteum must be kept to a minimum. Traction and gentle direct manipulation of the fragments usually achieve a satisfactory reduction. Power-driven pin fixation is then used, employing the fracture clamp as a vise to maintain reduction temporarily.

Complications of proximal phalangeal fractures include malrotation, PIP stiffness, and flexion and extension contractures.

Middle Phalangeal Fractures

Fractures of the middle phalanx are similar in mechanism of injury and configuration to those of the proximal phalanx. They are, however, less frequent than proximal phalangeal fractures because of the tendency for the PIP joint to dislocate before the fracture occurs. Deformity will be similar to proximal phalangeal fractures, with the proximal fragment flexed by the flexor digitorum superficialis, and the distal fragment extended by the extensor tendon mechanism.

These fractures are easily reduced by traction and flexion of the finger. Most reductions are stable; if instability is a problem, for spiral or oblique fractures, transverse pins may be placed across the phalanx; for transverse fractures use longitudinal or oblique pins. If possible, pinning across the PIP joint should be avoided. Because of the denseness of cortical bone, these fractures are somewhat slower to heal and usually require immobilization for 4 weeks. The plaster should extend to the fingertip.

Distal Phalangeal Fractures

Fractures of the distal phalanx are usually transverse or comminuted and are almost invariably the result of a crush injury. When these fractures are closed, they are often associated with a subungual hematoma that may cause considerable pain. If drainage is necessary, use a red-hot paper clip or a #11 blade. With

Fig. 33-2. A, radiogram shows three views of a spiral oblique fracture of the proximal phalanx with comminution into the proximal interphalangeal joint. B, closed reduction is maintained by the percutaneous application of a fracture clamp. Radiogram confirms good reduction. The tips of the clamp serve as markers for the percutaneous insertion of transverse Kirschner wires. C, reduction securely held by three fine transverse Kirschner wires.

open fractures, the proximal nail matrix will often be avulsed from its cul-de-sac. Accurate replacement of the nail matrix in these injuries is essential for regrowth of a normal nail. One horizontal mattress suture exiting well back on the dorsum of the distal phalanx will serve this purpose. Lacerations of the nail matrix must also be meticulously repaired. Too often, attention is focused entirely on the accurate alignment of the distal phalangeal fracture, while nail bed injuries are neglected. It must be emphasized that many patients regard a deformed nail as a significant cosmetic problem. Surgical correction of the post-injury nail deformity is frequently imperfect, and the surgeon would be well advised to take steps for its prevention.

The fracture is usually not significantly displaced, but if necessary, gentle molding will accomplish a more satisfactory reduction. Interposed nail matrix may occasionally block reduction and must be removed. A gap of greater than 2 mm. in the lateral x-ray usually suggests the presence of interposed nail matrix until disproved. Internal fixation is rarely necessary but may be accomplished with oblique or longitudinal Kirschner wires. A dorsal splint may suffice for immobilization, and the PIP joint is left free. Immobilization is for 3 weeks.

JOINT INJURIES

Joint injuries of the hand, from simple sprains to serious derangements, are among the most common injuries to the upper arm, and account for thousands of hours lost from work each year as well as significant personal disability. The evaluation and treatment of most joint injuries is straightforward; it depends on the application of a few basic principles and maneuvers, the precise adherence to which is critical. Improper diagnosis, incorrect splint position, or prolonged immobilization can turn a minor problem into a long-term disability.

The acutely injured joint may result in pain, fusiform swelling, or hemarthrosis. Tenderness is usually present circumferentially around the joint. X-rays are required; they may show an avulsion fracture or associated pathological condition, including some preexisting joint disease or tumor that might alter the course of therapy, as well as account for the degree and type of dislocation. However, stress films are not necessary, since the clinical stress examination will usually demonstrate whether ligamentous disruption has occurred. An accurate assessment of joint stability is essential; this assessment will determine the type of treatment. This includes testing stability to active as well as passive stretching under regional (digital, or wrist block where appropriate) anesthesia. Pain triggers extrinsic flexor and extensor muscle spasm, which may, by impacting the joint surfaces, give a false impression of stability. *Active* stability is assessed by having the patient move the injured finger through a full range of motion. Recurring dorsal displacement, if it occurs during the last 15 to 20 degrees of extension, indicates volar plate disruption. *Passive* stability is tested by applying gentle lateral stress to the fully extended joint to test each collateral ligament and posteroanterior stress to test the volar plate. The injured finger joint must always be compared with the same joint on the opposite hand. Angulation, hypermobility, or redisplacement indicates major disruption of the structure being tested. Stability to full active motion suggests that sufficient critical joint support is present to permit healing with minimal immobilization. It must be emphasized that a sprain is a diagnosis of exclusion, made after complete ligamentous disruption is ruled out. Nevertheless, a ligament may have a disruption of 99 percent of its fibers and its joint can still show stability. Since it is not possible to estimate the extent of an incomplete disruption, every sprain must be treated as if 99 percent of its ligament were torn.

Stable, acutely injured joints are immobilized for 10 to 14 days, while those demonstrating instability but not requiring open reduction are immobilized for 21 days. Interphalangeal joints may be adequately immobilized with dorsal aluminum splints; however, the more proximal metacarpophalangeal joints or carpometacarpal joints require a plaster cast. Following immobilization for the designated period, active motion is begun with the injured finger taped to an adjacent one for another week. Immobilization must always be for the minimum time necessary to achieve healing. A subsequent displacement or instability is rare if an acutely injured joint has been immobilized properly. On the contrary, persistent limited motion and stiffness are frequent sequelae.

Interphalangeal Joints

Anatomy

The proximal and distal interphalangeal joints are ginglymus or hinge joints; they differ in size but are alike in structure. On the proximal side of the joint the articular contours are broad and bicondylar; on the distal side the contour is just the opposite – two shallow, concave surfaces with a central tongue between which fits into the intercondylar groove (Fig. 33-3). The resultant structure allows free motion in the sagittal plane while resisting rotation. Basic support of the joint, however, is provided by a remarkable efficient boxlike confluence of ligaments (Fig. 33-4). Lateral stability is mainly provided by the paired collateral–accessory collateral ligament complex on each side of the joint. They arise from a

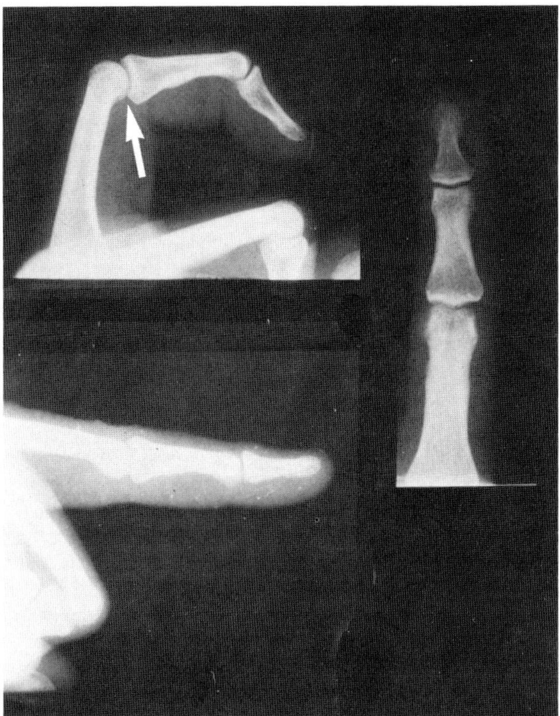

Fig. 33-3. Radiogram of normal interphalangeal joints. In the lateral views (upper and lower left), note how the middle phalanx maintains total contact with the concentric arc of the condyle of the proximal phalanx in all positions. In full flexion (upper left), the volar base of the middle phalanx fits perfectly into the retrocondylar fossa (arrow) of the proximal phalanx; obliteration of this fossa by scarring or a bone spicule will cause a great loss of flexion. In the posteroanterior projection (right), note how tongue and groove contour of articular surfaces increases joint stability.

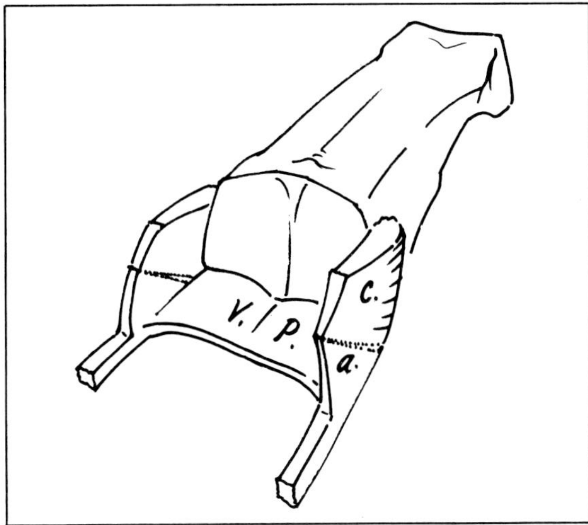

Fig. 33-4. The three-dimensional ligament support of interphalangeal joints. The volar plate (VP) *and paired collateral* (c) *and accessory collateral* (a) *ligaments insert into the base of the middle phalanx. They form a mobile boxlike configuration which has great strength with a minimum of bulk. Displacement cannot occur unless two sides of this box have been completely disrupted.*

concavity on the proximal condlye and insert into the lateral margins of the volar plate and base of the more distal phalanx. The floor of the joint is formed by the volar plate, which is broadly inserted into the distal side of the joint and continues laterally with the collateral ligaments. Proximally, the volar plate tapers into a thin central sheet that permits full interphalangeal flexion, while it thickens laterally to form a pair of tough check ligaments that are anchored to the volar periosteum, providing a firm restraint to hyperextension. This three-dimensional concept of a ligamentous box consisting of volar plate, collateral ligaments, and articular contours is the basis of interphalangeal joint stability. *For significant displacement to occur, two adjacent sides of the box must be disrupted.*

Proximal Interphalangeal Joints

Most PIP dislocations are of either the dorsal or the lateral type. Dorsal dislocation (Fig. 33-5) may result from hyperextension or vertical compression applied to the tip of a semiflexed digit [14]. The middle phalanx may hyperextend with its articular contours still in contact, undergo complete dorsal dislocation and sit astride the proximal phalanx like a bayonet, or even avulse a triangular fragment of bone from the base of the middle phalanx, depending on the severity of the force applied. The major ligamentous disruption is through the volar plate insertion with the tear extending dorsally from the point of rupture to split the collateral ligament in the line of its fibers. Note that the accessory collateral ligament–volar plate complex, restrained by the check ligaments, remains with the proximal phalanx. The collateral ligament proper, though torn, retains attachment both to its origin and to the base of the middle phalanx. It is the integrity of these displaced but attached collateral ligaments that is the key to a stable reduction, for with traction and flexion they allow the middle phalanx to pivot volarly and guide it back to an anatomical position. If, however, the dislocation is associated with an avulsion fracture from the base of the middle phalanx, varying amounts of the collateral ligament will, depending on the size of the fragment, remain with the avulsed phalangeal base,

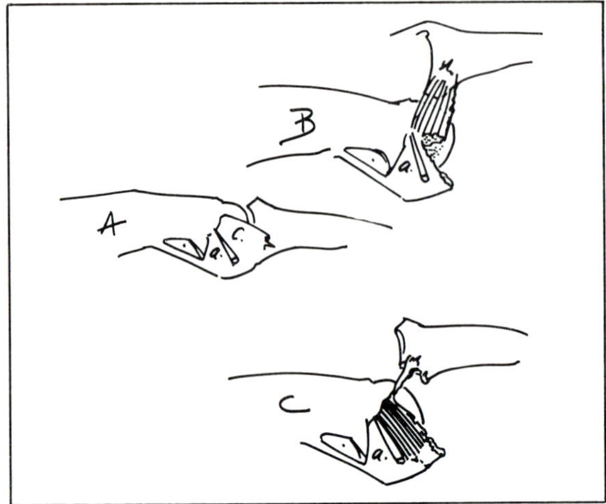

Fig. 33-5. Dorsal interphalangeal dislocation. A, normal interphalangeal joint relationship, with collateral (c) *and accessory collateral* (a) *ligaments shown separated for emphasis. The lateral capsule is normally continuous, having maximum thickness at its distal insertion and tapering proximally. B, simple dorsal dislocation. A longitudinal split between the collateral and accessory collateral ligaments permits dorsal displacement of the middle phalanx while the volar plate is securely anchored by the accessory portion of the collateral ligament and flexor sheath. C, pathomechanics of an unstable fracture-dislocation. There is avulsion of a large fragment from the base of the middle phalanx. Since this fragment contains most of the site of insertion for the collateral ligament as well as the volar plate, closed reduction is usually difficult and unstable. Smaller fragments which contain less than 40 percent of the articular surface retain sufficient collateral ligament attachment to be stable.*

since this is the insertion site of the collateral ligament. When the size of the fragment exceeds approximately 40 percent of the articular surface in the lateral projection, the entire collateral ligament may remain with the fragment, depriving the digit of the means for achieving or maintaining reduction. In such cases the joint will redisplace during the active motion test, and open reduction is indicated. Most dorsal dislocations, including those associated with avulsion of less than 40 percent of the volar articular surface, are stable when reduced.

Lateral dislocations result from torque, shear, or angulatory stress rupturing one collateral ligament and the volar plate insertion, thereby allowing the middle phalanx to pivot laterally on the opposite collateral ligament complex. Reduction is usually spontaneous and stable. Both dorsal and lateral dislocations are immobilized using dorsal metal splints with the PIP joint flexed 25 to 30 degrees. If the joint is stable to passive stress, as seen with minor tears, immobilization is for 2 weeks; if it is unstable to passive stress but stable to active motion, immobilization is for 3 weeks. Following this, the injured digit is taped to an adjacent digit for another week.

Open reduction is indicated (1) when the joint redislocates during the active motion test, (2) when the reduced parts slip during adequate immobilization and redislocate, or (3) when the dislocation cannot be reduced initially. The first two indications are usually seen in a complete dorsal dislocation with avulsion of a large fragment from the base of the middle phalanx. Although anatomical replacement of the fragment with a Kirschner wire is possible, it is difficult and the fragment may splinter. Less than anatomical replacement is unsatisfactory, since disabling osteoarthritis will be the likely result. Our preference is a volar plate arthroplasty, excising the fragment and advancing the volar plate into the defect, thereby resurfacing the middle phalangeal articular contour and reducing the dislocation (Fig. 33-6).

Distal Interphalangeal Joints

DIP dislocations are uncommon because of the stabilizing contribution of adjacent anatomical structures. These dislocations may be of the dorsal or lateral type, with the mechanism of injury similar to the PIP injuries (discussed earlier). Here, however, the volar plate, reinforced at its insertion by the expanded insertion of the flexor digitorum profundus, remains attached to the distal phalanx, with the tear occurring at the check ligaments. Likewise, the collateral ligaments are usually torn at their proximal condylar attachment and remain with the distal phalanx. The skin of the distal phalanx, firmly anchored by periosteal-dermal fascial fibers, may rupture rather than stretch in response to the deforming force, producing an open dislocation. Open wounds demand meticulous debridement and irrigation prior to reduction, as well as antibiotics and tetanus prophylaxis. Reduction is usually simple and quite stable for the same anatomical reasons that made dislocation difficult. In the unusual instance in which the reduced joint appears unstable, the proximal corners of the volar plate may be reattached with sutures and the joint transfixed in slight flexion (10 to 20 degrees) with a Kirschner wire. For both open and closed injuries, immobilization is for 3 weeks with a dorsal splint in 10 to 20 degrees of flexion.

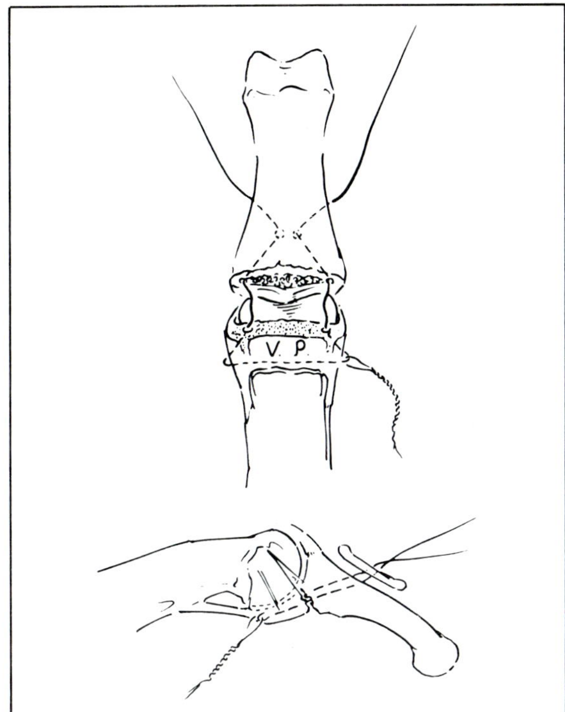

Fig. 33-6. Technique for reducing an unstable dorsal fracture-dislocation of the proximal interphalangeal joint. The volar fragment is usually comminuted and should be removed. The volar plate (VP) *is advanced into the defect. Using a lateral whip stitch with a pullout wire, the distal ends of the suture are passed from the dorsolateral margins of the defect to emerge through the dorsal skin. Traction on these sutures simultaneously reduces the middle phalanx as well as the joint and resurfaces the defect in the articular contour. Active* flexion *can be started in 2 weeks.*

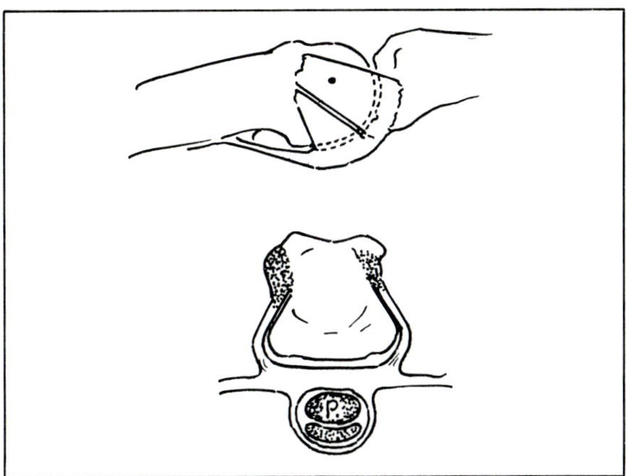

*Fig. 33-7. Ligaments of the metacarpophalangeal joint. The ligaments arise dorsal to the axis of rotation (see dot) and thus are relaxed in extension and progressively tightened with flexion. The lower diagram shows that their distal insertion is not only into the proximal phalanx and volar plate but also into the transverse intermetacarpal intervolarplate ligament. Immobilization of these joints should be in moderate flexion in order to maintain the length of these ligaments. (*P *is profundus tendon.)*

Metacarpophalangeal Joints

Anatomy

The structure of the MP joints differs significantly from that of the interphalangeal joints. The MP joints are condyloid rather than ginglymus, and their bony architecture does not confer upon them the stability inherent in the interphalangeal design. Unchecked by supporting structures, these joints are capable of abduction, adduction, and rotation as well as flexion and extension. The supporting ligaments govern the large potential versatility of the joint, limiting abduction, adduction, and rotation to approximately 30 degrees each when the joint is in extension. Each joint is flanked by a pair of collateral ligaments that arise from a condylar concavity dorsal to the axis of rotation and insert on the volar lateral base of the proximal phalanx (Fig. 33-7).

A unique anatomical design tightens the collateral ligaments and stabilizes the joint to lateral stress in flexion. The eccentric dorsal origin of the collateral ligaments combines with the elongated volar articular surface of the condyle to create a cam effect whereby the collateral ligament is progressively tightened with flexion. In addition, flexion must stretch the collateral ligaments over the flare of the condyle, a structure that in cross section approximates a volar-based triangle. In extension the collateral ligaments flank the condyle near the narrow apex of this triangle and are quite relaxed, thus permitting significant lateral motion. The thinner accessory collateral ligament arises from the condylar concavity just volar to the collateral ligament origin to insert into the lateral borders of the volar plate. The volar plate is membranous proximally, allowing MP flexion; it is thickened distally at its insertion. The volar plates are connected through a transverse linkage, the intervolar plate ligament (Fig. 33-8); this transverse linkage plays an important role in stability of the hand. It limits metacarpophalangeal rotation and hyperextension, and maintains the transverse metacarpal arch of the hand.

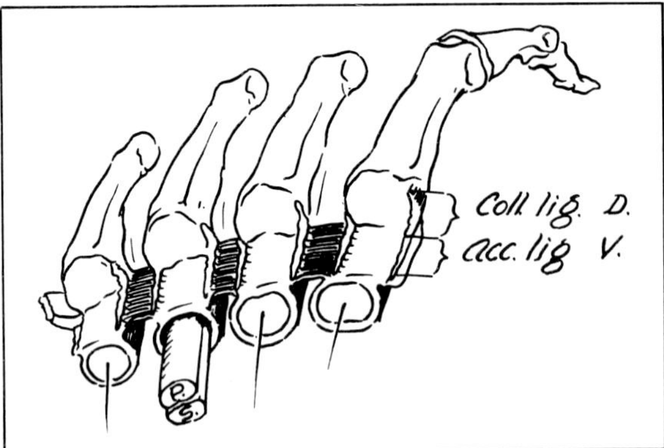

Fig. 33-8. Intervolar plate ligament, with metacarpal heads and collateral ligaments removed. This tough three-dimensional linkage provides maximum support with minimal bulk. Note attachment to flexor tendon sheath containing profundus tendon (P) *and superficialis tendon* (S). D = *dorsal,* V = *volar.*

Metacarpophalangeal Dislocations
MP dislocation is infrequent compared with interphalangeal dislocation. The middle and ring fingers, supported on both sides by the intervolar plate ligament, rarely undergo dislocation. The flanking digits, especially the index finger, are more vulnerable. Dorsal dislocation of the index metacarpophalangeal joint has been rightly termed the irreducible dislocation. It is usually caused by severe MP hyperextension, often the result of a fall on the outstretched hand. The membranous portion of the volar plate and the radial collateral ligament rupture, and the proximal phalanx rests atop the metacarpal in a bayonet configuration, shortened, slightly extended, and ulnar deviated. The metacarpal head, perforating the radial base of the volar plate, is volarly displaced and palpable subcutaneously in the palm. The situation must not be confused with MP joint subluxation, in which the proximal phalanx is hyperextended 60 to 90 degrees with the articular surfaces still in contact and a normal width to the joint space on radiograph. MP joint subluxation is amenable to closed reduction by traction and flexion; however, if the joint is hyperextended further by the examiner in an attempt to achieve reduction, the injury may easily be converted to an irreducible dislocation [10]. The volar plate remains with the proximal phalanx and lies wedged between the joint surfaces. The volarly displaced metacarpal head is held trapped by the taut flexor tendons flanking its neck on the ulnar side and the lumbrical on its radial side. Attempts at reduction by traction and flexion serve only to tighten the soft tissue noose around the metacarpal neck. Open reduction is required. Our preferred exposure is through a volar oblique incision parallel to the distal palmar crease. It will be found that reduction is blocked by the tautness of the flexor tendons passing around the ulnar side of the metacarpal neck. If a short length of flexor tendon sheath along the proximal phalanx is incised, the tendons can be retracted, and the entrapment relaxed. The interposed volar plate is then withdrawn from the joint space, and the dislocation reduced. Usually the reduction is stable. The volar plate may be reattached with one suture anchoring its proximal radial corner to the deep fascia. The use of a Kirschner wire is optional. The joint is immobilized in slight flexion (40 to 45 degrees) for 3 weeks with plaster extending just short of the PIP joint. Active flexion is begun at 3 weeks and active extension at 4 weeks.

Collateral Ligament Tears
Isolated MP collateral ligament tears are uncommon but occasionally result from a torque or angulatory stress applied to the flexed proximal phalanx. The extent of the injury may be ascertained by applying lateral stress to the fully flexed MP joint. Pain without lateral displacement indicates a partial tear, while lateral displacement indicates complete disruption. An adjacent supporting ligamentous structure must be torn before displacement occurs, as is true of interphalangeal joints. Immobilization in 50 degrees of flexion for 3 weeks is usually sufficient.

Other Injuries
Metacarpophalangeal hyperextension injuries without dislocation are common and may result in severe prolonged disability. Multiple digits are usually involved. The precise pathology in this injury in unknown but may represent momentary subluxation of the entire proximal phalangeal row, with accompanying tears of the volar plates, intervolar plate ligament, and even the palmar fascia. Pain is severe and associated with massive swelling and ecchymosis of palmar and dorsal aspects of the hand. Treatment should consist of elevation and gentle compressive dressings from midforearm to the PIP joints, with the MP joints immobilized in the position of function for a period of 2 to 3 weeks. A plaster shell should encase the dressings. As the enormous swelling recedes, it may be necessary to change the dressing at weekly intervals or it will become loose and ineffectual. Disability varies with the severity of the injury, but it may persist 4 to 6 months.

The Thumb
Because the thumb has unique anatomical and functional features that distinguish its joints from those of the other digits, joint injuries of the thumb are considered as a separate category.

Interphalangeal Joint of the Thumb
The interphalangeal joint of the thumb strongly resembles the DIP joints of the other digits. Dislocation is unusual but may be dorsal or lateral. Since the tear occurs through the proximal origin of the volar plate and collateral ligaments, the volar plate usually remains with the distal phalanx. A small sesamoid bone is incorporated within the volar plate, which may serve as a radiograph marker to determine volar plate position. Reduction is simple unless the flexor pollicis longus tendon becomes trapped lateral to one condyle, which often requires open reduction. Immobilization is for 3 weeks in a dorsal splint maintaining the joint in 15 to 20 degree flexion, leaving the MP joint free.

Metacarpophalangeal Joint of the Thumb
The MP joint of the thumb has features of both condyloid and ginglymus joints, and a highly variable normal range of motion [2]. The joint retains the basic ligamentous box configuration, although the structure of the volar plate is more complex. Two sesamoids are incorporated within its substance; the sesamoids, into which the thenar intrinsic muscles insert, articulate with the metacarpal condyle. The adductor pollicis inserts into the ulnar sesamoid, and the flexor pollicis brevis inserts into the radial.

Dislocations of the MP joint of the thumb occur with significantly greater frequency than digital MP dislocations [5, 6]. Dorsal and lateral displacements occur with equal frequency [8]. In dorsal dislocations, the entire volar plate and a major portion of the collateral ligament must rupture before the proximal phalanx assumes a bayonet configuration [9]. The volar plate ruptures proximal to the sesamoids, remaining with the proximal phalanx dorsal to the metacarpal head. The metacarpal head is displaced volarly. In contradistinction to the index MP dorsal dislocation, reduction is usually easily accomplished with traction and flexion to relax the intrinsic flexor-adductor muscles. The intrinsics, which retain their attachments to the sesamoids within the volar plate, serve to guide the phalanx back into position. Immobilization in 15 to 20 degrees of flexion for 3 weeks is recommended. In fresh injuries, open reduction is rarely necessary; however, it is indicated when the metacarpal head has become irreducibly buttonholed through the thenar muscle mass, or when the dislocation is complex and associated with lateral instability [13].

Lateral dislocations may present difficult problems in evaluation. The dislocation is usually momentary and is spontaneously reduced before it is seen by the physician. Ruptures of the ulnar collateral ligament are more common than ones on the radial side. The collateral ligament usually ruptures near its insertion on the proximal phalanx and may avulse a portion of the ulnar base of the phalanx. With complete ulnar collateral ligament rupture, the ligament may displace proximal to the adductor aponeurotic expansion into the extensor mechanism (Fig. 33-9). Realignment will now be blocked by the interposed adductor aponeurosis, and the ulnar collateral ligament, which normally lies deep to the aponeurosis, will lie superficial. Approximately two-thirds of complete ulnar collateral ligament disruptions will fit this pattern [15].

Diagnosis is made by applying lateral stress to the anesthetized fully extended MP joint. If the joint opens more than 40 degrees, significant ligamentous disruption has occurred, and operative repair is indicated. Treatment in cases where the joint opens less than 40 degrees involves immobilization in plaster for 3 weeks with the thumb in the position of function. Where reasonable doubt exists, exploration and repair are indicated, since inadequately treated ulnar collateral ligament tears may be progressively disabling and result in chronic weak and painful pinch

Fig. 33-9. A, dorsal view shows the mechanism of ulnar collateral ligament (u. coll. lig.) *disruption during forceful abduction. The proximal edge of the adductor aponeurosis sweeps distally across the metacarpal head. B, with spontaneous realignment the torn end of the collateral ligament is displaced superficially and proximally as the aponeurosis slides beneath it. This separates the proximal torn end from its distal insertion. Imperfect healing, with ligament laxity, is inevitable with such displacement.* (a. coll. lig. = *accessory collateral ligament;* add. expan. = *insertion of the adductor muscle into the extensor expansion;* EPL = *extensor pollicis longus.)*

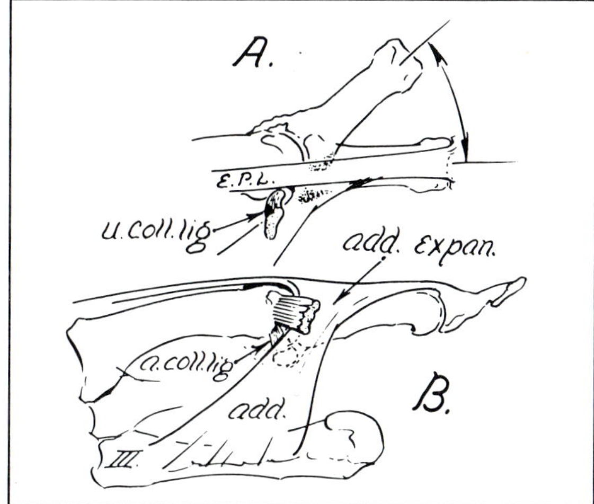

[12]. Ligament repair is best done within the 2 weeks following injury [7]; beyond that time the ligament becomes shortened, edematous, and difficult to reapproximate.

Exposure is through an ulnar oblique incision over the MP joint. Care must be taken here to preserve a small branch of the radial nerve to the dorsoulnar side of the digit. The adductor aponeurosis is divided dorsally parallel to the extensor pollicis longus. With the reflection of the divided adductor aponeurosis, the collateral ligament and base of the proximal phalanx are exposed. The ligament is reattached to the base of the proximal phalanx with a pullout wire. If small bone fragments are present, they are removed and the ligament is advanced into the defect. If a large fragment (particularly one containing articular surface) remains with the ligament, it is retained and reattached with pins or a pullout wire. At the conclusion of the procedure it is desirable to pin the joint in slight flexion and ulnar deviation, since the molding of the cast frequently places the MP joint in an abducted extended position that could jeopardize the repair.

Immobilization in plaster that extends to the thumb tip should be for 4 weeks. At that time the pins and pullout wire are removed and gentle active thumb motion is begun, while the MP joint is protected with an aluminum splint for an additional week.

Ulnar collateral ligament tears that are seen more than 3 weeks after the injury and chronic attenuations of the ulnar supporting structures (the so-called gamekeeper's thumb) require a ligament reconstruction using a tendon graft (Fig. 33-10).

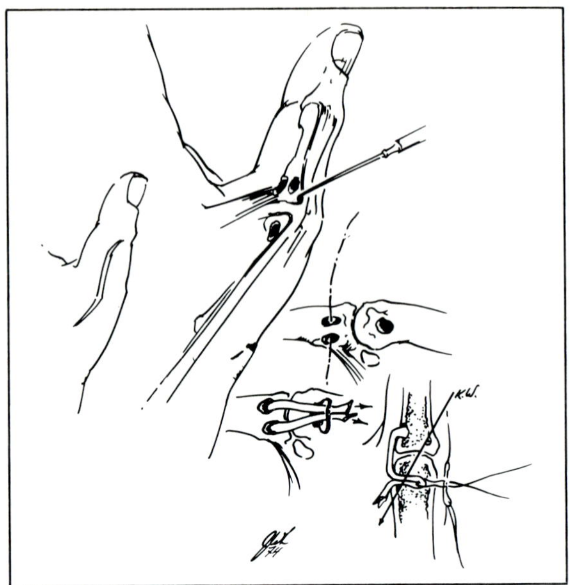

Fig. 33-10. Reconstruction of the ulnar collateral ligament using a tendon graft. An intramedullary channel is gouged in the proximal phalanx parallel to the joint surface. An oblique channel is then gouged in the metacarpal head. The graft is passed through the proximal phalanx channel and the paired ends are drawn into the metacarpal head channel with the aid of a wire loop. The free distal ends may then be sutured back to the volar plate. A Kirschner Wire (K.W.) *is then placed across the joint to immobilize it during healing.*

Carpometacarpal Joint of the Thumb

The basal joint of the thumb, a classic saddle joint, consists of reciprocally biconcave articular contours that allow thumb motion in more than a single plane. Its principal support is the volar ligament, which anchors the volar beak of the metacarpal to the trapezium. The volar ligament imparts to the basal joint the stability that the volar plate provides to the interphalangeal joint. Dorsal support is provided by the thin posterior oblique trapeziometacarpal ligament, reinforced by the tendinous insertion of the abductor pollicis longus.

Two types of injuries occur at this joint [3, 4]. The more common is the Bennett's fracture – dislocation produced by axial compression with the thumb ray in flexion-adduction, shearing off the volar beak of the thumb metacarpal. This triangular fragment remains attached to the volar ligament as the metacarpal shaft displaces dorsally. The degree of injury ranges between minimal displacement and complete dorsal dislocation. The second type of injury is a pure dorsal dislocation of the metacarpal caused by hyperextension of the entire ray, with rupture of the volar ligament and dorsal displacement of the thumb metacarpal base. Instability may vary from hypermobility following a partial tear to complete dislocation of the metacarpal base.

The Bennett's fracture may leave a significant defect in the articular surface of the metacarpal. A step of less than 1 mm. may be accepted, provided that the dislocation is well reduced. Occasionally a percutaneous Kirschner wire to maintain reduction is helpful, since pressure applied through the cast upon the usually swollen fracture area risks skin necrosis or loss of reduction when the swelling subsides.

Open reduction through a Wagner incision affords excellent exposure [16]. The maneuver for both closed and open reduction is traction with pronation in slight extension-abduction. The open reduction is stabilized with a fracture clamp and the fracture is transfixed with Kirschner wires.

Ligament tears of this joint vary in their degree of instability. Unless obvious joint incongruity exists or

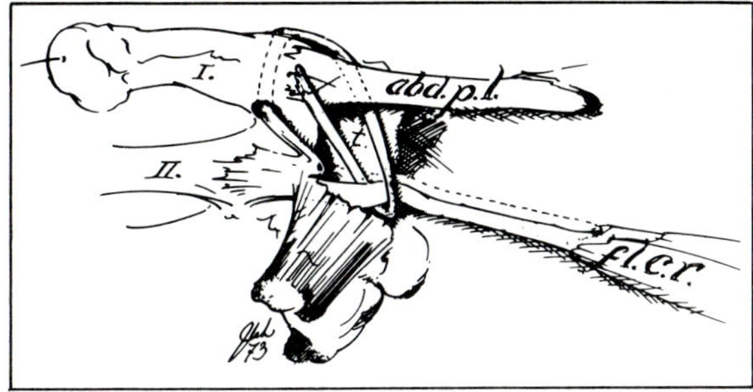

Fig. 33-11. Reconstruction of the basal ligament and capsule of the thumb carpometacarpal joint. A distally attached strip of the subjacent flexor carpi radialis (fl. c. r.) *is passed through a sagittal channel parallel to the articular surface of the metacarpal. The free end of the tendon strip is then passed beneath the abductor pollicis longus* (abd. p. 1.), *around the remaining flexor radialis, and back across the radial capsule.* t = *trapezium;* I = *1st metacarpal;* II = *2nd metacarpal. (Reproduced from R. G. Eaton and J. W. Littler, Ligament reconstruction for the painful thumb carpometacarpal joint.* J. Bone Joint Surg. *[Am.] 55:1655, 1973.)*

displacement occurs while the joint is immobilized, a 4-week period of plaster immobilization will suffice. If incongruity or dislocation is present, reconstruction of the essential volar ligament is indicated (Fig. 33-11).

REFERENCES

1. Arzimanoglou, A., and Skiadaressis, S. M. A study of internal fixation by screws of oblique fractures in long bones. *J. Bone Joint Surg.* [Am.] 34:219, 1952.
2. Coonrad, R. W., and Goldner, J. L. A study of the pathological findings and treatment in soft-tissue injury of the thumb metacarpophalangeal joint. *J. Bone Joint Surg.* [Am.] 50:439, 1968.
3. Eaton, R. G. *Joint Injuries of the Hand.* Springfield, Ill.: Thomas, 1971.
4. Eaton, R. G., and Littler, J. W. A study of the basal joint of the thumb. *J. Bone Joint Surg.* [Am.] 51:661, 1971.
5. Eaton, R. G., and Littler, J. W. Ligament reconstruction for the painful thumb carpometacarpal joint. *J. Bone Joint Surg.* [Am.] 55:1655, 1973.
6. Eaton, R. G., and Littler, J. W. Joint injuries and their sequelae. *Clin. Plast. Surg.* 3:85, 1976.
7. Gedda, K. O. Studies on Bennett's fracture, anatomy, roentgenology, and therapy. *Acta Chir. Scand.* [Suppl. 193]:5, 1954.
8. Green, D. P., and Terry, G. C. Complex dislocation of the metacarpophalangeal joint. Correlative pathological anatomy. *J. Bone Joint Surg.* [Am.] 55:1480, 1973.
9. Kaplan, E. B. Dorsal dislocation of the metacarpophalangeal joint of the index finger. *J. Bone Joint Surg.* [Am.] 39:1081, 1957.
10. McLaughlin, H. L. Complex "locked" dislocations of the metacarpophalangeal joints. *J. Trauma* 5:683, 1965.
11. Moberg, E. Fractures and ligamentous injuries of the thumb and fingers. *Surg. Clin. North Am.* 40:297, 1960.
12. Pollen, A. G. The conservative treatment of Bennett's fracture-subluxation of the thumb metacarpal. *J. Bone Joint Surg.* [Br.] 50:91, 1968.
13. Smith, R. J. Lateral instability of the metacarpophalangeal joint of the thumb. *J. Bone Joint Surg.* [Am.] 57:729, 1975.
14. Spinner, M., and Choi, B. Y. Anterior dislocation of the proximal interphalangeal joint. A cause of rupture of the central slip of the extensor mechanism. *J. Bone Joint Surg.* [Am.] 52:1329, 1970.
15. Stener, B. Displacement of the ruptured ulnar collateral ligament of the metacarpophalangeal joint of the thumb. *J. Bone Joint Surg.* [Br.] 44:869, 1962.
16. Wagner, C. J. Method of treatment of Bennett's fracture-dislocation. *Am. J. Surg.* 80:230, 1950.

34

Stiff Finger Joints

RAYMOND M. CURTIS

ANKYLOSIS OF THE INTERPHALANGEAL JOINTS OF THE FINGERS

The crippled hand frequently functions improperly because of limited flexion or extension in the interphalangeal joints. Dr. Sterling Bunnell [2] has pointed out that motion will become limited when the interphalangeal joint space is narrowed by even the slightest shortening of the capsular ligaments, as might be produced by disease or edema of the ligaments and subsequent fibrosis. This shortening, with limitation in motion, may occur despite the most rigid attention to proper splinting and to physical and occupational therapy, but more often it follows their improper application [1].

Mechanical Factors Limiting Flexion of Interphalangeal Joints

The surgeon who intends to correct a limitation of flexion of the interphalangeal joints must analyze the various anatomical factors that might cause it. These are:

1. Scar contracture of the skin over the dorsum of the finger.
2. A contracted long extensor muscle or adherent extensor tendon.
3. A contracted interosseous muscle or adherent interosseous tendon.
4. The retinacular ligament adherent to the lateral capsular ligament.
5. Contracted collateral ligaments.
6. Volar capsular ligament adherent to proximal phalanx.
7. Bony block or exostosis.
8. Flexor tendons adherent within sheath.

Preoperative Clinical Evaluation

Before embarking on surgery to correct the lack of flexion of the interphalangeal joints, it is important to determine by clinical examination and roentgenography just which anatomical structures are limiting flexion and to exclude the possibility of a true ankylosis by bony fusion or block. Bunnell, Doherty, and Curtis [3] have described various test positions for the hand and fingers that will aid in this determination. This is particularly helpful in the finger that does not flex, for it may be possible to determine before operation that, for example, the primary limiting factor is the *collateral ligaments*; then the operative approach would be directed first to a release of these ligaments [8, 10, 12]. On the other hand, if the defect was found to be primarily one of lack of flexion in the interphalangeal joints because of an *ischemic contracture of the interosseous muscles* [13], the first operative procedure would be their release in order to achieve flexion. While limitation of flexion may be due to a single, isolated structure such as the collateral ligament, it may also be due to pathological changes in all of the structures – that is, a finger may be limited in its degree of flexion as a result of collateral ligament thickening, a contracture of the interosseous muscles, and an adherence of the extensor tendon. To achieve flexion operatively in such a situation, all three abnormalities must be corrected.

If the joint passively flexes to 75 degrees, then efforts should be directed toward physical therapy and splinting to achieve further flexion rather than to operation.

Operative Technique and Postoperative Treatment

The interphalangeal joint is approached by a dorsal curvilinear incision (Fig. 34-1). (It may also be approached by a lateral incision on both its sides.) This incision is deepened through the skin and subcutaneous tissue to expose the extensor tendon over the dorsum of the finger. The skin flaps are reflected laterally to allow exposure of the retinacular ligaments on either side of the joint. The retinacular ligament is preserved so that joint stability may be maintained after the collateral ligaments have been excised. The *collateral ligament* of the proximal interphalangeal joint is best demonstrated by approaching the joint from the base of the middle phalanx after elevating the retinacular ligament and retracting it proximally [4]. As much of the collateral ligament as possible should be excised from its attachments to the base of the middle phalanx and to the distal end of the proximal phalanx on both sides of the joint. A small portion of the distal edge of the retinacular ligament can be excised, if necessary, in order to better expose either collateral ligament. In some long-standing cases, the volar synovial pouch becomes obliterated and must be re-formed with a small curved elevator or by forcing the base of the middle phalanx into flexion.

In some instances, it may be necessary to incise the retinacular ligament in a zigzag fashion to expose the joint completely so that a small exostosis, for

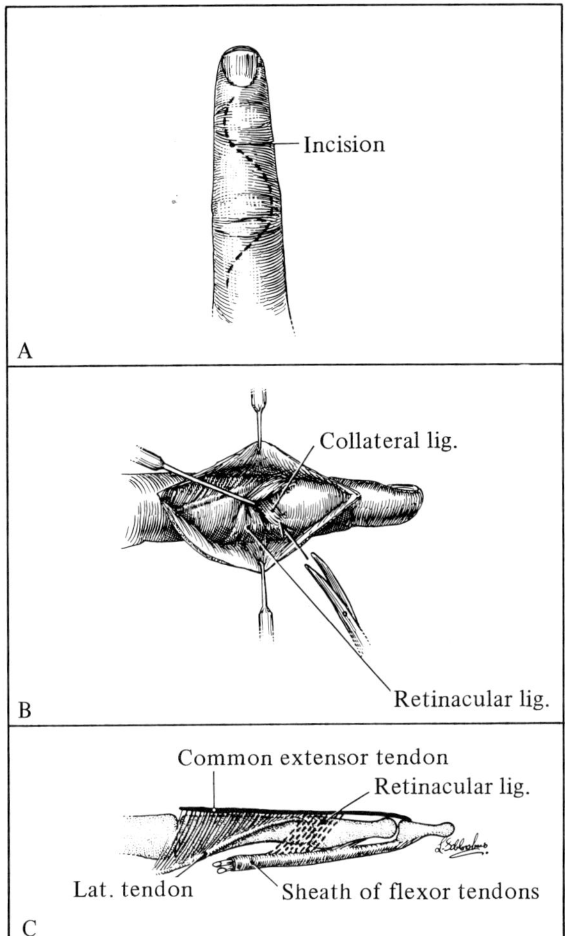

Fig. 34-1. Capsulectomy of the proximal interphalangeal joint. A, dorsal excision; the dorsal skin is elevated and retracted. B, retracted skin, with elevation of the retinacular ligament, exposes the collateral ligament, which is totally excised. C, relationship of the retinacular ligament to the joint capsule and the flexor and extensor tendons.

example, can be removed from the distal end of the proximal phalanx to achieve complete flexion. When this is required, the ligament should be resutured at the end of surgery to preserve joint stability.

Once the collateral ligament has been excised, the finger should be tested to determine whether the joint can be completely flexed. If it cannot, then some other structure within the finger is still limiting flexion. When there is an associated *contracture of the interosseous muscle,* it is lengthened by tenotomy at the juncture of the longitudinal fibers with the middle slip of the extensor tendon and allowed to slide proximally, where it is sutured to the extensor aponeurosis. Another effective procedure involves excising a triangular portion from the lateral band on both sides of the finger at the level of the proximal phalanx, as suggested by Littler and Howorth [11]. Such a tenotomy or excision relieves the mild contracture, but in more severe cases, tenotomy of the tendon must be carried out just proximal to the metacarpophalangeal joint in order to gain an adequate release.

When the *extensor tendon is adherent* dorsally, it can be freed if necessary. In some instances there is a thickening dorsally of the synovium of the proximal interphalangeal joint, and it may be necessary to excise it with the use of a small curved osteotome* in order to achieve flexion.

When surgery is completed, it should be easy to flex the joint passively. If the obstructing structures all have been released to the point where the finger can be carried into flexion with the same ease as the normal adjacent finger, a good result can be anticipated.

Once the finger has been stiff in extension, the flexor tendons frequently become adherent in their bed. The operator should routinely check function of these tendons by identifying them through a small incision in the palm of the hand and by placing traction on them in order to be certain that, with the joint freed surgically, they will completely flex the finger passively. It is sometimes necessary to free them not only through the palmar incision but also by exposing them in the finger by reflecting the original skin flaps laterally over the proximal phalanx.

An injection of 2 mg. of triamcinolone acetonide into the interphalangeal joint before wound closure sometimes seems to be of value.

Following wound closure, the hand is placed in a routine compression pressure dressing, with the fingers in moderate flexion, for the first 72 hours to prevent excessive swelling and to achieve perfect wound healing. Seventy-two hours postoperatively, rubber bands are attached to the fingertips with adhesive tape, and traction is started to pull the fingers slowly into the completely flexed position. This treatment is coupled with active extension and flexion of the fingers, but this is limited to the amount that can be carried out without producing undue swelling of the hand and fingers. The rubber-band traction to carry the fingers into flexion must sometimes be alternated with similar traction to carry the fingers into extension.

*Dental DeExcavators, Stock No. 845, item No. 13, 15, 18, 20, Friedman Dental Supply Company, Baltimore, Md. 21208.

Splinting is continued until the patient can maintain, by active and passive exercise, the range of motion achieved at surgery. In some instances, this has necessitated part-time splinting for as long as 3 or 4 months. Physical therapy, with active motion and careful passive motion, also is begun as soon as wound healing will permit. Of particular value in the late postoperative care is intermittent compression therapy using the Jobst unit, in which the hand, with fingers flexed, is slipped into a bag that is alternately inflated and deflated by a small compressor.

Mechanical Factors Limiting Extension of Interphalangeal Joints

The surgeon intending to correct a limitation of extension of the interphalangeal joints must consider the anatomical factors within a finger that may limit extension. These are:

1. Scar of skin on the volar surface of the finger.
2. Contraction of the superficial fascia in the finger, as in Dupuytren's contracture.
3. Contraction of the flexor tendon sheath within the finger.
4. Contraction of the flexor muscle or adherent flexor tendon.
5. Contraction or adherence of the volar plate of the capsular ligament.
6. Adherence of the retinacular ligament to the collateral ligaments.
7. Contracture of the accessory volar collateral ligaments.
8. Adherence of the collateral ligaments, with the finger in the flexed position, to the lateral aspect of the proximal phalanx.
9. Bony block or exostosis.

Preoperative Clinical Evaluation

Before attempting to correct the lack of extension of the interphalangeal joints surgically, it is important if possible to determine by clinical examination and roentgenography just which anatomical structures are limiting extension, and to exclude the possibility of a true ankylosis by bony fusion.

Palpation of the skin should permit the examiner to determine whether there is adequate skin to allow extension. Thickened strands of fascia such as found in Dupuytren's contracture can also be palpated. It may also be possible to determine that the fixation in the flexed position is due to an adherent flexor tendon. However, it is very difficult to be certain whether a contracture of the flexor tendon sheath or a contracture of the capsular ligament is causing the deformity.

In patients with a congenital flexion contracture of the finger, the problem is one of inadequate skin; as a rule there is a contracture both of the flexor superficialis tendon and of the volar capsule of the proximal interphalangeal joint.

Operative Technique and Postoperative Treatment

If the flexion contracture is due to inadequate soft tissue, this must be corrected by the addition of a cross finger pedicle flap if both skin and subcutaneous tissue are needed, or by the application of a partial-thickness skin graft if there is a good bed of subcutaneous tissue on which to place this graft. With a flexion contracture due to the thickened strand of fascia as in Dupuytren's contracture, local excision of the strand itself will usually correct the flexion contracture, although it is often necessary to add a Z-plasty to provide additional skin length. If the problem is of long duration, it also will be necessary to perform a volar capsulectomy with a partial resection of the accessory collateral ligaments on each side of the proximal interphalangeal joint. In some instances the retinacular ligaments have to be sectioned on both sides of the finger.

A finger fixed in flexion following trauma, but having adequate skin coverage, is best approached through a midlateral incision through the skin and subcutaneous tissue to expose the flexor tendons over the proximal and middle phalanges. A portion of the flexor tendon sheath over the proximal interphalangeal joint is then excised directly. In some instances the contraction and fixation of the sheath itself may be all that is limiting extension. If excision of the sheath fails to improve the degree of extension, it should be determined whether the flexor tendons are adherent within the finger; if this is the case, they are tendolysed. However, when the flexor tendon sheath and the flexor tendons themselves are not at fault, the problem is one of an adherent and contracted volar capsular ligament with adherence of the accessory collateral ligaments to the sides of the distal portion of the proximal phalanx. Merely freeing the volar plate from where it has become adherent to the distal end of the proximal phalanx may permit extension of the finger. In more advanced cases, on the other hand, it is necessary to excise the entire volar plate and to section a portion of the accessory collateral ligament on either side of the proximal interphalangeal joint through a small additional lateral incision on the opposite side of the joint (Fig. 34-2). It may also be necessary to free the retinacular ligaments from the lateral aspect of the lateral capsule. With this much of the volar capsule and the accessory collateral ligament released, the operator must be careful as he attempts to extend the proximal interphalangeal joint, since hyperextension following this degree of release will cause the cord portion of the collateral ligament to tear in two suddenly, and the joint will

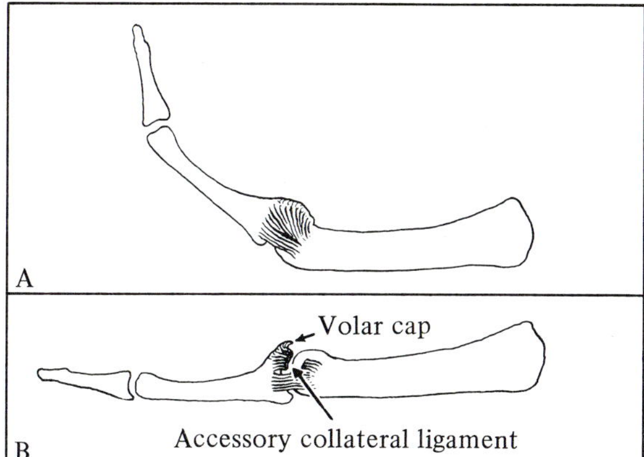

Fig. 34-2. Capsulectomy for release of flexion contracture of the finger. A, fixed flexion contracture. B, excision of a portion of the volar capsule and release of the accessory collateral ligament, leaving the cord portion to maintain stability of the joint. (From R. M. Curtis, as reported in J. P. Adams [Ed.], Current Practice in Orthopedic Surgery, *Vol. 2, St. Louis: Mosby, 1964.)*

subluxate. This creates a real postoperative problem, because the finger must then be held in a flexed position until adequate scarring heals the torn ligament.

In order to achieve extension, in some instances it has been necessary as a single operative procedure to excise the scar over the flexor surface of the finger, release the tendon sheath and the flexor tendons, excise the volar capsule and incise the accessory collateral ligament, hold the finger in moderate extension by a Kirschner wire across the proximal interphalangeal joint, and then cover the wound with a cross finger pedicle flap from an adjacent finger.

In a long-standing flexion contracture, it may also be necessary to free the extensor tendon over the dorsum of the finger, since adhesions here of the extensor tendon to the phalanx would prevent active extension.

To hold the finger in moderate extension, the Kirschner wire is inserted across the proximal interphalangeal joint with the finger in moderate but not extreme extension, so that an abnormal amount of pull is not placed on the digital nerve and vessel. This pin is left in place for 7 days. On the seventh day the Kirschner wire is removed and rubber-band traction begun on the tip of the finger in order to achieve further passive extension of the finger, at the same time allowing active motion of a graded type.

ANKYLOSIS OF THE METACARPOPHALANGEAL JOINTS OF THE FINGERS

Immobility of the metacarpophalangeal joints, for whatever reason, particularly if there is swelling with deposition of edema fluid in the ligamentous tissue itself, leads to adhesions of the extensor mechanism, contracture of the collateral ligaments, and thickening of the entire capsular ligamentous structure, with the consequent ankylosis so commonly seen in the metacarpophalangeal joints [6].

The anatomical factors that may limit metacarpophalangeal joint flexion are:

1. Insufficient skin coverage or scarring over the dorsum of the hand.
2. Adherence of the extensor tendons over the dorsum of the hand or of the extensor hood mechanism over the metacarpophalangeal joints.
3. Thickening of the dorsal capsule of the metacarpophalangeal joints.
4. Contracture of the collateral ligament (cord portion).
5. Bony block within the joint.

Ankylosis of the metacarpophalangeal joints is seen in hands that have been infected; it follows trauma of all types to the hands (including burns with burn scar contracture over the dorsum of the hand), accompanies congenital aplasia of the metacarpophalangeal joints, and is present in certain systemic diseases such as rheumatoid arthritis and dermatomyositis.

This very disabling abnormality can best be prevented by (1) early motion of the metacarpophalangeal joints; (2) elevation of the injured extremity to minimize edema; (3) using *no* plaster cast that immobilizes the metacarpophalangeal joints; (4) early elastic-band traction in patients who are developing this clinical entity; and (5) early active motion of all of the finger joints.

If progress is being made with conservative treatment, operative release should be delayed. If, on the other hand, several months of conservative treatment produce no improvement in the range of active or passive motion in the metacarpophalangeal joints, surgical release is indicated.

When the metacarpophalangeal joint is intrinsically good but cannot be flexed actively or passively, a good result can be anticipated from the release of the tight capsular ligaments and the extensor tendon mechanism. On the other hand, if 75 degrees of active motion is present in the metacarpophalangeal joint, there is less indication for surgical intervention. The patient who can flex these joints as much as 65 degrees should continue on physical therapy and special splinting. For patients whose hands are fixed in full extension or have a range of motion less than 65 degrees of flexion, sufficient improvement can be expected to warrant operative intervention.

Capsulectomy of the Metacarpophalangeal Joints

If the operative approach to the collateral ligaments is too radical, an initial improvement in flexion will frequently be obtained, but the ultimate result will be ulnar deviation of the fingers similar to that encountered in patients with rheumatoid arthritis who have complete destruction of the collateral ligaments on the radial side. Because this may also occur in patients with ulnar nerve paralysis, the procedure of capsulectomy illustrated in Figures 34-4 and 34-5 seems preferable. The technique permits release of the cordlike portion of the collateral ligament from the tubercle of the metacarpal on either side of the metacarpophalangeal joint after excision of the dorsal capsule. As a result of maintaining continuity between the cordlike portion of the collateral ligament and the accessory collateral ligament, there is still in essence an attachment of the cordlike portion of the collateral ligament to the metacarpal itself, which is enough to prevent the ulnar deviation [5, 6].

Operative Technique

The extensor tendon is exposed by a straight longitudinal incision over the metacarpal and then split longitudinally for a distance of approximately 2.5 cm. on either side of the metacarpophalangeal joint [9] (Fig. 34-3). The extensor aponeurosis or hood is then retracted to either side, and any attachments of the extensor tendon to the base of the proximal phalanx are severed. The synovium that lies between the base of the phalanx and the head of the metacarpal and forms the dorsal part of the capsule of the joint is excised, since this may be greatly thickened in severe cases. This excision of the dorsal capsule extends from one collateral ligament across to the opposite collateral ligament (Fig. 34-4).

Since it is the cordlike portion of the collateral ligament that limits flexion, it can be released from its attachment to the tubercle on either side of the head of the metacarpal. This cord is left attached to the accessory collateral ligament but freed of any adhesions that may have formed between the collateral ligament and the head of the metacarpal (Fig. 34-5B). The same type of release is carried out on both the radial and the ulnar aspects of the metacarpal head.

In those patients with greatly thickened collateral ligaments, a section of the cordlike portion of the ligament should be excised near the tubercle on either side of the head of the metacarpal. The remainder of the cordlike portion should be left attached to the accessory collateral ligament. This prevents ulnar deviation of the finger, which is seen when too much of it and the accessory ligament are removed. This deviation is particularly likely to occur in the patient with ulnar nerve palsy. Care must be exercised not to

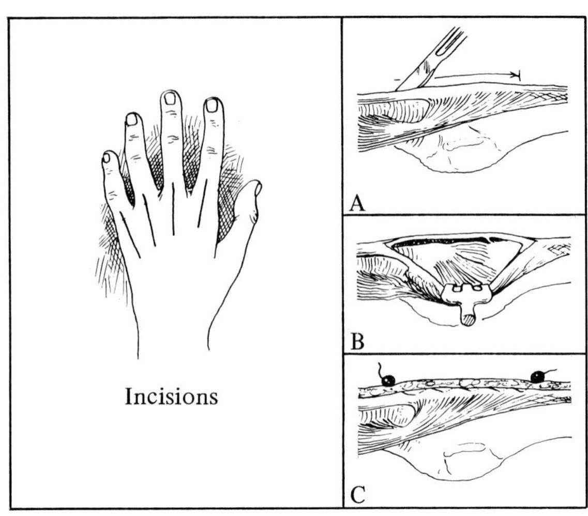

Fig. 34-3. Incisions for exposure of the capsular ligaments of the metacarpophalangeal joints of the fingers for capsulectomy [9]. A, splitting the extensor tendon, B, retraction of the extensor hood to expose the capsular ligament. C, closure of the extensor tendon with running 4-0 stainless-steel wire. (From R. M. Curtis as reported in J. E. Flynn, Hand Surgery. *Baltimore: Williams & Wilkins, 1975.)*

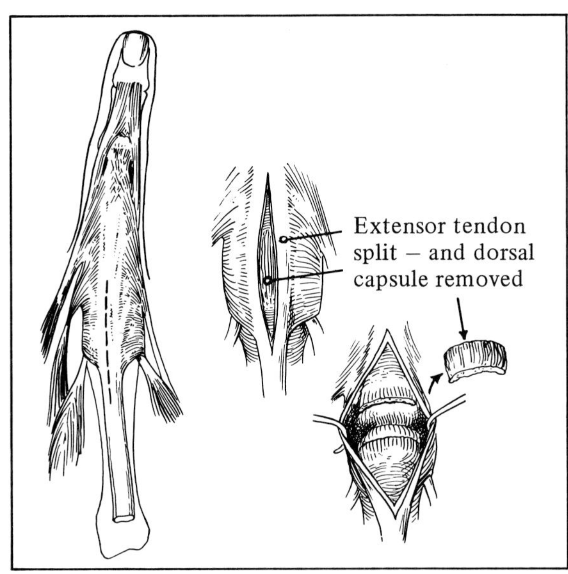

Fig. 34-4. Exposure of the joint by dorsal approach through the extensor tendon, with excision of thickened synovium, which forms the dorsal part of the capsule. (From R. M. Curtis, as reported in J. E. Flynn, Hand Surgery. *Baltimore: Williams & Wilkins, 1975.)*

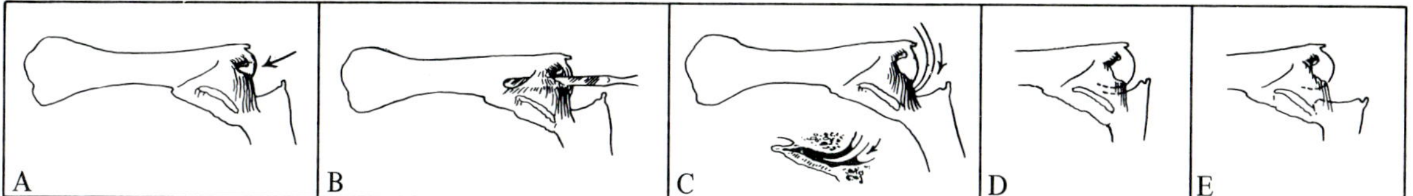

Fig. 34-5. Technique for capsulectomy with the release of the cordlike portion of the ligament. Continuity is maintained between the distal portion of the cordlike ligament and the accessory collateral ligament to prevent ulnar deviation even when a small wedge of the cordlike portion of ligament is excised. A, the dorsal capsule is excised and cordlike portion released at the point of attachment to the metacarpal; the accessory collateral ligament is still intact. B, elevator frees adhesions between the ligament and the head of the metacarpal. C, elevator releases the adherent volar capsule and re-creates a normal pouch beneath the metacarpal head. D, proper relation of the phalanx to the metacarpal. E, with inadequate release of the volar capsule, the phalanx does not rest beneath the head of the metacarpal. (From R. M. Curtis, as reported in J. E. Flynn, Hand Surgery. *Baltimore: Williams & Wilkins, 1975.)*

sever the attachment of the interosseous tendon into the base of the phalanx just distal to the attachment of the collateral ligament to the phalanx, because this may also lead to ulnar deviation of the fingers.

If the phalanx does not drop into flexion beneath the head of the metacarpal, then a curved periosteal elevator should be inserted around the head of the metacarpal to re-create the volar pouch, since in long-standing cases this pouch becomes obliterated when the volar plate becomes adherent to the metacarpal head (Fig. 34-5).

The excursion of the extensor tendons over the dorsum of the hand should also be checked. If these are not gliding freely, they should be freed over the dorsum of the hand, and if necessary over the dorsum of the wrist and into the forearm. In addition, it may be necessary to free the extensor hood well on either side of the metacarpophalangeal joint.

The extensor tendon is closed with a running suture of 4-0 stainless-steel wire, as illustrated in Figure 34-3. The hand is bandaged in a pressure dressing with the metacarpophalangeal joints in moderate flexion, but not to such a severe degree as to cause the extensor tendons to open over the metacarpophalangeal joint. The pressure dressing is left in place for 72 hours; then it is removed and a volar plaster splint applied so leather loops can be placed about the proximal phalanges and rubber-band traction started to aid flexion. The running 4-0 stainless-steel wire suture is removed from the extensor tendon in 3 weeks.

The elastic splinting must be continued as long as necessary, both day and night. After 4 to 6 weeks, a Bunnell knuckle-bender splint may be used. During the period of elastic splinting, some active extension should also be allowed. There is rarely any difficulty in achieving complete active extension following this procedure, although after traction for 2 or 3 weeks the question frequently arises whether the patient will ever again be able to extend the fingers completely. In some cases it may be necessary, for this reason, to alternate the rubber-band traction for flexion with rubber-band traction for extension of the fingers.

REFERENCES

1. Adams, J. P. *Current Practice in Orthopaedic Surgery,* Vol. 2. St. Louis: Mosby, 1964.
2. Boyes, J. H. *Bunnell's Surgery of the Hand* (4th ed.). Philadelphia: Lippincott, 1964.
3. Bunnell, S., Doherty, E. W., and Curtis, R. M. Ischemic contracture, local, in the hand. *Plast. Reconstr. Surg.* 3:424, 1948.
4. Curtis, R. M. Capsulectomy of the interphalangeal joints of the fingers. *J. Bone Joint Surg.* [Am.] 36:1219, 1954.
5. Flynn, J. E. *Hand Surgery* (2nd ed.). Baltimore: Williams & Wilkins, 1975.
6. Fowler, S. B. Mobilization of metacarpophalangeal joint. *J. Bone Joint Surg.* [Am.] 29:193, 1947.
7. Grant, J. C. B. *A Method of Anatomy* (4th ed.). Baltimore: Williams & Wilkins, 1948.
8. Harrison, D. H. The stiff interphalangeal joint. *Hand* 9:102, 1977.
9. Howard, L. D. Cited by Bunnell, S., in *Surgery of the Hand* (2nd ed.). Philadelphia: Lippincott, 1948.
10. Landsmeer, J. M. F. The anatomy of the dorsal aponeurosis of the human finger and its functional significance. *Anat. Rec.* 104:31, 1949.
11. Littler, J. W., and Howorth, M. B. *A Textbook of Orthopedics.* Philadelphia: Saunders, 1952.
12. Sprague, B. L. The proximal interphalangeal joint contractures and their treatment. *J. Trauma* 16:259, 1976.
13. Stack, H. G. Muscle function in the fingers. *J. Bone Joint Surg.* [Br.] 44:899, 1962.

Tendon Injuries in the Forearm and Hand

JAMES W. SMITH

The initial treatment of an injured hand is often determined by the mode of injury, the extent and type of tissue damage, the time lapse, and the degree of wound contamination. These factors may require even more careful consideration when immediate tendon repair is contemplated. Many attempts have been made to establish a classification for treatment, but no stereotyped set of rules can substitute for good common sense and a knowledge of fundamental surgical principles. The importance of individualized care cannot be overemphasized. No two injuries are exactly alike, nor are the abilities of the surgeons treating them. These are major reasons why the best primary care will vary with each case. Thus, ideal care may be defined as the most effective treatment that can be rendered under existing circumstances without appreciably increasing the risk of complications.

Treatment must always be directed toward restoring the greatest possible function in the shortest time. In some cases these goals can be accomplished by a single operative procedure. Others will require multiple stages of reconstruction. All must be planned systematically and methodically. Last to be considered in nearly any plan of reconstruction for a complicated injury will be the repair of tendons, because many prerequisites are necessary for proper tendon function. They include, in their order of priority, adequate circulation, satisfactory skin coverage, a well-aligned skeletal framework, good joint function, and the restoration of nerve continuity. Since all these factors are necessary for optimum tendon function, the repair of damaged tendons should be considered only after these prerequisites have been satisfied.

The most important initial consideration in treating an injured hand is to gain primary wound healing. Only when this and the other tissue requirements listed above can be met without seriously increasing the risk of a complication should restoration of tendon continuity be considered at the time of primary treatment.

As an aid to discussing treatment, extensor and flexor tendon injuries are considered separately.

EXTENSOR TENDON INJURIES

Extensor tendon injuries have been divided into five groups (Fig. 35-1) according to anatomical location: (1) insertion injuries (mallet finger), (2) middle slip injuries (boutonnière deformity), (3) extensor hood injuries, (4) tendon injuries over the dorsum of the hand, and (5) tendon injuries in the forearm and wrist.

Mallet Finger

The mallet or baseball finger deformity [1, 2, 31, 36–38] results from a disruption in the continuity of the extensor tendon mechanism at or near its site of insertion into the distal phalanx. This disruption may complicate an open laceration or may be found as a closed rupture of the extensor tendon from its site of insertion. When the tendon has been cut by a sharp instrument, it can be repaired by carefully reapproximating its ends (Fig. 35-2). One good technique is to run a continuous suture of 34 gauge wire or 4-0 nylon from one side of the finger to the other, weaving it back and forth through the tendon. With closed injuries that result in rupture there is usually extensive fraying of the tendon at the point of separation, making surgical repair more difficult and giving results that are less satisfactory than can be obtained by splinting alone. The exception to this statement occurs when a chip of bone adjacent to the site of tendon insertion is avulsed from the distal phalanx along with the tendon. A preoperative x-ray film will identify this type of case, which should be repaired surgically by reattaching the bony fragment to its former site [4, 30, 35]. Some surgeons feel that, if less than 30 percent of the articular surface of the distal interphalangeal joint is fractured off, it should not be opened. At most, the residual disability will be some slight swelling of the dorsum of the joint and perhaps a 10-degree deficit in extension. In other cases of closed disruption it is far better to immobilize the finger in either plaster or a metal splint, which will hold the distal joint in nearly maximum hyperextension and the proximal interphalangeal joint in moderate flexion [38]. This relaxes the lateral bands of the extensor mechanism and permits scar tissue to bridge the gap for the restoration of extensor tendon continuity. Splinting should be continuous for 6 weeks (Table 35-1). In closed disruptions this treatment is superior to other methods.

Another technique that has also been reported as satisfactory employs Kirschner pins to fix the distal interphalangeal joint or both the distal and proximal interphalangeal joints [31]. However, unless the operator is experienced with the placement of these pins,

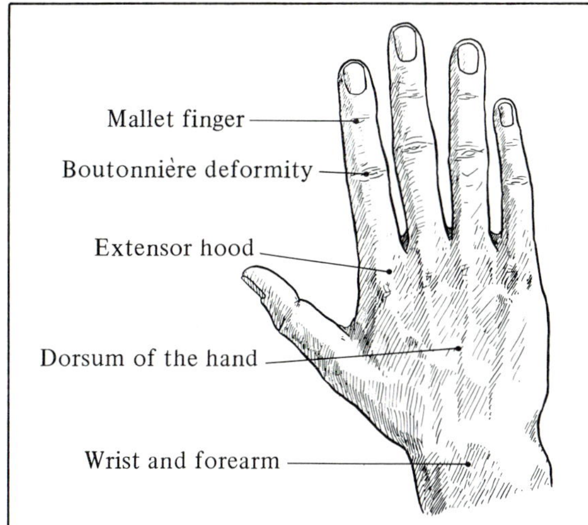

Fig. 35-1. Extensor tendon injuries are divided into five groups according to anatomical location for the purposes of discussion in this section.

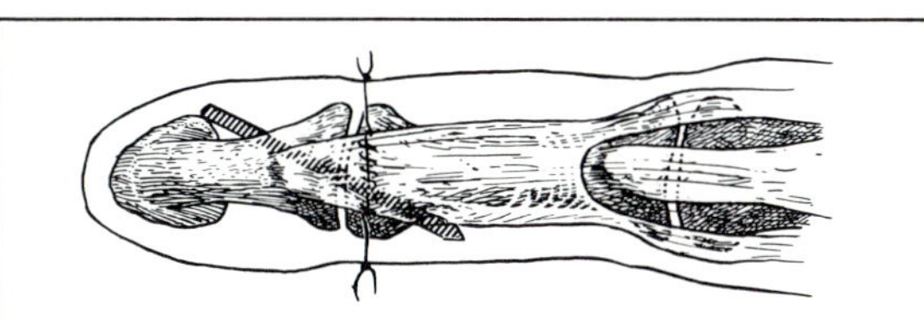

Fig. 35-2. A technique for the repair of mallet finger deformity. An extensor tendon divided at or near its site of insertion can be repaired by approximating the two ends with a wire or nylon suture. The two edges are woven back together with a continuous wire or nylon suture, which is passed through the skin on one side of the finger, through the tendon, and then out onto the skin on the other side. The suture can be tied to itself or fixed to the skin on either side for 3 weeks, then cut and removed by gradual tension. Also shown is cross-pin fixation of the distal interphalangeal joint to maintain some degree of hyperextension. If the pin is placed longitudinally so that it protrudes through the tip of the finger, there is great discomfort with use.

Table 35-1. Routine Periods of Immobilization[a]

Site	Tendon Injury	Time (weeks)
Finger	Flexor tendons	3
	Extensor tendons	4
Forearm	Wrist flexors & extensors (larger tendons)	5
Others	Mallet finger	6
	Boutonnière	6

[a]It is easier to remember the periods of immobilization by thinking of them as the "3, 4, 5, 6" rule; to each period should be added an additional week of guarded motion before normal activity is resumed.

the complications of further tendon damage, loss of soft tissue, and joint contracture may result.

Boutonnière Deformity

The boutonnière deformity [4, 21, 38] results from a disruption in the continuity of the central (middle) slip at the level of the proximal interphalangeal joint (Fig. 35-3). Here the extensor mechanism is made up of two lateral bands and a central slip, which, because of its dorsal location, is frequently damaged. When it is divided, the proximal interphalangeal joint may at first be capable of partial extension because the lateral bands, if not displaced, still aid in extension of this joint. With continued use, however, they slip volarward on either side of the joint and become less effective as extensors. If their displacement is extreme, they lie below the axis of joint rotation and can actually increase the flexion deformity. In such a circumstance the angle of approach of these lateral slips is altered at the distal interphalangeal joint and thus may cause its hyperextension.

When boutonnière deformities are of the closed type, repair is difficult because of the associated tendon fraying. Good results can be achieved by splinting the metacarpophalangeal and proximal interphalangeal joints in hyperextension for 6 weeks (Fig. 35-4). During the last 3 weeks of treatment, the splint can be removed for short periods to permit moderate flexion of the joints so that they do not become permanently stiff. If the central slip has been divided in an open injury, its proximal end is identified and resutured back into its normal location. The Bunnell technique is used, with 34 gauge stainless-steel wire. The pullout wire is used for its later removal. When old boutonnière deformities are complicated by volar displacement of the lateral tendon

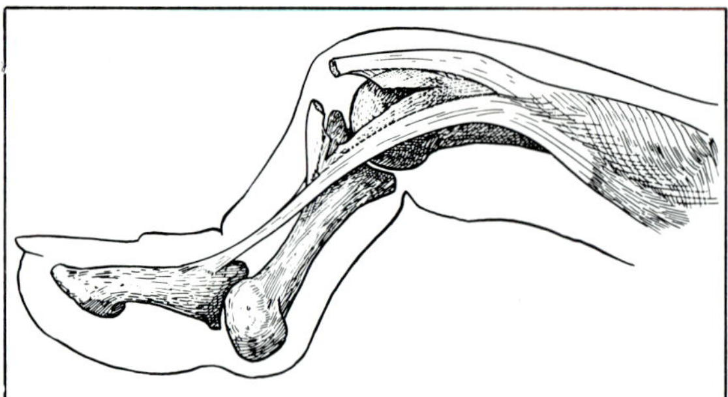

Fig. 35-3. In the boutonnière deformity, lacerations at the level of the proximal interphalangeal joint frequently divide the middle slip of the extensor tendon mechanism. Unless these injuries are quite wide and deep, the lateral bonds will frequently be spared. The potential gravity of the problem may not be appreciated if some extension remains at this joint. Finally the lateral bands slip volarward to a point where they lie below the axis of rotation and begin to act as joint flexors. They then begin to aid the development of a typical boutonnière deformity. Note that the distal interphalangeal joint falls into hyperextension with this deformity.

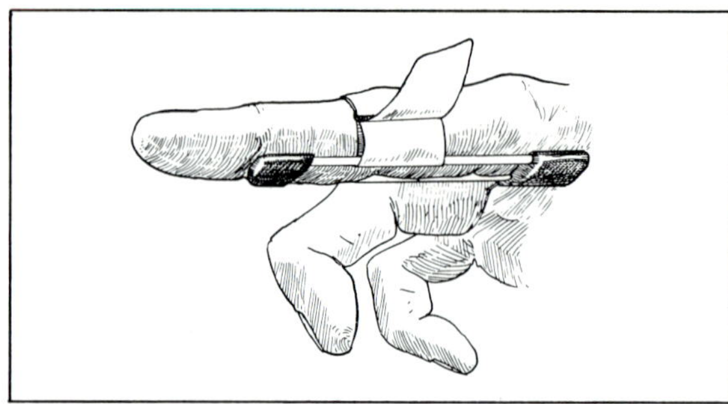

Fig. 35-4. Safety-pin splint holding the metacarpophalangeal and proximal interphalangeal joints in hyperextension during the 6-week period of treatment. Flexion of the distal joint should be encouraged during this time.

slips, it may be necessary to reposition these slips surgically to a more dorsal position.

Verdan suggests that, in the injury of long standing, the middle slip of the extensor tendon should be shortened over the middle third of the proximal phalanx [38]. With the finger in full extension, enough of the scar is resected to permit an end-to-end suture of the central slip. The lateral bands are then replaced in their physiological positions and held there by a few fine catgut sutures.

Another method for treating long-standing injuries has proved extremely satisfactory. Sometimes it becomes impossible to get the proximal interphalangeal joint into full extension, even passively, without some form of stretching. At the distal interphalangeal joint, the opposite deformity is present. This joint is hyperextended, and initially it appears impossible to get it into any degree of flexion because of the tightness of the lateral bands; there seems to be a shortening of the intrinsic tendons in these long-standing boutonnière deformities, which must be corrected prior to surgery. If a safety-pin splint and a strap are used to hold the metacarpophalangeal joint in extension and the strap is slowly tightened to gain extension at the proximal interphalangeal joint, the deformity can be partially corrected (Fig. 35-4). Making the splint of such a length that the patient can actively flex the distal interphalangeal joint further aids in obtaining the necessary preoperative correction. The main result of this maneuver seems to be some stretching of the shortened lateral bands, which allows them to reposition themselves more dorsally. To be effective, such splinting often requires 3 to 6 weeks of hard work on the part of the patient. Once complete passive extension has been gained at the proximal interphalangeal joint in conjunction with good active flexion of the distal joint, the central slip can be repaired.

Through a zigzag skin incision on the dorsum of the finger, the tubercle at the base of the middle phalanx is identified and a transverse tunnel established through it. It may be necessary to split the site where the lateral slips join beyond the proximal interphalangeal joint in a distal direction to gain a sufficiently good exposure to tunnel this anchoring site for the tendon. The original insertion of the middle slip is nearly always gone or has degenerated in long-standing injuries, and a suture of the tendon to the periosteum will not be strong enough to meet the needs of the repair. Neither will the central slip be long enough for the repair. Once it has been found and dissected out, a tendon graft is inserted as a loop between the end of the central slip and the bony tunnel while the fingers are held in extension. The tendon is sutured into place with 34 gauge wire or 4-0 nylon, either as a permanent suture or by the pullout technique.

For long-standing cases with marked hyperextension of the distal phalanx, Dolphin [4a] has suggested transecting the central part of the extensor tendon apparatus over the middle phalanx. This transection permits the patient to regain flexion of the distal phalanx and often some better extension of the proximal interphalangeal joint.

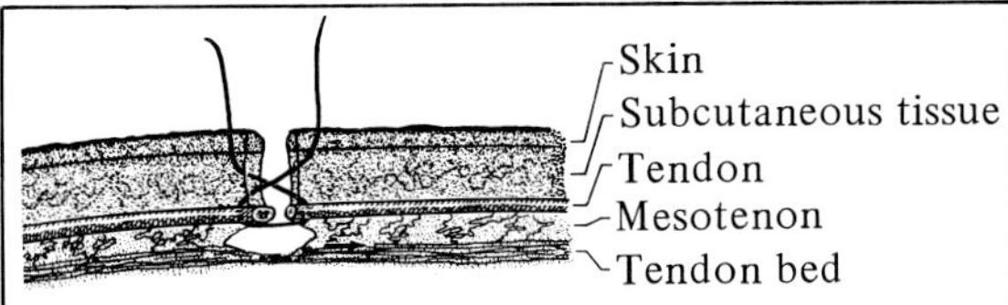

Fig. 35-5. Figure-of-eight suture. Suture is begun by passing one end through each side of the tendon, then crisscrossing the ends and bringing them out through the subcutaneous tissue and skin. Closing the wound by tying sutures also approximates the ends of the tendon. Later the sutures can be removed so that no buried suture material is left in tendon.

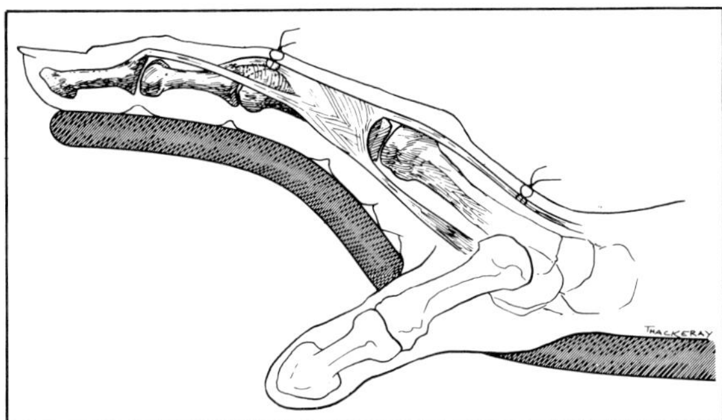

Fig. 35-6. Figure-of-eight sutures and splinting in repair of extensor tendon injury. If division of the middle slip is recognized at the time of injury, it can be repaired by several simple figure-of-eight sutures as shown here, or by weaving a suture transversely back and forth between the two ends of the tendon. It is important to the final healing that the wrist and fingers be placed in extension postoperatively for 6 weeks.

Any division of extensor tendons proximal to the metacarpophalangeal joint can be repaired in a similar fashion. These tendon repairs should be splinted for 4 weeks in complete extension before beginning a final week of guarded motion.

Extensor Hood Injuries

Injuries at the metacarpophalangeal joint level [30, 38] frequently damage the extensor tendon mechanism and expose the underlying joint. In these cases it is important to close the joint before repairing the tendon. This closure restores the architecture of the joint and provides a soft tissue bed on which the tendon can glide. Continuity of the extensor mechanism is restored by weaving a suture of stainless steel or 4-0 nylon back and forth between the two cut edges of the tendon. Each end of the suture is passed through the skin beyond the site of repair and tied

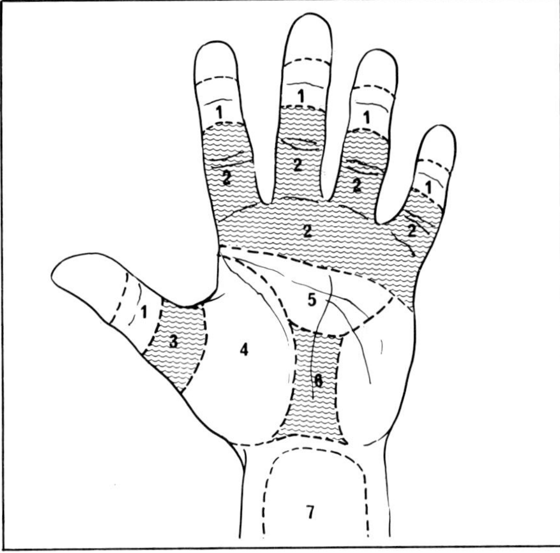

Fig. 35-7. Flexor tendon injuries can be classified topographically into seven zones. See text.

to itself. As an alternative, lead shot can be fixed onto the suture to maintain the proper tension necessary to hold the tendon ends together. The suture can be removed by cutting off one lead shot and pulling on the other end.

Extensor Tendon on Dorsum of Hand

Over the dorsum of the hand, the simple figure-of-eight suture, as suggested by Bunnell [4], provides a good means for either primary or secondary approximation of divided extensor tendons (Fig. 35-5). This suture, however, has no holding power, and splinting is necessary for some 4 weeks as an aid to immobilization and proper tendon healing (Fig. 35-6). This suture can also be used effectively for reapproximating divided extensor tendons in the forearm. If the point of suture is expected to pass beneath the dorsal carpal ligament once healing is complete and motion restored, it may be necessary to sacrifice part or all of this structure to prevent it from limiting tendon amplitude.

Extensor Tendon in Forearm

Tendons in the forearm can be injured either at their musculotendinous junction or within the substance of the muscle. Primary care should always include restoration of musculotendinous continuity when feasible. Its omission can result in a contracture of the substance of the muscle and a gap difficult to bridge at a later date because the end of the tendon slips distally. Even where there is not too much of a gap between the tendon end and its muscle, an interposition of scar tissue with healing will prevent tendon motion more distally. Before the musculotendinous repair is performed in these cases, all scar tissue should be completely removed. It is important to make a satisfactory soft tissue bed in which the repaired muscles or musculotendinous units can glide.

FLEXOR TENDON INJURIES

Verdan [38] classified flexor tendon injuries into seven surgical topographical zones to facilitate discussions of their treatment (Fig. 35-7).

Zone 1. The area between the proximal interphalangeal joint and the point where the profundus tendon inserts into the base of the distal phalanx.
Zone 2. The area between the distal palmar crease and the proximal interphalangeal joint.
Zone 3. The area of the fibroosseous sheath in the thumb.
Zone 4. The area at the base of the thumb where the thenar musculature surrounds the long flexor tendon.
Zone 5. The midportion of the palm.
Zone 6. The carpal tunnel area.
Zone 7. The area proximal to the carpal tunnel, including the forearm.

Zone 1

Zone 1 represents that part of the fibroosseous canal between the proximal interphalangeal joint and the insertion of the flexor profundus tendon occupied by this tendon alone. When the flexor profundus tendon is divided, there is naturally a loss of active flexion of the distal phalanx and a hyperextension instability of the distal interphalangeal joint [38]. This can result in a great deal of disability, particularly in the index and middle finger, because, with an unstable pinch, patients tend to drop things easily.

With these profundus tendon injuries in Zone 1, function of the proximal interphalangeal joint can be altered too. If the proximal end of the flexor profundus retracts backward, active flexion of the proximal interphalangeal joint can be markedly decreased. This often becomes worse as time goes on, because as the end of the tendon undergoes degenerative changes, contracting adhesions develop to the surrounding tissues. These changes are usually more marked in the ring and little fingers than they are in the index and middle fingers.

Profundus tendon injuries in this zone can be treated by either primary or secondary tendon repair. In the past these tendon junctures have frequently adhered to the underlying bed at the point of repair. Perhaps if careful suturing is done following the suggestions of Ketchum [14], this is less likely to happen.

Another method of treatment can be considered when profundus tendons are divided near their point of insertion. If the short broad vinculum over the distal joint is still intact, the distal tendon stump can be excised to a point just beyond the distal interphalangeal joint and the suturing done there. The proximal end of the cut tendon can often be found after a fresh injury by flexing the wrist and fingers; it is then advanced to the site of the distal tendon stump and sutured. In the thumb and index finger, as much as 2 cm. of tendon advancement is possible. Smaller advancements are advised for the other fingers if a flexion contracture is to be avoided. Before the cut proximal end of the tendon is advanced, the residual insertion, sheath, and surrounding tissue are excised. Greater advancement is possible if the more proximal vinculum of the profundus tendon is sectioned.

While these techniques have been recommended for a long time, one questions whether the blood supply to the flexor tendons is damaged significantly by dividing the vincula. It may be better simply to carry out the repair rather than divide a portion of the vincular system and possibly make a segment of the flexor profundus tendon avascular, since this can result in additional adhesions.

Zone 2 – No-Man's Land (Critical Zone)

Tendons are frequently injured within an anatomical area that in the past was labeled "the critical zone" or "no-man's land." This area lies between the distal palmar crease and the proximal interphalangeal joint. It is in the zone where the superficialis and profundus tendons are both enclosed by the fibroosseous sheath and lie in close proximity to one another. Since the repair of tendons lacerated in this region is often followed by their adherence to the adjacent fixed structures, most textbooks consider it best primarily to suture the skin only, and attempt to restore active flexion at a later date by tendon grafting [4, 21].

However, recent reports have renewed interest in the primary suture of tendons in this region [5, 16, 18, 38]. Verdan [38] and Kleinert and co-workers [16, 18], believe primary suturing can be accomplished successfully, which represents the best solution when undertaken by surgeons skilled in the techniques of hand surgery. However, if this primary tendon repair is performed badly, the additional scarring that follows can be so extensive that it compromises the whole future of the patient.

In a recent report, Lister and Kleinert [18] repaired both the profundus and superficialis tendons in selected cases to prevent retraction of the tendon ends and to preserve the local blood supply to the injured tendon segments. They used either a midlateral or Bruner zigzag incision to extend the original laceration. A flap of tendon sheath is elevated for the repair, with care taken to preserve the essential pulleys. Following the repair the tendon sheath is replaced; it must be carefully preserved [6]. Lister & Kleinert [18] believe that replacing the sheath may reduce adhesions. Furthermore, the site of the repair and the tendon juncture are less likely to catch on the edge of the sheath window with the start of finger mobilization.

The proximal end of the lacerated tendon has usually retracted proximally and can be retrieved by flexing all of the joints and "milking" the tendon back from the palm. Extending the incision proximally in order to find the tendon end is sometimes necessary.

Once retrieved, the two ends are abutted by flexing all joints. The proximal tendon is transfixed about 2 cm. from its cut end by passing a straight needle through the skin and tendon sheath of the finger from one side to the other, being careful to avoid the neurovascular structures. The cut edges of the tendon should be small and regular. If they are not, or if a part of the tendon is frayed, these fragments should be removed to square off the tendon.

Suturing is performed without tension; exacting approximation of the tendon ends is essential if fine sutures are to be used. The accordion-like effect that Bunnell shows in all of his drawings must be avoided when the tendon suture is tied, in order to minimize the intratendinous damage (Fig. 35-8). The Kessler modification of the Mason-Allen suture is preferred by some because it reduces longitudinal compression and at the same time increases longitudinal alignment [11, 12]. It is thought this should help to deter separation of the tendon ends (Fig. 35-9).

Either Ethiflex or Mersilene (4-0 or 5-0) is used, depending on the size of the tendon. It is best not to handle the outer surface of the tendon with instruments, because this is likely to cause additional adhesions. Instead, the cut end of the tendon should be grasped with a fine-tooth dissecting forceps. The suture can be passed through the tendon with greater ease and more control if the tendon is pressed against the adjacent soft tissues while inserting the suture.

After the Kessler suture has been tied, the margins of the tendon juncture are more accurately approximated with a running suture of 6-0 or 7-0 Dexon or monofilament nylon (Fig. 35-10). To prevent later adhesions, each part of the suture should help to enclose any exposed area of raw tendon, since this also could produce adhesions that later in healing might limit tendon movement within the tendon sheath.

When both the profundus and superficialis tendons have been divided, Lister and Kleinert [18] feel they both should be repaired. If both slips of the superficialis tendon have been divided, they should be

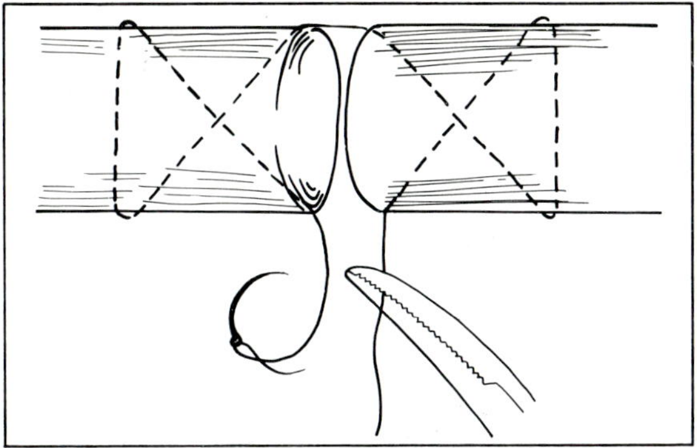

Fig. 35-8. The modified Bunnell suture. When tying suture, approximate ends without producing accordion effect or undue tension.

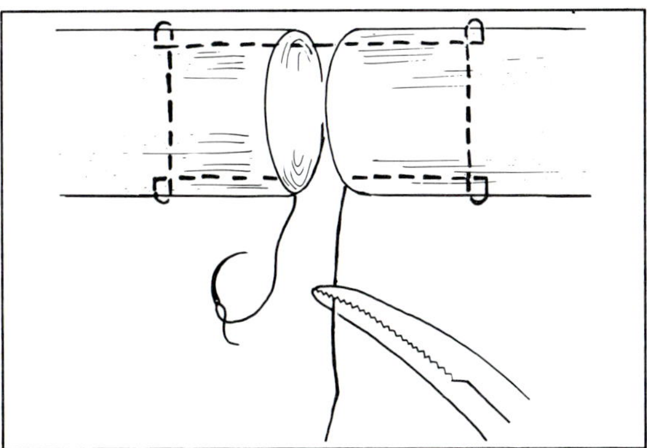

Fig. 35-9. The modified Kessler-Mason-Allen suture.

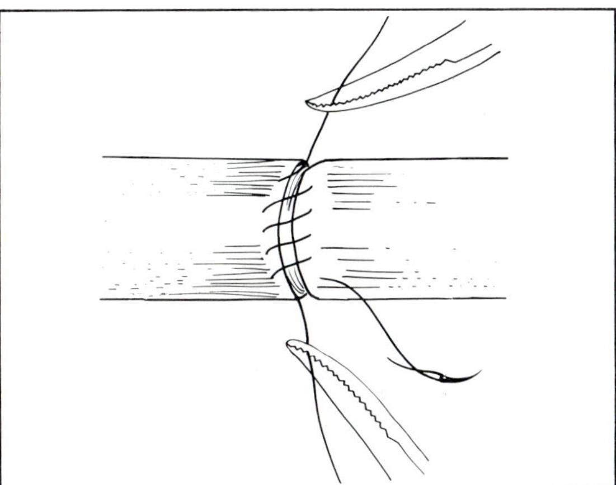

Fig. 35-10. The tenorrhaphy is completed by placing a running suture of fine material around the periphery of the tendon. Try to approximate the margins, eliminate raw surfaces, and invaginate any protruding tendon fibers.

repaired separately. Once suturing is completed some surgeons attempt to close the fibrous sheath loosely using a 6-0 nonabsorbable synthetic suture. Recent evidence suggests that preserving the sheath reduces the subsequent formation of adhesions.

At the end of surgery the extremity is elevated and gentle pressure placed over the area of repair while the tourniquet is released. A bipolar coagulator is used to help gain exacting hemostasis after the hyperemia has subsided. The wound is irrigated with Ringer's lactate solution to ensure that all blood clots have been removed. The wound is closed with 6-0 monofilament nylon. The straight needle that was placed in the tendon earlier can be removed at this point.

Dressings are applied and a dorsal plaster splint is applied that extends from the upper forearm to reach just beyond the tips of the fingers. The plaster holds the wrist in about 60 to 70 degrees of flexion, which represents a position about 20 degrees less than full flexion. The metacarpophalangeal joints are flexed 20 degrees and the interphalangeal joints about 10 degrees. The cast is molded to prevent finger extension. Since controlled mobilization of repaired tendons is begun immediately, rubber bands are attached to the nails of the fingers with transfixing sutures or by fastening a seamstress's hook and eye to the nail of the finger with acrocynalate glue.

Once the cast is hardened the rubber bands are attached to the nails and the other end is fastened to the dressing at the wrist level with a safety pin. This sort of attachment should hold the fingers at rest but with slight positive flexion toward the forearm. The rubber bands should be of a strength that will allow the patient to extend his fingers against resistance as far as the dorsal guard. The patient is encouraged to do this as often as possible during the 3 weeks until the splint is removed. After the splint has been removed, the rubber bands from the injured finger are attached to an Ace bandage at the wrist for an additional 2 weeks. Kleinert and colleagues [16] have shown that this method of controlled mobilization is effective in part because when one group of muscles contract against resistance it results in a synergistic relaxation of antagonist muscles. So, during sustained extension there is no activity in the flexor digitorum profundus or flexor digitorum superficialis tendons. As the fingers are relaxed and returned to full flexion, some power of contraction returns to the flexor units, but in this position little force can be generated because of the position of the tendon.

Kleinert and colleagues [18] describe six essential elements that are necessary for the technique of primary tendon suture in Zone 2 to be successful:

1. Avoiding tension at the suture line both during the repair and following it.
2. Careful handling of tissues.
3. Selection of proper suture materials. Nonreactive suture material should be used, because any swelling of the tendon increases its volume and, for success, swelling must be minimal.
4. Meticulous hemostasis. Hematomas cause pain and edema and prevent free movement in the tendon during the period of dynamic splinting.
5. Immediate controlled mobilization. To do this use a light dressing and select rubber bands to fill the needed requirements: long enough to hold the fingers down to the wrist and long enough to permit full extension to the plaster guard without stressing the hand. Emphasis is placed on being sure that the patient repeatedly exercises his fingers in the dynamic splint and that this exercise carries the fingers out to almost full extension at the interphalangeal joint. If this is not done, a severe flexion contracture can result that might compromise all subsequent attempts at salvage by secondary tendon grafting.
6. The final emphasis is placed on the element of practice. When the results using this technique were analyzed and compared with the results obtained by other techniques, Lister and Kleinert [18] found that the results were comparable with others used in Zone 2.

Flexor Tendon Grafts

In less than ideal circumstances, it is better to accept primary wound repair alone and then perform a secondary tendon graft. Factors important to the success of tendon grafting are complete wound healing, an absence of edema and induration, satisfactory skeletal alignment, and a full range of passive motion in the joints (Fig. 35-11). The ease with which this passive joint motion can be accomplished should be comparable to that in a normal finger.

Fig. 35-11. Web strap and buckle worn nearly all the time during the preparation for tendon grafting. It is necessary to have the joints of the injured finger as supple as those in adjacent normal fingers.

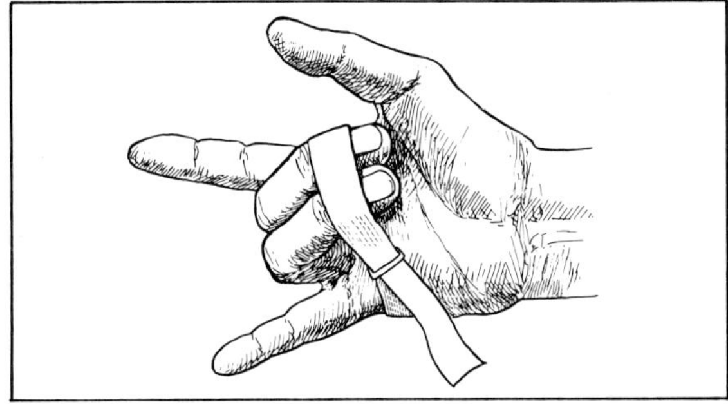

Technique of Flexor Tendon Grafting
A midlateral or midaxial incision or the zigzag volar-digital incision described by Bruner provides good exposure for the surgical procedure of tendon grafting [1, 2, 19, 20, 21, 32, 33, 38, 40]. The exact site for this midlateral incision can be determined by flexing the finger and identifying the point at each joint where the flexion crease ends (Fig. 35-12). If the points are connected, they will lie on a line that passes through the axis of rotation of each joint (mid-axial line) and therefore remains the same whether the finger is flexed or extended. After the skin has been incised along this line, it is best to continue to gain exposure in the central portion of any one finger segment, for here the fat is more plentiful than it is over the joints, which thus allows a greater margin of safety. As deeper dissection is begun, the first structure encountered will be Cleland's ligament [21]. This contains fibers that run almost in a volar-dorsal direction and connect the thinner fascial layers surrounding the digital nerve and artery with the skin.

The digital nerve and artery lie approximately 2 mm. volar to the margin of the incision, so it is best to preserve the thickness of fat on the volar flap (Fig. 35-13). Cleland's ligament may be isolated from the adjacent fat at the level of the proximal interphalangeal joint to a degree sufficient that it can be identified later and resutured. Such resuturing appears to prevent hyperextension deformities at the proximal interphalangeal joint following tendon grafting.

Once Cleland's ligament has been divided, deeper dissection will expose the side of the phalanx, with the margin of the flexor sheath extending forward along the volar surface much like the vista dome on the roof of a sightseeing bus. The tendon sheath can best be identified in an area away from the site of previous injury where the scar tissue will be minimal, and it can be readily separated away from the fat. As the dissection is continued near the tip of the finger, it is important that the skin incision lie adjacent to the side of the fingernail and that most of the fat be left on the flap, because beyond the distal interphalangeal joint the digital nerve divides and some branches lie on the side of the finger very close to the nail. It is easy to cut them at this location, if the surgeon is not careful. Once the "vista dome" of the flexor tendon sheath has been identified in the midphalangeal portion of each segment, the dissected segments can be connected over the areas of the joints. It is best to preserve at least two small pulleys in the finger, and these must be selected before the sheath is excised. The natural location of the pulleys can be noted by determining the points where the flexor tendon sheath is thickest. They are usually located in the proximal third of the middle phalanx and in the midportion of the proximal phalanx (Fig. 35-14). Such pulleys can be left about 3-mm. wide in order to prevent later "spanning" of the tendon graft. If a tendon injury has damaged the sheath at these levels, it is worthwhile to relocate them either more proximal or more distal, depending on the location of the scar, so that a suitable pulley will remain. All other remnants of the flexor tendon sheath can be excised along with the profundus and all scar tissue.

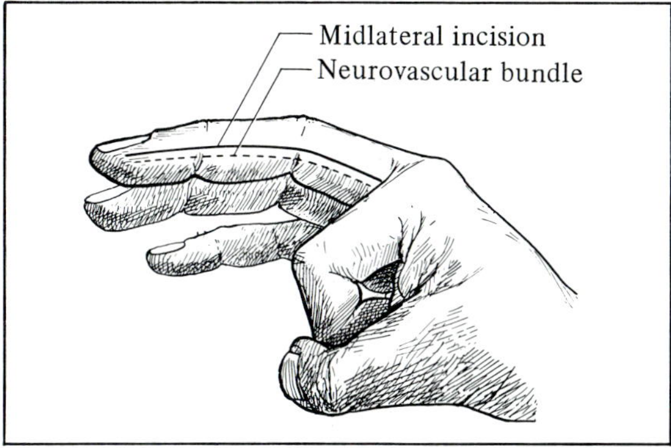

Fig. 35-12. The midlateral line or midaxial line passes through the axis of rotation of each joint.

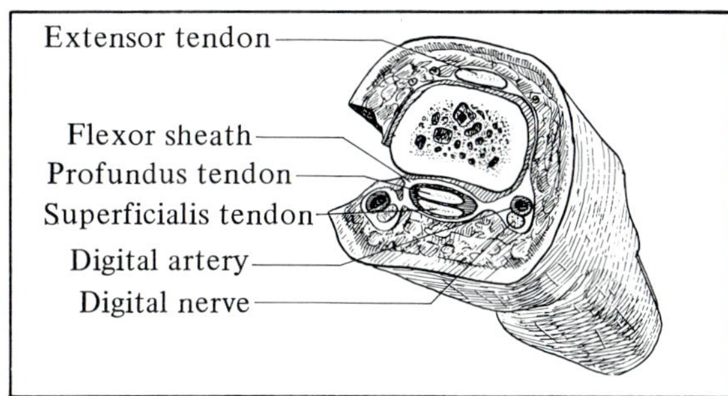

Fig. 35-13. Cross-sectional view of approach to the flexor tendon sheath. Note that the digital nerve and artery in the volar flap are preserved by this method.

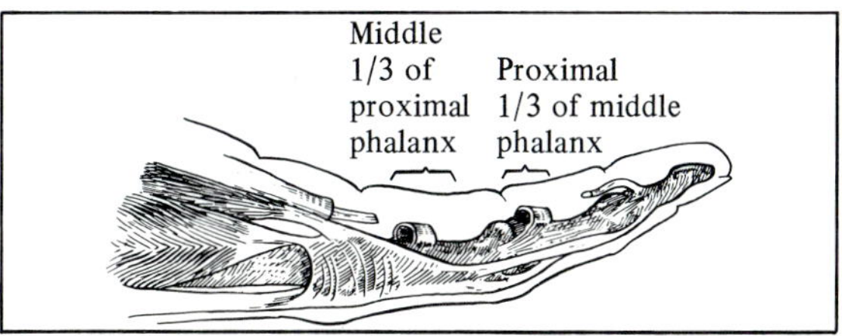

Fig. 35-14. Pulleys for tendon graft. When it is possible to place pulleys in the proximal one-third of the middle phalanx and the middle portion of the proximal phalanx, there will be little or no "spanning" of the tendon graft.

This will create a better bed through which a tendon graft can glide. In the joint areas the vincula of the superficialis and profundus tendons are preserved because it lessens tissue reactions during the time of tendon healing.

Distally, preparation must be made either for fixing the tendon graft to the remnant of the profundus tendon or for inserting it beneath a bone flap in the distal phalanx. Bone flaps [3, 4] are developed at the usual site of the profundus tendon insertion with a chisel (Fig. 35-15). The chisel perforates the volar surface of the cortical bone, and a little trapdoor of bone is elevated. A small drill bit is used to establish a tunnel between the overlying nail and the site where the bone flap has been elevated. A loop of 34 gauge wire is threaded through this tunnel and used as an aid for later placement of the tendon graft beneath the bone flap.

In the palm, a separate incision is used to identify and elevate a window of the palmar fascia so that the more proximal segments of the divided tendons can be freed. In identifying the superficialis and profundus tendons, it should be remembered that the superficialis is more volar and the attachment of lumbrical muscle to the profundus tendon helps identify it and usually prevents its proximal end from slipping back beyond this point.

When both tendons have been divided in a finger injury, the thin filmy covering (paratenon) overlying the tendons proximal to the metacarpophalangeal joint usually thickens during the several weeks elapsing between injury and repair. This thickened paratenon should be incised and a large amount removed so that the superficialis tendon can be identified and separated from the profundus tendon. Straight clamps are placed on each proximal tendon end, and the superficialis is identified so that if the wrist incision is performed later to obtain the palmaris tendon for a graft, the superficialis can be removed back to this level. The profundus tendon is best sutured to the tendon graft either at the level of the lumbrical muscle or just distal to it. Parkes [25a] as well as Littler [21] has emphasized the disastrous role the lumbrical may play; if it becomes shortened, it can exert a force on the finger in the wrong direction through the extensor tendon mechanism (Fig. 35-16). For this reason it may be better to section or resect the lumbrical if it appears damaged. Finally, before taking the graft, it is worthwhile to thread a suture through the pulleys and into the palm in preparation for sliding the tendon graft through the finger and into place. If the proximal end of this suture is attached to the cut end of the proximal portion of the superficialis tendon, it will later benefit the transfer of the tendon graft into the finger.

Fig. 35-15. Technique for elevating a bone flap in preparation for distal fixation of the tendon graft. Some surgeons prefer to suture the graft to the remnant of the profundus tendon.

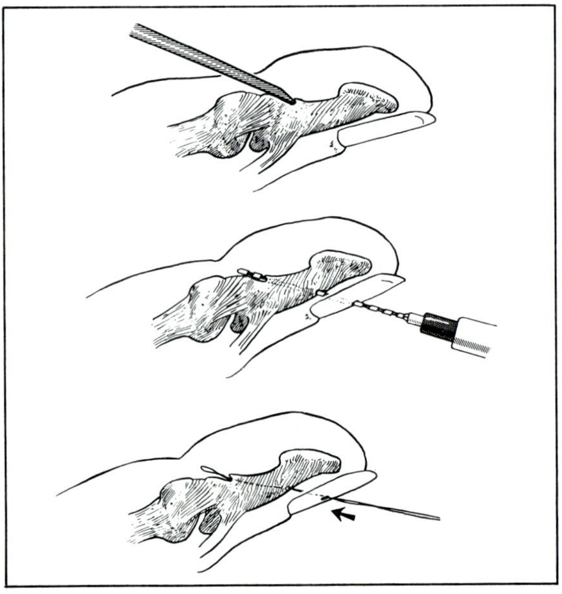

The palmaris longus tendon is available for use as a graft in 85 percent of cases [40]. Its presence should be determined before operation, if possible, so that the leg can be prepared if it is absent. The palmaris longus tendon can be removed through several small parallel incisions in the forearm. The procedure is as follows: The distal end of the palmaris longus tendon is identified at the wrist through a transverse incision. Tension is placed on its course to identify the point of its muscle juncture. A second transverse incision is made at this level and the skin and subcutaneous tissue are separated until the tendon can be identified in the filmy tissue beneath. The distal end of the tendon should be isolated at the point of its attachment to the palmar fascia at the wrist level and a double right-angle suture or some similar suture inserted through it for the purpose of handling and later transfer. In the proximal end of the tendon, another double right-angle suture is placed. Then the tendon is carefully separated from its paratenon and mesotendon so that it is free and no attachments remain. To accomplish this it may be necessary to make a third small transverse incision. If any residual fibers of paratenon are intact, they will prevent mobilizing of the tendon. With sutures in each end, the tendon graft is free so that it can be transferred to the finger.

The proximal end of the superficialis tendon is placed under tension to aid in its identification at the

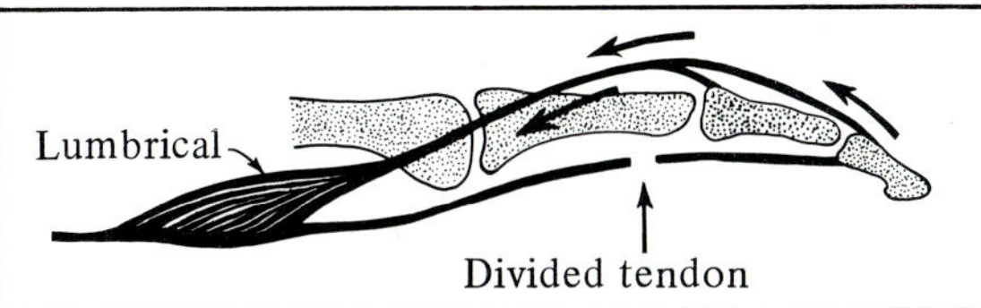

Fig. 33-16. The flexor profundus muscle can become a finger extensor if its tendon is divided or becomes lengthened distal to the lumbrical muscle origin.

wrist level. Through the wrist incision, a clamp is placed beneath the superficialis tendon and the tendon is withdrawn back at this level. As it is pulled out at the wrist level, the suture previously placed beneath the pulleys comes out with it. Some surgeons feel it is advantageous to slide the tendon graft from the forearm to the finger through the existing incisions, without actually removing it from the body. This decreases the possibility of injury to the surface of the tendon and keeps it from drying out. If this seems worthwhile, tie the distal end of the double right-angle suture to the proximal end of this suture. As it is pulled distally, the tendon graft will slide from the wrist incision through the superficialis tunnel and into the digit until its proximal end is in juxtaposition to the distal end of the profundus tendon and ready for an end-to-end suture of the modified Bunnell type (Figs. 35-8 and 35-17). Some surgeons prefer the Kessler suture because they feel it damages the tendon less (Fig. 35-9).

With a #11 knife blade, a small stab wound is made in the tip of the finger just beneath the nail (Fig. 35-18). A mosquito clamp or tendon passer is used to establish a channel from this point to the site of profundus insertion, and the distal end of the tendon graft is pulled back through to the tip of the finger to determine the point at which it will be under the desired degree of tension. A small, curved, empty needle can be placed through the tendon to keep it from retracting back into the finger, and the needle is repositioned until the proper tension in the graft appears to correspond to that of tendons in the adjacent fingers. Through the midlateral incision the point is noted at which the tendon graft under proper tension approximates to the profundus remnant or the bone flap window. The point is marked on the tendon graft and the distal suture is placed. If the tendon end is threaded into the bone flap with a modified Bunnell suture, it is held in its position beneath the volar bone flap by tying the ends of the tendon suture over a button on top of the fingernail. A pullout wire on the proximal end of this suture will permit its later removal; the pullout wire can be drawn through the volar flap, preferably in the fatty tissue in the midportion of the phalanx.

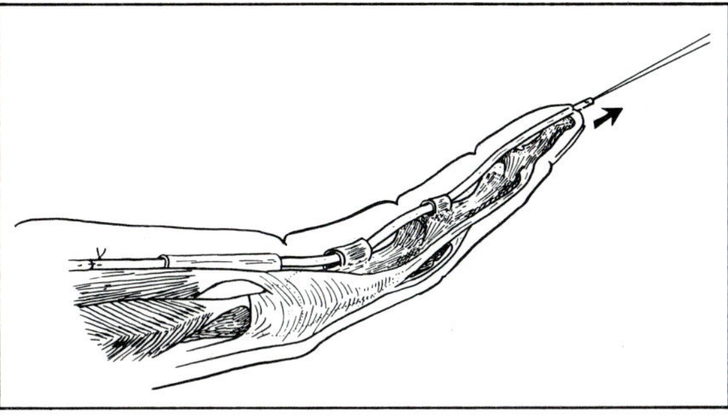

Fig. 35-17. End-to-end suture of the tendon graft to the motor unit at the base of the palm after tendon graft has been placed in tendon bed.

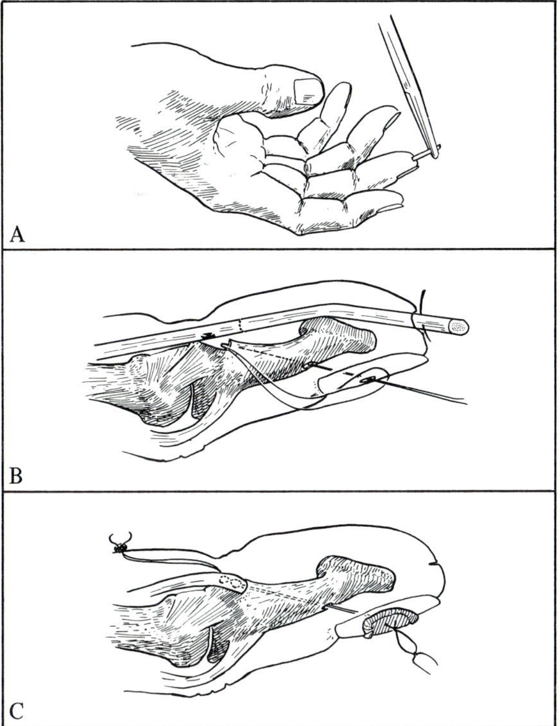

Fig. 35-18. Insertion of tendon graft. A, the tendon graft pulled through a stab wound in fingertip to determine the point where it will be under the desired degree of tension. B, a small curved needle placed through tendon to keep it from retracting back into the finger as tension is evaluated. Once proper tension is achieved and the length of the graft is known, the point where the graft lies adjacent to the bone flap can be marked on the tendon. C, the distal end of the tendon is fixed beneath the bone flap and tied over a button on the end of the finger.

When the palmaris tendon is absent, the superficialis, the plantaris tendon, or an extensor digitorum longus tendon will prove a satisfactory substitute. If the latter is selected, it must be removed from the second, third, or fourth toes and not from the great toe or little toe. Removal of the long extensor from the great toe jeopardizes too important a function. In the little toe, of course, there is no short extensor to substitute for the function of the long extensor if it is removed.

Where the time between injury and tendon grafting is long, the tendon graft should be a little shorter so that the finger will be under slightly greater flexor tension than an adjacent normal finger as a general rule. Some surgeons have suggested that the tendon be interwoven in the palm in order to decrease the chances of its becoming fixed at the point of juncture. This could be detrimental if the bulkiness of a tendon juncture prevents it from sliding beneath the carpal tunnel and thus limits the degree of flexion. In many cases it may be preferable to perform an end-to-end suture of the tendons (Fig. 35-17).

It is important to release the tourniquet before closing the wounds in order to establish good hemostasis. If the tendon graft were not vascularized because of a hematoma, a portion might undergo necrosis and become adherent to the scar. The hand is usually elevated for 10 minutes after release of the tourniquet to allow the hyperemia to subside before trying to establish hemostasis.

After hemostasis has been achieved, the arm is again elevated for a minute's time to allow venous blood to drain from the arm. Then the tourniquet is reinflated to avoid the accumulation of additional blood in the wound while it is being sutured. The small forearm incisions can be closed by a running suture, but perhaps it is better to put interrupted sutures in the fingers and palm to permit any serum or blood that might accumulate to leak out through the suture line during the early postoperative period.

The wrist is immobilized with a plaster splint in a position of 10 to 15 degrees less than maximum flexion, the fingers being allowed to fall into some degree of extension to compensate for the wrist flexion (Fig. 35-19). This type of immobilization is maintained for 3 weeks after operation. Active but guarded motion can be started during the fourth postoperative week, and the splint reapplied between exercise periods. No passive motion should be carried out before the end of the fourth week.

During the period of mobilization it is important to concentrate initially on gaining full flexion rather than be concerned about extension. The patient should be encouraged to flex the proximal and distal interphalangeal joints, and the metacarpophalangeal joints can be positioned in extension with a small exercise block placed in the palm. In this way the tendon graft must produce the finger movement, rather than having the metacarpophalangeal joint flex through the action of the lumbricals and interossei without necessitating movement of the tendon graft. The patient should be warned that it may require 2 or 3 months to achieve full flexion. At the same time all attempts to extend the fingers by strong passive force should be discouraged, because the result may be an overstretching of the tendon juncture; if it becomes too long, full flexion will never be possible.

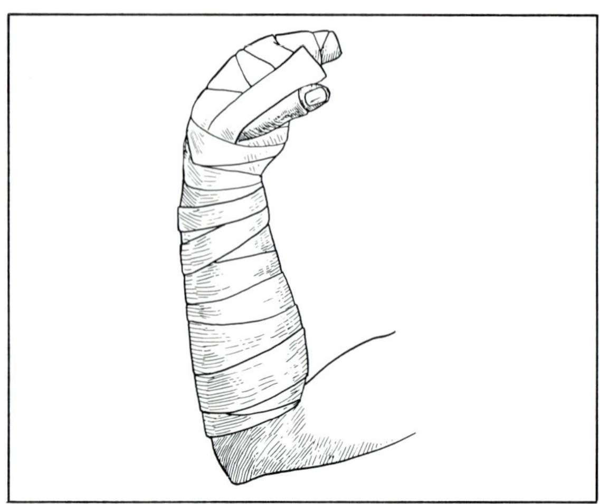

Fig. 35-19. A plaster splint is used to immobilize the hand with the wrist in some degree of flexion for 3 weeks. In the fourth week, guarded active motion is suggested before the cast is discarded. It is important not to place a bolus dressing in the palm at the time of wound closure, since this would not permit the tendon graft to move with the finger in case any unexpected muscle contraction occurs during the healing period.

Zones 3 and 4 – The Thumb

Tendon wounds in Zone 1 of the thumb usually occur at the interphalangeal crease. So long as the wound is clean, the flexor profundus tendon can be repaired either primarily or secondarily. It should be immobilized for three weeks' time postoperatively and a fourth week should be spent limbering up the finger carefully to prevent too much strain being placed on the tendon's suture line. Recovery should be excellent.

Wounds in Zone 3 lie in the region where the flexor tendon pulley is attached to the proximal phalanx and at the level of the sesamoid bones. Tendon injuries at the proximal phalanx level may be repaired either primarily or secondarily. At the time of tendon surgery the flexor tendon sheath must be resected widely so that the extent of the resection lies about 1 cm. beyond the excursion of the thickened area of sutured tendon.

Those Zone 3 tendon injuries more proximal – at the level of the sesamoids and metacarpal pulley – should be evaluated carefully when considering primary repair. Secondary repair would be preferable unless circumstances are ideal for primary repair. Remember, the metacarpal pulley is widely excised in either case.

Injuries to the flexor pollicus longus in Zone 4 are likely to occur in conjunction with injuries to the thenar muscles and recurrent branch of the median nerve because all these structures lie so close together. These possibilities should be considered in examining injuries to this area. Flexor pollicus longus repairs can be performed in this area either primarily or secondarily.

Zone 5 – Flexor Tendons in the Palm

Tendons are damaged less frequently with injuries in the palm, because of the protection of the palmar fascia and the fact that the tendons lie farther away from the surface. When only the superficialis tendon is divided in the midpalmar area, its repair is unnecessary. When both tendons are divided in ideal circumstances, and when the juncture does not appear to glide beneath the carpal ligament with full flexion, both of the tendons can be repaired with a fairly good chance that some independence of action can be achieved. In less tidy circumstances, perhaps only the profundus should be repaired and the adjacent parts of the superficialis resected. Because the mesentery-like arrangement that carries their segmental blood supply to them lies between the two tendons, it is well not to do any more freeing than necessary in preparation for their repair. It is much better merely to place sutures through the tendon ends and bring them into proper approximation.

Zones 6 and 7 – Flexor Tendons in the Wrist

Restoration of good hand function may prove difficult after tendon lacerations at the wrist because usually more than one tendon is divided; the proximity of their junctures after repair results in cross-adherence between them. In cases in which the sutured tendons will pass beneath the transverse carpal ligament with finger movement, a reapproximation of the profundus tendons alone may be advantageous. Since tendon junctures nearly always have a greater circumference than a normal tendon, this may produce an increased volume in the limited space of the carpal ligament, making the space through which these junctures must pass less confining. Tendon suturing further proximal in the forearm will not be accompanied by this mechanical problem, and under proper circumstances all tendons can be repaired primarily.

Injuries more proximal in the forearm can divide the muscles. They should be repaired primarily if at all possible, before muscle contractures create a gap and make later approximation more difficult. The fascia covering each muscle should be carefully sutured after hemostasis has been achieved. Draining the would helps to decrease skin tension. It is amazing what good results can be gained in these cases.

A division of the median and ulnar nerves frequently accompanies tendon lacerations in the forearm and wrist. Regardless of the technique chosen, some means of nerve approximation should be employed to prevent the retraction of their ends. Failure in this regard makes any secondary suture a great deal more difficult.

Postoperative splinting of the wrist in the position of flexion should be continued for 4 weeks after tendon repairs in the wrist and forearm level.

It is important to reemphasize that there is little evidence that the repair of a tendon at the time of injury results in any better function than a properly performed secondary repair or reconstruction. In dealing with acute injuries in which there has been tendon damage, the primary task is treatment of the wound itself. Immediate tendon repair should be considered only when it does not endanger the future function of the hand.

SILASTIC RODS

Nonreactive Silastic rods, popularized by Hunter and Salisbury [8], can sometimes serve as a valuable aid in tendon surgery. The term *space maintainer* seems to best describe their potential function. Sometimes when both tendons have been divided in no-man's land, tendon grafting can be performed as a delayed procedure, 7 to 10 days later. Before the overlying skin is closed, a small segment of Silastic rod is inserted into the tendon sheath so that it will span across the site of the injury to prevent the collapse of this structure. Then at the time of the grafting it is removed.

These rods are also helpful in severely scarred fingers with stiff joints and no flexor tendon function. After all possible scarring is removed from the finger, a Silastic rod is inserted beneath old pulleys and anchored distally to the stump of the profundus tendon at the terminal phalanx. Proximally it can extend into the palm or to the wrist. After 3 or more months, when the tissue reaction has subsided and joint mobility has reached a maximum, the rod is replaced with a tendon graft.

REFERENCES

1. Boyes, J. H. Flexor tendon grafts in the fingers

and thumb: An evaluation of end results. *J. Bone Joint Surg.* [Am.] 32:489, 1950.

2. Boyes, J. H. Evaluation of results of digital flexor tendon grafts. *Am. J. Surg.* 89:1116, 1955.
3. Boyes, J. H., and Stark, H. H. Flexor-tendon grafts in the fingers and thumb. *J. Bone Joint Surg.* [Am.] 53:1332, 1971.
4. Bunnell, S. Tendon Injuries. In Boyes, J. H. (Ed.), *Surgery of the Hand* (5th ed.). Philadelphia: Lippincott, 1970.

4a. Dolphin, J. A. Extensor tenotomy for boutonnière deformity of the finger. Presented at the American Society for Surgery of the Hand, 18th annual meeting, Jan. 18, 1963.

5. Duran, R. J. Controlled Passive Motion Following Flexor Tendon Repair in Zones Two and Three. In *AAOS Symposium on Tendon Surgery in the Hand.* St. Louis: Mosby, 1975.
6. Eiken, O., Lundborg, G., and Rank, F. The role of the digital synovial sheath in tendon grafting. *Scand. J. Plast. Reconstr. Surg.* 9:182, 1975.
7. Furlow, L. T. The role of tendon tissues in tendon healing. *Plast. Reconstr. Surg.* 57:39, 1976.
8. Hunter, J. M., and Salisbury, R. E. Flexor-tendon reconstruction in severely damaged hands. *J. Bone Joint Surg.* [Am.] 53:829, 1971.
9. Hurst, L. N., McCain, W. G., and Lindsay, W. K. Results of tenolysis. *Plast. Reconstr. Surg.* 52:171, 1973.
10. Kaplan, E. B. *Functional and Surgical Anatomy of the Hand.* Philadelphia: Lippincott, 1953.
11. Kessler, I. The grasping technique for tendon repair. *Hand* 5:253, 1973.
12. Kessler, I., and Nissim, F. Primary repair without immobilization of flexor tendon division within the flexor tendon sheath. An experimental and clinical study. *Acta Orthop. Scand.* 40:587, 1969.
13. Ketchum, L. D. Effects of triamcinolone on tendon healing and function. *Plast. Reconstr. Surg.* 47:471, 1971.
14. Ketchum, L. D. Primary tendon healing: A review. *J. Hand Surg.* 2:428, 1977.
15. Ketchum, L. D., Martin, N., and Kappel, D. Factors affecting tendon gap and tendon strength at the site of tendon repair. *Plast. Reconstr. Surg.* 59:708, 1977.
16. Kleinert, H. E., Kutz, J. E., Atasoy, E., and Stormo, A. Primary repair of flexor tendons. *Orthop. Clin. North Am.* 4:865, 1973.
17. Leffert, R. D., Weiss, C., and Athanasoulis, C. A. The vincula. *J. Bone Joint Surg.* [Am.] 56:1191, 1974.
18. Lister, G. D., Kleinert, H. E., Kutz, J. E., and Atasoy, E. Primary flexor tendon repair followed by immediate controlled mobilization. *J. Hand Surg.* 2:441, 1977.
19. Littler, J. W. Free tendon grafts in secondary tendon repair. *Am. J. Surg.* 74:315, 1947.
20. Littler, J. W. The severed flexor tendon. *Surg. Clin. North Am.* 39:435, 1959.
21. Littler, J. W. Principles of Reconstructive Surgery of the Hand. In Converse, J. M. (Ed.), *Reconstructive Plastic Surgery* (2nd ed.). Philadelphia: Saunders, 1977.
22. Lundborg, G., Myrhage, R., and Rydevik, B. The vascularization of human flexor tendons within the digital synovial sheath region – structural and functional aspects. *J. Hand Surg.* 2:417, 1977.
23. Mason, M. L., and Allen, H. S. The rate of healing of tendons: An experimental study of tensile strength. *Ann. Surg.* 113:424, 1941.
24. Matthews, P., and Richards, H. The repair potential of digital flexor tendons. *J. Bone Joint Surg.* [Br.] 56:618, 1974.
25. Matthews, P., and Richards, H. Factors in the adherence of flexor tendon after repair. *J. Bone Joint Surg.* [Br.] 58:230, 1976.

25a. Parkes, A. The "lumbricalis plus" finger. *J. Bone Joint Surg.* 53:236, 1971.

26. Peacock, E. E., Jr. A study of circulation in normal tendons and healing grafts. *Ann. Surg.* 149:415, 1959.
27. Peacock, E. E., Jr. Biological principles in the healing of long tendons. *Surg. Clin. North Am.* 45:461, 1965.
28. Peacock, E. E., Jr., and Hartrampf, C. R. The repair of flexor tendons in the hand. *Surg. Gynecol. Obstet.* 113:411, 1961.
29. Potenza, A. D. Tendon healing within the flexor digital sheath in the dog. *J. Bone Joint Surg.* [Am.] 44:49, 1962.
30. Potenza, A. D. The healing of autogenous tendon grafts within the flexor digital sheath in dogs. *J. Bone Joint Surg.* [Am.] 46:1462, 1964.
31. Pratt, D. R. Internal splint for closed and open treatment of injuries of the extensor tendon. *J. Bone Joint Surg.* [Am.] 34:785, 1952.
32. Pulvertaft, R. G. Tendon grafts for flexor tendon injuries in the fingers and thumb. *J. Bone Joint Surg.* [Br.] 38:175, 1956.
33. Pulvertaft, R. G. Suture materials and tendon junctures. *Am. J. Surg.* 109:346, 1965.
34. Smith, J. W. Blood supply of tendons. *Am. J. Surg.* 109:272, 1965.
35. Stark, H. H., Boyes, J. H., and Wilson, J. N. Mallet finger. *J. Bone Joint Surg.* [Am.] 44:1061, 1962.
36. Stark, H. H., Zemel, N. P., Boyes, J. H., and

Ashworth, C. R. Flexor tendon graft through intact superficialis tendon. *J. Hand Surg.* 2:456, 1977.

37. Verdan, C. E. Half a century of flexor-tendon surgery. *J. Bone Joint Surg.* [Am.] 54:472, 1972.
38. Verdan, C. E. Primary and Secondary Repair of Flexor and Extensor Tendon Injuries. In Flynn, J. E. (Ed.), *Hand Surgery* (2nd ed.). Baltimore: Williams & Wilkins, 1975.
39. Weeks, P. M., and Wray, R. C. Rate and extent of functional recovery after flexor tendon grafting with and without silicone rod preparation. *J. Hand Surg.* 1:174, 1976.
40. White, W. L. The unique, accessible and useful plantaris tendon. *Plast. Reconstr. Surg.* 25:133, 1960.

Nerve Injuries in the Forearm and Hand

JAMES W. SMITH

The traditional method of repairing peripheral nerves has been through the use of the epineurial suture (Fig. 36-1) [6, 25, 26, 29, 31, 32, 37, 39, 40, 41, 54, 55]. More recently, there has been an increasing volume of evidence to support the belief that fascicular suturing improves the results of nerve repair [1, 12, 14, 15, 19]. The return of motor and sensory function is less than satisfactory following epineurial repair, probably because the fasciculi can easily be deflected, kinked, or misdirected (Fig. 36-2) [10, 27]. If this happens, many of them can grow blindly into the interfascicular tissue or be deflected away from their corresponding fascicle, while the exterior appearance of the nerve is excellent. In contrast, fascicular sutures support the contact between the approximated fascicles, so that regenerating axons have a far better chance to grow across the site of nerve repair and straight down into the corresponding distal fascicles (Fig. 36-3).

Since nerves bear such strong similarities to electrical wires and cables, it is important to understand their anatomy and how it is affected by injury (Fig. 36-4).

ANATOMY

Each peripheral nerve contains a great number of nerve fibers or axons, individually enclosed within an enormous sheath. These units are in turn bound together into bundles of fasciculi by a condensation of adjacent connective tissue, the perineurium. Surrounding a group of the bundles is a loose areolar connective tissue framework called the *epineurium.* The epineurium also has an area of condensed connective tissue around the periphery of nerve that allows it to serve as a definitive external sheath separating the nerve from surrounding tissues. The epineurium contains collagen and elastin fibers, most of which run longitudinally. The endoneurium, perineurium, and epineurium constitute the connective tissue component of a peripheral nerve, and each aids in isolating or insulating one part from another. Each also has specific architectural or structural characteristics that deserve consideration.

In his study of the comparative amounts of connective tissue in cross-sectional areas of nerves, Sunderland [51] found the smallest amount to be about 22 percent; the greatest, 88 percent. In general, then, anywhere from 30 to 75 percent of a peripheral nerve is made up of connective tissue, depending upon the nerve and specific level being examined. There appears to be more connective tissue when the neural components are small and numerous and less when the bundles are few or of a larger size. There is also more at those sites where peripheral nerves pass across joints.

The endoneurium that surrounds each axon–Schwann cell complex is mostly composed of collagenous tissue. This supporting connective tissue also forms the fine, intrafascicular septa that separate and subdivide nerve fibers inside a fasciculus into even smaller groups of components. These septa contain the interfascicular blood supply.

The perineurium invests each bundle or fasciculus with a relatively thin but dense and distinctive sheath of fibrous tissue. It contains elastin and collagen fibers that intermesh by passing circularly, obliquely, and longitudinally. The fibrils form from 7 to 15 concentric lamellae or tubes; the number depends on the size of the fasciculus or bundle. When one carefully examines the fasciculus in the end of a freshly cut nerve, one sees that it has the ability to move back and forth independently within the epineurium. The external layers of the epineurium also have an independence of motion in relation to the other structures. Thus the entire unit is an unstable composite of about the quality of well-cooked spaghetti. Each piece of spaghetti looks like a fasciculus and has just about as much slipperiness and ability to bend and kink. Injection studies show the microcirculation to each fasciculus runs in the adjacent epineural connective tissue.

The internal circulation of the nerve is piped to it through the mesoneurium in a relationship similar to that of the intestine. All the nutrient vessels enter the nerve along the line where the mesoneurium attaches to the nerve. No vessels enter the nerve around the remainder of its circumference. Blood is supplied in a segmental fashion, being both dispersed and collected through a series of arcades within the mesoneurium. The grouping of arcades seems to change from one area to another to meet needs and requirements imposed by local anatomical variations. In areas such as the shoulder, elbow, and wrist, where great degrees of mobility are required of the nerve, the mesoneurium is longer, is more complex, and contains more vessels. When there is little or no tension on these vessels, they contract in an accordion-like arrangement. As tension increases with movement, the vessels within

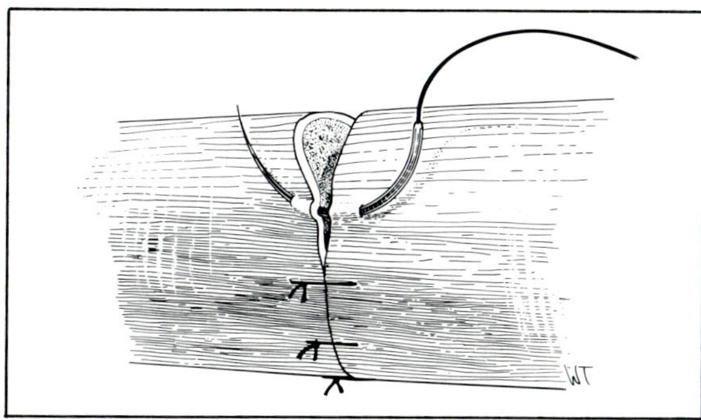

Fig. 36-1. *Epineurial suture. This suture is supposed to close all gaps in the epineurium so that no fascicles protrude or escape and form neuromas.*

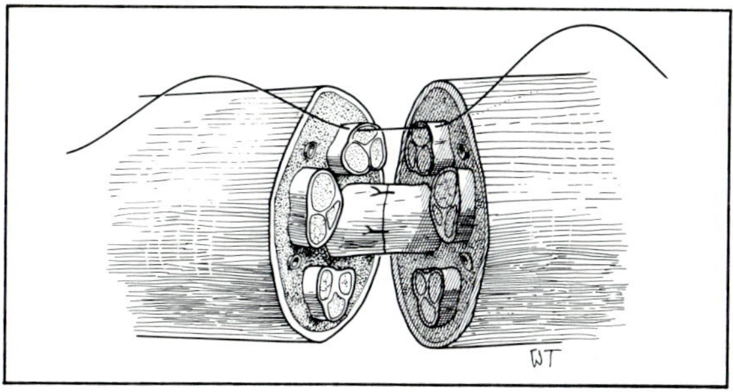

Fig. 36-3. *Corresponding fascicles are approximated by a perineurial suture in order to bring the nerve ends into proper alignment. No more than one or two sutures are required for each fasciculus or group of fasciculi.*

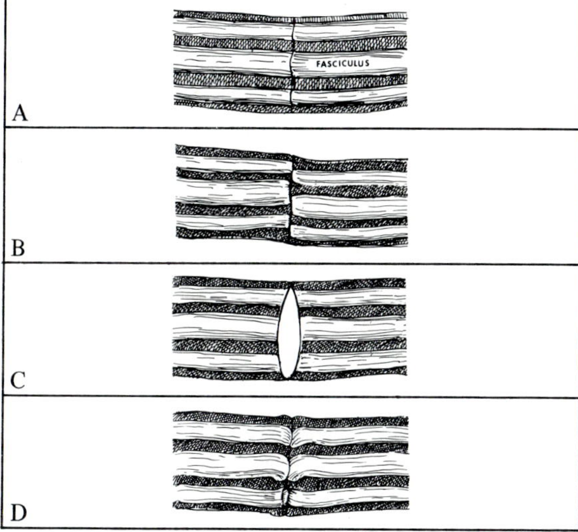

Fig. 36-2. *The findings of Edshage [10] demonstrated. A good epineurial closure does not mean that all of the internal architecture of the nerve has been restored. Consequently, even though the epineurium appears well approximated, the fascicles within may not be correctly aligned. A, properly aligned fascicles. B, misdirected alignment. C, if a dead space exists, this may result in excessive scar and poor axonal growth across the juncture. D, there may be kinking of the fascicles.*

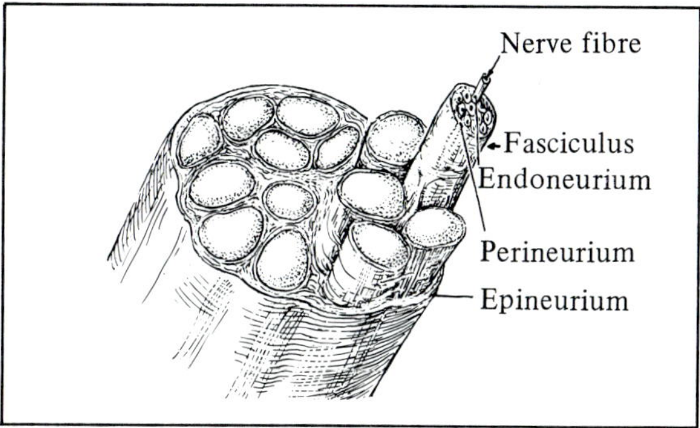

Fig. 36-4. *The nomenclature used in describing component parts of a peripheral nerve.*

the mesoneurium uncoil to accommodate for the changing position of the nerve. The nutrient vessels entering a given portion of nerve through the mesoneurium will, therefore, appear to vary in number depending on the position of the limb and the degree to which they are stretched. Peripheral nerves possess considerable strength and elasticity. Though it is not possible to isolate and separate the mechanical properties of each component part of a peripheral nerve, much of the tensile strength and elasticity of nerve trunks is supplied by the perineurium. It plays a major role in maintaining the integrity of the nerve trunk under tension.

NERVES OF THE HAND

The dorsal antebrachial cutaneous nerves and the medial and lateral antebrachial cutaneous nerves assist in supplying sensibility to the forearm, while the median, ulnar, and radial nerves furnish most of the motor and sensory control to the hand itself (Fig. 36-5). The motor nerves of the hand, except for those to the extrinsic muscles, are the ulnar and median. Since these nerves are not the sole manipulators of the hand, the *radial nerve* (Fig. 36-6), which assists in supplying the extensor muscles of the wrist and fingers, must also be considered. These muscles lie on the posterior or dorsal side of the forearm and are usually called the extensor group [11, 20, 24].

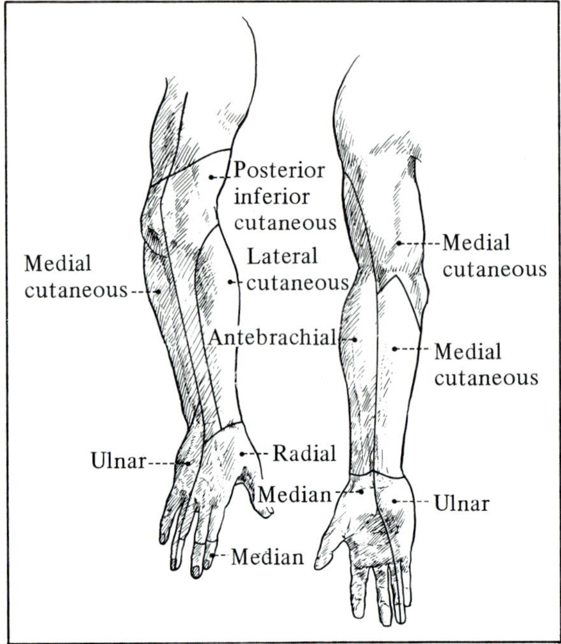

Fig. 36-5. General distribution of sensory nerves in the upper extremity. There is a great deal of variation in the area supplied by an individual peripheral nerve as well as in the extent of overlapping. (After Bing, as reproduced in Bunnell's Surgery of the Hand *[5th ed.]. Philadelphia: Lippincott, 1970).*

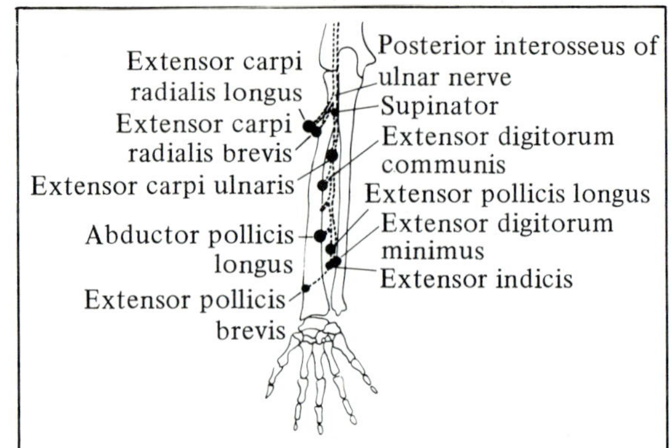

Fig. 36-6. Muscles supplied by dorsal interosseous branch of radial nerve. The radial nerve supplies the extensors of the wrist and fingers, through the dorsal interosseous branch. This chart can aid in determining whether any functional loss is more likely the result of a nerve or a muscle injury. If it is due to an injury of the dorsal interosseous nerve, function will be lost in the muscles listed here in a progressive fashion downward from the top of the diagram. (After D. P. Quiring, The Extremities *[3rd ed.]. Philadelphia: Lea & Febiger, 1967.)*

The muscles on the anterior or volar surface are referred to as the flexor group. If a line is drawn longitudinally across the center of the palm and onto the midportion of the ring finger, it in essence divides the hand into median and ulnar sensory components. Boyes [2] has termed this the "water-shed line". On the ulnar or medial side of the line, sensory innervation is provided by the ulnar nerve, and on the radial or lateral side, by the median nerve. Actually, both the median and ulnar nerves are mixed nerves, with the latter having a greater number of muscle funiculi than the median nerve, which has a larger sensory component.

The *ulnar nerve* (Fig. 36-7) innervates certain muscles that flex the wrist and fingers (flexor carpi ulnaris, and the ulnar half of the flexor digitorum profundus to the ring and little fingers. It also supplies all the intrinsic muscles of the hand except for the flexor pollicis brevis, abductor pollicis brevis, and opponens muscle in the thenar eminence and the lumbrical muscle to the index and middle fingers. Thus the usual test for ulnar nerve palsy is to alternately spread and approximate the fingers, whereas the test for median nerve palsy is to approximate

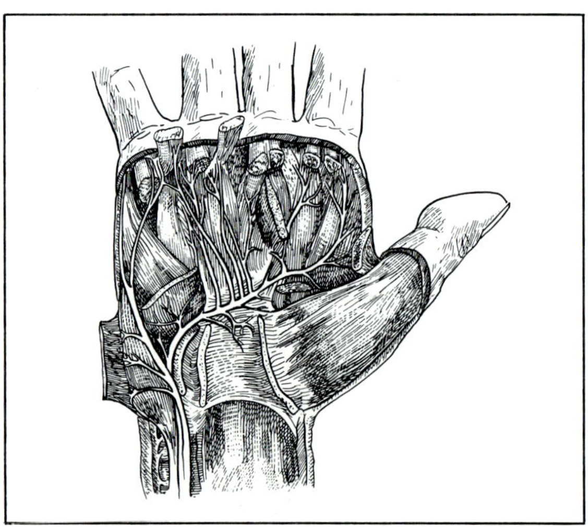

Fig. 36-7. The ulnar nerve supplies sensation to the little finger and half of the ring finger. It also has a motor branch that supplies all of the interosseous muscles and the lumbrical muscles to the ring and little fingers.

successively the tip of the thumb to the tips of the fingers in the form of an O. Since the interosseous muscles, which spread and approximate the fingers, are exclusively controlled by the ulnar nerve, this action of the interossei can serve as a test of ulnar nerve function. It is well known that if the ulnar nerve is damaged, the patient will have difficulty holding a piece of paper between adjacent fingers when they are fully extended. Another test of ulnar nerve function is to have the patient abduct the index finger away from the middle finger. If the first dorsal interosseous, the muscle used along with the thumb in pinching actions, contracts, it indicates that the last in a long string of muscles innervated by the ulnar nerve is functioning. Such a test is similar to troubleshooting complex electronic circuits that fail to function distal to the point of difficulty. By checking the first dorsal interosseous one is checking the last group of circuits to see if electricity or, in this case, nerve impulses are reaching this point.

The *median nerve* (Fig. 36-8) controls the remaining flexors: palmaris longus, flexor carpi radialis, flexor pollicis longus, all the muscles of the flexor superficialis group, the flexor digitorum profundus muscles for the index and middle fingers, and the pronator group. The one and a half muscles already mentioned (the flexor carpi ulnaris and ulnar half of the flexor digitorum profundus) are usually under ulnar nerve control. Thus, in the hand, the motor median nerve innervates the radial two lumbrical muscles and the thenar eminence. Among the muscles of the thenar eminence are the flexor pollicis brevis, the abductor pollicis brevis, and the opponens muscle. The last is highly overrated in importance for approximating the thumb tip successively to the fingertips. Actually, anomalous innervations of these flexor muscles, as well as the compensatory mechanisms that patients develop to minimize functional loss, often make it difficult to recognize the case in which only opponens function has been lost. It can be worthwhile, certainly in some cases, to test sensibility over the radial three and a half fingers, as a means of more easily identifying the median nerve injury. Since the median nerve distribution lies on the radial or lateral side of the "water-shed area," three and one-half fingers (the thumb, index, middle, and the radial half of the ring finger) will be supplied by the median nerve. It is often possible to determine whether the median nerve is intact by lightly passing an examining finger over the surface of one of the fingertips whose sensibility is in question and eliciting the patient's response as to whether the finger is numb or asleep when compared to the same finger on the opposite extremity. Of course, the use of pinprick and studies of temperature and touch will further aid in establishing the diagnosis in more difficult cases. The ninhydrin test is sometimes worthwhile because immediately after division, the sweat glands in the area supplied by the injured sensory nerve no longer function and dryness results. Sometimes the ninhydrin test will not be needed because the examiner can detect the comparative dryness of the anesthetic fingers in relation to adjacent ones that show sweating of a significant degree.

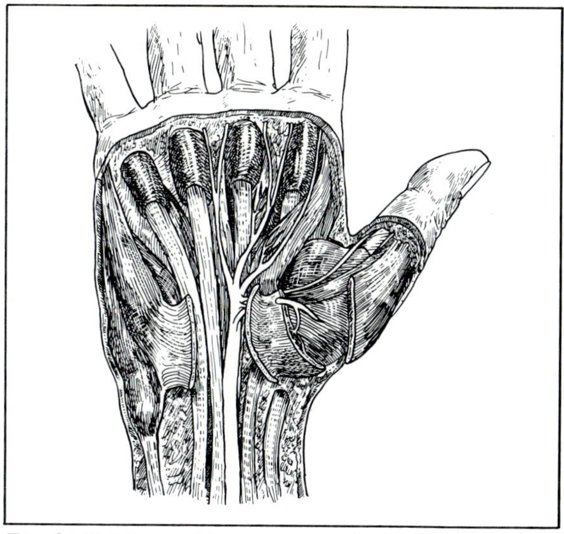

Fig. 36-8. The median nerve supplies sensation to the thumb, the index and middle fingers, and half of the ring finger. Its motor median branch goes to the thenar eminence.

Remember that the median nerve distribution to the dorsum goes only to the distal two phalanges of the thumb, index, middle, and half of the ring fingers [20]. In contrast, the dorsal branch of the ulnar nerve supplies sensibility to all of the dorsal surface on the ulnar half of the ring and little fingers. The dorsal radial sensory nerve provides feeling over the lateral two-thirds of the dorsum of the hand, a portion of the thenar eminence, and the proximal portions of the dorsum on the thumb, the index and middle fingers, and half of the ring finger. It is important to realize, however, that there is quite a variation in the sensory distribution of these three nerves. The sensory distribution on the volar surface of the palm is far more consistent.

Some people find it difficult to remember which fingers are innervated by the ulnar nerve and how many are innervated by the median nerve. One way is to remember the water-shed area, which has been previously mentioned. Another is to realize that the distribution of sensation by both the median and the ulnar nerve is through a cleft branching system.

As peripheral nerves approach the clefts between fingers, each divides so it can provide sensation for either side of the cleft. Thus, in all instances, the two sides of a finger cleft are innervated by the same nerve. However, the radial side of the index and the ulnar side of the little finger have no cleft nerve, and single nerve branches go to these areas. The thumb, of course, is innervated on each side by a separate branch coming out from the median nerve.

FACTORS AFFECTING NERVE REPAIR

Type of Injury

In peripheral nerve injuries, the type of damage greatly influences treatment, rate of regeneration, and quality of return [38, 45]. Generally speaking, the best prognosis for recovery is found in cases of contusion, compressions of short duration, and injuries associated with joint dislocations and fractures (Fig. 36-9). In these cases, when the framework of the nerve is preserved, recovery is rapid even though the damage may be severe enough to cause wallerian degeneration. Results are less satisfactory when the nerve has been subjected to stretching, ischemia, or division. Such stretch injuries as occur at birth or from severe traction may be accompanied by axonal ruptures and damage over an extensive area. Volkmann's ischemic contracture is an example of damage to the segmental blood supply of the nerve and replacement by scar tissue. Division of a nerve also carries with it a comparatively poor prognosis because the complex framework of a nerve, once destroyed, can never be restored.

Fig. 36-9. The percentage of impairment that might result from any nerve injury producing sensory loss in the hand. Many authorities consider 50 percent of hand function to be related to the ability to feel and the other 50 percent to movement. (Prepared by the Committee on Disability of The American Society for Surgery of the Hand.)

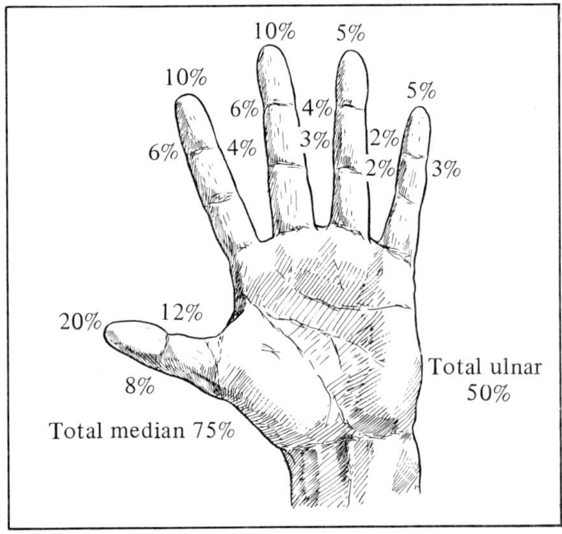

Accuracy of Repair

To understand the problems resulting from a nerve injury and the limitations that accompany repair requires an appreciation of neural complexity and a realization of the fact that nerves are not unlike vast cables. They contain bundles of funiculi, each well insulated from all the others. Each funiculus comprises about 10,000 fibers. The median nerve, for example, has from 20 to 30 funiculi; thus its division results in a disruption of continuity for somewhere between a quarter and a third of a million axons. In such a nerve, with a diameter the size of a pencil, there is no way of approximating single axons, no color code to distinguish one funiculus from another, and no technique that permits the proper repair and insulation of each individual bundle (Fig. 36-10). Thus far, from a surgical point of view, it has only been possible to approximate the ends of a nerve by

Fig. 36-10. This simplified drawing suggests how, at the periphery, fascicles are directed to specific areas and are usually primarily sensory or motor.

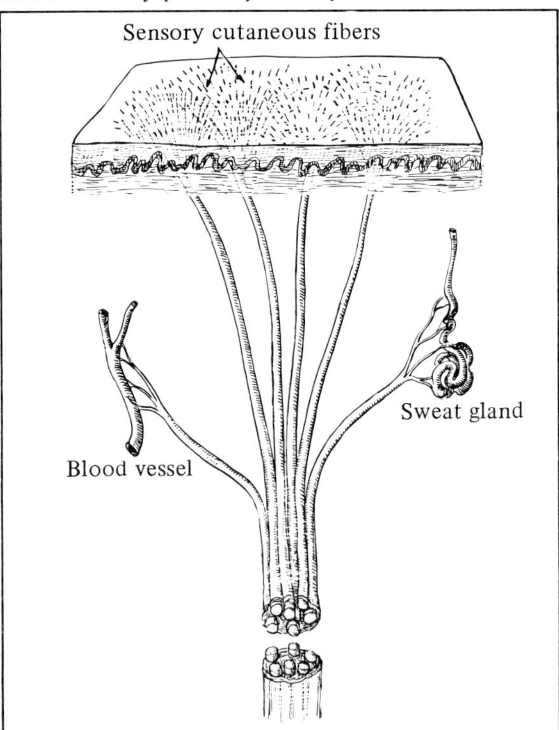

suturing its surrounding sheath and hope that healing will restore proper continuity of the wiring, prevent short circuits, and provide the necessary insulation between bundles. In mixed nerves containing both sensory and motor fibers, the problem is compounded. Loss of function may become exaggerated by any rotation of nerve ends. Such an error can result in sensory axons growing down motor pathways and vice versa. These misdirected axons are lost for function; there can be no mix and match in this type of problem.

Even when the epineural covering of a nerve has been closed accurately and proper care has been taken to prevent rotational errors, the funiculi within may still be poorly aligned. Any kinking or overriding of an enclosed funiculus can prevent the axons located proximally within it from finding their corresponding tubes in the distal interface of the repaired nerve; instead, they may grow into the interposed perineurium or become entrapped by scar tissue at the site of nerve juncture. Sometimes, even when there is an initially good approximation of funiculi, they can become distorted with bleeding or formation of a hematoma at the site of nerve juncture. It is therefore necessary to inspect every site of repair carefully after the tourniquet has been released for a period sufficiently long to allow circulation to return before closing the wound.

Age of the Patient

The prognosis is known to be much better in young children than in adults, but no one is quite certain why, aside from the greater powers of regeneration in children. Nerve repairs in children under 15 years of age are far more likely to be successful than those in older patients. Seddon [42] has said that after the age of 60 the stimulus responsible for initiating and maintaining the process of regeneration may be so poor that in some patients the repair is hardly worth doing.

Level of the Lesion

The more peripheral the injury, the greater the chance of success. After a divided motor nerve has been repaired, the rate of regeneration is so slow (1 mm. a day) that sometimes before regenerating axons can reach it the muscle has become atrophic. Another problem is that the slower the regeneration, the thicker the collagenous membrane lying between the returning nerve fibers and the end-plates becomes, and this may limit the degree of reinnervation and muscle activity that ultimately appears. Furthermore, Schwann tubes undergo a progressive atrophy, so that the longer the time before they are reinflated by myelin and axons, the less chance they will have of being restored to their original diameter.

Time Lapse Between Injury and Repair

The quality of sensation diminishes progressively as the time between injury and repair increases. However, it never falls to zero, and some degree of sensation, if only protective, can be achieved even years after the original injury. The same cannot be said of motor function, because of muscle atrophy. When the time between injury and repair of a motor nerve is long and the muscles innervated by it are not stimulated or functioning for 2 years, the degree of scarring in the muscle becomes so severe that muscle function is impossible.

State of Local Nutrition

The state of local nutrition is known to be important both to normal nerve function and to any regenerative activity [2]. It is probably related to either a localized or a generalized effect of ischemia on the segmental blood supply of a peripheral nerve.

Under normal circumstances the mesoneurium of a nerve (Fig. 36-11) appears to transport the entire volume of its circulating blood to and from the nerve [43, 44]. This arrangement allows the nerve to move in relation to its fixed bed and yet to maintain a continuous flow of blood. The ulnar nerve, for example, as the elbow flexes and extends, increases and decreases the length of the course over which the nerve passes. When this segmental distribution of a peripheral nerve's circulating blood and degree of collateral circulation are taken into account, nerves the size of the median or ulnar probably require complete isolation of a 10- to 16-cm. segment before they become avascular. This conclusion is based on postmorten injection studies, which show that isolating

Fig. 36-11. Cross section of the nerve, showing blood supply. The mesoneurium of the nerve, under normal circumstances, appears to transport the entire volume of circulating blood to and from a nerve. Such an arrangement allows the nerve to move in relationship to its fixed bed and yet maintain a continuous flow of blood. When a nerve is cut and its two ends spring apart, creating a gap, the separation is primarily due to a recoiling action of the mesoneurium and is not the result of the elasticity within the nerve tissue itself.

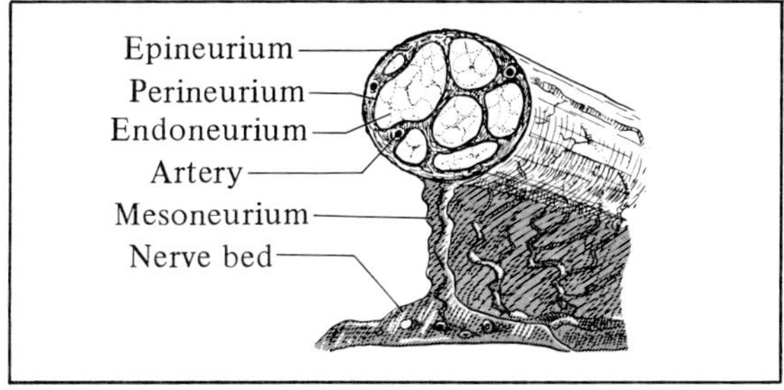

a divided nerve from its bed for 5 to 8 cm. results in insufficient collateral circulation to maintain blood flow to the cut end. If blood were entering an intact nerve from either end, as it might in the case of Volkmann's ischemic contracture of the forearm, the distance would be doubled, or in the range of 10 to 16 cm.

Amount of Scar

The amount of scar is probably related both to ischemia and to the fact that axoplasmal flow is impeded by compression [53]. When nerve gaps are studied by postmortem injection techniques, it appears that as a nerve is freed, and its length-to-width ratio increases, circulation becomes progressively compromised. This may be one reason why there is a poor prognosis in cases in which the nerve gap is large and approximation of the two ends can be gained only by extensive freeing.

Also detrimental to recovery would be the stretching that results following the mobilization of any joints placed in hyperflexion to facilitate the repair. This might either exert a pull at the suture line or result in a traction type of injury. When Highet and Sanders [17] studied the effects of stretching nerves after extensive mobilization to overcome a gap before suture, they found, when the area of surgery was later reexplored: extensive, abnormal degeneration in the central stump; separation of the stump when the suture line was not bound down by scar tissue; ruptured axonal tubes in the regions where the stretching was severest; and extensive edema and fibrosis both outside and inside nerve bundles.

Signs and Symptoms of Nerve Injury

Sensibility Changes

Sensibility is most highly developed over the median nerve distribution that supplies the skin of the thumb, the index and middle fingertips, and half of the ring finger [30]. For diagnostic purposes in the emergency room, it is often sufficient to quickly map out losses of sensibility by testing light touch and pinprick. While the tip of the examiner's finger may be used to lightly stroke the area in question, probably a cotton wisp is more sensitive and accurate. The fact that it touches a point on the hand or finger is verified by the patient with his eyes closed and head turned away. Similar tests with a sharp pinpoint sometimes are advantageous in distinguishing malingerers from those who really have a loss of sensibility.

Of course, once a nerve has been repaired and the extent of recovery is to be evaluated, such refined tests as the coin test, two-point discrimination, or a ninhydrin paper test are best for a true, accurate evaluation of the degree of recovery and remaining disability [29, 30, 35].

Changes in Motor Function

As soon as the nerve is divided, the muscles it innervates are completely paralyzed and will begin to undergo a progressive atrophy that can proceed so rapidly it may become marked within a month. Total fibrous degeneration requires 1 or 2 years; thereafter it is usually so marked that restoration of function is impossible, even though biopsy shows the presence of muscle tissue. To test function of a muscle requires identifying muscle contraction. Clinically, this evaluation can be undertaken by simply placing a fingertip on the muscle and noting whether it contracts or not. Motion of a part can also serve as evidence of muscle contraction when the musculotendinous unit in question is the only one capable of producing the movement as the patient attempts to contract it. Such testing obviously requires a knowledge of anatomy and the motions that can be performed by each muscle.

After a nerve has been divided, any muscle deinnervated will still react temporarily to stimulation with both faradic and galvanic current. The response to faradic stimulation disappears after 4 to 7 days, while galvanic stimulation will continue to produce a sluggish contraction followed by slow relaxation for a long time. Such galvanic stimulation has been shown by Seddon [40, 41] and others to slow the rate and lesson the degree of muscular atrophy and fibrous degeneration.

Electromyography is another way of determining whether a nerve has been completely severed. As early as 2 weeks after an injury, the reaction of degeneration becomes evident by this examination.

NERVE REPAIR

Type of Injury

The type of injury often is the major factor in determining the time of repair. With contusions, compression from external sources such as will occur when the extremity is held in an abnormal position, fractures, and dislocations, the chances of spontaneous recovery are extremely good, and immediate exploration is therefore not advised. In fact, such exploration may be detrimental to returning recovery. Seddon [39] reports, for instance, that when the radial nerve is injured in conjunction with a fracture of the humerus there is spontaneous recovery in 82 percent of cases. The best plan of treatment for injuries such as these is to plot out the amount of time that might be expected to elapse until a regenerating nerve would reinnervate the next lower muscle or sensation should return to a specific area. After the given period of time has elapsed, based on an anticipated rate of return of 1 mm. per day, determine whether or not regeneration can be noted and if recovery is proceeding satisfactorily. If it is not, then exploration is required.

Degree of Nerve Damage

Often with lesions in continuity or with incomplete divisions of the nerve, even direct examination of the area at surgery will not provide a simple, cut-and-dried solution to the problem of selection of the correct treatment [40]; judgment and experience may be the final important factors in making a decision [42]. Several suggestions on this type of problem may prove beneficial:

1. If a lesion in continuity is slightly enlarged and the nerve does not feel too firm, the prognosis is often good and no additional treatment may be required (Fig. 36-12A).
2. When the swelling is extensive and the nerve feels hard on palpation (Fig. 36-12B), a great degree of scar tissue is probably present within the nerve complex itself. In such an instance, it might be well to consider a transverse biopsy to determine the extent of the scar in relation to the amount of neural tissue present. If no real funiculi are encountered immediately, it is worthwhile to continue cutting deeper, even through the remainder of the nerve if necessary, in order to establish more positively the state of scarring and the chances of satisfactory recovery.
3. If the nerve is cut half to three-quarters of the way through and examination shows that there is little or no neural tissue present, probably resection of the neuroma (Fig. 36-12C) and a suture of the two ends is indicated. With partial division of nerves, there is often greater damage inside than would be suspected from direct examination, and nerves that have associated notching frequently require resection of the damaged segment and end-to-end approximation.
4. In all injuries of the dumbbell type (Fig. 36-12D), when neuroma and glioma are connected by a thin intervening thread or segment of tissue, resection of the damaged segment and end-to-end approximation are required.

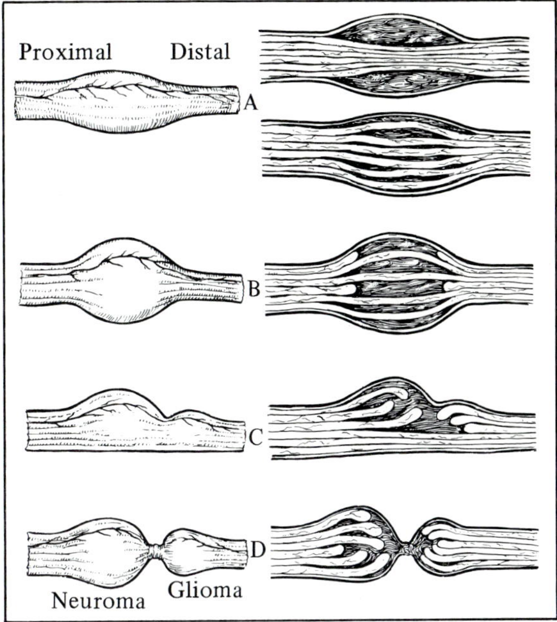

Fig. 36-12. The significance of a neuroma is often difficult to ascertain, and can make the surgical management a problem. The diagrams present some generalized categories that can be of help. A, the nerve is slightly enlarged and only slightly firmer than normal; the prognosis is often good and repair may not be necessary. B, extensive swelling and firmness of nerve, which often indicates extensive scarring within the nerve and a destruction of the intraneural architecture; resection of neuroma and nerve repair may be necessary. C, neuroma in partially transected nerve. Nerves cut as much as one-half or three-quarters of the way through often require resection and repair; however, if some important segment of the nerve seems to be intact and functioning, it may be necessary to dissect apart the neuroma under magnification and repair only the divided elements, preserving the intact portion of the nerve. D, the dumbbell configuration, which usually suggests that the nerve has been completely transected and the ends are being held in approximation only by scar tissue. A proper resection and repair will usually be necessary.

Local Tissue Conditions

Nearly everyone seems to agree that the more severe nerve injuries of the military type should be repaired as a secondary procedure. However, most civilian injuries are caused by glass or sharp knives (94 percent). A primary nerve repair is favored by many when these injuries are located in the distal part of an extremity and the trauma is localized.

Yet Nicholson and Seddon [32], in reviewing their series of cases, found that an early secondary suture offered as good an opportunity for recovery as a primary repair. Nicholson feels that secondary suturing is more reliable because at the time of secondary repair the epineurium is two to four times its normal thickness and the sutures seem more secure.

Grabb's fine experimental study [13] supports those who believe that in civilian wounds, when circumstances permit, the primary repair of a divided nerve yields the best results. Still, most surgeons experienced in this type of work will agree that an inexperienced surgeon will have a much greater chance of getting a poor result after a primary repair than he will with a secondary repair. Part of the reason for this is that the connective tissues in and around the freshly cut nerve are normally quite filmy. Their appearance and holding power are far less than they would be at the time of a secondary repair. Furthermore, the fasciculi themselves are more flexible immediately after a nerve injury. They also can be pulled in and out of the exposed end of the cut nerve with a great deal more independent mobility than at the time of the secondary repair. Thus, the inexperienced surgeon trying to do a primary repair more easily shreds and fragments the nerve end into a number of separate fasciculi. When an insufficient amount of connective tissue remains between these fasciculi, the only thing to do to relieve frustrations and complete the repair is to place sutures right through the fasciculi. If the sutures being used in the repair are not sufficiently small, the prognosis will be jeopardized even more severely than it was by the injury alone.

These circumstances are quite a contrast to the strong thickened perineurium and epineurium usually found at the time of the second repair. The fasciculi seem to be "stiffer," to have less independent movement, and to be more fixed in position in the interface. Their tendency to kink or get angulated at the time of suturing is therefore diminished, and a better holding surface is produced for the sutures being used in repair.

Metabolic Considerations in Nerve Repair

Advocates of a delayed primary repair have emphasized in recent years the need to postpone the repair of any injured nerve for at least 4 to 21 days [9]. They felt that the cell body and its axons were better primed for the repair and outgrowth of axons if sufficient time was allowed for the cell body to hypertrophy. Experimental and clinical studies, however, have failed to show that a delay in repair results in any significant increase in the return of function or sensibility [8].

Technique for Repair of Peripheral Nerves

If a peripheral nerve has been divided, it may be difficult to find the ends. They tend to retract back from the wound edge because of the elasticity of the mesoneurium and perineurium. Perhaps the easiest way to find the ends of a divided nerve, especially at the time of injury, is to look in the normal tissues proximal and distal to the wound, where the anatomical relationships are intact. The surgeon must identify the nerve ends at this level and then trace each back into the area of injury. Once located, the cut ends should be tagged with a suture so that they will be easy to recognize.

Naturally when the viability of a part is in jeopardy, vascular repair takes precedence over nerve repair. The latter should be considered only when it will not decrease the chances for survival of the part or appreciably increase the chances of an infection or some other complication arising.

When a nerve repair is to be deferred until a later date, it is important to approximate the nerve ends with a single suture to aid in their later identification and prevent retraction. If a small segment of nerve is missing so that the ends cannot be approximated, the ends should be tacked to the bed or some other fixed structure to keep them from retracting. This procedure will minimize one of the great problems that often makes secondary nerve repair more difficult – the gap between the two ends. In a fresh nerve injury, even though there has been no loss of nerve substance, this gap is present because the nerve ends retract because of the elasticity in the mesoneurium. In order to restore continuity, it is often necessary initially to place gentle traction on both ends of the nerve to get them together. If primary nerve repair is to be undertaken, the next step is to prepare the cut ends.

Funiculi can be seen protruding slightly from the ends of the nervelike wires extending from a section of cable; the epineurium slips back and forth over the bundles. Seddon and Medewar [39] call this the "prepuce test." Each individual fasciculus also has an independence of movement from its surrounding epineurium (Fig. 36-13). This independent mobility of each fasciculus is a prominent feature of normal nerve tissue. It is diminished or almost absent in the nerve stump being freshened for a secondary repair because of the increased amount of fibrosis present. This difference makes the primary repair of a peripheral nerve an entirely different problem, from a technical point of view, from that of a secondary repair.

In a primary repair the mobility of each fasciculus has to be controlled to keep it from retracting, protruding too far, kinking, or being displaced in one direction or another. Consequently, I insert "skewer" sutures or guide sutures to bolster the internal architecture and help make an orderly preparation for the biological repair (Fig. 36-14).

As the suturing is begun, it is important to try to reestablish the original relationships of the nerve ends. There are at least four ways in which proper alignment can be restored and rotational error minimized:

1. The blood vessels on the outer surface of each nerve stump should be studied and then lined up as the nerve ends are approximated.
2. The cut ends of the nerve bundles resemble mirror images that can be used as a guide in matching up the ends.

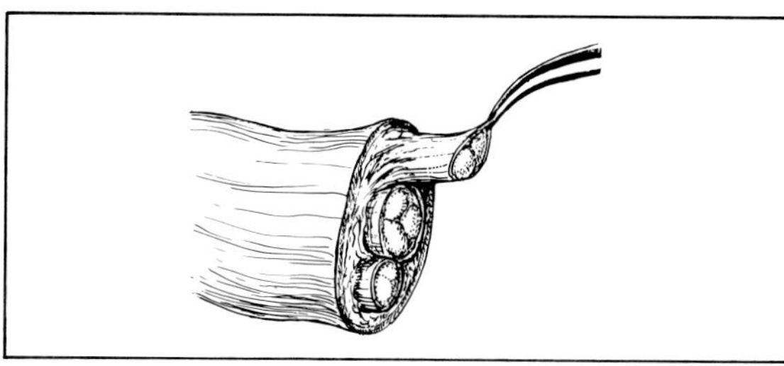

Fig. 36-13. Independent movement of each fasciculus within the interface of a divided nerve is greatest in fresh injuries.

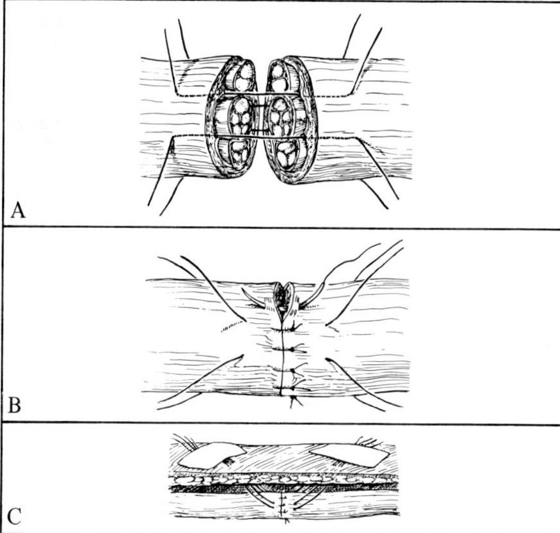

Fig. 36-14. Combined fascicular-epineurial repair. A, several small "skewer" sutures are placed adjacent to and parallel with the course of more major fasciculi; these perineurial fascicular sutures help to align the internal fasciculi. B, epineurial approximation is achieved with a few epineurial sutures. C, the skewer sutures can be brought through the skin and fixed to it with adhesive tape. One end of the skewer sutures can be released from the skin about a week later. Tension on the other end pulls them out to minimize the number of foreign bodies at the site of the nerve juncture. The remaining epineurial sutures maintain the integrity of the repair.

3. A small groove or other difference in the contour on either side should be found that will help establish the proper alignment.
4. The mesoneurium normally extends downward from the underside of a nerve to its underlying bed. Even if the mesoneurium is not intact at the site of nerve injury, remnants of it can be identified and used as a guide in correcting rotational error.

The surgeon should ascertain that all damaged and devitalized tissue has been removed from each nerve end before starting the repair. Magnification can be of help. The extent of damage may be difficult to evaluate if the pneumatic tourniquet is being used and the tissues have no color contrast. Many surgeons use a somewhat diluted mixture of methylene blue (1%) to improve contrast along the cut margin of the nerve. Very little is needed, and it can be applied to the cut nerve end with a sterile toothpick; the excess dye is washed away with saline. This helps to outline the epineurium and the nerve bundles more clearly.

The surgeon inserts funicular guide sutures of nylon as the initial step before approximating nerve ends. These sutures are placed through the epineurium about 1 cm. back from the cut end and run horizontally down the nerve through the perineurium to the cut surface of the nerve. A corresponding site is selected on the other cut end of the nerve and the guide suture is passed down along the perineurium and out through the epineurium in just the reverse order from which it was inserted. If two to four sutures of this type (7-0 nylon) are accurately inserted, they can be used in the realigning and will also serve well as traction or stay sutures to pull the ends together for the repair.

Epineurial guide sutures are placed accurately, one on each side of the nerve, but slightly more on its anterior surface, about 120 degrees apart. For the palm or the finger in an adult, a 7-0 nylon suture might be needed to overcome the tension. If 7-0 silk is used for the repair, it should be lubricated by running it through adjacent fat. Attention should again be directed to aligning the funiculi by using the mirror image—patterns as a guide, so that any discrepancy in rotation is corrected as these sutures are placed into the epineurial sheath. Once they are tied, light tension is placed upon them by clamping the ends of the suture with small mosquito clamps or a small lead weight. This will aid in spreading out the epineurium at the site of repair and lining it up so that suturing is easier. The anterior repair should be performed first with a 7-0 or 8-0 microsurgical suture; then the posterior repair is performed as follows: After the suturing is completed anteriorly, one of the epineurial guide sutures is drawn beneath the nerve and the other over the top so that the nerve repair on the posterior side can be finished. If these epineurial guide sutures have been placed 120 degrees apart, the posterior margins of the sheath will remain slightly separated, a technical factor that greatly aids in identifying and more accurately closing the sheath on this side.

At the completion of the suturing, it is important to inspect the line of juncture to be sure that there are no defects in the epineurium through which funiculi can protrude. If the suture line is rolled between the fingers as one rolls a cigarette, the lining up of the funiculi will be further facilitated. The funicular guide sutures on each side of the repair can be threaded onto a large cutting needle and passed out through the skin. They can be tied to one another after the wound is closed. Funicular guide sutures are removed at 7 days when the edema and early stages of healing have fixed the funiculi to one another at the site of nerve juncture.

Splinting of the extremity should hold it in such a position that there will be no tension on the nerve ends during the 3 to 6 weeks of healing.

Secondary Nerve Repair

The ends of the nerve are identified by gross vision and dissected out. Each is sectioned serially backward until a pattern of funiculi can be seen protruding slightly from the end. In secondary nerve repairs each interface must be prepared so that it will be flat and approximate to the other one without causing distortion, twisting, or protrusion of any of the funiculi. For some of the larger nerves it is worthwhile to hold the nerve in a fixed position while cutting it so that the interface will be absolutely perpendicular to the long axis of the nerve (Fig. 36-15). One way to do so is to wrap a narrow thin sheet of plastic (such as Vi-Drape) around the cut end of the nerve. The ends are immobilized by tightening the plastic noose around the nerve and applying a straight clamp along the base of the plastic to hold it firm. With a razor blade or dermatome blade, a good, clean transverse cut is made. The freshly prepared interface should then be studied with magnification to be certain that it is beyond the area of scar and neuroma and that it is satisfactory for approximation to the other end. Once the other end has been prepared, the repair can be undertaken (Fig. 36-16).

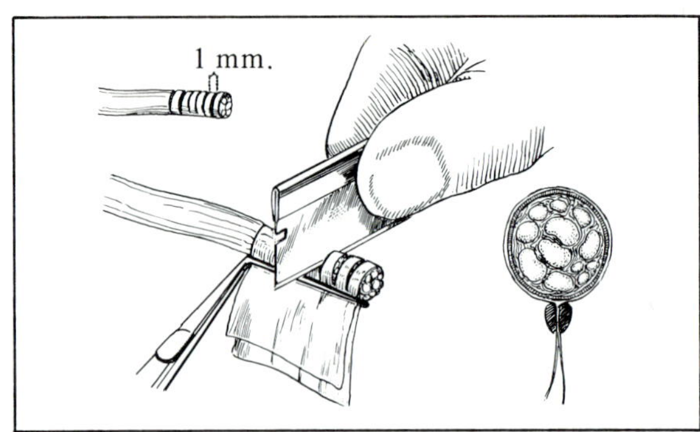

Fig. 36-15. Preparing the nerve ends for repair. At the neuroma site, a narrow strip of plastic (such as polyethylene or Vi-Drape) can be placed around the nerve end and tightened in a nooselike fashion with a right-angle clamp as the plastic is put under slight tension. A razor blade or a dermatome blade is used to cut it in 1-mm. sections, which can be studied to ensure that all severely damaged areas are removed prior to suturing. An excellent interface is also established by this technique.

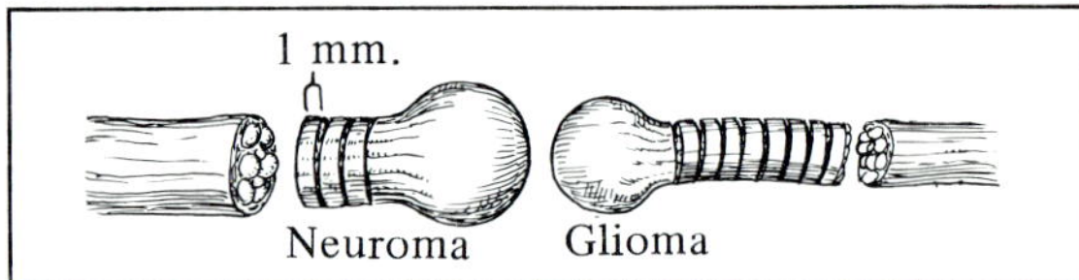

Fig. 36-16. Magnification is often of great aid in studying the surfaces of the freshened nerve ends after the neuroma and glioma are cut away. Once a level is found where the fascicular components appear normal, the two ends are ready for nerve suture.

Sometimes, in secondary nerve repairs, the fascicular bundles seem small compared to the extensive amount of epineurium between them. The epineurium may further confuse the microsurgeon, for if it is thick and somewhat laminated, it can lessen the accuracy of the fascicular approximation. If it becomes a problem, some of this epineurial connective tissue can be stripped away from the site for repair.

Resecting a segment of epineurium from either side of the repair also helps to reduce scarring. Eliminating tension reduces the amount of endoneurial fibrosis that might subsequently develop in the proximal and distal nerve stumps. Moreover, it prevents the adverse effect of connective tissue proliferation and shrinkage at the suture line that affects regenerating axons in the distal stump long after they have crossed the gap. Millesi, Meissl, and Berger [28] have shown both experimentally and clinically that axons can more easily cross the two tensionless lines of a fascicular nerve graft than penetrate the scar that will form at a site of nerve repair carried out under tension.

Sometimes simple epineurial sutures will hold the two nerve ends in proper approximation. In other instances, however, they will not produce a sufficiently accurate degree of alignment to satisfy the operating surgeon. In such cases, the usual problem is that the fasciculi in the two ends do not approximate because of atrophy or scar. To hold them in a more proper relation may require skewer sutures at the site of intended juncture. A double-armed monofilament nylon, placed adjacent to the fasciculus to be aligned, should help facilitate the approximation. When multiple fasciculi are being approximated, additional skewer sutures may be advantageous. I find that the use of these sutures cuts down tremendously on the need for epineurial sutures to maintain accuracy of approximation.

Nerve Grafts
When a loss of nerve substance or a gap from the retraction of the nerve ends makes approximation of the nerve ends impossible without tension, a nerve graft should be considered.

REFERENCES

1. Bora, F. W. Peripheral nerve repair in cats: The fascicular stitch. *J. Bone Joint Surg.* [Am.] 49:659, 1967.
2. Boyes, J. H. *Bunnell's Surgery of the Hand* (5th ed.). Philadelphia: Lippincott, 1974.
3. Brown, P. W. Factors influencing the success of surgical repair of peripheral nerves. *Surg. Clin. North Am.* 52:1137, 1972.
4. Buncke, H. J., Jr. Digital nerve repairs. *Surg. Clin. North Am.* 52:1267, 1972.
5. Denny-Brown, D. Electromyography and Other Electrical Aids to Diagnosis. In Flynn, J. E. (Ed.), *Hand Surgery* (2nd ed.). Baltimore: Williams & Wilkins, 1975.
6. Ducker, T. B., and Hayes, G. J. A comparative study of the technique of nerve repair. *Surg. Forum* 18:443, 1967.
7. Ducker, T. B., and Hayes, G. J. Experimental improvements in the use of Silastic cuff for peripheral nerve repair. *J. Neurosurg.* 28:582, 1968.
8. Ducker, T. B., and Kauffman, F. C. Metabolic factors in surgery of peripheral nerves. *Clin. Neurosurg.* 24:406, 1976.
9. Ducker, T. B., Kempe, L. G., and Hayes, G. J. The metabolic background for peripheral nerve surgery. *J. Neurosurg.* 30:270, 1969.
10. Edshage, S. Peripheral nerve suture. *Acta Chir. Scand.* [Suppl.] 331:7, 1964.
11. Flynn, W. F. Peripheral Nerve Injuries in the Hand: General Considerations. In Flynn, J. E. (Ed.), *Hand Surgery* (2nd ed.). Baltimore: Williams & Wilkins, 1975.
12. Goto, Y. Experimental study of nerve autografting by funicular suture. *Arch. Jap. Chir.* 36:478, 1967.
13. Grabb, W. C. Median and ulnar nerve suture. Experimental study comparing primary and secondary repair in monkeys. *J. Bone Joint Surg.* [Am.] 50:964, 1968.
14. Grabb, W. C., BeMent, S. L., Koepke, G. H., and Green, R. A. Comparison of methods of peripheral nerve suture in monkeys. *Plast. Reconstr. Surg.* 46:31, 1970.
15. Hakstian, R. W. Funicular orientation by direct stimulation. *J. Bone Joint Surg.* [Am.] 50:1178, 1968.
16. Henderson, A. R., and Hunter, D. Timing of peripheral nerve repair. Important local neuropathological factors. *Clin. Neurosurg.* 24:391, 1977.
17. Highet, W. B., and Sanders, F. K. The effects of stretching nerves after suture. *Br. J. Surg.* 30–31:355, 1942–1944.
18. Hubbard, J. H. The quality of nerve regeneration: Factors independent of the most skillful repair. *Surg. Clin. North Am.* 52:1099, 1972.
19. Ito, T., Hirotani, H., Goto, Y., and Tamura, T. A study of funicular suture. Personal communication, 1967.
20. Kaplan, E. B. *Functional and Surgical Anatomy of the Hand* (2nd ed.). Philadelphia: Lippincott, 1965.
21. Kline, D. G. Physiological and clinical factors contributing to the timing of nerve repair. *Clin. Neurosurg.* 24:425, 1977.
22. Kline, D. G., and Hackett, E. Reappraisal of timing for exploration of civilian peripheral nerve injuries. *Surgery* 78:54, 1975.
23. Kline, D. G., Hayes, G. J., and Morse, A. S. A comparative study of response of species to peripheral nerve injury: II. Crush and severence with primary suture. *J. Neurosurg.* 21:980, 1964.
24. Lampe, E. W. Surgical anatomy of the hand. *Ciba Found. Symp.* 9:17, 1957.
25. Madden, J. W., and Peacock, E. E., Jr. Some thoughts on repair of peripheral nerves. *South Med. J.* 64:17, 1971.
26. McEwan, L. E. Median and ulnar nerve injuries. *Aust. N.Z. J. Surg.* 32:89, 1962.
27. Millesi, H. Fascicular Peripheral Nerve Repair Using Cutaneous Nerve Grafts. In Daniller, A. I., and Strauch, B. (Eds.), *Symposium on Microsurgery.* St. Louis: Mosby, 1976.
28. Millesi, H., Meissl, G., and Berger, A. The interfascicular nerve grafting of the median and ulnar nerves. *J. Bone Joint Surg.* [Am.] 54:727, 1972.
29. Moberg, E. Evaluation and management of nerve injuries in the hand. *Surg. Clin. North Am.* 44:1019, 1964.
30. Moberg, E. Methods for Examining Sensibility of the Hand. In Flynn, J. E. (Ed.), *Hand Surgery* (2nd ed.). Baltimore: Williams & Wilkins, 1966.
31. Moberg, E. Nerve repair in hand surgery: An analysis. *Surg. Clin. North Am.* 48:985, 1968.
32. Nicholson, O. R., and Seddon, H. J. Nerve repair in civil practice. *Br. Med. J.* 2:1065, 1957.
33. Nulsen, F. E., and Kline, D. G. Acute Injuries of

Peripheral Nerves. In Youmans, J. R. (Ed.), *Neurological Surgery,* Vol. 2. Philadelphia: Saunders, 1973.
34. Omer, G., and Spinner, M. Peripheral Nerve Testing and Suture Techniques. In *American Academy of Orthopedic Surgeons Instructional Course Lectures.* Vol. 24. St. Louis: Mosby, 1975.
35. Onne, L. Recovery of sensibility and sudomotor activity in the hand after nerve suture. *Acta Chir. Scand.* [Suppl.] 300:1, 1962.
36. Peacock, E. E., Jr. Some studies on restoration of sensation in hands with an extensive defect in the median nerve. *J. Bone Joint Surg.* [Am.] 44:1036, 1962.
37. Sakellarides, H. A follow-up study of 172 peripheral nerve injuries in the upper extremity in civilians. *J. Bone Joint Surg.* [Am.] 44:140, 1962.
38. Seddon, H. J. Three types of nerve injury. *Brain* 66:237, 1943.
39. Seddon, H. J. War injuries of peripheral nerves. *Br. J. Surg.* [War Surg. Suppl. No. 2]: 325, 1948.
40. Seddon, H. J. *Peripheral Nerve Injuries.* London: Her Majesty's Stationery Office, 1954.
41. Seddon, H. J. Primary Suture. In *Surgical Disorders of the Peripheral Nerves.* Baltimore: Williams & Wilkins, 1972.
42. Smith, J. W. Personal correspondence, 1979.
43. Smith, J. W. Factors influencing nerve repair: I. Blood supply of peripheral nerves. *Arch. Surg.* (Chicago) 93:335, 1966.
44. Smith, J. W. Factors influencing nerve repair: II. Collateral circulation of peripheral nerves. *Arch. Surg.* (Chicago) 93:433, 1966.
45. Smith, J. W. Microsurgery of peripheral nerves. *Plast. Reconstr. Surg.* 33:317, 1964.
46. Smith, J. W. Surgical Repair of Peripheral Nerves. In Cooper, P. (Ed.), *The Craft of Surgery.* Boston: Little, Brown, 1970.
47. Smith, J. W. Newer techniques in peripheral nerve repair. *Clin. Neurosurg.* 24:456, 1977.
48. Smith, J. W. Peripheral Nerves. In Rand, R. W. (Ed.), *Microneurosurgery* (2nd ed.). St. Louis: Mosby, 1977.
49. Smith, J. W., and Grabb, W. C. Microsurgical Repair of Nerves. In Converse, J. M. (Ed.), *Reconstructive Plastic Surgery* (2nd ed.). Philadelphia: Saunders, 1977.
50. Smith, J. W., and Jacobson, J. Microsurgical Repair of Blood Vessels and Peripheral Nerves. In Flynn, J. E. (Ed.), *Hand Surgery.* Baltimore: Williams & Wilkins, 1966.
51. Sunderland, S. *Nerves and Nerve Injuries.* Edinburgh: Livingstone, 1968.
52. Weiss, P. A. Neuronal Dynamics and Neuroplasmic Flow. In Schmitt, F. O. (Ed.), *The Neurosciences* (Second Study Program). New York: Rockefeller Press, 1970.
53. Weiss, P. A., and Taylor, A. C. Impairment of growth and myelinization in regenerating nerve fibers subject to constriction. *Proc. Soc. Exp. Biol. Med.* 55:77, 1944.
54. Woodhall, B., Nulse, F. E., White, J. C., and Davis, L. Neurosurgical Implications. In Woodhall, B., and Beebe, G. W. (Eds.), *Peripheral Nerve Regeneration* (V.A. Medical Monograph). Washington, D.C.: U.S. Government Printing Office, 1957.
55. Zachary, R. B., and Holmes, W. Primary suture of nerves. *Surg. Gynecol. Obstet.* 82:632, 1946.

37

Rheumatoid Arthritis of the Hand

JEROME E. ADAMSON AND AUSTIN D. POTENZA

Advances in surgical technique have enabled the properly trained hand surgeon to apply the basic principles of reconstruction to improve the function and appearance of the extensive deformities of the hand that occur with rheumatoid arthritis. This insidious disease of mesenchymal tissues affects over five million people in the United States alone, and 94 percent of these individuals have involvement of their hands. Reconstruction of the arthritic hand has yielded heartening results and is a definite addition to the armamentarium available to all physicians caring for these persons.

Treatment must be organized with a multidisciplinary team approach. The treatment team for rheumatoid arthritis of the hand should consist of a rheumatologist, a hand surgeon, an orthopedic surgeon, and a physiotherapist. The team must work together in a well-coordinated effort to outline a specific medical, surgical, and rehabilitative program with ongoing consultation to ensure appropriate modifications depending upon response to treatment or varying activity of the disease. Surgical treatment should be well planned and well coordinated for the total functional benefit of the patient. It is ridiculous, for example, for the hand surgeon to perform wrist arthroplasty or arthrodesis with extensive reconstructive finger surgery designed to maintain or restore fine manipulative digital function if the patient is totally dependent upon crutches for ambulation in the postoperative period. The continued use of crutches will impose destructive forces on the operated hands and defeat the purposes of reconstructive hand surgery. The patient's ambulatory functional needs should first be analyzed and an attempt should be made to make the patient independently ambulatory prior to reconstructive hand surgery. This may require reconstructive hip or knee surgery (e.g., joint replacement, ligament reconstruction, long bone corrective osteotomies to overcome angular deformities, arthrodesis of selected weight bearing joints).

Reconstructive hand surgery must take full cognizance of the patient's functional deficits and anatomical deformities and limitations; these factors must be balanced against the patient's needs and desires.

PATHOLOGICAL CHANGES

Rheumatoid arthritis progressively destroys the joints of the hand. Initially, the articular surfaces are involved with a synovitis. This inflammatory process invades the adjacent tissues, damaging cartilage, ligaments, and pericapsular structures. The rheumatoid inflammatory process attacks the joint cartilage directly and also destroys the subchondral bone of the joint by invading the vascular channels in the metaphysis of the bones at sites of capsular and ligamentus attachment; subchondral cysts are formed. Joint cartilage is destroyed from both surfaces – within the joint itself and from the underlying subchondral bone. The joint space may be obliterated with an intense granulomatous-like inflammation. Tendons are involved. The intrinsic musculature is involved in the inflammatory rheumatoid process by a vasculitis, and it undergoes fibrotic contracture as a healing response to the inflammation. Tendon rupture, joint destruction, muscle atrophy, and a marked imbalance of function develop. Eventually total destruction of the functional capabilities of the hand occurs.

Frequently, in over 90 percent of patients, the initial symptom of rheumatoid arthritis occurs in the hand. Usually periarticular swelling, with redness and tenderness, is the primary symptom. From an extensive tenosynovitis, such difficulties as "trigger finger," de Quervain's syndrome, or carpal tunnel syndrome with median nerve compression from the synovial inflammation of the flexor compartment will be the initial complaints. The usual surgical treatment for these problems is accompanied by synovectomy of the diseased and proliferative synovium. Rarely, a rheumatoid nodule within a tendon will cause either of these problems. Occasionally spontaneous rupture of extensor or flexor tendons will occur with a boutonnière deformity, mallet finger deformity, or loss of functional flexor of the finger as a result of the disease.

The balance of the digit is destroyed by the synovitis and subsequent fibrotic shortening of the muscle-tendon units of the intrinsic and extrinsic mechanisms. This contracture causes a dislocation of the bony parts, e.g., subluxation of the carpal row beneath the base of the metacarpal; a compensatory hyperextension deformity, as in the "swan neck" deformity, at the proximal interphalangeal joint; and the mallet finger deformity with compensatory flexion at the distal interphalangeal joint. At the same time ulnar drift occurs. This is related to a combination of factors; the most important one is the anatomical relationship of the articular surfaces at the metacarpophalangeal joint. Gravity, the angle of approach of the flexor tendons, the constant push toward the ulnar side by the pinch mechanism, and the imbalance that often occurs in the intrinsic muscle systems also play a part in the development of ulnar drift.

Because the wrist joint is the key to dynamic balance of the hand, the metacarpophalangeal joint is the key to dynamic functional balance of the fingers. For every given force of pinch exerted by the flexor tendons at the tip of the finger there is a force three times as great exerted by the flexor tendons at the metacarpophalangeal joint working to produce volar dislocation of the proximal phalanx; in a joint whose capsular, ligamentous and other supporting structures are weakened by rheumatoid arthritis, this volar dislocation occurs, producing imbalance of intrinsic and extrinsic muscles with resultant weakness and dynamic deformities. These deformities include boutonnière deformity or swan neck deformity of the proximal interphalangeal joint and/or mallet finger or a fixed hyperextension deformity of the distal interphalangeal joint. When one joint shows gross deformity (i.e., subluxation-flexion deformity of the metacarpophalangeal joint), a neighboring joint will manifest a compensatory opposite dynamic deformity (i.e., swan neck deformity of the proximal interphalangeal joint). In simplest terms, in a biarticular linked-joint system, when one joint "zigs" the other joint will "zag," producing a dynamic zigzag deformity (i.e., flexion deformity of the metacarpophalangeal joint and swan neck deformity of the proximal interphalangeal joint; another example is the boutonnière deformity of the proximal interphalangeal joint with fixed hyperextension deformity of the distal interphalangeal joint). Similar deformities can also occur in the thumb, producing the classic zigzag collapse.

TREATMENT IN THE ACUTE STAGE

The early stages of the disease should be surgically treated if medical treatment fails after 90 days. Prophylactic resection of the involved synovial tissues is performed at the level of the metacarpophalangeal joint, the keystone joint of the digit, thus preventing the development of disabling swan neck deformities and severe ulnar drift.

If involvement of the intrinsic extensor mechanism is very early, it may be corrected with an intrinsic release. This is done on the ulnar side in early cases and on both radial and ulnar sides in those that are more advanced. The release should always accompany synovectomy; it involves resection of the oblique fibers of the lateral bands. Proximally, the vertical fibers and, more distally, the horizontal fibers are preserved to maintain intrinsic extensor function. By this relative lengthening of the involved joints, function is improved and further deformity is prevented.

Prophylactic night splints and vigorous therapy with antirheumatic medications are indicated, but frequently the disease will progress. Hand deformities will usually develop unless synovectomy and intrinsic release are performed at this early stage. Acute activity of rheumatoid arthritis is not contraindication to early reconstruction.

Intraarticular injection of antiinflammatory agents, such as thiotepa, nitrogen mustard, and cortisone, is given by many. Improvement is sometimes noted, but has not been striking. No long-term effects or "cures" of synovitis in a specific joint have been reported. Synovectomy is indicated. All involved flexor sheaths should be excised.

TREATMENT IN THE CHRONIC STAGE

In the later stages of the disease, when previously mentioned complications (e.g., ulnar drift) have occurred, treatment is aimed at restoring the normal balance of the extensor, intrinsic, and flexor tendon systems, placing the fingers in a more functional position, obtaining joint stability, and improving muscle strength.

A careful preoperative evaluation and preparation of the patient is mandatory to obtain ideal results. It is ridiculous for any surgeon to attempt to achieve a good functional result with a rheumatoid patient who has been psychologically and physically destroyed by the chronic pain and increasing disability the rheumatoid arthritis so typically produces. Forearm and intrinsic muscle atrophy will have occurred in practically all patients because of the disuse of these muscle systems. This atrophy results from the voluntary limitation of any motion that will cause pain. In all chronic rheumatoid patients this problem will be seen. As an effective test for the candidacy of a patient who may desire operative reconstruction, a series of preoperative forearm and hand strengthening muscle exercises is instituted. The circumferential measurement of forearm muscle bulk serves as a useful guide of their motivation and ability to utilize the reconstruction that may be available to them. If after 3 to 4 months no improvement in forearm size or strength has been noted, it is likely that these patients will not be good candidates for rheumatoid hand reconstruction. They may be well motivated psychologically, but may have progressed to the point physically that reconstruction may be markedly compromised. One cannot make a silk purse from a sow's ear and should not try.

Arthroplasty at the Metacarpophalangeal Joint

Bunnell [1], recognizing the abnormal length of the bony framework of the digital ray relative to the contracted interosseous muscles, initially detached the origins of the intrinsic muscles from their metacarpal insertions and shifted them distally to a more normal and relaxed position. Balance to the contracted system was thus restored. The extensive muscle fibrosis that developed made this approach impractical. Bunnell [1] then resected a portion of the midshaft of the metacarpal, indirectly lengthening the contracted intrinsic system. He shortened the bony arch and thus relatively lengthened the contracted, damaged intrinsic mechanism. This same approach has been modified by the present technique of shortening the "too long" metacarpal at the metacarpal head level. Synovectomy is performed simultaneously.

Since then many have advocated techniques for correcting the basic deformity at the metacarpophalangeal joint. In the less deformed hand, we recommend a conservative metacarpophalangeal arthroplasty consisting of resection of the diseased metacarpal head and synovial tissues, plus a Littler-type release or some modification of it (Fig. 37-1A). This improves the imbalance of intrinsic contracture. Synovectomy aids in preventing further damage, and a more normal joint is restored. Balance to the finger is restored by the bony resection and the intrinsic release. In the severely deformed, extensively damaged, and more frequently seen type of rheumatoid hand, a more radical metacarpophalangeal arthroplasty consisting of resection of the bony arch is necessary to correct the intrinsic contracture completely (Fig. 37-1B, C). If the bony arch is adequately shortened, it is not necessary, and indeed is harmful, to remove a portion of the intrinsic extensor mechanism (i.e., at the lateral band level). The operation for radical resection of the metacarpal head and neck is carried out through a transverse, wavy, dorsal skin incision proximal to the region of the metacarpal heads so as not to involve the dorsum of the web space by a transverse scar contracture. All dorsal veins and sensory nerves are preserved. The extensor hood is incised longitudinally on the radial side. Bony attachments of all the capsular structures are carefully detached from their insertion on the neck of the metacarpal, preserving them intact. A slightly curved resection of the metacarpal head and distal shaft is performed with a small sagittal saw or air drill. A radial dorsal angle of 5 to 8 degrees is established to aid in preventing the recurrence of ulnar drift. Usually, 1.5 to 2 cm. of the head and neck of

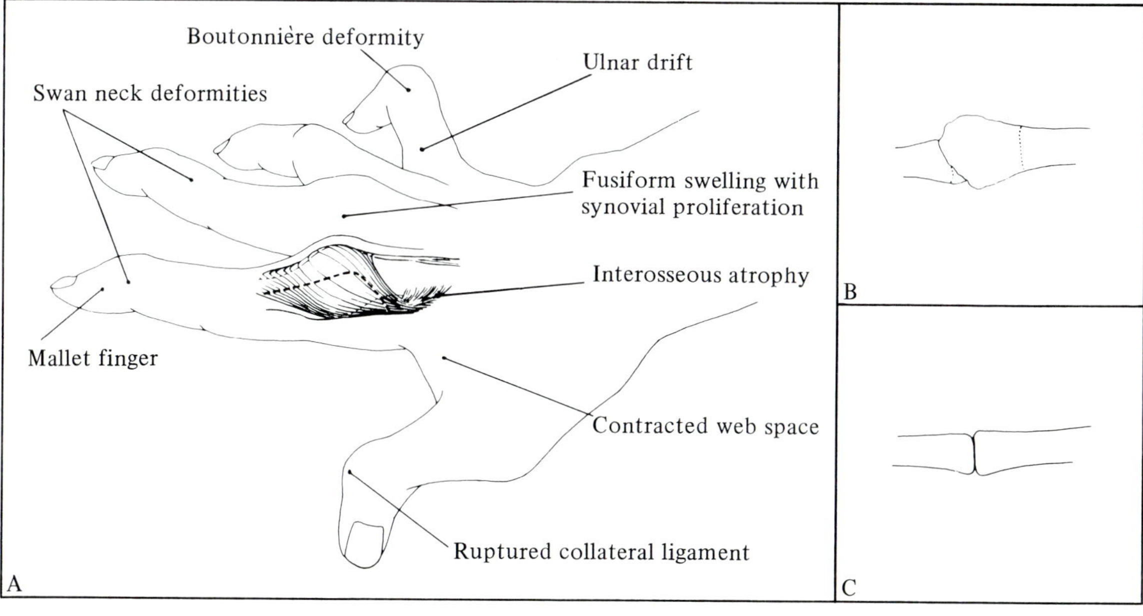

Fig. 37-1. Deformities of the rheumatoid hand. A, the usual deformities seen in the rheumatoid hand, i.e., swan neck deformity, mallet finger, periarticular swelling, boutonnière deformity, and subluxation of the distal joint of the thumb. In the phantom view of the metacarpophalangeal joint, the markedly attenuated fibers of the intrinsic extensor hood mechanism are displayed. The distortion of this joint with volar subluxation of the base of the proximal phalanx is noted. Dotted lines indicate the usual line of resection in performing the Littler intrinsic release. B, area of minimal bony resection (dotted lines) in the radical metacarpophalangeal arthroplasty. Removal of more of the shaft may be necessary to provide adequate shortening of the bony arch. C, the joint following a radical metacarpophalangeal arthroplasty functions as a hinge joint.

the metacarpal is removed to restore balance in the digit. Adequacy of resection is evaluated at operation by being able to hyperextend the metacarpophalangeal joint to proximally 200 degrees, i.e., 20 degrees more than normal. Any osteophytic lip or deformity at the base of the proximal phalanx should be excised to make a smooth, butt-type joint. Collateral ligaments, volar plate, and capsule that have been detached shift to new areas of insertion on the distal stump of the metacarpal shaft.

The use of the silicone metacarpophalangeal joint prostheses has gained widespread acceptance. It appears, despite such rare shortcomings as fracture, dislocation, and, in some instances, a secondary tissue reaction with secondary axillary adenopathy due to silicone particles, that artificial joint prosthesis of the silicone rubber–type will remain as an effective adjunct to the multifaceted operation for rheumatoid hand reconstruction. It is extremely important to utilize a joint prosthesis that fits exactly. The base of the proximal phalanx and the distal shaft of the metacarpal are drilled to receive the prosthesis. To prevent fracture, it is helpful to round off the distal ends of the metacarpal shaft stump. The prosthesis should be handled delicately – for example, its surface should not be pierced by forceps. Correction of intrinsic contracture by shortening the metacarpal is still absolutely necessary. One cannot restore balance by an inadequate bony resection, since ulnar drift will almost certainly recur.

The ulnar-deviated extensor tendon is shifted to a new, more midline position by suturing with nonabsorbable sutures in an imbricating manner the extensor hood mechanism on the radial side. Occasionally, synovectomy does not relax the attenuated hood structures on the ulnar side sufficiently to allow for complete shift of the ulnar-deviated extensor tendon to the midline. In such instances a horizontal incision through these ulnar fibers may be necessary. This defect is not sutured. Slight redundancy of the extensor and flexor systems will be compensated for by forearm muscle retraction postoperatively.

Transfer of the intrinsic extensor tendons at the lateral band level from the ulnar side of one finger to the radial side of the adjacent finger may be helpful in preventing recurrence of ulnar drift. Usually this is not necessary if balance between the bony arch and muscle-tendon systems has been achieved by adequate bony shortening.

A transfer of the extensor indicis proprius tendon to the first dorsal interosseous tendon will provide greater stability of pinch and will assist in prevention of ulnar drift. The tendon is detached from its distal insertion, withdrawn at the wrist, and passed subcutaneously to the insertion of the usually atrophic first dorsal interosseous muscle. This tendon should not be anchored under much tension, as is usually performed with tendon transfers, since a flexion contracture or a supination deformity of the index finger at the metacarpophalangeal joint may develop.

Tenotomy of the abductor digiti minimi, or, in rare instances, a transfer of this tendon from the ulnar to the radial side of the little finger will assist in maintaining position of the little finger after a radical arthroplasty. A similar tenotomy of the flexor digiti minimi further prevents ulnar drift of the little finger.

Reconstruction of the Interphalangeal Joints

Proximal Interphalangeal Joint

If extensive synovitis is present in the proximal interphalangeal joint, synovectomy may be performed through a dorsal wavy midline incision. The oblique retinacular ligament is elevated on either side of the joint. The collateral ligaments are excised from beneath the oblique ligament. A synovectomy and detachment of any adhesions in the volar plate pouch are carried out. Maintaining the retinacular ligaments intact preserves lateral stability of the joint. Prompt postoperative motion prevents the formation of limiting adhesions.

In the rheumatoid hand with a severe swan neck deformity, after a radical metacarpophalangeal arthroplasty with or without prosthesis has been performed, a scar tenodesis can be effected in the hyperextended, unstable, proximal interphalangeal joint to provide more stability. This is done at the time of synovectomy by roughening the volar plate and immobilizing the finger for approximately 10 days in a slightly flexed position of 15 to 20 degrees.

Insertion of a silicone joint prosthesis is helpful to reconstruct a badly damaged and often stiffened proximal interphalangeal joint. A midline incision splits the extensor mechanism. Care is taken to preserve the midline slip insertion at the base of the middle phalanx. The joint surfaces are resected, distal and proximal defects in the shafts are made, and the prosthesis is fitted into place. Resection of the collateral ligaments is not advisable unless they are contracted. These are usually allowed to remain intact, providing lateral stability with the oblique retinacular ligaments. The dorsal tendon mechanism is carefully sutured with nonabsorbable interrupted sutures. Motion is started in 2 days as pain permits.

Boutonnière deformities from rupture of the middle extensor slip respond poorly to standard attempts at correction because in the rheumatoid hand the severe tenosynovitis has caused so much damage to all adjacent structures. Fusion in the position of function usually gives best results, but occasionally it may be helpful to reinsert the ruptured middle extensor slip, utilizing a graft from the palmaris tendon, and insert, as needed, a proximal interphalangeal joint prosthesis.

Distal Interphalangeal Joint

If at the distal interphalangeal joint a mallet finger deformity has occurred as the result of rupture of the extensor tendon, fusion of this joint in 20 to 30 degrees of flexion is indicated. More flexion is needed as one proceeds from the index to the little finger. Resection of both joint surfaces with the sagittal saw or air drill and cross-joint Kirschner wire fixation will give adequate stability. Wire loop fixation is not satisfactory in the usual rheumatoid patient because of the extensive bony damage that is usually present. If bony fusion has not occurred after 2½ to 3 months, a bone graft across the joint space may be necessary. However, a satisfactory painless fibrous ankylosis will frequently develop.

Reconstruction of the Thumb

Stabilization of either one or two of the three joints (the proximal and distal interphalangeal joints and the carpometacarpal joint) of an unstable thumb by fusion will improve pinch. It is best to leave one of the three joints unfused. In patients with severe joint destruction and either marked instability or joint ankylosis, fusion of the interphalangeal joints in a position of function and resection of the trapezius will usually improve function. In those individuals with destruction of the carpometacarpal joint, resection of the carpal bone and insertion of the appropriate Silastic preformed prosthesis will frequently provide improvement in motion; relief of pain is usually best along the dorsal aspect of the joint. Care should be taken to avoid injury to the branches of the superficial radial nerve. The joint prosthesis must be carefully selected to obtain an exact size replacement. Use of a joint prosthesis in the metacarpophalangeal joint of the thumb has not been as successful as it has been in other joints, probably because of the greater range of motion in the thumb as compared with any finger. Dislocation may occur frequently if the prosthesis is not exactly fitted into position.

Deepening of a contracted thumb web by Z-plasty or double Z-plasty may be helpful. When the contracture is marked, a proximally based dorsal flap can be elevated from the region of the second and third metacarpals and rotated into the thumb web to give satisfactory improvement. The doner area is closed by a split-thickness skin graft. Partial release of the abductor and short flexor insertions on the metacarpal of the thumb should be performed at the same time if needed.

Treatment of Tendon Rupture and Wrist Deformity

Flexor or extensor tendon rupture in patients with rheumatoid arthritis usually occurs at the level of the wrist. If the stability of the wrist joint has not been too badly compromised by synovitis, ruptured tendons should ideally be repaired, but usually transfer of the distal ends to adjacent functioning tendons is most expedient. A synovectomy of the radial carpal joint should be performed. Frequently, resection of the distal ulna at this time prevents further deformity and provides a greater range of supination and pronation. As a synovectomy is performed, relocation of the transverse retinacular ligament of the wrist to a position beneath the common extensor tendons as they pass through the multiple (usually six) constricting channels of the dorsal wrist ligament will prevent future tendon rupture. The slight bowstringing that may develop is usually not significant. Bony projections from the carpus should be removed to prevent tendon erosion.

If wrist joint involvement is severe and subluxation of the carpus appears imminent, the wrists should be fused with one hand at 180 degrees and the other in slight hyperextension before any other reconstruction is undertaken. In long-standing deformities with wrist subluxation, it may be necessary to resect the proximal row of carpal bones in addition to the distal head of the ulna. Bone grafting with Steinmann pin cross-fixation at the fusion site gives best results if accompanied by appropriate plaster cast immobilization for approximately 3 months. Often the best functional result in a rheumatoid wrist is a moderately stiff fibrous ankylosis with a 25- to 35-degree range of useful motion about the neutral axis of the wrist. Such wrists are often pain-free, and their limited range of useful motion enhances finger function and still allows for feeding and perineal care. Such a wrist can often be achieved by radical intercarpal and radiocarpal synovectomy followed by Steinmann pin cross fixation for 6 to 8 weeks.

In a wrist that is undergoing volar carpal subluxation, an arthroplasty achieved by creating a volar supporting shelf of the distal radius and displacing the carpus dorsal to the shelf will often provide stability and increase the strength of the hand. When chronic massive destruction of the carpus occurs with progressive volar subluxation and especially with ulnar subluxation, arthrodesis provides the best result – a stable, pain-free, and strong wrist. The role of replacement arthroplasty of the wrist in rheumatoid arthritis is not clearly defined at this time.

The tendons most frequently ruptured by rheumatoid disease are the common extensor tendons to the fingers. The long extensor and long abductor tendons to the thumb are often ruptured by the constrictive tenosynovitis that occurs as a result of synovial involvement of the tendon sheaths at the wrist level. After the wrist joint has been stabilized by fusion, function of the fingers and thumb can be restored by transfer of appropriate tendons to reactivate those that have been ruptured. We have had most success utilizing the flexor sublimis tendon of the ring finger routed subcutaneously in an ulnaward direction and attached to the common extensors in the middorsum of the hand. Occasionally the flexor carpi ulnaris may be prolonged with a "split-tailed" palmaris graft for a common extensor transfer. However, the flexor sublimis tendon has a greater range of excursion and will provide more adequate power for extensors.

To restore function to the ruptured long extensor of the thumb, the flexor sublimis of the middle finger routed radially at a subcutaneous level across the wrist gives good results when attached to the intact tendon at the metacarpal level. The extensor indicis proprius is not as good a motor because it does not have an adequate range of excursion or power. Repair of the extensor pollicis longus to the thumb after rupture is not indicated because of atrophy of the muscle, which occurs rapidly (by 2 months), destroying its effectiveness as a functional motor.

Rarely, the flexor tendons rupture either from a stenosing tenosynovitis at the proximal pulley level or from direct involvement of the tendon with the rheumatoid process. Transfer of an adjacent flexor superficialis tendon as a motor will improve function. Frequently tenodesis of the distal interphalangeal joint is all that is indicated if only the flexor profundus is involved. Excision of the compromising tendon sheath is absolutely essential to prevent further damage.

Dorsal Rhytidectomy

Because of extensive wrinkling of the skin in some patients, an incision on the ulnar border of the hand can be made, the skin of the dorsum undermined, and excess skin excised. It will frequently be necessary to remove redundancy by making a "hockey stick" extension along the wrist crease toward the dorsum. Care should be taken not to damage the dorsal veins or sensory nerves. This procedure improves the appearance of the hand.

Reconstructive surgery of the rheumatoid hand should restore the hand to a functional working unit in the shortest possible time. As much reconstructive surgery as is needed to restore the hand to overall optimal functional status should be performed in the shortest possible time, preferably in one operative sitting. Operative trauma, anesthetic dangers, and potential postoperative complications and postoperative discomfort are thus confined to one relatively short period. Importantly, the hand can be rehabilitated postoperatively as a functional grasping, manipulative unit. Piecemeal surgery that does not restore overall capacity to the hand until after many individual operations is to be condemned. Such surgery is discouraging and disheartening to the patient by prolonging surgery over many months and often turning the patient into a social, emotional, and economic cripple rather than restoring him to functional capacity in the shortest possible time. A total surgical approach to the patient facilitates postoperative physiotherapy and rehabilitation by directing such treatments to functional hand activities, such as grasping, manipulative functions, and work tasks in patterns rather than to isolated range of motion exercises for one or two operated joints or digits.

POSTOPERATIVE CARE

After basic corrections at the metacarpophalangeal, interphalangeal, and wrist joints have been achieved, dorsal and volar plaster splints are applied with the hand in the position of function. If Silastic joint prostheses are utilized, early mobilization is valuable in obtaining effective function. Usually a dorsal outrigger attached to a forearm splint with slings to the proximal phalanges of the four fingers pulling in a slight radial direction will give adequate mobilization. Patients are instructed in simple flexion and extension; the hand is constantly elevated for 2½ to 3 weeks until adequate healing of the underlying capsular and pericapsular structures is achieved. Skin sutures are then removed, and a vigorous program of active and passive exercises is instituted. The goals of the preoperative exercise program are finally achieved, with the patient easily slipping into the already established and understood program for rehabilitation. Improvement is gradual; the maximal result is usually not reached for 9 to 12 months because of the slowness with which the average patient improves the total power of the forearm and intrinsic musculature. The importance of maintaining a full range of active and passive joint motion until muscle rehabilitation is complete cannot be overemphasized.

In those individuals with very severe rheumatoid disease, fusion of the metacarpal and proximal interphalangeal joints will often result not in improvement in the function of the hand, but in markedly improved appearance of the hand. This treatment is reserved for only those individuals who have such severe disability with extensive damage to the forearm and intrinsic musculature that no other improvement in function can be achieved. The importance of careful selection of the suitable patient and the specific group of operations cannot be overemphasized.

REFERENCE

1. Bunnell, S. *Bunnell's Surgery of the Hand* (5th ed.). Philadelphia: Lippincott, 1970.

Dupuytren's Contracture

JOHN T. HUESTON

The primary lesion in this hereditary condition is a nodule of hyperplastic fibroblasts in the subcutaneous space of the palm or digits. This nodule becomes fixed to the volar aspect of the palmar aponeurosis or its dermal and digital extensions, and subsequent contraction at the level of the nodule produces deformity of the dermis or digits [7a, 8]. The rate of progression of the hyperplastic nodule varies between individuals, and in many victims the condition does not proceed to the stage of deformity. Also, histologically similar nodules can occur in ectopic sites such as over the proximal interphalangeal joints and on the plantar fascia without producing deformity. Thus, since clinical contraction is not an essential feature for diagnosis, many prefer to call this simply Dupuytren's Disease.

The origin of the proliferating fibroblasts appears to be from the perivascular cellular cuff of the small arterioles and capillaries in the fine septa between the fat loculi of the palm [8, 18a]. The mechanism of actual contraction has recently been clarified by the identification within these hyperplastic nodules of the contracting fibroblasts or "myofibroblasts." Myofibroblasts appear to represent a phase of development of the fibroblasts in which the cells share some important nuclear and cytoplasmic features with smooth muscle cells [5]. That these myofibroblasts are formed only within the nodules and not in the bands of Dupuytren's contracture [14] confirms the essential pathology of this condition – namely, that the primary focus is the hyperplastic nodule and that the bands are secondarily produced by simple work hypertrophy due to the tension induced by the contracting foci in the nodules [18, 18a].

The patterns of fascial contraction conform to involvement of normally occurring fascial strands within the palm and digits [6, 20, 24]. Displacement of digital neurovascular bundles into surgically vulnerable situations is most common with bands drawn up from Cleland's ligaments [20].

The freedom from contraction found in ectopic deposits in the extensor paratenon of the fingers and in the plantar fascia may be due to the regular stretching of these areas in daily activity and may indeed thus confirm the value of the traditional advice for controlling early palmar lesions – namely, to stretch the palm passively by sitting on the hand with the palm downward.

Operative statistics have given the impression that the process affects men 10 times more frequently than women, but population studies suggest that a two or three times greater frequency is a closer estimation. People of unmixed dark-skinned races do not incur the disorder, and people of Mediterranean extraction are less often affected than northern Europeans. Although the condition is inherited, a patient's report on his family is rarely accurate. It has been found to be more severely manifested in epileptics, alcoholics, diabetics, and patients with pulmonary tuberculosis.

A single episode of injury is often soon followed by the appearance or progression of the proliferative palmar process, even though the hand is only secondarily involved by a proximal injury such as a nerve lesion or the swelling and immobilization after a Colles fracture or dislocation of the shoulder [9]. Recurrence or extension soon after fasciectomy can be interpreted likewise as a post-traumatic exacerbation of this process.

Heavy manual labor has never been proven to have an injurious effect on deep palmar structures [26]. However, the fact that Dupuytrens has a greater frequency in invalids than manual workers, suggests it is best to stress the physiological efficiency of this region. Incidence of the condition is not related to handedness [1, 26], and clerical workers are if anything slightly more often affected [4, 8]. Pressure may cause tenderness in a nodule (just as skin callosity often results from heavy manual labor), but this occurs as an effect rather than being a cause of the underlying pathology.

DUPUYTREN'S DIATHESIS

The inherited potential of any particular patient for this order – that is, Dupuytren's diathesis – can be assessed from the extent and severity of general factors and ectopic sites. The strength of the diathesis as assessed in a particular patient will influence the timing and extent of surgical intervention [13].

Dupuytren's diathesis serves as a guide to prognosticate the likelihood of further progression by either recurrence (i.e., within the operated field) or extension (i.e., beyond the operated field) of the disease process in the hand. The diathesis, or constitutional tendency to the disease, increases proportionally with increases in these factors: (1) the youth of the patient, (2) the strength of the family history, (3) the extent of ectopic deposits as knuckle pads and plantar lesions, and (4) the presence of the predisposing factors of alcoholism and epilepsy. The stronger the diathesis is, the more likely it is that there will be recurrences at the operative site and that secondary surgery will become necessary – in particular, skin graft replacement may become necessary, because this is the sole reliable means of preventing recurrence in a patient with a strong diathesis. Lesser degrees of diathesis may not result in true recurrence but merely extension elsewhere, and the patient with the lowest diathesis will show no evidence of the process in other areas [8].

SURGICAL MANAGEMENT

Preoperative Planning

The aim in management is to retain hand function. The mere presence of a palmar nodule is not an indication for an operation. Progressive deformity is an indication for surgery, and the optimum time for operation is when metacarpophalangeal flexion is present but before interphalangeal flexion has developed.

The *table top test* is a useful guide in timing surgery. Thus, when the hand cannot be placed flat on a table top, surgery is indicated [11]. Individuals with only nodules or minimal contracture can be advised to return later when the digital deformity has progressed to a positive table top test. If they follow this advice, it is thus possible to prevent the progression of the deformity to uncorrectable proximal interphalangeal flexion, which might otherwise result from ignorance or neglect of the condition.

In principle the operation should be restricted to restoring hand function by the correction of the deformity. If, however, recurrence has occurred or is anticipated from an assessment of a strong Dupuytren diathesis, then the operation should be directed to a permanent local cure of the disease by skin grafting. It is empirically known that the hyperplastic process of Dupuytren's disease does not occur under skin introduced from elsewhere [10]. Probably the palmar skin itself carries the ingredients that induce deeper fibroplasia and contraction, but there is as yet no explanation of the mechanism that causes this phenomenon.

SELECTION OF OPERATION

It is hard to select an operation for Dupuytren because the published results of the different surgical approaches are not strictly comparable unless the procedures are performed by the same surgeon; in addition, different opinions based on the results of surgery in different parts of the world may be explained on the different ethnic population of the patients.

Fasciotomy

Simple palmar fasciotomy is sufficient to correct most of the metacarpophalangeal deformities and some of the proximal interphalangeal deformities. In some elderly patients with a low diathesis and limited life expectancy, this treatment is recommended. In such patients the chances are slight that the ends of the divided band will reunite, causing a recurrence of the deformity. A 1-cm. longitudinal incision is used beside the band in the palm – the incision is never placed in the finger because of the risk of dividing a digital nerve.

Regional Fasciectomy

The most common operation is the regional removal of all the macroscopically involved tissues of the band-nodule deforming mechanism. This is usually performed through a longitudinal incision with Z-plasty rearrangements to provide lengthening of the overlying skin to prevent longitudinal scar contracture. This operation is advisable when the interphalangeal joints are deformed and when simple palmar fasciotomy would result in early recurrence of a metacarpophalangeal joint deformity. The operation is limited only in the extent of palmar resection; all the diseased tissue is excised, but resection is not followed back into the proximal portion of the palm, because there is little risk of recurrence from leaving proximal segments of bands in the palm. This residual tissue, lying proximal to the metacarpophalangeal joints, usually atrophies because it is no longer stretched during joint movement. Moreover, the risk of hematoma is greatly reduced if the skin is not elevated from the hollow of the proximal portion of the palm. Fasciectomy of more than one finger is commonly needed at the same operation. Longitudinal incisions are favored for all digital dissections, because the operation of fasciectomy is essentially a dissection of the digital nerves. Once they are located in the palm, these digital nerves can be carefully followed throughout the most tortuous course down the digit. When the flexor tendon sheath in the palm has been located, the fascia can be lifted from the medial to the lateral side; it is safer to find the common digital nerve by incising the lateral paratendinous septum. This exposes the common digital nerve and its bifurcation just anterior and parallel to the lumbrical muscle belly. The value of longitudinal exposure is still obtained by sinuous or angled incisions; the only advantage of Z-plasties is to provide some skin lengthening [12]. Interphalangeal joint stiffness is the greatest disability after operation, and it appears to be unrelated to the extent of the dissection.

Extensive Fasciectomy

Extensive fasciectomy requires excision of the whole width of the palmar aponeurosis from the palm. In the fingers the same degree of dissection is required to correct the interphalangeal deformity regardless of the extent of the palmar dissection. This approach is warranted in young people with multifocal palmar lesions and a strong diathesis. In this specific group of patients, the chance of further palmar deposits is high, but excision of the anatomical longitudinal fascial strands will prevent new nodules from drawing up new deforming bands. There are added risks of palmar hematoma and wound margin necrosis associated with this more radical surgery. Hence the extensive palmar dissection is not justified in young people with localized disease and a low diathesis, in middle-aged or elderly patients, and in women. Closure of a long transverse palmar incision after radical fasciectomy may be executed in one of three ways:

1. Direct suture, with flexion at the metacarpophalangeal joints and subsequent stretching of the dermal contraction after healing.
2. The open palm method, as described by McCash [19], relies on wound contraction to close the palmar defect and rapidly unravels dermal contractions. The healing phase is comfortable and free of hematoma, even though the healing may require several weeks to reach its completion.
3. A free skin graft into the defect, allowing early resumption of the full range of movement. Healing after skin grafting takes no longer than after wound closure by suture.

Dermofasciectomy and Skin Graft

Skin grafts prevent the recurrence of Dupuytren's contracture in the grafted area, although of course new disease may appear elsewhere in the hand and even beneath the adjacent replaced palmar skin flaps. The immunity from recurrence enjoyed by skin-grafted areas in the hand has led to the use of full-thickness free skin grafts (Wolfe grafts) in the digits when there has already been a recurrence or when the age and the strong diathesis of the patient suggest that later recurrence is likely. In selected cases it is being increasingly used as a primary prophylaxis against recurrence [10]. Thus while in most cases the *area* of dissection is reasonably limited to that of the deforming mechanism, a more radical excision in *depth* to include the overlying skin may be warranted if prophylaxis against recurrence is the aim.

A midline longitudinal incision is used for the safe exposure of the digital nerves throughout the digit; this ensures the preservation of an intact fibrous flexor sheath [13]. The two longitudinal lateral skin flaps are preserved until it is clear that the flexor sheath has been left completely intact as a safe bed for the free skin to be applied. If a portion of the flexor tendon is exposed the skin on either side of the midline can be converted to small local flaps to cover the tendon in those areas where there is no sheath present. The exposed tendons would not provide a satisfactory bed for the free skin grafts. Thus after total excision of the volar integument of the finger from midlateral line to midlateral line, a full-thickness (Wolfe) graft is taken, usually from the inner aspect of the upper arm (or from the trunk if several digits require resurfacing); the graft is carefully sutured into place. Care should be taken to ensure that the darts in the lateral suture line conform with the principles of correction of burn scar contractures. A gentle pressure dressing is applied for 5 days. A plaster volar slab is used for 5 days after every operation for Dupuytren's contracture.

REFERENCES

1. Boyes, J. H. Dupuytren's contracture. *Am. J. Surg.* 88:147, 1954.
2. Brickley Parsons, D., Albin, R., Smith, R., Adams, J., and Glimcher, M. J. Biosynthesis of the Cross Linkages of Collagen of Dupuytren's Contracture and Normal Palmar Fascia Grown in Organ Culture. In *Transactions of the 22nd Annual Meeting of the Orthopaedic Research Society,* January, 1976. Vol. 1, p. 91.
3. Conway, H. Dupuytren's contracture. *Am. J. Surg.* 87:101, 1954.
4. Early, P. F. Dupuytren's contracture. *J. Bone Joint Surg.* [Br.] 44:602, 1962.
5. Gabbiani, G., and Majno, G. Dupuytren's contracture: Fibroblast contraction. *Am. J. Pathol.* 66:131, 1972.
6. Gosset, J. The Development and the Anatomy of the Palmodigital Aponeurosis. In Hueston, J. T., and Tubiana, R. (Eds.), *Dupuytren's Disease.* London: Churchill-Livingstone, 1974.
7. Harrison, S. H., and Morris, A. Dupuytren's contracture: The dorsal transposition flap. *Hand* 7:145, 1975.

7a. Hueston, J. T. Aetiological Questions in Dupuytren's Contracture. In Hueston, J. T., and Tubiana, R. (Eds.), *Dupuytren's Disease.* London: Churchill-Livingstone, 1974. P. 33.

8. Hueston, J. T. *Dupuytren's Contracture.* London: Livingstone, 1963.
9. Hueston, J. T. Dupuytren's contracture and specific injury. *Med. J. Aust.* 1:1084, 1968.
10. Hueston, J. T. The control of recurrent Dupuytren's contracture by skin replacement. *Br. J. Plast. Surg.* 22:152, 1969.
11. Hueston, J. T. The table top test. *Med. J. Aust.* 2:189, 1976.
12. Hueston, J. T. Dupuytren's Contracture. In Converse, J. M. (Ed.), *Reconstructive Plastic Surgery* (2nd ed.). Philadelphia: Saunders, 1977.
13. Hueston, J. T. Dupuytren's Disease. In Pulvertaft,

C. (Ed.), *Robb and Smith Operative Surgery* (3rd ed.). London: Butterworths, 1977.

14. Hueston, J. T., Hurley, J. V., and Whittingham, S. The contracting fibroblast as a clue to Dupuytren's contracture. *Hand* 8:10, 1976.
15. Hunter, J. A. A., and Ogden, C. Dupuytren's contracture: II. Scanning electron microscope observations. *Br. J. Plast. Surg.* 28:19, 1975.
16. Hunter, J. A. A., Ogden, C., and Norris, M. G. Dupuytren's contracture: I. Chemical pathology. *Br. J. Plast. Surg.* 28:10, 1975.
17. James, J. I. P. The Genetic Pattern of Dupuytren's Contracture and Idiopathic Epilepsy. In Hueston, J. T., and Tubiana, R. (Eds.), *Dupuytren's Disease.* Edinburgh and London: Churchill-Livingstone, 1974.
18. Luck, J. V. Dupuytren's contracture; a new concept of the pathogenesis correlated with the surgical management. *J. Bone Joint Surg.* [Am.] 41:635, 1959.

18a. MacCallum, P., and Hueston, J. T. The pathology of Dupuytren's contracture. *Aust. N.Z. J. Surg.* 31:241, 1962.

19. McCash, C. R. The open palm technique in Dupuytren's contracture. *Br. J. Plast. Surg.* 17:271, 1964.
20. McFarlane, R. M. Patterns of the diseased fascia in the fingers in Dupuytren's contracture. *Plast. Reconstr. Surg.* 54:31, 1974.
21. Orlando, J. C., Smith, J. W., and Goulian, D. Dupuytren's contracture; a review of 100 patients. *Br. J. Plast. Surg.* 27:211, 1974.
22. Peacock, E. E., Jr. Dupuytren's disease: controversial aspects of management. *Clin. Plast. Surg.* 3:29, 1976.
23. Skoog, T. Management of Dupuytren's Contracture – A Rational Approach Based on Its Pathogenesis. *Transactions of the Fifth International Congress of Plastic and Reconstructive Surgery.* Melbourne, Australia: Butterworth, 1971.
24. Stack, H. G. The Palmar Fascia and the Development of Deformities and Displacements in Dupuytren's Contracture. In Hueston, J. T., and Tubiana, R. (Eds.), *Dupuytren's Disease.* London: Churchill-Livingstone, 1974.
25. Wilflingseder, P., Bauer, M., and Ioannovich, I. Venous-Occlusion Plethysmography in Dupuytren's Contracture. *Transactions of the Fifth International Congress of Plastic and Reconstructive Surgery.* Melbourne, Australia: Butterworth, 1971.
26. Zachariae, L. Dupuytren's contracture: The aetiological role of trauma. *Scand. J. Plast. Reconstr. Surg.* (Dedication volume to K. B. Rasmusson.) P. 29, 1971.

39

Tumors of the Hand

JAMES W. SMITH AND RANDOLPH H. GUTHRIE

Tumors of the hand can prove to be a challenge in differential diagnosis. Boyes [1], Mason and Wheelock [11], Posch [15], Pack [13, 14], Stack [18], and others [7] who have reviewed the subject emphasize that tumors may arise from any of the tissues in the hand.

BENIGN TUMORS

Ganglia

The ganglion is by far the most common tumor found in the hand; it nearly always appears at one of three sites: (1) the dorsum of the wrist, (2) the volar radial aspect of the wrist, and (3) the volar surface of a finger near its base. Ganglia develop more frequently in women than in men; they are rarely found in children. Trauma, either in the form of direct injury or repeated minor trauma, is often reported by the patient to have preceded the swelling [10].

When they appear on the dorsum of the wrist, ganglia are frequently accompanied by complaints of weakness or pain. They usually arise from the scaphoid-lunate ligament and protrude from between the common digital extensor tendon of the index finger and the long extensor tendon of the thumb. Then a swelling is observed under the skin; it becomes more apparent and firmer as the wrist is volar-flexed.

Ganglia on the volar surface of the wrist appear to arise from the synovial tissue of the radiotrapezial joint or from the adjacent ligamentous tissues.

Both volar and dorsal ganglia appear to have their origin in the connective tissue near joints, but they do not communicate with the synovial spaces. Most contain a thick gelatinous fluid high in mucin content. The floor of the ganglion often appears contiguous with the joint lining; at this site there will be an area several millimeters in diameter where the tissues seem transparent and almost look like a window between the ganglion and the joint.

Although ganglia at the base of the finger contain the same type of gelatinous fluid as the others, they nearly always seem to arise from the flexor tendon sheath (Fig. 39-1). They appear after the local tissues have become pinched, compressed, or injured in some manner. Because of their intimate relationship with the flexor tendon sheath, these small, round, fixed masses can often be identified by the fact that they do not move back and forth with the underlying tendon as the finger moves. While tenderness may be associated with these ganglia on direct pressure, they seldom seem accompanied by the severe complaints of pain produced by ganglia on the dorsum of the hand.

TREATMENT. Among the many forms of treatment recommended for ganglia is rupture of the cyst with a heavy book. Down through the years the Bible has been considered the book that gave the best results. However, nearly all ganglia recur after this form of therapy.

Another technique currently popular is to aspirate the thick, gelatinous fluid after anesthetizing the overlying skin, and to replace the fluid with a mixture of lidocaine (1%) and a synthetic corticosteroid such as triamcinolone (40 mg./ml.) in equal parts instilled into the cystic cavity. At the same time, some physicians try to perforate the wall of the ganglia at several sites with the injecting needle. While a small percentage of ganglia appear to diminish in size or disappear following this treatment, it should not be used repeatedly to treat recurrences.

Complete excision is probably the best treatment. It is best to use a pneumatic tourniquet so that the site of origin can be properly identified and the ganglion completely excised. In the best of circumstances, recurrence is common even when the lesion appears to have been completely excised.

Mucous Cysts

Mucous cysts are typically found on the side of the dorsal skin of a distal phalanx (Fig. 39-2). Seventy-five percent of these lesions occur in females, and the middle finger is most commonly involved. They often result from an underlying bony spur. The covering skin is so thin that the clear, mucoid fluid can be seen inside the cyst. They rarely grow larger than 5 mm., but the distension of the dorsal finger tissues often renders them extremely painful. Compression of the surrounding tissue may also groove the adjacent fingernail. Aspiration of the fluid with instillation of triamcinolone (Kenalog; 40 mg./ml.) or methylprednisolone (Depo-Medrol; 40 mg./ml.) is worth a trial, and patients often are relieved of symptoms for many months. Definitive treatment involves opening the cyst and rongeuring off the bony spur. We no longer use a split-thickness or full-thickness skin graft from the antecubital fossa or a local rotation flap for closure. If no skin is excised, the area will close spontaneously after the bony spur is eliminated.

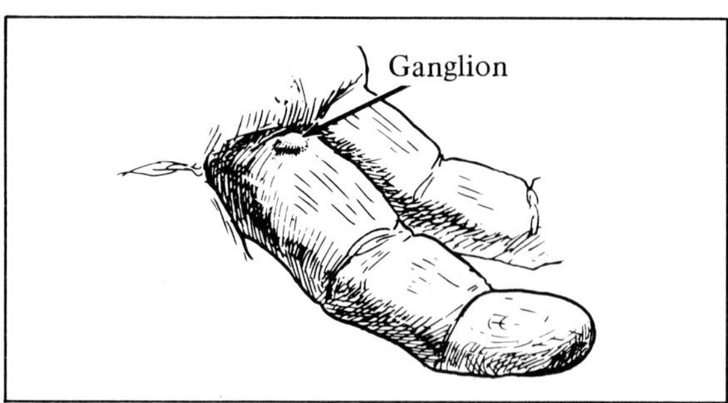

Fig. 39-1. Ganglion at the base of the finger. Any small, round, fixed mass at the base of the finger, on its volar surface, may be a ganglion. It does not move back and forth with the underlying tendon as the finger moves.

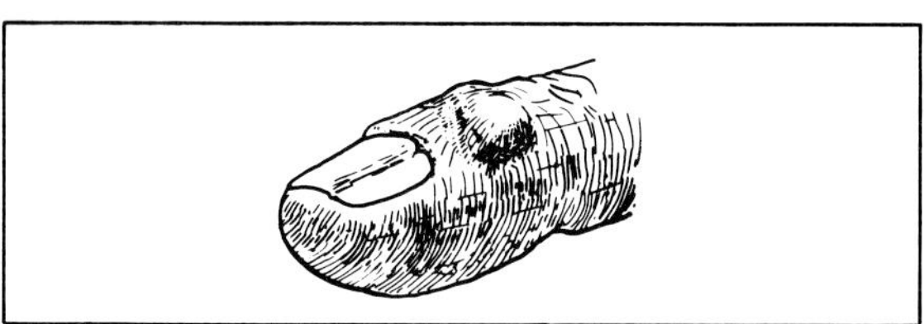

Fig. 39-2. Mucous cyst. This cyst is located on the dorsum of the finger near the base of the nail. Because the cyst is intimately involved with the overlying skin, excision requires the removal of both skin and cyst. The defect can be resurfaced with either a split-thickness or a full-thickness skin graft.

Epidermoid Cysts

Traumatic puncture wounds may drive small pieces of skin into the subdermal tissues where the implanted glandular elements continue to function. The resultant accumulations of sebaceous-like material produce a round, rubbery, freely movable, sometimes tender mass. The distal phalanx is the most common site, and, because of the tightness of the tissues, bone erosion may occur. If symptomatic, these cysts must be removed; the surgeon must include the entire capsule to prevent recurrence. Involved bone must be curetted.

Sebaceous Cysts

There are no sebaceous glands in palmar skin, but they do occur in the dorsal skin. A blockage of sebaceous gland ducts, presumably from injury, infection, or irritation, causes a cyst to form. It is typically about 1 cm. in size, well circumscribed, movable, and slow growing. Its characteristic sign is a small dimple in the center of the dome, which is an expanded duct. Such a cyst frequently becomes infected, and patients often delay seeing a physician until the infection has occurred. Malignancies rarely develop.

Treatment is surgical removal. A small ellipse of skin is taken, including the dimple and the entire cyst wall, to prevent recurrences. If the cyst is infected when first seen, initial therapy involves the application of moist compresses. If much erythema surrounds the infected cyst, an antibiotic may be given. If the infection does not subside, the cyst should be incised and drained.

Verrucae (Warts)

Verrucae are caused by a contagious virus that may be passed from one person to another, or from one place in the body to another. They are found most commonly in children but can occur at all ages. Verrucae are discrete, circumscribed, and raised, have rough surfaces, and are usually found around the fingernails [5]. If transected, they disclose many fine blood vessels arising from the base, which appear as tiny puncta. Verrucae around the fingernails are notorious for their propensity to recur, often because of inadequate removal for fear of permanent injury to the nail bed.

Warts have been the object of home-invented remedies and old wives' tales more than any other disease. Because the spontaneous disappearance of warts is not uncommon, fanciful remedies are frequently rewarded with success. In actuality, spontaneous disappearance is probably the result of autoimmunization. More standard realistic treatments include the following:

1. Various acids, applied with a dropper directly onto the warts once or twice a day, have been used with success. The most popular of these is trichloroacetic acid. The process takes several months and must be continued until the deep root of the wart has been completely burned out.
2. Radiation has been used and is reported to be highly effective, but we strongly advise against it since the dosage necessary to destroy the wart may permanently damage the skin.
3. Surgical removal of warts is effective if there is enough adjacent skin to allow closure. Otherwise, a skin graft may be needed. Tightness of skin usually precludes surgical excision around the fingernail.
4. Electrodesiccation is the most common method of treatment. The wart is burned until a thin black crust is formed. The crust is removed with forceps and a knife, and the electrodesiccation is again applied. The process is repeated until the entire wart and its deep base are removed. This can be done easily in an office under local anesthesia. The resultant wound heals rapidly under a simple

Band-Aid, and the scar is usually unnoticeable and asymptomatic.

Keratoses

Keratoses usually are benign but occasionally undergo malignant degeneration. Keratoses are of two types: senile, and seborrheic. Microscopically, both types show hypertrophy of the epidermis. and they are probably both caused by irritation.

The *senile keratoses* are formed in people with fair complexions who are frequently exposed to the irritating effects of sun, wind, and salt water. Usually these dark-gray or brown spots on the skin are less than 1 cm. in diameter and may be rough or covered with scales. Occasionally they are flat. Ulceration, inflammation, or sudden growth suggest malignant change.

Seborrheic keratoses are greasy, crusted, flat or raised lesions. They may grow as large as 5 cm. in diameter but are usually about 1 cm., and are covered with yellow, brown, or black horny masses, overlying a small, central wartlike core. Malignant degeneration is uncommon but does occur.

Treatment of keratoses is much the same as for warts. They can be removed with dry ice or electrocoagulation, or by surgical excision. Another acceptable form of treatment is with 5-fluorouracil cream, which effectively removes senile keratoses. It is particularly useful when an area has multiple small lesions, since this treatment may avoid multiple excisions and also removes microscopic growths. We have found that the best results come from a 5 percent concentration of the cream applied twice a day until marked erythema results, usually in 10 to 21 days. The skin affected by the cream sloughs superficially within 2 weeks after cessation of the treatment, removing the lesions with the slough. If a lesion persists, it must be surgically excised, and a biopsy should be performed.

Scraping of a keratosis is commonly done when the cosmetic result is especially important. A sharp scalpel is used. The lesion with a small margin of surrounding epidermis is abraded until a clean dermal base is produced. The scrapings are sent to the pathology laboratory for examination; if they prove malignant, excisional surgery is done.

Nevi

Nevi (or moles) are classified into types, depending on the location of the nevus cells within different layers of the skin. *Compound nevi* are about 5 mm. in diameter; they are slightly raised, light brown, and hair-bearing. *Intradermal nevi* are usually flat and hairless; they may be brown, black, or colorless. A *blue nevus* is usually flat, dark blue or black, and hairless. The *junctional nevus* is usually flat, dark brown, and hairless. It is probably the most important of all the nevi to both patient and physician because it can degenerate into malignant melanoma. The telltale signs of degeneration are sudden enlargement, elevation, ulceration, bleeding, darkening, and induration. Moles in the palmar skin of the hand are almost always junctional, and removal of these is frequently recommended.

When a mole is being excised, the incision should entirely encompass the lesion, including a definite margin of normal skin around it. The margins of the specimen must be labeled; if the tumor is malignant, the diagnosis can be made and it can be determined where in the wound there may still be malignant tissue.

One-half the patients in a large series with malignant melanoma had a history of previous treatment by acids, dry ice, or electrodesiccation. An accurate diagnosis had never been made. If a nevus needs treatment, surgical excision is warranted, a point that cannot be made too strongly.

Angiomas

The category of lesions termed *angiomas* includes malformations of both the blood and lymph channels. These lesions are almost entirely congenital in origin and may or may not connect with the normal blood or lymph system. If they do connect, they are enlarged at birth. If they do not, they may not become apparent until later life, at which time an angioma may suddenly grow to enormous size.

Xanthomas

Often referred to as *giant-cell tumors* or *localized nodular tenosynovitis,* these tumors represent the second most common subcutaneous tumors of the hand (Fig. 39-3). They are found with equal frequency in both hands, but appear more often in the index and middle fingers. Xanthomas are most commonly seen in patients between the ages of 40 and 60 years, but are not predominant in either sex. Though frequently found near joints, their origin is unknown. They can fill an interphalangeal joint space or erode a bone by pressure. An x-ray film that demonstrates such an erosion strongly supports the diagnosis of xanthoma. When a xanthoma arises from joint capsule or lies near to it, it may begin to cause such symptoms of mechanical interference as limitation of motion. These tumors may surround the digital nerves and can produce symptoms of numbness or discomfort. They are characterized by firmness, irregularity, and good encapsulation even though they can be palpated as multiple, adjacent nodules. The firmness of the tumors frequently aids in distinguishing them from lipomas and angiomas. The diagnosis of ganglion or one of the other tumors that might be considered is

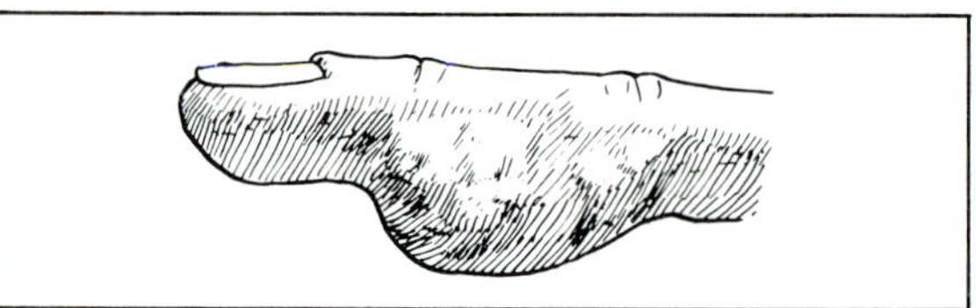

Fig. 39-3. Xanthoma. Xanthomas are found near joints, and very often an x-ray examination reveals an area of erosion in the adjacent bone. At the time of surgery the variegated appearance confirms the diagnosis.

less likely when the xanthoma is lying near a joint, when it is asymmetrically located, and when its tension does not change with position [16].

TREATMENT. Treatment should consist of carefully excising the mass in the operating room. A pneumatic tourniquet should be used because of the frequency with which these tumors extend into joints or around nerves. At the time of surgery, the variegated gray-yellow and brownish areas immediately confirm the diagnosis. On pathological examination, these tumors will be found to contain round cells and multinucleated giant cells in some specific areas, while in others there will be decreased cellularity, increased collagen, and fibrosis. Scattered groups of macrophages and foam cells are also seen.

Lipomas

Lipomas are fatty tumors that are usually soft, generally lobulated, and surrounded by a thin but definite capsule. The capsule sometimes creates a sense of fluctuation on palpation; this can make it difficult to differentiate the lipoma from a hemangioma. If the area becomes firmer when it is cooled with ice, the lesion is more likely to be a lipoma; the consistency of a hemangioma usually remains about the same [8].

Lipomas are found on both the dorsal and the volar aspects of the hand and may arise in subcutaneous tissues or in such deep sites as beneath the muscles of the thenar eminence. In some cases they seem to involve tendon sheaths. At the thenar eminence, a lipoma can lie hidden beneath the thenar muscles for a long time until suddenly trauma causes it to herniate through a weak point in the fascia and appear almost as if by magic.

TREATMENT. Treatment should consist of surgical removal. Such surgery is best performed with the use of a pneumatic tourniquet to be certain that all components of a multilobulated lipoma are identified and completely removed. It may be necessary to tease them from around any peripheral nerve that might pass through the center; care should be exercised not to injure the nerve.

Fibromas and Neurofibromas

Fibromas are rare in the hand and consist of a collection of fibrous tissue in the subcutaneous layer of the skin. Occasionally a fibroma grows through the skin to become a surface mass or even pedunculated. Fibromas are usually single but may be multiple. The lesions are very firm in most cases but may be soft, particularly in children. They are not known to undergo malignant degeneration [5].

Neurofibromas consist of the same collection of fibrous tissue but intermingled with nerve tissue. These lesions are often associated with von Recklinghausen's disease, where they may be multiple over the entire body [5]. Treatment of a single neurofibroma, as of simple fibromas, is surgical excision. The multiple neurofibromas accompanying von Recklinghausen's disease are usually too numerous to resect, and in any event new ones constantly appear. However, 13 percent of neurofibromas found in this disease are reported to undergo malignant degeneration, and suspicious lesions should, therefore, be excised.

The origins of fibromas and neurofibromas are unknown. Neurofibroma is frequently seen in conjunction with gigantism of the finger. In such cases there are often neurofibromas involving the nerves of the forearm and palm.

Tumors of Peripheral Nerve

Neuromas

Neuromas are benign tumors of nerve tissue. They usually result from trauma to a peripheral nerve, where some or all of the nerve fibers, or axons, have been severed. As these axons attempt to regenerate, some of them become adherent to adjacent scar tissue and form a neuroma. If sensory fibers are present, the neuroma may become quite sensitive and painful.

A neuroma can make the end of an amputated finger quite painful if it is in a spot where it is repeatedly bumped. In this instance, the pain may be lessened by repeatedly striking the finger against a firm surface. If symptoms do not improve sufficiently, the neuroma can be identified by surgery and its nerve transected at a more proximal level. Then it will lie in an area away from the scar tissue; the new neuroma that forms will then be at a site where it will be subjected to trauma less frequently. Other forms of treatment include injecting it with alcohol, covering it with a silicone cap, and tying off the end. No treatment to date has proved totally effective for solving this problem. (This problem is discussed in greater detail in Chapter 36.)

Neurilemomas (Schwannomas)

Neurilemomas arise from the Schwann cells of peripheral nerve sheaths [3]. They are rarely found in the hand but one may appear as a painful swelling in the forearm along the course of the median or ulnar nerve. Tapping over neurilemomas will produce a sensation described as "pins and needles" or "an electric shock." The neurilemoma will usually shell out of the nerve sheath readily when the overlying epineurium over it has been incised. At times the tumor is adherent to the nerve; removal necessitates sectioning of the nerve followed by primary anastomosis.

Glomus Tumors

Glomus tumors [6] arise from a normal glomus, a structure that is believed, under normal circumstances, to control blood pressure and temperature by regulating peripheral blood flow. They are seen more frequently in women than in men, and in about half the cases they are located subungually (Fig. 39-4). Such lesions are known for the unusually severe, radiating pain that can be triggered by pressure, by impact, or often by temperature change. Application of cold water or ice to the area produces discomfort, while heat tends to relieve it. When such a lesion is located subungually, it appears as a bluish or cyanotic discoloration beneath the fingernail. The lunula of the nail may be blurred and the nail may be raised or have a transverse convexity. If located in the terminal phalanx, the glomus tumor can have a cystic appearance that permits roentgenological detection. When found just under the skin, it may be reported as an exquisitely tender nodule.

TREATMENT. At exploration the glomus tumor can appear as a salmon-colored or flesh-colored spongy mass or as a purple mass of varicosities, depending on its vascular composition. It can be so small that magnification will be needed for its identification.

The best surgical incision for removing a glomus located beneath the fingernail will in part depend upon its actual location. However, since most of these lesions actually lie beneath the nail bed, an incision that permits elevation of the bed from the underlying phalanx is preferable. Those lying under the proximal end of the nail can be removed through an incision placed about halfway between the joint and the base of the nail. At this site neither the extensor tendon insertion nor the nail root is damaged if the incision is carried down to the phalanx so that the nail root and nail bed can be elevated as a unit.

Microscopic examination shows the tumor to consist of many nonmyelinated nerve fibers and blood vessels; the walls of the blood vessels are thickened by layers of round cells. These cells have clear cytoplasm around the nucleus and have been identified as pericytes.

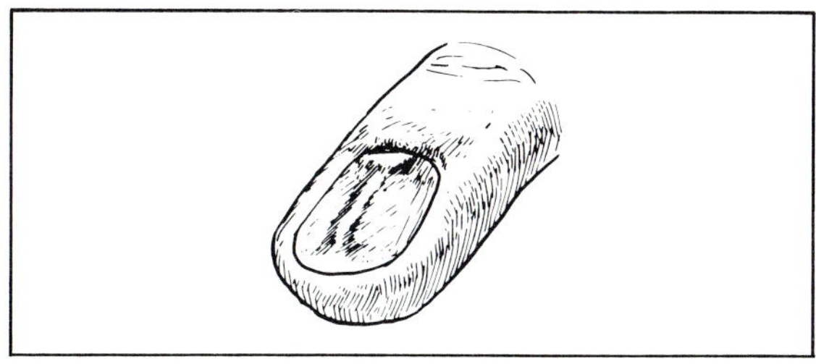

Fig. 39-4. Glomus tumor. A bluish or cyanotic streak beneath the fingernail, accompanied by pain, suggests the presence of a glomus tumor. These tumors are also sensitive to changes in temperature.

Aneurysms

False aneurysms of the palmar arteries usually follow a penetrating wound complicated by direct arterial injury [17]. Their walls are formed by the organization of fibrous tissue, a feature that distinguishes them from the "true" aneurysm.

The *true aneurysm* develops by fusiform dilation of the arterial wall once it has been weakened by idiopathic, mycotic, or traumatic processes. Its walls still retain the basic features of an artery even though they may be distorted. Special histological preparations are often required to demonstrate the presence of smooth muscle or elastic fibers. When no definite history of a blunt injury or of repetitive minor trauma can be obtained, the terms *idiopathic* and *spontaneous* aneurysm have been employed.

True aneurysms develop at three specific sites: (1) near the hamate bone, (2) at the base of the thenar eminence, and (3) in the deep palmar arterial arch.

The hamate bone is by far the most common site of true aneurysm (Fig. 39-5). The hamate probably functions as an anvil, and any cushioning effect of the adjacent soft tissue is lessened by the nearness of the bone. This makes repeated trauma to the ulnar artery overlying it especially damaging.

SIGNS AND SYMPTOMS. The signs and symptoms produced by palmar aneurysms are related to their location, size, and direction of protrusion. They often start as a soreness that has the characteristics of a bruise or ache. Discomfort is accentuated by any local pressure or trauma, regardless of how slight. This discomfort increases with the appearance of a tender swelling. The presence of pulsations corresponding to those of arteries elsewhere, a thrill, and a bruit are all of great help in establishing the diagnosis. However, any or all may be absent, especially if the aneurysmal sac is filled with an organizing

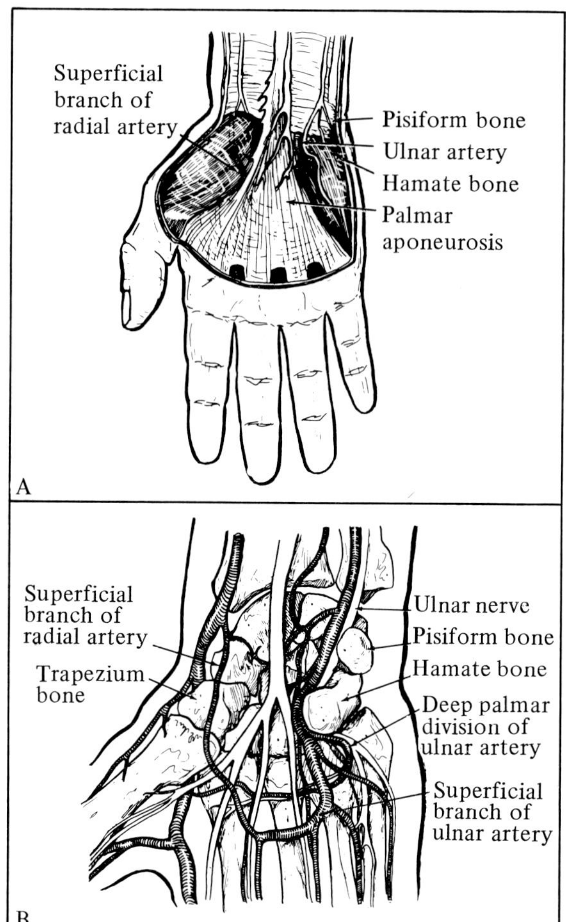

Fig. 39-5. Aneurysms of the hand. A, the two sites where the superficial arterial arch appears most vulnerable to injury: on the hypothenar eminence adjacent to the hamate bone and on the thenar eminence where the trapezium lies beneath the superficial branch of the radial artery; neither location has the protection of the palmar aponeurosis. They are the most common sites for "true palmar aneurysms." B, anatomical relationships of the two component branches of the superficial arterial palmar arch to the underlying bony structures. Note that the ulnar artery is relatively fixed at the level of the hamate bone by the course of its deep arterial branch. The superficial radial artery is held to a definite course over the trapezium by its passage between the abductor brevis and opponens muscles. Repeated trauma to these sites causes more damage because of the arterial fixation and underlying bony anvils. (From J. W. Smith Am. J. Surg. *104:7, 1962.)*

thrombus. This fact has resulted in the mistaken diagnosis of abscess on several occasions. The true nature of the swelling, however, becomes apparent at the time of operative intervention.

TREATMENT. The treatment of palmar aneurysms is surgical excision. It is recommended that a pneumatic tourniquet be employed. Those aneurysms that involve the ulnar artery can most easily be approached through an incision paralleling the flexion crease at the base of the hypothenar eminence.

Those aneurysms located on the thenar eminence should be approached through an incision paralleling the flexion crease at the base of the thumb.

Enchondromas

Enchondromas are solitary, benign bone tumors of congenital origin that are almost always found in the hand [4]. Such lesions are believed to arise from cartilagenous rests; they are frequently not identified or called to the attention of a physician until a pathological fracture occurs through the site of the tumor. Enchondromas are easy to identify because they appear on x-ray examination as eccentrically located, radiolucent areas in the bone covered with a distended thin cortex (Fig. 39-6). Such lesions result in pathological fracture in almost 25 percent of cases.

Microscopic examination of this bone tumor shows it to consist of hyaline cartilage with a lobulated pattern. The chondrocytes tend to be uniformly small, with dark-staining nuclei. Such a tumor is probably best treated by surgical curettage, the resultant cavity being filled with bone chips. Malignant degeneration, although extremely rare, has been reported.

Osteoid Osteomas

The osteoid osteoma is rare in the hand. The patient is almost always in the 15- to 30-year-old age group, and the condition presents as localized pain and swelling. The pathological picture on x-ray is one of a small nidus involving both cortex and medulla of bone. The lesion is usually less than 1 cm. in diameter and is filled with fibrous tissue mixed with osteoid material but without calcified trabeculae. The etiology is unknown. When the lesion is symptomatic, the entire nodule can be removed and replaced with an iliac bone graft or bone chips.

Exostoses

Exostoses grow outwardly from the cortex of bones and are usually capped by a covering of cartilage. They are also known as osteochondromas, chondromas, or exostoses cartilaginea. It is not known whether these lesions are congenital or neoplastic. When multiple, they may be hereditary. Symptoms are rare, and treatment is usually requested for cos-

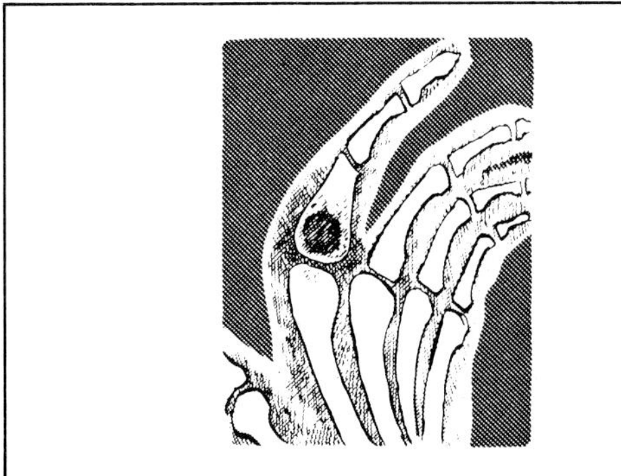

Fig. 39-6. Enchondroma. These lesions are easily identified on x-ray study as eccentrically located, radiolucent areas in bone, covered by a thin distended cortex. An associated pathological fracture is often encountered and first calls attention to the lesion.

metic improvement. The tumor can be simply removed with a chisel and rongeur, the bone being shaped to a normal contour.

MALIGNANT TUMORS

Both basal cell carcinomas and squamous cell carcinomas are common on the backs of the hands. Sixty percent of skin cancers of the hand occur in persons older than 60, and only 1 percent in those under the age of 30. Males predominate over females by two to one, and three-quarters of the malignant skin lesions are of the basal cell type.

Malignant tumors of the skin are most often the result of radiation; they can result from a number of common irritative agents including radiation, sunlight, burns, and chronic infections with resulting scars and ulcerations, chemical irritants, and chronic arsenical poisoning. They are often small lesions that appear innocuous, and they are frequently mistaken for nevi or keratoses. These lesions are often ignored and allowed to grow larger or to metastasize. They may be treated with electrodesiccation or caustic agents; at best, this delays the diagnosis of malignancy, while at worst, the tumor may spread or be converted into a more virulent form. All skin tumors must be viewed with a high degree of suspicion for malignancy, and the slightest doubt warrants an excisional biopsy.

Basal Cell Carcinoma

The typical patient with a basal cell carcinoma is an elderly, light-complexioned blond with thin, dry, wrinkled skin. The patient has a slowly growing, burrowing "rodent-ulcer" that begins as a small, beaded, discrete nodule, often with telangiectases just under its surface. As the tumor grows, it usually ulcerates centrally, producing a crater surrounded by an irregular rim. If it is neglected, growth will continue through a burrowing attack on the surrounding normal skin, leaving a widening crater in the center. It is dangerous to life only if it invades important neighboring structures. There have been reports of metastases, but these are exceedingly rare.

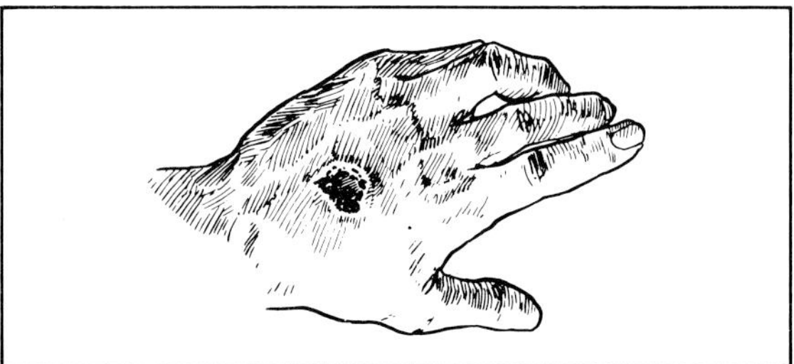

Fig. 39-7. Squamous cell carcinoma of the hand. Most of these tumors are found on the back of the hand, have a somewhat irregular umbilicated appearance, and are ulcerated in the center.

Squamous Cell Carcinoma (Epidermoid Carcinoma)

Squamous cell carcinomas typically develop at a younger age in patients who have light, sensitive skin and a history of exposure to sun, wind, and salt water; significant radiation or irritating chemicals; or persistent dermatoses, warts, moles, or long-standing scars.

The lesion may closely resemble basal cell carcinoma, appearing as a small papule and spreading centrifugally with an advancing rim surrounding a central ulcerated crater (Fig. 39-7). However, this lesion is always more indurated than basal cell types, and the rim is not as discrete. Sometimes squamous cell carcinoma assumes an entirely different form and is then seen as a flat, dry keratosis blending into the surrounding skin. In both cases its rapid rate of growth gives away the diagnosis. Squamous cell carcinoma is much more dangerous than basal cell carcinoma because it has the capacity not only to invade neighboring structures but also to metastasize early to regional lymph nodes.

If nodes are obviously involved, they too must be removed at operation. If they are not visibly enlarged and no evidence is seen of their involvement at operation for the primary tumor, prophylactic resections are not routinely done. These lesions are separated by the pathologist, on the basis of their appearance, into four grades: Grade I the least and Grade IV the most malignant. Statistically, Grade I lesions recur in 10 percent of cases and Grade IV in 90 percent. The overall mortality is 19 percent. With lesions over 5 cm. in diameter, it is 82 percent; with lesions under 1 cm., 7 percent.

Malignant Melanoma

The term *malignant melanoma* is unnecessary because the single word *melanoma* suffices to describe this disease fully; it was known historically as "black cancer." It results from the malignant degeneration of a nevus. Usually, and fortunately for ease of detection, the lesions are pigmented. However, the primary lesion and its metastases may contain no pigment and have no dark color, in which case it is known as *amelanotic* melanoma.

Melanoma may spread both by lymph channels and through the blood stream [12]. It often does so by either route early in its course. There are numerous examples that show a relation of the initial complaint with liver metastases. The primary tumor is sometimes difficult to find. It is thought that melanomas arise only from nevi with "junctional changes," those with a disruption of the basal layer of the skin. Since nevi occurring on the palms of the hands are almost always junctional, particular attention should be paid to them.

This disease occurs in one out of every 50,000 people and represents 2 percent of all malignant tumors and 20 percent of all skin cancers [14]. Paradoxically, it is very rare in blacks. The average age of incidence is around 50 years. The typical melanoma at first looks like a blue-black or brown-black nevus. It is usually firm, smooth, and hairless. With the onset of malignant change there is sudden growth, darkening of color, ulceration, bleeding, or the appearance of an erythematous, inflammatory halo around the tumor. Any one of these signs means that the nevus should be removed immediately.

If the tumor is diagnosed microscopically as a melanoma, then regardless of whether or not the pathology report shows the margins to be clear, a second surgical resection must be done, taking enough additional normal skin so that the margin of resection from the original tumor is 5 cm. or equal to the tumor diameter, whichever is greater. All the underlying subcutaneous tissue and fascia must be excised. This procedure usually necessitates coverage of the defect with a skin graft. In addition, a prophylactic lymph node dissection is normally done in continuity with the resection. If a finger is involved, amputation of the finger and its metacarpal (ray resection) is performed. In spite of these radical procedures, death is all too common from this disease. Of persons with lymph nodes microscopically free of disease, 40 percent are dead in 10 years; of those with involved nodes, 60 percent are dead in 10 years; and of those with palpable nodes that were not removed, 95 percent are dead in 10 years.

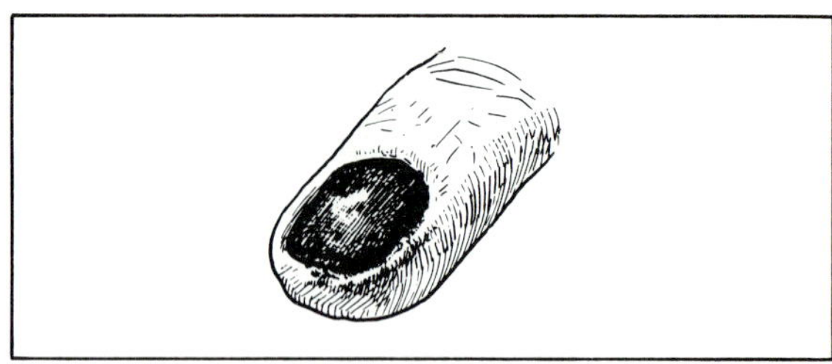

Fig. 39-8. Subungual melanoma. This appears initially as a black spot underneath the fingernail and is accompanied by a history of trauma in more than 60 percent of cases

Malignant Bone Tumors

Malignant bone tumors include osteogenic sarcoma, chondrosarcoma, fibrosarcoma, and metastatic tumors, principally from bronchogenic carcinoma. All are very rare in the hand, and instances of the first two are reportable [4]. In general, wide local resection of the tumors offers a good prognosis. Recurrence warrants amputation of the hand.

REFERENCES

1. Boyes, J. H. *Bunnell's Surgery of the Hand* (5th ed.). Philadelphia: Lippincott, 1970.
2. Butler, E. D., Hamill, J. P., Seipel, R. S., and de Lormier, A. A. Tumors of the hand. *Am. J. Surg.* 100:293, 1960.
3. Byrne, J. J. Nerve Tumors. In Flynn, J. E. (Ed.), *Hand Surgery* (2nd ed.). Baltimore: Williams & Wilkins, 1975. Pp. 693–701.
4. Carroll, R. E. Tumors of the Hand Skeleton. In Flynn, J. E. (Ed.), *Hand Surgery* (2nd ed.). Baltimore: Williams & Wilkins, 1975. Pp. 668–678.
5. Conway, H. *Surgery of Tumors of the Skin.* Springfield, Ill.: Thomas, 1966.
6. Curtis, R. E. Tumors of the Blood and Lymphatic Vessels. In Flynn, J. E. (Ed.), *Hand Surgery* (2nd ed.). Baltimore: Williams & Wilkins, 1975. Pp. 679–692.
7. Flynn, J. E. *Hand Surgery* (2nd ed.). Baltimore: Williams & Wilkins, 1975.
8. Gaisford, J. C. Tumors of the hand. *Surg. Clin. North Am.* 40:549, 1960.
9. Haber, H. H., Alter, A. H., and Wheelock, M. C. Tumors of the hand. *Surg. Gynecol. Obstet.* 121:1073, 1965.
10. Mason, M. L. Tumors of the hand. *Minn. Med.* 37:600, 1954.
11. Mason, M. L., and Wheelock, M. C. Aneurysmal bone cyst of the hand. *Q. Bull. Northwest. Univ. Med. School* 32:268, 1958.
12. Pack, G. T. *Tumors of the Hands and Feet.* St. Louis: Mosby, 1939.
13. Pack, G. T. Symposium: Tumors of the hands and feet. *Surgery* 5:1, 1939.

14. Pack, G. T., Gerber, D. M., and Scharnagel, I. M. End results in treatment of malignant melanoma: A report of 1190 cases. *Ann. Surg.* 136:905, 1952.
15. Posch, J. L. Tumors of the hand. *J. Bone Joint Surg.* [Am.] 38:517, 1956.
16. Posch, J. L. Soft Tissue Tumors of the Hand. In Flynn, J. E. (Ed.), *Hand Surgery* (2nd ed.). Baltimore: Williams & Wilkins, 1975. Pp. 642–667.
17. Smith, J. W. True aneurysms of traumatic origin in the palm. *Am. J. Surg.* 104:7, 1962.
18. Stack, H. G. Tumours of the hand. *Br. Med. J.* 1:919, 1960.

V

Microsurgery

Introduction to Microsurgery

HARRY J. BUNCKE, Jr., AND ZOLTAN SZABO

A new field of replantation and transplantation surgery has been opened by the successful anastomosis or repair of blood vessels having an external diameter of 1.0 mm. or less. It is now possible to replant amputated fingers, transplant toes to the hand, and transplant large composite blocks of tissue in the form of free microvascular flaps, microneurovascular flaps, micromyocutaneous flaps, and microosteocutaneous flaps – thus bypassing the classic techniques of delayed transfer using tubed pedicles and flaps. To perform these intricate procedures one must be able to use the operating microscope with dexterity. Practice is necessary, and the microsurgical laboratory is the backbone of any replantation or transplantation service or team. This training laboratory or training area may take the form of a single microscope near the main operating room where an individual can practice in his or her spare time; or it may be a formal laboratory containing several microscopes for research, training, and practice. The latter organized laboratory requires three basic ingredients:

1. A full-time laboratory supervisor and technical director.
2. Adequate equipment.
3. Funding and support from the institution and staff.

Given these ingredients, an environment can be created where surgeons can gain these microsurgical skills.

The operating microscope now found in almost all hospital operating rooms must be available in the laboratory (preferably in the form of diploscope so that two individuals can work together in the same operating field) for instruction and acquisition of joint operating skills and for the repair of small vessels and nerves. The instruments used in microvascular tissue transplantation are not elaborate. Most of these tools have been borrowed from other medical specialties or adapted from the field of electronics or jewelry assembly. Forceps for suture tying and dissection must be very fine pointed. The jaws should be delicately rounded on their edges so that they do not break the suture material. The flat handles of these instruments should be built up with silicone rubber or some other material to create a cylinder that can be rolled 45 to 90 degrees, thus increasing the range of manipulation under the microscope. Microscissors should be curved or straight for suture cutting and microdissection. Probably the most important instrument is the microvascular clamp of the single and double variety. These clamps are now available commercially with a blade-closing pressure of 30 to 50 gm. Pressure greater than this produces endothelial crushing leading to microvascular thrombosis. Needle holders also should be round-handled and without a lock (the release of a lock produces uncontrollable traumatic movement of the instrument tip). Microsutures are now available commercially in adequate supply, with needles varying from 30 to 140 microns; the needles are mounted on suture material of 15 to 30 microns. The very fine 30-micron needle is used for microlymphatic anastomoses and for the repair of vessels in the realm of 0.5 mm. The 70-micron needle is acceptable for vessels about 1.0 mm. in size, and the 140-micron needle is acceptable for vessels of 1.5 to 2.0 mm.

All of these delicate instruments must be carefully maintained. The points must be aligned and ground down and checked repeatedly under the microscope. The blade pressure of microvascular clamps should be calibrated and color coded. In addition, aneurysmal clamps with a crushing blade pressure of over 100 mg. per square millimeter must not become mixed with microvascular clamps used for temporary small vessel occlusion. The maintenance and checking of these instruments should be the responsibility of a trained technician either in the operating room or in the microsurgical laboratory.

BASIC PRINCIPLES FOR LABORATORY MICROSURGERY

Basic microsurgical manipulative skills are best acquired working on live experimental animals, preferably under supervision. The femoral artery and vein of a 300- to 400-gm. rat measures about 1.0 mm. in external diameter; such an animal provides an inexpensive training model. These basic maneuvers will be outlined in a steplike fashion in Figures 40-1 through 40-24.

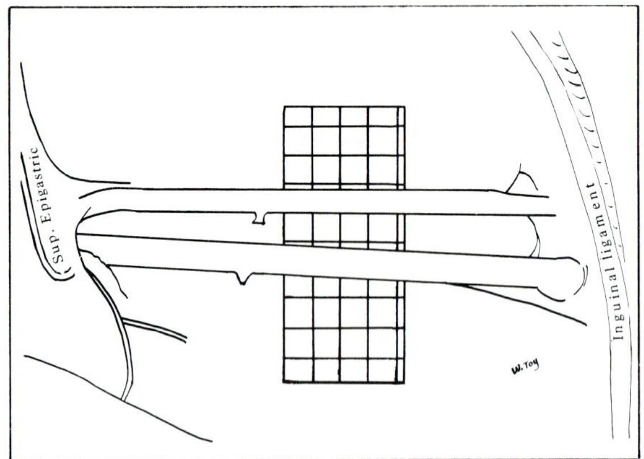

Fig. 40-1. Dissected vascular bundle of the rat femoral area. The groin area of the animal should be shaved and cleared from the inguinal ligament to the knee joint. The artery and vein are exposed through a liberal skin incision and by gentle dissection using sharp forceps from the femoral nerve and the perivascular aureolar tissue. Muscle branches from the artery and vein arising from the deeper surface should be coagulated, providing a vessel 3.0 to 4.0 cm. in length for the area of repair. The arterial repair will be described first.

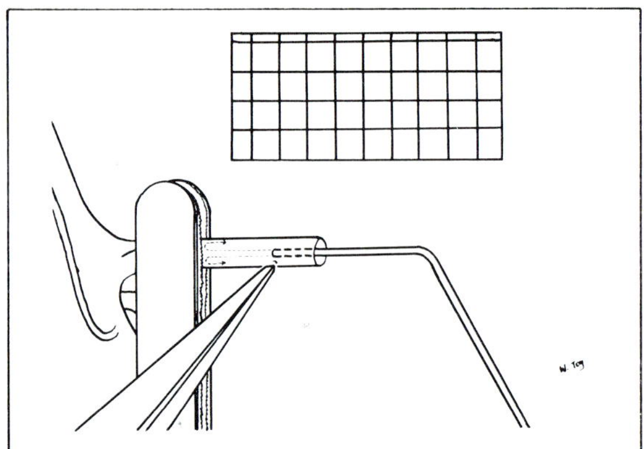

Fig. 40-2. Irrigation. The vessels once transected can be dilated hydrostatically by inserting a blunt 30-gauge needle and injecting sterile saline under pressure. Atraumatic dilatation can also be accomplished by inserting very fine tipped forceps into the lumen and gently separating the blades.

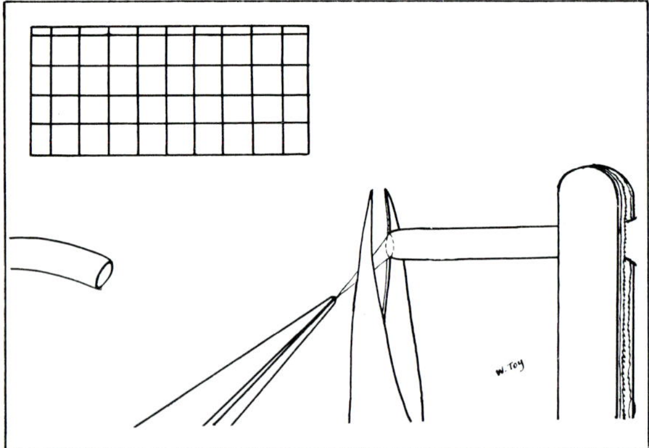

Fig. 40-3. Stripping of the adventitia. The adventitia need not be stripped over a great distance from the vessel ends. It can be easily removed by pulling it gently over the end of the vessel and debriding this adventitia with sharp scissors. Years ago, Jacobson described this as "circumcising the vessel." After the vessel has been stabilized in a double atraumatic clamp, the vessel ends should be brought together so that they can be approximated without tension. In a clinical situation if this cannot be achieved, one must consider the use of a vascular interpositional graft. It is sometimes possible to relieve some of this tension by dissecting the vessel proximally and distally free from the surrounding tissues. Occasionally a small branch can be mobilized and ligated. The ligating suture is left long and traction placed on this branch to relieve tension at the proposed site of anastomosis.

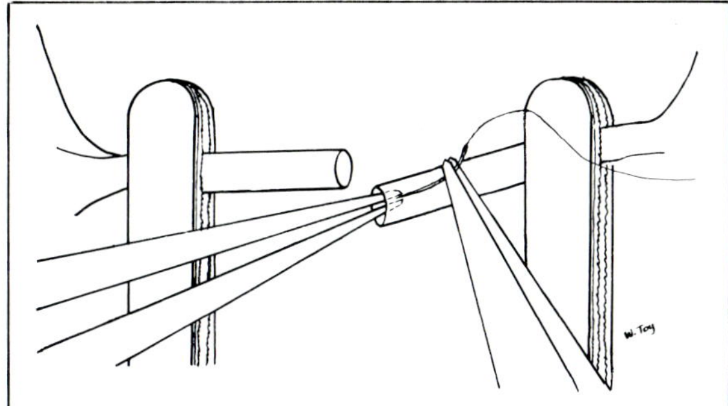

Fig. 40-4. First stitch, entrance bite. It is preferable to place the first stitch in the very top portion of the vessel using fine-tipped atraumatic forceps for counterpressure. The tip of the needle should be thrust through the wall between the assisting forceps blades with gentle but steady pressure. The present commercially available needles have fine tips; minimal vessel wall trauma is produced if the tip of the needle remains sharp. The microfine point of the needle can be completely blunted by the smallest of burs; therefore, one should be careful to avoid touching the tip of the needle with the instruments. The size of the bite should be varied according to the size of the vessel and the wall thickness. Too large a bite will cause inversion at the anastomosis line, while too small a bite will produce tearing and leakage. Once the needle is withdrawn with the assisting forceps, the lumen should be examined to be certain that the posterior wall has not been picked up.

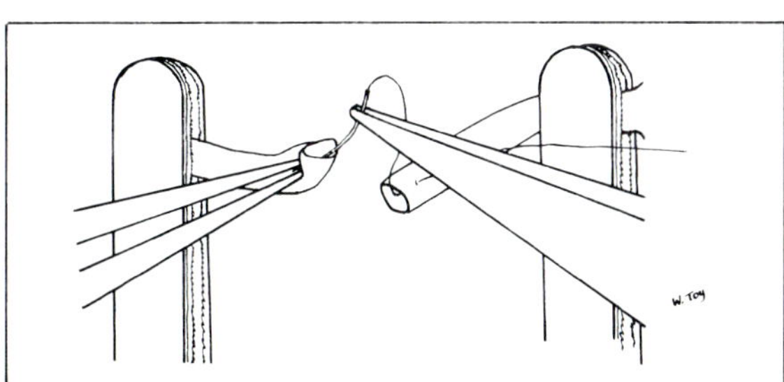

Fig. 40-5. First stitch, exit bite. The needle is then returned to the needle holder and the distal lumen cannulated with the needle. This is usually a simple maneuver with an artery but can prove challenging with a vein. Flooding the field with saline or even dilating the distal vessel with a blunt hypodermic needle is helpful. Once the lumen has been cannulated, the needle is withdrawn to the proposed exit site. Again, the assisting forceps is brought into position and the needle thrust between the blades, providing gentle counterpressure.

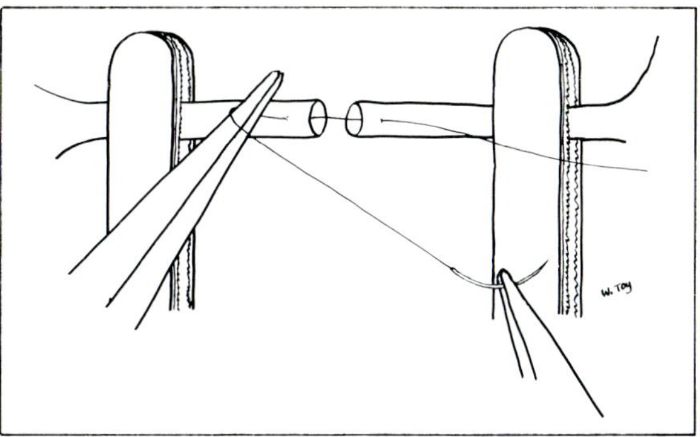

Fig. 40-6. Pulling the thread. The extracted needle is then returned to the needle holder and the assisting forceps is used as a pulley so that the suture material is pulled in a longitudinal fashion through the two puncture wounds. Failure to do this converts the thread into a saw, which increases the size of the needle hole and produces subsequent bleeding and platelet thrombosis. The suture end should be pulled int. the microscopic field so that the short tail is easily visible. There is a tendency to leave the short tail of the suture too long, which complicates the manipulation necessary for knot tying. If the free end can be positioned so that it lies on one of the clamp blades or background material, it can be picked up easily. If the short end lies on the vessel wall it is trapped by surface tension, where it sticks tenaciously. The tying forceps usually picks up shreds of the adventitia with the suture material, and the entire maneuver must be abandoned. One should slide the loose end of the suture off the vessel wall either onto smooth, colored background material or into the clamp blade.

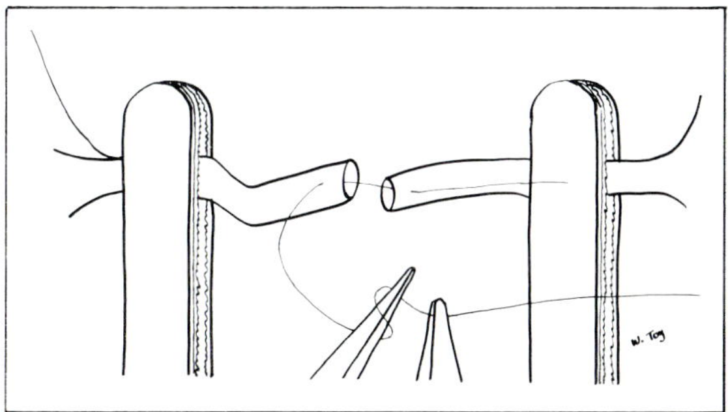

Fig. 40-7. Beginning of the knot-tying sequence. Knot tying. In order to lay the knots absolutely flat and square, it is sometimes easier to tie the first knot holding the long end of the suture with the needle holder; the second knot is tied holding the long end with the assisting forceps.

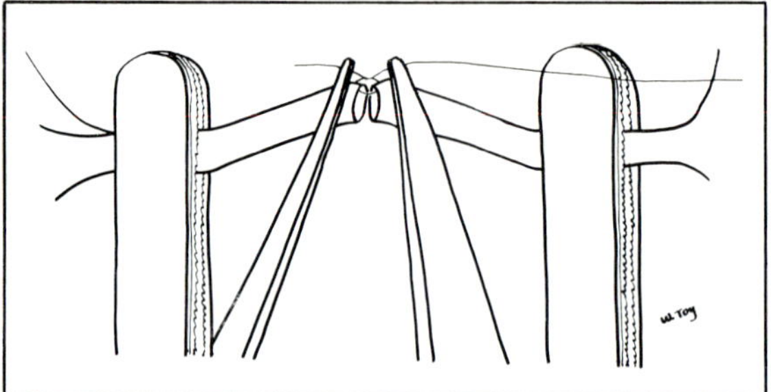

Fig. 40-8. The first knot is brought down snugly, lifting it up slightly so that the vessel edges are brought together accurately. The knot may be positioned somewhat in this fashion.

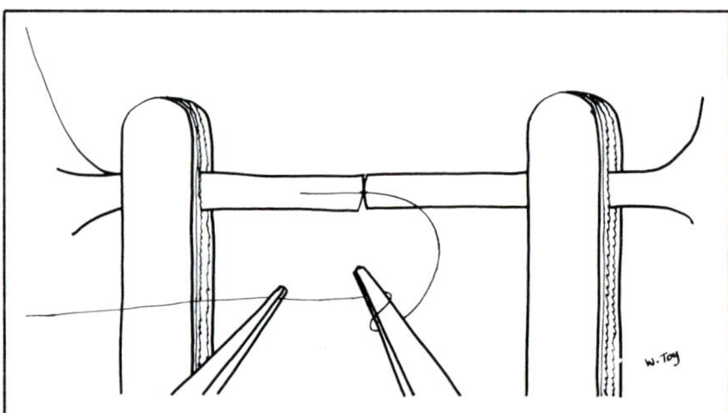

Fig. 40-9. The second knot is now thrown, holding the long end of the suture with the assisting forceps and tying with the needle holder. The short end is here visualized lying on the vessel wall where it will be extremely difficult to pick up. It should be slid off superiorly-inferiorly so that it can be picked up from the background material.

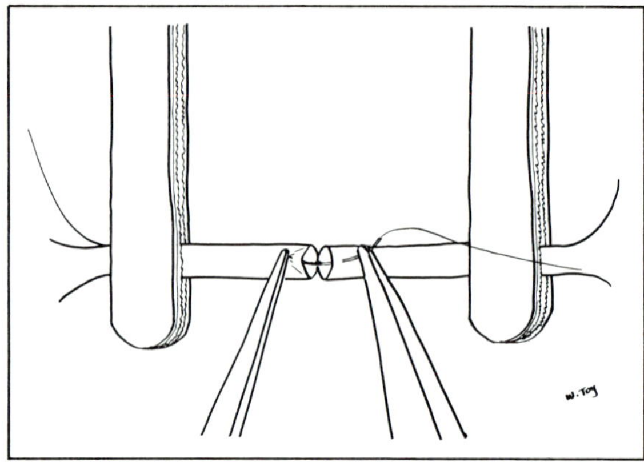

Fig. 40-10. Second stitch. The immobilizing double clamp is now rotated 180 degrees and the second suture placed directly opposite the first. The exit bite shown here is being performed using the assisting forceps for gentle counterpressure.

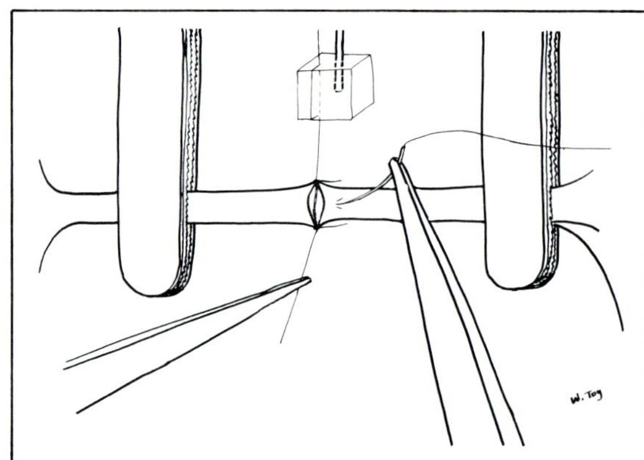

Fig. 40-11. Third stitch. The posterior stay suture has been immobilized in a small silicone block mounted on a bar extending from the double clamp. Gentle traction on the second suture aligns the vessel wall so that the third suture can be placed halfway in between. One may have to insert the assisting forceps into the lumen to provide counterpressure once the exact position of the third suture has been sighted.

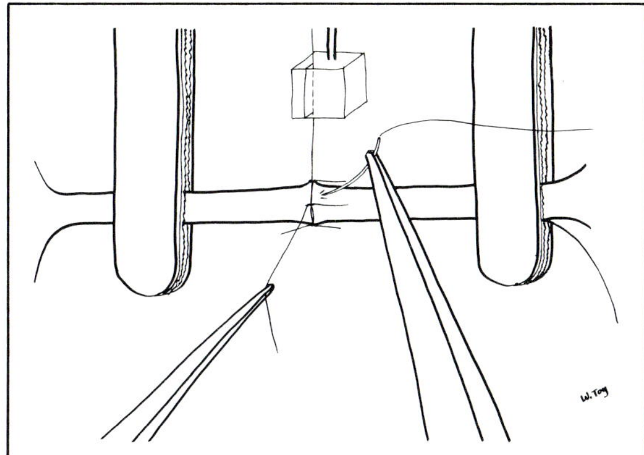

Fig. 40-12. Fourth stitch (deep thrust). The fourth suture is placed, halving the distance between the third suture and the stay secured in the silicone block. It is wise to examine each suture before the needle is brought through to be certain that the back wall has not been trapped. One can accomplish this by gently pulling on the previously inserted sutures or by dilating the vessel with heparinized saline. Once patency has been confirmed, the needle can be extracted and the knot completed.

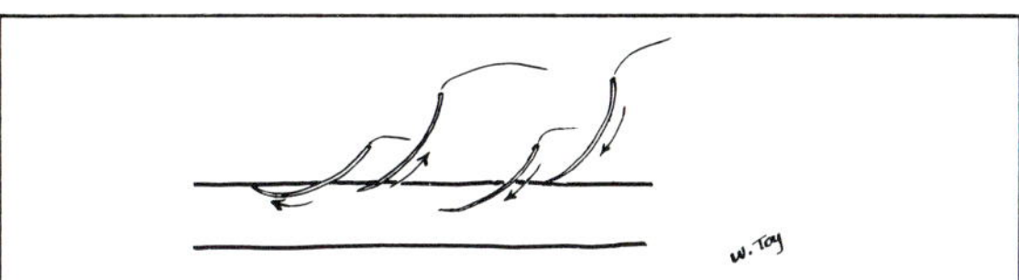

Fig. 40-13. This side view shows the deep thrust technique of passing the needle through the wall, retracting it slightly to be sure that the posterior wall has not been picked up, and then proceeding to extract the needle or complete the exit bite.

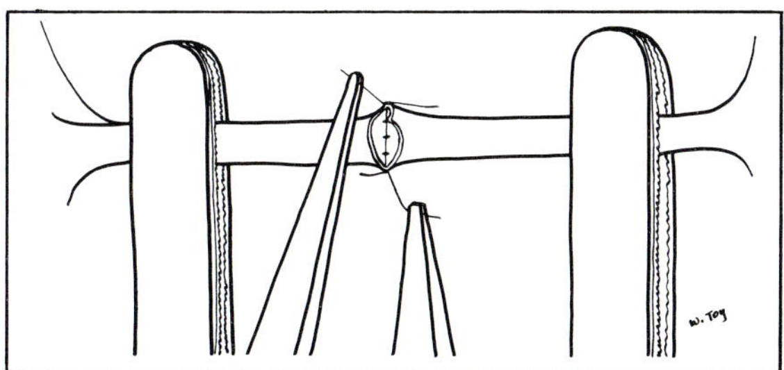

Fig. 40-14. Direct visual inspection of the luminal suture line (first half); the posterior wall has been picked up. The double clamp has now been rotated back to its original position, exposing the interior of the vessel. Suture placement and patency can be checked at this time.

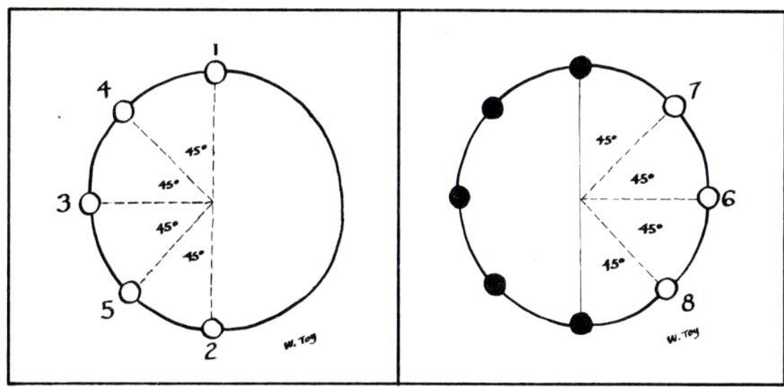

Fig. 40-15. Review of the suture placement sequence. One may have to vary the sequence in a clinical situation where the clamp cannot be rotated or the field cannot be oriented in an ideal fashion.

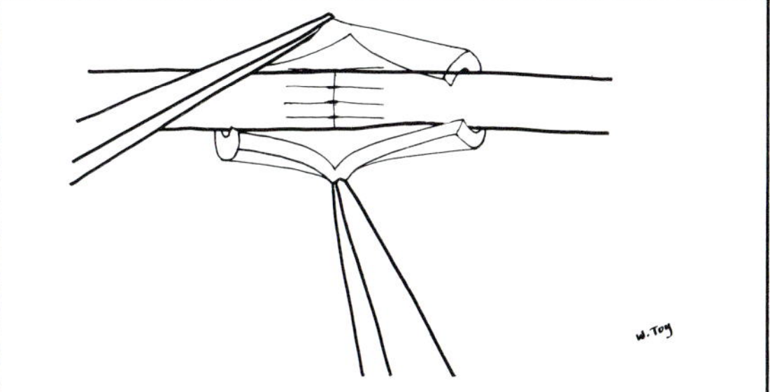

Fig. 40-16. The placement of a small segment of silicone tube cut longitudinally creates a hemostatic cuff around the vessel. (The silicone cuff is placed around the completed anastomosis before releasing the clamps. The distal clamp is released before the proximal clamp.) This additional external support helps to minimize the initial bleeding that occurs through the suture hole and the suture intervals. Eight sutures and a cuff are sufficient for 1.0-mm. vessels. A completely hemostatic repair can be performed with multiple small sutures but the additional trauma and foreign material make this type of repair unjustified.

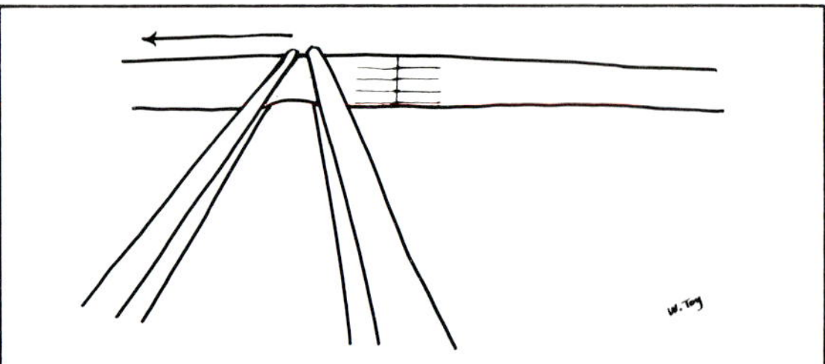

Fig. 40-17. Starting position of radical pressure test. The silicone cuff is removed after 4 or 5 minutes and the patency of flow confirmed downstream beyond the site of anastomosis, using two forceps in the radical patency test described by Acland. Pulsation in the region of the anastomosis does not necessarily mean patency. Pulsation several centimeters beyond the site of anastomosis in a clinical situation is certainly good evidence of patency.

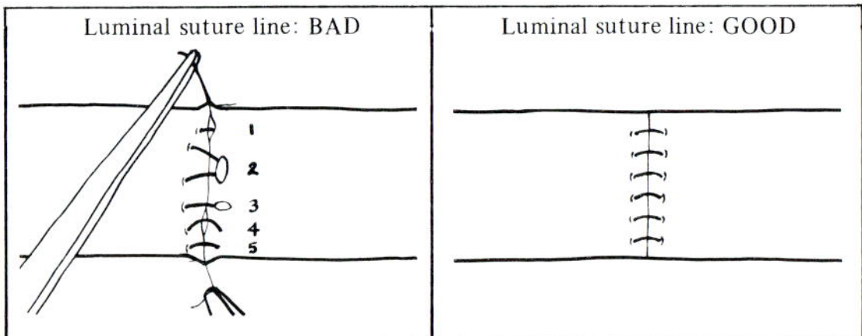

Fig. 40-18. Some of the common mistakes made in microvascular repairs are shown at top. Suture 1: small bite; the intimal layer was not included. Suture 2: converging neighboring stitches have created a large tear. Suture 3: unequal bites have caused a tear on the smaller side. Suture 4: a loose stitch has left a gap. Suture 5: a correct stitch. At the bottom, it can be seen that ideal repair has a finely tailored appearance; such a repair is attended with minimal platelet agglutination. Patency rates of almost 100 percent should be attained.

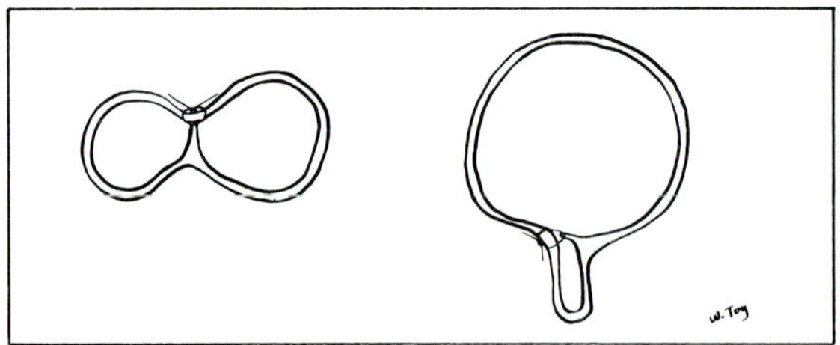

Fig. 40-19. Cross section of the most frequent error – picking up the posterior or lateral wall. Picking up the posterior wall produces a band across the vessel lumen, which inevitably leads to thrombosis.

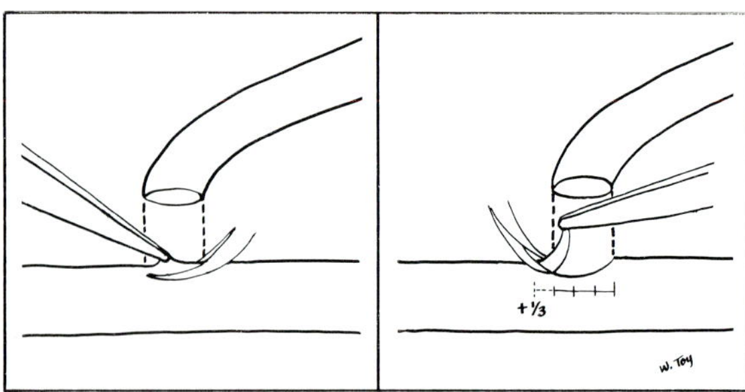

Fig. 40-20. End-to-side repairs must also be mastered, since they may be needed frequently in clinical situations. Cutting a hole of the proper size for an end-to-side anastomosis is often difficult and requires extremely sharp small curved scissors. This oval window should be about one-third larger than the diameter of the vessel to be anastomosed. In this manner the vessel lumen is held open in a somewhat fusiform fashion. The most important principle in an end-to-side repair is to have enough vessel length so that the repair can be completed without tension and the vessels can be manipulated anteriorly and posteriorly.

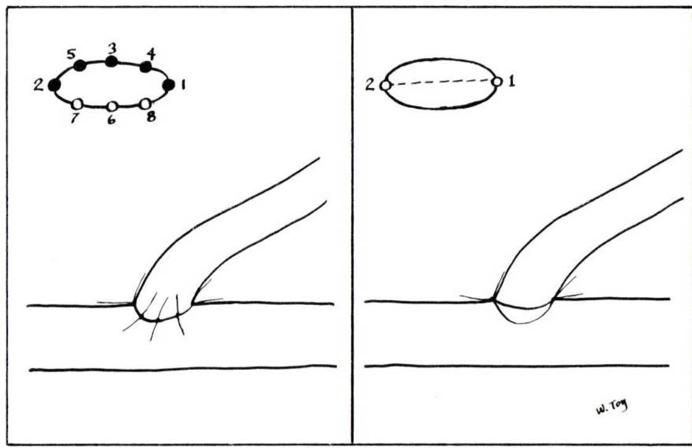

Fig. 40-21. The first two sutures stabilize the anastomotic area; sutures 3, 4, and 5 can then be placed in the posterior wall, with the lumen visualized at all times to prevent catching the anterior edge. (It is somehow easier to make this mistake with the end-to-side repair than it is with an end-to-end repair.)

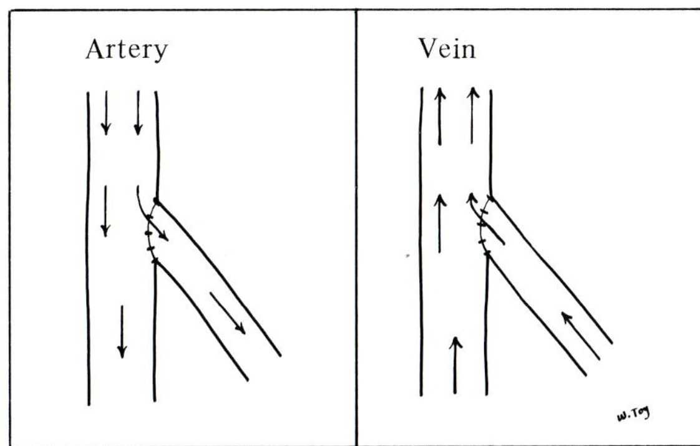

Fig. 40-22. The arrows show the flow dynamics in an ideal 45-degree end-to-side repair for an artery and a vein.

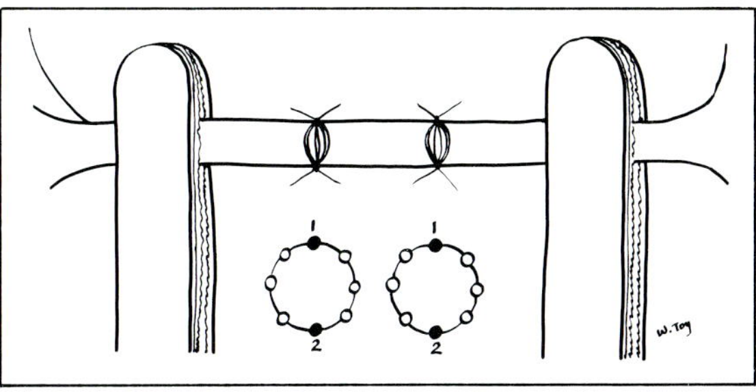

Fig. 40-24. Initial anchoring of interpositioned graft. Segmental microvascular grafts are often required clinically, especially when replanting digits. The rat femoral model again can be used to perfect this technique. The graft should be stabilized proximally and distally with two sutures to ensure proper length and alignment.

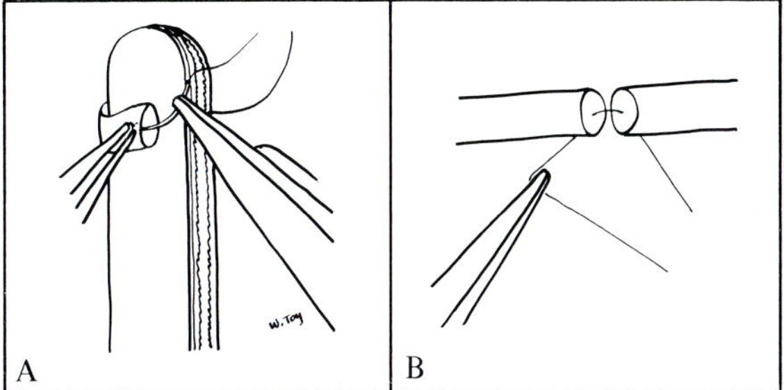

Fig. 40-23. A, the starting position in an end-to-end anastomosis of a vein. B, in a clinical situation where double clamps cannot be used or when the vessel cannot be rotated, one is forced to perform the anastomosis starting with the back wall first. In this instance the first suture is placed directly in the middle of the posterior wall, and subsequent sutures are added above and below it in a circumferential fashion. From a practical standpoint one is faced with this situation in half of clinical microvascular repairs.

Clinical Microvascular Surgery and Free Tissue Transfers

ROLLIN K. DANIEL

Microsurgical techniques have been adopted and adapted by many surgical specialties; in each specialty a similar evolutionary pattern occurs. The first generation of workers develops in the research laboratory the essential microsurgical techniques for that particular specialty; these are translated to clinical cases by the second generation and accepted as standard procedures by the third generation [76, 78]. Plastic surgery is now witnessing its third generation of microsurgeons who are principally interested in clinical microsurgery and consider the teaching laboratory to be only a transitory first step. This chapter emphasizes the important technical considerations that are essential in a successful transition from the microsurgical teaching laboratory to the clinical operating room. Thus, I assume that the reader will review standard microsurgical texts and achieve proficiency with experimental microvascular techniques in the laboratory prior to clinical application [23].

The enthusiast must realize that a few weeks of practice does *not* make an "instant microsurgeon." A standard 1-mm. arterial anastomosis performed under ideal laboratory conditions is totally different from anastomosing a 1-mm. artery to a 3-mm. artery in a deep cavity during a free flap transfer. In the latter situation, one must choose between an end-to-end anastomosis with adjustment for vessel size discrepancy, an end-to-side anastomosis, or an interposition vein graft. The decision is often difficult, the actual execution is technically demanding, and success is totally dependent on the result. Whereas vascular thrombosis is a part of the learning process in the teaching laboratory, it is catastrophic in the clinical setting and must be corrected immediately. Thus prior to attempting elective clinical microvascular surgery, the surgeon must obtain extensive experience with a variety of anastomotic techniques in the microsurgical teaching laboratory followed by initial clinical experience in upper extremity surgery for traumatic injuries (replantations).

EQUIPMENT

Magnification Systems

Magnification systems, including ocular loupes and an operating microscope, are essential for microsurgery. Most surgeons have at least one pair of loupes with a 2.5 X magnification useful for routine dissection; an optional 3.5 to 4.0 X loupe is used for more difficult dissections. Loupes should provide adequate magnification with a wide field of view and depth of focus, plus adjustable interpupillary distance and optional insertion of corrective lenses. Many novices purchase an inexpensive pair of 2.0 X Occulus loupes with "caps" that increase magnification to 4.0 X when required. As one progresses to more complicated cases with long operative times, comfort becomes more important and a lightweight pair of loupes mounted in the bifocal area of the glasses' frame is desirable. A head lamp provides requisite additional illumination, which is often necessary with increased magnification.

Although microsurgical research can be done with table-mounted and/or portable microscopes, clinical microsurgery is best done with a sophisticated operating microscope including variable zoom magnification, motorized focusing, and a fiberoptic or halogen light source [37]. We generally prefer a multipurpose Zeiss OpMi 7P/H, which can be adjusted to various body regions and operative techniques. One should gain initial experience with the operating microscope in the teaching laboratory. Otherwise, the instant microsurgeon will become confined by the microscope's restrictive operative field rather than liberated by its increased magnification.

Microinstruments

During the past decade, microinstruments have progressed from homemade prototypes to complex externally powered devices and currently to commercially available precision instruments [14]. A basic microinstrument set for clinical microvascular surgery is as follows:

1 microneedle holder (extra fine, round tips)
1 microscissors, Wescott type (curved, round tips)
1 microscissors, Vannes type (straight, sharp tips)
4 #5 jewellers forceps
2 #2 jewellers forceps
1 vessel dilator
1 Louisville clamp approximator
4 Kleinert-Kutz 15-mm.-long clamps (including 1 angulated clamp)
1 clamp applying forcep
1 bipolar coagulator with jewellers forceps
2 #28 blunt needles for irrigation
1 combination suction–irrigation tip
1 hemoclip applicator (small size)
1 sterilizable instrument case

Assorted background material
Absorbent "spears" and applicator sticks

The most important choices involve the selection of microvascular clamps and clamp approximators. The clamps must be atraumatic, with a known closing pressure, and they must be easy to apply. The ideal clamp approximator consists of two removable clamps sliding along an intervening bar with optional cleats mounted on a surrounding frame. The cleats serve to hold stay sutures and are most valuable in the experimental laboratory [4]. I generally prefer the Louisville clamp and clamp approximators for 1.0- to 1.5-mm. vessels but rely on a Henderson [35, 56] or Gilbert-O'Brien clamp approximator for larger vessels. Frequently, one encounters "slippage" of vessels out of the clamps and incorrectly blames the clamp approximator, However, the problem is rarely mechanical, but rather due to excessive tension caused by retraction of the vessels, which exceeds the closing pressure of the clamp. Instead of increasing the clamps' pressure, one should do additional dissection (thereby facilitating vessel mobilization) or insert a vein graft.

A bipolar coagulator remains critical in the dissection and preparation of vessels for microvascular anastomoses. Because of the smallness of the vessels, a spring-handle needle holder is essential for clinical microvascular surgery, instead of simple forceps, which do not provide adequate needle purchase. In addition, a wide variety of microscissors are necessary. I generally prefer basic Wescott scissors for dissection, a smaller Vannes scissors for removal of sutures, and a large straight-bladed scissors for single-cut transection of larger vessels. The importance of maintaining microinstruments in good condition cannot be overemphasized.

Microsutures

At the present time, nylon suture material (size 10-0 and 11-0) swaged to atraumatic needles (100 micron, 70 micron, or 50 micron) is commercially available [1, 60]. In general, I prefer the stronger 100-micron needle with a 3/8 or 1/8 circle curvature for clinical microvascular surgery and only rarely use other sizes [10]. Virgin silk, which retains its highly inflammatory seracin gums and resins, has no place in reconstructive microsurgery. When larger sutures are required, one should use 8-0 Prolene swaged to 100-micron needles.*

ACQUISITION OF MICROSURGICAL SKILLS

Although many avenues are available, clinical microvascular surgery is best perfected over several months and should be considered a three-stage progression. First, basic microsurgical skills should be acquired in the teaching laboratory. Second, in-depth microsurgical experience should be obtained via replantation surgery or complex experimental free tissue transfers, the latter a less suitable alternative. Third, preparation for elective reconstructive microsurgery should be completed, including the following: in-depth studies of the vascular anatomy of common donor sites, establishment of dissection techniques in fresh cadavers, and careful case selection to ensure minimal morbidity.

Laboratory Exercises

A series of step-by-step graded laboratory exercises for the would-be microsurgeon are detailed in *Reconstructive Microsurgery* [23] by Daniel and Terzis. Essentially, one masters microscopes, microinstruments, and microsutures while suturing together the cut edge of a rubber glove and partially severed cadaver vessels. Next one evolves an anastomotic technique utilizing cadaver vessels; this particular exercise is extremely valuable even for the experienced microsurgeon, because it allows a rapid comparison of different anastomotic techniques within a standardized setting. As a third exercise, one dissects out the peripheral vessels in the rat and then progresses to end-to-end arterial anastomoses.

As noted in many microsurgical manuals, the rat remains the ideal experimental animal in which to perfect microvascular techniques. The femoral vessels are isolated from the inguinal ligament to their bifurcation into the saphenous and popliteal branches, with severance of the circumflex and superficial epigastric branches. The femoral artery measures 0.8 to 1.0 mm. and the femoral vein 1.1 mm. Multiple anastomotic techniques are then performed.

Clinical Progression

Although current methods and results of digital replantation are discussed elsewhere, these cases represent one of the most demanding applications of clinical microvascular surgery [77]. One is frequently obligated to determine the exact extent of vessel damage and the adequacy of arterial perfusion pressure in a traumatized vessel, and to select the optimal microvascular anastomotic technique. Errors in judgment are punished by failing fingers that require immediate anastomotic revision. Therefore, one quickly learns to excise greater lengths of damaged vessels and to insert a vein graft rather than follow the painful progression of suture removal with thrombectomy, revision of the anastomosis, and hours later insertion of a vein graft. Since several hundred rat vessel anastomoses can never equal the difficulty of replanting four amputated fingers [45],

*Ethicon, Inc., Somerville, N.J. 08876

one should make every effort to acquire clinical microsurgical experience via traumatic extremity surgery [46].

To some surgeons, this approach may not be possible; they are obligated to acquire the necessary skills either by attaining extensive laboratory experience dealing with complex experimental free flap transfers or (preferably) by undergoing a 6-month fellowship at a center specializing in reconstructive microsurgery. Ultimately, one is ready to progress from traumatic cases to the more demanding realm of elective operations. Whereas replantation surgery is a salvage procedure, free tissue transfers are often single-stage alternatives to conventional techniques; therefore a low failure rate is necessary to justify the complexity of these procedures.

MICROVASCULAR ANASTOMOTIC TECHNIQUES

Despite extensive experience in the microsurgical laboratory, I have found that the following principles have acquired greater importance in the clinical setting. During isolation and preparation of vessels for anastomosis, it is critical to achieve absolute hemostasis, to minimize trauma to the vessels, and to select arteries with a strong arterial perfusion pressure and veins with adequate drainage. A pulsatile jet of blood in a transected artery is the sine qua non of adequate perfusion pressure; mere oozing from the vessel is not acceptable. One resects any venous valves that are encountered. Often, a short common arterial origin must be converted into its two separate branches, followed by insertion of a reversed Y-shaped vein graft.

Suturing with 10-0 nylon is a complex art that requires repeated practice. As one achieves proficiency, the number of suture tail pull-throughs and anterior to posterior wall sutures decreases. However, there still remain in the clinical setting the problems of poor suture tail placement, inadequate adventitial resection, and insertion of too few sutures. Suture tails should be carefully "placed" rather than abandoned, allowing them to hide beneath the vessel or to stick to the adventitia. If the needle disappears, it can easily be retrieved by pulling the suture through the jaws of a forceps. The wound must be kept constantly moist to keep the suture from sticking to tissue. Some of the most common suture errors include (1) failing to cut the suture to an optimal short length, (2) a small entrance bite coupled with a large exit bite, and (3) microneedles bent because the needle is held too close to the swage or held at the tip following limited penetration of the vessel.

Utilization of a trained assistant has been one of the principal reasons for the dramatic rise in patency rates for 1-mm. vascular anastomoses (Table 41-1). The ideal situation is to have two experienced micro-

Table 41-1. Series of End-to-End Microvascular Suture Anastomoses

Surgeon	Date	Experimental Model (Arteries)	Vessel Diameter (mm.)	Patency Rate (%)
Jacobson	1960	Rabbit and dog; carotid	1.4–3.2	100 (26/26)
Urschel	1961	Dog; ulnar	1.5–2.0	81 (30/37)
Chase	1962	Dog; brachial	1.2–1.7	100 (34/34)
Man	1962	Dog; brachial, carotid, thyroid	1.0–2.5	65 (40/62)
Mozes	1963	Dog; multiple vessels	0.6–2.0	69 (47/68)
Salmon	1964	Dog; femoral, brachial	1.1–3.0	75 (9/12)
Stahl	1964	Dog; brachial	1.5–2.5	75 (15/20)
Collins	1964	Dog; multiple vessels	1.0–2.0	86 93
Green	1966	Rat; aorta	0.8–1.5	90 (18/20)
Cobbett	1967	Rat; aorta	1.5	100 (6/6)
Jenkins	1967	Dog; dorsalis pedis	1.0–2.0	98 (49/50)
Yasargil	1967	Dog; superficial temporal to middle cerebral	0.8–1.1	69 (9/13)
Ikuta	1968	Rabbit; femoral, brachial	0.5–1.0	29 (19/65)
		Dog; femoral, brachial	1.1–2.0	57 (28/49)
O'Brien	1970	Rabbit; femoral	0.9	81 (47/58)
Acland	1972	Rat; superficial epigastric	0.5	95 (19/20)
Nomoto	1974	Rat; femoral	0.7–0.9	95 (19/20)
Hayhurst	1975	Rabbit; femoral	0.9	98 (49/50)

vascular surgeons who alternate anastomoses, each assisting the other. However, a novice microsurgeon can be an extremely valuable assistant, while learning a great deal about microvascular techniques at the same time. During dissection and preparation, the assistant provides effective countertraction, removes debris, irrigates the wound, and suctions away excess fluid. During suturing, the assistant may have the limited role of stabilizing the vessel, retrieving the suture tail, and cutting sutures. Ultimately, the assistant may become increasingly active and tie the sutures once they are inserted by the surgeon. Unfortunately, trained assistants are not always available; it is far better to do an anastomosis alone than to accept the fumbling attempts of an untrained assistant, who can easily create chaos rather than convenience. In the final analysis, one must be prepared to do microvascular surgery without an assistant, even though his presence dramatically increases the ease and rapidity of most anastomoses.

Certain microsurgical fundamentals must be repeatedly emphasized:

1. The *work plane* of the microscope is horizontal; if one lifts structures out of this horizontal plane, they will be out of focus.
2. Since the *visualization plane* is vertical, instruments should always be inserted from an angled approach.
3. One must realize that if one cannot *see* then one should not continue. Errors are often irreparable; one must make every effort to visualize critical structures *before* manipulating them.
4. If one is struggling, then something is wrong. At such a time, stop to identify and correct the difficulty, and then proceed.
5. Instrument tips must be frequently washed and all coagulum removed. One should operate only with instruments in perfect condition.

There are as many methods for anastomosing blood vessels as there are microsurgeons; in turn, there are clinical situations in which each technique would be the "optimal" one to employ. The novice microsurgeon will do well to try various methods, but he should perfect a specific technique that he can rely on in critical situations and only later practice the numerous variations.

Fundamental microvascular anastomotic technique originally consisted of three guide sutures plus the appropriate number of coapting sutures [8, 16]. However, one may vary the critical guide sutures as to location (10–2–4 o'clock position versus 12–4–8 o'clock position), distance apart (120 versus 180 degrees), sequence of insertion (all guide sutures inserted versus anterior wall completion), and even number (triangular versus quadrangular) [17]. In certain difficult clinical situations, every suture is left long and used as a guide for placement of the next suture. The following descriptions are offered only as a starting point for the reader and should *not* be accepted as the only way or even the best technique, but rather as one surgeon's current preference, subject to revision as experience dictates.

End-to-End Anastomoses

Arterial Anastomoses

An end-to-end anastomosis may be conceived of as an inverted triangle set within a luminal circle. It is produced by insertion of three equidistant guide sutures, followed by the appropriate number of intervening interrupted coaption sutures (Fig. 41-1). The guide sutures ensure correct orientation and approximation of vessels ends. Since traction is periodically placed on the guide sutures to improve luminal visibility, their bites must be 1½ to 2 times vessel wall thickness, with an initial double-throw knot; one suture tail should be left long. The intervening interrupted coaption sutures differ from guide sutures in the following ways: their function is coaption rather than approximation, the needle bites are smaller, a single-throw first knot is used, and both tails are cut short.

There is no "correct" number of sutures for a specific vessel diameter – the number varies with suture technique. For example, the surgeon who takes minimal bites (a bite approximately equal to a 70-micron needle) will require far more sutures than a surgeon who takes larger bites (a bite approximately equal to 1½ to 2 times vessel wall thickness) [7, 35]. The former justifies his method as minimizing direct vessel damage, but at the price of a greater number of sutures, which increases anastomotic time, the amount of interluminal foreign body, and chances for suture error. As a general rule, 9 sutures (3 guide sutures and 6 coaption sutures) are adequate for a 1-mm. vessel, 12 sutures for a 1.5-mm. vessel, and 15 sutures for a 2.0-mm. vessel. However, one must always strive for the "perfect" anastomosis, regardless of the number of sutures [3]. In most clinical situations, it is far better to insert an extra coaption suture with the clamp approximator in place than to have to return once the clamps are removed [53]. Removal of the clamps should be done while observing under the microscope to check for immediate flow, luminal distention, and any significant leaks. Slight oozing at an anastomosis is inevitable and unnecessary to correct. However, a jet of blood from the anastomosis indicates a significant leak; it should be corrected immediately by the insertion of an additional suture.

Venous Anastomoses

Human veins have thicker walls and are easier to anastomose than the femoral vein of the rat. However, the

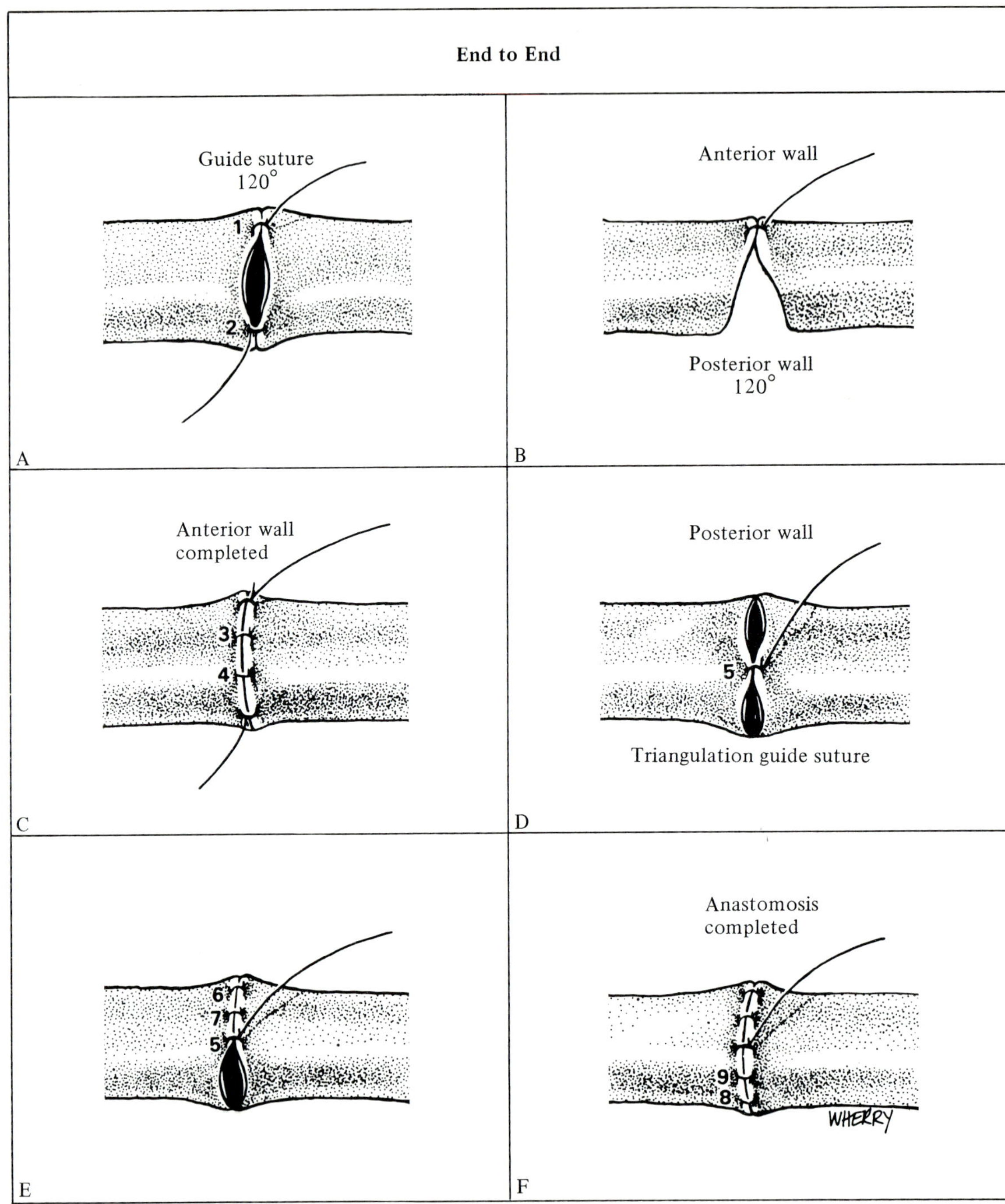

Fig. 41-1. End-to-end anastomosis (artery or vein). A triangulation technique is employed utilizing three guide sutures placed 120 degrees apart, plus additional interrupted coaption sutures as required.

same meticulous technique is required if disasters are to be avoided. Periadventitial tissue is excised from the vein and any adventitial fluff removed while the vein is submerged in a pool of saline. Mechanical dilatation is performed with polished forceps. With preparations complete, the vein is carefully inspected under saline irrigation and the first guide suture inserted. A standard end-to-end anastomosis is done, with constant visualization of the needle tip. Frequent irrigation and luminal identification are mandatory throughout to prevent the most common and devastating error – a suture through both the anterior and posterior walls.

The number of sutures required for a venous anastomosis, as compared to that for an arterial anastomosis, has been reviewed by many surgeons; the conclusion is that more sutures are required in a vein because its vessel walls are expansile, as well as to ensure perfect coaption of the vessel edges [34].

Differences in Luminal Diameter

Anastomosis of arteries with significantly different luminal diameters is a very real technical problem. Traditionally, the solution was an end-to-side anastomosis. Since most end-to-side anastomoses are often technically more difficult, an end-to-end anastomosis is preferred whenever possible. Within the spectrum of 0.5- to 4.0-mm. vessels, these general guidelines are followed:

1. Discrepancies less than 50 percent (1.0:1.4) require only mechanical dilatation of the smaller vessel.
2. Discrepancies greater than 50 percent but less than 100 percent (1.0:2.0) require both an angled cut (30 degrees) and mechanical dilatation of the smaller vessel.
3. Discrepancies greater than twofold (1.0:3.0) mandate an end-to-side anastomosis or occasionally insertion of a vein graft.

The following technique is employed for end-to-end anastomoses where significant luminal diameter differences exist (Fig. 41-2). Vessel preparation is critical. The larger vessel must be severed transversely in a single cut using scissors with blades sufficiently long to transect the vessel cleanly. The smaller vessel is cut at a 30-degree angle to permit a smooth funnel-shaped orifice rather than the skewed orifice that results when the angle cut exceeds 45 degrees. Two guide sutures are inserted 140 to 180 degrees apart to ensure maximum expansion of the smaller vessel and its equal distribution along the larger vessel. The vessels are then turned over and the third or "triangulation" guide suture is inserted. The posterior wall is completed with equal distribution of the small vessel along the larger vessel. The vessel is turned back over and the anterior wall completed. Differences in venous luminal diameter that do not exceed threefold (1.0:4.0) can be accommodated in an end-to-end anastomosis because veins have expansile walls.

End-to-Side Anastomoses

The end-to-side anastomosis, which is rarely utilized in replantation surgery, is frequently employed in free tissue transfers to establish an artificial branch from a critical vessel or when vessel size discrepancy cannot be accommodated by an end-to-end anastomosis. Although many experimental techniques exist, the clinical situation often dictates a very precise and difficult end-to-side anastomotic technique. In contrast to experimental models, in which both vessels are mobile (permitting easy visibility and access of both walls), clinical vessels are often fixed, which forces one to work outward from the posterior wall. For purposes of discussion, the larger vessel will be termed the recipient or primary vessel and the smaller vessel will be the donor or secondary vessel. The following sequential technique is utilized (Fig. 41-3):

An elliptical excision in the recipient vessel is made, since a longitudinal or transverse slit might collapse. In large vessels, one can easily create too large an excision or too superficial a cut, resulting in a transmedial dissection. One must make a precise and definitive single cut; multiple bites will result in an irregular-shaped orifice. If an adequate length of donor vessel is available, it is cut on an angle to ensure a low angle of union with the recipient vessel. The donor vessel is then mechanically dilated into an expanded funnel-shaped orifice. The recipient vessel may be immobile because of critical branches or the donor vessel may be fixed due to anchoring of the free tissue transfer; thus, one must use an approach that does not "roll over" the vessels being connected. The central back wall suture is inserted first and then coaption sutures are placed until the superior guide suture is secured. Next, the inferior portion of the posterior wall is completed. On the back wall, the entrance bite is taken on the large vessel, which permits cannulation of the lumen of the smaller vessel on the exit bite. On the front wall, the entrance bite is on the smaller vessel, which is thus expanded to fit the larger recipient vessel. This maneuver ensures careful approximation of the endothelial margins without relying on external adventitial appearance. Similar techniques are used for both arteries and veins.

Vascular Grafts

Perhaps the greatest single reason for the increasing survival rates in digital replantation and salvage of failing free flaps has been the early utilization of vein grafts in both arterial and venous systems. The use of

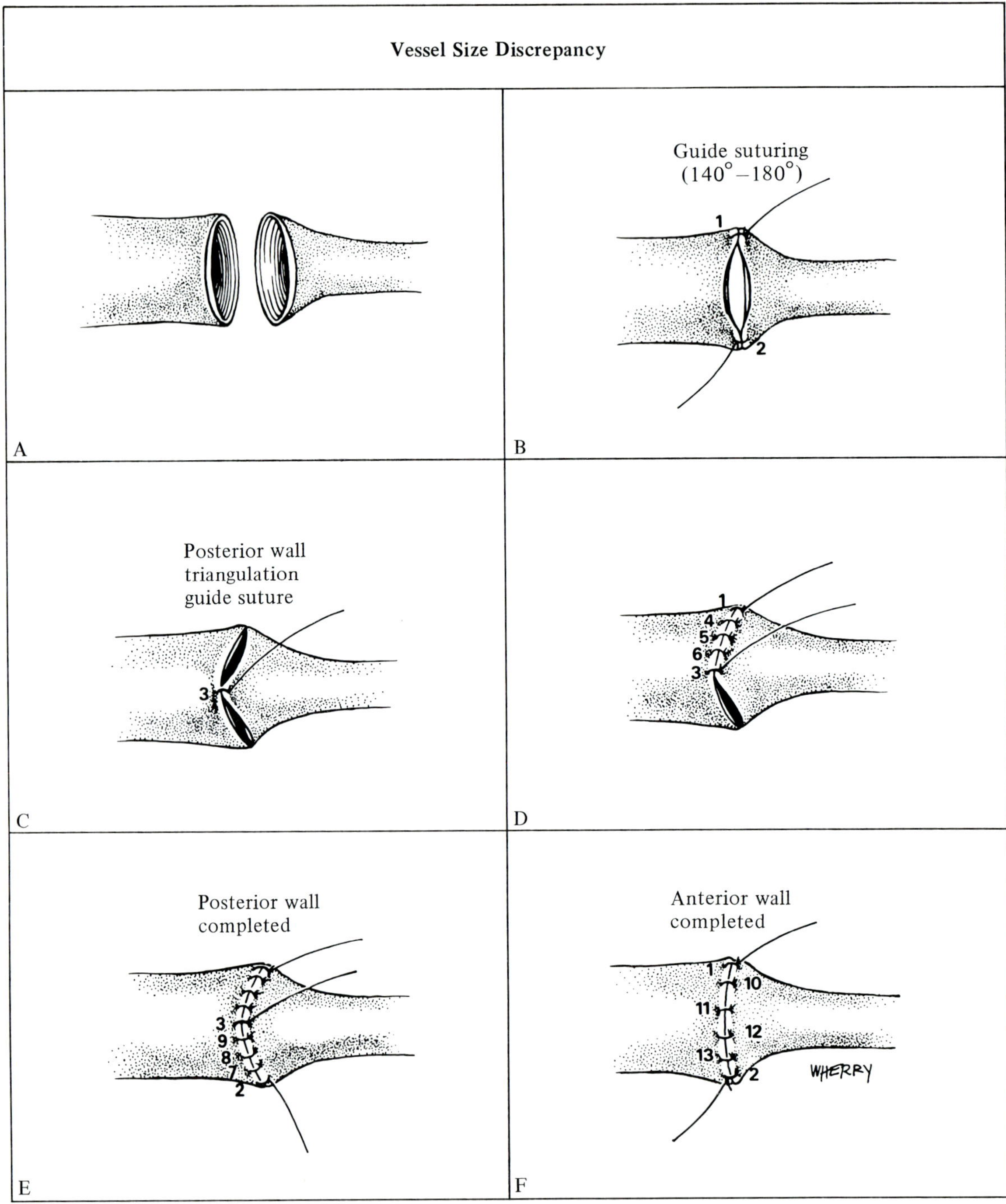

Fig. 41-2. Anastomosis of vessels with significant diameter discrepancy. Two guide sutures are inserted 140 to 180 degrees apart followed by completion of the posterior wall and then the anterior wall.

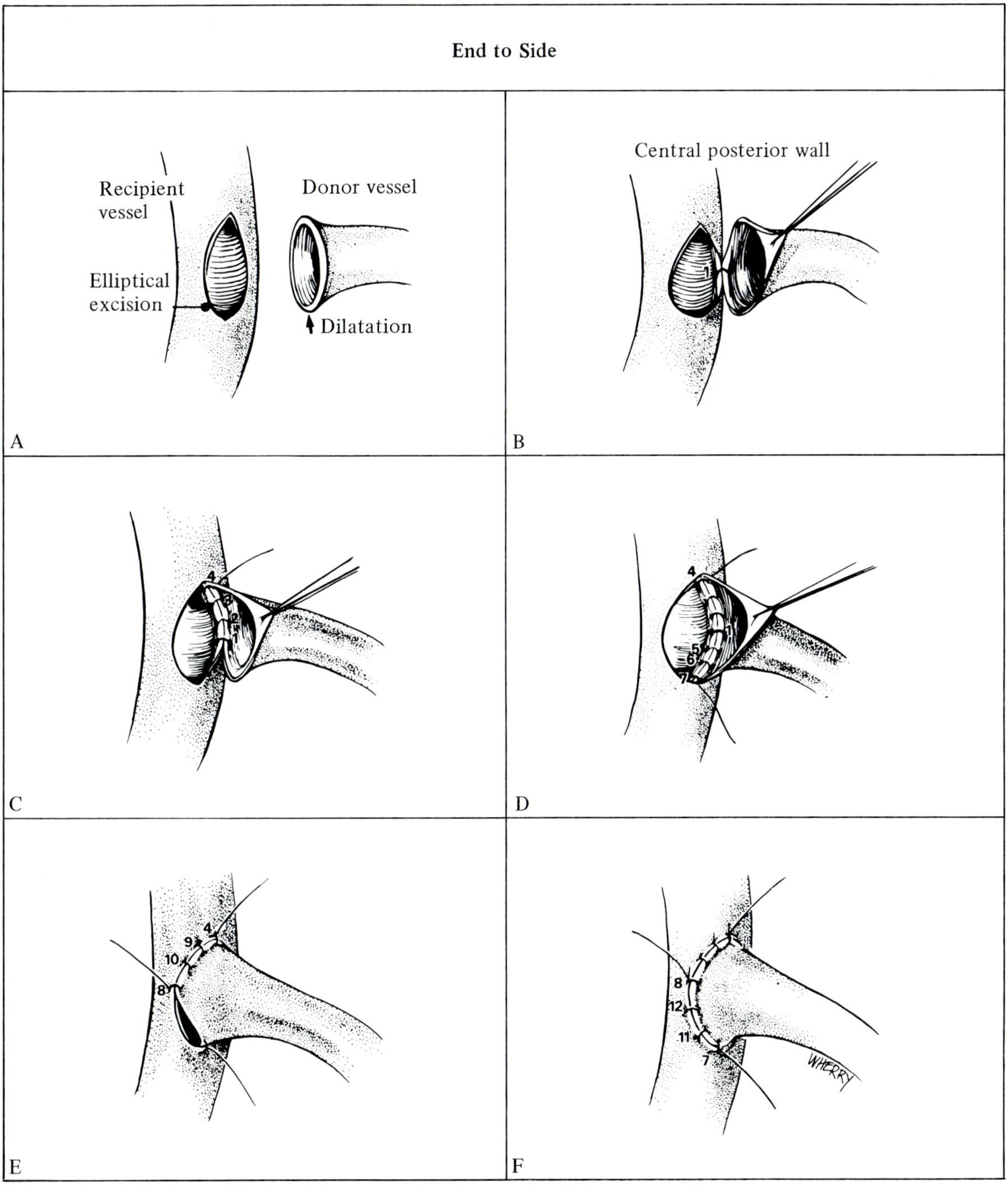

End to Side

Recipient vessel

Donor vessel

Elliptical excision

Dilatation

A

Central posterior wall

B

C

D

E

F

WHERRY

Fig. 41-3. End-to-side anastomosis. An elliptical incision is made in the recipient vessel and the donor vessel dilated. Clinically, one is frequently obligated to complete the posterior wall anastomosis first, followed by that of the anterior wall.

vein grafts reduces tension at the anastomotic site and permits a more liberal resection of damaged vessels. Rather than accept a segment of damaged artery albeit that would permit an end-to-end anastomosis, one is more frequently resecting the damaged vessel, thereby necessitating an interposition vein graft.

The following clinical considerations have become apparent with greater employment of vein grafts:

1. Resistance to the use of a vein graft diminishes greatly if a supply of vein grafts is immediately available. Therefore, I have an assistant harvest the vein grafts quite early when revision of an anastomosis is contemplated or reoperation is necessary.
2. The dorsal venous arch of the foot extending distally into the toe web spaces is the ideal donor site. The dorsum of the hand is cosmetically unacceptable in many patients. The forearm veins are often too few and selection too limited.
3. Contraction of the graft following its removal from the donor site easily approaches 30 percent; one must obtain a length of graft greater than the defect.
4. Veins have extensive perivascular tissue that must be removed in the anastomotic area; otherwise suture tails become repeatedly entrapped and tissue will slide over the luminal orifice.
5. Most grafts are inserted too long and will kink when the retracted wound margins are released. Therefore, one should check graft length early and release the retracting sutures if necessary. Diameter is rarely a critical problem, although isodiametric grafts are preferred.
6. In most clinical situations, a long graft is taken and the more difficult anastomosis done first. Length is checked and any excessive graft resected, followed by completion of the second anastomosis. Flow is reestablished once both anastomoses are done.
7. Vascular segments of both arteries and veins work equally well in either the arterial or venous system, provided that one is cognizant of both blood flow and valvular direction. Arterial grafts are rarely utilized, because dispensable donor sites do not exist, except in amputated parts unsuitable for replantation [13].

In summary, the end-to-end anastomosis is the most frequently employed anastomotic technique in clinical microvascular surgery and must be totally mastered. However, one must increasingly rely on end-to-side anastomoses and vein grafts. These anastomoses must be practiced repeatedly, because their implementation will occur at critical moments in complex cases (Fig. 41-4). The most common errors in clinical microvascular surgery include the following:

1. There may be inadequate preparation of the vessel, including insufficient mobilization and periadventitial tissue excision. Therefore, one should extend the dissection, coagulate the collateral branches, and remove all perivascular tissue, especially on the back wall.
2. Inadequate exposure frequently makes anastomoses difficult. Rather than attempting an anastomosis in a deep dark hole, one should reflect the wound margins and suture them out of the way. Alternatively, one can extend the incision in both directions.
3. In order to minimize ischemia time, a small error is often accepted in the rush to finish the anastomosis, thereby triggering a series of increasing technical difficulties. Such an error would have been easy to correct initially, but becomes impossible later on. Consequently, one should accept a certain amount of ischemia time and do a perfect anastomosis starting with the first guide suture.
4. Significant oozing or a jet of blood is often allowed to cease spontaneously; it subsequently progresses to a thrombus in 15 to 20 minutes. One must always evaluate the quality of an anastomosis under the microscope immediately following the removal of the clamps and insert additional sutures as required.
5. An immediately patent anastomosis is often accepted as a "fait accompli" and attention is directed elsewhere while a clot develops. One must do patency tests on all vascular anastomoses prior to wound closure [2].

It must be emphasized that basic microsurgical skills may come easily to many, but surgical judgment emerges only through repetitive experience. One must never equate the controlled simplicity of most experimental models with the highly variable complexity of clinical cases. *It is only when one can "guarantee" patent microvascular anastomoses – irrespective of the specific technique that must be utilized – that one can consider undertaking clinical reconstructive microsurgery.*

FREE TISSUE TRANSFERS

Free tissue transfer by microvascular anastomoses is rapidly revolutionizing reconstructive surgery (Fig. 41-5). Free tissue transfers can be classified as follows:

A. Single free tissue transfers
   1. Free flap
      a. Free skin flap
      b. Free myocutaneous flap
   2. Free bone transfer
   3. Free muscle transfer
   4. Free nerve transfer
   5. Free intestinal transfer

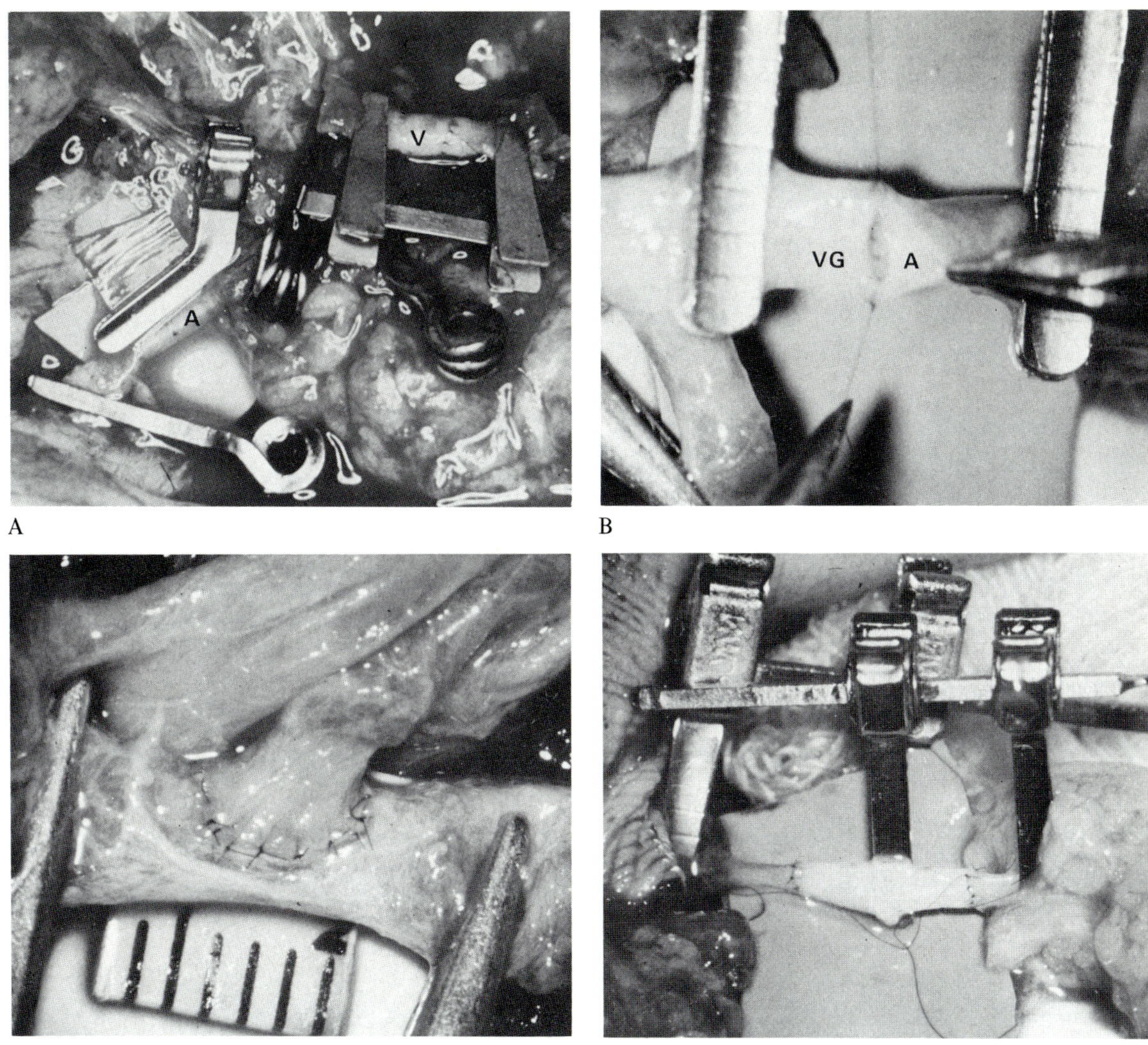

Fig. 41-4. Clinical microvascular anastomoses in free tissue transfers. A, end-to-end anastomosis of an artery (A) *(plastic wrapper) and vein* (V). *B, end-to-end anastomosis requiring adjustment of significant vessel discrepancy between a 2-mm. vein graft* (VG) *and a 1-mm. artery* (A). *C, an end-to-side arterial anastomosis. D, insertion of an 8-mm.-long vein graft.*

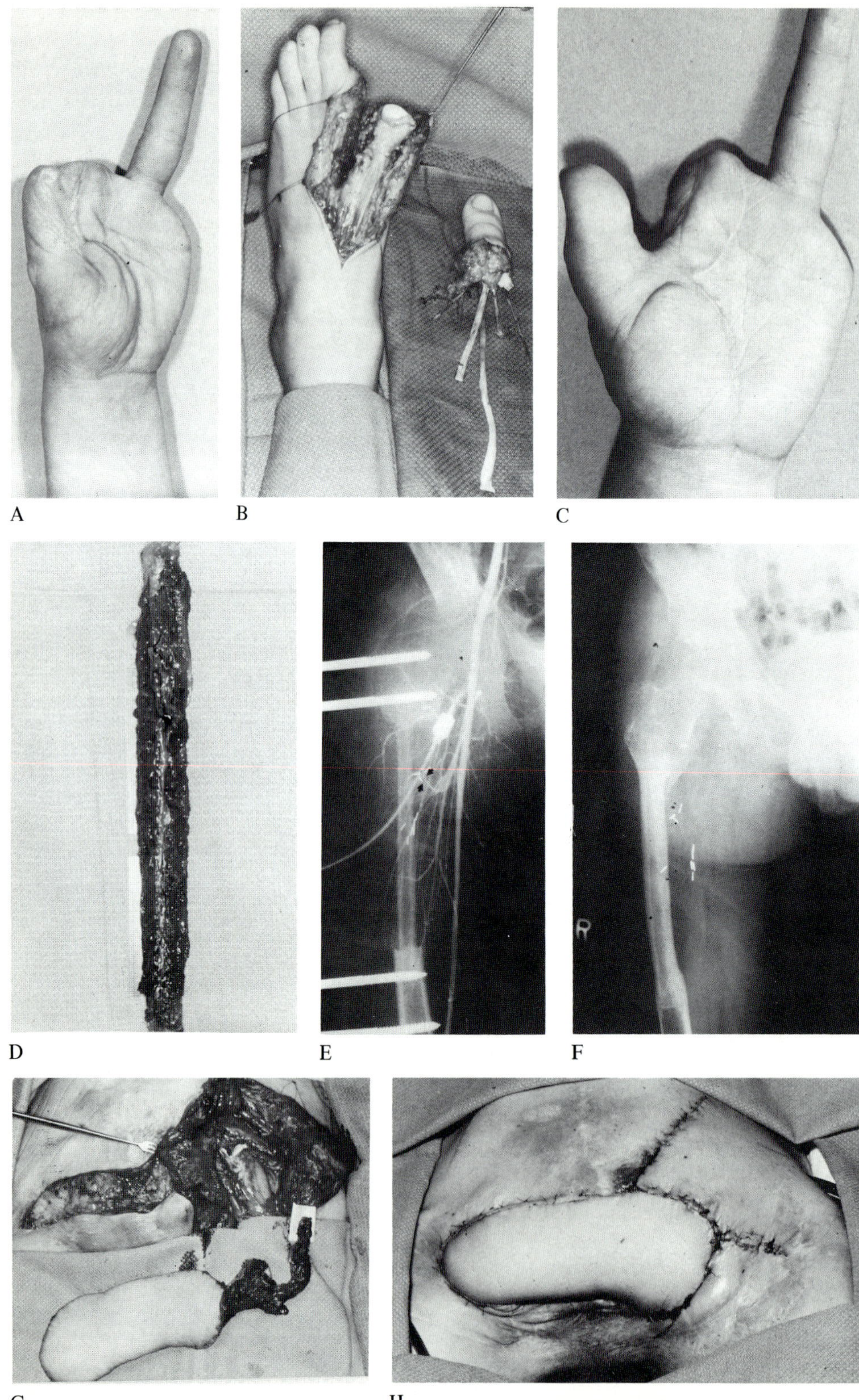
A
B
C
D
E
F
R
G
H

6. Free omental transfer

B. Compound free tissue transfers
   1. Free neurovascular flap
   2. Free osteocutaneous flap
   3. Free musculocutaneous flap
   4. Free toe-to-hand transfer

Previously, the patient with a nonunion of the tibia and inadequate skin cover was obligated to undergo multiple operations including skin grafting, flap coverage, and bone grafting over several months. Today, one can provide both skin flap coverage and a vascularized bone graft in a single operation utilizing a free composite osteocutaneous groin flap [21]. However, utilization of free tissue transfers must be based on extensive experience with numerous microvascular anastomotic techniques, a detailed knowledge of the vascular anatomy of the different donor sites, and fundamental training in reconstructive surgery. Principles common to all free tissue transfers will be discussed in depth followed by a review of current clinical application (Fig. 41-6). During the past 2 years we have performed 45 free tissue transfers consisting of the following:

1. Free skin grafts. There were 18 of these grafts: groin (10); dorsalis pedis (6); intercostal (1); first foot web space (1)
2. Latissimus dorsi myocutaneous free flaps (2)
3. Free osteocutaneous flaps (11)
4. Free muscle transfers (1)
5. Free toe-to-hand (3)
6. Free fibula transfers (10)

The overall success rate has been 91% (41/45) with a reoperation rate of 7% (3/45) – all successful. The reader interested in actual operative techniques is referred elsewhere (*Reconstructive Microsurgery* [23] by Daniel and Terzis).

Fig. 41-5. The spectrum of free tissue transfers. A, B, C, a toe-to-hand transfer in a 9-year-old girl. A, complete amputation of all digits except for a normal ring finger. B, dissection of the great toe with the preservation of all critical neurovascular structures. C, the hand at 4 months, with the new "thumb" in good position; there is a normal range of motion plus a two-point discrimination of 12 mm. which decreased to 6 mm. at 1 year. D, E, F, free fibula transfer in a 9-year-old boy. D, a 22-cm. segment of isolated fibula. E, the fibula inserted in the femur at 6 weeks; an arteriogram shows patency of the arterial anastomosis. F, the bone at 11 months, with hypertrophy of the fibula and complete mobilization of the patient. G, H, a neurovascular free flap transfer in a paraplegic. G, the isolated intercostal neurovascular free flap, with exposure of the recipient vessels. H, complete survival of the flap 10 days postoperatively prior to reinnervation with nerve grafts.

Preoperative Preparations

With increasing emphasis on composite free tissue transfers, one should ask the following questions when confronted with difficult clinical problems. What tissues are missing and what is required to achieve optimal reconstruction in one stage? What donor tissues, both locally and from a distance, are available to achieve these goals? For example, a severe upper-extremity injury might be corrected by resection of scar tissue followed by appropriate tendon transfers and restoration of sensory skin coverage with a neurovascular free flap. Once basic objectives are ascertained, one can determine the specific tissue transfers required and "design" the ideal operative technique for the individual patient.

Prior to operation, the surgeon must evolve an operative technique and identify potential pitfalls, both of which are primarily related to the vascular supply in the donor and recipient areas. One must assess the quality of the recipient artery, especially in traumatized extremities in which collateral blood flow may be limited. Contrary to some recommendations, arteriography remains the only *direct* method for evaluating arterial flow in traumatized extremities. Doppler probes are frequently unreliable and offer only indirect evidence, which in turn requires an "act of faith" that the "swish" heard correlates with specific vessels [44]. Superficial veins can be rotated into the recipient site, or the deep paired venae comitantes can be found paralleling the recipient artery. Following preliminary selection of the recipient vessels, the approximate size of the recipient defect is measured. Next, various donor sites are evaluated to determine: (1) whether they can provide the required tissues, (2) the adequacy of their blood supply, and (3) the extent of donor site morbidity.

Once recipient site requirements and donor site potential are reconciled, then an operative sequence can be evolved, usually working in reverse. From a technical viewpoint, the critical factor is overlap of both sets of vessels, which will permit tension-free anastomoses. Initially, one should write out a step-by-step protocol for the entire operation. This plan is then taken first to the anatomical dissection room, where operative approaches are evaluated, and then to the autopsy room, where "dress rehearsals" are performed. Following numerous modifications, the ideal operative technique is evolved. One must never forget to work out a planned retreat and explain it to the patient.

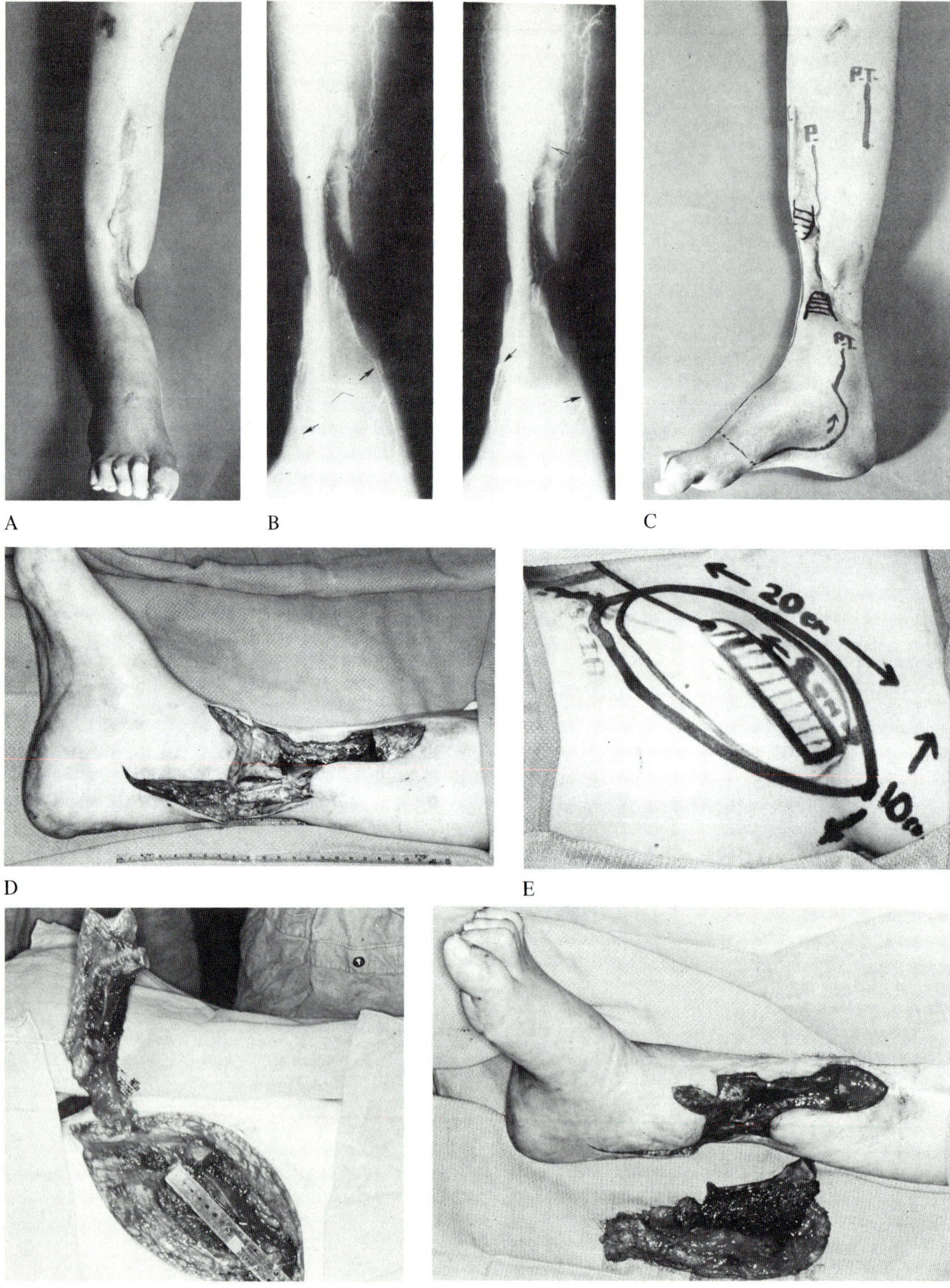
A
B
C
P.T.
P.
P.T.
20cm
10cm
D
E
F
G

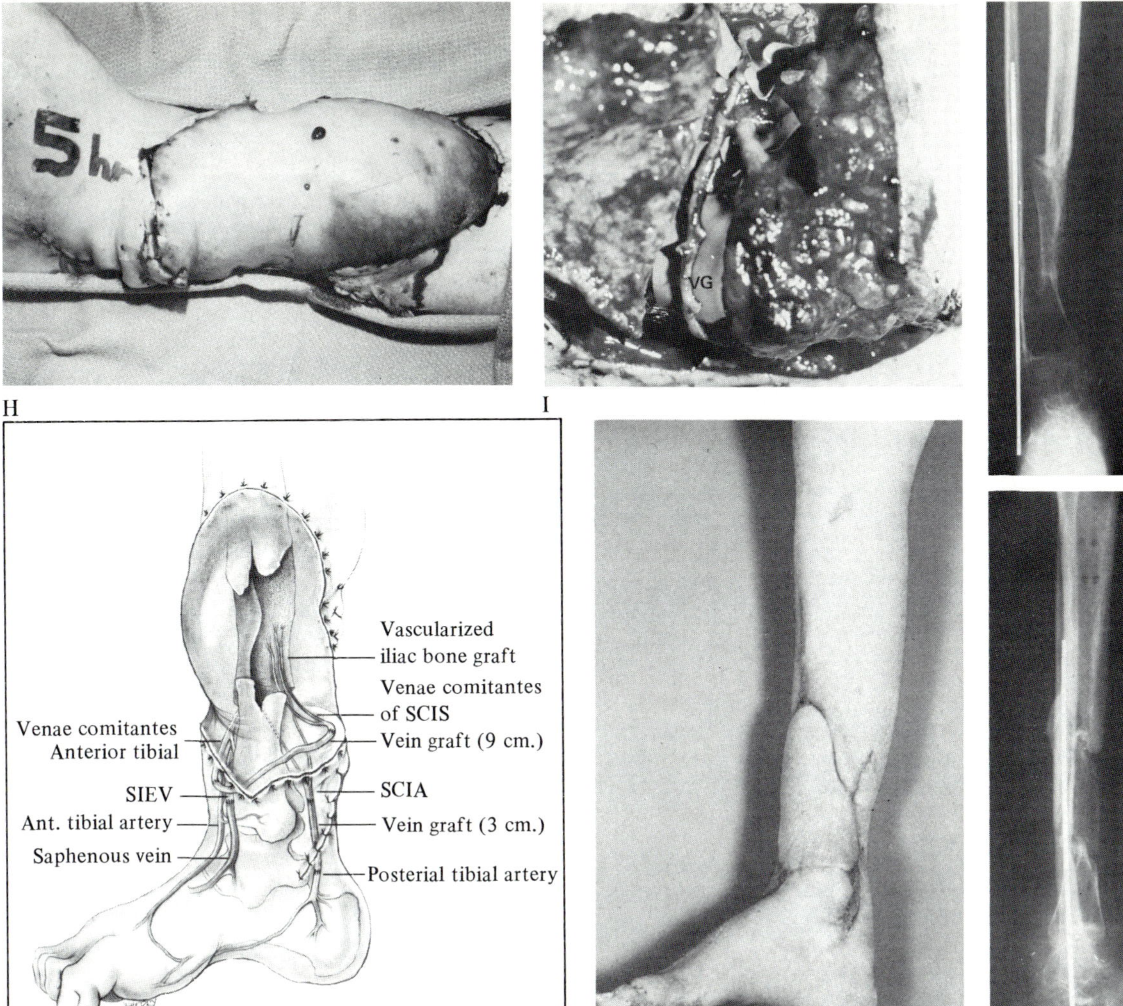

Fig. 41-6. One-stage reconstruction of an anterior tibial defect utilizing a compound osteocutaneous free groin flap transferred by microvascular anastomosis. A, severe compound defect of the lower tibia secondary to a motor vehicle accident. At 8 months, the patient had neither stable skin coverage nor bony union. B, arteriogram demonstrating the 8-cm. defect in the tibia, a nonunion of the fibula, and preservation of the anterior tibial artery as the only artery to the foot with complete interruption of the posterior tibial and peroneal arteries. Note the retrograde perfusion of the posterior tibial artery via the anterior tibial. C, the tibial defect (marked in hatch marks) and the retrograde flow in the posterior tibial artery, which had a palpable pulse. D, the defect in the leg following isolation of the distal posterior tibial artery and saphenous vein, as well as the recreation of the bony defect. E, the groin flap outlined with a 20-cm. × 10-cm. skin flap, including an 8-cm. segment of the iliac crest. F, free groin flap completely isolated onto its vascular stalk, with preservation of the anterior superior iliac spine. G, undersurface view of the flap next to the leg prior to insertion. H, 5 hours postoperatively, the flap shows venous congestion in approximately 20 percent of the flap and a dark purple blood oozing from simple stab wound incision. I, insertion of a 9-cm.-long vein graft (VG) from the venae comitantes of the superficial circumflex iliac artery to a vena comitans of the anterior tibial artery. J, the vascularized iliac bone graft and

Operative Technique

Free tissue transfers are often long operations (6 to 18 hours) which are best conceived of as a series of separate steps, each of which must be flawlessly executed to ensure a perfect result.

Recipient Vessels

The first critical step is evaluation and preparation of the recipient vessels. Appropriate skin flaps are elevated and the recipient vessels isolated. If the recipient artery is undamaged, it is stripped of its collateral branches and mobilized for several centimeters with its accompanying venae comitantes. However, if the artery was previously traumatized, it must be divided and resected back to *healthy* vessel with strong perfusion pressure (mere oozing is insufficient – *the blood must spurt for several feet*). Once one is satisfied with the recipient artery, the recipient veins –either the deep venae comitantes or large superficial veins – are selected. The former are most frequently used in the extremities while the latter are relied upon in the head and neck region.

Recipient Site Preparation

With the assurance that healthy recipient vessels are available, one can complete preparations in the recipient site; additionally, one can perform other reconstructive procedures – i.e., release of scar contracture, wound debridement, tendon transfer, or bony tumor resection. Following their completion, the exact recipient site requirements are determined and the donor tissue isolated accordingly. This sequence of complete recipient site preparation allows for more of a rapid operation without multiple positional changes, but it is recommended only for experienced microsurgeons. More conservatively, the novice should first isolate the recipient vessels followed by isolation of the vascular supply to the donor tissue; this approach ensures satisfactory donor vessels before extending operative morbidity in recipient site.

Isolation of Donor Tissue

Selection of the donor tissue must satisfy recipient site requirements while maintaining the tissue's intrinsic vascular integrity. The nutrient vascular stalk incorporates as many vessels with as great a diameter and length as possible, thereby facilitating the number, type, and location of the vascular anastomoses. The actual isolation technique will vary according to the donor site and the surgeon's preference. In most cases, the donor site is subsequently closed primarily with minimal patient morbidity.

Tissue Transfer

The donor tissue is then transferred to and inserted in the recipient site. The complexity of this step will vary with the type of tissue utilized; the procedure may vary from simple skin anchoring sutures for a free skin flap to compression plate fixation for a free bone transfer. The donor tissue is placed in the desired position to achieve the basic reconstructive goal while making certain that both the donor and recipient vessels overlap, thereby facilitating the vascular anastomoses. One should not rush through this step to minimize ischemia time, because this would only compromise final functional reconstruction. The donor tissue is *not* perfused intravascularly.

Microvascular Anastomoses

The actual technique and sequence of the vascular anastomoses will depend upon the specific conditions of each case [41, 61]. Therefore, one must be prepared to modify the preoperative plan depending upon the final situation as seen under the operating microscope. In general, I prefer to do the arterial anastomosis first, then a venous anastomosis followed by reestablishment of blood flow to the free tissue transfer. The circulation is allowed to equilibrate for 15 minutes. Then an additional donor vein is opened, the quantity of outflow is assessed as an indication of tissue perfusion, and a second venous anastomosis is done. Ischemia time averages 2 to 3 hours since the donor tissue must be fixed in the recipient site and the vessels carefully anastomosed. Anticoagulants and antiplatelet agents are not used, with the exception of aspirin suppositories postoperatively.

Although immediate tissue revascularization is usually achieved, vascular complications can occur intraoperatively. They must be dealt with immediately and effectively, by revision of a thrombosed anastomosis or insertion of a vein graft if tension is present.

---

the free flap. The vascular anastomoses required suturing the posterior tibial artery, with its retrograde arterial flow to the superficial circumflex iliac artery (SCIA) *with a 3-cm. interposition vein graft. The superficial interior epigastric vein* (SIEV) *was anastomosed to the saphenous vein based on retrograde flow through the short saphenous vein into the deep venous system. Augmentation of these patent anastomoses required insertion of a 9-cm. vein graft between the venae comitantes of the superficial circumflex iliac artery in a vena comitans of the anterior tibial artery some 5 hours postoperatively. All vascular anastomoses were patent. K, the patient at 4 months, with complete survival of the free flap. L, x-ray studies at 4 months, demonstrating union of the iliac bone graft in the tibial defect.*

Wound Closure
The wound is closed once the free tissue transfer has been revascularized and the patency of the anastomoses proved. The wound should be closed with minimal tension, because compression of the vessels can occur; if necessary, a skin graft can be inserted to minimize tension. Drainage catheters are always inserted under direct vision and sutured into place far away from the vascular anastomoses.

Postoperative Management
The postoperative period consists of general patient care and monitoring of the free tissue transfer.

Patient Care
Because of the prolonged operative times, the following complications must be anticipated: wound infection, pneumonia, pressure sores, and pulmonary emboli. The following precautionary measures are recommended:

1. The patient is begun intraoperatively on a broad-spectrum antibiotic (such as cephalothin), which is continued for 5 days postoperatively.
2. Pulmonary care includes preoperative pulmonary function studies, periodic maximal pulmonary expansion intraoperatively, and frequent tracheal suction postoperatively.
3. The patient is placed on a water-filled cooling mattress intraoperatively and on a standard water mattress postoperatively, to protect all bony prominences including the heels and occiput.
4. The patient's lower extremities are wrapped preoperatively, the legs are moved every 2 hours intraoperatively, and early mobilization is begun postoperatively.

Monitoring Free Tissue Transfers
Evaluation of free tissue transfers varies from simple direct inspection of free skin flaps to complex "washout" scans in free bone transfers. One can subjectively assess color, capillary refill, and temperature; incisional bleeding and systemic fluoroscein are more objective signs (Table 41-2). In general, the arterial and venous failure patterns are similar to those seen in digital replantation. Arterial failure, which is the more common problem, is recognized by absence of bleeding on incision and by nonfluorescence following systemic injection of fluoroscein. The most common causes of arterial failure are selection of a damaged recipient artery, tension at the anastomosis, and suture error. Venous failure, characterized by increasing cyanosis and tissue turgor, is usually due to a suture error or external compression. Its occurrence is markedly reduced if two venous anastomoses are done at the time of free tissue transfer. The treatment of vascular complications requires careful selection and execution of the following alternatives: (1) suture removal with thrombectomy, (2) revision of the anastomosis, (3) interposition vein graft, and (4) rotation of new recipient vessel. For the experienced microsurgeon, the most common solution is an interposition vein graft.

Table 41-2. Vascular Complications

Clinical Sign	Arterial Complication	Venous Complication
Color	Pale white	Cyanotic to purple
Bleeding on incision	Absent	Purple ooze
Systemic fluoroscein	No fluorescence	Fluorescence
Capillary refill	Decreased	Rapid
Tissue turgor	Decreased	Increased
Temperature	Decreased	Minimal change

In an arterial failure, the arterial anastomosis and one venous anastomosis are excised. The arterial anastomosis is redone, utilizing the appropriate technique. Circulation is restored, outflow through the open vein is assessed, and then the venous anastomosis is redone. In a venous failure, only the venous anastomosis is excised; after the outflow through the open vein is assessed, systemic fluorescein is injected to validate arterial perfusion, and then the venous anastomosis is redone. Other complications include hematoma formation, infection, and external compression.

FREE SKIN FLAPS

A free flap may be defined as a composite tissue transfer composed of skin and subcutaneous tissue that is transferred in one stage to a distant recipient site and revascularized via microvascular anastomoses. The *critical* factor is that its survival is totally dependent upon a functioning intravascular circulation, both arterial and venous; in comparison, a skin graft can survive on plasmatic circulation from the recipient bed. The evolution of free flaps was dependent upon the introduction of microvascular techniques and an improved understanding of the blood supply to the cutaneous circulation [20, 66]. The pioneering efforts of Jacobson [42, 43] in developing microvascular surgery were extrapolated by Buncke [8, 14] to 1-mm. vessel repairs. This advance stimulated Goldwyn and colleagues' [29] initial efforts at free skin flap transfers, which in turn were perfected by Krizek and co-workers [47] and extended by Strauch and Murray [68] to nutrient vessels 1 mm. in diameter. However, these experimental series were done in loose-skin animals; the essential validation in fixed-skin animals was subsequently provided by Daniel [19, 25].

The blood supply to the skin can be divided into direct cutaneous and musculocutaneous arteries. Direct cutaneous arteries course parallel to the skin for vast distances and can nourish large free skin flaps. Musculocutaneous arteries are short perpendicular vessels that individually nourish small areas of skin; they can be collectively maintained via a muscle cuff to supply a large free flap (i.e., free myocutaneous flap). With this information, it becomes possible to identify many free flap donor sites [72]. The first report of a successful free flap transfer in man was published in 1973 by Daniel and Taylor [22, 71].

At the present time, a free skin flap is considered whenever a multistaged pedicle flap or a complex direct flap is planned or has previously failed. Standard free flaps have been used to provide skin coverage following trauma, to reconstruct defects following release of scar contractures secondary to burns, to restore surface contours, and to provide skin coverage with permanent blood supply in the treatment of radiation ulcers [31]. Specialized free flaps can be used to restore critical sensation or to reconstruct compound defects. In the final analysis, free skin flaps represent a dramatic advance over conventional techniques of distant skin flap migration and permit new specialized reconstructive procedures.

Donor Sites

Free skin flap donor sites are numerous, allowing the surgeon to select the optimal free flap for each case. (The various free flap donor sites are compared and discussed in Table 41-3.) Undoubtedly, the free iliofemoral (groin) flap remains the most commonly utilized donor site, while the dorsalis pedis flap is a distant second [6, 22, 24, 32, 57]. It should be noted that the dorsum of the foot remains a privileged donor site, one that should *not* be used indiscriminately since significant donor site morbidity may occur. If critical sensation is required, the first web flap has finer sensation with minimal morbidity [50]. The axillary [26], deltopectoral [28, 32], and scalp donor sites are occasionally used while the forehead, gluteal [27], gracilis, and postauricular sites are rarely considered. Recently myocutaneous free flaps (latissimus dorsi, tensor fascia lata) have become popular due to the ease of dissection, large size, long vascular pedicle, large diameter vessels, and generally acceptable morbidity.

Results

Large series of free flap transfers are being reported from numerous microsurgical centers around the world. Harii and Ohmorii [30] have done over 200 free skin flaps, with a 92 percent survival rate. O'Brien [55] has performed 42 free skin flaps with 33 survivals (a 78 percent success rate). Serafin and co-workers [65] reported 38 free groin flaps with 6 total failures and partial loss in 4. Serafin and associates [64] have compared free flap transfers with conventional cross leg flaps and jump flaps for coverage of lower extremity defects. He found that free flaps provided excellent skin coverage with shorter hospitalization, reduced costs, and comparable survival rates (Table 41-4). Thus, free flap transfers have a survival rate comparable to tubed pedicle flaps, but with definite advantages in terms of decreased hospitalization and patient morbidity [67].

An analysis of our own initial experience with 12 free flaps (10 groin flaps, 2 dorsalis pedis flaps) has demonstrated the following (Table 41-5): (1) success was achieved in 11 cases (92 percent), with the only failure being a buried free flap; (2) there was a wide range of application from the oral cavity to the lower extremity; (3) numerous microvascular anastomotic techniques were used, including 4 vein grafts and 2 end-to-side anastomoses; and (4) a failing free flap was successfully salvaged.

Complications

The most significant complications of free skin flaps are vascular in origin; their frequency varies from a high of 40 percent to a low of 7 percent. In 42 free skin flaps O'Brien [55] experienced 16 postoperative vascular complications (38 percent) that required immediate reoperation. These complications involved 13 arterial and 3 venous thromboses; in the latter cases, the flaps were salvaged by simple anastomotic revision. In 8 of the patients with arterial thromboses, the flaps were lost, probably due to selection of damaged recipient arteries with poor flow. Thus far, I have had to reoperate in only 1 case (8 percent), a low complication rate that I attribute to the following maneuvers: (1) utilization of only those recipient arteries that have a strong pulsatile perfusion pressure, (2) careful assessment of anastomotic patency prior to wound closure, (3) early insertion of vein grafts rather than repeated anastomotic revisions, and (4) the use of multiple arterial and venous anastomoses whenever possible. As repeatedly emphasized, most vascular complications are postoperative confirmations of intraoperative suspicions – they should be recognized and corrected at the initial operation, not 6 to 12 hours later.

Table 41-3. Free Flap Donor Sites

Location	Flap Vessels: Vessels	Flap Vessels: Diameter of Artery (mm.)	Flap Vessels: Stalk	Maximal Size (cm.)	Donor Site Closure	Options
Regional flaps						
Iliofemoral	Superficial circumflex iliac Superficial inferior epigastric	0.8–3.0	Moderate (2–10 cm.)	30 X 20	Primary	Iliac crest Twelfth intercostal nerve
Deltopectoral	Anterior thoracic perforators	0.8–1.2	Short (1–2 cm.)	19 X 19	Primary	Limited neural innervation
Axillary	Direct cutaneous artery from subscapular	2.0–5.0	Moderate	20 X 15	Primary	None
Arterial flaps						
Scalp	Superficial temporal	1.0–1.8	Short (2–3 cm.)	15 X 3	Primary	Hair growth
Forehead	Superficial temporal	1.0–1.8	Long (0–10 cm.)	7 X 5	Skin graft	None
Dorsum of foot	Dorsalis pedis	2.0–4.0	Long (0–10 cm.)	10 X 10	Skin graft	Neural innervation (15–20 mm. two-point)
First web space	First metatarsal	1.0–2.0	Long (0–10 cm.)	8 X 3	Skin graft	Neural innervation (10–15 mm. two-point)
Myocutaneous flaps						
Intercostal	Posterior intercostal	1.5–2.5	Long (0–20 cm.)	25 X 12	Primary	Neural innervation, rib, and muscle
Gluteus	Superior gluteal	1.5–2.5	Medium (0–6 cm.)	15 X 10	Primary	Muscle for padding or possible reinnervation
Gracilis	Dominant muscle artery (or retrograde dissection)	1.2–1.8	Short (0–4 cm.)	33 X 10	Primary	Muscle
Latissimus dorsi	Thoracodorsal	2.0–3.0	Long (0–10 cm.)	40 X 22	Primary	Rib and muscle
Tensor fascia lata	Lat. femoral circumflex	1.5–2.5	Moderate (0–6 cm.)	40 X 12	Primary	Neural innervation and muscle

Table 41-4. Comparison of Skin Flap Coverage Techniques*

Type of Flap (No. of Cases)	Survival			Number of General Anesthetics	Hours of General Anesthesia	Days of Immobilization	Days of Hospitalization	Total Cost
	Complete	Partial	Failure					
Cross Leg (18)	14	3	1	3.7	9.1	32.8	62.3	$10,325.00
Jump (6)	2	3	1	9	21.7	120.8	121.2	$21,731.00
Free (17)	10	3	4	1.7	12.7	15.7	36.2	$ 9,071.00

*From Serafin, Georgiade, and Smith [64].

Advantages and Disadvantages

The advantages of free flaps are numerous and include the following:

1. A one-stage operation providing essential skin coverage.
2. Retention of permanent intrinsic circulation.
3. Minimal flap fibrosis with maximal flexibility.
4. Excellent survival rate, with shorter hospitalization and a reduced cost.
5. More comfortable patient position and shorter immobilization.
6. Primary donor site closure.
7. Specialized single-stage reconstruction with restoration of sensation, incorporation of a vascularized bone graft, or incorporation of functional muscle.

The disadvantages of free flaps are few but formidable, and include the following:

1. Difficult and tedious operations of long duration (6 to 18 hours).
2. Perilous vascular complications requiring immediate reoperation.
3. Variable donor site morbidity.

FREE VASCULARIZED BONE TRANSFERS

Free vascularized bone transfers were pioneered experimentally by Östrup [58, 59], who demonstrated that osteocyte survival could be achieved following distant transfer if the nutrient blood supply was reestablished by microvascular anastomoses. Thus, a vascularized bone graft would unite quickly at both ends by normal fracture healing, as opposed to prolonged incorporation by the creeping substitution that follows routine bone grafting of cortical bone [13]. Documented clinical success was first achieved by Taylor and co-workers [74], who transferred a 22-cm. fibula segment to reconstruct a long tibial defect. Buncke and associates [11] pioneered the free rib transfer including associated skin to provide dramatic one-stage reconstruction of compound pretibial defects.

Free vascularized bone transfers are most often used to restore bony continuity following trauma, infection, tumor resection, or radiation necrosis. The length, location, structural characteristics, and associated requirements determine selection of the donor site (Table 41-6). The fibula is most valuable for long defects in the femur, tibia, humerus, radius, or ulna. Free fibula transfers represent the best alternative for reconstruction of long bone deformities; this is particularly the case in comparison with autogenous cancellous bone grafts, which provide viability but not stability. Short bone defects with associated skin coverage problems are best reconstructed with a free composite osteocutaneous groin flap, in which the iliac crest acts as a vascularized bone graft and skin coverage is provided by the attached iliofemoral flap; both the iliac crest and the flap are supplied preferentially by the deep circumflex iliac artery. Free rib transfers are valuable for mandibular reconstruction, but they present technical difficulties. I have performed 24 free bone transfers – 10 free fibula transfers, 7 free composite osteocutaneous groin flaps, 4 free osteocutaneous foot flaps, and, 3 free rib transfers [79, 80]. Thus far the initial survival rate has been 100 percent for the free fibula transfers with two subsequent losses due to infection and vascular compromise. The free composite groin free foot flaps have all survived. None of the free rib transfers have survived. Complications have been few in free fibular transfers because the vessels were of large diameter and because there was adequate venous

Table 41-5. An Analysis of 12 Consecutive Free Flap Transfers

Patient	Defect	Free Flap	Anastomoses		Vascular Complications	Results
H.M.	Ankle (trauma)	Groin	A SCIA:RT V VC:VC V SIEV:GSV	E-E/SD E-E E-E	None	Survival
R.V.	Left hand (trauma)	Foot	A DP:PP V VC:DM V GSV:DM	E-E E-E E-E	None	Survival
E.H.	Floor of mouth hypopharynx (tumor resection)	Groin	A SCIA:FA A SIEA:FA V SIEV:IJ	E-E E-E/SD E-E	None	Survival
V.W.	Total nose (tumor, radiation)	Foot (lined FSTSG)	A DP:FA V SV:FV/Y-VG V VC:FV/Y-VG	E-E	Intraoperative revision of arterial anastomosis	Survival
K.K.	Rhomberg's syndrome	Groin (deepithelialized)	A SCIA:FA V SIEV:FV	E-E E-E	Compression of venous anastomosis	Failure
C.C.	Left forearm (trauma)	Groin	A SCIA:UA V VC:VC	E-E E-E	None	Survival
P.V.	Left leg (trauma)	Groin plus iliac crest	A SCIA:AT V SIEV:VC	E-E E-E	None	Survival
M.R.	Oral lining (commando resection)	Groin plus iliac crest	A SCIA:EC/Y- VG A SIEA:EC/Y- VG		None	Survival
M.H.	Right ankle (trauma)	Groin plus iliac crest	A SCIA:PT/VG V SIEV:GSV	 E-E	Venous congestion Anastomosis patent, insertion vein graft (VC:VC/VG)	Survival
G.H.	Left face (trauma)	Groin plus iliac crest	A SCIA:LA/ V SIEV:EJ/	E-E E-E	None	Survival
T.D.	Left cheek (commando resection following radiation)	Groin plus iliac crest	A SCIA:FA/ V SIEV:FV/	E-E E-E	None	Survival
C.D.	Right leg (trauma)	Groin	A SCIA:PT/ V SIEV:SV/ V VC:VC/VG	E-E E-E	None	Survival

A = artery; V = vein; SCIA = superficial circumflex iliac artery; SIEV = superficial inferior epigastric vein; SIEA = superficial inferior epigastric artery; VC = venae comitantes; DP = dorsalis pedis; PP = princeps pollicis; FA = facial artery; FV = facial vein; AT = anterior tibial; SV = saphenous vein; EC = external carotid; PT = posterior tibial; E-E = end-to-end anastomosis; E-E/SD = end-to-end discrepancy; Y-VG = "Y" vein graft; VG = vein graft; EJ = external jugular; L = lingual artery; UA = ulnar artery.

Table 41-6. Free Bone Transfers

Characteristics	Fibula	Rib	Iliac Crest
Bone			
Length (maximum)	22–26 cm.	30 cm.	10 cm.
Shape	Straight	Curved	Slight curve
Structure	Cortical, straight	Membranous, malleable	Corticocancellous, fixed
Vessels			
Artery	Peroneal (1.5–2.5 mm.)	Posterior intercostal (1.0–1.5 mm.)	Superficial, circumflex iliac (0.8–3.0 mm.)
Vein	2 venae comitantes (2.0–3.0 mm.)	1 intercostal (0.8–1.5 mm.)	Superficial inferior epigastric (1.5–3.0 mm.)
Vascular stalk	Short (1.0–3.0 cm.)	Long (3.0–5.0 cm.)	Moderate (1.0–10 cm.)
Dissection	Simple, tedious, superficial	Difficult, quick, deep	Slow, superficial
Options			
Articular surface	Yes	Yes	No
Epiphysis	Yes	No	No
Functional muscle	Yes	Yes	No
Overlying skin	No	Yes	Yes
Nerve	No	Yes	Yes
Complications	Minimum	Thoracotomy Venous difficulties	Abdominal wall hernia
Applications	Long bone defects (extremities)	Mandibular reconstruction, composite bone-skin replacement	Short bone defects (extremity), mandibular reconstruction, composite bone-skin replacement

drainage. Problems with free composite groin flaps are similar to those of standard free groin flap transfers and are largely avoidable. Free rib transfers present the following technical difficulties: (1) difficult donor site dissection, (2) limited venous drainage through a single vein, and (3) restricted malleability. The free composite groin flap is currently finding wide application both in mandibular reconstruction and in reconstruction of compound lower extremity defects; as a result there is limited indication for free rib transfers. The free fibula transfer is rapidly becoming the best method available for reconstruction of long bone defects, especially in the extremities.

FREE TOE-TO-HAND TRANSFERS

The free toe-to-hand transfer is now one of the best methods for reconstructing traumatically damaged or congenitally deformed hands. The great toe can be transferred to replace the thumb, and the second toe to replace other digits or even partial digital amputations. The pioneering experimental work of Buncke and colleagues [9] was confirmed clinically by Cobbett [18] and Yang [5]. The following technical refinements have contributed to the increasing survival rate and final function of free toe-to-hand transfers:

1. Isolation of the toe on the first dorsal metatarsal–dorsalis pedis arterial system and the dorsal venous arch–greater saphenous vein venous system.
2. Careful anastomosis of both volar metatarsal nerves and the deep peroneal nerve.
3. Repair of long flexor and extensor tendons proximal to the wrist.

However, isolation of the donor toe remains a tedious difficult dissection that is best perfected during repeated "dress rehearsals" in fresh cadavers.

Buncke and Furnas [10] have reported a series of 14 free toe-to-hand transfers, with an 85 percent survival rate. Functional recovery has been good, with an almost normal range of motion in the interphalangeal joint and a two-point discrimination of 10 to 20 mm. O'Brien [55] reported complete survival of 9 free toe-to-hand transfers (3 great toes, 5 second toes, 1 third toe).

Complications are potentially numerous and include the following: (1) vascular thrombosis, either arterial or venous, (2) donor site morbidity with delayed healing and compromised gait, (3) limited reinnervation, and (4) restricted motion. The vascular difficulties have been largely eliminated by isolation of the toes on a long dorsal pedicle, which allows vascular anastomoses between 2-mm. vessels proximal to the original trauma site. Donor site morbidity can be minimized by careful placement of incisions and preservation of the metatarsal head. Reinnervation and active motion remain a challenge; the best results have been achieved in younger patients [51].

In the final analysis, free toe-to-hand transfers are applicable in the following situations:

1. Following multiple-digit trauma – the great toe may be utilized to replace the thumb and the second toe to replace other digits.
2. Congential aphalangia affecting either the thumb or multiple digits.
3. Partial single-digit amputation when cosmetic replacement is desired.

FREE MUSCLE TRANSFER

During the past decade, free muscle transfers have progressed from an experimental curiosity to a clinical reality. Initial investigations were begun by Tamai and associates [69, 70] and subsequently confirmed by Ikuta [40] and Terzis and colleagues [75]. They have convincingly demonstrated that free muscle transfers will survive and will be functionally reinnervated, provided that the microneurovascular anastomoses are flawless. Reinnervation of the muscle usually occurs by 5 months; the final function is determined in part by muscle insertion under the correct tension.

Clinical success has been reported by Ch'en [15], Harii, Ohmori, and Tarii [33], Ikuta [40], and Manktelow [48]. These muscle transfers were utilized to reconstruct traumatic forearm defects and even facial paralysis [62]. The gracilis muscle and the lateral portion of the pectoralis major are the principal donor sites; the latter is favored in the restoration of multiple flexor tendons. With clinical confirmation, one can expect increasing utilization of free muscle transfers in the future.

FREE INTESTINAL TRANSFERS

Free intestinal transfers were pioneered by Seidenberg and co-workers [63] and were perfected by Hiebert and Cummings [36] and Nakayama and associates [54]. Various segments of the alimentary tract have been used to replace the esophagus, with the current preference being for the jejunum or colon. For many years, free intestinal transfers were considered to have an unacceptable risk of vascular thrombosis, when compared to more reliable local flaps. However, local flaps require controlled pharyngostomes with multistage reconstruction. Recent improvements in microvascular techniques, with a near 100-percent patency rate for the requisite 2- to 3-mm. vessels, have caused renewed interest in intestinal transfers. May and Bunting [49] currently favor the jejunum as a donor site for esophageal replacement, while others prefer the colon. With either method, success rates for single stage intestinal transfer are now close to 100 percent, as compared to Nakayama's original 76 percent (16 of 21).

FREE NERVE TRANSFERS

The free nerve transfer is a method of maintaining circulation to a large whole nerve graft in which the survival of Schwann cells would be compromised in a scarred recipient bed. Essentially, the donor nerve is isolated with careful preservation of its vasa nervorum, which in turn are traced to their origin from larger nutrient vessels. The complete nerve and its intact blood supply are inserted into the recipient nerve defect and the essential intrinsic circulation is reestablished through microvascular anastomoses. Since the Schwann cells survive, the endoneural tubular architecture is preserved and axonal reinnervation will occur more rapidly. Taylor and Ham [73], who developed this technique, have found the rate of reinnervation in 3 cases to be much faster than would be expected with conventional nerve grafting techniques.

FREE OMENTAL TRANSFER

Free omental transfers were originally conceived of by McLean and Buncke [52] in 1972 as viable malleable clinical building blocks for auricular reconstruction; subsequently the technique was considered as a substitute for the then unproved free skin flap. The omentum is harvested from the abdomen and transferred to a distant site; its supplying gastroepiploic vessels (either right or left) are then anastomosed to the recipient vessels. Free omental transfers can be buried beneath the skin to correct contour deformities or covered with a split-thickness skin graft to provide essential skin coverage [39]. With perfection of free skin flap transfers, the indications for and incidence of free omental transfers have decreased dramatically. However, they can be extremely valuable for revascularizing the irradiated brachial plexus.

RECONSTRUCTIVE MICROSURGERY: TO DO OR NOT TO DO?

Many practicing plastic surgeons and virtually all plastic surgery residents are now confronted with the reality of reconstructive microsurgery. Specifically, it is no longer acceptable to deny the patient with a clean-cut multiple-digit amputation the chance of replantation or to submit a patient to a tube flap migration simply because the surgeon is not trained in microsurgical techniques. It is equally unfair for the enthusiastic but untrained microsurgeon to attempt these cases when referral to a microsurgical center would be possible. Therefore, plastic surgeons must decide their individual commitment to reconstructive microsurgery.

First, it would benefit every plastic surgeon, in any stage of training, to acquire basic microsurgical skills. Initial emphasis should be placed on familiarization with ocular loupes, operating microscopes, microinstruments, and microsutures. Applications would involve the precise suturing of small structures, including cleft lip surgery, pediatric plastic surgery, hypospadias repair, and numerous other types of clinical cases.

Second, surgeons involved in upper extremity surgery must be trained in microsurgical techniques, both microneural and microvascular. Traumatic hand surgery frequently involves peripheral nerve repairs and occasionally mandates revascularization of ischemic digits. Therefore, a high level of microsurgical expertise is mandatory regardless of one's interest in replantation surgery. Realistically, replantation surgery requires the constant availability of many surgeons and is probably best done in regional or state centers.

Third, free tissue transfers are difficult, complex elective procedures that demand nearly perfect results. Therefore, most cases will be performed within large regional medical centers by surgeons who are particularly interested in microvascular surgery and who have a sufficient number of cases that they can acquire meaningful experience. Free tissue transfers should *not* be done by the occasional microsurgeon. One must remember that proficiency in the microsurgical teaching laboratory and familiarization with vascular anatomy from a few cadaver dissections are inadequate preparation for clinical free tissue transfers. Rather, the surgeon wanting to learn reconstructive microsurgery must be prepared to take a 6-month fellowship at a specialized center following his training in plastic and reconstructive surgery.

Reconstructive microsurgery remains in its infancy. Current operations are often considered unusual and viewed as "salvage" procedures. With increasing experience and a decreasing complication rate, these radical procedures will become routine and new operative techniques will emerge to revolutionize all of reconstructive surgery.

REFERENCES

1. Acland, R. D. A new needle for microvascular surgery. *Surgery* 71:130, 1972.
2. Acland, R. D. Signs of patency in small vessel anastomosis. *Surgery* 72:744, 1972.
3. Acland, R. D. Thrombus formation in microvascular surgery: An experimental study of the effects of surgical trauma. *Surgery* 73:766, 1973.
4. Acland, R. D. Microvascular anastomosis: A device for holding stay sutures and a new vascular clamp. *Surgery* 75:185, 1974.
5. American Replantation Mission to China. Replantation surgery in China. *Plast. Reconstr. Surg.* 52:476, 1973.
6. Baudet, J., Le Maire, J.-M., and Guimberteau, J.-C. Ten free groin flaps. *Plast. Reconstr. Surg.* 57:577, 1976.
7. Baxter, T. J., O'Brien, B. McC., Henderson, P. N., and Bennett, R. C. The histopathology of small vessels following microvascular repair. *Br. J. Surg.* 59:617, 1972.
8. Buncke, H. J. The Suture Repair of 1 Millimeter Vessels. In Donoghy, R. M. P., and Yasargil, M. G. (Eds.), *Microvascular Surgery*. St. Louis: Mosby, 1967.
9. Buncke, H. J., Buncke, C. M., and Schulz, W. P. Immediate Nicaladoni procedure in the rhesus monkey, or hallux-to-hand transplantation, utilizing microminiature vascular anastomoses. *Br. J. Plast. Surg.* 19:332, 1966.
10. Buncke, H. J., and Furnas, D. W. Free Compound Bone–Skin Flap Transfer. In Daniel, R. K., and Terzis, J. K. (Eds.), *Reconstructive Microsurgery*. Boston: Little, Brown, 1977.
11. Buncke, H. J., Furnas, D. W., Gordon, L., and Achauer, B. M. Free osteocutaneous flap from a rib to the tibia. *Plast. Reconstr. Surg.* 59:799, 1977.
12. Buncke, H. J., and McLean, D. H. The advantage of a straight needle in microsurgery. *Plast. Reconstr. Surg.* 47:602, 1971.
13. Buncke, H. J., and Murray, D. E. Autogenous Arterial Interposition of Grafts of Less Than 1 mm in External Diameter in Rats. *Transactions of the Sixth International Congress of Plastic and Reconstructive Surgery*. London: Butterworth, 1971.
14. Buncke, H. J., and Schulz, W. P. Total ear reimplantation in the rabbit utilizing microminiature vascular anastomoses. *Br. J. Plast. Surg.* 10;15, 1966.
15. Ch'en, C. W. *Zhonghua Yixue Zazhi* 8:530, 1975.
16. Cobbett, J. Small vessel anastomosis: A compari-

son of suture techniques. *Br. J. Plast. Surg.* 22:16, 1967.

17. Cobbett, J. Microvascular surgery. *Surg. Clin. North Am.* 47:521, 1967.
18. Cobbett, J. R. Free digital transfer; report of a case of transfer of a great toe to replace an amputated thumb. *J. Bone Joint Surg.* [Br.] 51:677, 1969.
19. Daniel, R. K. Direct Transfer of Skin Flaps by Microvascular Anastomoses. M. Sc. Thesis, McGill University, 1973.
20. Daniel, R. K. The Anatomical and Hemodynamic Characteristics of the Cutaneous Circulation and Their Influence on Skin Flap Design. In Grabb, W. C., and Myers, B. (Eds.), *Skin Flaps.* Boston: Little, Brown, 1975.
21. Daniel, R. K., and May, J. W., Jr. Free flaps: An overview. *Clin. Orthop.* 133:122, 1978.
22. Daniel, R. K., and Taylor, G. I. Distant transfer of an island flap by microvascular anastomoses. *Plast. Reconstr. Surg.* 52:111, 1973.
23. Daniel, R. K., and Terzis, J. K. *Reconstructive Microsurgery.* Boston: Little, Brown, 1977.
24. Daniel, R. K., Terzis, J., and Midgley, R. D. Restoration of sensation to anesthetic hand by free neurovascular flap from foot. *Plast. Reconstr. Surg.* 57:275, 1976.
25. Daniel, R. K., and Williams, H. B. The free transfer of skin flaps by microvascular anastomoses. *Plast. Reconstr. Surg.* 52:16, 1973.
26. Dessart, B. Les transpositions de lambeaux cutanes par microanastomoses des pedicules vasculaires. Monograph, Lyon, 1975.
27. Fujino, T., Harashina, T., and Aoyagi, F. Reconstruction for a plasia of the breast and pectoral region by microvascular transfer of a free flap from the buttock. *Plast. Reconstr. Surg.* 56:178, 1975.
28. Fujino, T., Tanino, R., and Sugimoto, C. Microvascular transfer of free deltopectoral dermal-fat flap. *Plast. Reconstr. Surg.* 55:428, 1975.
29. Goldwyn, R. M., Lamb, D. L., and White, W. L. An experimental study of large island flaps in dogs. *Plast. Reconstr. Surg.* 31:528, 1963.
30. Harii, K., and Ohmori, K. Free skin flap transfer. *Clin. Plast. Surg.* 3:111, 1976.
31. Harii, K., Ohmori, K., and Ohmori, S. Successful clinical transfer of ten free flaps by microvascular anastomoses. *Plast. Reconstr. Surg.* 53:259, 1974.
32. Harii, K., Ohmori, K., and Ohmori, S. Free deltopectoral skin flaps. *Br. J. Plast. Surg.* 27:231, 1974.
33. Harii, K., Ohmori, K., and Tarii, S. Free gracilis muscle transplantation, with microneurovascular anastomoses for the treatment of facial paralysis: A preliminary report. *Plast. Reconstr. Surg.* 57:133, 1976.
34. Hayhurst, J. W., and O'Brien, M. McC. An experimental study of microvascular technique, patency rates, and related factors. *Br. J. Plast. Surg.* 28:128, 1975.
35. Henderson, P. N., O'Brien, B. McC., and Parel, J. M. An adjustable double microvascular clamp. *Med. J. Aust.* 1:715, 1970.
36. Hiebert, C. A., and Cummings, G. O., Jr. Successful replacement of the cervical esophagus by transplantation and revascularization of free graft of gastric antrum. *Ann. Surg.* 154:103, 1961.
37. Hoerenz, P. The design of the surgical microscope. *Ophthalmic Surg.* 4:40, 89, 1973.
38. Ikuta, Y. Studies on small vessel anastomosis. *Hiroshima J. Med. Sci.* 17:285, 1968.
39. Ikuta, Y. Autotransplant of omentum to cover large denudation of the scalp. *Plast. Reconstr. Surg.* 55:490, 1975.
40. Ikuta, Y. Free Muscle Transfer. In Daniel, R. K., and Terzis, J. K. (Eds.), *Reconstructive Microsurgery.* Boston: Little, Brown, 1977.
41. Ikuta, Y., Watari, S., Kawamura, K., Shima, R., Matsuishi, Y., Miyoshi, K., and Tsuge, K. Free flap transfers by end-to-side arterial anastomosis. *Br. J. Plast. Surg.* 28:1, 1975.
42. Jacobson, J. H. Microsurgery. *Curr. Probl. Surg.* February, 1971.
43. Jacobson, J. H., and Suarez, E. L. Microsurgery in anastomosis of small vessels. *Surg. Forum* 11:243, 1960.
44. Karkowski, J., and Buncke, H. J. A simplified technique for free transfer of groin flaps, by use of a Doppler probe. *Plast. Reconstr. Surg.* 55:682, 1975.
45. Kleinert, H. E., Juhala, C. A., Tsai, T.-M., and Van Beek, A. Digital replantation – selection, technique, and results. *Orthop. Clin. North Am.* 8:309, 1977.
46. Kleinert, H. E., Serafin, D., and Daniel, R. K. The place of microsurgery in hand surgery. *Orthop. Clin. North Am.* 4:929, 1973.
47. Krizek, T. J., Tani, T., Des Prez, J. D., and Kiehn, C. L. Experimental transplantation of composite grafts by microsurgical anastomoses. *Plast. Reconstr. Surg.* 36:538, 1965.
48. Manktelow, R. Free Muscle Transfer. In Serafin, D. E., and Buncke, H. J. (Eds.), *Microsurgical Composite Tissue Transplantation.* St. Louis: Mosby, 1979. Pp. 369–390.
49. May, J. W., Jr., and Bunting, P. D. Free Jejunal Transfer for Irradiated Esophageal Reconstruction. In Daniel, R. K., and Terzis, J. K. (Eds.), *Reconstructive Microsurgery.* Boston: Little, Brown, 1977.
50. May, J. W., Jr., Chait, C. A., Cohen, B. E., and

O'Brien, B. McC. Free neurovascular flap from the first web of the foot in hand reconstruction. *J. Hand Surg.* 2:387, 1977.
51. May, J. W., Jr., and Daniel, R. K. Great Toe-to-Hand Free Tissue Transfers. *Clin. Orthop.* 133:140, 1978.
52. McLean, D. H., and Buncke, H. J. Autotransplant of omentum to a large scalp defect with microsurgical revascularization. *Plast. Reconstr. Surg.* 49:268, 1972.
53. McLean, D. H., and Buncke, H. J. Use of the Saran wrap cuff in microsurgical arterial repairs. *Plast. Reconstr. Surg.* 51:624, 1973.
54. Nakayama, K., Tamiya, T., Yamamoto, K., and Akimoto, S. A simple new apparatus for small vessel anastomosis (free autograft of the sigmoid included). *Surgery* 52:918, 1962.
55. O'Brien, B. McC. *Microvascular Reconstructive Surgery.* Edinburgh: Churchill-Livingstone, 1977.
56. O'Brien, B. McC., Henderson, P. N., Bennett, R. C., and Crock, G. W. Microvascular surgical technique. *Med. J. Aust.* 1:722, 1970.
57. O'Brien, B. McC., Morrison, W. A., Ishida, H., MacLeod, A. M., and Gilbert, A. Free flap transfers with microvascular anastomoses. *Br. J. Plast. Surg.* 27:220, 1974.
58. Östrup, L. T. *The Free, Living Bone Graft.* Linköping University Medical Dissertations, No. 31, Linköping (Sweden), 1975.
59. Östrup, L. T., and Fredrickson, J. M. Distant transfer of free, living bone graft by microvascular anastomoses. *Plast. Reconstr. Surg.* 54:274, 1974.
60. Polack, F. M., Sanchez, J., and Eve, F. R. Microsurgical sutures: I. Evaluation of various types of needles and sutures for anterior segment surgery. *Can. J. Ophthalmol.* 9:42, 1974.
61. Rigg, B. M. Transfer of a free groin flap to the heel by microvascular anastomoses. *Plast. Reconstr. Surg.* 55:36, 1975.
62. Schenck, R. R. Free muscle and composite skin transplantation by microneurovascular anastomoses. *Orthop. Clin. North Am.* 8:367, 1977.
63. Seidenberg, G., Rosevak, S. S., Hurwitt, E. S., and Som, M. L. Immediate reconstruction of the cervical esophagus by a revascularized isolated jejunal segment. *Ann. Surg.* 149:162, 1959.
64. Serafin, D., Georgiade, N. G., and Smith, D. H. Comparison of free flaps with pedicled flaps for coverage of defects of the leg or foot. *Plast. Reconstr. Surg.* 59:492, 1977.
65. Serafin, D., Shearin, J. C., and Georgiade, N. G. The vascularization of free flaps. *Plast. Reconstr. Surg.* 60:233, 1977.
66. Smith, J. W. Microsurgery: Review of the literature and discussion of microtechnique. *Plast. Reconstr. Surg.* 37:277, 1966.
67. Stranc, M. F., Labandter, H., and Roy, A. A review of 196 tube pedicles. *Br. J. Plast. Surg.* 28:54, 1975.
68. Strauch, B., and Murray, D. E. Transfer of composite graft with immediate suture anastomosis. *Plast. Reconstr. Surg.* 40:325, 1967.
69. Tamai, S., Komatsu, S., Sakamoto, H., Sano, S., Sasauchi, N., Hori, Y., Tatsumi, Y., and Okuda, H. Free muscle transplants in dogs with microsurgical neurovascular anastomoses. *Plast. Reconstr. Surg.* 46:219, 1970.
70. Tamai, S., Sasauchi, N., Hori, Y., Tatsumi, Y., and Okuda, H. Microvascular surgery in orthopaedics and traumatology. *J. Bone Joint Surg.* [Br.] 54:637, 1972.
71. Taylor, G. I., and Daniel, R. K. The free flap: Composite tissue transfer by vascular anastomoses. *Aust. N.Z. J. Surg.* 43:1, 1973.
72. Taylor, G. I., and Daniel, R. K. The anatomy of several free flap donor sites. *Plast. Reconstr. Surg.* 56:243, 1975.
73. Taylor, G. I., and Ham, F. J. The free vascularized nerve graft. *Plast. Reconstr. Surg.* 57:413, 1976.
74. Taylor, G. I., Miller, G. D. H., and Ham, F. J. The free vascularized bone graft: A clinical extension of microvascular techniques. *Plast. Reconstr. Surg.* 55:533, 1975.
75. Terzis, J. K., Dykes, R. W., and Williams, H. B. Functional recovery in free muscle transfers by microneurovascular anastomoses. *J. Hand Surg.* (In press).
76. Troutman, R. C. *Microsurgery of the Anterior Segment of the Eye,* Vol. 1. *Introduction and Basic Techniques.* St. Louis: Mosby, 1974.
77. Tsai, T.-M. Experimental and clinical application of microvascular surgery. *Ann. Surg.* 181:169, 1975.
78. Yasargil, M. G. *Microsurgery: As Applied to Neurosurgery.* Stuttgart: Verlag, 1969.
79. Weiland, A. J., Daniel, R. K., and Reilly, L. H., Jr. Application of the free vascularized bone graft in the treatment of malignant or aggressive bone tumors. *Johns Hopkins Med. J.* 140:85, 1977.
80. Weiland, A., Kleinert, H. E., Kutz, J. W., and Daniel, R. K. Free vascularized bone transfers for upper extremity reconstruction. In Serafin, D. E., and Buncke, H. J. (Eds.), *Microsurgical Composite Tissue Transplantation.* St. Louis: Mosby, 1979. Pp. 605–625.

Microsurgical Repair of Peripheral Nerves

HANNO MILLESI

With the use of fine suture material and proper instruments, the surgery of peripheral nerves has become less and less traumatic. For many years, magnification was obtained by the use of loupes. Microscopes for operative use have been available since 1963 [23]. By magnification the extent of damage to the nerve tissue can be better recognized; in secondary repairs, when dissecting the neuroma, it is easier to achieve a sufficient resection if the surgeon has a better view. The magnifying power of a microscope allows one to proceed with a dissection into tissue layers that can be handled otherwise only with much greater difficulties. The main advantage is the really atraumatic surgical technique, which results not only from the magnification but even more from the development of new instruments. The stable position of the microscope and the excellent illumination, along with the possibility of increasing the magnification, are significant advantages over the use of simple loupes, even if the magnifying power applied during the major part of the operation does not differ very greatly.

EQUIPMENT

For microsurgery of peripheral nerves, rather simple equipment is needed. Of course one must have a good microscope that provides magnifications between 4 and 25 times. It is a real advantage if the microscope provides motorized focusing. A diploscope is not necessary because the assistant can do his job without magnification. A set of fine-pointed watchmaker's forceps, a fine forceps with teeth, a needle holder, and scissors that are opened by a spring, are all one needs.

There are two ways to transect a nerve, and the different methods involve the use of different equipment. If one end of the nerve is fixed and the nerve can be easily pulled and brought under tension, a sharp knife can be used. A diamond knife was developed to provide sharp cutting. If the nerve cannot be easily extended sufficiently, the cutting can be done best with a scissors having ondulated blades, to avoid shifting the nerve tissue. If the nerve is cut fascicle by fascicle, the trauma caused by such a transection is acceptable. As stitches, 10-0 nylon sutures have proved extremely useful. Hemostasis can be easily achieved by bipolar coagulation.

GENERAL CONSIDERATIONS ON THE SURGICAL TECHNIQUE

A wide exposure facilitates the whole operation. In secondary repairs the nerve to be repaired should be exposed in the same tissue proximally and distally to the site of lesion. The dissection then proceeds from the scar tissue towards the lesion. If from the primary operation it is known that the nerve is not only completely transected but has suffered a long defect, an exposure of the whole field can be avoided. Under these conditions it is sufficient to expose the proximal and the distal stump and to create a tunnel. Continuity of the nerve is reestablished by putting nerve grafts across the tunnel and performing the proximal and distal coaptation at the separate incisions. In the forearm and the hand, the operation is usually performed under tourniquet in a bloodless field. The tourniquet is kept until the exposure is completed and the nerve stumps are prepared. Thereafter the tourniquet is released and complete hemostasis performed, using bipolar coagulation. If a nerve graft is needed, the time allotted for hemostasis can be used to provide the nerve graft.

Wound closure is carried out in the usual way. It is extremely important to avoid shearing forces that might dislocate the repaired nerves when the skin edges are united. After the operation careful immobilization is essential. In a case of an end-to-end nerve repair, the adjacent joints are immobilized in flexed position for 3 to 4 weeks; thereafter gradual mobilization is encouraged. If a graft was used and longitudinal tension is avoided completely, immobilization is maintained in exactly the position the limb had during the operation; this immobilization is continued for only 10 days, after which free motion is allowed.

INTRANEURAL INTERFASCICULAR DISSECTION

In brachial plexus surgery, Bateman [1] and Pecinka [20] recommended interneural neurolysis; however, this suggestion was rejected by a majority of the authors because of the tissue trauma and the damage that might be inflicted to the nerve tissue when operating within the nerve. Under microscopic vision and using microsurgical techniques, it is possible to perform dissections within the nerves with minimal tissue trauma. In areas with a high rate of fiber exchange between fascicle groups, some of these connections are transected during interfascicular dissection, but this will not lead to a clinically significant functional loss.

The epineurium is incised longitudinally; again it is favorable to start the dissection in healthy tissue and proceed towards the damaged area. The epineurium can be reflected easily. Following the intraneural vessels as guidelines, the dissection proceeds into the depth of the nerve between the individual fascicles and fascicle groups (Fig. 42-1).

In minor degrees of damage the fibrosis is limited to the epineurium, which can be thickened and which compresses the nerve like an overly tight stocking. The fibrosis can involve the interfascicular tissue and in severe cases even the perineurium and the fascicle itself. The perineurium is incised (starting from healthy tissue), undermined, and resected. If the epineurectomy brings sufficient relief, one can watch the fascicles expanding after relief of compression (Fig. 42-2, center fascicle (C)). If the interfascicular tissue has also developed a fibrosis, the epineurectomy does not relieve the compression; then the dissection has to proceed between the fascicles into the depth of the nerve, isolating the fascicle groups and the individual fascicles (Fig. 42-2, fascicles on top (A)). Major interconnections between fascicles and fascicle groups can be saved. Minor connections are necessarily lost. If the resection of the interfascicular tissue relieves the compression, the fascicles expand. However, when fibrosis involves the perineurium or the whole fascicle, this expansion does not occur. In that case the best way to solve the problem is resection and restoration of continuity by nerve grafts (Fig. 42-2, lower fascicles (D, E)).

After the resection of the interfascicular tissue and the epineurium, the individual fascicles are isolated but there is no danger as far as blood supply is concerned. Of course scar tissue will develop; this formation of scar tissue between the isolated fascicles is one of the arguments held against interfascicular dissection. The situation is similar to the correction of a cosmetic scar in the face. One can correct the scar only by producing another scar, but it is hoped that the surgical scar after the operation will be better and less prominent than the original scar. The same is true with interfascicular dissection; if there is a great deal of fibrosis, the resultant scar will be less troublesome. But for this reason one should use the interfascicular dissection step by step, starting with the epineurectomy, and do only what is really necessary to relieve the compression of the fascicles.

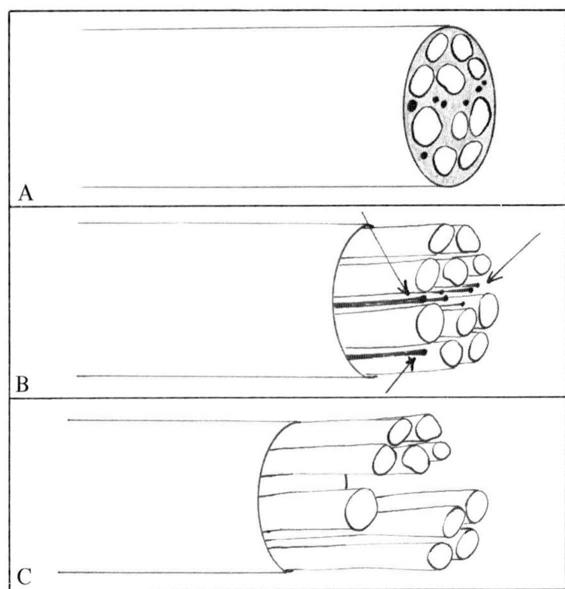

Fig. 42-1. A, a peripheral nerve consists of a number of fascicles, each of which is surrounded by perineurium. The perineurium forms a tube of dense connective tissue, which provides tensile strength and maintains the pressure inside the fascicles; this tube acts as a fluid barrier. The fascicles are kept together by the epineurium, which expands between the fascicles (interfascicular tissue) (gray tissue). B, the major intraneural vessels are located in the interfascicular spaces (arrows point to vessels). After resection of the outer epineurium one can dissect between the fascicles, following the course of the vessels. C, in the peripheral sections of the nerves, groups of fascicles can be separated.

Clinical Applications of Interfascicular Dissection

Lesion in Continuity due to Intraneural Fibrosis
Intraneural fibrosis develops after traction lesion, if the nerve is exposed to chronic irritation and after ischemic or chemical (injection) damage.

Compression Syndromes
Interfascicular fibrosis is quite common in cases of compression syndromes like carpal tunnel syndrome or irritation of the ulnar nerve in the cubital area. Certainly some of these patients with compression syndromes get great benefit from an interfascicular dissection [5].

Nerve Tumors
Different tumors can develop within the peripheral nerve. Only the most common ones will be listed here. A *ganglion* can develop within a nerve, compressing and dislocating the fascicles. By use of the microscope the ganglion with all its extensions can be excised easily, without doing harm to the fascicles. A *neurofibroma* is usually encapsulated and can be excised easily. But again the use of a microscope helps to avoid damaging the fascicular tissue. Since *neurinomas* (schwannomas) originate from the nerve fascicles, the involved fascicles have to be resected; the amount

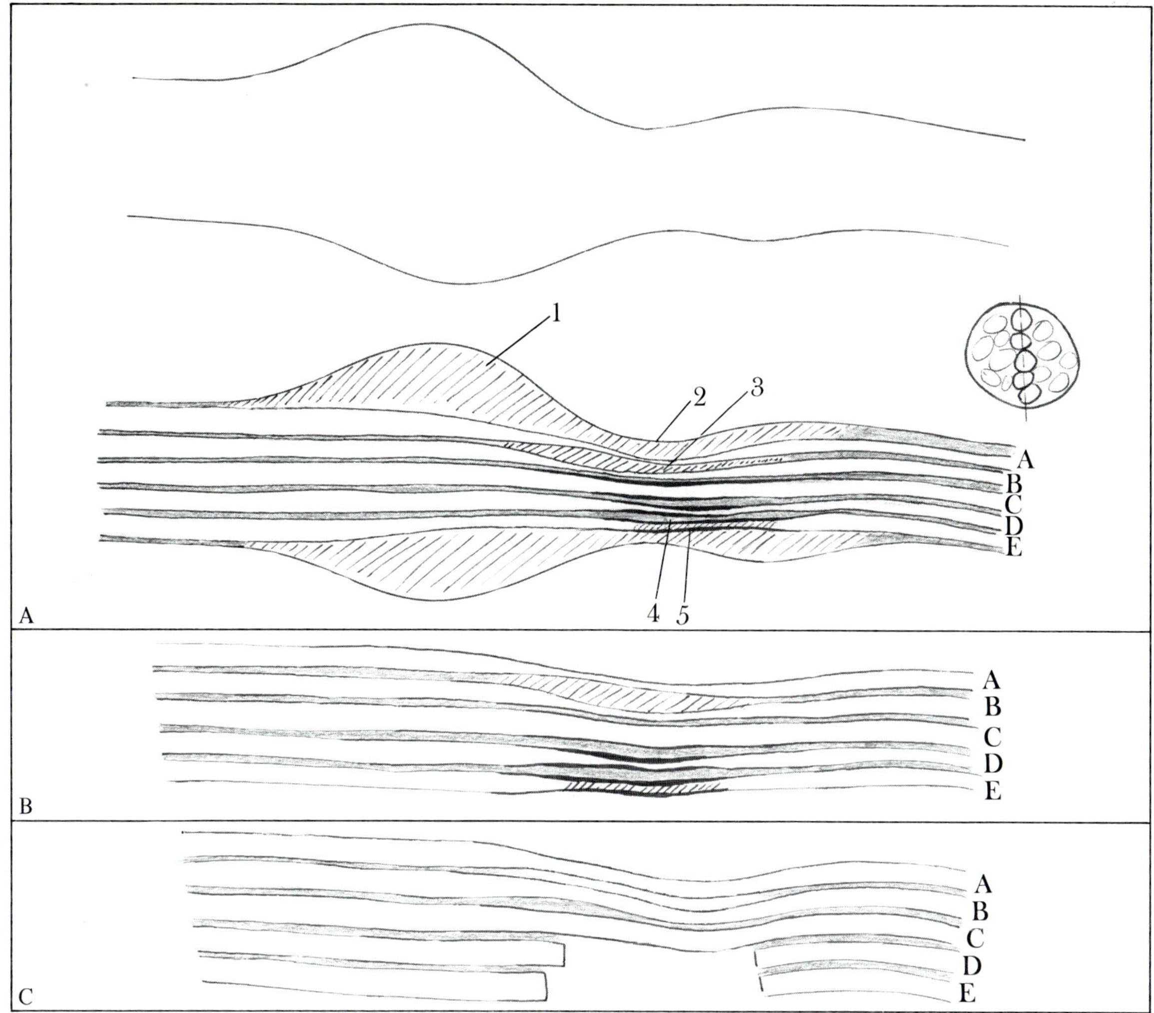

Fig. 42-2. Lesion in continuity. A, irregular appearance of the nerve. In a cross section, different possibilities of tissue reaction are illustrated schematically. 1, proliferation of the epineurium. 2, constriction of the nerve by tight epineurium, causing compression of fascicle C. *3, intraneural fibrosis with compression of fascicles* A *and* B. *4, perineural fibrosis compresses fascicle* D. *5, fascicle* E *has become completely fibrotic.*

B, after epineurectomy, fascicle C *has expanded, due to sufficient relief of compression. Fascicles* A *and* B *could not expand because of interfascicular fibrosis. As a result of the perineural and interfascicular changes, the fascicles* D *and* E *cannot expand at all.*

C, after removal of interfascicular fibrous tissue, fascicles A *and* B *are relieved and can recover. Recovery of fascicles* D *and* E *is not likely to occur; these fascicles are therefore resected and the defect is bridged by nerve grafts.*

of resection can be better judged by microscopic view. The defects are bridged by nerve grafts. Neighboring fascicles that are not involved in the tumor can be easily saved.

Interfascicular Dissection after Loss of Continuity
Interfascicular dissection is used in the same way as described above for the repair of two nerve stumps after transection if fascicular or interfascicular nerve repair is planned.

The dissection of the lesion is started proximally and distally in healthy tissue and proceeds toward the neuroma and the glioma, respectively. Each fascicle group is transected exactly at the point where it loses the normal appearance and disappears in the neuroma. A much more thorough resection of neuroma and scar tissue is achieved compared to the consecutive resection of tissue slices beginning at the end of the stump.

To prepare the stumps, a strip of epineurium is resected. This is done not only to facilitate interfascicular dissection but also to avoid early invasion of the gap between the two stumps by proliferating connective tissue, which originates to a large extent from the epineurium.

RESTORATION OF CONTINUITY

Primary versus Secondary Nerve Repair

There is a continuous discussion about whether primary or early secondary nerve repair should be the treatment of choice.

Time Factor
It is evident that if primary nerve repair is performed time is gained and a second operation avoided. If satisfactory regeneration occurs this is a significant advantage; however, if regeneration does not occur a dilemma develops as far as time is concerned. Sufficient time has to elapse until return of function can be expected. On the other hand, it is well known that the chances of a good regeneration start to decrease after about 6 months have elapsed since the original injury. If one waits too long, the optimal time for reexploration might be lost. Therefore, at about 6 months after the primary nerve repair one has to decide if sufficient regeneration can be expected or if a reintervention has to be considered, and this decision is very often extremely difficult. In many instances the patient is not aware of the fact that loss of time might be harmful; it is, therefore, the responsibility of the surgeon who performed the primary nerve repair to ensure that the patient is seen regularly and the decision of an eventual reexploration is done in time.

Quality of Regeneration
Primary nerve repair does not offer any advantage over secondary repair as far as the quality of regeneration is concerned. On the contrary, there are arguments that the reaction of the ganglion cells and the increase of axon plasma flow would favor an early secondary repair during the second or third week after the injury.

Anatomy
In a clean transection the anatomical relationship of the transected part can be easily defined at the time of primary repair because no scar tissue has formed yet. There is no fibrous retraction of the stumps and end-to-end nerve repair can be performed more easily because only the elastic retraction of the nerve tissue has to be overcome. But if the nerve stumps had retracted due to elasticity of the nerve tissue, additional incisions might be necessary to locate the retracted stumps; this leads to the danger of spreading an eventual infection. In the case of secondary repair one always will start the dissection from the healthy tissue, where the anatomy is still well-preserved. If fibrous retraction has already occurred within the nerve stumps, nerve grafting offers a good solution of the problem. This means that in secondary repairs, nerve grafts will be used more often.

Evaluation of Stumps
The forces acting on the nerve during the injury cause a certain damage to the nerve stumps. The damaged parts all become fibrotic, and this fibrosis will impede the nerve regeneration in both the proximal and the distal stump. One key to proper nerve repair is sufficient resection of the damaged part. In secondary nerve repairs the amount of damage can be easily recognized because the damaged part has already become fibrotic. At primary nerve repair this evaluation is extremely difficult, and thus there is the risk of uniting two fibrotic stumps.

Local Factors
If the injury causes not only the transection of the peripheral nerve but also other injuries to muscles, tendons, and bone, or if a skin defect is present, there is an increased risk of postoperative complications that might interfere with proper nerve regeneration. It is evident that in such a case early secondary nerve repair offers a safer solution.

General Condition of the Patient
The general status of the patient is an important factor when making the decision of whether a primary nerve repair should be performed or the repair of the nerves delayed.

Factors Regarding Personnel and Equipment
The chances of good regeneration after nerve repair

will be increased if the nerve repair was performed by an experienced surgeon with modern equipment and sufficient time to perform the repair as exactly as possible. If experienced personnel and equipment are not provided or if the operation is performed under time pressure in an emergency situation, it is much more favorable to delay the repair to a later date.

Other Factors in the Decision Between Primary and Secondary Repair

Whether primary nerve repair should be performed or not will be an individual decision according to local and general factors regarding the patient. The training and the experience of the surgeon will influence the decision. The surgeon who is very much involved with emergency surgery will always tend to perform primary repairs. Another surgeon, who does reconstructive surgery and thus tends to see cases of failed primary nerve repairs, will decide instead in favor of early secondary repair.

The main guideline in handling the case should be the principle of not inflicting any additional damage on the patient. If there is a clean cut without further complications and without defect of nerve tissue, the primary nerve repair can save time and cannot cause much harm. In such a case a primary nerve repair should be performed but the patient has to be followed closely so that in case of failure the decision for reexploration is done in time. If there is a loss of nerve substance or a skin defect, it is much wiser to delay the nerve repair. In such a case the optimal time for the early secondary repair would be when the original wound has healed well, the edema has disappeared, and the general status of the patient is good. This could be after as little as 2 weeks or as much as 6 weeks; 2 to 3 weeks after the original injury would be the optimal time from the theoretical point of view regarding nerve regeneration. But more decisive are the local and general conditions of the patient – if they are not favorable the theoretical arguments are not strong enough to force an earlier date for the secondary repair.

End-to-End Nerve Repair versus Nerve Graft

There is no question about the fact that an end-to-end nerve repair offers the best chances of nerve regeneration. If there is no nerve defect, the fascicular pattern of the two stumps is compatible and the corresponding fascicles can be reunited. The regenerating axons have to cross only one suture line to reach the peripheral stump. There is also no question about the fact that end-to-end nerve repair has its limits. If there is a loss of nerve substance, the structure of the fascicular pattern is different. The two stumps have to be approximated under tension and coaptation has to be maintained against tension. It is true that by flexing the adjacent joints, relief of tension can be achieved as long as immobilization is maintained. But when mobilization commences the suture site is exposed to longitudinal tension; even if the flexed position is relieved gradually the permanent tension has its consequences on the suture site. As is the case with scar reaction in other tissues, hypertrophy of scar tissue or stretching of the scar tissue might develop. There is clinical and experimental evidence that these changes at the suture site can damage axons that had already crossed the suture line and reached the distal stump. In such cases it is better to avoid tension by the use of nerve grafts. The disadvantage of the nerve graft – having two suture lines – is compensated for by the fact that these suture lines are in optimal shape. Regenerating axons are able to cross two optimal suture lines more easily than one very bad one.

In the past the majority of surgeons regarded grafts as not very useful. But thanks to modern techniques and especially techniques based on microsurgery, the results of nerve grafting have been improved. The value of nerve grafts is not generally accepted. The discussion continues as to what size of defect would be an indication to perform a nerve graft rather than to force an end-to-end nerve repair. There are surgeons who are confident that a median nerve defect of 3 to 4 cm. could be easily overcome by mobilization and flexing of the adjacent joints. Other surgeons, including myself, would regard a defect of 1.5 or 2 cm. already big enough to consider nerve grafting. Of course there are again individual differences, because some patients have much laxer tissues and a defect can be overcome more easily than with other patients. Age plays a role, because in children a longer gap can be closed by end-to-end nerve repair with likelihood of recovery than in adults. One must exploit any chances to shorten a defect by rerouting – for example, the transposition of the ulnar nerve to the volar side of the elbow joint. There are basically two ways to apply a nerve graft to handle a nerve defect. A given loss of nerve substance leads to a defect that can be minimized by mobilizing the nerve stumps and flexing the adjacent joints (minimal defects). If the nerve stumps are allowed to retract according to the elasticity and the joints are in neutral position, we can measure a maximum distance between the two stumps. If the graft bridges the maximum defect, tension can be completely avoided, but a longer graft has to be used. In a case of a smaller defect, there is tension at the two suture lines but a shorter graft can be adopted. Since the length of the graft within certain limits does not influence the final results, it is much better to use longer grafts, thus avoiding tension, rather than to minimize the defect by other means.

Intraneural Topography As It Relates to Nerve Repair

In very proximal levels the fibers of individual functions are distributed rather diffusely over the cross section of the nerve. More distally the fibers tend to be arranged according to a division into the branches. Even in monofascicular nerves, sectors with preference for fibers of certain functions can be defined. The facial nerve at the stylomastoid foramen represents a monofascicular nerve. But by studying the fiber distribution using serial section [14], it was possible to distinguish sectors of preference of fibers going to the forehead, the eyelids, the cheek, the upper lip, the lower lip, and the neck. At the root level of the brachial plexus and in the proximal portions of the peripheral nerves, the structure is monofascicular, oligofascicular, or polyfascicular without group arrangement.

In the periphery – and this is the area where the majority of nerve lesions occur – the peripheral nerves have a polyfascicular structure with group arrangement. The fascicular pattern of peripheral nerves changes very much because of fiber connections and because of the adjustment of the nerve structure to the functional stress. In areas of more mechanical irritation, the nerves consist of smaller fascicles with more interfascicular tissue than in other areas. The pattern of the fascicle groups remains more stable and does not change as much as the pattern of the individual fascicles. To define the corresponding fascicle groups at operation, a sketch is made of the fascicular pattern of the two cross sections. In a peripheral lesion the exposure is extended until the division of the nerve is exposed; there the individual branches can be defined easily. In a retrograde way the fascicles of the individual branches are followed until the distal stump is reached. In this way the function of the fascicle groups is easily defined. Next a comparison is done between the two sketches; according to the size and distribution a guess is made as to which part of the proximal stump corresponds with the distal stump. It is possible to differentiate between motor and sensory nerve fibers by direct stimulation [8]. By a special staining technique [7], motor fibers can be recognized (unfortunately it takes 2 days to get the result). An evaluation of the long-term results demonstrates that in the majority of my cases the guess as to which group of the proximal stump corresponds with which group of the distal stump (without further help) was correct. In more proximal levels without group arrangement the differentiation is not so important because of the diffuse distribution of the fibers. Studies of the intraneural topography [25], which were intensified during recent years, provide information showing that preference of fibers for a certain function can be expected.

TECHNIQUE OF END-TO-END NERVE REPAIR

Epineural Nerve Repair

The classic epineural nerve repair [9] achieves a coaptation of the two stumps by suturing the circumferential layers of the epineurium without touching the fascicular or interfascicular tissue. Another advantage is that the epineural sutures are able to accept some tension. If there is tension in a longitudinal direction, each stitch approximates only one point (Fig. 42-3A) and many circumferential stitches are needed. It is a great disadvantage if one loses any control of the behavior of the fascicular structures within the nerve. This is not important in peripheral nerves, which consist of a few large fascicles (Fig. 42-3B). In such nerves epineural nerve repair provides very good fascicular adaptation; a fascicular (perineural) repair cannot offer an advantage. Experiments on such a model, as performed by Bora and co-workers [3], do not provide any information about whether epineural or perineural nerve repairs are more favorable. In multifascicular nerves, a lack of control of coaptation of the individual fascicles might lead to improper alignment and buckling (Fig. 42-3C) if the stitches are tight, or to separation of the fascicles if the epineural sutures have been done loosely (Fig. 42-3D). Improper fascicular alignment has more severe consequences in a nerve carrying many nerve fibers with different functions. Improper fascicular alignment can also be the result of malrotation (Fig. 42-4B). In nerves having a rather high percentage of interfascicular tissue, there is a certain probability that the fascicles will come into contact with interfascicular tissue.

Guide Sutures

To avoid malrotation, guide sutures can be used [15, 16, 23]. These stitches are located in the interfascicular tissue at exactly the corresponding points of the cross section (Fig. 42-4C).

Intrafascicular Sutures

To secure a proper alignment of the individual fascicles, Hakstian [8] suggested the use of sutures that penetrate the nerve and the individual fascicles, emerging intrafascicularly and entering the corresponding fascicle of the distal stump to leave a nerve again at some distance distally. The ends of these very fine stitches can be brought across the skin to the surface, to be removed a few days after the nerve repair in order to avoid a foreign body reaction (Fig. 42-5). However, Brunelli [4] reported disappointing results with this technique.

Perineural Nerve Repair

Langley and Hashimoto [12] as early as 1917 tried to unite the individual fascicles by the use of perineural stitches. This technique did not become popular because at that time the technique was unrefined and the suture material too coarse. Bora [2] recommended this technique again, but later reported dis-

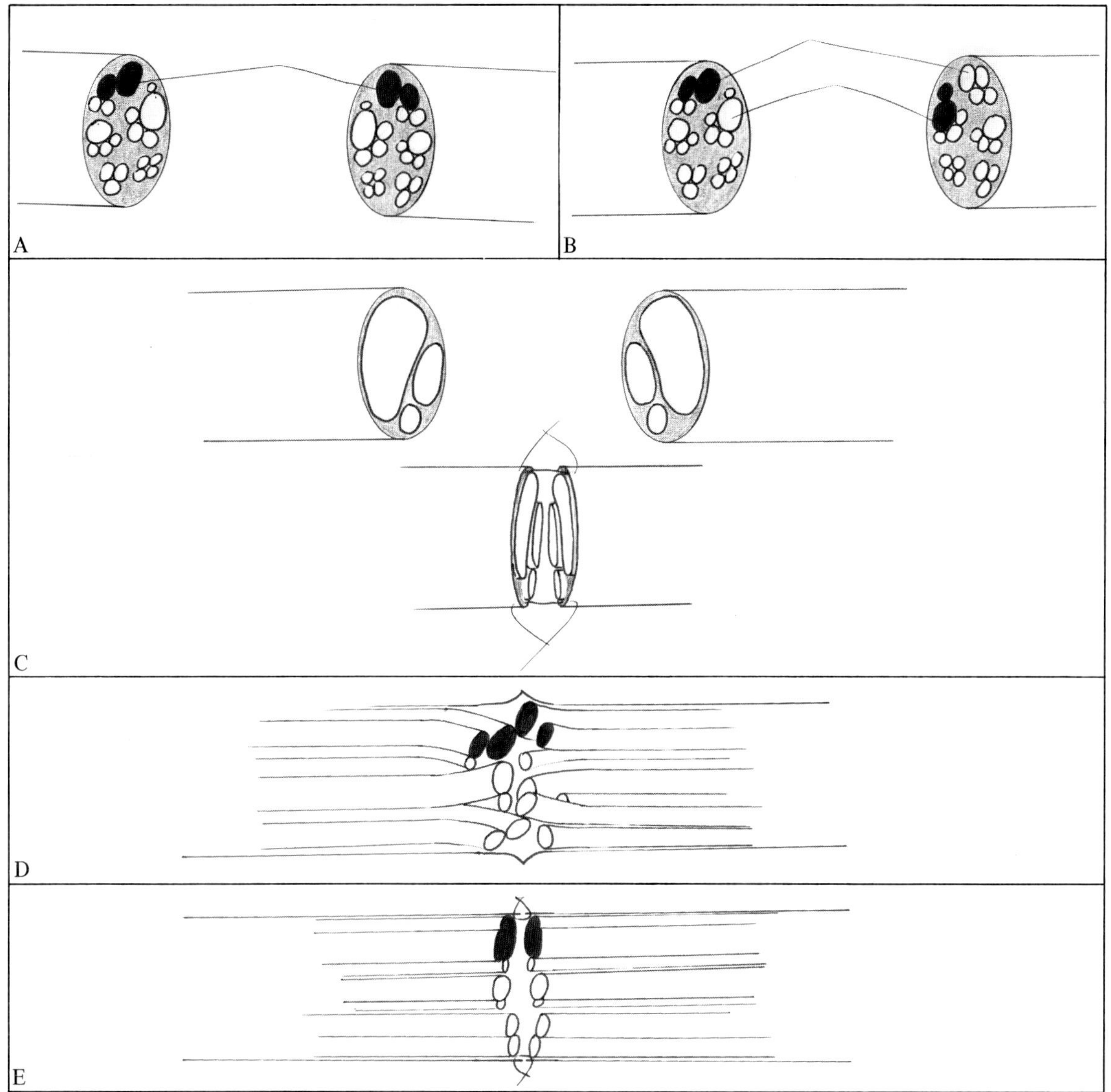

Fig. 42-3. Epineural suture. Nerve repair under tension. A, each stitch approximates the area where the stitch is located. The remaining cross section tends to separate. B, many stitches are necessary. C, in an oligofascicular nerve, epineural repair provides satisfactory fascicular alignment. D, E, in polyfascicular nerves, buckling of the fascicles (D) or inner separation (E) can occur.

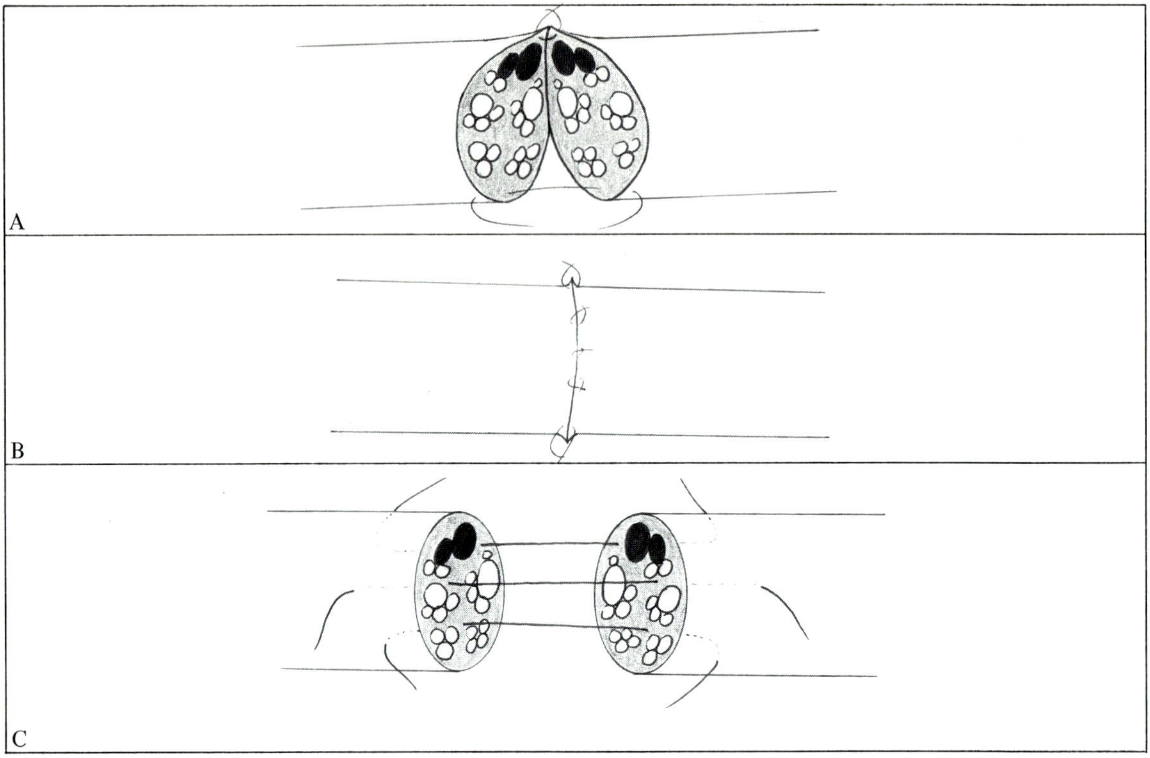

Fig. 42-4. Epineural repair with guide sutures. A, exact alignment of the corresponding fascicles is essential in polyfascicular nerves containing many nerve fibers of many different functions. B, malrotation brings the motor fibers in the fascicles (black) into contact with sensory fascicles (white) or with interfascicular tissue. C, guide sutures prevent malrotation.

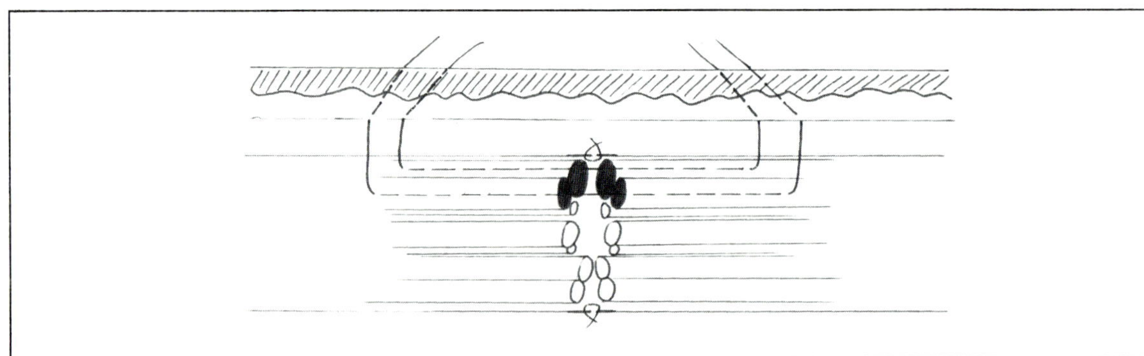

Fig. 42-5. Exact fascicular alignment is achieved by interfascicular sutures at the expense of increased surgical trauma. The stitches are brought across the skin to the surface, to allow removal.

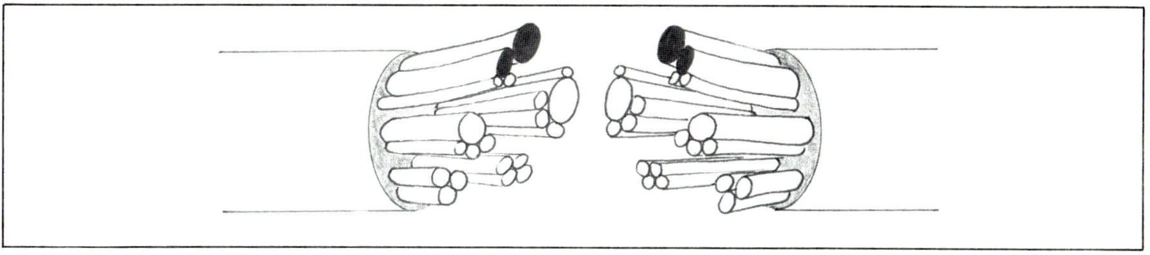

Fig. 42-6. Interfascicular coaptation. After resection of a strip of epineurium and interfascicular dissection in a nerve with group arrangement of the fascicles, the fascicle groups are isolated and coapted with the corresponding fascicle group. Approximation is achieved by one or two very fine stitches (nylon 10-0), which are anchored in the remaining interfascicular tissue. Coaptation is maintained by natural fibrin clotting. No tension can be accepted. Further separation is not favorable. In nerves with a few major fascicles, the individual fascicles are isolated and coapted (fascicular coaptation).

couraging experimental results in 1976. The great advantage of an exact fascicular coaptation is neutralized by the surgical trauma of the several perineural stitches.

Fascicular Coaptation

The technique of fascicular coaptation attempts to approximate individual fascicles of a peripheral nerve without tight union of the perineurium. One or two perineural stitches are inserted only to approximate the fascicles and to achieve broad contact of the cross sections. The final coaptation is provided by natural fibrin clotting and not by stitches, reducing surgical trauma to a minimum. A small gap between the edges of the perineurium is bridged in a short time by a fibrin clot. This technique cannot accept any tension and can be used only if complete tensionless coaptation is possible. It is evident that this technique can be used only with nerves consisting of only a few rather large fascicles.

Interfascicular Coaptation

The majority of the perineural nerves consist of many fascicles. In their peripheral portion, the peripheral nerves very often show arrangement of these fascicles in fascicle groups. The stumps of such nerves can be easily dissected into these fascicle groups, and coaptation of the corresponding fascicle groups is achieved (Fig. 42-6). The additional surgical trauma of isolating each individual fascicle is avoided. The approximation of the fascicle groups is achieved by one or two stitches that are placed into the remaining interfascicular tissue between the fascicles of the fascicle group. As in the case of fascicular approximation, the coaptation is finally provided by fibrin clotting; therefore tension in longitudinal direction has to be avoided.

Wrapping of Suture Sites

Results have not proved favorable from the wrapping of the suture site with foreign material (Silastic membrane, collagen membrane, millipore) to avoid invasion of the suture site by proliferating connective tissue from the surroundings and from aberrant axon sprouts. In spite of the good external appearance of the suture sites, invasion of the suture line by connective tissue cannot be avoided. One of the main sources for proliferating connective tissue is the epineurium, and this remains inside the tube. Foreign body reaction against the tube can occur, especially if the site of the nerve repair is located in an area of constant motion.

TECHNIQUE OF NERVE GRAFTING

The relative merits of nerve grafting (Fig. 42-7) compared with end-to-end nerve repair have been stressed previously. The indications for the use of a nerve graft vary with the individual surgeon. Increasing satisfactory experience with nerve grafting over the past 14 years has led me to expand my use of nerve grafting. If the two stumps of a transected nerve cannot be approximated easily after gentle mobilization without flexion of the adjacent joint, a nerve graft is preferred to an end-to-end nerve repair. This technique has resulted in a significant improvement of my results. Other surgeons report satisfactory results with end-to-end nerve repair, overcoming gaps of several centimeters. In such instances wider mobilization and flexion of the adjacent joint with immobilization in flexed position are used. As it is extremely difficult to compare the results of nerve repairs, the decision to use a nerve graft with defects between 2 and 4 cm. will be open to discussion. In cases with defects greater than 4 cm., the majority of the authors of today prefer nerve grafts. No matter which technique one uses, there should not be a compromise between the different approaches. If one is ready to accept tension, one has to use a technique that is able to bear the tension – this is conventional epineural nerve repair. If one chooses to use a nerve graft, the graft has to be long enough and tension must be

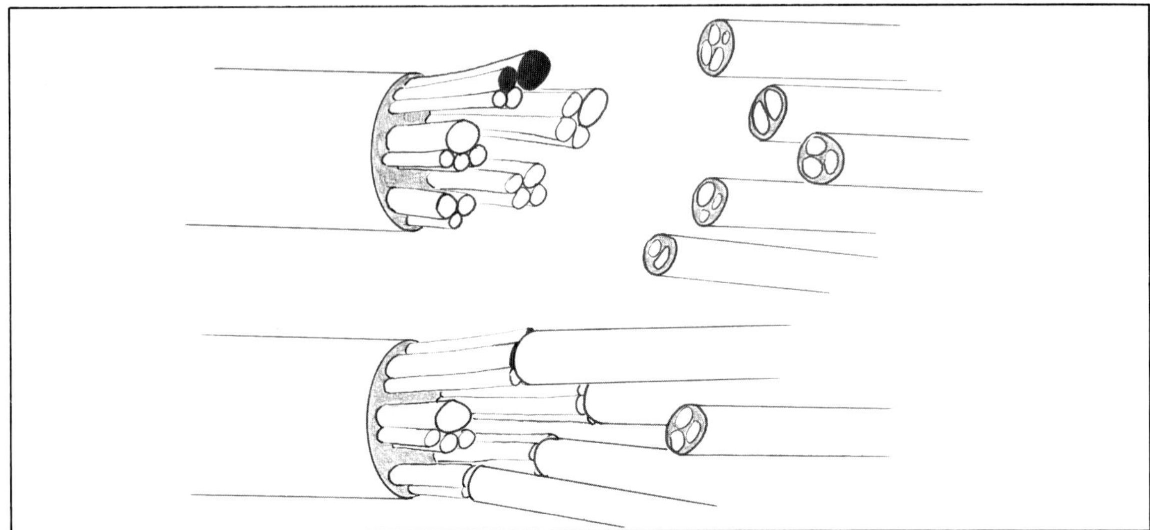

Fig. 42-7. Polyfascicular nerve with group arrangement. After resection of the epineurium and interfascicular dissection, each fascicle group is coapted with one graft (interfascicular grafting).

avoided completely. Therefore it is wrong to attempt to minimize the defect to be able to use a shorter graft. One of the reasons for the bad reputation of nerve grafting in the past is due to tension on the nerve graft.

The result of nerve grafting decreases with the length of the nerve defect to be bridged; this is due to the different fascicular pattern and not to the length of the graft. Within certain limits the length of the graft does not influence the result. It is evident that a nerve graft of 2 cm. will yield a better result than a graft of 15 cm., but there is not very much difference between grafts of 6 and 9 cm. On the contrary, a longer graft placed into well-vascularized soft tissue will yield a better result than a shorter graft that was embedded in scar tissue. It is therefore better to bypass an area of scar tissue, even if a longer nerve graft is needed.

To date only autografts give predictably satisfactory results. Fresh and preserved homografts (by irradiation, lyophilization, cialite solution) have not proved successful. Early optimistic reports by Jacoby and associates [10] could not be confirmed [11].

Donor Nerves

There are many different nerves available as donors for nerve grafting.

Sural Nerve

This nerve is my first choice. It is easily defined by a small transverse incision behind the lateral ankle. With a gentle pull, the course of the nerve can be palpated; the whole nerve can be excised with several additional transverse incisions. One must have in mind the fact that in the area of the lateral ankle the sural nerve divides into several branches. All these branches have to be transected; if this is done, the nerve can be extracted easily. Other surgeons prefer a longitudinal incision to excise the whole nerve under vision. Nerve strippers can be used, but in about 15 percent of the cases the sural nerve gets additional sources, and this might be destroyed by stripping. In proximal levels the sural nerve can be monofascicular, but during its course it becomes more and more polyfascicular. It offers the possibility of selecting an optimal portion if only a short graft is needed.

Nervus Cutaneous Antebrachii Medialis

This nerve provides a rather thick graft in its proximal level. It divides into two branches in the distal part of the upper arm. This nerve should not be used if the ulnar nerve of the same extremity has to be repaired.

Nervus Cutaneous Antebrachii Dorsalis

The use of this nerve was suggested by McFarlane [13].

Ramus Superficialis Nervi Radialis

This nerve is known for the frequent occurrence of painful neuromas after traumatic lesions; therefore, its use is not recommended. It should not be used if the median nerve of the same extremity is involved because of the overlapping of sensory function. But in a brachial plexus lesion, when the nerve is already not functioning and many grafts are needed, its use can be necessary.

Ramus Dorsalis Nervis Ulnaris
A rather short but thick graft of this nerve can be utilized. It should not be used in a median or ulnar nerve lesion of the same extremity, to avoid a larger sensory loss resulting from possible overlapping.

Intercostal Nerves
The intercostal nerves contain motor fibers, which was an argument in favor of the use of these nerves; however, they show extensive branching, which might lead to a loss of axons.

Nervus Cutaneous Femoris Lateralis
This nerve can be easily found below the iliac spine. It can be exposed into the pelvis, which has the advantage that the proximal neuroma is buried very deep within the pelvis. For this reason this nerve is used when the indication for nerve grafting is a painful neuroma. Any neuroma formed at the site of transection of this nerve would not be exposed to mechanical irritation.

Nervus Saphenous
This nerve should not be excised as a graft if the sural nerve of the same site is used.

Nerves of the Cervical Plexus
These nerves are easily available and often used to graft defects of the facial nerve.

The functional loss after excision of a donor nerve is minimal and can be neglected. However, it is evident that the patient has to be warned about possible complications and must agree to the excision of a donor nerve.

Distal Suture Site
After nerve grafting the regenerating axons have to cross two suture lines. It is possible that at the distal end of the graft a dense scar has formed when the regenerating axons arrive. The further progress of the axons might be impeded. This situation can be recognized by the fact that the Tinel-Hoffmann sign, which advances from the proximal stump along the graft, stops at the distal end of the graft and does not proceed. If this failure of the Tinel-Hoffmann sign to progress persists for several months, an exposure of the distal suture site is indicated. There might be an external compression that can be corrected; if scar tissue blocks the distal suture site, this segment is resected and an end-to-end nerve repair performed. In the first 50 cases of my series this occurred in 7 (14 percent). With increasing technical skill the incidence of blockage at the distal suture site has dropped greatly.

REEXPLORATION AFTER FAILURES OF CONVENTIONAL NERVE REPAIR

One of the problems in primary repair is the fact that in case of failure reexploration in proper time has to be undertaken. If there is no return of function at all, the decision to explore and resect the suture site is easily made. But if there is some indication that function might return but in an unsatisfactory way, the surgeon who performs the reexploration accepts great responsibility. On the other hand, waiting might mean that all chances of a useful recovery will be lost. A painful neuroma at the suture site and paresthesias are good arguments in favor of a reexploration. After exposure a thickening at the suture site is usually seen, mostly as a result of proliferation of epineural tissue. The operation starts with an epineurectomy proximally and distally of the suture site and resection of the epineurium at that site. The stitches from the first operation are usually found underneath this epineural thickening. Starting from the healthy tissue an interfascicular dissection is performed. Fascicles or fascicle groups that are in good contact with the corresponding fascicles of the distal stump are isolated and saved. Fascicles or fascicle groups forming a neuroma without contact are resected and are then reunited by nerve grafts.

REFERENCES

1. Bateman, J. E. An operative approach to supraclavicular plexus injuries. *J. Bone Joint Surg.* [Br.] 31:34, 1949.
2. Bora, F. W., Jr., Pleasure, D. E., and Noubar, A. A study of nerve regeneration and neuroma formation after nerve suture by various techniques. *J. Hand Surg.* 1:138, 1976.
3. Bora, F. W. Peripheral nerve repair in cats. *J. Bone Joint Surg.* [Am.] 49:659, 1967.
4. Brunelli, G. Lecture. Symposium on Microsurgery of Peripheral Nerves and Vessels, Vienna, October 1972.
5. Curtis, R. M., and Eversman, W. W. Internal neurolysis as an adjunct to the treatment of the carpal tunnel syndrome. *J. Bone Joint Surg.* [Am.] 55:733, 1973.
6. Förster, O. Vortrag gehalten an der ausserordentlichen Tagung der Deutschen Orthopädischen Gesellschaft am 8. u.9.2. 1916 in Berlin.
7. Freilinger, G., Gruber, H., Holle, J., and Mandl, W. Zur Methodik der 'sensomotorisch' differenzierten Faszikelnaht peripherer Nerven. *Handchirurgie* 7:133, 1975.
8. Hakstian, R. W. Funicular orientation by direct stimulation: An aid to peripheral nerve repair. *J. Bone Joint Surg.* [Am.] 50:1178, 1968.

9. Hueter, K. *Die Allgemeine Chirurgie.* Leipzig: Vogel Verlag, 1873.
10. Jacoby, W., Fahlbusch, R., and Mackert, B. Indikation und Technik der Überbrückung von Nervendefekten mit homologen lyophilisierten Nerven. *Melsunger Med. Mittlg.* 116:209, 1972.
11. Kuhlendahl, H., Mumenthaler, M., Penzholz, H., Röttgen, P., Schliack, H., and Struppler, A. Behandlung peripherer Nervenverletzungen mit homologen Nervenimplantaten. *Z. Neurol.* 202:251, 1972.
12. Langley, J. N., and Hashimoto, M. On the suture of separate nerve bundles in a nerve trunk and on internal nerve plexuses. *J. Physiol.* [Lond.] 51:318, 1917.
13. McFarlane, R. M., and Mayer, J. R. Digital nerve grafts using the lateral antebrachial cutaneous nerve. *Hand Surg.* 1:81, 1976.
14. Meissl, G. Intraneurale topographie des n. facialis. Personal communication, 1976.
15. Michon, J. Les sutures nerveuses. Presented at the Tenth Congress of the SICOT, Paris, 1966.
16. Michon, J. Etat actual des techniques de réparation des nerfs péripheriques. *Orthop. Traumatol.* 1970. P. 273.
17. Millesi, H. Zum Problem der Überbrückung von Defekten peripherer Nerven. *Wien. Med. Wochenschr.* 118:182, 1968.
18. Millesi, H., Berger, A., and Meissl, G. The interfascicular nerve grafting of the median ulnar nerves. *J. Bone Joint Surg.* [Am.] 54:727, 1972.
19. Millesi, H., Ganglberger, J., and Berger, A. Erfahrungen mit der Mikrochirurgie peripherer Nerven. *Chir. Plast. Reconstr.* 3:47, 1967.
20. Pecinka, H. Die operative Behandlung der traumatischen Lähmungen des Plexus brachialis. *Zentralbl. Chir.* 85:1678, 1960.
21. Seddon, H. J. Restoration of function in peripheral nerve injuries. *Lancet* 1:418, 1947.
22. Seddon, H. J. *Surgical Disorders of the Peripheral Nerves.* Edinburgh and London: Churchill-Livingstone, 1972.
23. Smith, J. W. Microsurgery of peripheral nerves. *Plast. Reconstr. Surg.* 33:317, 1964.
24. Strange, F. G. St. C. An operation for nerve pedicle grafting. Preliminary communication. *Br. J. Surg.* 34:423, 1947.
25. Sunderland, S. Blood supply of the nerves of the upper limb in man. *Arch. Neurol. Psychiatry* (Chicago) 53:91, 1945.
26. Taylor, G. I., and Ham, F. J. The free vacularized nerve graft. *Plast. Reconstr. Surg.* 57:413, 1976.

Replantation

GRAHAM D. LISTER AND HAROLD E. KLEINERT

The first successful replantation of an amputated arm was reported in 1962 by Malt and McKhann [21]. Komatsu and Tamai [14] performed the first successful digital replantation in 1968. Since then a large number of replantations have been attempted; the number of centers equipped to perform revascularizations [10, 11] and replantations [6, 27, 30, 35] has increased greatly. When the improved techniques that are detailed in this chapter are employed, and when cases are selected properly, it is now possible to achieve a survival rate of over 95 percent in ideal replantations and over 40 percent in salvage cases. With an increased number of parts surviving, the surgeon has rightly turned his attention to function – the foremost consideration in all surgery of the hand [16]. The functional outcome is as yet less impressive than the survival rates [22, 36], but it is now improving as confidence in our microsurgery permits us to concentrate increasingly on those aspects that will better restore to the amputated extremity its former unique capabilities.

SELECTION

Although the number of surgeons willing to attempt replantation is increasing rapidly, they are still far removed, in most cases, from the potential beneficiary of their skills. Clear rules regarding suitability for replantation are therefore necessary if undue hope and unnecessary expenditure are to be avoided. Ideally, these rules should be known to all emergency room physicians, but this is impossible in practice. It is obviously best that the referring physician speak directly to the replantation surgeon and imperative that whoever does take the referring call be well versed in the rules of selection [28].

Absolute Contraindications

Significant Associated Injuries

There are rarely other major injuries in cases of digital amputation, but injuries involving the trunk and head frequently occur in conjunction with loss of an arm. These other injuries may have been overlooked in the understandable preoccupation with the more dramatic amputation. Time must be taken to eliminate or treat such injuries, since they may be life-threatening.

Extensive Injury to the Affected Limb

Successful repairs are uncommon when injuries involve multiple levels. Extensive degloving and crush injuries involving much of the extremity are even less likely to be repaired successfully.

Severe Crush or Multiple Injuries of the Amputated Part

Success in replantation depends upon blood flow, which cannot be achieved without an adequate "run-off." Major injuries to the amputated part such as crush injuries (Fig. 43-1A) will compromise this run-off. An adequate evaluation may be made simply, or a more sophisticated study may be required. X-ray studies of the part may reveal multiple fractures, which can be used as a measure of the severity of the crush (Fig. 43-1B). Avulsion of the branches of the digital arteries may be suspected from the presence of "Chinese red streaks" – patches of bruising along the sides of the fingers due to an extravasation of blood. They usually indicate that attempts at vascular repair will fail.

Chronic Illness

Chronic illness sufficient to make transportation or prolonged surgery hazardous is a contraindication. We have had one potential candidate for replantation admitted from an airport in left heart failure and two patients who developed myocardial infarctions during replantation.

Relative Contraindications

Relative contraindications are often encountered in combination, in which case the bar to replantation is appropriately greater.

Single-Digit Amputations

The functional results have thus far made the replantation of a single digit an unrewarding exercise. The index finger, unless it functions almost perfectly, will not be used, while poor function in any of the ulnar three digits will hamper motion in the others due to the common origin of the profundus tendons. Nonetheless sensory return is predictably satisfactory after microscopic digital nerve repair following a clean injury. Therefore, replantation is justifiable if the amputation of a single digit is through the middle phalanx or beyond, and if the patient or relatives still want to proceed after being made aware of the problems of replantation.

Patients Over 50 Years of Age

The amount of degenerative change in the vascular

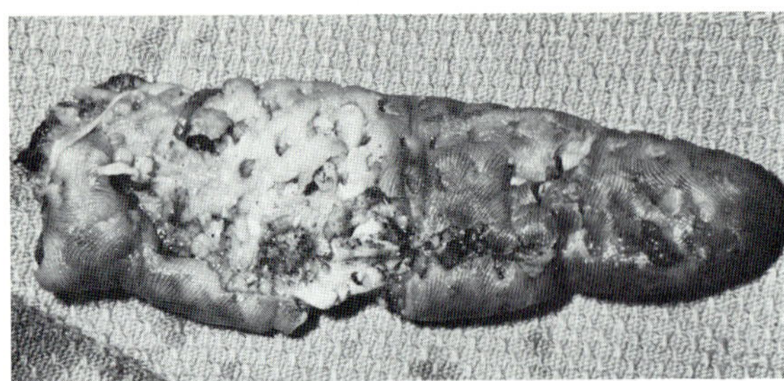

A

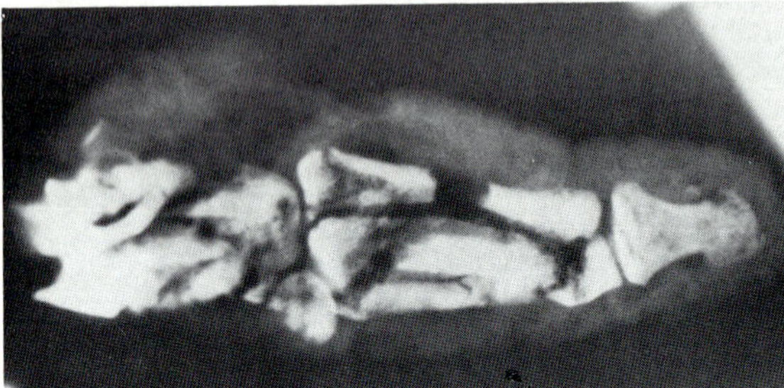

B

Fig. 43-1. A, the severe crush which has been sustained by this right ring finger was evident on clinical examination. B, the impression gained clinically was confirmed forcibly by x-ray examination, showing multiple comminuted fractures.

tree is very variable but, if the degeneration is advanced, the survival rate will be reduced. More importantly, recovery of function is not as good in the older patient. When this is considered in conjunction with the greater likelihood of stiffness in the uninjured fingers, the surgeon must be more circumspect in choosing the course to follow.

Avulsion Injuries

In avulsion injuries the damage done to both vessels and nerves usually is not limited to the site of amputation, but often extends for some distance both proximally and distally. Such damage may result in vascular failure or in poor nerve regeneration. The mechanism of injury often signals this type of avulsion, an obvious example of which is the ring degloving injury. In other instances the less experienced examiner may feel initially that the amputation has been fairly sharp, but on closer inspection of the part he may discover structures dangling from its cut end (Fig. 43-2). These may be tendons or (more commonly) nerves, but rarely vessels. Although this may suggest that the vessels at least are in good condition, that is usually not the case; the reason for the absence of the vessels is that they are more commonly avulsed more distally. Sometimes an apparently suitable distal

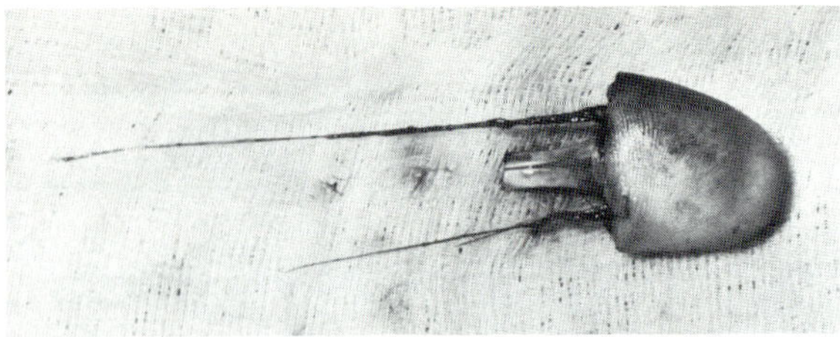

Fig. 43-2. This amputation of the left index finger shows avulsion injury, as evidenced by the significant length of tendon and nerve, which can be seen dangling from the amputated part. This was not fit for replantation.

stump can be found. Viability can be successfully restored with the use of vein grafts, but sensory return is less than ideal.

Lengthy Warm Ischemia Time

Muscle undergoes irreversible changes after 6 hours at room temperature, whereas connective tissues, nerves, tendon, skin, and bone remain viable for varying periods in excess of 12 hours. With immediate cooling of the part, we have successfully restored circulation to a digit 27 hours after injury. The Chinese have successfully replanted extremities after more than 30 hours.

Extreme Contamination

Extreme contamination rarely prevents replantation, because amputations present an unusual opportunity for radical surgical debridement. However, occasionally oil or grease will be driven into the tissues to an extent that makes debridement impossible.

Previous Injury or Surgery

On occasion a digit may have been previously injured, which might be evident from old scars or x-ray changes, or it might not be noted initially. Such an injury might be suspected only after the surgeon encounters a thrombosed artery, scarred veins, or a digital neuroma.

Salvage Replantations

If the surgeon follows these rules of selection, then the patient whose case he feels should be undertaken can be called an *ideal replantation* candidate. In three instances, as described below, relative contraindications should be disregarded. Such cases undertaken despite the presence of such contraindications can be termed *salvage replantations.*

Children

Relative contraindications may be set aside in children, not only because the results of primary repair

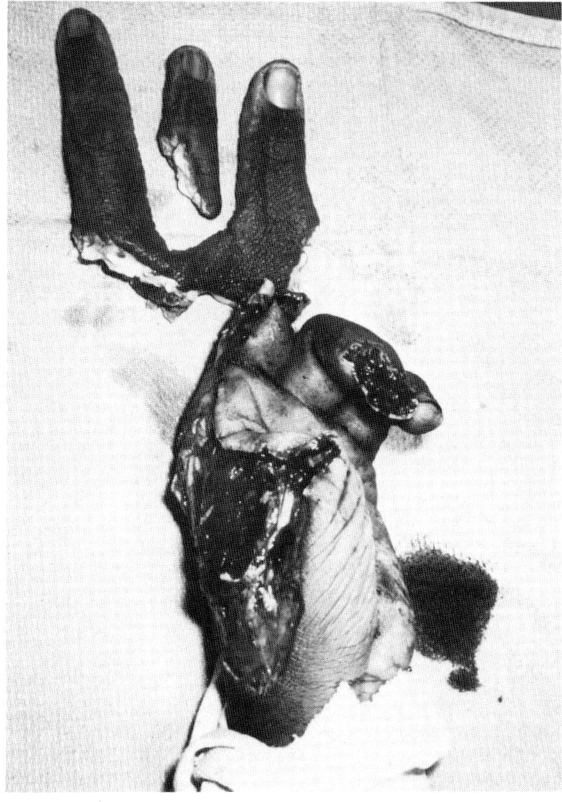

A

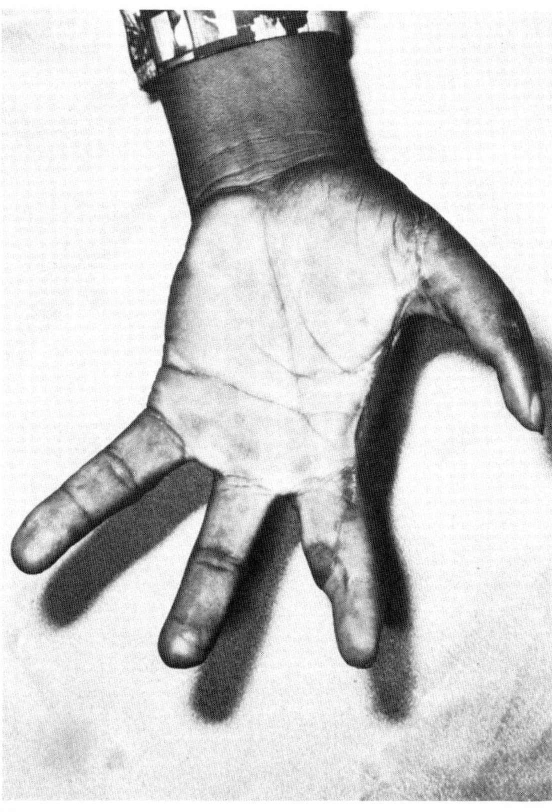

B

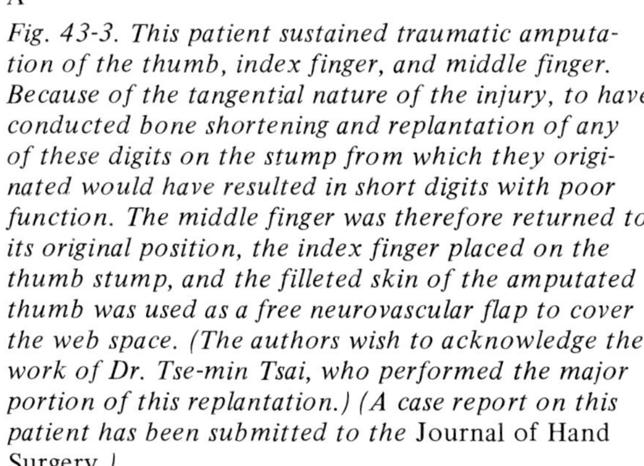

Fig. 43-3. This patient sustained traumatic amputation of the thumb, index finger, and middle finger. Because of the tangential nature of the injury, to have conducted bone shortening and replantation of any of these digits on the stump from which they originated would have resulted in short digits with poor function. The middle finger was therefore returned to its original position, the index finger placed on the thumb stump, and the filleted skin of the amputated thumb was used as a free neurovascular flap to cover the web space. (The authors wish to acknowledge the work of Dr. Tse-min Tsai, who performed the major portion of this replantation.) (A case report on this patient has been submitted to the Journal of Hand Surgery.*)*

are so much better, but also (and more importantly) because the eventual vocation of any child is unknown and his skills may require all the digits that can be saved. Normal growth in replanted extremities can be anticipated [9].

Multiple Digit Loss

When faced with loss of a patient's hand or arm, or of more than two digits, the surgeon must attempt replantation except when the prospects are quite hopeless. If several digits have been amputated in an unsuitable fashion, replantation should be attempted on each of them, since the surgeon cannot predict which of the digits is likely to survive. The replantations should not, however, be done in a slavishly anatomical fashion. Rather, the operator should recall his prime concern of restoring function, which may be best achieved by putting one digit on a different stump in order to maintain appropriate length or important joint motion, or to restore significant sensation (Fig. 43-3).

The Thumb

The thumb is of much greater functional importance than any other digit and should be replaced. It also functions well when it is deprived of all motion except that at the basal joint, provided that good sensation is restored. However, the injunction to replant all thumbs should not be pursued to a foolish extreme. A thumb that is amputated at the level of the interphalangeal joint with good local skin cover is preferable to a crushed, insensitive, dysesthetic replant that shows severe cold intolerance.

TRANSPORTATION

Having decided that both patient and part are fit for transfer, the replantation surgeon should give clear instructions regarding transportation. Customary precautions for the evacuation of any patient are necessary, including the following:

1. The appropriate management of other injuries or illnesses.
2. Arrest of hemorrhage. This can usually be achieved by application of a pressure dressing and elevation of the involved extremity. No further treatment of the stump is needed. Time spent on meticulous cleaning and debridement is time lost in restoring circulation.
3. Assurance of normovolemia and normotension during travel. This may require preliminary transfusion but can usually be achieved by starting an intravenous infusion.
4. Adequate analgesia. There is no cause to deny the patient relief from pain, provided that a record is kept and passed on to the receiving anesthesiologist.
5. Preventive antibiotics. While not favoring prophylactic antibiotics as a general rule, we believe they have benefit for the patient being moved over long distances for lengthy surgical procedures. Cephalothin intravenously is appropriate.
6. Qualified company on the journey is highly desirable; it is mandatory for patients in whom intravenous fluids are being administered.

Care of the Amputated Part

The amputated part requires little treatment. Any gross contaminant can be washed off, but lengthy irrigation of the exposed tissues should *not* be done, because it can make the identification of structures more difficult. The amputated part should be placed *dry* in a dry polyethylene bag, and the bag should be placed in *regular ice.*

PREPARATION FOR SURGERY

The History

When the patient comes to replantation, he does so only after a full evaluation. The history taken from the patient and/or relatives includes not only details of the injury but (even more important) information about other injuries and about preexisting illness.

Mechanism of Injury

The patient is often accompanied by someone who knows about the circumstances of the amputation. When it was the result of an instrument other than a straightforward sharp edge or power saw, a detailed description of the mechanism can be of assistance in determining the degree of shortening necessary or the desirability of vein grafting.

Associated Injuries

Since the amputated extremity captures one's attention, other injuries may have been missed. The receiving surgeon must pursue any other complaints and conduct a swift but complete physical examination.

Preexisting Illness

It must be remembered that the patient is about to spend a long time on an operating table and that replantation never justifies risking the patient's general health. Standard investigations should include electrocardiogram, chest x-ray, and complete blood count. Consultation with specialists may be necessary if there is any doubt about the patient's fitness for surgery. The anesthesia department should always be encouraged to take part in this assessment.

Monitoring and Maintenance of the Patient

The patient should come to replantation with the following aids to his continued general health: (1) electrocardiography, (2) pulse monitor, (3) intravenous therapy, with antibiotics and/or transfusion when indicated, (4) urinary catheter (with volume recorded hourly), (5) central venous pressure catheter, and (6) rectal thermometer.

Preoccupation with restoring circulation to the amputated part may cause the surgeon to overlook the welfare of the patient during a lengthy procedure. This can be avoided by the presence of a competent anesthesiologist. However when one cannot be in constant attendance, attention should be directed at controlling certain important areas.

Cardiovascular Status

Some estimate of blood loss prior to arrival may be obtained from observers, but it is most reliably indicated by the usual compensatory mechanisms of tachycardia, sympathetic overactivity (as evidenced by peripheral vasoconstriction and sweating), and hypotension. If such trends are present, they should be reversed by typing and cross matching, intravenous therapy (dextran has been shown to restore renal blood flow most swiftly [19]), and transfusion. Circulating blood volume can be assessed during surgery by measuring the hourly urinary output through the catheter, by frequent estimation of the microhematocrit, and by the use of a pulse monitor. The height of the wave on a pulse monitor is an index of pulse pressure and therefore of peripheral perfusion. Excess transfusion can be as great a problem as hypovolemia in children and the elderly; it can best be avoided by placing a central venous pressure line. The pulse monitor and central venous pressure line, together with continuous electrocardiography, aid in observing the patient who has preexisting cardiac problems or who develops them during surgery.

Temperature
A common cause of pyrexia during long surgical procedures is hyperthermia in infants and children. This should be prevented by exposing as much of the child as possible; the temperature is monitored by using a rectal probe in patients under regional anesthesia and an esophageal thermometer in those under general anesthetic.

Anesthesia and Sedation
The majority of our replantations are performed under axillary block using bupivacaine (Marcaine) 0.5% with epinephrine. The block lasts for 12 to 16 hours and may thereafter be supplemented by further block or by the induction of general anesthesia. Sedation is given as required in the form of diazepam (Valium) and pentobarbital (Nembutal).

Preparation of the Part
Once the patient arrives at the replantation center, the replantation surgeon should confirm that the criteria for selection have been met. Then, while another physician readies the patient for surgery, the replantation surgeon should take the amputated part and the x-ray studies to the operating room and immediately commence preparation. This preparation involves several steps:

Skeletal Management
The x-rays should be studied and decisions made.

BONE SHORTENING. Whenever bone shortening can be achieved without sacrificing function, it should be done. The surgeon should decide from the x-rays and from subsequent inspection of the part in what proportion the shortening can be done on the part and on the patient. If shortening would destroy salvageable and significant function, vein grafts are likely to be necessary.

PRIMARY ARTHRODESIS. When the amputation passes through a joint and damages the articular surfaces, immediate fusion in the correct position with respect to the joint and the digit will give the required bone shortening and result in the quickest return to maximum function.

CHOICE OF FIXATION. In order to prepare the skeleton appropriately, the surgeon should select the means of fixation after studying the x-rays. Firm internal fixation will ensure bony union and permit early motion. Thus, wherever possible, compression plates are used for the humerus, radius, ulna, and metacarpals, and intraosseous wiring is used for the phalanges [18].

Inspection of the Part
Having made these decisions, the surgeon should commence work on the amputated part, which is laid on a sterile sheet with an operating microscope available. The amputated part is inspected to ensure that replantation is appropriate.

Skin Incisions
The identification of neurovascular structures can be simplified by making three longitudinal incisions in the digit, two over the neurovascular bundles and one over the midline dorsally. If similar incisions are later made on the stump of the digit and if bone shortening has been performed, the corresponding cuts should be placed some 5 to 10 mm. out of alignment. When the wounds are closed at the end of the procedure, the flaps can be transposed as small 90-degree Z plasties; this lengthens the circumferential scar, which may otherwise become constrictive, and also takes up much of the tissue made redundant by skeletal shortening (Fig. 43-4). Certainly, at no time prior to closure should any potentially viable skin be excised. Edema can cause a remarkable reduction in available skin, and there are few situations in which the surgeon finds himself more powerless than when he is faced with a circumferential defect overlying vascular repairs.

Preparation of Neurovascular Structures
The dissection should be performed beneath the operating microscope, the amputated part being held by an assistant or by stay sutures attached to the table. As in all dissections, structures are mostly easily identified away from the site of injury. Hence the longitudinal incisions enable the surgeon to identify the arteries, nerves, and veins, and to trace them back to the site of amputation. What is more important, he can inspect the tissues away from the primary wound for evidence of extravasation of blood. Such extravasation indicates significant crush or avulsion, which will probably have damaged the main vessels; in such cases, vein grafts may well be required. Damaged branches should be identified and coagulated by bipolar diathermy, because bleeding from such branches may give flow across the anastomosis without perfusion of the distal part. As each neurovascular structure is dissected out and identified, a marking suture of 7-0 nylon should be placed in its end (Fig. 43-5). The vessels and nerves can be easily seen at this stage; however, hours later when the part has been replanted and the tissues are bloodstained, the structures will have retracted into an amorphous mass

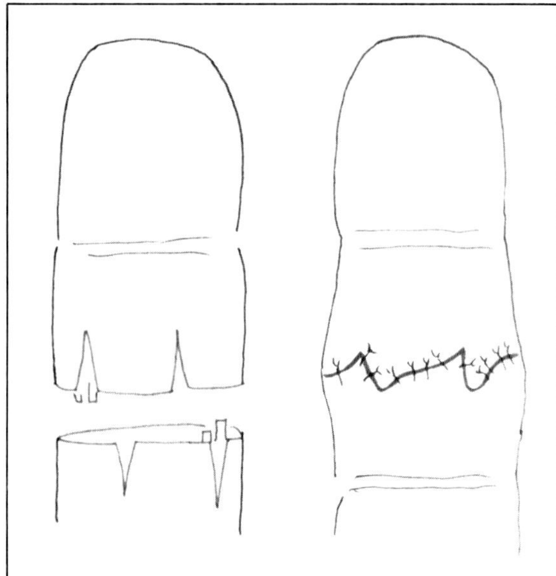

Fig. 43-4. This drawing illustrates the positioning of longitudinal incisions on the amputated part and on the stump. The incisions are placed out of alignment by some 5 to 10 mm., so that closure after bone shortening can be performed as a Z plasty. The circumferential wound is thereby lengthened, preventing later constriction and also taking up the redundancy of soft tissue present in the longitudinal axis of the digit.

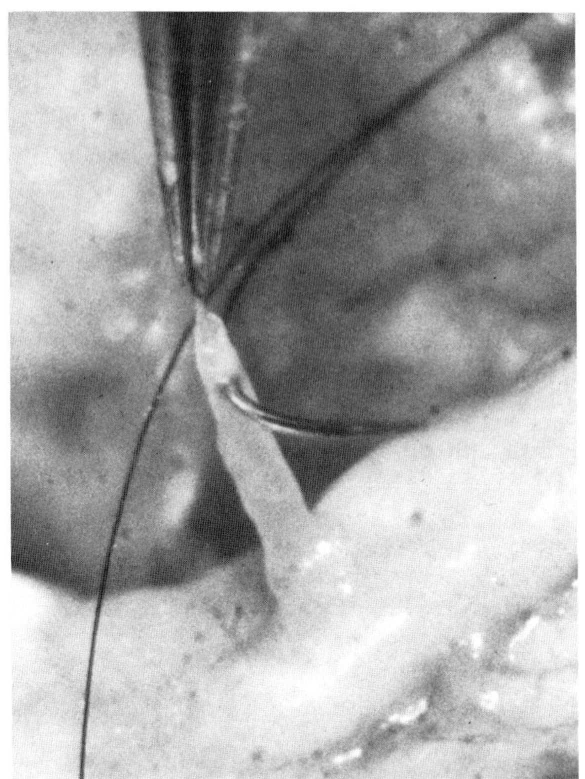

A

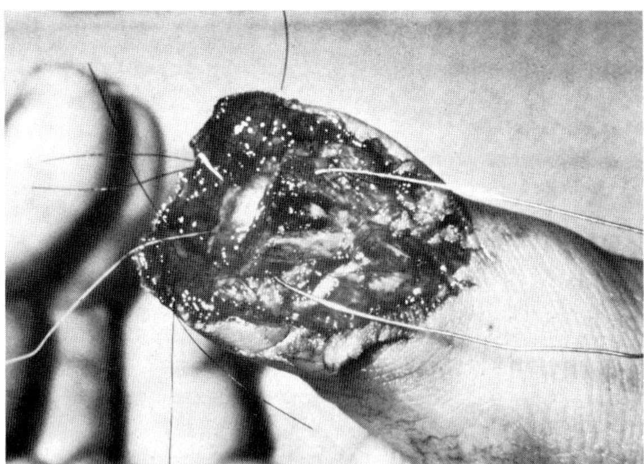

B

Fig. 43-5. The marking of vessels and nerves for subsequent repair. A, in this very distal replantation, an 8-0 nylon suture is placed through the very end of a small branch of the digital artery later used for replantation. B, marking sutures can be seen in the proximal stump of a thumb amputation, the double ends identifying arteries and the single ends identifying nerves. Note that the intraosseous wire for fixation has already been placed.

of soft tissue. It is our practice to tag each vessel with two ends of equal length, while the nerve is tagged with only one long end. Microvascular clamps should *not* be used for identification for three reasons: (1) they may slip off in the course of subsequent manipulations; (2) if left on for a considerable time, they can cause intimal damage; (3) if the vessel is for some reason not used, the clamp may be forgotten in the course of a long case with several changes of scrub nurse, only to be revealed (to the surgeon's embarrassment) on the postoperative x-ray studies.

Tendon Exposure

Depending upon the position of the hand at the time of injury, the distal tendon ends may lie at the amputation site or further distally. Appropriate incisions should be made in the sheath to display the tendon ends, taking special care to preserve the pulleys over the proximal ends of the proximal and middle phalanges and to leave a cuff of sheath attached to bone for subsequent closure.

Bone Resection
In those cases in which the surgeon has chosen to shorten the amputated part, the periosteum should be carefully stripped away from the bone end for subsequent closure and the bone resected with a power saw. Care must be taken at this point, since it is difficult to control the part adequately while also guarding the soft tissues. At this point, the surgeon should undertake any other preparation for fixation that can be done, such as the retrograde insertion of a Kirschner wire and the drilling of transverse holes for intraosseous wiring.

Hemostasis
It is strange to write of hemostasis in an amputated part, but bleeding after replantation can be a significant problem that can be reduced by bipolar coagulation of vessels encountered while preparing the amputated part. Such vessels may be obscured after replantation and may be difficult to locate without the risk of damage to the vascular anastomoses. Of particular importance are the vessels in a transmetacarpal amputation. The metacarpal arteries, which are the branches of the deep palmar arch, are of significant size but are rarely if ever used in revascularizing the extremity. They connect, more often than not, with the common digital arteries at the point of their bifurcation. Herein lies their importance, because after the superficial arch and its branches have been repaired, back bleeding may occur along the metacarpal arteries; this reduces digital perfusion and often causes a significantly large hematoma in the palm. Such a hematoma further reduces flow distally both by pressure and by inducing vascular spasm. These vessels must therefore be sought on the amputated part and ligated.

By the time the amputated part has been prepared, the patient should be ready. The extremity should be returned to the ice pack while the stump is attended to.

Preparation of the Stump
In preparing the stump the same techniques are used (as detailed under the heading Preparation of the Part) with respect to skeleton, periosteum, skin incisions, and identification of nerves and veins. Two structures require additional attention.

Tendons
The flexor tendons will have retracted proximally and should be retrieved by flexing the wrist and "milking" the palm of the hand. Once retrieved they should be held out at a level suitable for later repair by transfixing them proximally with Keith or Bunnell straight needles. If left until after bony fixation has been performed, retrieval is more difficult.

Arteries
By seeking out the arteries before elevating the tourniquet, the surgeon can often locate them all simply by inspecting the stump through operating loupes for the tell-tale pulsations. The arteries, like the nerves and veins, should be tagged with 7-0 nylon as previously described (Fig. 43-5B). However, before this is done, the presence of adequate proximal flow should be confirmed by gripping the very end of the vessel with jeweller's forceps and cutting through three-fourths of the vessel circumference with microsurgical scissors. If good flow is not encountered, steps should be taken to improve the flow. As a crude guide, flow from a digital artery should reach the end of the hand table, while flow from the ulnar or radial artery should reach the near side of the scrub nurse's table! Steps to be taken are as follows:

DILATATION OF THE VESSEL. Much has been made in the past of the sanctity of the vessel lumen. Certainly the lumen must be treated with delicate respect, but dilatation performed as described below not only confirms the presence of flow but also overcomes vascular spasm for some time. In larger vessels, dilatation can be performed using loupes and plastic intravenous cannulas of increasing dimension – a bougienage of the vessel. In smaller vessels this step should await introduction of the microscope; the initial dilatation is performed with carefully selected jeweller's forceps or specially designed dilatation forceps [1].

MORE PROXIMAL SECTION OF THE VESSEL. By choosing to resect more vessel to obtain acceptable flow the surgeon often commits himself to the use of vein grafts.

Hemostasis in the Stump
Having identified appropriate vessels carrying good flow, the surgeon should take time with the tourniquet released to achieve hemostasis. Bleeding should be deliberately provoked by mechanical debridement. Otherwise, after replantation when vessel spasm abates, significant hemorrhage may ensue. This problem is especially likely in transmetacarpal amputations; in such cases, the branches of the deep palmar arch should receive particular attention.

REPLANTATION
When the preparation of all structures in the stump and the amputated part (or parts) is complete, the amputated part can be taken off ice and replantation commenced [7, 12, 13, 17, 26, 29, 31]. In amputations of the arm or forearm, however, the replantation can be performed with the distal part still

encased in ice packs, which gives a better chance of preserving muscle viability.

Use of Tourniquet
If continued oozing obscures the surgeon's view, the tourniquet should be used after exsanguination of the extremity. The tourniquet should be released after 90 to 120 minutes, but can be reapplied without hesitation [15] provided that (1) it has been left off for more than 20 minutes, (2) flow has been observed in any anastomoses for 20 minutes before reapplication, and (3) the patient has received aspirin, 650 mg. before reapplication.

Sequence of Repair
Structures are repaired in the following sequence under normal circumstances:

Bone
Firm skeletal fixation by internal methods is desirable because it promotes early union. Whenever possible, joints should not be fixed, thereby permitting early motion. Thus compression plates are recommended for humerus, radius, ulna, and metacarpals, and intraosseous wiring is recommended for phalanges (Fig. 43-6). As in all osteosyntheses, attention must be given to alignment, rotation, and angulation, because subsequent correctional osteotomy is a tiresome and unnecessary procedure. In multiple digital replantations, the skeleton of all digits should be fixed at this stage except (1) when ischemia time has been long (in excess of 6 hours at the stage of osteosynthesis) or (2) when arthrodesis of one digit is necessary, because appropriate angulation may impede the access to adjacent digits during the microsurgical stages (Fig. 43-7).

Periosteum
When the bone has been shortened and the periosteum carefully preserved, the periosteum can be repaired with benefit because its presence speeds union and also probably helps to prevent tendon adhesions. A 5-0 or 6-0 suture is usually employed.

Extensor Tendons
The extensor tendons are repaired with 4-0 or 5-0 synthetic nonabsorbable suture, using a series of interrupted figure-of-eight stitches. At this juncture, some replantation surgeons repair at least one or two veins. This has the advantage of reducing blood loss after arterial repair, but it also has the disadvantages of prolonging ischemia and of requiring the introduction and removal of the microscope.

Flexor Tendons
All flexor tendons are repaired by the technique we have described [20]. We do not agree with the recommendation [15] that tendons be left for secondary repair, because the tendons are more difficult to handle secondarily and (more important) because secondary repair necessitates operating in the region of the vascular repairs at a stage when they are still vulnerable. The tendons are sutured with as much care as in a straightforward laceration to give the best chance of good functional return. Whenever possible the sheath is closed, since this has been shown to decrease the incidence of tendon adhesions [23].

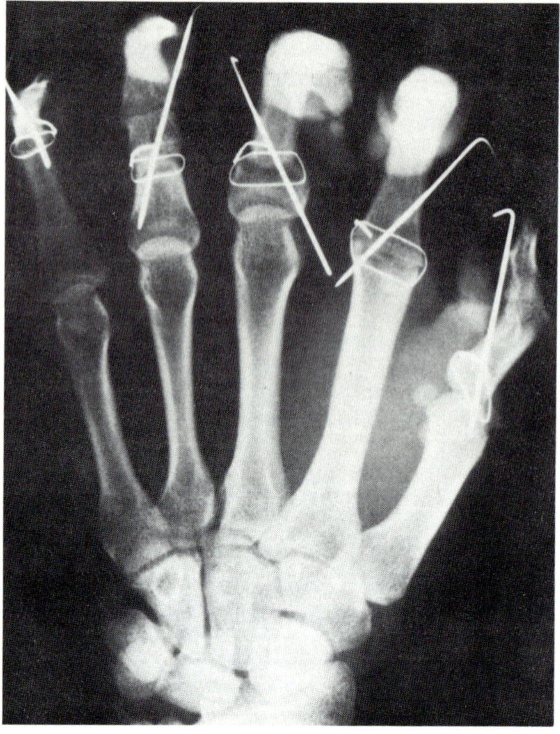

Fig. 43-6. In this five-finger replantation, intraosseous wiring and oblique Kirschner wires have been employed to obtain osteosynthesis in the thumb and middle and ring fingers as well as arthrodesis of the metacarpophalangeal joint of the index finger and proximal interphalangeal joint of the small finger.

The Introduction of the Microscope
At this juncture, if the tourniquet has been in use, it is released. The microscope is now introduced. The instrument employed should have the following capabilities: (1) *magnification* from 3.5 X to 16 X or 25 X; (2) *powerful independent lighting* with a reserve lamp; (3) *foot pedal controls* for zoom magnification and focusing; and (4) *two binocular operating positions,*

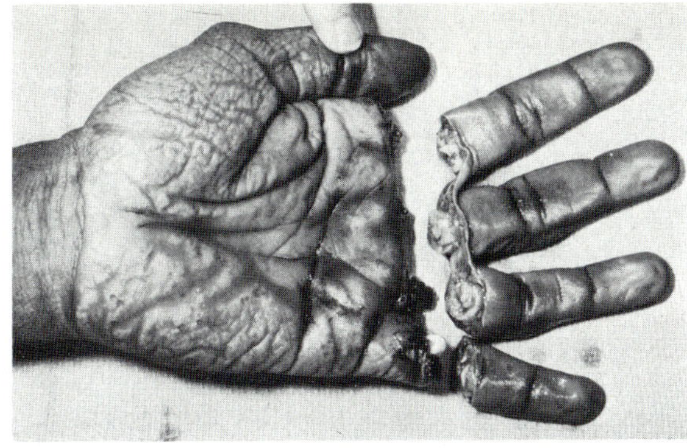

A

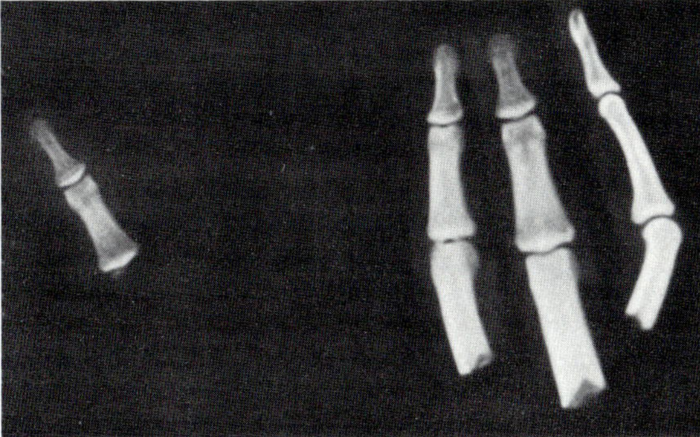

B

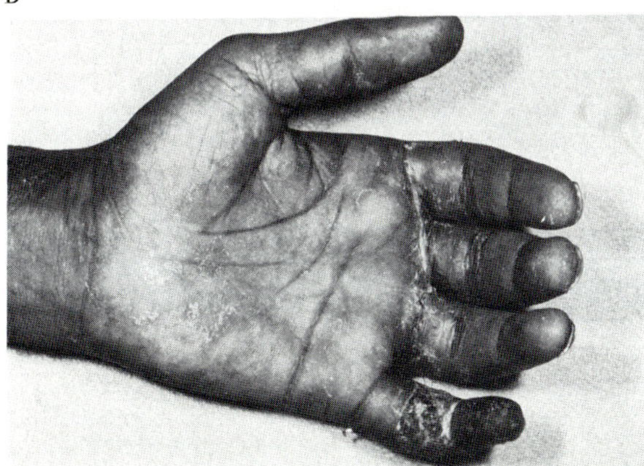

C

Fig. 43-7. A, this four-finger amputation with a power saw was deemed suitable for replantation after inspection of the x-rays. B, these x-rays, however, confirmed the need for arthrodesis of the small finger; for this reason the index, middle, and ring fingers were replanted before arthrodesis and replantation of the small finger were undertaken. C, the eventual ischemia time for the small finger was over 24 hours (the patient had arrived at the replantation center 12 hours after the original injury). As can be seen in this photograph, the replantation of the small finger failed.

the angles of which can be adjusted. If possible, the microscope should also have (1) *traverse capability* – that is, the possibility of moving the field longitudinally and transversely by use of either a tilting head or an X-Y coupling; (2) *an observer scope,* of value in teaching and in allaying nurse boredom; and (3) a *photographic attachment.*

The microscope should be positioned by the surgeon in such a way that it can be swung into place over the hand when required with no further handling. This positioning should be done immediately after the patient is prepared and draped. The surgeon should at that time make a final check that the instrument is functioning properly and should ensure that the eyepieces are correctly positioned and focused for both himself and his assistant.

Positioning for Microsurgery

The patient's hand should be held immobile by some device (such as a hand made of lead) in a position that gives clear exposure of the vessels to be repaired. This is most difficult to achieve in the case of the ulnar digital artery of the thumb over the metacarpal and proximal phalanx. To display this properly, the patient would be best placed prone; however, this is not practical. If adequate visualization cannot be achieved then it is quite justifiable to resort to a vein graft between two points that are better exposed (see information on vein grafts). The hand should be sufficiently far away from the microsurgeon to permit him to rest his forearms comfortably on the hand table. His wrists and the ulnar border of his hands should also be supported, often by placing stacked towels beneath them. Thus tremor is largely eliminated. We do *not* subscribe to the view that the microsurgeon should eschew coffee, alcohol, nicotine, or whatever other pleasurable pursuits may take his fancy; what little tremor they provoke can be overcome. Nor do we consider it necessary for the experienced microsurgeon, on hearing of a pending replantation, to hasten to the animal laboratory to sharpen his skills. This would seem only to add to his burden and accelerate the onset of fatigue. He would do better to sleep as best he can on a nearby stretcher.

Arteries

Looking through the microscope, the surgeon should relocate the two vessels ends previously tagged with 7-0 nylon. He should ensure that his view of them is *perfect,* performing any adjustments or additional incisions or skin stay sutures that are required. Repair can then be undertaken in the following order.

Preparation of the Vessel
A length of vessel on either side of the division sufficient to permit the application of the approximating microvascular clamp should be prepared, stripping off the adventitia by gripping the very end of the vessel (later to be excised) and peeling back the adventitia and attached fat with jeweller's forceps and microsurgical scissors. Any tethering branches should be coagulated with bipolar microforceps.

Excision of the Vessel End
The end of the vessel which has been handled should be excised with scissors. After the walls have been eased apart with microforceps, a clean, smooth lumen should be revealed. Dilatation as previously described should be repeated if necessary, and the vessel end thoroughly irrigated with warm heparin solution. Never again should the vessel end be gripped with forceps.

Confirmation of Flow
Proximal flow should be confirmed yet again as previously described. Once confirmed it can be controlled by applying a double approximating vascular clamp and, if necessary because of adjacent bleeding, by reapplying the tourniquet.

Correction of Tension
The surgeon should ensure that no undue tension will be necessary to bring the vessel together. Vessel ends that cannot be approximated by double microvascular clamps or by the use of a 10-0 nylon suture are under excessive tension. To repair them despite such tension, either by traction on the vessel or by the use of a larger suture, will result in an unsatisfactory, difficult, and leaking anastomosis that, if left uncorrected, will lead to a failed replant. *Undue tension can be easily overcome by use of a vein graft.*

Suturing the Vessel
The technique for microvascular repair has been described in Chapter 40.

Observation for Arterial Flow
The vessel should be observed for a period of 20 minutes after it has been sutured to ensure that flow continues [3]. The criteria of continued flow are as follows:

1. Bleeding from the amputated part, especially its veins.
2. Swift refill of the artery. This is tested by carefully emptying a segment distal to the anastomosis, which involves moving two forceps apart while occluding the vessel and then releasing the *proximal* forceps (Fig. 43-8).
3. Pinkness of the extremity. This sign is not necessarily present immediately in digits replanted after a long cold ischemia time; such digits may remain pale for up to 45 minutes in the face of good flow as assessed by the first two criteria.

Poor or absent flow may be due to (1) a lack of proximal flow, (2) technically incorrect anastomosis, (3) poor run-off, or (4) spasm. The first three of these problems have already been discussed. Spasm is a normal homeostatic mechanism and is always encountered; it should be overcome before repair by dilatation. After repair spasm may recur, most commonly as the result of one or more of three causes [4]:

1. Unhealthy vessel – the cure for this is resection and reanastomosis or insertion of a vein graft.
2. Whole blood in contact with the vessel.
3. Cold.

Irrigation
The second and third causes of spasm can be avoided by thorough irrigation with warm fluids after completion of the anastomosis. The irrigating fluids must be kept in a warming bath; we have found a blood warmer with a sterile liner to be most useful. The choice of irrigating fluid [33] has in the past included:

1. Magnesium sulphate. Acland [2] demonstrated the merits of this solution in preventing platelet aggregation in *experimental animals,* but he has frequently denied that it has any value in thicker-walled human vessels.
2. Bupivacaine (Marcaine). Used in high doses, this will induce bleeding from vessels adjacent to the repaired artery and thereby increase hematoma formation.
3. Heparin. Heparin has no drawbacks when used for irrigation, but it does not have advantages when applied to the outside of the vessel.

For irrigation we currently use heparin inside the lumen before the anastomosis and warm Ringer's lactate externally after vessel repair. While the artery is being observed, the veins should be permitted to bleed freely. This is especially true in arm or forearm amputations and when there is associated crush of the part, because perfusion of the part by arterial blood that does not recirculate reverses lactic acidosis in the extremity while avoiding a sudden fall in systemic pH [34]. During the period of observation, the adjacent nerve can be repaired.

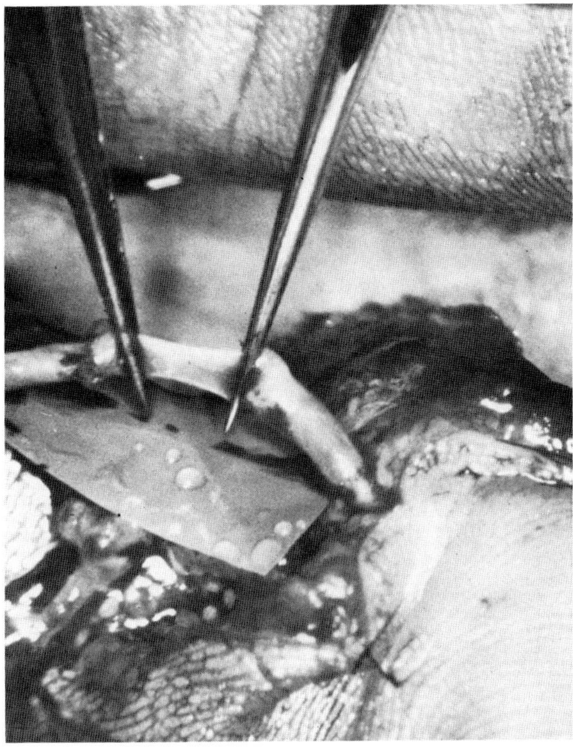

A

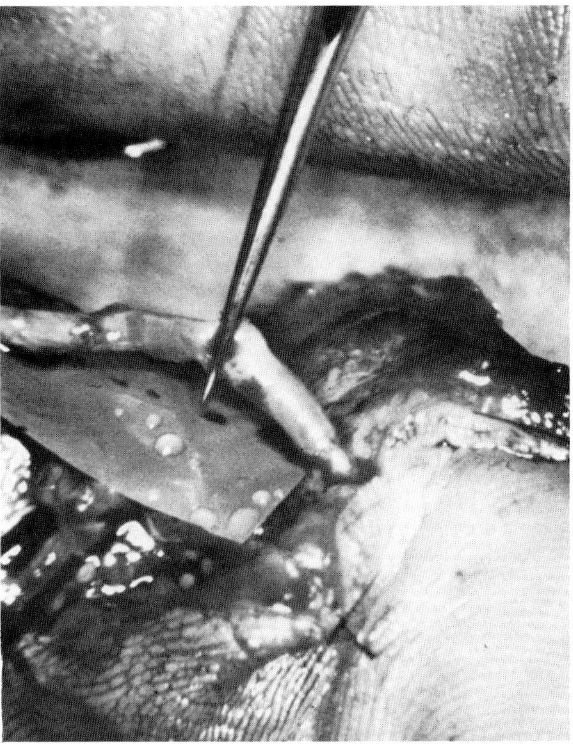

B

Fig. 43-8. The technique of testing for flow is shown in this vein graft inserted following ring avulsion. A, the proximal microforceps (on the left in the photograph) occludes flow from the artery proximally, and the distal forceps sweeps the blood out of the segment distal to the first forceps. B, on release of the first forceps, swift flow into the intervening segment indicates rapid refilling distal to the proximal anastomosis in this vein graft.

Nerve

The arguments for and against fascicular and epineurial repair have been presented elsewhere [8, 17]. Suffice it to say that we believe that the best results are obtained when the fascicles are aligned without distortion or strangulation or excess use of suture material. It is possible to achieve either good or bad results according to these criteria using either technique. Attention should therefore be directed less at the choice of technique but rather at its execution with respect to the fascicles on completion of the repair. We repair groups of fascicles on forearm major nerves and perform either fascicular or epineurial repair on digital nerves.

After one artery and nerve are repaired on a digital replantation, the procedure is repeated on the other digital artery and nerve. Whatever patency rate one has following arterial repair (unless it is 100 percent), repair of a second artery must increase one's replantation survival figures.

Veins

If the surgeon has ensured good arterial inflow by repairing all arteries, the only potential cause of failure in an ideal replant is congestion due to venous insufficiency, with a resultant rise in resistance to arterial run-off and later arterial thrombosis. The more veins that are repaired, therefore, the higher survival will be. All veins that can be found should be repaired; four is the minimum number acceptable if success without reexploration is to be ensured. Before removing the microscope to turn the hand and explore the dorsum, some time should be spent seeking volar veins in the digits. Although usually of smaller caliber, these veins can be quickly prepared and repaired.

Localization

Localization presents little or no problem in the hand and arm. In the digit, longitudinal incisions offset for later Z plasty (as already described under the heading, Preparation of the Part) are of great help. A common error is to search too superficially in the region of the dermis. The veins lie in a distinct plane, which the surgeon can ascertain in routine elective incisions. If the flaps are reflected from the extensor tendon, this plane will lie on the undersurface of the flap, to which the veins often have a tenacious hold.

Removal of Adventitia

The adventitia of the vein is more difficult to remove than that of the artery, partly because the vein itself is more flimsy. The removal can best be done by teasing the adventitia free, using two forceps pulling on it in opposite directions.

Suturing

A technique is employed similar to that used in arterial repair. It is much more likely that the back wall will be caught during a venous anastomosis, a tendency that can be overcome only by repeated irrigation and careful identification of the lumen with each suture. Usually six sutures per vein are sufficient. Before proceeding with skin closure, flow through both arterial repairs should finally be confirmed.

Skin Closure

The skin should be closed in such a way as to avoid all compression that would compromise venous return. This can usually be achieved, especially if Z plasties have been incorporated. In all cases, however, a critical eye should be kept on the color of the digital pulps. Any duskiness or increase in speed of refill after blanching should be corrected by releasing appropriate skin sutures. Occasionally significant skin defects may be left, especially in crush amputations or following prolonged ischemia. In such instances, free split-thickness skin grafts should be applied. Exposure of any of the repaired vessels, even of vein grafts, should not cause concern because skin grafts will take well in such circumstances.

SPECIAL OPERATIVE CONSIDERATIONS

Vein Grafts

Failure to employ vein grafts when they are indicated is usually due to inexperience and often causes more technical difficulty for the surgeon than does their use.

Indications for Vein Grafts

RELUCTANCE TO SHORTEN THE SKELETON. This may result from the need to preserve a significant joint such as the metacarpophalangeal joint of any of the digits.

FAILURE TO SHORTEN THE SKELETON ADEQUATELY. Even if shortening has been done in an attempt to avoid the need for vein grafts the surgeon must not stubbornly persist in attempting anastomoses under tension.

RESECTION OF A DAMAGED VESSEL. As emphasized previously, only ideal vessels should be repaired; the operator must remember, however, that resection of long segments involves sacrificing their branches also. This may result in loss of skin overlying the graft or in localized ischemia in bones, joints, or tendons, with effects that are still to be determined.

SHUNTING OF FLOW. Although rarely necessary, shunting of the flow may be indicated when one artery to the limb or digit is damaged proximally and the other distally. This is encountered only in salvage replantation following previous trauma or multiple level injuries.

A DESIRE TO LENGTHEN THE COURSE OF THE ARTERY. The surgeon may wish to avoid an obvious skin defect, especially over a bed unlikely to take a free skin graft. Such defects require flap cover, but a delay of a few days may be prudent after replantation.

THE NEED TO IMPROVE EXPOSURE FOR MICROSURGICAL REPAIR. Such a situation arises in the thumb amputation just distal to the metacarpophalangeal joint. Often the princeps pollicis is the only important artery at this level, but it is extremely difficult to position the hand to allow a good view of the vessel through the microscope, since the vessel lies on the ulnar aspect of the thumb. This problem can be overcome by placing a vein graft between the radial artery on the dorsum of the first web space and the digital artery over the proximal phalanx. These are both positions relatively accessible to the microscope. If the radial artery of the index finger is to be sacrificed in this procedure, it should first be occluded with a vascular clamp; the tourniquet is then released and flow to the index finger confirmed.

Sources of Vein Grafts

Veins have a remarkable capability to vary their caliber, far exceeding that of arteries. Within reason, they can often therefore be dilated enough that they almost exactly match the vessel to which they are being attached. However, if they are thereafter subjected to arterial pressure they will assume their maximum diameter, which may be disproportionately large. A vein of roughly equivalent dimension in the undisturbed state should therefore be selected from the following sites.

FOR DIGITAL VESSELS. Veins of the anterior forearm in its distal half are used.

FOR FOREARM VESSELS. Dorsal forearm veins are used, or, if it appears unwise to harvest veins from the injured arm, those from the opposite arm or from the lower part of the leg are used. Leg veins, if not varicose, are particularly suitable for major artery repairs, since their walls are somewhat thicker than those of the arm.

Harvesting Vein Grafts

Harvesting vein grafts should be done under tourniquet control, since only then can small tributaries be identified and coagulated with bipolar forceps. Where it is intended to use a vein graft to join one artery proximally to two or more distally, as in injuries to the superficial palmar arch, a vein with an adequate number of proximal branches should be selected. Since an incision directly over the vein increases the possibility of inadvertent injury, so a lazy S cut is made with the vein as its axis. The caliber of the vein should be checked immediately after skin incision, because the vein will go into spasm during dissection. All branches should be ligated or coagulated. Because of the great elasticity of veins, the necessary length of graft (as previously measured) should be marked off before sectioning either end; this is most conveniently done with 10-0 nylon sutures in the wall. If a great length is required, the sutures should be placed on the same aspect of the vein to aid in avoiding torsion. Some convention should be employed to indicate the direction of flow so that the venous valves are not an impediment. We place a ligature on the proximal end of the vein and none on the distal end. More graft than is required should be taken.

The graft should be correctly oriented for flow.

Anastomosis

The technique of anastomosis is similar to that described above; only a few additional points need to be made. The first end to be anastomosed should be that from which flow is to come. It should be noted that while the double clamp will hold the vessels for repair, the vessels can be further stabilized by applying distal traction to the graft.

SIZE DISCREPANCY. There is often a discrepancy in caliber between graft and vessel. If this does not exceed 2:1, it presents few problems. Sutures are inserted as already described, first dividing the circumference of each side of the repair into thirds, and then dividing each third into thirds. The discrepancy will thus be distributed evenly around the repair. When such a discrepancy exceeds 2:1, a new graft of better fit should be taken.

BLOOD FLOW IN THE GRAFT. After the first anastomosis is completed, there are benefits in allowing flow through the graft:

1. Torsion is avoided, since the flow straightens out the graft.
2. Flow can be confirmed; this confirmation should be made, because the open vein graft offers a unique opportunity to overcome proximal spasm. With care a catheter can safely be passed along the graft past the anastomosis to overcome inadequate flow. If the catheter is arrested at the proximal repair, the anastomosis is faulty and should be revised. Using this method, the revision can be done before the graft is cut to length.
3. The length of graft required can be more accurately judged. Vein grafts lengthen marvelously under the influence of arterial pressure.
4. Leaks can be repaired both at the proximal anastomosis and along the graft, allowing the surgeon to concentrate on distal leaks after the second repair.

If the surgeon is concerned about leaving blood static in the graft while the second repair is done, a clamp can be reapplied proximal to the first anastomosis and the graft washed out with heparin saline. However, we find this unnecessary.

CHECKING GRAFT SIZE. Despite all efforts to prevent it, the graft may be too long once flow is fully established through a vein graft. This will result in kinking, with a significant reduction in perfusion. The surgeon should not hesitate to take out a segment of vessel at the site of repair and redo it; 15 to 20 minutes spent on another anastomosis seems especially inconsequential when one is faced with an underperfused replantation on the following day.

Levels of Amputation

Certain factors are peculiar to replantations at different levels of amputation.

Arm and Forearm

In the arm and forearm, there is a significant bulk of ischemic muscle. For this reason, arterial repair should, in most cases, follow bone fixation in order to reestablish circulation at the earliest moment. The vessels are sturdy and can be repaired with 8-0 nylon, which will withstand the disturbance caused by subsequent muscle and nerve repair. During the period of bone fixation, metabolism in the extremity can be lowered by keeping it packed in ice. Even with these precautions, fasciotomy of the forearm and intrinsic muscular compartments should be performed.

After bone fixation it is beneficial if two surgeons can work simultaneously; one starts with the ulnar artery repair and works across the anterior aspect of the arm, while the other commences with the radial artery and then moves on to the tendons of the thumb, the radial nerve, and the extensors.

Wrist

In addition to the considerations discussed above, the wrist presents the problem of bone shortening at the level of an important joint. This can be resolved by any one of three methods.

EXCISION OF THE JOINT AND PRIMARY ARTHRODESIS. This procedure is particularly appropriate when the joint surfaces have been damaged, and it has distinct merit in the person who does heavy manual labor.

PROXIMAL ROW CARPECTOMY. Most appropriate in sedentary workers, this procedure has drawbacks that are well recognized.

SHORTENING OSTEOTOMY OF THE RADIUS AND A DARRACH PROCEDURE. Recently described in Japan, this is a modification that preserves function while facilitating the repair of all structures.

Transmetacarpal Area

As stated already, the prevention of hematoma is of great importance in the transmetacarpal area; consequently, special precautions must be taken *before* replantation. Here most of all, postoperative anticoagulant therapy is probably contraindicated (Fig. 43-9).

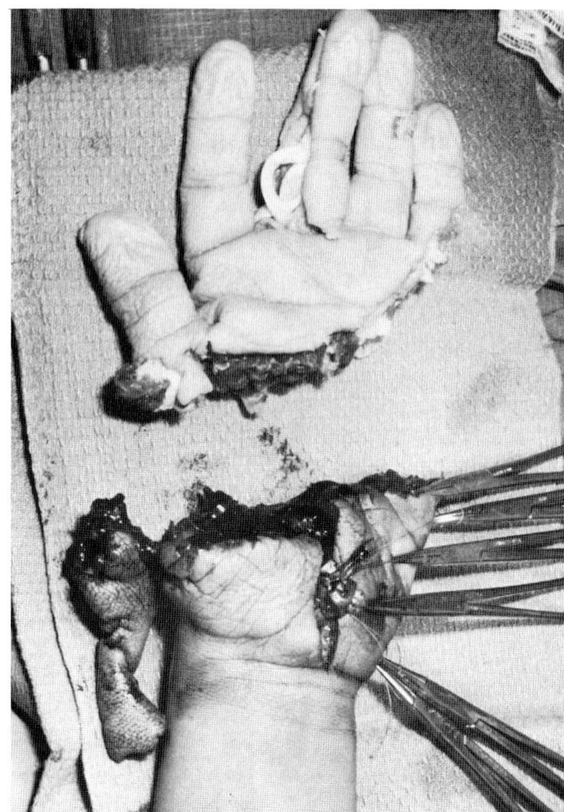

Fig. 43-9. In this type of transmetacarpal amputation, particular care must be taken to ensure hemostasis by ligating the ends of the metacarpal arteries in the amputated part prior to replantation. If this is not done, significant bleeding can seriously hamper the chances of survival of the amputated part. (The authors are grateful to Dr. Joseph Kutz for permission to publish the photograph of his patient.)

Proximal Phalanx

In the proximal phalanx (the "no man's land" of Bunnell), tendon repairs are all-important. The consequences of prolonged ischemia are much less devastating in digital replantation; therefore time can be devoted to a careful primary tendon repair. Whenever possible the joints should be left free, and active motion should commence within the first few days after replantation. Rubber band traction is not indicated because of the extensor tendon repair.

Proximal Interphalangeal Joint

If the proximal interphalangeal joint is destroyed, the arthrodesis must be in the most functional position. In the index finger, this is the position in which the pulp can be most readily approximated to that of the thumb – 0 to 20 degrees, according to the amount of shortening. In the other fingers, it is the greatest angle that can be achieved at the joint while still allowing the tip of the finger to extend to the plane of the palm of the hand by hyperextension of the metacarpophalangeal joint. This is usually an angle of 30, 40, and 50 degrees in the middle, ring, and small fingers respectively.

Middle Phalanx

Beyond the superficialis insertion in the middle phalanx, sensation is all-important and the chances of excellent sensory recovery are high. Although apparently unnecessary, replantation at this level is relatively straightforward and gives good functional results.

Distal Phalanx

Replantation at the level of the distal phalanx is largely cosmetic (and none the worse for that), with the notable exception of the thumb; in the thumb the

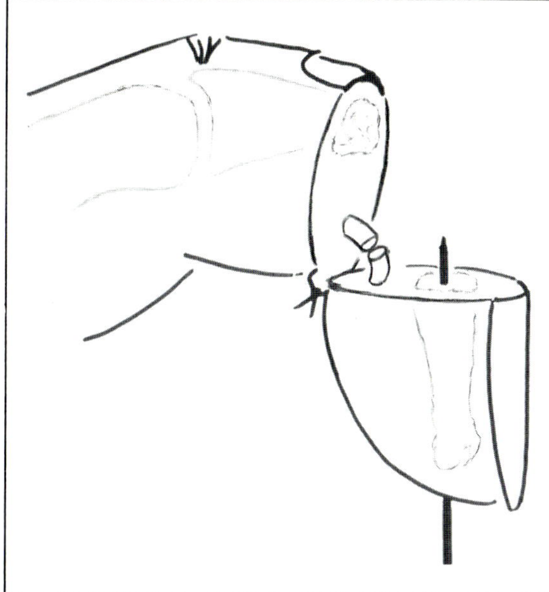

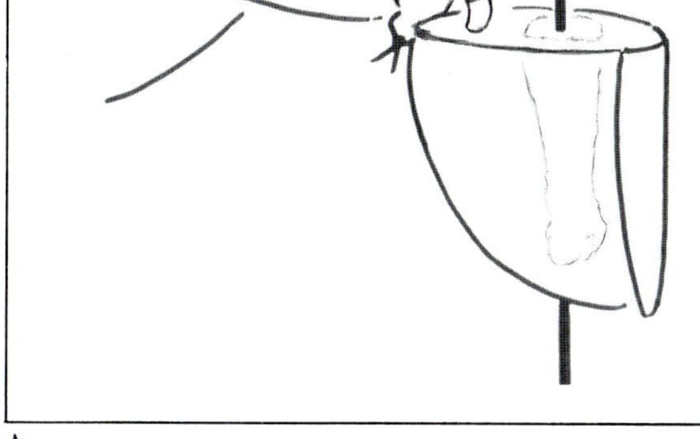

A

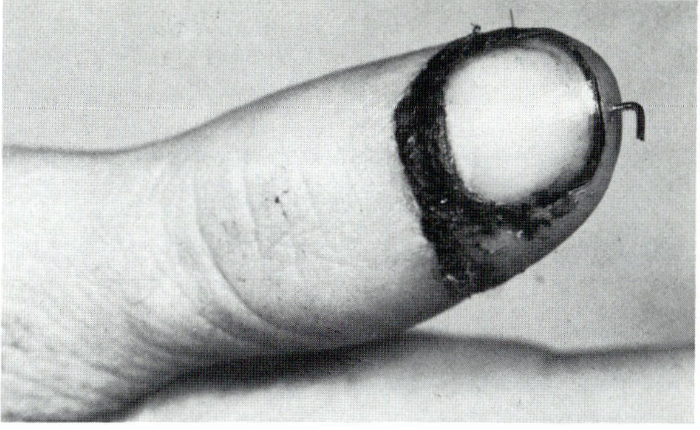

B

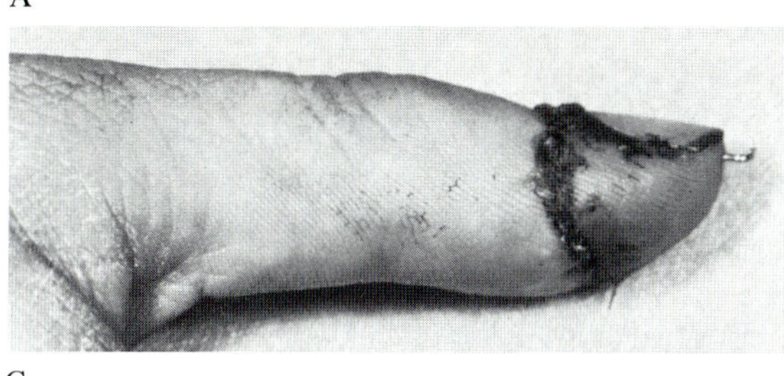

C

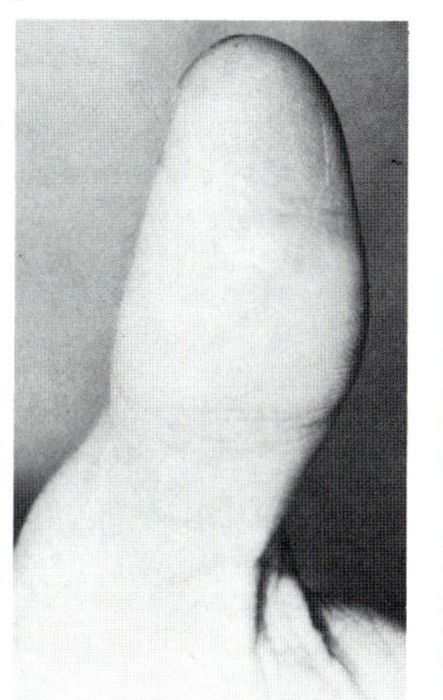

D

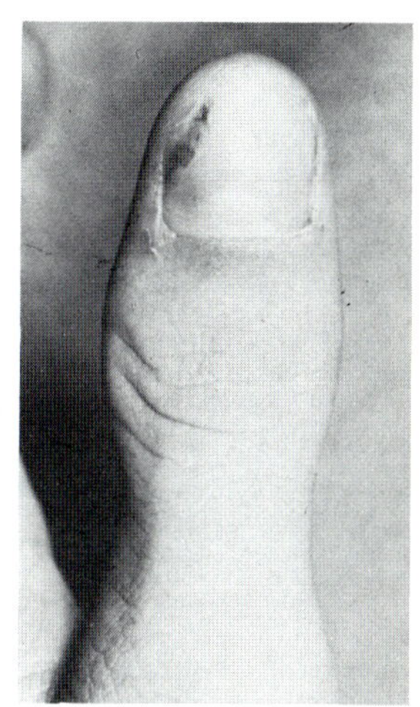

E

Fig. 43-10. Replantation at the level of the distal phalanx. A, this drawing illustrates the essential elements of the technique in which the Kirschner wire is passed retrograde out through the stump of the thumb. The palmar skin is sutured before arterial anastomosis is undertaken. B, C, the dorsal wound was left open and survival of the digit (shown here 10 days after replantation) is good. D, E, the significant function of the thumbnail has thus been preserved in a patient who was treated in under 2 hours and was permitted to go home immediately after replantation.

absence of the nail seriously hinders the ability to pick up thin flat objects. If the amputation is through the nailbed, the sequence of repair is unique (Fig. 43-10). The tip of the nail is stabilized by a Kirschner wire placed retrograde through the amputated phalanx and by suture of the palmar skin. Arterial repair is performed looking from dorsally past the unreduced bone; there are five or six arteries on the palmar periosteum, any one of which requires only three to six 10-0 sutures. Reduction and pinning of bone are performed. No venous repairs are possible [32], and the nailbed is left open and dressed with fluffs. The whole procedure takes less than 2 hours, and can be done on an outpatient basis.

Dressings

Although understandably fatigued, the replantation surgeon will ensure better results if he applies or supervises the dressing of the hand (Fig. 43-11).

1. The initial dressing of paraffin gauze should be laid in longitudinal strips on to the wound with fluffed dry gauze applied in abundance over it, again longitudinally. No circumferential dressings are applied below the next layer, which is of plastic sponge.
2. A plastic sponge 1 to 3 cm. thick is wrapped once around the entire limb, leaving a gap down one side; it is held in place by a circumferential stretch

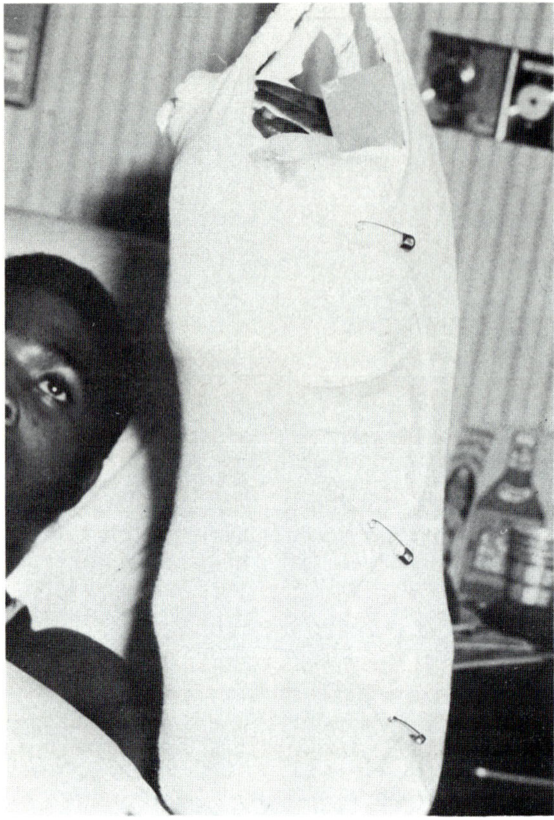

A

B

gauze bandage. The sponge should extend out as far as the tips of the fingers.

3. Plaster of Paris is then applied over the customary paper felt bandage. This plaster is again laid on longitudinally; it should pass around the flexed elbow in "sugar tong" fashion and incorporate a plaster sling beyond the fingertips, from which the limb is suspended.
4. The fingers should be checked on one final occasion for circulation and for the absence of constrictive dressings.
5. The arm should be elevated using the plaster sling or a 15-cm. stockinette above the elbow.

POSTOPERATIVE CARE

Medication

Over the past 5 years we have at various times employed all the drugs that have been recommended to assist microvascular repairs. We have dispensed with most of them and will probably discard the remainder in the near future. Antibiotics are given until 2 days after replantation unless some indication exists to continue therapy. Other medications we use are detailed below.

In the Ideal Replantation

Aspirin, 650 mg., is given twice daily, and dextran 40, 500 ml. over 12 hours, is given every day for 3 days.

In the Salvage Replantation

HEPARIN. In certain cases, especially when it has not been possible to ensure that all vessels employed are in perfect condition (as in crush injuries), we still administer heparin in continuous intravenous infusion. The initial dose, given before flow is permitted to pass through the first anastomosis, is 100 mg. (or 10,000 IU) in the adult. Thereafter doses are titrated against 6-hourly estimations of the activated partial thromboplastin time, which should be kept at a level two and one-half times that of the control. As our confidence in the technique of replantation has increased, however, we have used heparin less, because it has the disadvantages [5] that it can cause allergic reactions; internal hemorrhage; uncontrolled bleeding from the extremity, requiring transfusion (with its attendant dangers), protamine neutralization (with a possibility of increased clotting by the elimination of endogenous heparin); and hemorrhage at the site of

Fig. 43-11. A, the dressing that is applied contains no circumferential dressings deep to the plastic foam, which can be seen in both of these photographs. The circumferential dressings are applied outside the plastic foam; suspension of the limb is achieved by placing the suspending dressing above the elbow, thereby exerting no distal compressive force on the replanted hand. B, in another patient, the dressing leaves the fingers exposed so that their color and temperature can be compared.

replant, which in turn causes vasospasm acutely and organization and fibrosis chronically.

PROTHROMBIN DEPRESSANTS. In those cases in which heparin has been employed, prothrombin depressants are substituted; they are introduced on the third day in doses sufficient to reduce prothrombin activity to 20 to 30 percent of normal.

Observation

Circulation Checks

Initially circulation checks [15] should be performed at hourly intervals. *Color of the nailbed and return of blood after blanching* are the criteria we employ (Fig. 43-11B). If the color is pale, with slow return, arterial insufficiency is present, while if the color is dark red, with very swift return, there is venous congestion. The perfect response exists when the color is pink with return comparable to adjacent digits. The pinkness of a good replantation will tend to diminish after 4 or 5 days, which should not cause concern.

Other Methods of Checking Flow

TEMPERATURE. Using a thermocouple, temperature is a most useful guide [29], especially when the adjacent fingers were not injured and can be used for comparison. A fall of temperature below 30°C is an indication for immediate exploration.

DIGITAL PULSE MONITOR AND ULTRASOUND. When these aids are required because there is doubt regarding color and refill, then reexploration is usually already indicated.

BLEEDING. More commonly employed in black patients undergoing free flap transfer where no nailbed is available, bleeding from a stab wound is the ultimate reassurance of flow. However, it does not warn the surgeon of venous congestion.

DRESSING CHECKS. Even when circumferential dressings are not used, dressings soaked in blood that then congeals can be a potent source of constriction. When dressings are adherent or heavily bloodstained, they should be carefully removed and replaced. With the dressing described above, this can be done easily without changing the outer sponge and plaster casing.

REEXPLORATION. Like fasciotomy and tracheostomy, exploration of a replantation is necessary if the surgeon even considers it. The situation will invariably prove to be worse than anticipated. Provided that it is undertaken in good time, reexploration is a worthwhile procedure, often necessitating the use of vein grafts. With experience, our rate of reexploration has fallen steadily, which is almost certainly due to the fact that at least two healthy arteries and four healthy veins are repaired correctly in each replanted extremity.

LATE COMPLICATIONS

Nonunion and Malunion

Originally not uncommon, skeletal problems such as nonunion and malunion have been virtually eliminated by the use of greater care in obtaining rigid internal fixation of congruous bone ends.

Muscle Contractures

Wherever significant muscle bulk has remained ischemic for more than 6 hours, contractures are probable. Intrinsic contractures can be released, and when necessary their function can be taken over by tendon transfers. Ischemic contracture of the forearm muscles presents a much greater problem, which is dealt with elsewhere.

Inadequate Sensation

The higher the amputation, the more this becomes a problem. However if the limb is well vascularized, we have found the results of nerve repair in replantation to be at least as good as those of a conventional primary repair.

Joint Stiffness

Every effort should be made to avoid transfixing joints with the internal fixation necessary for replantation. If this has been successfully avoided, limited range-of-motion exercises should be commenced on the first or second postoperative day and the joints should be passively manipulated when the dressing is first changed at 10 days.

Tendon Adhesions

The single greatest cause of poor function in replantation, tendon adhesions can be somewhat reduced by meticulous repair and early active exercise. Active exercise is commenced despite the obvious hazards of possible rupture, since they are outweighed by the problem of adhesion. When adhesions have occurred, tenolysis or tendon graft (with or without preliminary rods) has thus far given only limited improvement.

ORGANIZATION

Successful replantation requires organization.

Surgeons

Replantation should be undertaken by the lone surgeon only after careful consideration of the consequences. It is not the single digit tonight that will seriously disrupt his practice but the three-finger amputation on the following night. Regular replantation requires at least three surgeons capable of such work, with skilled assistance. It is of significance that Munich and Louisville, the two centers probably doing the most cases, have eleven and six replantation surgeons respectively, with the latter having at least four Fellows in hand surgery sufficiently well trained to undertake microvascular work.

Nurses

In the emergency and operating rooms, smooth progress is possible only with the presence of nurses knowledgeable in the management of amputated parts, operating microscopes, and microsurgical instruments. In the ward, nurses practiced in evaluation of circulation and handling of dressings are essential if otherwise salvageable extremities are not to be lost. Our recent acquisition of a hand ward has made us very aware of these benefits.

Planning

When confronted with a multiple digit replantation, the surgeon must plan the procedure to ensure maximum efficiency. With the involvement of three or four surgeons and assistants, the operation can proceed swiftly in stages, each done by different pairs. Thus no surgeon need operate for more than 4 to 6 hours without rest during a case that may take up to 20 hours.

Changing Gear

Microsurgery is a precise and exacting skill, which of necessity is done at a relatively slow pace. There is a danger that the whole replantation may be conducted at that pace, partly through fatigue. The surgeon must cultivate the ability to "change gear," working quickly when it is possible without marring the quality of his techniques.

REFERENCES

1. Acland, R. New instruments for microvascular surgery. *Br. J. Surg.* 59:181, 1972.
2. Acland, R. Prevention of thrombosis in microvascular surgery by the use of magnesium sulphate. *Br. J. Plast. Surg.* 25:292, 1972.
3. Acland, R. Signs of patency in small vessel anastomosis. *Surgery* 72:744, 1972.
4. Acland, R. Thrombus formation in microvascular surgery: An experimental study of the effects of surgical trauma. *Surgery* 73:766, 1973.
5. Ariyan, S., and Stansel, H. C. Further hazards of heparin therapy in vascular surgery. *Arch. Surg.* 111:120, 1976.
6. Biemer, E., Duspiva, W., Herndl, E., Stock, W., and Ramatschi, P. Early experiences in organizing and running a replantation service. *Br. J. Plast. Surg.* 31:9, 1978.
7. Buncke, H. J., and Schulz, W. P. Experimental digital amputation and reimplantation. *Plast. Reconstr. Surg.* 36:62, 1965.
8. Cabaud, H. E., Rodkey, W. G., McCarroll, H. R., Mutz, S. B., and Niebauer, J. J. Epineurial and perineurial fascicular nerve repairs: A critical comparison. *J. Hand Surg.* 1:131, 1976.
9. Furnas, D. W. Growth and development in replanted forelimbs. *Plast. Reconstr. Surg.* 46:445, 1970.
10. Kleinert, H. E., and Kasdan, M. L. Restoration of blood flow in upper extremity injuries. *J. Trauma* 3:461, 1963.
11. Kleinert, H. E., Kasdan, M. L., and Romero, J. L. Small blood vessel anastomosis for salvage of severely injured upper extremity. *J. Bone Joint Surg.* [Am.] 45:788, 1963.
12. Kleinert, H. E., Kutz, J. E., Atasoy, E., Neale, H. W., and Serafin, D. Replantation of nonviable digits – ten years' experience. *J. Bone Joint Surg.* [Am.] 56:1092, 1974.
13. Kleinert, H. E., Serafin, D., Kutz, J. E., and Atasoy, E. Reimplantation of amputated digits and hands. *Orthop. Clin. North Am.* 4:957, 1973.
14. Komatsu, S., and Tamai, S. Successful replantation of a completely cut-off thumb. *Plast. Reconstr. Surg.* 43:374, 1968.
15. Lendvay, P. G. Replacement of the amputated digit. *Br. J. Plast. Surg.* 26:398, 1973.
16. Lister, G. D. Mikrochirurgisch Probleme der Replantation, *Handchirurgie* 9(2):45, 1977.
17. Lister, G. D. Techniques in Replantation. Nerve Grafting and Microsurgery. In Lamb and Kuczynski (Eds.), *A Practice of Hand Surgery.* Edinburgh: Blackwell (in press).
18. Lister, G. D. Intraosseus wiring of the digital skeleton. *J. Hand Surg.* 3:427, 1978.
19. Lister, G. D., and Bell, G. The relative efficacy of whole blood, normal saline and dextran 110 in restoring renal cortical blood flow following haemorrhage. Proceedings of the Joint Meeting of the American Association of University Surgeons, the European Society of Surgical Research, and the Surgical Research Society, London, 1969.
20. Lister, G. D., Kleinert, H. E., Kutz, J. E., and Atasoy, E. Primary flexor tendon repair followed by immediate controlled mobilization. *J. Hand Surg.* 2:441, 1977.
21. Malt, R. A., and McKhann, C. F. Replantation of severed arms. *J.A.M.A.* 189:716, 1964.
22. Malt, R. A., Remensnyder, J. P., and Harris, W. H. Long-term utility of replanted arms. *Ann. Surg.* 176:334, 1972.

176:334, 1972.
23. Matthews, P., and Richards, H. Factors in the adherence of flexor tendon after repair. *J. Bone Joint Surg.* [Br.] 58:230, 1976.
24. McLean, D. H., and Buncke, H. J. Use of the Saran Wrap cuff in microsurgical arterial repairs. *Plast. Reconstr. Surg.* 51:624, 1973.
25. Nomoto, H., Buncke, H. J., and Chater, N. L. Improved patency rates in microvascular surgery when using magnesium sulfate and a silicone rubber vascular cuff. *Plast. Reconstr. Surg.* 54:157, 1974.
26. O'Brien, B. McC. Replantation surgery. *Clin. Plast. Surg.* 1:3, 1974.
27. O'Brien, B. McC. Replantation and reconstructive microvascular surgery: Part 1. *Ann. R. Coll. Surg. Engl.* 58:87, 1976.
28. O'Brien, B. McC. Replantation and reconstructive microvascular surgery: Part 2. *Ann. R. Coll. Surg. Engl.* 58:171, 1976.
29. O'Brien, B. McC. *Microvascular Reconstructive Surgery.* Edinburgh: Churchill-Livingstone, 1977.
30. O'Brien, B. McC., MacLeod, A. M., and Miller, G. D. H. Clinical replantation of digits. *Plast. Reconstr. Surg.* 52:490, 1973.
31. O'Brien, B. McC., and Miller, G. D. H. Digital reattachment and revascularization. *J. Bone Joint Surg.* [Am.] 55:714, 1973.
32. Serafin, D., Kutz, J. E., and Kleinert, H. E. Replantation of a completely amputated distal thumb without venous anastomosis. *Plast. Reconstr. Surg.* 52:579, 1973.
33. Swartz, W. M., Brink, R. R., and Buncke, H. J. Prevention of thrombosis in arterial and venous microanastomoses by using topical agents. *Plast. Reconstr. Surg.* 58:478, 1976.
34. Tamai, S., Tatsumi, Y., Shimizu, T., Hori, Y., Okuda, H., Takita, T., Sakamoto, H., and Fukui, A. Traumatic amputations of digits: The fate of remaining blood. An experimental and clinical study. *J. Hand Surg.* 2:13, 1977.
35. Weiland, A. J., Villarreal-Rios, A., Kleinert, H. E., Kutz, J. E., Atasoy, E., and Lister, G. D. Replantation of digits and hands: Analysis of surgical techniques and functional results in 71 patients with 86 replantations. *J. Hand Surg.* 2:1, 1977.
36. White, J. C. Nerve regeneration after replantation of severed arms. *Ann. Surg.* 170:715, 1969.

Breast

Augmentation Mammoplasty

JAMES L. BAKER, JR.

From earliest times [37, 46], the breast has been the symbol of femininity. Often the woman with small breasts feels inferior and less desirable than her better endowed "sister." In recent years, because of improvements in breast prostheses and safe surgical techniques, breast augmentation has become one of the most requested cosmetic operations. It has been estimated that several hundred thousand augmentation mammoplasties have been performed to date, with an annual increase of 30 percent [53, 54]. Even though cultural and biological pressures play an important role in encouraging women to seek mammary augmentation, studies show that the personal symbolic representation of the breast is the most important stimulus to the woman requesting surgery [19, 20, [34]. The size and shape of a woman's breast are extremely important to her body image and self concept [6].

The typical female requesting augmentation is an educated, upper-middle-class mother of two children, in her early thirties. She has considered augmentation for many years but felt that the operation involved serious medical risk or was unobtainable. Learning of the feasibility of augmentation from a friend who had undergone the procedure, she made the appointment with a surgeon [6].

A study of the psychosexual dynamics of 132 patients who underwent breast augmentation revealed that some women feel that it is unacceptable to use an external means (padded brassiere) to produce the illusion of adequate breast size, no matter how natural in feel or appearance. For an artificial device to be effective for these women, it must be implanted beneath the skin, so that it can become incorporated as part of their body image. (The psychological mechanism by which this is accomplished involves the tactile and visual exploration of self [6].)

Incorporation of the implant into the body image occurred within 60 days in most of these patients, but was delayed in those patients who developed complications. (All incorporated the implant after the complications cleared.) When the patients were asked to evaluate their own feelings of self-esteem, 93 percent reported increased self-confidence, 84 percent reported a strong feeling of increased adequacy, 84 percent had an increased feeling of elation and joy, and 80 percent had increased feelings of equality and self-worth. When they were questioned about sexual response, 79 percent reported that the increase in breast size had been followed by an increased interest in sexual relations, 53 percent reported increased frequency of intercourse, 69 percent reported a better quality of sexual relations, 52 percent had an increased frequency of orgasm, and 78 percent had an increased desire for breast play. Apparently, many of these women had feelings of inadequacy because of their small breasts; increased sexual satisfaction presumably results from the release of sexual inhibitions caused by these feelings [6].

HISTORICAL BACKGROUND

The silicone rubber prosthesis represents only the present state of the art of breast augmentation in the twentieth century. In seeking the ultimate of total patient satisfaction, the plastic surgeon's climb has traversed three main stages: autogenous tissue transplantation, injectable materials, and prosthetic devices. Although we have paused at each plateau, hoping that ours was the answer, we found it represented only a stepping stone. The climb must continue, a stage at a time, until we can solve our final problem (i.e., capsular contracture of the augmented breast) and obtain the goal of a breast that looks and feels natural today and will remain so throughout a lifetime.

Czerny [16] began the development of breast augmentation in 1895 when he transplanted a lipoma from a patient's thigh to fill out a breast defect resulting from removal of a fibroadenoma. Gersuny [26, 27] followed in 1899, utilizing percutaneous injections of paraffin. Surgeons continued the advance throughout this century. In 1925 Lexer [40] introduced free fat grafts. Schwarzmann in 1930 and Thorek in 1942 [62] recommended inserting glass balls into the breasts for augmentation.

In an attempt to avoid resorption and liquefaction of the free fat grafts, Berson [8] in 1945 suggested dermal fat grafts. Bames [7] and Maliniac [43–45] expanded this work in 1950, while Longacre [41, 42] utilized local upper abdominal dermal fat flaps rotated superiorly and inserted beneath each breast.

Pangman [48, 49] introduced the Ivalon (polyvinyl alcohol–formaldehyde) polymer sponge in 1951. This sponge was carved to shape, soaked in water for 24 hours, and then sterilized. Fibrous ingrowth invaded the sponge postoperatively, causing firmness and contracture. To prevent this, the sponge was coated with polyethylene or polyurethane [9, 11,

18, 19]. However, fluid accumulation in the sac and infections were not uncommon. Etheron (polyether) sponge was introduced in the early 1960s [12, 28, 55]; although it caused fewer problems than Ivalon sponge, excessive contracture of the material remained a problem.

Despite the terrifying complications reported from the use of other injectable materials earlier in the century [33, 38], during the 1950s and 1960s some physicians turned to silicone injections for breast augmentation. Products were initially available in Japan, as Elicon (heat-treated, vulcanized silicone gel) and Zeflon (a fluid mixed with an organic salt of tin at room temperature) [47]. Some of the complications seen from liquid silicone injection into the breast include: nodularity, granulomatous hepatitis, migration along fascial planes, embolism, and death [17, 19, 58]. It is now generally accepted that liquid silicone should not be utilized in breast augmentation.

In 1963, Cronin and Gerow [14, 25] introduced the silicone "natural-feel" breast prosthesis, which was constructed of a silicone rubber shell containing soft silicone gel and backed with a Dacron mesh. It was this advancement that brought us to our present stage of development.

CHEMICAL COMPOSITION OF THE IMPLANTS

Medical grade silicones used in surgical implants include elastomers and gels [56, 62]. These materials contain no toxic additives and are compatible with body tissues following implantation. Silicones are polymers with molecular backbones that consist of silicon and oxygen.

The mammary prosthesis is a silicone elastomer shell containing a silicone gel. The shell is made from silicone polymers of moderate to high molecular weight; these polymers have been reinforced with silica filler and cross-linked via an addition reaction at moderate temperatures. The silicone polymers used to form the elastomer are a mixture, with the dominant species being polydimethylsiloxane. Polymethylvinylsiloxane and polymethylhydrogen-siloxane are present in lesser amounts. The vinyl and hydrogen groups are necessary for the addition reaction. This reaction creates networks that transform the silicones from a soft putty to an elastic, rubber-like material [57].

The gel that fills the envelope consists of a mixture of polymers similar to that used for the envelope, but the polymers are of moderate molecular weight and no reinforcing filler is used. Gelation of the mixture is effected by the cross-linking of the polymers. The addition reaction that accomplishes this network formation employs the same chemistry as that used in the formation of the elastomeric envelope. (For additional information on silicones, see Chapter 3.)

PREOPERATIVE PLANNING

Aesthetic Goals

The surgeon's responsibility to the patient is to give her, whenever possible, the type of breast she desires. However, the opinions of the surgeon and the patient can vary greatly, depending upon cultural, regional, or individual factors. The present fashions and the mass media have contributed greatly to the image women have of the "ideal" breast. If maximal postoperative patient satisfaction is to be attained, the patient's expectations and motivations must be fully appreciated preoperatively. Full cognizance should be given to the patient's desires concerning her body image during consultation. It should be kept in mind that the surgery is being performed to satisfy the patient, and the surgeon's satisfaction is secondary. If she desires breasts that are "as large as possible," a prosthesis should be used that will afford her a rich, full appearance without appearing grotesque [2]. If she requests only a slight increase in size, despite the fact that the surgeon may feel she could easily accommodate a larger implant, a smaller prosthesis should be provided. If the surgeon finds anatomical limitations that may modify his patient's expectations, these must be discussed thoroughly with the patient preoperatively, so that postoperative misunderstandings and disappointment are avoided. The psychosexual dynamics of breast augmentation must be understood by the surgeon and should play an important role in his preoperative planning [1, 6].

Indications

The patient presenting with micromastia, either unilateral or bilateral, is the ideal candidate for mammary augmentation. The other important group of patients involves those with postpartum involution of breasts that were adequate prior to pregnancy. Drastic weight reduction also takes its toll on the breast. Ptosis, either idiopathic or postpartum, should be carefully evaluated. If the nipple is 1 cm. or more below the inframammary crease, augmentation will only accentuate the ptotic condition, yielding a highly unaesthetic result. Under these circumstances, mastopexy combined with augmentation should be considered. Postsurgical deformity can frequently be corrected by breast augmentation, either unilateral or bilateral, utilizing different size prostheses. Psychological indications are as important as any obvious physical deficiency of breast tissue. Not infrequently, the surgeon will examine a patient in whom he feels the breast mass is adequate by any normal standard. However, the patient has feelings of inferiority and inadequacy since in her own body image she sees herself as having deficient breast mass. This patient should be evaluated very carefully by the surgeon. If her motivation and psychological condition appear normal, surgery is indicated; however, if any doubts exist in the surgeon's mind, she should be referred for psychiatric counseling prior to undertaking the surgery. The final group of patients who are frequently overlooked are those seeking larger breasts for economic motives – i.e., professional dancers or entertainers who want to attain large breasts to enhance their desirability for jobs that may afford increased incomes. Their needs are as real as those of a woman with severe micromastia who wants only to "look better in my clothing," and should not be disregarded by the surgeon.

Preoperative Evaluation
A routine history is taken. The patient should be asked about previous pregnancies, breast feeding, and breast pathology; a family history of breast cancer should be inquired about, and she should be asked whether she takes any hormones, including birth control pills. The motivation for surgery is discussed in detail. The patient is asked why she wants to have her breasts made larger. The patient who responds "I feel inferior and inadequate due to my small breast size," or "I want to look better in my clothing" should have an excellent postoperative result both physically and psychologically. Another significant positive prognostic finding is seen in the woman who has experienced pleasurable feelings associated with breast enlargement during a previous pregnancy. If she was unhappy with the breast enlargement of pregnancy, she will also be dissatisfied with the enlargement produced by augmentation. The patient who desires increased breast size because of a marital problem (for example, a straying husband) or because the husband desires her to have larger breasts should be considered a poor candidate for surgery; she should instead be referred for psychiatric and/or marital counseling.

The expectations of the patient are then questioned. It is important to listen to the patient; if the surgeon can create the breasts that the patient desires, the unhappy postoperative patient will be avoided. An attempt should be made in every case to provide the patient with a breast size that she desires and that will fit her basic anatomy.

Physical examination of the breasts is then carefully performed, and any questionable masses are evaluated with preoperative xerograms and/or consultation with a general surgeon when indicated. Any breast size or chest wall discrepancies that will cause the breasts to attain a different appearance postoperatively are pointed out to the patient. She is warned that the surgeon can only work around her anatomical framework. This will eliminate the unhappy postoperative patient who may have been unaware of these preoperative findings. Photographs are taken of all patients.

There should be a detailed discussion of the possible complications, including hematoma; infection; wide scars; loss of sensation over the skin and/or nipple areolar complex (which could be permanent); and capsular contracture, resulting in firmness of the breast. Special consent forms, listing each of the complications, are signed and witnessed in the office. The patient takes a copy of this consent home with her.

Despite our efforts to fully inform each patient of all the ordinary risks of her surgery, most of them demonstrated marked repression and denial of any serious complications; they could not recall these risks. This denial mechanism may be responsible for some of the unfounded legal suits that are occasionally instituted after aesthetic surgical procedures [6].

If the patient raises any question regarding sensory loss of the nipple, the surgeon should stress that there is no guarantee that sensation will be retained; if nipple sensation is important to her sexual satisfaction, she must consider the operation carefully. It is much better to have a patient leave the office disappointed before an operation than to have her leave the office in search of an attorney after the operation, stating that "If I had known I would have a numb nipple, I never would have had the operation!"

Preoperative Preparation
The procedure may be performed under general or local anesthesia, as a hospital or office procedure. Because of rising costs of hospitalization (an aesthetic procedure is unlikely to be covered by insurance), and because safe, simplified surgical techniques are available, more and more breast augmentations are being performed as office procedures.

An angiocath is inserted in an antecubital vein and 10 to 30 mg. of diazepam (Valium) is injected slowly just prior to the injection of local anesthesia into the breast. The angiocath is then rinsed with sterile saline, administered through a disposable 10-ml. syringe; several milliliters of the solution are left in the angiocath with the syringe attached to facilitate later administration of intravenous medication if that becomes necessary.

SURGICAL PROCEDURE

The three basic surgical approaches are the inframammary, periareolar, and transaxillary (Fig. 44-1). Another less common technique transects the nipple and areolar from three o'clock to nine o'clock transversely, as advocated by Pitanguy [56] and Cronin [15].

Inframammary Technique
The most common surgical approach for breast aug-

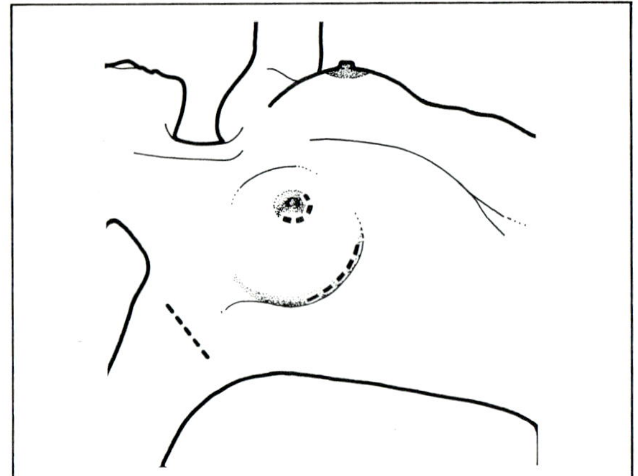

Fig. 44-1. Broken lines illustrate the three standard approaches to breast augmentation – the inframammary, periareolar, and transaxillary techniques.

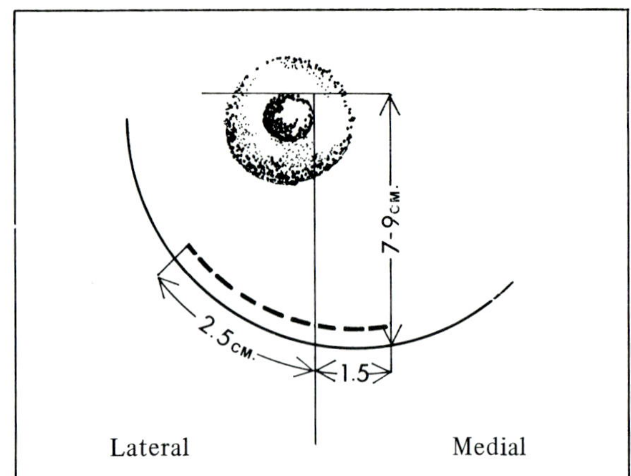

Fig. 44-2. The location of the incision for the inframammary approach. The curvilinear incision is placed 7 to 9 cm. from the top of the nipple.

mentation utilizes a 3- to 4-cm. incision placed approximately 1 cm. above the inframammary crease [30]. This allows easy access and excellent exposure in the field of dissection, as well as simple reentry into the retromammary space in the event that reexploration operation is necessary for drainage of hematoma or surgical capsulotomy. It is the procecure that I prefer and utilize almost exclusively.

This approach is initiated with the patient lying in the supine position with the arms extended. As in all procedures, the chest wall is prepared with alcohol.

A vertical line is drawn with gentian violet from the medial aspect of the nipple inferiorly, crossing the inframammary crease. Beginning 1.5 cm. medial to this reference line, a curvilinear line is drawn 3 to 4 cm. in length and placed 6 to 9 cm. below the top of the nipple, depending on implant size (Fig. 44-2).

Intravenous Valium 10 to 30 mg. is slowly administered for its amnesic effect. Infiltration anesthesia utilizing lidocaine 0.5% with epinephrine 1:200,000 is administered through a 20 gauge spinal needle. This solution is injected into the tissue plane between pectoralis fascia and posterior capsule of the breast, covering the area necessary for dissection. The large gauge needle is preferred, since a finer gauge needle could accidentally deflect upon striking a bony prominence, producing a pneumothorax. Also for prevention of pneumothorax, great care is taken to keep the needle at right angles to the ribs during the injection phase (Fig. 44-3). Disposable paper drapes are utilized for the office procedures.

The opening incision is made with a #15 blade, and a 2-cm. percutaneous flap is developed inferiorly down to the pectoralis fascia. At this point the dissection turns cephalad (Fig. 44-4). Care is taken to stay

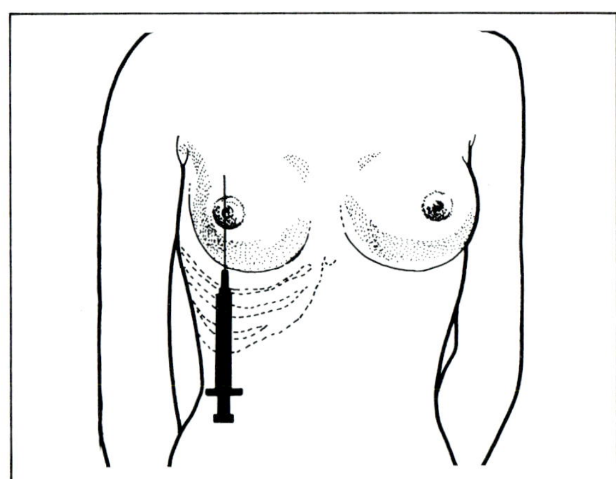

Fig. 44-3. For infiltrative anesthesia the needle should be inserted at a right angle to the ribs to avoid accidental penetration of the intercostal space, which could result in pneumothorax.

in the correct plane between pectoralis fascia and posterior capsule of the breast. Sharp dissection is utilized for several centimeters; once the proper plane has been identified, the finger is inserted and the breast capsule freed from the pectoralis fascia by blunt dissection. The pocket is developed – a large pocket is dissected to accommodate the implant. I feel that adequate space is necessary to allow the implant to glide, which will help produce a "bursal" type space and allow for some degree of capsular contraction without encroaching on the implant. Care is taken to avoid the dissection being carried too far laterally, which can produce numbness of the

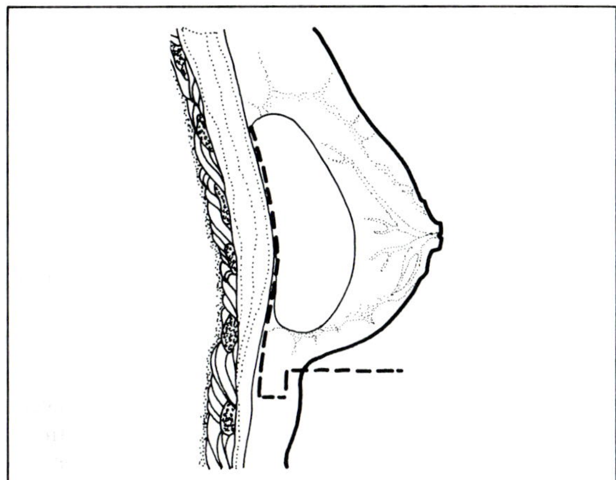

Fig. 44-4. In the inframammary approach a subcutaneous flap is developed prior to beginning the retromammary dissection.

nipple due to intercostal nerve damage in this area [13]. Meticulous hemostasis is mandatory; it can be accomplished in most cases by electrocoagulation. If major arteries are injured, they are suture ligated. Sterile saline is utilized to irrigate the cavity; after a final check for hemostasis, 40 mg. of triamcinolone in 3 ml. of saline is instilled into the cavity. If the patient is not allergic to penicillin, 0.5 gm. of cephalothin (Keflin Neutral) in 3 ml. of diluent is also instilled. The solutions are dispersed throughout the cavity to avoid pooling of the steroid which could result in localized atrophy. With the aid of a small Dever retractor, the implant is inserted. A subcutaneous flap is reapproximated with 3-0 Surgilon (this has avoided ptosis of the prosthesis, which was noted in 1 percent of the patients when absorbable suture was utilized for this retaining flap). The skin incision is closed with a running 5-0 Vicryl subcuticular suture. No external sutures are required and Steri-Strips are utilized to reinforce the wound. These are left in place for 2 weeks postoperatively. A brassiere one cup size larger than that normally worn is utilized as a final dressing. The patient is discharged following the surgery.

Periareolar Approach

The periareolar approach is the second most common technique utilized for breast augmentation.

With the patient lying supine on the operating table with arms abducted at 90 degrees or at the patient's side, the incision lines are drawn circumferentially just inside the areolar border from three o'clock to the nine o'clock position. Valium is administered intravenously and local infiltration anesthesia accomplished in the same manner as described for the inframammary approach; however, the areolar skin is infiltrated with a 27 gauge short needle with 1% lidocaine with epinephrine 1:100,000. The subcutaneous and breast tissue that will be involved in the plane of dissection is also infiltrated with the spinal needle. Care must be taken to avoid penetration of the thoracic cavity with the needle. With this surgical approach, two planes of dissection can be utilized. The approach I use, which avoids violation of the mammary gland, is a subcutaneous dissection to the inferior border of the breast, where the dissection turns cephalad and the retromammary space is enlarged for the prosthesis. A fiberoptic retractor greatly aids in visualization of the cavity.

After hemostasis has been accomplished, the cavity is irrigated with saline; triamcinolone and an antibiotic solution (when not contraindicated by allergy) are instilled. A small Dever or 2 Army-Navy retractors are utilized to aid in insertion of the desired prosthesis. Care is taken to suture the inferior border of the breast to the pectoralis fascia with nonabsorbable suture to prevent the implant from slipping and to ensure that it remains in the retromammary space. If this is not done, implant migration into the subcutaneous space anterior to the breast can occur. The periareolar incision is closed with subcuticular inverted 6-0 Vicryl sutures and Steri-Strips are applied. No external sutures are utilized. A piece of Telfa is placed over the incision, and the brassiere is utilized as a final dressing.

In the other periareolar approach, the incision is carried straight down through the breast (Fig. 44-5). Bleeders are suture ligated and/or coagulated. The full extent of the incision is utilized and a skin hook is placed at the angle of each skin edge to allow better visualization of the dissection. After the pectoralis fascis has been identified, the pocket is developed superiorly and inferiorly from this point to the necessary dimensions. After complete hemostasis, the cavity is irrigated and the steroid and antibiotic solutions indicated are instilled. Insertion of the prosthesis is aided by the retractors. The breast tissue is reapproximated with interrupted 3-0 Dexon sutures on a cutting needle. Skin incisions are closed as noted above.

The disadvantage of this technique is that it transects the ductal systems to the lower portion of the gland and produces scarring within the breast; this scarring may later be difficult to distinguish from a possible tumor. However, many surgeons utilize this technique and do not find this a disadvantage.

In my experience, when the periareolar approach has been utilized, there is a greater incidence of sensory loss to the lower portion of the nipple-areolar complex than when other techniques are utilized.

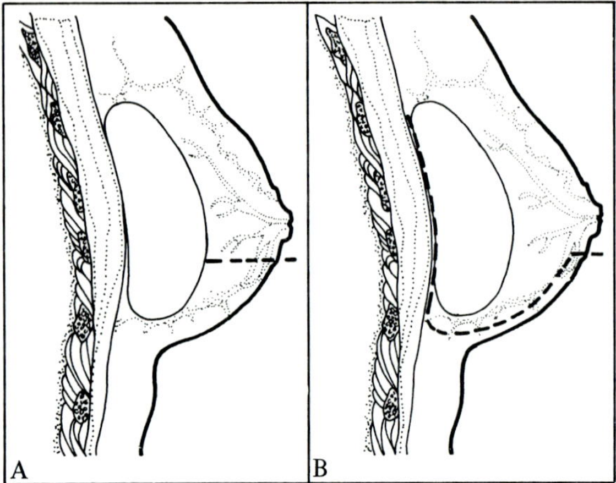

Fig. 44-5. A, the more common periareolar approach cleaves the gland. B, when using the periareolar approach it is possible to avoid cleaving the gland by means of subcutaneous dissection.

Although this is usually temporary, it can frequently be of concern to the patient.

Transaxillary Approach

The patient is placed on the operating table in a semi-sitting position with arms and forearms abducted at right angles. The incision is marked in the hair-bearing portion of the axilla, 4 cm. in length, either vertically or obliquely. While the vertical incision provides easier exposure to the pectoralis, the oblique incision placed in a natural crease imparts a more pleasant cosmetic result.

After intravenous administration of Valium, infiltration anesthesia is accomplished with a 27 gauge needle and 1% lidocaine with epinephrine 1:100,000 in the axillary skin up to the border of the pectoralis muscle. The remaining infiltration anesthesia is accomplished with 0.5% lidocaine and epinephrine 1:200,000 as previously described for the inframammary approach.

The incision is made with a #15 blade and carried down to the subcutaneous tissue. The incision is pulled superiorly with a double hook. With the vertical incision, the rim of the muscle is easily identified; utilizing sharp dissection, a short tunnel is made over the superior portion of the pectoralis major and the dissection plane is visualized. This is to ensure that the remaining blunt dissection is superficial to the muscle. If the surgeon is careful to keep the dissection above the rim of the pectoralis muscle at all times, there is no danger of injury to the axillary contents. The surgeon uses a finger to dissect a pocket over the upper pole of the breast to the lateral border of the sternum. This plane is easily developed, since the pectoralis fascia is thick at the upper half and the plane separates easily. As much dissection as possible is carried out with the finger. Further dissection is carried out utilizing a 4-cm. malleable retractor. Care is taken to ensure that the insertion of the retractor is over the rim of the muscle. Grasping the breast in the opposite hand, the surgeon pushes the retractor inferiorly to separate the lower pole of the gland from the chest wall. If any restrictive bands of tissue remain, a #32 Guyan urethral sound is inserted and the bands are broken. The cover of the sound is used to lift the breast up and aid in identification of the dimensions of the dissection. A sponge stick is helpful in completing the peripheral dissection deep in the pocket. The retromammary space is inspected to ascertain that there is no active bleeding. (Fortunately this almost never occurs in the transaxillary approach.) After the pocket is irrigated, the steroid and appropriate antibiotic solutions are instilled and the prosthesis is inserted and pushed inferiorly to help seat the implant in the lowest portion of the dissection. The incision is closed in a single layer of 5-0 Vicryl vertical mattress sutures. The axilla is sprayed with Neosporin aerosol, which is prescribed postoperatively as well. A brassiere is utilized as a final dressing.

The transaxillary approach was first described by Viñas [63] in 1962 and later by others [21, 32, 51]; it has the advantage of leaving no telltale scar on the breast. The incision, which is placed either vertically or obliquely in the hair-bearing portion of the axilla, provides difficulty from the standpoint of exposure and hemostasis. After having performed 138 transaxillary augmentations, I have discontinued the approach for two reasons. First, if capsular contracture occurs, the prosthesis will be pushed up and out, producing a severe deformity that necessitates surgical intervention for correction (Fig. 44-6). Second, reentry for surgical capsulotomy or hemostasis (in case of hematoma) is extremely difficult through the transaxillary incision; not infrequently an additional inframammary incision is necessary for correction of the problem. This then leaves the patient with three or four scars instead of two.

TYPES OF PROSTHESES

All breast prostheses utilized today are made of silicone rubber. There are three basic types: prostheses that are gel filled, inflatable, or filled with a combination of gel and saline. Most prostheses available in the United States are manufactured by Cox-Uphoff, Dow Corning Corporation, Heyer Schulte, McGhan Medical Corporation, Roger Kline Ltd., and Surgitek (Medical Engineering Corporation). There are a wide variety of sizes and shapes to meet the needs of the individual patient. The gel implants come in contour, round, low profile, and underfill varieties, as well as

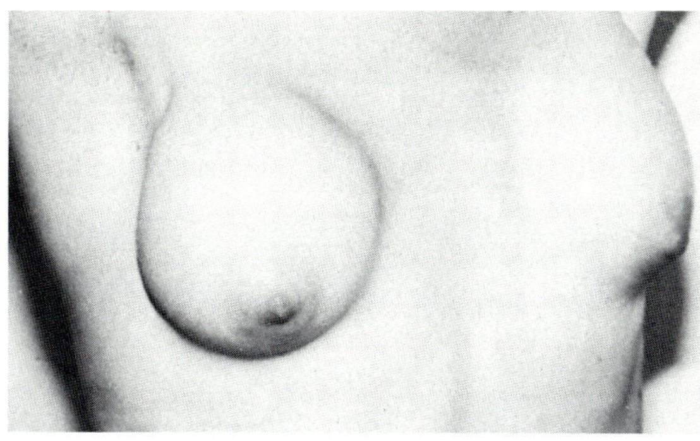

Fig. 44-6. Elevation and distortion of both breast implants caused by capsular contracture following augmentation mammoplasty by the transaxillary technique.

in various shapes named after the surgeons who developed them. The inflatable prostheses are either a contour design or round. The various valve mechanisms of the inflatable prostheses have positions that involve filling and sealing from the side, anterior surface, or posterior wall of the prosthesis. The newer combination prostheses have an inner core of gel with an outer ring of saline (or vice versa); these combine the advantages and/or disadvantages of both components. (See the appendix listing currently available implants at the end of this chapter.)

The implants are fixed to the chest wall by either Dacron patches or small silicone tabs that can be sutured into the pectoralis fascia.

Since surgeons will frequently defend the use of their favorite type of implant, it is futile to attempt to elucidate the merits of these at this time. It is enough to say that any of the inflatable implants are particularly useful to correct asymmetries of the breast, and they can be inserted through smaller incisions. Each surgeon must find the prosthesis that he considers best and that attains uniform results for him.

In a patient evaluation I undertook several years ago with three other surgeons (Bass, Greer, and Obi) [4], 59 volunteer patients in a double blind study underwent breast augmentation, with a random assignment by computer of the various types of prostheses. No differences regarding feel or appearance of the breast could be found in any of the patients who had an inflatable prosthesis on one side and a gel-filled prosthesis on the other. There was also no difference between the sides when patients had one contour and one round-shaped gel prosthesis. The capsular contracture rate was evaluated, and inflatable implants demonstrated a 10 percent lower incidence than gel prostheses. However, I have had a 6 percent deflation rate when inflatables were utilized (in most instances from faulty valves), necessitating reoperation. For this reason, I utilize gel prostheses in most cases; the inflatables or combination gel-inflatable implants are reserved for patients who request them and for those who have marked breast asymmetry. All these patients are warned that deflation is possible at some time in their life, and reoperation for correction would then be necessary.

POSTOPERATIVE ORDERS

Achievement of a problem-free healing period depends largely on the patient's thorough understanding and execution of the surgeon's postoperative orders. Since almost all breast augmentation is done as an outpatient procedure, there is severe limitation of the surgeon's control over the activity of the patient. It is necessary for the patient to be thoroughly familiarized with the modifications in routine and activity that should be observed postoperatively. Instructions are given to the patient on printed forms to avoid confusion.

Prevention of Infection

A broad-spectrum antibiotic, doxycycline hyclate (Vibramycin) 200 mg., is administered orally the day prior to surgery, followed by 100 mg. daily for 8 days postoperatively. If allergy exists, another broad-spectrum antibiotic is given in therapeutic doses. Vibramycin is preferred because it has a high degree of lipoid solubility (the area of dissection involves making a pocket in a mostly adipose environment), it is highly stable in normal human serum, it is active against a wide range of gram-positive and gram-negative organisms, and it needs to be administered only once a day. If infection occurs following augmentation, it almost always results in loss of the prosthesis, causing added expense and inconvenience (not to mention the psychological effect of having a long-desired breast removed, even if only temporarily). Subclinical infection may also play a role in the formation of early capsular contracture.

Home Care

The patient is instructed to go directly to bed upon arrival at her destination, and to take the prescribed pain medication at that time, even if no discomfort is being experienced. Two pillows cushioned behind the upper portion of the back will place the patient in a desirable semireclining position. Aspirin and aspirin-containing compounds (because of their anticoagulant effect) should be avoided beginning 2 weeks prior to operation.

Since hematoma is most common in the first 48 hours following surgery, the patient is directed to rest; she should limit the use of the arms to only routine acts such as eating, brushing teeth, and combing hair.

She should strictly avoid vigorous arm motion and using the arms to push or pull. The elastic brassiere secured following surgery should not be removed.

Provided that no narcotics are being taken, the patient may resume driving her car on the third or fourth day following surgery. She is seen in the surgeon's office on the fourth postoperative day. During this office visit, the patient is instructed in proper massage technique, which allows for movement of the implant in the pocket and helps create a bursal effect. The breast is massaged in a rotary fashion, squeezing and flattening it with the hand (Fig. 44-7). As the breast loses postoperative tenderness, the massage should become more vigorous. The regimen should be executed as often as possible in the immediate postoperative period, and at least daily thereafter. The patient may begin showering at this point and may sleep in the prone position the following week. The Steri-Strips applied at the completion of surgery are left intact, and the patient is instructed to remove them 2 weeks later. She is also instructed to wear a brassiere night and day, but she may sleep without it after 3 days. The second week she may go braless if she wishes; however, she is cautioned that this may encourage later ptosis of the breast. Unlimited physical activity may resume 20 days postoperatively. A summary of instructions about postoperative care follows:

Immediate postoperative care:
1. Immediate mobilization is encouraged.
2. A regular brassiere is used as the final dressing.

Three days postoperatively:
1. The patient should massage her breasts twice daily for several minutes.
2. The patient may sleep without a brassiere.
3. The patient may drive an automobile.

Ten days postoperatively:
1. The patient may go braless.

Twenty days postoperatively:
1. The patient may resume unrestricted physical activity.

The patient is reexamined by the surgeon at the third, sixth, and twelfth months postoperatively. The breasts are examined annually thereafter. To encourage the patient to return for breast evaluation by the surgeon, all follow-up care is performed without additional charge.

POSTOPERATIVE COMPLICATIONS

Early Complications

Although capsular contracture is the most common complication following breast augmentation, it is not usually seen in the immediate postoperative period.

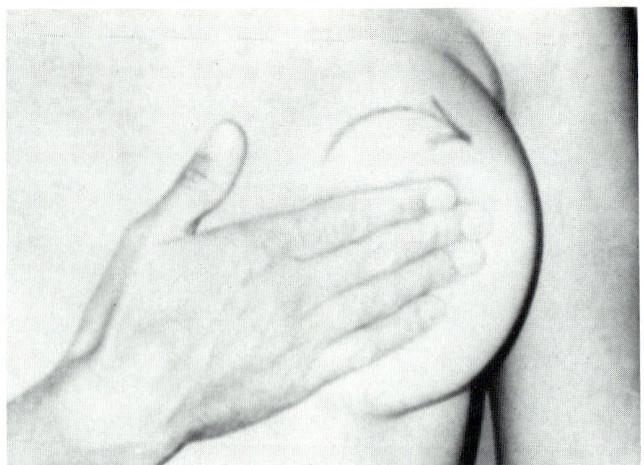

Fig. 44-7. The arrow shows the direction of rotary motion of the breast in the recommended technique of postoperative daily massage.

The most common complications encountered in this period are anesthesia/paresthesia of the nipple, hematoma, infection, wound dehiscence, ptosis of the prosthesis, leakage (of inflatable implants), and Mondor's disease (phlebitis of superficial epigastric vein).

Statistical analysis was performed on 1,282 patients who underwent augmentation as an office outpatient procedure under local anesthesia. The findings are listed in Table 44-1.

CHANGES IN BREAST OR NIPPLE SENSATION. Approximately 15 percent of these patients reported postoperative changes in breast or nipple sensation [13]. Anesthesia can occur in an area of breast skin, in the nipple, or in the areolar complex. Although this condition usually exists temporarily (6 months to 2 years postoperatively), it can be permanent. Therefore all

Table 44-1. Postoperative Complications in 1,282 Breast Augmentations

Complication	Incidence (percent)
Capsular contracture	27
Alteration in nipple sensation	15
Leakage of inflatable prosthesis	6
Hematoma formation	2
Wound separation (suture reaction)	1.5
Ptosis of prosthesis	1
Mondor's disease	1[a]
Infection	0
Implant erosion	0

[a]Approximate.

patients should be made aware of this possibility prior to surgery. Paresthesia, a much more common condition, usually disappears by the sixth postoperative month.

HEMATOMAS. Most hematomas will occur within the first 24 hours. The patient should be warned preoperatively that any undue swelling of the breasts or unusual discomfort, especially on one side, should be reported to her surgeon immediately for evaluation. I believe that all hematomas should be evacuated as soon as possible after diagnosis. This can be performed under local anesthesia in the office. Hematomas permitted to resorb can not only cause severe capsular contracture, but also impose upon the patient possible weeks of discomfort and asymmetry.

INFECTION. If overt infection with contamination of the prosthesis occurs, the implant should be removed, culture of the wound taken, and appropriate antibiotic therapy begun. It is usually preferable to wait a minimum of 3 to 4 months before attempting reinsertion of the prosthesis.

WOUND SEPARATION. This is usually due to suture reaction; as long as there is no exposure of the implant, the separation can usually be resutured successfully.

PTOSIS OF THE PROSTHESIS. This problem is more common when inflatable implants are utilized (since saline solutions are heavier than the silicone gel); it can be due to loosening of the flap, more commonly noted when resorbable suture is used or when there is atrophy of the subcutaneous flap from steroid pooling. The ptosis can usually be corrected simply by opening the incision and reapproximating the remaining subcutaneous flap to the pectoralis fascia with nonabsorbable suture.

LEAKAGE OF THE PROSTHESIS. The leakage can be a slow process with gradual diminution in the volume of the augmented breast or rapid deflation. Most frequently, a faulty valve mechanism will be the cause. As soon as it is diagnosed, the implant should be replaced. The faulty prosthesis should be returned to the manufacturer for evaluation.

MONDOR'S DISEASE. This is an idiopathic phlebitis affecting the large subcutaneous veins normally crossing the lateral chest region and breast from the epigastric or hypochondriac region. It appears as a tender band usually beginning at the inframammary crease and is a benign, self-limiting condition that requires no specific therapy. The patient should be assured that the disease is of no consequence.

EROSION OF THE PROSTHESIS. Erosion of the implant through the skin is extremely rare in breast augmentation. It could occur from a pressure point on the breast as a result of capsular contracture that produced undue tension on the skin surface. This could result in ulceration with eventual slough of the overlying skin and subsequent loss of the prosthesis. When this occurs, the prosthesis must be removed and the area allowed to heal before the implant can be reinserted.

Capsular Contracture

Excessive firmness of the breast is the most common complication of breast augmentation [2, 3, 24, 29, 61, 65, 67]. Statistical analysis has shown that it occurred to some degree in 27 percent of my cases. (Some authors have reported contractures in up to 40 percent of their cases.) I utilize the following grading system for follow-up of all patients:

Grade I. Absolutely natural – no one could tell that the breast was augmented.
Grade II. Minimal – I can tell that surgery was performed, but the patient has no complaint.
Grade III. Moderate – the patient feels some firmness.
Grade IV. Severe – the implant is obvious just from observation.

Excessive firmness is usually noted in the first 6 months following surgery (Table 44-2). It can occur either bilaterally or unilaterally at any time, even years following surgery. The firmness usually results from contracture of the fibrous capsule; as the capsule contracts, there is a decrease in the ratio of its surface area to the volume it contains, producing an increase in pressure within the capsule. In accordance with Archimedes' theory, this produces a more spherical configuration of the prosthesis because the sphere is the geometric shape that has the least surface area for a given volume [24]. The firmness and distorted shape of the resulting spherical breast cause discomfort and often embarrassment to the patient [31].

Table 44-2. Onset of Capsular Contracture in 1,282 Breast Augmentations

Time of Onset	Number of Cases	Percentage of Contracture Cases
0– 6 months	215	62
6–12 months	104	30
More than 12 months	28	8
Total	347	100

Etiology
Although the exact cause of capsular contracture remains obscure, the basic problem of scar contracture appears to be the most likely culprit [50]. Various causative factors have been implicated, including hematoma, seroma, the type of implant utilized, impurities in the silicone rubber, fiberogenic drugs applied locally, and overt or subclinical local infection [24, 29, 35, 36]. Although the medical literature provides little information as to what agents in silicone implants may cause problems, I feel this area holds the key that will someday open the door to the control of capsular contracture. These agents that are suspect include surface contaminants, unreacted monomers, catalyst residues, silica filler, or impurities not yet identified [60].

Prophylaxis
Various methods have been advocated to prevent capsular contracture [10, 29, 59, 67]. Steroids can be placed either in the pocket, or in an inflatable prosthesis, or both. In the case of inflatable or combination gel-inflatable prostheses, methylprednisolone (Solu-Medrol) has been advocated [52]. Inflatable implants, massage, pressure bandages, replacement with a smaller prosthesis, long immobilization, and early mobilization all have believers and nonbelievers.

I now utilize steroids (40 mg. triamcinolone) in all cases. In a study I conducted in 1974 on 122 patients who received soft-gel implants, various amounts of different steroids were instilled at the time of surgery in 60 patients, both unilaterally and bilaterally in random selection; 62 patients received no steroids and acted as controls. The breasts that were treated with 40 mg. triamcinolone at the time of surgery had a 10 percent lower incidence of capsular contracture than occurred in the control group [2]. That dosage of triamcinolone was found to be safe and most effective.

Although these measures may reduce the incidence of contracture, they are far from infallible. Capsular contracture will not be controlled until we learn how to control scar contracture or the etiological factors that produce it.

Treatment
When capsular contracture has occurred and treatment is indicated, the techniques that have been utilized include steroid injections into the fibrous tissue surrounding the prosthesis; closed "squeeze" capsulotomy; and open surgical capsulotomy with or without capsulectomy, either total or subtotal. Any of the surgical procedures may be combined with exchange of the prosthesis with a new unit of the same type, replacement of the same undamaged unit, replacement with a smaller implant, or changing from a gel prosthesis to an inflatable or a combination implant.

STEROID INJECTION. This technique has been partially successful in only a minority of cases [66]. Steroid solution (usually triamcinolone 40 to 80 mg. diluted to 10 ml. with saline) is injected percutaneously with a 22 gauge spinal needle into the fibrous tissues surrounding the prosthesis. The patient is instructed to massage the breast frequently after the injection. While improvement can occur in a number of patients, complications can be frequent and severe.

In my own experience, 130 breasts with contracture were treated in this way. Approximately 35 percent experienced some softening within 3 weeks. Others were injected at 3- to 6-week intervals for a maximum of three series of injections. During the 9 months following injection, many complications were observed. Tissue atrophy with unsightly depressions, telangiectasia, and depigmentation was not uncommon. Several patients presented with severe atrophy of overlying breast and subcutaneous tissue in the area of what was thought to be a blue dome cyst; in fact it was the prosthesis seen through a thin dermal covering. This evidence of pending prosthesis erosion was corrected by immediate surgical intervention, with surgical capsulotomy and rotation of capsular flaps to reinforce the defect from within. Because of the complications arising from percutaneous steroid injection and because there was minimal improvement in the condition, I have discontinued this treatment for the problem of capsular contracture [1].

NONSURGICAL "SQUEEZE" CAPSULOTOMY. Closed nonsurgical "squeeze" compression of the breast has been found to be highly successful and is associated with a small complication rate [3, 64]. The technique may be employed as soon as firmness is noted in the augmented breast. With the patient lying supine, arms at her sides, the breast is grasped at its base with both hands and circumferential compression is administered until a popping noise is heard and softening of the breast is felt (Fig. 44-8). The hands are turned 90 degrees and another squeeze is applied to complete the capsular tear. Flat compression of the breast with the palm of the hand, in a circular motion, completes the procedure. The patient is instructed to massage the breast vigorously and frequently for several weeks and several times a day thereafter.

In over 400 squeeze capsulotomies [5], we have observed a recurrence rate of 30 percent. As in all procedures, complications can occur. Soreness and bruising are not uncommon for several days after the squeeze capsulotomy. Hematomas that required surgical evacuation were encountered in 2 percent of the

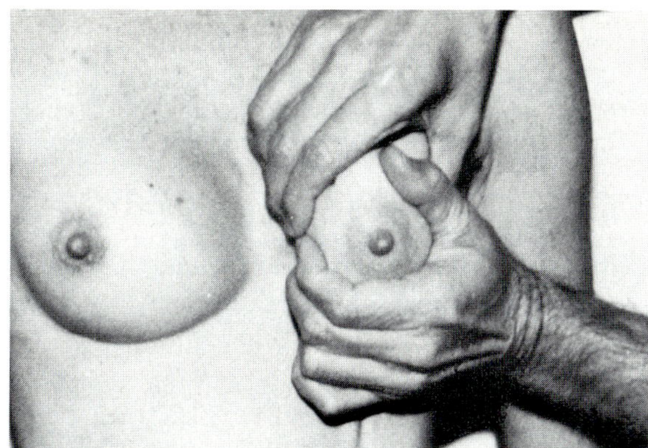

Fig. 44-8. The technique of grasping the breast in the "squeeze" capsulotomy.

breasts treated by this technique. Some cases did not respond or had incomplete tears in the capsular wall, resulting in bizarre shapes that required surgical capsulotomy. Damage of the prosthesis has also been reported [22, 23]. The procedure has been repeated in all cases of recurrence.

Ninety percent of these procedures are performed without sedation or analgesia; however, 10 mg. of intravenous Valium is utilized for patients exhibiting apprehension or discomfort. Before the procedure, the possible complications are discussed; the ingestion of aspirin is prohibited for 72 hours before and after the procedure. Surgical capsulotomy is recommended in patients with recurring firmness after five squeeze procedures.

SURGICAL CAPSULOTOMY. Surgical capsulotomy is usually performed under local anesthesia, as an outpatient procedure. The incision is reentered. If the transaxillary method was utilized during augmentation, an inframammary incision is now required. After dissection of the subcutaneous flap, by cold knife, the capsular wall is approached. An electrosurgical knife is utilized to split the capsule. (Fortunately, this electrocautery will not perforate the silicone membrane when it comes in light contact with the prosthesis.) The implant is removed. The capsule is incised at its base 360 degrees with the electrosurgical knife, and the pocket is expanded to large proportions by sharp and blunt dissection [1, 2, 15, 24, 68]. If the capsule is very thick, either subtotal or total capsulectomy is performed. Steroids and antibiotics (when indicated) are instilled, and the original or a new prosthesis is inserted. The wound is closed in layers and the same postoperative regimen is followed as in primary breast augmentation.

REFERENCES

1. Baker, J. L., Jr. Techniques and complications of augmentation mammaplasty; 4 year survey. Presented at the Symposium on Plastic Surgery of the Breast, Scottsdale, Arizona, November 1975.
2. Baker, J. L., Jr. Augmentation Mammoplasty. In Owsley, J. Q., Jr., and Peterson, R. A. (Eds.), *Symposium on Aesthetic Surgery of the Breast.* St. Louis: Mosby, 1978.
3. Baker, J. L., Jr., Bartels, R. J., and Douglas, W. M. Closed compression technique for rupturing a contracted capsule around a breast implant. *Plast. Reconstr. Surg.* 58:137, 1976.
4. Baker, J. L., Jr., Bass, C. B., Obi, L. J., and Greer, D. M. Evaluation of various breast prostheses. Presented at the American Society of Plastic and Reconstructive Surgery meeting, Toronto, Canada, 1975.
5. Baker, J. L., Jr., Douglas, W. M., and Bartels, R. J. Personal series, 1977.
6. Baker, J. L., Jr., Kolin, I. S., and Bartlett, E. S. Psychosexual dynamics of patients undergoing mammary augmentation. *Plast. Reconstr. Surg.* 53:652, 1974.
7. Bames, H. Augmentation mammaplasty by lipotransplant. *Plast. Reconstr. Surg.* 11:404, 1953.
8. Berson, M. I. Derma-fat-fascia transplant used in building up the breasts. *Surgery* 15:451, 1944.
9. Blumbert, J. B., Griffith, P. C., and Merendino, K. A. The effect of specific compression on soft-tissue response to foralinized polyvinyl alcohol (Ivalon) sponge. *Ann. Surg.* 151:409, 1960.
10. Broadbent, T. R., and Woolf, R. M. Augmentation mammaplasty. *Plast. Reconstr. Surg.* 40:517, 1967.
11. Brown, J. B., Fryer, M. P., and Lu, M. Polyvinyl and silicone compounds as subcutaneous prostheses. *Arch. Surg.* 68:744, 1954.
12. Conway, H. Mammaplasty: Analysis of 110 consecutive cases with end results. *Plast. Reconstr. Surg.* 10:303, 1952.
13. Courtiss, E. H., and Goldwyn, R. M. Breast sensation before and after plastic surgery. *Plast. Reconstr. Surg.* 58:1, 1976.
14. Cronin, T. D., and Gerow, F. J. Augmentation mammaplasty; a new "natural feel" prosthesis. Transactions of the Third International Congress of Plastic Surgery. Amsterdam: Excerpta Medica, 1963.
15. Cronin, T. D., and Greenberg, R. L. Our experiences with the Silastic gel breast prosthesis. *Plast. Reconstr. Surg.* 46:1, 1970.
16. Czerny, V. Plasticher Ersatz der Brust drüse durch ein lipom. *Zentralbl. Chir.* 27:72, 1895.
17. Delage, C., Shane, J., and Johnson, F. Mammary

silicone granuloma. *Arch. Dermatol.* 108:104, 1973.

18. Dukes, C. E., and Mitchley, B. C. V. Polyvinyl sponge implants: Experimental and clinical observations. *Br. J. Plast. Surg.* 15:225, 1962.
19. Edgerton, M. T., and McClary, A. R. Augmentation mammaplasty. Psychiatric implications and surgical indications. *Plast. Reconstr. Surg.* 21:279, 1958.
20. Edgerton, M. T., Meyer, E., and Jacobson, W. E. Augmentation mammaplasty: II. Further surgical and psychiatric evaluation. *Plast. Reconstr. Surg.* 27:279, 1961.
21. Eiseman, G. Augmentation mammaplasty by the transaxillary approach. *Plast. Reconstr. Surg.* 54:229, 1973.
22. Eisenberg, H. V., and Bartels, R. J. Rupture of a silicone bag gel breast implant by closed compression capsulotomy. *Plast. Reconstr. Surg.* 59:6, 1977.
23. Feliberti, M. G., Arrillage, A., and Conon, G. A. Rupture of inflated breast implants in closed compression capsulotomy. *Plast. Reconstr. Surg.* 59:6, 1977.
24. Freeman, B. S. Successful treatment of some fibrous envelope contractures around breast implants. *Plast. Reconstr. Surg.* 50:107, 1972.
25. Gerow, F. J. Breast implants. In Georgiade, N. (Ed.), *Reconstructive Breast Surgery.* St. Louis: Mosby, 1976. Chap. 3.
26. Gersuny, R. Ueber eine subcutane Prosthese. *Z. Heilkde.* 21:199, 1900.
27. Gersuny, R. Harte und weiche Paraffinprosthesen. *Zentralbl. Chir.* 30:1, 1903.
28. Giacomelli, M. Substitutive prosthesis by means of polystan sponge following mastectomy. *Minerva Chir.* 9:584, 1963.
29. Grossman, A. R. The current status of augmentation mammaplasty. *Plast. Reconstr. Surg.* 52:1, 1973.
30. Grossman, A. R. *Augmentation Mammaplasty.* Springfield, Ill.: Thomas, 1976.
31. Gurdin, M., and Carlin, G. A. Complications of breast implantations. *Plast. Reconstr. Surg.* 40:530, 1967.
32. Hoehler, H. Breast augmentation: The axillary approach, *Br. J. Plast. Surg.* 26:373, 1973.
33. Hollander. Abstract from Berliner Gesellschaft fur Chirurgie (Eigener Bericht), Sitzung von 9 December, 1912. *Munch. Med. Wochenschr.* 59:2842, 1912.
34. Hoopes, J. E., and Knorr, N. J. Psychology of the Flat-Chested Woman. In Masters, F. W., and Lewis, J. R. (Eds.), *Symposium on Aesthetic Surgery of the Face, Eyelid and Breast,* Vol. 5. St. Louis: Mosby, 1972. Chap. 22.
35. Imber, G. Fibrous capsule formation after subcutaneous implantation of synthetic materials in experimental animals. *Plast. Reconstr. Surg.* 54:183, 1974.
36. Johnson, H. A. Silastic breast implants: Coping with complications. *Plast. Reconstr. Surg.* 44:588, 1969.
37. Kay, B. D. Micromastia vs. macromastia. *Med. Aspects Hum. Sex.* 7: 1973.
38. Kolle, F. *Plastic and Cosmetic Surgery.* New York: Appleton, 1911.
39. Letterman, G., and Schurter, M. A. Personal communication, 1977.
40. Lexer, E. 20 Hahre Transplantations for chung. *Munch. Med. Wochenschr.* 72:830, 1925.
41. Longacre, J. Correction of the hypoplastic breast with special reference to reconstruction of the "nipple type breast" with local dermo-fat pedicle flaps. *Plast. Reconstr. Surg.* 14:431, 1954.
42. Longacre, J. Surgical reconstruction of the flat discoid breast. *Plast. Reconstr. Surg.* 17:358, 1956.
43. Maliniac, J. W. A mammaplastic substitute for amputation in hypertrophy. *Surgery* 26:573, 1949.
44. Maliniac, J. W. *Breast Deformities and Their Repair.* Baltimore: Waverly Press, 1950.
45. Maliniac, J. W. Use of pedicle dermo-fat flap in mammaplasty. *Plast. Reconstr. Surg.* 12:110, 1953.
46. Morris, D. *The Naked Ape.* New York: McGraw-Hill, 1968.
47. Ohmori, S. Personal communication, 1978.
48. Pangman, W. J., II. Experiences with the use of Ivalon sponge in breast and soft tissue augmentation. Presented at the Annual Meeting of the California Society of Plastic Surgeons, Carmel, Calif., April 1953.
49. Pangman, W. J., II, and Wallace, R. The use of a plastic prosthesis in breast plastic and other soft tissue surgery. *West J. Surg. Obstet. Gynecol.* 63:503, 1955.
50. Peacock, E. E., Jr., and Van Winkle, W. *Biology of Wound Repair.* Philadelphia: Saunders, 1970.
51. Penn, J. Personal correspondence, 1973.
52. Perrin, E. R. The use of soluble steroids within inflatable breast prostheses. *Plast. Reconstr. Surg.* 52:163. February 1979.
53. Peters, S. Personal communication, 1977.
54. Peterson, R. A. Directions in plastic surgery. *PRS Newsletter,* May 1977.
55. Pickrell, D. An Evaluation of Etheron as an Augmentation Material in Plastic and Reconstructive Surgery; A Long-Term Clinical and Experimental Study. Presented at annual meeting of American Society of Plastic and Reconstructive Surgeons, Hawaii, October 1962.

56. Pitanguy, I. Personal communication, 1977.
57. Rathjen, A. Personal communication, 1977.
58. Rees, T. D. Plastic Surgery of the Breast. In Converse, J. M. (Ed.), *Reconstruction and Plastic Surgery: Principles and Procedures in Correction, Reconstruction and Transplantation,* Vol. 5. Philadelphia: Saunders, 1964.
59. Rees, T. D., Guy, C. L., and Coburn, R. J. The use of inflatable breast implants. *Plast. Reconstr. Surg.* 52:609, 1973.
60. Sevinor, S. J. Personal communication, 1977.
61. Snyder, G. B. Augmentation Mammoplasty. In Grabb, W. C., and Smith, J. W., *Plastic Surgery, A Concise Guide to Clinical Practice* (2nd ed.), Boston: Little, Brown, 1973.
62. Thorek, M. *Plastic Surgery of the Breast and Abdominal Wall.* Springfield, Ill.: Thomas, 1942.
63. Viñas, Jose C. Surgical experience with silicone rubber implants; transaxillary approach to augmentation mammoplasty. *Quints Journadas Rioplantenses de Cirugia Plastica,* October 12, 1962.
64. Vinnik, C. A. Spherical contracture of fibrous capsules around breast implants. *Plast. Reconstr. Surg.* 58:555, 1976.
65. Weiner, D. L., Aiache, A. E., and Silver, L. A new soft round silicone gel breast implant. *Plast. Reconstr. Surg.* 53:174, 1974.
66. Wilkinson, T. S. Personal communication, 1976.
67. Williams, J. E. Experience with a large series of Silastic breast implants. *Plast. Reconstr. Surg.* 49:253, 1972.
68. Williams, J. E. Personal communication, 1976.

APPENDIX. AVAILABLE STYLES OF BREAST PROSTHESES MANUFACTURED IN THE UNITED STATES

Dow Corning Corp., Midland, MI 48640

Contour design Silastic mammary prosthesis, available in singles or pairs, sterile, with or without patches.

Volume	*Base Diameter*	*Projection*
120 cc.	7.3 cm.	3.7 cm.
145 cc.	8.5 cm.	3.4 cm.
175 cc.	8.5 cm.	3.4 cm.
200 cc.	9.7 cm.	3.6 cm.
225 cc.	9.7 cm.	3.6 cm.
250 cc.	9.7 cm.	4.7 cm.
310 cc.	11.3 cm.	4.4 cm.
350 cc.	11.3 cm.	4.6 cm.

Low-profile contour design Silastic mammary prosthesis, available in singles or pairs, sterile, with or without patches.

Volume	*Base Diameter*	*Projection*
150 cc.	9.4 cm.	2.3 cm.
175 cc.	10.0 cm.	2.5 cm.
200 cc.	10.5 cm.	2.6 cm.
225 cc.	11.3 cm.	2.7 cm.
250 cc.	11.6 cm.	2.8 cm.
275 cc.	11.8 cm.	2.9 cm.
300 cc.	11.8 cm.	3.2 cm.

Round design Silastic mammary prosthesis, available in singles or pairs, sterile, with or without patches.

Volume	*Base Diameter*	*Projection*
130 cc.	8.6 cm.	2.6 cm.
175 cc.	8.8 cm.	3.0 cm.
200 cc.	10.2 cm.	3.1 cm.
235 cc.	10.5 cm.	3.3 cm.
270 cc.	10.7 cm.	3.6 cm.
305 cc.	11.0 cm.	3.7 cm.
340 cc.	12.7 cm.	3.7 cm.

Low-profile round design Silastic mammary prosthesis, available in singles or pairs, sterile, with or without patches.

*Volume**	*Base Diameter*	*Projection*
165 cc.	11.3 cm.	2.4 cm.
200 cc.	12.0 cm.	2.5 cm.
235 cc.	12.7 cm.	2.7 cm.
270 cc.	13.3 cm.	2.8 cm.
305 cc.	13.8 cm.	2.9 cm.
340 cc.	14.3 cm.	3.0 cm.

Surgitek, Medical Engineering Corp., 3037 Mt. Pleasant, Racine, WI 53404

Round self-sealing inflatable mammary prosthesis, available in singles or pairs, sterile or unsterile, without patches, valve on apex, posterior, or side.

Volume	*Base Diameter*	*Projection*
100 cc.	7.6 cm.	3.7 cm.
150 cc.	8.6 cm.	3.8 cm.
200 cc.	10.8 cm.	4.2 cm.
250 cc.	11.5 cm.	4.3 cm.
300 cc.	12.1 cm.	4.4 cm.
400 cc.	13.3 cm.	4.5 cm.
550 cc.	14.8 cm.	5.0 cm.

Modified tear-drop self-sealing inflatable mammary prosthesis, available in singles or pairs, sterile or unsterile, without patches, valve on posterior or apex.

*New volumes now available: 130 cc., 180 cc., 220 cc.

Volume	*Base Diameter*	*Projection*
140 cc.	8.5 cm.	5.7 cm.
185 cc.	9.0 cm.	6.0 cm.
240 cc.	9.5 cm.	6.5 cm.
275 cc.	10.0 cm.	6.6 cm.
300 cc.	10.5 cm.	7.0 cm.
340 cc.	11.5 cm.	7.3 cm.

Gel-filled low-profile round mammary prosthesis, available in pairs or singles, sterile* or unsterile, without patches.

Volume	*Base Diameter*	*Projection*
70 cc.	8.0 cm.	–
90 cc.	8.5 cm.	–
110 cc.	9.5 cm.	2.2 cm.
130 cc.	10.0 cm.	2.3 cm.
150 cc.	10.5 cm.	2.3 cm.
170 cc.	11.0 cm.	2.3 cm.
190 cc.	11.5 cm.	2.3 cm.
205 cc.	12.0 cm.	2.3 cm.
220 cc.	12.2 cm.	2.4 cm.
235 cc.	12.5 cm.	2.4 cm.
255 cc.	13.0 cm.	2.4 cm.
285 cc.	13.5 cm.	2.5 cm.
300 cc.	13.7 cm.	2.5 cm.
320 cc.	14.0 cm.	2.6 cm.
340 cc.	14.5 cm.	2.6 cm.
365 cc.	15.0 cm.	2.7 cm.
400 cc.	15.3 cm.	2.7 cm.
440 cc.	15.6 cm.	2.8 cm.
485 cc.	16.0 cm.	2.9 cm.
600 cc.	18.0 cm.	3.2 cm.

Round inflatable mammary prosthesis, available in pairs or singles, sterile, with valve that can be placed on anterior or posterior varifil valve.

Volume	*Base Diameter*	*Projection*
110–150 cc.	9.7 cm.	2.3 cm.
140–180 cc.	10.3 cm.	2.4 cm.
160–200 cc.	10.9 cm.	2.5 cm.
180–220 cc.	11.5 cm.	2.6 cm.
210–250 cc.	12.0 cm.	2.7 cm.
230–290 cc.	12.4 cm.	2.8 cm.

G. B. Snyder implant (modified tear-drop gel-filled), available in singles or pairs, sterile† or unsterile, without patches.

Volume	*Base Diameter*	*Projection*
130 cc.	8.5 cm.	4.7 cm.
165 cc.	9.0 cm.	4.9 cm.
180 cc.	9.5 cm.	5.0 cm.
200 cc.	10.0 cm.	5.1 cm.
235 cc.	10.5 cm.	5.5 cm.
255 cc.	11.0 cm.	5.7 cm.
280 cc.	11.3 cm.	5.9 cm.
300 cc.	11.5 cm.	6.0 cm.
330 cc.	12.0 cm.	6.2 cm.
365 cc.	12.5 cm.	6.4 cm.
400 cc.	13.0 cm.	6.6 cm.
500 cc.	15.5 cm.	7.2 cm.

*Round implants are available in sterile pack in standard sizes of 365 cc. or less.
†Sterile packs available in standard sizes of 365 cc. or less.

Low-profile gel-filled oval implants, available in singles or pairs, sterile or unsterile, without patches.

Volume	*Base Diameter*	*Projection*
150 cc.	9.5 cm.	3.3 cm.
180 cc.	10.0 cm.	3.5 cm.
210 cc.	10.3 cm.	3.6 cm.
225 cc.	10.6 cm.	3.7 cm.
245 cc.	10.8 cm.	3.7 cm.
265 cc.	11.0 cm.	3.8 cm.
310 cc.	11.8 cm.	4.0 cm.

Oval gel-filled mammary implants, available in singles or pairs, unsterile only, without patches.

Volume	*Base Diameter*	*Projection*
200 cc.	10.2 cm.	4.5 cm.
215 cc.	10.4 cm.	4.6 cm.
235 cc.	10.5 cm.	4.8 cm.
255 cc.	10.7 cm.	5.0 cm.

Georgiade prosthesis contour gel-filled, available in singles or pairs, unsterile only, with or without patches.

Volume	*Base Diameter*	*Projection*
100 cc.	8.0 cm.	4.5 cm.
140 cc.	8.5 cm.	4.6 cm.
165 cc.	8.9 cm.	4.8 cm.
185 cc.	9.4 cm.	5.4 cm.
225 cc.	10.0 cm.	6.1 cm.

Perras-Papillon design (short-tail axillary prolongation), available in singles or pairs, unsterile only, with or without patches.

Volume	*Base Diameter*	*Projection*
140 cc.	9.0 cm.	5.0 cm.
175 cc.	10.0 cm.	5.1 cm.

Perras-Papillon extra soft shell (modified) with axillary prolongation, available in singles or pairs, unsterile, with or without patches.

Volume	*Base Diameter*	*Projection*
150 cc.	8.7 cm.	5.0 cm.
175 cc.	9.0 cm.	5.1 cm.

225 cc.	9.8 cm.	5.5 cm.
265 cc.	10.5 cm.	6.0 cm.

McGhan Medical Corp., P.O. Box 6447, Santa Barbara, CA 93111

Round gel-filled mammary implant, available in singles or pairs, sterile, with or without patches.

Volume	*Base Diameter*	*Projection*
100 cc.	9.7 cm.	3.0 cm.
120 cc.	10.0 cm.	3.5 cm.
140 cc.	10.9 cm.	3.9 cm.
160 cc.	11.3 cm.	4.1 cm.
180 cc.	11.6 cm.	4.3 cm.
200 cc.	11.8 cm.	4.6 cm.
220 cc.	12.1 cm.	4.8 cm.
240 cc.	12.4 cm.	5.0 cm.
260 cc.	12.7 cm.	5.1 cm.
280 cc.	13.2 cm.	5.2 cm.
300 cc.	13.6 cm.	5.3 cm.
320 cc.	14.0 cm.	5.4 cm.
340 cc.	14.5 cm.	5.6 cm.
360 cc.	14.7 cm.	5.7 cm.
400 cc.	14.9 cm.	5.8 cm.
460 cc.	15.1 cm.	5.8 cm.
500 cc.	15.3 cm.	5.9 cm.
560 cc.	15.6 cm.	6.2 cm.

Tear-drop gel-filled mammary implant, available in singles or pairs, sterile, with orientation tab, with or without patches.

Volume	*Base Diameter*	*Projection*
105 cc.	8.5 cm.	4.0 cm.
125 cc.	8.8 cm.	4.2 cm.
145 cc.	9.1 cm.	4.5 cm.
165 cc.	9.3 cm.	5.2 cm.
185 cc.	10.0 cm.	5.5 cm.
205 cc.	10.2 cm.	5.6 cm.
225 cc.	10.4 cm.	5.7 cm.
245 cc.	10.9 cm.	5.9 cm.
265 cc.	11.2 cm.	6.1 cm.
285 cc.	11.4 cm.	6.3 cm.
315 cc.	11.7 cm.	6.6 cm.
345 cc.	11.9 cm.	6.8 cm.
375 cc.	12.1 cm.	7.2 cm.

Oval low-profile gel-filled mammary implant, available in singles or pairs, sterile, with orientation tab, with or without patches.

Volume	*Base Diameter*	*Projection*
130 cc.	10.0 cm.	3.6 cm.
150 cc.	10.1 cm.	3.8 cm.
170 cc.	10.2 cm.	4.7 cm.
190 cc.	10.4 cm.	4.9 cm.
210 cc.	10.6 cm.	5.0 cm.
230 cc.	11.2 cm.	5.2 cm.
250 cc.	11.3 cm.	5.3 cm.
270 cc.	12.0 cm.	5.5 cm.
290 cc.	12.2 cm.	5.6 cm.
310 cc.	12.3 cm.	5.7 cm.
350 cc.	13.0 cm.	6.0 cm.
400 cc.	13.4 cm.	6.2 cm.

Round inflatable mammary implant with leaf valve, available in singles or pairs, unsterile, with or without patches, valve on apex or posterior.

Volume	*Base Diameter*	*Projection*
100–140 cc.	10.1 cm.	2.7 cm.
140–180 cc.	10.5 cm.	3.1 cm.
180–220 cc.	11.0 cm.	3.6 cm.
220–260 cc.	11.5 cm.	4.2 cm.
260–300 cc.	12.2 cm.	4.4 cm.
300–340 cc.	12.7 cm.	4.8 cm.
340–380 cc.	13.2 cm.	5.2 cm.

Round inflatable mammary implant with retention valve, available in singles or pairs, sterile, with or without patches, valve on apex or posterior.

Volume	*Base Diameter*	*Projection*
100–140 cc.	9.6 cm.	4.4 cm.
140–180 cc.	10.2 cm.	5.0 cm.
180–220 cc.	10.5 cm.	5.5 cm.
220–260 cc.	11.0 cm.	5.8 cm.
260–300 cc.	11.7 cm.	6.1 cm.
300–340 cc.	12.1 cm.	6.7 cm.
340–380 cc.	12.8 cm.	7.2 cm.

Tear-drop inflatable mammary implant with leaf or retention valves, available in singles or pairs, unsterile, with or without patches, valve on apex or posterior.

Volume	*Base Diameter*	*Projection*
165–185 cc.	9.1 cm.	5.5 cm.
205–225 cc.	9.2 cm.	6.2 cm.
245–265 cc.	9.8 cm.	6.2 cm.
285–305 cc.	10.3 cm.	6.5 cm.
315–335 cc.	10.6 cm.	6.8 cm.
345–365 cc.	10.9 cm.	7.2 cm.

Round inflatable mammary implant with diaphragm valve, available in singles or pairs, unsterile, with or without patches, valve on apex or posterior.

Volume	*Base Diameter*	*Projection*
100–140 cc.	9.6 cm.	4.4 cm.
140–180 cc.	10.2 cm.	5.0 cm.
180–220 cc.	10.5 cm.	5.5 cm.
220–260 cc.	11.0 cm.	5.8 cm.
260–300 cc.	11.7 cm.	6.1 cm.

300–340 cc.	12.1 cm.	6.7 cm.
340–380 cc.	12.8 cm.	7.2 cm.

Round two-lumen (gel inner sack, inflatable outer envelope) mammary implant with retention valve, available in singles or pairs, unsterile, with or without patches, posterior valve.

Volume	*Base Diameter*	*Projection*
120/220 cc.	11.0 cm.	3.6 cm.
140/240 cc.	11.3 cm.	4.0 cm.
160/260 cc.	11.5 cm.	4.2 cm.
180/280 cc.	11.8 cm.	4.4 cm.
220/340 cc.	12.7 cm.	4.9 cm.
240/360 cc.	13.0 cm.	5.1 cm.

Tear-drop two-lumen (gel inner sack, inflatable outer envelope) mammary implant with retention valve, available in singles or pairs, unsterile, with or without patches, posterior valve.

Volume	*Base Diameter*	*Projection*
125/225 cc.	9.2 cm.	6.2 cm.
145/245 cc.	9.5 cm.	6.2 cm.
165/265 cc.	9.8 cm.	6.2 cm.
185/285 cc.	10.0 cm.	6.4 cm.
205/315 cc.	10.3 cm.	6.7 cm.
225/345 cc.	10.6 cm.	6.8 cm.
265/375 cc.	10.9 cm.	7.2 cm.

Oval low-profile two-lumen (gel inner sac, inflatable outer envelope) mammary implant with retention valve, available in singles or pairs, unsterile, with or without patches, posterior valve.

Volume	*Base Diameter*	*Projection*
150/250 cc.	11.0 cm.	5.3 cm.
170/270 cc.	11.7 cm.	5.5 cm.
190/290 cc.	12.0 cm.	5.6 cm.
210/310 cc.	12.1 cm.	5.7 cm.
230/350 cc.	12.6 cm.	6.0 cm.

Round two-lumen (gel inner sac, inflatable outer envelope) mammary implant with modified leaf valve, available in singles or pairs, unsterile, with or without patches, posterior valve.

Volume	*Base Diameter*	*Projection*
120/140 cc.	10.9 cm.	2.7 cm.
140/160 cc.	11.0 cm.	2.9 cm.
160/180 cc.	11.3 cm.	3.1 cm.
180/200 cc.	11.5 cm.	3.4 cm.
200/220 cc.	11.8 cm.	3.6 cm.
220/260 cc.	12.4 cm.	4.2 cm.
240/280 cc.	12.8 cm.	4.3 cm.
260/300 cc.	13.2 cm.	4.4 cm.
280/320 cc.	13.4 cm.	4.5 cm.

Heyer-Schulte Corp., 600 Pine Ave., Goleta, CA 93017

Round inflatable mammary prosthesis with diaphragm valve, available in singles, unsterile, with or without patches, valve on apex.

Volume	*Base Diameter*	*Projection*
120–170 cc. (small)	9.5 cm.	3.0 cm.
170–250 cc. (medium)	11.0 cm.	3.5 cm.
250–350 cc. (large)	12.5 cm.	4.0 cm.

Contour inflatable mammary prosthesis with diaphragm valve, available in singles, unsterile, with or without patches, valve on apex.

Volume	*Base Diameter*	*Projection*
160–200 cc. (small)	8.4 cm.	5.0 cm.
200–260 cc. (medium)	9.1 cm.	5.6 cm.
260–350 cc. (large)	9.6 cm.	6.3 cm.

Round inflatable mammary prosthesis with retention valve, available in singles, sterile, with or without patches, valve on posterior.

Volume	*Base Diameter*	*Projection*
120–170 cc. (small)	9.5 cm.	3.0 cm.
170–250 cc. (medium)	11.0 cm.	3.5 cm.
250–350 cc. (large)	12.5 cm.	4.0 cm.

Contour inflatable mammary prosthesis with retention valve, available in singles, sterile, with or without patches, valve on posterior.

Volume	*Base Diameter*	*Projection*
160–200 cc. (small)	8.4 cm.	5.0 cm.
200–260 cc. (medium)	9.1 cm.	5.6 cm.
260–350 cc. (large)	9.6 cm.	6.3 cm.

Oval moderate-profile gel-filled mammary prosthesis, available in singles, sterile, with or without patches.

Volume	*Base Diameter*	*Projection*
125 cc.	8.3 cm.	3.1 cm.
150 cc.	8.6 cm.	3.2 cm.
175 cc.	9.2 cm.	3.3 cm.
200 cc.	10.1 cm.	3.4 cm.
225 cc.	10.3 cm.	3.5 cm.
250 cc.	10.8 cm.	3.6 cm.
275 cc.	11.2 cm.	3.7 cm.
300 cc.	11.6 cm.	3.8 cm.
350 cc.	12.0 cm.	4.0 cm.
400 cc.	12.4 cm.	4.2 cm.
450 cc.	12.6 cm.	4.2 cm.

Round moderate-profile gel-filled mammary prosthesis, available in singles, sterile, with or without patches.

Volume	Base Diameter	Projection
100 cc.	9.3 cm.	1.9 cm.
125 cc.	9.6 cm.	1.9 cm.
150 cc.	10.3 cm.	1.9 cm.
175 cc.	11.0 cm.	2.3 cm.
200 cc.	11.9 cm.	2.6 cm.
225 cc.	12.1 cm.	2.7 cm.
250 cc.	12.3 cm.	2.7 cm.
275 cc.	12.6 cm.	2.8 cm.
300 cc.	13.1 cm.	2.9 cm.
325 cc.	13.5 cm.	2.9 cm.
350 cc.	14.1 cm.	3.0 cm.
400 cc.	14.3 cm.	3.1 cm.
450 cc.	14.7 cm.	3.4 cm.

Round Hartley combination gel-inflatable, available in singles, unsterile, without patches, valve on posterior.

Volume	Base Diameter	Projection
125–175 cc.	10.3 cm.	2.8 cm.
150–200 cc.	10.6 cm.	3.0 cm.
200–250 cc.	11.3 cm.	3.2 cm.
250–300 cc.	12.9 cm.	3.6 cm.
300–350 cc.	13.3 cm.	3.7 cm.
375–475 cc.	14.3 cm.	3.9 cm.

Oval moderate-profile combination gel-inflatable, available in singles, unsterile, without patches, valve on posterior.

Volume	Base Diameter	Projection
150–200 cc.	9.3 cm.	3.6 cm.
175–225 cc.	9.6 cm.	3.7 cm.
200–250 cc.	10.2 cm.	3.8 cm.
275–325 cc.	11.3 cm.	4.0 cm.
325–375 cc.	12.2 cm.	4.2 cm.
400–500 cc.	13.0 cm.	4.5 cm.

Cox-Uphoff Co., 725 East Yononali St., Santa Barbara, CA 93101

Round gel-filled mammary prosthesis, available in singles, with or without suture loops and patches.

Volume	Base Diameter	Projection
120 cc.	9.7 cm.	3.0 cm.
140 cc.	10.2 cm.	3.2 cm.
160 cc.	10.3 cm.	3.5 cm.
180 cc.	11.1 cm.	3.5 cm.
200 cc.	11.5 cm.	3.6 cm.
220 cc.	11.6 cm.	3.7 cm.
240 cc.	11.8 cm.	3.9 cm.
260 cc.	12.0 cm.	4.1 cm.
280 cc.	12.2 cm.	4.3 cm.
300 cc.	12.4 cm.	4.5 cm.
320 cc.	12.6 cm.	4.6 cm.
340 cc.	12.7 cm.	4.7 cm.
360 cc.	12.8 cm.	4.8 cm.

Conical design mammary prosthesis, available in singles, with or without suture loops and patches.

Volume	Base Diameter	Projection
130 cc.	9.0 cm.	3.7 cm.
170 cc.	9.7 cm.	3.9 cm.
210 cc.	10.3 cm.	4.5 cm.
250 cc.	10.6 cm.	4.9 cm.

Oval design mammary prosthesis, available in singles, with or without suture loops and patches.

Volume	Base Diameter	Projection
115 cc.	7.7 cm.	3.8 cm.
135 cc.	8.2 cm.	4.0 cm.
155 cc.	8.7 cm.	4.1 cm.
175 cc.	9.0 cm.	4.2 cm.
195 cc.	9.3 cm.	4.5 cm.
215 cc.	9.6 cm.	4.7 cm.
235 cc.	10.3 cm.	4.9 cm.
255 cc.	10.6 cm.	5.1 cm.
275 cc.	10.7 cm.	5.3 cm.
295 cc.	10.8 cm.	5.5 cm.

Low-profile oval-design mammary prosthesis, available in singles, with or without suture loops and patches.

Volume	Base Diameter	Projection
145 cc.	9.4 cm.	3.5 cm.
180 cc.	10.0 cm.	3.8 cm.
215 cc.	10.9 cm.	4.0 cm.
250 cc.	11.6 cm.	4.1 cm.
285 cc.	12.1 cm.	4.3 cm.
320 cc.	12.2 cm.	4.6 cm.
355 cc.	12.8 cm.	4.9 cm.

Round inflatable mammary prosthesis, available in singles, sterile or unsterile, self-sealing valve, valve on posterior or anterior.

Volume	Base Diameter	Projection
110–130 cc.	8.9 cm.	3.6 cm.
130–150 cc.	9.5 cm.	4.1 cm.
150–170 cc.	9.8 cm.	4.2 cm.
170–190 cc.	10.3 cm.	4.4 cm.
185–215 cc.	10.4 cm.	4.5 cm.
205–235 cc.	10.8 cm.	4.6 cm.
225–255 cc.	10.9 cm.	4.9 cm.
245–275 cc.	11.4 cm.	4.9 cm.
265–295 cc.	11.7 cm.	5.1 cm.
285–315 cc.	11.8 cm.	5.1 cm.
325–355 cc.	11.9 cm.	5.4 cm.

Oval low-profile inflatable mammary prosthesis, available in singles, sterile or unsterile, self-sealing valve, valve on posterior or anterior.

Volume	*Base Diameter*	*Projection*
150–170 cc.	8.9 cm.	4.5 cm.
190–210 cc.	9.8 cm.	4.9 cm.
225–255 cc.	9.9 cm.	5.3 cm.
265–295 cc.	10.6 cm.	5.3 cm.
305–335 cc.	10.9 cm.	5.6 cm.
345–375 cc.	11.3 cm.	6.4 cm.
385–415 cc.	11.9 cm.	6.5 cm.

Roger Klein, Ltd., 61 Sprain Rd., Scarsdale, N.Y. 10583

Round inflatable mammary prosthesis (Mammatech) available in sterile packs, with valve on apex or posterior.

Mammatech periareolar inverted center tube (CT model)

Volume	*Base Diameter*	*Projection*
125 cc.	8.5 cm.	3.0 cm.
150 cc.	9.5 cm.	3.0 cm.
200 cc.	10.5 cm.	3.5 cm.
250 cc.	12.0 cm.	2.5 cm.

Mammatech inframammary inverted side tube (IT model)

Volume	*Base Diameter*	*Projection*
135 cc.	8.5 cm.	3.0 cm.
170 cc.	9.5 cm.	3.0 cm.
200 cc.	10.0 cm.	3.5 cm.
250 cc.	12.0 cm.	2.5 cm.

Reduction Mammoplasty and Correction of Ptosis of the Breast

PAUL K. McKISSOCK

Few operations in plastic surgery have provoked more diversified ideas than those for the treatment of hypertrophic and ptotic breasts. Yet, despite this heritage, modern reduction mammoplasty and mastopexy still largely consist of an expanding stockpile of individual techniques from which an orderly code of principles has yet to emerge. Although reduction mammoplasty and mastopexy have important fundamental differences, their similarities are greater than their differences, and most plastic surgeons will seek a technique that, by minor modification, can be adapted to both conditions.

REDUCTION MAMMOPLASTY

The usual reduction mammoplasty involves repositioning of the nipple-areolar complex, reduction of the areolar diameter, a partial resection of parenchyma, and a contouring resection of excess skin. The modern era of reduction mammoplasty might be characterized by the obsolescence of the multistaged approach and of wide skin undermining, and by the reservation of the free nipple graft to special situations such as extreme macromastia and the borderline patient with high medical risks. The modern-day mammoplasty would also seem to invariably feature a segment of deepithelialized skin somewhere for vascular protection of the nipple.

Historically, while earlier techniques seemed to emphasize the area of glandular resection as the most critical variable [2, 28, 32, 33], the decade of the 1960s was characterized by variable techniques of nipple transport using some sort of deepithelialized dermal flap [35, 36, 53, 64, 70]. If the 1970s have an identifying characteristic for this procedure, it would seem to be in the area and design of the skin resection and the resulting scar pattern [9, 13, 40, 59, 69]. The reduction of the excessive skin envelope is the part of mammoplasty in which a measure of artistry is required; thus, in this regard at least, reduction mammoplasty has become a more difficult problem for the surgeon.

Prevention of avascular necrosis of the nipple, once considered the overriding hallmark of success in any technique, is now generally accepted as a matter of course, and the surgeon is obliged to concentrate upon contour and scarring, previously considered as frivolous details. If one can speculate on a continuation of this trend, it would seem reasonable to expect the surgeons of the next decade to be preoccupied with such things as the permanence of shape and the preservation of nipple sensibility.

Etiology

The normal breast is so obviously an endocrine-dependent end organ that it is tempting to assign an endocrine etiology to all of its pathological states. While this may in fact be true, the mode of hormonal interaction affecting the organ is so complex and the relevant information is still so sparse that no valid conclusions regarding the cause of parenchymal hypertrophy can be made.

Endocrine Physiology of the Normal Breast

The normal growth and development of the female breast, which is generally the first evidence of puberty, occurs primarily as a response to rising levels of estradiol in the absence of effective levels of testosterone. Once ovulatory cycles have been established, progesterone from the corpus luteum and pituitary prolactin join into a complex interaction with estradiol; these hormones presumably act on hormone receptors in the breast tissue to effect normal ductal, lobuloalveolar, and stromal development, and the deposition of fat. Normal breast growth, then, proceeds in the presence of these three hormones to a certain point at which it customarily ceases abruptly without any measurable change in hormone levels. No negative hormonal feedback system is known to exist for breast growth; the mechanism that acts to stop breast growth is uncertain. Most authorities speculate [61, 76] that the regulating factor exists in the breast tissue itself; for example, a finite number of available receptor sites may be genetically determined or otherwise influenced by factors as yet unknown.

Pregnancy adds a fourth hormone, human placental lactogen [72], which results in dramatic breast growth and lobuloalveolar differentiation; the rising levels of estrogen and progesterone are also involved in these changes. At the termination of pregnancy, all the hormone levels but that of prolactin fall precipitously; although the breast engorges with milk, stromal growth and epithelial differentiation cease for the moment. Following lactation, an involutional process occurs that is predictable only qualitatively, and it will leave behind an organ with greater or lesser quantities of any of its structural elements (including skin) than existed prior to the pregnancy.

Pathophysiology of the Hyperplastic Breast

With the exception of pregnancy states and recognizable endocrinopathies, macromastia has never been associated with measurable abnormalities in hormone levels. Just as the etiology of breast hypertrophy varies, so will the histological picture. There appears to be no pathological common denominator to breast hypertrophy. Several types are recognized:

ENDOCRINE HYPERTROPHY. This is associated with a variety of endocrine abnormalities along with other generalized changes, such as abnormal hair distribution and precocious puberty. The histological picture would be that of hyperplasia of ductal and stromal elements and increased fat deposition.

VIRGINAL HYPERTROPHY. This probably represents an abnormal end organ response, but is not associated with abnormal hormonal effects elsewhere in the body. The onset is usually in the second decade and may be unilateral or bilateral to an enormous degree. Progesterone therapy will often inhibit further growth but will not induce remission. The histological picture is usually that of stromal and ductal proliferation with little lobular reaction; in many ways it is not dissimilar to the histological picture seen in gynecomastia.

OBESE HYPERTROPHY. This condition is associated with generalized exogenous obesity, but it is usually not sufficiently diminished by weight reduction. Histologically, increased fat deposition occurs.

INVOLUTIONAL HYPERTROPHY. Characterized by breast growth at middle age around the menopausal period, involutional hypertrophy usually has a histological picture of lobular atrophy and fatty replacement.

GRAVID HYPERTROPHY. This condition results from the hormonal changes in pregnancy, involving the interaction of estradiol, progesterone, prolactin, and human placental lactogen.

POSTGRAVID HYPERTROPHY. This condition of relative macromastia, which is characterized by a larger breast after pregnancy than existed before, results from incomplete involution and from the persistence of stromal, ductal, and fatty hypertrophy of pregnancy.

Breast Pathology Associated with Macromastia

With the exception of the uncommon "malignant" variety of virginal hypertrophy, most plastic surgeons visualize the hypertrophic breast simply as an oversized but otherwise normal organ. The histological criteria of normalcy in adult breast tissue seem vague to the nonpathologist, but normal breast tissue could be considered that which is free of both malignancy and fibrocystic disease. In one sense, the normal breast is, or in time will become, a fibrocystic organ. The extent to which it can be considered to harbor fibrocystic "disease" seems mainly related to the degree of prevalence of certain specific characteristics as well as being a reflection of the pathologist's personal criteria. Some pathologists have come to regard the term "fibrocystic disease" as inaccurately broad and obsolete, and they have therefore discarded it in favor of more specific designations.

Several authors [50, 51, 55, 65] have reported the incidence of chronic mastopathy found in large series of patients operated upon for breast hypertrophy. The reported incidence varies from 50 to 75 percent and encompasses the full spectrum of histopathological entities, often ill defined, that together comprise the potpourri of "fibrocystic disease." The specific microscopic diagnoses will include: stromal fibrosis, fibroadenomatosis, ductal ectasia, lobular atrophy, sclerosing adenosis, intraductal hyperplasia and papillomatosis, microcystic and macrocystic disease, blunt duct adenosis, apocrine metaplasia, adenosis, and adenofibrosis, to name but a few. In addition, the student is further confounded by the persistence of vaguely descriptive terminology such as mammary dysplasia, chronic cystic mastitis, and mazoplasia.

In my own series, 75 percent of the specimens submitted to the pathologist for routine examination and description were returned with a report bearing the label "fibrocystic disease," which would seem to correlate well with other reported series. None of these data, however, involved a comparison with the same pathological entities in a random sampling of the general female population not operated upon for clinically suspicious conditions. In a study of 100 apparently normal breasts obtained at postmortem examinations, Sloss and associates [63] were able to find histopathological changes, usually regarded as representing "significant mastopathy," present in almost all of the specimens. They concluded on this basis that the histological elements of fibrocystic disease occur so commonly that their mere presence does not signify a disease. If this is even partially true, it would imply that fibrocystic disease and macromastia bear no specific causal relationship despite this 75 percent coincidence.

The finding of an occult carcinoma in a specimen removed for breast reduction has been reported on many occasions, but no statistical evidence exists linking breast hypertrophy per se with malignancy.

Indications

The principal indication for reduction mammoplasty is the alleviation of symptoms associated with breast weight; of almost equal importance are complaints that relate to obtaining and wearing clothing normally. In a study that I performed [9], only 25 percent of patients listed cosmetic improvement in the appearance of the undraped breast as their principal goal in seeking the surgery.

Within certain limits, macromastia can be a subjective judgment on the part of the patient. Ideal breast size seems to vary to a degree among contemporary cultures at any given time, and from decade to decade in western culture. Changing fads in clothing styles have even influenced women's concept of what constitutes an ideal breast size. The current movement of social liberation among women has resulted in an increased definition of what is ideal in terms of their own values as opposed to those of men. The result has been some increased demand by women for reduction of their breast size for a variety of personal reasons. For the most part, however, reduction mammoplasty deals with hypertrophy of the organ to a degree that warrants description of it as a pathological state. Strömbeck [65] has observed that most women will consider their breasts too large when the volume of one breast exceeds 400 cc. (approximately 1 pound).

Principal Methods of Breast Reduction

Innumerable techniques that have been described over the years are effective in breast reduction; however, features such as wide skin undermining or multistaged planning render many of them obsolete according to present-day interests. In addition, the literature abounds with innovative ideas often presented as unique approaches, but which in fact should be considered as modifications of a recognized basic operation. The following discussion will be limited to a description of the basic operations in which most surgeons seem to be expressing a continued interest.

According to present-day thinking, it would seem reasonable to classify these various techniques according to their differences in skin resection and resulting scar patterns. Two categories are recognized: lateralizing operations (in which no scar is left medial to the breast meridian) and the operations that result in an inverted-T scar pattern. Each category presents its own set of advantages and disadvantages.

Lateralizing Operations for Breast Reduction

The lateralizing operations have the advantages that there is no scarring of the intermammary area, there is less linear scarring and a decreased likelihood of skin necrosis, and the operation is more easily adapted to cases of minor skin excess (i.e., mastopexy). The disadvantages of this procedure are that it is progressively more difficult to perform as the size of the skin envelope increases, the surgeon is unable to predetermine new nipple position accurately because a new inframammary fold will be creasted, and there are less definite guidelines – more guesswork and judgment are needed during surgery.

Technique of Dufourmentel and Mouly

A technique that was previously described by Marc [34] and Hollander [24] was perfected and popularized by Dufourmentel and Mouly. It stands as the prototype of all lateral approaches (Fig. 45-1).

PREOPERATIVE PLANNING. This involves the determination of points A, B, C, and D. Point A is best determined with the patient in the erect position; points B, C, and D are established with the patient recumbent.

Point A: At the junction of the inframammary crease with the anterior axillary line.
Point B: Along the line joining the suprasternal notch and the point of the nipple, 16 to 20 cm. from the suprasternal notch.
Point C: At the nipple level, 8 to 9 cm. from midsternum.
Point D: On the breast meridian, 6 cm. above the inframammary crease.

Straight lines are drawn from point A to the ends of an arc tangential to the remaining points when the breast mass is pushed downward and upward respectively.

RESECTION. Full-thickness wedge resection of the skin and gland is performed as outlined by points A, P, and Q; the parenchyma beneath and inferior to the areola is included if necessary.

CLOSURE. A single straight-line oblique scar results.

Technique of Regnault

The technique of Regnault is defined by its originator as the "B technique" because of the resemblance of the skin resection to the capital letter B. The unique features of this technique are that (1) the segment of skin resected is principally circumareolar, where the excess is most likely to exist, and (2) the procedure uses the Z-plasty type of closure, involving interdigitating skin flaps (Fig. 45-2).

PREOPERATIVE PLANNING. With the patient erect, points M, X, A, and B are established.

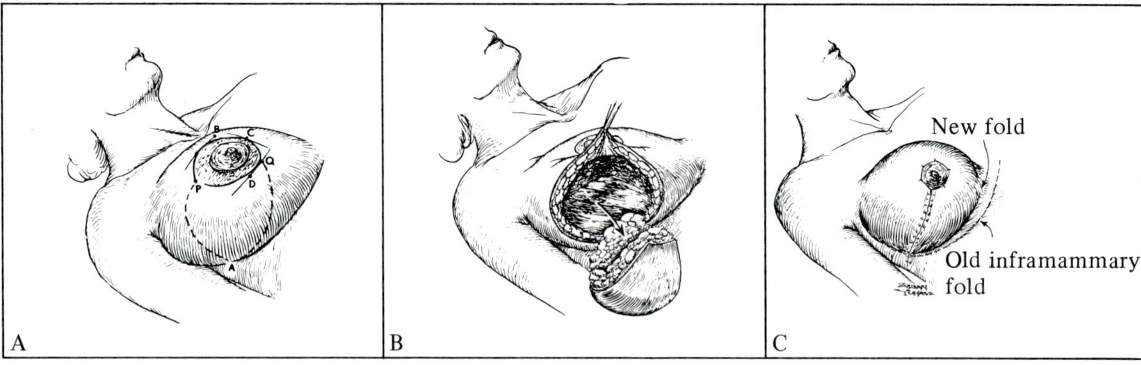

Fig. 45-1. The technique of Dufourmentel and Mouly. A, preoperative plan. B, resection. C, closure.

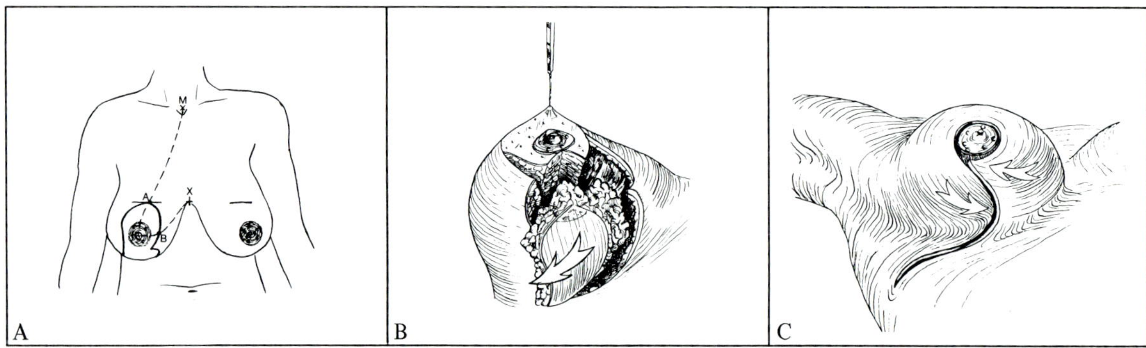

Fig. 45-2. The technique of Regnault. A, preoperative plan. B, resection. C, closure.

Point M: At the sternal notch.
Point A: On a line joining point M with the nipple, 15 to 20 cm. from point M.
Point X: The point at which a horizontal line joining points A of both breasts intersects the midsternal line.
Point B: On a line joining point X with the nipple, 7.5 to 10 cm. from point X.

With the patient supine, the skin to be resected is estimated and outlined by a B-shaped pattern of arcs passing through points A and B and 1 to 2 cm. above the existing inframammary fold.

RESECTION. The areola is reduced as needed and the circumareolar skin is deepithelialized. A full-thickness wedge of skin and gland is resected from the inferior part of the breast including some of the gland beneath the medial skin edge and some from the upper portion of the breast if necessary.

CLOSURE. The medial flap is rotated upward and laterally and the lateral flap downward and medially, interdigitating them as in a Z-plasty. The resulting scar has the configuration of the letter J.

Related Lateralizing Techniques

TECHNIQUE OF ELBAZ AND VERHEEKE. This technique [3] is similar to the technique of Dufourmentel and Mouly. The glandular resection is principally lateral, and the skin resection extends to the breast meridian inferiorly resulting in an L-shaped scar pattern.

TECHNIQUE OF MEYER AND KESSELRING. This technique [40] is similar to the technique of Regnault. The glandular resection is principally inferior; skin resection follows a keyhole pattern with the medial limb near the breast meridian. An L-shaped scar pattern results.

Operations for Breast Reduction Resulting in an Inverted-T Scar Pattern

The operations that result in an inverted-T scar pattern have the advantages that they are applicable with equal facility to all degrees of skin excess, they allow

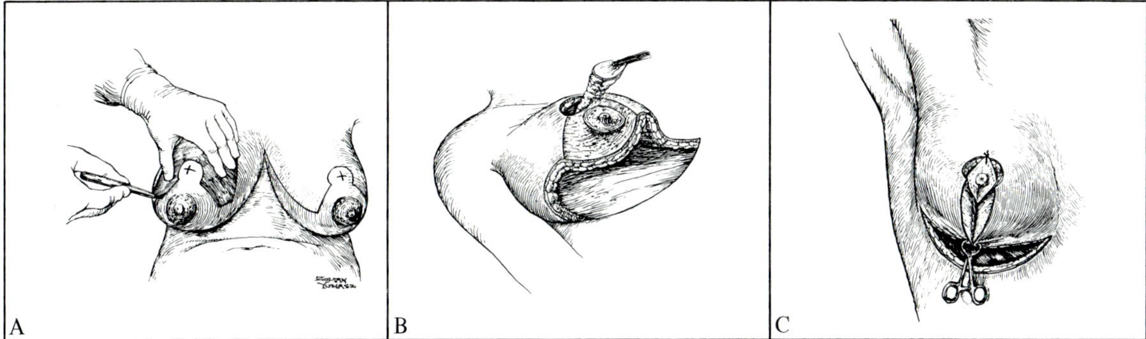

Fig. 45-3. Technique of Strömbeck. A, preoperative plan. B, resection. C, closure.

more accurate and complete pattern design preoperatively, they necessitate less guesswork and fewer decisions at surgery, and the scars are in a more desirable location, except for scars in the medial inframammary limb. The disadvantages of these operations are that the scar in the intermammary area may be visible, there is a greater possibility of skin flap necrosis, and the most stretched (circumareolar) skin is the least resected.

Technique of Strömbeck

Strömbeck is generally credited with application of the Schwartzmann [60] maneuver to modern mammoplasty. In his technique, the breast is reduced to a horizontally directed, bipedicle flap bearing the nipple-areolar complex at its midpoint, and extending between the medial and lateral skin flaps (Fig. 45-3).

PREOPERATIVE PLANNING. This utilizes a fixed keyhole pattern of celluloid, with a 135-degree spread. The new nipple position is established along the breast meridian, 22 cm. from the sternal notch, or in relationship to the inframammary level.

RESECTION. The horizontal flap is deepithelialized except for the areola, and the areola is reduced in diameter as needed. A full-thickness wedge of skin and gland inferior to the pedicle and skin flaps is resected, along with a full-thickness cylinder beneath the new areolar window.

CLOSURE. The horizontal flap is infolded so that the areola protrudes into the new areolar window, and the medial and lateral skin flaps are approximated in midline. If infolding is difficult, the lateral pedicle may be sectioned to facilitate closure.

Technique of Pitanguy

Although the approach is different, the ultimate resection in the technique of Pitanguy is not unlike that in the Strömbeck procedure. The resection is all done from below upward to the upper gland in the shape of a keel; then the areolar window is excised after closure to exteriorize the nipple. The medial and lateral glandular pillars are sutured together to enhance the shape (Fig. 45-4).

PREOPERATIVE PLANNING. The marking is performed with the patient supine but elevated 15 degrees. Points A, B, and C are established as follows:

Point A: At midmammary line slightly lower than the inframammary sulcus as projected to the face of the breast by the index finger.

Points B and C: On a line transversely through the nipple, equidistant from it, and 6 to 7 cm. from point A.

Lines are drawn joining points B and C with point A and with the medial and lateral ends of the inframammary fold (points D and E).

RESECTION. The triangular area outlined by points A, B, and C is deepithelialized except for the areola. An incision is made from point D to point E along the inframammary crease, and a second incision along line E–B–C–D, which will outline the area of skin resection. This elliptical wedge is resected superiorly from the deep aspect of the gland in a keel shape extending to the upper gland as needed, leaving stout glandular pillars medially and laterally to preserve nerve and blood supply.

CLOSURE. The medial and lateral glandular pillars are sutured together and the skin flaps are approximated in the midline. The areolar window is excised where desired and the areola is exteriorized.

Technique of Skoog

The technique of Skoog is essentially Strömbeck's procedure when one pedicle is sectioned. It differs in that (1) the medial pedicle is the one sectioned, (2) the resection is performed en bloc, and (3) Skoog

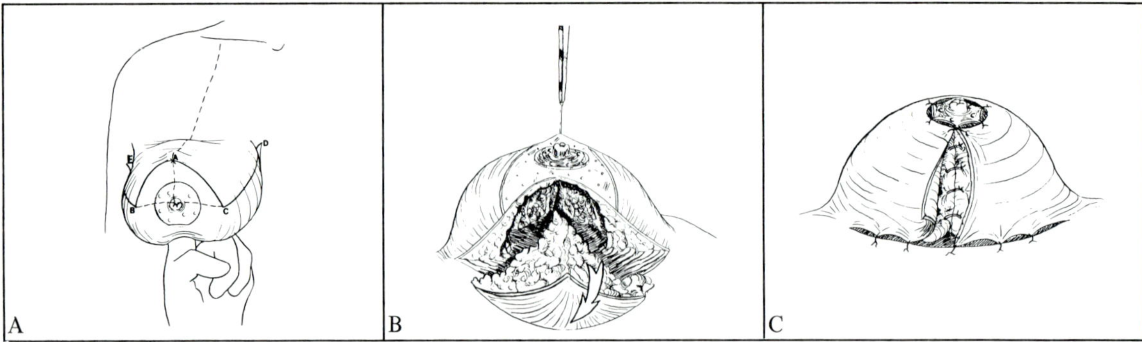

Fig. 45-4. Technique of Pitanguy. A, preoperative plan. B, resection. C, closure.

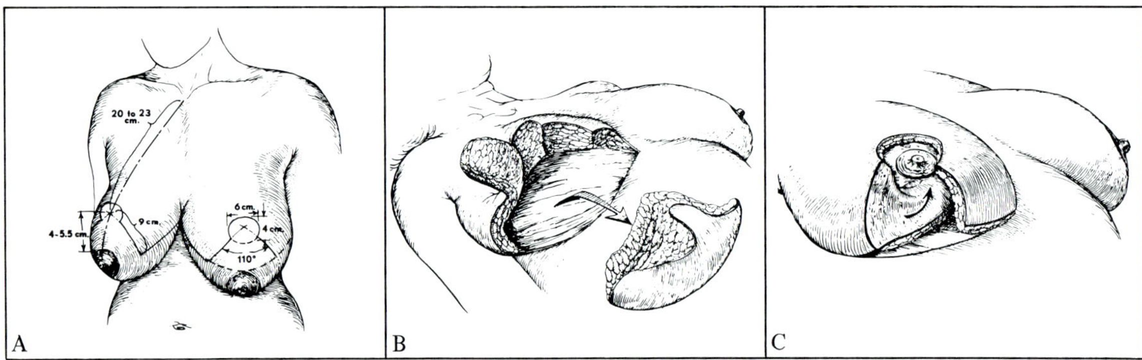

Fig. 45-5. Technique of Skoog. A, preoperative plan. B, resection. C, closure.

visualizes the principal blood supply of the nipple-bearing flap to be cuticular rather than parenchymal (Fig. 45-5).

PREOPERATIVE PLANNING. A fixed pattern is not used; the pattern is custom designed for each breast according to an exact system of measurements. The nipple height is related to inframammary level, 5.5 cm. above that level when accurately transposed to the face of the breast. The skin flap separation is 110 degrees, and the distance between the flaps is established 7.0 to 9.0 cm. from the new nipple point. An oval-shaped areolar window is predetermined 4 X 6 cm. in dimension. The nipple-bearing flap is designed as an extension of the lateral skin flap generously encompassing the areola.

RESECTION. The nipple-bearing flap is deepithelialized and elevated about 1.0 cm. in thickness back to its lateral skin flap base. All remaining excess skin and gland are resected en bloc as indicated by the case.

CLOSURE. The deepithelialized flap is rotated upward, placing the areolar into its window, and the skin flaps are approximated in the midline.

Author's Technique

The breast is reduced to a vertically directed, bipedicle flap based superiorly on the upper rim of the new areolar window and inferiorly on the thoracic wall in the inframammary area. The flap bears the nipple near its upper third and is prepared as a deepithelialized flap, although the principal blood supply should be visualized as parenchymal rather than dermal. The skin pattern is totally designed preoperatively and rigidly adhered to, leaving a minimum of decisions to be made at surgery.

PREOPERATIVE PLANNING. With the patient erect, the breast meridian is established by dropping a line from midclavicle to the nipple (Fig. 45-6A). The inframammary level is measured in relation to the clavicle utilizing a pair of obstetrical calipers (Fig. 45-6B). This level is transposed to the face of the breast and marked at the meridian (Fig. 45-6C).

The midpoint of the new nipple site is determined (Fig. 45-6D) by the use of the lower edge of the

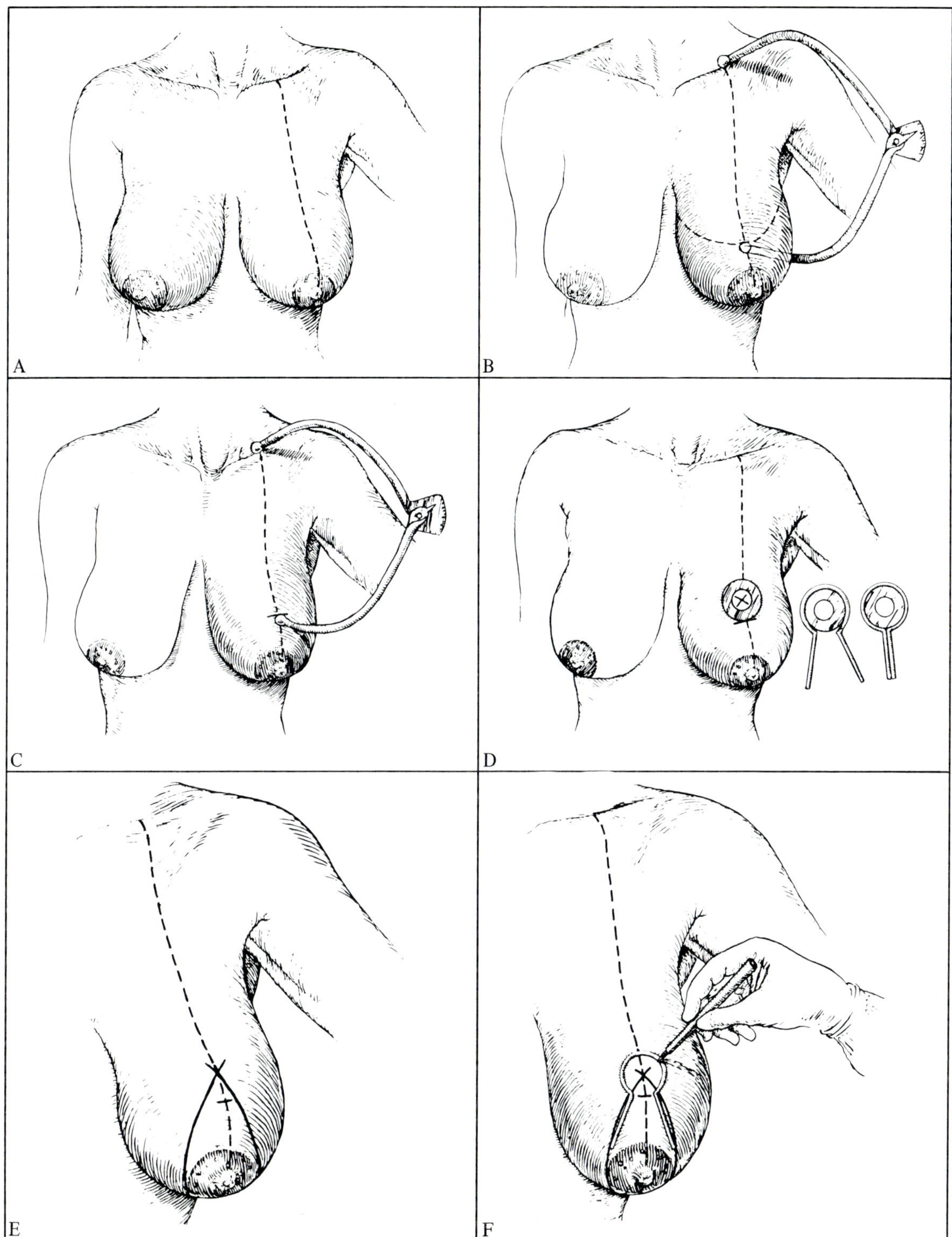

Fig. 45-6. The author's technique: preoperative planning. (See text for details.)

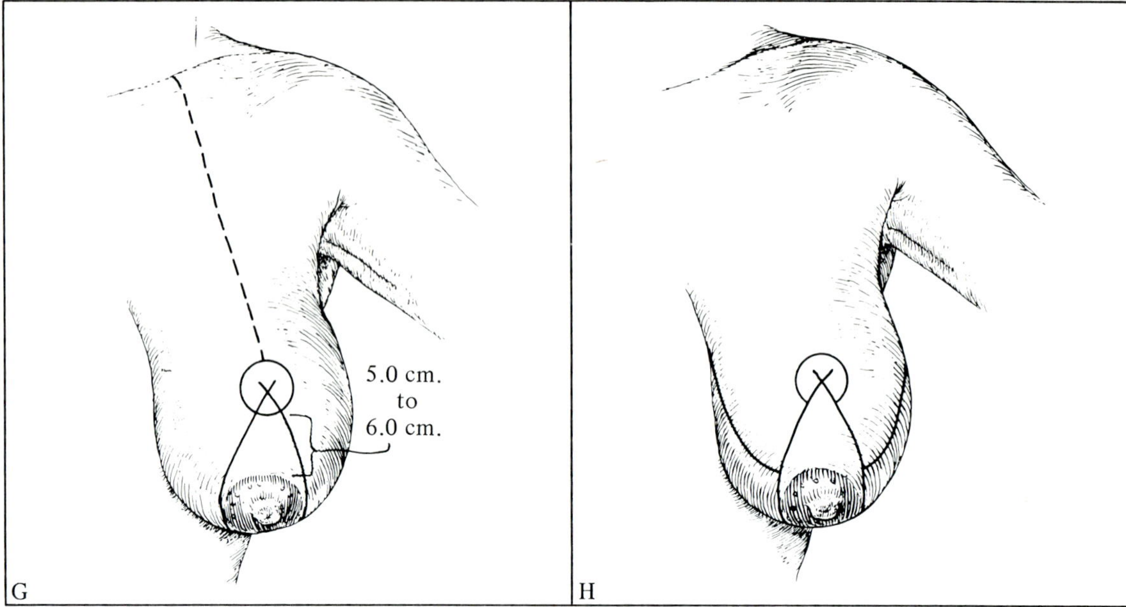

Fig. 45-6 (Cont.)

areolar template that will be used at surgery; the template is placed at the inframammary level and the center of this circle is marked (Fig. 45-6D). A metallic washer 37 mm. in diameter can be used as a template to circumcise the areolar at surgery; a length of malleable wire that is fashioned to fit the washer will retain the same circumference when opened. Two lines are drawn downward from the new nipple point tangential to the point where the areolar pigmentation disappears (Fig. 45-6E). The wire keyhole pattern marker is applied to the breast and the areolar window is traced while the wire is opened to fit the spread of the diverging lines (Fig. 45-6F). From the intersection of the areolar window with the diverging lines, a distance of 5.0 to 6.0 cm. is measured downward to establish the width of the skin flaps; this distance will vary with the intended size of the new breast (Fig. 45-6G). From these points, lines are drawn medially and laterally to the ends of the inframammary fold (Fig. 45-6H). These lines should have a slight "lazy-S" configuration, particularly laterally, to contour the breast properly.

OPERATIVE TECHNIQUE. The areola is circumcised to a diameter of 37 mm. using the metal template; the vertical flap is outlined by extending the lines of the skin flap ends downward to the inframammary fold (Fig. 45-7A). The vertical flap is deepithelialized (Fig. 45-7B).

The medial and lateral dermoglandular wedges are resected down to, but not including, the pectoral fascia (Fig. 45-7C and D). The preservation of a thin layer of the fatty tissue immediately overlying the fascia, particularly laterally, may safeguard against injury to the fourth anterolateral cutaneous nerve on its course to the nipple.

Additional tissue is resected from beneath the vertical flap and from beneath the adjacent skin flaps (Fig. 45-7E). This resection will convert the vertical flap into a true "bucket handle" bipedicle flap (Fig. 45-7F). The resection should not extend above the upper rim of the new areolar window. The flap is folded upward upon itself, placing the areola into its window (Fig. 45-7G). The skin flaps are draped around the bulk of the folded flap, closing from medial and lateral with the ends toward the center; any discrepancy in flap length is adjusted at this time (Fig. 45-7H).

After the flap ends have been trimmed, final closure is performed using subcuticular sutures (Fig. 45-7I) reinforced by adhesive tape strips. A Penrose drain is left across the full width of each breast and out the lateral end of the inframammary wound.

Free Nipple Graft

Of less use today than in previous years, the free nipple graft has always been described as a variant of a straightforward wedge amputation resulting in an inverted-T scar [71, 75]. In my opinion it should be reserved for (1) patients with extreme macromastia (i.e., resections exceeding 2 kg. per breast), (2) elderly patients and patients with borderline medial

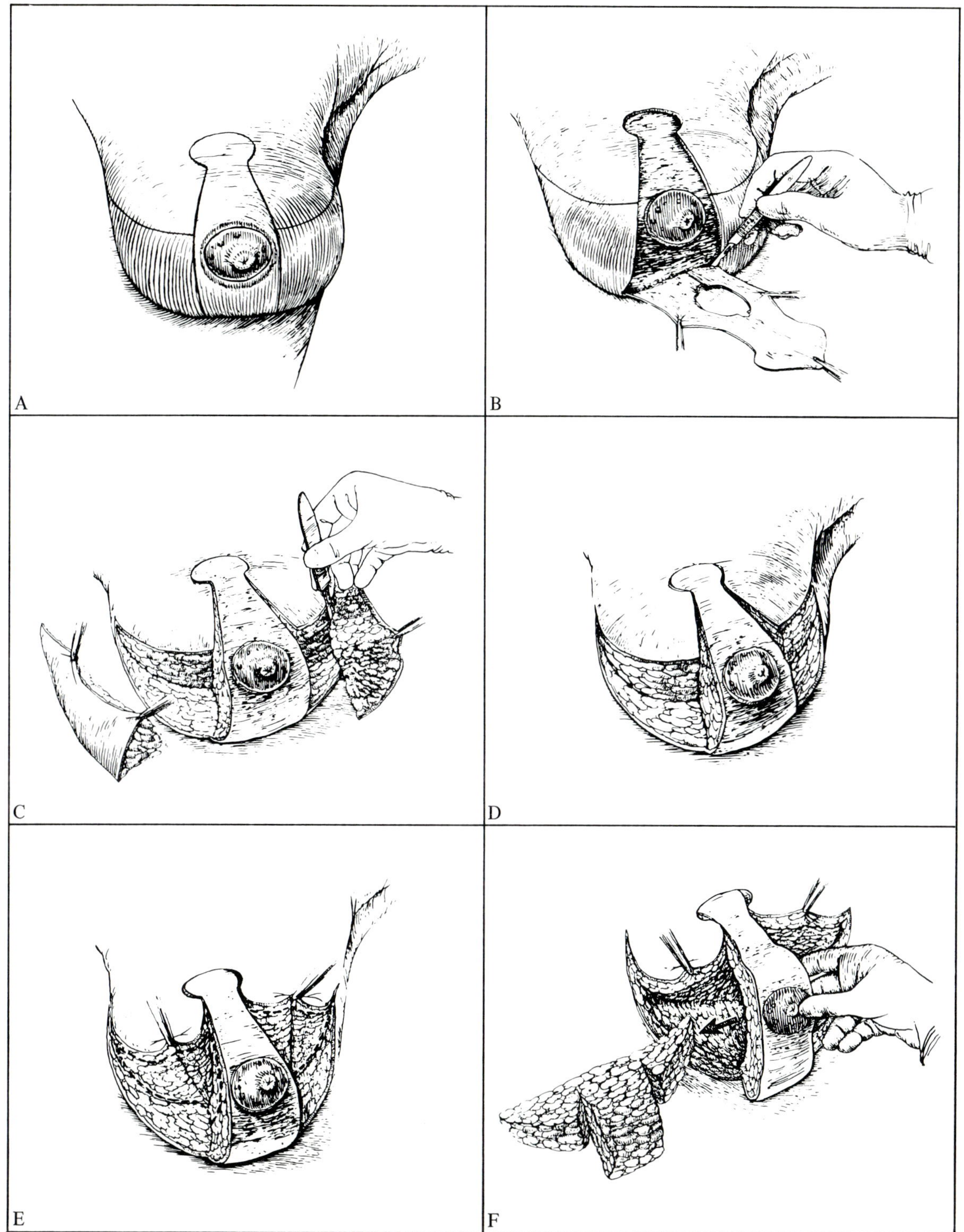

Fig. 45-7. The author's technique: the operative technique. (See text for details.)

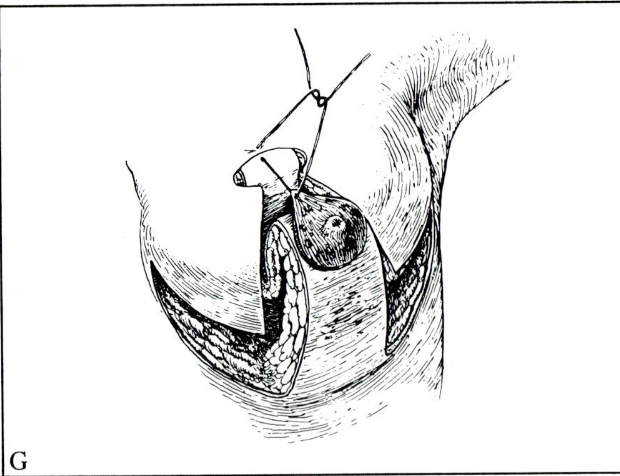

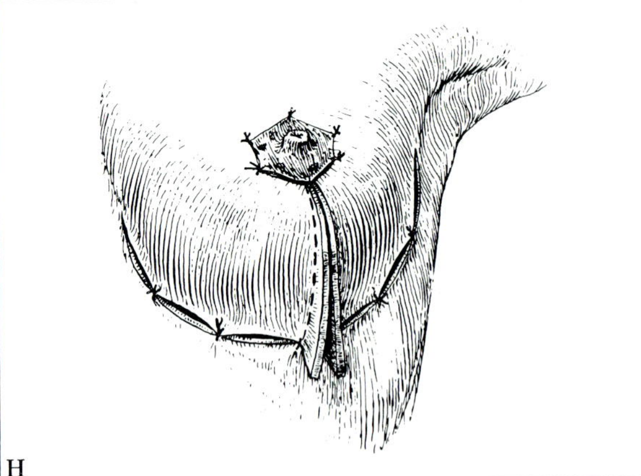

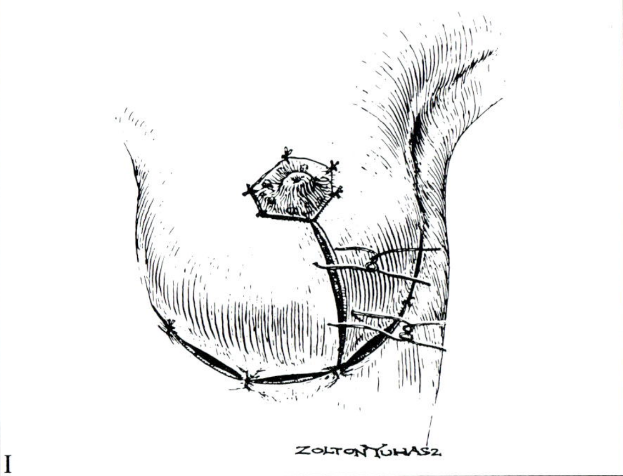

Fig. 45-7 (Cont.)

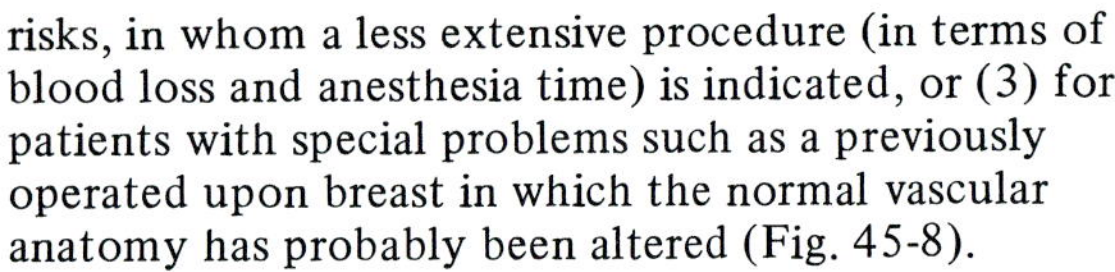

risks, in whom a less extensive procedure (in terms of blood loss and anesthesia time) is indicated, or (3) for patients with special problems such as a previously operated upon breast in which the normal vascular anatomy has probably been altered (Fig. 45-8).

PREOPERATIVE PLANNING. The pattern marking as described on page 742 under "Author's Technique" can be used without alteration.

RESECTION. The areola is reduced to 37 mm. in diameter and is removed as a full-thickness graft. Only the areolar window is deepithelialized. A simple through-and-through wedge amputation is performed from the pattern marking anteriorly to the thoracic wall. Additional tissue may be resected from the deep aspect of the gland if necessary.

CLOSURE. A direct skin closure will usually result in obliteration of all dead space, but the use of a Penrose drain is still wise. The areola is "defatted" and reapplied as a full-thickness graft including the usual tie-over bolus dressing.

Postoperative Care

The suture lines are dressed with a grease-impregnated gauze (such as Xeroform) and bulky absorbent pads are placed over only the drain sites. The breasts are dressed with a wraparound halter-type dressing, crisscrossing the breasts and around the neck to provide support but not compression. The drains are removed after 48 hours; the patient may be discharged from the hospital on the third postoperative day, if her general condition permits. Prior to discharge, a review of the pathologist's report of the resected specimen would be in order. The patient is instructed to wear a well-fitting brassiere day and night for 6 weeks postoperatively to provide support and immobilization during the early phases of wound healing.

The Four-Hour Check

Within 4 to 6 hours following the end of the operation, the surgeon should reexamine his patient, removing all dressings to allow proper inspection and palpation of the breasts. Hematoma and/or impending vascular complications should be apparent at this point, and treatment without fear of irreversible damage should still be possible.

HEMATOMA. In any procedure in which the nipple has been moved on a buried pedicle, hematoma is an emergency requiring prompt evacuation; a second general anesthetic is usually necessary.

IMPENDING VASCULAR COMPLICATIONS. If there is any suspicion of impending vascular complications of the areola and/or skin flaps, they should be treated at

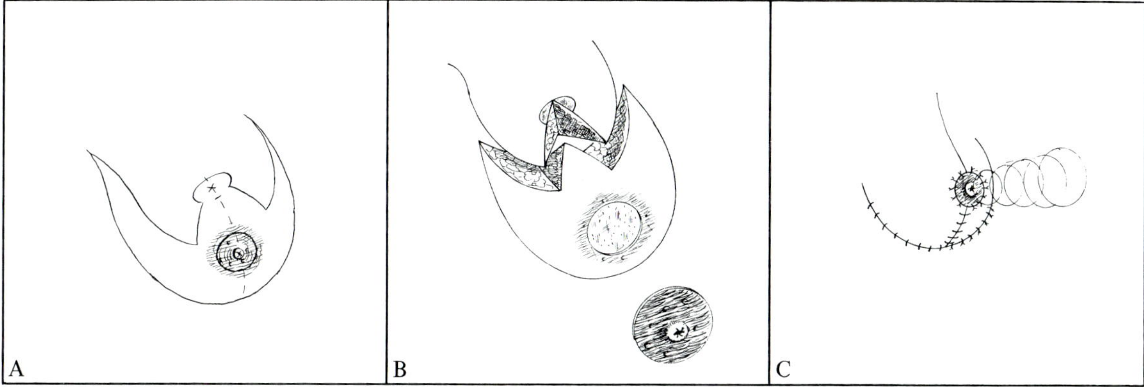

Fig. 45-8. Free areolar graft technique. A, preoperative plan. B, resection. C, closure.

this point. Initial treatment should be directed at decompression of the breast by releasing the inframammary and vertical suture lines while retaining the general integrity of the breast with adhesive tape straps and moist compresses over the dehisced wounds. This treatment can usually be done without a secondary anesthetic, and it will grant the surgeon 1 or 2 hours continuance before more aggressive measures are necessary.

If the areola distinctly responds by improved perfusion, the breast may be left in this state for several days until the resolution of edema will allow a delayed secondary closure, or until the defect is closed by skin grafting.

If, on the other hand, the areola fails to respond and the surgeon perceives the perfusion to be deteriorating, the vascular integrity of the nipple-bearing pedicle must be inadequate; this approach must then be aborted in favor of a free nipple graft. The early use of intravenous fluorescein testing, as advocated by Grabb [19], can be helpful in confirming the status of areolar perfusion in doubtful cases, sparing the surgeon hours of procrastination and delay. The patient must be returned to the operating room, the areola removed, and the vertical pedicle amputated by sectioning the superior pedicle at the level of the lower edge of the areolar window. The inferior pedicle is amputated at whatever level appears to be safely viable. The areola is then reapplied as a free, full-thickness graft on the dermal bed of the stump of the superior pedicle, which has been inset back into the closed areolar window. This procedure has been done as late as 24 hours postoperatively with survival of the free areolar graft. In any event, decompression of the tense breast alone is about all that can be done to assist the skin flaps.

Results

If the criteria for evaluating postoperative results were to be based solely upon patient satisfaction and alleviation of preoperative symptoms, the success rate of reduction mammoplasty would be extremely high. However, the surgeon is frequently more critical of the result than the patient, particularly when substantial degrees of hypertrophy have been involved. Beyond patient satisfaction, any evaluation of results will customarily amount to an analysis of medical complications and artistic errors in craftsmanship.

Complications

Postoperative complications may be classified as early (necrosis, hematoma, infection, and wound dehiscence) and late (abnormal scarring, permanent sensory changes, loss of shape, recurrent hypertrophy, and interference with the capacity for lactation). Late tumor formation, in my experience, has always proved to be a dysplastic condition in the residual breast tissue not felt to be specifically related to the surgery and has therefore not been considered as a complication per se. Strömbeck [70], reporting on a very large series of cases, has indicated that a correlation exists between exogenous obesity and the rate of local vascular complications. The incidence of nipple necrosis (in particular, fat necrosis) seemed as related to the patient's generalized obesity as to the weight of specimen resected.

My reportable series includes 184 patients; the data are classified by the breast rather than by the patient. The type of dissection I have described was performed on 362 breasts in 184 patients; 6 cases involved unilateral reductions. The patients varied in age from 15 to 65 years, with an average age of 34 years. The weight of specimen resected from each breast varied from 85 gm. to 2,265 gm., with an average weight of 724 gm. per breast. The complications encountered in this group of patients are described next.

Necrosis

NIPPLE AND AREOLA. There have been no cases of total loss of the nipple-areolar complex in my series. Partial loss of the areola occurred in 5 breasts (1.4 percent); this usually manifests itself as a cyanotic areola that gradually improves in color, but ulitmately results in a melting away of 3 to 4 mm. of the areolar circumference often as late as 3 to 4 weeks following surgery. The final deformity is often not as severe as initially feared, and if the resulting circumareolar scar remains spread rather than hypertrophic, the result may be better left as such instead of revising it at the expense of an asymmetry in circumference.

SKIN. A significant loss of skin occurred in 3 breasts, and a minor loss of the tip of a flap in another 4 breasts. None were extensive enough to require skin graft closure, but all resulted in unsightly scarring requiring a secondary revision.

PARENCHYMA. A transient episode of asymmetrical pain and induration that recedes spontaneously without drainage can be presumed to represent focal fat necrosis of a minor degree, which may be common. This is more likely to be a manifestation of poor wound toilet and pedunculated fat left behind after an untidy resection. A major infarction of a portion of the parenchyma, however, will appear as an indurated, tender area with erythema of the overlying skin. It may be associated with fever and eventually results in the massive drainage of an oily liquid; the fluid is sterile to culture or will grow out minor skin contaminants. Treatment is directed at improved drainage, irrigation, and antibiotics to discourage secondary bacterial infection. The condition usually responds rapidly to proper treatment and ultimately results in a disrupted scar at the site of drainage and a reduced breast volume. This complication occurred in 6 breasts in my series and was bilateral in one case.

Hematoma

Hematomas large enough to require evacuation occurred 8 times, 3 of these in the same patient (bilaterally the night of surgery and in 1 breast 9 days postoperatively). In another patient a massive hematoma occurred 1 week after the operation. In no case was a coagulation disorder evident. In 3 cases, the evacuated and drained hematoma eventually led to a deep wound infection.

Infection

Except as a complication following hematoma or fat necrosis, the development of a deep wound abscess has been a surprisingly uncommon problem, even though prophylactic antibiotic therapy has not been used. This probably is mainly the result of the use of a Penrose drain for 48 hours postoperatively, preventing space-occupying fluid accumulations. In my series, there was only one case of deep primary infection that was not directly associated with fat necrosis or hematoma.

Wound Dehiscence

Unintentional wound dehiscence occurred in 4 breasts; 1 was a result of premature suture removal and the others were related to concomitant steroid therapy. Skin flaps developed by the keyhole pattern require suture (or adhesive tape) support for 12 to 14 days. An intentional wound dehiscence was induced in an additional 2 breasts for decompression as prophylaxis against an impending vascular complication. One case required skin graft closure. Reduction mammoplasty should obviously not be performed upon patients who have been taking therapeutic doses of steroids. A history of previous long-term steroid therapy should alert the surgeon to the possibility of a forced resumption of therapy if the patient's adrenal response proves inadequate.

Late Complications

Abnormal Scarring

Hypertrophic scarring, particularly involving the inframammary scar, has been the single most distressing complication in my experience. A hypertrophic scar developed somewhere, at some time during the healing period, in 65 percent of patients. Of those patients demonstrating hypertrophic changes, the inframammary scar was involved 80 percent of the time. The circumareolar scar was the next most commonly involved, although it should be the scar least affected by closure tension (which is often presumed to be related etiologically to scar hypertrophy). The younger patients manifested a greater tendency to hypertrophic scarring, a lesser tendency to resolve with time, and a greater tendency to recurrent scar hypertrophy with secondary revision. I have not yet discovered a particular suture material or type of wound management that seems to offer a distinctly reduced incidence of hypertrophic scarring.

Permanent Sensory Changes

Evaluation of areolar sensibility based upon subjective testing is difficult and unreliable even preoperatively, and it has generally not been seriously studied nor honestly reported. A recent study performed by Courtiss and Goldwyn [5] attempted a controlled and objective evaluation of areolar sensibility. They used a sensitive dental nerve stimulator, and found far greater apparent sensory effects from all sorts of breast surgery than have been previously recognized. Even operations, such as augmentation mammoplasty, that are thought to interfere only minimally with the anatomical integrity of the breast resulted in measurable changes in areolar innervation. In reduction mammoplasty, a substantial decrease in nipple-areolar sensibility was reported, regardless of the particular technique of glandular resection used. One would expect that, when the areola is circumcised and a major portion of the gland parenchyma is resected, the likelihood of denervation of the areola would be high. One would further expect that the risk of nipple denervation would to a degree vary directly with the percentage of parenchyma that had been resected. Thus the reduction of a 1,700-cc. breast to a 300-cc. volume would involve substantially different risks to areolar sensibility than the reduction of a 550-cc. breast to a 300-cc. volume. However, while this seems generally true, it does not correlate uniformly with clinical experience. I have observed on more than one occasion, for instance, the near total denervation of a nipple-areolar complex following a simple mastopexy dissection involving no glandular resection whatsoever.

Several publications over the years [5, 11, 12] have implied the existence of a special "nerve to the nipple," usually identified as the anterior branch of the fourth lateral cutaneous nerve. This nerve, so far best demonstrated in cadaver dissections by Edwards [12], is described as coursing around the lateral border of the pectoralis major muscle, then medially along the surface of the muscle to enter the deep aspect of the gland somewhere near the mid-breast meridian. It traverses the parenchyma deeply through the substance of the gland to end in the nipple. Although formal documentation of its course is as yet sparse, and a clinical definition of its actual sensory territory is only speculative, there appears to be a growing acceptance of its importance. Grabb [20] feels that a special attempt to protect the nerve has effectively reduced the incidence of areolar denervation. The protection of the nerve is accomplished by leaving behind 1 cm. of prepectoral soft tissue during glandular resection.

My technique for reduction mammoplasty markedly disrupts the normal anatomy of the breast, and a high degree of nipple sensory change is to be expected. In my series, 92 percent of breasts subjected to this type of dissection demonstrated some degree of reduction in nipple sensibility with the loss ranging from slight to total) immediately postoperatively. During the 6-month period following surgery, 80 percent of those breasts appeared to regain a variable amount of sensation; in the end, 22 percent of the total group were found to have normal or nearly normal sensibility. Eight percent of breasts remained totally and permanently anesthetic, while the remainder were left with varying degrees of reduced sensation. In a study that I performed utilizing anonymous questionnaires [39], it was of interest that of the group reporting an alteration in nipple sensibility, 65 percent stated that the change was of no concern to them whatsoever.

Late Loss of Shape

If the attractive classic breast shape is attained following reduction mammoplasty, it is almost never permanent. Despite numerous claims to the contrary, it has not yet been established that the tendency to late loss of shape varies with the technique of resection employed. The areola is more securely fixed to its surroundings than the gland bulk is to its surroundings despite scarring or any special techniques of parenchymal suspension. The result is a gravitational descent of the gland bulk, leaving the fixed areola behind as the infraareolar skin sling gives way under the weight. This produces the typical picture of the "dropped-out" breast, as illustrated in Figure 45-9. In my experience, this change occurred to a significant degree in 50 percent of cases after 1 year. It probably happens to some degree in all cases. If this tendency to secondary ptosis can be correlated to any single factor, it would likely be to postoperative breast size. Its best prevention, then, would lie in performing an adequate reduction so as to produce a smaller breast. Late loss of shape will form an infrequent complaint among a group of typical reduction mammoplasty patients, who have enjoyed a substantial reduction in their breast weight.

Recurrent Hypertrophy

Continued breast growth following reduction surgery has been reported [3], usually in association with rapidly progressive cases of virginal hypertrophy in whom surgical intervention was necessary at a younger age than usual. Whenever possible, reduction mammoplasty should be delayed until after the age of 16 years.

Interference with Capacity for Lactation

Reduction mammoplasty will generally eliminate the breast's ability to lactate, regardless of the surgical technique used, if a substantial amount of the parenchyma is resected. This should be considered as an inevitable consequence of the surgery rather than a complication. The surgeon is well advised to inform potential candidates of this fact if they are of child-bearing age.

Artistic Errors in Craftmanship

Of far greater incidence than postoperative medical complications is a heterogenous group of undesirable

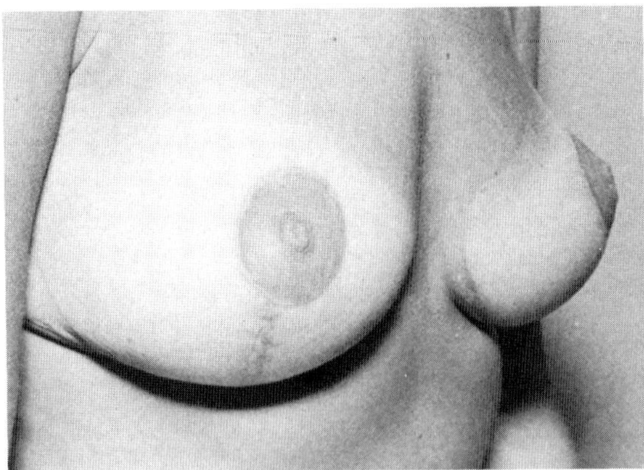

Fig. 45-9. Typical example of late loss of shape after 1 year. Distance from lower areolar edge to inframammary crease has increased from 5.5 cm. to 7.0 cm.

features that detract from the quality of the result and tend to reflect upon the artistry and judgment of the surgeon. This category includes errors such as the following:

1. *Symmetry.* The breasts may be asymmetric in size, shape, or nipple location.
2. *Contour.* There may be a square breast, medial and/or lateral fullness, a flat breast, or a cylindrical breast.
3. *Resection.* The procedure may have involved an inadequate or excessive resection, or an excessive resection in relation to the capacity of the skin envelope.
4. *Nipple malposition.* The nipple may have been placed too high, low, medial, or lateral.
5. *Areolar shape.* The areola may be a tear drop or oblique oval shape, tethered, too large or small, or asymmetrical in size.

A detailed analysis of the causes or prevention of each of these problems is beyond the scope of this chapter. Breast reduction surgery necessarily involves a continuous struggle with each of these elements, which constitutes the challenge of mammoplasty. Absolute mastery over them all would result in consistent perfection of results; this is a position only to be strived for but realistically never achieved. Beyond experience and an artistic aptitude on the part of the surgeon, I believe that the most effective means of limiting these errors lies in the utilization of total preoperative planning and a rigid adherence to that plan throughout surgery, reducing intraoperative decisions to a minimum.

CORRECTION OF PTOSIS OF THE BREAST

Mastopexy is classically the operation for the correction of mammary ptosis when no volume alteration is indicated. To be more in line with current practices, it might be more accurate to define the operation as one used for ptosis when no volume *reduction* is indicated. It is becoming increasingly popular to combine the repositioning of the nipple and uptake of excessive skin with augmentation mammoplasty in the treatment of the sagging, deflated breast. Under these circumstances the operation is still popularly referred to as a mastopexy (but in this case the procedure is a mastopexy with an implant). Etymologically, the word "mastopexy" implies a suspension of the breast; actually this is only one of its goals, but it is probably its least achieved goal.

The ingredients of a mastopexy include an elevation of the nipple-areolar complex, a contouring resection of excess skin, and sometimes an attempt to affix the gland bulk to its thoracic foundation. From a practical standpoint, the operation's most commonly realized objective is a recontouring of the breast; therefore it is, in the end, a mammoplasty. From a technical standpoint, it is a reduction mammoplasty in which no glandular resection is performed. The procedure employs the same basic maneuvers of nipple elevation and skin resection that are used in reduction mammoplasty, and the preoperative rules of design are the same. Beyond that, the two procedures diverge. In most cases, the surgical manipulation of the organ is done to a lesser extent than in breast reduction. The needed nipple elevation is usually less, the amount of skin resected is less, and the gland is not surgically violated. These differences in procedure lead to a corresponding decrease in the risk of vascular and sensory nerve injury to the areola and skin, the length of the inframammary scar, the operating time, the amount of blood loss, and the scope of postoperative complications. On the surface then, it would appear as though mastopexy is the lesser of the two procedures in terms of the needed investment of surgical craftsmanship. However, this is not so clearly the case. Mastopexy is a purely aesthetic operation, and the type of patient and her motive in seeking the surgery vary accordingly. The surgeon will sense a greater responsibility toward the artistic demands of the procedure. The patient will be more demanding in terms of the preciseness of contouring and symmetry; more concerned over the quality, location, and extent of the scars; and less willing to accept any functional alterations such as interference with sensibility and capacity for lactation. Perhaps most of all, the permanence of the result assumes a higher level of importance in the minds of both patient and surgeon than it does in reduction mammoplasty. In view of these differences, many surgeons consider mastopexy to be the more difficult of the two procedures.

Mastopexy and Augmentation Mammoplasty

The emergence of prosthetic implantation in the breast as a practical operation over the past two decades has probably affected the incidence of mastopexy and its place in plastic surgery. Some surgeons whose active practices have extended from the preimplant era to the present feel that mastopexy as a solitary procedure is less called for now than in the past. There are a significant number of patients presenting with simple ptosis who would have previously been subjected to mastopexy; today many of these patients, whether correctly or not, are being treated by breast implant alone. The mechanism for this procedure involves inflating rather than reducing an excessive skin envelope without the surgical repositioning of the nipple. The average patient will more readily accept the inherent drawbacks of a breast implant than the scars of a mastopexy, at least preoperatively, and the average surgeon will be subject to the same lure. In those patients in whom the skin envelope is not markedly excessive, and in whom *the nipple is not below the inframammary level,* this may be a practical and satisfactory solution to the problem. In the remaining majority of patients it will not.

The relationship of nipple height to the inframammary level is generally recognized as defining the indication for mastopexy. If the midpoint of the nipple distinctly falls below the inframammary level when the patient is erect, a proper breast contour cannot be accomplished by implantation of the breast alone. Attempts to treat borderline cases by the lower-than-usual placement of a larger-than-usual implant will usually result in borderline results at best. When the indications for mastopexy are present and an augmentation of volume is needed as well, the two procedures can safely be done at the same operation. The inclusion of a breast implant into the operative plan will introduce a special set of advantages and disadvantages not present in mastopexy alone. The advantages to be realized lie in the area of improved contour and its permanence. The ballooning of the skin envelope by a centrally placed bolus will accomplish what the surgeon is attempting to accomplish by glandular shaping and intraparenchymal suturing procedures. More important, perhaps, there is the possibility that the implant capsule firmly based upon the pectoral fascia will provide a balcony-like support for the implant, which will affect the longevity of the result. It is my opinion that it is easier to achieve a good breast contour with mastopexy than it is to keep it, and the inclusion of a breast implant into the operative plan, if otherwise indicated, will do more to combat late loss of shape than any of the many technique modifications described.

At the same time, the inclusion of a breast implant will introduce a disadvantage that must be weighed against this theoretical advantage. The breast now becomes subject to all of the possible complications inherent in augmentation mammoplasty, the most significant being capsular contracture causing a firm breast. The incidence of clinically significant capsular contracture in breast implant surgery is probably higher than anyone has yet been inclined to admit, presenting a real drawback to the procedure. Until the high incidence of this undesirable phenomenon becomes substantially reduced, these advantages and disadvantages must be fully discussed with the patient before deciding upon the combined operation.

The decision of whether or not to use an implant and of the appropriate size of implant will depend upon the surgeon's judgment of the adequacy of existing parenchymal volume measured against the patient's expressed desire for a particular final breast size. In my experience, a 140-cc. implant has been the most frequently used size.

Breast Suspension

Goulian [16] coined the term "dermal mastopexy," which has become popularly accepted for reasons not intended by its author. Many surgeons have felt that this term simply described the "skin brassiere" nature of gland shaping and suspension in mastopexy. Actually, the term was intended to imply a dermis-to-dermis adhesion between buried, deepithelialized surfaces that, it was hoped, would provide support of the gland weight. The concept is appealing and has caught the fancy of other authors as well. Lalardrie [30] visualizes a similar phenomenon, which forms the basis for his "dermic vault" operation for reduction mammoplasty. Buried, deepithelialized dermal strips interlaced through the pectoral muscle form the principal feature of Hinderer's approach to reduction mammoplasty and mastopexy [21–23]. I initially [35] visualized the buried dermal surface of the inferior pedicle of my reduction mammoplasty technique as persisting and forming a suspensory hammock for the breast mass above it. However, I now feel that, in my operation at least, this phenomenon simply does not occur. The inability of normal intact skin to support relatively minor amounts of weight over a period of time is clearly apparent in a multitude of clinical situations observed in daily practice. The fate of buried dermis that has been deepithelialized by freehand dissection has not been objectively studied; in my opinion, its persistence as an unyielding collagenous sling is at least suspect.

The principal causative factor underlying mammary ptosis as well as secondary loss of shape following mastopexy is gravity, which despite many well-intended technical efforts designed to combat it, will probably win out in the long run if given sufficient mass to work upon. Many authors claim that a specific pattern of skin resection possesses a unique ability to maintain breast shape, but these claims, along with the value of glandular shaping and retromammary suspensory techniques, have yet to be validated. Meanwhile, it must be concluded that the basis for breast contouring and support is the skin brassiere; its permanence is more related to the bulk of the breast than any other single factor.

Techniques of Mastopexy

Since most hypertrophic breasts are also ptotic, reduction mammoplasty and mastopexy share a close relationship in method. Reduction mammoplasty can be considered to be a mastopexy in which a reduction in parenchymal mass is included. Most commonly used techniques for breast reduction can be used for mastopexy by simply eliminating the glandular resection. The lateralizing techniques as described previously (see pp. 739–740) may be used in this regard without substantial alteration. These techniques function best when smaller amounts of skin resection and nipple elevation are needed. This fact plus their advantage in eliminating scarring in the intermammary area makes the lateralizing techniques particularly well suited to mastopexy.

Technique of Dufourmentel and Mouly

The technique of Dufourmentel and Mouly was originally introduced as a modification of the "periwinkle-shell operation" [8] for the correction of mammary ptosis, and was later expanded into a method of breast reduction. When used as a mastopexy, no gland is resected, but an inferiorly based dermoglandular flap of lateral breast tissue is rotated superiorly and medially into a retromammary pocket; that flap is then sutured to the posterior aspect of the gland. The nipple is moved slightly upward and medially, and closure results in the same oblique scar that is found in the breast reduction operation. Schatten and coworkers [57, 58] have popularized the technique in the United States, and they have introduced modifications, including fixation of the rotated flap to the periosteum of the third rib.

Technique of Regnault

This is performed essentially as described previously (p. 739) except that only the skin is resected from the lower part of the B. This technique would seem to possess the added advantage of a relatively greater resection of skin from the circumareolar area, where the skin is most stretched, rather than from the periphery of the breast.

Techniques Involving Resection of Circumareolar Skin

Numerous authors over the years [4, 27, 42, 43, 59], perhaps recognizing the fact that the excessive skin envelope is relatively more stretched centrally than peripherally, or more probably in an effort to avoid scarring elsewhere on the breast, have attempted to reduce the skin envelope by resection of principally circumareolar skin. The advantages to this technique are as obvious as its limitations. It is generally applicable only to minor degrees of skin excess. Primary closure after excision of a circumareolar cuff of skin requires the approximation of concentric skin edges of unequal circumferences. This can be accomplished up to a point, relying upon the contraction of the greater circle of thinner skin, and/or the expansion of the areolar circumference. Beyond this point equalization of the two excisional edges is necessary. Multiple V excisions from the peripheral skin edge (as described by Noël and Lopez-Martinez [42] and Claoué [4]) result in a radial pattern of scarring that most will consider unacceptable by present-day standards. The excision of a single V wedge from the inferior margin of the outer circle will result in a most acceptable vertical linear scar from areola to inframammary fold, as stressed by Regnault [53]. When the length of this scar exceeds the ideal 5 to 6 cm., however, Morgan [41] has found that a compensating horizontal excision is needed. Beyond the moderate degrees of mammary ptosis, the skin excision must extend to include peripheral portions of the envelope.

The Author's Technique

I make no claim of originality in the technique to be described. It is a technique that most resembles that described by Goulian [16], and bears no relationship to the technique of breast reduction that I have described except in the preoperative planning and skin marking. The rationale underlying my approach to mastopexy is based upon the following points, which I feel are true although they are not necessarily accepted as axiomatic:

1. The most ideal location for breast scars are: down the inferior breast meridian and along the inframammary sulcus, so long as the latter scar does not extend beyond the overhang of the breast medially.
2. The smaller the breast envelope to be reduced, the less extensive the inframammary scar will be, medially and laterally.
3. When the vascular pedicles of the breast are respected and the gland is not surgically violated by incisions into it or excisions from it, there is no justification for the creation of a deepithelialized dermal bridge for vascular protection of the nipple.
4. Some skin undermining is necessary, as shown in

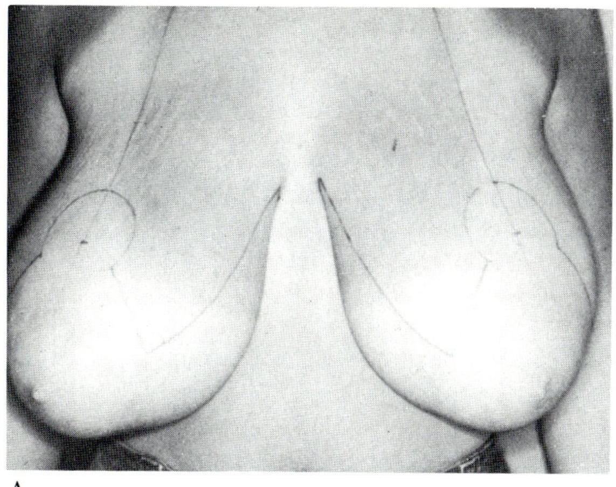
A

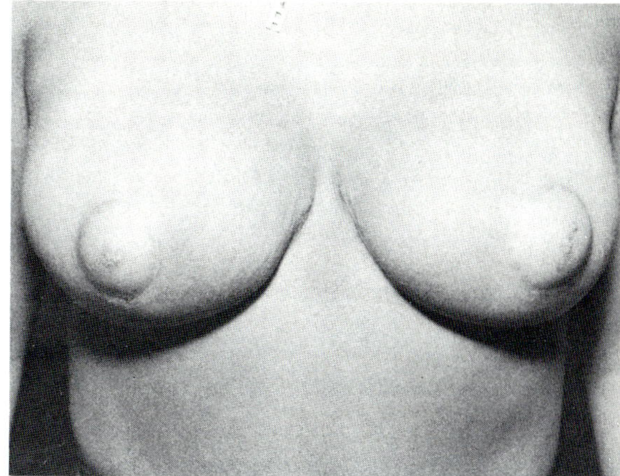
B

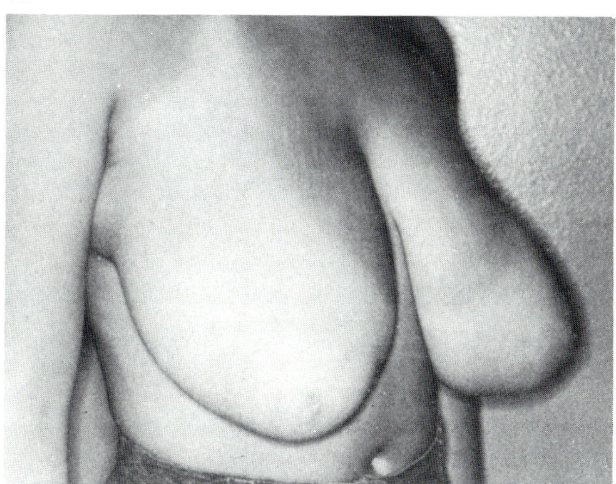
C

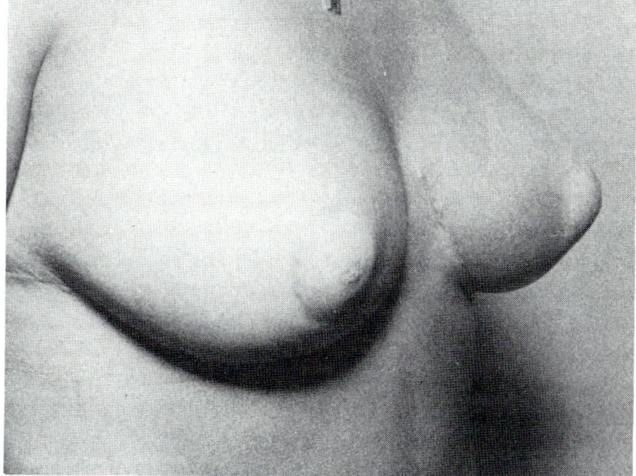
D

Fig. 45-10. Representative case using the author's technique of reduction mammoplasty. A, preoperative frontal view, showing pattern markings. B, postoperative frontal view after resections of 900 gm. and 1,040 gm. from the left and right breasts respectively, C, preoperative oblique view. D, postoperative oblique view.

Figure 45-10, to accomplish adequate repositioning of the gland mass with respect to skin, and to facilitate closure.

5. Some retromammary undermining is necessary posteriorly in order to accomplish adequate repositioning of the gland mass with respect to its thoracic foundation.
6. The axillary tail must be mobilized and repositioned in order to attain a proper contour.

PREOPERATIVE PLANNING AND PATTERN DESIGN. The planning and marking procedure is identical to that done for my technique of reduction mammoplasty (Fig. 45-6). All measurements and markings are performed with the patient fully erect, and the nipple height is determined in relation to the inframammary fold transposed to the face of the breast (Fig. 45-11A). The inframammary fold should be marked for reference to its medial termination, but the inferior edge of the medial skin flap need not be drawn preoperatively, because this will be determined at closure (Fig. 45-11B).

OPERATIVE TECHNIQUE. Surgery may be performed under local or general anesthesia with the patient in a semisitting position. The circumareolar incision site is marked around its natural pigmentary border or according to a template 37 mm. in diameter, whichever is the smaller. The areola is circumcised along this marking either for its full thickness or part of the way into the dermis if the proximity of the skin pattern will allow a narrow collar of deepithelialized

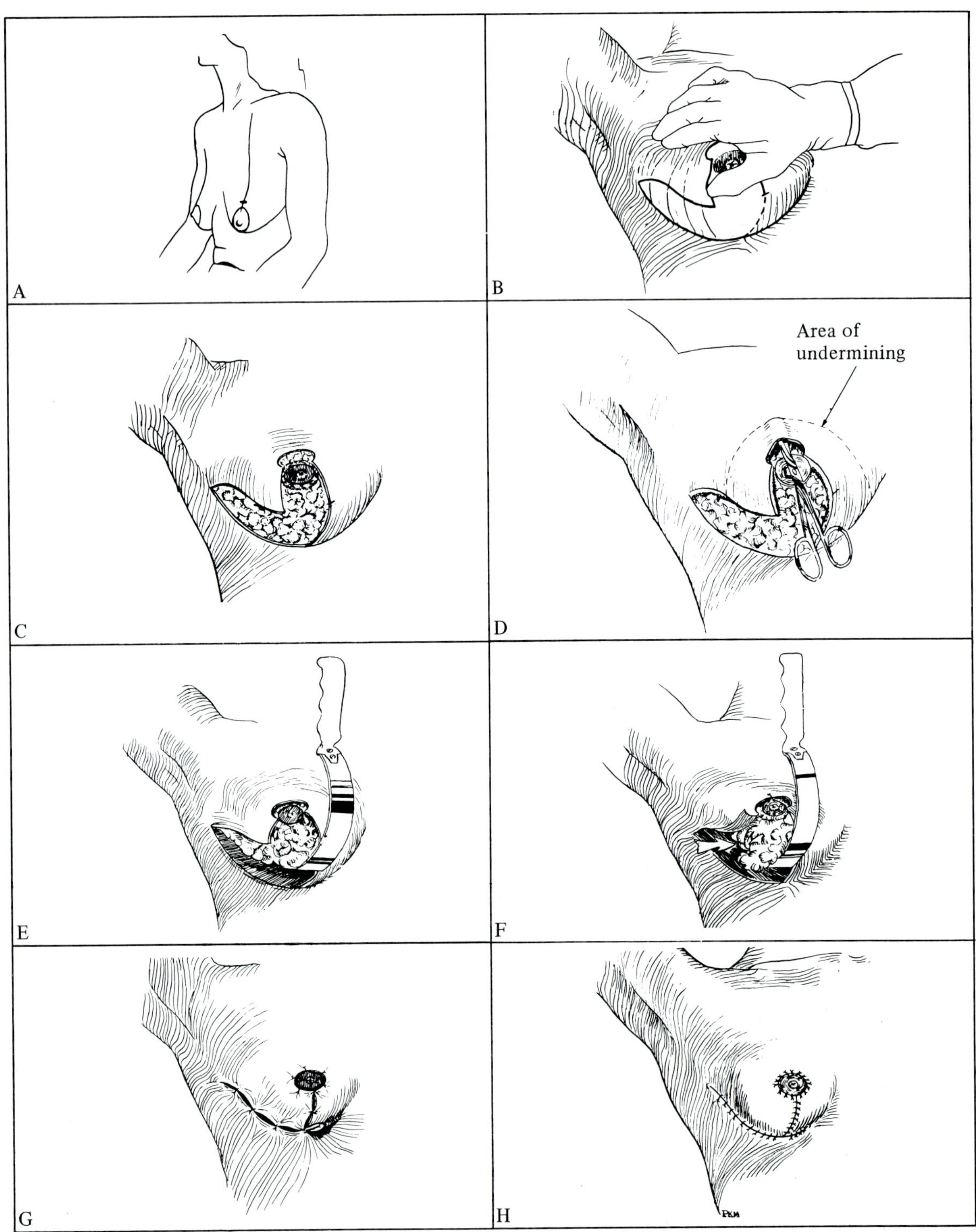

Fig. 45-11. The author's technique of mastopexy. (See text for further explanation.)

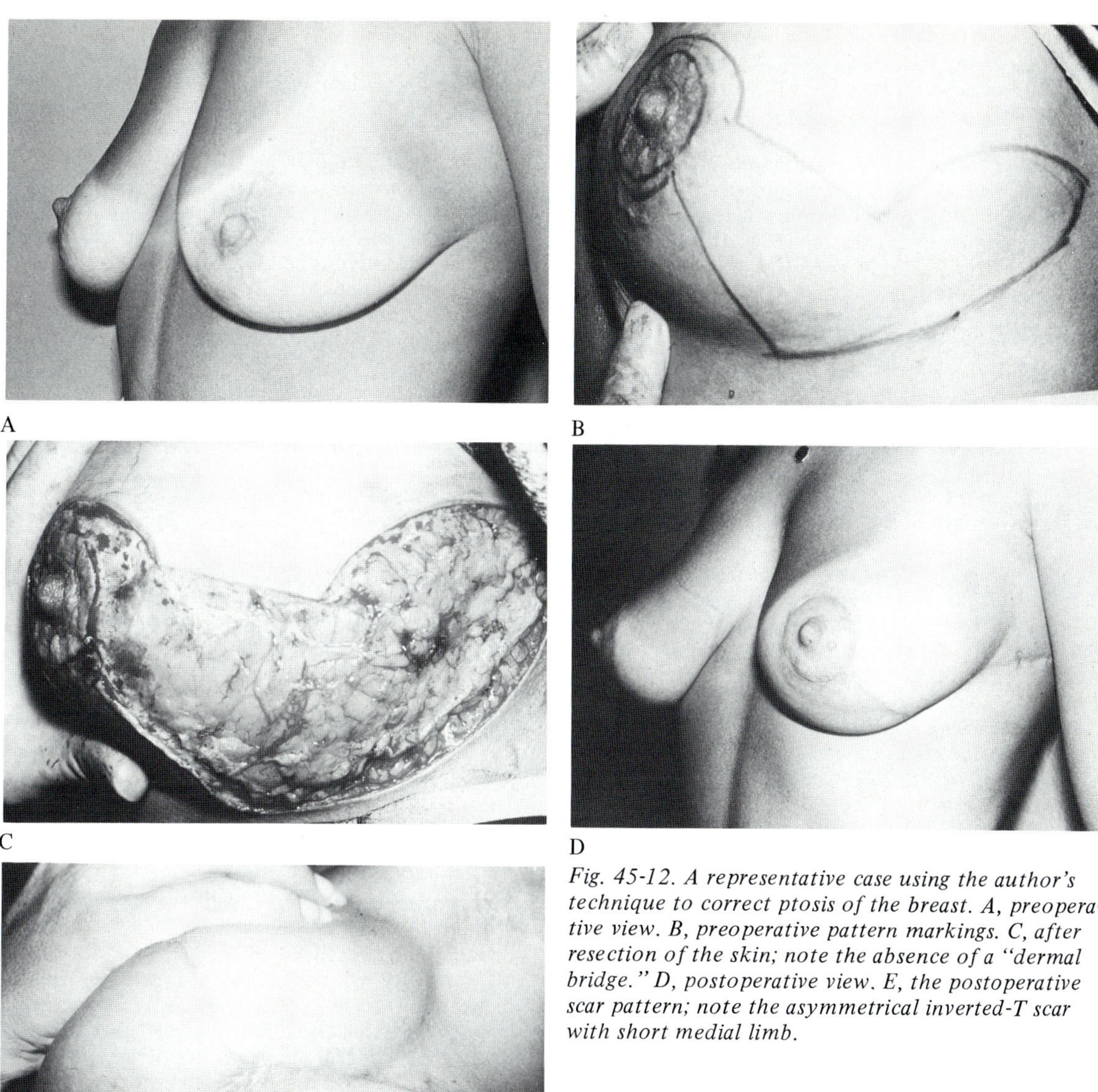

Fig. 45-12. A representative case using the author's technique to correct ptosis of the breast. A, preoperative view. B, preoperative pattern markings. C, after resection of the skin; note the absence of a "dermal bridge." D, postoperative view. E, the postoperative scar pattern; note the asymmetrical inverted-T scar with short medial limb.

circumareolar skin (Fig. 45-11C). The full thickness of the remaining skin inside the pattern is resected down to the subcutaneous fat. The skin beneath the medial flap is not excised at this point.

The skin is undermined enough to allow easy flap closure and elevation of the gland mass inside the skin envelope (Fig. 45-11D). The gland is separated from the pectoral fascia enough to allow elevation of its mass along the thorax (Fig. 45-11E). If a prosthetic implant is included in the operative plan, this undermining (as in "simple" augmentation mammoplasty) should be extensive enough to provide a pocket substantially larger than the implant to be used. The axillary tail is mobilized and rotated into the retromammary space and sutured to the posterior aspect of the gland (Fig. 45-11F). If an implant is to be used, it is inserted at this point while the breast is widely open (so it will exert its ballooning effect upon closure) and prior to dog-ear adjustment. The skin flaps are approximated in the midline and to the inframammary edge laterally, and the areola is sutured into its window. A "dog ear" will form medially, defining the extent of the medial skin excision (Fig. 45-11G). The operation is completed by excision of the medial dog ear along the medial inframammary fold marking, but only to the extent dictated by the size of the dog ear (Fig. 45-11H).

Wound closure is performed in two layers in all areas, using absorbable suture material such as 3-0 or 4-0 Dexon or Vicryl in the subcutaneous layer and a running, removable 4-0 Prolene subcuticular suture in the skin. A running, subcuticular suture of absorbable material simply left in place is preferred by many surgeons because it will eliminate the later discomfort of suture removal, but the possibility that it could cause some increased scar hypertrophy is still a matter of dispute. In any event, it seems widely agreed that any technique which avoids sutures penetrating the skin anywhere on the breast will be worth the extra effort invested.

The use of sterile Micropore paper adhesive tape strips (Steri-Strips) as a primary method of surface skin closure has a growing following today in many areas of plastic surgery. Its effectiveness in mammoplasty may be somewhat less than when used in the closure of flat surface defects, but the technique offers enough advantages to warrant further trial.

POSTOPERATIVE CARE. The suture lines are dressed with grease-impregnated gauze, and a snug, but not compressive, halter-type wraparound dressing is applied. After 48 hours, a dressing change is usually indicated; a simpler dressing is reapplied, just covering the suture lines and held in place by a comfortable commercial brassiere. The patient is encouraged to wear the brassiere continuously, day and night, for 6 weeks. Beyond this time, the advantage of the regular use of a supportive brassiere during the daytime is stressed to the patient. All removable subcuticular sutures are customarily removed 2 weeks following surgery, and the suture lines are reinforced by adhesive tape strips for an additional week or 10 days. Shoulder and arm motion is not felt to be detrimental enough to wound healing in the breast to warrant special restrictive rituals. The patient should avoid the direct pressure on the breasts that occurs when sleeping prone. Otherwise, most customary activities will not be injurious to the breast even during the early postoperative period; these activities are allowed if kept within the limits dictated by the discomfort they cause. The patient is simply instructed to stay within the limits of her discomfort but also to eliminate unnecessary vigorous exertion such as athletic activities for a few weeks.

If a prosthetic implant has been used in association with the mastopexy, mobilization of the implant throughout its cavity during the early postoperative period is currently in vogue, and it may be important in terms of preserving the size of the cavity larger than the implant. In the implanted breast, once the scar capsule has formed, it may well function as a supportive device and render the wearing of a brassiere obsolete, at least for the maintenance of shape. In the nonimplanted breast that has undergone mastopexy, a brassiere remains the last line of defense against gravity [Fig. 45-12).

REFERENCES

1. Bames, H. O. Reduction of massive breast hypertrophy. *Plast. Reconstr. Surg.* 3:560, 1948.
2. Biesenberger, H. *Deformitaten und Kosmetische Operationen der Weiblichen Brust.* Wien: Mandrich, 1931.
3. Castro, C. C. Subcutaneous mastectomy for gigantomastia in an adolescent girl. Case report. *Plast. Reconstr. Surg.* 59:575, 1977.
4. Claoué, C. Chirurgie réparatrice mammaire. Distribution de la peau sur le sein néoforme. *Bull. Soc. Med. Paris* 418, 1936.
5. Courtiss, E. H., and Goldwyn, R. M. Breast sensation before and after plastic surgery. *Plast. Reconstr. Surg.* 58:1, 1976.
6. Dufourmentel, C., and Mouly, R. Plastie mammaire par la méthode oblique. *Ann. Chir. Plast.* 6:45, 1961.
7. Dufourmentel, C., and Mouly, R. Developments récents de la plastie mammaire par la méthode oblique laterale. *Ann. Chir. Plast.* 10:227, 1965.
8. Dufourmentel, C., and Mouly, R. Modification of the periwinkle shell operation for small ptotic breasts. *Plast. Reconstr. Surg.* 41:523, 1968.
9. Dufourmentel, C., and Mouly, R. Mammaplasty

by the Lateral Method. *Transactions of the Fifth International Congress of Plastic and Reconstructive Surgery.* Melbourne, Australia: Butterworth, 1971.

10. Dufourmentel, C., and Mouly, R. Reduction Mammaplasty by the Lateral Approach. In Goldwyn, R. M. (Ed.), *Plastic and Reconstructive Surgery of the Breast.* Boston: Little, Brown, 1976.
11. Edgerton, M. T., and McClary, A. R. Augmentation mammaplasty, with special reference to use of polyvinyl alcohol sponge (Ivalon). Psychiatric implications and surgical indications. *Plast. Reconstr. Surg.* 21:279, 1958.
12. Edwards, E. A. Surgical Anatomy of the Breast. In Goldwyn, R. M. (Ed.), *Plastic and Reconstructive Surgery of the Breast.* Boston: Little, Brown, 1976.
13. Elbaz, J. S., and Verheeke, G. La cicatrice en L dans les plasties mammaires. *Ann. Chir. Plast.* 17:283, 1972.
14. Frantz, V. K., Pickren, J. W., Melcher, G. W., and Auchincloss, H., Jr. Incidence of chronic cystic disease in so-called "normal breasts": A study based on 225 post-mortem examinations. *Cancer* 4:762, 1951.
15. Gillies, H., and McIndoe, A. H. The technique of mammoplasty in conditions of hypertrophy of the breast. *Surg. Gynecol. Obstet.* 68:658, 1939.
16. Goulian, D., Jr. Dermal mastopexy. *Plast. Reconstr. Surg.* 47:105, 1971.
17. Goulian, D., Jr. Ptosis and Its Correction. In Goldwyn, R. M. (Ed.), *Plastic and Reconstructive Surgery of the Breast.* Boston: Little, Brown, 1976.
18. Goulian, D., Jr. Dermal Mastopexy. In Perras, C. (Ed.), *Clinics in Plastic Surgery,* Vol. 3. Philadelphia: Saunders, 1976.
19. Grabb, W. C. Comment on McKissock, P. K. Correction of Macromastia by the Bipedicle Vertical Dermal Flap. In Goldwyn, R. M. (Ed.), *Plastic and Reconstructive Surgery of the Breast.* Boston: Little, Brown, 1976.
20. Grabb, W. C. Personal communication, 1977.
21. Hinderer, U. T. Plastia mamaria modelante de dermopexia superficial y retromamaria. *Rev. Esp. Cir. Plast.* 5:65, 1972.
22. Hinderer, U. Remodeling Mammaplasty with Superficial and Retromammary Dermopexy. *Transacta der 3 Tagung der Vereinigung der Deutschen Plastichen Chirurgen,* Koln, 1972.
23. Hinderer, U. T. The Dermal Brassiere Mammaplasty. In Perras, C. (Ed.), *Clinics in Plastic Surgery,* Vol. 2. Philadelphia: Saunders, 1976.
24. Hollander, E. Die Operation der Mammahytrophie und der Hangebrust. *Dtsch. Med. Wochenschr.* 50:1400, 1924.
25. Hseuh, A. J., Peck, E. J., Jr., and Clark, J. H. Oestrogen receptors in the mammary gland of the lactating rat. *J. Endocrinol.* 58:503, 1973.
26. Joseph, J. *Nasenplastik und Sonstige Gesichtsplastik, nebst Mammaplastik.* Leipzig: C. Kabitsch. 1928.
27. Kausch, W. Die operation der mammahypertrophie. *Zentralbl. Chir.* 43:713, 1916.
28. Kraske, H. Dier Operation der Atrophischen und hypertrophischen Hangebrust. *Munch. Med. Wochenschr.* 70:672, 1923.
29. Lalardrie, J.-P. Reduction Mammaplasty for Hypertrophy with Ptosis. *Transacta der 3 Tagung der Vereinigung der Deutschen Plastichen Chirurgen,* Koln, 1972.
30. Lalardrie, J.-P. Technique de la Voute Dermique. In Lalardrie, J.-P., and Jouglard, J.-P. (Eds.), *Chirurgie Plastique du Sein.* Paris: Masson, 1974.
31. Lalardrie, J.-P., and Jouglard, J.-P. *Chirurgie Plastique du Sein.* Paris: Masson, 1974.
32. Lexer, E. Ptosis operation. *Klin. Monatsbl. Augenheilkd.* 70:464, 1923.
33. Maliniac, J. W. Arterial blood supply of the breast: Revised anatomic data relating to reconstructive surgery. *Arch. Surg.* 47:329, 1943.
34. Marc, H. La plastique mammaire par la méthode oblique. *Rev. Port. Obstét.* 5:363, 1952.
35. McKissock, P. K. A new approach to reduction mammaplasty: Preliminary report. Presented at the annual meeting of the California Society of Plastic Surgeons, Palm Desert, Calif., 1968.
36. McKissock, P. K. Reduction mammaplasty with a vertical dermal flap. *Plast. Reconstr. Surg.* 49:245, 1971.
37. McKissock, P. K. Correction of Macromastia by the Bipedicle Vertical Dermal Flap. In Goldwyn, R. M. (Ed.), *Plastic and Reconstructive Surgery of the Breast.* Boston: Little, Brown, 1976.
38. McKissock, P. K. Reduction Mammaplasty by the Vertical Bipedicle Flap Technique: Rationale and Results. In Perras, C. (Ed.), *Clinics in Plastic Surgery,* Vol. 3. Philadelphia: Saunders, 1976.
39. McKissock, P. K., and Barrett, B. Long-term results following reduction mammaplasty. Presented at the annual meeting of the California Society of Plastic Surgeons, Scottsdale, Ariz., 1974.
40. Meyer, R., and Kesselring, U. K. Reduction mammaplasty with an L-shaped suture line. *Plast. Reconstr. Surg.* 55:139, 1975.
41. Morgan, S. Mastopexy, the V-technique. Presented at the annual meeting of the California Society of Plastic Surgeons, Guadelajara, Mexico, 1977.
42. Noël, A., and Lopez-Martinez, M. Nouveaux

procédés chirurgicaux de correction du prolapsus mammaire. *Arch. Franco-Belg. Chir.* 31:138, 1928.
43. Padron, J. G. Mammareduktionsplastik. *Transacta der 3 Tagung der Vereinigung der Deutschen Plastichen Chirurgen,* Koln, 1972.
44. Penn, J. Breast reduction. *Br. J. Plast. Surg.* 7:357, 1954.
45. Penn, J. A Perspective and Technique for Breast Reduction. In Goldwyn, R. M. (Ed.), *Plastic and Reconstructive Surgery of the Breast.* Boston: Little, Brown, 1976.
46. Pitanguy, I. Breast Hypertrophy. *Transactions of the Second International Congress of Plastic Surgery,* London, 1959.
47. Pitanguy, I. Surgical treatment of breast hypertrophy. *Br. J. Plast. Surg.* 20:78, 1967.
48. Pitanguy, I. Breast Hypertrophy. *Transactions of the Fifth International Congress of Plastic and Reconstructive Surgery.* Melbourne, Australia: Butterworth, 1971.
49. Pitanguy, I. Personal Preferences for Reduction Mammaplasty. In Goldwyn, R. M. (Ed.), *Plastic and Reconstructive Surgery of the Breast.* Boston: Little, Brown, 1976.
50. Pitanguy, I., and Torres, E. T. Histopathological aspects of mammary gland tissue in cases of plastic surgery of the breast. *Br. J. Plast. Surg.* 17:297, 1964.
51. Ragnell, A. Operative correction of hypertrophy and ptosis of the female breast. *Acta Chir. Scand.* 94:113, 1946.
52. Regnault, P. Reduction mammaplasty by the "B" technique. *Plast. Reconstr. Surg.* 53:19, 1974.
53. Regnault, P. Reduction Mammaplasty by the "B" Technique. In Goldwyn, R. M. (Ed.), *Plastic and Reconstructive Surgery of the Breast.* Boston: Little, Brown, 1976.
54. Regnault, P. Breast Ptosis: Definition and Treatment. In Perras, C. (Ed.), *Clinics in Plastic Surgery,* Vol. 3. Philadelphia: Saunders, 1976.
55. Regnault, P., Hakstian, R. W., and Lauxon, G. Mammary Dysplasia, Total and Partial Subcutaneous Mastectomy. *Transactions of the Fifth International Congress of Plastic and Reconstructive Surgery.* Melbourne, Australia: Butterworth, 1971. P. 1189.
56. Ribiero, L. A new technique for reduction mammaplasty. *Plast. Reconstr. Surg.* 55:330, 1975.
57. Schatten, W. E., Hartley, J. H., Jr., Crow, R. W., and Griffen, J. M. Further experience with lateral wedge resection mammaplasties. *Br. J. Plast. Surg.* 28:37, 1975.
58. Schatten, W. E., Hartley, J. H., Jr., and Hamm, W. G. Reduction mammaplasty by the Dufourmentel-Mouly method. *Plast. Reconstr. Surg.* 48:306, 1971.
59. Schrudde, J. Eine Methode der Mammaplastik. *Transacta der 3 Tagung der Vereinigung der Deutschen Plastichen Chirurgen,* Koln, 1972.
60. Schwartzmann, E. Uber Ein Neue Methode der Mammaplastik. *Wien. Med. Wochenschr.* 86:100, 1936.
61. Shyamala, G., and Nandi, S. Interactions of $6{,}7\text{-}^{3}H$ 17B – estradiol with the mouse lactating mammary tissue in vivo and in vitro. *Endocrinology* 91:861, 1972.
62. Skoog, T. A technique of breast reduction; transposition of the nipple on a cutaneous vascular pedicle. *Acta Chir. Scand.* 126:453, 1963.
63. Sloss, P. T., Bennett, W. A., and Clagett, O. T. Incidence in normal breasts of features associated with chronic cystic mastitis. *Proc. Mayo Clin.* 33:1181, 1957.
64. Strömbeck, J. O. Mammoplasty: Report of a new technique based on the two pedicle procedure. *Br. J. Plast. Surg.* 13:79, 1960.
65. Strömbeck, J. O. Macromastia in women and its surgical treatment. *Acta Chir. Scand.* [Suppl. 341] 1964.
66. Strömbeck, J. O. Reduction Mammoplasty. In Gibson, T. (Ed.), *Modern Trends in Plastic Surgery.* London: Butterworth, 1964.
67. Strömbeck, J. O. Reduction Mammoplasty for Television Demonstration. *Transactions of the Fifth International Congress of Plastic and Reconstructive Surgery.* Melbourne, Australia: Butterworth, 1971.
68. Strömbeck, J. O. Reduction mammoplasty. *Surg. Clin. North Am.* 51:453, 1971.
69. Strömbeck, J. O. Reduction Mammoplasty. In Grabb, W. C., and Smith, J. W. (Eds.), *Plastic Surgery: A Concise Guide to Clinical Practice* (2nd ed.). Boston: Little, Brown, 1973.
70. Strömbeck, J. O. Reduction Mammoplasty by Upper and Lower Glandular Resections. In Goldwyn, R. M. (Ed.), *Plastic and Reconstructive Surgery of the Breast.* Boston: Little, Brown, 1976.
71. Thorek, M. *Plastic Surgery of the Breast and Abdominal Wall.* Springfield, Ill.: Thomas, 1942.
72. Varma, K., Driscoll, S. G., Emerson, K., Jr., and Selenkow, H. A. Clinical and pathologic evaluation of serum immuno-reactive human placental lactogen (IR-HPL) in abnormal pregnancy. *Obstet. Gynecol.* 38:487, 1971.
73. Wise, R. L. Preliminary report on a method of planning the mammaplasty. *Plast. Reconstr. Surg.* 17:367, 1956.
74. Wise, R. L. Further experience with reduction mammaplasty. *Plast. Reconstr. Surg.* 32:12, 1963.
75. Wise, R. J. Breast Reduction with Nipple Trans-

plantation. In Goldwyn, R. M. (Ed.), *Plastic and Reconstructive Surgery of the Breast.* Boston: Little, Brown, 1976.

76. Wittliff, J. L., Hilf, R., Brooks, W. F., Jr., Savlov, E. D., Hall, T. C., and Orlando, R. A. Specific estrogen-binding capacity of the cytoplasmic receptor in normal and neoplastic breast tissues of humans. *Cancer Res.* 32:1983, 1972.

Management of Benign and Premalignant Disease of the Female Breast

ROBERT M. ONEAL AND WILLIAM W. BLACKBURN II

Cancer of the breast is the most common neoplasm in females. Approximately 7 percent, or 1 out of every 13 women, will develop breast cancer during her lifetime. In 1975, there were nearly 90,000 new cases reported in the United States. Breast cancer is also the leading cause of *cancer deaths* in women as well as the leading cause of deaths from all causes in women age 40 to 44. Nearly 33,000 deaths in the United States during 1975 can be attributed to breast cancer. Another way of appreciating its significance is that approximately every 15 minutes one women in the United States dies of cancer of the breast [76]. There is general agreement that the earlier the diagnosis, the more favorable should be the long-term survival rate. However, the age-adjusted death rate has not improved appreciably over the last 20 years [36a, 76]. By the time present technology can detect a breast cancer, the carcinoma may have been present for a significant period of time and microscopic metastases may have already occurred [52].

Obviously, these startling statistics point up the importance of finding a preventative approach to breast cancer.

IDENTIFYING THE HIGH-RISK PATIENT

The Pap test, associated with massive public and physician education leading to early diagnosis of preinvasive lesions, has been associated with the decrease in mortality due to cancer of the uterine cervix from 28 to 11 per 100,000 during the last 30 years [109]. Unfortunately a single diagnostic screening test to identify premalignant precursors of cancer of the breast is not yet available, so that it has been difficult to select those patients who should be candidates for prophylactic removal of breasts involved with premalignant change as a means of cancer prevention.

Mammography has emerged as an extremely valuable noninvasive tool for diagnosis of early nonpalpable breast cancers, but its predictability to identify premalignant changes has not been established [48]. Modern techniques of mammography have reduced the radiation dose to a fraction of what it was 10 years ago. The present state of the art would indicate that the risk of mammography, if any, is minimal when contrasted with the results of early diagnosis and treatment of breast cancer [30]. This should reduce the concern over its cancer-inducing potential. Recent guidelines have been proposed for the rational nonroutine diagnostic use in women under 50 years of age [76]. Hopefully additional refinements in xeromammography, thermography, and ultrasound will add to their diagnostic value. Wolfe's [122] approach of grading mammograms in terms of risk factors may be one promising means of identifying high-risk patients. In a retrospective study of 7,214 patients, he showed that by classifying mammograms according to the prominence of their duct pattern he can sort out a small group he calls *dysplastic* (DYS). That group constitutes 7 percent of the study population but it may have as many as 30 percent of the carcinomas [122]. When he included those patients with slightly less dysplasia but a very *prominent duct pattern* (P2), the two groups together contained as many as 80 percent of the patients who develop carcinoma. Since the dysplastic findings normally disappear with aging, their presence after the age of 40 is most significant. There is still controversy over the interpretation of these findings, but the work seems quite important. It may indicate that the stimulus for the development of cancer also produces (or is associated with) a prominent duct pattern and acts to prevent the normal regression of mammary dysplasia. To date there has not been a prospective study of the relationship between the radiological findings in the high-risk group and specific pathological features which constitute their breast tissue.

Techniques of breast duct cytology and contrast mammography are beginning to be evaluated and may be useful adjuncts in the future [109]. Promising investigations into breast tissue immunology may lead to the development of skin or blood diagnostic tests [109]. McDivitt has provided an excellent review of current concepts of factors associated with increased risk of breast cancer [81a].

Leis [74] has stated that the development of breast cancer does not appear to be a chance event or to occur randomly. A variety of interrelated genetic, environmental, sociobiological, and physiological factors appear to be associated with an increased risk of breast cancer, but no single factor or combination of variables presently known is sufficient to explain the etiology of the disease [74]. Carcinogenesis appears to involve a constellation of risk factors, with environmental and genetic forces exerting influence in the duel between the potential for tumor growth and the resistance of the host [74].

Based on our assessment of the literature we have concluded that the following seem to be the most significant of the high-risk factors:

1. Previous cancer in one breast.
2. Strong family history of breast cancer. Particular significance is attached to the premenopausal or bilateral cancer in a mother or sister [2, 79a, 95].
3. Histological changes defined as *precancerous mastopathy* [14, 15] (see the discussion of pathological classification, pp. 761–765).
4. Infertility or age greater than 30 at first pregnancy [74].
5. A classification of DYS or P2 in Wolfe's [122] method of grading mammograms.

As McDowell [82] has pointed out, it seems reasonable to assume that the prophylactic removal of 95 to 99 percent of the breast tissue in those women with an expected higher incidence of breast cancer would significantly reduce the incidence of and thereby deaths from cancer of the breast. It seems reasonable and justified to follow this course even though irrefutable evidence is not available. Long-term prospective studies should help delineate more accurately the high-risk patient and provide us with the evidence we need to establish a more sound scientific basis for the prevention of breast cancer. At the present state of the art, prophylactic reconstructive mastectomy cannot be considered a cancer operation, and it is certainly not primarily an aesthetic one. It is simply an attempt to remove as much breast tissue as possible in a susceptible high-risk patient group and to provide prosthetic reconstruction to an acceptable aesthetic level as a compromise women will accept [50a].

BASIC BIOLOGY AND HORMONAL ACTIONS

The breast is composed of three types of tissue: epithelium, fibrous tissue, and fat. The epithelium is found in large and small ducts and terminal lobular acini. There are normal variations in the proportion of these elements; these variations seem to be influenced by the interaction of hormones during the menstrual cycle, in pregnancy, and even in the postmenopausal period [89]. These effects are not uniform and may vary from cycle to cycle in the same female.

An excellent review of the hormonal actions on the female breast has been presented by Sawin [105]. Although the major hormones and their action have been identified, many of the details of their regulation and specific action a e as yet unclear.

Among other actions, the *estrogens* stimulate proliferation of the ducts and fibrous tissue. Of the three fractions *estradiol* is a stronger estrogen than *estrone.* Both may stimulate ductal epithelial hyperplasia, both have been considered etiological factors in atypical hyperplasia [74, 76], and both are powerful promoters of carcinogenesis [75]. The third fraction, *estriol,* has a minimal estrogenic effect; it is believed to be antagonistic to the carcinogenic effects of the other two fractions [78].

Progesterone, produced by the corpus luteum, influences the maturation of acini and the development of the alveolar lobules. These actions depend on the estrogens for their priming effect on the ductal system. Progesterone also appears to exert a direct antagonistic effect on estradiol [74].

Prolactin, secreted by the anterior pituitary, causes milk secretion and further acinar maturation. It seems to enhance the tissue binding of estradiol.

Kirschner [69], in a recent review on the role of hormones in the etiology of breast cancer, stated that in spite of some limited data linking breast cancer development with possible alterations in endocrine function, no comprehensible or clear-cut patterns are yet evident.

PATHOLOGICAL CLASSIFICATION

A classification of benign and premalignant diseases of the female breast appears in the following outline.

- I. Benign proliferative breast disease.
  - A. Fibrocystic disease.
    - 1. Cysts, due to dilatation of ducts; they may be solitary or multiple, gross or microscopic.
    - 2. Fibrosis of stroma, perilobular and/or intralobular.
    - 3. Adenosis, which represents *elongation* of lobular ducts rather than *intraductal* hyperplasia.
      - a. Blunt duct, with small ducts that end blindly.
      - b. Florid, involving a lobular pattern in small scattered foci.
      - c. Sclerosing, involving a lobular pattern with invasion of fibrous stroma and marked secondary fibrosis.
    - 4. Apocrine metaplasia, with transformation of normal cuboidal epithelium that lines ducts into columnar type.
    - 5. Intraductal epithelial hyperplasia, with proliferation of normal cuboidal epithelium that lines the ducts and acini; this may occur in solid or circumferential forms or may be a result of cell layering transition into a papillary variety. (Both apocrine metaplasia and intraductal epithelial hyperplasia can show progressive proliferative changes going on to atypia.)
  - B. Adenofibroma.
  - C. Cystosarcoma phylloides.

D. Intraductal papilloma.

II. Noninvasive carcinoma.

A. Intraductal (in situ) carcinoma.

1. Papillary type.
2. Comedo type.

B. Lobular carcinoma in situ (lobular neoplasia).

Benign Proliferative Breast Disease

Benign Fibrocystic Disease

Benign fibrocystic disease of the breast appears to be a variabion of the *normal* amounts of epithelium, fibrous tissue, and fat in the breast. These changes are reported to be present in 50 percent of all female breasts microscopically and 20 percent clinically. Much of the confusion surrounding the significance of fibrocystic disease and its etiological relationship to developing breast cancer is due to the confusion in terminology [60].

Clinicopathological studies of the relationship of fibrocystic disease to cancer of the breast have included retrospective and prospective studies, analysis of noncancerous areas of cancerous breasts, and autopsy comparisons of cancerous and noncancerous breasts [60]. In analyzing any study, it is important to know the pathological classification used and whether noninvasive foci of breast cancer were included with other forms of benign disease. Although some studies have concluded that there is an increased incidence of carcinoma associated with cystic disease [27, 115], many others disagree [81a]; Devitt [29] strongly decried "terrorizing women by insisting on this relationship."

Haagensen has recently noted that there is four times the normal incidence of breast cancer in long-term follow-up of patients with gross cystic disease [54]. The observation that the subsequent carcinomas were not related to the location of the previous cysts and that they were as common on the contralateral side suggests there may be a more specific etiological factor. The simultaneous incidence of carcinoma in gross cysts is low [103].

The search for a definite *precancerous lesion* has been long, diligent, and progressive [60]. Charteris [20] in 1930 and many others have concluded that atypical epithelial hyperplasia of both large and small ducts is the *lesion of significance* [14, 29, 36, 44, 84]. The observation that epithelial atypical hyperplasia of large ducts may be precursors to the development of invasive carcinoma [68, 114] lends special significance to the practice of deliberately leaving ductal tissue associated with the nipple-areolar complex at the time of prophylactic breast gland removal [89]. Gallagher and Martin [44], on the basis of whole organ studies, showed that every breast containing a primary cancer showed epithelial hyperplasia in ducts or lobules or both. However, they felt that the progressive change in ductal epithelium from normal to hyperplastic to atypical hyperplasia to malignancy was *nonobligatory* and that the progression could terminate at any point or might even regress [44, 45]. The qualification placed on atypical hyperplasia by Gallagher limiting it to the status of a nonobligate precursor stimulates speculation about the relative risks of various types of hyperplasia [71]. Jensen and associates [64a] suggested there was indirect evidence supporting atypical lobules as a premalignant marker after finding a higher association with carcinomatous breasts than with breasts having routine biopsies in similar age women. Some doubt was raised regarding the predictive value of these atypical changes as a marker when Cramer and Rush [71] found an incidence of 40 percent of atypical epithelial change in routine autopsies of elderly women not associated with breast cancer. Black and Chabon [15] have developed a classification allowing for specific pathological description of the type of ducts, the extent of disease, and the grading of proliferative variants [14, 15]. This has been well described by Leis [74]. The outline that follows gives the proposed progression of premalignant cellular changes, modified from Black and Chabron [15].

I. Types of cellular changes.

A. Normal cellular structure.

B. Hyperplasia; the multilayering of epithelium includes both myoepithelial and epithelial lining cells with and without intraductal papillation. (The groups in which atypia is seen, namely groups 2, 3, and 4 below, constitute precancerous mastopathy.)

1. No atypia.
2. Distinct but minimal atypia; the cellular proliferation is typically monomorphic with some loss of polarity and increased nuclear/cytoplasmic ratio.
3. Atypia suggestive of in situ carcinoma, with progressive loss of cellular and nuclear polarity.
4. Atypia consistent with in situ carcinoma.

II. Specific duct transformation.

A. Large primary, major interlobular ducts → intraductal papillary or comedo carcinoma.

B. Terminal interlobular ducts → in situ ductular carcinoma.

C. Preterminal intralobular ducts → in situ lobular carcinoma.

D. Terminal intralobular ducts and acinar ductules → in situ lobular carcinoma.

Black and associates [14] studied patients with benign biopsies and compared those who later developed invasive cancer to patients who did not. Using this grading system, they found that patients with more than a moderate amount of atypia (but not at the level of in situ carcinoma) had a *five times* greater risk of developing invasive cancer than those without such atypia. If apocrine metaplasia was present, the relative risk was somewhat smaller.

Black and his co-workers combined cases of *moderate* and *severe cellular atypical hyperplasia* with cases of *in situ carcinoma* and called the entire group of lesions *precancerous mastopathy.* Interestingly, they felt that these changes also represented a favorable host response, since when cancer coexists with precancerous changes, the patients generally have a more favorable clinical stage and prognosis than patients with cancers that develop without the precancerous changes. This has also been suggested by the studies of Silverberg and associates [108].

Another study demonstrated that there is an upward trend in breast cancer incidence as the atypia score rises [70]. Askikari and co-workers [5], in a follow-up study of patients with atypical epithelial changes, found a risk of subsequent breast cancer of 4 percent at 30 months and 9 percent at 4 years. Also to be considered is that almost half of the later cancers that arose in a precancerous setting arose in the opposite breast [14, 60]. Recent studies resectioning breasts removed prophylactically in patients with contralateral breast cancer showed a high incidence of epithelial hyperplasia and cellular atypia, and occasional occult cancers [48a, 80b]. Gallagher [45] has also shown with his whole organ studies that as a histological lesion *bilaterality* of breast cancer may approach 100 percent. This suggest any prophylactic treatment logically needs to be bilateral.

There is experimental evidence to suggest that when estriol and progesterone are present in adequate amounts, the effect of estradiol in causing hyperplastic changes in breast epithelium is modified [74]. Also pregnancy, possibly through the increased levels of estriol and progesterone, exerts a protective influence on the development of premalignant lesions [74]. It is still not known whether the development of hyperplastic changes is due to an increase in estradiol, a decrease in estriol and/or progesterone, or some other imbalance between these factors [69, 74]. Peacock [89] suggests that in some cases atypical changes may be reversible with progesterone therapy. Only when the atypical changes are unresponsive does he feel that operation is indicated. He relies on four-quadrant needle biopsies for baseline evaluation and documentation. In our experience routine needle biopsies have not produced a specimen that can be reliably interpreted by the pathologists that we work with and a better method of diffusely sampling the breast is needed. The use of the drill biopsy (previously reported with tumors) should be evaluated [107].

It is now reasonably clear that there can be a progression from precancerous mastopathy to infiltrative cancer. Recent rodent studies have offered definite proof of the neoplastic potential of atypical tissue by demonstrating development of transplanted lesions into cancers [18]. This may show a way for further experimental work with human tissue. Not all premalignant lesions progress to malignancy; therefore there is still the question of which women (if any) with the diagnosis of premalignancy should be subjected to prophylactic surgery [81a]. A very significant study along this line by Gullino [52] has demonstrated that the progression from hyperplasia to neoplasia can be evaluated by determining whether human mammary tissue has acquired the capacity to induce angiogenesis (new blood vessel formation) in the iris of rabbits. Gullino states, "If angiogenic propensity of hyperplastic epithelium can identify a population of women with mammary parenchyma at higher risk of developing breast cancer, a powerful tool is available for predicting neoplastic transformation before clinical manifestations" [52]. It is obvious that multiple lines of evidence must converge to more definitely identify a cellular marker or precursor [80a]. When this marker can be more equivocally defined it can then be combined with multifactorial profiles of clinical risk factors and may help to more accurately define which women would really benefit from prophylactic mastectomy.

Adenofibroma

The adenofibroma is an extremely common lesion that frequently presents as a dominant mass with a peak incidence in the third decade of life. It consists of both proliferating fibrous and epithelial components. There are scattered reports of malignant degeneration but they are almost always benign [109]. Treatment by enucleation is satisfactory even when the lesion is quite large [24].

Cystosarcoma Phylloides

Cystosarcoma phylloides is a fibroepithelial tumor that may grow rapidly and to large proportions. The average age at onset is 45 years. The lesion may be related to fibroadenoma but transformation has not been shown [109]. Cystosarcomas are not truly encapsulated and require local excision with a margin of normal breast tissue. There are reports of malignant degeneration in approximately 6 percent of the cases [53]. The neoplasm acts like a sarcoma, and metastases are usually blood borne. In treatment of the large benign lesions, subcutaneous mastectomy with reconstruction may be indicated.

Intraductal Papilloma

Intraductal papillomas commonly involve a large

duct in the subareolar area; half of the time, the patient presents with a bloody discharge from the nipple. There seems to be an increased malignant potential after the age of 50 [74].

Treatment involves identification (aided by contrast mammography) [109] of the involved duct and complete local excision with margin of normal breast tissue when breast function is to be preserved. In older women complete excision of the central ducts and preservation of the nipple and areola are indicated [74]. Multiple intraductal papillomas may fill the ducts, and this process is usually peripheral to the central ducts. Although some feel that there is an increase in the malignant potential for this lesion [70], the increase is thought to be related to the degree of atypicality of the epithelial changes.

Noninvasive Carcinoma

Ductal Carcinoma in Situ (Intraductal Carcinoma)
Ashihari, Hajdu, and Robbins [4] reported 112 patients in whom they found no focus of invasive cancer. A dominant mass was found in 54 percent, some mammographic findings were seen in 74 percent, atypical hyperplasia was found in 75 percent, and multifocal in situ carcinoma was found in 32 percent. Most patients were treated with standard, modified mastectomy. Only one patient had positive axillary nodes (Level I), but 5 patients ultimately died of disseminated breast cancer; 4 of these 5 had advanced breast cancer on the other side.

One of the major problems in dealing with lesions regarded as intraductal carcinomas is the uncertainty about the presence of invasion. In one series of 38 patients, unexpected invasion was found at the time of mastectomy in 18 percent; 13 percent of the whole group had positive lymph nodes [19]. Residual intraductal carcinoma was found in 66 percent. Paget's disease was present in 5 patients. The logical surgical treatment, if the biopsy proves intraductal carcinoma, seems to be modified radical mastectomy [4, 19]. Even though the evidence of bilaterality is less than with lobular carcinoma in situ [4, 5], the fact that it does occur suggests the need for contralateral biopsy, close follow-up, and possibly simple mastectomy with reconstruction.

Lobular Carcinoma in Situ
Lobular carcinoma in situ has been termed *lobular neoplasia* by Haagensen [53] and in situ small cell lesion by Toker and Goldberg [115a]. The changes are usually found incidentally at the time of breast biopsy for other indications. It is most common in premenopausal women in their early forties [5]. There are no specific mammographic findings and there is almost never a palpable mass.

There is general agreement that the lesion is premalignant (although it may regress), it is clearly nonobligate, and it has a relatively slow expressivity to invasive carcinoma [63, 109]. McDivitt and associates [81] followed 40 patients treated by local excision and calculated the cumulative risk for subsequent development of invasive carcinoma as 15 percent at 10 years, 27 percent at 15 years, and 35 percent at 20 years. Hutter, Foote, and Farrow [63] followed a group of patients for 4 to 27 years; they suggest that excisions less than mastectomy would result in an increased risk of invasive carcinoma.

Ashikari, Huvos, and Snyder [5] found a 36 percent incidence of *multifocal lesions,* suggesting that a total mastectomy was the only logical surgical therapy. This view is supported by Lambird and Sheely [72], who noted that 48 percent of the in situ foci were close to the nipple and areola; they felt that removal of the nipple and underlying ducts is indicated.

Carter and Smith [19] found a 36 percent incidence of *bilaterality* of the in situ lesions; they contended that when the lesions were bilateral, there was a significant increase in synchronous invasive carcinoma. Anderson [3], in a follow-up of 44 patients with lobular carcinoma in situ, noted invasive cancer developing at 12 times the expected incidence. This was confirmed by Toker and Goldberg [115a]. He also noted a statistically similar ipsilateral and contralateral occurrence of the invasive carcinomas. Haagensen [53] and Wheeler and associates [119] share this view that both breasts should be treated in the same way, whatever treatment program is advised.

In a recent review Fisher and Fisher [35] propose an alternative view. They feel that there is uncertain significance of the multicentricity and a still unproved relationship between the in situ carcinoma and the invasive form. They recommend segmental mastectomy in the involved breast with low axillary lymph node dissection (axillary "sampling") and biopsy of the opposite breast based on mammographic and clinical findings. Similar recommendation is also advocated by Rosen and associates [102a]. Others, such as Wanebo, Huros, and Urban [117], have advocated modified radical mastectomy.

Several authors [3, 53, 119] have suggested that close clinical follow-up may be a better course than surgical ablation. Their reasons for this view include the relative youth of the patients, the nonobligate nature of the in situ lesions, the necessity of bilateral procedures, the long interval before invasive carcinoma develops, and the better prognosis if it does. However, it has also been shown that there may be as high as a 5 percent ten-year mortality from invasive carcinoma in patients followed with lobular carcinoma in situ [3]. In another series, when compared to the general population the deaths due to breast carcinoma were eleven times more frequent than expected [102a]. Many patients, when they are presented with the data regarding the risk of lobular carcinoma in situ, and they and their physicians are faced with the responsibility of lifetime surveillance [115a], may ask for an alternative course. It seems reasonable to us that if a patient could be offered a prophylactic removal of all the breast tissue possible (including the nipple and underlying ducts) and be assured of a reasonable reconstruction, this would be a satisfactory resolution of the dilemma for many of these patients. We also feel that at the time of the surgical procedure the areola could be free grafted; if the specimen mammography shows no suspicious lesion, then it seems reasonable to go ahead with prosthesis insertion as part of the same procedure when that seems indicated. From the foregoing discussion it seems obvious that none of the recommended choices are entirely satisfactory for all patients [102a] and the final answer may have to await more extensive prospective studies.

"MINIMAL" BREAST CANCER

There have been reports [24, 40, 41] that subcutaneous mastectomy could be considered an appropriate treatment for "minimal" breast cancer. Others [61, 111] have pointed out the dangers of leaving foci of breast cancer or potentially malignant tissue behind in the effort to leave a defect that can be more easily reconstructed [61]. It has also been pointed out that an invasive lesion as small as 1.0 cm. may represent 30 doubling times of a cancer and a certain percentage will have already disseminated [52, 61, 111]. We agree with Ackerman and Katzenstein [1] that the pathologist must be able to distinguish between in situ and invasive lesions. We feel that invasive carcinoma regardless of size should not be considered minimal and cannot be subjected to "minimal" surgery, but should be considered as any other invasive carcinoma.

SELECTION OF PATIENTS

Team Approach

A *team approach* is mandatory in the selection of patients for prophylactic breast surgery [85]. This approach should include an adequate consultation with a *general surgeon* experienced in the management of breast cancer. Current mammograms should be reviewed with an experienced *radiologist,* and any suspicious lesions should be thoroughly discussed as to the necessity of preliminary biopsy. In some breasts with diffuse changes, total breast tissue extirpation may be the only practical approach to analysis of this suspicious area. An experienced *pathologist* should review all of the previous biopsy material in light of the current pathological terminology.

Evaluation of the Patient

Each patient must be considered individually and her specific circumstances evaluated. Time must be taken with the patient to assess her understanding of the problem, the reasonableness of her expectations, and her psychological stability. Frequently, patients have become overwhelmed with the fear of having cancer that can't be controlled even with radical therapy including mastectomy. Thus, they easily become enamored with magical thoughts of having all their breast tissue removed and the idea that the prosthetic reconstruction will cause them to end up "better than ever." However, the patient must be resigned to the fact that all the breast tissue cannot be removed; since this is true, the operation cannot be considered 100 percent prophylactic. She must understand that it will be necessary to have *periodic clinical* and *radiological follow-up examinations* [50a]. She should also be made aware that in a large group of patients undergoing "prophylactic mastectomy" there has been reported a 6 percent incidence of occult breast cancer [93]. This unsuspected finding may necessitate a more radical procedure for that breast than the one that was originally described. The patient must understand that there is a high incidence of postoperative complications. She, and her husband, must be psychologically prepared for a possible delay of 3 to 6 months before prosthetic reconstruction. They must also understand that it is not realistic to anticipate a normal-looking or normal-feeling breast. An occasional patient may need a thorough psychological evaluation prior to arriving at a decision.

Indications for Prophylactic Mastectomy

Indications for operation have been proposed by many authors [8, 37, 42, 50, 50a, 85, 91, 92]. The following list includes indications that are considered the most significant. They become even more significant when there is more than one or when associated with one or more of the supportive indications in the list following this one.

1. *Biopsy proved precancerous mastopathy.*
2. *History of breast cancer in the maternal side of the family.*
3. *Previous invasive cancer of the other breast.* The risk is considered five times that of the general female population and women who developed their original cancer prior to age 50 had twice the risk of older women [81a]. Particularly significant is lobular cancer. If a patient survives cancer-free for ten years after the initial cancer, the risk of contralateral cancer may become greater than the risk of recurrence from the initial one [87].
4. *Multiple persistent or recurrent breast nodules*

requiring frequent biopsy. Particularly important if the nodularity or scarring from previous biopsy precludes adequate clinical assessment by an experienced *breast cancer surgeon*.

The following less definitive but supportive indications present frequently either singly or in combination are associated with the more definitive indications listed above.

1. Patient's age greater than 40.
2. Late onset of menses.
3. Infertility or first pregnancy after the age of 30.
4. Increasing anxiety of patient and her physician over the persistent increasing nodularity of the breasts. This can present as cancerophobia.
5. Mammographic density secondary to fibrous tissue proliferation associated with fibrocystic disease severe enough to obscure detection of early minimal breast cancer.
6. Xeroradiographic findings of Wolfe's P2 or PYS classification [122].
7. Severe mastodynia that is unresponsive to short courses of specific hormonal derivatives and other conservative medical management (such as diuretics and antihistamines) [89]. These patients must be thoroughly evaluated for other physical and psychological reasons for unremitting pain. According to Leis [74], the differential diagnosis of mastodynia should be pursued. Cervical or dorsal radiculitis, herpes zoster, duct ectasia and comedo mastitis, costochondral chondritis, and even breast cancer should be included in the differential diagnosis. We feel patients who meet criteria for operation with this condition are relatively rare. In those patients who do, *delayed prosthetic placement* is indicated so that both the patient and the surgeon can be convinced that the mastectomy has alleviated the pain before the variable of an implant is added (particularly when the implant is placed under the pectoralis major muscle).

PREOPERATIVE EVALUATION AND GENERAL TECHNICAL CONSIDERATIONS

The size of the breasts and the degree of ptosis and asymmetry must be accounted for in the operative plans. Since previous scars may determine where the incisions will be made, their presence, locations, and age should be noted. The thickness of the subcutaneous layer should be estimated as a help in determining the possibility of thin flaps and the likelihood of vascular impairment necessitating delayed implantation.

Since there is frequently a need for transfusion in these operations, autotransfusion is recommended. To eliminate the hazards of homologous transfusion, 1 or 2 units of blood are drawn from the patient during the 2 to 3 weeks prior to operation, and she is then placed on iron therapy. Cutler [26] recommends the use of hypotensive anesthesia.

Anatomical Considerations

An excellent review has been provided by Edwards [32]. The breast is a modified cutaneous appendage situated between the superficial and deep layers of the superficial fascia on the anterior chest wall. The gland extends from the second and third ribs to the sixth or seventh costal cartilage and from near the sternum to the anterior axillary line. In some patients thin layers of mammary tissue continue as far as the clavicle above, to the midline medially, to beyond the edge of the latissimus dorsi muscle laterally, and very close to the axillary skin. The connective tissue and epithelial elements of the breast are so closely interrelated that there is no plane of dissection within the substance of the gland itself.

Cooper's ligaments are peripheral projections of fibrous tissue that fuse with the superficial layer of the superficial fascia; they contain breast tissue reaching almost to the dermis [56]. Likewise, breast tissue may fuse with the muscle fascia and *may* extend between the muscle bundles of the pectoralis major.

To achieve the goal of carcinoma prophylaxis, resection of the breast tissue must be as complete as possible. But how well can this goal of breast tissue resection be met? Several studies have noted the futility of attempting a total removal of breast tissue by any procedure short of complete ablation and skin grafting [39, 49, 56]. Hicken [56], in a study of simple mastectomy, was able to demonstrate residual breast tissue in the majority of cases. With radiopaque injections he found mammary ducts present over the entire anterolateral chest. In 95 percent the ducts ascended into the axilla, and frequently followed the brachial plexus and blood vessels into the axillary fossa. In 15 percent some ducts passed downward and medially into the epigastric space and in 2 percent a few ducts extended beyond the anterior border of the latissimus dorsi muscle. Rubin [104a] reported finding additional breast tissue after standard mastectomies for cancer in 16 percent of the patients he biopsied. Areas vulnerable to incomplete removal were the axillary extensions, subcutaneous zones, sternal segments, and epigastric area. Hicken [56] showed quite clearly that skin flaps must be practically devoid of subcutaneous tissue if breast tissue is to be totally resected. Goldman and Goldwyn [49], in performing subcutaneous mastectomies on 6 cadavers (including flaps of full-thickness skin only and resection of pectoralis fascia), found residual breast tissue under the areola in all, and elsewhere in 5 of the 6 specimens. Therefore, subcutaneous mastectomy procedures must of necessity represent a compromise between elimination of breast tissue and the necessity for leaving a reconstructible defect.

There is general agreement that an attempt should be made to remove all the breast tissue from the skin flaps. It has been shown that it is easy to miss areas peripherally [49, 56] but ideally this can be minimized by a more meticulous dissection. There is some confusion in the literature regarding the thickness of the skin flaps to allow the removal of breast tissue while leaving viable flaps that are thick enough for reconstruction [40, 112, 118]. Some authors feel it is important to have uniformity of thickness of skin and subcutaneous flaps to ensure a good aesthetic result [117]. Snyderman [112] answered this in 1974, making a strong and justifiable plea that the surgeon "must make a strenuous effort to remove as much breast tissue as possible without being overly concerned about the appearance or viability of the remaining flaps." The breast-subcutaneous tissue interface is frequently very irregular and its surgical delineation is complicated by a prominent Cooper's ligament and preexisting scars. It is relatively easy, particularly for the inexperienced, to thin out the flaps too vigorously. It is our opinion that it is unreasonable to leave a scattering of breast tissue attached to skin flaps as a result of either poor surgical technique or ignorance of the purpose of the procedure. It is very aggravating to the patient to return several months postoperatively with a new nodule of fibrocystic disease in a peripheral island of retained breast tissue.

There is major disagreement about whether it is justified to leave the nipple-areolar complex as part of the skin flaps. Retention of the nipple-areolar complex has been thought to necessitate leaving the underlying, intimately associated ductal tissue to maintain vascularity to the nipple and areola. The alternative is an attempt at a "total" mastectomy with removal of all the subareolar breast tissue and the accompanying ductal tissue and nipple, regrafting the areola as a full-thickness skin graft. The importance of as complete removal as possible is underlined by reports of carcinoma occurring after subcutaneous mastectomy in the retained subareolar breast tissue or axillary tail [16, 74, 91]. Pennisi [90], reporting a survey that was conducted in 1974, reported a 0.5 percent incidence of carcinoma after subcutaneous mastectomy in 4,179 operations (long-term follow-up may increase that percentage). Whether the small but definite risk justifies the more extensive operation is still a controversial point.

GENERAL OPERATIVE TECHNIQUE

Surgical gloves should be washed free of powder using a dilute alcohol solution followed by copious saline irrigations. If the operation is planned as a bilateral simultaneous procedure, it may be safer to use separate instruments for each breast because of the possibility that an occult carcinoma may be found [93]. Posterior dissection is generally done first, and a decision about the necessity of removing the pectoralis fascia must be made. If the posterior breast tissue is quite adherent to the fascia, it should be removed with the specimen. However, it should be remembered that stripping the fascia from the muscle can complicate certain techniques in the later use of the pectoralis major muscle for coverage of the implant [64, 121]. The fascial connections of the lateral border of the pectoralis major and the serratus anterior are particularly vulnerable. Occasionally, only a small area of fascia needs to be included with the specimen. Peripherally the dissection should be superficial to the muscle fascia but carried beyond the limits of where breast tissue is likely to extend. Medially, the perforating arteries need to be identified, clamped, and divided. If not carefully controlled, these easily retract into the muscle and can be quite troublesome. The superficial dissection is complicated by the fact that the junction of the breast tissue and subcutaneous layer is quite variable and must be dissected sharply and meticulously. Subcutaneous instillation of a dilute epinephrine solution (no less than 1:500,000) usually reduces bleeding and aids visibility; however, this precludes the use of intravenous fluorescein as a check on skin flap viability, which may be an important factor if primary reconstruction is contemplated [86, 109a].

It is important to dissect out Cooper's ligaments because they are accompanied by breast tissue and to resect them as close to the dermis as possible, and then return back to the plane between the subcutaneous tissue and the breast tissue (see Fig. 46-2A). This dissection is aided by gentle upward traction on the flaps and countertraction on the specimen. This creates an irregular flap but one that will retain more subcutaneous tissue than if a deliberate plane is selected just at the subdermal level. This dissection can be quite frustrating and difficult for the conscientious surgeon. The ideal dissection should leave no breast tissue on the flap and minimal fat on the specimen [12]. Dissection should proceed peripherally beyond all visible breast tissue and then connect up with a deeper dissection. The dissection will frequently extend to the midline, to the clavicle, beyond the preexisting inframmary fold and onto the rectus fascia, and to the anterior border of the latissimus dorsi muscle, as well as under the upper axillary border of the pectoralis major muscle up to the axillary skin. This latter part of the dissection can be accompanied by rather brisk bleeding. Bleeders must be carefully identified, clamped, and ligated. Superiorly, the clavipectoral fascia, which is sometimes quite prominent, will have to be clamped and divided inferior to the clavicle [42]. Goldwyn and Goldman [50] have suggested that peripheral frozen section biopsies may be helpful in determining the adequacy of mastectomy as a guide for additional excisions at the time of delayed prosthesis insertion. Adequate thickness must be left under preexisting scars, and frozen section biopsy may assist the differentiation between scar tissue and breast tissue.

Hemostasis is very important; it is aided by the use of electrocoagulation, insulated forceps, and a fiberoptic retractor or headlight. Particular attention must be paid to residual bleeding on the skin flaps, particularly in the axillary area. We recommend systemic antibiotics started preoperatively if a prosthesis is to be inserted [80b, 102]. The pocket should be copiously irrigated with a physiological solution, and handling the tissues with rough gauze or sponges should be minimized. Postoperative suction drains are used routinely; light pressure dressings with Telfa, soft padding, and elastic bandages are applied. We close all these wounds when possible with a double subcuticular suture of 4-0 nylon, after placing some deep sutures in the subcutaneous tissue, using absorbable suture material. The first layer of subcuticular suture is placed in the deepest layer of the dermis, and the second one in the superficial epidermis for accurate approximation of the wound edges. Steri-Strips are used to support the wound closure; they are frequently left on for 2 weeks, until the sutures are removed. If a prosthesis is placed, a sterile brassiere is usually used for a dressing, or a very light compression dressing with foam rubber and elastic bandages may be applied. We try to avoid the use of elastic tape or excessive pressure. The adjustable Jobst support* as recommended by Fredricks [38] may be very useful.

Management of the Pathological Specimen

Immediately upon removal, the breast tissue should be marked with a suture for orientation, and the specimens from each breast should carefully be kept separate. Particular attention should be paid to marking the subareolar area in a *subtotal* mastectomy so that this area can be carefully identified pathologically. The specimens can be weighed, which may be helpful in estimating the size of the prosthesis to be placed. *Specimen mammography* should be obtained and interpreted by an experienced radiologist and correlated with the preoperative mammogram. The specimen and radiographs should be personally correlated by the surgeon, and any suspicious area should be marked for a detailed gross examination by the responsible pathologist before fixation of the tissue. We do not usually rely on frozen sections but await careful analysis of permanent tissue sections. Occult carcinomas are difficult to detect except with meticulous examination of the entire specimen. After fixation, the specimen should be sectioned carefully at no less than 1.0-cm. intervals and examined grossly. Any radiologically or grossly suspicious areas warrant special attention, and extra sections should be taken from them. It may be wise to delay the placement of a prosthesis, particularly if a submuscular location is planned, if there is any suspicion of a carcinoma [84a].

*Jobst, Box 653, Toledo, OH 43694.

CHOICES OF SPECIFIC OPERATIVE TECHNIQUE

In an excellent essay, Freeman [42] outlined the range of choices available to the surgeon faced with a patient needing some type of breast tissue ablation. The following discussion is an expanded adaptation of his outline to include all the proposed approaches that seem reasonable. Because there is not as yet any scientific evidence to support one approach or another, the surgeon will have to be guided by such factors as his own conscience, his concept of what the objectives of the procedure are, the size of the breasts, the degree of ptosis, the amount of excess skin, the thickness of the subcutaneous layers, any preexisting scars, and (perhaps most important) the underlying seriousness of the breast pathology.

Adenomammectomy with Retained Continuity of Skin and Nipple-Areolar Complex

This operation, commonly known as a subcutaneous mastectomy, is designed to leave a cushion of breast tissue beneath the nipple-areolar complex but to remove the rest of the breast tissue.

Techniques for the Small Breast without Skin Redundancy or Nipple Ptosis

The use of the *inframammary* incision was described by Freeman [42], Goldwyn and Goldman [50], and Molenaar [85]. The incision needs to be longer than that used for routine augmentation, and the visibility and access can be difficult in the axillary and subclavicular areas, particularly in patients with large or wide chests. A small counterincision in the anterior axillary fold has often proved necessary to adequately remove the axillary tail of the breast. When possible, it is advisable to stagger the subcutaneous incision below the skin incision to offset the wound closure. A more laterally oriented peripheral incision is advocated by Fredricks [38] and Dodenoff [31] (Fig. 46-1C) and is frequently used on our service. We feel it gives better access to the more difficult areas such as the axilla and the superior reaches of the excision.

The *lateral incision* (Fig. 46-1E) from the

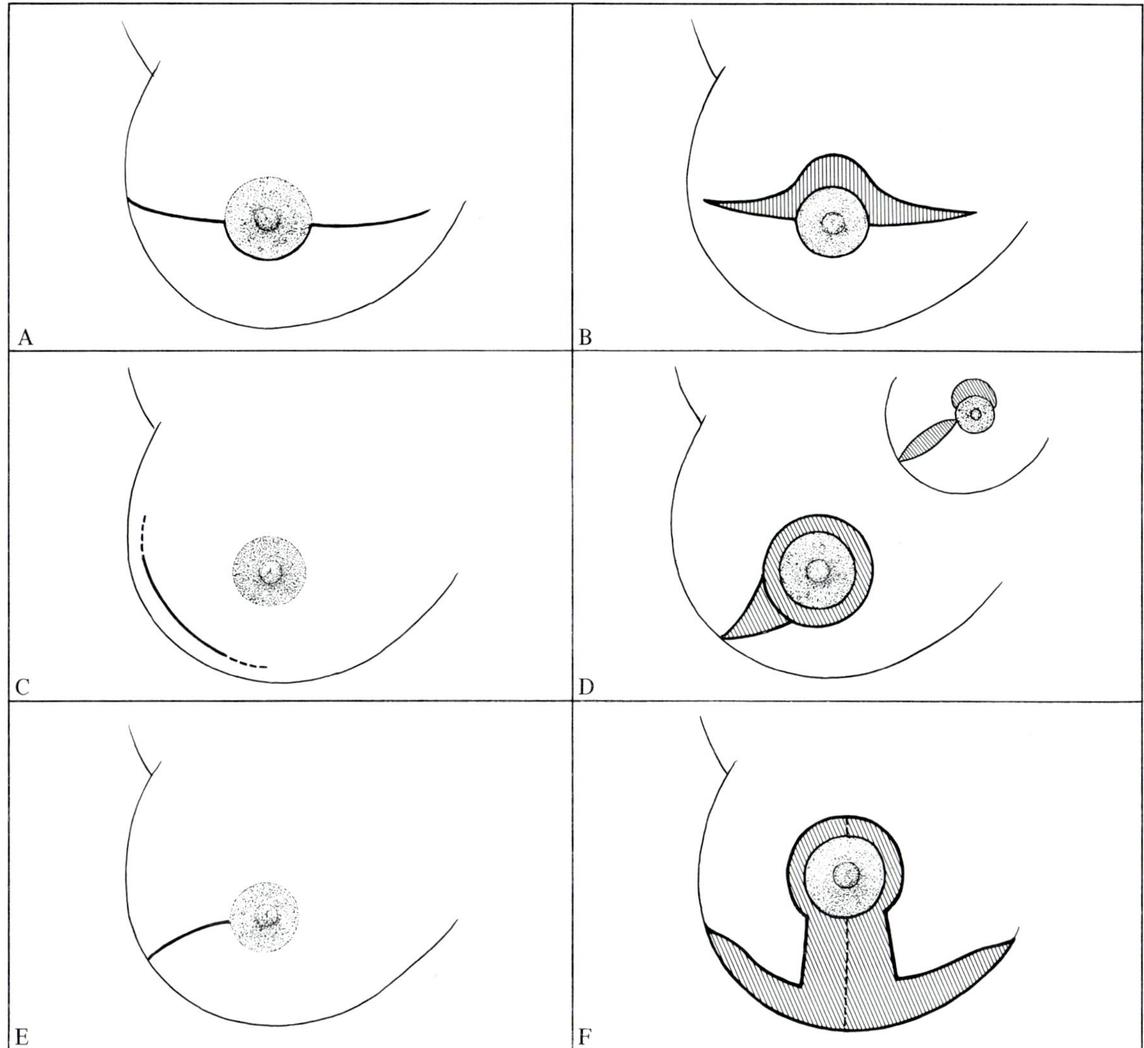

Fig. 46-1. Various incisions for subcutaneous mastectomy. A, breast-halving incision. B, breast-halving incision oriented superiorly for correction of ptosis; the shaded areas are deepithelialized. C, laterally oriented inframammary incision. D, lateral approach for ptosis correction. The inset shows a modification limiting the deepithelialization and incisions. E, lateral radial incision. F, incisions patterned after reduction mammoplasty for the reduction of ptosis in larger breasts. The dotted line shows the incision through the dermal pedicle for removal of the breast tissue.

lateral border of the areola to the lateral inferior margin of the breast gives excellent exposure. It does leave a scar laterally and may be best used when an area of excess skin can be deepithelialized.

Corso and Zubiri [23] have described a breast-halving incision that gives excellent exposure (Fig. 46-1A). It can be designed so that the medial or lateral limbs will include old scars. The incision is placed inferiorly so that the nipple-areolar complex is based on a superior pedicle. If there is mild ptosis, the incision is made superior to the areola, and the skin is deepithelialized to allow upward movement of the nipple-areolar complex (Fig. 46-1B). In a recent communication, Corso [22] continues to recommend the operation but cautions that the risk of areolar edge necrosis can approach 10 to 15 percent. This is more likely to occur if the flaps are too long or excessively scarred by previous surgery.

Techniques for Medium-sized Breasts with Moderate Ptosis

Fredricks [38] has shown that if there is excess skin but not excessive ptosis of the nipple, the skin envelope may shrink after resection of the gland. Kern and Binns [67] described a lateral skin excision without repositioning the areola to achieve a satisfactory reduction of the skin brassiere.

Most techniques for ptosis include a method of repositioning the nipple-areolar complex on a dermal pedicle and utilizing deepithelialized flaps of excess skin to reinforce suture lines. Alternatives include the V-Q technique and the B technique of Regnault [98, 99], the dermomastopexy technique of Goulian and McDivitt [51], the superior pedicle as reported by Georgiade and Hyland [47], breast halving by Corso [23], and the inferior dermal reinforcing flap as described by Biggs, Brauer, and Wolf [13]. A similar technique was reported by Baroudi and associates [9]. The lateral approach as adopted by Hartley and coworkers [55] (Fig. 46-1D) is also useful. The modification of Wilkinson [121] (Fig. 46-1D, inset) can also be very useful. The periareolar deepithelialization is limited to the superior area, minimizing the possibility of vascular impairment of the nipple and areola but still correcting nipple ptosis and skin ptosis by the reinforcement of the lateral suture line.

Techniques for Breasts with Excessive Skin and Nipple Ptosis

Freeman [42] described a Strömbeck-type approach similar to that used in reduction mammoplasty. Zbylski and Parsons [123], Letterman and Schurter [79], and Molenaar [85] have all additionally advocated using the excess tissue as a dermal-fat flap based on the inframammary fold, as originally described by Longacre [80] and de Cholnoky [28], to reinforce the vertical suture line. Although Freeman [42] suggests that this flap may lead to misinterpretation in postoperative clinical examination and mammography, in practical experience this has not been a problem. In some patients, as pointed out by Goulian and McDivitt [51], the dermal-fat flap provides enough bulk, when infolded behind the superior skin flaps, to produce a breast of adequate volume *without* requiring an implant. In some of the cases, when the swelling has reduced or some fat has been resorbed, an implant may later be required as a secondary procedure.

Both Hoopes and Ryan [57] and Georgiade [46] have advocated the use of a McKissock approach (Fig. 46-1F) [83]. The vertical bipedical flap supports the circulation of the nipple-areolar complex and protects the suture line of the vertical flap closure inferior to the areola.

Adenomammectomy with Retention of Areola in Continuity with Skin Flaps

Freeman [43] has described total glandular removal that still leaves the areola attached to the skin flap. He dissects the breast tissue off the underside of the areola and removes the ductal tissue and nipple in continuity with the gland. To minimize trauma to the retained areola and subdermal vasculature, he uses magnification and bipolar cautery during a very careful dissection. He has not reported any areolar necrosis in 9 cases in which this technique has been used. Crile [24] has endorsed the potential validity of this concept. We have had no experience with this procedure but question whether the maintenance of the areola in continuity with the skin flaps has any advantage over the modified total mastectomy.

Modified Total Mastectomy

This operation is also known as simple mastectomy with free areolar graft.

Techniques in the Breast without Skin Redundancy

These techniques are illustrated in Figure 46-2. Minimal skin resection is done and the areola and cuff of skin at the base of the nipple (Fig. 46-2C) are removed as a free full-thickness skin graft; the nipple and all ductal tissue are removed with the specimen (Fig. 46-2B). After closure, the nipple opening in the graft is purse-string sutured and the areolar graft is then placed on a circular deepithelialized dermal bed in an appropriate location (Fig. 46-2E, F, G).

Techniques in Larger Breasts with More Ptosis

Three techniques can be used in breasts with more ptosis. Rubin [104] described dermal-fat flaps on the inferior edge of the reduction mammoplasty-

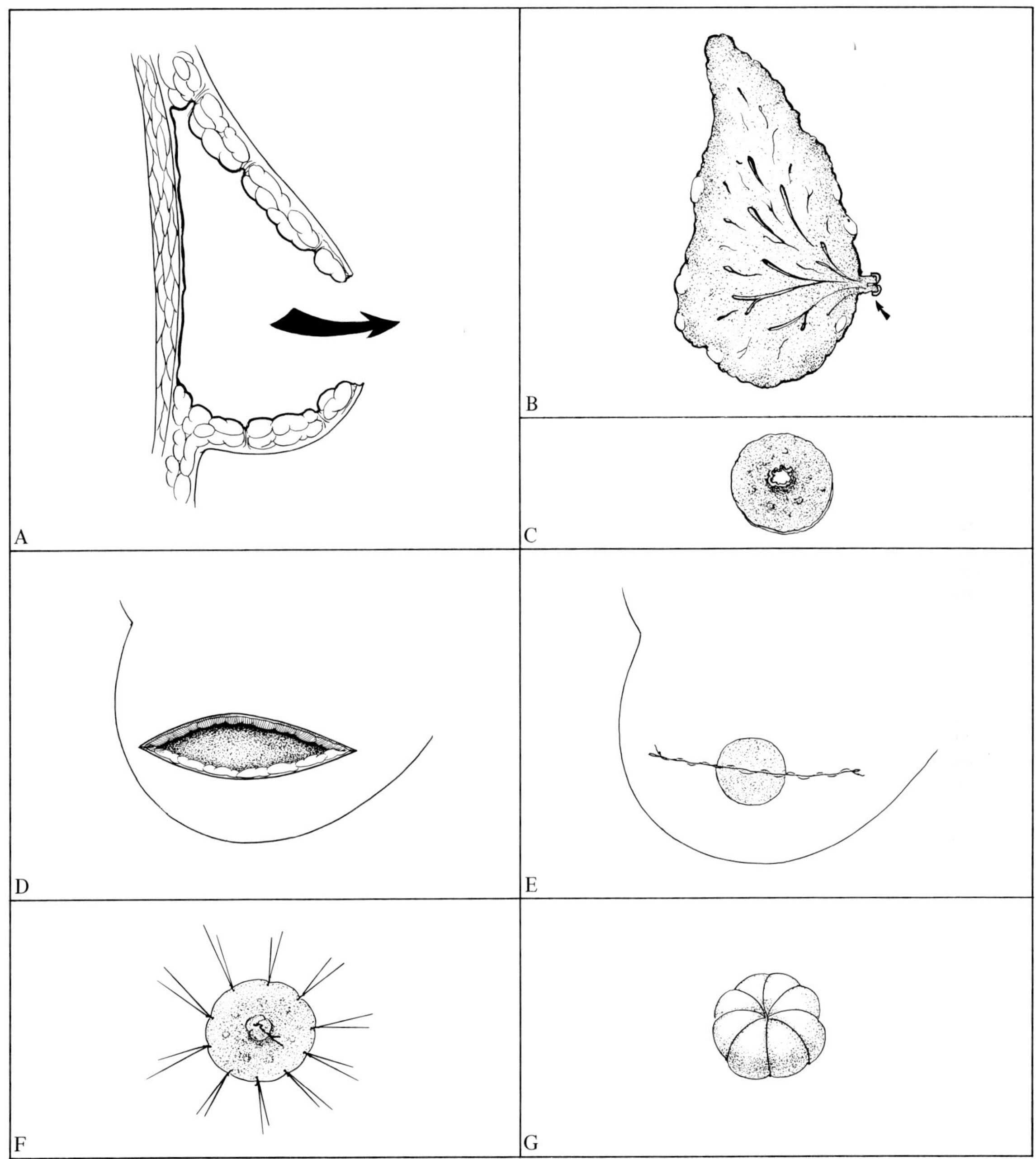

Fig. 46-2. Modified total mastectomy. A, showing the level of dissection and emphasizing irregularities of the flaps due to the necessity of resecting the Cooper's ligament. B, the specimen with the retained ductal tissue and cuff of nipple skin (see arrow). C, an excised full-thickness graft of areola and cuff of the base of nipple skin. E, defect closed with subcuticular sutures and a deepithelialized zone for the areolar graft. F and G, the nipple is reconstructed with a purse-string suture and the areola is sutured with a stent dressing.

type skin flaps, and they are folded under to cushion the skin flaps from the prosthesis.

Horton and associates, using a lateral approach in a smaller breast [58] or a transverse approach in a large breast [59], use an inferiorly based dermal-fat flap that reinforces the skin flap. In the case of a large breast, the flap will frequently come up over to cover the implant completely and attach to the pectoral fascia superiorly [59].

Shaping of the upper flaps into a more conical form is possible using the technique of Spira [113], in which the upper flap is transposed with a keyhole pattern similar to that used with reduction mammoplasties (Fig. 46-3). The deepithelialized inferior flap is sutured to the pectoralis major muscle along its inferior and medial border. This provides a completely separate pocket for the implant. The musculodermal interface creates a protective barrier from any necrosis or wound separation that might occur, and may allow retention of the implant under these circumstances.

In some cases, if the breasts are large enough and the fatty layers are thick enough, the inferior dermal-fat flap can create enough volume so that the breast can be reconstructed *without* the use of an implant (Fig. 46-4). We have utilized this technique with very satisfactory results in 6 patients. D'Assumpcaõ [26a] has reported a series of 30 patients showing good results.

TIMING OF THE INSERTION OF THE IMPLANT

Immediate Insertion of Implant

Immediate intraoperative replacement of the resected breast tissue with a prosthesis is certainly the most efficient, convenient, and gratifying procedure for both the patient and the surgeon. However, the following is a list of problems that may complicate the simultaneous insertion of the prosthesis into the subcutaneous space.

1. Hemostasis is frequently difficult.
2. The pocket created by a wide resection of breast tissue is frequently too large for the implant.
3. There is frequently concern about the tension on suture lines, viability of skin flaps, and the likelihood that the areolar graft will take [50b].
4. There is the uncertainty of a pathological diagnosis of the resected tissue [84a].
5. The patient never has an opportunity to visualize the deformity and may have difficulty being objective about the ultimate result.

Certain techniques are available for controlling some of these potential problems:

1. Buried dermal flaps can be used to reinforce the suture lines or thinned areas of the flaps.
2. Intravenous fluorescein can be used to delineate possible nonvascular areas of skin flaps [86].
3. Pocket size can be controlled by recontouring the skin flaps by circumferential suturing [21, 38], or by placing the implant in a submuscular pocket [64].

Delayed Primary Insertion of Implant (3 to 7 Days)

Deliberately postponing the placement of the prosthesis offers these advantages: The viability of the skin flaps is known; a more accurate recreation of the pocket in the subcutaneous space is possible; the final pathological report is known; additional removal of breast tissue as dictated by intraoperative biopsies can be carried out; and the patient has an opportunity to see the preprosthetic deformity. The second operation can be done relatively quickly, utilizing only a portion of the original incision (unless a submuscular insertion is planned). If there is worry about prolonging the hospitalization, the operation can be accomplished under local anesthesia and sedation on an outpatient basis, as described by Goldwyn and Goldman [50]. Postoperative drainage is frequently not necessary under these circumstances. In our experience with operations that preserve the nipple-areolar complex, this seems to be a reasonable plan for the prosthesis insertion. However, Goldwyn [50b] states that he has seen an occasional skin slough in cases of delayed primary reconstruction.

One of the few complications that we have seen specifically related to the use of a primary delayed implant was the unrecognized dehiscence of the wound closure under a fresh areolar full-thickness skin graft, partial graft loss, and subsequent infection necessitating the removal of the implant. We feel that either simultaneous or delayed secondary insertion of the implant is the method of choice in total mastectomy with an areolar graft.

Delayed Secondary Prosthesis Insertion (3 to 6 Months)

After a delay of more than 2 to 3 weeks, the scar and induration in the wound usually make it advisable to wait 3 to 6 months before attempting prosthesis insertion. Periodic examinations are necessary to evaluate the pliability of the skin. Some of the common indications for the delay of the implant are:

1. Resolution of complications of skin necrosis and slough.
2. Failure of the immediate implant.
3. Indecision on the part of the patient or the surgeon regarding the need or the desirability of prosthetic reconstruction.

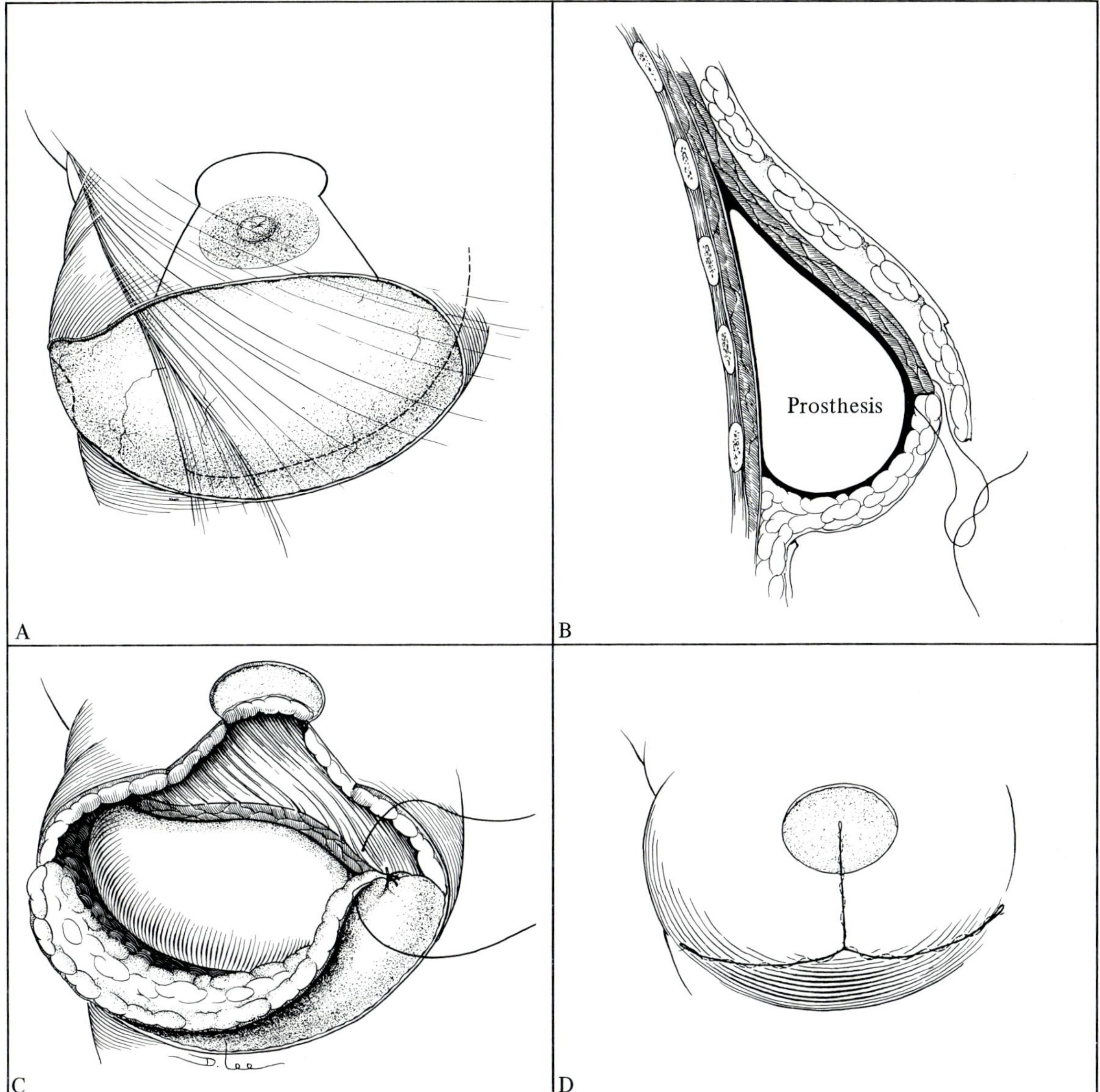

Fig. 46-3. The Spira procedure. A, stippled area is a deepithelialized dermal-fat flap. The dotted line shows the level of detachment of the inferior medial insertion of pectoralis muscle. B and C, after a simple mastectomy is done similar to Figure 1 A and B the mammary prosthesis is placed in the pocket created by the cut edge of the pectoralis muscle to the upper edge of the dermal-fat flap. D, the skin is then closed in inverted-T fashion, and the deepithelialized area is a recipient of a full-thickness areolar graft similar to Figure 2 F and G.

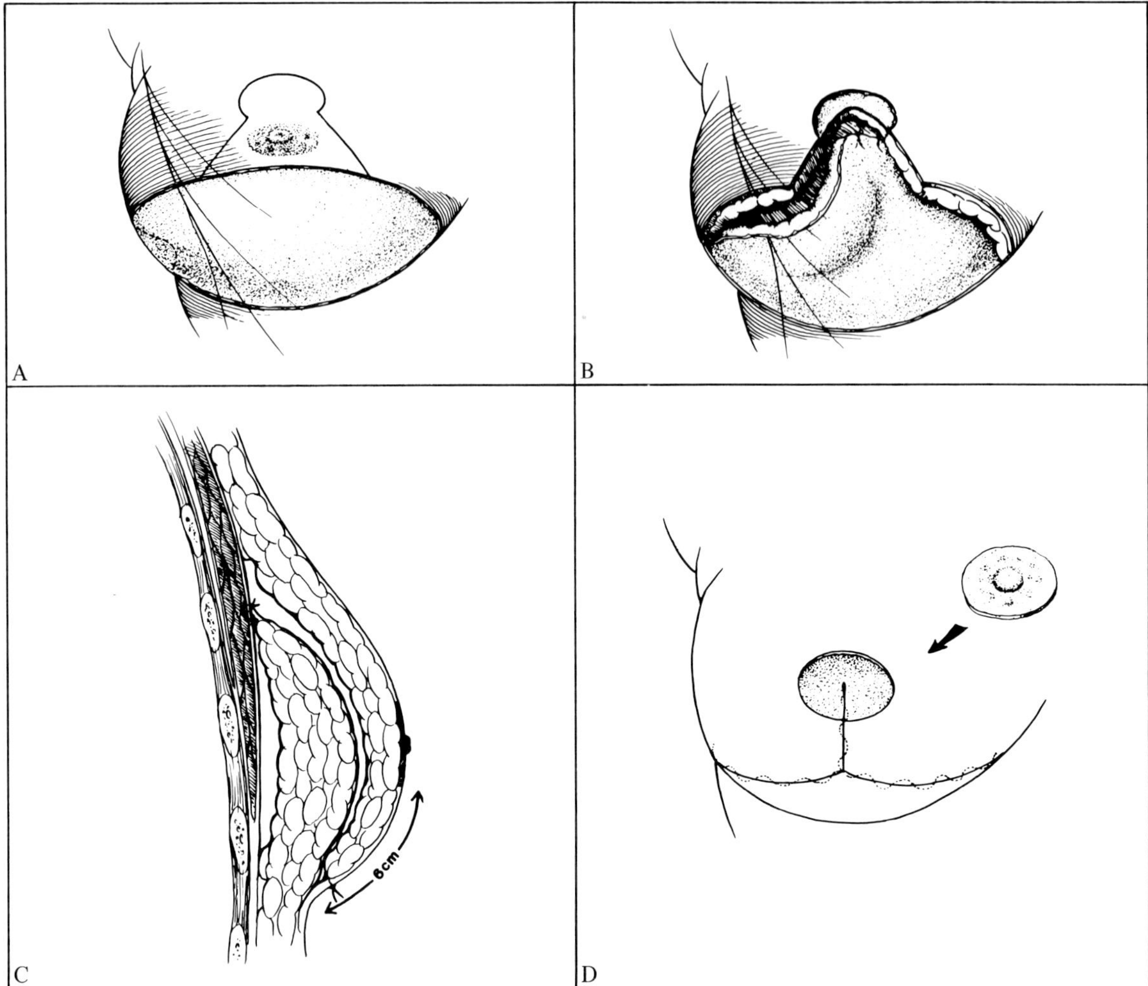

Fig. 46-4. The use of excess tissue in dermal-fat flaps for reconstruction in hypertrophied breasts. A, outline of keyhole incisions and inferiorly based deepithelialized flap. B, after total glandular removal, a dermal-fat flap is shaped and sutured to the pectoralis muscle. C, overlays of superiorly posed skin flaps and inferiorly based dermal-fat prosthesis. D, closure of skin flaps and deepithelialized area for full-thickness areolar graft (see Fig. 46-2 for technique in placing areolar graft).

4. Mastodynia as a primary indication for the operation.

In our experience the severe mastodynia is one of the few *absolute* indications for delayed implantation. Both the patient *and* the surgeon must be convinced that resection of the breast tissue will alleviate the preoperative pain. Molenaar [85] reported 16 patients with mastodynia in his series of 23 patients. Postoperatively 8 of these patients had significant persistent pain that inevitably resolved, but frequently this took 6 weeks to 6 months. Our findings agree with this and support the idea that the patient needs to be convinced that the preoperative pain has been alleviated before the variable of the implant is introduced.

One of the major problems with this delayed technique is the subcutaneous scarring that occurs secondary to the healing process. Tissue spacers (such as a Silastic disc or Teflon spacer) have been advocated [92], but they can cause problems such as fluid collection. If one is to use such a spacer, the diameter of the two-dimensional discs must be much larger than the diameter of the proposed three-dimensional implant to allow retention of a space large enough for free movement of the implant. Perhaps an expansile implant would function well in selected cases.

At the time of delayed implantation we have usually developed a surgical plane deep to the initial dissection. This implies a pocket deep to the pectoralis major muscle and frequently deep to the fascia of the serratus anterior, the upper portion of the rectus abdominis and external oblique muscles. Goldwyn and Goldman [50] described an intermediate level of dissection that included some of the fibers of the pectoralis major muscle (they remove the pectoralis fascia with their initial dissection) under areas that are thinned and/or excessively scarred. Probably these fibers become devitalized, but they do provide some protection between troublesome areas of the skin flap and the breast prosthesis.

Usually the secondary procedure can be accomplished through a limited portion of the original scar; frequently the scar can be deepithelialized and this portion used as dermal flap to reinforce the wound closure.

SIZE AND TYPE OF IMPLANT

Since the original description by Cronin and Gerow [25] of the silicone breast prosthesis, the technological advances in a variety of implants have provided the surgeon with a wide range of choices for reconstruction (see Chapter 44).

The objective of the reconstructive part of the procedure is the replacement of the tissue removed rather than the enlargement or improvement of the original shape of the breast. Consequently, modest-sized implants are usually indicated, although this is not universally agreed upon.

Size of Implant

The weight of the resected breast tissue can be used as a guide for the size of the implant if simultaneous implantation is indicated. An inflatable implant in the range of 150 to 250 cc. can be used as a test spacer, which is very helpful in confirming the estimate [101]. The size of the pocket and the tension of the wound closure are the factors that frequently control the final decision. It is much safer to err on the side of too small an implant, and the patient should be told of this preoperatively. When the implant is delayed, the size of the implant can be determined with the use of a modest-sized unpadded brassiere (usually a B cup) and available gel breast implant sizers. Although we prefer to make an accurate preoperative estimate of the size, this may have to be modified at the time of prosthesis insertion. Because of this need for flexibility, the use of at least an inflatable component provides some advantages. We rarely use implants larger than 300 cc., and we favor those in the 185- to 250-cc. range.

Type of Implant

There are a variety of implants available (see listing in Chapter 44). There is no general agreement among surgeons as to the best type of implant. The major advantages of the inflatable variety are that there is a minimum of foreign material, there is an adjustable volume, and there may be a lower rate of capsular contracture [55a] and infection [106] than with gel-containing implants. The major disadvantage is a possibility of deflation as a result of dehiscence of the outer lumen and leakage of the saline. However, this disadvantage may be outweighed by the potential danger of rupture of the shell surrounding the gel implant and migration of the gel. Huang and associates [59a] have reported such ruptures after closed capsulotomy. We have also seen a patient in whom spontaneous rupture of a gel implant occurred; this was associated with an enlarged axillary lymph node containing what appeared to be silicone [87a]. Considering these facts we are currently recommending using the inflatable implant.

METHODS TO DECREASE INCIDENCE OF FIBROUS CAPSULE CONTRACTURE

Although the early results with the various silicone mammary implants are satisfactory, many observers (including ourselves) feel that a fibrous capsular contracture is the *inevitable* result of a smooth-walled implant being placed in a subcutaneous pocket after a prophylactic mastectomy [12, 17, 34, 64, 97]. Several techniques have been introduced to reduce this occurrence so that the result will be a softer breast mound that feels more natural.

Use of Steroids

As pointed out by Baker (see Chapter 44), there is a mild influence on capsular contracture by the use of 40 mg. of triamcinolone (Kenalog) instilled in the pocket at the time the implant is placed. Wilkinson [121] uses 10 mg. of triamcinolone hexacetonide (Aristospan) instilled on the second or third post-operative day through an operatively placed suction catheter before its removal. Ellenberg [34] is following a series of 50 patients using a combined gel-inflatable prosthesis, with approximately 75 to 100 ml. saline in the inflatable portion; the saline aliquot contains 10 mg. of methylprednisolone sodium succinate (Solu-Medrol). (This method was originally described by Perrin [94].) Ellenberg now has follow-up of 2 years, and he feels that the softness in his series is comparable to that obtained in routine augmentation. However, long-term follow-up studies are not yet available. He did, however, report severe complications of implant ptosis and overlying skin thinning with the use of Kenalog placed in the implant [33]. It has become quite clear that the use of an insoluble steroid within the implant is definitely *contraindicated.* We have also noticed that with higher doses of Solu-Medrol, between 30 and 60 mg. within an implant, a high incidence of atrophy, thinning, and implant ptosis will be observed. These effects seem to be reversible by exchanging the implant for one not containing steroids. Capsular contracture has not been universally prevented.

Postoperative Massage

Many have advocated the vigorous movement of the implant as a means of maintaining adequate size of the pocket. According to Wilkinson [121], instillation of bupivacaine (Marcaine) 0.25% in small increments through a retained catheter (at the same time as the instillation of the Aristospan) facilitates early movement. A new stretch garment manufactured by Surgitek* flattens the implant against the chest wall and may be helpful as an adjunct in prevention of capsular contracture.

Partial Covering of the Implant with Polyurethane

In an effort to alleviate the problem of capsular contracture and wrinkling, Capozzi [17] has been using a soft, low-profile gel implant covered with polyurethane except on its anterior two-thirds [91]. (This implant is custom made by the Heyer-Schulte Corp.†). The implant is not compartmentalized, thus differing from the originally described polyurethane covered prosthesis reported by Ashley [7]. The implant is inserted at the time of breast tissue resection in the subcutaneous space superficial to the muscles. Capozzi is now following 48 patients with 95 implants. With the exception of 1 patient, the implants in all these patients have remained acceptably soft on follow-up to at least 1 year. In 2 patients, exposure of the implant occurred; however, because of adhesions to the polyurethane around the area of exposure, the implant was salvaged by rotation of local skin flaps. Another recent follow-up study reported that in a small series of 8 patients with polyurethane covered gel implants 2 patients' implants required removal because of infection. However, Horton and associates [59a] have reported a larger series of over 70 implants placed subpectorally with no loss of implant. Capozzi [17] reports that the edge of the polyurethane anteriorly may be palpable but has not been visible. There have been recent reports studying the histological detail of the capsule secondary to the polyurethane [110, 116]. These studies have shown an intense foreign body reaction and slow degradation of the polyurethane over a period of 2 years. The capsule was very difficult to remove, which proves to be a distinct disadvantage if persistent infection necessitates removal of the implant. There does not seem to be any correlation with the foreign body reaction and the remaining softness of the implant; thus it appears that only continued long-term follow-up will delineate whether there are any adverse effects of the subcutaneously implanted polyurethane.

Submuscular Site for Prosthesis Implantation

The pectoral muscle is an available structure that has been utilized in a variety of ways to enhance the results of prosthesis implantation following mastectomy for benign disease. Placing the implant under the muscle has the following advantages.

1. It forms a barrier to well-vascularized tissue between the scarred or irregular skin flap and the implant. It can also protect an implant from minor wound breakdowns or areolar necrosis.
2. In subtotal mastectomy it provides a barrier between the remaining subareolar breast tissue and the implant, allowing biopsy and/or later removal of this tissue with less chance of exposing the implant.
3. It adds opacity, warmth, and improved contour.
4. When this procedure is used with delayed implantation or in secondary operations for complications, the prosthesis can be implanted in a plane separate fromthe original scarred subcutaneous plane or previous unsatisfactory prosthesis pocket.

*Medical Engineering Corp., 3037 Mt. Pleasant St., Racine, WI 53404.

†600 Pine Ave., Box 946, Goleta CA 93017.

5. There is a reported lower incidence of significant capsular contracture with subpectoral implantation [96, 100, 120].
6. Localized pectoral flaps may help solve difficult complications occurring in the cutaneous cover over the prosthesis [120].

Anatomical Considerations

The pectoralis major muscle is encased in a fascia of varying thickness. The superficial fascia blends with the rectus abdominis fascia inferiorly and the serratus anterior fascia laterally. The primary neurovascular supply to the muscle enters the undersurface of the muscle superiorly and is covered by a pad of fat and the deep layer of fascia. The entire muscle can survive on the superior vascular pedicle even if all the peripheral attachments are divided. There the prosthesis can be inserted into the relatively avascular plane between the deep surface of the muscle and the deeper structures including the pectoralis, minor muscle, and the serratus anterior muscles which are both closely adherent to ribs. However, there is a great deal of variability in the size and thickness of the muscle as well as in the position of the lateral border and the inferior attachments relative to the location of the inframammary fold and the overlying breast tissue. This is not always emphasized in current anatomical descriptions.

In 1977, Pickrell, Pluckett, and Given [96] reported on the use of small implants (less than 165 cc. in volume) placed in the subpectoral space without detaching the muscle medially. In order to create enough space for a larger implant, the muscle must be detached across its inferior attachments and one-third to one-half of the way up the sternal attachments [88, 100]. Care is taken to leave enough stump of muscle against the chest wall to allow control of perforating arteries as well as to blend in with the periphery of the pocket. This more extensive mobilization is necessary to allow proper position and mobility of the implant. If this is done as a delayed procedure, the subpectoral space can be reached by minimal dissection, leaving the superficial attachments of the muscle fascia to the subcutaneous scarred layer intact, and the muscle will not retract.

We have recently used a direct approach, using the lateral portion of the previous horizontal incision (extended inferior or superior to the areola if necessary), splitting the inferior-lateral fibers of the pectoralis major muscle, and dissecting an extended subpectoral pocket in a plane that is both deep to and separate from the previous subcutaneous dissection [101a]. A similar extended subpectoral pocket using serratus muscle fascia has been successfully used by Horton and associates [59a].

Wilkinson [120] described a superiorly based muscle flap for use in simultaneous implantation. In order to enlarge the area that the prosthesis covers, he recommends filleting the muscle fascia and the superficial muscle fibers to allow the muscle to fan out laterally. He also detaches it inferiorly and medially and reattaches the inferior portion to the subcutaneous tissue with permanent sutures to prevent retraction. Some degree of ptosis can be corrected simultaneously by suspending the skin flaps on the fanned-out muscle, creating an "internal mastopexy" [120, 121]. This radically mobilized muscle will usually cover the upper one-half to two-thirds of the implant. According to Spira [113], it can be combined with an inferiorly based dermal flap in the ptotic breast to produce a completely separate pocket for the implant. Wilkinson [120, 121] feels that the use of this pectoralis major muscle flap (in combination with instillation of Kenalog, as previously described) and the employment of early vigorous pressure massage have reduced capsule formation in a recent series to approximately 4 percent.

When there is cutaneous thinning and impending extrusion postoperatively, Wilkinson [120] uses a muscle flap incorporating the lower one-third of the pectoralis major muscle based on its inferior attachments and rotated down to lie beneath the thin skin. This has been a useful adjunct in combination with mobilization of the posterior fibrous capsule to reinforce the inferior cutaneous thinning when there is impending extrusion of the implant. He feels that this secondary procedure can be done through a circumareolar incision. He has successfully salvaged six implants in this manner.

Jarrett, Cutler, and Teal [64] have recently reported impressive results in terms of the appearance of the breast in 70 patients. They dissected a submuscular pocket using the serratus anterior muscle, the rectus abdominis muscle, and the external oblique muscle dissected off the chest wall in conjunction with the pectoralis major all in one layer (Fig. 46-5). The integrity of the connections of the muscle fascia between the pectoralis and serratus is crucial to this technique. They are careful to leave some muscular attachments peripherally, so that when the muscular layer is closed over the implant there should be continuous "internal massage" as a result of the muscles contracting during normal activity. These authors usually use a 230- to 260-cc. smooth-gel implant. This technique is also applicable where there is mild ptosis or when skin reduction and/or a free areolar graft is used. They have noted no serious complications or extrusion. They find that the incidence of unsatisfactory results due to significant capsular contracture has been reduced to 10 percent. Initially the breasts are flattened, but they assume a more natural shape as muscles stretch. This appears to be a most promising technique and one we are

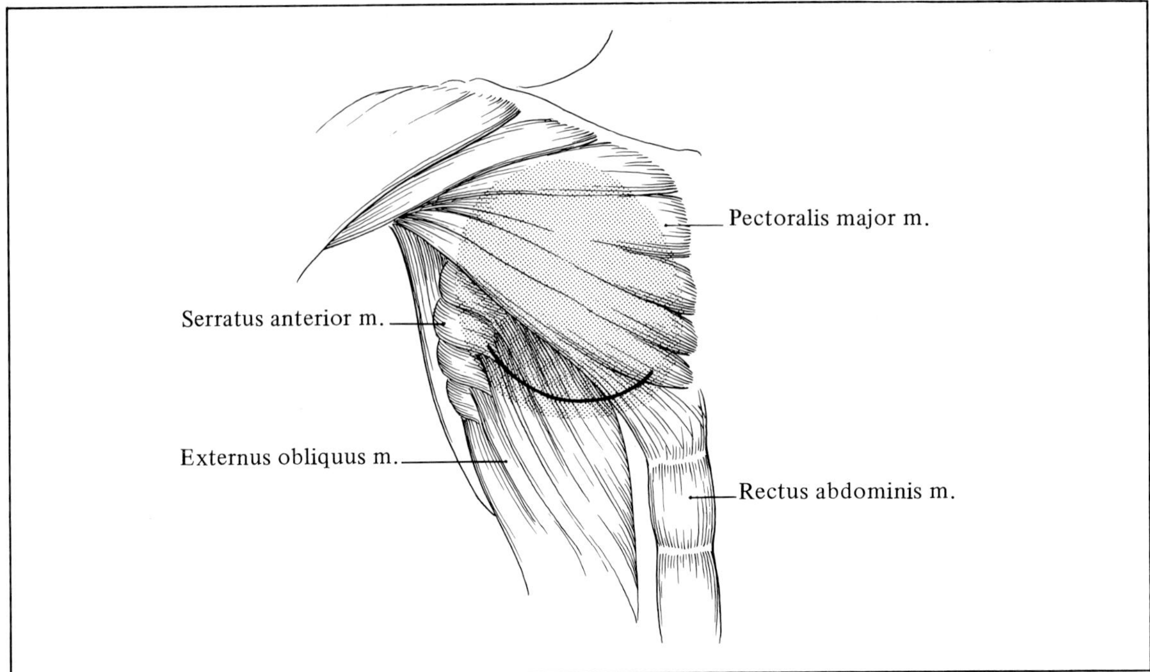

Fig. 46-5. A submuscular prosthesis implantation. The black line is the incision through the muscle placed 1–2 cm. above the proposed inframammary fold. The shaded area is a large submuscular pocket.

presently using with enthusiasm in primary reconstruction.

Disadvantages of Subpectoral Implantation
Subpectoral implantation has the following disadvantages:

1. In simultaneous breast excision and prosthesis insertion, subpectoral implantation violates the subpectoral space before the possibility of occult cancer is ruled out. This may only be a theoretical disadvantage but it should be considered [84a].
2. In our personal group of patients (in whom only the pectoralis major muscle was utilized), we felt that the postoperative discomfort was increased. There was a slightly slower occupational rehabilitation, although others have not reported this difficulty [100, 120].
3. The submuscular dissection is more tedious and time-consuming, and it increases the blood loss.
4. The puckering of the skin that is seen with the attachment of the pectoralis major to the skin flap may be avoidable using a totally submuscular technique [64].
5. Before we started using the totally submuscular approach, when we were placing the implants under the pectoralis major alone, we had not noted a dramatic decrease in capsule formation. We hope the excellent results of Jarrett and co-workers [64] can be duplicated, and we are presently evaluating their technique.

POSTOPERATIVE PROBLEMS

Most of the problems associated with prophylactic mastectomy are a result of thin, partially devascularized skin flaps, or are due to complications of the implant itself. Severe postoperative problems are common and produce a high percentage of unsatisfactory results. A classification of problems is presented in Table 46-1.

An early report in 1966 by Kelly and associates [66] described 25 problems in 11 patients. Study of two more recent reports [97, 106] suggests that solutions to these problems are still elusive. Redfern and Hoopes [97] reported 25 patients with a 28-month follow-up. They found a 59 percent incidence of problems significant enough to require secondary operations. A review of 40 of our patients revealed a 50 percent complication rate. Complications from these two series included incidence of hematoma of 7–9 percent, early wound or flap necrosis of 15 percent, and delayed flap necrosis and implant extrusion of 15 percent. We noted that 32 percent of our patients ultimately lost their implants compared to the

Table 46-1. Postoperative Problems

Time of Onset	Complications	Unfavorable Results
Early problems (up to 2 weeks) postoperative)	Hematoma Infection Necrosis of skin or nipple Wound dehisence, frequently leading to exposure of implant	Superficial loss of skin in nipple or areola Shift of implant Improper size of implant
Delayed problems (2 weeks to 6 months)	Pain Shift of implant Infection and late extrusion	Superficial thrombophlebitis Loss of sensation of the skin or nipple Evanescent hyperemia or discoloration of skin
Late problems (beyond 6 months)	Severe fibrous capsular contracture Late extrusion or implant removal Significant pain, usually related to capsular contracture Carcinoma Recurrent fibrocystic disease requiring the need for further resectional surgery Complications from the use of steroids to prevent contracture	Unsatisfactory appearance, including asymmetry, loss of sensation, wrinkling and ptosis of the implant.

incidence in other recent series of 28 percent [106] and 22 percent [97]. It should be noted that in these three series a very small percentage of the implants were placed subpectorally. A small but significant number developed problems many months to more than a year after the original surgical procedure.

Although there seems to be no statistical evidence to support the improvement in results by delayed reconstruction [106], it is recognized that in most series the patients selected for delayed implantation carried an increased risk of complications such as thin skin flaps, more extensive dissections, and previous scars. In reality, an even higher rate of complications may have been avoided by delaying the reconstruction. Goldwyn [50b], in responding to the report of Redfern and Hoopes [99], not only felt that delay was necessary for reducing complications but also stressed the importance of subpectoral placement. We have seen, as Schlenker and associates have reported [106], complications even with a delayed submuscular approach. However, Horton and associates [59a] have submitted an encouraging report of 79 successful subpectoral implants with a 3-year follow-up.

Infection, as a cause of implant extrusion, continues to be a persistent problem. Schlenker and associates [106] reported a dramatic decreased incidence of infection from 25 percent to 2 percent with preoperative and 2-day postoperative systemic antibiotics. They used either a penicillinase-resistant penicillin or a cephalosporin. We have observed several infections in our series caused by gram-negative or staph epidermitis so we favor the broader spectrum cephalosporins. Schlenker and associates also noted a lesser incidence of infection with inflatable implants (2 percent) compared to gel-filled ones (21 percent).

Satisfactory results, as judged by the surgeon, in those patients who retained their implants was 60 percent in one series [106]. Another study [97] noted that though there was a high incidence of capsule contracture, patient satisfaction was high, underscoring the disparity between objective and subjective patient evaluation. The significant incidence of late complications indicates the need for more long-term follow-up reports.

REFERENCES

1. Ackerman, L. V., and Katzenstein, A. L. Concept of minimal breast cancer and the pathologist's role in diagnosis of "early carcinoma." *Cancer* 39:2755, 1977.
2. Anderson, D. E. Breast cancer in families. *Cancer* 40:1885, 1977.
3. Anderson, J. A. Lobular carcinoma in situ of the breast. *Cancer* 39:2597, 1977.
4. Ashikari, R., Hajdu, S., and Robbins, G. Intraductal carcinoma of the breast. *Cancer* 28:1182, 1971.
5. Ashikari, R., Huvos, A. G., and Snyder, R. E. Prospective study of non-infiltrating carcinoma of the breast. *Cancer* 39:435, 1977.
6. Ashikari, R., Huvos, A. G., Snyder, R. E., Lucas, J., Hutter, R. V. P., McDivitt, R. W., and Schottenfield, D. A clinicopathologic study of atypical lesions of the breast. *Cancer* 33:310, 1974.
7. Ashley, F. L. A new type of breast prosthesis. *Plast. Reconstr. Surg.* 45:421, 1970.
8. Bader, K., Pellettiere, E., and Curtin, J. W. Definitive surgical therapy for the "premalignant" or equivocal breast lesion. *Plast. Reconstr. Surg.* 46:120, 1970.
9. Baroudi, R., Keppke, E. M., and Carvalho, C. Breast modeling after subcutaneous mastectomy. *Aesthetic Plast. Surg.* 2:235, 1978.
10. Benfield, J. R., Fingerhut, A. F., and Warner, N. E. A multidiscipline view of lobular breast carcinoma. *Am. Surg.* 38:115, 1972.
11. Benfield, J. R., Jacobson, M., and Warner, N. E. In situ lobular carcinoma of the breast. *Arch. Surg.* 91:130, 1965.
12. Biggs, T. M. Mastopexy in conjunction with subcutaneous mastectomy (reply to letter by Dr. Vecchione). *Plast. Reconstr. Surg.* 61:103, 1978.
13. Biggs, T. M., Brauer, R. O., and Wolf, L. E. Mastopexy in conjunction with subcutaneous mastectomy. *Plast. Reconstr. Surg.* 60:1, 1977.
14. Black, M. M., Barclay, T. H. C., Cutler, S. J., Hankey, B. F., and Asire, A. J. Association of atypical characteristics of benign breast lesions with subsequent risk of breast cancer. *Cancer* 29:338, 1972.
15. Black, M. M., and Chabon, A. B. In Situ Carcinoma of the Breast. In Sommers, S. C. (Ed.), *Pathology Annual.* New York: Appleton, Century, and Crofts, 1969.
16. Bowers, D. G., Jr., and Ridlauer, C. B. Breast cancer after prophylactic subcutaneous mastectomy and reconstruction with Silastic prostheses. *Plast. Reconstr. Surg.* 44:541, 1969.
17. Capozzi, A. Personal communication, 1977.
18. Cardiff, R. D., Wellings, S. R., and Faulkin, L. H. Biology of breast preneoplasia. *Cancer* 39:2734, 1977.
19. Carter, D., and Smith, R. R. L. Carcinoma in situ of the breast. *Cancer* 40:1189, 1977.
20. Charteris, A. A. On the changes in the mammary gland preceding carcinoma. *J. Pathol. Bacteriol.* 33:101, 1930.
21. Conroy, W. C. Reducing the pocket in the subcutaneous mastectomy to accommodate a smaller implant. *Plast. Reconstr. Surg.* 59:446, 1977.
22. Corso, P. F. Personal communication, 1977.
23. Corso, P. F., and Zubiri, J. S. A breast halving incision for subcutaneous mastectomy. *Plast. Reconstr. Surg.* 56:1, 1975.
24. Crile, G., Jr. The voice of polite dissent re: Subcutaneous mastectomy for central tumors of the breast with immediate reconstruction. *Plast. Reconstr. Surg.* 51:447, 1973.
25. Cronin, T. D., and Gerow, F. J. Augmentation Mammoplasty: A New "Natural Feel" Prosthesis. *Transactions of the Third International Congress of Plastic Surgery* (1963). Amsterdam: Exerpta Medica, 1964, P. 41.
26. Cutler, R. G. Personal communication, 1977.

26a. D'Assumpçaõ, E. A. Immediate reconstruction without prostheses following subcutaneous mastectomy in large breasts. *Br. J. Plast. Surg.* 31:24, 1978.

27. Davis, H. H., Simons, M., and Davis, J. B. Cystic disease of the breast; relationship to carcinoma. *Cancer* 17:957, 1964.
28. de Cholnoky, T. Reconstruction of breast following mastectomy. *Plast. Reconstr. Surg.* 16:226, 1955.
29. Devitt, J. E. Fibrocystic disease of the breast is not premalignant. *Surg. Gynecol. Obstet.* 134:803, 1972.
30. Dodd, G. D. Present status of thermography, ultrasound, and mammography in breast cancer detection. *Cancer* 39:2796, 1977.
31. Dodenoff, T. Personal communication. 1976.
32. Edwards, E. A. Surgical Anatomy of the Breast. In Goldwyn, R. M. (Ed.), *Plastic and Reconstructive Surgery of the Breast.* Boston: Little, Brown, 1976.
33. Ellenberg, A. H. Marked thinning of the breast skin flaps after insertion of implants containing triamcinolone. *Plast. Reconstr. Surg.* 60:755, 1977.
34. Ellenberg, A. H. Personal communication, 1977.
35. Fisher, E. R., and Fisher, B. Lobular carcinoma

of the breast: An overview. *Ann. Surg.* 185:377, 1977.

36. Foote, F. W., and Stewart, F. W. Comparative studies of cancerous versus noncancerous breasts. *Ann. Surg.* 121:197, 1945.

36a. Fox, M. S. On the diagnosis and treatment of breast cancer. *J.A.M.A.* 241:489, 1979.

37. Fredricks, S. Subcutaneous mastectomy, a prophylactic and cosmetic operation. *Panminerva Med.* 4:137, 1969.

38. Fredricks, S. A 10-year experience with subcutaneous mastectomy. *Clin. Plast. Surg.* 2:347, 1975.

39. Freeman, B. S. Complications of subcutaneous mastectomy with prosthetic replacement, immediate or delayed. *South. Med. J.* 60:1277, 1967.

40. Freeman, B. S. Subcutaneous mastectomy for central tumors of the breast with immediate reconstruction. *Plast. Reconstr. Surg.* 51:263, 1973.

41. Freeman, B. S. Subcutaneous Mastectomy: A Treatment of Minimal Breast Cancer. In Snyderman, R. K. (Ed.), *Symposium on Neoplastic and Reconstructive Problems of the Female Breast.* St. Louis: Mosby, 1973.

42. Freeman, B. S. Subcutaneous Mastectomy. In Georgiade, N. B. (Ed.), *Reconstructive Breast Surgery.* St. Louis: Mosby, 1976. Chap. 19.

43. Freeman, B. S., and Weimer, D. R. Total glandular mastectomy. *Plast. Reconstr. Surg.* 62:167, 1978.

44. Gallager, H. S., and Martin, J. E. Early phases in the development of breast cancer. *Cancer* 24:1170, 1969.

45. Gallager, H. S., and Martin, J. E. The study of mammary carcinoma by mammography and whole organ sectioning. *Cancer* 23:855, 1969.

46. Georgiade, N. G. Immediate Reconstruction of the Breast Following Subcutaneous Mastectomy. In Georgiade, N. G. (Ed.), *Reconstructive Breast Surgery.* St. Louis: Mosby, 1976.

47. Georgiade, N. G., and Hyland, W. Technique for subcutaneous mastectomy and immediate reconstruction in the ptotic breast. *Plast. Reconstr. Surg.* 56:121, 1975.

48. Gershon-Cohen, J., and Hermel, M. B. Modalities in breast cancer detection: Xeroradiography, mammography, thermography and mammometry. *Cancer* 34:1226, 1969.

48a. Goin, J. M., and Kern, W. H. Multicentric ductal and lobular atypia and occult carcinoma in prophylactic subcutaneous mastectomies: A preliminary report. *Ann. Plast. Surg.* 2:121, 1979.

49. Goldman, L. D., and Goldwyn, R. M. Some anatomic considerations of subcutaneous mastectomy. *Plast. Reconstr. Surg.* 51:501, 1973.

50. Goldwyn, R. M., and Goldman, L. D. Subcutaneous Mastectomy and Breast Replacement. In Goldwyn, R. M. (Ed.), *Plastic and Reconstructive Surgery of the Breast.* Boston: Little, Brown, 1976.

50a. Goldwyn, R. M. Subcutaneous mastectomy (Editorial). *N. Engl. J. Med.* 297:503, 1977.

50b. Goldwyn, R. M. Voice of polite dissent. Subcutaneous mastectomy: A plea for conservatism. *Plast. Reconstr. Surg.* 62:888, 1978.

51. Goulian, O., Jr., and McDivitt, R. W. Subcutaneous mastectomy with immediate reconstruction of the breasts using dermal mastopexy technique. *Plast. Reconstr. Surg.* 50:211, 1972.

52. Gullino, P. M. Natural history of breast cancer progression from hyperplasia to neoplasia as predicted by angiogenesis. *Cancer* 39:2697, 1977.

53. Haagensen, C. D., Lane, N., Lattes, R., and Bodian, C. Lobular neoplasia (so-called lobular carcinoma in situ) of the breast. *Cancer* 42:737, 1978.

54. Haagensen, C. D. The relationship of gross cystic disease of the breast and carcinoma (Editorial). *Ann. Surg.* 185:375, 1977.

55. Hartley, J. H., Jr., Schatten, W. E., and Griffin, J. M. Subcutaneous mastectomy. The excess skin problem. *Plast. Reconstr. Surg.* 56:5, 1975.

55a. Hetter, G. P. Augmentation Mammaplasty. In *Plastic Surgery Forum,* Vol. I. Chicago: American Society of Plastic and Reconstructive Surgeons, 1978. P. 122.

56. Hicken, N. F. Mastectomy. *Arch. Surg.* 40:6, 1940.

57. Hoopes, J. E., and Ryan, J. R. The McKissock approach to subcutaneous mastectomy and immediate prosthesis implantation. *Br. J. Plast. Surg.* 28:171, 1975.

58. Horton, C. E., Adamson, J. E., Mladick, R. A., and Carraway, J. H. Simple mastectomy with immediate reconstruction. *Plast. Reconst. Surg.* 53:42, 1974.

59. Horton, C. E., and Carraway, J. H. Total Mastectomy with Immediate Reconstruction for Premalignant Disease. In Goldwyn, R. M. (Ed.), *Plastic and Reconstructive Surgery of the Breast.* Boston: Little, Brown, 1976.

59a. Horton, C. E., Rosato, F. E., Schuler, F. A., and McGraw, J. Postmastectomy reconstruction. *Ann. Surg.* 188:773, 1978.

59b. Huang, T. T., Blackwell, S. J., and Lewis, S. R. Migration of silicone gel after the "squeeze technique" to rupture a contracted breast capsule. *Plast. Reconstr. Surg.* 61:277, 1978.

60. Hutter, R. V. P. The Precancerous Breast. In Snyderman, R. K. (Ed.), *Symposium on Neo-*

plastic and Reconstructive Problems of the Female Breast. St. Louis: Mosby, 1973.

61. Hutter, R. V. P. The voice of polite dissent re: Subcutaneous mastectomy for central tumors of the breast with immediate reconstruction. *Plast. Reconstr. Surg.* 51:445, 1973.
62. Hutter, R. V. P., and Foote, F. W., Jr. Lobular carcinoma, in situ. *Cancer* 24:1081, 1969.
63. Hutter, R. V. P., Foote, F. W., Jr., and Farrow, J. H. In Situ Lobular Carcinoma of the Female Breast, 1939–1968. In *Breast Cancer, Early and Late.* Chicago: Year Book, 1970. Pp. 201–226.
64. Jarrett, J. R., Cutler, R. G., and Teal, D. F. Subcutaneous mastectomy in small, large or ptotic breasts with immediate submuscular placement of implants. *Plast. Reconstr. Surg.* 62:702, 1978.
64a. Jensen, H. M., Rice, J. R., and Wellings, S. R. Preneoplastic lesions in the human breast. *Science* 191:295, 1976.
65. Karpas, C. M., Leis, H. P., Jr., Oppenheim, A., and Mersheimer, W. L. Relationship of fibrocystic disease to carcinoma of the breast. *Ann. Surg.* 162:1, 1965.
66. Kelly, A. P., Jacobson, H. S., Fox, J. I., and Jenny, H. Complications of subcutaneous mastectomy and replacement by the Cronin Silastic mammary prosthesis. *Plast. Reconstr. Surg.* 37:438, 1966.
67. Kern, F. B., and Binns, J. H. Subcutaneous mastectomy and reconstruction in large breasts. *Plast. Reconstr. Surg.* 54:648, 1974.
68. Kern, W. M., and Brooks, R. N. Atypical epithelial hyperplasia associated with breast cancer and fibrocystic disease. *Cancer* 24:668, 1969.
69. Kirschner, M. The role of hormones in the etiology of human breast cancer. *Cancer* 39:2716, 1977.
70. Kodlin, D., Wenger, E. E., Morgenstern, N. L., and Chen, U. Chronic mastopathy and breast cancer. A follow-up study. *Cancer* 39:2603, 1977.
71. Kramer, W. M., and Rush, B. F. Mammary duct proliferation in the elderly. A histopathologic study. *Cancer* 31:130, 1973.
72. Lambird, P. A., and Sheely, W. M. The spatial distribution of lobular in situ carcinoma. *J.A.M.A.* 210:689, 1969.
73. Leis, H. P., Jr. Diagnosis and Treatment of Breast Lesions. Flushing, N. Y.: Medical Examination Publishing, 1970.
74. Leis, H. P., Jr. Premalignant Breast Lesions. In Snyderman, R. K. (Ed.), *Symposium on Neoplastic and Reconstructive Problems of the Female Breast.* St. Louis: Mosby, 1973.
75. Leis, H. P., Jr. Risk factors in breast cancer. *AORN J.* 22:723, 1975.
76. Leis, H. P., Jr. The diagnosis of breast cancer. *CA, a cancer journal for clinicians.* 27:209, 1977.
77. Leis, H. P., Jr., and Bowen, W. F. Premalignant lesions of the breast. *West. J. Surg. Obstet. Gynecol.* 72:171, 1964.
78. Lemon, H. M. Abnormal estrogen metabolism and tissue receptor proteins in breast cancer. *Cancer* 25:423, 1970.
79. Letterman, G., and Schurter, M. Inframammary based dermal fat flaps in mammary reconstruction following a subcutaneous mastectomy. *Plast. Reconstr. Surg.* 55:156, 1975.
80. Longacre, J. J. The use of local pedicle flaps for reconstruction of the breast after subtotal or total extirpation of the mammary gland and for correction of distortion and atrophy of the breast due to excessive scar. *Plast. Reconstr. Surg.* 11:380, 1953.
80a. Lynch, H. T., Harris, R. E., Organ, C. H., and Lynch, J. F. Management of familial breast cancer. *Arch. Surg.* 113:1053, 1978.
80b. McCarty, K. S., Kesterson, G. H. D., Wilkinson. W. E., and Georgiade, N. Histopathologic study of subcutaneous mastectomy specimens from patients with carcinoma of the contralateral breast. *Surg. Gynecol. Obstet.* 147:682, 1978.
81. McDivitt, R. W., Hutter, R. V. P., Foote, F. W., Jr., and Stewart, F. W. In situ lobular carcinoma. A prospective follow-up study indicating cumulative patient risks. *J.A.M.A.* 201:82, 1969.
81a. McDivitt, R. W. Breast carcinoma (progress in human pathology). *Hum. Pathol.* 9:3, 1978.
82. McDowell, F. Subcutaneous mastectomy, syntax and seat belts (Editorial). *Plast. Reconstr. Surg.* 51:575, 1973.
83. McKissock, P. K. Reduction mammoplasty with a vertical dermal flap. *Plast. Reconstr. Surg.* 49:245, 1972.
84. McLaughin, C. W., Jr., Schenken, J. R., and Tomisica, J. X. A study of precancerous epithelial hyperplasia and noninvasive papillary carcinoma of the breast. *Ann. Surg.* 153:735, 1961.
84a. Mladick, R. A. Possible danger of placing implants subpectorally immediately after subcutaneous mastectomy (Letter to the Editor). *Plast. Reconstr. Surg.* 62:289, 1978.
85. Molenaar, A. Subcutaneous mastectomy. *Clin. Plast. Surg.* 1:427, 1974.
86. Myers, M. B. Prediction of skin slough at the time of operation with use of fluorescein dye. *Surgery* 51:158, 1962.
87. Niederhuber, J. Personal communication, 1977.

87a. Oneal, R. M. Unpublished letter to editor. *Plast. Reconstr. Surg.* 1979.
88. Papillon, J. Pros and cons of subpectoral implantation. *Clin. Plast. Surg.* 3:321, 1976.
89. Peacock, E. E. Biological basis for management of benign disease of the breast. *Plast. Reconstr. Surg.* 55:14, 1975.
90. Pennisi, V. R. Incidence of obscure carcinoma in subcutaneous mastectomy. Results of a national survey. *Plast. Reconstr. Surg.* 56:9, 1975.
91. Pennisi, V. R. Subcutaneous mastectomy and fibrocystic disease of the breast. *Clin. Plast. Surg.* 3:205, 1976.
92. Pennisi, V. R., and Capozzi, A. Treatment of chronic cystic disease of the breast by subcutaneous mastectomy. *Plast. Reconstr. Surg.* 53:520, 1973.
93. Pennisi, V. R., Capozzi, A., and Perez, F. M. Subcutaneous mastectomy data. *Plast. Reconstr. Surg.* 59:53, 1977.
94. Perrin, E. R. Use of soluble steroids within inflatable breast prosthesis. *Plast. Reconstr. Surg.* 57:163, 1976.
95. Petrakis, N. L. Genetic factors in the etiology of breast cancer. *Cancer* 39:2709, 1977.
96. Pickrell, K. L., Puckett, C. L., and Given, K. S. Subpectoral augmentation mammoplasty. *Plast. Reconstr. Surg.* 60:622, 1977.
97. Redfern, A. B., and Hoopes, J. E. Subcutaneous mastectomy: A plea for conservatism. *Plast. Reconstr. Surg.* 62:706, 1978.
98. Regnault, P. Breast ptosis. *Clin. Plast. Surg.* 3:193, 1976.
99. Regnault, P. Reduction Mammoplasty by the "B" Technique. In Goldwyn, R. M. (Ed.), *Plastic and Reconstructive Surgery of the Breast.* Boston: Little, Brown, 1976.
100. Regnault, P. Partially submuscular breast augmentation. *Plast. Reconstr. Surg.* 59:72, 1977.
101. Rigg, B. M. A method for the intraoperative selection of the best size for a mammary prosthesis. *Plast. Reconstr. Surg.* 52:589, 1973.
101a. Robles, J. M., Zimman, O. A., and Lee, J. C. A larger subpectoral pocket for breast implants. *Plast. Reconstr. Surg.* 62:78, 1978.
102. Robson, M. C., Krizek, T. J., and Heggers, J. P. Biology of surgical infection. *Curr. Probl. Surg.* 1:62, 1973.
102a. Rosen, P. P., Lieberman, P. H., Braun, D. W., Kosloff, C., and Adair, F. Lobular carcinoma in situ of the breast. *Am. J. Surg. Pathol.* 2:225, 1978.
103. Roth, J. A., Feinberg, M., and McAvoy, J. M. Carcinoma arising in the wall of a breast cyst during pregnancy. *Ann. Surg.* 185:279, 1977.
104. Rubin, L. R. Cushioned augmentation repair after a subcutaneous mastectomy. *Plast. Reconstr. Surg.* 57:23, 1976.
104a. Rubin, L. R. A preventative mastectomy with immediate reconstruction for high-risk cancer patient. *Clin. Plast. Surg.* 6:107, 1979.
105. Sawin, C. T. Endocrine Physiology and Pathophysiology of the Breast. In Goldwyn, R. M. (Ed.), *Plastic and Reconstructive Surgery of the Breast.* Boston: Little, Brown, 1976.
106. Schlenker, J. D., Bueno, R. A., Ricketson, G., and Lynch, J. B. Loss of silicone implants after subcutaneous mastectomy and reconstruction. *Plast. Reconstr. Surg.* 62:853, 1978.
107. Sieninski, W., and Dobska, M. Usefulness of drill biopsy in diagnosis of breast tumors. *Cancer* 38:2567, 1976.
108. Silverberg, S. G., Chetab, A. R., and Levitt, S. H. Prognostic implications of fibrocystic dysplasia in breasts removed for mammary carcinoma. *Cancer* 29:574, 1972.
109. Silverstein, M. J., Sartorius, O. W., and Zarem, H. A. Pathology of the Breast for Ptotic and Reconstructive Surgeons. In Goldwyn, R. M. (Ed.), *Plastic and Reconstructive Surgery of the Breast.* Boston: Little, Brown, 1976.
109a. Singer, R., Lewis, C. M., Franklin, J. D., and Lynch, J. B. Fluorescein test for prediction of flap viability during breast reconstruction. *Plast. Reconstr. Surg.* 61:371, 1978.
110. Smahel, J. Tissue reactions to breast implants coated with polyurethane. *Plast. Reconstr. Surg.* 61:80, 1978.
111. Snyderman, R. K. The voice of polite dissent re: Subcutaneous mastectomy for central tumors of the breast with immediate reconstruction. *Plast. Reconstr. Surg.* 51:448, 1973.
112. Snyderman, R. K. Subcutaneous mastectomy with immediate prosthetic reconstruction – an operation in search of patients (Letter to the Editor). *Plast. Reconstr. Surg.* 53:582, 1974.
113. Spira, M. Subcutaneous mastectomy in the large ptotic breast. *Plast. Reconstr. Surg.* 59:200, 1977.
114. Swerdlow, M., and Humphrey, L. J. Fibrocystic disease and carcinoma of the breast. *Arch. Surg.* 87:457, 1963.
115. Tellem, M., Prive, L., and Meranze, D. R. Four quadrant study of breasts removed for carcinoma. *Cancer* 15:10, 1962.
115a. Toker, C., and Goldberg, J. D. The small cell lesion of mammary ducts and lobules. *Pathol. Annu.* 12:217, 1977.

116. Wagner, H., Beller, F. K., and Pfautsch, M. Electron and light microscopy examination of capsules around breast implants. *Plast. Reconstr. Surg.* 60:49, 1977.
117. Wanebo, H. J., Huros, A. G., and Urban, J. A. Treatment of minimal breast cancer. *Cancer* 33:349, 1974.
118. Weiner, D. L., Volk, H., Frater, R. W., Alpert, S., Pauporle, J., Silver, L., and Alache, A. E. Subcutaneous mastectomy with reconstruction. From the combined breast/surgical clinics of the Albert Einstein College of Medicine, New York, N.Y., and Dow Corning Corp., Midland, Mich., 1973.
119. Wheeler, J. E., Enterline, H. T., Roseman, J. M., Tomasulo, J. P., McIlvaine, C. H., Fitts, W. J., Jr., and Kirshenbaum, J. Lobular carcinoma of the breast: Long term follow-up. *Cancer* 34:554, 1974.
120. Wilkinson, T. S. The use of the pectoralis major in destructive and reconstructive breast surgery. Presented at the annual meeting of the American Society of Plastic and Reconstructive Surgeons, Boston, Mass., 1976.
121. Wilkinson, T. S. Personal communication, 1977.
122. Wolfe, J. N. Breast patterns as an index of risk for developing breast cancer. *Am. J. Roentgenol. Radium Ther. Nucl. Med.* 126:1130, 1976.
123. Zbylski, J. R., and Parsons, R. W. A method of adenectomy and breast reconstruction for benign disease. *Plast. Reconstr. Surg.* 37:38, 1966.

Reconstruction of the Breast after Mastectomy

THOMAS D. CRONIN

It is safe to say that all women subjected to a radical mastectomy suffer psychological and emotional shock, often of a marked degree, with effects that may persist for years. Knowing that reconstruction may be possible, especially if a modified radical mastectomy has been done, may ease the reaction somewhat. Although Snyderman [67] emphasizes the simple creation of a mound that will fill out a brassiere or a bathing suit, I believe that we, as plastic surgeons, should strive for more realism by constructing a nipple-areolar complex and the use of skin flaps when there is a gross deficiency of skin on the chest wall; this allows the construction of a more pleasingly shaped breast.

When a reasonable aesthetic result has been obtained by reconstruction, the reaction of my patients has varied from pleased satisfaction to real ecstasy. I recall only one patient who, because of unrealistic expectations in a particularly difficult reconstruction, was not entirely satisfied. It is important not to arouse false expectations. The plastic surgeon would do well to show examples of his *own* reconstructions to the patient.

SELECTION OF PATIENTS

Indications

Most important in the selection of patients is that the local disease has been eradicated. Thus, the best candidates are patients classified as Class A in the Columbia Clinical Classification system (no skin edema, ulceration, or solid fixation of the tumor to the chest wall; no involvement of the axillary nodes; this is comparable to Class I of the International Classification). Other patients who had more advanced disease but who have survived 3 years or more are also favorable candidates, since 70 percent of recurrences take place within the first three years [6]. Motivation of the patient is important if multiple stages are required. The fact that some patients may eventually succumb to distant metastasis is no reason to deny them the satisfaction of reconstruction in the intervening years.

Contraindications

The main contraindications are inflammatory cancer and large, aggressive lesions with questionable local eradication. Relative contraindications include large skin-grafted areas; large, extremely thin flaps with absent pectoralis muscle; and severe radiation changes.

PREOPERATIVE PLANNING

Timing of Reconstruction

Cronin and associates [19] advocate a delay of 2 to 4 months (or until the tissues have returned to normal) after a radical mastectomy or when the prosthesis is to be placed on top of a retained pectoral muscle. However, if subpectoral implantation is intended in association with a modified radical or simple mastectomy, it might be done at the same time or within a few days. Hueston and McKenzie [41], working with the general surgeon, have advocated insertion of a Silastic-gel implant (on top of muscle) about 4 days after mastectomy. Horton [39], working with the general surgeon, has done immediate reconstruction with subpectoral implants.

Choosing a Prosthesis

The absence of breast tissue usually makes it necessary to use a larger prosthesis than would be used for an augmentation in the same patient. A broad-based implant with edges that will blend into the chest is preferable to a narrow-based implant that may rest on the chest like an orange. Considering the width of the chest, the amount of skin available, the size of the other breast, and the woman's desires, a prosthesis is selected. I prefer the Dow Corning prostheses. When the pectoralis major muscle is absent, a 310-c.c. contour-shape prosthesis has been a frequent choice, because it has somewhat more projection than the low-profile round design. When the muscle is present and subpectoral implantation is planned, the following low-profile, round prostheses have been used: 235 c.c., 270 c.c., and 305 c.c.; rarely, larger sizes up to 350 to 400 c.c. might be used.

OPERATIVE TECHNIQUES

Techniques in Patients with Adequate Soft Tissue Coverage

If the skin flaps are sufficiently thick and loose enough to cover a Silastic-gel prosthesis, the lateral end of a transverse or inferior end of a vertical scar is incised, and a pocket created into which a Silastic-gel implant of suitable size can be inserted (Fig. 47-1). If the pectoralis major muscle is present it is probably better to do a subpectoral dissection, especially if the skin flaps are thin (Fig. 47-2). The muscle should be relaxed by incising it from its origin on the rib cage. On the left side, the dissection is from 5 to 9 o'clock,

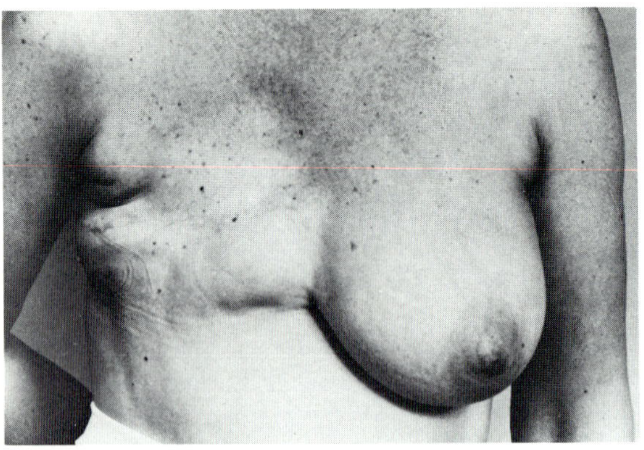

A

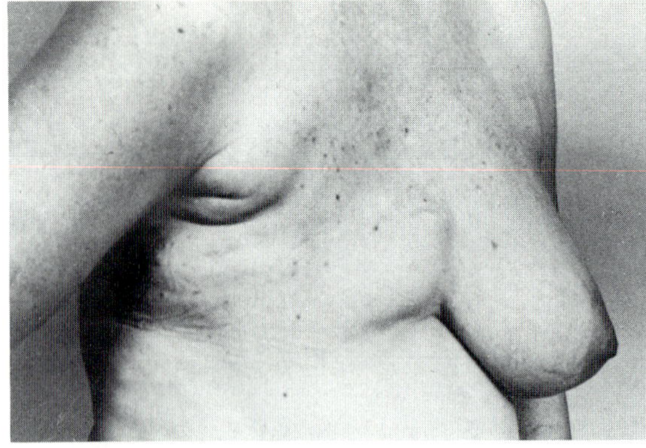

B

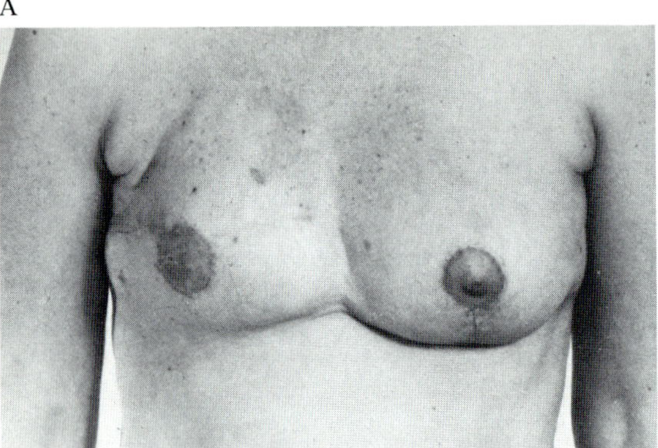

C

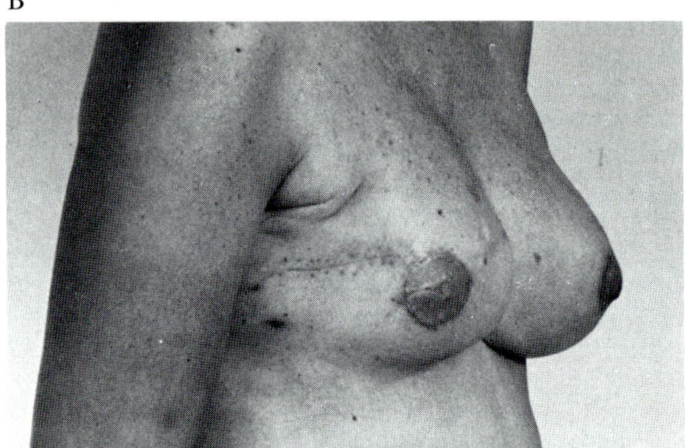

D

Fig. 47-1. A, B, a 52-year-old woman, 10 years after a total mastectomy for fibrocystic disease with focal intraductal papillomatosis and cellular atypia. C, D, appearance after a single operation in which a 400-c.c. Silastic-gel "tear drop" implant was inserted through an incision in the lateral end of the old scar, into a suprapectoral pocket. At the same time the areola was reconstructed by the conjoined-circle method of nipple sharing, and the other breast was reduced by the Strömbeck method. (From T. D. Cronin, J. Upton, and J. M. McDonough. Reconstruction of the breast after mastectomy. Plast. Reconstr. Surg. *59:1, 1977.)*

and on the right from 3 to 7 o'clock [60]. A gel implant of suitable size is inserted. A nipple-areolar complex may be added at this time, but it can be located and matched more accurately at a later time when the other breast is modified, if it is to be modified.

Guthrie [31] attempts reconstruction without additional skin flaps even when the skin flaps are extremely thin and adherent. Through a 10-cm. incision, 3 cm. below the opposite inframammary fold he dissects a pocket widely and inserts an Ashley prosthesis, which is in three compartments and covered by a layer of polyurethane. Because of its rigid construction this implant tends to retain its shape, but it produces a firm-to-hard breast.

Techniques in Patients with Inadequate Soft Tissue Coverage

The following is an outline of the techniques used in patients with inadequate skin coverage:

A. Skin and myocutaneous flaps.
   1. Transverse thoracoepigastric flaps, which are especially suitable when a vertical scar is present (Figs. 47-3 and 47-4).
   2. Latissimus dorsi myocutaneous flap [9] (Fig. 47-5).
   3. Large, local rotational flap from the anterior chest and the abdominal wall (Cronin [19]), when the scar is transverse (Fig. 47-6).
   4. Reverse abdominoplasty flap (Peterson [55]) when the scar is transverse (Figs. 47-7 and 47-8).
   5. A transverse lower abdominal tube flap (Millard [47]).

B. Flaps from the other breast.
   1. One-half of the other breast (Pontes [57]; Fig. 47-9).

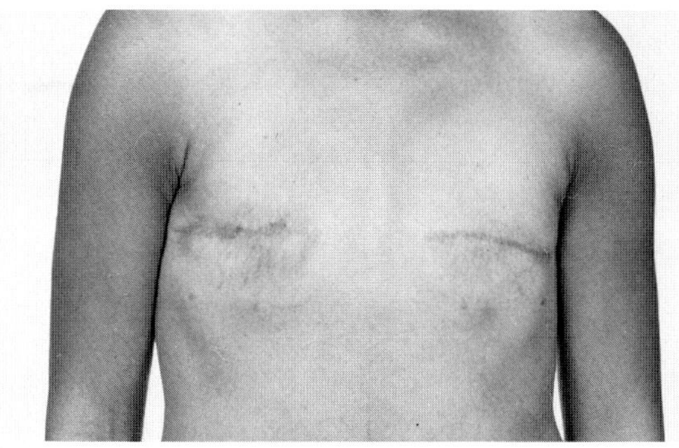

A

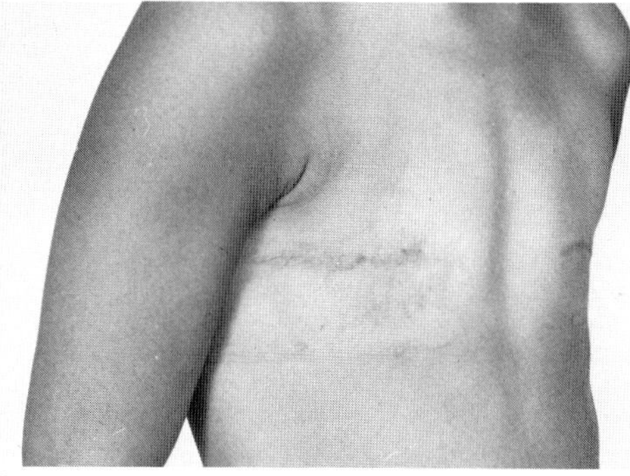

B

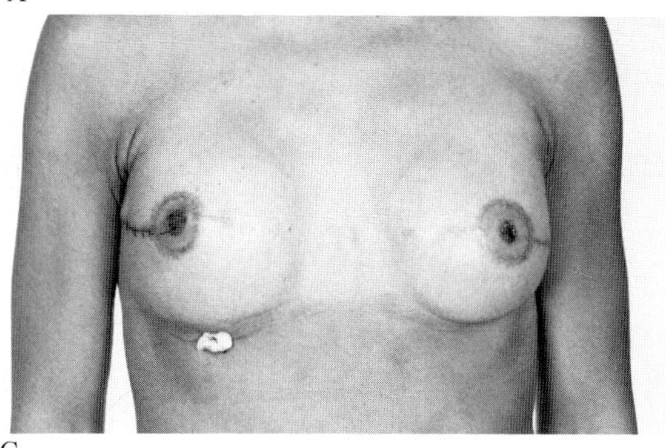

C

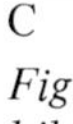

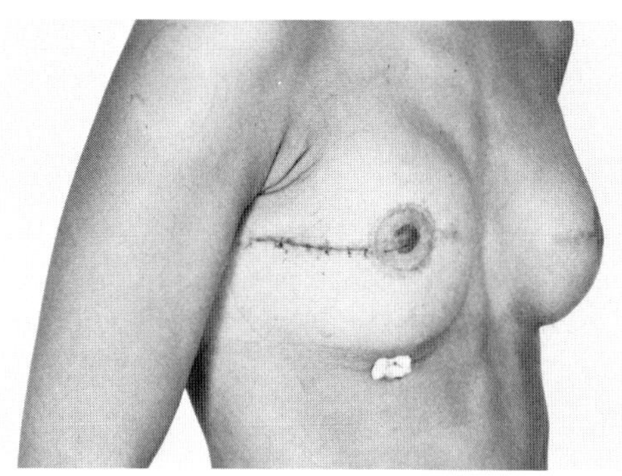

D

Fig. 47-2. A, B, a 29-year-old woman who had had bilateral total mastectomies 3 years previously because her mother and two sisters had cancer of the breast. C, D, appearance after breast reconstruction by subpectoral insertion of a 270-cc. Silastic-gel implant on the left and a 340-cc. on the right (an unusual hollow of the rib cage on the right required this larger size to equalize the appearance of the breasts). Diminutive labia minora directed attention elsewhere, and hemorrhoidal skin was used for the nipples. The areolae were made from full-thickness skin grafts of lightly pigmented skin of upper, inner thighs.

2. Transverse tube flap from the other breast (Holdsworth [38] and Alexander and Block [2]).

C. Reconstruction using the omentum with split-thickness skin flaps [3, 23].

Skin and Myocutaneous Flaps

THE TRANSVERSE THORACOEPIGASTRIC FLAP. I have found that a thoracoepigastric flap [18] is the most convenient and useful flap in patients with inadequate soft tissue coverage, when there is a vertical scar. It is based on the internal mammary and superior epigastric vessels (Figs. 47-3 and 47-4). This flap, if it is made with a wide base (10 to 14 cm.) and if it does not extend beyond the midaxillary line, can be transposed without delay; if the flap extends beyond the posterior axillary line, delay would be necessary. The implant may be inserted at the time of transfer unless the circulation is questionable, in which case insertion should be delayed for 1 or 2 weeks.

The donor site can usually be closed by flexing the table with the patient on her side and undermining inferiorly – if necessary, beyond the iliac crest, according to Davis and colleagues [20].

LATISSIMUS DORSI MYOCUTANEOUS FLAP. The latissimus dorsi muscle is a large flat muscle arising from the midline of the back from the lower six thoracic vertebrae down to the posterior crest of the ilium. From its very broad origin it narrows and is inserted into the intertubercular sulcus of the humerus. The vascular supply (the thoracodorsal branch of the subscapular artery) and nerve (thoracodorsal nerve) supply of the latissimus muscle enter the axilla near its insertion, which makes it ideal for transposition on this narrow pedicle.

The use of this arterialized muscle gives the best correction for the infraclavicular hollow area, but it is also valuable because the skin overlying the latissimus is supplied by muscular perforators; therefore, that skin can be moved with the muscle (Fig. 47-5).

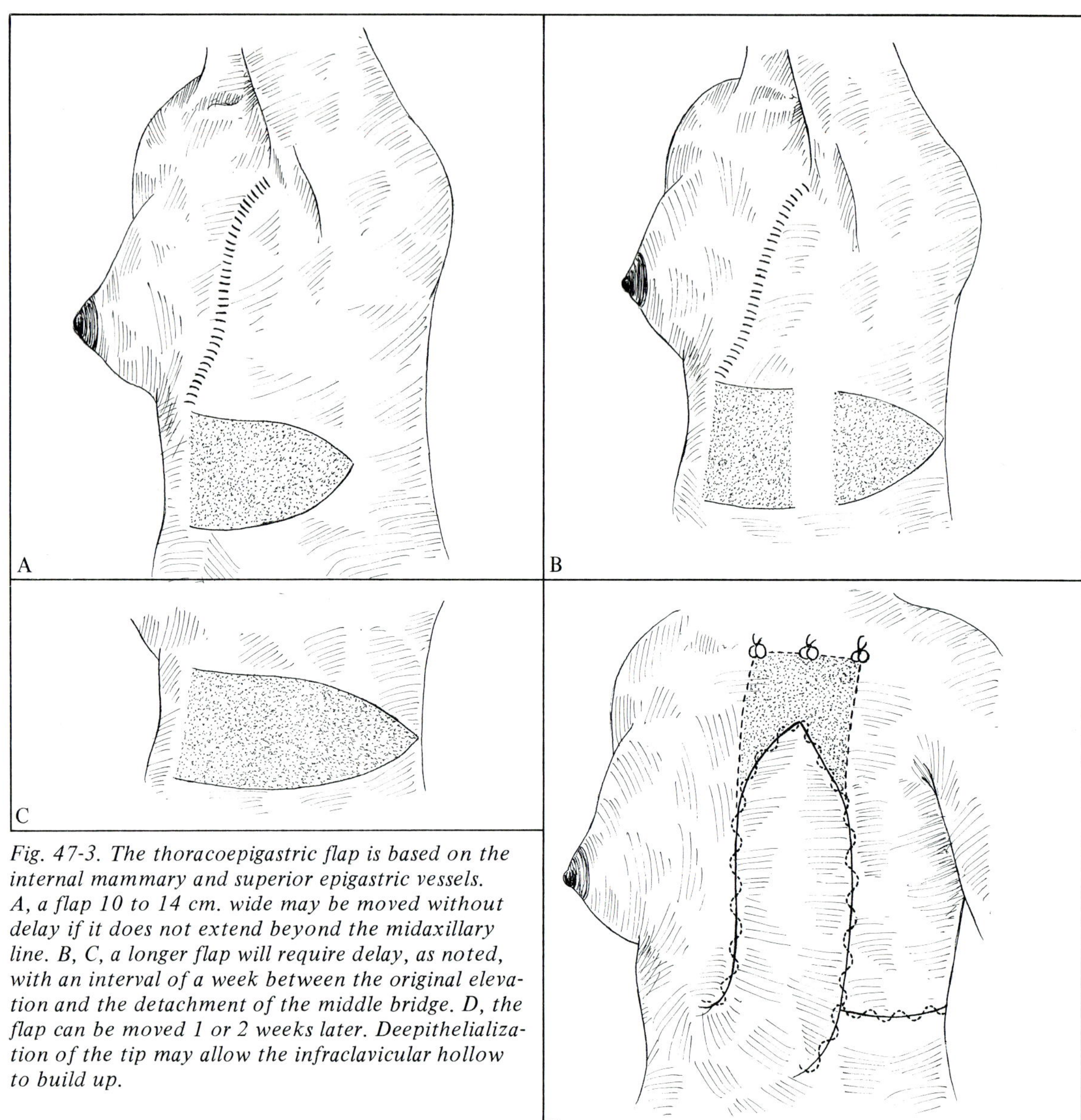

Fig. 47-3. The thoracoepigastric flap is based on the internal mammary and superior epigastric vessels. A, a flap 10 to 14 cm. wide may be moved without delay if it does not extend beyond the midaxillary line. B, C, a longer flap will require delay, as noted, with an interval of a week between the original elevation and the detachment of the middle bridge. D, the flap can be moved 1 or 2 weeks later. Deepithelialization of the tip may allow the infraclavicular hollow to build up.

Fig. 47-4. A, a 51-year-old physician 7 years after a classic radical mastectomy for a 2.9-cm. intraductal carcinoma in the upper outer quadrant. Her 21 axillary nodes were negative, and she received 7,000 R. B, C, D, appearance at 9 months after reconstruction with a thoracoepigastric flap and a 235-cc. Silastic-gel round prosthesis. The left breast was treated by subcutaneous mastectomy and insertion of the same sized implant; later a mastopexy was done on the left. The nipple-areolar complex was constructed by the conjoined-spiral method of sharing. E, incisions for conjoined-spiral nipple sharing. F, the recipient nipple and areola at 9 months. G, the donor nipple and areola. (From T. D. Cronin, J. Upton, and J. M. McDonough. Reconstruction of the breast after mastectomy. Plast. Reconstr. Surg. *59:1, 1977.)*

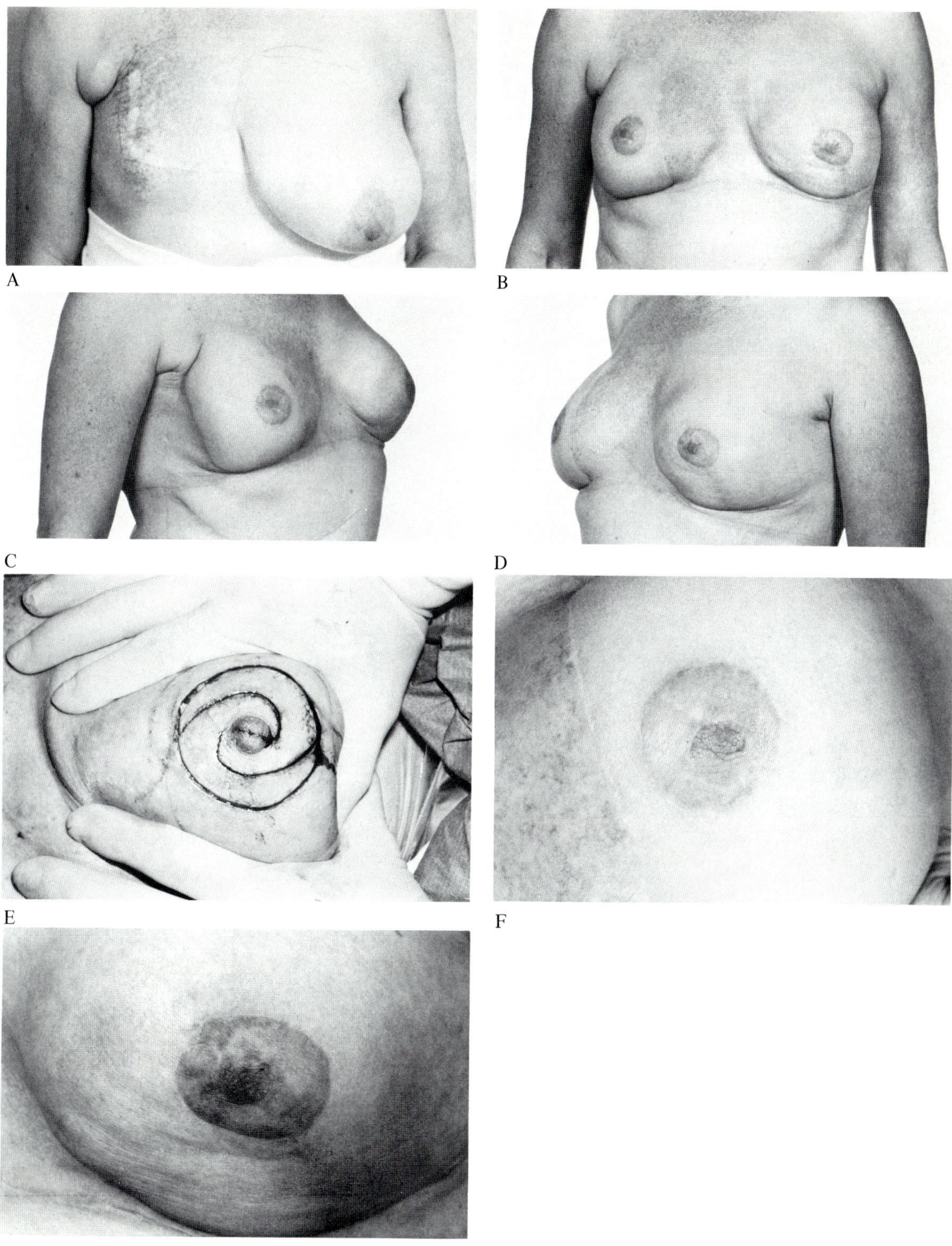
A
B
C
D
E
F
G

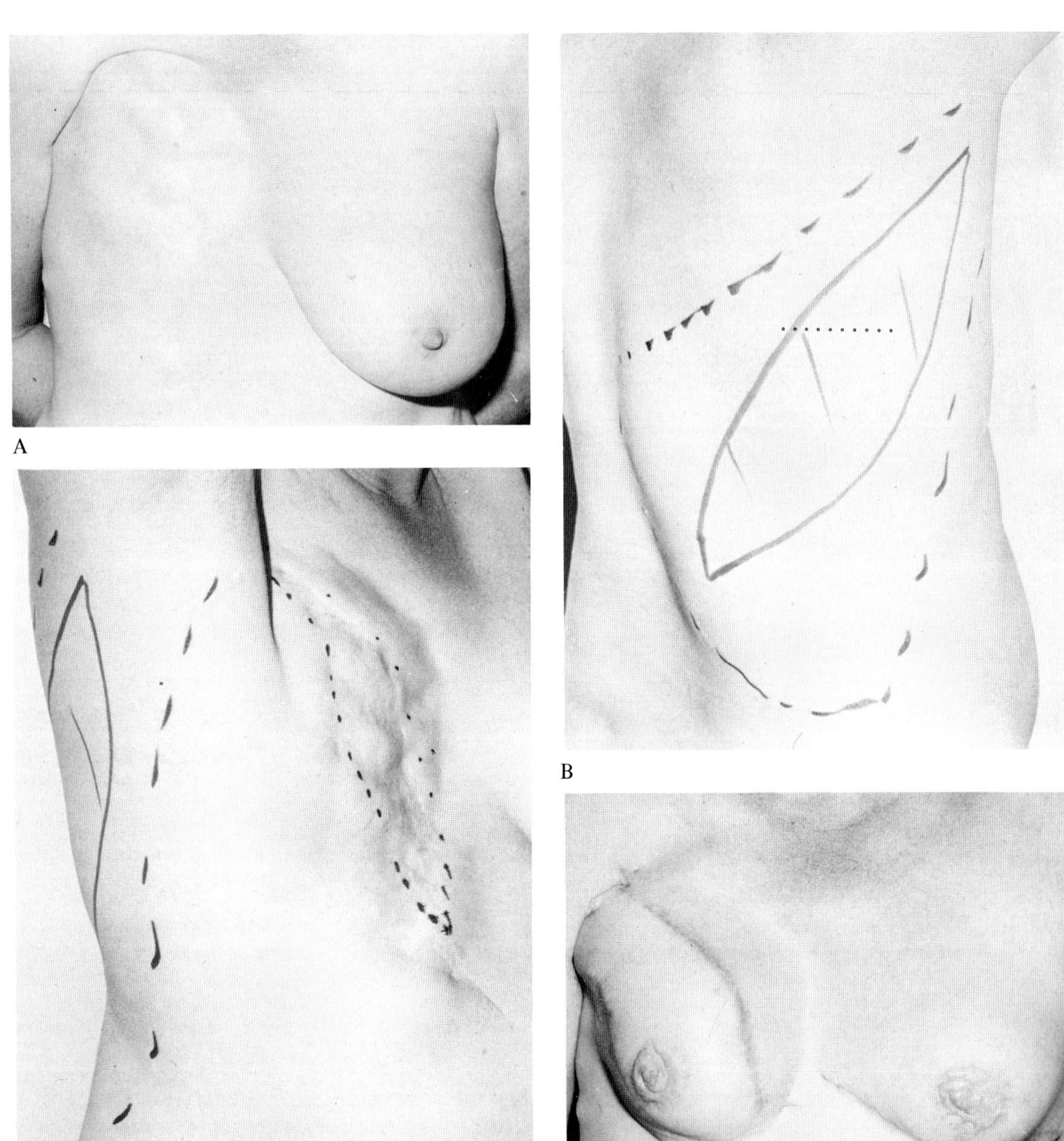

Fig. 47-5. The latissimus dorsi myocutaneous flap. A, note the unsightly infraclavicular hollow with ribs visible under the thin skin flaps. B, the dashed lines indicate the extent of the latissimus dorsi muscle. The solid lines show the skin that will be left attached to the muscle. The dotted line shows the 10-cm, incision in the line of the brassiere through which the muscle can be dissected, if no skin is to be transferred with it. C, in this view both the proposed myocutaneous flap and the scarred area on the anterior chest can be seen. D, the myocutaneous flap is delivered anteriorly through the upper end of the anterior incision, or through a separate one across the axilla. The skin of the anterior chest wall is elevated and the latissimus dorsi muscle is pulled under the skin and sutured to the clavicle and sternal border, while the skin portion is sutured to the edges of the remaining chest skin. The prosthesis can be inserted at this time, or later. (From J. Bostwick, III, et al. Breast reconstruction after a radical mastectomy. Plast. Reconstr. Surg. 61:682, 1978.)

ANTERIOR CHEST AND ABDOMINAL WALL ROTATION FLAP. Sometimes, particularly in the presence of a transverse scar, with tightness of skin in a vertical direction, a large, posteriorly based flap may be rotated upward from the anterior chest and abdominal wall (Fig. 47-6).

REVERSE ABDOMINOPLASTY FLAP. Peterson [55] has demonstrated the possibility of doing, in effect, a reverse abdominoplasty by advancing the skin flap upward (Figs. 47-7 and 47-8).

TRANSVERSE LOWER ABDOMINAL TUBE FLAP. When local tissues are scant or unavailable, Millard's [47] procedure involves a large transverse tube flap that can be constructed across the lower abdomen just above the pubic hair line, the abdominal skin above being brought down as in a typical lipectomy. This method leaves an inconspicuous scar, but it requires many stages to transfer and shape the breast. However, if it is used as a source of skin, I believe it is best to open up the scar on the chest widely and simply fill in with the flap. An implant can be inserted later, which is easier and more satisfactory than attempting to shape a breast on the chest wall by coiling or folding the tube flap.

Flaps from the Other Breast
The chief objection to the use of the remaining breast is the fact that there is an increased incidence of carcinoma developing in this breast. It has been used, nevertheless.

ONE-HALF OF THE OTHER BREAST. Pontes [57], in a one-stage procedure, splits a pendulous breast down the middle and swings it across to the other side. In his hands, excellent results have been obtained (Fig. 47-9).

TRANSVERSE TUBE FLAP FROM THE OTHER BREAST. Transverse tube flaps from the opposite breast have been used [2, 38] (Fig. 47-10).

Reconstruction Using the Omentum with Skin Graft
Arnold, Hartrampf, and Jurkiewicz [3] and others [24] have done a one-stage reconstruction of the breast, or repair of radiation necrosis, by subcutaneous passage of the omentum to replace the deficiency of skin flaps. After inserting the implant and covering it with the omentum, a thick, split-thickness skin graft is applied.

NIPPLE-AREOLAR COMPLEX

Although some surgeons and some women may be satisfied with the mere construction of a mound, I feel that the realism achieved by construction of the nipple-areolar complex is well worth the effort.

Methods Used to Construct the Nipple-Areolar Complex

Nipple Sharing from the Other Breast
When employing the concentric-circle or conjoined-spiral (Fig. 47-11) methods of nipple sharing, Table 47-1 can be used to find the diameters of two equal circles, each of which is one-half of the area of the donor areola. The same information is determined by taking 70% of donor areola diameter. Example: 10.7 X 7 cm. = 4.9 cm.

CONCENTRIC CIRCLE WITH OR WITHOUT COMPOSITE NIPPLE GRAFT. This technique [19] involves trimming the circle of areola in the course of a reduction mammoplasty or mastopexy. A 3- to 4-mm. thickness of the nipple is cut off as a graft (see Table 47-1).

CONJOINED-SPIRAL METHOD. This procedure [18] is illustrated in Figure 47-11 (see also Table 47-1).

SPLIT-THICKNESS GRAFT FROM THE AREOLA AND COMPOSITE GRAFT FROM THE NIPPLE. A thin, split graft of areola is obtained freehand with a scalpel in this technique [18].

Use of Labium Minus and Majus
In Adams' [1] procedure a full thickness of the labium minus alone is used. Wiemer and Freeman [77] use split-thickness grafts from the inner side of the labium majus for the areola and a full-thickness graft from the labium minus for the nipple. Cronin [18] uses a full-thickness graft from the labium minus for the nipple and a full-thickness skin graft from the inner thigh for the areola.

Use of Hemorrhoidal Tissue
Full-thickness external hemorrhoidal skin tags are used by Cronin [18] for the nipple; a full-thickness skin graft from inner thighs is used for the areola.

Table 47-1. Relation between Diameter of Areola and Diameter of Half Its Area

Diameter of Donor Areola	Diameter of Half of Areolar Area
7 cm.	4.9 cm.
6.5 cm.	4.6 cm.
6 cm.	4.2 cm.
5.5 cm.	3.8 cm.
5 cm.	3.5 cm.
4.5 cm.	3.2 cm.
4 cm.	2.8 cm.
3.5 cm.	2.5 cm.
3 cm.	2.1 cm.

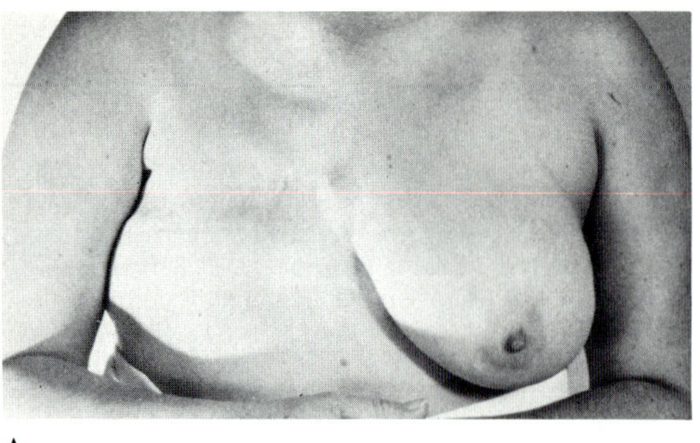

A

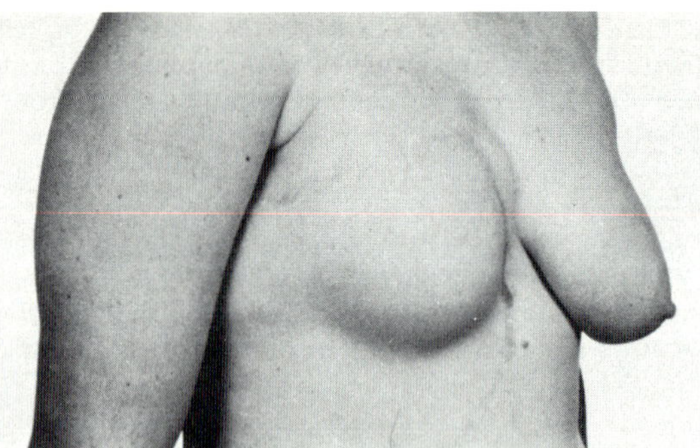

B

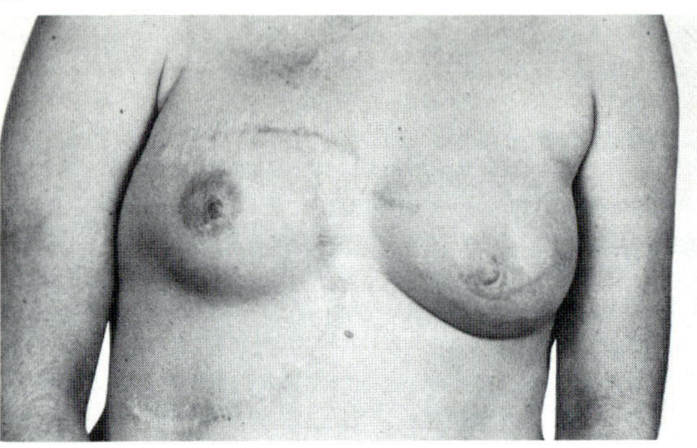

C

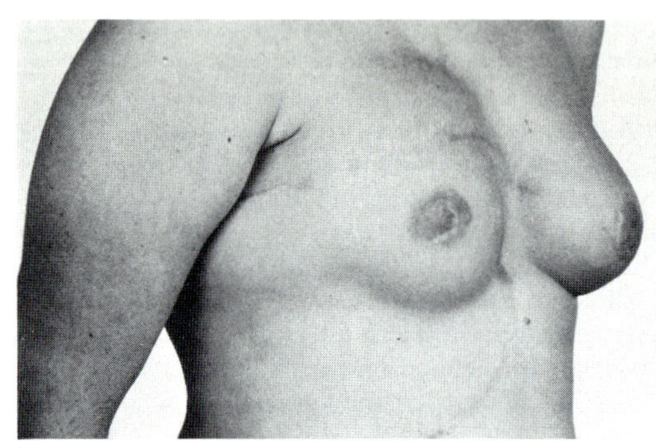

D

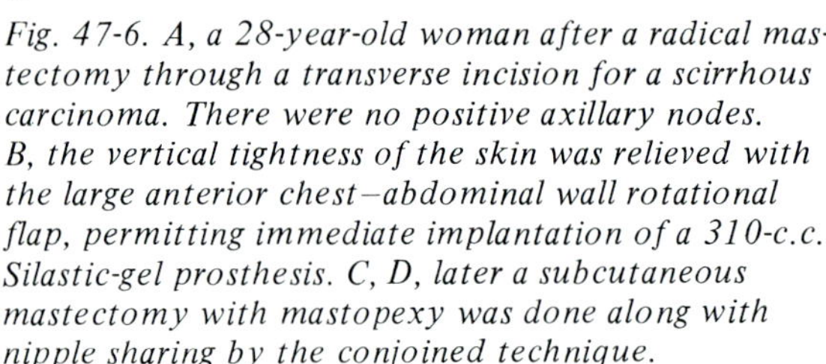

Fig. 47-6. A, a 28-year-old woman after a radical mastectomy through a transverse incision for a scirrhous carcinoma. There were no positive axillary nodes. B, the vertical tightness of the skin was relieved with the large anterior chest–abdominal wall rotational flap, permitting immediate implantation of a 310-c.c. Silastic-gel prosthesis. C, D, later a subcutaneous mastectomy with mastopexy was done along with nipple sharing by the conjoined technique.

Use of Auricular Cartilage

Brent and Bostwick [10] describe the use of a composite graft from an ear lobule and a free full-thickness postauricular skin graft with bits of ear cartilage as Montgomery's glands (Fig. 47-12). This method is useful when a light colored nipple-areolar complex is desired.

Use of Conchal Cartilage

Greater nipple projection can be attained in the procedures using the labium or hemorrhoidal tissue by the insertion of two discs of conchal cartilage. The discs are sewed one on top of the other and inserted as a second stage beneath the center of the graft. They are obtained through a postauricular incision with the use of a dermal punch 8 to 10 mm. in diameter [10].

Other Techniques Used for the Nipple-Areolar Complex

When a pink nipple-areolar complex is desired, a full-thickness buccal mucosal graft may be satisfactory, but it should be kept lubricated for a time until it adjusts to the new dry environment.

The nipple-areolar complex, or at least the areola, can be stored at the time of mastectomy (but the base of the nipple should be checked for cancer). A dermal bed is prepared in the groin to receive the nipple-areolar complex until it is needed.

Tattooing the areola is also possible.

Location of the Nipple-Areolar Complex

Determination of the precise location of the nipple-areolar complex may be exasperatingly difficult because of the mobility of the remaining breast from supine to upright positions, while the reconstructed breast has limited mobility. It is usually better to delay the placement of the nipple until the remaining breast has been modified, if it is to be modified. The site is measured from fixed points – the sternal notch, midline, midclavicular line, and inframammary crease. The measurements should be made with the patient in both sitting and supine positions. Such measurements on occasion may not look just right, and an "eyeball" compromise may finally be chosen as the most symmetrical location.

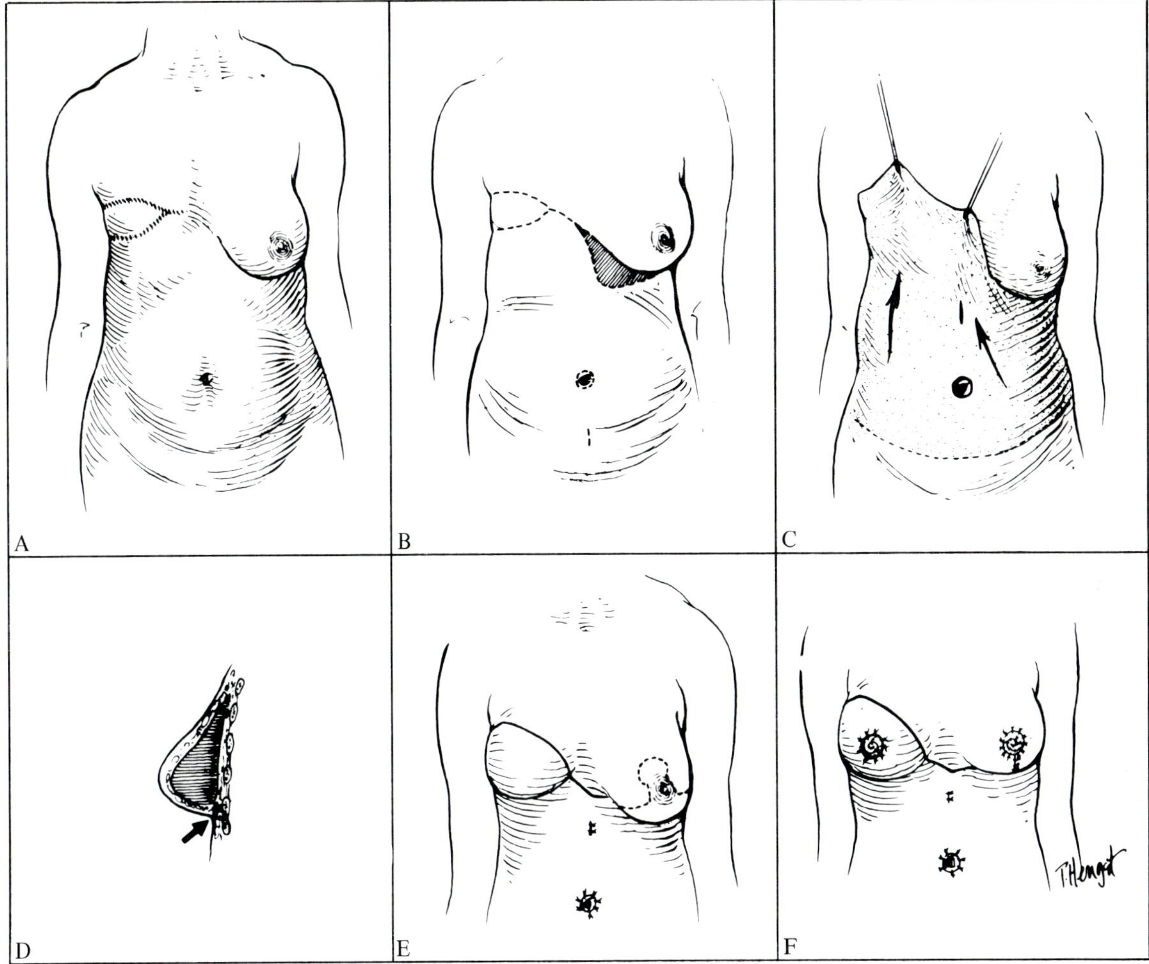

Fig. 47-7. Reverse abdominoplasty of Peterson. A, transverse scar and skin graft after mastectomy. B, lines of incision for removal of the graft and excision of excess skin under the left breast. C, the dotted area is to be undermined and advanced upward. Note the release of the umbilicus. D, the skin flap has been advanced and the gel prosthesis inserted; the remaining breast is now modified by one of the techniques mentioned in the text. ↗ the skin flap is anchored to form a new inframammary crease. E, the completed reconstruction with conjoined-spiral nipple sharing. F. Postoperative appearance. (From R. Peterson. Presented at the Symposium on Aesthetic Surgery of the Breast, Scottsdale, Arizona, November 1975.)

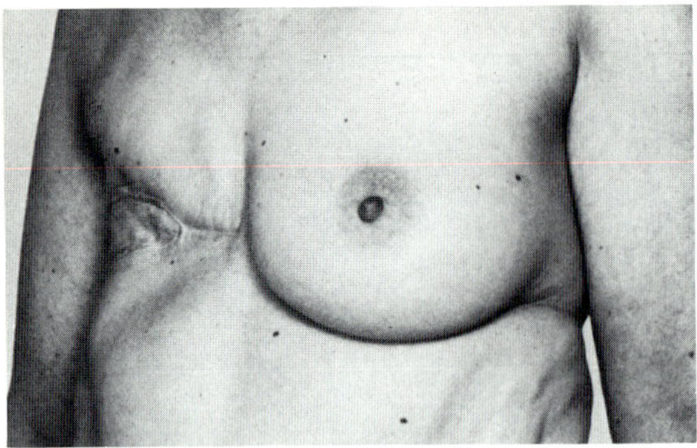

A

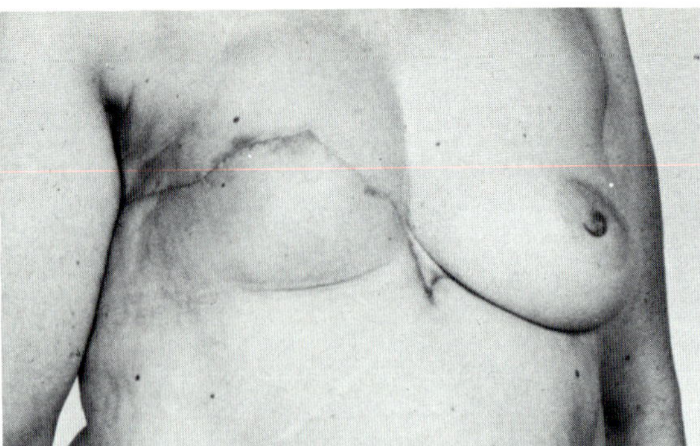

B

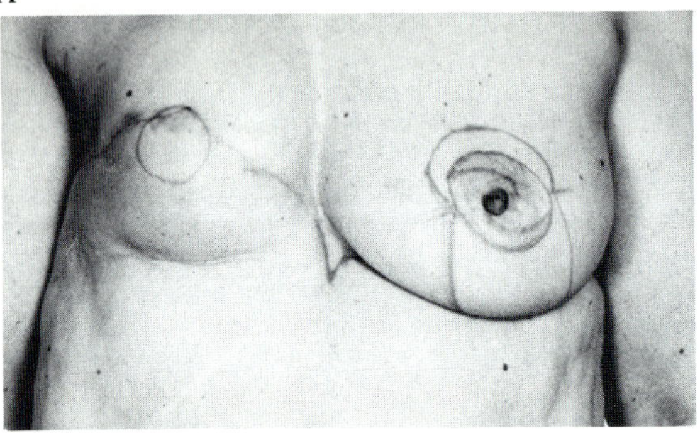

C

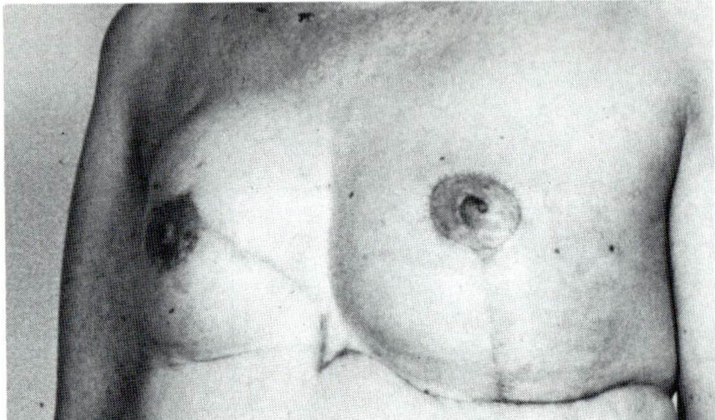

D

Fig. 47-8. A, a 65-year-old woman after a right modified radical mastectomy, using a transverse incision with skin graft. B, the appearance after the advancement of the abdominal flap and the insertion of a 310-c.c. gel implant. C, the lines of incision for subcutaneous mastectomy with mastopexy of left breast and conjoined-spiral nipple sharing procedure for right breast. D, the appearance after reconstruction was complete. (Courtesy J. M. McDonough.)

PROCEDURES FOR THE REMAINING BREAST

Usually something must be done to the remaining breast to improve its match with the reconstructed one. The following procedures have been used:

1. Mastopexy
2. Reduction mammoplasty
3. Subcutaneous mastectomy
4. Subcutaneous mastectomy with mastopexy
5. Simple mastectomy
6. Augmentation mammoplasty.

In all cases, periodic reexamination is performed, including xerograms.

The best symmetry in both upright and supine positions is attained when silicone implants are used in both breasts, as in 3, 4, 5, and 6 above.

COOPERATION WITH THE GENERAL SURGEON

The cancer surgeon can contribute greatly to the reconstructive effort when he is able to:

1. Preserve the pectoralis muscle.
2. Use a transverse incision.
3. Leave thicker skin flaps.
4. Avoid excessive skin excision.
5. Bank the nipple-areolar complex, or at least the areola.

COMPLICATIONS

In the reconstruction of 55 breasts by the Cronin, Brauer, and Biggs Clinic, the following complications were noted:

Necrosis of the tip of the flap	8
Fluid accumulation beneath flap donor site	7
Malposition of implant	5
Hematoma	3
Infection	2
Fat necrosis of tubed pedicle	1
Palsy of the long thoracic nerve	1
Extrusion of implant	1
Brachian injury	1

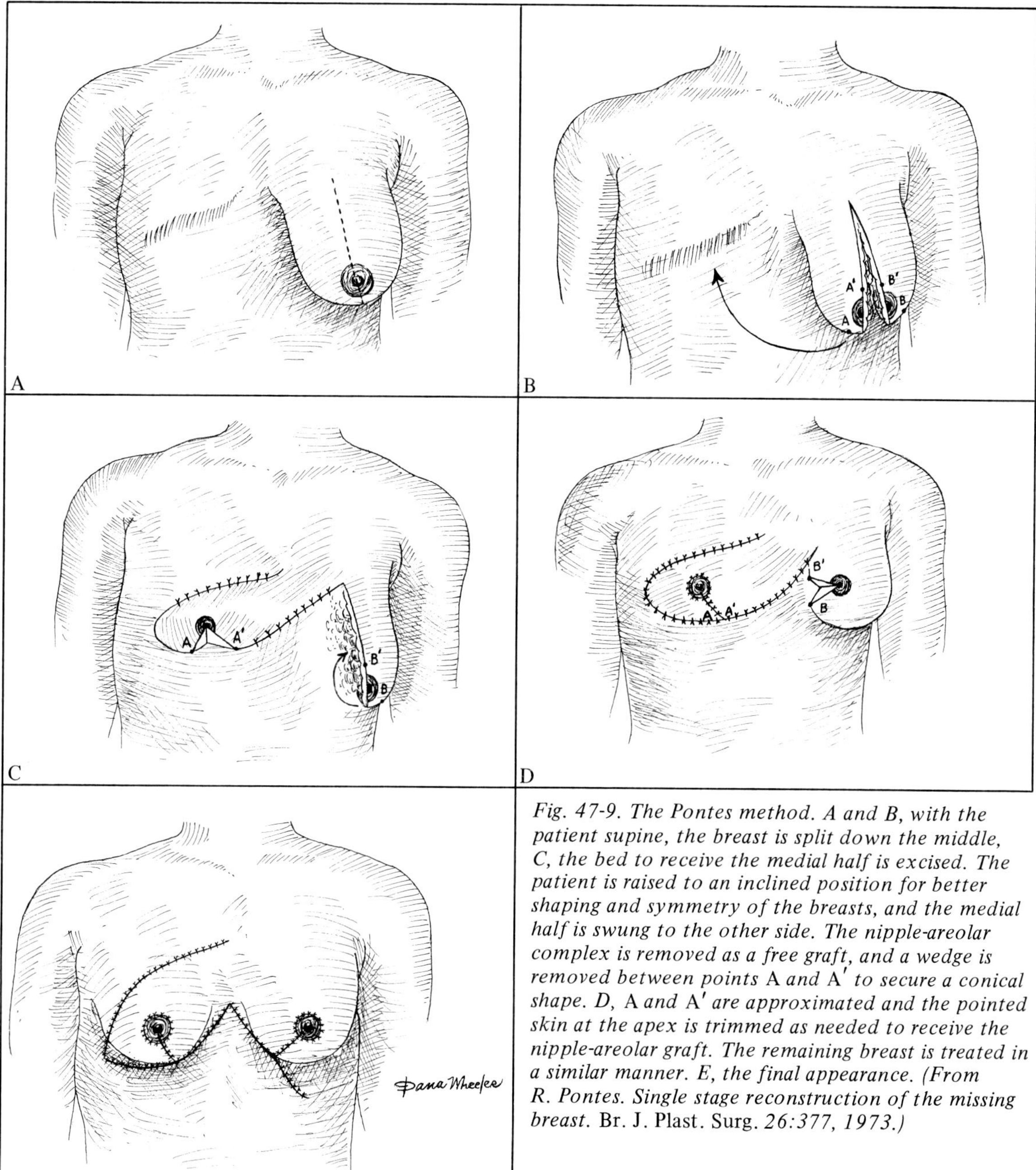

Fig. 47-9. The Pontes method. A and B, with the patient supine, the breast is split down the middle, C, the bed to receive the medial half is excised. The patient is raised to an inclined position for better shaping and symmetry of the breasts, and the medial half is swung to the other side. The nipple-areolar complex is removed as a free graft, and a wedge is removed between points A *and* A′ *to secure a conical shape. D,* A *and* A′ *are approximated and the pointed skin at the apex is trimmed as needed to receive the nipple-areolar graft. The remaining breast is treated in a similar manner. E, the final appearance. (From R. Pontes. Single stage reconstruction of the missing breast.* Br. J. Plast. Surg. *26:377, 1973.)*

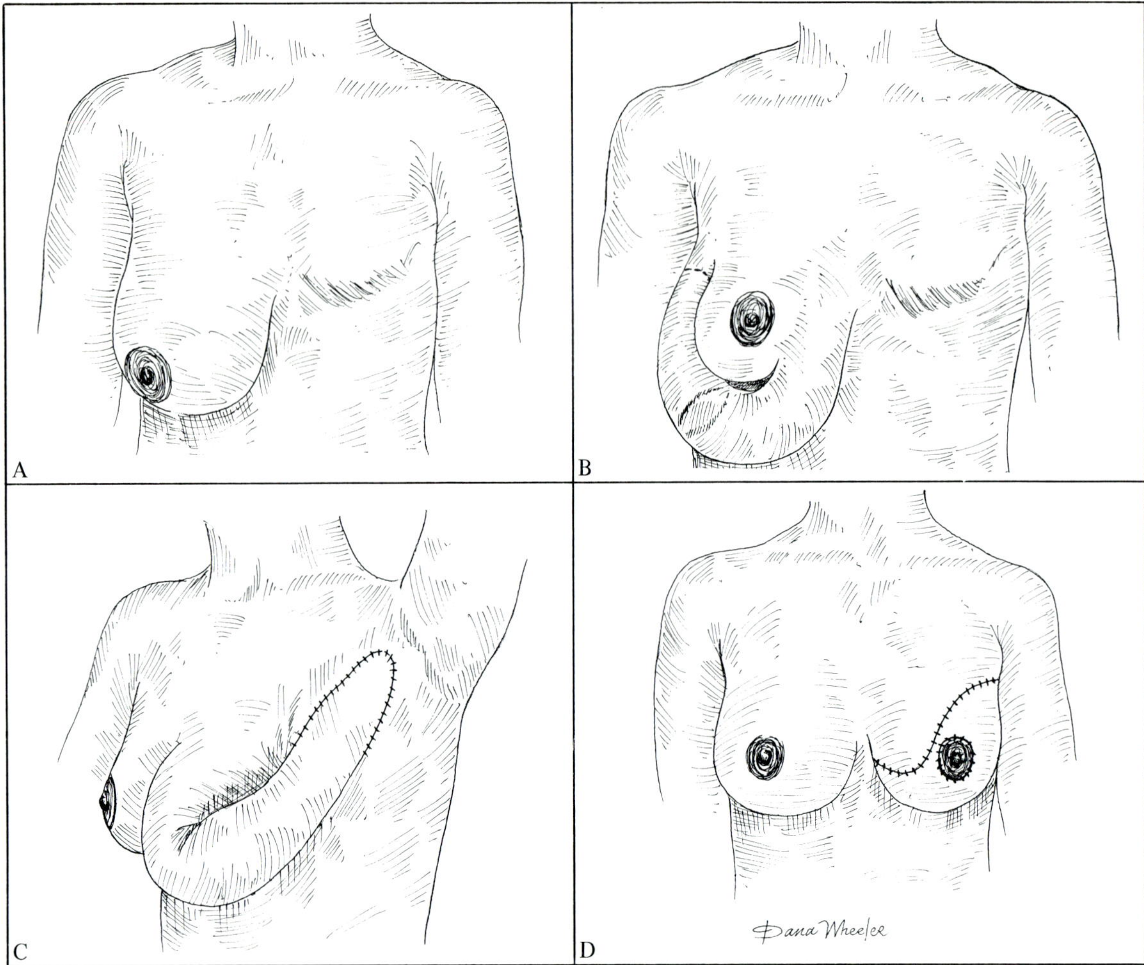

Fig. 47-10. The Holdsworth method. A, postmastectomy scar with pendulous remaining breast. B, a large tube flap has been made from the pendant portion of the breast. The nipple that was on the tube was transferred as a free graft to the breast and the disc of skin from the breast was transplanted to the tube. C, several months later the axillary end of the tube was transferred to a site high on the anterior axillary fold. D, about a month later the medial end of the tube was severed, opened, and inset along a crescentric incision. The skin and fat were excised as needed to conform to the other breast. Later the areola was simulated with a split graft, while the nipple was represented by a full-thickness skin graft. (Adapted from W. G. Holdsworth. A method of reconstructing the breast. Br. J. Plast. Surg. *9:161, 1956.)*

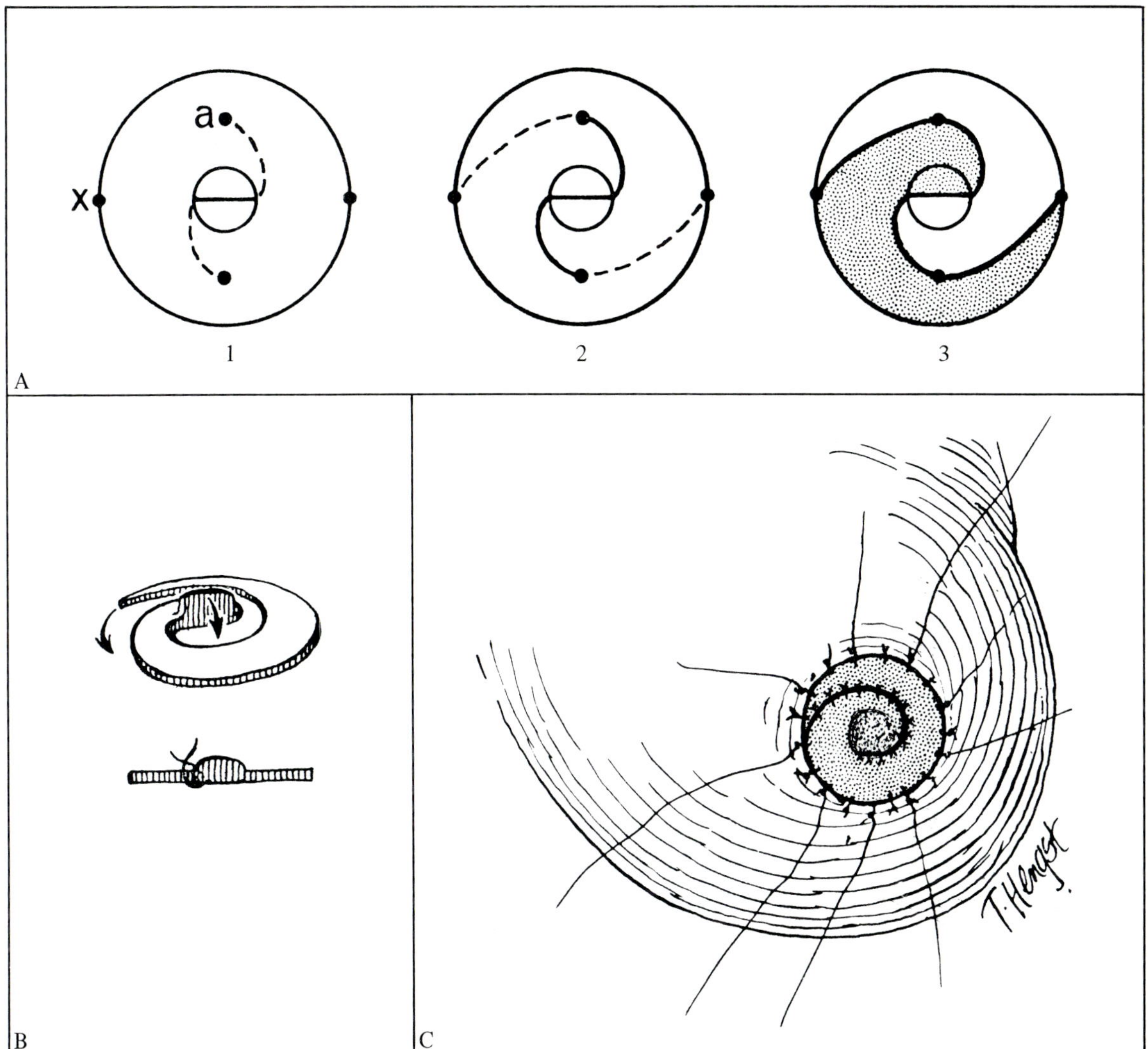

Fig. 47-11. The conjoined-spiral method of nipple sharing. A, the nipple is divided transversely and point a *is marked midway between the margin of the nipple and the edge of the areola. A curving line then connects the end of the line dividing the nipple and goes through point* a *and on to the areolar margin at* x, *which is opposite the nipple splitting line. B, formation of new nipple-areolar complex by coiling. C, the new half-size nipple-areolar complex with sutures left long to tie over a bolster. (See Table 47-1.)*

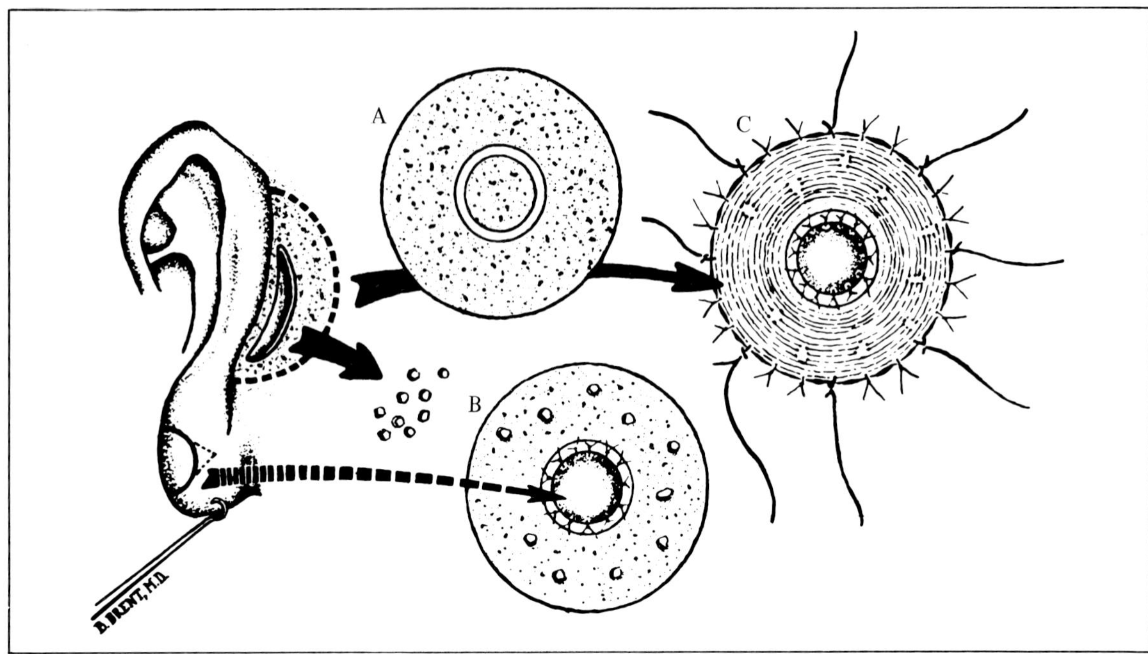

Fig. 47-12. Use of ear tissues for the reconstruction of the nipple and areola by the method of Brent and Bostwick. A, the nipple site is deepithelialized except for a 1.5-mm.-wide ring with an inside diameter of 8 to 12 mm. B, a composite graft of skin and fat from the ear lobe is sutured inside the ring of skin. A small strip of conchal cartilage is cut up into small bits and scattered under the areolar graft to simulate Montgomery glands. C, a full-thickness postauricular skin graft forms the areola. The postauricular donor site can be covered with the skin removed from the nipple site. (From B. Brent, and J. Bostwick, III. Nipple areolar reconstruction with auricular tissues. Plast. Reconstr. Surg. *60:353, 1977.)*

Fluid accumulation beneath the thoracoepigastric flaps was common, sometimes requiring repeated aspirations. If necrosis of the tip of a flap extended through the full thickness, further advancement of the flap was necessary, but the extent of necrosis was hard to determine immediately; a wait-and-see attitude often revealed only superficial loss that recovered spontaneously. Palsy of the long thoracic nerve, with winging of the scapula, was the most serious complication. Recovery occurred slowly after a partial brachial plexus injury, which apparently resulted from the stretching of the nerves when the arm was fixed in an abducted position of about 90 to 100 degrees during the surgery. Malposition was mainly the difficulty of locating the reconstructed breast at the same level as the remaining breast.

REFERENCES

1. Adams, W. M. Labial transplant for correction of loss of nipple. *Plast. Reconstr. Surg.* 4:195, 1949.
2. Alexander, J. E., and Block, L. I. Breast reconstruction following radical mastectomy. *Plast. Reconstr. Surg.* 40:175, 1967.
3. Arnold, P. G., Hartrampf, L. R., and Jurkiewicz, M. J. One-stage reconstruction of the breast using the transposed greater omentum. *Plast. Reconstr. Surg.* 57:520, 1976.
4. Auchincloss, H. Local recurrence after radical mastectomy. *Cancer* 11:611, 1958.
5. Berson, M. Construction of pseudoareola. *Surgery* 20:808, 1946.
6. Biggs, T. M., Cronin, T. D., and Upton, J. Breast reconstruction: How the general surgeon can help the plastic surgeon. *Tex. Med.* 74:53, 1978.
7. Bohmert, H. Personal Method for Reconstruction of the Female Breast Following Radical Mastectomy. *Transactions of the Sixth International Congress of Plastic and Reconstructive Surgery,* Paris, 1975. Paris: Masson, 1976.
8. Bohmert, H. Cited in Reconstruction of the Breasts Following Mastectomy. In Georgiade, N. G. (Ed.), *Reconstructive Breast Surgery.*

St. Louis: Mosby, 1976.

9. Bostwick, J., III, Vasconez, L. O., and Jurkiewicz, M. J. Breast reconstruction following a radical mastectomy. *Plast. Reconstr. Surg.* 61:682, 1978.
10. Brent, B., and Bostwick, J., III. Nipple-areolar reconstruction with auricular tissues. *Plast. Reconstr. Surg.* 60:353, 1977.
11. Chong, G. C., Masson, J. K., and Woods, J. E. Breast reconstruction for cancer. *Proc. Mayo Clin.* 50:453, 1975.
12. Cocke, W. M. Reconstruction of the breast following radical mastectomy. *J. Tenn. Med. Assoc.* 68:15, 1975.
13. Conway, H. and Neumann, C. G. Evaluation of skin grafting in the technique of radical mastectomy in relation to local recurrence of carcinoma. *Surg. Gynecol. Obstet.* 88:45, 1949.
14. Crile, G., Jr. Rationale for cutting thick skin flaps and not grafting skin in operations for cancer of the breast. *Cancer* 18:795, 1965.
15. Crile, G., Jr., and Hoehn, S. Results of treatment of carcinoma of the breast by local excision. *Surg. Gynecol. Obstet.* 132:780, 1971.
16. Cronin, T. D., and Gerow, F. Augmentation Mammaplasty: A New "Natural Feel" Prosthesis. *Transactions of the Third International Congress of Plastic Surgery.* Amsterdam: Excerpta Medica, 1964.
17. Cronin, T. D., and Freeman, B. S. Reconstruction in cystic breast disease. In Saad, M. N., and Lichtveld, P. (Eds.), *Reviews in Plastic Surgery.* Amsterdam: Exerpta Medica, 1974.
18. Cronin, T. D., Upton, J., and McDonough, J. M. Reconstruction of the breast after mastectomy. *Plast. Reconstr. Surg.* 59:1, 1977.
19. Cronin, T. D., and Upton, J. Reconstruction of the Breast After Mastectomy. In Peterson, R., and Owsley, J. (Eds.), *Proceedings of the Symposium on Aesthetic Surgery of the Breast.* Vol. 18. St. Louis: Mosby, 1978.P. 202–217.
20. Davis, W. M., McCraw, J. B., and Carraway, J. H. Immediate use of the thoraco-epigastric flap for difficult wounds of the thorax and upper extremity. Presented at the annual meeting of the American Society of Plastic and Reconstructive Surgeons, Boston, Mass. September 1976.
21. de Cholnoky, T. Breast reconstruction after radical mastectomy: Formation of missing nipple by everted navel. *Plast. Reconstr. Surg.* 38:577, 1966.
22. Donegan, W. L. Local and Regional Recurrence in Cancer of the Breast. In Spratt, J. S., and Donegan, W. L. (Eds.), *Cancer of the Breast.* Philadelphia: Saunders, 1967.
23. Drever, J. M. Total breast reconstruction with either of two abdominal flaps. *Plast. Reconstr. Surg.* 59:185, 1977.
24. Dupont, C., and Menard, Y. Transportation of the greater omentum for reconstruction of the chest wall. *Plast. Reconstr. Surg.* 49:263, 1972.
25. Edgerton, M. T. Breast reconstruction after radical mastectomy for cancer. *South. Med. J.* 60:719, 1967.
26. Freeman, B. S. Experiences in reconstruction of the breast after mastectomy. *Clin. Plast. Surg.* 3:277, 1976.
27. Fujino, T., Harashina, T., and Enomoto, K. Primary breast reconstruction after a standard radical mastectomy by a free flap transfer: A case report. *Plast. Reconstr. Surg.* 58:372, 1976.
28. Gibson, E. W. Reconstruction of the breast after mastectomy for cancer. *Clin. Plast. Surg.* 3:371, 1976.
29. Gillies, H. Surgical replacement of the breast. *Proc. R. Soc. Med.* 52:597, 1959.
30. Goldwyn, R. M. Reconstruction after mastectomy. *Arch. Surg.* 110:246, 1975.
31. Guthrie, R. J. Breast reconstruction after radical mastectomy. *Plast. Reconstr. Surg.* 57:14, 1976.
32. Haaschild, W. A. Reconstruction of the female breast after bilateral simple mastectomy. *Br. J. Plast. Surg.* 23:54, 1970.
33. Halsted, W. W. The results of radical operations for cure of cancer of the breast. *Trans. Am. Surg. Assoc.* 25:61, 1907.
34. Handley, R. S., Patey, D. H., and Hand, B. H. Observations and reflections on breast cancer. *J. R. Coll. Surg. Edinb.* 6:1, 1960.
35. Hartwell, S. W., Anderson, R., Hall, N. D., and Esselstyn, C. Reconstruction of the breast after mastectomy for cancer. *Plast. Reconstr. Surg.* 57:152, 1976.
36. Hoehler, H. Reconstruction of the breast after radical mastectomy. *Langenbecks Arch. Chir.* 339:756, 1975.
37. Hoehler, H. Further progress in the technique of reconstruction of the female breast after radical mastectomy. Presented at the annual meeting of the American Society of Plastic and Reconstructive Surgeons, Boston, Mass., September 1976.
38. Holdsworth, W. G. A method of reconstructing the breast. *Br. J. Plast. Surg.* 9:161, 1956.
39. Horton, C. E. Total mastectomy and immediate reconstruction. Presented at the annual meeting of the Texas Medical Association, Houston, Texas, May 1977.
40. Horton, C. E., Adamson, J. E., and Mladick, R. A. Breast Reconstruction after Surgery and Trauma. In Masters, F. W., and Lewis, J. R. (Eds.), *Symposium on Aesthetic Surgery of the Face, Eyelid and Breast.* St. Louis: Mosby, 1972.

41. Hueston, J., and McKenzie, W. Breast reconstruction after radical mastectomy. *Aust. N.Z. J. Surg.* 39:367, 1970.
42. Kiskadden, W. S. Case report on skin grafting of nipple. *Plast. Reconstr. Surg.* 5:184, 1950.
43. Losken, H. W. Breast Reconstruction by Breast Augmentation and Nipple/Areola Reconstruction. *Transactions of the Sixth International Congress of Plastic and Reconstructive Surgery*. Paris: (1975). Paris: Masson, 1976.
44. McCraw, J. B., Moyers, B., Shanklin, K. The value of Fluorescein in predicting the viability of arterialized flaps. *Plast. Reconstr. Surg.* 60:710, 1977.
45. Madden, J. L., Kandaloft, B., and Bourque, R. Modified Radical Mastectomy. In *Breast Cancer; Early and Late.* (Collection of Papers Presented at 13th Annual Clinical Conference on Cancer by M. D. Anderson Hospital.) Chicago: Year Book, 1970.
46. Millard, D. R., Jr. Nipple and areola reconstruction by split skin graft from the normal side. *Plast. Reconstr. Surg.* 50:350, 1972.
47. Millard, D. R., Jr. Breast reconstruction after a radical mastectomy. *Plast. Reconstr. Surg.* 58:283, 1976.
48. Millard, D. R., Jr., Devine, J., Jr., and Warren, E. D. Breast reconstruction: A plea for saving the uninvolved nipple. *Am. J. Surg.* 122:763, 1971.
49. Miller, S., and Graham, W., III. Breast reconstruction after radical mastectomy. *Am. Fam. Physician* May 1975. Pp. 97–101.
50. Millesi, H. Breast reconstruxtion nach Mammaamputation. *Dtsch. Med. Wochenschr.* 97:785, 1972.
51. Mir y Mir, L. Reconstruction mamaria tras mastectomia. *Acta Chir. Plast.* 7:9, 1965.
52. Orticochea, M. Use of buttock to reconstruct the breast. *Br. J. Plast. Surg.* 26:304, 1973.
53. Perel, L. Reconstruction de sein après exérèse pour cancer: Indications et techniques. *J. Chir.* 94:53, 1967.
54. Perras, C. The creation of a twin breast following radical mastectomy: A report of 50 consecutive cases, 1959–1975. *Clin. Plast. Surg.* 3:265, 1976.
55. Peterson, R. Reverse abdominoplasty: Operation performed at the Symposium on Aesthetic Surgery of the Breast. Scottsdale, Ariz., November 1975.
56. Picaud, A. J., and Lotte, J. Est-ce licité de récontruire un sein à l'aide de prothèse après mastectomie pour cancer? Quand et comment? *Ann. Chir. Plast.* 27:278, 1972.
57. Pontes, R. Single stage reconstruction of the missing breast. *Br. J. Plast. Surg.* 26:377, 1973.
58. Rapin, M. Reconstruction of the nipple. *Br. J. Plast. Surg.* 7:372, 1955.
59. Rees, T. D. Reconstruction of breast areola by intradermal tattooing and transfer. *Plast. Reconstr. Surg.* 55:620, 1975.
60. Regnault, P. Reconstruction After Radical Mastectomy. *Proceedings, Symposium on Aesthetic Surgery of the Breast.* Vol. 18. St. Louis: Mosby, 1978.
61. Romsdahl, M., Slar, M., and Eckles, N. Post-treatment Evaluation of Breast Cancer. In *Breast Cancer, Early and Late.* Chicago: Year Book, 1970.
62. Rosato, R. E., Fink, P. J., Horton, E. E., and Paine, R. L., Jr. Immediate post-mastectomy reconstruction. *J. Surg. Oncol.* 8:277, 1976.
63. Silsby, J. J. Nipple reconstruction. *Plast. Reconstr. Surg.* 57:667, 1976.
64. Snyder, C. C., Perkens, J. E., and Slater, P. V. Surgery of the Areola-Nipple Complex. In Masters, F. W., and Lewis, J. R. (Eds.), *Symposium on Aesthetic Surgery of the Face, Eyelid and Breast.* St. Louis: Mosby, 1972.
65. Snyderman, R. K. (Ed.). *Symposium on Neoplastic and Reconstructive Problems of the Female Breast.* St. Louis: Mosby, 1973.
66. Snyderman, R. K. What the Plastic Surgeon Has to Offer in the Management of Breast Tumors. In Gallager, H. S. (Ed.), *Early Breast Cancer.* New York: Wiley, 1976.
67. Snyderman, R. K., and Guthrie, R. H. Reconstruction of the female breast following radical mastectomy. *Plast. Reconstr. Surg.* 47:565, 1971.
68. Spina, J. Neoareoloplasty with labial transplant: Symmetrical correction of the shape and volume of the breast. *Plast. Reconstr. Surg.* 6:400, 1950.
69. Tai, Y., and Hasegawa, H. A transverse abdominal flap for reconstruction after radical operations for recurrent breast cancer. *Plast. Reconstr. Surg.* 53:52, 1974.
70. Thorek, M. Plastic reconstruction of the female breast and abdomen. *Am. J. Surg.* 43:268, 1939.
71. Thorek, M. P. Twenty-five years experience with plastic reconstruction of the breast and transplantation of the nipple. *Am. J. Surg.* 67:445, 1945.
72. Urban, J. A. Bilateral Breast Cancer. In *Breast Cancer, Early and Late.* Chicago: Year Book, 1970.
73. Urban, J. A., and Castro, E. D. Selecting variations in extent of surgical procedure for breast cancer. *Cancer* 28:615, 1971.
74. Van Dongen. J. A., and Lichtveld, P. Mammareconstrücte na ablative therajsie; afgensing van de indicatie. *Ned. Tijdschr. Geneeskd.* 119: 997, 1975.

75. Watts, C. T. Restorative prosthetic mammaplasty in mastectomy for carcinoma and benign lesions. *Clin. Plast. Surg.* 3:177, 1976.
76. Wexler, M. R., and O'Neal, R. M. Areolar sharing to reconstruct the absent nipple. *Plast. Reconstr. Surg.* 51:176, 1973.
77. Wiemer, D. R., and Freeman, B. S. Bilateral reconstruction of the nipple-areolar complex. *Plast. Reconstr. Surg.* 58:310, 1976.
78. Woods, J. E., and Payne, S. Contour restoration following simple or modified radical mastectomy. *J.A.M.A.* 235:5588, 1976.
79. Yoshiaki, J., and Hasegawa, H. A transverse abdominal flap for reconstruction after radical operations for recurrent breast cancer. *Plast. Reconstr. Surg.* 53:53, 1974.

Gynecomastia

BERNARD E. SIMON

Gynecomastia, or enlargement of the male breast, may occur in a variety of diseases and clinical settings. The first description of the surgical treatment may be found in the writings of Paulus of Aegina [22] (A.D. 635–690). The majority of the cases seen by plastic surgeons that require surgical treatment occur in adolescent or young adult males and are without obvious etiology. Embarrassment due to the female contour of the chest is the main concern since, except for the earliest stages, there is no pain or tenderness or, indeed, any symptoms except for the abnormal appearance.

Developmentally, transient enlargement of the breast may be seen in young males at birth lasting for a few days, presumably due to the stimulation of maternal and placental hormones. Prepubertal enlargement is rare, only 23 cases having been reported by 1972 [2]. The appearance of gynecomastia before puberty should prompt a careful search for an endocrine tumor.

During puberty, the incidence of breast enlargement, consisting usually of a small, firm, rubbery, subareolar nodule, has been reported as ranging between 38.7 [21] and 73 percent [14]. It occurs most often between 14 and 15 years of age and ordinarily regresses completely within 18 months of its initial appearance.

ETIOLOGY

Although the etiology of breast enlargement in the male is not as yet clear, there can be no doubt that it is basically a result of the actions of circulating hormones on specific receptors in the target cell. The importance of the receptors in these target cells is pointed up by the not infrequent appearance of unilateral gynecomastia. Workers in the field, notably Gabrilove [11], Sawin [26], and others, point out that rational explanations for observed phenomena should result from the introduction into endocrine research of (1) radioimmunoassays capable of measuring small amounts of hormones in the circulating blood, (2) tissue cultures of breast cells, and (3) assays capable of demonstrating hormone receptors or binding sites in the breasts of individuals. There is increasing evidence that the estrogen-androgen ratio rather than the absolute level of these hormones is critical in causing enlargement of the male breast, a theory first suggested by Lewin [19] in 1941. Gabrilove [12, 13] has enlarged on this concept, presenting overwhelming evidence in its support. It is also known that the pituitary and some functioning Leydig cells are necessary since gynecomastia does not appear in castrated men or in those with total hypopituitarism.

Gynecomastia is seen in a remarkably wide variety of clinical settings, including hepatic disease, hyperthyroidism and hypothyroidism, hypogonadism (such as Klinefelter's syndrome), endocrine-secreting tumors of the testes and the adrenal gland, adrenal hyperplasia, endocrine-secreting tumors of nonendocrine tissues (such as certain pulmonary tumors), paraplegia, and refeeding after starvation. A not uncommon etiological agent is the use of estrogenic hormones in the treatment of prostatic cancer. This distressing complication may be prevented by the administration of small amounts of radiation to the breast [1]. A wide variety of drugs are also responsible for gynecomastia. Among the most important ones which may cause enlargement of the male breast are spironolactone, reserpine, the phenothiazines, and methyldopa, as well as marijuana in large amounts.

Obesity may stimulate gynecomastia of endocrine origin [7, 27], and this body configuration may continue into adolescence and adulthood. Recently, Ryan and Hoopes [25] reemphasized the role of obesity and other causes of breast prominence in the male in producing a gynecomastia-like clinical picture.

One of the most interesting endocrine syndromes in which gynecomastia is seen is the entity described by Klinefelter and his associates [15] in 1942; the syndrome involves gynecomastia, small testes, azospermia, aspermatogenesis with aleydigism, and increased urinary excretion of follicle-stimulating hormone. Because of the frequent and important association of Klinefelter's syndrome with cancer of the breast [8], prophylactic mastectomy has been advised [5].

PATHOLOGICAL CHANGES IN GYNECOMASTIA

Stromal changes are predominant over ductal proliferation in gynecomastia. *True acinar lobules, such as are noted in the female breast, are not seen.* The stromal changes include hypervascularity and proliferation of fibroblasts, periductal "cuffs" of loose connective tissue, deposition of collagen, and hyalinization of connective tissue. The ductal changes include proliferation (an increase in number, an increase in length, and branching), budding and pseudolobule formation, and an increase in layers with formation of intraluminal papillae and sprouts.

No one specimen will demonstrate all the pathological changes described above. The picture ranges from what has been called by Williams [31] Type I (or florid), with striking ductal proliferation, a loose cellular stroma, and periductal cuffs, to Type II (or quiescent fibrous) hyalinized stroma, with little or no ductal proliferation. Nicolis and co-workers [20] showed that this variation in appearance *correlates with the duration of the breast hypertrophy regardless of its etiology.*

SURGICAL TREATMENT

The incisions and approaches to the treatment of gynecomastia have been many and varied. They are described and illustrated in more complete accounts [18, 28]. Modern treatment begins in 1946 with Webster's [30] classic paper describing the very inconspicuous intraareolar incision. Actually, the incision was originally described in 1928 by Dufourmentel [10], who used it in one case of gynecomastia while emphasizing its use in other breast conditions.

The object of treatment is to restore normal male contour and appearance, while leaving scars that are either concealed or quite inconspicuous. The use of the intraareolar approach enables the achievement of this ideal in 75 percent of the cases seen. The scar heals in a most satisfactory fashion, almost never hypertrophies, and is usually not noticed by even critical observers. The J.P. Webster-Dufourmental approach uses a semicircular incision placed just within the skin-areolar junction. The transverse transareolar variant of Pitanguy [24] is also useful and satisfactory.

A rough clinical classification that was proposed in 1973 [29] has been found useful both in selection of operative approaches and in prediction of results (Table 48-1).

It will be noted that all cases in Grade 1 and 2A – i.e., the small enlargements and moderate enlargements without skin redundancy – do very well with the simple procedure performed through the areola. This applies to many of the cases in Grade 2B (Fig. 48-1) as well – i.e., cases with moderate enlargement and some skin redundancy. However, cases in Grade 3, the pendulous female type of configuration, will be left with residual and visible skin redundancy (Fig. 48-1C). (This group will be discussed later.)

Table 48-1. Grading of Gynecomastia (77 Cases)

Grade	Description	Number of Cases
Grade 1	Small, visible breast enlargement without skin redundancy	26
Grade 2	Moderate breast enlargement without skin redundancy	24
Grade 2B	Moderate breast enlargement with skin redundancy	17
Grade 3	Marked breast enlargement with marked skin redundancy (i.e., pendulous female breasts)	10

Intraareolar Operation for Gynecomastia

A semicircular (180-degree) incision just within the skin-areolar junction is made down to the capsule of the breast (Fig. 48-2A). It is usually placed between 3 and 9 o'clock, but its position may be varied to secure the best possible exposure. When the areola is small and the breast mass large, additional exposure may be obtained by making a short (1 cm.) radial incision at each end of the intraareolar incision – the so-called inverted omega [3]. The surrounding skin below the incision is dissected from the face of the breast to a point beyond the periphery (Fig. 48-2B). The nipple and areola are now undercut, leaving an attached button of breast tissue (Fig. 48-2C); the face of the breast above the nipple is released from the overlying skin and subcutaneous tissue (Fig. 48-2D). In obese patients with fatty breasts, there may not be a well-defined breast capsule and the dissection is made at a depth of 10 to 15 mm. below the skin surface. Visualization at that depth is facilitated by the use of a fiberoptic headlight or retractor (Fig. 48-2E). Hemostasis is secured by the use of the Malis bipolar coagulator [4].

The gland, having now been completely exposed on its outer face, may be removed from the underlying pectoral fascia by grasping its periphery and dissecting it free (Fig. 48-2F). If the skin opening is small and the gland bulky, it may be necessary to halve or quarter the breast and remove it successively piece by piece, as described by Webster [30]. It is important to "feather" or taper the edges of the dissection so as to avoid a "drop off" visible externally (Fig. 48-2E). Failure to do this will result in an obvious dishlike deformity. Before closing, careful hemostasis is secured.

The cavity, including its roof and floor, is trimmed free of any irregularities and the space is irrigated copiously. A suction drain of the Hemavac or Jackson-Pratt variety is placed through a lateral stab incision and the wound is closed in layers (Fig. 48-2G). A light dressing permits inspection of the skin and nipple for circulation and enables the detection of an expanding hematoma.

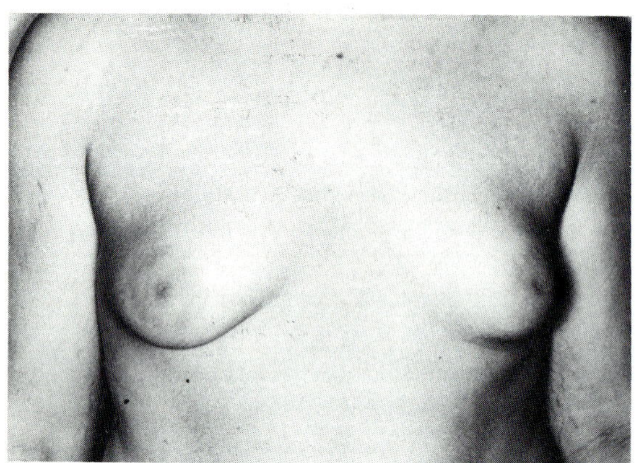
A

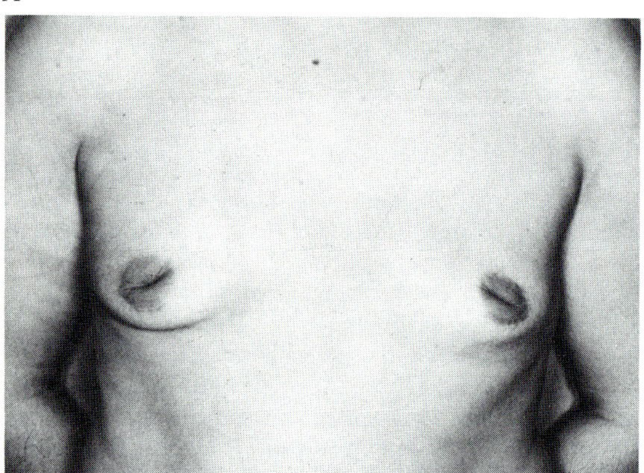
B

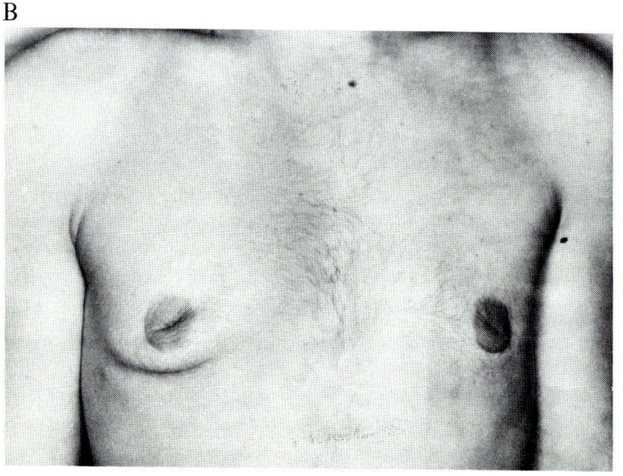
C

Fig. 48-1. This patient with asymmetrical gynecomastia exhibited Grade 2B enlargement on the left and Grade 3 on the right. A, preoperative view. B, the appearance 6 months following a subcutaneous mastectomy by the standard intraareolar method; note the skin excess and nipple inversion. C, the appearance 1 year after the operation. The result is satisfactory on the left, where the skin excess has disappeared, but there is persistence of the skin excess on the right side. This illustrates the importance of waiting at least 1 year before secondary surgery. (From B. E. Simon, and S. Hoffman, Correction of Gynecomastia. In R. Goldwyn [Ed.], Plastic and Reconstructive Surgery of the Breast. *Boston: Little Brown, 1976.)*

Fig. 48-2. The classic operation for gynecomastia through intraareolar approach. A, the incision. B, the separation of the skin from the anterior face of the breast. C, undercutting of the nipple and areola; note that a thick button of breast tissue must be left. D, dissection of superior portion of anterior face of breast. E, the periphery of the breast mass is tapered, using a fiberoptic illuminated retractor. F, the deep surface of the breast mass is separated from the pectoral fascia. G, the incision is sutured; a suction catheter is left in place. (From B. E. Simon, and S. Hoffman, Correction of Gynecomastia. In R. Goldwyn [Ed.], Plastic and Reconstructive Surgery of the Breast. *Boston: Little Brown, 1976.)*

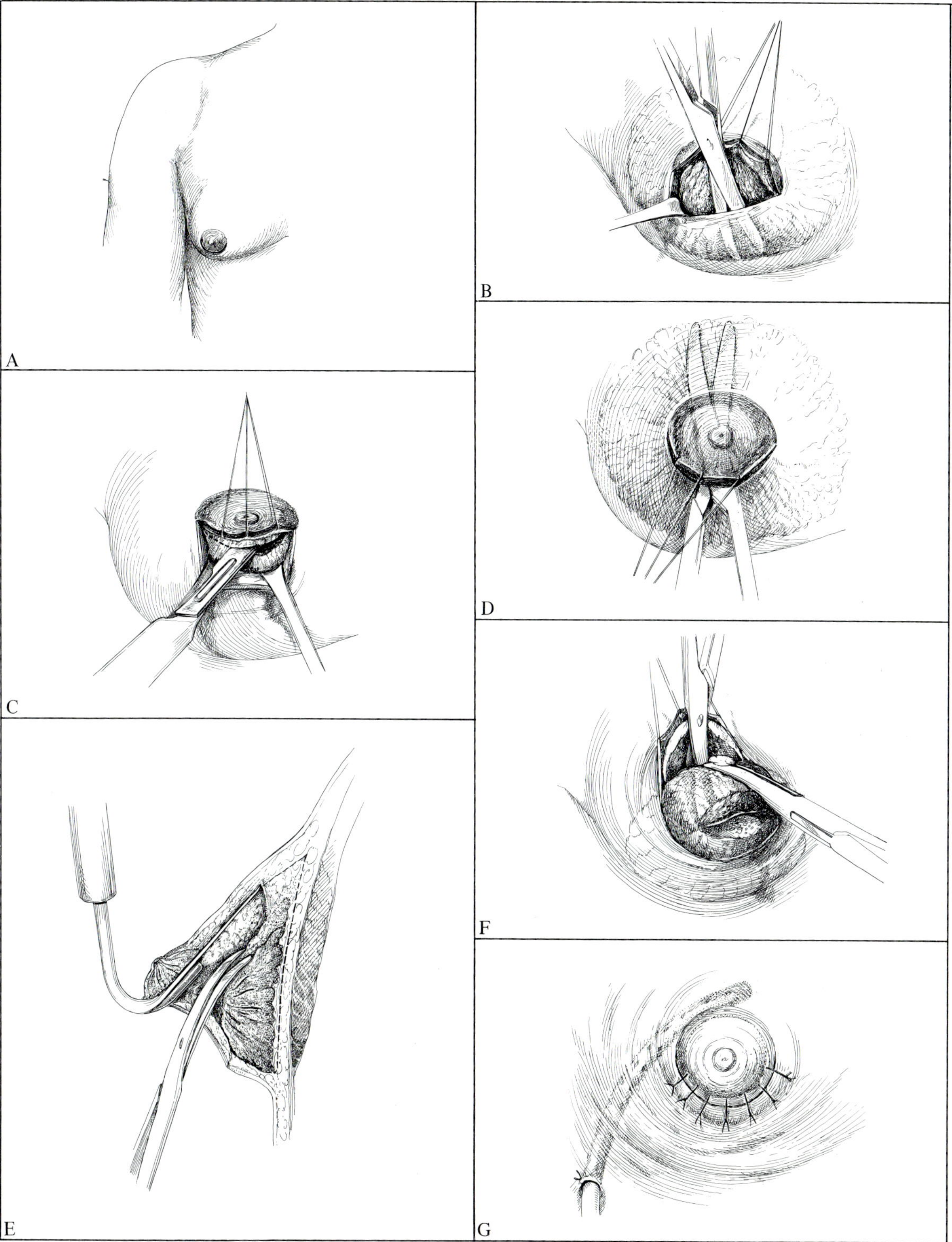
A
B
C
D
E
F
G

Management of Gynecomastia with Significant Skin Redundancy
Cases of moderate breast enlargement with skin redundancy (Grade 2B) and of marked enlargement with considerable skin redundancy (Grade 3) may not obtain a good result when the intraareolar procedure is used. This is especially true in those patients in whom the hypertrophy has existed for a long while and the skin has become permanently stretched out. In the younger patient with borderline skin redundancy, it is best to proceed with the intraareolar procedure informing the patient that contraction and flattening of the skin envelope will require at least a year (Fig. 48-1). It is preferable to do an intraareolar procedure and wait a year rather than put a scar in the skin outside the areola at the initial procedure. The patient should be informed that a second operation with one or more scars on the skin of the chest wall may be required if the skin envelope does not flatten sufficiently.

In cases of mild skin redundancy, the simple crescentic excision of skin above the nipple as described by Letterman and Schurter [16] may be effective, although this procedure is usually best used to correct or to prevent downward folding of the nipple postoperatively.

For patients with greater redundancy, a number of operations have been described. Among the procedures available is the operation of Letterman and Schurter [17], which is based on the oblique mammoplasty of C. Dufourmentel and Mouly [9]. For larger hypertrophies, simple excision (much like a limited simple mastectomy) with free graft of the nipple has been described by Simon and Hoffman [28]. Also useful in the larger hypertrophies is the procedure of Wray, Hoopes, and Davis [32], which involves a wide excision of skin and subcutaneous tissue; the margins along the inframammary crease and the lateral border of the pectoralis major muscle are removed en bloc, and the nipple is replaced as a free graft. More recently (in 1975) Bretteville-Jensen [6] added two procedures for the correction of marked redundancy; the first is another modification of the Dufourmentel-Mouly method, and the second, for even larger hypertrophies, is a modification of the Pers and Bretteville-Jensen [23] method of mammoplasty. In the second method, the nipple is carried on a deepithelialized, thin vertical bipedicle, and large amounts of skin with the underlying breast are removed medially and laterally. The wound is then closed transversely.

In all these procedures, a scar is visible in the skin outside the areola. Scar hypertrophy or true keloid may develop and may require treatment. It is important that the patient be aware of this possibility before he agrees to the operation.

TREATMENT OF EARLY COMPLICATIONS

In 2 of my 77 cases, there was acute postoperative bleeding into the large dead space despite suction drainage. An expanding hematoma requires an immediate return to the operating room, evacuation of clots, and ligation or electrocoagulation of the bleeding vessels. Minor fluid collections occur, and they should be aspirated under sterile conditions. Infection and loss of skin have not been a problem in gynecomastia surgery.

PREVENTION AND TREATMENT OF UNSATISFACTORY RESULTS

Nipple Abnormalities
Inversion, retraction, and folding of the nipples will result when the surgeon does not leave an adequate button of breast tissue or fat beneath the nipple. A downward folded nipple can sometimes be corrected by use of the superior crescentic excision described by Letterman and Schurter [16].

Depression of Contour
Depression of contour resulting from overenthusiastic removal of subcutaneous tissue can be prevented by leaving an adequate pad of subcutaneous tissue on the undersurface of the skin flaps and by tapering the periphery so as to obviate the "drop off." Most patients will not object to a slight concavity, being only too happy to get rid of the protuberance of the abnormal breast. Correction of late depression is difficult; attempts at correction using dermal-fat grafts or alloplastic materials are apt to be disappointing. Extending the tapering of the subcutaneous tissue at the periphery may be sufficient to render the central depression inconspicuous.

Inadequate Removal of Fat and/or Breast
Reoperation and additional excision of tissue are necessary when there has been inadequate removal of fat and/or breast.

Residual Skin Redundancy
Residual skin redundancy can best be managed by modifying one of the more extensive procedures described above. It must again be emphasized that at least 1 year should elapse before reoperation, to permit maximal foreshortening of the excess skin (Fig. 48-1).

Scar Hypertrophy
Scar hypertrophy is most often seen in incisions that extend beyond the areola onto the pectoral skin. Those segments of the scar medial to the areola are more apt to hypertrophy than the lateral portions. Intralesional injections of corticosteroids, such as

triamcinolone acetonide (Kenalog, Aristocort), are usually helpful.

REFERENCES

1. Alfthan, O., and Holstoi, L. R. Prevention of gynecomastia by local roentgen irradiation in estrogen-treated prostatic carcinoma. *Scand. J. Urol. Nephrol.* 3:183, 1969.
2. August, G. P., Chandra, R., and Hung, W. Prepubertal male gynecomastia. *J. Pediatr.* 80:259, 1972.
3. Barsky, A. J., Kahn, S., and Simon, B. E. (Eds.). The Breast. In *Principles and Practice of Plastic Surgery* (2nd ed.). New York: McGraw-Hill, 1964.
4. Barsky, A. J., Kahn, S., and Simon, B. E. (Eds.). Free Skin Grafts. In *Principles and Practice of Plastic Surgery* (2nd ed.). New York: McGraw-Hill, 1964.
5. Becker, K. L. Clinical and therapeutic experiences with Klinefelter's syndrome. *Fertil. Steril.* 23:568, 1972.
6. Bretteville-Jensen, M. B. Surgical treatment of gynecomastia. *Br. J. Plast. Surg.* 28:177, 1975.
7. Bruch, H. Obesity. *Pediatr. Clin. North Am.* 5:613, 1958.
8. Cuenca, C. R., and Becker, K. L. Klinefelter's syndrome and cancer of the breast. *Arch. Intern. Med.* 121:159, 1968.
9. Dufourmentel, C., and Mouly, R. Plastie mammaire par la méthode oblique. *Ann. Chir. Plast.* 6:45, 1961.
10. Dufourmentel, L. L'incision aréolaire dans la chirurgie du sein. *Bull. Mem. Soc. Chir. Paris* 20:9, 1928.
11. Gabrilove, J. L. Personal communication, 1974.
12. Gabrilove, J. L. Some recent advances in virilizing and feminizing syndromes and hirsutism. *Mt. Sinai J. Med.* 41:636, 1974.
13. Gabrilove, J. L., Nicolis, G. L., Mitty, H. A., and Sohval, A. R. Feminizing interstitial cell tumor of the testis: Personal observations and a review of the literature. *Cancer* 35:1184, 1975.
14. Jung, F. T., and Shafton, A. L. The mammary gland in the normal adolescent male. *Proc. Soc. Exp. Biol. Med.* 33:455, 1935.
15. Klinefelter, H. F., Jr., Reifenstein, E. C., Jr., and Albright, F. Syndrome characterized by gynecomastia, aspermatogenesis without aleydigism, and increased excretion of follicle-stimulating hormone. *J. Clin. Endocrinol.* 2:615, 1942.
16. Letterman, G., and Schurter, M. The surgical correction of gynecomastia. *Am. Surg.* 35:322, 1969.
17. Letterman, G., and Schurter, M. Surgical correction of massive gynecomastia. *Plast. Reconstr. Surg.* 49:259, 1972.
18. Letterman, G., and Schurter, M. Gynecomastia. In Georgiade, N. (Ed.), *Reconstructive Breast Surgery*. St. Louis: Mosby, 1976.
19. Lewin, M. L. Gynecomastia – the hypertrophy of the male breast. *J. Clin. Endocrinol.* 1:511, 1941.
20. Nicolis, G. L., Modlinger, R. S., and Gabrilove, J. L. A study of the histopathology of human gynecomastia. *J. Clin Endocrinol. Metab.* 32:173, 1971.
21. Nydick, M., Bustos, J., Dale, J. H., Jr., and Rawson, R. W. Gynecomastia in adolescent boys. *J.A.M.A.* 178:449, 1961.
22. Paulus A. On Male Breasts Resembling the Female. In Adams, F. (translator), *The Seven Books of Paulus Aegineta.* London: Sydenham Society, 1846. Vol. 2, Book 6, Sect. 46.
23. Pers, M., and Bretteville-Jensen, G. Reduction mammoplasty based on vertical vascular pedicle and "tennis ball" assembly. *Scand. J. Plast. Reconstr. Surg.* 6:61, 1972.
24. Pitanguy, I. Transareolar incision for gynecomastia. *Plast. Reconstr. Surg.* 38:414, 1966.
25. Ryan, J. J., and Hoopes, J. E. Prominence – more than gynecomastia. Presented at American Association of Plastic Surgeons meeting, Chicago, May 10, 1977.
26. Sawin, C. T. Endocrine Physiology and Pathophysiology of the Breast. In Goldwyn, R. M. (Ed.), *Plastic and Reconstructive Surgery of the Breast.* Boston: Little, Brown, 1976.
27. Schonfeld, W. A. Body-image disturbances in adolescents with inappropriate sexual development. *Am. J. Orthopsychiatry* 34:493, 1964.
28. Simon, B. E., and Hoffman, S. Correction of Gynecomastia. In Goldwyn, R. M. (Ed.), *Plastic and Reconstructive Surgery of the Breast.* Boston: Little, Brown, 1976.
29. Simon, B. E., Hoffman, S., and Kahn, S. Classification and surgical correction of gynecomastia. *Plast. Reconstr. Surg.* 51:48, 1973.
30. Webster, J. P. Mastectomy for gynecomastia through a semicircular intra-areolar incision. *Ann. Surg.* 124:557, 1946.
31. Williams, M. J. Gynecomastia: Its incidence, recognition and host characterization in 447 autopsy cases. *Am. J. Med.* 34:103, 1963.
32. Wray, R. C., Jr., Hoopes, J. E., and Davis, G. M. Correction of extreme gynecomastia. *Br. J. Plast. Surg.* 27:39, 1974.

VII

Trunk and Lower Extremity

Reconstructive Procedures of the Lower Extremity

LUIS O. VASCONEZ AND JOHN B. McCRAW

Locomotion is the most important function of the lower extremities. As man developed and acquired the erect posture, the distribution of his weight changed significantly, applying a considerable amount of pressure over a relatively small cross-sectional area – the feet. The support for the body is provided by the rigid bony skeleton, and walking and running are effected by very powerful muscles under voluntary control.

Proprioception and protective sensation are essential for locomotion. An insensitive foot eventually ulcerates and a progressive loss of the extremity can follow. Therefore, an important aim in the reconstructive surgery of the lower extremity should be to provide sensation whenever possible to the weight-bearing surfaces. The loss of one extremity for any reason puts an excessive burden on the opposite one. This burden on the remaining extremity is well tolerated in the young, healthy patient who has suffered a traumatic loss, but is a severe problem in patients with diabetes, peripheral vascular disease, or one of the neuropathies; in such patients, amputation of one extremity may provoke an accelerated degeneration in the remaining leg.

CAUSES OF SKIN LOSS

Reconstruction of the lower extremity usually involves soft tissue coverage to repair skin loss. This chapter mainly deals with the use of muscle flap transposition for such coverage. The skin loss can result from vascular disease, trauma, or prolonged pressure. Prolonged pressure, an important factor in the formation of ulcers, is discussed in Chapter 50.

Vascular Disease

Ulcerations in the lower extremities occur from a variety of causes, some of which are discussed below.

Arterial Insufficiency

Ulcerations secondary to arterial insufficiency require, as primary treatment, arterial revascularization of the extremity. On occasion an adjacent muscle may be used to cover an exposed vein graft or a graft of synthetic material as a salvage procedure; however, as a rule, peripheral arterial insufficiency is a relative contraindication to muscle flaps.

Venous Stasis

In treating ulcers caused by venous stasis, the aim should be to diminish venous tension; this can be accomplished by competent valves and eradicating the incompetent perforators of the deep venous system, or by the use of an external elastic support. The former is only partly successful at this stage, while external elastic support is a cumbersome and palliative procedure that is effective if properly used. Muscle flaps have been successfully used to cover venous ulcers, particularly if a concomitant decrease in venous pressure can be achieved by the subfascial ligation of the incompetent perforators.

Diabetes

Ulcerations in the diabetic patients, particularly if there is associated peripheral neuropathy, are most difficult to treat and tend to break down again. It is important to maintain meticulous care, with particular attention to bacteriological control, as described by Robson and Edstrom [6]. This measure, along with the use of skin grafts and limited amputations of necrotic tissues, has resulted in the salvage of a number of extremities.

Vasculitis

Small, punched-out ulcerations, commonly seen in the extremities of patients with vasculitis (particularly secondary to collagen diseases), are best left to heal by the slow processes of wound contraction and epithelialization. Excision and grafting of these ulcerations are usually not indicated unless there is subcutaneous necrosis or undermining, as these procedures can result in a larger ulcer.

Sickle Cell Anemia

Ulcerations in the patient with sickle cell anemia need careful hematological control with frequent and continued blood transfusions. It is our feeling, after observing a few selected patients, that future breakdown is diminished if the ulcer is excised and covered with a muscle flap and skin graft or (perhaps even better) with a musculocutaneous flap.

Concurrent Steroid Therapy

Special problems are presented by ulcerations in patients who have been treated with steroids on a long-term basis. They usually have very thin skin, and delayed healing of the skin graft donor site is not uncommon. A useful maneuver has been to mesh a thin split-thickness skin graft to increase its area by 50 percent (1½:1); the graft is then used to cover the area of the excised ulcer and most of the donor site.

Traumatic Loss of Skin

Avulsions of skin and subcutaneous tissue in the lower extremity can be easily replaced by the application of split-thickness skin grafts, provided that there is a suitable recipient site. Even on the sole of the foot, split-thickness skin grafts are durable and functional. This is not the case when bone is exposed, particularly if it has lost its periosteal cover.

COVERAGE OF EXPOSED BONE

One of the most challenging problems for the plastic surgeon is the coverage of exposed bone devoid of its periosteum. This problem, which is usually caused by trauma, is particularly severe in the lower extremity where the tibia is located subcutaneously in a most vulnerable position throughout its length. Classically, ulcerations exposing the tibia have been treated by decortication of the bone and delayed application of split-thickness skin grafts, by reverse dermis grafts, or by cross leg flaps. Recently, two new techniques have been introduced: the use of free skin flaps (with the aid of microvascular surgery) and the use of transposition muscle or musculocutaneous flaps.

Decortication and Skin Grafting

Decortication down to bleeding bone and secondary skin grafting after the appearance of granulation tissue is a time-honored procedure but it requires prolonged hospitalization. Moreover, the coverage provided is quite thin and prone to injury and reulceration because the skin is fixed to the bone. Several points should be mentioned when considering this technique. Decortication with a curved chisel down to bleeding bone is preferable to the technique of drilling holes down to the marrow cavity. It is quite possible that a split-thickness skin graft, particularly if it is meshed, may be placed immediately over the bleeding bone, since there are sufficient capillaries from the haversian canals to revascularize the graft. The resulting thin coverage over the bone can be thickened by dermal overgrafting; this is accomplished by dermabrading the split-thickness skin graft or by removing a very thin layer from this graft and applying a thicker graft over it. The overgrafting procedure can be carried out more than one time.

Reverse Dermis Graft

The reverse dermis graft is another method for covering exposed bone or for increasing the thickness of the skin over the bone. This graft has the advantages of a skin graft that is relatively thick and probably is similar to a flap in its ability to withstand pressures. The following is a description of the technique. A thin, 0.012-inch split-thickness skin graft is raised from the donor area with a Brown dermatome. The underlying dermis is then removed with the same device, this time set between 0.030 and 0.040 inch. The split-thickness skin graft is then replaced on the donor site as a free graft. Next, the dermis graft is reversed, and the deepithelialized surface is applied face down on the prepared recipient area. The greater number of vascular channels on the surface of the graft, which is now in contact with the wound, permits rapid revascularization by inosculation with vessels from the host site. The thick dermis graft takes better than does a skin graft of the same thickness. The exposed portion of the graft is covered with a thin 0.012-inch split-thickness skin graft from another donor site, which serves as a temporary dressing or as a permanent graft (in around 50 percent of the cases). If it fails, one can regraft the area in about 10 to 14 days.

Cross Leg Flaps

Transferring tissue from one extremity to another by the cross leg flap technique is an appropriate method for coverage of ulcerations over the tibia. The disadvantages include the secondary donor defect as well as the prolonged hospitalization and significant morbidity. The cross leg flap is being relegated into history as is discussed in Chapter 1.

Free Skin Flaps

Free skin flaps are an alternative for surface coverage of some of the most challenging defects. In fact, Serafin, Georgiade, and Smith [7] have demonstrated that the morbidity and total effort were decreased with the use of free skin flaps for coverage of defects in the lower extremity, as compared with cross leg skin flaps. In our experience they are especially useful for the treatment of defects around the ankle. Chapter 41 includes additional information on free flaps.

Coverage of Defects by Muscle Transposition

A significant advance in the coverage of exposed bone in the lower extremity was the demonstration by Ger [1–3] of the principle of muscle transposition. This technique involves the transposition of an adjacent and appropriate muscle with its intact neurovascular bundle to cover the defect and the application of a split-thickness skin graft over the muscle [4, 5, 8–10].

Prerequisites for Muscle Transposition

To be suitable for transposition, a muscle must have a belly of reasonable size and must be of sufficient length. The site of the main arterial source and venous return equally influences the feasibility of using a particular muscle as a flap. If the vascular pedicle is located close to the origin, the muscle then can be extensively rotated with safety. When there are multiple arterial muscular branches, these branches in the proximal third of the muscle must be dominant or the muscle will not survive as an immediate transposition flap. It is essential to have exact knowledge of the location of the neurovascular bundle, since it must be preserved intact.

A lower extremity muscle used in transfer can no longer serve its original locomotor function. Consequently, there should be an ample number of synergistic muscles to compensate for this decrease in muscular function. Preservation of motor innervation is not an absolute requirement in the muscle flaps since muscular contractions in the rotated position serve no function. In fact, in some circumstances the eventual decrease of denervated muscle bulk may well be a desirable feature. Even a normally innervated muscle will undergo a diminution of its muscle bulk to about 50 percent of normal in all cases if its insertion has been divided. Significant experience has been accumulated now to enable us to know the appropriate muscle that may be used to cover a particular defect over the lower extremity.

General Plan for Muscle Transposition Plus a Skin Graft

If one chooses to cover exposed bone over the tibia with transposition of a muscle, the following plan is recommended. The site of the ulceration determines which muscle is chosen. Incisions are planned so that there is not any excessive undermining of the skin. The pneumatic tourniquet is elevated during the dissection to minimize bleeding and to allow for a more accurate dissection. The ulceration is excised as a unit with a small rim of normal skin and includes the exposed cortical portion of the bone. This is accomplished by using a curved osteotome to get down to bleeding bone. Bleeding should be controlled by the compression of the marrow cavity (by gentle tapping with a mallet) or by individual cauterization of the larger bleeders with a needle electrode rather than by the use of bone wax. The proper muscle is then dissected free, preserving the proximal neurovascular bundle. It is then elevated sufficiently to cover the entire ulceration without any tension. If necessary, the muscle may be spread moderately in order to expand the area of coverage. It is important to anchor the muscle through its tendinous insertion or through the fascia to the underlying dermis at the rim of the ulceration with nylon sutures to prevent disruption from muscle contractions. Finally, an unexpanded meshed (1½:1) split-thickness skin graft is applied immediately.

We do not believe that there is any reason for performing this operation in stages, even in patients with osteomyelitis. Specifically, the ulceration and the exposed necrotic and infected bone are excised, radically if necessary, and the entire surface is covered

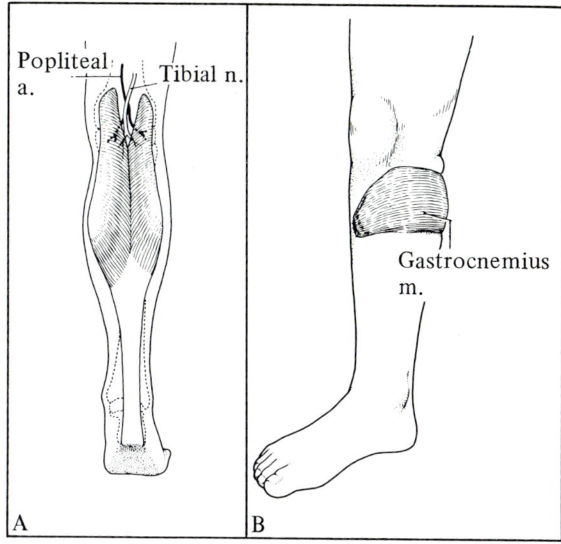

Fig. 49-1. A, posterior view of the leg showing the two bellies of the gastrocnemius muscle. Note that the vascular bundles enter at the proximal third of the muscle. B, the medial head has been transposed, and it will cover defects over the proximal third of the tibia. The medial head of the gastrocnemius muscle is preferred over the lateral head because it is longer and in closer proximity to the tibia.

with an adjacent, well-vascularized muscle flap. To leave the bone exposed again will only produce further desiccation and necrosis.

The Use of Muscle Transposition in Specific Defects

DEFECTS OVER THE KNEE JOINT AND UPPER THIRD OF THE TIBIA. These defects can easily be covered by transposing the *medial head of the gastrocnemius muscle* (Fig. 49-1). The gastrocnemius is a superficial posterior leg muscle composed of medial and lateral bellies that merge midway in the leg to form a common tendon. The longer medial belly is used because of its length as well as its location, which is closer to the usual defect on the proximal third of the tibia. The neurovascular bundle to the medial head enters at the proximal aspect near its origin (Fig. 49-1). The muscle can usually be exposed by a midposterior incision. Sometimes it is only necessary to extend the ends of the primary defect through oblique incisions both superiorly and inferiorly to expose the muscle. A technical point of importance is the division of the medial head with a portion of its tendinous insertion, which is used for handling. The muscle is freed up in a normal plane from the lateral head as well as from the underlying soleus as long as the posterior fascial coverage is divided. A different plane of dissection is encountered if this is not done. The muscle can then be transposed by simple rotation on the neurovascular axis; on occasion, transposition is facilitated by turning the muscle over completely, placing the superficial aspect to form the deep surface. As long as the dominant neurovascular bundle is identified, the origin of the gastrocnemius muscle can be divided from the medial femoral condyle and the muscle transposed as an island, gaining additional mobility and coverage. In performing this maneuver, the surgeon must protect the neurovascular bundle with the finger, and he should keep in mind the location of the popliteal vessels and nerves, which must be protected from injury. By transposing the muscle flap as an island, it can be used to cover the knee joint.

For the occasional defect on the lateral aspect of the proximal tibia, the peroneus longus muscle can be divided distally along its tendinous insertion and transposed to cover the defect as long as the proximal neurovascular bundle from the peroneal artery is preserved (Fig. 49-2).

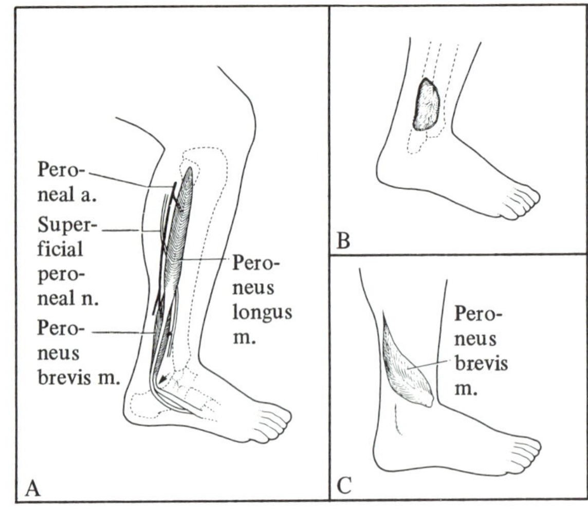

Fig. 49-2. A, the peroneal musculature and their correspondent neurovascular bundles. B, defect of distal third of leg. C, the peroneal brevis can at times be transposed to cover defects on the distal third of the leg, particularly over the lateral aspect.

DEFECTS IN THE MIDDLE THIRD OF THE TIBIA. The *soleus muscle,* as well as the *flexor digitorum longus,* can be utilized alone or together for coverage of defects in the middle third of the tibia (Fig. 49-3). When the tibial defect is long and narrow, the *anterior tibialis muscle* can be used. The soleus is a broad, flat muscle that arises from the upper posterior surface of the tibia and fibula and lies deep to the gastrocnemius. Its broad muscle belly is admirably suited for transfer procedures. This muscle is exposed through a posterior medial incision; because it inserts as part of the Achilles tendon, it must be sharply separated from it. Following the skin incision in the posteromedial aspect of the leg, the Achilles tendon is identified and its medial border retracted with traction sutures. Then the muscle fibers of the soleus are separated from the overlying tendon, using sharp dissection. The dominant arterial vessels to the muscle enter at the proximal third of the muscle. There are one or two additional inferior branches that may be transected to allow further mobilization of the muscle. The flexor digitorum longus is a deep posterior leg muscle with a moderate-sized belly; it can provide supplementary tissue to fill larger defects in the middle third of the tibia. This muscle lies immediately posterior and adjacent to the soleus muscle. There are constant arterial branches entering its proximal third from the posterior tibial artery. There is also an arterial branch to the distal third of the muscle which may be critical in certain cases when the artery is large. Temporarily clamping this artery while using the I.V. fluorescein test can be helpful in determining

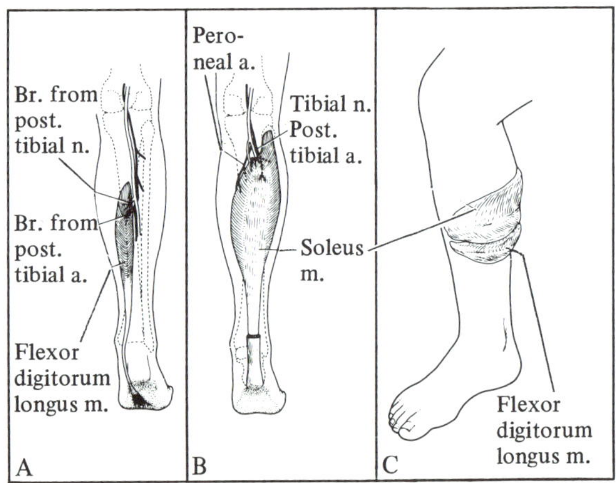

Fig. 49-3. The flexor digitorum longus (A) and soleus (B) with the corresponding neurovascular bundles. C, the soleus and flexor digitorum longus muscles have been transferred to cover defects over the middle third of the tibia.

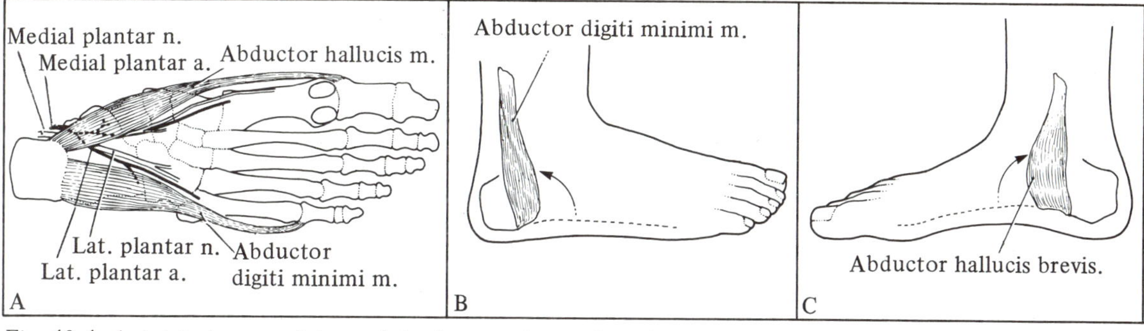

Fig. 49-4. A, intrinsic musculature of the foot used for coverage of defects on the medial and lateral malleolus Note the location of the neurovascular bundles. B, the abductor digiti quinti can cover an ulcer over the lateral malleolus. C, the abductor hallucis is divided from its insertion near the great toe and rotated 90 degrees to cover an ulcer over the medial malleolus.

whether this artery can be divided (see Chapter 1).

For long and narrow ulcerations over the tibia, one should consider the use of the anterior tibialis muscle, which has a segmental blood supply and is most important functionally. However, on occasion, the muscle can be divided at its tendinous end; its muscular belly is spread over to bridge the exposed bone.

DEFECTS IN THE DISTAL THIRD OF THE LEG. Muscle tissue for coverage of this area is less readily available, primarily because the motor units are predominantly tendinous at this level. In particular, defects above the ankle joints are almost impossible to close by muscle transposition; alternative methods must be considered.

The following muscles can at times be used to close defects in the distal third of the tibia: the *flexor digitorum longus,* which will cover defects in the upper part of the lower third of the tibia (Fig. 49-3); and the *abductor hallucis brevis* (with its vascular pedicle entering the proximal third of the muscle) which may be transposed to fill defects on the lower medial aspect of the leg (Fig. 49-4C).

DEFECTS ON THE MEDIAL MALLEOLUS. The *abductor hallucis brevis,* an intrinsic muscle of the foot, can be used to cover defects of the medial malleolus (Fig. 49-4C). It has a large muscle belly, which can be reached by an incision in the medial aspect of the foot. Its insertion is divided and the muscle is rotated superiorly 90 degrees. It is preferable to divide or excise the bridge of skin between the ulceration and the approach incision, rather than attempt to tunnel the muscle under it. The arterial source originates from branches of the medial plantar artery. A large proximal branch consistently enters near the origin of the muscle. There may be two or three smaller branches entering along the muscle belly, and they can usually be sacrificed.

DEFECTS ON THE LATERAL MALLEOLUS. For defects that cannot be covered by spreading out the peroneal musculature on the lateral aspect of the foot, the *abductor digiti minimi muscle* should be considered (Fig. 49-4B). Its muscle bulk is diminutive; although access to the muscle is easily accomplished through an incision on the lateral aspect of the foot, transposition requires an extensive dissection extending to the undersurface of the calcaneus. The arterial supply comes from the lateral plantar artery, which enters very close to the origin of the muscle belly. On occasion, this muscle can be made to cover small defects on the most distal portion of the Achilles tendon [3].

DEFECTS OVER THE CALCANEUS. Defects over the calcaneus or over both the calcaneus and the distal portion of the Achilles tendon can be covered by transposing the *flexor digitorum brevis muscle* (Fig. 49-5). This muscle originates from the distal calcaneus beneath the plantar fascia. Its insertion is in four tendinous slips that extend to the plantar aspects of the phalanges. The innervation and blood supply are from the medial plantar nerve and artery, which enter at its most proximal aspect. The muscle may be detached from its insertion on the toes by exposing it through a midplantar incision. It is then turned back 180 degrees to cover the calcaneus. There is also an arterial branch of the medial plantar artery, which enters the midbelly of the muscle; it can be sacrificed with safety. In dissecting this muscle, extreme care must be observed during the folding procedure in order to preserve the plantar and digital nerves.

Functional Deficits from Muscle Transposition

Loss of the medial head of the gastrocnemius is not critical since plantar flexion can be performed by the

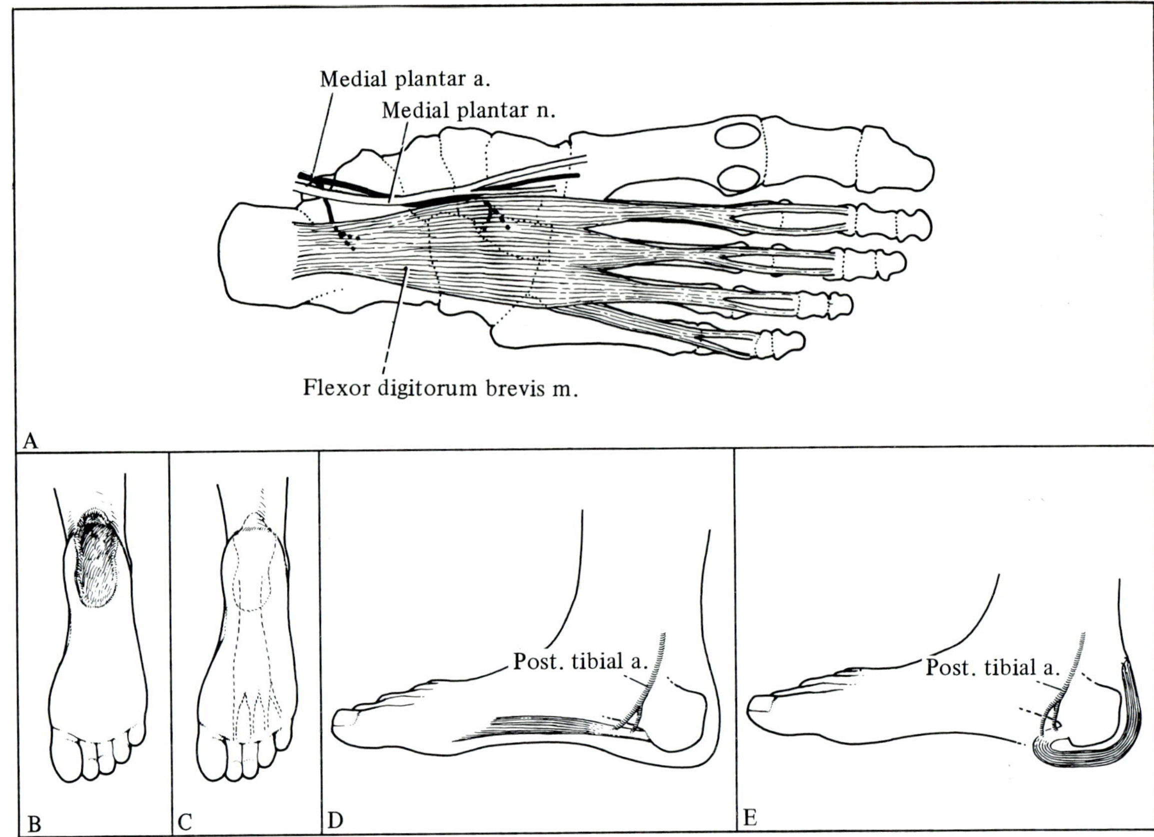

Fig. 49-5. A, plantar view of the flexor digitorum brevis showing its insertion into the toes and the two neurovascular bundles. The muscle will survive on the most proximal bundle alone. B, the position of the ulcer. C, the position of the muscle that is freed of its insertion through an approach incision on the medial aspect of the foot. D, E, the muscle is folded over 180 degrees to cover the ulcer over the calcaneus, and it may even reach the distal insertion of the Achilles tendon.

soleus, flexor digitorum longus, flexor hallucis longus, tibialis posterior, and peroneus muscles. No functional deficit has been noted from any transfer of either head of the gastrocnemius muscle alone. When the soleus and flexor digitorum longus are transposed for middle third tibial defects, plantar flexion of the ankle is rapidly taken over by the strong gastrocnemius. If all three muscles are used there is a significant impairment of plantar flexion. The loss of the flexor digitorum longus is easily tolerated, since phalangeal flexion will be performed by the flexor digitorum brevis. Loss of the peroneus longus muscle alone does not pose a significant deficit, since plantar flexion and foot eversion persist when the foot flexors and the peroneus brevis muscle remain intact. If both the peroneus longus and brevis muscles are used, the foot will lose eversion, which in some circumstances may be an acceptable disability. Loss of function of the peroneal muscles is not significant when the muscles of the anterior compartment are intact – especially when the extensor digitorum longus is intact, since it acts as an evertor of the foot.

The abductor digiti minimi produces abduction and flexion of the fifth toe, and its loss is of little significance. Loss of the flexor digitorum brevis is unimportant, since interphalangeal flexion will be preserved by the action of the flexor digitorum longus.

Complications

Complications of muscle transposition procedures involve the loss of the skin graft or, rarely, the loss of the muscle. The loss of skin graft has been minimized with the use of a meshed split-thickness skin graft, which avoids an underlying hematoma. On occasion, the muscle may be lost (although the loss is usually partial), particularly if it is transposed under a considerable amount of tension or if it disrupts from its attachment to the rim of the ulceration, thus offering only partial coverage. This problem can be avoided by a tension-free transposition. Needless to say, injury to the main neurovascular bundle results in necrosis of the entire muscle, and it must be avoided. In one patient, the medial tibial nerve was injured during dissection of the soleus muscle, but this can be easily avoided. Injury to adjacent structures is almost totally avoidable if basic anatomical considerations are observed.

REFERENCES

1. Ger, R. New operative approach in the treatment of chronic osteomyelitis of the tibial diaphysis: A preliminary report. *Clin. Orthop.* 70:165, 1970.
2. Ger, R. Surgical treatment of the ulcerative lesions of the lower extremity. *Curr. Probl. Surg.* 1:52, 1972.
3. Ger, R. The surgical management of ulcers of the heel. *Surg. Gynecol. Obstet.* 140:909, 1975.
4. Mathes, S. J., McCraw, J. B., and Vasconez, L. O. Muscle transposition flaps for coverage of lower extremity defects: Anatomic considerations. *Surg. Clin. North Am.* 54:1337, 1974.
5. Pers, M., and Medgyesi, S. Pedicle muscle flaps and their applications in the surgery of repair. *Br. J. Plast. Surg.* 26:313, 1975.
6. Robson, M. C., and Edstrom, L. E. Conservative management of the ulcerated diabetic foot. *Plast. Reconstr. Surg.* 59:551, 1977.
7. Serafin, D., Georgiade, N. G., and Smith, D. H. Comparison of free flaps with pedicled flaps for coverage of defects of the leg or foot. *Plast. Reconstr. Surg.* 59:551, 1977.
8. Vasconez, L.O., Bostwick, J., and McCraw, J. B. Coverage of exposed bone by muscle transposition and skin grafting. *Plast. Reconstr. Surg.* 53:526, 1974.
9. Vasconez, L. O., and McCraw, J. B. The Use of Muscle in Plastic and Reconstructive Surgery. In Krizek, T. J., and Hoopes, J. E. (Eds.), *Symposium on Basic Science: Applications to Plastic Surgery.* St. Louis: Mosby, 1976.
10. Vasconez, L. O., Schneider, W. B., and Jurkiewicz, M. J. The treatment of "pressure sores." *Curr. Probl. Surg.* April, 1977.

Pressure Sores

B. HEROLD GRIFFITH

In the years that have elapsed since operative procedures were first applied to the repair of pressure sores in 1945 [1], many improvements have been made in the management of these common problems [3, 4, 7, 8, 9, 10]. The techniques outlined in this chapter have evolved from personal experience with, and follow-up studies on, approximately 1,750 cases [6].

CAUSE

A pressure sore usually results from excessively long compression of the soft tissues between a bony prominence and the bed or chair upon which the patient is resting. The patient who has anesthesia of the skin because of paraplegia has no discomfort to warn him that he has been in one position for too long. The nonparaplegic patient may be too ill or weak to change his position, even though he is uncomfortable.

Prolonged pressure causes anoxia of the soft tissues and thrombosis of the small blood vessels within them; necrosis is then inevitable. When the necrotic tissue sloughs or is debrided away, an ulcer is left. Secondary infection causes acceleration and progression of the process. If external drainage of the infection is inadequate, as is common when a bursa is involved, serious systemic infection may occur. As the necrosis and infection extend more deeply, the underlying bony prominence becomes exposed and infected. A neurogenic trophic factor, first suggested by Charcot in 1879, has never been satisfactorily demonstrated.

Contributing factors are friction, contusion, uncontrolled spasticity, and malnutrition (with anemia, hypoproteinemia, and vitamin deficiencies). Alcoholism, drug addiction, and a desire for self-destruction may contribute to the malnutrition.

The ulcers that develop while the patient is recumbent occur over the sacrum, the greater trochanter of the femur, the anterior superior iliac spine, the patella, the heel, and the anterior edge of the tibia. These might properly be called *decubitus ulcers,* since "decubitus" is the Latin adjective meaning "lying down." Ulcers that develop over the ischial tuberosity or coccyx while the patient is sitting up are not "decubitus" ulcers in the true sense of the word. It is better, therefore, to call all ulcers that result from excessive pressure, *pressure sores.* Certainly, the use of the word "decubitus" as a noun should be avoided.

Cultures of the wound may reveal the presence of any organism or a combination of several. *Staphylococcus aureus, Escherichia coli, Streptococcus pyogenes, Pseudomonas aeruginosa, Aerobacter aerogenes,* and *Proteus vulgaris* are common offenders.

PREVENTION

AVOIDANCE OF PRESSURE. Avoidance of excessive pressure in any one area is obviously essential. The recumbent patient must turn or be turned at least every 2 hours, day and night. A Foster or Stryker frame or a CircOlectric bed is very useful, especially in the severely handicapped patient. In a conventional bed, a firm, noncored, foam rubber mattress distributes the patient's weight quite well. Synthetic sheepskin, kept directly under the skin, has merit. For the past several years, we have been using an air mattress with multiple communicating sections, partially filled with water. It is placed between the patient and his regular mattress, and it distributes his weight extremely well. An inexpensive (about $15.00) air mattress, which is readily available in sporting goods stores, has proved as good as more expensive types. Its filling spout can be easily fitted with a standard brass stopcock for ease in filling and emptying and for protection against leakage.

When the patient is sitting, he should raise himself up for at least a few seconds every half hour to allow some blood to flow into the tissues. In addition, he should lie down, or in some way get his weight completely off the ischia, for at least 10 minutes every 2 hours. Ischial pressure sores are extremely common in patients who sit up continuously for 4 to 6 hours or more.

A good cushion is essential. One made of 7- to 10-cm. thick, firm, noncored foam rubber distributes the weight fairly evenly. An inflatable cushion with interconnecting air cells (such as Roho) has been used and serves well for some patients. Before either of these types is chosen, the patient's adaptation to it should be thoroughly tested. A "flotation" cushion filled with semiliquid silicone has proved to be quite useful for many patients, although it is somewhat expensive and heavy.

The canvas seat of a folding wheelchair tends to sag under the occupant's weight, and pressure sores over the posterior edges of the greater trochanters have been seen from pressure on the side bars of the frame, even when a thick cushion has been used. It is therefore important to place a board under the cushion to prevent sagging. This may be of light, strong plywood, and may be incorporated in the plastic cover of a foam cushion. The board should be square and, except in very rare circumstances, should not have a cutout on the posterior edge. We have seen several ischial ulcers that resulted from pressure against the edge of a cutout area.

SKIN CARE. The skin should be washed, dried, and lightly dusted with talcum powder at least twice daily. Careful inspection of the skin for areas of redness should be routine. Soilage of the skin must be prevented by routine bowel care and by the use of a catheter, condom ("Texas catheter"), rubber urinal, or by automatic bladder function. Too many problems result from injudicious cystectomy and ileal conduit replacement for this procedure to be warranted, except in extreme circumstances. We have had no experience with cutaneous vesicostomy, but have reservations about its value.

EARLY AMBULATION. Whenever possible, early ambulation, using braces, crutches, and parallel bars, is helpful in getting the patient off his "pressure points" for a while each day and in preventing soft tissue calcification around the hip and knee joints. Ischial weight-bearing calipers are contraindicated. The use of braces or crutches requires the expenditure of a considerable amount of physical effort, and is of course possible only for patients who are highly motivated and have strong upper extremity musculature.

ELIMINATION OF FLEXOR SPASMS. Flexor spasms contribute to the development and persistence of pressure sores, especially over the greater trochanters, since they cause friction of the hips against the bed and make it difficult for the patient to lie prone or supine. For a long time, surgical rhizotomy from the tenth thoracic to the second sacral level was the most satisfactory means of relieving spasm. In the past few years, however, intrathecal phenol injections have been found to be as effective as rhizotomy in most patients, and do not involve a major operative procedure. Obviously in paraplegic patients, no destructive procedure, whether surgical or chemical, should be performed until all hope for further recovery of neurological function has been abandoned – usually 18 months after the injury to the spinal cord, unless the cord is known to have been completely severed and no motor or sensory return is possible.

Patients who have sensation or some motor function are not usually candidates for rhizotomy or phenol injection. Drugs have not proved to be totally effective in abolishing spasms, although meprobamate and diazepam (Valium) are of some value. Dantrolene (Dantrium) is showing great promise in reducing spasticity in some patients, so that surgery is possible with good expectation of success. Although narcotics are effective, it is obvious that they cannot be used for long periods.

The relief of spasticity is mandatory before surgical closure of an ulcer in the trochanteric or ischial area, since the wound that results from postoperative dehiscence is invariably much larger than the initial ulcer. It is also obviously impossible to turn a patient from front to back on a turning frame if his hips are flexed by spasticity or contractures.

TREATMENT

Preoperative Care

At the first sign of redness over a bony prominence, all pressure must be taken off the area and kept off until the skin returns to normal. If necrosis occurs, surgical debridement should be carried out as soon as demarcation is complete. After debridement, continuous, room-temperature, moist (not wet) saline dressings are applied; they are changed completely every 2 to 4 hours. Acetic acid (1%), substituted for saline solution, is usually effective in eradicating most strains of *Pseudomonas*.

The wound is cultured, and the sensitivity of the organisms to various antibiotics is determined. Systemic antibiotics are not administered preoperatively except when there is a systemic infection or when the wound is infected by beta-hemolytic *Streptococcus*. Topical streptomycin solution is usually more effective against beta-hemolytic *Streptococcus* than is systemic penicillin unless there is systemic as well as local infection

Laboratory studies include complete blood count and hematocrit, bleeding time, partial thromboplastin time, prothrombin time, total proteins and albumin-globulin ratio, and blood urea nitrogen. The involved bone is examined by x-ray.

The patient is given a high-protein diet, multiple vitamin supplements, and iron, when indicated. Transfusions of whole blood may be required, but they should be avoided if possible. The operation is postponed until the hemoglobin is above 12 gm. per 100 ml. Bladder calculi are removed and other genitourinary problems are corrected as completely as possible by the urology service. Flexor spasms and contractures are eliminated.

The operation is carried out as soon as the above requirements are met, and when the ulcer is clean and beginning to show spontaneous healing at the edges.

Surgical Procedure in Patients with Paraplegia

Principles of Surgical Closure

The ulcer is excised, along with the surrounding scar and the underlying bursa (when one is present) (Fig. 50-1).

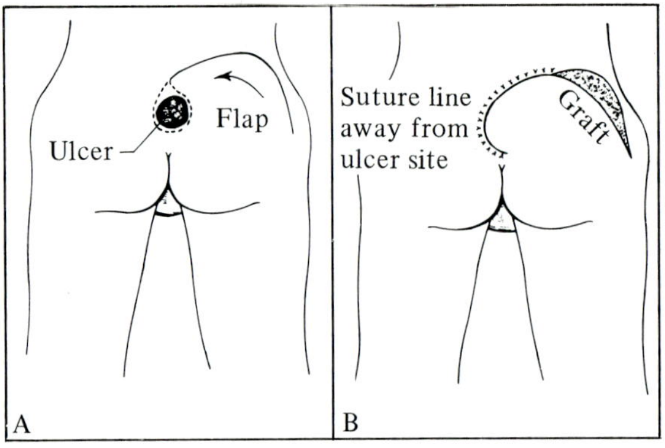

Fig. 50-1. A, the dotted line indicates the area of excision of the scar and ulcer over the sacrum. A flap of full-thickness skin and subcutaneous fat is raised from the buttock. Note that the base of the flap is wide and distally located so that the scar will not be traumatized by sitting. B, the flap is rotated over the sacrum. A split-thickness skin graft is placed over the muscle of the upper outer quadrant of the buttock. Note that the sutures do not go through the skin of the flap.

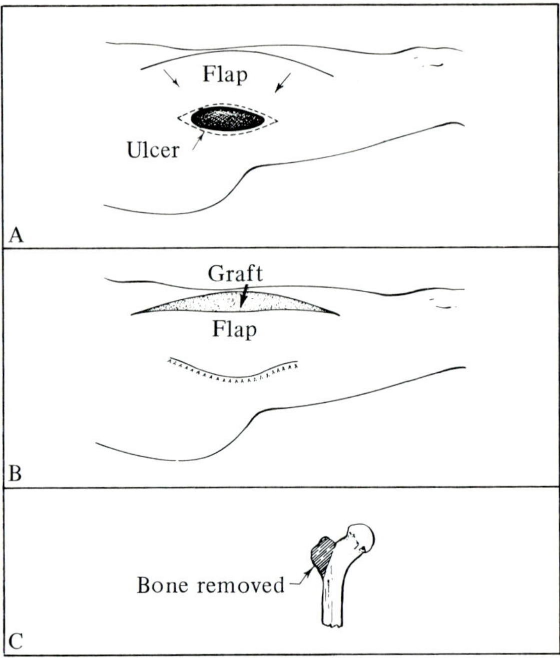

Fig. 50-2. A, a large double-pedicle flap, shifted laterally from the anterior thigh, is used to close a trochanteric ulcer. The anterior relaxing incision is really much farther around the anterior thigh than can be shown in the drawing and actually is just lateral to the iliac crest and femoral triangle. B, a free split-thickness skin graft is used to close the relaxing wound. C, the entire trochanter is removed in addition to a small amount of the upper lateral cortex of the shaft.

The underlying bony prominence is removed. In the sacral area, the medial and lateral sacral crests, the posterior superior iliac spines, and the coccyx are removed. In the trochanteric area, the greater trochanter of the femur and the upper lateral cortex of the shaft adjacent to the trochanter (Fig. 50-2) are excised. In the ischial area, the entire ischium from the pubis to the acetabular rim is usually resected (Fig. 50-3). The periosteum must be removed to prevent the bony prominence forming again. Although perineal ulcers have occurred in rare instances following bilateral total ischiectomy, the total removal of the ischium has been conclusively found in our patients to be far more satisfactory than partial ischiectomy, since the latter procedure is followed by a high incidence of recurrent ulceration [5, 6, 18].

Any soft tissue calcification that may be present in the area *is removed.*

Meticulous hemostasis is achieved by means of electrocoagulation and ligation with 4-0 plain catgut.

The stump of the bone is covered with a flap of soft tissue. In the sacral area, flaps of fascia are turned over from the gluteus maximus, while in the trochanteric wound, fascia lata or tensor fasciae latae is used. The biceps femoris muscle is divided in the distal thigh and folded back into the defect made by the ischiectomy to obliterate dead space and form a pad for sitting (Fig. 50-3).

The wound is covered with a large regional flap of full-thickness skin and fat. For a sacral or ischial ulcer, a rotation flap is usually employed. A large flap is used for several reasons:

1. The larger the flap, the better the blood supply, provided that the length does not greatly exceed the width; since delay is usually not necessary, the entire operation can be done in one stage.
2. The suture line of a large flap is distant from the site of the ulcer. In the event that the ulcer should recur, there is abundant unscarred tissue close at hand to rotate a second time. In the planning of a flap, the scar should always be placed in a position where it will not be over a bony prominence and will not interfere with the construction of another flap that might be required later to close an ulcer in a different site.
3. A large rotation flap will often stretch enough to permit closure of its donor wound by simple suturing. If there is tension on the suture line, a free graft is essential (Figs. 50-1, 50-2, and 50-3), and

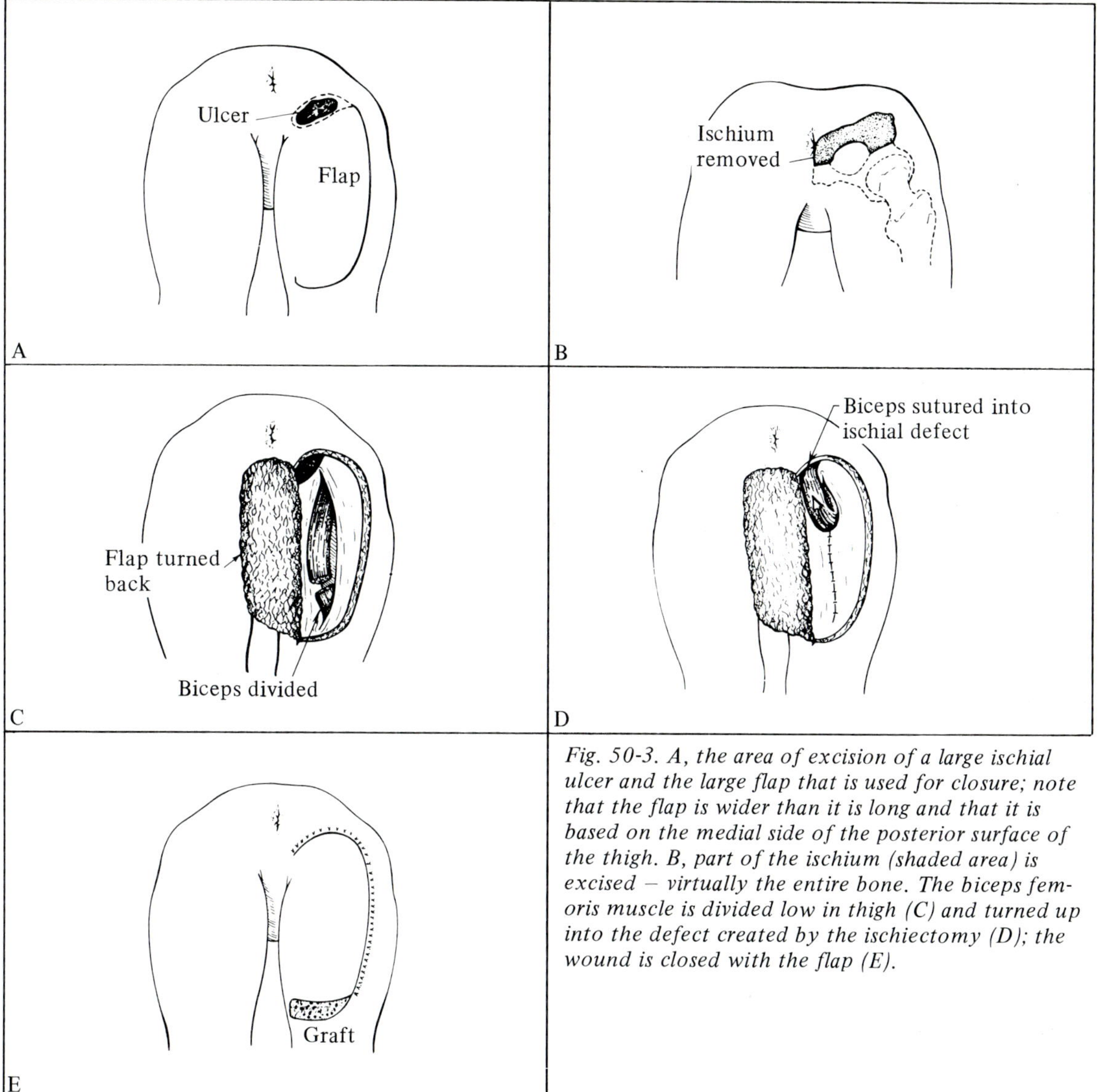

Fig. 50-3. A, the area of excision of a large ischial ulcer and the large flap that is used for closure; note that the flap is wider than it is long and that it is based on the medial side of the posterior surface of the thigh. B, part of the ischium (shaded area) is excised – virtually the entire bone. The biceps femoris muscle is divided low in thigh (C) and turned up into the defect created by the ischiectomy (D); the wound is closed with the flap (E).

should be placed over muscle, well away from the site of the ulcer.

The wound is carefully sutured, using 3-0 chromic catgut in the deeper layers, 3-0 or 4-0 plain catgut or Dexon in the subcutaneous tissue, and horizontal half-buried mattress sutures of 4-0 nylon or polypropylene in the skin. The suture sutures are left in for 14 days.

Wound Suction
Multiperforated, siliconized polyethylene (Hemovac) catheters are placed in the depths of the wound in the area of the ostectomy and in the subcutaneous space, and are brought out through separate stab wounds. They are kept connected to a continuously functioning suction pump for 14 days, regardless of the volume of fluid evacuated [15].

Miscellaneous Details
The operation is carried out under sedation if the operative area is without sensation; otherwise, general anesthesia is used. Even if the patient is awake for the procedure, an anesthetist is in constant attendance to monitor the patient's vital signs and general condition and to administer intravenous fluids and blood as required. The operating table is padded to prevent ulceration over a dependent bony prominence. For closure of a sacral ulcer, the patient is placed prone with a pillow under the pelvis; for an ischial ulcer, he is prone with the hips slightly flexed. The lateral decubitus position is usually best for a trochanteric ulcer. The urethral catheter or other device is connected to gravity drainage throughout the procedure.

Postoperative Care
A dressing of Xeroform gauze and large abdominal pads is placed over the operative site and held in place with nonallergenic adhesive tape or a circumferentially wrapped Kerlix* bandage. The patient is kept on a Stryker frame, and is turned from front to back every 2 hours. Pressure is kept off sacral flaps for at least 48 hours. The use of the frame permits frequent turning, good general care, and normal bowel care, without the danger of flexion of the hips, which might tear the wound open. The patient is given a high-protein diet, vitamin C (1 gm. daily), multivitamins, and the appropriate antibiotic. After 2 weeks passive range-of-motion exercises are begun. The patient can usually be up in his wheelchair on his cushion by the end of the third week. It has been suggested that monitoring the temperature in pressure areas helps to avoid recurrences, but I have had no personal experience with this technique as yet.

*Kendall Company, Bauer & Black Division, Chicago, IL 60606.

Closure of Specific Ulcers

Sacral Ulcers
For closure of an ulcer over the sacrum, a large rotation flap is usually best. This flap consists of the skin and the subcutaneous fat of almost one entire buttock, and is based inferiorly, so that the scar will not be irritated by sitting (Fig. 50-1). The donor site of the flap is closed by a split-thickness skin graft placed over the upper outer quadrant of the gluteus maximus. If one flap is inadequate to repair the sacral defect, a second flap, also based inferiorly, is rotated from the other buttock.

A very large sacral ulcer can occasionally be more satisfactorily closed by a double-pedicle flap, which can be constructed transversely in the lumbar area and shifted distally or formed obliquely on the buttock and flank and shifted inferomedially. It usually must be "delayed" at least once. If disarticulation of the hip should be necessary for other reasons, the filleted soft tissues of the buttock can be used to resurface the sacrum, but disarticulation is not justified solely for the repair of a sacral ulcer. Too many problems result from a change in the patient's center of gravity and the faulty distribution of weight after disarticulation to make this a desirable procedure, except in extreme circumstances [11].

Split-thickness skin grafts are usually much too thin for satisfactory permanent coverage of the sacrum, but multilayered split-thickness skin grafts (overgrafting) or the Hynes reverse dermis graft (see Chapter 1) may be utilized when local tissue for a flap is not available and a tubed skin pedicle would not be practical. The procedure can be repeated three or four times if necessary.

Trochanteric Ulcers
In the past, a large inferoposteriorly based rotation flap was favored for the closure of a trochanteric wound. This type of flap is still used at times, but necrosis of the upper edge of the flap has occurred often enough to make it a second choice. A large, double-pedicle flap has proved to be almost universally successful. This flap is shifted laterally from the anterior thigh; the oblique anterior relaxing incision is made just lateral to the iliac crest and the femoral triangle. The free skin graft, which must be used for coverage of the donor wound, is actually much farther around on the anterior thigh than it appears to be in Figure 50-2.

For the closure of a small trochanteric defect, when there is abundant soft tissue over the hip and thigh, the wound edges can occasionally be sutured together without tension, without the need for a relaxing incision anteriorly.

In the case of a combination of inadequate soft tissue for any local flap and intractable infection of the bone and joint beneath, amputation of the extremity may be considered. If this is done, the abundant soft tissues of the deboned thigh are preserved and swung up for coverage of the ischial, trochanteric, and sacral areas as required. Amputation should be only a last resort, since it introduces additional serious problems in balance, distribution of weight, and recurrent ulceration.

Ischial Ulcers

For the closure of a large ischial defect, the most satisfactory operation is total ischiectomy, biceps muscle flap, and upward rotation of a very large flap of skin and fat, based on the posteromedial surface of the thigh (Fig. 50-3). The length-to-width ratio of the skin flap is 1:2 or 1:3. A free skin graft, if required to avoid tension, is placed over the muscle in the lower third of the thigh.

In the case of a small ischial ulcer, it is sometimes possible, following total ischiectomy, to approximate the local muscles, subcutaneous tissue, and skin, in layers, without tension, and without the need for a biceps muscle flap or rotation flap of skin. This procedure was virtually abandoned some years ago because of the high incidence of recurrence due to postoperative hematoma. In selected cases, however, it has definite usefulness, owing largely to the fact that continuous postoperative wound suction can usually be depended on to prevent the formation of a hematoma, and primary healing is thus ensured.

OTHER ULCERS. Pressure sores in other locations that do not heal under conservative treatment (e.g., debridement, moist dressings, and avoidance of pressure), can be treated as follows:

1. *Coccyx* – Coccygectomy and two advancement skin flaps (primary suture).
2. *Knee* – Patellectomy and double-pedicle or rotation skin flap from the anterior thigh.
3. *Shin* – A skin graft, or two double-pedicle skin flaps, with a split-thickness graft to cover the donor site on the calf.
4. *Heel* – A skin graft, or excision of the ulcer, and a portion of the os calcis and primary suture.
5. *Malleolus* – A local rotation skin flap after excision of the bony prominence.
6. *Anterior superior iliac spine* – Excision of the bone and primary suture.
7. *Chest wall* – Resection of the underlying rib and primary suture.
8. *Dorsal spine* – Resection of the spinous processes of the vertebrae and a large rotation skin flap.
9. *Soft tissues of the buttock* – A skin graft.
10. *Elbow* – Excision of the prominent edge of the olecranon process, excision of the olecranon bursa, and closure by primary suture.

New Techniques of Closure

In the last few years, several alternative methods of closure of pressure sores have been reported, especially *muscle flaps covered by split-thickness skin grafts* [12, 13] (see also Chapter 49). In essence each of these procedures consists of covering the stump of the resected bone with a turnover flap or rotation flap of adjacent muscle, and then covering the well-padded muscle flap with a meshed skin graft instead of with a flap of skin and fat, as had been the standard for many years. The gluteus maximus muscle is recommended for sacral and ischial wounds and the rectus femoris, sartorius, and vastus lateralis muscles for trochanteric ulcers [19]. The results that have been published indicate a reasonable degree of success. However, in the sacral and ischial areas, the skin incisions that are used for access to the muscles can leave scars in areas that may be subjected to trauma later; such scars may also interfere with the construction of skin flaps that may be needed later for the repair of ulcers in other locations.

It appears that the muscle flaps covered by skin grafts have their greatest usefulness in the repair of recurrent ulcers in which there is insufficient normal adjacent skin and subcutaneous tissue to allow coverage by conventional methods. These muscle flaps covered with skin grafts provide good pads over trimmed-off bony prominences, and they should prove more satisfactory than multiple dermal overgrafts for the coverage of difficult-to-close recurrent sores. In my opinion muscle flaps covered by skin grafts are *not* the treatment of choice for primary repairs of pressure sores in most cases.

In addition, *myocutaneous flaps* using the gracilis and other muscles have been tried in some centers [19, 20]. Here, too, the padding that these flaps provide offers a great advantage. However, the scarring that results from obtaining the muscle is often highly undesirable, since it is likely to be in an anesthetic area that is subject to trauma and may well interfere with necessary subsequent operations. Free myocutaneous flaps at present appear to offer little help because of the lack of suitable vessels for anastomosis and because unwanted scars are created in the donor areas.

TREATMENT IN NONPARAPLEGIC PATIENTS

The pressure sore that develops in the nonparalyzed patient usually results from a sheet burn, maceration of the skin, infrequent turning in bed, or pressure from a poorly padded operating table or plaster cast. The patient is likely to be elderly and debilitated. Conservative measures may be sufficient for the healing of small ulcers; these measures include moist dressings, avoidance of pressure, ambulation, and improvement of the general nutritional state.

A superficial ulcer without exposed bone may be closed with a split-thickness skin graft. If the ulcer is deep, closure with a flap is indicated as soon as the patient's general condition permits. Partial ostectomy is generally better than total ischiectomy in the nonparaplegic patient. A functioning muscle should not be sacrificed for use as a muscle flap. Sensation is a great help in preventing recurrence of the ulcer following rehabilitation. The patient who is terminally ill from cancer should not be subjected to a major surgical procedure to close the ulcer, but should receive general supportive care and local conservative treatment as described above.

REHABILITATION OF PARAPLEGIC PATIENTS

The rehabilitation of the patient with paraplegia is an involved process that requires the dedicated services of several disciplines, but particularly the department of physical medicine. Countless articles and books have been written on the subject, but none is more useful for the plastic surgeon than Betts and Rosen's chapter [2] in Ruge's book on spinal cord injuries. They point out that from the time of injury "each patient must be treated as if no neurological return will occur," since it is impossible at that time to predict which patients will have complete return of function, who will have partial return, and who will have none. Each must be started on a thorough program as soon as his general condition will permit – with an aim toward future independence with or without externally powered devices.

In the *early phase,* turning every two hours on a frame is essential, along with the other measures outlined above. Joints should be kept limber by passive range-of-motion exercises, and strengthening of all remaining functioning muscles must be started early and continued indefinitely. Occupational therapy, education, and emotional support are of enormous importance. A realistic presentation of possible future disability is given, with the goal of maximum cooperation of the patient in his program of rehabilitation.

In the *comprehensive phase,* when the injured part is stable and the patient can enter the rehabilitation center, a tilt table may help in getting him from the horizontal to the vertical position without hypotensive episides. A program is started to help the patient achieve mobility in a wheelchair; as mentioned previously, a proper cushion should be used and the patient should raise himself up periodically. Range-of-motion and progressive resistive exercises are continued. Caution is needed to avoid fracturing osteoporotic bones. Bracing and ambulation are begun for patients who have a strong desire for braces and who possess sufficient muscle innervation and stability to use them effectively. The patient is taught skills such as transferring from bed to chair and personal grooming. Vocational counseling helps the patient set realistic goals for the future. Considerable education and/or reeducation is often needed to prepare the patient for at least partial self-reliance in a new life geared to his physical capabilities. Psychiatric help and family counseling are frequently needed. Sexual adjustments are difficult; frank, realistic, and sympathetic advice is required. Therapeutic recreation often affords a helpful means of muscle-building and readjustment to society.

After discharge from the rehabilitation center, the patient must be followed closely and encouraged to return for any advice or assistance that may be required. Periodic physical evaluations are essential to avoid urological problems and pressure sores, to monitor neurological improvement (or worsening), to provide replacement of worn-out appliances (such as wheelchairs, braces, and supports), to keep the patient apprised of new developments in the field of research on paraplegia, and to provide the stabilizing influence of a continuing relationship with interested, knowledgeable, and caring health professionals. Paraplegia is more than a condition, it is a way of life that no one chooses but to which many must adjust.

REFERENCES

1. Barker, D. E. Surgical treatment of decubitus ulcers. *J.A.M.A.* 129:160, 1945.
2. Betts, H. B., and Rosen, J. Rehabilitation. In Ruge, D. (Ed.), *Spinal Cord Injuries.* Springfield, Ill.: Thomas, 1969.
3. Blocksma, R., Kostrubala, J., and Greeley, P. W. The surgical repair of decubitus ulcer in paraplegics: Further observations. *Plast. Reconstr. Surg.* 4:123, 1949.
4. Cannon, B., O'Leary, J. J., O'Neil, J. W., and Steinsieck, R. An approach to the treatment of pressure sores. *Ann. Surg.* 132:760, 1950.
5. Comarr, A. E., and Bors, E. Radical ischialectomy in decubitus ischial ulcers complicating paraplegia. *Ann. West. Med. Surg.* 5:210, 1951.
6. Conway, H., and Griffith, B. H. Plastic surgery for closure of decubitus ulcers in patients with paraplegia: Based on experience with 1000 cases. *Am. J. Surg.* 91:946, 1956.
7. Conway, H., Kraissl, C. J., Clifford, R. H., Gelb, J., Joseph, J. M., and Leveridge, L. L. The plastic surgical closure of decubitus ulcers in patients

with paraplegia. *Surg. Gynecol. Obstet.* 85:321, 1947.

8. Conway, H., Stark. R. B., Weeter, J. C., Garcia, F. A., and Kavanaugh, J. D. Complications of decubitus ulcers in patients with paraplegia. *Plast. Reconstr. Surg.* 7:117, 1951.
9. Croce, E. J., Schullinger, R. N., and Shearer, T. P. The operative treatment of decubitus ulcer. *Ann. Surg.* 123:53, 1946.
10. Gelb, J. Plastic surgical closure of decubitus ulcers in paraplegics as result of civilian injuries. *Plast. Reconstr. Surg.* 9:525, 1952.
11. Georgiade, N., Pickrell, K., and Maguire, C. Total thigh flaps for extensive decubitus ulcers. *Plast. Reconstr. Surg.* 17:220, 1956.
12. Ger, R. The surgical management of decubitus ulcers by muscle transposition. *Surgery* 69:100, 1971.
13. Ger, R., and Levine, S. A. The management of decubitus ulcers by muscle transposition. *Plast. Reconstr. Surg.* 58:419, 1976.
14. Griffith, B. H. Advances in the treatment of decubitus ulcers. *Surg. Clin. North Am.* 43:245, 1963.
15. Griffith, B. H. An improved method of postoperative wound suction. *Plast. Reconstr. Surg.* 31: 294, 1963.
16. Griffith, B. H. Pressure Sores. In Ruge, D. (Ed.), *Spinal Cord Injuries.* Springfield, Ill.: Thomas, 1969. Chapter 16.
17. Griffith, B. H. Pressure Sores. In Goldwyn, R. M. (Ed.), *The Unfavorable Result in Plastic Surgery: Avoidance and Treatment.* Boston: Little, Brown, 1972.
18. Griffith, B. H., and Schultz, R. C. The prevention and surgical treatment of recurrent decubitus ulcers in patients with paraplegia. *Plast. Reconstr. Surg.* 27:248, 1961.
19. Minami, R. T., Hentz, V. R., and Vistnes, L. M. Use of vastus lateralis muscle flap for repair of trochanteric pressure sores. *Plast. Reconstr. Surg.* 60:364, 1977.
20. Minami, R. T., Mills, R., and Pardoe, R. Gluteus maximus myocutaneous flaps for repair of pressure sores. *Plast. Reconstr. Surg.* 60:242, 1977.
21. Rogers, J., and Wilson, L. F. Preventing recurrent tissue breakdowns after "pressure sore" closures. *Plast. Reconstr. Surg.* 56:419, 1975.
22. Sloan, D. F., Brown, R. D., and Larson, D. L. Evaluation of a simplified water mattress in the prevention and treatment of pressure sores. *Plast. Reconstr. Surg.* 60:596, 1977.

51

Lymphedema

TIMOTHY A. MILLER

edema . . . the presence of abnormally large amounts of fluid in the intercellular tissue spaces of the body; usually applied to demonstrable accumulation of excessive fluid in the subcutaneous tissues.

Dorland's Illustrated Medical Dictionary
Twenty-fifth ed., 1974

Lymphedema is characterized by the accumulation of protein-rich fluid within the subcutaneous space tissues of the extremity. For reasons that are not entirely clear, the deep muscle compartment is not involved. Lymphedema can be caused by surgical removal or destruction by disease of regional lymph nodes *(acquired lymphedema)* or it can presumably result from an inborn error in the anatomy and/or function of the lymphatic vessels *(primary lymphedema)*. Primary lymphedema probably includes several different conditions involving lymphatic malfunction in which the cause of the swelling is incompletely understood.

ANATOMY OF THE LYMPHATIC SYSTEM

A significant portion of lymphedema is due to some embryological aberration in the development of lymphatics. It is generally agreed that lymphatics and lymph nodes arise from endothelial sprouting of the primordial venous system [3, 10]. This development begins in four areas: the paired jugular and iliac systems, the cysterna chyli and retroperitoneal systems. These sacs develop peripherally and invade almost all tissues of the body with the major exceptions of the central nervous system, bone marrow, and coats of the eye. The thoracic duct results from a fusion of the cysterna chyli and left jugular buds. Lymphatic channels and regional nodes of each extremity are eventually formed by this peripheral growth and drain either into the cysterna chyli (lower extremities) or directly into the thoracic ducts (upper extremities), which return lymph to the venous system. Variations in the communications between the major lymphatic trunks and the subclavian veins are relatively common [3].

Leg Lymphatics

The subcutaneous compartment (in which lymphedema occurs) is drained by three groups of lymphatics: a dermal plexus, collecting channels, and superficial lymphatic trunks. Intradermal lymphatics which do not have valves drain into a valved system lying in the deepest dermal level at the subcutaneous junction [3]. (This entire system would therefore be preserved in any pedicle flap.) By means of collecting channels, the dermal plexus drains into main lymphatic trunks located slightly superficial to the investing muscle fascia. It is these lymphatics that are seen in lymphangiograms.

In 1954 Kinmonth [4] introduced lymphangiography as a radiological means of visualizing the lymphatic system, and information about lymphatic drainage has largely been obtained by this method (see under the heading, Technique of Lymphangiography). There is general agreement that the superficial (subcutaneous) and deep (muscle) lymphatic systems are separate and communicate only under abnormal conditions, such as proximal obstruction [6, 13].

The deep lymphatic system consists of several channels deeply located near bone. In the leg, vessels can be cannulated posterior to the medial malleolus [5]. As the vessels ascend, they maintain a constant diameter, and valves can be seen at relatively regular 1-cm. intervals indicated by a beaded pattern. About four vessels normally drain into the popliteal lymph nodes in the posterior knee and ascend the thigh medially to drain into the deep inguinal nodes.

The superficial lymphatic system, which is best studied by lymphangiography, drains in two pathways closely corresponding to the venous drainage of the leg. In the routine lymphangiogram a soluble blue dye is injected into the web space. The dye enters the dermal lymphatics and eventually outlines the superficial trunks which are identified through a small incision, cannulated, and injected with contrast material. About five vessels are usually seen along the medial aspect of the extremity, generally following the course of the saphenous vein. A drainage system that parallels the lesser saphenous system can also be seen along the lateral aspect of the leg. These trunks are valved, they bifurcate and rejoin, and they maintain the same diameter as they ascend the extremity. Some evidence exists that lymphatic channels draining the lower leg do not receive tributaries from the thigh. Lymphangiographic studies have shown that the thigh drains into the superior inguinal lymph nodes, while the lower leg drains into the more inferior inguinal nodes [8]. Because of this, in some patients with acquired lymphedema the swelling may be limited to the lower leg.

The inguinal nodes are divided into two groups: superficial (around the fossa ovalis) and deep (within the fatty tissue of the femoral sheath). These nodes (approximately 15) drain into the nodes surrounding the iliac vessels. Although virtually all lymphatic flow passes through the inguinal nodes, it has been shown that lymph drainage can bypass these nodes and drain directly into the iliac area [11].

Arm Lymphatics

The superficial lymphatic channels appear anatomically similar to those in the leg, coursing along the general pattern of the basilic (medial aspect) and cephalic (lateral aspect) veins. At times they join each other, but normally they course separately until they drain into the axillary nodes.

TECHNIQUE OF LYMPHANGIOGRAPHY

The technique involves injecting 5 ml. of a 1:1 mixture of methylene blue and 1% lidocaine into each of the web spaces of the involved extremity. In the normal individual, dermal lymphatic channels are outlined by this concentration of the dye. Upon visualizing these channels, a transverse incision is made, the lymphatic channels are identified and cannulated, and contrast medium is injected to perform the actual lymphangiogram. Considerable information, however, can be gained from the rate of diffusion and pattern of the methylene blue dye alone.

PHYSIOLOGY OF THE LYMPHATIC SYSTEM

The lymphatic system serves a number of functions: drainage of a fraction of the macromolecular protein loss from the capillary circulation, removal of bacteria and foreign material, and transport of specific substances (e.g., vitamin K and long-chain fatty acids) from the gastrointestinal tract.

Lymphatics at the capillary level have no basement membrane and are therefore extremely permeable [11, 14]. Because of this permeability, the low hydrostatic pressure within lymphatics (as compared to interstitial fluid), and the valves that encourage unidirectional flow, lymph passes proximally and does not normally accumulate within the interstitium. Lymph is essentially an ultrafiltrate somewhat similar to plasma; it forms as a transudate resulting from the relatively high hydrostatic pressure of the arterial system. According to Starling's law, the osmotic pressure within the blood partially balances this loss. The protein loss from this process is substantial, however; in any 24-hour period, over 50 percent of the circulating albumin can be lost [14]. Although the major portion of that loss is resorbed into the venules by a combination of osmotic and hydrostatic forces, a minimal amount (approximately 0.1 percent) is not resorbed [8]. The lymphatic system is responsible for the return of this fraction of the macromolecular capillary loss. Lymph normally contains 0.1 to 0.5 gm. total protein per 100 ml. in the extremities (as compared to 6 gm. protein per 100 ml. in blood). In this more dilute protein concentration, there is a disproportionately high ratio of albumin to globulin owing to the higher molecular weight of globulin, again emphasizing the fact that lymph results from an ultrafiltration process across a semipermeable membrane. Once lymph enters a lymphatic space, it is not appreciably altered or concentrated [12].

Lymph flow is comparatively slow and results from a combination of factors: interstitial pressure; the negative and positive fluctuation in intraabdominal and intrathoracic cavities; and the adjacent compression of arterial pulsation and muscular activity. The valves promote proximally directed flow. It is likely that the compression of arterial pulsation and muscular contraction are particularly influential in the flow within the deep lymphatic system.

There has been some question as to whether lymphatic flow is also due to an intrinsic contractile mechanism within the vessels themselves. Several investigators have shown that lymphatics respond to a variety of hormonal and chemical influences, and it seems likely that some function similar to peristalsis does exist [1, 9, 16, 25]. If so, it would most critically affect the subcutaneous lymphatics, which are not surrounded by muscle (unlike those in the deep compartment).

Clinical lymphedema probably has several causes and involves impaired transcapillary fluid exchange or impaired transport of lymph, or both conditions. While different factors obviously characterize the primary (congenital) and acquired types of this condition, in both forms, lymph drainage fails to keep up with production, generating the accumulation of relatively protein-rich interstitial fluid. Edema owing to cardiac failure rarely contains more than 0.9 gm. of total protein per 100 ml. edema fluid, whereas in chronic lymphedema total protein may be as high as 5 gm. per 100 ml. [26]. According to the concept of Donnan's equilibrium, the resultant high osmotic pressure secondary to the high protein concentration will attract and obligate even greater amounts of fluid. It has also been observed that in lymphedematous extremities there is a 20 to 30 percent increase in venous flow, presumably as a compensatory mechanism [23].

In lymphedema, a new balance of pressures is established, and the increase in interstitial pressure and surrounding tissue compliance tends to increase lymph flow. Elastic stockings encourage this aspect of lymphatic drainage.

SYMPTOMS OF LYMPHEDEMA

The severity of symptoms can vary from mild extremity swelling to seriously disabling or life-threatening complications such as recurrent cellulitis and lymphangiosarcoma.

Early edema fluid accumulation results in a soft,

pitting type of edema usually beginning in the ankle and gradually ascending. Although measurement may reveal only a modest increase in extremity diameter, the associated weight increase can be substantial (e.g., an increase of 9 cm. around the thigh results in approximately a 2-kg. increase in weight). Such patients typically complain of fatigue in the involved extremity. As swelling increases, normal function can be compromised and there can be significant discomfort, presumably from the distention of the tissues. Corresponding with the duration of the process, the protein concentration of the edema fluid gradually increases [26]. This, combined with lymphatic stasis, serves as an ideal culture medium for bacteria. As many as 25 percent of patients have recurrent episodes of lymphangitis [24], usually not preceded by trauma, that can have an extremely rapid onset. Such attacks account for a significant morbidity in some patients and can occur several times in a year.

In time, there is increased fibrosis of the connective tissue elements within the subcutaneous tissue and skin, a process that accelerates with each episode of infection. In chronic lymphedema (elephantiasis), the skin is thick and hyperkeratotic, and the entire extremity is indurated with a nonpitting edema.

Lymphangiosarcoma is an unusual, highly malignant endothelial tumor that can occur in any patient with lymphedema [17], although it is most common in the acquired form, particularly in postmastectomy patients. Similar to Kaposi's sarcoma, it is characterized by the appearance of papular bluish lesions that often ascend the extremity. It occurs infrequently and only after lymphedema has been present for several years. Although it can be treated by a combination of surgery and radiotherapy, the condition is rarely cured.

Primary Lymphedema

Perhaps more accurately termed "idiopathic lymphedema," the classification of primary lymphedema can be subdivided by the age of onset or by lymphangiographic findings. In general, these factors are related.

Classification by Age of Onset

Milroy's disease is a specific congenital form of lymphedema first described in 1891 [22]. A hereditary form of extremity edema present at birth, it is characterized by marked hypoplasia of the lymphatic trunks and a familial, sex-linked incidence [19].

There is general agreement that primary lymphedema stems from some anatomical abnormality of the lymphatics resulting from developmental and/or functional disorders. Primary lymphedema probably encompasses several conditions with varying and incompletely understood etiologies. Edema may appear at any time, from birth *(lymphedema congenita)* to middle age *(lymphedema tarda)*, but the highest incidence occurs during adolescence *(lymphedema praecox)* and accounts for approximately 80 percent of patients. The remaining 20 percent of cases are equally divided between the remaining two groups.

Classification by Lymphangiographic Findings

Three general lymphatic patterns have been described in primary lymphedema: aplasia, hypoplasia, and hyperplasia (varicose) [4]. The most common lymphangiographic finding is *hypoplasia*, seen in 70 percent of cases of patients with primary lymphedema. In this form of lymphedema, following initial injection of blue dye into the web space there is slow spread over the dorsum of the foot. Occasionally a single superficial lymphatic channel can be visually identified. On radiographic examination there is typically a single, slightly enlarged lymphatic vessel. In the *aplastic* form (approximately 15 percent) the blue dye diffuses readily through the dermal plexus but remains confined to the dorsum of the foot and rarely extends above the ankle. Upon exploration no lymphatic trunks can be identified. The blue dye can remain for months in such patients. In the *hyperplastic* or *varicose* pattern (15 percent), blue dye diffuses over the dorsum of the foot and several trunks can be visualized along the anterior aspect of the ankle. Numerous dilated, tortuous channels that easily fill with contrast medium can be seen radiologically. Moreover, dermal backflow (retrograde filling of the dermal plexus) is almost always evident. The varicose type is thought to be the consequence of incompetent lymphatic valves [4]. Also seen in other forms of lymphedeam, dermal backflow is considered evidence of some form of lymphatic obstruction.

Lymphangiographic findings generally correlate with the age of onset [25]. In those individuals who have the congenital form or an early onset of edema, the aplastic lymphangiographic form is usually found. The hypoplastic form predominates in patients with an onset in adolescence.

The uncertainties regarding the etiology of primary lymphedema derive from its many unusual features: women are afflicted at least three times more frequently, the left leg is affected significantly more often than the right, but the upper extremity is rarely involved. No single pathophysiological concept seems to encompass the entire spectrum of this condition. The tendency for symptoms to appear during the menarche and pregnancy suggests a hormonal cause, yet there is no explanation for the significant incidence in males. A particularly difficult aspect is the identification of a precipitating factor. It is completely unknown why a normal middle-aged adult would develop lymphedema without any known predisposing cause.

Although most evidence seems to indicate that some anatomical abnormality is likely to be present in patients who have lymphedema, it is becoming apparent that this correlation is not absolute. In a lymphangiographic study of 200 patients, it was impossible to correlate the pathological lymphatic patterns (seen on contrast medium radiological examination) and the clinical severity of the condition [23]. In patients who have unilateral lymphedema, abnormal lymphangiographic findings on the clinically normal side are characteristic [15]. Although a substantial number of these patients eventually develop bilateral swelling, others do not [18, 21]. It is therefore possible that in addition to an anatomical abnormality, some functional derangement within the lymphatics must exist.

Acquired Lymphedema

While the basic pathology inherent in primary lymphedema undoubtedly resides in the lymphatics, the regional lymph nodes are the pathological site in the acquired form. The axillary or inguinal nodes can be destroyed or damaged by surgery, radiation, infection (e.g., filariasis, tuberculosis, lymphogranuloma, actinmycosis, and cat scratch fever), tumor invasion, or inflammatory process (from a snake or insect bite or from chronic lymphangitis). Perhaps the most common worldwide cause is direct infestation of the lymph nodes by the parasite *Filaria bancrofti*, estimated to have been the source in 200 million documented cases of lymphedema [17, 25]. However, the occurrence of permanent lymphedema complicating other infectious or inflammatory processes is unusual.

The other common cause of this condition is radical axillary or groin excision in the treatment of malignant tumors. Approximately 10 to 15 percent of patients undergoing radical mastectomy will develop significant postoperative arm swelling [20, 27]. Radiotherapy, obesity, and postoperative problems with wound healing are associated with a higher incidence. The swelling may not begin immediately and may be delayed for as long as a year, particularly following irradiation. This delay is the result of the ongoing fibrotic process, which further constricts and obstructs lymphatic drainage. The swelling generally begins in the upper arm and eventually may become massive.

DIFFERENTIAL DIAGNOSIS

In the vast majority of patients the diagnosis of lymphedema can be made by history and physical examination. The gradual ascent of edema from the ankle proximally during a period of several months, unassociated with other symptoms, is characteristic. Classically, the swelling occurs in females at the time of the menarche or pregnancy. In other instances it can be traced to a preceding trauma, although whether this incident actually precipitated the lymphedematous process is often not clear. In a large proportion of patients, no apparent cause can be identified. While unilateral enlargement of an extremity always raises the possibility of malignancy, lymphedema from this cause is rather unusual and frequently accompanied by many clinical signs pointing to the malignant process.

A major diagnostic problem is determining whether leg swelling is due to *lymphatic or venous etiologies*. This distinction can, in all but a few patients, be made on clinical evidence. Chronic edema secondary to venous disease is usually due to incompetent valves, a condition that increases capillary pressure. As a result, capillary perfusion is decreased, and in time a characteristic dark, brawny edema occurs. When the problem is long-standing, ulceration of the skin results from the impaired perfusion and tissue anoxia. In lymphedema, however, capillary perfusion is unimpaired and ulceration is extremely rare. Although either can increase fibrous content within the skin, the deep brown discoloration typical of venous problems is very unusual in lymphedema.

Left leg swelling has been claimed to be the result of obstruction of the left vein by the crossing of the right iliac artery. This has been termed the *iliac compression syndrome* and has been proposed as an etiology for lymphedema [29]. However, few of these patients demonstrate any classic evidence of peripheral venous disease, and it is difficult to see how venous hypertension can be reflected as lymphedema without a high incidence of chronic skin changes and ulceration. Venography in such cases is useful but not always easily interpreted [14]. When *acute venous thrombosis* is a possible cause, Doppler findings may be valuable [28].

Following a period of bed rest, lymphedema typically resolves in several days, whereas venous edema tends to improve within hours. In very difficult diagnostic situations, *venography* is generally more informative than lymphangiography and considerably easier and safer to perform. Indeed, *lymphangiography* is tedious, difficult, and hazardous (Fairbairn and associates [30] reported 16 fatalities in 16,000 studies), and it offers little information that is not available on clinical examination. Moreover, it is associated with numerous wound healing problems; except in rare instances, the lymphangiographic findings will not influence the eventual surgical management.

Lymphangiomas are localized endothelial-lined spaces that can appear in the extremity as soft tumors. They are not uncommon, and 90 percent appear before the second year of life [27]. Like congenital lymphedema and cystic hygromas, they are believed to be inborn malformations of the lymphatic system. Although they can occur anywhere in the body, the hands, feet, and tongue are the most frequent locations. They do not spontaneously regress. Their localized nature, spongy nonpitting texture, and failure to resolve on bed rest distinguish them from lymphedema. Treatment is surgical, usually postponed until the child has grown to allow the anatomical extent of the tumor to be defined more easily. Recurrence from inadequate excision is high [31].

The relatively rare condition of *lipedema,* seen generally in women, is considered a lipodystrophy; it is characterized by diffuse, symmetrical, nonpitting enlargement of the subcutaneous tissue of the extremity. A weight-reduction regimen may be helpful, but surgery should be undertaken only in selected cases.

MEDICAL MANAGEMENT

Most patients with lymphedema are adequately managed without surgical intervention. Unfortunately, however, neither the medical nor surgical approach can provide a cure, and it is therefore imperative that the patient completely understand the chronicity of this condition as well as the importance of *controlling the edema* and *preventing infection.* Medical management can only attempt to improve lymphatic drainage by periodic elevation of the extremity, external compression, and the use of diuretics.

Certain measures can be taken by the patient. It is important to avoid unnecessary standing for long periods, to elevate the foot of the bed with 15-cm. blocks, and to wear elastic stockings conscientiously. The stockings should fit tightly, and the measurements of the individual patient should be taken *after* a period of bed rest, when the extremity is smallest in diameter. New stockings should be obtained every few months to maintain firm compression. A full-length stocking or the leotard type of stocking often proves to be too inconvenient, and as a result it is often discarded. For most patients, a knee-length stocking is an excellent compromise because it is considerably easier to use. While the intermittent compression machine has been recommended by many, lymphedema characteristically resolves slowly, and short periods of using this device can never substitute for conscientious attention to daily activities.

Diuretics are often initially effective, and in rare instances they can completely resolve the swelling; unfortunately, the improvement is usually not permanent. To be most beneficial, diuretics should be taken intermittently, particularly in the premenstrual period. It is recommended that the patient be given one of the longer acting thiazides combined with a potassium-sparing diuretic over a 4-day period.

Generally, infection cannot be avoided. Although in many patients no predisposing injury can be identified, other patients have fungal infections of the web space that precipitate skin breakdown and an ascending lymphangitis. Meticulous skin care and antifungal treatment frequently prove successful without additional measures. In patients with recurrent infectious episodes of unknown origin, prophylactic penicillin is the drug of choice, because Streptococcus is the most common etiological agent.

When infection occurs, it must be treated early and aggressively. The patient should be restricted to bed rest and the extremity elevated until the infection has resolved. This urgency is explained by the fact that the infection can be fulminant, and each inflammatory process exacerbates fibrosis.

It must be emphasized that in this chronic, incurable condition, education of the patient and support by the physician are perhaps the most significant features of management.

SURGICAL MANAGEMENT

Surgical intervention should be considered only after medical management has been attempted and has failed. *Functional impairment* caused by inability to control the size of the extremity represents the predominant indication for surgery. Patients frequently complain of fatigue related to the weight of the swollen extremity. Indeed edema can account for 10 or more pounds of additional weight. Despite the fact that *cosmetic indications* have in the past been minimized, it should be remembered that this condition frequently affects adolescent females, and the associated physiological problems must be considered. Finally, in some patients, regardless of conscientious medical management, *recurrent lymphangitis* cannot be controlled.

The frustration encountered in the surgical management of lymphedema is reflected in the numerous procedures described over the last 70 years.

The surgical procedures are divided into categories in the following outline.

I. *Physiological operations.* These procedures attempt to reconstruct lymphatic drainage either by introducing distant or local pedicled tissue, or by microvascular techniques. The dermal flap and omental flap combine physiological and excisional components, in that significant excision of subcutaneous fat is involved.
   A. Direct lymphatic reconstruction.
      1. Alloplastic implants.
      2. Microlymphatic repair.
      3. Lymph node–venous anastomosis.
   B. Pedical flaps.
      1. Local skin flap.

2. Burred dermis flap.
3. Omental flap.

II. *Excisional operations.* These procedures remove varying amounts of the subcutaneous tissue and skin.
   A. Total subcutaneous excision and skin grafting.
   B. Subcutaneous excision beneath flaps.

It must be emphasized that normal lymphatic function cannot be achieved and some swelling recurs following all of the currently available procedures. The postoperative evaluation of each procedure is therefore often highly subjective. Indeed, we lack objective, reproducible standards by which we can assess a patient's progress and judge operative results. While *circumferential measurements* are frequently used to estimate the magnitude of swelling, they are subject to considerable variations. To be meaningful, the same measurement must be carefully reproduced on each occasion. Ideally, this should be done in the afternoon after a full day's activity, utilizing a bone landmark for reference. As previously mentioned, comparatively small variations in extremity diameter can represent substantial changes in fluid accumulation and weight. A more accurate but cumbersome method of documenting changes in size is *water volume displacement* [35]. Another technique involves the use of a *radioisotope,* particularly gold (^{198}Au) or radioiodinated (^{131}I) human serum albumin (RIHSA), to quantify lymphatic function. In normal individuals, approximately 80 percent of RIHSA injected into the web space will be cleared in 24 hours [46], but in those with lymphedema the percentage is approximately halved [13, 35, 52]. RIHSA clearance has been used to document postoperative improvement in lymphatic function subsequent to the dermal flap procedure [13, 35, 44] and subcutaneous excision [52]. The contralateral extremity should not be used as a control in primary lymphedema because of the high incidence of bilateral lymphatic abnormalities. Variables such as the volume of radioisotope injected, activity during the test, position of the extremity, and monitoring techniques (size of counter, time) must be rigidly controlled and standardized.

Physiological Operations

Direct Lymphatic Reconstruction

Perhaps one of the earliest procedures advocated for lymphedema was the subcutaneous implantation of silk threads (lymphangioplasty) described by Handley [42] in 1908. A wide variety of other materials were subsequently used, but such techniques have proved totally unsuccessful because of the incidence of infection and extrusion [13, 17, 25, 43]. Theoretically, it is difficult to conceive how valveless channels formed around a foreign body can drain lymph against gravity; nevertheless, this technique has recently been reproposed [59].

The intimate relationship between the lymphatic and venous systems was used by Rivero and coworkers [58] in 1967 when he surgically approximated a hemisectioned lymph node to the side of a vein. Early results were encouraging, and this technique was repeated by others, who also achieved initial patency [53, 57]. However, fibrous ingrowth eventually occluded the communication several months later [32].

O'Brien [55], who obtained limited success with microvascular repair of lymphatics in patients with postmastectomy edema, advocates a minimum of three lymphatic anastomoses. This approach is obviously the most direct method of lymphatic reconstruction, but long-term evaluation and increasing experience will be necessary. Nevertheless, with the astounding progress of microsurgery, this technique offers realistic hope for patients suffering from the acquired form of lymphedema.

Pedicle Flap Reconstruction

Local skin flaps have been used [38, 61] but they have not been successful, probably because the dermal lymphatic plexus is transferred.

Kondoleon [47] originally proposed the excision of deep muscle fascia so that the involved subcutaneous tissue would drain into the normal muscle compartment. This was unsuccessful because of rapid fascial regrowth [56]. In 1962 Thompson [62] introduced a procedure in which a deepithelialized *dermal flap* was buried into the muscle with the expectation of achieving a permanent lymphatic communication between the edematous subcutaneous tissue and uninvolved muscle compartment (Fig. 51-1). A favorable outcome of this operation in both primary and secondary forms of lymphedema has been reported [13, 25, 48]. Moreover, RIHSA clearance studies have documented improvement postoperatively [13]. Although the success of this operation was credited to the reconstructed lymphatic drainage within the dermal flap, there has been no lymphangiographic documentation of function of this flap. The procedure is performed in two (or occasionally three) stages, and in each a substantial amount of subcutaneous tissue is excised (Fig. 51-1A). Almost identical improvement in RIHSA clearance was noted following completion of subcutaneous and skin excision alone, suggesting that it is the excision of the subcutaneous tissue rather than the dermal flap that accounts for the improvement [52].

A pedicle of *omentum* has been employed to serve as a new conduit of lymphatic flow (Fig. 51-2) [40, 41]. Although initial reports of this innovative procedure were encouraging, its long-term value

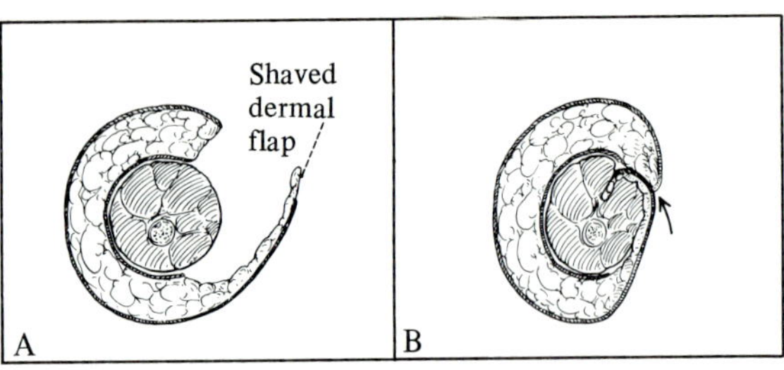

Fig. 51-1. A, the deepithelialized dermal flap following excision of subcutaneous tissue. B, the flap buried into the muscle compartment.

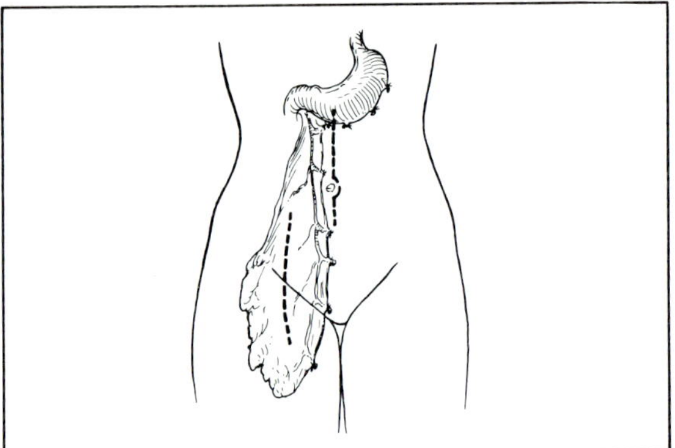

Fig. 51-2. Omental flap transferred into the lower extremity.

and theoretical basis have been seriously questioned. Experimental studies have shown that no communications between the omentum and the extremity develop [34]. Similar observations have been noted clinically at the time of reoperation and the omentum was found to be surrounded by a smooth bursa-like sac [52]. Although the omentum is rich in lymphatics, its resorptive capacity is low [54]. In view of this and considering the fact that the omental lymphatics do not contain valves, it seems unlikely that substantial lymphatic drainage could be achieved. Moreover, a high rate of postoperative complication following omental transposition has been noted [39].

Excisional Operations

Total Subcutaneous Excision

Originally described by Charles [33] in 1912, and commonly used since then, this operation is an extensive procedure that removes all of the skin, subcutaneous tissue (except in the foot and region overlying the calcaneal tendon) and deep fascia. The bared muscle is covered by split- or full-thickness grafts (Fig. 51-3). Although split-thickness grafts are technically easier and initially appear satisfactory,

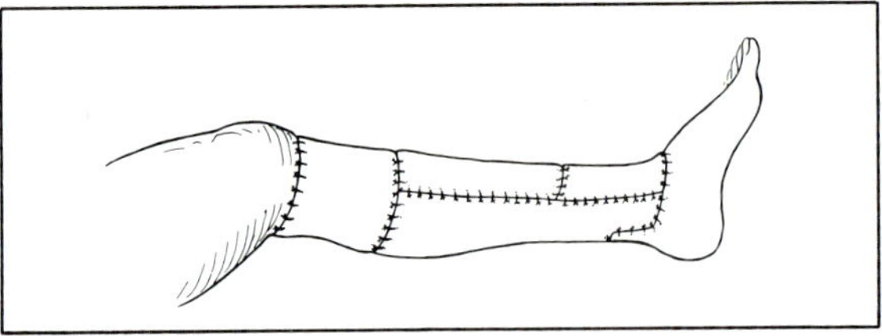

Fig. 51-3. Total subcutaneous excision followed by skin grafting.

late scarring is marked and the grafts are likely to be injured easily; they ulcerate frequently and develop a severe hyperkeratotic, weeping, chronically infected dermatitis. The end result is often far worse than the original problem of lymphedema and therefore we strongly oppose the use of split-thickness graft resurfacing after subcutaneous excision.

On the other hand, full-thickness grafts taken from the excised tissue are considerably more durable [37, 49, 50] although it is admittedly a formidable technical challenge to achieve a complete take of full-thickness grafts over such a large area. Moreover, if a problem with graft vascularization arises, the situation is exacerbated and morbidity is prolonged. Even when the grafts are successful, substantial scarring and chronic breakdown of these areas are not uncommon. In chronic longstanding lymphedema, however, where there is a substantial element of fibrosis, this may be the only technically feasible procedure available.

Staged Subcutaneous Excision Beneath Flaps

This procedure was first described by Sistrunk [60] in 1917 and later popularized by Homans [45]. In my opinion this approach provides the most reasonable surgical compromise – reliable improvement and a minimum of unfavorable postoperative complications. Improvement is directly related to the amount of skin and subcutaneous tissue removed and to the personal care and attitude of each patient. The surgical procedure is described to patients as a means of facilitating management of their lymphedema and not as a cure [51]. During the operation, as much subcutaneous tissue and skin are removed as possible while attempting to maintain skin flap viability and achieve primary wound healing [36, 51].

PREOPERATIVE CARE. All patients are placed at bed rest and the extremity elevated until the edema has subsided. Although this can initially be done at home, the patient should be admitted to the hospital 3 or 4 days preoperatively. A modified Thomas orthopedic splint suspended from an overhead frame may help patients with leg involvement. The edema resolves over 5 to 14 days; the rate of resolution is dependent on the chronicity of the condition and amount of fibrous tissue present. While the patient is in bed, the extremity should be washed daily. Preoperative antibiotics are not routinely used. One week preoperatively, one or two units of blood can be taken from the patient to be used as an autotransfusion.

OPERATIVE TECHNIQUE. All procedures are performed by utilizing a pneumatic tourniquet placed as proximally as possible. In both the leg and the arm, more tissue can be removed from the medial than from the lateral aspect.

PROCEDURES IN THE LEG. The subcutaneous excision in the leg is shown in Figure 51-4. In this procedure, flaps 1.5 cm. thick (2 cm. in the thigh) are elevated from a midmedial incision, anteriorly and posteriorly to the midsagittal plane of the calf. The dissection is less extensive in the thigh and ankle. All subcutaneous tissue beneath the flaps is removed. After excising the subcutaneous fat from the periosteum of the tibia, the deep fascial compartment of the calf is entered, affording a relatively avascular and easy plane of dissection just above the gastrocnemius muscle. Posteriorly the sural nerve is identified and preserved. All of the attached subcutaneous fat and deep fascia along the medial aspect of the calf are removed. Dissection proceeds superiorly over the knee joint and inferiorly in the ankle region above the fascia. As much subcutaneous fat as possible is removed. The flap should not be developed beyond the anterior border of the malleolus. Because of the potential for avascular necrosis, flaps in the ankle are rarely longer than 6 cm. Substantial amounts of redundant skin can be excised (often 6 to 10 cm.) (Fig. 51-5) after removal of subcutaneous fat (usually 450 to 900 gm.). A rubber suction catheter is placed at the dependent portion of the posterior flap and left in place a minimum of 5 days. Interrupted and continuous 4-0 nylon is employed for skin closure; no subcutaneous or dermal sutures are used. The extremity is immobilized by a gauze dressing reinforced with a posterior splint and is kept elevated. Sutures are removed on the eighth day and the wound is secured by benzoin and tape. The patient is then measured for a form-fitting elastic stocking. Dependency of the leg is begun on the ninth day, ambulation by the eleventh postoperative day, but *only* when the leg is firmly wrapped.

The second stage is performed on the lateral aspect of the leg, 2 or 3 months later. The operative technique is essentially the same except that fascia is not removed and care is taken to avoid damaging the peroneal nerve or the sensory branches (superficial peroneal nerve) leading to the dorsum of the foot, which pierce the deep fascia approximately 4 to 6 cm. above the extensor retinaculum of the ankle. Several months later, specific areas of swelling in the ankle can be excised through separate incisions.

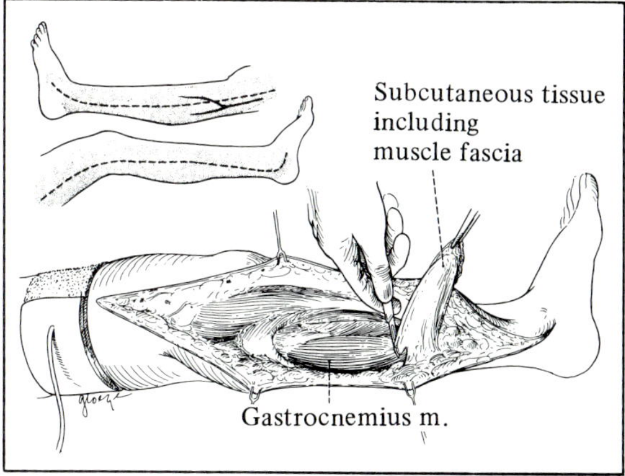

Fig. 51-4. Subcutaneous excision in the medial aspect of the leg. The medial and lateral incisions are shown, and the area of subcutaneous tissue excision is indicated by stippling.

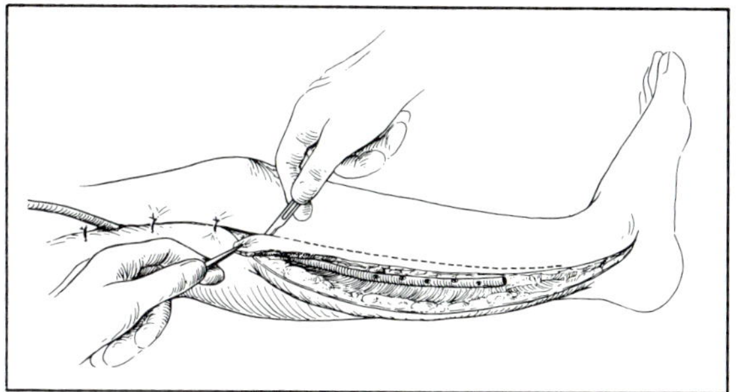

Fig. 51-5. Closure following the excision of redundant skin.

PROCEDURES IN THE ARM. In postmastectomy patients, medial excision is carried out from an incision extending from the distal ulna across the medial epicondyle through the posteromedial upper arm. Flaps approximately 1 cm. thick are elevated to the midsagittal aspect of the forearm, and the dissection is tapered distally and proximally. The deep fascia is left undisturbed. During lateral dissection, the dorsal sensory branches of the ulnar and radial nerves are identified and preserved. If possible, the medial antebrachial cutaneous nerve is specifically identified and preserved. Considerable amounts of fat can be excised from the upper arm. Flaps should be somewhat thicker in this area (approximately 1.5 to 2 cm.); the ulnar nerve is identified in the region of the medial

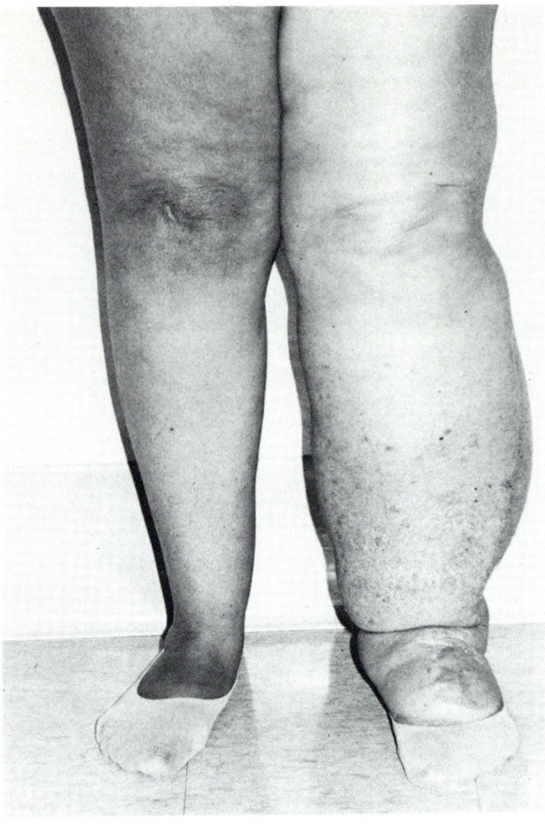

A

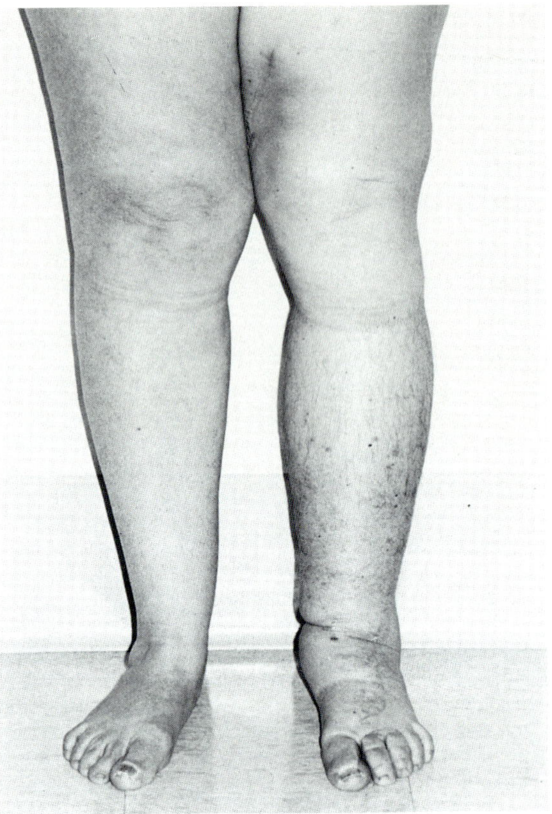

B

Fig. 51-6. A, the legs of a 42-year-old woman with lymphedema of 18 years' duration following radical gross dissection. Two dermal flap procedures had been performed 5 years earlier. B, the patient's legs 1 year following lateral and medial skin excision and excision of subcutaneous tissue.

epicondyle and traced proximally. Wide bands of redundant skin can be excised. If necessary, the tourniquet can be removed, the area reprepped, and skin and subcutaneous tissue excised up to the axilla. A suction catheter is used for at least 3 days. The arm is immobilized and elevated for 5 days and thereafter can be placed in a sling. Otherwise, the postoperative management is similar to that described for the leg.

Results Following Skin and Subcutaneous Excision
A total of 49 operative procedures have been performed on 25 patients, 20 of whom have been followed for periods longer than 2 years. There have been 3 postoperative complications related to ischemic necrosis of the flap, all of which healed by secondary intention and did not require further surgery. Although these patients have experienced varying degrees of decreased sensation approximately 3 cm. on either side of the line of incision, this has not been a source of complaint. No alteration in hand or foot sensation has been observed. All patients have some recurrence of swelling after a full day's activity. At least a 50 percent reduction in extremity size and entirely normal function resulted in 17 of the 20 patients currently followed (Figs. 51-6, 7). All wear elastic support stockings. Progressive swelling has occurred in the postoperative period in 3 patients, and in 1 the swelling has exceeded preoperative size. Whereas 9 patients had complained of repeated (more than two) episodes of cellulitis postoperatively, only 2 patients have experienced postoperative infection.

One year after surgery, a two-fold increase in the clearance of RIHSA has been documented, suggesting that the excision of substantial amounts of subcutaneous tissue somehow improves lymphatic function. The mechanism and explanation of this improvement are unclear at this time; several possible explanations, singly or in combination, exist. Extensive surgical dissection may establish lymphatic-venous anasto-

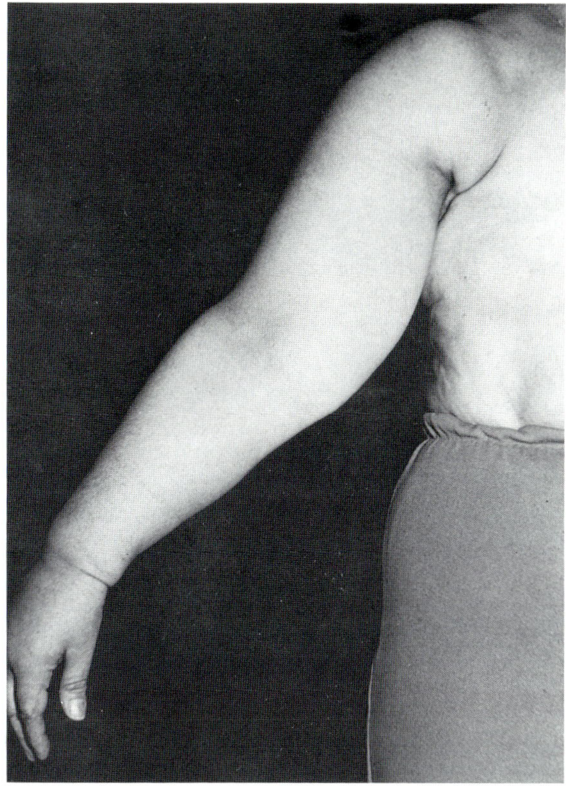

A

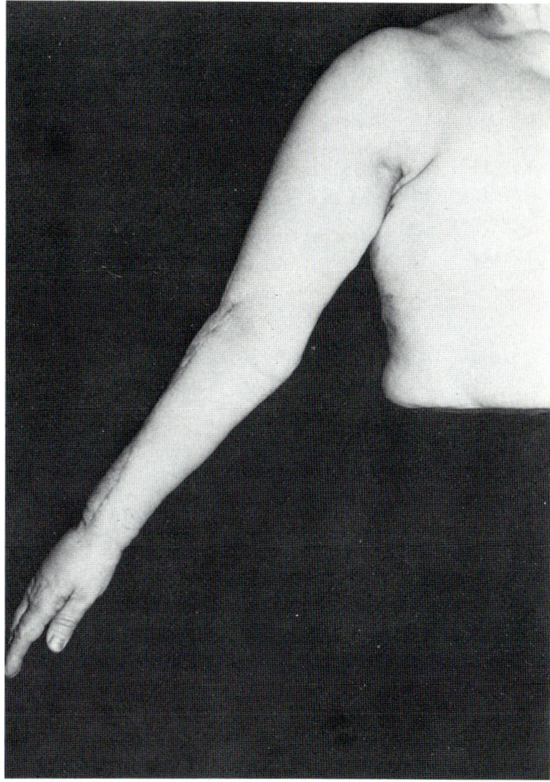

B

Fig. 51-7. A, the arm of a 58-year-old woman 8 years after a radical mastectomy. B, the patient's arm 1 year following two-staged excisions of subcutaneous tissue.

mosis during the process of healing [13]; the procedure may favorably alter the balance of lymph flow by effectively reducing the amount of lymph-forming tissue; the excision of substantial subcutaneous tissue and skin may result in external compression effecting an increase in interstitial pressure (much like elastic stocking), thus improving lymph flow.

Perhaps because there is always some recurrence of edema, this approach has been almost abandoned in recent years. Other more theoretically appealing and innovative procedures, previously discussed, seem more attractive. Nevertheless, the discouraging fact remains that no procedure cures lymphedema; a degree of edema inevitably follows any operative procedure. In my opinion, compared to all available methods of surgical management, skin and subcutaneous excision is the most reliable, consistently beneficial, and uncomplicated means of managing the symptoms of lymphedema.

REFERENCES

Anatomy and Physiology

1. Acevedo, D. Motor control of the thoracic duct. *Am. J. Physiol.* 139:600, 1943.
2. Anson, B. J. *Atlas of Human Anatomy.* Philadelphia: Saunders, 1950.
3. Crockett, D. J. Lymphatic anatomy and lymphoedema. *Br. J. Plast. Surg.* 18:12, 1965.
4. Kinmonth, J. B., Taylor, G. W., Tracey, G. D., and Marsh, J. D. Primary lymphedema: Clinical and lymphangiographic studies of a series of 107 patients in which the lower limbs were affected. *Br. J. Surg.* 45:1, 1957.
5. Larson, D. L. Deep lymphatic system of the lower extremity. *Am. J. Surg.* 2:217, 1967.
6. Malek, P., Belan, A., and Kocandrle, V. L. The superficial and deep lymphatic system of the lower extremities and their mutual relationship under physiological and pathological conditions. *J. Cardiovasc. Surg.* 5:686, 1964.
7. Ngu, V. A. Lymph drainage of the leg and its implications. *Clin. Radiol.* 15:197, 1964.
8. Rodbard, S., and Feldman, P. Functional anatomy of the lymphatic fluids and pathways. *Lymphology* 8:49, 1975.

9. Rusznyak, I. Recent experiments on the physiology and pathology of the lymphatic circulation. *Minerva Med.* 43:1468, 1954.
10. Sabin, F. R. The Development of the Lymphatic System. In Keibel, F., and Mall, F. P. (Eds.), *Manual of Human Embryology,* Vol. 2. Philadelphia: Lippincott, 1912.
11. Selkurt, E. (Ed.). *Physiology.* Boston: Little, Brown, 1966.
12. Taylor, A., and Gibson, H. Concentrating ability of lymphatic vessels. *Lymphology* 8:43, 1975.
13. Thompson, N. The surgical treatment of chronic lymphoedema of the extremities. *Surg. Clin. North Am.* 47:445, 1967.
14. Yoffey, J. M., and Courtice, F. C. *Lymphatics, Lymph and Lymphoid Tissue.* Cambridge: Harvard University Press, 1956.

Lymphedema: Primary and Acquired

15. Buonocore, E., and Young, J. R. Lymphangiographic evaluation of lymphedema and lymphatic flow. *Am. J. Roentgenol. Radium Ther. Nucl. Med.* 95:751, 1965.
16. Calnan, J. Lymphoedema: The case for doubt. *Br. J. Plast. Surg.* 21:32, 1968.
17. Dale, A. The swollen leg. *Curr. Probl. Surg.* Sept., 1973.
18. de Rooe, T. The value of lymphography in lymphedema. *Surg. Gynecol. Obstet.* 124:755, 1967.
19. Ersek, R. A., Danese, C. A., and Howard, J. M. Hereditary congenital lymphedema (Milroy's disease). *Surgery* 50:1098, 1966.
20. Fitts, W. T., Keuhnelian, J. G., Ravdin, I. S., and Schor, S. Swelling of the arm after radical mastectomy. *Surgery* 35:460, 1954.
21. Gough, M. H. Primary lymphedema: Clinical and lymphangiographic studies. *Br. J. Surg.* 53:917, 1966.
22. Milroy, W. F. An undescribed variety of hereditary oedema. *N.Y. Med. J.* 56:505, 1892.
23. Pflug, J. J., and Calnan, J. S. The normal anatomy of the lymphatic system in the human leg. *Br. J. Surg.* 58:925, 1971.
24. Schirger, A., Harrison, E. G., and Janes, J. M. Idiopathic lymphedema: Review of 131 cases. *J.A.M.A.* 182:14, 1962.
25. Stone, E. J., and Hugo, N. E. Lymphedema. *Surg. Gynecol. Obstet.* 135:625, 1972.
26. Taylor, G. W., Kinmonth, J. B., Rollinson, E., Rotblat, J., and Frances, G. E. Lymphatic circulation studied with radioactive plasma protein. *Br. Med. J.* 1:133, 1957.
27. Treves, N. An evaluation of the etiological factors of lymphedema following radical mastectomy. *Cancer* 10:444, 1957.

Differential Diagnosis

28. Barnes, R. W., Wu, K. K., and Hoak, J. C. Differentiation of superficial thrombophlebitis from lymphangitis by Doppler ultrasound. *Surg. Gynecol. Obstet.* 143:23, 1976.
29. Crockett, F. The iliac compression syndrome. *Br. J. Surg.* 52:391, 1967.
30. Fairbairn, J. F., Juergens, J. L., and Spittell, J. A. *Peripheral Vascular Diseases* (4th ed.). Philadelphia: Saunders, 1972.
31. Fonkalsrud, E. W. Surgical management of congenital malformations of the lymphatic system. *Am. J. Surg.* 128:152, 1974.

Surgical Therapy

32. Calnan, J. S., Reis, N. D., Rivero, O. R., Copenhagen, H. F., and Taylor, L. M. The natural history of lymph node-to-vein anastomosis. *Br. J. Plast. Surg.* 20:134, 1967.
33. Charles, R. H. *A System of Treatment,* Vol. 3. London: Churchill, 1912.
34. Danese, C. A., Papaioannou, A. N., Morales, L. E., and Mitsuda, S. Surgical approaches to lymphatic blocks. *Surgery* 56:821, 1968.
35. Emmett, A. J., Barron, J. N., and Veall, N. The use of I^{131} albumin tissue clearance measurements and other physiological tests for the clinical assessment of patients with lymphoedema. *Br. J. Plast. Surg.* 20:1, 1967.
36. Fonkalsrud, E. W., and Coulson, W. F. Management of congenital lymphedema in infants and children. *Ann. Surg.* 177:280, 1973.
37. Gibson, T., and Tough, J. S. A simplified one-stage operation for the correction of lymphedema of the leg. *Arch. Surg.* 71:809, 1955.
38. Gillies, H., and Fraser, F. R. The treatment of lymphoedema by plastic operation: A preliminary report. *Br. Med. J.* 1:96, 1935.
39. Goldsmith, H. S. Long term evaluation of omental transposition for chronic lymphedema. *Ann. Surg.* 180:847, 1974.
40. Goldsmith, H. S., and de los Santos, R. Omental transposition in primary lymphedema. *Surg. Gynecol. Obstet.* 125:607, 1967.
41. Goldsmith, H. S., de los Santos, R., and Beattie, E. J. Relief of chronic lymphedema by omental transposition. *Ann. Surg.* 166:572, 1967.
42. Handley, W. S. Lymphangioplasty: A new method for the relief of the brawn arm of breast cancer and for similar conditions of lymphatic oedema: Preliminary note. *Lancet* 1:783, 1908.
43. Handley, W. S. Hunterian lectures on the surgery of the lymphatic system. *Br. Med. J.* 1:922, 1910.
44. Harvey, R. F. The use of I^{131} labelled human serum albumin in the assessment of improved

lymph flow following buried dermis flap operation in cases of post-mastectomy lymphoedema of the arm. *Br. J. Radiol.* 42:260, 1969.
45. Homans, J. The treatment of elephantiasis of the legs: A preliminary report. *N. Engl. J. Med.* 215: 1099, 1936.
46. Ju, D. M. C., Blakemore, A., and Stevenson, T. W. A lymphatic function test. *Surg. Forum* 5:697, 1954.
47. Kondoleon, E. Die operative Behandlung der elephantiastischen Oedeme. *Zentralbl. Chir.* 39:1022, 1912.
48. Larson, D. L., Coers, C. R., Doyle, J. E., Rappaport, A. S., Kloehn, R., and Lewis, S. R. Lymphedema of the lower extremity. *Plast. Reconstr. Surg.* 38:293, 1966.
49. McCormack, R. M. Surgical treatment of post-mastectomy lymphedema. *Plast. Reconstr. Surg.* 14:62, 1954.
50. McKee, D. M., and Edgerton, M. T. Surgical treatment of lymphedema of the lower extremities. *Plast. Reconstr. Surg.* 23:480, 1959.
51. Miller, T. A. Surgical management of lymphedema of the extremity. *Plast. Reconstr. Surg.* 56:633, 1975.
52. Miller, T. A., Harper, J. D., and Longmire, W. P., Jr. The management of lymphedema by staged subcutaneous excision. *Surg. Gynecol. Obstet.* 136·1, 1973.
53. Nielubowicz, J., Olszewski, W., and Sokolowski, J. Surgical lymphovenous shunts. *J. Cardiovasc. Surg.* 9:262, 1968.
54. Nylander, G., and Tjernberg, B. The lymphatics of the greater omentum; an experimental study in the dog. *Lymphology* 2:3, 1969.
55. O'Brien, B. Replantation and reconstructive microvascular surgery. *Ann. R. Coll. Surg. Engl.* 58:87, 171, 1976.
56. Peer, L. A., Shahgholi, M., Walker, J. D., Jr., and Mancusi-Ungaro, A. Modified operation for lymphedema of leg and arm. *Plast. Reconstr. Surg.* 14:347, 1954.
57. Politowski, M., Bartkowski, S., and Dynowski, J. Treatment of lymphedema of the limbs by lymphatic-venous fistula. *Surgery* 66:639, 1969.
58. Rivero, O. R., Calnan, J. S., Reis, N. D., and Taylor, L. M. Experimental peripheral lymphovenous communication. *Br. J. Plast. Surg.* 20:124, 1967.
59. Silver, D., and Puckett, C. Lymphangioplasty: A ten year evaluation. *Surgery* 80:748, 1976.
60. Sistrunk, W. E. Further experiences with the Kondoleon operation for elephantiasis. *J.A.M.A.* 71:800, 1918.
61. Smith, J. W., and Conway, H. Selection of appropriate surgical procedures in lymphedema; introduction of hinged pedicle. *Plast. Reconstr. Surg.* 30:10, 1962.
62. Thompson, N. Surgical treatment of chronic lymphoedema of the lower limb. *Br. Med. J.* 5319:1567, 1962.

Lipectomy

PAULE REGNAULT

Although overall obesity should be treated medically before any surgical treatment can be attempted, some patients, discouraged after several unsuccessful attempts to lose weight, may be encouraged if one operation is performed. They may then seriously follow a drastic diet to permit further surgical corrections.

Massive weight loss creates very loose skin and subcutaneous tissue, which is greater when the loss happens in older persons rather than younger ones; the more extensive the loss is, the more severe are the deformities. Some of these deformities may be operated on at the same stage, but some should be treated separately. At the same time as an abdominal lipectomy, a breast ptosis, an arm reduction, or a face lift is possible, but not a thigh reduction because of the patient's position on the operating table when the abdomen is sutured (and same position in the bed later on), and because both are major operations.

For the same reason, at the time a thigh reduction is done, one can perform any other correction except an abdominoplasty. When procedures are planned for the breast, arms, or face, the thigh reduction is started in the back and finished in front, and the other surgery is then performed.

All the cases of multiple procedures should be most carefully evaluated, and preparation should be made for blood transfusion. These are serious operations with a loss of large amounts of tissue and the risk of a major blood loss. Furthermore, these operations are lengthy procedures.

ABDOMINAL DERMOLIPECTOMIES

To treat all of the various abdominal wall deformities surgically, one should consider several surgical techniques. The indications for the right technique to be used in each case should be carefully evaluated and discussed. The amount of fat removal and the final scar location depend on the operation selected.

Two main categories of deformities are considered: (1) excess fat (abdominal obesity) and (2) excess skin (abdominal dermochalasis or dermolysis).

Abdominal Obesity

The excess fat tissue in the abdomen may be isolated to the abdomen or may be part of a general obesity. When the patient's general condition is satisfactory enough for surgery, the operation may be undertaken even if weight loss does not seem to be possible. It relieves the local condition and may encourage the patient to achieve weight reduction later on.

The goal in the treatment of abdominal adiposity is to remove the greatest possible amount of fat tissue, where it lies, with no undermining, and without concern for the final scars.

Treatment of Lower and Medial Abdominal Obesity

The technique indicated in lower and medial abdominal obesity is the "fleur de lys" operation (Figs. 52-1 and 52-2), a three-branched excision (modified Castanares [5]) technique. The amount of the excision is roughly estimated by pinching the soft tissues when the patient is standing up, and it is marked on the skin with a felt pen. It is verified later on the operating table, after the patient is prepared and draped. The lower incision follows a W design and is located about 2 cm. above the inguinal folds laterally and above the pubic hair medially. The upper limits of the lateral excisions are traced by pinching the tissues from above. The vertical branch of the fleur de lys design is also traced by pinching the tissues from each side of the body midline. The umbilicus is incised in a diamond shape.

The operation is started at the lower (W) incision and progresses upward. The dissection is done leaving a fine layer of areolar tissue over the fascia. Each lateral branch of tissue is then excised. The right lateral incision of the vertical branch is made, extended down to the level of areola fascia, and dissected from the right to the left. One should carefully estimate the amount of possible removal before complete resection so that the defect can be closed with moderate tension.

After complete resection of the specimen of skin and fat, a diastasis of the rectus abdominus muscles, a large ventral hernia, or an umbilical hernia may become very obvious. In case of a major umbilical hernia, the umbilicus should be sacrificed. The average diastasis of the recti muscles may be closed by simple plication and closure of the aponeurosis with heavy nonabsorbable material. In a large ventral hernia, when the recti cannot be safely approximated, a sheath of synthetic mesh is sewn around the hernia.

Although no undermining or defatting is done, it may be useful to remove a small amount of fat at the upper end of the vertical branch to avoid an unaesthetic redundancy. Suturing is done in two layers: heavy absorbable material on the deep fat layer and

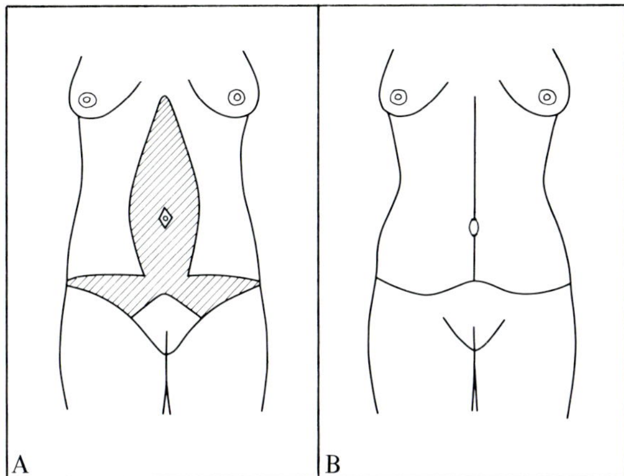

Fig. 52-1. *A, the fleur de lys excision (the pubic area is respected). The excision is estimated by pinching the cutaneous fat layer. B, the resulting scar.*

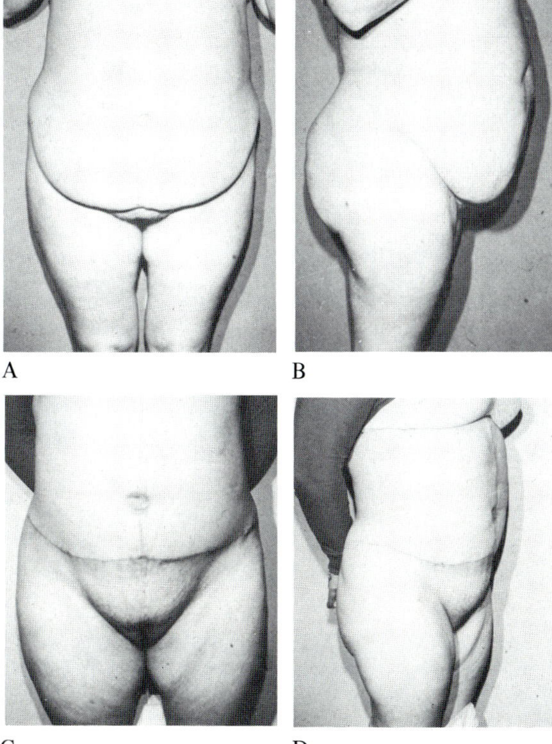

Fig. 52-2. *A, B, localized abdominal obesity at the lower and medial areas, with large diastasis of the recti. C, D, the appearance several months after a fleur de lys excision and fascia plication.*

subcuticular running suture on the skin. It is started on the vertical branch first and then extends laterally from each end of the horizontal branches. The umbilicus is located in the vertical scar. The table may be placed in a jackknife position when the lateral incisions are closed, in case there seems to be some tension. Drainage is rarely necessary, since no dead space remains. The final position of the lower scar is horizontal most of the time because the lower angles exert an upward pull (Fig. 52-2C, D).

Treatment of Upper and Medial Abdominal Obesity
A three-wing excision with the horizontal portion at the waistline and the vertical portion downward gives excellent results; it is a modified Weinhold technique resulting in a T scar (Fig. 52-3). When the adiposity extends onto the lateral portions and the back, the horizontal incisions may be continued to the spinal area.

The technique for estimating the amount of tissue excess, the method of marking, and the excision are exactly the same as in the fleur de lys technique. No undermining is done. In these cases the removal of fat should be started at the back and the patient turned on the table so that the anterior portion of the operation can be completed.

The umbilicus may be placed in the horizontal scar, at the junction of the three branches of the T, or in the vertical scar, according to the location of the fat removed and according to tissue elasticity. In the pubic area, a small horizontal excision prevents disfiguring redundancy. Drainage is useful at the back and laterally.

Abdominal Dermochalasis
The excess skin in abdominal dermochalasis is often associated with striae. This problem appears in younger women after pregnancy; an extensive undermining is necessary to remove enough skin and to locate the scar in a low position [3, 10, 14]. The W technique seems to give best results in these cases.

W Technique of Abdominoplasty
The W technique differs from some methods developed in the past in that the W incision is located at the inguinal fold or slightly above, but it is never on the thighs (Fig. 52-4). No pattern should be used because the bodies of women are not standard and a woman's skin is more elastic than any pattern. The excision takes advantage of the skin's elasticity. Since the skin is more supple laterally than in the midline, the basic goal of this method is to release tension in the midline and bring more tension laterally.

The placement of the lower incision is inside the pubic hair when the tissues are very loose, or slightly above that level when skin elasticity seems only moderate.

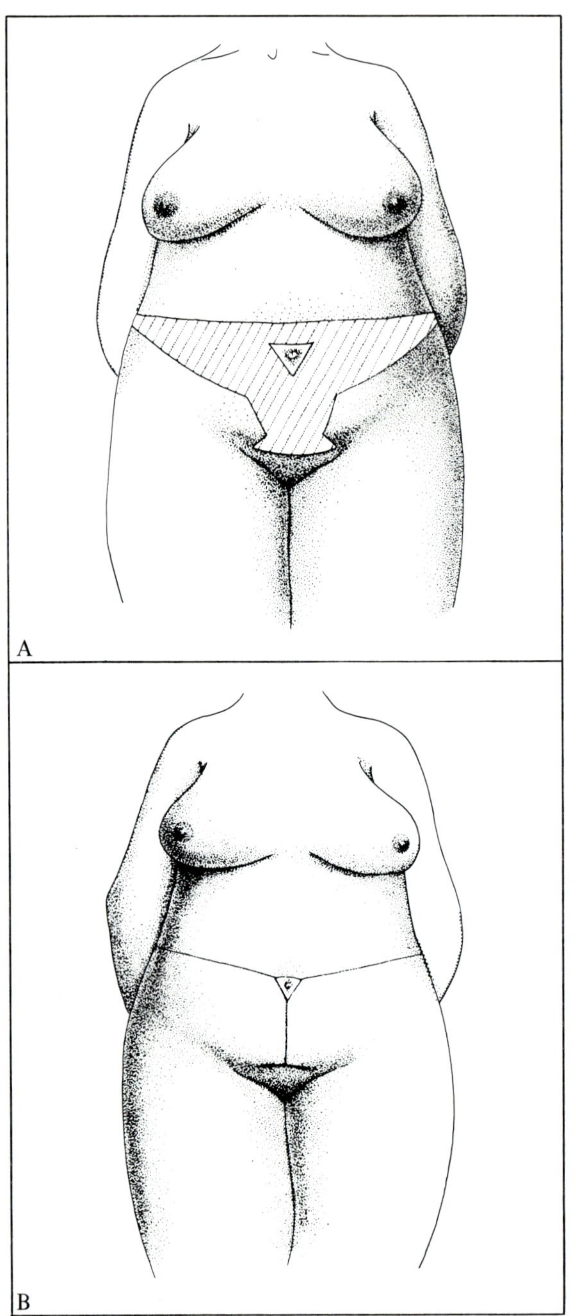

Fig. 52-3. *A, the T excision is recommended when the maximum adiposity is at or above the waist line. B, the resulting scars.*

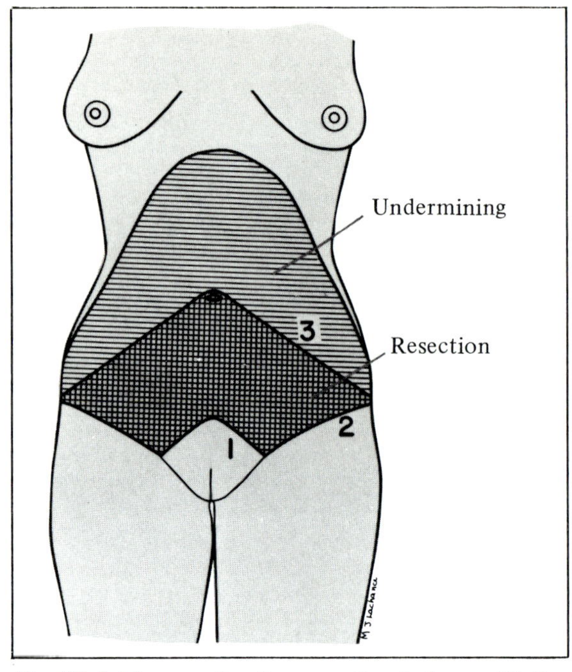

Fig. 52-4. Planning for the operation is done with the patient standing up. The lower incision in the shape of a W may be at the inguinal folds at the upper limit of pubic hair, or slightly above these when there is poor elasticity. The central limb of the W is usually half the length of the lateral limb. The upper limit is from the umbilicus to the end of the lower lateral limb. The upper line of the excision should be the sum of the W lines or a little less (i.e., the length of line 3 in this drawing is equal to the sum of the lengths of line 1 and line 2).

From the midline the incision goes downward to reach the inguinal fold either at the fold or slightly above it, depending on the elasticity of the skin. The incision then goes upward and laterally, following the direction of the fold. The central limb of the W is usually half the length of the lateral one, but this varies according to the patient's build and the tissues to be excised (Fig. 52-4).

The incision of the umbilicus is in a horizontal spindle shape (in the manner of a marquise cut) [2]. The upper line of the excision is also marked with the patient standing up. It is a straight line joining the umbilicus to the lateral ends of the lower incision, and its length should be equal to or less than the sum of the two lower lines. The upper line should never be longer than the lower lines if dog ears are to be avoided at the time of closure.

After the patient is prepared and draped, the amount of tissue to be removed is estimated again by pinching the soft tissues, and the draping may be adjusted accordingly. The upper portion of the excision is only scratched with the scalpel; it should not be completely incised at this moment but only after the undermining has been completed. When tissue elasticity is poor, the amount of skin excised may be less than previously planned.

The lower incision is made through the skin and then taken obliquely upward to avoid the inguinal lymph nodes. When the fascia is reached, the very fine cellular layer covering the fascia should be completely avoided over the whole undermined area. This layer seems to have an important action on fluid resorption. and its retention leads to reduced pain postoperatively. The undermining may be done with blunt dissection very gently.

Hemostasis is accomplished by clamping all perforating vessels. When the umbilicus is reached, the flap is cut in the midline, the umbilicus is freed, and the undermining is continued upward to the xyphoid process and over the lower ribs.

Repair of the diastasis of the recti muscles (if present) is done by plication of the fascia sutured with nonabsorbable material. This shortens the umbilical stem and will result in a pleasing umbilical dimple after closure (Fig. 52-5). The resection of the flap is then performed; this resection usually follows the preoperative marking but it may be larger if pulling on the flap proves that a greater amount of tissue may safely be removed. In case of poor elasticity (which is rare), the amount may be less than previously planned, and a small vertical scar will have to remain at the lower midline.

The umbilical location in the flap is then estimated, placing a finger on the umbilicus. A straight horizontal incision, about 2 cm. wide, is made in the midline between the iliac crest and lower costal margin, below the waistline. This area is defatted, to leave enough room for the umbilicus and to contribute to the umbilical dimple. A thread is left on the umbilicus and passed through this wound to allow easy suturing of the umbilicus after the lower suture has been done.

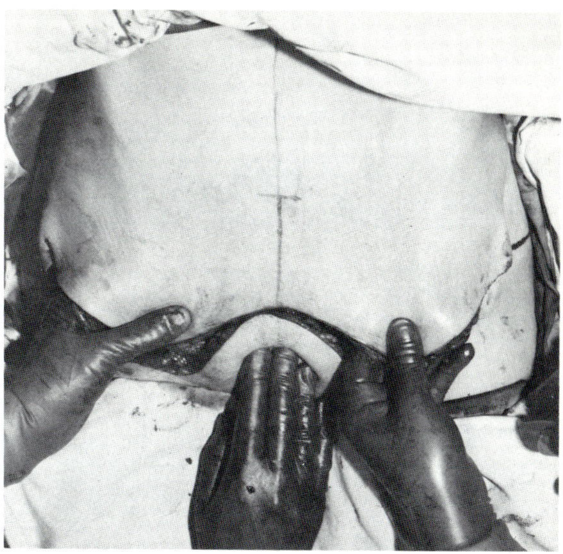

Fig. 52-5. While the table is still horizontal, the surgeon pulls on the upper flaps and pushes on the pubic area, which gives the final estimate of the possible removal.

The operating table is then put in a jackknife position, so that the wound edges come together easily. The angle of the table may be 90 to 120 degrees (Fig. 52-6). This position is the key to easy closure without tension.

Suturing is done in two layers; heavy absorbable material is used on fat and fascia, and subcuticular running suture is used on the skin. When the midportion of the pubis seems to form an unaesthetic sharp angle, it may be rounded. After the midline deep suture has been placed, if the closure seems to leave too much redundancy laterally, a small excision may be done in the prolongation of the lateral branches of the W. Adhesive paper strips are left on all sutures (Fig. 52-7). Drains are left for 48 hours.

The appearance of the resulting scar will vary according to the skin elasticity; it may look like either a W or an almost horizontal line (Fig. 52-8).

Dressing and Postoperative Care

In all types of abdominoplasty, adhesive paper strips should be applied to the skin over all the sutures. A moderate pressure dressing is applied, using pads covered by elastic adhesive bandages in an X forma-

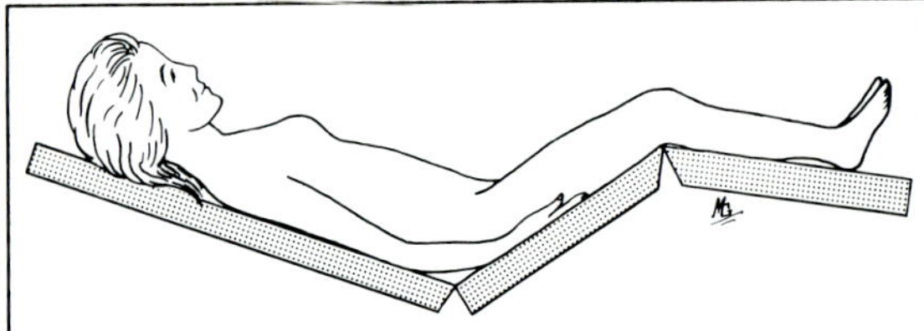

Fig. 52-6. The operating table in the jackknife position, which facilitates the approximation of wound edges.

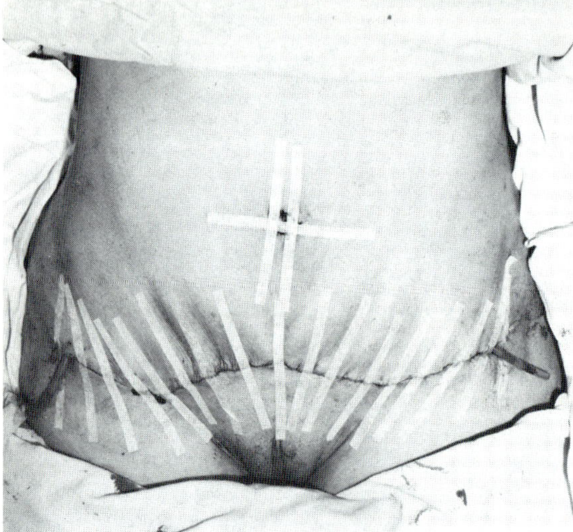

Fig. 52-7. Suturing is done in two layers, and adhesive strips are used.

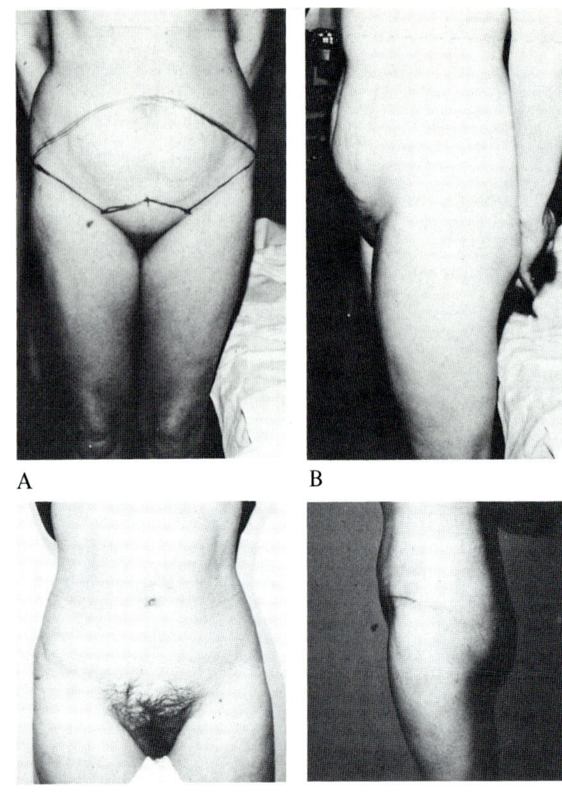

Fig. 52-8. A, B, a young, 30-year-old patient with striae, moderately localized fat, and diastasis of the recti. C, D, the appearance 3 months postoperative, after the W technique was applied.

tion (Fig. 52-9). No cast or sandbag is ever used. The patient is transported to bed in the same position used on the operating table at the time of suturing and remains in that position for 48 hours. At the end of that time, the drains and bandages are removed; the adhesive strips are left for 2 to 4 weeks. The patient is then allowed to get up. After having undergone a W procedure, the patient should wear a soft elastic girdle for a few weeks.

Complications of Abdominal Lipectomies

Complications are rare when the operative technique has been selected correctly. Nevertheless, several factors may result in complications, including: postoperative bleeding, excessively tight pressure bandages, poor vascularization, too much tension, a reaction to the suture material, mistakes in postoperative care, and failure to maintain the jackknife position in bed. These problems can lead to the following results:

HEMATOMA. This may often be avoided by adequate drainage. If hematoma occurs, it should be evacuated as soon as detected; otherwise it may provoke skin necrosis and infection.

SKIN NECROSIS. This always appears at the midline, whatever the cause. The necrotic area should be excised as soon as the limit is well defined, and it is replaced with a skin graft, which can be removed 6 months later.

INFECTION. Whether a result of hematoma or reaction to suture material, infection is treated by antibiotics and wet dressings; when there is no necrosis the wound will close.

SCAR FORMATION. Hypertrophic scars and keloids are treated by local injections of triamcinolone

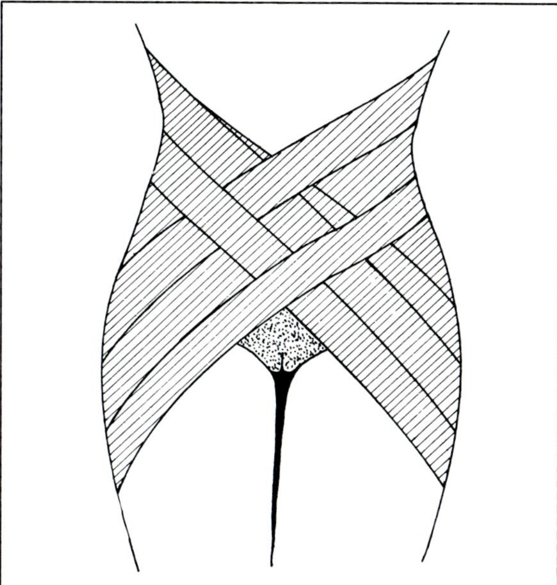

Fig. 52-9. Elastic adhesive bandages are applied in X formation.

(Kenalog) 10 mg/ml. These scars may be followed by atrophic scars, which are corrected secondarily.

EDEMA. Lasting edema (more than 1 to 6 months) may lead to disappointment with the W technique, since the large undermining and the long lower scar may retard normal vascularization and lymphatic drainage of the flap. This condition may be somewhat prevented or diminished by the use of a soft girdle during the day as soon as the first dressing has been removed.

ABNORMAL UMBILICAL POSITION. The umbilical position may be too lateral if the midline has not been marked before the undermining; it may be displaced upward if the umbilical site has been incised too high. In the latter case, a horizontal incision may be made at a lower location, and the umbilicus retransposed.

THIGH REDUCTION

In each case a special technique should be applied in order to get the best aesthetic results. The following are the techniques that will be discussed: semicircular reduction; circular reduction; vertical reduction; combined circular and vertical reduction; trochanteric defatting procedure (correction of riding breeches deformity); correction of lower medial thigh deformities; and corrections of complications of thigh reduction and secondary thigh deformities.

Overweight patients showing firm adiposity are not good candidates for surgery, since the amount of tissue that can be removed safely is relatively small. These patients are advised to lose weight. They may be encouraged to do so if they are convinced that surgery will be possible for the tissue redundancy that follows weight reduction.

Patients with firm adiposity may be accepted only when it is localized, as in those with trochanteric adiposity or buttock adiposity; in these patients a fairly substantial amount of tissue may be removed safely.

Semicircular Reduction

The operations described in the past are certainly excellent when dealing with upper medial or upper lateral defects [22, 24, 25, 26, 27].

Planning

The evaluation of and marking for the removal should be made with the patient standing, which helps in planning for an adequate excision (Figs. 52-10 and 52-11). The upper line of the excision is marked first; then by pushing upward on the thigh tissues, one can judge what width of tissue removal will give a reasonably good correction, and the lower incision is then marked. The marking is continued at the back and laterally. One should be cautious not to plan too large a removal of the buttocks, or a flat unpleasant contour might result. The planned excision is usually larger laterally than it is posteriorly and should end slightly higher or more lateral than the anterior marking.

The marking may be facilitated by having the patient wear a bikini pantie; the upper line of the marking should remain about 2 or 3 cm. above the lower edges of the pantie.

Operative Technique

FIRST PART OF THE OPERATION – ANTERIOR EXCISION. The patient is in the supine position with the legs slightly apart. The lithotomy position is not recommended because it pulls on lower tissues and makes suturing very difficult. The planned excision is verified and measured to ensure symmetry.

The incisions follow the markings, going through skin and fat down to the superficial fascia, which is preserved along with the large veins and nerves. The specimen can be separated from the superficial fascia by simply pulling (stripping). Dissection is carried as far as the medial part of the thigh, where the specimen is severed medially and removed. The same procedure is done on the other thigh. The thigh tissues are mobilized slightly medially to obtain a moderate rotation. Closure is done with interrupted absorbable

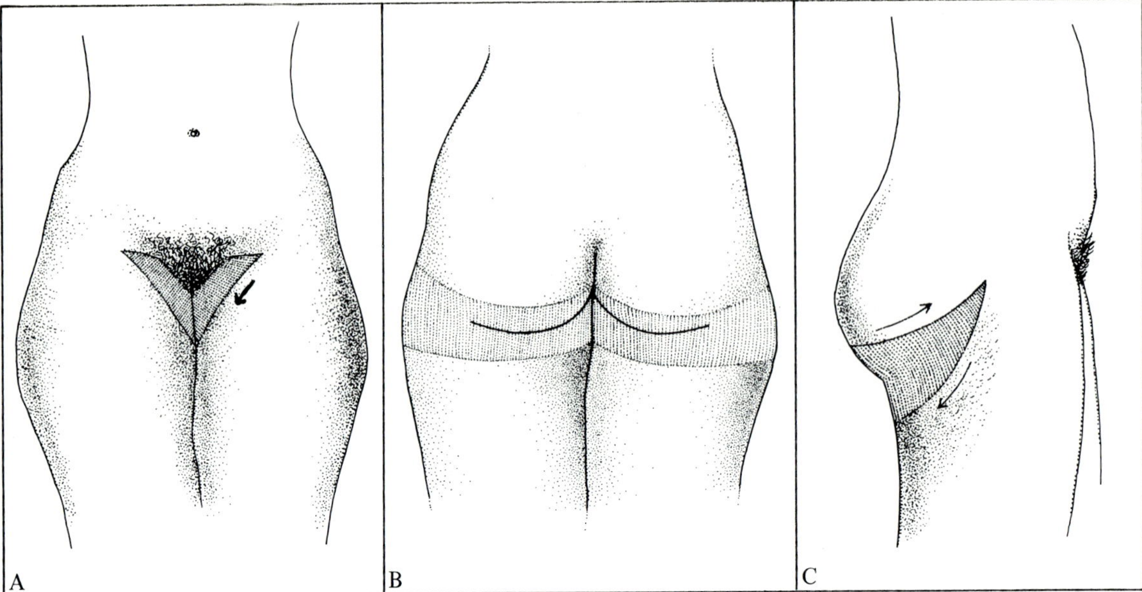

Fig. 52-10. Preoperative planning for semicircular thigh reduction. Note the arrows indicating slight rotations of the lower edge.

suture and a subcuticular continuous absorbable suture. A temporary dressing is left over the suture lines, and a sterile drape is applied.

SECOND PART OF THE OPERATION – POSTERIOR EXCISION. The patient is then turned over, employing the technique recommended by Pitanguy [26]: the arms are lifted above the head and the patient is placed near the edge of the operating table and then rolled around 180 degrees. A pillow should be placed under the anterior thorax. Skin preparation and draping are then done. The markings made before the operation are verified or modified accordingly.

The incisions follow the markings down to the musculoaponeurotic plane. On the posterior side there is no plane of dissection and stripping dissection is not possible. A small layer of fat should be left over the musculoaponeurotic plane. No undermining is done medially. The rotation of tissues is continued in the same rotary axis on the posterior thigh as was done in the front, but laterally it is done in the opposite direction to avoid secondary riding breeches deformity. Closure is performed using the same suture material as employed on the front. Adhesive strips and a light dressing are used. The patient is then turned again to the supine position. A catheter is left in the urethra to facilitate postoperative care. The temporary dressing is removed and adhesive strips are left on the anterior suture, but no other dressing is used.

The patient is allowed to get up the next day and walk. The catheter is removed. Sitting down is not permitted for 2 to 3 weeks to prevent stretching of the posterior suture line.

Circular Reduction

Circular reduction of the thigh is indicated when a large amount of excess skin and/or excess fat appears not only medially and laterally but also in the front of the thigh. With the patient standing up, one can lift the excess tissue upward and medially with both hands; the same excess tissue makes folds at the anterior part of the inguinal fold and all around the root of the thigh when the tissue is pushed upward with both hands (Figs. 52-12 and 52-13).

Operative Technique

ANTERIOR EXCISION. The technique is basically the same as the technique described for the semicircular operation. The anterior tissue is removed first, and the specimen is divided laterally and medially as far as it is possible, being limited by the surface of the table. The thigh tissues are rotated medially (as is done in the semicircular thigh reduction). The wound may seem temporarily to close under some tension at the lateral portion of the excision because of the unexcised tissues remaining at the back. After closure of both thighs, a temporary sterile dressing is left covering the incision and the patient is turned to the front position (as in the semicircular operation).

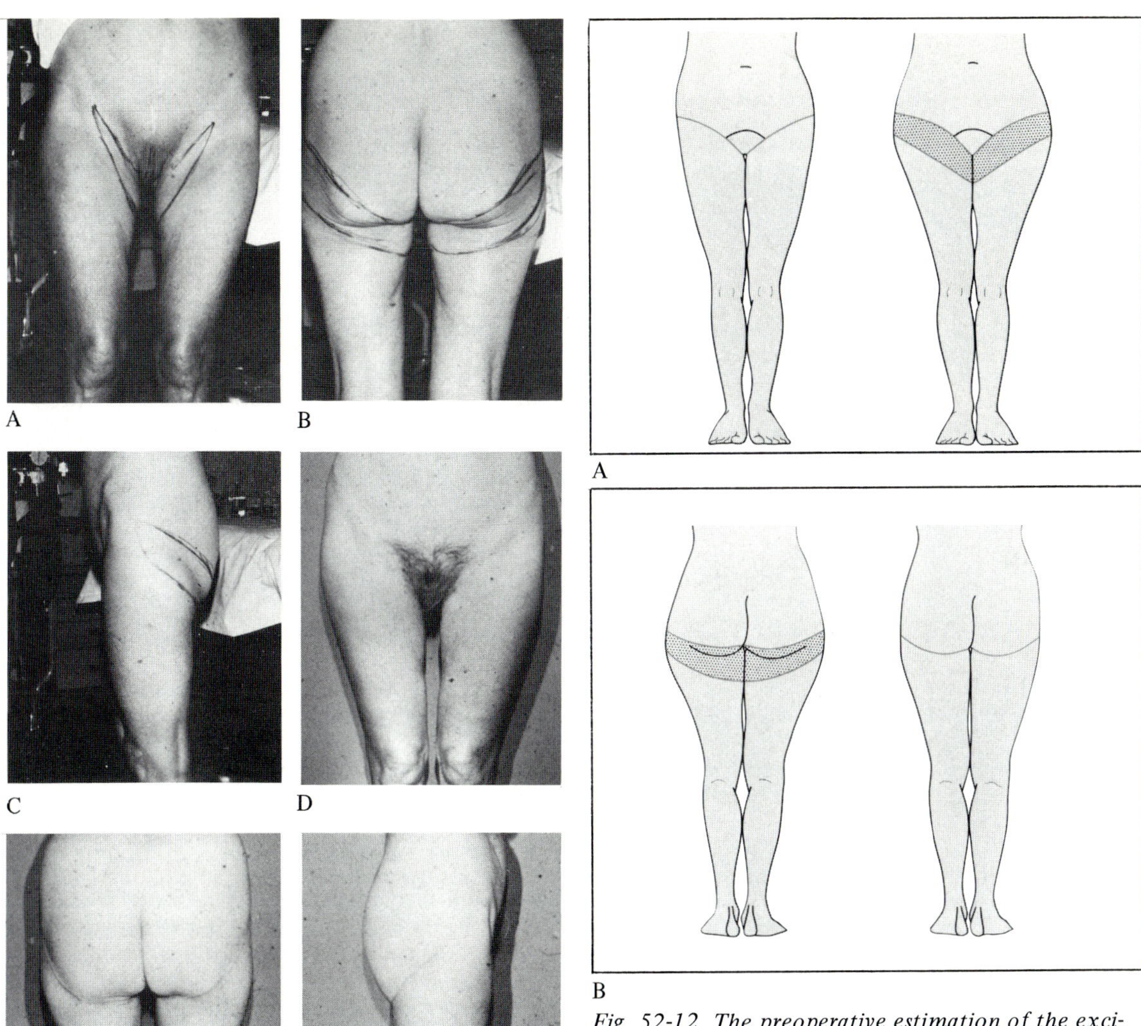

Fig. 52-11. A, B, C, a patient with moderate lipodystrophy of the thighs, showing preoperative markings. D, E, F, the postoperative result after a semicircular thigh correction.

Fig. 52-12. The preoperative estimation of the excisions for a circular thigh reduction.

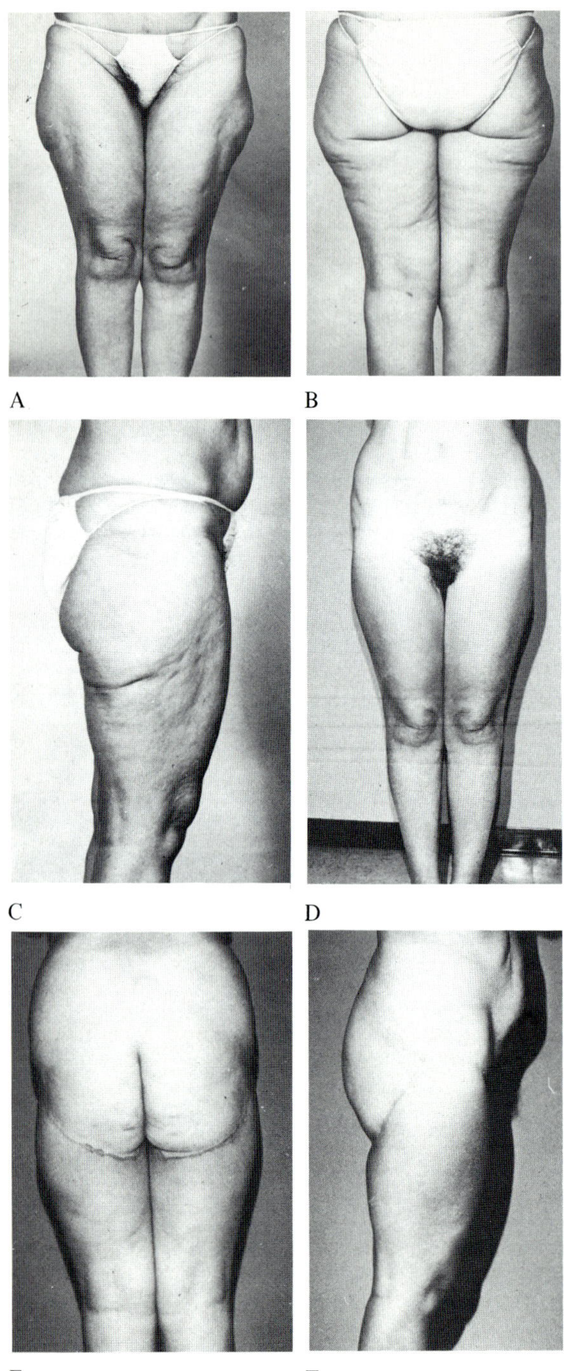

Fig. 52-13. A, B, C, a patient with typical massive circular deformity and skin hyperelasticity. D, E, F, the result 1 year after a circular thigh reduction.

POSTERIOR EXCISION. After the skin has been prepared and drapes have been applied, the preoperative plan is verified by mobilizing the tissue and measuring the width of the excision necessary to make the operation symmetrical on both sides.

The incisions follow the preoperative marking, and the dissection is started laterally going progressively upward, removing skin and fat, leaving a fine layer of fat tissue over the musculoaponeurotic plane. Before suturing is started, the medial tissues on the lower flap are rotated outward and the lateral lower flap tissues rotated inward, while upper tissues are left in position. This antagonistic rotation may seem illogical, but the gathering of lower tissues at the back prevents a secondary riding breeches deformity. The same type of suturing is done as for the semicircular thigh reduction. Adhesive strips and a light dressing are used on the back side. A urethral catheter is inserted after the patient has been turned again to the supine position, and adhesive strips are put on the frontal suture line; no other dressing is used in the front.

Vertical Reduction

The use of vertical reduction is rarely indicated. Most deformities can be reduced with the preceding procedures. However in particular patients, such as those with the Simons-Barraquer syndrome (lipodystrophia progressiva), it is the only procedure that can bring a valuable result (Fig. 52-14). It may also be used in older persons when a major reduction is needed and when the vertical scar will not be a cosmetic problem (for example, at the beach).

The best technique for vertical reduction is a posterolateral vertical excision, turning above the popliteal region. The deep aponeurosis is preserved, and no undermining is done. When reduction should be drastic and the tissue is not supple, a lateral vertical excision may be added to the posteromedial excision at a separate procedure.

Combined Circular and Vertical Reduction

Reduction using both the circular and vertical approaches is excellent for massive reductions (Fig. 52-15). The principle is the same as for the previously described techniques.

The operation is started in front; then the patient is turned and the circular and posteromedial excisions are done without undermining. Where the line of the vertical excision meets the horizontal line of closure, a Z-plasty is utilized to prevent scar retraction at this location (Fig. 52-15).

Trochanteric Defatting Procedure

Correction of the trochanteric fat pad (riding breeches deformity) is usually done at the same time as a semicircular or circular operation (Figs. 52-16 and 52-17).

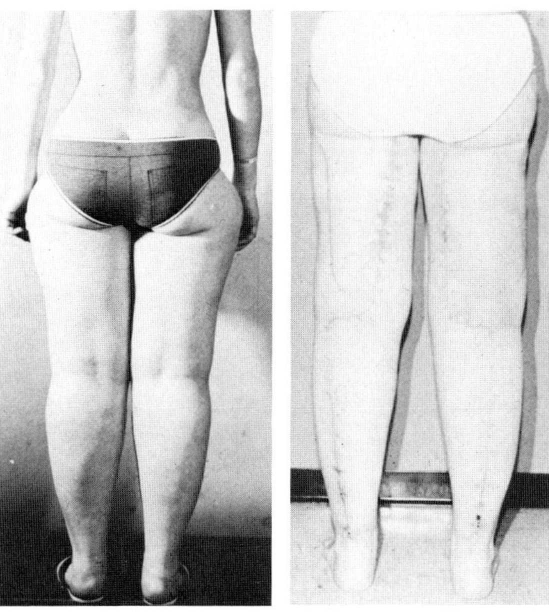

A B

Fig. 52-14. A, in the typical patient with Simons-Barraquer's deformity, it is impossible to wear pants or boots. B, vertical excisions were done in two stages – first laterally, and then medially down to the ankles 2 weeks after the first procedure.

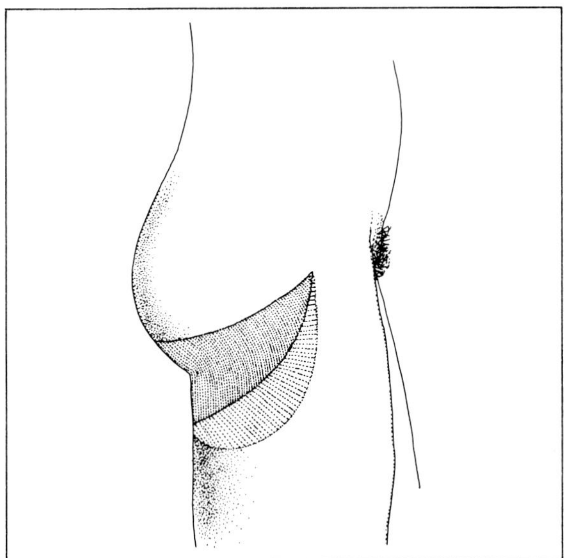

Fig. 52-16. Preoperative planning for trochanteric fat removal.

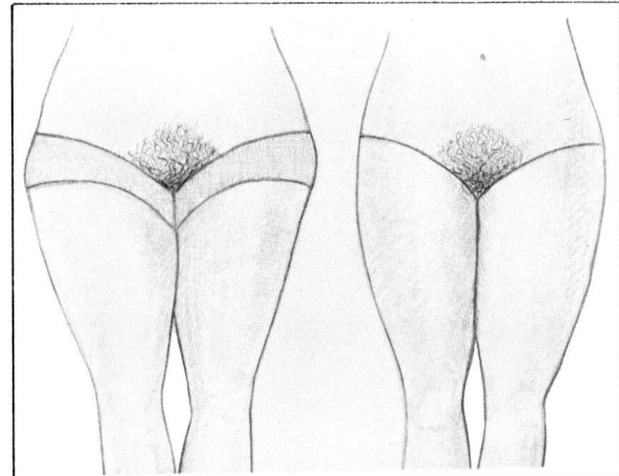

A

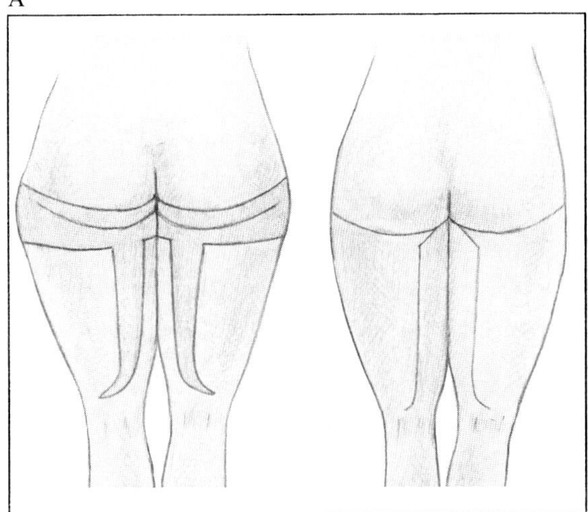

B

Fig. 52-15. Preoperative planning for the combined circular and vertical thigh reduction. The angular flaps are placed using a Z-plasty technique to prevent retraction.

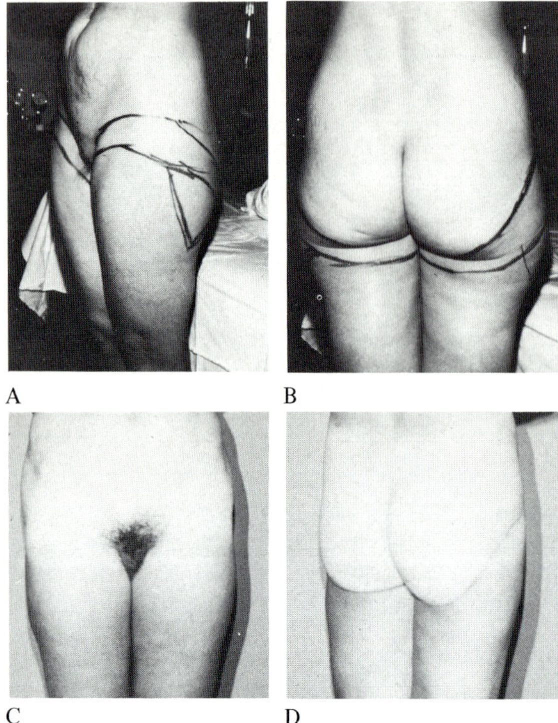

Fig. 52-17. *A, B, a typical patient with trochanteric fat pad and circular deformity. C, D, the appearance 1 year after circular thigh reduction and associated trochanteric defatting.*

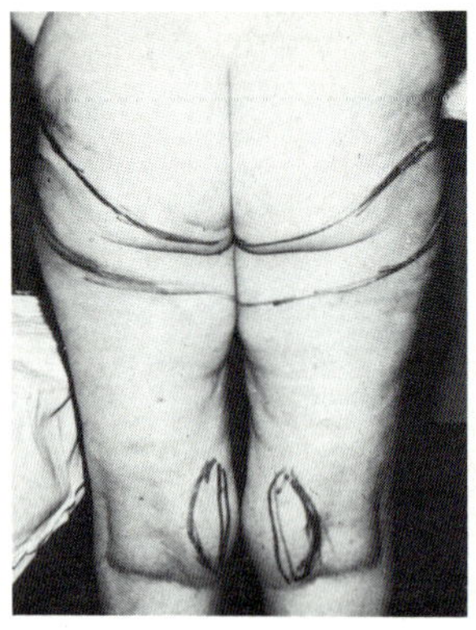

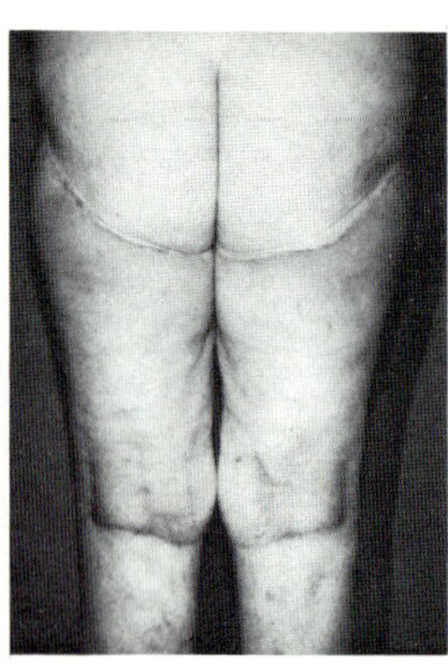

Fig. 52-18. *A, a patient with deformity of the medial lower aspect of the thighs, showing preoperative marking. B, the result after lower semilunar excision.*

It may be done alone, most of the time as a secondary procedure when it was not done at the time of the thigh reduction.

The area to be defatted is marked before operation with the patient standing up (because the supine position corrects almost everything by itself). The procedure should be done with the patient prone. After the previously described excision has been completed on the back side, undermining of the trochanteric area is done. Care should be taken to leave the subcutaneous layer of fat, which averages 15 mm. in thickness.

The fat pad is dissected from the fascia, leaving a small layer of fat above the fascia to help reestablish normal vascularization more easily and to enable reabsorption of any fluid or blood that might collect. When this defatting procedure is done, a drain is necessary. A small stab wound incision is made at the lowest part of the undermining, and a semicircular drain or suction drain is left for at least 48 hours.

In spite of excellent hemostasis and good drainage, trochanteric defatting is often complicated by hematoma. The blood should be evacuated as often as necessary until the pocket remains dry. The hematoma may last for about a month; if it is correctly treated from the beginning, no necrosis will occur.

Correction of Lower Medial Thigh Deformities

Occasionally a vertical semilunar excision is done at the posteromedial aspect of the lower part of the thigh to correct a redundancy of the lower medial thigh (Fig. 52-18). No undermining or defatting is done; closure is performed in two layers, and adhesive strips are left. No drainage or dressing is used.

Corrections of Secondary Thigh Deformities

After a semicircular or circular thigh reduction, an unpleasant exaggeration of the trochanteric fat pad may appear when it has not been removed. Above this fat pad there is an iliac depression. This secondary riding breeches deformity can be corrected by the excision of skin at the level of the depression, with no fat removal at this level; defatting is done at the site of the trochanteric area, as in a primary defatting.

Complications

Immediate Complications

HEMATOMA. This is rare in the usual thigh reduction when hemostasis has been well performed and no dead space has been left, but bleeding is common in trochanteric defatting procedures. The patients should be warned about this problem. Good drainage and repeated evacuations are necessary, and the bleeding may last for several weeks before it is completely cured.

INFECTION. Infection of the suture line is also common at the medial aspect of the thighs; it is probably the result of maceration and possible friction, and it is treated with local and systemic antibiotics. The patient is asked to keep the thighs apart as much as possible. Infection following a hematoma is less common but may occur. It may be prevented by the use of antibiotics as soon as the hematoma is detected. It usually disappears in a short time with daily evacuation of the pus and wet dressings as well as local and systemic antibiotics.

NECROSIS. Necrosis is very rare; it should not occur with the techniques previously described. It is a complication of those cases in which undermining was done. However, after a severe hematoma that was not detected early enough or after a serious infection, some localized areas of skin sloughing may appear; these areas should be excised. If necessary, skin grafting should be done, and a secondary revision can be done at a later time.

EDEMA. Edema of the lower limbs should be of short duration if the large veins and lymphatic vessels have been left in place. The use of elastic stockings for a few weeks or months will help to relieve this condition; it is also helpful for the patient to keep the legs elevated whenever possible. Walking and exercises are recommended.

SCARS. Scars are rarely a problem except after infections. Hypertrophic scars are treated by injections of triamcinolone. Visible scars that appear lower than the bathing suit result from too wide an excision and from downward pulling on the suture line. They should not be corrected until at least 1 year after operation. At that time the correction is done by excision and by trying to elevate the scar as much as possible. This complication should not happen when good preoperative planning has been done (keeping in mind the possible downward dislocation of the scars) and when the rotation has been performed as described.

DEFORMITY OF THE VULVA AND LABIA MAJORIS. This deformity may appear temporarily if too much tension has been applied on the medial side. This problem can be avoided by more carefully evaluating the amount of skin and fat for removal. It is also helpful to insert deep sutures that go through the deep aponeurosis on the medial and posteromedial aspect. The problem can also be avoided by spirally rotating the anteromedial aspect posteriorly instead of pulling the tissues directly upward.

LIPECTOMY OF THE LOWER LEG

Lipectomy is performed on the lower leg only for functional reasons, because it leaves such visible scars. The excision may be done posteromedially following the same principles used in the vertical thigh reduction. If both the thigh and the leg need reduction, a continuous excision can be made, with a horizontal line or step placed at the level of the popliteal area.

Limited defatting may be done in the calf and ankle area as long as enough subcutaneous fat is left with the skin. Elastic stockings should be used in the postoperative period.

LIPECTOMY OF THE ARM

Whatever the case and the technique used, the expected result may be very satisfactory for the aesthetic shape obtained; but the patient should be warned that there will be a permanent scar that is more or less visible when the arms are lifted [30, 33].

Most patients who request aesthetic arm surgery are women who have lost weight and present with pendulous upper arms. Rarely does the surgeon encounter women who have simple, firm, nonpendulous adiposity of the arm. When such a patient does come for consultation, general weight reduction must be advised first.

Minor, moderate, or major arm reduction may be performed, according to the seriousness of the deformity.

Minor Arm Reduction

Minor arm lipectomy is done when the defect is located in the upper third of the arm. Such defects are accepted by most women, but correction may be required by a perfectionist.

Arm lipectomy is easily done under local anesthesia with a low percentage of anesthetic – 0.20% lidocaine with epinephrine 1:500,000 – so that a large amount may be used with no toxicity.

The planning of the operation is done with the patient sitting up. The excision should be done so as to avoid scarring in the axilla; however the excision should remain close to the axilla with an angular marking with a fish-tail shape (M-plasty). Following the lower contour of the medial side of the arm, the convexity varies with the flaccidity. The medial line is straight or slightly curved parallel to the lateral line [30, 33]. The amount of tissue to be excised is decided upon by gentle pinching.

For minor arm reduction, the patient should be positioned on the table with the hands elevated at the level of the head.

Preparation and draping are done as in other procedures. After local or general anesthesia has been administered, the incision is started at the medial end of the line marked previously in the axilla. Dissection of the fat layer should be done carefully to leave the superficial fascia and the large superficial vein intact. The plane of dissection is usually found easily. Dissection is continued to the level of the posterior line of the markings and tissue elasticity is then tested. The resection is done according to the needs of the individual patient, more or less following the preoperative marking of the posterior line. Undermining is usually not done. Closure is done in three layers of suture, with fat, subcutaneous, and continuous subcuticular closures, starting at each end. Adhesive strips are the only dressing used.

Moderate Arm Reduction

Moderate arm lipectomy is done in the same way as in minor arm lipectomy except that the excision is longer and the removal of tissue is more extensive. The planning is done as usual, with the patient sitting up.

The position on the table is selected in order to get an easy field of operation (Fig. 52-19). The forearms are taped, and the hands are elevated above the patient's head, attached to intravenous stands or poles. The technique follows the same order as for the minor arm reduction.

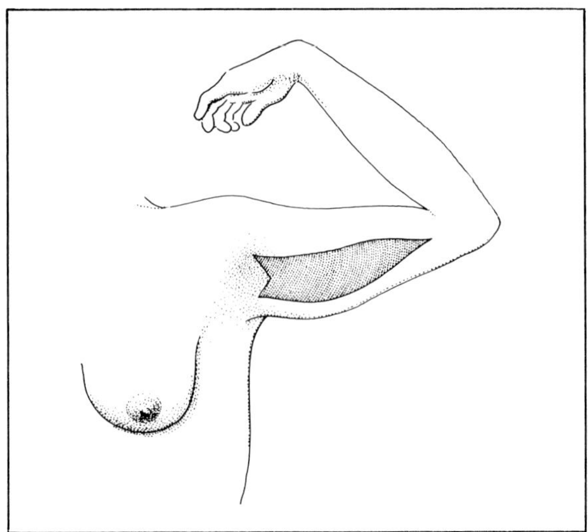

Fig. 52-19. The position of the patient on the operating table. The arms may be lifted and operated on separately.

Major Arm Reduction

Major reduction is necessary when a large amount of tissue has to be removed. The marking is similar to that for the moderate arm flaccidity at the level of the axilla and arm, but it is continued to the back of the elbow, permitting the removal of the folds above the elbow, which often constitute a problem. In patients undergoing major arm reduction, it would not give a satisfactory result to end the excision at the epitrochlear level [35].

The operation is performed in the same way as in the other procedures, except that the arms may be elevated more. Because the operation takes longer, the second arm is placed in the operative position only after the first arm is completely done, unless two teams are performing the surgery simultaneously.

In cases of major arm reduction, the suturing may be started at the elbow to get a perfect line with no redundancy. At the axilla, care should be taken to avoid traction on the axillary angle; otherwise a retraction might occur.

Postoperative Care

However extensive the procedure, adhesive strips are left as long as 3 weeks, but they may be changed at the second day if necessary. The use of absorbable 4-0 material for the subcuticular running suture avoids the need for suture removal; otherwise, nonabsorbable sutures should remain in place for 10 days. The scars will remain pink for a few months.

Complications

Hematoma and necrosis are unusual because there is no dead space left. Infection of the suture lines is rare but should be treated immediately with systemic and local antibiotics. An unsatisfactory scar is the most common complication. If the scars become hypertrophic and painful, they should be treated with triamcinolone injections. With time the scars may widen. A revision is not performed earlier than 6 months after the operation.

REFERENCES

Abdominal Lipectomy

1. Babcock, W. Plastic reconstruction of the female breasts and abdomen. *Am. J. Surg.* 43:260, 1939.
2. Baroudi, R. Umbilicaplasty. *Clin. Plast. Surg.* 2:431, 1975.
3. Baroudi, R., Keppke, E. M., and Tozzi Netto, F. Abdominoplasty. *Plast. Reconstr. Surg.* 54:161, 1974.
4. Callia, E. P. *Dermolipectomia Abdominal (Operacao de Callia).* Sao Paulo, Brazil: Carlo Erba, 1965.
5. Castanares, S., and Goethel, J. Abdominal lipectomy: A modification in technique. *Plast. Reconstr. Surg.* 40:378, 1967.
6. Dufourmentel, C., and Mouly, R. *Chirurgie Plastique.* Paris: Flammarion, 1959. P. 381.

7. Galtier, M. Traitement chirurgical de l'obésité de la paroi abdominale avec ptose. *Mem. Acad. Chir.* 81:341, 1955.
8. Gonzalez-Ulloa, M. Belt lipectomy. *Br. J. Plast. Surg.* 13:179, 1960.
9. *Gray's Anatomy*. Philadelphia: Lea & Febiger, 1959. Pp. 462, 651, 998, 1033, 1157.
10. Grazer, F. M. Abdominoplasty. *Plast. Reconstr. Surg.* 51:617, 1973.
11. Hinderer, U. T. The dermolipectomy approach for augmentation mammaplasty. *Clin. Plast. Surg.* 2:359, 1975.
12. Kelly, H. A. Excision of the fat of the abdominal wall. *Surg. Gynecol. Obstet.* 10:229, 1910.
13. Pitanguy, I. Abdominal lipectomy: An approach to it through an analysis of 300 consecutive cases. *Plast. Reconstr. Surg.* 40:384, 1967.
14. Pitanguy, I. Surgical reduction of the abdomen, thighs and buttocks. *Surg. Clin. North Am.* 51: 479, 1971.
15. Regnault, P. Abdominal dermolipectomies. *Clin. Plast. Surg.* 2:411, 1975.
16. Serson, D. Geometric Planning for Abdominal Dermolipectomy. In Stephenson, K. L. (Ed.), *Year Book of Plastic and Reconstructive Surgery, 1972*. Chicago: Year Book, 1973.
17. Somalo, M. Dermolipectomia circular del tronco. *Sem. Med.* 1:1435, 1940.
18. Tai, Y., and Hasegawa, H. A transverse abdominal flap for reconstruction after radical operations for recurrent breast cancer. *Plast. Reconstr. Surg.* 53:52, 1974.
19. Thorek, M. Plastic reconstruction of the female breasts and abdomen. *Am. J. Surg.* 43:268, 1939.
20. Vernon, S. Umbilical transplantation upward and abdominal contouring in lipectomy. *Am. J. Surg.* 94:490, 1957.

Thigh Lipectomy

21. Delerm. A., and Girotteau, Y. Plastie cruro-fémoro-fessière ou circum fessière. *Ann. Chir. Plast.* 18:31, 1973.
22. Farina, R., Baroudi, R., Golcman, B., and De Castro, O. Riding trousers-like type of pelvicrural lipodystrophy (trochanteric lipomatosis). *Br. J. Plast. Surg.* 13:174, 1960.
23. Hoffman, S., and Simon, B. E. Experiences with the Pitanguy method of correction of trochanteric lipodystrophy. *Plast. Reconstr. Surg.* 55:551, 1975.
24. Lewis, J. R., Jr. Correction of ptosis of the thighs: The thigh lift. *Plast. Reconstr. Surg.* 37:494, 1966.
25. Lewis, J. R., Jr. *Atlas of Aesthetic Plastic Surgery.* Boston: Little, Brown, 1973.
26. Pitanguy, I. Surgical reduction of the abdomen, thigh and buttocks. *Surg. Clin. North Am.* 51:479, 1971.
27. Planas, J. The crural meloplasty for lifting of the thighs. *Clin. Plast. Surg.* 2:495, 1975.
28. Vilain, R. Surgical correction of steatomeries. *Clin. Plast. Surg.* 2:467, 1975.
29. Vilain, R. Some considerations in surgical alterations of the feminine silhouette. *Clin. Plast. Surg.* 2:449, 1975.

Arm Lipectomy

30. Baroudi, R. Dermatolipectomy of the upper arm. *Clin. Plast. Surg.* 2:485, 1975.
31. Clarkson, P. Lipodystrophies. *Plast. Reconstr. Surg.* 37:499, 1966.
32. McCraw, L. H. Surgical rehabilitation after massive weight reduction: Case report. *Plast. Reconstr. Surg.* 53:349, 1974.
33. Pitanguy, I. Correction of lipodystrophy of the lateral thoracic aspect and inner side of the arm and elbow dermosenescence. *Clin. Plast. Surg.* 2:477, 1975.
34. Vilain, R. Surgical correction of steatomeries. *Clin. Plast. Surg.* 2:467, 1975.
35. Zook, E. G. The massive weight loss patient. *Clin. Plast. Surg.* 2:457, 1975.

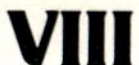

Genitalia

Hypospadias, Epispadias, and Exstrophy of the Bladder

CHARLES E. HORTON, CHARLES J. DEVINE, JR., JEROME E. ADAMSON, AND JAMES H. CARRAWAY

HYPOSPADIAS

Hypospadias is a congenital anomaly in which the urethra ends on the ventral surface of the penile shaft or in the perineum. It occurs in 1 of 300 live male births and ranges in severity from the most frequent type involving the glans, through the less frequent penile shaft types, to the rarer and more severe scrotal or perineal forms [2]. Various classifications of hypospadias have been described; however, elaborate classifications are not essential. We have used the following categories: glanular, distal penile, penile, penoscrotal junction, scrotal, and perineal. In most patients with hypospadias there is a downward curvature of the penis, especially during erection. This *chordee,* as it is called, is caused by fibrous tissue that extends from the hypospadiac meatus to the glans penis. Rarely chordee may occur without hypospadias. In these patients fibrous tissue around the urethra causes the bending.

An intravenous pyelogram and complete systemic evaluation of the patient are essential in every case. Undescended testicles, kidney abnormalities, hernias, and other congenital anomalies are found more frequently in patients with hypospadias than in the general population. In severe cases of hypospadias, the external appearance may leave the sex in doubt; if so, sex chromatin studies, cystoscopy, and occasionally laparotomy may be necessary for a definite diagnosis.

Embryology

The sex of the developing embryo is determined at the time of conception by the chromosome content of the spermatozoon that fertilizes the ovum. A sperm containing an X chromosome will yield an XX individual (female). A Y-containing spermatozoon will result in an XY (male). At 2 weeks of development the embryonic disc consists of ectoderm and entoderm. A midline groove has formed, and a third cell layer (the embryonic mesoderm) formed there begins to migrate peripherally, separating the ectoderm and entoderm layers. Caudal to this primitive streak, the ectoderm and entoderm remain fused and form the cloacal membrane. The embryonic disc buckles upward and begins to overgrow its slower growing margins. As the head and tail folds form, the cloacal membrane becomes part of the ventral wall. During the second month the embryo begins to assume human form as the limbs and facial structures become developed. Cranial to the cloacal membrane the genital tubercle is formed with a midline depression, which is called the urethral groove. The tubercle lengthens with growth of the embryo. This stage is an indifferent period and is the same for both sexes. If the testes did not develop, the external genitalia would grow into a normal female configuration. The genital tubercle would become the clitoris, the urogenital folds would become the labia minora, and the labia scrotal swellings would enlarge to form the labia majora.

The developing testes secrete a substance that causes the external genitalia to develop a male configuration from this indifferent stage. The genital tubercle grows rapidly and assumes a more cylindrical shape until it can be identified as a phallus. A definite groove appears at the distal end demarcating the glans. As the phallus elongates, the urethral groove deepens from the open urogenital ostium to extend distally onto the shaft. The urethral folds become prominent and at the end of 3 months begin to close. The edges proliferate around the deepening groove and the urethral grooves seam together from the proximal opening extending in a distal direction. The seam remains as a prominent midline raphe. Closure of the urethra continues to the glans, where the urethral groove deepens but does not fuse at this stage. At about the third month, a roll of skin arises on either side of the urethral opening and extends to encircle the shaft of the penis. This skin forms the prepuce, which, as it grows, covers the edges of the glans; the glans seals the glanular urethra until the urethral meatus reaches its final location at the tip of the glans.

At about 8 weeks, the labioscrotal swellings appear and then migrate posteriorly around the phallus, forming the scrotum. The median raphe and septum act as a divider and maintain two separate compartments to hold the testicles. The testicles descend into the scrotum, usually at 9 months, completing development of the male external genitalia.

Hypospadias is a form of incomplete masculinization of the genitalia caused by premature involution of the interstitial cells of the testicle. Masculine development ceases at the stage that exists when the involution occurs. Because this is a function of time, the more nearly developed cases are seen more often than the less well developed.

Pathological Anatomy

The structures that form the bulk of the substance of the penis are the three erectile bodies consisting of the paired corpora cavernosa and the corpus spongiosum, which lies ventrally in the groove between the two corpora cavernosa. Each is surrounded by a fascial covering known as the tunica albuginea. Central arteries are located in the corpora cavernosa and bring blood into these structures. The urethra traverses the penis through the corpus spongiosum and emerges at the distal end of the conical enlargement of the corpus called the glans penis. Below the penile skin is found the dartos fascia, a loose layer of connective tissue in which run superficial lymphatics and the superficial dorsal veins. Buck's fascia is located beneath the dartos fascia and extends distally to the free margins of the prepuce. It surrounds the corpora cavernosa and splits to contain the corpus spongiosum separately.

The hypospadiac penis differs from the normal in the absence of the urethra and corpus spongiosum. The abnormal tissue causing chordee is composed of fibrous tissue that encircles the opening of the existing urethra and extends distally as a fan-shaped sheet to the base of the glans. The lateral margins meet the edges of the prepuce. This fibrous tissue causes an angulation of the glans on the shaft and ordinarily extends beneath the abnormally shaped glans. Some feel that growth of the penis may be inhibited by this tough fibrous tissue on the ventral surface. The glans of the hypospadiac penis is usually spatulate and flattened, and the prepuce is deficient ventrally. The midline raphe of the penis may deviate to one side or the other, associated with torsion or twisting of the penile skin. Blind urethral channels may be found distal to the existing meatus, and congenital urethral fistulas have been reported in association with hypospadias. Occasionally the scrotum may be found anterior to the base of the penis (engulfment), and in proximal cases the scrotum is cleft with a deep groove present at the midline.

Treatment of Hypospadias

Two-Stage Repair

CORRECTION OF CHORDEE. The first requisite of a good hypospadias repair is to straighten the penis by resecting all of the tissues causing the chordee. For many years surgeons felt that this fibrous tissue causing the chordee had a potential of new growth and that the penis must be watched for recurrence of the chordee before urethroplasty was attempted at a later date. We believe that the fibrous tissue of the chordee does not regrow, that once it is removed the condition is permanently corrected, and that recurrence is due to an incomplete primary resection, except that postoperative hematoma or infection can cause new fibrous tissue to be deposited.

To remove this fibrous tissue, we recommend an incision around the meatus extending distally in the midline of the shaft of the penis to the coronal sulcus. The lateral skin flaps are elevated and all abnormal tissue in this area is removed down to the normal tunica albuginea. Bleeding from the venae profundae penis, which lies immediately adjacent to Buck's fascia, may lead the surgeon to feel that he has inadvertently entered the corpora. These veins are, in fact, some distance from the tunica albuginea, and the dissection should be continued to a deeper plane until the blue and glistening tunica albuginea has been completely uncovered. Dissection must be carried around the existing meatus only to the tip of the corpus spongiosum. If this structure is entered, excessive bleeding will be encountered. We recommend extending the dissection under the glans where the abnormal fibrous tissue inserts into the glanular tissue. If the tunica albuginea of the corpora cavernosa is inadvertently entered in this dissection, it is repaired using 6-0 chromic gut sutures.

Acute dorsiflexion of the penis over an assistant's finger will aid in the dissection and in controlling bleeding while resecting the fibrous tissue causing the chordee. Palpation of the tunica albuginea may reveal small strands of fibrous tissue that may be hard to visualize but that must be resected. Bleeding can best be controlled with the coagulation current, using fine-tipped forceps to grasp each individual bleeding point. Once all abnormal fibrous tissue is removed, the penile shaft should remain straight and have no visible ventral curvature. We are firmly committed to the principle that hypospadias is best repaired in one stage of surgery. However, if a multistaged repair is planned, the ventral defect is closed with either an Ombrédanne-type hood in which a buttonhole is made in the unfolded prepuce and the prepuce is transferred to the ventral surface of the penis; preferably, the repair may be done by unfolding the prepuce, splitting it in the middle, and transferring the two flaps of prepuce ventrally [2]. The buttonhole flap produces unsightly dog ears laterally, and has not been used as a procedure of choice for many years. Skin closure can be performed with any type of suture material, such as nylon, silk, steel, or gut. We prefer 6-0 chromic gut sutures, which do not require later removal.

URETHROPLASTY. The second stage of the two-stage repair is carried out after allowing at least 6 months for healing. A new urethra can be reconstructed in this second stage either by using a free graft or by using local flaps. A full-thickness graft will have normal growth potential and will not contract. If a split-thickness graft is used, it must be splinted for at least 6 months to overcome a tendency for contracture. Either graft can be inserted through a subcutaneous tunnel to the tip of the glans, where it can be anastomosed to a V-shaped glanular flap. The anastomosis between the graft and the urethra can be completed

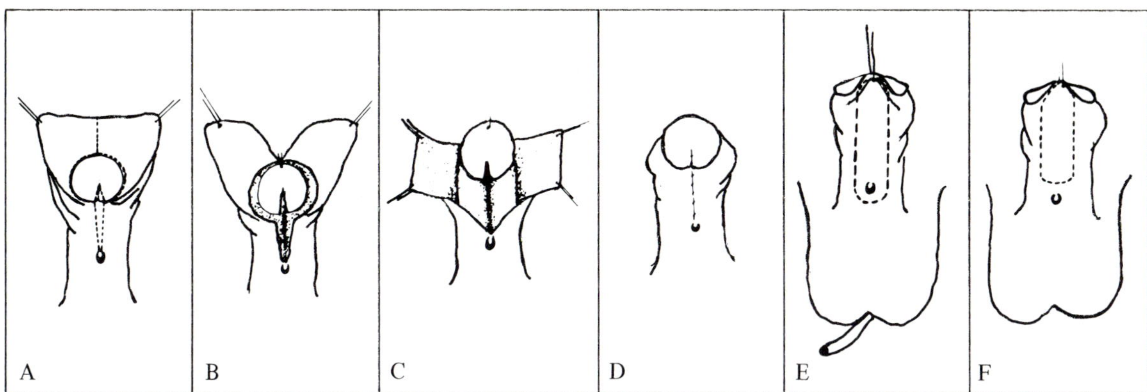

Fig. 53-1. Byars' (1951–1955) two- or three-stage repair for hypospadias. E, two-stage design; F, three-stage design. The urethral channel is connected at third stage. (From L. T. Byars, A technique for consistently satisfactory repair of hypospadias. Surg. Gynecol. Obstet. *92:149, 1951.)*

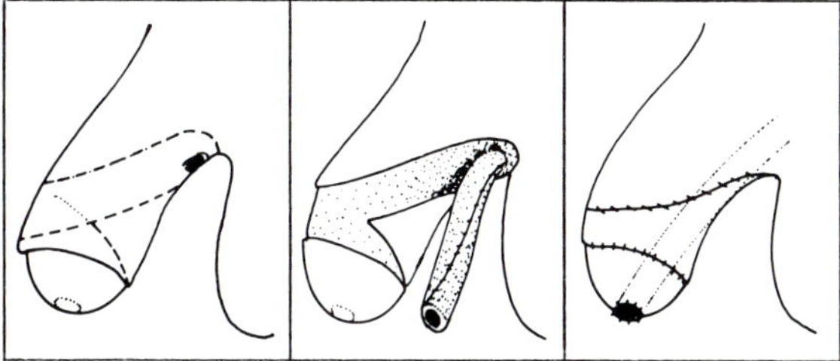

Fig. 53-3. Broadbent's (1960) one-stage repair for hypospadias. (From T. R. Broadbent, R. Woolf, and E. Toksu, Hypospadias, one-stage repair. Plast. Reconstr. Surg. *27:154, 1961.)*

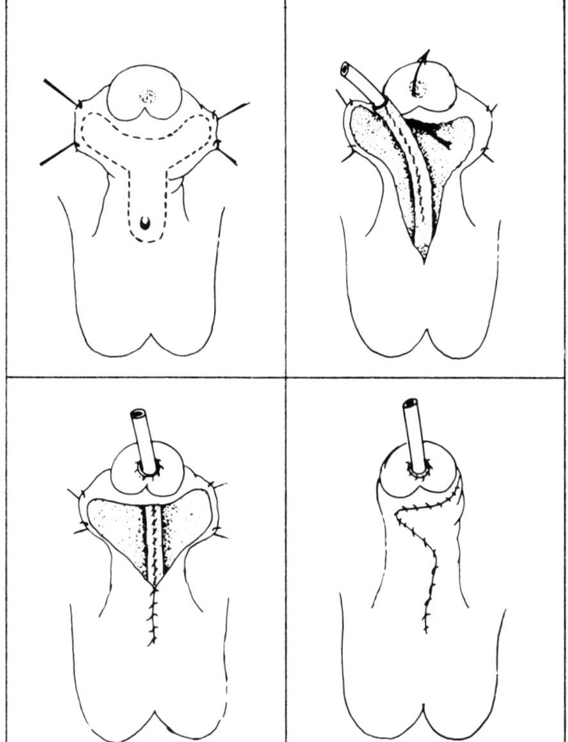

Fig. 53-2. Ricketson's (1958) two-stage repair for hypospadias. Chordee has been released previously. (From G. Ricketson, A method for repair of hypospadias. Am. J. Surg. *95:279, 1958.)*

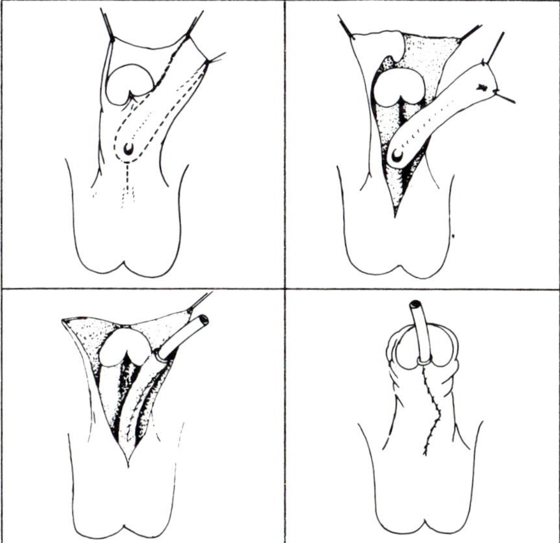

Fig. 53-4. Des Prez and Persky's (1961) one-stage repair for hypospadias. (From J. D. Des Prez, L. Persky, and C. L. Kichn, One-stage repair of hypospadias by island flap technique. Plast. Reconstr. Surg. *28:405, 1961.)*

at this second stage of surgery or can be deferred for a third stage.

If local flaps are to be used, the Byars modification of the Duplay technique is recommended (Fig. 53-1). Parallel incisions are made around the existing meatus distally to the glans. This central strip of skin is undermined at the edges and is formed into a tube [7]. The lateral penile skin is then undermined widely and is used to cover the newly formed urethral tube. It is difficult to get the meatus to extend to the exact tip of the glans with this technique, and many operators prefer to construct the new urethra only to the coronal sulcus. The Ricketson repair also has great merit (Fig. 53-2).

In patients whose lateral penile skin is deemed insufficient for ventral coverage, the penis may be buried in the scrotum for 3 to 4 weeks, and later scrotal skin flaps can be used for ventral penile resurfacing (Cecil-Culp operation) [4].

One of the most popular techniques for hypospadias repair was devised by Denis Browne; in it, a strip of skin is outlined by two parallel incisions from the existing meatus to the glans [3]. This strip of skin is not elevated at its edges. The lateral penile skin is widely undermined and then closed over the buried strip of skin. In the process of healing, the epithelium grows from the edges of the strip and forms a tube. In principle this technique is simple, but execution must be meticulous, or multiple fistulas and strictures may result.

One-Stage Repairs

In 1955 we [10] started a series of one-stage hypospadias repairs, using full-thickness skin grafts from the prepuce. Many surgical techniques have recently been described to complete hypospadias repair in one stage. The evolution of the one-stage repair for hypospadias seems assured as Broadbent and Woolf, Des Prez and Persky, Toksu, Hodgson, Hinderer, Mustardé, and others have reported one-stage operations for this congenital anomaly (Figs. 53-3 to 53-7).

The advantage of completely correcting the chordee and reconstructing the urethra in a single operation is responsible for the growing acceptance of various one-stage repairs for hypospadias. Satisfactory function and appearance with a normal urinary stream and sexual function should be obtainable in every case.

One-stage repairs are preferable to multiple-stage repairs because they reduce hospitalization, minimize physical and mental trauma, and allow completion of repair prior to the age of memory recall. Successful one-stage operations require more attention to detail and more delicate surgical technique than multiple-stage procedures and are offered as a better, not an easier way to repair hypospadias.

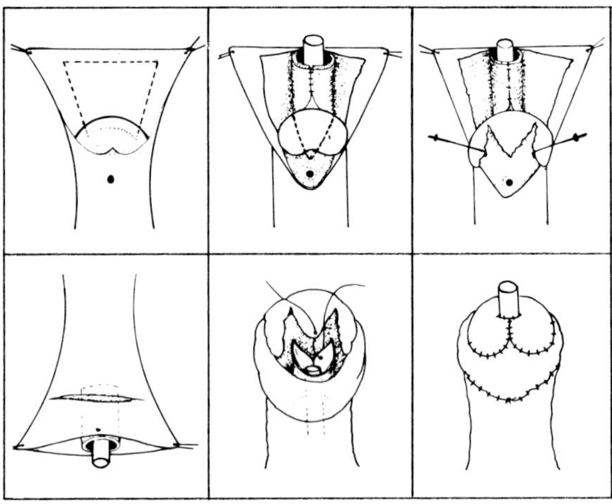

Fig. 53-5. Toksu's (1970) one-stage repair for hypospadias. (From E. Toksu, Hypospadias: A one-stage repair. Plast. Reconstr. Surg. *45:365, 1970.)*

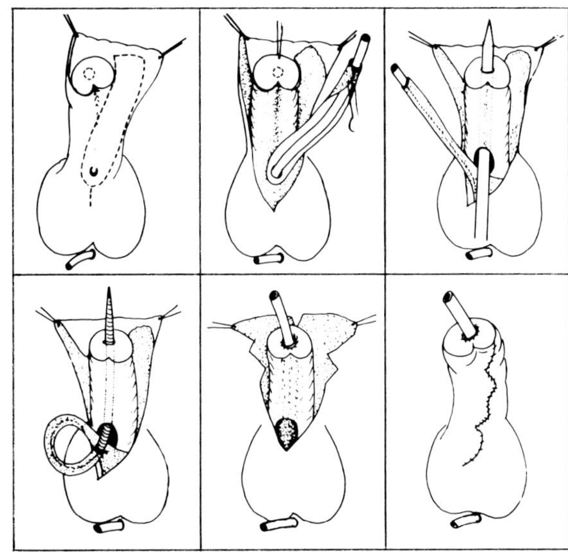

Fig. 53-6. Hinderer's (1970) one-stage repair for hypospadias. (From U. Hinderer, Hypospadias. Plast. Reconstr. Surg. *43:434, 1969.)*

In our experience, no one operation is suitable for every case of hypospadias. The surgeon is obligated to have a variety of techniques available for use in each particular situation where circumstances demand. Over a period of years we have evolved three one-stage techniques that have been useful for (1) distal shaft hypospadias, (2) proximal shaft hypospadias, and (3) scrotal or perineal hypospadias.

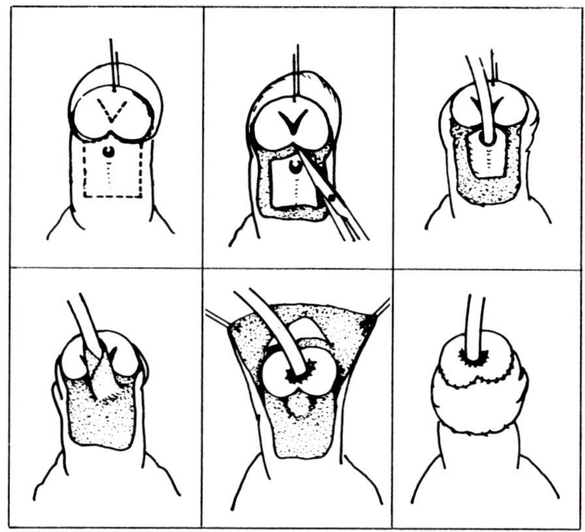

Fig. 53-7. Mustardé's (1965) one-stage repair for hypospadias. (From J. C. Mustardé, One-stage correction of distal hypospadias; and other people's fistulae. Br. J. Plast. Surg. *18:413, 1965.)*

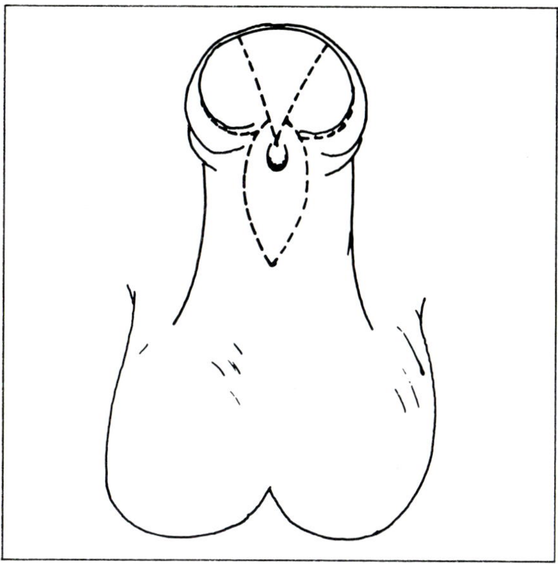

Fig. 53-8. An incision to develop "flip flap" operation for distal hypospadias.

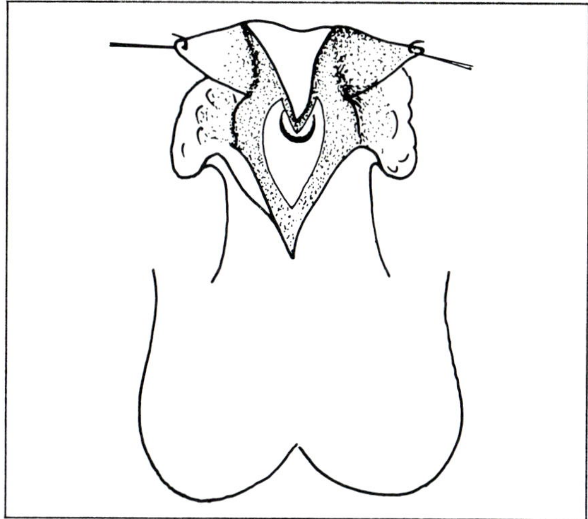

Fig. 53-9. The incisions are opened.

THE AUTHORS' ONE-STAGE REPAIR OF DISTAL SHAFT HYPOSPADIAS. To plan the operation, a triangular flap with a broad base located at the exact tip of the penis is marked on the glans. If a urethral groove is present, the flap should include this area, because the epithelium will flatten when the flap is elevated. Prior to surgery, 0.5 to 1 ml. of lidocaine with 1:200,000 epinephrine is injected into the area to aid hemostasis. An incision is marked, beginning at the meatus and continued distally to the coronal sulcus where it encircles the glans. The incisions are made in the skin of the shaft and the fibrous tissue causing the chordee is resected (Fig. 53-8). This tissue extends from the urethral meatus to the glans, and dissection must be continued beneath the glans. The triangular glanular flap is elevated, and the lateral wings of the glans are freed with sharp dissection. A long penile skin flap based distally on the urethral meatus is then outlined on the ventral surface of the penis. This flap is elevated, taking care to protect the urethra, which lies immediately beneath the flap. The dorsal roof of the existing urethra is incised for a distance of 0.5 cm. so that the triangular flap taken from the glans can be inserted into the groove (Figs. 53-9 and 53-10). The glans flap is used to reconstruct the roof of the urethra. It should be sutured to both the tunica albuginea and the urethral epithelium, using 6-0 chromic gut sutures. The retrograde flap based on the meatus is then flipped forward to form the ventral surface of the urethra. It is sutured to the triangular flap and anchored to the tunica albuginea with multiple interrupted sutures to complete the urethral reconstruction to the tip of the glans (Fig. 53-11). The lateral glanular wings are now brought around the new urethra to the midline and are sutured together, changing the spatulate shape of the glans to a more conical, normal shape (Fig. 53-12). The uncovered ventral surface should now be resurfaced, either using an Ombrédanne hood or preferably splitting the prepuce in the midline to bring the

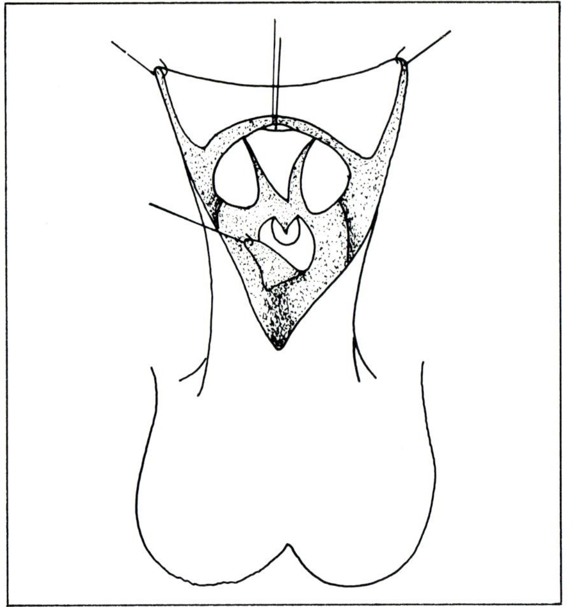

Fig. 53-10. A midline glanular flap is inserted in dorsal meatotomy incision, and the lateral glanular wings are mobilized.

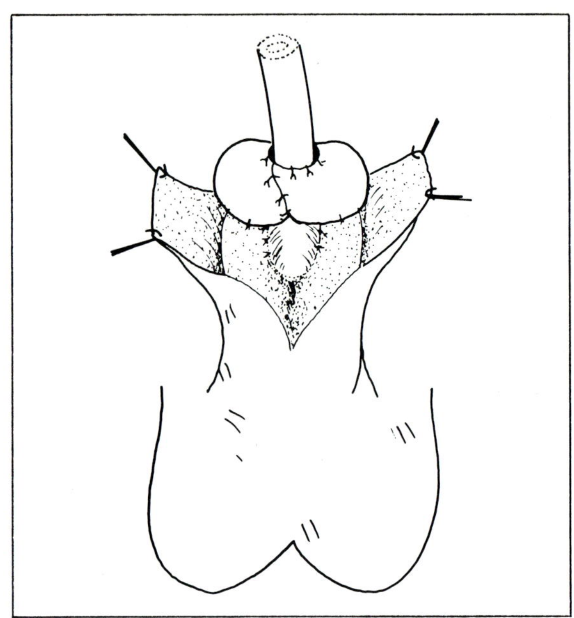

Fig. 53-12. The glanular wings are approximated to form a normal-shape glans.

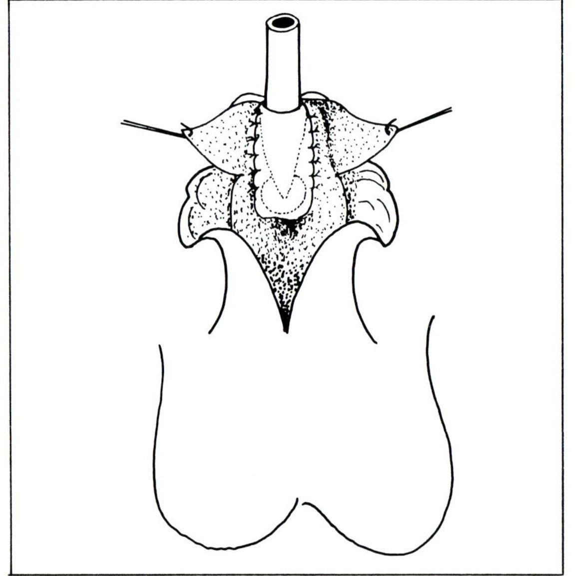

Fig. 53-11. The "flip flap" of penile skin is sutured to the midline glanular flap to form the urethra.

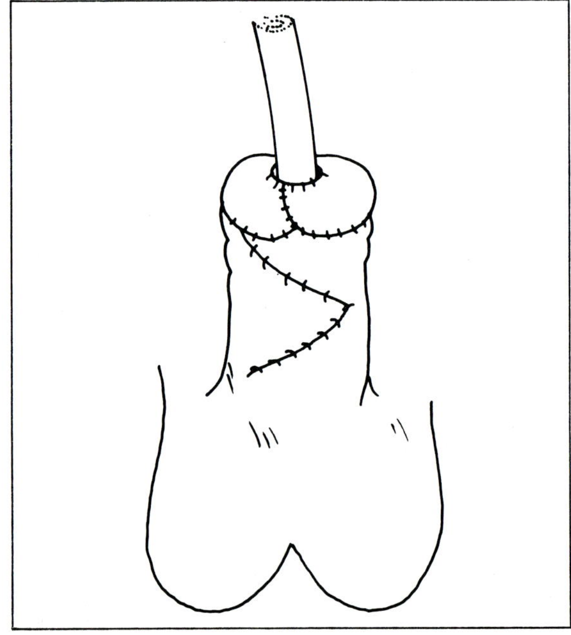

Fig. 53-13. The vertical skin deficit is closed with preputial flaps.

lateral flaps of the prepuce inferiorly [2] (Fig. 53-13). An indwelling Foley catheter or small feeding tube is left in place for 3 days after surgery.

ONE-STAGE REPAIR OF PROXIMAL SHAFT HYPOSPADIAS. In this type of hypospadias the glanular triangle flap will not reach to the existing urethral meatus. It is, therefore, necessary to construct a tube of skin from a free full-thickness preputial graft that will bridge the area between the meatus and the triangular flap. In this technique an incision is made around the existing urethral meatus, down the midline of the ventral surface of the penis to the coronal sulcus where the incision is carried completely around the glans. The penile skin flaps are elevated and the tissues causing chordee are resected as previously described. The usual triangular midline glanular flap is constructed and the lateral glanular wings are mobilized (Fig. 53-14). The existing urethral meatus is incised dorsally to create a groove into which a tongue of the new skin graft urethra will fit. The prepuce is then unfolded into a single layer. A graft of proper length is obtained from the most distal portion of the prepuce. The graft is thinned by removing the excess subcutaneous tissue and is then sutured into a tube with the raw surface outward over a red rubber catheter stent of proper size. The caliber of the skin graft tube is determined by gently calibrating the existing urethra. If a #10, #12, or #14 sound can be passed with ease, then the skin graft urethra should be constructed to be approximately 10, 12, or 14 mm. in circumference. Suture material is 6-0 chromic gut. A pointed tongue of the graft is left at the proximal end to fit into the incision in the normal urethral meatus. The distal end of the seam is stopped short of the end of the skin graft tube, and the tongue of the glanular flap is fitted into this gap, preventing a distal circular anastomosis line. Both anastomoses are completed with 6-0 chromic gut sutures (Fig. 53-15). The lateral glanular wings are brought to the midline around the graft and sutured with 6-0 gut interrupted sutures. Once the urethra has been reconstructed, the ventral surface defect must be covered. This is resurfaced with either an Ombrédanne-type hood or a Byars-type midline incision in the remaining prepuce, bringing the prepuce to the ventral side of the penis. The prepuce is usually ample enough that what remains of it can be used to resurface to the base of the penis after removal of sufficient tissue for the graft (Figs. 53-16 and 53-17).

ONE-STAGE REPAIR OF PERINEAL OR SCROTAL HYPOSPADIAS. This hypospadias repair differs in that the scrotum is cleft and there is an unusually severe chordee present. Usually, the prepuce is long enough to resurface only to the base of the penis. To build

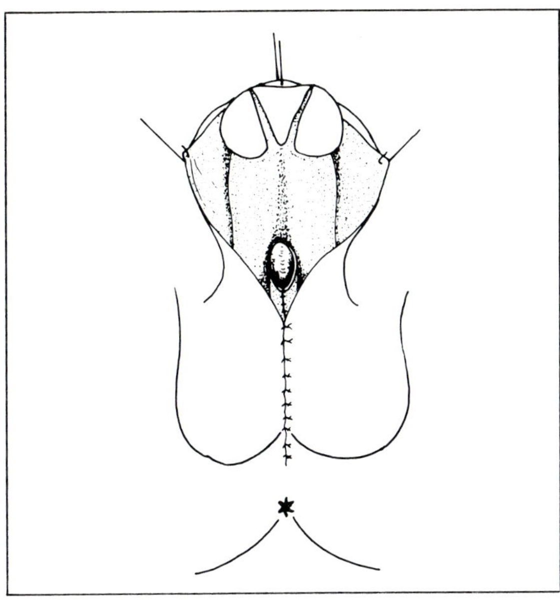

Fig. 53-14. The procedure is carried out in three steps: (1) the midline incision is carried around the urethra proximally and around the glans distally; (2) a midline glanular flap is formed; (3) all abnormal fibrous tissue is excised to expose the corpora.

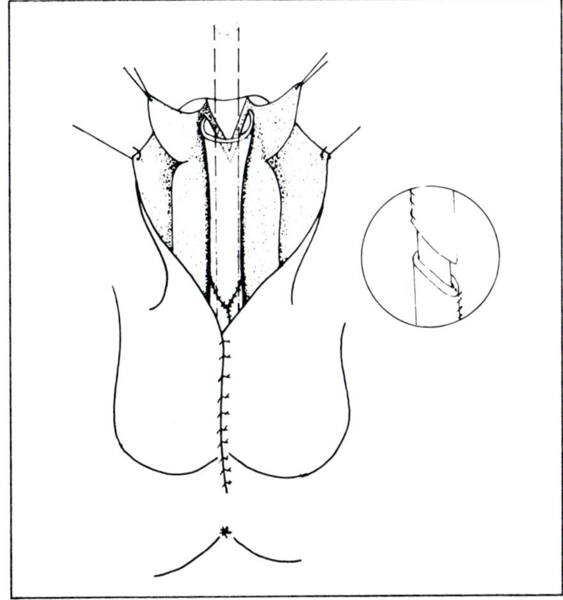

Fig. 53-15. A preputial full-thickness skin graft tube is anastomosed to the distal midline glanular flap and the proximal new urethra.

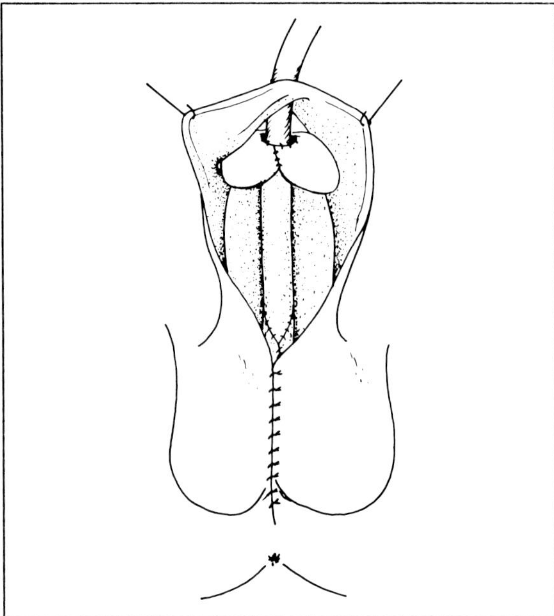

Fig. 53-16. The lateral glanular wings are sutured over the distal urethra. A buttonhole incision is made to transfer the prepuce ventrally.

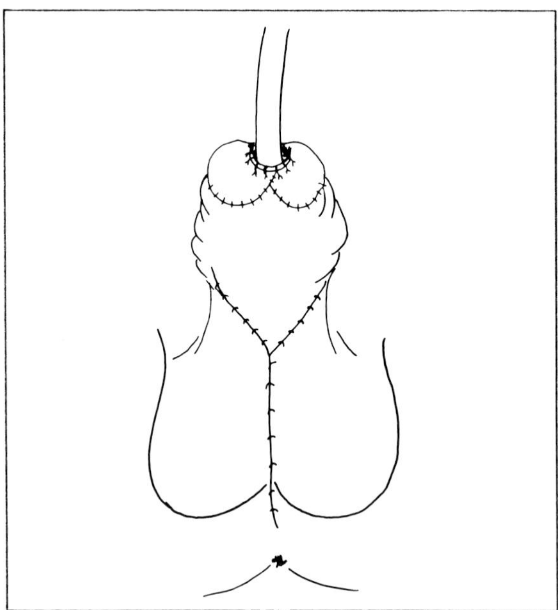

Fig. 53-17. The preputial hood is brought to the ventral surface to complete skin coverage.

the urethra to reach to the base of the penis, a flap is outlined on the hairless skin area within the cleft of the scrotum by making parallel incisions from around the meatus distally to the base of the penis (Fig. 53-18). This flap is elevated, leaving the base attached at the urethral meatus. It is formed into a tube, using 6-0 chromic gut sutures (Fig. 53-19). This maneuver extends the meatus distally to the base of the penis by utilizing the good skin within the cleft of the scrotum (Figs. 53-20 and 53-21). As the scrotal tube is constructed, the tissue causing the chordee is dissected from beneath it. The chordee present in the shaft of the penis is handled as previously described. A preputial skin graft is obtained, tubed over a red rubber catheter stent, and sutured, using an elliptical anastomosis, to the tube of skin constructed from the scrotal cleft. A distal elliptical anastomosis is completed with a glanular triangular flap, and resurfacing to the base of the penis is completed by using either an Ombrédanne-type hood or a Byars midline division of the prepuce. The scrotum is sutured together in the midline to cover the proximal part of the repair and to reconstruct the bifid scrotum.

URINARY DIVERSION. We prefer the use of a #8 Silastic feeding tube taped and sutured into position through the new urethra into the bladder for 3 to 4 days postoperatively to prevent direct urinary contact with the healing suture line in patients with *distal hypospadias* in whom no graft has been necessary. In patients with *proximal penile shaft* or *scrotal* or *perineal hypospadias,* we prefer either a perineal diversion or, if there is not room in the perineal urethra, a suprapubic catheter. After the catheter has been removed, we urge the patient to void frequently so that small volumes are passed and great pressures are not generated by the bladder. We recommend that postoperatively the patient be soaked three times a day in a sterile tub to help decrease edema and to clean the area. We do not remove bandages manually but allow them to soak off in the tubbing process. In shaft or perineal cases, the catheter stent is removed on the seventh postoperative day, and the perineal or suprapubic diversionary catheter is removed in 10 days. The meatus should be cleaned frequently with an antibiotic ointment in an ophthalmic tipped tube. The tip of the tube is gently placed in the meatus to remove all crusts so that plugging of the urethral meatus will not occur. Postoperative calibration or instrumentation is not necessary in the absence of urinary symptoms. If symptoms indicative of stricture or infection occur, the urethra should be calibrated and dilated as necessary.

Complications of Hypospadias Treatment

PREOPERATIVE COMPLICATIONS. If the sex is misdiagnosed prior to surgery or if associated anomalies

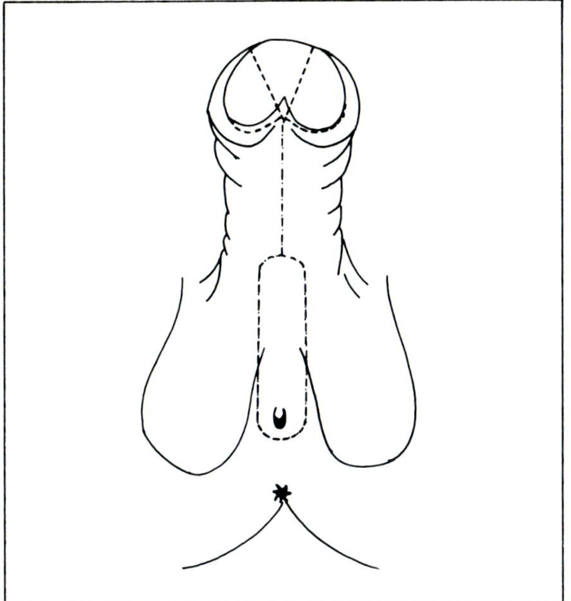

Fig. 53-18. Incisions for scrotal or perineal hypospadias with bifid scrotum.

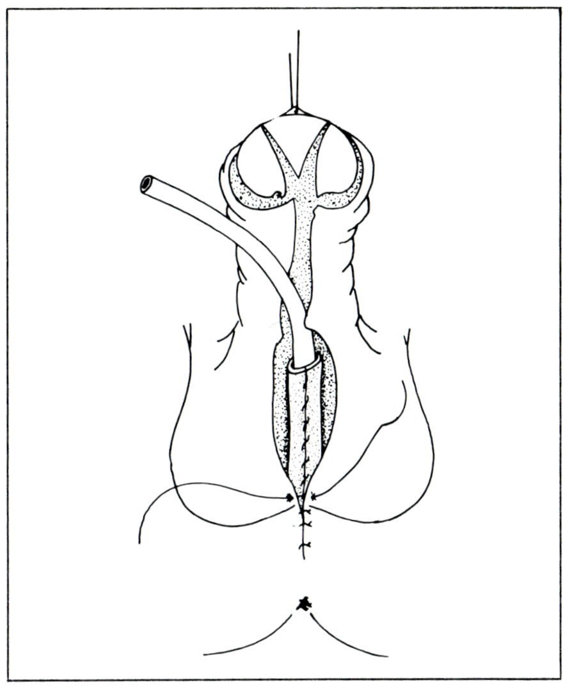

Fig. 53-20. The urethra is elongated with a tube of hairless skin from the cleft of the scrotum.

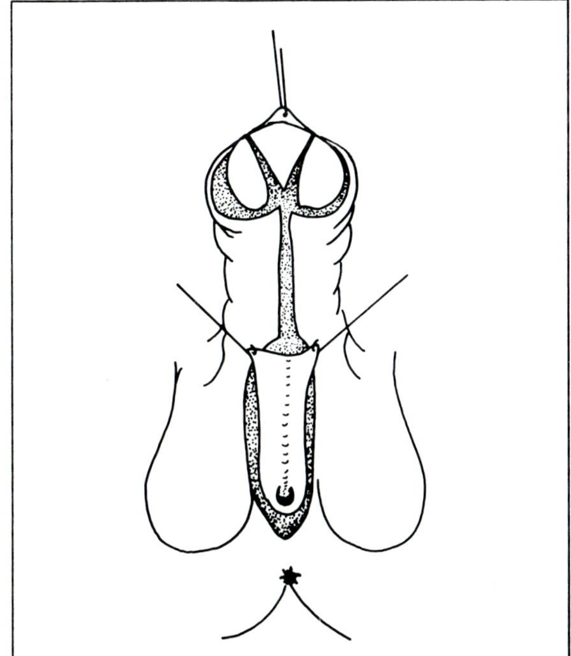

Fig. 53-19. The completed incisions.

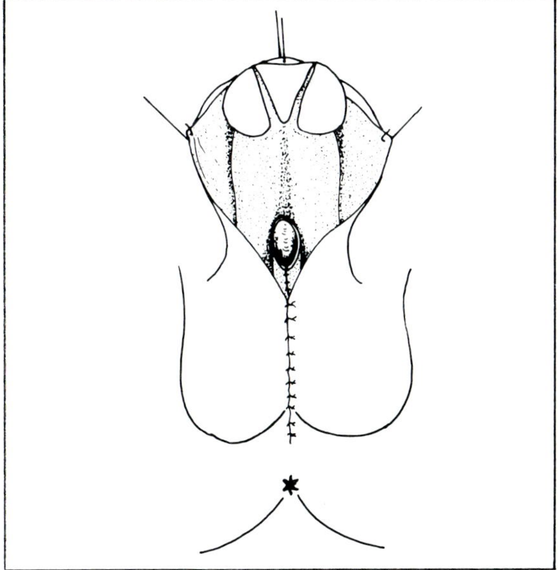

Fig. 53-21. The bifid scrotum is closed to cover the skin tube. The urethral defect is now confined to the penile shaft and can be repaired with the usual technique, utilizing a free, full-thickness preputial skin graft tube.

are undetected, the patient can have irreparable harm done by indiscriminate surgery. All obstructuve uropathy should be corrected, and plans should be formulated for the correction of other anomalies at appropriate times. Circumcision should never be done in cases of hypospadias, even though the degree of hypospadias may be slight. Occasionally more chordee will become evident as the penis grows, and patients who were initially felt not to require surgery may later need correction. This hazard should have been resolved by age 4 years.

The urethral meatus in hypospadiac patients is usually patulous and allows a good urinary stream. Occasionally, however, meatal stenosis occurs. A ventral meatotomy should not be done, because this will cause the meatus to recede further down the penile shaft. A dorsal slit meatotomy may be sufficient in some cases; however, we have found that inserting a triangular flap of glans epithelium into a dorsal meatal slit is the most efficient way to correct meatal stenosis.

POSTOPERATIVE COMPLICATIONS. In our series of one-stage hypospadias repairs, approximately 90 percent of all cases have healed primarily and required no further surgery. No complication has ensued from a one-stage hypospadias repair that would not be expected in a comparable series of multiple-stage repairs. No irreversible results have occurred in our series. Immediate complications are concerned either with infection or skin necrosis due to avascularity of flaps. Should infection or wound dehiscence occur, local and symptomatic treatment should be carried out; but no attempt to resuture the damaged tissue should be made in the immediate healing phase. The wound should be allowed to heal and secondary surgical procedures performed several months later. If hematoma occurs in the immediate postoperative phase, the flaps should be opened and the hematoma evacuated.

Erection after surgery can be a serious problem. We prefer to operate on children 1½ to 2 years of age so that erections will cause little concern. In the teenager or adult, however, postoperative bleeding and pulling apart of sutures can occur as a result of an erection. Amyl nitrate pearls are kept at the bedside so the patient can crush them and inhale the fumes; this seems to control erection immediately. Erotic material should be avoided. Nocturnal erections without conscious control by the patient present a serious problem. Diazepam (Valium) given by mouth may help sedate the patient.

Regardless of the type of surgery utilized, urethrocutaneous fistulas and strictures occur following all hypospadias repairs. The basic principles of atraumatic tissue handling must be observed to prevent crushing of the skin edges and delayed healing. All flaps and grafts used in the formation of the urethra should be adequate in width and should not be stretched. The original urethral meatus must be patulous prior to the construction of the new urethra. Any anastomosis should be constructed with a long ellipse, because a circular anastomosis will contract and cause a stricture.

Postoperative pain caused by bladder spasm is a distressing complication. If the catheter is placed too far into the bladder, it may touch the trigone, which is the most sensitive area of the bladder. In an effort to prevent bladder spasm, we insert the urethrostomy catheter into the bladder, after which we pull it out until the urine flow stops, thus locating the neck of the bladder. The catheter is then inserted 2 cm. further into the bladder and sewn in place so that the point of the catheter will not touch the trigone area. If postoperative spasm occurs, tincture of belladonna and opium rectal suppositories may be indicated. Hot baths may also be of some assistance. The patient must be carefully evaluated for possible urinary infection.

Meatal stenosis had been a common complication in procedures that attempted to bring the urethra to the tip of the penis. We believe stenosis to be caused by the circular anastomosis of the urethral tube and the glans epithelium; additionally, in most procedures a core of glanular tissue is not removed. With the use of our V-shaped glanular flap we have not been troubled by meatal stenosis. This glanular flap can be modified and adapted to many types of hypospadias repair, enabling the operator to place the meatus at the tip of the penis. It is important that all sutures in this flap also catch the tunica of the corpora cavernosa to prevent its being pulled out of the meatus as healing occurs. If postoperative meatal obstruction occurs, a V-shaped glanular flap can be advanced on the dorsal side of the meatus as far internally as necessary to correct the stenosis. As the wider portion of the triangle is advanced into the stenotic area, the caliber of the meatus increases.

Complete breakdown of the hypospadias repair has not occurred in our series. Our most frequent complication of one-stage repairs consisted of small fistulas, usually measuring 1 to 2 mm. in size. Occasionally these fistulas will heal spontaneously without surgical intervention. We recommend that no attempt at fistula repair be made until 6 months after the initial surgery to allow tissue softening and healing. Local treatment with silver nitrate or trichloroacetic acid sometimes stimulates healing. If surgical repair of the fistula is required, the urethra should be calibrated gently to make certain that there is no obstruction distal to the fistula. If a distal obstruction is present, it must be corrected prior to the fistula repair.

Fistula repair is accomplished by careful dissection of the tract to the uroepithelium; the uroepithelium is closed with multiple gut sutures that are placed extraluminally. If the channel of the urethra is diminished by direct closure of the fistulous opening, a small flap based on the side of the fistula can be turned to provide epithelial lining for the urethra. When the uroepithelial surface has been reestablished, the surrounding skin should be undermined widely and closed in multiple layers over the urethra. If excess tissue is present on the ventral surface of the penis, we prefer to sacrifice normal skin from around the fistula repair and to rotate a wide flap over the repair, taking care not to impose the suture lines in the flap over the uroepithelial closure.

Rarely diminution in the size of the urethra will occur postoperatively with a structure formation. These patients should be observed for graft growth maturation, because occasionally as softening occurs the strictures may be dilated adequately by the physiological stretching of voiding. In the event that an intractable stricture occurs, a direct incision should be made over the area and the strictured segment opened. Reconstruction of an adequate urethral channel can be accomplished by a patch graft of full-thickness skin with the epithelial surface placed inside the lumen of the urethra. After wide undermining, the skin can be closed in layers over this repair.

Another rare complication is the development of a diverticulum. When distal obstruction occurs, the proximal urethra may dilate with formation of small epithelial pockets. If this occurs, the distal obstruction should be corrected prior to excision of the diverticulum. The entire sac of diverticulum can be excised and the uroepithelium closed. The overlying tissues should be closed in layers and a catheter kept indwelling for approximately 5 days for urinary diversion.

Hypospadias repair is difficult even in the most experienced hands. While many multiple-stage repairs give excellent results, we feel that the one-stage hypospadias repair is reliable and should be considered by more surgeons. Each operator should be familiar with many types of hypospadias repair, and each procedure must be tailored to the existing condition in a given case. We feel that a normally functioning and appearing penis is possible for all patients with hypospadias. In this area of the body where function of the organ is so dependent on the psyche of the patient (which in turn is influenced by the appearance of the penis), perfection in surgical planning and technique is mandatory.

EPISPADIAS AND EXSTROPHY OF THE BLADDER

Epispadias and exstrophy of the bladder may be defined as congenital deformities of the external genitalia and bladder in which there is failure or blockage of normal development of the dorsal surface of the penis, abdomen, and anterior bladder wall (Figs. 53-22 to 53-24). Although they are not completely understood embryologically, it is essential to consider these defects as varying degrees of a single disorder. It is not known whether the disorder results from a developmental arrest of the lower portion of the urogenital tract or because of an abnormal development of the cloacal membrane. Exstrophy rarely occurs in more than one member of a family, so the parents of children with this unfortunate anomaly can be reassured with some certainty that the chances of future offspring having this disorder are slight.

Exstrophy of the bladder with complete epispadias is the form of the anomaly most commonly seen, occurring in approximately 1 per 30,000 to 40,000 births. It is three to four times more common in males; probably 100 to 150 newborn infants are seen each year in the United States with exstrophy [9]. Complete epispadias or bifid clitoris almost always accompanies exstrophy, but cases of exstrophy with a normal penis have been reported. Exstrophy of the bladder is seen four times more frequently than epispadias alone.

Even though the exstrophy is almost always complete, minor variations of an abdominal wall defect with a superior or inferior vesical fissure may be seen. Simple layered closure of these defects is usually considered adequate treatment.

Repair of Epispadias

In epispadiac deformities distal to the bladder neck, urinary continence is not a problem, so a cosmetically satisfactory and anatomically functional reconstruction should be possible. The abnormal urethral plate is mobilized, all tissues causing chordee are resected, and a U-shaped glans flap is constructed in the midline, to attach to the distal urethra, and lateral glanular wings are used to cover the end of the urethra while reshaping the flat glans into a more normal conical one. It is not necessary to take the urethra to the ventral surface of the penis, if the meatus is placed centrally in the glans. Adequate dissection of the urethra may provide adequate length to the penis, but occasionally the crura of the penis will have to be detached partially from the pubic rami and approximated in the midline to give more length and to restore a more normal angle. This deformity is more difficult to reconstruct than hypospadias, but the same principles may be applied. Additional urethral length may be gained with a full thickness skin graft so that the meatus can be located at the tip of the glans penis. The same catheter-stent technique as suggested for hypospadias cases is used. The corpora are sutured over the graft. Once reconstruction is completed, adequate coverage is achieved by mobilizing local skin flaps as in the hypospadias repair. Postoper-

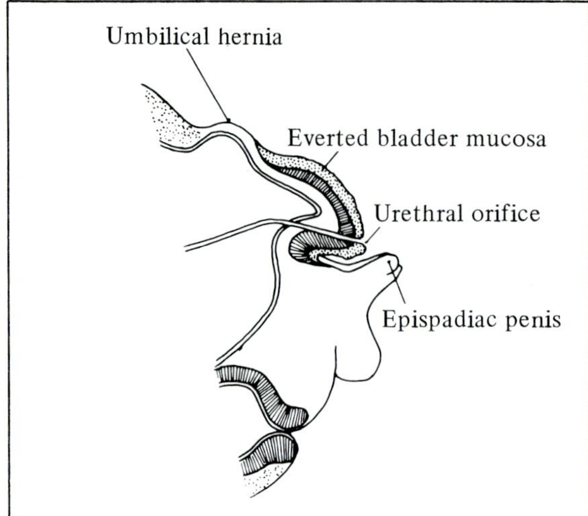

Fig. 53-22. Diagrammatic representation of an epispadiac deformity with associated exstrophy of the bladder.

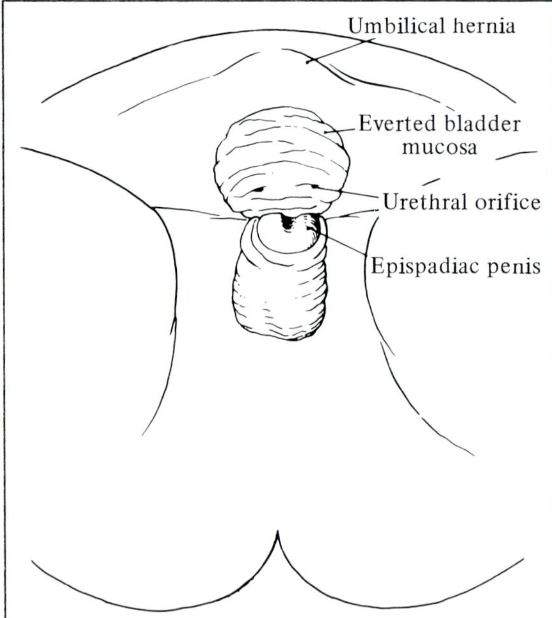

Fig. 53-23. In the usual case of exstrophy of the bladder, the penis is small and almost hidden beneath the painful, tender, exposed bladder mucosa.

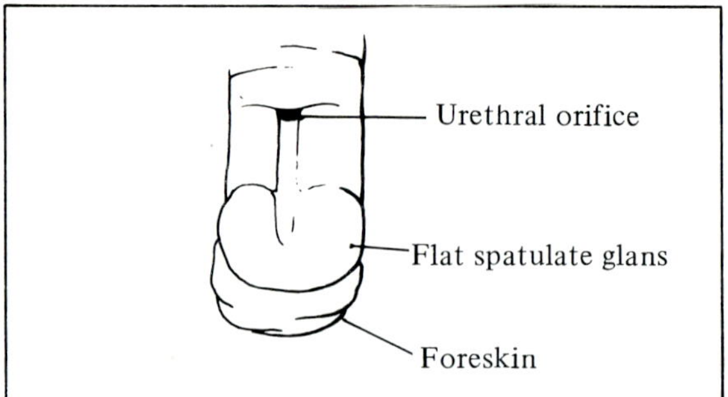

Fig. 53-24. The typical spade penis with a dorsal urethral opening as seen in a moderate epispadiac deformity.

ative management is the same as for hypospadias.

This technique is similar to many other procedures used to repair mild forms of epispadias, except that a full-thickness graft of preputial skin is used to gain additional length in the urethra. It is essential to correct any stenotic portion of the urethra far enough proximally to reach an area of maximal diameter so that the oblique graft-urethra anastomosis can be performed as in the hypospadias technique.

Epispadias associated with bladder-neck and urinary incontinence can usually be repaired functionally by releasing the bladder from the symphysis pubis and resecting a wedge of the anterior bladder neck. This portion of the urethra is closed, and the surrounding tissues that contain the sphincter muscle fibers are imbricated about it. After the sphincter has been reconstructed, the distal urethral deformity is treated as in lesser degrees of epispadias.

Repair of Exstrophy of the Bladder

Exstrophy of the bladder represents a more serious abnormality; there is separation of the symphysis pubis, with widening of the linea alba, and a defect in the abdominal wall. The anterior bladder wall is absent, and the bladder is everted. This is accompanied by incompetence of the upper urinary tract. If this condition is not corrected it results in infection, ureteral dilatation, and renal destruction. An occasional patient whose exstrophy has not been corrected has lived to adult life, but this is unusual. Carcinoma of the bladder frequently develops in older untreated patients [8].

The best treatment for exstrophy of the bladder remains a controversial subject. There are two schools of thought. One advocates urinary diversion, excision of the bladder mucosa, and closure of the abdominal wall defect using bladder muscle with local flaps of striated muscle, fascia, and skin, as well as correction of the deformity of the external genitalia [18]. The other advocates an attempt to gain functional closure of the bladder and provide some degree of continence without obstruction and without causing vesicoureteral reflux along with a repair of deformities of the external genitalia [13].

Urinary Diversion, Excision of Bladder Mucosa, and Closure of Abdominal Wall
No method of treatment for this congenital anomaly is entirely satisfactory. Urinary diversion by ureterocolic anastomosis may provide continence, but a moderate percentage of patients with exstrophy of the bladder also have rectal incontinence. (However, incontinence cannot be assessed in infants.) Long-term results of this procedure have shown that it is not always satisfactory even in those who are continent. Many die early from infection and its complications. Ileal diversion is an alternative, because it provides better protection to the kidneys, but it requires an external collection device. There is still strong feeling that sigmoid diversion is better tolerated in the young patient than in the older. Recently an isolated sigmoid loop diversion has been recommended. This has the advantage that it can be replaced as the patient becomes older if the anal sphincter works adequately.

Functional Closure of Exstrophy of the Bladder
In recent years, surgeons have described a "functional closure" for exstrophy of the bladder. They recommend that this procedure be done either immediately after birth or at approximately 1 year of age. It may be preceded by bilateral iliac osteotomy to bring the symphysis pubis together at the midline, thus reducing the size of the abdominal wall defect and simplifying the closure [16]. Some consider that osteotomy shortens the penis and is unnecessary. The everted bladder is freed from its attachment to the abdominal wall and the edges are approximated with a two-layer closure. The abdominal wall is closed in layers. Flaps of muscle and fascia can be raised to provide anterior wall support. A catheter is left in as a suprapubic drain. Any deformities of the external genitalia are also repaired.

Vesicoureteral reflux is frequent in these reconstructed cases. It is often necessary to do an anti-reflux procedure either at the time of primary closure or later. Because of the distorted nature of the bladder wall and the irregularity of the mucosa, it may be better to delay this procedure. If it is done at the primary stage, reimplanting the ureter would be preferable to an intravesical reinforcing procedure. When the repair is carried out primarily, it is necessary to continue the suprapubic drainage for 6 to 8 weeks to avoid damage to the ureteral repair by increasing intravesical pressure. The suprapubic catheter is then removed, and if necessary, a urethral catheter is inserted until the suprapubic sinus heals.

Snyder [17] has reported an ingenious technique of dividing the sigmoid colon and attaching the distal segment to the posterior bladder wall to serve as a urinary receptacle. The defect of the anterior abdominal wall is closed in layers and the epispadias repaired. The intact anal sphincter provides voluntary control. Preservation of the normal ureterovesical junction decreases the possibility of recurrent complications of reflux. The distal end of transected sigmoid colon is brought through the anal sphincter posterior to the normal anus, thus restoring fecal continence. Although long-term results have not been reported, initial results have been excellent.

In all patients with exstrophy, the degree of continence to be expected depends on the sex of the patient. It is unusual for male patients to become continent. Females have a better chance of being continent after functional closure. All patients develop urinary tract infection and must be maintained on urinary antiseptics or antibiotics. If obstruction becomes a problem – with the sequelae of severe, uncontrollable infection and dilatation and destruction of the upper urinary tract – a diversionary procedure, usually with an ileal loop, should be undertaken.

No current treatment of exstrophy of the bladder is giving good results in all patients. The immediate urinary diversionary procedures, with excision of the exstrophic bladder mucosa and repair of the abdominal defect and external genitalia, can give immediate good results, but the long-term results leave much to be desired. Functional repair of the bladder has also not proved to be an ideal solution. The patient is generally still incontinent and requires constant treatment for urinary infection. However, it seems that this may be the initial treatment of choice, particularly in females. If it fails, a urinary diversionary operation can be carried out. It must be emphasized that protection of renal function is the primary objective of treatment, and all other considerations are secondary [15].

REFERENCES

1. Bialas, R. F., Horton, C. E., and Devine, C. J., Jr. The adaptability of the glans flap in hypospadias repair. *Plast. Reconstr. Surg.* 60:416, 1977.
2. Blair, V. P., and Byars, L. T. Hypospadias and epispadias. *J. Urol.* 40:814, 1938.
3. Browne, D. An operation for hypospadias. *Proc. R. Soc. Med.* 42:466, 1949.
4. Cecil, A. B. Surgery of hypospadias and epispadias in the male. *J. Urol.* 27:507, 1932.
5. Devine, C. J., Jr., and Horton, C. E. Hypospadias repair. *J. Urol.* 118:188, 1977.
6. Devine, C. J., Jr., and Horton, C. E. Surgery of

the Male Genitalia. In Devine, C. J., Jr., and Stecker, J. F., Jr. (Eds.), *Urology in Practice.* Boston: Little, Brown, 1978.

7. Duplay, S. Sur le traitment chirurgical de l'hypospadias et de l'epispadias. *Arch. Gen. Med.* 5:257, 1880.
8. Higgins, C. C. An evaluation of cystectomy: For exstrophy, for papillomatosis, and for carcinoma of the bladder. *J. Urol.* 80:279, 1958.
9. Hoffman, W. W., and Spence, H. M. Management of exstrophy of the bladder. *Southern Med. J.* 58:436, 1965.
10. Horton, C. E. (Ed.). *Plastic and Reconstructive Surgery of the Genital Area.* Boston: Little, Brown, 1973.
11. Horton, C. E., and Carraway, J. H. Plastic Surgery Technique, Wound Healing, Grafts and Flaps in Urology, In Devine, C. J., Jr., and Stecker, J. F., Jr. (Eds.), *Urology in Practice.* Boston: Little, Brown, 1978.
12. Horton, C. E., and Devine, C. J., Jr. Simulated erection of the penis with saline injection; a diagnostic maneuver. *Plast. Reconstr. Surg.* 59:670, 1977.
13. Marshall, V. F., and Muecke, E. C. Variations in exstrophy of the bladder. *J. Urol.* 88:766, 1962.
14. McIndoe, A. The treatment of hypospadias. *Am. J. Surg.* 28:176, 1937.
15. Panel discussion: Anomalies of external genitalia in infancy and childhood. (Harry M. Spence, Moderator; Victor F. Marshall, Discussant.) *J. Urol.* 93:1, 1965.
16. Shultz, W. G. Plastic repair of exstrophy of bladder combined with bilateral osteotomy of ilia. *J. Urol.* 79:453, 1958.
17. Snyder, C. C. A new therapeutic concept of the exstrophied bladder. *Plast. Reconstr. Surg.* 22:1, 1958.
18. Sweetser, T. H., Chisholm, T. C., Thompson, W. H., Berglund, E. B., Wesolowski, S. P., and Sweetser, T. H., Jr. Exstrophy of the urinary bladder: Its treatment by plastic surgery. *J. Urol.* 75:448, 1956.

Injuries of the Male Genitalia

JULIUS A. HOWELL

Injuries of the male genitalia such as contusions, lacerations, avulsion wounds, and burns are not encountered very often. Avulsion wounds are by far the most common, and are usually caused when a patient's clothing becomes entangled in moving machinery. As the clothing is torn from the body, the skin covering the shaft of the penis, the scrotum, and sometimes the perineum is partially or completely avulsed. Other injuries to this area result from automobile accidents, war wounds, surgical procedures, and the trouser zipper. Occasionally, the shaft of the penis may be partially or completely amputated.

Burns of this region can be thermal, electrical, or chemical. Chemical burns should be thoroughly washed to remove all of the offending agents. Such injuries frequently cause only a superficial or second-degree skin loss, which heals without the necessity of skin grafting. Electrical burns are often the full-thickness type and require cleaning, debriding, and skin grafting by the usual technique. In deeper burns of the penis, it may be necessary to wait for demarcation if viable tissue cannot be distinguished from nonviable.

INJURIES OF THE PENIS

Lacerations

Simple lacerations of the male genitalia are rare. The skin around them should be washed thoroughly and the wounds sutured with either absorbable sutures (i.e., 4-0 Dexon) or nonabsorbable sutures (i.e., 4-0 silk). A dressing can be held in position with an athletic supporter, which provides mild compression.

Salvatierra and others [22], reporting on a large series of urological war injuries in Vietnam, believed that anatomical approximation of Buck's fascia was possible in most cases and that such early repair was important in preventing later deformity. The penile skin was closed in about half of their series of patients, but where the defect was large it was left open, the skin closing being carried out secondarily at a later date.

The "zipper syndrome" has been noted by Lapidus and Graham [18]. Although not serious it is most painful. It occurs most often in juveniles and more often in uncircumcised than in circumcised patients. Nylon zippers have caused an increase in the incidence of this injury.

Strangulation Injuries

Strangulation injuries of the penis are caused by encircling bands, such as rings or rubber bands. These injuries should be treated conservatively after all obviously necrotic tissue has been removed and a catheter passed through an external urethrotomy [10].

A rather rare penile injury is a fracture that occurs from a direct blow to the erect penis. The characteristic pathology is a tear in the tunica albuginea with hemorrhage, hematoma, and distortion of the penis [5]. Hudson [14] has described a case of rupture of the corpus cavernosum. Early surgical repair rather than conservative management is the treatment of choice today; however, in some cases it has been necessary to delay the operation, and erectile difficulty with bending during erection has occurred [5, 24, 25]. Waterhouse and Gross [9, 25] stress the evacuation of the hematoma and the repair of the corpora in all cases of rupture of the corpora cavernosa.

Avulsion of Skin

In avulsion injuries, skin at the base of the penis may be partially or completely torn away, along with a varying amount of the skin of the scrotum and perineum. In such cases the patient does not usually experience much pain, and blood loss is not great owing to the fact that the tissue separates in a relatively bloodless plane. By contrast, injuries involving the body of the penis may bleed so profusely as to require a tourniquet for control. The skin over the glans, being firmly attached, is not avulsed easily.

Psychological and endocrinological evaluations done at intervals are of value from both the diagnostic and therapeutic standpoints. Baxter and others [2] outline the surgical requirements: (1) a soft flexible cover for the penis to facilitate return of sensation; and (2) adequate protective covering for the testes to preserve their physiological function and permit normal activity.

If the patient is seen within the first few hours after injury, the penis will be in erection. Emergency care includes the use of warm saline compresses, antibiotics, and gas and tetanus antitoxin. To prevent wound sepsis, the denuded penile shaft should be grafted as soon as possible, preferably within the first 6 to 12 hours. Avulsed penile skin should not be reapplied as a full-thickness skin graft because of its tendency to slough. It is better to discard it and to resurface the defect with a fresh, thick split-thickness skin graft. According to Hawtrey and others [12], a split-thickness graft possesses antibacterial properties that tend to sterilize granulation tissue or to protect the wound from being colonized by bacteria. He and his group used split-thickness skin grafts almost exclusively when large surface areas were involved, but used heterografts otherwise. Impotence was not encountered and patients in whom the testes had been placed in thigh pockets were able to father children. May [19], on the other hand, suggests the use of the torn penile skin unless it is too dirty and ragged for resurfacing the avulsion defect. Kendall [17] recommends use of scrotal skin to cover the denuded penis, although, if the defect is large or if adequate scrotal skin is not available, a thick split-thickness graft can be used. Huffman and co-workers [15] report that marked edema, which persists for a long time, will follow the reapplication of partly avulsed skin to the penis. Other surgeons have used abdominal flaps, but these are likely to produce an organ that is excessively large, bizarre in shape, and hairy [15]. Surgical procedures such as this require a series of operations and do not provide the best coverage for the penis [7].

When skin has been partially denuded from an area near the base of the penis, the defect can be covered with a pedicle flap from the adjacent scrotal skin [3]. Goodwin and Thelen [8] recommend closing raw areas on the shaft by implanting the denuded surface under the elastic tissue of the scrotum.

Treatment of Avulsion of the Penile Skin

For repairing avulsion injuries of the penis, the patient is given a general anesthesia and the penile shaft is thoroughly washed with a soapy solution and flushed copiously with saline solution. Debridement is carried out and complete hemostasis obtained. A split-thickness skin graft, 10 × 20 cm. in area and 0.020 to 0.024 inch in thickness, is removed from the thigh or the abdomen with a Reese or Padgett dermatome and draped around the penis so that the suture line will lie on the dorsum (Fig. 54-1). The edges of the graft are trimmed to make a zigzag closure along the dorsum, and it is sutured with interrupted 4-0 chromic cargut. Interrupted 3-0 silk sutures are used to attach the graft to adjacent skin proximally and distally; the ends of the sutures are left long so that they can be tied over a bolus of sponge rubber. These sutures are tied in a longitudinal direction under sufficient tension to hold the dressing snugly in place [11]. The glans penis remains exposed to allow frequent observation for circulatory impairment. Some surgeons use bromides or diethylstilbestrol to reduce the erection; however, I agree with Huffman and others [16] that this has never caused a problem.

The initial dressing is not changed for 10 to 14 days, and the indwelling urethral catheter is removed only after 2 weeks. Such catheters are irrigated daily with sterile water or saline solution to prevent any

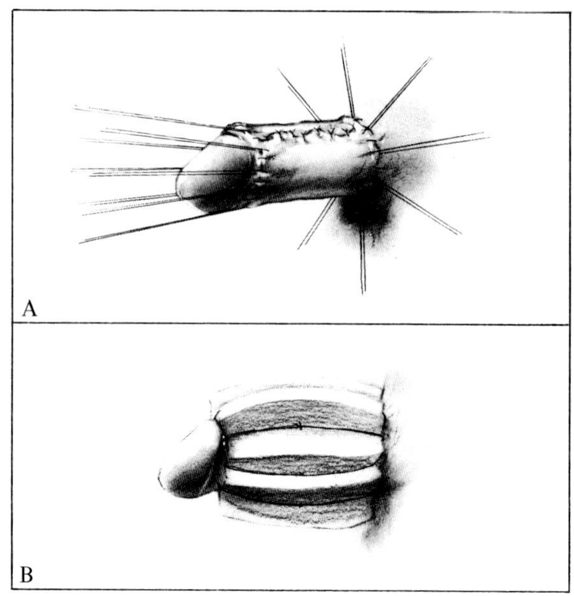

Fig. 54-1. Skin graft to replace avulsed penile skin. A, split-thickness skin graft, 0.020 to 0.024 inch thick, is placed around the penis so that the suture line lies on the dorsum. The edges of the graft are trimmed to make a zigzag closure around the dorsum. B, a tie-over dressing with a bolus of sponge rubber holds the skin graft in place.

accumulation of deposits that would interfere with drainage of urine. Urinary chemotherapy is given while the catheter is in place.

The patient should remain in bed for 5 to 7 days except for a few minutes daily when he can sit in a chair or on the edge of the bed. The entire dressing is removed in 10 to 14 days; thereafter a dressing over the newly grafted skin is usually not necessary. The graft is firmly adherent after 4 weeks, but sexual intercourse is not permitted until after 6 weeks. There have been no reports of the patient's sexual life being altered by skin grafting of the shaft. Early postoperative erections pose no problem [15]. The split-thickness skin grafts expand sufficiently to allow unrestricted erection within a few weeks following surgery.

Amputation

Partial amputation of the penile shaft and glans penis is associated with considerable bleeding. After debridement and control of hemorrhage, a skin graft is applied to the denuded portion; it is sutured to the urethra distally and to the remaining margin of the penile skin proximally. The sutures are tied over a bolus, as described before. Sutures placed in the urethra have not pulled out or posed any problem. In the rare case of complete amputation, reanastomosis is technically possible but extremely difficult. Schulman [23], in 1973, reported the eighth successful case of reanastomosis of a traumatically amputated penis; however in that case the amputation was partial. When reanastomosis is not attempted in cases of complete amputation, the stump is oversewn with 3-0 sutures to close the wound and preserve as much tissue as possible.

INJURIES OF THE SCROTUM

Penetrating Scrotal Wound

Penetrating wounds of the scrotum are most often seen in war injuries [22]. The scrotum has an elastic expansile capacity that allows it to hold a large amount of blood with no tamponade effect. Extreme conservatism is emphasized by Salvatierra and associates [22] in the treatment of testicular injuries.

Avulsion of Scrotal Skin

Partial or complete avulsion of the scrotal skin is usually accompanied by severe trauma to the penis. Complete loss of the scrotum is also often associated with varying degrees of perineal avulsion; since the rectal sphincter is occasionally torn, digital examination is important to test its function [4]. Millard [20] suggests use of a split-thickness skin graft. The vas deferens and the neurovascular pedicles are partially retracted up into the inguinal canals, and the testicles are sutured to each other and to the Colles fascia in order to present one reasonably regular mass to receive the skin graft. Others [19] believe that the irregularity of the testicles and the inadvisability of applying proper pressure do not favor regeneration of a free graft; therefore, the simplest way to provide coverage would be the formation of a subcutaneous pocket on the medial surface of the thighs to receive the structures. Robinson and Masters [21] have pointed out that in the rare instance in which neither local thigh nor inguinal skin is available, the denuded shaft and testicles should be resurfaced with split-thickness skin grafts. Contraction of the skin grafts, however, is likely to produce severe distortion and reproductive function is destroyed.

Treatment of Avulsed Scrotal Skin

After evaluating an injury involving the scrotum, securing hemostasis, and debriding the wound, closure can be carried out. When there is sufficient skin, the deeper tissues can be closed with interrupted sutures of 4-0 plain catgut, and the skin is closed with interrupted sutures of 4-0 silk. A firm supportive dressing is applied using an athletic supporter. It is surprising how little skin is required to completely close a wound of the scrotum after partial avulsion, and often a small patch of remaining skin may be sufficient to cover the testes. Although initially tight, the skin stretches and the scrotum will expand to nearly normal size.

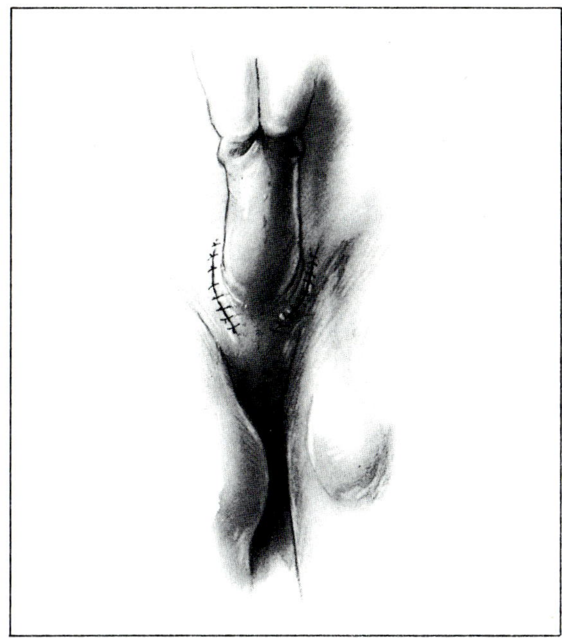

Fig. 54-2. The testicles and their spermatic cords are buried beneath the skin of the upper thigh following avulsion of scrotal skin. Through an incision just lateral to the base of the penis, a pocket is made beneath the skin of the medial thigh, with dissection as far posterior as the length of the spermatic cord permits. One pocket is placed slightly below the other to prevent friction between the two.

When there is insufficient scrotal skin to close an avulsion wound, the usual method of management is to bury the testicles and their spermatic cords in an adjacent pocket beneath the skin of the upper thigh [7]. The best position on the thigh is as far posterior as the length of the spermatic cord permits. The testicles should be embedded at different levels so they do not lie opposite each other; then there will be little or no discomfort even when the patient abducts his thighs or crosses his legs.

An incision is made just lateral to the base of the penis, on either side, and pockets are created just beneath the skin by blunt dissection (Fig. 54-2). The testicles are buried in them and held there by silk traction sutures [7].

Culp and Huffman [6] carried out studies to determine the advisability of burying exposed testes at this site. Their findings indicated that such implantations just beneath the skin provided an environment sufficiently cool to permit normal spermatogenesis, whereas the higher temperatures beneath the subcutaneous fat might be expected to lead to regression and disorganization of spermatogenesis.

Injuries of the Urethra

Trauma to the male urethra is fairly frequent and usually results from a "straddle" type of injury in which the urethra is crushed against the pubic arch in fractures of the pelvis. The urethra may also be injured by avulsions and penetrating wounds.

When the injury is only a simple contusion of the urethra or a minimal tear of the urethral mucosa, the diagnosis is made by passing a Foley catheter into the bladder. Treatment involves bed rest, the application of cold compresses, and catheter drainage of the bladder for 5 to 7 days.

Discoloration of the skin of the penis and immediate local swelling are indicative of rupture of the urethra, with blood escaping from the tear into the adjacent tissues. It is imperative that all extravasated blood and urine be drained promptly, and the urinary stream should be diverted by either a perineal urethrostomy or a suprapubic cystostomy.

A fairly high percentage of patients who have sustained urethral injury will develop strictures. Conservative therapy for this complication is indicated, at least at first, with the urethra being dilated at frequent intervals. Later, dilations may be carried out at intervals of 4 months or longer until the stricture no longer obstructs urinary drainage.

REFERENCES

1. Anderson, B. L., and Pless, J. Fracture of the penis. *Plastikkir. Afd. Odense Syngch. Odense Ugenkrloeg.* 138:1034, 1976.
2. Baxter, H., Hoffman, M., Smith, E., and Stern, K. Complete avulsion of skin of penis and scrotum; surgical, endocrinological and psychological treatment. *Plast. Reconstr. Surg.* 4:508, 1949.
3. Brown, J. B., and Fryer, M. P. Surgical reconstruction of the penis. *G.P.* 17:104, 1958.
4. Bruner, J. Traumatic avulsion of the skin of the external male genitalia. *Plast. Reconstr. Surg.* 6:334, 1950.
5. Creecy, A. A., and Beazlie, R. S., Jr. Fracture of the penis: Traumatic rupture of the corpora cavernosa. *J. Urol.* 78:620, 1957.
6. Culp, D. A., and Huffman, W. C. Temperature determination in the thigh with regard to burying the traumatically exposed testis. *J. Urol.* 76:436, 1956.
7. Davis, A. D., and Berner, R. E. Primary repair of total avulsion of skin from the penis and scrotum. *Plast. Reconstr. Surg.* 3:417, 1948.
8. Goodwin, W. E., and Thelen, H. M. Plastic reconstruction of the penile skin: Implantation of the penis into the scrotum. *J.A.M.A.* 144:384, 1950.
9. Gross, M., Arnold, T. L., and Waterhouse, K. Fracture of the penis: Rationale of surgical management. *J. Urol.* 106:708, 1971.
10. Hamm, F. C., and Waterhouse, K. Injuries of the Genital Tract. In Campbell, J. (Ed.), *Urology.* Philadelphia: Saunders, 1963.
11. Hand, J. R. Surgery of the Penis and Urethra. In Campbell, J. (Ed.), *Urology.* Philadelphia: Saunders, 1963.
12. Hawtrey, C. E., Culp, D. A., and Hartford, C. E. The management of severe inflammatory and traumatic injuries to the genital skin. *J. Urol.* 108:431, 1972.
13. Horton, C. E. (Ed.). *Plastic and Reconstructive Surgery of the Genital Area.* Boston: Little, Brown, 1973.
14. Hudson, M. J. K. Rupture of the corpus cavernosum of the penis. *Br. J. Clin. Pract.* 29:191, 1975.
15. Huffman, W. C., Culp, D. A., and Flocks, R. H. Injuries of the External Male Genitalia. In Converse, J. M. (Ed.), *Reconstructive Plastic Surgery.* Philadelphia: Saunders, 1964.
16. Huffman, W. C., Culp, D. A., Greenleaf, J. S., Flocks, R. H., and Grintnall, E. S. Injuries of male genitalia. *Plast. Reconstr. Surg.* 18:344, 1956.
17. Kendall, A. R., and Karafin, L. Repair of the denuded penis. *J. Urol.* 98:484, 1967.
18. Lapidus, S. M., and Graham, W. P. Complete avulsion of the genital skin. *Pa. Med.* 76:38, 1973.
19. May, H. Reconstruction of scrotum and skin of penis. *Plast. Reconstr. Surg.* 6:134, 1950.
20. Millard, D. R., Jr. Scrotal construction and reconstruction. *Plast. Reconstr. Surg.* 38:10, 1966.
21. Robinson, D. W., and Masters, F. W. The treatment of avulsion of the male genitalia. *J. Trauma* 8:436, 1968.
22. Salvatierra, O., Jr., Rigdon, W. O., Norris, D. M., and Brady, T. W. Vietnam experience with 252 urological war injuries. *J. Urol.* 101:615, 1969.
23. Schulman, M. L. Reanastomosis of the amputated penis. *J. Urol.* 109:432, 1973.
24. Thompson, R. F. Rupture (fracture) of the penis. *J. Urol.* 71:226, 1954.
25. Waterhouse, L., and Gross, M. Trauma to the genitourinary tract: A 5-year experience with 251 cases. *J. Urol.* 101:241, 1969.

Vaginal Agenesis

DONALD R. LAUB AND BRUCE J. DUBIN

A woman born without a functioning vagina is deprived of both coitus and childbearing. The body image is disturbed and the patient develops deep-seated doubts about her femininity. The resultant psychological discord may be reflected in all aspects of her life. In addition, a certain subgroup of patients may develop severe physiological derangements, secondary to intact cyclical ovarian function.

This entity is by no means rare and is a frequent cause of primary amenorrhea [18]. The incidence of congenital absence of the vagina is usually stated to be 1 out of 4,000 to 5,000 females [6, 8, 18], but estimates in the literature vary from 1 out of 1,500 to 1 out of 80,000 [11]. Partial or complete absence of the vagina requiring surgical reconstruction may be part of several distinct syndromes.

In this chapter we will discuss the relevant embryology of the female reproductive tract, the differential diagnosis of partial and complete vaginal absence, the work-up of such a patient, and the methods currently available for reconstruction.

EMBRYOLOGY

In order to understand the possible etiologies of this condition, one must have a knowledge of the normal development of the genitourinary tract (Fig. 55-1). At about 5 weeks of gestation, sexually indifferent gonads begin to differentiate from the urogenital ridges, which are posterior thickenings of the coelomic epithelium. Differentiation into ovary or testis is determined by the sex chromosomes of the embryo. If the sex karyotype is XX, ovaries are formed; if the sex karyotype is XY, testes are formed. At about the same time that the gonads are differentiating, the mesonephroi develop from the nephrogenic cord. These primitive excretory organs consist of a series of tubules that join the mesonephric or wolffian ducts, which extend down to the cloaca. The mesonephric ducts open into the urogenital sinus. The ureters develop as diverticulae from the caudal portions of the mesonephric ducts near the urogenital sinus. The ureter, in turn, induces development of the metanephros, which will become the definitive adult kidney. The metanephros originally develops in the pelvis and then later ascends to the adult position. (This will be helpful in understanding some of the renal anomalies associated with vaginal atresias.)

If the embryo is female and hence has a primitive ovary, the absence of the two testicular-derived compounds leads to growth and development of the müllerian ducts and regression of the wolffian ducts, which in the adult female are represented by the epoophoron, the paraoophoron, and Gartner's duct.

The solid cords of proliferating mesothelial cells that make up the müllerian ducts grow caudally and canalize. When they contact the dorsal wall of the urogenital sinus, they elevate it to form the müllerian tubercle. The two müllerian ducts fuse above this level to form a single duct with two lumens. By 16 weeks of gestation, this septum disappears, forming a single uterus. The fallopian tubes are derived from the cephalic unfused portions of the müllerian ducts. Epithelium next to the müllerian tubercle proliferates at 8 weeks to form the paired sinovaginal bulbs, which form a solid cord – the vaginal plate – connecting the urogenital sinus to the fused müllerian ducts. This vaginal plate canalizes by 22 weeks to form the vagina.

The conventional embryological teaching is that the müllerian ducts give origin to the tubes, uterus, and cervix and the proximal 70 to 80 percent of the vagina, while the remaining distal external portion of the vagina is derived from the urogenital sinus. The junction of these two parts is represented by the hymen. Recently, an alternate hypothesis has been suggested, in which müllerian-derived tissues extend to the level of the hymen but are invaded and replaced by cells from the urogenital sinus up to the level of the external os [28]. Thus, according to this hypothesis, the vagina consists of tissue derived from both müllerian and urogenital sinus origins. This theory helps to explain the condition of vaginal adenosis found in girls who were exposed in utero to diethylstilbestrol. The adenosis extending for variable distances below the cervix is thought to represent rests of müllerian-derived lining that fail to be replaced by advancing lining derived from the urogenital sinus [28]. Interestingly, the prenatal influence of estrogen is related to adenocarcinoma of the vagina in young women.

The external genitalia of both sexes are derived from a common genital eminence that differentiates into male or female external genitalia under the influence of androgens or estrogens, respectively. The development of the external genitalia, illustrated in Figure 55-2, is beyond the scope of this discussion.

DIFFERENTIAL DIAGNOSIS

Congenital Absence of the Vagina

Congenital absence of the vagina is also known as the

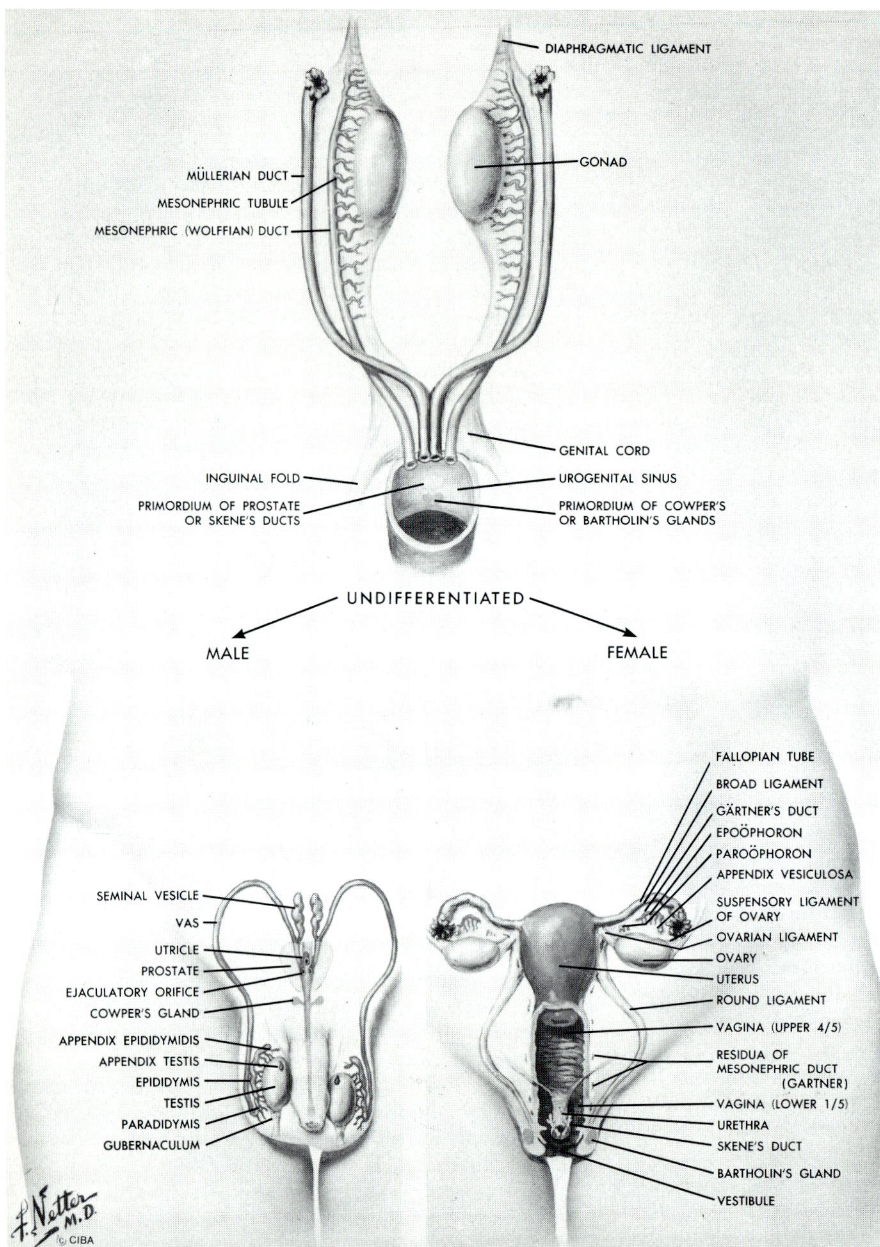

Fig. 55-1. Development of the male and female internal genitalia. In the male, the wolffian ducts give rise to the adult structures while the müllerian ducts regress. The opposite occurs in the female. (©1954-1965 CIBA Pharmaceutical Company, Division of CIBA-GEIGY Corporation. From The CIBA Collection of Medical Illustrations *by Frank H. Netter, M.D. All rights reserved.)*

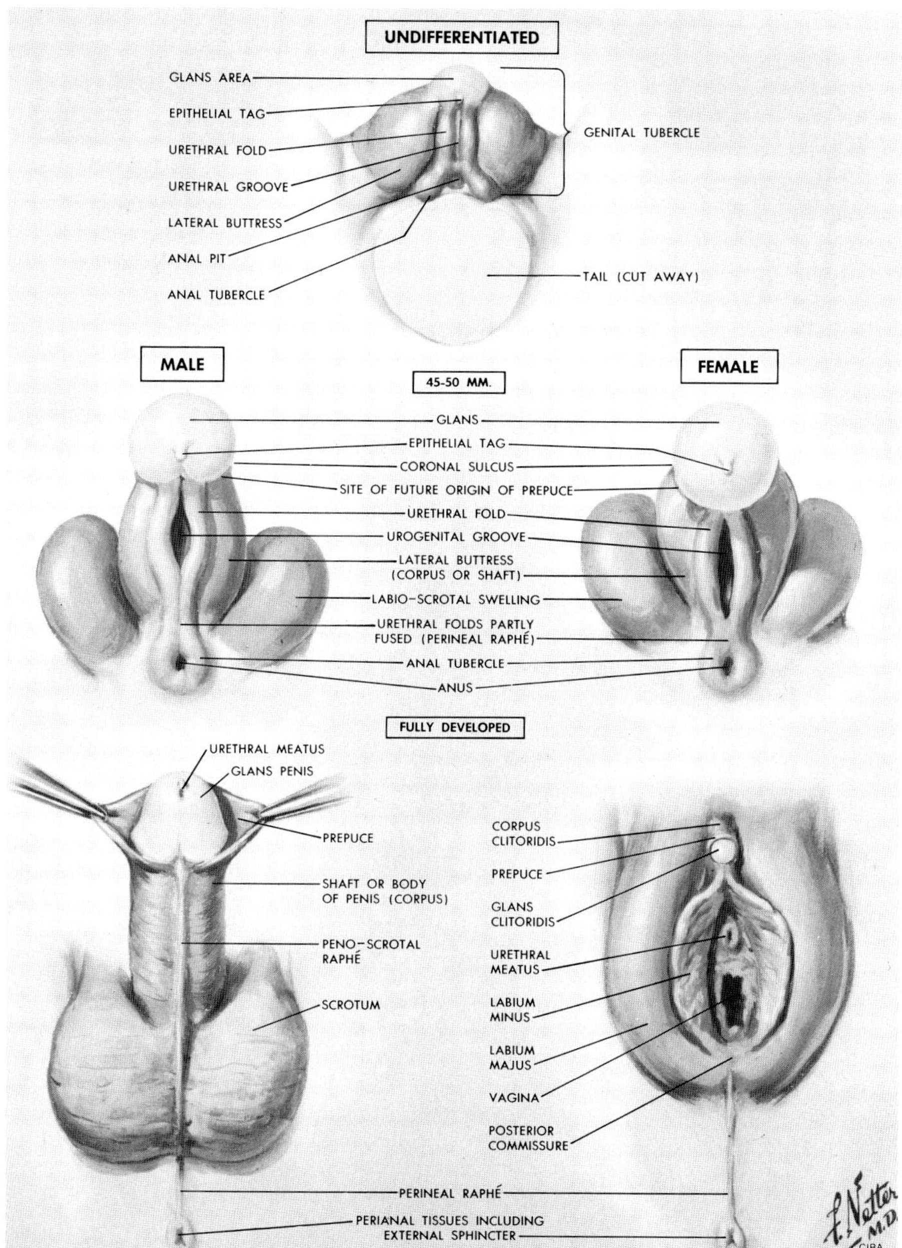

Fig. 55-2. Development of the male and female external genitalia. There is a homologous development of the male and female structures from the embryologic anlage. (©1954-1965 CIBA Pharmaceutical Company, Division of CIBA-GEIGY Corporation. From The CIBA Collection of Medical Illustrations *by Frank H. Netter, M.D. All rights reserved.)*

Rokitansky-Kuster-Hauser syndrome [18]. Patients with this disorder have a normal female karyotype and typically present at the age of menarche or later because of primary amenorrhea. Some patients present because of the inability to accomplish intercourse. Rarely is the anomaly discovered at birth. The findings include a normal vulva with an absent vagina or a vagina that is represented by a shallow 1- to 2-cm. dimple. There is usually absence of the uterus and cervix, which are represented by bilateral noncanalized muscular bands. The ovaries are normal and there is normal cyclical ovarian function as reflected by circulating hormone levels and by ovulation. The fallopian tubes may or may not be normal, but complete absence is rare [15]. The female breasts, pubic and axillary hair, and female body habitus develop normally. In less than 10 percent of the patients, a functioning uterus and cervix and an upper vaginal segment are present [15, 17]. These patients present with hematometra, hematocolpos, monthly episodes of abdominal pain, and an increasing abdominal mass due to the accumulation of menstrual products. After the surgical construction of a vagina, these patients may become pregnant.

There is a very high association of renal anomalies, ranging from 34 to 49 percent, depending on the series [5, 11, 13, 18]. Skeletal abnormalities occur in 10 to 15 percent of patients [11, 18].

It appears that the occurrence of this condition is sporadic. Lischke and co-workers [22] have demonstrated a lack of concordance in a series of 3 pairs of monozygotic twins. Despite a report by Jones and Mermut [20] of a high incidence in a particular family, most authors feel that there is generally not a familial incidence [33] but that there is a multifactorial etiology.

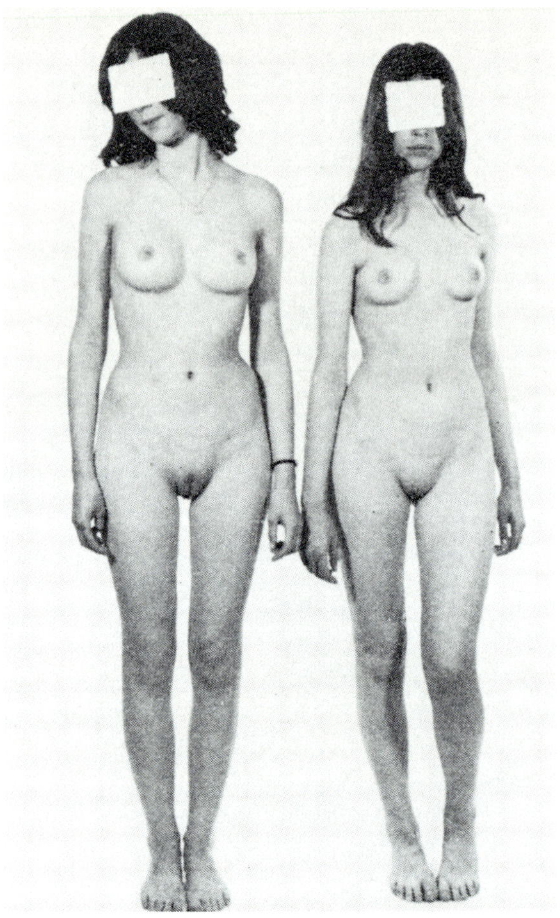

Fig. 55-3. Testicular feminization syndrome. These "sisters" have normal female phenotypes despite male karyotypes. (From C. J. Dewhurst, Clin. Endocrinol. *4:625, 2975.)*

Testicular Feminization Syndrome

Patients with the testicular feminization syndrome (also known as the androgen insensitivity syndrome) superficially resemble those with congenital absence of the vagina but the two are really quite different, as the patients with testicular feminization syndrome are actually genetic males. Initial presentation is at puberty or thereafter because of primary amenorrhea. Examination reveals an individual with a normal female body habitus, normal female breast development, and normal external female genitalia (Fig. 55-3). In most of the patients, there is sparse development of axillary and pubic hair [14]. The vagina may be of variable length but ends in a blind pouch without a cervix. Often there are bilateral inguinal hernias. The physician's suspicion should be aroused as to the possible presence of this syndrome when confronted with a female infant with bilateral inguinal hernias. Further evaluation shows that there is an absence of internal female genitalia except for rudimentary anlage of müllerian structures, and the patients are therefore sterile. Intraabdominal or inguinal gonads are present in the form of testes. Histological examination of these testes shows an absence of spermatogenesis but an increase in Leydig cells. Hormonal analysis reveals that these testes secrete both androgens and estrogens. Chromosomal analysis demonstrates a male karyotype. Unlike congenital absence of the vagina, testicular feminization syndrome has a high familial incidence [14, 15]. Genetic transmission is by way of maternal carriers, but the exact mechanism still has not been determined [24].

Currently, the most likely explanation for this syndrome is that there is a deficiency in the androgen receptors and therefore an inability to concentrate

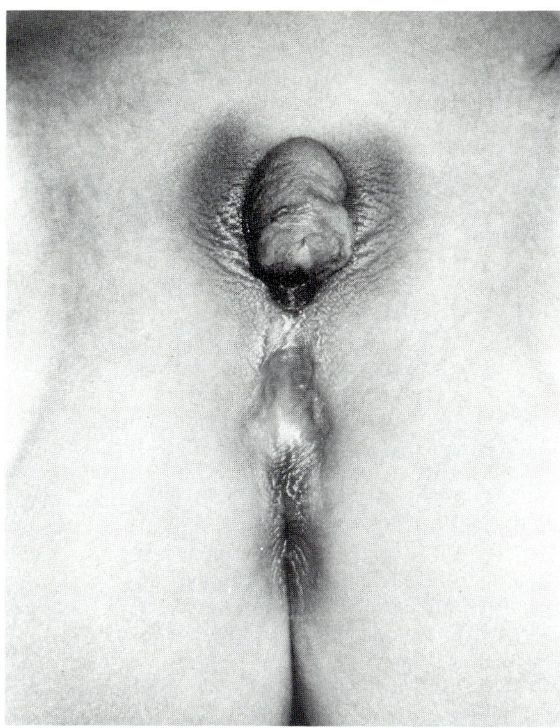

Fig. 55-4. Adrenogenital syndrome. The external genitalia of this female infant are masculinized and ambiguous as a result of the influence of adrenal androgens. (Photograph courtesy of Luigi Luzzati, M.D.)

androgens at the active sites in the cell nucleus. Thus, the testes secrete normal amounts of androgens but because the cells of the body are not able to respond to them, no virilization takes place and the body develops a female phenotype in response to the testicular estrogens that are produced.

For the sake of completeness, it should be noted that there are several incomplete forms of testicular feminization syndrome; the interested reader is referred to the articles by Glenn [14] and by Dewhurst [9].

Those patients with testicular feminization syndrome who have markedly underdeveloped vaginas will need surgical construction of a serviceable vagina. There is a relatively high incidence, as high as 33 percent according to Federman [10], of malignant degeneration of the testes, which are therefore best removed after puberty. The patient will then need exogenous estrogens to avoid menopause-like symptoms.

The Adrenogenital Syndrome

The adrenogenital syndrome is due to a genetically determined defect in the metabolic pathway of cortisol synthesis [10]. The resulting impaired cortisol production leads to overstimulation of the adrenal by ACTH, causing overproduction of adrenal androgens. In the female fetus, this leads to virilization of the external genitalia, manifested by varying degrees of clitoral hypertrophy, labial fusion, and underdevelopment of the vagina (Fig. 55-4). The internal genitalia develop normally, because there are no testes to produce müllerian-inhibiting substance. These girls are potentially fertile.

The diagnosis of this condition should be made at birth or shortly thereafter and the patient treated with exogenous corticosteroids. The physician caring for these infants should be alert to those forms of the syndrome that are characterized by severe salt-wasting, which may lead to severe dehydration and shock in the infant. These children should be raised as females; those who are more extensively virilized will need corrective genital surgery that may include vaginal construction.

Gonadal Dysgenesis

Patients with gonadal dysgenesis (Turner's syndrome) are characterized by a female phenotype, an XO karyotype, short stature, streak gonads, and various other congenital anomalies such as webbing of the neck and shortness of the fourth and fifth metacarpals. Despite the gonadal dysgenesis, these patients have female internal and external genitalia, although the genitalia remain infantile and amenorrhea is the rule. Some of these patients will need vaginal reconstruction to create a serviceable vagina. Various forms of mosaicism (the most common ix XO/XX) may also exist; these patients generally have a greater degree of feminization.

Hermaphroditism and Other Intersex Conditions

By definition, a true hermaphrodite has gonadal tissue of both sexes; it may be separate or combined as an ovotestis. Most true hermaphrodites have an XX karyotype, Pseudohermaphroditism includes a variety of intersex conditions involving ambiguous external genitalia but with only one type of gonadal tissue. A full discussion of these conditions is beyond the scope of this chapter. In general terms, the sex of assignment and rearing should be based on the external anatomy so that the patient will be most likely to attain normal adult sexual function. If the phallus appears inadequate, the patient should be assigned as a female and reared as such, regardless of the chromosomal or gonadal sex. However, caution must be exercised in cases of microphallus, as a surprising growth potential may be present. For example, in severe perineal hypospadias, the penis may grow to adequate size following early release of the chordee. The sex assignment must be made as early as possible to allow appropriate gender identification.

Iatrogenic Causes
Although it is far less common today than formerly, various forms of anomalous sexual development can arise from maternal ingestion of drugs. For example, women who became pregnant while taking androgenic contraceptives or who took androgenic progestins to prevent abortion gave birth to female children who were partially virilized. A similar situation may occur in the presence of an androgenic tumor in the mother. Such children may later require vaginal reconstruction at the time of sexual maturity, in addition to other reconstructive work on the external genitalia. Male children who lose the penis as a result of complications of circumcision are best reared as females, with early external genital reconstruction and later vaginal reconstruction at the time of sexual maturity. A similar decision should be made in the case of microphallus. Again, these decisions are predicated on the attainment of a normal adult sexual function regardless of chromosomal or gonadal sex.

HISTORY, PHYSICAL EXAMINATION, AND DIAGNOSTIC TESTS

It is very complicated to differentiate definitively which intersex condition is involved when a child has ambiguous external genitalia; this differentiation is beyond the scope of this chapter. However, the diagnosis among the conditions involving vaginal agenesis is relatively simple. Obviously, the first step is a good history. One must specifically inquire about possible maternal drug ingestion. A careful family history must be taken, looking for similar conditions in family members. Monthly episodes of abdominal discomfort are highly significant.

A complete physical examination should be done, with emphasis on the external genitalia, the distribution of body hair, evidence of secondary sex characteristics such as breast development, and the presence of abdominal or inguinal masses. The rectal examination is most important, for a carefully done examination will reveal the presence or absence of derivatives of the müllerian system. Williams [31] has described a very characteristic finding on rectal examination in cases of congenital absence of the vagina – the uterosacral ligaments can be felt in front of the rectum continuously from one pelvic side wall to the other because there is no midline uterus or cervix.

Buccal smears should be obtained for karyotypes; they are key to the differential between congenital absence of the vagina and testicular feminization syndrome. Hormonal assays, including those for androgens, estrogens, corticosteroids, and gonadotropins, may be obtained as needed. Because of the high association of renal tract anomalies, an intravenous pyelogram is mandatory; it may suggest that further studies such as cystoscopy and retrograde pyelography are needed. Gynecography (pelvic x-rays after gas insufflation), sonography, and laparoscopy will elucidate the nature of internal sex organs.

The information obtained from the history, physical examination, and diagnostic tests should lead to the correct diagnosis in the vast majority of cases. It should not be necessary except in the very complicated case to resort to diagnostic laparotomy.

David and associates [8] have called attention to the patient's need for emotional support from her physicians. Capraro and Gallego [6] have stressed the importance of reinforcing the positive and normal aspects of her condition. It should be emphasized that she will be able to marry and participate in sexual intercourse, and she may become a mother through adoption. In patients with testicular feminization syndrome, it is best to refer to the "gonads" or "sex glands" rather than to "testes."

TREATMENT OF VAGINAL AGENESIS

This history of attempts to form a vagina is a fascinating and colorful chapter in the history of medicine that begins in ancient times. The interested reader is referred to the excellent review by Goldwyn [16]. Our discussion will be limited to those methods that are in use today.

Use of Inlay Split-Thickness Skin Grafting (McIndoe Operation)
The use of a split-thickness skin graft to line the vaginal space was first pioneered by Robert Abbe, best known for his cross lip flap. The use of the split-thickness skin graft was later popularized by Counsellor [7] and by Sir Archibald McIndoe [23], whose name has since been associated with this procedure. This is perhaps the most commonly performed operation for the correction of vaginal atresia and the standard against which other procedures must be compared. Our method of performing the McIndoe operation is similar to our technique for neocolporrhaphy in the transsexual patient (see Chapter 56).

Surgery is undertaken at the time the patient wishes to become sexually active. Some patients will request surgery even though they do not plan to become sexually active at the time of surgery, because of psychological feelings of inadequacy and the desire to be a "complete woman." In most cases, surgery is undertaken after the age of 16 and after full physical growth, because the newly constructed vagina will not subsequently grow. Regardless of the patient's age, she must be well motivated because it will be necessary for her to use a vaginal stent postoperatively for at least 6 months and possibly longer to prevent contraction of the skin graft. The procedure is doomed to failure in the patient who will not diligently cooperate in the postoperative management.

Preoperatively, the patient uses a mechanical bowel preparation, and postoperatively she is kept constipated with diphenoxylate with atropine (Lomotil) or tincture of opium to prevent fecal contamination. The operation is performed with the patient under general anesthesia; hypotensive techniques may be helpful during the perineal dissection. The procedure is begun by harvesting a full Reese dermatome drum of split-thickness skin from the lateral hip or buttock. A thickness of 0.016 or 0.018 inch is used. This graft is then sewn raw side out around an inflatable Silastic vaginal stent,* which we feel is superior to some of the firmer stents formerly used. The graft is sewn in a spiral fashion to minimize later straight line contraction; 4-0 chromic catgut sutures are used.

The patient is then placed in an exaggerated lithotomy position and a Foley catheter is placed in the bladder. The O'Connor drape is used to allow the surgeon to place a finger in the rectum during the dissection. The labia are retracted, revealing the site of the vaginal dimple. An inverted U-shaped incision is then made across the region of the dimple between the urethral meatus anteriorly and the anus posteriorly. By a combination of blunt and sharp dissection, the vaginal space is created up to the level of the peritoneal reflection between the urinary structures anteriorly and the rectum posteriorly. The dissection is very easy if the fibromuscular remnant of the müllerian ducts is present. If this is not present, the dissection may be difficult; in this situation, we have found it very helpful to have the gynecologist perform a "minilaparotomy" and place his hand in the pouch of Douglas to guide the simultaneous perineal dissection. The urethral catheter and the finger in the rectum aid in preventing inadvertent injury to adjacent structures. After the space has been dissected, absolute hemostasis is obtained by the use of electrocautery and packing. This step is critical to ensure good take of the split-thickness skin graft. The previously prepared stent covered with the skin graft is then introduced into the vaginal space, and the stent is inflated and fixed in place by sutures to the perineal skin. A suprapubic Bonnano catheter is placed, and the Foley catheter is removed. The perineum is then dressed with silver sulfadiazine (Silvadene) cream, perineal pads, and a T binder. The patient is taken out of the lithotomy position and a specially designed abduction pillow is placed between the knees to provide immobilization.

The patient is kept supine at absolute bed rest for 5 to 7 days. After this period, the stent is removed by the physician and the graft is inspected. We have not found it necessary to do this first dressing change under any anesthesia other than intramuscular analgesics. Generally, inspection at this stage reveals excellent graft take. The patient is then begun on a program involving douches with a dilute solution of povidone-iodine (Betadine) and sitz baths 3 times a day; she is instructed on the placement and care of the stent. Once the patient feels confident in caring for herself, she is discharged. Sexual intercourse is permitted after 6 weeks. The patient is instructed to wear the stent continuously except for changes and intercourse for the first 6 months. Thereafter, it may be discontinued if the patient has frequent intercourse. If intercourse is infrequent, the intermittent use of the stent is continued to prevent contraction.

The McIndoe procedure [23] is not without potential complications, including loss of portions of the skin graft (with resultant stenosis of the newly constructed vagina), rectovaginal fistula, and urethrovaginal fistula. The management of these complications is described in reference to neocolporrhaphy (see Chapter 56).

Several large series of patients treated by the McIndoe technique have been reported with generally excellent results. Ortiz-Monasterio and colleagues [25] have reported a series of 21 patients who had vaginal construction by the McIndoe method. The patients were followed for periods ranging from 1 to 16 years. One patient developed a rectovaginal fistula, which was felt to be due to pressure from a firm vaginal mold. Partial loss of the skin graft requiring regrafting occurred in 1 patient. There was no evidence of stenosis of the vagina in 17 patients; 3 patients had some contracture, and 1 patient had marked stenosis. Of the 21 patients, 19 reported excellent sexual function.

Garcia and Jones [13] have reported a 100 percent take of the skin graft in 47 of 64 patients, and an 80 to 90 percent take in 13 other patients. Dyspareunia occurred postoperatively in only 5 patients, and it was felt that in 3 of these the problem was related to the presence of widespread condyloma acuminata [13]. Cali and Pratt [5] reported an extensive series of 123 patients treated by the McIndoe operation who were followed for periods ranging from 1 to 37 years. There were 10 failures that required reoperation and another 20 patients judged as anatomical failures, making a total of 30 failures (22 percent). With respect to the long-term results, 42 percent of the patients had some degree of vaginal contraction but 90 percent reported good sexual function [5]. Most of these patients were happily married.

It is interesting to note that with time, the split-thickness skin graft assumes the appearance both histologically and physiologically of normal vaginal mucosa.

*Available from Heyer-Schulte Co.

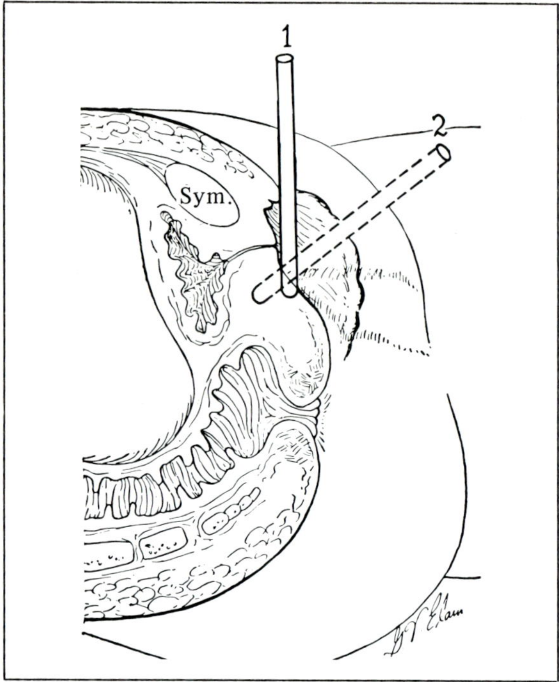

Fig. 55-5. Nonoperative method of Frank. Progressively larger dilators are used to gradually enlarge the vaginal dimple. The dilator is inserted into the vaginal dimple as shown at position 1. The dilator is then rotated to position 2 and pressure applied until mild discomfort is experienced. (From H. W. Jones and W. M. Scott [Eds.], Hermaphroditism, Genital Anomalies, and Related Endocrine Disorders. *© 1971, Williams & Wilkins Co., Baltimore.)*

Nonoperative Method of Frank

In 1938, Frank [12] reported on a method by which serviceable vagina could be constructed without surgery by repeated application of pressure to the septum between the urethra and rectum using graduated glass tubes. Many authors have reported inconsistent or disappointing results with this method [6, 15, 19], but recently Broadbent and Woolf [4] have renewed interest in this method and have reported excellent results in 8 patients. These authors used Silastic molds of graduated sizes. The smallest dilator is used first and the tip is applied to the vaginal dimple (Fig. 55-5). The patient is instructed to apply pressure until mild discomfort is experienced. Pressure is alternately applied and released for 15 minutes twice daily. The size is progressively increased; by the end of 2 months, all but 1 of the patients were using the largest dilator. After 1 month's use of the largest dilator, the patient begins intercourse. If intercourse then occurs at least twice a week, the use of a dilator is abandoned. A normal appearing vaginal mucosa is reported. These authors advocate that this method be tried first in all cases. If the method fails, operative construction may still be carried out.

The Williams Vulvovaginoplasty

In 1964, Williams [32] described a simplified operative approach that he termed vulvovaginoplasty (Fig. 55-6). The operation is simple to perform and does not require the use of dilating stents to prevent contraction of the cavity. The operation is done in the lithotomy position and may be performed using local anesthesia. A Foley catheter is placed in the bladder. The labia majora are grasped with Allis clamps and traction is exerted to spread them widely apart to expose the area. A U-shaped incision is made beginning 4 cm. lateral to the urethra on the medial aspect of the labia majora near the pubic hairline, and it continues down and around to split the fourchette and ends at the same starting level on the opposite labia. The incision is carried down to the level of perineal muscles; then, after appropriate mobilization, the medial skin margins are joined together, beginning posteriorly and extending forward. The knots are tied so that they will lie on the inside of the new cavity. The lateral skin and subcutaneous tissues are then closed over the new vagina. Immediately after the operation, the new vagina will usually admit two fingers but its axis is perpendicular to the ground and pointing anteriorly. Postoperatively, the patient is kept at bed rest for 1 week. The catheter is removed at 4 or 5 days. The patient is then instructed on the use of dilators to enlarge the cavity and also to change its axis. This process is also aided by sexual intercourse. Williams [31] has stated that neither the patients nor their partners have complained about the slight misplacement of the new vagina and he further states that the patients are "often particularly successful at coitus" because of the sensibility of the tissue used.

Use of Bowel Form of Vagina

The use of various portions of bowel to construct the vagina is not a new technique; in fact, it antedates the methods that have been previously discussed. European surgeons reported the use of various segments of bowel to replace the vagina at the turn of the century. In the United States, Baldwin [2] in 1904 used an ileal loop. Subsequently, this became known as the Baldwin operation. Because of the increased mortality and morbidity associated with the intraabdominal surgery, especially in the preantibiotic era, the Baldwin procedure was generally abandoned in favor of the safer and simpler McIndoe operation. Other dis-

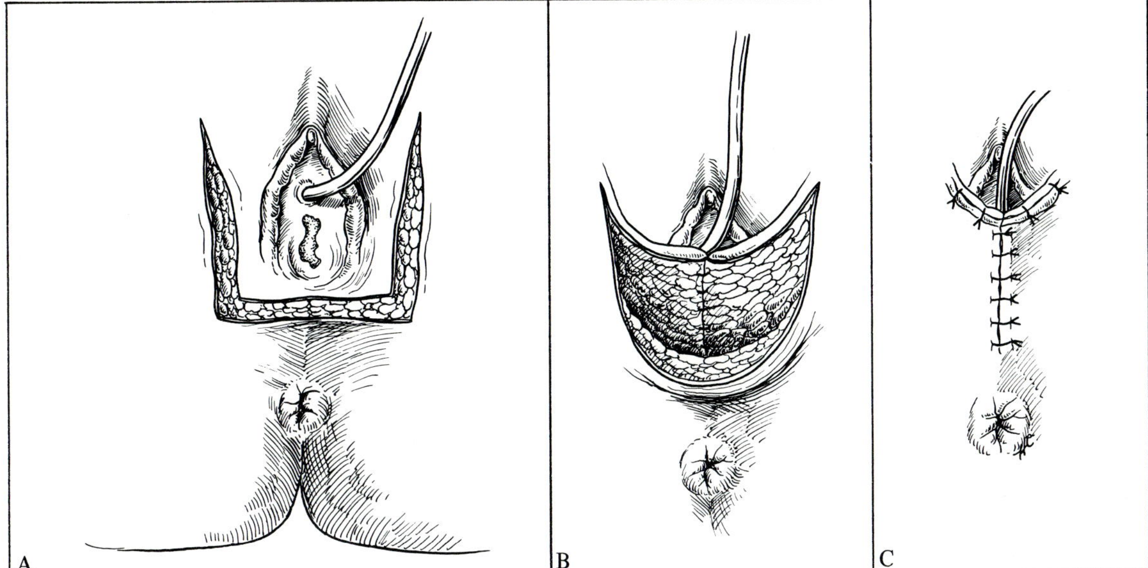

Fig. 55-6. The Williams vulvovaginoplasty. A, the skin incision has been made. B, the inner mucosa has been sutured. C, the skin is sutured over the inner closure. (From E. A. Williams, Am. R. Coll. Surg. Engl. *58:266, 1976.)*

advantages to the use of ileum included bleeding with coital trauma to the thin mucosa, excessive mucous secretion, periumbilical pain with intercourse, and a tendency to prolapse. Pratt [26] has reported good results in a series of patients in whom he used a segment of sigmoid colon for vaginal construction. This is a one-stage operation that required minimal postoperative care. Mucous secretion does not seem to be a problem when sigmoid is used.

We have generally used the bowel for vaginal construction only in those cases that have been treated unsuccessfully by the McIndoe procedure.

REFERENCES

1. Akinkugbe, A. Vaginal atresia and cryptomenorrhea. *Obstet. Gynecol.* 46:317, 1975.
2. Baldwin, J. F. The formation of an artificial vagina by intestinal transplantation. *Ann. Surg.* 40:398, 1904.
3. Baramki, T. A. Embryology of the urogenital system in man and genetic factors in intersex problems and transsexualism. *Clin. Plast. Surg.* 1:201, 1974.
4. Broadbent, T. R., and Woolf, R. M. Congenital absence of the vagina: Reconstruction without operation. *Br. J. Plast. Surg.* 30:118, 1977.
5. Cali, R. W., and Pratt, J. H. Congenital absence of the vagina. *Am. J. Obstet. Gynecol.* 100:752, 1968.
6. Capraro, V. J., and Gallego, M. B. Vaginal agenesis. *Am. J. Obstet. Gynecol.* 124:98, 1976.
7. Counsellor, V. S. Congenital absence of the vagina. *J.A.M.A.* 136:861, 1948.
8. David, A., Carmil, D., Bar-David, E., and Serr, D. M. Congenital absence of the vagina: Clinical and psychologic aspects. *Obstet. Gynecol.* 46:407, 1975.
9. Dewhurst, C. J. The aetiology and management of intersexuality. *Clin. Endocrinol.* 4:625, 1975.
10. Federman, D. D. *Abnormal Sexual Development: A Genetic and Endocrine Approach to Differential Diagnosis.* Philadelphia: Saunders, 1967.
11. Fore, S. R., Hammond, C. B., Partan, R. T., and Anderson, E. E. Urologic and genital anomalies in patients with congenital absence of the vagina. *Obstet. Gynecol.* 46:410, 1975.
12. Frank, R. T. The formation of an artificial vagina without operation. *Am. J. Obstet. Gynecol.* 35:1053, 1938.
13. Garcia, J., and Jones, H. W. The split thickness graft technique for vaginal agenesis. *Obstet. Gynecol.* 49:328, 1977.
14. Glenn, J. F. Testicular feminization syndrome. *Urology* 7:569, 1976.
15. Golditch, I. M. Vaginal aplasia. *Surg. Gynecol. Obstet.* 129:361, 1969.
16. Goldwyn, R. M. History of attempts to form a vagina. *Plast. Reconstr. Surg.* 59:319, 1977.
17. Green, T. H., Jr. *Gynecology* (3rd ed.). Boston: Little, Brown, 1977.

18. Griffin, J. E., Edwards, C., Madden, J. D., Harrod, M., and Wilson, J. D. Congenital absence of the vagina. *Ann. Intern. Med.* 85:224, 1976.
19. Hueston, J. T., and McDonald, I. A. Congenital Absence of the Vagina. In Horton, C. (Ed.), *Plastic and Reconstructive Surgery of the Genital Area.* Boston: Little, Brown, 1973.
20. Jones, H. W., and Mermut, S. Familial occurrence of congenital absence of the vagina. *Am. J. Obstet. Gynecol.* 114:1100, 1972.
21. Jost, A. Intersexuality. In Jones, H. W., and Scott, W. W. (Eds.), *Hermaphroditism, Genital Anomalies and Related Endocrine Disorders* (2nd ed.). Baltimore: Williams & Wilkins, 1971.
22. Lischke, J., Curtis, C. H., and Lamb, D. J. Discordance of the vaginal agenesis in monozygotic terms. *Obstet. Gynecol.* 41:920, 1973.
23. McIndoe, A. Treatment of congenital absence and obliterative conditions of the vagina. *Br. J. Plast. Surg.* 2:254, 1950.
24. Money, J. Intersexual problems. *Clin. Obstet. Gynecol.* 16:169, 1973.
25. Ortiz-Monasterie, F., Serrano, A., Barrera, G., and Aralco, J. Congenital absence of the vagina – long-term follow-up of 21 patients treated with skin grafts. *Plast. Reconstr. Surg.* 49:165, 1972.
26. Pratt, J. H. Vaginal atresia corrected by use of small and large bowel. *Clin. Obstet. Gynecol.* 15:639, 1972.
27. Steffanoff, D. N. Late development of squamous cell carcinoma in a split-skin graft lining a vagina. *Plast. Reconstr. Surg.* 51:454, 1973.
28. Ulfelder, H., and Robboy, S. J. The embryologic development of the human vagina. *Am. J. Obstet. Gynecol.* 126:769, 1976.
29. Wharton, L. R. A simple method of constructing a vagina. *Ann. Surg.* 107:842, 1938.
30. Wilfingseder, P. Presented at the *5th International Congress of Plastic Surgery,* Paris, 1974.
31. Williams, E. A. A Simple Method of Vaginal Construction. In Taymor, M. L., and Grun, T. H., Jr. (Eds.), *Progress in Gynecology,* Vol. 6. New York: Grune & Stratton, 1975.
32. Williams, E. A. Congenital absence of the vagina: A simple operation for its relief. *J. Obstet. Gynecol. Br. Commonw.* 71:511, 1964.
33. Williams, E. A. Uterovaginal agenesis. *Ann. R. Coll. Surg. Engl.* 58:266, 1976.
34. Yves. J. *Transactions of the Fifth International Congress of Plastic Surgery,* Paris, 1974.

Gender Dysphoria

DONALD R. LAUB AND BRUCE J. DUBIN

I would like to remind everyone of an important fundamental fact – the difference between sex and gender. Sex is what you see. Gender is what you feel. Harmony between the two is essential for human happiness.

Harry Benjamin, M.D.
New York City, June 1976

A definition of plastic surgery is the application of surgical modalities to improve function and appearance. This chapter discusses perhaps the most dramatic and controversial example of the application of plastic surgery – the alteration of the sex of the body to meet the body image. Furthermore this profound alteration of a healthy body is considered for a purely behavioral disorder. Many people, particularly the surgeons who do the work, find this disturbing, especially because it may be uncertain in individual cases whether surgery is the treatment of choice. We hope that the reader will critically evaluate the information that will be presented.

While the etiology of gender dysphoria syndrome is unclear and therefore specific prevention and treatment are unknown, much can be done to palliate individuals with this form of disturbed behavior. The available data suggest that properly selected patients who participate in a well-organized gender dysphoria program demonstrate significant improvements in lifestyle, social relationships, sense of self-esteem and body image, employment status, and sexual adjustment. Surgery is only one part of such a rehabilitation program, which must include attention to the economic, social, and psychological needs of the patient in addition to anatomical requirements. It does little good to perform a technically perfect operation and still have a patient who is isolated from society, maladjusted, and receiving public assistance. A multidisciplinary approach is needed and strict criteria must be met prior to any surgery if serious errors in patient selection are to be avoided.

A dividend of gender dysphoria surgery is that the same surgical procedures may be adapted for use in patients who have suffered loss of either the vagina or penis from trauma, cancer, infection, or radiation.

HISTORICAL BACKGROUND

References to cross-gender behavior can be found in early Greek and Roman literature, and examples of cross-gender identification can be found among diverse cultural and racial groups [21]. Despite isolated reports in the 1930s of "sex conversion operations," the interest of the lay public and medical profession was not aroused until the well-publicized story of Christine Jorgensen was reported by Hamburger and associates [23] in 1953. Since then, interest in this phenomenon has steadily increased.

Although the term "transsexual" was coined earlier by Caldwell [8], it was the pioneer sexologist Harry Benjamin who popularized this term and delineated the clinical aspects of transsexualism in his book, *The Transsexual Phenomenon.* Benjamin [4] listed these four characteristics: (1) a lifelong sense of being a member of the opposite sex, (2) gender behavior of the opposite sex and early and persistent cross-dressing without erotic feeling, (3) repugnance and disgust for one's genitalia without deriving pleasure from them, and (4) disdain for any homosexual behavior.

In 1963, Edgerton, Jones, Knorr, and Money established the first gender identity clinic at Johns Hopkins University. This represented the first multidisciplinary attempt to study and treat disorders of gender identification. Subsequently other groups were formed at major medical institutions across the country. In 1969, Green and Money [21] published *Transsexualism and Sex Reassignment,* which was the first truly scientific book that dealt with this problem.

As more experience was gained by these groups, it became clear that not all of the patients who presented themselves requesting sex change surgery conformed to the classic definition of transsexualism, although many patients had consciously or unconsciously developed congruous histories in their attempt to gain acceptance for surgery. To circumvent this problem, Fisk [14] proposed the new descriptive term "gender dysphoria syndrome." Meyer [41] has suggested that the term "transsexual" be used in the broad sense to describe any patient who has completed sex change surgery; he prefers the term "eonist" for the classic transsexual as described by Benjamin. In this chapter, the nomenclature outlined by Fisk (as discussed below) will be followed.

DIFFERENTIAL DIAGNOSIS

The gender dysphoria syndrome includes all patients who are so dissatisfied with their body that they demand gender-altering surgery. The syndrome includes the following diagnostic categories:

1. Classic transsexualism. It is estimated that only 15 to 20 percent of all patients with gender dysphoria fall into this category (the characteristics

of this group have already been described).

2. Former effeminate homosexuality. Male patients in this category are sexually attracted to other men and initially derive pleasure from their penis. With time, they gradually assume a more feminine lifestyle and evolve into seeking surgery as a means of avoiding the moral, financial, and social stigmata of homosexuality. Furthermore, under hormonal therapy, the penis becomes inactive as a source of pleasure. An analogous situation may exist for masculine lesbians.
3. Former transvestitism. Transvestites derive erotic stimulation from cross-dressing. These men generally start out with a heterosexual orientation; often they are married and have children. Gradually some may evolve into the gender dysphoria syndrome for reasons similar to those of the homosexual group. Transvestitism appears to be purely a male phenomenon, and there is no analogous situation for genetic females.
4. Psychosis. Many psychotic patients suffer from some delusion in their sexual identity, but these patients must be distinguished from transsexuals who develop psychoses secondary to the stress associated with their gender dysphoria. Psychotic patients may present after having made attempts at accomplishing gender conversion on themselves.
5. Psychoneurotic sociopathy. These patients are frankly exhibitionists and seek sex change as a means of obtaining notoriety, such as newspaper and television publicity.
6. Inadequate and schizoid personality. These individuals do not have a well-developed sense of gender and they request gender change in an attempt to minimize stress associated with functioning in society.

In general, patients from the first three categories may be suitable for surgery, while those from the last three categories are not.

We have found that the above classification scheme is helpful in two respects: (1) By allowing for other entities in addition to the classic transsexual of Benjamin, it encourages honesty in the patient and physician during the preliminary evaluation process and therefore it should lead to better preoperative screening. (2) It allows the indications for surgery to be determined on the basis of successful preoperative self-rehabilitation rather than on the basis of predetermined diagnostic categories.

It is virtually impossible to obtain reliable statistics pertaining to the incidence of gender dysphoria syndrome. The incidence cited in the literature for male-to-female transsexualism ranges from 1 per 100,000 to 1 per 40,000 men [46]. Estimations of the ratio of female-to-male (anatomical female) transsexuals to male-to-female transsexuals range from as low as one to one to as high as eight to one [46]. In all the reported surgical series, the number of anatomical males obtaining surgery always exceeds the number of females. This may reflect the fact that it is generally easier and more socially acceptable for a female to pass as a male than for a male to pass as a female. Also, the results of surgery for male-to-female conversion are more satisfactory than those for female-to-male conversion.

ETIOLOGY

The sex of an organism may be defined according to several possible parameters including: chromosomes, gonads, sex hormone patterns, internal sex organs, external sex organs, secondary sex characteristics, sex-rearing, sex roles and behavior, and sexual object choice [4]. According to Meyer [42], gender identity is an "amalgam" of the various influences that determine the sense of being male or female. In most individuals all of these variables are consistent, and there is no gender identification problem.

Except for a few patients with Klinefelter's syndrome and gonadal dysgenesis [46], patients with gender dysphoria have no recognized abnormalities of chromosomes, external or internal anatomy, or adult hormonal patterns [16, 42]. Hypotheses as to the origin of this condition have generally fallen into two broad categories [32]: (1) the prenatal influence of sex hormones on the developing fetal nervous system and (2) postnatal social and psychological influences.

Evidence for the first category comes from experimental work with mammals and lower primates. In at least four of these species (rat, hamster, dog, and rhesus monkey), it has been demonstrated that manipulation of the fetal or neonatal hormonal environment can produce transsexual behavior. It appears that the hypothalamus of the developing nervous system plays a key role in mediating these hormonal effects. Money and Ehrhardt [45] have summarized much of this intriguing experimental work. Despite this evidence in experimental animals, there is no evidence that such fetal hormonal factors have an effect on human adult sexual behavior [43]. Ehrhardt and Money [13] followed 10 normal female children whose mothers received androgenic progestins during pregnancy. While most of these girls exhibited "tomboyish" behavior, none of them had any problem with developing an adult female gender identification. Similarly, Yalom and co-workers [57] followed male children who were exposed to high levels of female hormones in utero. While many of these boys exhibited definitely effeminate behavior, none exhibited any transsexual behavior.

The second broad etiological category is that of postnatal sociological and psychological influences.

Green, Newman, and Soller [22] have followed a population of young boys who manifested definite feminine behavior, including cross-dressing and improvising feminine attire, preference for playing with girls and for feminine games, and statements indicating their desire to be girls or women. This group may well represent a "pretranssexual" population. On detailed family evaluation several common traits were noted, including an abnormal physical closeness with the mother (who often had anxiety regarding her own gender identification and who unconsciously would reinforce the feminine behavior) and an absent or distant father. Green and associates have been able in some cases to reverse the feminine behavior in these boys by intense psychiatric intervention involving not only the boy but the entire family. Meyer [42] has reported similar experiences with adolescents.

Money [44] has done extensive studies of gender identification in both intersex patients and transsexual patients. He feels that there is a critical time period during which "core gender identity" is established, usually by the third year, and after which this identity cannot be changed. He feels that this identification is basically a learned phenomenon and in general corresponds to the same period during which language is developed. Meyer [43] feels that this gender identity is largely determined by early rearing experiences within the family.

Regardless of the basic etiology, which must be considered unknown at present, the fact remains that once gender identity has been established, it is virtually impossible to change it. Attempts by psychiatrists to reverse adult transsexualism have been generally unsuccessful. Barlow and associates [2] have reported one case in which a young adult was successfully treated with behavior modification techniques. Kirkpatrick and Friedman [31] have reported a few cases. Levine [34] has also reported that some patients have at least temporarily given up their desire for sex change surgery after intense psychotherapy, but he cautions that these patients should not be considered cured. Hastings [24] has summarized the situation well:

> Since the gender role seems to be laid down in indelible fashion during the first forty months of life, it is not surprising that attempts to change it in later life by whatever treatment modality have been found to be an exercise in futility. The only avenue of therapy, if one wishes to do anything to help these unfortunate people, seems to be that of the surgical route.

GENERAL MANAGEMENT

The plastic surgeon cannot manage this complex behavior disorder alone. Furthermore, the goal of a gender dysphoria program must be total rehabilitation of the patient, not just surgical change (which is only one part of the whole picture). Just as not all patients who request aesthetic surgical procedures are appropriate candidates, similarly, surgery should not be performed at the demand of patients claiming to be transsexuals and desiring sex reassignment. Proper patient selection is paramount if the surgeon is to adhere to the basic tenet of "primum non nocere." Many other disciplines must be brought into evaluation and therapy if these unfortunate people are to be truly helped. The team should include not only psychiatrists, plastic surgeons, and other medical specialists, but also vocational rehabilitation counselors, social workers, attorneys, and other nonmedical advisors.

To avoid disaster, the criteria for selecting patients for surgery must be strict. The criteria at the Stanford Gender Dysphoria Program are typical of many programs across the country. These requirements are as follows:

1. A documented history of gender dysphoria must be present.
2. The patient must not be psychotic when seen.
3. The patient must not be married in his anatomical sex.
4. No medical contraindications to the surgery must exist.
5. The patient must agree to postoperative follow-up.
6. Appropriate exogenous hormonal therapy must be administered for 12 to 24 months. In general, after 6 months of hormone therapy, the female-to-male patients are able to pass as male quite successfully. This is not the case for male-to-female patients.
7. There must be a 12- to 24-month trial period of total cross-gender living.

The last requirement is perhaps the most important. Patients may come into the program with very unrealistic expectations about what it is like to live in the opposite gender. The required period of cross-living makes the patient realize that this change may impose very real hardships. Frequently the patients must move and change jobs, often with a loss of earning potential. They often suffer rejection by family and friends and must establish new social relationships in the gender of choice. To be able to pass successfully in their new gender, patients often need advice regarding the most basic aspects of grooming and deportment. A professional model can teach grooming to the male-to-female patients, and a body-building program may be helpful for the female-to-male patients. Vocational rehabilitation counselors can suggest new avenues of employment and perhaps assist in job retraining. Attorneys can help in obtaining new birth certificates and change of name on school records, and they can give advice about how to avoid trouble with the law. Supervision of the hormonal therapy by an endocrinologist or an internist is necessary. General supportive psychiatric therapy may help the patient resolve or adjust to psychiatric problems unrelated to the gender dysphoria, and it allows the psychiatrist more time to fully assess the patient prior to surgery. Contact with successful postoperative patients may help the patient's motivation and be a source of encouragement. A "half-way house" may also help motivate the patient.

By establishing certain goals that must be met to achieve the "reward" of surgery, the program becomes a means of behavior modification aimed at total rehabilitation of the patient. We have found that holding a steady job is the most important single measure of success. Indeed, virtually all of the criteria are met if the patient can maintain gainful employment. Not only does it allow the patient to function in our society, but also it provides the associated reinforcement of self-dignity and self-esteem by others, which serves to lessen the quest for perfection of the body by surgery. Strict prerequisites yield the dividend to the surgeon that only successful patients will receive surgery, as poor candidates are selected out. Even the patients who never meet all the criteria and therefore do not qualify for surgery are often benefited by the behavior modification inherent in their attempts to qualify. In our series, only about 10 percent of the patients screened and evaluated actually qualify for surgery. Edgerton [11] has reported a similar experience.

The surgeon should be aware that there is a marked difference in behavior between the male-to-female patients and the female-to-male patients that must be reflected in their management. The male-to-female patients have been described as hysterical, narcissistic, demanding, manipulative, psychopathic, perfectionistic, exhibitionistic, seductive, sociopathic, and destructively competitive among their peer group. On the other hand, the female-to-male patients have been described as stoic, independent, reliable, diligent, accepting of authority, and more cooperative among their peer group. The reader will note that the qualities ascribed to the male-to-female patients are the undesirable attributes of stereotyped femininity, while those characteristics associated with the female-to-male patients are the most desirable qualities associated with stereotyped masculinity. We are unaware of any explanation for this polarization.

SURGERY FOR THE MALE-TO-FEMALE TRANSSEXUAL

Preoperative evaluation involves a complete history and physical examination and appropriate laboratory studies, as for any patient undergoing a major operative procedure. The patients begin a complete bowel preparation prior to entering the hospital. We have used a separate special operative consent form, which is usually signed by the patient in the presence of the patient's attorney as well as the surgeon prior to the hospitalization. A full discussion of the procedure and its risks and complications is conducted.

Neocolporrhaphy

Hypotensive anesthesia has been used to minimize intraoperative bleeding, especially for the perineal dissection. This is usually accomplished by the combination of halothane and a sympathetic ganglion-blocking agent. Of course, it requires the participation of an expert anesthesiologist well versed in this technique.

The patient is positioned in a somewhat exaggerated lithotomy position. The O'Connor rectal drape and a Foley catheter placed into the bladder facilitate the dissection. The goal of surgery is the construction of a cosmetically acceptable vulva and a functionally satisfactory neovagina [11, 19]. Specifically, the neovagina must be large enough to permit comfortable intercourse. Ideally there should be no hair-bearing skin within the neovagina; the perineum must not only look realistic, but also be free of a painful penile stump and neuromas. The reconstructed urethral meatus must not be stenotic and must be directed at an angle such that the patient can sit to void. There should be no postoperative incontinence or fistula. If skin grafts are used, they should be taken from inconspicuous donor sites.

A number of specific operations have been described in an attempt to achieve these goals. A step common to all of the operations is the dissection of a perineal pocket for the neovagina. This step of the procedure is similar to a perineal prostatectomy (Fig. 56-1). After identifying the bulb of the urethra, the central tendon of the perineum is divided; using sharp dissection, the surgeon develops the space between the prostate and bladder anteriorly and the rectum posteriorly. The Foley catheter and the surgeon's finger placed in the rectum aid in the dissection. The rectourethralis muscle should be carefully identified and sharply divided as the dissection proceeds, because blunt separation may lead into the muscle planes of the bowel or urinary structures. Usually it is necessary to divide part of the levator ani muscle to insure adequate width. Denonvilliers' fascia is identified by its shiny white appearance, and the layers are sharply separated. The dissection beyond this landmark may involve blunt separation and may proceed rapidly in the now avascular plane. The dissection is completed at the level of the peritoneal reflection (Fig. 56-2). The surgeon must be

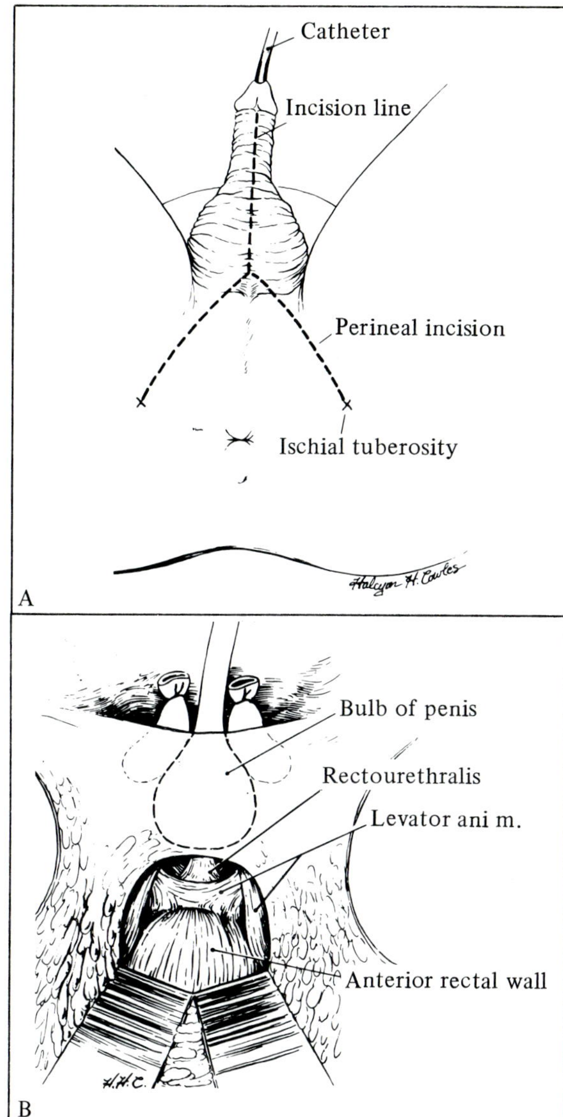

Fig. 56-1. Perineal dissection. A, typical incision. B, the rectourethralis muscle and a portion of the levator ani muscle must be divided to deepen the dissection. (From D. R. Laub and N. Fisk, Plast. Reconstr. Surg. *53:388, 1974.)*

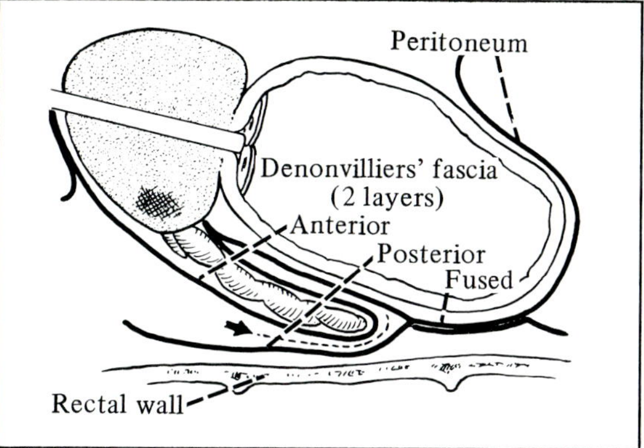

Fig. 56-2. The completed perineal dissection. A raw space has been created between the urinary structures anteriorly and the rectum posteriorly. (From W. L. Parry and C. B. Dawson. In J. F. Glenn and W. H. Boyce [Eds.], Urologic Surgery. *New York: Hoeber Medical Div., Harper & Row, 1969.)*

sure that the pocket is of adequate size, because failure to accomplish this is a common error with this portion of the procedure [11].

Another step that is common to all techniques is the shortening and repositioning of the urethra. In general, the corpus spongiosum and the contained urethra are dissected free from the corpora cavernosa, which are subsequently freed to the level of their separation into crura and then amputated at the pubic rami. The urethra is then shortened and retrodisplaced to an appropriate position for the female perineum, where it is brought to the surface and sutured to the skin. In some techniques, the urethra is placed posterior to the superficial transverse perineal muscle prior to being brought to the surface. It is important that the anastomosis to skin be done in a way that prevents the later development of cicatricial meatal stenosis. This is most simply accomplished by enlarging the urethral meatal circumference with a "fish-mouthing" technique or a Z-plasty.

All procedures also include bilateral orchiectomies with high ligations of the spermatic cords. Inguinal hernias must be discovered and repaired prior to surgery.

Lining for the Neovagina and Creation of the Vulva

The specific procedures that are currently described basically differ in how the lining is provided for the neovagina and how the vulva is constructed from the remaining available tissues.

Jones and co-workers [29] describe the procedure that was used in the first surgery at Johns Hopkins Hospital. In this technique, an inverted U-shaped incision is made across the scrotum, developing a posterior scrotal and perineal flap. The testes are removed, and an anterior flap is then made of penile skin by incising along the ventral midline of the penis and then circumferentially just proximal to the coronal sulcus. The penectomy is then performed. The two skin flaps are then sutured together and placed into the neovagina. A stent is needed to maintain the space. A similar technique has been employed by Flowers [15] with good results and also by Biber [5]. According to Edgerton [11], this technique suffers from two principal disadvantages: it results in hair-bearing scrotal skin being placed in the neovagina, and there is often insufficient penile and scrotal skin to provide a neovagina of adequate depth.

Edgerton and Bull [12] have advocated a two-stage procedure that utilizes an inverted penile tube pedicle based posteriorly (Fig. 56-3). The first stage consists of an inverted U-shaped incision around the superior aspect of the scrotum and base of the penis with the remaining posterior attachment of the scrotum to the perineum being the vascular pedicle of the penile flap. The erectile bodies of the penis are then separated from the penile skin which is left intact as a tube. The glans is left attached to the penile skin tube and later serves to simulate a cervix. After the perineal pocket is dissected, the penile skin tube is inverted into the raw space. Packing is used to maintain the skin in the proper position. A split-thickness skin graft is used to cover the anterior perineal wound. Four weeks later at the second stage, the pedicle of the penile skin tube is divided and the remaining scrotal skin is used to make the labia. The urethra is also shortened and placed in the proper position. While this technique has the disadvantage of requiring two stages, Edgerton and Bull feel that it leads to a better vaginal and perineal reconstruction.

Burou [7] has described a method using a one-stage penile tube pedicle that he has employed in over 700 cases, which represents the largest single series by any one surgeon. In his method a midline vertical incision is made beginning near the anus and extending through the midline of the scrotum to the base of the penis. After the orchiectomies and the perineal dissection are completed, the erectile tissues of the penis are shelled out of the penile skin, which is left as a tube attached by an anterior pedicle. The penile skin tube is then inverted and placed in the neovagina and held in proper position by a vaginal mold. Pandya and Stuteville [50] and Granato [20] have described one-stage procedures that are virtually identical to Burou's method.

Barbosa [1] has described a procedure that uses the penile skin as a free full-thickness skin graft. Jayaram [28] also uses a similar method.

We have used a different technique from those described above (Fig. 56-4). A full Reese dermatome drum of thick split-thickness skin is harvested from the thigh and then sewn (with the raw side out) over a specially designed pneumatically inflatable silicone vaginal stent.* An inverted U-shaped incision is made in the perineal skin and a posteriorly based perineal skin flap is developed. An anteriorly based penile skin flap is then made by incising along the ventral aspect of the penis and then circumferentially around the penis just proximal to the coronal sulcus. The perineal pocket is developed in the usual manner. The posterior perineal flap is introduced for a few centimeters into the neovagina and affixed there under no tension. The anterior penile skin flap is used for the first few centimeters of the anterior neovaginal wall and also used to reconstruct the labia minora. The urethra is brought through an appropriately placed buttonhole incision in the penile skin flap. The urethral mucosa is everted as it is sutured to the skin, and this sensitive exposed mucosa serves as a neoclitoris. After the perineal and penile skin flaps have been sewn in place, the skin graft and the stent it covers are then introduced into the neovagina and carefully secured in place by sutures to the perineal skin. Using this technique, we have seldom had deficient neovaginas, although these patients must use a vaginal stent for at least 6 months postoperatively to prevent subsequent contraction of the graft. The use of a split-thickness skin graft ensures that there is enough tissue for adequate lining without having to use the hair-bearing scrotum and without placing undue tension on a penile skin flap. It also allows more of the scrotum to be used in reconstructing the labia majora. Figure 56-5 shows the postoperative appearance of a typical patient.

Complications

Complications are listed in Table 56-1. One of the most common complications that may occur with any of the above operations is *neovaginal stenosis.* According to Markland [37], this occurs in 10 to 20 percent of patients. Markland has described a technique to deal with this problem that employs a segment of either cecum or sigmoid colon (the sigmoid colon is preferred because of the ease of mobilization). A segment of sigmoid colon is isolated, with its blood supply preserved. The distal end of the segment is closed and the proximal end is brought down through an extensive perineal dissection and then anastomosed to the perineal skin. The colon functions well as a neovagina, with the possible exception of the presence of excess mucus secretion.

Another significant complication that can occur is *rectovaginal fistula;* if these fistulas are small, they

*Available from Heyer-Schulte Corp., 600 Pine Ave., Goleta, Ca. 93017.

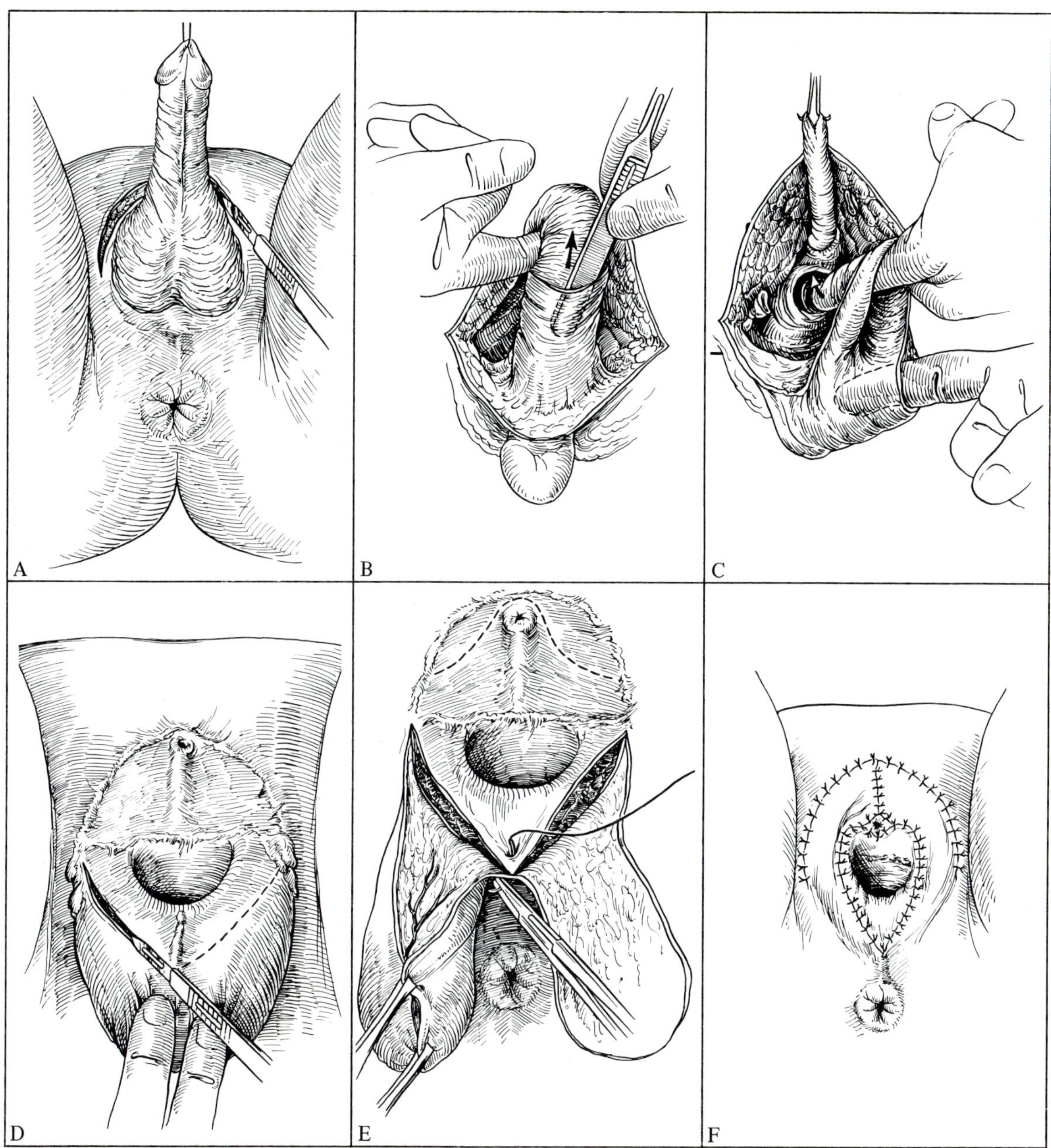

Fig. 56-3. Neocolporrhaphy according to Edgerton and Bull. A, the initial incision. B, the penile skin is dissected off along Buck's fascia. C, the everted penile skin is introduced into the raw neovaginal space. D, the incision for the second stage; note that a skin graft was applied at the first stage to cover the perineal defect. E, the scrotum has been split to construct labia and the urethra is released anteriorly. F, the completed second stage. (From M. Edgerton, Clin. Plast. Surg. *1:285, 1974. Courtesy of the W. B. Saunders Co., Philadelphia.)*

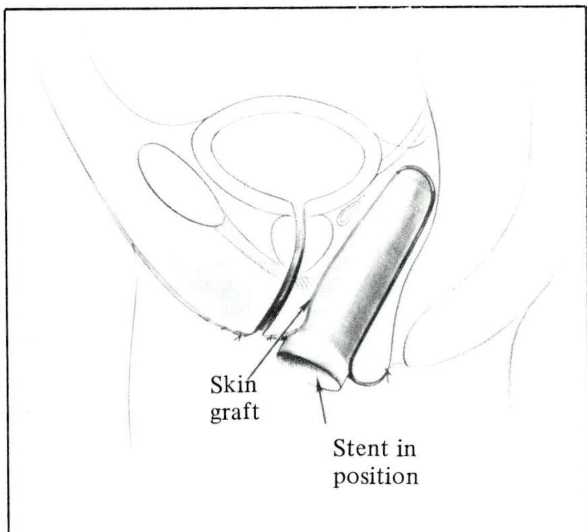

Fig. 56-4. Neocolporrhaphy using split-thickness skin graft. A split-thickness skin graft is sutured around a soft vaginal stent. (From C. Markland, Obstet. Gynecol. Annu. *4:309, 1975.)*

Table 56-1. Operative Complications of 97 Male-to-Female Patients (Standord Gender Dysphoria Program)

Complication	Number
Urethral stenosis	6
Urethrovaginal fistula	4
Vaginal stenosis	3
Rectovaginal fistula	5
Contracture secondary to skin graft loss	11
Pulmonary embolus	2
Delayed healing	2
Hemorrhage with regrafting and take	4
Total	37[a]

[a]These complications occurred in 33 patients; several patients had more than one complication.

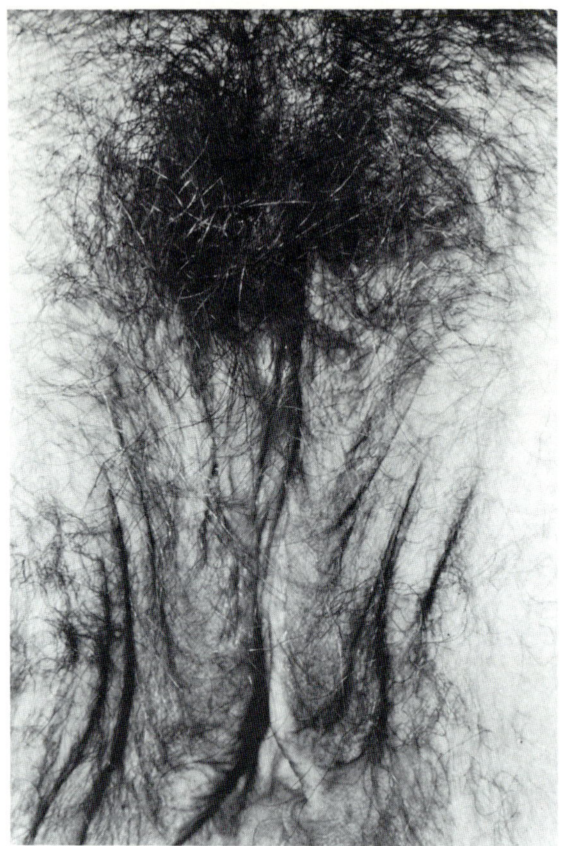

Fig. 56-5. The appearance of the external genitalia following one-stage neocolporrhaphy.

may heal spontaneously but often with accompanying stenosis of the neovagina. If these fistulas fail to heal spontaneously, surgical repair must be done and a diverting colostomy may be needed to help effect closure [3]. Once healing has occurred, the perineal pocket must be redeveloped; it may be lined with a split-thickness skin graft or, in persistent cases, with a vascularized segment of sigmoid colon, as described above. *Urethrovaginal fistulas* are also possible but are uncommon in most authors' experience, perhaps occurring in 2 or 3 out of each 100 cases. The use of an indwelling suprapubic cystostomy is important in preventing this complication.

Other complications include a *prominent corpus spongiosum stump,* which may become erect during sexual stimulation and may cause the patient insecurity about her femininity. Urethroplasty will be needed to remedy this. Since the male pelvis is very narrow and the male levator ani is strong, *prominent levator spasm* may be a barrier to penetration; this must be distinguished from neovaginal stenosis. Biofeedback exercises to encourage relaxation may be helpful to relieve this spasm; in severe cases, section of the levator may be needed. Because much of the patient's feminine body image is invested in the appearance of the perineum, the surgeon must be prepared to respond to the patient's request for revision of relatively minor anatomical inaccuracies.

Perhaps the most disturbing and distressing complication to the surgeon is *the patient who postoperatively decides to revert to his original gender.* The patients seem to adjust to this turn of events much better than their doctors.

Ancillary Surgery for the Male-to-Female Transsexual

Augmentation Mammoplasty

While the administration of female hormones produces adequate breast development in some patients, many will need additional augmentation. Since the width of the male chest is greater than the female, broad-based implants should be used. One should be aware that the nipples will appear to be more laterally placed in the transsexual patients. We have limited lateral dissection of the submammary pockets in order to place the implants more medially and thus provide more cleavage.

Rhinoplasty

Very often a large, masculine-appearing nose (especially if there is a prominent dorsal hump) will lessen the patient's ability to pass as a female. In these cases, a rhinoplasty can improve the feminine body image. This procedure is often done during the cross-living period prior to genital surgery, to aid the patient in being accepted as a female. It is interesting to note that not as much of the body image appears to be invested in the nose in these patients as in the genetic female requesting rhinoplasty.

Mentoplasty

The patient with either a jutting chin or a square chin may benefit from sculpting the prominence to achieve a more feminine facial contour. This can conveniently be done through an intraoral approach, thereby leaving no external scars. The guidelines of Gonzales-Ulloa and Stevens [17] are used in shaping the profile.

Chondroplasty

A very prominent "Adam's apple" due to the ala of the thyroid cartilage can be a source of concern for the patient and interfere with acceptance as female. The technique for chondroplasty is straightforward and has been described by Good [18] and also by Wolfort and Pany [56] (Fig. 56-6). A horizontal neck incision is made in an inconspicuous natural crease that does not necessarily have to overlie the cartilage (the cervicomental angle is often the least conspicuous place). Through this incision the thyroid cartilage is exposed after retraction of the strap muscles laterally. The mucosa of the larynx is gently teased away from the inner aspect of the offending cartilage and subperichondreal shaving of the cartilage is performed. This procedure can be performed on an outpatient basis. Rarely a few patients have been hoarse following this technique [11].

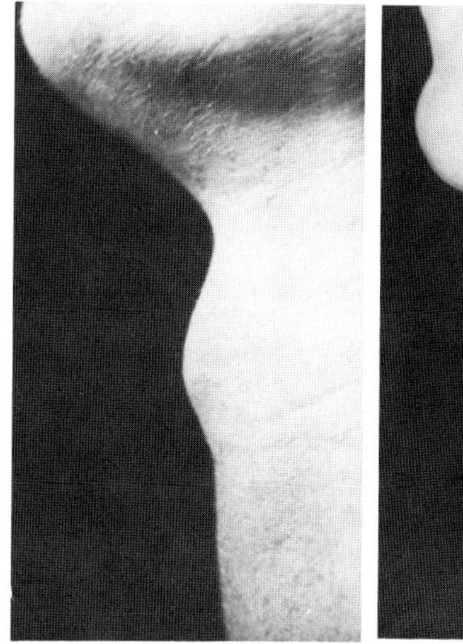

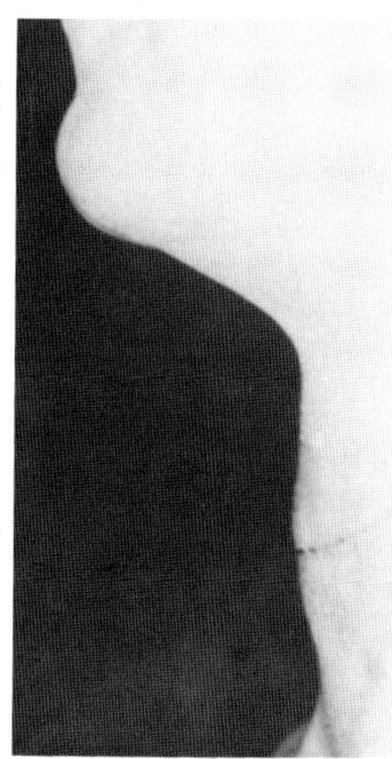

A B

Fig. 56-6. Laryngeal chondroplasty. A, the preoperative appearance. B, the postoperative appearance. (Photographs courtesy of Richard Good, M.D.)

Voice

Many patients have inquired about operations to raise the pitch of the voice. We are unaware of any reliable procedure to accomplish this. Furthermore, with the aid of a voice coach many patients are able to modulate their voices to obtain a more pleasing pitch. Speech therapists also remind us that more than pitch is involved in feminine speech. Choice of words and other speech mannerisms are also important and can be cultivated by the patients.

Electrolysis

A skilled electrologist can be of inestimable value in helping these patients rid themselves of beard and other unwanted hair. This ordinarily requires many sessions and causes the patient some pain, which may lead to the use of habituating drugs. It may also entail considerable expense.

Hormones

These patients will generally require female hormonal support, which is aimed at simulating the hormonal levels found in normal females. Surgeons should be aware that this is not without potential complications. Symmers [55] has reported 2 cases of breast cancer developing in male-to-female transsexuals. Lehrman [33] has reported a massive pulmonary embolus in a transsexual patient who was receiving high doses of estrogen. It is also important to remember that these patients still have their prostate glands. Markland [36] has followed a patient who at the age of 54 developed prostate carcinoma. These facts serve to emphasize that these patients require lifelong follow-up.

SURGERY FOR THE FEMALE-TO-MALE TRANSSEXUAL

The goals of altering the body image of the female-to-male transsexual include (1) the removal of the most conspicuous and symbolic female secondary sex characteristics, which are the breasts and menstruation, and (2) the acquisition of the appurtenances of masculinity, including beard and body hair, muscle bulk, masculine mannerisms, and, of course, the penis.

The use of hormones in the female-to-male patient is a very powerful tool. Testosterone 200 mg. given intramuscularly every 2 weeks induces cessation of menses in almost all patients, and it produces the growth of luxuriant body hair and an increase in muscle mass with the redistribution of body fat to a more masculine configuration. After 6 months of such therapy, many of these patients are able to pass quite successfully as males.

Mastectomy

In the patient with small or medium-sized breasts, this procedure can be performed by a periareolar incision as described in Chapter 48. A prominent areola may also be reduced by a wedge, concentric, or stellate-shaped excision prior to closing the wound. Excess skin is not resected or only minimally resected in this approach. Over time, the excess skin shrinks to the new contour in properly selected patients. Sometimes, one can misjudge the amount of skin shrinkage that will occur, and subsequent excision of excess skin may be needed; however, it is surprising how well the skin envelope of the young patient will recontour even after the removal of considerable breast tissue.

In larger breasts, the mastectomy is performed by amputating the breast and then replacing the reduced nipple and areolar complex as full-thickness grafts. The incision can be planned so that the scar will conform to the inferior border of the pectoralis major muscle. In positioning the nipple grafts, it is important to remember that the normal male nipple is situated more laterally than the female nipple. Hoopes [26] states that the nipple should be placed not less than 11 cm. from the midsternum in the fifth intercostal space.

Hysterectomy and Salpingo-oophorectomy

Many patients request hysterectomy and salpingo-oophorectomy, especially those patients who continue to have menstrual discharge despite androgenic hormones. We have combined this procedure with the phalloplasty (as will be described subsequently), but in patients who do not desire phalloplasty, the hysterectomy can be performed as a separate procedure. An ill-timed hysterectomy that results in abdominal scarring can significantly complicate later attempts at phalloplasty. While many patients initially inquire about removal of the vagina, few patients persist in demanding vaginectomy after the cessation of menses and phalloplasty.

Phalloplasty

Surgical attempts to construct a phallus are generally disappointing when compared with the excellent functional and cosmetic result obtainable with neocolporrhaphy. This discrepancy is due to the unique erectile tissue of the penis, for which there is no good substitute. The methods that are available for phalloplasty have been derived largely from techniques for the treatment of traumatic loss of the penis. Noe, Birdsell, and Laub [47] have stated that the objectives should be the construction of a neophallus that is satisfactory cosmetically, psychologically, and functionally. The third objective includes the capability for coitus, the presence of sensibility, and the ability to function as a urinary conduit so that the patient can urinate in the standing position.

Gillies' method of penile reconstruction has been applied to phalloplasty by Hoopes [26] (Fig. 56-7). This technique involves making three parallel oblique lateral abdominal incisions such that *two separate tubed flaps are developed*: a narrower medial flap that will be used to make the neourethra and a wider lateral flap that will make the neophallus. The second stage, performed at least 3 weeks after the first stage, involves raising the abdominal flap (including the contained neourethra) and then tubing this flap. Thus one has a tubed flap containing another smaller tubed flap. At a third stage, the superior pedicle is divided and implanted into a position in the midline inferior to the pubic symphysis. This will be the base of the neophallus. The fourth stage, preceded by an appropriate delay procedure, involves dividing the original inferior pedicle, which then becomes the distal end of the neophallus. Hoopes [26] also points out that if urethral continuity is going to be established between the female urethra and the neourethra, the normal female urethra must be lengthened. This involves a separate procedure that may be combined with the first or second stage of the phalloplasty.

Davies [9] and Birdsell [47] have developed a technique based on a modification of a procedure originally described by McIndoe [39], utilizing a *midline lower abdominal tubed flap*. This method, which we have adopted, involves only two stages (Fig. 56-8). At the first stage, two parallel paramedian incisions are made 8 to 10 cm. apart, extending from the level of the umbilicus to the pubic symphysis. The blood supply to this flap comes from the superior external pudendal arteries, which enter the base of

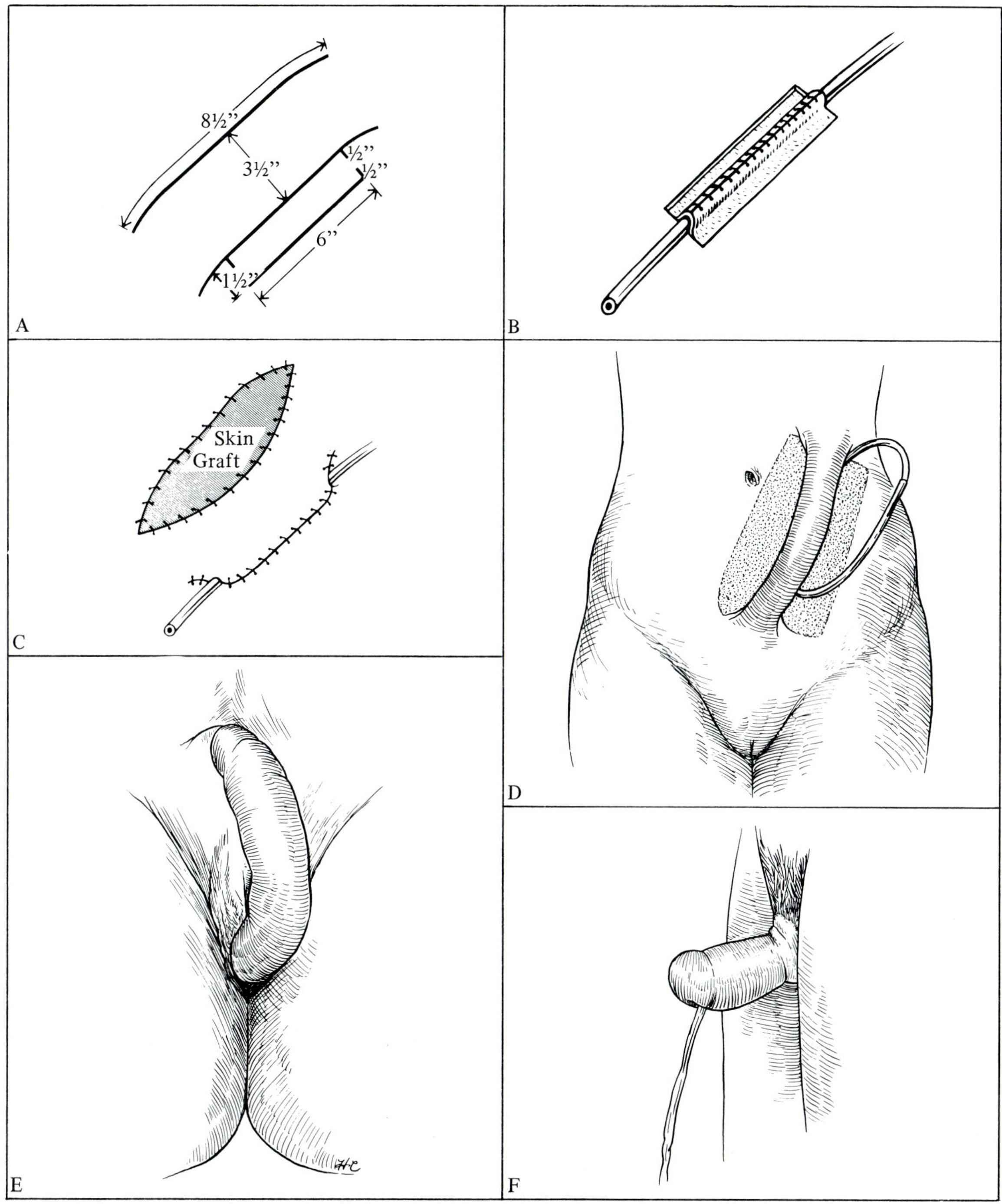

Fig. 56-7. Phalloplasty after the Gillies method. A, the incisions. B, the urethral flap is sutured (raw side out) over the catheter, C, the neourethra is covered by a skin flap. D, at the end of the second stage, the flap containing the neourethra has been tubed. E, at the third stage, the upper end of the pedicle has been inset into the perineum. F, the final result after a cartilage graft has been inserted, showing the angle of urine flow. (From A. J. Evans. In C. E. Horton [Ed.], Plastic and Reconstructive Surgery of the Genital Area. *Boston: Little, Brown, 1973.)*

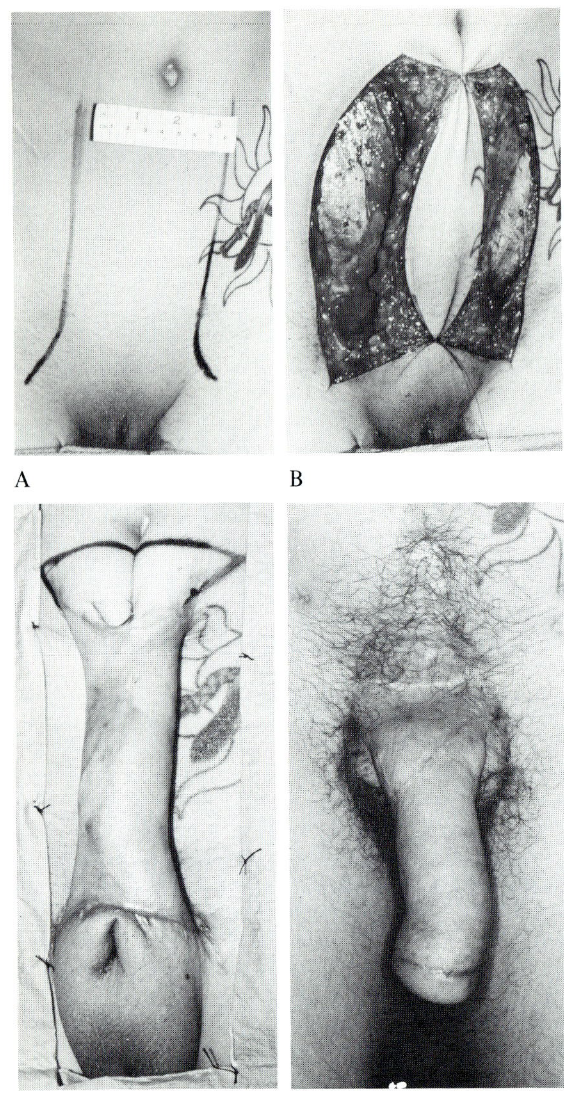

Fig. 56-8. Phalloplasty after Davies and Birdsell. A, the incisions for the first stage. B, the bipedicle flap is raised and tubed. C, at the second stage, the superior pedicle is divided and a neoglans fashioned. D, the final result. (From J. Noe, D. Birdsell, and D. Laub, Plast. Reconstr. Surg. *53:511, 1974.)*

the flap. The bipedicle flap is then undermined at the level of Scarpa's fascia, and it is tubed with the skin turned inside. A split-thickness skin graft taken from the buttock or hip is then sewn around the tube in a spiral fashion to avoid a single longitudinal scar. A split-thickness skin graft is also used to line the base of the inferior pedicle; this facilitates subsequent mobilization at the second stage. The donor site for the tube is closed primarily under tension, employing large retention sutures as needed. Postoperatively the patient is not allowed to flex at the hips, and the tube is supported by a carefully applied dressing for several days. Once the grafts are completely healed, the patient is instructed to use a tourniquet around the superior pedicle to condition the flap. The second stage, which is done a minimum of 3 months after the first stage, involves releasing the superior pedicle along with an elliptical extension from which the neoglans is fashioned. After the superior pedicle has been released, the old abdominal scar is excised and hysterectomy and bilateral salpingo-oophorectomy can be conveniently performed.

This procedure results in a neophallus with a skin-lined tube running through it that is open at both ends. Stiffening is provided by a special Teflon rod or baculum that can be placed into this channel by the patient when sexual intercourse is desired. The proximal end of the baculum rests under the pubic symphysis in the region of the patient's clitoris; therefore, it can serve as a source of erotic stimulation during the act of coitus.

We have not attempted to establish urinary continuity through the neophallus because of the possible complications. However, tissue is available for this extension of the urethra. To circumvent the need for urinary reconstruction and yet still allow the patient to void in a standing posture, Schultz [54] has developed a "urinary assist device," which consists of a small cup that fits over the normal female urethral meatus with a long silicone tube placed through the channel in the neophallus. This device then serves as a passive conduit for urine, which exits from the neoglans.

At the time of the second-stage procedure, the anterior portions of the labia majora may be fused in the midline to simulate a scrotum; then at an optional third-stage procedure, testicular prostheses may be placed. Another optional revision involves transposing hair-bearing pedicle tissue from the labia majora to the suprapubic location. This helps to camouflage scars and also simulates a male escutcheon.

Horton [27] has recently described a one-stage method that utilizes a gracilis myocutaneous flap. He emphasizes that a key requirement in neophallus construction is the provision of adequate sensibility. To achieve this goal, he uses a superiorly and inferiorly based vaginal flap as a sensory surface combined with a gracilis myocutaneous flap. The urethra is lengthened at the same operation. While the neophallus is constructed in one stage, Horton admits that many subsequent revisions are necessary to achieve the best results. The patient can voluntarily contract the gracilis muscle and thereby make the neophallus firm, but it does not elongate. Horton thinks that the patient will require a penile implant to facilitate intercourse.

Durfee and Roland [10] have described a procedure that involves lengthening the hypertrophied clitoris. After many months of therapy with high doses of androgen, the patient undergoes two procedures. In the first procedure the labia minora is used to extend the urethra to the tip of the clitoris. At a second stage, the base of the clitoris is mobilized and advanced downward 2 or 3 cm. This reportedly produces a phallus-like structure 7½ cm. long; no erectile capability is present. It is reported that some patients are satisfied with this result.

Some patients will decide against phalloplasty; for these patients a number of prosthetic penile substitutes are available. Those patients who have elected to proceed with phalloplasty have in general been pleased with the results.

RESULTS OF SURGERY FOR THE TRANSSEXUAL PATIENT

The Stanford Gender Dysphoria Program has recently conducted an in-depth review of 97 patients who have had surgical treatment for transsexualism [48]. This included 75 male-to-female patients and 22 female-to-male patients. Follow-up periods ranged from 6 months to 8 years. In general, surgery had a favorable effect on sexual adjustment. All but 11 of the 75 male-to-female patients had functioned sexually, and 20 of the patients were married. Among the 22 female-to-male patients, 16 were having satisfactory sexual intercourse. Economic adjustment as measured by employment status was relatively unchanged by surgery. Two-thirds of the patients were felt to have improved social adjustment as assessed by family relationships and the lack of association with the transsexual community. Psychologically, most patients had acquired positive self-attitudes postoperatively. However, patients who exhibited sociopathic behavior preoperatively tended to continue in this behavior pattern postoperatively. Some surgical complication occurred in 33 of the 75 male-to-female patients (as seen in Table 56-1). There were 2 patients who committed suicide postoperatively, and 2 patients who underwent neocolporrhaphy returned to living as males.

In our long-term follow-up the findings were in accord with those of Meyer [42], who found that the patients experienced an initial period (2 to 5 years) of euphoria at achieving the goal of obtaining gender surgery. However, the patients eventually came to realize that, although they could pass in their new gender, they still were different from a genetic male or female and always would be. Furthermore, the basic psychological problems present before surgery often persisted.

REFERENCES

1. Barbosa, J. Surgery Experience with Large Series of Transsexual Patients. Harry Benjamin Fourth International Conference on Gender Identity. Stanford University, Palo Alto, February 1975.
2. Barlow, D., Reynolds, J., and Agras, S. Gender identity change in a transsexual. *Arch. Gen. Psychiatry* 28:569, 1973.
3. Bellinger, C., and Goulian, D. Secondary surgery in transsexuals. *Plast. Reconstr. Surg.* 51:628, 1973.
4. Benjamin, H. *The Transsexual Phenomenon.* New York: Julian Press, 1966.
5. Biber, S. Harry Benjamin Fourth International Conference on Gender Identity. Stanford University, Palo Alto, February 1975.
6. Block, N., and Tessler, A. Transsexualism and surgical procedures. *Surg. Gynecol. Obstet.* 132: 517, 1971.
7. Burou, G. Male to Female Transformation. *Proceedings of the Second Interdisciplinary Symposium on Gender Dysphoria Syndrome.* Stanford University School of Medicine, Palo Alto, 1973.
8. Caldwell, D. O. Psychopathis transsexualis. *Sexology* 16:274, 1949.
9. Davies, D. Presented at the Third International Confederation of Plastic Surgery, Washington, D.C., 1962.
10. Durfee, R., and Roland, W. Penile Substitution with Clitoral Enlargement and Urethral Transfer. *Proceedings of the Second Interdisciplinary Symposium on Gender Dysphoria Syndrome.* Stanford University School of Medicine, Palo Alto, 1973.
11. Edgerton, M. The surgical treatment of male transsexuals. *Clin. Plast. Surg.* 1:285, 1974.
12. Edgerton, M., and Bull, J. Surgical construction of a vagina and labia in male transsexuals. *Plast. Reconstr. Surg.* 46:529, 1970.
13. Ehrhardt, A. The Etiology of Transsexualism. *Proceedings of the Second Interdisciplinary Symposium on Gender Dysphoria Syndrome.* Stanford University School of Medicine, Palo Alto, 1973.
14. Fisk, N. Gender Dysphoria Syndrome – The How, Why and What of a Condition. *Proceedings of the Second Interdisciplinary Symposium on Gender Dysphoria Syndrome.* Stanford University School

of Medicine, Palo Alto, 1973.
15. Flowers, R. One Stage Operation for Male Transsexuals. *Proceedings of the Second Interdisciplinary Symposium on Gender Dysphoria Syndrome.* Stanford University School of Medicine, Palo Alto, 1973.
16. Friedman, R., Green, R., and Spitzer, R. Reassessment of homosexuality and transsexualism. *Annu. Rev. Med.* 27:57, 1976.
17. Gonzales-Ulloa, M., and Stevens, E. The role of chin correction in profileplasty. *Plast. Reconstr. Surg.* 41:477, 1968.
18. Good, R. Thyroid Cartilage Shaved. *Proceedings of the Second Interdisciplinary Symposium on Gender Dysphoria Syndrome.* Stanford University School of Medicine, Palo Alto, 1973.
19. Govan, D., and Hentz, V. A Surgical Program and Technique for Male to Female Patients. *Proceedings of the Second Interdisciplinary Symposium on Gender Dysphoria Syndrome.* Stanford University School of Medicine, Palo Alto, 1973.
20. Granato, R. Surgical approach to male transsexuals. *Urology* 3:792, 1974.
21. Green, R., and Money, J. (Eds.). *Transsexualism and Sex Reassignment.* Baltimore: Johns Hopkins University Press, 1969.
22. Green, R., Newman, L., and Soller, R. Treatment of boyhood transsexualism. *Arch. Gen. Psychiatry* 26:213, 1972.
23. Hamburger, C., Sturup, J. K., and Dahl-Iverson, E. Transvestism: Hormonal, psychiatric and surgical treatment. *J.A.M.A.* 152:391, 1953.
24. Hastings, D. The surgical route. *Int. J. Psychoanal.* 9:273, 1970–71.
25. Hastings, D. Post surgical adjustment of male transsexual patients. *Clin. Plast. Surg.* 1:335, 1974.
26. Hoopes, J. E. Surgical correction of the male external genitalia. *Clin. Plast. Surg.* 1:325, 1974.
27. Horton, C. Presented at the annual meeting of the American Society of Plastic and Reconstructive Surgeons, San Francisco, 1977.
28. Jayaram, D. Personal communication, 1977.
29. Jones, H., Schrimer, H., and Hoopes, J. E. A sex conversion operation for males with transsexualism. *Am. J. Obstet. Gynecol.* 100:101, 1968.
30. Kaplan, I. A rapid method for constructing a functional sensitive penis. *Br. J. Plast. Reconstr. Surg.* 24:342, 1971.
31. Kirkpatrick, M., and Friedman, C. Treatment of request for sex change surgery with psychotherapy. *Am. J. Psychiatry* 133:1194, 1976.
32. Laub, D. R., and Fisk, N. A rehabilitation program for gender dysphoria syndrome by surgical sex change. *Plast. Reconstr. Surg.* 53:388, 1974.
33. Lehrman, K. Pulmonary embolism in a transsexual man taking diethylstilbestrol. *J.A.M.A.* 235:532, 1976.
34. Levine, S. Personal communication, 1977.
35. Malloy, T., Noone, B., and Morgan, J. Experience with the one-stage surgical approach for constructing female genitalia in male transsexuals. *J. Urol.* 116:335, 1976.
36. Markland, C. Complications in Male Transsexual Surgery. *Proceedings of the Second Interdisciplinary Symposium on Gender Dysphoria Syndrome.* Stanford University School of Medicine, Palo Alto, 1973.
37. Markland, C. Vaginal reconstruction using cecal and sigmoid bowel segments in transsexual patients. *J. Urol.* 111:217, 1974.
38. Markland, C. Transsexual surgery. *Obstet. Gynecol. Annu.* 4:309, 1975.
39. McIndoe, A. Deformities of the male urethra. *Br. J. Plast. Surg.* 1:29, 1948–49.
40. McRoberts, J. Sex Conversion Surgery for Biological Male Transsexuals. *Proceedings of the Second Interdisciplinary Symposium on Gender Dysphoria Syndrome.* Stanford University School of Medicine, Palo Alto, 1973.
41. Meyer, J. Some Thoughts on Nosology and Motivation among Transsexuals. *Proceedings of the Second Interdisciplinary Symposium on Gender Dysphoria Syndrome.* Stanford University School of Medicine, Palo Alto, 1973.
42. Meyer, J. Psychiatric considerations in the sexual reassignment of non-intersex individuals. *Clin. Plast. Surg.* 1:275, 1974.
43. Meyer, J., and Hoopes, J. E. The gender dysphoria syndrome. *Plast. Reconstr. Surg.* 54:444, 1974.
44. Money, J. Long-term psychological follow-up of intersexed patients. *Clin. Plast. Surg.* 1:271, 1974.
45. Money, J., and Ehrhardt, A. *Man and Woman, Boy and Girl.* Baltimore: Johns Hopkins University Press, 1972.
46. Montague, D. K. Transsexualism. *Urology* 2:1, 1973.
47. Noe, J., Birdsell, D., and Laub, D. The surgical construction of male genitalia for the female to male transsexual. *Plast. Reconstr. Surg.* 53:511, 1974.
48. Norberg, M., and Laub, D. Harry Benjamin Fourth International Conference on Gender Identity, Stanford University, Palo Alto, February 1975.
49. Orticochea, M. A new method of total reconstruction of the penis. *Br. J. Plast. Surg.* 25:347, 1972.
50. Pandya, M., and Stuteville, O. A one-stage technique for constructing female external genitalia in male transsexuals. *Br. J. Plast. Surg.* 26:277, 1973.

51. Pauley, I. B. Male psychosexual inversion: Transsexualism. *Arch. Gen. Psychiatry* 13:172, 1965.
52. Randall, J. Preoperative and Postoperative Status of Male and Female Transsexuals. In Green, R., and Money, J. (Eds.), *Transsexualism and Sex Reassignment*. Baltimore: Johns Hopkins University Press, 1969.
53. Rish, B. Technique of Male to Female Surgery. *Proceedings of the Second Interdisciplinary Symposium on Gender Dysphoria Syndrome.* Stanford University School of Medicine, Palo Alto, 1973.
54. Schultz, W. Personal communication, 1977.
55. Symmers, W. Carcinoma of the breast in transsexual individuals after surgical and hormonal interference with primary and secondary sex characteristics. *Br. Med. J.* 2:82, 1968.
56. Wolfort, F., and Pany, R. Laryngeal chondroplasty for appearance. *Plast. Reconstr. Surg.* 56:371, 1975.
57. Yalom, I., Green, R., and Fisk, N. Prenatal exposure to female hormones: Effect on psychosocial development in boys. *Arch. Gen. Psychiatry* 28:554, 1973.

Selected Reading List

Selected Reading List*

General References

Borges, A. F. *Elective Incisions and Scar Revisions.* Boston: Little, Brown, 1973.

Converse, J. M. *Reconstructive Plastic Surgery* (2nd ed.). Vols. 1–7. Philadelphia: Saunders, 1977.

Fitzpatrick, T. B., Eisen, A. Z., Wolff, K., Freedberg, I. M., and Austen, K. F. *Dermatology in General Medicine.* New York: McGraw-Hill, 1979.

Goldwyn, R. M. *The Unfavorable Result in Plastic Surgery.* Boston: Little, Brown, 1972.

Kernahan, D. A., and Vistnes, L. M. *Biological Aspects of Reconstructive Surgery.* Boston: Little, Brown, 1977.

McGregor, I. A. *Fundamental Techniques of Plastic Surgery* (6th ed.). London: Churchill Livingstone, 1975.

Peacock, E. E., Jr., and Van Winckle, W., Jr. *Wound Repair* (2nd ed.). Philadelphia: Saunders, 1976.

Trauma; Aesthetic and Reconstructive Surgery

Artz, C. P., Moncrief, J. A., and Pruitt, B. A. *Burns: A Team Approach.* Philadelphia: Saunders, 1979.

Daniel, R. K., and Terzis, J. K. *Reconstructive Microsurgery.* Boston: Little, Brown, 1976.

Dingman, R. O., and Natvig, P. *Surgery of Facial Fractures.* Philadelphia: Saunders, 1964.

Georgiade, N. *Reconstructive Breast Surgery.* St. Louis: Mosby, 1976.

Goldwyn, R. M. *Plastic and Reconstructive Surgery of the Breast.* Boston: Little, Brown, 1976.

Grabb, W. C., and Myers, M. B. *Skin Flaps.* Boston: Little, Brown, 1975.

Kazanjian, V. H., and Converse, J. M. *Surgical Treatment of Facial Fractures.* Baltimore: Williams & Wilkins, 1974.

Mustardé, J. C. *Repair and Reconstruction of the Orbital Region* (2nd ed.). Baltimore: Williams & Wilkins, 1979.

Reeh, M. J., Beyer, C. K., and Shannon, G. M. *Practical Ophthalmic Plastic and Reconstructive Surgery.* Philadelphia: Lea & Febiger, 1976.

Rees, T. D., and Wood-Smith, D. *Cosmetic Facial Surgery.* Philadelphia: Saunders, 1973.

Serafin, D., and Buncke, H. J. *Microsurgical Composite Tissue Transplantation.* St. Louis: Mosby, 1979.

Sheen, J. H. *Aesthetic Rhinoplasty.* St. Louis: Mosby, 1978.

Hand Surgery

Boyes, J. H. *Bunnell's Surgery of the Hand* (5th ed.). Philadelphia: Lippincott, 1970.

Flatt, A. E. *The Care of Minor Hand Injuries.* St. Louis: Mosby, 1972.

Flynn, J. E. *Hand Surgery* (2nd ed.). Baltimore: Williams and Wilkins, 1975.

Henry, A. K. *Extensile Exposure Applied to Limb Surgery.* Baltimore: Longman, 1970.

Lister, G. *The Hand: Diagnosis and Indications.* London: Churchill/Livingstone, 1977.

Littler, J. W. Volume 6 in *Reconstructive Plastic Surgery* by J. M. Converse. Philadelphia: Saunders, 1977.

Rank, B. K., Wakefield, A. R., and Hueston, J. T. *Surgery of Repair as Applied to Hand Injuries* (4th ed.). Edinburgh: Churchill/Livingstone, 1973.

Spinner, M. *Injuries to the Major Branches of Peripheral Nerves of the Forearm* (2nd ed.). Philadelphia: Saunders, 1978.

Congenital Defects

Grabb, W. C., Rosenstein, S. W., and Bzoch, K. R. *Cleft Lip and Palate Surgical, Dental and Speech Aspects.* Boston: Little, Brown, 1971.

Millard, D. R., Jr., *Cleft Craft - The Evolution of its Surgery,* Vols. I and II. Boston: Little, Brown, 1977.

Mustardé, J. C. *Plastic Surgery in Infancy and Childhood* (2nd ed.). London: Churchill/Livingstone, 1979.

Oncology

Andrade, R., Cumport, S. L., Popkin, G. I., and Rees, T. D. *Cancer of the Skin: Biology, Diagnosis and Management.* Philadelphia: Saunders, 1976.

Batsakis, J. G. *Tumors of the Head and Neck* (2nd ed.). Baltimore: Williams & Wilkins, 1979.

Haagensen, C. D. *Diseases of the Breast.* Philadelphia: Saunders, 1974.

Loré, J. M. *An Atlas of Head and Neck Surgery* (2nd ed.). Philadelphia: Saunders, 1973.

*Compiled with the assistance of Kenneth Rothaus

Index

Index

Abbe flap (vermillion-bordered lip flap)
division time, 44
in lip reconstruction, 7, 345, 348
secondary, after cleft lip closure, 198
Abdominal dermolipectomy, 838–843
complications, 842–843
in dermochalasis, 839–841
W-technique, 839, 840, 841, 842
dressings and postoperative care, 841–842, 843
in obesity, 838–839
"fleur de lys" technique for lower and medial, 838–839
modified Weinhold technique with T scar, 839, 840
Abdominal wall
abdominoplasty in breast reconstruction, 786, 791, 793, 794. *See also* Abdominal dermolipectomy
closure of mucosal excision in exstrophy of bladder, 867
skin flaps from, 56
in breast reconstruction, 786, 791, 792
for cheek defects, 349
tubed, in phalloplasty, 892, 893, 894
skin grafts from, 21, 25, 56
Abductor digiti minimi transposition for ankle defects, 815
Abductor hallucis brevis transposition for leg defects, 815
Abrasion
adventitious tattooing and, 559
facial, 227, 229
hand, 580–581
Absorbable sutures
described, 10–11
wound infection and, 12
Accessory salivary gland tumors, 395, 396
Acetabulum reconstruction, 106
Achilles tendon
defects
muscle transposition in, 815, 816
skin flaps in reverse in, 46, 47
pressure sore closure, 823

By Helene K. Marer

Acne rosacea, 544–545
Acne vulgaris, 543–544
Acquired digital fibrokeratoma, 537
Acracephalosyndactyly. *See* Apert's syndrome
Acrochordon, 536
Acrospiroma, accrine, 534
ACTH, adrenogenital syndrome and, 877
Actinic (senile) keratosis, 532, 643
Adenocarcinoma(s)
forehead and scalp, 275
jaw, 361
Adenoid cystic carcinoma of oral floor, 363
Adenoidectomy, 217
Adenofibroma of breast, 761, 763
Adenoma(s)
benign, of parotid gland, 391
defined, 533
sebaceous, 535, 537
Adenomammectomy. *See* Mastectomy, subcutaneous
Adhesive(s), 98
dressings
after abdominal dermolipectomy, 841–842, 843
after arm reduction, 850
in skin graft fixation, 29–30
in wound closure, 15–16, 756, 768
Adrenogenital syndrome, 877
Advancement flaps, 52–54
in helical rim defects, 311
limitations in use of, 54
in lip reconstruction, 345, 346, 348
multiple Y-V, 53
volar, in fingertip injury, 572, 573, 575
Advancement of wound edges in radiation injury, 487
Adventitious (traumatic) tattoos
defined, 559
treatment, 559–560
Aesthetic surgery. *See* Cosmetic surgery; *and specific topic, e.g.,* Blepharoplasty
Agenesis, vaginal, 873, 881
Airway maintenance
in burns, 463, 475, 477
in cleft palate, 209
in cystic hygroma, 523
in facial trauma, 227, 242
postoperative
maxillary hypoplasia, 173
velopharyngeal incompetence, 221
Alar cartilages
composite grafts for closure of, 18, 324
in rhinoplasty
incisions and sculpturing, 424, 426, 427–429, 433, 545
wedge resection of base, 431–432
Allograft(s), 75–85
acquired transplantation tolerance, 81–82
allograft reaction, 75–82
clonal selection theory, 79
histologic change and, 75–76
immune mechanism and, 76–77
immunologic enhancement and, 77–78
lymphocytes and, 78–79
prolongation of allograft survival, 79–82
in burn wound closure, 18, 474
defined, 75
donor selection, 82–84
graft-versus-host reaction and, 82
immune mechanism and, 76–78, 79, 80
allograft survival, 79–80, 81–82
immunological enhancement, 77–78
specific immunological tolerance, 80
immunological inaccessibility of, 79–80
immunosuppressive agents and, 80–81
isogenic transplants, 84
in nasal reconstruction, 323
nerve, 694
as skin graft donor site dressing, 33
survival, 79–82
factors prolonging, 79–80
methods of prolonging, 80–82
tissue selection for, 79, 84, 85
tissue typing for, 82–84
wound bacteria and, 24
Allopathic implantation. *See* Breast implants and prostheses. Implants and prostheses
Alopecia, 275–277, 545–546
differential diagnosis, 545
incidence, 275
treatment, 275–277, 545–546
hair plugs in, 275–276, 545–546
patient selection for, 275
scalp flaps in, 276–277, 545–546
strip grafts in, 276, 545–546
Alopecia areata, 545
Alveolus, dental
bone grafts in clefts, 211
cleft
cleft lip and, 205
repair, 210, 211–212, 213, 214

Alveolus, dental –*Continued*
preprosthetic surgery, 178
tumors, 361, 362
Ambiguous external genitalia, differential diagnosis, 878
Ameloblastomas of jaw, 361, 362
Ambulation in pressure sore prevention, 819
Amputation, therapeutic
digital ray (metacarpal), 577–578
fingers, 575–578, 648
fingernail management, 577, 578
functional losses, 575–576
high-voltage electrical burns, 493
multiple digit losses, 576
techniques of, 576–577, 578
Amputation, traumatic
of ear, 307
of penis, 870–871, 878
replantation in, 699. *See also* Replantation
care of part for replantation, 700
operative technique and level of, 709–711
Amputation neuroma, 107
digit, 577
excision of, 107
hand, 577, 644
Anastomoses in microvascular surgery, 658, 659, 660, 663–665, 666, 667, 668, 669–670
end-to-end, 660, 663–665, 666, 668, 669–670
end-to-side, 660, 665, 667, 668, 669–670
in free tissue transfer, 674
hemostasis in, 662, 668
luminal diameter differences and, 665, 666, 669–670
patency rates, 662, 668
principles of, 662–663
suturing, 662, 663
of vein grafts in replantation, 709
Anastomotic arteries, 37–38
Androgen insensitivity syndrome (testicular feminization syndrome, 876–877, 878)
Androgens
adrenogenital syndrome and, 877
external genitalia development and, 873
female-to-male patients and, 892
gynecomastia and, 802
in pregnancy
gender dysphoria and, 884–885
sexual development and, 878
receptors, testicular feminization syndrome and, 876–877
Anesthesia. *See under specific procedure*
Angiofibromas, 537
Angioleiomyomas, 535
Angiomas, 643
Animal bites, 229, 237–238
contamination of, 237
rabies vaccination in, 237–238
Ankle defects, muscle transposition in, 815, 816
Ankylosis
of finger joints
interphalangeal joints, 598–601
metacarpophalangeal joints, 601–603
of temperomandibular joint
described, 182, 183, 186–187
management, 182, 187–188
Anophthalmia, orbit in, 155
Antecubital region as skin graft donor site, 20
Antibiotics
in avulsion injuries of penis, 869
in burns, 460, 467, 469, 476
electrical burns, 491, 492, 493
in facial wounds, 238
in hand infections, 579, 581
intraoperative, in combined radical neck dissection, 369
preoperative, prosthesis insertion after mastectomy and, 768
in pressure sores, 819, 822
in pyoderma gangrenosum, 547
after replantation, 713
in septicemia, 478
in skin graft infection, 31
in temperomandibular joint infection, 182
topical, bacteria in open wounds and, 24
Apert's syndrome, 120, 145–150
combined Le Fort III and I osteotomy in, 148, 149
coronal craniectomy in, 154–155
differential diagnosis, 119, 120
etiology, 120
Le Fort III maxillary advancement in, 145–148
orbital hypertelorism correction, 148, 149
physical signs, 120, 144
subcranial hypertelorism correction, 148–149
total correction, 153–154
Apertognathia, 140, 172, 182
Aplastic lymphedema, 828
Apocrine cystadenomas, 535
Apocrine tumors, 535
Areola-nipple complex
abnormalities after gynecomastia surgery, 806
Areola-nipple complex – *Continued*
construction
areola and nipple grafts in, 791
areola sharing procedures, 21
auricular cartilage in, 792, 798
composite nipple graft, 791
concentric-circle or conjoined spiral nipple sharing, 791, 797
conchal cartilage in, 792
hemorrhoidal tissue in, 791
labia majora or minora in, 791
nipple sharing in, 791–797
position and shape errors, 750
split-thickness skin grafts in, 791
continuity with skin or skin flaps, 768, 770
determination of location of, 792
free grafts
in gynecomastia, 806
in reduction mammoplasty, 744, 746, 747
medical tattooing in loss of, 560, 792
necrosis after reduction mammoplasty, 737, 746–747, 748
sensation
after augmentation mammoplasty, 721, 723, 726–727
evaluation, 748–749
after reduction mammoplasty, 748–749
in skin flaps in mastectomy, 767
as skin graft donor site, 21
special innervation of, 749
storage during mastectomy, 792
timing placement of, 786, 792
Arms. *See also* Finger(s); Hand; Thumb
constricting scars, Z-plasty for, 64
direct flaps from, 54–56
direct flaps from trunk to, 54–55
innervation, 619, 620
lipectomy, 849–850
lymphatic system, 827
lymphedema, subcutaneous excision in, 833–834
replantation, operative technique, 703–704, 709–710
split-thickness skin graft cutting on, 25
tendon injuries
extensor tendon, 604, 607
flexor tendons, 615
Arterial flaps. *See* Axial pattern flaps
Arteries. *See also* Blood vessels
aneurysms in hand, 645–646
insufficiency, ulceration and, 811
microvascular anastomoses
end-to-end, 660, 663, 664, 665

Arteries, microvascular anastomoses – *Continued*
end-to-side, 660, 665, 667, 668, 669–670
luminal diameter differences and, 665, 666, 669–670
postoperative problems
free skin grafts and, 676
free tissue transfer and, 675
in replantation, 705–706, 707
correction of tension, 706
excision of end, 706
flow confirmation and observation, 706, 707, 713
irrigation, 706
preparation of, 703, 706
suturing, 706
Arteriovenous fistulas, 229, 524
Arteriovenous malformations, 524
Arthrodesis in replantation
amputated part, 701
wrist, 710
Arthroplasty
in rheumatoid arthritis
metacarpophalangeal joint, 632–634
wrist volar carpal subluxation, 635
temperomandibular joint, 185, 187, 188
Atraumatic technique of excision of skin lesions, 3
Atropine as circulation test, 45
Atypical fibroxanthomas, 537
Augmentation mammoplasty, 719–729, 731–736
aesthetic goals, 720, 721
complications, 105, 722, 723, 724, 725, 726–729
capsular contraction, 722, 724, 725, 727–729. *See also* Breast, postoperative capsular contraction
erosion of prosthesis, 727
hematoma, 722, 724, 725, 727
infection, 725, 727
leakage of prosthesis, 727
Monder's disease, 727
ptosis of prosthesis, 727
scarring, 723, 724
sensation changes, 721, 723, 726–727
wound separation, 727
dressings, 726
fat grafts in, 89, 719
history of, 719–720
indications for, 720–721
after male-to-female surgery, 891
mastopexy plus, in ptosis, 720, 751
operative technique, 721–724
inframammary technique, 721–723
Augmentation mammoplasty, operative technique – *Continued*
periareolar technique, 721, 722, 723–724
transaxillary technique, 721, 722, 724, 725
postoperative home care, 725–726
postoperative orders, 725–726
preoperative breast examination and evaluation, 721
preoperative preparation, 721
prostheses and implants, 105, 751
chemical composition of, 720
evaluation of inflatable vs. gel-filled, 725
fluid, 103
history of, 719–720
implant fixation, 725
types, described, 724–725, 731–736
psychological factors and, 719, 720–721
reexamination after, 726
typical patient, described, 719
Augmentation mentoplasty
implants and prostheses in, 100–101
operative technique of, 166–167
profile and, 432–433
Augmentation of nasal tip in rhinoplasty, 428–429, 433, 436, 437
Auricle. *See also* Auricle reconstruction
anatomy and embryology of normal, 440, 441
anomalies in hemifacial microsomia, 116, 117
avulsion, 307
burns, 307–308
cartilage of
in auricle reconstruction, 308–309, 310, 311, 313
in helical defects, 311
marsilization in otoplasty, 441–442
definition and elevation in auricle reconstruction, 305–306
prostheses for, 300–301, 303, 307
trauma, 307–308
Auricle reconstruction, 299–316
in acquired defects, 308–316
cutaneous pocket construction, 307
external auditory canal, 309
helical rim loss management, 309, 312, 313, 314, 315
in lower-third auricular defects, 310, 312, 315
in middle-third auricular defects, 311, 312, 314
Auricle reconstruction, in acquired defects – *Continued*
problems in, 306–308
residual tissue utilization in, 308–309, 310, 311
support materials in, 308–309, 310, 311, 314
in upper-third defects, 310, 311–312, 313
galeal flap in, 305
helical rim reconstruction in, 309, 311, 312, 313, 314, 315
hemostasis in, 302, 303
in microtia, 299–306
coadaptation of skin to framework, 303, 304
elevation of upper auricular region, 306
framework fabrication, 300, 301–302
framework implantation, 302–303, 304
framework materials, 299, 300–301, 302, 303
lobule rotation, 300, 305
location of reconstructed ear, 300
optimum time for, 299
planning and preparation, 300, 301, 302
postoperative management and complications, 303, 304, 305
preoperative consultation, 299
touch-up and secondary reconstruction, 306
tragal construction and conchal definition, 305–306
postoperative infection, 303, 305
primary vs. secondary, 233
prostheses and implants in, 300–301, 303, 307
problems with, 307
psychological factors and, 299
in satyr ear, 448
skin flaps in, 448
coadaptation to framework, 303, 304
limitation of, 299
skin grafts in auricle definition, 303, 306
"valise handle" technique, 305–306, 310, 316
Autograft(s), 85–90
bone, 87–88, 94
in burn closure, 18
cartilage, 88–89, 94
collagen, 87
defined, 75
dermis, 86–87
fascia, 89, 94
fat, 89
indications and advantages, 94
muscle, 89–90
nerve, 694

Avulsion injuries
  auricle, 307
  chin, 237
  eyelid, 233, 235
  face, 222, 230–232, 239–240
    excision and dressing, 230, 231
    mechanisms of, 230, 231
    skin flaps for, 235
    skin grafts for, 232
  fingernail, 575
  lower extremity, 812
  male urethra, 872
  penis, 869–870
  perineal, with scrotal loss, 871
  replantation in, 698
  scalp, 267, 268, 269
  scrotal skin, 871–872
Axial arteries, 37–38
Axial pattern flaps
  blood supply, 38, 39, 40, 48
  delay procedure, 38
  design and size, 38, 40
  free flaps, 39, 41
  island flaps, 38–39
  in nasal reconstruction, 326, 329
  peninsular flaps, 38
  survival of, 35, 36
Axilla
  as free flap donor site, 676, 677
  hidradenitis suppurativa, 546
  hyperhydrosis, 546
  lymph nodes of, 827

Bakamjian flap, 40, 51–52, 374. *See also* Deltopectoral flaps
Baldness. *See* Alopecia
Baldwin technique for vaginal construction, 880
Banner flap
  in auricle reconstruction, 313
  in nasal reconstruction, 325
Basal cell carcinoma
  external ear, 502
  eyelid, 505
  hand, 647
  scalp, 274, 275
  skin, 504–506
    clinical types, 504–505
    limits of excision of, 499
    recurrence, 505
    site and incidence, 504
    terebrating (boring), 503–504
    treatment, 504, 505
Basal cell epitheliomas, 535
Baseball (mallet) finger, 604–605
BCG vaccine
  as immune-response stimulant in cancer, 368
  in malignant melanoma, 515
Bell's palsy, 337, 338
Benign juvenile melanoma, 530
Benign mixed salivary gland tumors, 391, 392–393, 395
Bennett's fracture of thumb, 596
Bifid clitoris, 865
Bifid nose with median cleft lip, 122–123
Bifid uvula, 209
Bilobed flap for donor site closure, 49, 50
Biological dressings, 24, 85, 95
Biopsy punch in tattoo removal, 562, 563
Bipedicle flaps
  advancement, 54
  dividing base of, 36
  in phalloplasty, 894
  tubed, on neck, 56
  from upper lip in eyelid reconstruction, 284
Bites, 229, 237–238
Bladder
  carcinoma, exstrophy and, 866
  exstrophy, 865, 866–867. *See also* Exstrophy of bladder
  mucosa excision, 867
  spasm 864
Blascowicz technique for eyelid ptosis, 293, 295
Bleeding. *See* Hemorrhage
Blepharochalasis, 404
Blepharophimosis, ptosis with, 297
Blepharoplasty, 404–408
  anesthesia in, 404
  approach to protruding fat, 404, 405, 406, 407, 408
  closure and postoperative care, 408
  skin excision and incisions in, 404, 405, 406
Blood vessels. *See also* Arteries; Circulation and blood supply; Vein(s)
  angiomas, 643
  lymphatic system physiology and, 827
  in replantation
    arteries, 705–706, 707
    preoperative preparation, 701–702, 703
    veins, 707–708
  skin loss in extremities and, 811
  surgery. *See* Anastomoses in microvascular surgery; Microvascular surgery
Blowout fracture(s), 251–259
  associated injuries, 254
  common sites, 251, 253
  defined, 251
  diplopia in, 251–252, 257
  enophthalmos in, 252, 254, 257
  implants in, 102
    postoperative extrusion of, 258
  indications for surgery, 254–255
Blowout fracture(s) – *Continued*
  infraorbital nerve and, 254, 259
  postoperative complications
    asymmetrical inferior scleral exposure, 257–258
    damage to lacrimal pump, 259
    enophthalmos over or under correction, 257
    eyelid lymphedema, 258–259
    implant extrusion, 258
    infection, 258
    infraorbital nerve hyperesthesia or anesthesia, 259
    residual diplopia, 257
  production of, 251, 253
  surgical therapy, 255–257
    anterior infraorbital approach, 255–257
    Caldwell-Luc approach, 257
Blue nevi, 531–532, 643
Bone. *See also* Bone grafts; Osteotomy
  acute trauma, surgical management, 155
  dust in skull reconstruction, 271–272
  exposed, covering, 479
    cranial, 267, 268, 269
    muscle flaps in, 89
    muscle transposition in, 812–817
    reverse dermis grafts in, 812
    skin flaps in, 41, 56–57
    skin grafts in, 17, 22
  finger
    management of end in amputation, 577
    shortening and closure in injury, 574, 576
  free bone transfer for defects, 678, 680
  periosteal membrane and regeneration of, 88
  prosthetic replacement of, 106
  radiation injury, 486
    management, 487–488
  removal in pressure sore management, 820, 821, 823, 824
  in replantation
    fixation, 704, 705, 709, 710
    resection in amputated part, 701, 703
  structure of, 87
  tumors
    hand, 646–647, 648
    surgical management of, 155–156
Bone dust in skull reconstruction, 271–272
Bone flaps with flexor tendon grafting, 612

Bone grafts. *See also* Iliac bone grafts; Split-rib grafts
allografts, 84
in alveolar clefts, 211
autografts, 94
avascular necrosis of, 86
cancellous, 87–88
in cleft palate repair, 213–214
cortical, 87, 88
in craniofacial contour irregularities, 134, 155, 270
in cranioplasty, 269–272
contour restoration after, 270
iliac bone, 269, 271
prostheses plus, 102
securing graft, 270–271
split-rib grafts, 269–270
donor sites, 87–88
in fractures, 155
free vascularized, 678, 680
fate of, 87–88
growth of, 88
immobilization of, 87, 88
mandible, 103, 175–176, 177
in asymmetry, 171, 172
in malunion, 175–176
soft tissue damage and, 176
in stabilization, 386–387, 394
in underdevelopment, 117, 118
in microgenia, 166
in micrognathia, 165
in nasal reconstruction, 322
cantilever grafts, 323
fixation of, 323
transfer guidelines, 322
in palpebral fissure slant, 119
in short face syndrome, 173
surgical techniques in use of, 173
xenografts, 84
Bony cavernous hemangiomas, 521
Bourneville's disease, 537
Boutonnière deformity
described, 604, 605–606
in rheumatoid arthritis, 632, 633, 634–635
Bowel segments
in cervical esophagus construction, 401
in vaginal construction, 880–881
Bowen's disease, 507–508, 532–533
Boxer's fracture, 586–587
Brachial plexus
free omental transfer for revascularizing, 681
interneural neurolysis, 685
nerve grafts in injuries, 694
Branchial arch deformities, 103
Branchial arch syndrome (hemifacial microsomia), 115–118
etiology, 115–116
management, 117–118
physical signs, 116–117
Branchial cleft cysts
described, 126
squamous cell carcinoma in congenital, 401
Branchial fistulas, 126
Branchial sinuses, 126
Branchiogenic carcinoma
branchial embryonic remnants and, 126
primary, 401
Breast. *See also* Breast cancer; Breast implants and prostheses; Breast ptosis; Breast reconstruction after mastectomy; Mammoplasty; Mastopexy
anatomy, mastectomy related to, 766–767
benign and primary disease, 760–764
adenofibroma, 761, 763
cystosarcoma phylloides, 761, 763
ductal carcinoma in situ, 762, 764
fibrocystic disease, 738, 761, 762–763
identification of patients at risk for cancer development, 760–761
intraductal papilloma, 762, 763–764
lobular carcinoma in situ, 762, 764–765
pathologic classification, 761–762
contour
depression after gynecomastia surgery, 806
after mastopexy, 751–752
after reduction mammoplasty, 749–750
endocrine physiology of, 737, 761
extent of tissue resection in mastectomy, 766–767, 768
gynecomastia, 802–807. *See also* Gynecomastia
hypertrophy
in cancer, 738
etiology, 737
recurrence after reduction mammoplasty, 749
types, 738
pathologic specimen management after mastectomy, 768
postoperative capsular contraction, 722, 724, 725, 727–729
etiology, 728
incidence, 727
nonsurgical "squeeze" capsulotomy for, 728–729
prophylaxis, 738
steroid injections for, 728
surgical capsulotomy for, 729
Breast – *Continued*
pregnancy and, 737, 738, 763
preoperative examination for augmentation mammoplasty, 721
symbolism of, 719
tissue types, 761
tissues and flaps in breast reconstruction, 486–487, 791, 795, 796
Breast cancer
classification, reconstruction after mastectomy and, 785
development in second breast, 791
fibrocystic disease and, 762–763
identification of high-risk patients, 760–761
incidence and mortality, 760
invasive, related to lobular carcinoma in situ, 764–765
Klinefelter's syndrome and, 802
"minimal," subcutaneous mastectomy in, 765
noninvasive, 762, 764–765
ductal carcinoma in situ (intraductal carcinoma), 762, 764
lobular carcinoma in situ, 762, 764–765
psychological factors and, 765
surgery. *See* Mastectomy
Breast implants and prostheses
Ashley prosthesis, 786
in augmentation mammoplasty, 100–101, 105
chemical composition of, 720
erosion of, 727
evaluation of inflatable vs. gel filled, 725
history of, 719–720
implant fixation, 725
injectable or Ivalon sponge, 719–720
leakage of, 727
ptosis of, 720
silicone fluids, 103
types and manufacturers, 724–725, 731–736
in breast reconstruction, 765
postoperative massage, 776
submuscular implantation, 767, 775, 776–778, 785–786, 797
timing implantation of, 772, 775, 779, 785
types of, 775
capsule contraction, 775–778, 779
partial implant coverage with polyurethane and, 776

Breast implants and prostheses, capsule contraction – *Continued*
postoperative massage and, 776
steroids and, 776
submuscular implantation and, 776–778
choosing, 785
dermal fat flaps as, 770, 772, 774
extrusion of, 778–779
implant fixation, 725
implantation
pocket for, 785, 786
preoperative antibiotics, 768
submuscular, 767, 776–778, 785–786, 787
timing, 772, 775, 779, 785
inflatable vs. gel, 725, 775
injectables, 719, 720
Ivalon sponge, 719–720
leakage of, 727
in mastopexy, 751, 756
partial coverage with polyurethane, 776
pectoralis coverage, 767, 777–778, 785–786, 797
postoperative massage, 776
ptosis of, 727
size of, 775
types and manufacturers, 103, 105, 724–725, 731–736, 751, 775
Breast ptosis, 720, 750–756
after augmentation mammoplasty, 727
augmentation plus mastopexy in, 720, 751
breast suspension in, 751–752
causative factors, 751–752
mastectomy techniques in
modified total mastectomy, 770–772, 773, 774
subcutaneous mastectomy, 768, 769, 770
mastopexy in, 750–751, 752–756
augmentation mammoplasty plus, 720, 751
breast suspension in, 751–752
postoperative care, 756
techniques, 750–751, 752–756
secondary, after mammoplasty, 727, 749
Breast reconstruction after mastectomy, 765, 772, 775–778, 785–798
breast tissues and flaps in, 486–487, 791, 795, 796
from other breast, 786–787, 791, 795, 796
choosing prosthesis, 775, 785
size of prosthesis, 775
classification of tumor and, 785
Breast reconstruction after mastectomy – *Continued*
dermal fat flaps in, 772, 774
latissimus dorsi myocutaneous flap in, 786, 787, 790
local rotation flaps from chest and abdominal wall in, 786, 791, 792
mastectomy technique and, 795
pectoralis dissection and implant coverage, 767
nipple-areolar complex addition. *See also* Areola-nipple complex, construction
techniques, 791–792, 797, 798
timing, 786
omentum with split-thickness skin flaps in, 787, 791
operative techniques
in patients with adequate soft tissue coverage, 785–786, 787
in patients with inadequate soft tissue coverage, 786–791
pocket for prosthesis implantation, 785, 786
postoperative complications, 772, 778–780, 794, 798
fibrous capsule contraction, 775–778, 779. *See also* Capsular contraction of breast
hematoma, 778, 779
implant loss, 778–779
infection, 779
malposition, 798
pain, 775, 779
procedures for remaining breast, 794
prostheses. *See* Breast implants and prostheses, in breast reconstruction
psychological factors and, 785
reverse abdominoplasty flaps in, 786, 791, 793, 794
selection of patients for, 785
submuscular prosthesis implantation, 776–778, 785–786, 787
timing, 785
implant insertion, 772, 775, 779, 785
nipple-areolar complex addition, 786
transverse lower abdominal tube flaps in, 786, 791
transverse thoracoepigastric flaps in, 786, 787, 788–789
Brent and Bostwick technique for nipple-areolar construction, 792, 798
Broadbent and Woolf technique for hypospadias, 857, 858
Brown electrical dermatome, 25, 27
Buccal mucosa
in nipple-areolar construction, 792
in cleft palate closure, 210, 214
Buccal sulcus, creating mandibular, 178, 179
Buccinator muscle, 336
Buck tooth deformity, 163, 174
Budinger-Müller technique for eyelid reconstruction, 291, 292
Bullet wounds, 227, 229, 559
Bunnell suture in hand flexor tendon injury, 609
Buried dermis flap in reconstruction in lymphedema, 831, 832
Buried sutures, 12
use with skin tapes, 14, 15
in wound closure in layers, 12–13
Burn(s), 453–481
acute, treatment summary, 475–477
age distribution of, 454, 455
agent related to severity of, 457–458
airway establishment and oxygen therapy in, 462, 475, 477
ambulation in, 474, 477
anemia in, 454, 469
antibiotics in, 460, 467, 469–470, 476
electrical burns, 491
associated injuries, 461, 493–494
bone exposure in, 479
cardiac complications, 455–456
prophylactic digitalization in, 468
catheterization in, 462, 475
circulatory response in, 454, 478
classification of, 457, 459, 461
contractures
flexion contractures, 479
prevention of, 469, 473
rehabilitation in, 481
Z-plasty for, 64, 65
CVP monitoring in, 466–467
dressings for outpatients, 460
dye tests in, 458
ear, 307–308, 311, 312
edema in, 454, 458, 477
electrical, 457, 489–494. *See also* Electrical burns
evaluation in, 456–459
area of burn, 455, 456–457, 458
associated injuries, 461
depth of burn, 457–459
patient, 461, 475
first aid and transportation in, 459–460
first-degree
classification of, 457, 459
first aid in, 459

Burn(s) – *Continued*
fluid-electrolyte therapy in, 455, 456, 462–465, 475–476
catheterization for, 462, 475
CVP as index of inadequate, 466
estimation of fluid requirements, 463–464, 475–476
fluid test load, 466
indications, 464
recommendations of fluid replacement, 464–465
scheduling rate of, 465
fourth-degree, 457, 459
gastrointestinal complications, 479
hand, management of, 471–472
head and neck, 462, 469
healing process related to severity of, 458–459
hypoproteinemia in, 453, 469
hypovolemia in, 454, 463, 466, 478
infections and, 478–479
electrical burns, 493
septicemia, 478–479
urinary tract infecions, 478
intubation in, 462, 475, 477
joint immobilization in, 469
laboratory studies in, 462–463, 476
lesion appearance in, 458
maintenance of IV pathway in, 462
of male genitalia, 869
metabolic response to, 453, 454–455, 469, 480–481
morbidity and mortality, 453
factors contributing to, 455–456
nutrition maintenance in, 480–481
oral feedings and fluids, 467–468, 469, 476
patient positioning in, 469, 475
physiologic response to acute vs. subacute phase, 453, 454–455
psychological support in, 462, 468
rehabilitation in, 481
renal function and, 454, 478, 493
diuretics and, 465
electrical burns, 490–491, 493, 494
urinary output maintenance and monitoring, 465–466, 476
respiratory complications, 477
scars
lip, 345, 346, 348
multiple excision of, 6
Z-plasty for contracture of, 64, 65
scalp and forehead, 272–273
second-degree
appearance of, 458
classification of, 457, 459
first aid in, 459
healing, 455, 457
sedation in, 462, 475

Burn(s) – *Continued*
sensation in, 458
septic arthritis and, 479–480
septicemia and, 469
shock in, 453, 454, 463, 477–478
hypovolemic, 463
skin flaps in, 18, 492, 493
skin grafts in, 18, 85, 455, 457
allografts, 474
applying, 473
donor sites, 20, 472–473
dressings and immobilization, 473, 474–475
face, 18, 272–273
healing, 455, 457
mesh expansion, 473
minor grafting, 460–461
postoperative care, 474–475
thickness of, 473, 492, 493
xenografts, 474
tetanus prophylaxis, 460, 467, 476
in electrical burns, 491
thermal plus electrical, 490, 491–492
third-degree
appearance of, 458
classification of, 457, 459
first aid in, 459–460
healing, 455, 457
skin grafts in, 455, 457, 460–461
toxic psychosis in, 481
tracheostomy in, 462, 475, 477
wounds
bacteriostatic dressings, 469–471
cleaning, 460, 469
closure. *See* skin flaps in; skin grafts in
decompression incisions, 469, 470, 471
enzymatic debridement, 472
excision, 470, 471–472, 491–492
initial management phase, 469–472
removal of necrotic tissue, 471–472
summary of care, 476–477
"Burn-lung" syndrome, 477
Burou technique of neovaginal construction, 888
Burrow's triangle excision in lip reconstruction, 345, 346, 347
Buschke-Lowenstein tumor, 549
Buttocks
pressure sore closure on, 823
as skin graft donor site, 21, 25
Buttonhole flap in chordee correction, 856
Byers technique for hypospadias, 857, 858, 861, 862

Calcaneous defects, muscle transposition in, 815, 816
Calcifying epitheliomas, 534
Caldwell-Luc technique for blowout fractures, 257
Calvaria (Calvarium)
anatomy and embryology, 265
congenital deformities, 265, 266. *See also* Apert's syndrome; Crouzon's syndrome
covering exposed bone on, 267, 268, 269
radiation injury, 272
reconstruction in skull defects, 269–272
Cancer. *See specific topic, e.g.,* Head and neck cancer; Sarcoma(s)
Cancrum oris (noma), 548
Candidiasis, 548
Canthal ligament
loss, 288–289
surgery
in facial palsy, 338, 339–340
in lower eyelid reconstruction, 281, 282, 283
Cantilever bone graft in nasal reconstruction, 323
Capillary cavernous hemangiomas, 521–522
Capillary hemangioma(s), 518–520, 521–522
cavernous, 521–522
port-wine stain, 273, 518–519, 560
pyogenic granuloma and, 520, 521
strawberry, 273, 519–520
Capsular contraction of breast, 722, 724, 725, 727–729
etiology, 728
incidence, 727
nonsurgical "squeeze" capsulotomy in, 728–729
prophylaxis, 728
steroids for, 728
surgical capsulotomy for, 729
Capsulectomy
in flexion contractures of finger, 600–601
interphalangeal joints, 598–600
in metacarpophalangeal joint ankylosis, 602–603
Capsulorrhaphy in temperomandibular joint hypermobility, 185
Capsulotomy in breast capsular contraction, 728–729
Carcinoma. *See specific topic, e.g.,* Carcinoma in situ; Squamous cell carcinoma
Carcinoma in situ
Bowen's disease as, 532
breast
ductal, 762, 764
lobular, 762, 764–765
larynx, 399

Carotid artery
  involvement in neck cancer, 400
  management in ear carcinoma resection, 502
Carotid body tumors, 401
Carpal tunnel syndrome, 631
Carriers in flap transfer, 56
Cartilage. *See also* Cartilage grafts
  areola-nipple construction with ear, 792, 798
  described, 85
  exposed
    skin flaps for, 41, 56–57
    skin grafts for, 17, 22
  metabolism of, 85–86
  structure of, 88
Cartilage grafts
  allografts, 85, 117, 118
  autografts, 94
  donor sites, 85, 88, 89
  in ear surgery
    auricle reconstruction, 299, 301–304, 308–309, 310, 311, 313
    helical defects, 311
  in eyelid reconstruction, 282–283, 284
  growth of, 89
  in mandibular underdevelopment, 117, 118
  in nasal reconstruction, 322, 324
    from ear, 435–436, 437
    fixation of, 322–323
    from nasal septum, 428–429, 434–435, 436–437, 438
    transfer guidelines, 322
  for palpebral fissure slants, 119
  survival of, 89
  xenografts, 85
Castroviejo dermatome, 27
Caterpillar method of flap migration, 56
Catgut sutures
  knotting, 14
  types of, 10
Catheterization
  in avulsion injuries of penis, 870
  bladder spasm and, 864
  in burns, 462, 475
  in functional closure of bladder exstrophy, 867
  for urinary diversion in hypospadias, 862, 864
Cautery. *See* Electrocautery
Cavernous hemangiomas, 273, 521
Cavernous lymphangiomas, 518, 523
Cecil-Culp technique for penile resurfacing, 858
Cell-mediated lympholysis (CML) test, 84
Cellulitis
  dissecting, of scalp, 545
Cellulitis – *Continued*
  in hand infections, 579
Central venous pressure (CVP) monitoring
  in burns, 466–467
  before replantation, 700–701
Cerebrospinal rhinorrhea in facial fractures, 243, 249
Cervical flaps for nasal reconstruction, 331, 332
Cervical lymph node metastases. *See* Lymph node(s), metastases
Cervical plexus
  management in radical neck dissection, 375, 380, 381
  as nerve graft donor site, 695
Cheek(s). *See also* Cheek flaps
  aging signs, 410
  anatomy of, 348
  animal bite wounds, 237
  avulsion injury, 237
  in facial palsy, autogenous fascia lata to suspend, 338, 340, 341
  implants for malar complex, 102
  laceration, 236–237
  multiple excision of skin lesions, 6
  reconstruction
    in contour defects, 349
    skin flaps in, 52, 348, 349
  scars related to skin lines of, 3
Cheek flaps
  advancement, 143, 144
  bilateral in nasal dorsum resurfacing, 328
  cutting mucosal, 27
  in lip reconstruction, 346
  in nasal reconstruction, 326, 327, 328
  rotation
    in loss of both eyelids, 290–291
    in lower eyelid reconstruction, 281, 282, 283, 284, 290
Chemical agents in decorative tattoo removal, 565
Chemical face peel (chemosurgery), 418, 421–422
Chemotherapy
  drugs for, described, 367, 368
  effectiveness of radiotherapy related to, 368
  in head and neck cancer, 366, 367, 368, 369
    radiotherapy plus, 389
  in malignant melanoma, 515
  in skin cancer, 497, 498
  systemic toxicity of, 366
Chest wall
  flaps for wounds of, 41, 58
  flaps from
    direct, to arm, 54
    rotation, in breast reconstruction, 786, 791, 792
Chest wall – *Continued*
  pressure sore closure on, 823
  prosthetic implants, 106
Chin. *See also specific topic, e.g.,* Micrognathia
  aging and, 410
  augmentation mentoplasty, 100–101, 166–167, 432–433. *See also* Augmentation mentoplasty
  lacerations, 237
  in Pierre Robin syndrome, 123, 124
  submental lipectomy, 417
  surgery after male-to-female surgery, 891
Chondritis in auricular burns, 307–308
Chondrocutaneous composite grafts in auricle reconstruction, 309, 312, 313
Chondrodermatitis nodularis chronica helicis, 538
Chondroid syringoma, 535
Chondromucosal flaps in nasal reconstruction, 322
Chondroplasty, laryngeal, after male-to-female surgery, 891
Chondrosarcomas of hand, 648
Chordee
  correction in hypospadias, 856
  penis growth and, 864
Chromic catgut sutures, 10
Cicatricial alopecia, 545
Cilia in eyelash provision, 119
Circular excision of skin wounds, 8, 9
Circular scar revision
  on face, 238
  Z-plasty in, 64
Circular thigh reduction, 844, 845, 846, 847
Circulation and blood supply
  burns and, 454, 463, 466, 478
  in fascial grafts, 89
  fingertip, 569
  high-voltage electrical injury and, 493
  peripheral nerves, 618–619
    injury repair and, 623–624
  replantation and, 697, 698
    observing and checking, 706, 707, 713
    preoperative monitoring, 700–701
    in vein grafts, 709
  skin, 36, 37–38
  in skin flaps
    anatomy and, 36, 37–38
    area of body and, 42
    classification of flaps by, 38–41, 46, 48
    design and survival and, 42

Circulation and blood supply, in
skin flaps – *Continued*
maintaining, 45–46
tests of, 44–45
in skin grafts
development of, 22–23
recipient bed vascularity and, 21–22
survival and, 21–23, 86
temperature as indicator of, 713
Cirsoid aneurysms of scalp, 274
Circumcision, 864, 878
Clavicular flaps in nasal reconstruction, 331
Cleaning adventitious tattoos, 559
Clear cell hidradenomas, 534
Cleft earlobes
Cleft lip. *See also* Cleft lip closure
alveolar clefts and, 205
anatomy of, 192, 193
bilateral, 192, 198–203
holoprosencephalopathy with, 121
median
bifid nose and, 122–123
hypertelorism with, 120–122
lower, 123
median facial defects associated with, 120
unilateral, 193–197
Cleft lip closure
anesthesia for, 192
bilateral
optimum time for, 192
orthodontia and, 192
rotation-advancement technique, 198–203
secondary revisions, 203
median, 123
plumping devices after, 350
postoperative care, 203
unilateral
Mirault technique, 194, 198
quadrilateral flap, 194
rotation-advancement in, 194–197
secondary revisions, 197–198
straight-line closure, 193, 198
triangular flaps for, 194
V-Y rolldown for mucosal defect, 197
Z-plasty in, 64
Cleft palate, 205–222. *See also* Cleft palate repair
airway maintenance in, 209
associated anomalies, 210
classification of, 208–209
embryology of, 207, 208
experimental production of, 208
feeding neonates with, 209
incidence, 208
maxillary retrusion and collapse in, 173, 174
Cleft palate – *Continued*
middle ear disease in, 209, 212
muscles in, 205, 206
palatal clefts, 205, 206
classification of, 208–209
embryology and etiology of, 208
in Pierre Robin syndrome, 123, 209
prepalatal clefts, 205, 206
alveolus in, 207, 211
classification of, 208
embryology and etiology, 207
questions from parents, 210
speech in, 207, 217
submucosal clefts, classification of, 209
vomer in, 205
Cleft palate repair
anesthesia in, 212
follow-up, 217
hard palate, 213
bone grafts in, 213–214
mucosal flaps in, 213–214
timing, 210, 213
vomer flaps in, 210, 213, 214
palatal clefts, 212–218
patient position and management in, 212–213
postoperative care, 217
postoperative ear problems, 215, 217
postoperative prostheses and orthodontia, 222
preoperative considerations, 212
prepalatal and alveolar clefts, 211–212, 213
alveolar bone grafts in, 211
dental occlusion in, 211–212
mucosal flaps in, 210, 214
timing, 210
secondary palatal procedures, 219
soft palate
intraalveolar veloplasty and palate lengthening, 214, 215–217
nasal mucosa management, 215, 216
prostheses in, 211, 222
speech in prosthetic vs. surgical repair, 211
timing, 211
velopharyngeal competence achievement, 214
speech considerations in, 207, 217
timetable, 210–211, 213
velopharyngeal function
postoperative competence, 214, 217
postoperative incompetence, 218
treatment of incompetence, 219–222
Clitoris
bifid, 865
lengthening in phalloplasty, 895
Clonal selection theory of allograft rejection, 79
Closure of wounds. *See* Wound closure
Coccyx, pressure sore closure on, 823
Collagen
injection for contour defects, 87
metabolism, abnormal scarring and, 552
Collar-button abscess of hand, 580
Colon
as urine receptacle in bladder exstrophy, 867
in vagina construction, 881
Color
of skin flaps, 34, 57
of skin grafts, 34, 86
matching to face, 19, 20
prevention of hyperpigmentation, 34
Columella
bilateral nasolabial flaps in reconstruction of, 327
management in rhinoplasty, 427, 431, 432
rotation-advancement technique for short, 200
Composite flaps, 57. *See also specific topic, e.g.,* Myocutaneous flaps
in cheek reconstruction, 349
in digit reconstruction, 42
Composite grafts
in auricle reconstruction, 309, 312, 313
bridging phenomenon and vascularization of, 21
in eyelid reconstruction, 291
in lip reconstruction, 345
in nasal reconstruction, 324, 325
Compound nevi, 530, 643
Compound skip flaps, described, 57
Compression syndromes, intraneural interfascicular dissection in, 686
Concealing scars, 3, 4, 5
Conchal cartilage
in ear reconstruction
auricle, 308–309, 310, 311, 313
tragus formation, 305, 306
excision in otoplasty, 441
Conchal-mastoid sutures in otoplasty, 441, 445, 446
Condylectomy
in hyperplasia of mandibular condyle, 172
of temperomandibular joint, 185, 187
Condyloma acuminata, 549
Condylomas of tongue, 357
Congenital absence of vagina, 873, 876, 878
Congenital fissured tongue, 356

Conjunctiva
  corneal covering in eyelid loss, 289, 290
  flaps from, in eyelid reconstruction, 285, 288
  mucosal grafts, 18–19
  repair in eyelid reconstruction, 283, 284
  transconjunctival exposure, 133
Connective tissue tumors of jaw, 361
Contamination
  of animal bite wounds, 237
  replantation in presence of, 698
Contour defects
  bone grafts for craniofacial, 134, 155, 270
  breast
    augmentation mammoplasty and, 432–433
    depression after gynecomastia repair, 806
    mastopexy and, 751–752
    reduction mammoplasty and, 749–750
  dermal grafts for, 87
  fat grafts for, 89
  fingertip injury repair and, 570
  free omental transfer in, 681
  implants for, 100, 102, 270, 349
  injectable collagen for, 87
  silicone fluid for, 103
Continuous over-and-under sutures, 13, 14
Continuous sutures, 13–14
Contour lines of skin, 4
Contraction
  of skin grafts
    growth and, 35
    immobilization in preventing, 31–32, 34
    primary vs. secondary, 33–34
  of wounds in fingertip injury, 571
Contracture(s)
  in burns
    flexion, 479
    prevention of, 469, 473
    rehabilitation in, 481
    Z-plasty for, 64, 65
  Dupuytren's, 53–54, 627–628, 637–639
  finger
    in fingertip injury, 571
    flexion, 600–601
    in rheumatoid arthritis, 631
  hand, 66
  muscle, after replantation, 713
  scar
    Y-V advancement flaps in, 53–54
    Z-plasty in lengthening, 62, 64, 65, 66
Contracture(s) – *Continued*
  skin, 60
  skin grafts, 32
    area related to, 31–32
    prevention of, 18
  Volkmann's ischemic, 622
  Z-plasty for, 60, 62, 64, 65–66
Contusions
  face, 227, 228–229
  male urethra, 872
  scalp, 267
Converse technique for cranioplasty, 271
Cooper's ligaments
  breast tissue in, 766, 767
  dissection in mastectomy, 767–768
Cornea, medical tattooing of, 560
Coronal craniectomy, 154–155
Coronal synostosis, 154–155
Corpora cavernosa rupture, 869
Corpus spongiosum stump in male-to-female surgery, 890
Corrugator muscle, 336
Cortical hyperostosis, 125
Corticosteroid therapy
  allograft reactions and, 80–81
  capsular breast contraction, 728, 776
  burns, 469, 477
  infantile cortical hyperostosis, 125
  hypertrophic scars and keloids, 556–557, 806–807, 842–843, 849, 850
  pyoderma gangrenosum, 547
  rheumatoid arthritis of hand, 632
  temperomandibular joint disorders, 182, 183
  treatment of ulcers and, 811
Cortisol, adrenogenital syndrome and, 877
Cosmetic surgery. *See also specific topic, e.g.,* Blepharoplasty
  abdominal dermolipectomy, 838–843
  arm lipectomy, 849–850
  blepharoplasty, 404–408
  chemical face peel (chemosurgery), 418, 421–422
  dermabrasion, 419–421
  ears, 440–448. *See also* Otoplasty
  lower leg lipectomy, 849
  rhinoplasty
    primary, 424–433
    secondary, 434–439
  rhytidectomy, 411–417, 418–419
  of scalp in baldness, 275–277
  thigh reduction, 838, 843–849
Costal cartilages
  in auricle reconstruction, 309
    framework fabrication, 301–302, 303
    framework implantation, 302–303, 304
Costal cartilages, in auricle reconstruction – *Continued*
    limitations of, 299
    obtaining cartilage, 301, 302, 303
  as cartilage graft donor site, 85, 88, 89
  shaping for insertion as free graft, 89
Cotton sutures, 10
Crane principle of skin flaps, 56–57
Cranial vault reshaping with jigsaw procedures
  anterior, jigsaw Type I, 149, 150
  hazards of, 131, 149
  total, 151–152
    jigsaw Type II, 151
    jigsaw Type III, 151–152
Craniectomy, coronal, 154–155
Craniofacial disjunciton, 248, 249
Craniofacial dislocation, 260
Craniofacial dysostosis. *See* Crouzon's syndrome
Craniofacial fibrous dysplasia, 362
Craniofacial microsomia
  etiology, 156
  mandibular laterognathism in, 171
  orthodontia in, 172
  sagittal split mandible and, 172
  surgical techniques in, 156–158, 171–172
Craniofacial surgery, 131–158. *See also specific topic, e.g.,* Hypertelorism; Maxillary osteotomy
  anesthesia in, 132
  in central facial anomalies, 142–144
  in coronal synostosis, 154–155
  cranial vault reshaping, 149–153
    anterior, 149, 150
    total, 151–152
  in Crouzon's or Apert's syndrome, 120, 145–150
  eye protection in, 134
  history of, 134
  in hypertelorism, 135–138
  jigsaw procedures
    hazards of, 131, 149
    Type I, 149, 150
    Type II, 151
    Type III, 151–152
  in orbital dystopia, 138
  radiography for, 132
  requirements for surgeons, 131
  surgical exposures in
    medial canthal ligament, 134
    Meisterschnitt, 133
    oral cavity, 133–134
    skull and facial bones, 133
    transcon junctival, 133

Craniofacial surgery – *Continued*
team approach in, 131–133
conference, 133
planning, 131–132
team members, 131–133
in Treacher Collins syndrome, 131, 138–142
Cranioplasty
alloplastic materials in, 269
bone dust in, 271–272
bone grafts in, 269–272
contour restoration after, 270
iliac bone, 269, 271
split-rib grafts, 269–270, 270–271
jigsaw procedures in
hazards of, 131, 149
Type I, 149, 150
Type II, 151
Type III, 151–152
soft tissue closure in, 272
Craniostenosis, 149, 150
Cranium. *See specific topic, e.g.,* Calvaria (Calvarium); Craniofacial surgery; Cranioplasty
Cronin technique for auricle reconstruction, 306
Cross arm flaps, use of, 54
Cross finger flaps, 54
division of, 44
in fingertip injury, 572, 573, 574
Cross-gender behavior. *See* Gender dysphoria
Cross leg flaps, 39, 40
division of, 36, 44, 55
in lower extremity reconstruction, 39
covering exposed bone, 812
in tibial defects, 812
myocutaneous flaps as, 58
transfer of, 55
results of use, 676, 678, 812
Crouzon's syndrome, 119–120, 144–150
differential diagnosis, 119, 120
etiology, 120
physical signs, 119–120, 144–145
treatment, 120, 145–150
combined Le Fort III and I osteotomy, 148, 149
coronal correction, 154–155
hypertelorism correction, 148–149
Le Fort III maxillary advancement, 145–148
maxillary hypoplasia and retrusion, 173, 174
"Crows feet," 410
Crush injuries, replantation in, 697, 698
Cryoglobulinemia, 543
Cryotherapy in head and neck cancer, 389
Cupid's bow
construction with Hagedorn-Le Mesurier quadrilateral flap, 198
described, 344
simulation of, 348
Curling's ulcer, 479
Cutaneous arteries, 37, 38
Cutaneous flaps. *See* Random pattern flaps
Cutaneous nerves as nerve graft donor, 694, 695
Cutaneous papillomas, 536
Cutaneous tags, 536
Cutis hyperelastica, 5, 541
Cutis laxa, 541
Cyanoacrylates
in skin graft fixation, 29–30
as wound adhesives, 16
Cylindromas (turban tumors), 274, 534–535
Cyst(s)
branchial, 126
dermoid, 536
epidermoid, 536, 642
hand, 641, 642
jaw, 361
mucous, 641, 642
myxoid, 537
pilar, 536
sebaceous, 642
thyroglossal duct, 126–127
Cystadenomas, apocrine, 535
Cystic hygroma, 518, 523–524
Cystosarcoma phylloides of breast, 761, 763
Cytoxic humoral antibodies, 77

Dacryocystorhinostomy
indications, 232
technique, 232–233, 234
Dacron implants, described, 95–96
Dacron sutures, 10, 11
Dal Pont's modified technique for mandibular sagittal split, 165, 170
Darier's disease (keratosis follicularis), 532
Davies and Birdsell phalloplasty, 892, 894
De Quervain's syndrome, 631
Debridement
in avulsion of penile skin, 870
in bacteria removal from wounds, 24
in burns, 472
electrical, 492
scalp, 272
of ear, 233
Debridement – *Continued*
in facial laceration, 229–230, 266
of infected skin grafts, 31
of mouth wounds, 237
Decompression incisions in escharotomy, 469, 470, 471
Decorative tattoos
defined and described, 560–562
overtattooing, 562, 563, 565
removal of
chemical agents in, 563, 565
choice of technique, 562
dermabrasion or silabrasion, 563–565
electrical devices in, 563, 565
surgical excision, 562, 563
Decubitus ulcers. *See* Pressure sores
Degloving injuries
repair of distal phalangeal, 573–574
replantation in, 697
Delayed skin flaps, 42–45
axial pattern flaps, 38
delay mechanism, 42–44
dividing base of, 36
double delay procedure, 44
indications of viability of, 36
in pressure sore closure, 822
staging technique, 43
surviving length, 36, 43–44
epinephrine and, 46
transfer timing, 44
vasodilation and, 42, 43
Delayed skin grafts
defined, 10
recipient bed and, 23, 28
Deltopectoral flaps
in cheek reconstruction, 349
described, 38, 40
free, 676
in head and neck reconstruction, 40, 51–52, 374
hypopharyngeal and cervical esophageal, 399, 401
Denis Browne technique for hypospadias, 858
Dentures
in alveolar and prepalatal clefts
expansion, 212
retaining, 211–212
insertion before prosthetic surgery, 178, 179
after mandible resection, 386, 387
in maxillary fracture malunion, 176
Dermabrasion, 419–421
of facial scars, 238
of hyperpigmented skin grafts, 34
indications, 419–420
of lip scars, 345
in patients susceptible to skin cancer, 498

Dermabrasion – *Continued*
postoperative care, 420, 421
in rhinophyma, 544, 545
in tattoo removal
accidental tattoos, 229, 559
decorative tattoos, 562–565
techniques, 420
Dermal fat grafts, 89, 94
in augmentation mammoplasty, 89, 719
in congenital facial asymmetry, 158
in vermillion reconstruction, 348
Dermal flaps
buried, in reconstruction in lymphedema, 831, 832
fat, in breast reconstruction, 770, 772, 774
Dermatofibromas, 536–537
Dermatofibrosarcoma protruberans, 537
Dermatomes for cutting skin grafts, 25, 26–27, 86
drum, 25, 26
electrical, 26–27
setting and graft thickness, 16
Dermis grafts
bulk
histologic changes in, 87
in pressure sore closure, 822
reverse, in covering exposed bone, 812
for soft tissue defects, 87, 158
taking, 86
Dermochalasis
abdominal, dermolipectomy in, 839, 840, 841, 842
of eyelids, 404
Dermoid cysts, 536
Dermolipectomy. *See* Abdominal dermolipectomy
Des Prez and Persky technique for hypospadias, 857, 858
Diabetes mellitus, 542
burns in, 456
hand infection in, 582
leg ulceration and, 811
peripheral neuropathy in, 582
Dieffenbach technique for lip reconstruction, 346
Digits. *See* Finger(s); Toes
Digital fibrokeratomas, 537
Digitate fibromas, 537
Dimethylpolysiloxane injections in progressive facial hemotrophy, 128
Diplopia
in blowout fractures, 251–252, 255
residual postoperative, 252
in facial fractures, 243
Direct flaps
bone shortening with, in fingertip injury, 574, 576
distant, 54–56
arm, 54
leg, 54–56
pedicle and facial avulsion, 235
trunk, 54
Discoid lupus erythematosus, 538
"Dishface" deformity, 173, 176
Dislocations
hand
carpometacarpal joint, 596–597
immobilization principles, 586
interphalangeal joints, 590, 591–592, 593, 595
metacarpophalangeal joints, 590, 593, 594, 595–596
thumb, 594–596
temperomandibular joint, 182, 183
management, 185, 186, 260, 262
Dissecting cellulitis of scalp, 547
Dissection technique in microvascular surgery, 654
Distal shaft hypospadias, repair of, 858, 859–861
Distant flaps, 54–56
in avulsion defects of face, 235
in cheek reconstruction, 348–349
from chest wall to arm, 54
direct, 54–56
in finger amputation, 576
indirect, 56
leg, 54–56
in nasal reconstruction, disadvantages of, 331–332
omentum, in reconstruction in lymphedema, 831–832
in resurfacing radiation injuries, 487
in scalp defects, 272
trunk, 54
Diuretics
in burns, 465, 491
in lymphedema, 830
Dog ears
formation at flap pivot point, 48–49
in skin lesion excision, 5–6
Donor sites
bone grafts, 87–88
iliac bone grafts, 134, 271. *See also* Iliac bone grafts
split-rib grafts, 134, 270–271. *See also* Split-rib grafts
cartilage grafts, 85, 88, 89
composite grafts, 18
free skin flaps, 676, 677
free tissue transfer, 671, 674
Donor sites – *Continued*
nerve grafts, 694–695
skin flaps, closure of, 14, 18, 48, 49
secondary flap, 49, 50
split-thickness skin grafts in, 17, 18, 28, 33, 48, 86, 273
skin graft storage on, 32
skin grafts, 33
anesthesia of, 27
areas for, described, 19–21
bleeding from, 16, 21
in burns, 472–473
closure, 17, 18, 28, 33, 86, 811
dressing, 33
epithelialization, 33
eyelids, 18
to face, 19, 20
fingertip injury, 572
healing, 33, 86, 811
matching grafts to recipient site, 19
meshed grafts for covering, 811
nose, 233
overgrafting, 19
thickness of graft and, 16, 86
Doppler flowmeter in circulation evaluation, 45
Dorsalis pedis flap, use of free, 676, 677
Drainage
auricle reconstruction, 303, 304
free tissue transfer, 675
hand infections, 579, 581
mastectomy, 768
Penrose drains in rhytidectomy, 414, 416, 417
pressure sore closure, 822
skin grafts, 29
suprapubic, in functional closure of bladder exstrophy, 867
Dressing(s)
abdominal dermolipectomy, 841–842, 843
acute radiodermatitis, 487
arm reduction, 850
augmentation mammoplasty, 726
avulsed scrotal skin, 871
avulsion flap healing and, 230, 232
avulsion injuries of penis, 870
biological, 24, 85, 95
blepharoplasty, 408
burns, 473, 474–475
bacteriostatic, 469–471
electrical burns, 492
hypertrophic scars, 481
outpatient, 460
capsulectomy, 599, 603
dermabrasion, 420–421
hand fractures, 586, 589

Dressing(s) – *Continued*
hand joint injuries, 590
hypertrophic scars, 556
in burns, 481
mastectomy, 768
mastopexy, 756
otoplasty, 444–445
pressure sore closure, 822
primary hand tendon suturing, 610
radical neck dissection, 380, 381
replantation, 711–712
checking for bleeding, 713
rhinoplasty, 432
rhytidectomy, 417
skin graft donor sites, 33
skin grafts, 31
bleeding and, 10
tie-over dressings, 23, 29, 30
tourniquet release and, 28
Ductal carcinoma in situ of breast, 762, 764
Dufourmentel flap, 51
Dufourmentel and Mouly technique for mastopexy, 752
Dufourmentel and Mouly technique for reduction mammoplasty, 739, 740
Dupuys-Dutemps-Hughes technique for lower eyelid reconstruction, 285
Dupuytren's contracture, 637–639
dermofasciectomy and skin grafts in, 639
Dupuytren's diathesis, 627–628
fasciectomy in, 638–639
fasciotomy in, 638
Y-V advancement flap in, 53–54
Dural defects, grafts and flaps for, 19, 493
Durfee and Roland phalloplasty, 895
Dye tests in burns, 458
Dystosis
craniofacial. *See* Crouzon's syndrome
mandibulofacial. *See* Treacher Collins syndrome
Dystopia, orbital, 138
Dystrophic epidermolysis bullosa, 540–541

Ear(s). *See also specific topic, e.g.,* Auricle; Earlobe(s); Otoplasty
amputation, 307
anatomy and embryology of normal, 440, 441
burns, 311, 312
infection and, 307–308
cartilage grafts from, 85
in areola-nipple construction, 792, 798

Ear(s), cartilage grafts from – *Continued*
in auricle reconstruction, 308–309, 310, 311, 313
in nasal reconstruction, 322, 324
in secondary rhinoplasty, 435–436, 437
composite grafts from, 18, 324
debridement, 233
disease of middle, in cleft palate, 209–210, 212, 217
in hemifacial microsomia, 116–117
implants and prostheses, 101–102, 350
invaginated, 446, 448
lop ears, 446, 447, 448
management of injuries, 233
otohematoma, 308
positioning opposite with constructed auricle, 306
postauricular flaps from, 331
prominent, 440–446
abnormal conchal depth, 445–446
definitions and terms for, 440–441
indications and timing correction, 441
otoplasty for, 441–446. *See also* Otoplasty
psychological effects of deformities, 441
reconstruction of microtic, 299–306. *See also* Auricle reconstruction, in microtia
resection in carcinoma, 502
satyr, 448
shell, 448
skin grafts from, for face, 19, 20
in Treacher Collins syndrome, 118, 139
wedge excision of skin lesions, 7
Earlobe(s)
cleft, 316
keloids, 316
reconstruction, 316
rotation in auricle reconstruction, 305
Ecchymosis in facial fractures, 243
Eccrine acrospiromas, 534
Eccrine hidrocystomas, 534
Eccrine poromas, 534
Eccrine spiradenomas, 534
Eccrine tumors, 534–535
Ectropion
eyelid, prevention in blepharoplasty, 404, 408
lip, 346
Edema. *See also* Lymphedema
after abdominal dermolipectomy, 843
in burns, 454, 458, 477

Edema –*Continued*
eyelid, 258–259
in fractures
blowout, 252
facial, 243
hand, 586
after gynecomastia surgery, 896
iliac compression syndrome and, 829
nerve, repair and, 625
after thigh reduction, 849
of venous disease, differential diagnosis lymphedema, 829
Edgerton and Bull technique for neocolporrhaphy, 889
Ehler-Danlos syndrome, 5, 541
Elastomer implants, 97
in contour defects, 102
in ear, 101
Elbaz and Verheeke technique for reduction mammoplasty, 740
Elbow, pressure sore closure on, 823
Electrical burns, 489–494
associated injuries, 490–491, 493–494
depth and severity of, 457
laboratory evaluation of, 490–491
male genitalia, 869
management, 490–493
antibiotics, 491, 492, 493
cleaning, 492
debridement, 492
dressings, 492
excision, 491–492, 493
high-voltage injury, 492–493
low-voltage injury, 492
thermal burns plus, 490, 491–492
vascular impairment, 493
pathogenesis, 489–490
Electrocautery
in decorative tattoo removal, 563, 565
in hemostasis, 9–10, 23, 768
in keratoses, 643
of warts, 642–643
Electrodessication of nevi, 273
Electrolysis after male-to-female surgery, 891
Elliptical incisions
in correction of inversion of wound edges, 12
in skin lesion excision, 5–7, 8, 9
dog ears and, 5–6
multiple excision technique, 5, 6–7
simple excision technique, 5–6
Enchondromas of hand, 646, 647

Endocrine breast hypertrophy, 738
Endotracheal intubation
  in burns, 462, 475, 477
  after maxillary hypoplasia correction, 173
  preoperative, in radical neck dissection, 369
End-to-end microvascular anastomoses, 660, 663–665, 668, 669–670
  arterial, 660, 663, 664, 665
  luminal diameter differences and, 665, 666, 669–670
  venous, 663, 664, 665
End-to-end nerve repair
  nerve grafts vs., in continuity restoration, 689, 693
  technique, 690–693
    epineural, 690–691, 692
    fascicular alignment, 690, 692
    fascicular coaptation, 693
    interfascicular coaptation, 693
    intrafascicular sutures, 690, 692
    perineural, 690, 693
    wrapping suture sites, 693
End-to-side microvascular anastomoses, 660, 665, 667, 668, 669–670
Enopthalmos in blowout fractures, 252, 254, 257
Entropion of lip, 346
Ephelis (freckle), 531
  benign, 531
  Hutchinson's melanotic, 510, 530, 531
Epidermoid carcinoma. *See also* Squamous cell carcinoma
  hand, 647
  jaw, 361, 362
  metastatic head and neck, 387
Epidermoid cysts, 536, 642
Epidermolysis bullosa dystrophica, 540–541
Epinephrine
  delayed flap, surviving length of, and, 46
  for hemostasis, 10, 21
Epineural sutures in peripheral nerve repair, 618, 619, 627, 628, 690, 691, 692, 707
Epispadias
  defined, 865
  exstrophy of bladder with, 865
  repair, 865–866
Epithelial cysts, 535–536
Epithelial inlay (stent) skin graft, 30
Epithelioma(s)
  basal cell, 535
  calcifying, of Malherbe, 534
  defined, 533
  sabaceous, 535
Epithelioma adenoides cysticum, 533–534
Eponychial marsupialization paronychia, 580, 581
Epulis of jaw, 361
Erection of penis, 855–856
  in avulsion injuries, 869, 870
  after hypospadias surgery, 864
Erythema after dermabrasion, 421
Erythroplasia of Queyrat, 532
Escharotomy. *See also* Scar(s)
  electrical high-voltage burns, 493
  incisions for, 469, 470
Esophagus
  cervical cancer and, 400–401
  implants, 105
  reconstruction
    after laryngeal cancer surgery, 399
    after resection, 399, 400–401
    silicone rubber tube in, 105
Estlander flap for lip reconstruction, 346, 347
Estrogens, 877
  breast and, 737, 763, 802
  complications of therapy, 891
  external genitalia development and, 873
  in pregnancy, development of gender dysphoria and, 884–885
  after surgery from male-to-female, 891–892
Ethmoid sinus fractures, 259–260
Everbusch technique for eyelid ptosis, 293
Excision. *See* Excision of skin lesions; Resection and excision
Excision of skin lesions, 3–10
  atraumatic technique, 3
  avulsion flap, 239–240
  circular excision, 8, 9
  elliptical excision, 5–7, 8, 9
    dog ear formation and, 5–6
    multiple excision technique, 5, 6–7
    simple excision, 5–6
  on face
    avulsion flaps, 239–240
    scar polarity altering, 239, 240
    scar revision, 238–239
    U-shaped scars, 238, 239–240
  hemostasis in, 9–10
  instruments for, 8
  on scalp, 266
  scar after, 3–5
    skin lines and, 3–4
  wedge excision, 7, 9
Exophthalmos in Apert's syndrome, 120
Exostoses
  hand, 646–647
  jaw, 361
Explosive adventitious tattooing, 559–560
Exstrophy of bladder
  defined, 865
  epispadias with, 865
  results of untreated, 866
  treatment, 866–867
    functional closure, 867
    urinary diversion, excision of bladder mucosa and abdominal wall closure, 867
Extensor tendon(s)
  extension limitation in interphalangeal joints
    clinical evaluation, 600
    operative management, 600–601
  injury in hand and forearm, 604–607
    boutonnière deformity, 604, 605–606
    immobilization in, 605, 606
    mallet finger, 604–605, 631, 632, 633, 635
    management in rheumatoid arthritis, 635–636
  repair in replantation, 704
External auditory canal
  anomalies in hemifacial microsomia, 116
  auricle reconstruction and, 309
  stenosis, 309
External genitalia. *See also specific topic, e.g.,* Penis
  ambiguous
    differential diagnosis, 878
    sex assignment in, 877, 878
  embryologic development of, 873, 875
  in gender dysphoria, 884
  in testicular feminization syndrome, 876, 877
  in Turner's syndrome, 877
Extremities. *See also specific topic, e.g.,* Finger(s); Hand; Toe(s)
  management of high-voltage electrical burns on, 493
  skin grafts to flexor surfaces, 18
  splinting, 23
Eye. *See also specific topic, e.g.,* Eyelid(s); Orbit
  blowout fractures and movement of, 251–252
  cataracts and electrical injuries, 494
  eyelid reconstruction in absence of, 290–292
    partial loss of both lids, 291–292
    total loss of both lids, 290–291
  protection in craniofacial surgery, 134
  transconjunctival exposure, 133

Eyebrow(s)
concealing scars in hair of, 4
considerations in surgery on, 232
hair bearing skin grafts from, 292, 293
incision in zygomatic fracture fixation, 250, 251, 252
medical advancement in hypertelorism, 122
ptosis correction and, 410, 417–418
raising in facial palsy, 338, 339
reconstruction, 292–293
Eyelashes
adding, in lower lid reconstruction, 281
grafts to provide, 119
Eyelid(s). *See also* Eyelid reconstruction
avulsion of skin of, 233, 235
baggy eyelid deformity correction, 404–408. *See also* Blepharoplasty
basal cell carcinoma of, 505
blepharochalasis, 404
compartments of fat in, 404
as donor site for grafts, 20, 280, 286, 287, 288
infections, 232
injury management, 232
Kuhnt–Szymanski technique for abnormalities of, 119, 340
lacerations, 232
lymphedema, 258–259
paralysis
facial nerve injury and, 236
free muscle grafts for lid closure in, 340, 341
muscle and fascia transfer in, 338–340
ptosis correction, 293–298. *See also* Eyelid ptosis
retraction of lower, 257–258
skin grafts for closure of, 18
suspension of lower, in facial palsy, 338, 339–340
suture scars on, 12
in Treacher Collins syndrome, 118, 119
wedge excision of skin lesions on, 7
xanthelasma palpebrum, 538
Eyelid ptosis, 293–298
acquired traumatic, 298
anterior route (Everbusch) correction, 293, 294
blepharophimosis with, 297
etiology of congenital, 293
frontalis sling procedures for, 296–297, 298
Eyelid ptosis – *Continued*
posterior route (Blascowicz) correction, 293, 295
problems in correction, 293–294
ptosis adiposa of Sichel, 404
split level lid resection in, 294, 295
levator hitch with, 296–297, 298
Eyelid reconstruction, 280–292
in basal cell carcinoma, 505
basic principles, 280–281
canthal loss
lateral, 288
medial, 288–289
cartilage grafts in, 291, 292
in eye absence, 290–292
in partial loss of both lids, 291–292
in total loss of both lids, 290–291
indications, 280
length and width needed for, 280, 286
loss of both lids, 289–290, 291–292
lower and part of upper lid, 289–290
partial loss of both lids, 291–292
skin flaps for, 289, 290, 291–292
total loss of both lids, 289, 290–291
upper and part of lower lid, 290, 291
lower lid, 281–286
adding eyelashes, 281
alternative techniques, 284–285
complications, 285–286
partial losses of lids, 281, 282–283
problems in, 280
rotation flaps in, 281, 282, 283, 284
"sharing" procedures in, 285–286
skin flaps in, 222, 281, 282, 283–285, 286–287, 288
skin grafts in, 284
total lid loss, 280, 283, 285–286
planning, 280
skin grafts for lining, 290–291, 291–292
upper lid, 286–288
partial loss, 286–287, 288
problems and goals, 280, 286
tissue for, 280, 284
total loss, 287, 288

Face. *See also specific topic, e.g.,* Craniofacial surgery; Eye; Facial muscles; Facial scars
aging signs in skin of, 410–411
Face – *Continued*
animal bites, 237–238
asymmetry (craniofacial microsomia), 156–158, 171–172
burns, grafts for, 18
cancrum oris of, 548
carcinoma excision, 18
chemical face peel (chemosurgery), 418, 421–422
clefts, 123
contour defects
rib grafts for, 134
silicone fluid for, 103, 104
dermabrasion, 238, 419, 420
excision of excess skin, 415, 416, 417, 418
excision of skin lesions, 6
female hirsutism, 546
flaps for reconstruction of, 41, 51, 54
bulkiness of, 57
myocutaneous flaps, 58
sickle flaps, 51
fractures, 242–262. *See also* Facial fractures
implants and prostheses for, 102, 349–350
injuries. *See* Facial fractures; Facial soft tissue injury
in leprosy, 548
lines of expression, 4
lipodystrophy, 103
median cleft face syndrome, 122
median facial dysgenesis, 120–122
osteoradionecrosis, 486, 487–488
port-wine stains, 273
rhytidectomy, 411–417, 418–419. *See also* Rhytidectomy
skin grafts to, 18, 238
in burns, 18
color match, 19, 20, 34
donor sites, 19, 20
full-thickness, 17
immobilization of, 23
in scars, 238
surgical exposure of bones of, 133
in Treacher Collins syndrome, 118
wrinkles, 3, 4
removal of deep forehead, 418
Facelift, 411–417, 418–419. *See also* Rhytidectomy
Facial fractures, 242–262. *See also specific topic, e.g.,* Maxillary fractures
blowout fractures, 251–259. *See also* Blowout fracture(s)
in children, 260
classification, 242, 247, 248, 249, 251
diagnosis, 242–243

Facial fractures – *Continued*
emergency treatment, 242
frontonasoethmoid region, 259–260
hemorrhage in, 242
mandible, 245–246, 246–248
maxilla, 245–246, 248–249
maxillary augmentation implants in, 102
nasal, 249–250
optimum repair time, 242
pain in, 227
postoperative care and complications, 262
roentgenograms in, 243
soft tissue injury in, 242
teeth and occlusion in, 242, 244–246
in fracture line, 244–245
intermaxillary fixation, 245–246
tracheostomy in, 243, 260
treatment of multiple, 260, 261
zygoma, 242, 250–251
Facial hemiatrophy (Romberg's disease), 103, 127–128, 349
Facial muscles, 336–344. *See also* Facial palsy
hemifacial microsomia, 117, 118, 172–173
hypertrophy of, 344
benign masseteric, 172–173
injury, 237
muscles of expression, 237, 336
muscles of mastication, 237, 336–337
progressive facial hemiatrophy, 127–128, 349
Facial nerve
course of mandibular branch, 414
crosses and grafts in palsy, 338, 339, 343
damage in chin lacerations, 237
management in surgery
for parotid gland tumors, 393
in radical neck dissection, 370, 375, 376, 377
paralysis, 337–344. *See also* Facial palsy
results of injury, 236
spontaneous regeneration of, 338
Facial palsy, 337–344
autogenous fascia lata for suspension in, 338, 340, 341
bilateral complete, 338
categories of reconstructive procedures, 338–339
characteristic defect of, 337–338
cross facial nerve graft and free muscle graft in, 342, 343
evaluation of treatment, 344
Facial palsy – *Continued*
fronto-palpebral (upper facial)
eyebrow raising in, 339
facial nerve neurectomy in, 338, 339
muscle and fascia grafts and transfers in, 338, 340, 341
palpebral fissure widening in, 339–340
hemifacial microsomia, 117, 118
indications for reconstruction, 338
lower
nonparalyzed side correction, 342–344
paralyzed side correction, 340, 342
Möbius syndrome, 125
muscle grafts in, 338, 340, 341, 342, 343
muscle transfer in, 338, 340, 342
myomectomy or neurectomy on nonparalyzed side, 342, 343, 344
nerve crosses and grafts in, 338, 339, 342, 343
after rhytidectomy, 419
Facial scars, 238
avulsion flap, 230, 232
dermabrasion in, 238
healing, 238
revision of, 238–240
altering scar polarity, 239, 240
U-shaped scars, 238, 239–240
V-Y plasty in, 238, 239, 240
W-plasty in, 238, 239, 240
Z-plasty in, 238, 239, 240
simple lacerations, 229–230
skin grafts for, 238
suture scars, 12
Facial soft tissue injury, 227–240
abrasion, 227, 229
accidental tattoo, 229
animal bites, 237–238
avulsion defects, 230–232, 235, 239–240
contusion, 227, 228–229
diagnosis and classification, 227–228
evaluation of associated injuries, 227
in facial fractures, 242
hematoma in, 227, 228–229
hemorrhage control in, 227, 228
infection in, 238
lacerations, 229–230
management
anesthesia for, 227, 228
in children, 228
immediate, 227–228
preparation for, 228
punctate wounds, 229
Facial soft tissue injury, management – *Continued*
skin grafts in, 18
timing, 227–228, 229
muscles in, 237
nasoorbital, 232–233, 234
pain in, 227
postoperative care, 238
psychological factors in, 238
puncture wounds, 229, 238
retained foreign bodies, 229
False aneurysms of palmar arteries, 645
Fan flaps in lip reconstruction, 345
Fascia grafts, 89
allografts, 85
autografts, 94
in facial palsy, 338, 340, 341
in meningeal defects, 269
in vermillion reconstruction, 348
Fascial space infection in hand, 581
Fasciectomy in Dupuytren's contracture, 638–639
Fasciotomy
in Dupuytren's contracture, 638
in high-voltage electrical burns, 493
Fascicular sutures in peripheral nerve repair, 618, 619, 627, 628–629, 707
Fat, as skin graft recipient bed, 22
Fat flap(s)
dermal, in breast reconstruction, 700, 772, 774
fat flip flap, 57
in pressure sore closure, 820, 822
Fat grafts, 17
absorption of, 89
allografts, 85
in augmentation mammoplasty, 89, 719
in contour defects, 89
full-thickness skin grafts plus, 17
Feeding
neonates with cleft palate, 209
oral, in burns, 467–468, 469, 470
Feet. *See also* Leg(s); Toe(s)
grafts vs. flaps for plantar surfaces, 18
hyperhidrosis, 546
sensation, importance of, 811
split-thickness skin grafts to, 812
use as graft donor site, 676
Felons, 580
Ferris-Smith knife for cutting skin grafts, 24, 25
Fibrin foam for hemostasis, 10
Fibrocystic disease of breast, 738, 761, 762–763
clinopathology, 761, 762
progression of premalignant cellular changes, 762–763

Fibroepithelial polyps, 536
Fibrokeratoma, acquired digital, 537
Fibroma durum, 536–537
Fibroma molle, 536
Fibroma molluscum, 536
Fibroma pendulum, 536
Fibroma simplex, 536–537
Fibromas, 536–537, 644
Fibrosarcoma(s)
  hand, 648
  head and neck, 401, 402
  jaw, 361
Fibromatosis, 537
Fibrosis, intraneural, 686
Fibrous dysplasia
  craniofacial bones, 362
  jaws, 125
Fibrous skin tumors, 536–537
Fibula
  free fibula transfers, 678, 680
  free tissue transfer to, 671, 672
Figure-of-eight sutures, 607
Finger(s). *See also* Fingernail(s); Fingertip(s); Hand; Thumb
  acquired fibrokeratoma, 537
  amputation, 575–578. *See also* replantation
    fingernail management in, 577, 578
    functional losses in, 575–576
    in malignant melanoma, 648
    multiple digit losses, 576, 699
    techniques for therapeutic, 576–577, 578
  avulsion injury management, 20, 34
  boutonnière deformity, 604, 605–606
  collateral ligament tears, 594
  contracture, in rheumatoid arthritis, 631
  degloving management, 574
  flaps in injuries of
    bulkiness of, 57
    sensation restoration and, 42
  flexor tendon injury, 607–615
    critical zone, 608–614
    flexor tendon grafts in, 610, 611–614
    primary tendon suturing in, 608–610
    thumb, 614–615
    zone 1, 607–608
  fractures, 586–590
  high-voltage electrical burns, 493
  infections, 579–581, 582
    goals of management, 578–579
    opportunistic, 582
  interphalangeal joint reconstruction, 634–635

Finger(s) – *Continued*
  joint ankylosis
    interphalangeal joints, 598–601
    metacarpophalangeal joints, 601–603
  joint injuries
    interphalangeal joints, 590, 591–592, 593, 595
    metacarpophalangeal joints, 590, 593, 594, 595–596
    thumb, 595–596
  mallet (baseball) finger, 604–605, 631, 632, 633, 635
  nerves, anatomy and function, 619–622
  prostheses for, 106, 576
  replantation
    amputation level and technique, 710–711
    in multiple amputation, 699
    vein grafts in, 665, 668
  skin grafts to
    donor sites, 20
    sensation restoration and, 34
    shrinkage of, 34
  transfer and reconstruction, 42
Fingernail(s)
  amputation, 577, 578
  anatomy, 569
  avulsion management, 575
  infections, 548, 580
  management in digit amputation, 577, 578
  reconstruction of nail bed, 575
Fingertip(s). *See also* Fingernail(s)
  anatomy, 569–570
  importance, 569
  injury repair, 570–575
    anesthesia for, 571
    bone shortening and direct flap closure, 574, 576
    degloving of distal phalanyx, 573–574
    flap techniques, 41, 572, 573, 574–575, 576
    goals of, 570–571
    split-thickness skin grafts in, 571–572, 573
    wound contraction, 571
  injury types, 570
Firearm wounds, 227, 229, 559
First aid in burns, 459–460
First branchial cleft sinus hemifacial microsomia, 117
Fistula(s)
  branchial, 126
  palatal, 219
  parotid gland, 236
  thyroglossal duct, 126–127
Flag flaps in fingertip injuries, 572, 574

Flap(s), 35–66. *See also specific topic, e.g.,* Muscle flaps; Myocutaneous flaps; Omental flaps; Skin flaps
  defined, 36
  indications for, 35, 36
  in pressure sore closure, 18, 41, 58, 820, 821, 822
    muscle covered by skin, 823
  skin graft attached to margin of, 29, 48
  skin graft replacement with, 19
Flat-face deformity, 103
"Fleur de lys" technique in abdominal obesity, 838–839
Flexion
  limitation in interphalangeal joints
    clinical evaluation, 598
    operative management, 598–600
  limitation in matacarpophalangeal joints, 601–603
    capsulectomy in, 602–603
    etiology, 601
Flexion contractures in burns, 479
Flexion crease scars, Z-plasty for, 64
Flexor digitorum brevis muscle transposition, 815, 816
Flexor digitorum longus muscle transposition, 814–815
Flexor pollicus longus tendon injuries, 615
Flexor profundus tendon injuries, 607–608
  primary repair, 608–610
  tendon grafting in, 610, 611–614
  thumb, 614, 615
Flexor spasms, pressure sores and, 819
Flexor superficialis tendon injuries
  primary repair, 608–610
  tendon grafting in, 611, 612–613, 614
Flexor surfaces, skin grafts on, 18
Flexor tendons of hand
  injuries, 607–608, 615
    critical zone, 608–614
    primary repair, 608–610
    tendon grafts in, 610, 611–614
    thumb, 614, 615
  rupture management, 635–636
  sheath
    excision in grafting, 611–612
    infection, 580–581
Flip flap of penile skin in hypospadias repair, 859, 860
Fluid-electrolyte balance in burns, 455, 456, 462–465, 475–476
  CVP as index of inadequate, 466
  electrical burns, 490, 491, 493–494
  fluid replacement, 463–465, 475–476

Fluid-electrolyte balance in burns
– *Continued*
catheterization for, 462, 475
estimation of fluid requirements, 463–464, 475–476
fluid test load, 466
indications, 464
recommendations on, 464–465
urinary output and, 465, 466
Fluoroscopy, radiation injury from, 485
5-Fluorouracil
for benign skin lesions, 532
for keratoses, 643
for skin carcinoma, 498
Foam for hemostasis, 10
Foot. *See* Feet; Toe(s)
Forearm. *See* Arms; Hand; Wrist
Forehead. *See also* Forehead flaps
advancement
jigsaw Type I with anterior cranial vault reshaping, 149, 150
jigsaw Type II, 151
jigsaw Type III, 151–152
Le Fort III maxillary advancement, 147–148
aging signs, 410
anatomy and embryology, 265
burns, 272–273
circoid aneurysms, 274
injury repair, 232, 272
rib bone grafts in, 134, 146–147
skin flaps and grafts in, 272–273
lacerations, 266–267
radiation injury, 273
removal of deep wrinkles, 418
tumors
benign, 273–274
malignant, 274–275
U-shaped scars, 266
Forehead flaps
advantages of, 329
in cheek reconstruction, 349
classification, 329
in eyelid reconstruction, 289, 290, 291
in lip reconstruction, 346
in nasal reconstruction, 329–331
scalping flap technique, 329, 331
Forehead lift, 418
Foreign material
removal
in adventitious tattooing, 559–560
from eye globus, 232
retained
facial, 227, 229
oral, 229
tattoos from, 419
Forked flaps in cleft lip repair, 200, 202–203
Four-flap Z-plasty, 62
Fractures. *See specific fracture, e.g.* Facial fractures
Frank nonoperative technique for vagina construction, 880
Freckle(s)
benign, 531
Hutchinson's melanotic, 510, 530, 531
Free bone transfer, 678, 680
Free flaps, 39
intestine, 681
in leg reconstruction, 39, 40
muscle, 676, 677, 681
omentum, 681
osteocutaneous groin
for short bone defects, 678, 680
for tibial defects, 673, 674
skin, 675–678, 679
advantages and disadvantages, 678
complications, 676
development of, 675–676
donor sites, 676, 677
for exposed leg bones, 812
monitoring, 675
results, 676, 678
uses, 676
transfer of, 39, 504, 681
vein grafts in salvaging, 665, 668
Free grafts
areola-nipple
in gynecomastia, 806
in reduction mammoplasty, 744, 746, 747
bone, 87–88, 678, 680
monitoring, 675
types and uses, 678, 680
in finger amputation, 576
in hypospadias repair, 861
nerve, 681
skin, 639
in pressure sore closure, 820, 822
thickness of, 86
tissue transplants as, 75. *See also* Free tissue transfer; Tissue transplantation
in urethroplasty in hypospadias repair, 856, 857, 858
Free tissue transfer, 75, 668, 671–675
complications, 675
fibula, 671, 672
monitoring tissue, 675
neurovascular free flaps, 671, 672
operative technique, 674–675
osteocutaneous free groin flap, 673, 674, 678, 680
postoperative management, 675
preoperative preparation, 671
Free tissue transfer – *Continued*
toe-to-hand, 671, 672, 680–681
types, 668–669
in wound closure, 675
Frické flap in eyelid reconstruction, 284, 290
Frontal bone
in cranioplasty, 269–272
spur in osteotomy, 137, 146–147
Frontalis muscle
anatomy, 336
sling procedures in eyelid ptosis, 296–297, 298
Frontonasoethmoid fractures, 259–260
Frown lines, 410
Full-thickness skin grafts, 17
contraction of, 31, 33
cutting, 27–28
defined, 16
in epispadias repair, 866
in external auditory canal stenosis, 309
in eyelid defects, 287, 288
for face, 17, 18
fat grafts plus, 17
in fingertip injury, 572
free, in Dupuytren's contracture, 639
in hypospadias repair, 858, 861
after multiple excision of skin lesions, 6–7
in nasal reconstruction, 324
in pressure sore closure, 820–821
size of, 27–28
split-thickness grafts in closure of donor sites of, 17, 18, 28, 33, 86
survival of, 86
after total subcutaneous excision in lymphedema, 832
vascularity of, 22
"Functional closure" in exstrophy of bladder, 867
Fungus infections
of fingernails, 548
of hand, 582

Galeal flap in auricle reconstruction, 305
Ganglion (Ganglia), in arm, 641, 642, 686
Gastrocnemius muscle transposition, 813–814
Gelatin foam for hemostasis, 10
Gender. *See also* Gender dysphoria
defined, 884
established, changing, 885
in intersex and transsexuals, 885
Gender dysphoria, 883–895
behavior modification in, 886
diagnostic categories, 883–884

Gender dysphoria – *Continued*
general management, 885–886
history of study, 883
incidence, 884
female-to-male changes, 892–895
mastectomy in, 892
hysterectomy and salpingo-oophorectomy in, 891
phalloplasty in, 892–895. *See also* Phalloplasty
results of, 895
scrotal and testicular prostheses for, 894
testosterone and, 892
urinary assist devices in, 894
male-to-female changes, 886–892
augmentation mammoplasty in, 891
chondroplasty in, 890
complications, 888, 890–891
decision to return to original gender, 890–891
electrolysis in, 890
hormone therapy in, 891–892
neocolporrhaphy in, 886–891. *See also* Neocolporrhaphy
penectomy in, 888
preoperative preparation, 886
results, 895
rhinoplasty in, 891
voice training in, 891
male-to-female vs. female-to-male patients, 886
postnatal sociological and psychological influences and, 884–885
postoperative team for achievement of goal in, 885–886
prenatal influences of sex hormones on, 884
preoperative period of total cross-gender living, 885–886
"pretranssexual" population, 884
psychological factors and, 883, 884–885
rehabilitation in, 883, 885–886
selecting patients for surgery, 884, 885–886
Genital leiomyomas, 535
Genitalia. *See specific topic, e.g.,* External genitalia; Penis
Genitourinary tract, development of normal, 873, 874, 875
Geographic tongue, 356
Giant-cell tumors (xanthomas)
hand, 643–644
jaw, 361
skin, 537–538
Giant pigmented nevus, 530–531
Gillies technique for phalloplasty, 892, 893
Gingival hyperplasia, 361
Glenoid fossa construction, 157, 158
Gliomas, 625
Glomus tumors (glomangiomas), 538, 645
Glossectomy
in cervical esophageal and hypopharyngeal carcinoma, 400
in laryngeal carcinoma, 399
in tongue carcinoma, 359
Glossitis rhomboidica medians, 356
Glossoptosis, 123
Gonadal dysgenesis, 884
Gracilis myocutaneous flap in phalloplasty, 894–895
Graft-to-host reaction, 82
Grafts. *See* Bone grafts; Cartilage grafts; Donor sites; Free grafts; Skin grafts
Granular cell myoblastomas, 357, 538
Granular cell schwannomas, 538
Granulation, skin grafts and, 21, 22
Granuloma(s)
pyogenic, 520, 521
silicone fluid injection and, 104
Gravid breast hypertrophy, 738
Groin flaps
described, 38, 39, 40–41
free, 676, 677
for short bone defects, 678, 680
for tibial defects, 673, 674
Growth
bone grafts, 88
cartilage grafts, 89
replanted extremities, 699
skin flaps, 35, 57
skin grafts, 35
Guérin fracture, 248, 249
Guide sutures in end-to-end nerve repair, 690, 692
Gunshot wounds
adventitious tattoos from, 559
hemorrhage in, 227
removal of bullet fragments, 229
treatment, 227
Guthrie technique for breast reconstruction, 786
Gynecomastia, 802–807
clinical classification of, 803, 804, 806
etiology, 802
intraareolar technique for, 803, 804–805, 806
pathological changes in, 802–803
postoperative complications, 806–807
in puberty, 802
skin redundancy management, 806
unilateral, 802

Hagedorn-LeMesurier quadrilateral flap for cupid's bow, 198
Hair
concealing scars in, 4
electrolysis after male-to-female surgery, 891
female hirsutism, 546
growth
in skin flaps, 57
in skin grafts, 34
hair-bearing tissue, 173–174
for baldness, 275–277, 545–546
for eyebrow reconstruction, 292, 293
for eyelashes, 119
in scalp defects, 272
loss
alopecia, 275–277, 545–546. *See also* Alopecia
after auricle reconstruction, 306
after rhytidectomy, 419
tumors with hair follicular differentiation, 534–535
Hair follicle nevus, 533
Hair plugs in alopecia, 275–276, 545–546
Hairy nevus, 273
Hairy tongue, 355, 356
Half-buried horizontal mattress sutures, 14
Halving procedure for eyelid defect closures, 281, 282
Hand. *See also* Finger(s); Thumb
in Apert's syndrome, 120
arterial aneurysm of, 645–646
burns
electrical, 493
excision and grafting in, 471–472
hypertrophic scarring and, 471
nerves and, 493
positioning in, 469
spontaneous healing, 417
cancer, 647
contracture
Dupuytren's, 53–54, 627–628, 637–639. *See also* Dupuytren's contracture
four-flap Z-plasty for, 62
digital ray (metacarpal) amputation, 577
flaps for, 54, 57
fractures, 586–590. *See also* Hand fractures
hyperhidrosis, 546
infections, 578–581, 582
goals of management, 578–579
opportunistic, 582
types, 579–581
joint injuries, 590–597. *See also* Hand joint injuries
in leprosy, 548
nerves, 618–629. *See also* Hand nerves

Hand – *Continued*
prostheses
joint, 634, 636
tendon, 615
radiation injury, 487
replantation. *See also* Replantation
amputation level and, 710–711
dressing, 711–712
rheumatoid arthritis, 631–636
arthroplasty in, 632–634
dorsal rhytidectomy in, 636
excess skin excision in, 636
interphalangeal joint reconstruction in, 634–635
pathology of, 631–632
tendon rupture and wrist deformity in, 635–636
thumb reconstruction in, 635
as skin graft donor site, 20
tendon injuries, 604–615. *See also* Hand tendon injuries
toe-to-hand free tissue transfer, 671, 672, 680–681
tumors, 641–648. *See also* Hand tumors
vascular gigantism, 525
Hand fractures, 586–590
edema in, 586
management principles, 586
metacarpal, 586–587
pharyngeal
distal, 589–590
middle, 589
proximal, 587–589
Hand joint injuries, 590–597
assessment and management principles, 590
immobilization principles, 590
interphalangeal joints, 590–592, 593
thumb, 595
metacarpophalangeal joints, 590, 593, 594
thumb, 595–596
prostheses in, 634, 636
thumb, 594–597
interphalangeal joints, 595
metacarpophalangeal joints, 595–596
Hand nerves, 618–629
anatomy and function, 619–622
injury repair related to, 622–623
burns and, 493
circulation and blood supply, 618–619
injury repair related to, 623–624
injury repair, 622–629
accuracy of, 622–623
amount of scar and, 624, 625
nerve grafts in, 629
Hand nerves, injury repair – *Continued*
primary, 625–626, 627–628
secondary, 625–626, 628–629
techniques, 626–629
time between injury and repair, 623, 626
motor function tests, 624
in median vs. ulnar palsy, 620–621
regeneration, 623
signs and symptoms of injury, 624
Hand tendon injuries, 604–615
burns and, 493
extensor tendon, 604–606
boutonnière deformity, 604, 605–606, 632, 633, 634–635
classification, 604, 605
dorsum of hand, 604, 607
extensor hood, 604, 606–607
mallet finger, 604–605, 631, 632, 633, 635
flexor tendon, 607–615
critical zone, 608–614
flexor tendon grafting in, 610, 611–614
palm, 615
primary tendon suturing in, 608–610
thumb, 614–615
topographic classification, 607, 608
wrist, 615
zone 1, 607–608
goal of initial treatment, 604
prostheses in, 615
in rheumatoid arthritis, 631–632
management of rupture, 635–636
Hand tumors, 641–648
angiomas, 643
bone
endochondromas, 646, 647
exostoses, 646–647
malignant, 648
osteoid osteomas, 646
carcinoma, 647
epidermoid cysts, 642
fibromas, 644
ganglia, 641, 642, 686
glomus tumors, 645
keratoses, 643
lipomas, 644
malignant melanoma, 648
mucous cysts, 641, 642
neuromas, 644
nevi, 643
sebaceous cysts, 642
verrucae (warts), 549, 642–643
xanthomas, 643–644
Hard palate closure
bone grafts in, 213–214
Hard palate closure – *Continued*
mucosal flaps in, 213–214
timing, 210, 213
vomer flaps in, 210, 213, 214
Harvesting vein grafts, 709
Head and neck. *See also specific topic, e.g.,* Cleft palate; Face; Head and neck cancer; Nose
burns, management, 462, 469
flaps for
advancement flaps, 52–53
deltopectoral flaps, 51–52
vascularity and survival of, 36
injury incidence, 266
Head and neck cancer. *See also specific topic, e.g.,* Mouth, cancer; parotid gland, tumors
chemotherapy, 366, 367, 368, 369, 389
combined therapy, 369, 389
results, 366, 367, 368
timing and planning, 366–367
excision in
necrotic masses, 388
primary lesion, 369
immune mechanism and, 368
immunotherapy, 368
mandible resection in, 386
metastatic, 388
operability of, 368
palliative neck dissection in, 388–389
postoperative tracheotomy in, 368
radical neck dissection in, 365–389. *See also* Radical neck dissection
radiotherapy
chemotherapy plus, 389
head and neck cancer after, 383, 384
postoperative, 383
radical neck dissection plus, 366, 367, 368, 369
results, 366, 369, 388–389
sarcomas, 401–402
supraomohyoid neck dissection in, 383–385
TNM clinical staging, 365
prognosis and, 365–366
treatment and, 367
treatment principles, 365–367
Heel. *See* Achilles tendon
Helix
lengthening in lop ears, 446, 448
in otoplasty
cartilage excision, 444
flattening and tubing antihelical fold, 441
in shell ears, 448
rim reconstruction, 309, 311, 312, 313, 314, 315
in satyr ear correction, 448

Hemangiolymphangiomas, 518, 523–524
Hemangioma(s)
capillary, 518–520, 521
port-wine stain, 273, 518–519, 560
pyogenic granuloma, 520, 521
strawberry, 273, 519–520
capillary-cavernous, 521–522
cavernous, 273, 521
clinical classification, 518
excision indications, 273
jaw, 361–362
keratotic, 522–523
scalp or forehead, 273
tongue, 356, 357
verrucous, 522–523
Hemangiomatous gigantism, 524–525
Hemangiopericytomas, 538
Hematoma(s)
ear, 307, 308
face, 227
in fractures, 243
management, 228–229
nasal septum, 233
postoperative
abdominal lipectomy, 842
arm reduction, 850
augmentation mammoplasty, 105, 722, 724, 725, 727
gynecomastia surgery, 806
hypospadias repair, 864
mastectomy and breast reduction, 778, 779
reduction mammoplasty, 746, 748
rhytidectomy, 419
thigh reduction, 848
in puncture wounds, 229
in skin flaps, 37–45
in skin graft recipient beds, 23
prevention, 87
removal, 22, 31
subgaleal, 267
subungual, 589–590
Hemifacial atrophy (Romberg's disease), 103, 127–128, 349
Hemifacial microsomia (branchial arch syndrome), 115–118
etiology, 115–116
management, 117–118
physical signs, 116–117
Hemorrhage. *See also* Hemostasis
in facial injuries, 227, 228
fractures, 242
gastrointestinal, in burns, 479
after gynecomastia surgery, 806
penile
in avulsion injuries, 869
in traumatic amputation, 870
in recipient bed for skin grafts, 10
Hemorrhoidal tissue in nipple-areolar construction, 791
Hemostasis
in augmentation mammoplasty, 723, 724
in auricle reconstruction, 302, 303
in chordee correction, 856
electrosurgery for, 9–10
epinephrine for, 10
in excision of skin lesions, 9–10
in facial injuries, 227, 228
in flexor tendon grafting, 614
implant materials for, 10
ligation for, 9
in mastectomy, 767, 768
in microvascular surgery, 657, 662
peripheral nerve repair, 685
in pressure sore closure, 820
in replantation, 704
amputated part, 703
checking postoperative, 713
stump, 703
in skin grafting, 23, 28
Henoch-Schönlein purpura, 542
Hermaphroditism, 877
Heterografts. *See* Xenografts
Hidradenitis suppurativa, 546–547
Hidradenomas, 534
High-voltage electrical injuries, 492–493
Hinderer technique for hypospadias, 858
Hip replacement, 106
Hirsutism, 546
Histamine wheal test of circulation, 45
Histiocytomas, 536–537
Histocompatibility tests, 83–84
Holdsworth technique of breast reconstruction, 787, 791, 796
Holoprosencephaly, 121
Homografts. *See* Allograft(s)
Homosexuality, gender dysphoria and, 884
Horizontal mattress sutures, 14
Horton technique for phalloplasty, 894–895
Hubbard tank for burn wound cleaning, 471, 477
Hueston volar transposition flap in finger injury, 575
Human leukocyte antigen (HL-A)
allograft reactions and, 76
tissue typing for transplantation and, 82–83
Human placental lactogen, breast and, 737
Humby knife for skin graft cutting, 24, 25
Hutchinson's melanotic freckle (lentigo maligna), 511, 530, 531
Hynes pharyngoplasty in velopharyngeal incompetence, 221
Hynes reverse dermis grafts in pressure sore closure, 822
Hyperbaric oxygen, skin graft survival and, 31
Hyperhidrosis, 546
Hypermobility syndromes of jaw, 185–186
Hyperplastic (varicose) lymphedema, 828
Hypertelorism
in Apert's and Crouzon's syndrome, 120, 145
defined, 122, 259
etiology, 122, 259
median cleft lip and bifid nose with, 120, 122
orbital, 134–138, 259. *See also* Orbital hypertelorism
surgical correction
combined Le Fort III and I osteotomy, 148, 149
intracranial approach (frontal bar), 135–138
medial wall osteotomy, 135, 136
subcranial orbital correction, 135, 136, 148, 149
telecanthus and, 122
traumatic interorbital, 259, 260
true vs. false, 122
Hypertrophic scars, 552–558. *See also* Keloids
from burns, 481
on hand, 471
chemical skin peeling and, 421
defined and described, 552, 553
diagnosis, 552
etiologic factors
age, 555
infection, 552, 553, 554, 555
pressure, 556
tension, 554–555
postoperative
abdominal dermolipectomy, 842–843
arm reduction, 850
gynecomastia surgery, 806–807
reduction mammoplasty, 748
thigh reduction, 849
prevention, 555
region of body related to incidence of, 4, 554–555
skin pigmentation and, 555
tendency towards, rhytidectomy and, 411–412
therapy
combination, 558
surgery, 555
triamcinolone, 556–557, 806–807, 842–843, 849, 850
Hypoglossal nerve
radical neck dissection and, 365, 380, 381, 382

Hypoglossal nerve – *Continued*
submaxillary gland tumors and, 394
Hypopharynx
cancer, 400–401
radical neck dissection in primary, 383
closure or reconstruction, 399, 400–401
Hypoproteinemia, burns and, 469, 480
Hypospadias, 855–865
circumcision in, 864
complete breakdown of repair of, 864
diagnosis and classification, 855
embryology of, 855
one-stage repairs, 857, 858–863
advantages of, 858
distal shaft hypospadias, 858, 859–861
perineal or scrotal hypospadias, 861–862, 863
proximal shaft hypospadias, 861, 862
reliability of, 865
pathologic anatomy of, 855–856
postoperative complications, 864–865
preoperative problems, 862, 864
two-stage repairs
chordee correction, 856
urethroplasty, 856, 857, 858
urinary diversion in, 862, 864
Hysterectomy in female-to-male conversion, 892, 894

Ileofemoral free flaps, 676, 677
Iliac bone grafts
in cranioplasty, 152, 269, 271
in mandible reconstruction, 176
in nasal reconstruction, 322
technique of taking, 134, 271
Iliac compression syndrome, 829
Iliac crest, free transfer of, 678, 680
Iliac osteotomy in exstrophy of bladder, 867
Immobilization
of bone grafts, 87, 88, 323
in burns, 473, 474
of joints, 469
of skin grafts, 473, 474–475
after capsulectomy, 599–600, 601, 603
of hand
in dislocations, 586, 590, 592, 593, 594, 595, 596, 597
in extensor tendon injury, 605, 606
in flexor tendon grafting, 614
in flexor tendon injury of wrist, 615
in flexor tendon suturing, 610

Immobilization, of hand – *Continued*
in fractures, 586, 587, 588, 589, 590
in infection, 579, 581
in radiation injury, 487
in rheumatoid arthritis, 632, 636
of mandible
in malpositioned fractures, 173
in stabilization, 386–387, 394
in peripheral nerve repair, 685
of skin grafts, 18, 23, 31–32, 34
in burns, 473, 474–475
on extremities, 18, 23, 31–32, 34
on joints, 32
in temperomandibular joint dislocations, 182
of zygomatic fractures, 250–251, 252
Immune mechanism
acquired transplant tolerance and, 81–82
allografts and, 76–80, 81–82
graft-versus-host reaction, 82
histocompatibility tests and, 83–84
immunologic enhancement and, 77–78
specific immunologic tolerance, 80
tissue typing and, 82–83
cancer and, 368
head and neck cancer, 368
malignant melanoma, 515
squamous cell carcinoma, 507
cytotoxic humoral antibodies against donor cells, 77
immunocompetence testing, 368
radiotherapy and, 368
tissue transplantation and, 76, 77, 82, 83
Implants and prostheses, 94–107. *See also* Breast implants and prostheses; Dentures
acceptability criteria, 95
in blowout fractures, 102, 255–256
postoperative extrusion of, 258
bone, 106, 107
chest wall, 106
chin, 100–101, 349, 433
in condylectomy, 185, 187, 188
ear, 101–102, 350
auditory canal stenosis prevention, 309
auricle reconstruction, 300–301, 303, 307
esophagus, 105
in eyelid reconstruction, 290
face, 102, 349–350. *See also specific topic, e.g.,* mandible
in contour deformities, 102, 270, 349
in progressive facial hemiatrophy, 128

Implants and prostheses, face – *Continued*
rationale for use of, 349–350
requirements for maxillofacial, 333
types of, 350
fluids, 95–96
general precautions with, 94
hand
finger, 576
joint, 634, 636
tendon, 615
thumb, 635
ideal soft tissue substitutes, 94
intraoral, after mandibular resection, 386, 387
joint, 106, 634, 636
lip, 200, 201, 350
in lymphatic reconstruction, 830, 831
in malar depression, 102
mandible, 102–103
in asymmetry, 171
in augmentation of mental symphysis, 166
bone grafts plus, 176, 177
in malpositioned fractures, 175
after resection, 386, 387
in underdevelopment, 117
maxilla, 102
inlay, 350
in meningeal defects, 269
in nasal reconstruction, 100, 321, 322, 323, 333
contraindications in secondary rhinoplasty, 434, 435
silicone rubber, 100
nerve, 107
orbit, 102, 350
palate, 211, 222
in palpebral fissure slant, 119
for penile stiffening, 894
pharynx, 104–105, 221, 222
plastics, described, 96
safeguards in surgical techniques with, 94–95
silicones
clinical advantages, 98, 99
described, 95, 97
handling, 99
inflatable bag, 56
rubber, 97–98, 100, 104–105
in skull and cranial defects, 102, 269
bone grafts plus, 102
in contour restoration, 270
stainless steel, 95
tendon, 107
hand, 615
silastic rods, 617
testes, 106
in female-to-male surgery, 894
textiles, 95–96
in urethral reconstruction, 106

Implants and prostheses – *Continued*
in velopharyngeal incompetence, 104–105, 221
vitallium, 95, 96
Incontinence
epispadias and, 865, 866
exstrophy of bladder and, 867
Indirect distant flaps, 56
Infantile cortical hyperostosis, 125
Infantile digital fibromatosis, 537
Infection(s)
avulsion injuries of penis, 869
burns, 478–479, 493
ear, 307–308
dermis grafts, 87
in exstrophy of bladder, 867
eyelid, 232
in facial injury, 238
fingernail, 548
after free tissue transfer, 675
hand, 578–581, 582
in diabetes, 582
in drug addiction, 582
goals of management, 578–579
opportunistic, 582
types, 579–581
host resistance and, 579
in hypertrophic scar etiology, 552, 553, 554, 555
joint, 582
lymphedema and, 828, 829, 830
organism virulence and, 579
postoperative
abdominal dermolipectomy, 842
arm reduction, 850
augmentation mammoplasty, 725, 727
auricle reconstruction, 303, 305
blowout fracture repair, 258
craniofacial surgery, 132
hypospadias repair, 864
mastectomy and breast reconstruction, 779
reduction mammoplasty, 748
thigh reduction, 848–849
pressure sores and, 818
skin, 546–549
dissecting cellulitis, 547
hidradenitis suppurativa, 546–547
leprosy, 548
lupus vulgaris, 548
molluscum contagiosum, 549
noma, 548
pyoderma gangrenosum, 547
wart virus, 549
in skin flaps, 37, 45–46
in skin grafts, 29, 31
recipient bed, 24
sutures and, 12
temperomandibular joint, 182
Inflammatory response, scar formation and, 552, 553, 554
Inframammary technique for augmentation mammoplasty, 721–727
Infraorbital technique for blowout fractures, 255–257
Infraorbital nerve, blowout fractures and, 254, 259
Inguinal region
lymph nodes of, 826–827
as skin graft donor site, 20
Inlay prostheses for maxilla, 166, 350
Inlay skin grafts
described, 30, 349
split-thickness, in vaginal agenesis, 878–879
Intercostal nerves as donor sites, 695
Interfascicular sutures in end-to-end nerve repair, 690, 692
Intermaxillary fixation of mandibular fractures, 245–246, 247, 248, 260, 261
Interorbital hypertelorism, 259, 260
Interphalangeal joints
amputation, replantation in, 710
anatomy, 590–591
ankylosis, 598–601
extension limitation in, 600–601
flexion limitation in, 598–600
dislocations and injuries, 590, 591–592, 593, 595
reconstruction in rheumatoid arthritis, 634–635
stabilization of thumb, 635
Interpolation flaps, 51–53
described, 51, 53
dog ears at pivot point, 48–49
Interrupted sutures, 14, 29
Intersex, 877. *See also* Gender dysphoria
differential diagnosis, 878
gender identification in, 885
iatrogenic causes, 878
psychological factors in, 878
Intestine
free transfer of, 681
segments
in esophagus construction, 401
in vagina construction, 880–881
Intraareolar technique for gynecomastia, 803, 804–805, 806
Intraalveolar veloplasty in soft palate closure, 214, 215–217
Intercapsular tuberculopasty in temperomandibular joint hypermobility, 186
Intracranial orbital correction (frontal bar), 135–138
complications, 138
Intracranial orbital correction – *Continued*
postoperative management, 137
surgical technique, 136–137
Intradermal nevi, 530, 643
Intraductal papillomas of breast, 762, 763–764
Intraneural fibrosis, 686
Intraneural interfascicular nerve dissection, 686–688
in compression syndromes, 686
in lesion in continuity, 686, 687
in nerve tumors, 686, 688
in restoration of continuity, 688
secondary, 695
Intravenous fluorescein test of skin flap viability, 44–45
Invaginated ears, 446, 448
Involutional breast hypertrophy, 738
Island flaps, 9
in avulsion defects of face, 235
converting peninsular flaps to, 39
described, 38–39, 52
eyebrow reconstruction with scalp, 292–293
in nasal reconstruction, 330
from forehead, 330
for nasal lining, 215
nasolabial flap, 326
neurovascular, in fingertip injury, 575
Ischeal pressure sores, 820, 821, 823, 824
Isograft, defined, 75

Jadassohn-Lewandowski syndrome, 548
Jaw(s). *See also* Mandible; Maxilla; Temperomandibular joint
augmentation mentoplasty, 100–101, 166–167, 432–433. *See also* Augmentation mentoplasty
cysts, 361
deformity
in Apert's syndrome, 120
cephalograms in diagnosis, 161, 162, 163
in Crouzon's syndrome, 120
malocclusion in, 161. *See also* Malocclusion
fibrous dysplasia of, 125
hypermobility syndrome management, 185–186
intermaxillary fixation in fractures, 245–246
osteoradionecrosis, 486
posttraumatic deformities, 175–179
preprosthetic surgery, 178, 179

Jaw(s) – *Continued*
tumors, 360–362
cancer, 360
classification, 361
hemangioma, 361–362
metastatic, 360, 361, 362
Jigsaw procedures
hazards of, 131, 149
Meisterschnitt approach, 152–153
Type I, 149, 150
Type II, 151
Type III, 151–152
Joint(s). *See also specific topic, e.g.,* Arthroplasty; Rheumatoid arthritis
ankylosis of finger
interphalangeal joints, 598–601
metacarpopalangeal joints, 601–603
Dupuytren's contracture, 53–54, 627–628, 637–639. *See also* Dupuytren's contracture
flexion contractures in burns, 479
immobilization of
in burns, 469
in skin grafting, 32
infections of, 582
injuries of hand, 590–597. *See also* Hand joint injuries
prosthetic replacement of, 106, 635
rheumatoid arthritis and, 631–632. *See also* Rheumatoid arthritis
stability assessment in hand injuries, 590
stiffness after replantation, 713
transplants in temperomandibular ankylosis, 187
Jump flaps
for leg reconstruction, 39, 676, 677
in scalp avulsion, 267, 268
Junctional nevi, 273, 530, 643

Kaposi's sarcoma, 532, 543, 828
Kasabach-Merritt syndrome, 519, 522
Keloids. *See also* Hypertrophic scars
after abdominal lipectomy, 842–843
butterfly-shaped sternal, 4
defined, 552, 553
diagnosis, 552
of earlobe, 316
etiology, 552
pressure as treatment of, 556
prevention, 555
region of body and incidence of, 4
skin pigmentation and, 555
tendency towards, rhytidectomy and, 411–412
sutures and, 12
therapy
combination, 558
radiotherapy, 555–556
Keloids, therapy – *Continued*
surgery, 555
triamcinolone, 556–557, 806–807, 842–843, 849, 850
Keratoacanthomas, 508, 533, 535
Keratoses
actinic, 532
chemical skin peeling for, 421
hand, 643
seborrheic, 532
Keratosis follicularis, 532
Keratosis palmaris et plantaris, 532
Keratotic hemangiomas, 522–523
Kussler-Mason-Allen suture for hand tendon injuries, 609
Kidney
embryologic development of, 873
function, burns and, 454, 478, 490–491, 493–494
Kinking of skin flaps, 37, 45, 46
Klinefelter's syndrome, 802, 884
Klippel-Feil syndrome, 126
Klippel-Trenaway-Weber syndrome, 524–525
Knee
muscle transposition in defects over, 813–814
pressure sore closure on, 823
Knot tying in sutures, 14, 655–656
Koenen's periungual tumors, 537
Kuhnt-Szymanowski techniques for eyelid surgery, 119, 340

Labia majora
deformity after thigh reduction, 849
grafts from, 20–21
in nipple-areolar construction, 791
in scrotum construction, 894
Labia minora grafts in nipple-areolar construction, 791
Laceration(s)
facial, 227, 229–230
chin, 237
cheek, 236–237
eyelid, 232
forehead, 266–267
wound toilet in, 229–230
fingertip, 570
penis, 869
scalp, 266, 267
Lacrimal system
injury
in blowout fracture repair, 259
dacryocystorhinostomy in, 232–233, 234
preservation in eyelid repair, 232
Landolt-Hughes technique for eyelid reconstruction, 285
Larynx
carcinoma, 398–400
diagnosis, 398
prognosis, 399–400
Larynx, carcinoma – *Continued*
treatment, 399
chrondroplasty after male-to-female surgery, 891
laryngectomy, 399, 400
Laser in decorative tattoo removal, 563, 565
Lateral canthotomy in eyelid reconstruction, 281, 282, 283
Lateral facial clefts, 123
Lateralizing procedures in reduction mammoplasty, 739–740
Laterognathism, 171–172
Latissimus dorsi muscle
anatomy and circulation, 787
myocutaneous flap in breast reconstruction, 790
Le Fort Type I maxillary osteotomy
in craniofacial microsomia, 156, 157
in mandibular asymmetry, 171
in maxillary fractures, 248, 249
in short face syndrome, 173
Le Fort Type III plus
in Crouzon's or Apert's syndrome, 148, 149
in subcranial hypertelorism, 148–149
Le Fort Type II maxillary osteotomy
in maxillary fractures, 248, 249
in perinasal flattening, 142
in retromaxillism, 143
winged, 143, 144
Le Fort Type III maxillary advancement, 145–148
with anterior open bite, 146, 147
forehead advancement plus, 147–148
with frontal spur and forehead rib grafts, 146–147
jigsaw Type III plus, 151–152
with lateral orbital wall split, 146
standard, 145–146
with zygomatic step cut, 146
Le Fort Type III maxillary fracture, 248, 249, 260
Le Fort Type III maxillary osteotomy
subperiosteal stripping in, 133
Type I plus
in Crouzon's or Apert's syndrome, 148, 149
subcranial hypertelorism correction and, 148–149
Leg(s). *See also* Leg flaps; Leg reconstruction
edema, 828
iliac compression syndrome and, 829
subcutaneous excision of lymphedema, 833
after thigh reduction, 849
lipectomy
lower leg, 849

Leg(s), lipectomy – *Continued*
thigh reduction, 838, 843–849. *See also* Thigh reduction
lymphatic system, 826–827
skin grafts to, 26, 27
immobilization of, 32
in ulcers, 30, 32
skin loss
traumatic, 812
vascular disease and, 811
ulceration, 30, 32, 811
Z-plasty for constricting scars on, 64
Leg flaps
cross leg flaps, 36, 39, 40, 44, 55, 58, 676, 678, 812
direct flaps, 54–56
free skin flaps, 676, 678, 812
jump flaps, 39, 40, 676, 678
muscle flaps, 41, 58
myocutaneous flaps, 41
Leg reconstruction, 811–817
aims of, 811
ankle, 815, 816
cross leg flaps in, 36, 39, 40, 44, 55, 58, 676, 678, 812
direct flaps in, 55–56
exposed bone coverage, 812–817
cross leg flaps for, 812
decortication and skin grafting in, 812
free skin flaps in, 676, 678, 812
muscle transposition in, 812–817
reverse dermis grafts in, 812
free skin flaps in, 676, 678, 812
functional defects after, 815–816
jump flaps in, 39, 40, 676, 678
knee joint, 813–814
muscle flaps in, 41, 58
muscle transposition in, 812–817
ankle, 815, 816
complications, 816–817
distal third of leg, 815
general plan of skin grafts plus, 813
meshed split-thickness grafts plus, 816
middle third of leg, 814–815
upper third of leg, 813–814
myocutaneous flaps in, 41
results of, 676, 678
tibia, 813–815
Leiomyomas, 535
Lentigo maligna, 510, 511, 530, 531
Lentigo senilis, 531
Leprosy, 548
Leukoplakia
jaw, 361
tongue, 356, 357, 358
Lidocaine (Xylocaine)
in facial injuries, 228
in temperomandibular joint disorders, 183
Limberg flap
described, 49, 51
in nasal reconstruction, 325–326
planning, 51, 52
Lines of dependency of skin, 4
Lingual nerves, submaxillary gland tumors and, 394
Lingual sulcus formation, 178, 179
Lingual tonsils, 356
Lip(s). *See also* Cleft lip; Lip reconstruction
anatomy, 192, 193, 344
burns
full-thickness, 492
management, 345, 346, 348, 492
cancer
radical neck dissection in, 382
squamous cell, 507
supraomohyoid neck dissection in, 384
in cheek and chin injuries, 235
dermabrasion vs. skin peeling around, 420
ectropion, 345
entropion, 346
implants, 350
in bilateral cleft lip, 200, 201
injury repair, 237
loss, 345–348
mucosal graft cutting from, 27
scars, management, 345
suspension in facial palsy, 338, 340, 341
wedge excision of skin lesions, 7
Lip reconstruction, 344–348. *See also* Cleft lip closure
Abbe flap in, 7, 345–346, 348
secondary, 198
commissure reconstruction, 346, 348
Estlander flap in, 346, 347
full-thickness defects, 345–346
lower lip, 346–348
mucosal flaps in, 345, 347, 348
mucosal surface defects, 345, 346
skin grafts in, 348, 349
skin surface defects, 345, 346
total loss, 346–348
upper lip, 345–346
vermillion reconstruction, 348
Lipectomy
abdominal, 838–843. *See also* Abdominal dermolipectomy
arm, 849–850
lower leg, 849
submental, 417
thigh, 838, 843–849. *See also* Thigh reduction
Lipedema, 830
Lipodystrophica progressiva, 846, 847
Lipomas of hand, 644
Liposarcomas of head and neck, 401, 402
Lobular carcinoma in situ of breast, 762, 764–765
Local flaps, 48–54. *See also specific flap, e.g.* Transposition flaps
advancement flaps, described, 52–54
advantages of, 48
in burn wound closure, 492, 493
in cheek reconstruction, 348, 349
in external audiotory canal stenosis, 309
in finger amputation, 575–576
in forehead defects, 272
interpolation, described, 51–52, 53
for lip scars, 345
in lymphedema reconstruction, 830, 831
in nasal reconstruction, 325–326, 327
open vs. closed, 48
pivot point of, 48–52
in radiation injuries, 273
in radical neck dissection, 368–369, 383, 384
rotation, described, 48–49
rotational, in breast reconstruction, 786, 791, 792
in scalp defects, 267
hair-bearing, 272
transposition, described, 49–51, 52
in urethroplasty for hypospadias, 856, 857, 858
Lop ears, 446, 447, 448
Lower extremities. *See* Feet; Leg(s); Toe(s)
Low-voltage electrical injuries, 492
Lupus erythematosus
discoid, 538
systemic, 539
Lupus vulgaris, 548
Luxation of temperomandibular joint, 262
Lymph node(s). *See also* Lymphadenectomy; Lymphatic system
acquired lymphedema and, 829
allograft reactions and, 76, 77
arm, 827
biopsy in head and neck cancer, 365
embryologic development of, 826
metastases
cervical esophageal carcinoma, 400
hypopharyngeal carcinoma, 400
parotidectomy for, 393
radical resection of negative, 488

Lymph node(s), metastases
– *Continued*
salivary gland tumors, 395
squamous cell carcinoma of hand, 647
thyroid carcinoma, 396–397, 398
tongue carcinoma, 355, 359
venous anastomosis in, in lymphedema, 830, 831
Lymphadenectomy, 488
axillary, in breast cancer, 764
in malignant melanoma, 513–514, 648
in radical neck dissection, 365
regional, 514
in squamous cell carcinoma, 506–507
supraomohyoid, 383–385, 386
in thyroid carcinoma, 397
Lymphangiography, 826, 827, 828, 829
Lymphangiohemangiomas, 518, 523–524
Lymphangioma(s), 643, 829–830
clinical classification, 518
scalp and forehead, 273–274
tongue, 356
types, described, 523–524
Lymphangioplasty, 831
Lymphangiosarcomas, 828
Lymphangitis, lymphedema and, 828, 829, 830
Lymphatic system. *See also* Lymph node(s); Lymphadenectomy; Lymphangioma(s); Lymphedema
anatomy
arms, 827
legs, 826–827
continuity development in skin grafts, 22, 23
embryologic development of, 826
lymphangiography, 826, 827, 828, 829
physiology, 827
reconstruction in lymphedema, 830, 831
Lymphedema, 826–835
acquired, 826, 827
etiology, 829
differential diagnosis, 829–830
eyelid, 258–259
infection and, 828, 829, 830
lymphangiosarcoma and, 828
lymphatic system physiology and, 827
medical management, 830
primary, 826, 827
age of onset, 828
etiology and precipitating factors, 828–829
Lymphedema – *Continued*
surgical management, 830–835
direct lymphatic reconstruction, 830, 831
indications, 830
pedicle flap reconstruction, 830–831, 831–832
postoperative evaluation, 831
staged subcutaneous excision, 831, 832–834, 834–835
total subcutaneous excision plus skin grafts, 831, 832, 834–835
symptoms, 827–829
acquired, 829
primary, 828–829
Lymphocyte-dependent antibody (LDA) test in allograft donor selection, 83–84
Lymphocytes
allograft rejection and, 78–79
HL-A test, 76, 82–83
LDA test, 83–84
subpopulations of, 78

McFee incision for radical neck dissection, 369, 374, 375
McIndoe technique for vaginal agenesis, 878
McKissock technique for mastopexy, 752–756
operative technique, 753, 754, 756
preoperative planning, 753, 754
principles, 752–753
McKissock technique for reduction mammoplasty, 742–746
operative technique, 744, 745, 746
preoperative planning, 742, 743, 744
Macrogenia,
prognathism vs., 167
transverse mental symphysis ostectomy in, 170–171
Macromastia. *See also* Reduction mammoplasty
etiology, 737
pathology associated with, 738
recurrence after reduction mammoplasty, 749
subjective nature of concept of, 739
types, 738
Macrostomia, 117, 118
Malar process
flap rotation from, 281
implants for depression of, 102
Malherbe calcifying epithelioma, 534
Malignant clear cell hidradenomas, 534
Malignant eccrine poromas, 534
Malignant melanoma(s), 511–515
clinical staging, 512
diagnosis, 511, 512
differential diagnosis, 530
of hand, 648
histopathology, 511–512
incidence and epidemiology, 511, 648
in infants and children, 530
metastases, 512, 513–514, 515
nodular, 511
origin from benign growths, 511, 530–532, 643, 648
recurrence, 513, 515
spread, 511, 648
treatment, 511–515
chemotherapy, 515
immunotherapy, 515
lymphadenectomy, 513–514, 515
resection and excision, 512–513, 648
Malleolus
muscle transposition in defects of, 815
pressure sore closure on, 823
Mallet (baseball) finger
described, 604–605
management, 635
in rheumatoid arthritis, 631, 632, 633, 635
Malocclusion, 161–163. *See also* Orthodontia
Angle's classification of, 161
apertognathia and, 140, 172, 182
cephalometric analysis in, 162, 163
Class II, 163, 174
Class III, 145
Le Fort maxillary osteotomy in, 143
mandibular prognathism in, 167
in Crouzon's or Apert's syndrome, 145, 146, 147
in facial fractures, 242, 244–245
managment in alveolar or palatal cleft repair, 211–212
in overdevelopment of maxilla, 174
in temperomandibular joint arthritis, 182
after temperomandibular joint surgery, 188
Malunion of fractures
mandibular, 175–176, 177
maxillary, 176
Malunion after replantation, 713
Mammography, 760, 761, 768
Mammoplasty
augmentation, 719–729, 731–736. *See also* Augmentation mammoplasty

Mammoplasty – *Continued*
reduction, 737, 739–750. *See also* Reduction mammoplasty
secondary ptosis after, 727, 749
Mandible. *See also* Alveolus, dental; Mandibular defects and deformities; Mandibular fractures; Mandibulectomy; Tempero-mandibular joint
augmentation of, 166–167
basic movements of, 180
in craniofacial microsomia, 172
hyperplasia of mandibular condyle, 172
muscles
benign masseteric hypertrophy, 172–173
functions of, 247
osteoradionecrosis, 486, 487–488
palpation, 243
primary malignant tumors of, 360
reconstruction
bone grafts in, 166, 176
compound flaps in, 57
implants in, 102–103, 166
of mandibular sulcus, 178, 179
skin flaps in, 176
skin grafts in, 178, 179
of symphyseal area, 177
scar revision on, 12
stabilization, 176, 394
surgical exposure of, 134
terms for positional relations of, 180
Mandibular defects and deformities. *See also specific topic, e.g.,* Micrognathia; Retrognathia
bone grafts in, 166, 175–176, 177
bony configuration, soft tissue profile and, 163
cartilage allografts, 117, 118
cephalometric analysis in, 161, 162, 163
in craniofacial microsomia, 156, 157
in Crouzon's or Apert's syndrome, 145
in hemifacial microsomia, 117–118
laterognathism or asymmetry, 171–172
overdevelopment, 167–171
unilateral, 172
in Pierre Robin syndrome, 163
prostheses for, 102–103, 117, 166
in Treacher Collins syndrome, 118, 140–141, 163
underdevelopment, 118, 140–141, 163–167
Mandibular fractures, 245–246, 246–248
classification and incidence, 242, 246, 247
closed reduction of, 248
Mandibular fractures – *Continued*
healing of malpositioned, 175
intermaxillary fixation of, 245–246, 247, 248, 260, 261
malunion correction, 175–176, 177
musculature and, 246, 247
open reduction of, 247, 248, 261
in multiple facial fractures, 260
of subcondylar region, 260
wiring teeth in occlusion in, 247–248
Mandibulectomy
arch restoration after, 386–387
buccal and lingual sulcus creation and, 178, 179
in head and neck cancer, 386–387
intraoral appliances after, 386
in osteoradionecrosis, 487–488
osteotomy in, 186
in parotid gland tumors, 393
Mandibulofacial dysostosis. *See* Treacher Collins syndrome
Marsupial flaps, 56
Masseter muscle
anatomy, 336
benign hypertrophy of, 344
transfers, in facial palsy, 338, 340, 342
Mastectomy
bilateral, separation of instruments for, 767
breast anatomy related to, 766–767
breast reconstruction after, 772, 775–778, 785–789. *See also* Breast reconstruction after mastectomy
procedures for remaining breast, 774
technique related to reconstruction, 767, 794
in carcinoma in situ, 764
in female-to-male surgery, 892
hemostasis in, 767, 768
modified total
in breast without skin redundancy, 770
dermal fat flap creation in, 770, 772, 774
in large breast with ptosis, 770–772, 773, 774
Spira technique, 772, 773
pathologic specimen management, 768
postoperative care, 768
postoperative complications, 765
hematoma, 778, 779
infection, 779
necrosis, 772, 778, 779
pain, 775, 779
prophylactic, 761, 765–780
Mastectomy, prophylactic – *Continued*
anatomy of breast related to technique, 766–767
autotransfusion in, 766
breast reconstruction after, 765, 772, 775–778
evaluation of patient for, 765
general operative approach, 766–767, 767–768
incidence of occult cancer in, 765
indications, 765–766
operative techniques, described, 768–772, 773, 774
postoperative complications, 765, 772, 778–779
preoperative evaluation, 765, 766–767
psychological factors and, 765
team approach in, 765
psychological factors and, 765, 785
reexamination and follow-up, 794
simple. *See* modified total
skin flaps in, nipple-areolar or breast tissue in, 767
subcutaneous
incisions in, 768, 769, 770
in "minimal" cancer, 765
residual breast tissue after, 766–767
retained continuity of skin and areola-nipple, 768–769
total
breast resection extent in, 766–767, 768
in lobular carcinoma in situ, 764
wound closure in, 768
Mastopexy
defined, 750
postoperative and home care, 756
prosthesis inclusion in, 751, 756
psychological factors and, 750
secondary loss of shape, 751–752
techniques, 750–751, 752–756
Dufourmental and Mouly, 752
McKissock, 752–756
Regnault, 752
resection of circumareolar skin, 752
Mattress sutures
for everting wound edges, 12
in otoplasty for prominent ears, 441, 443, 444
in skin closure, 12, 13, 14
Maxilla. *See also* Maxillary advancement; Maxillary defects and deformities; Maxillary fractures; Maxillary osteotomy
primary malignant tumors of, 360
skin flaps for open wounds of, 41
skin grafts in postoperative closure of, 18

Maxilla – *Continued*
stability determination, 243
surgical exposure of, 134
Maxillary advancement, 145–148
anterior open bite and, 146, 147
forehead advancement plus, 147–148
with frontal spur and forehead rib grafts, 146–147
jigsaw Type III procedures plus, 151–152
with lateral orbital wall split, 146
standard, 145–146
with zygomatic step cut, 146
Maxillary defects and deformities
anterior retrusion, 142
bony configuration, soft tissue profile and, 163
cephalometric analysis in, 162, 163
in craniofacial microsomia, 156, 157
in Crouzon's or Apert's syndromes, 145–148
in hemifacial microsomia, 117
hypoplasia, 103
retrusion plus, 173, 174
implants for, 102, 103
inlay prostheses, 350
overdevelopment and protrusion, 174–175
recession, 143
retromaxillism with Class III malocclusion, 143
retrusion
without cleft palate, 173, 174
management in cleft palate, 173, 174
in prognathism, 173
Maxillary fractures, 245–246, 248–249
classification, 242, 248–249
frontonasoethmoid region, 259–260
incidence and etiology, 248
intermaxillary fixation in, 245–246
Le Fort Type III, 248, 249, 260
malunion, management, 176
tooth suspension and arch bars in, 249, 261
Maxillary osteotomy
Le Fort Type I
in craniofacial microsomia, 156, 157
in Crouzon's or Apert's syndrome, 148, 149
in mandibular asymmetry, 171
in maxillary fractures, 248, 249
in short face syndrome, 173
Type III plus, 148–149
Maxillary osteotomy – *Continued*
Le Fort Type II
in maxillary fractures, 248, 249
in perinasal flattening, 142
in retromaxillism, 143
winged, 143, 144
Le Fort Type III
in Crouzon's or Apert's syndrome, 145–148
subperiosteal stripping and, 133
Type I plus, 148–149
Maxillofacial osteoradionecrosis, 486, 487–488
Maxillofacial surgery. *See* Craniofacial surgery; *and specific topic, e.g.,* Maxillary osteotomy
Maxillonasal dysplasia of Binder, 142
Medial orbital wall osteotomy, 135, 136
Median cerebrofacial dysgenesis, 120–122
Median nerve
injury, 615, 624
muscles innervated by, 620, 621–622
palsy, 548
test for, 620–621
Meisterschnitt approach
intracranial orbital correction, 136
jigsaw procedures, 152–153
mandibular condyle exposure, 134
medial canthal ligament, 134
for osteotomy, 133
Melanoma(s)
benign juvenile, 530
jaw, 361
malignant, 511–515, 530–532, 643, 648. *See also* Malignant melanoma(s)
oral floor, 363
Melanotic freckle of Hutchinson, 510, 511, 530, 531
Meningeal defect repair, 269
Menisectomy in temperomandibular joint surgery, 185, 186
Mental symphysis
augmentation
implants for, 100–101
operative technique, 166–167
profile and, 432–433
transverse ostectomy of, 170–171
Mesh expansion of skin grafts, 29
in burns, 473
leg muscle transposition plus, 816
in ulcers, 811
Metabolism, burns and, 453, 454–455, 455–456, 469, 480–481
Metacarpal fractures, 586–587
Metacarpophalangeal joints
anatomy, 593
ankylosis, 601–603
capsulectomy in, 602–603
arthroplasty in rheumatoid arthritis, 632–634
dislocations and injuries, 590, 593, 594
thumb, 595–596
silicone prostheses for, 634
Metastases. *See* Lymph node(s), metastases
Methylmethacrylate implants, 96
Meyer and Kesselring technique for reduction mammoplasty, 740
Microcrystalline collagen for hemostasis, 10
Microgenia
micrognathia vs., 163
surgical correction of, 166–167
Micrognathia, 163–164
bone plus skin grafts in, 165–166
implants in, 100
malocclusion in, 163, 164, 165
microgenia vs., 163
osteotomy in, 165
in Pierre Robin syndrome, 123, 124
retrognathia vs., 163
Microphallus, 877, 878
Microporous surgical adhesive tape, 14–15, 29–30
Microsurgical repair of peripheral nerves , 685–695
continuity restoration, 688–690
end-to-end repair vs. nerve grafts in, 689
intraneural interfascicular dissection in, 688
intraneural topography and, 689–690
primary vs. secondary, 688–689
end-to-end repair
nerve grafts vs., 689
technique, 690–693
equipment for, 685
general principles of, 685
hemostasis in, 685
immobilization in, 685
intraneural interfascicular dissection, 685–688
in compression syndrome, 686
in lesion in continuity, 686, 687
in nerve tumors, 686, 688
in restoration of continuity, 688
surgical technique, 685–686
nerve graft technique, 685, 693–695
distal suture site, 695
donor nerves, 694–695
primary vs. secondary repair, 688–689
reexploration after repair failure, 695

Microsurgical repair of peripheral nerves – *Continued*
timing, 688
wound closure, 685
Microtic ear, reconstruction of, 299–306. *See also* Auricle reconstruction, in microtia
Microvascular surgery, 653–659, 660, 663–670
anastomoses, 660, 662–665, 666, 667, 668, 669–670
end-to-end, 660, 663–665, 666, 669–670
end-to-side, 660, 665, 667, 668, 669–670
free tissue transfer, 674
hemostasis in, 662, 668
luminal diameter differences and, 665, 666, 669–670
patency rate, 662, 668
principles and fundamentals of, 662–663
suturing, 662, 663, 668
in congenital facial asymmetry, 158
equipment for, 653, 660–661, 704–705
instruments, 660–661
magnification systems and microscopes, 660, 685, 704–705
sutures, 661
in explosive adventitious tattooing, 560
free intestine transfer, 681
free muscle transfer, 681
free nerve transfer, 681
free omental transfer, 681
free skin flaps, 675–678, 679
advantages and disadvantages, 678
complications, 676
development of, 675–676
donor sites, 676, 677
results, 676, 678
free tissue transfer, 668, 671–675, 681
anastomoses, 674
complications, 675
donor sites, 671, 674
fibula, 671, 672
monitoring tissue, 675
neurovascular free flaps, 671, 672
operative technique, 674–675
osteocutaneous free groin flap, 673, 674, 678, 680
postoperative management, 675
preoperative preparation, 671
recipient bed, 671, 674
tissue transfer technique, 674
toe-to-hand, 671, 672, 680–681
types, 668–669
wound closure, 675

Microvascular surgery – *Continued*
free vascularized bone transfers, 678, 680
indications for reconstructive, 682
lymphatic anastomoses in lymphedema, 830, 831
in nasal reconstruction, 331
in oral and pharyngeal reconstruction, 349
in peripheral nerve repair, 685–695. *See also* Microsurgical repair of peripheral nerves
in replantation, 697–714. *See also* Replantation
in scalp defects, 267, 272
sutures in, 655–656, 661, 662, 663, 668, 685
techniques
clinical progression in, 661–662
common errors, 658
experimental work, 653–659
free tissue transfer, 671, 672
training and laboratory exercises, 653–659, 660, 661–662, 682
vein grafts in, 665, 668, 669–670
Midface degloving, 134
Midpalmar abscess, 581
Migration in flap transfer, 56
Milia, 536
Mirault-Blair-Brown method for cleft lip, 194, 198
Mixed leukocyte culture (MLC) test in allograft donor selection, 83
Mixed oblique facial clefts, 123
Möbius syndrome, 125–126
Mohs' chemosurgery in skin carcinoma, 497, 498
Moles. *See* Nevus (nevi)
Molluscum contagiosum, 549
Mondor's disease, 727
Monoblock neck dissection
in radial neck dissection, 365, 368, 369, 384
in supraomohyoid neck dissection, 383–384
Monostatic fibrous dysplasia of jaws, 125
Mouth
aging signs, 410
avulsion injury of chin and, 237
cancer, 363
of floor, 362–363, 383–384, 386
mandible resection in, 386
radical neck dissection in, 382–383
supraomohyoid neck dissection in, 383–384
TNM clinical staging, 365
tongue, 354–355, 357–360. *See also* Tongue, cancer
treatment related to stage, 367
exposure in osteotomy incisions, 133–134

Mouth – *Continued*
failure to remove foreign bodies, 229
full-thickness burns, 492
preprosthetic surgery, 178, 179
ranula, 362–363
skin grafts, 345
in micrognathia, 165–166
mucosal lining, 386, 394
after resection of mandible, 386
after submaxillary gland resection, 394
vestibuloplasty, 178
wound management, 237
Mucoceles of tongue, 356
Mucoepidermoid carcinoma of oral floor, 363
Mucosal flaps
in alveolar clefts, 210, 214
in bilateral cleft lip, 200, 201
in cheek reconstruction, 349
in cleft palate closure, 210, 213–214
in lip reconstruction, 345, 347, 348
"apron" in vermillion reconstruction, 348
mucosal surface defects, 345
Mucosal grafts, 18–19
buccal, in areola-nipple construction, 792
in eyelid reconstruction, 282–283, 284
in lip reconstruction
mucosal surface defects, 345
V-Y rolldown for vermillion, 197
nasal, 18–19, 215, 216
Mucous cysts of hand, 641, 642
Mucous membrane. *See also* Mucosal grafts
in nasal reconstruction, 233
removal, in frontal cranioplasty, 269
skin grafts in replacing, 18–19
suture scars on, 12
Mullerian ducts, genitourinary tract development and, 873, 874
Müller's muscle, eyelid ptosis and, 293, 294, 296
Multiple advancement flaps, 54
Multiple elliptical excision of skin lesions, 6–7
Multiple trichoepitheliomas, 533–534
Muscle(s). *See also specific topic, e.g.,* Facial muscles; Muscle flaps; Muscle transposition
contracture after replantation, 713
flexor spasms, pressure sores and, 819
free transfer of, 681
smooth muscle tumors, 535
transposition. *See also* Muscle transposition
in facial palsy, 338, 340, 341, 342, 343

Muscle(s), transposition
– *Continued*
in lower extremity, 812–817
Muscle flaps, 58, 89–90. *See also specific topic, e.g.,* Delto-pectoral flaps
in bilateral cleft lip, 200, 201
contractile power of, 89
for covering bone, 89
for covering breast prostheses, 777–778
described, 57–58
in leg reconstruction, 41
in pressure sore closure, 58, 823
in radical neck dissection, 383, 384
skeletal muscle as free, 89–90
skin grafts plus, 57–58
survival of, 35
in vermillion defects, 348
Muscle grafts in facial palsy, 338, 340, 341, 342, 343
Muscle transposition
in facial palsy, 338, 340, 341, 342, 343
free, 681
in lower extremity, 812–817
ankle, 815, 816
complications, 816–817
distal third of leg, 815
functional defects and, 815–816
general plan of skin grafts plus, 813
knee and upper third of tibia, 813–814
meshed split-thickness skin grafts plus, 816
middle third of tibia, 814–815
after parotid gland surgery, 393
Musculocutaneous arteries, 36, 37, 38
Musculocutaneous flaps, 89
Mustardé technique for hypospadias, 858–859
Mycobacterial infections of hand, 582
Mycosis fungoides, 542–543
Myocutaneous flaps, 58
in breast reconstruction, 790
free, 676
gracilis, in phalloplasty, 894–895
in leg reconstruction, 41
in pressure sore closure, 823
survival of, 35
Myofacial pain dysfunction syndrome, 181, 182–183
Myomectomy in facial palsy, 342, 343, 344
Myotomy in hypermobility of jaw, 186
Myxoid cysts, 537
Myxomas, 537
Nail(s). *See* Fingernail(s)
Nasal reconstruction, 321–334. *See also* Rhinoplasty
alternatives in, 321
anatomy of nose and, 321
basic problems in, 322
bone grafts in, 322, 323
cartilage grafts in, 322–323
cartilage repair, 233
composite grafts in, 324, 325
fixation in, 322–323
implants and prostheses for, 100, 321, 322, 333
in leprosy, 548
loss and deformity related to, 321
mucous membranes, 233
objectives of, 321
planning, 332–333
in rhinophyma, 544–545
skin flaps in, 324–332
cervical, 331, 332
clavicular, 331
direct flaps from arm, 54
forehead, 329–331
local flaps, 325–326, 327
nasolabial, 326, 327, 328, 329
postauricular, 331
subcutaneous pedicle island flaps, 326, 329
transfer of distant, 331–332
skin grafts in, 323–324
full-thickness, 324
guidelines for use of, 322, 323–324
split-thickness, 323–324
Nasolabial flaps
in cheek reconstruction, 349
in eyelid reconstruction
lower lid, 284–285
rotating, in loss of both lids, 290, 291
in lip scars, 345, 346
in nasal reconstruction, 326, 327, 328, 329
for lining and covering, 328
in nasal floor reconstruction, 327
optimum size, 326
tubing, 324
Nasolabial folds, 410, 418
Nasomaxillary osteotomy, 142
Naso-ocular clefts, 123
Nasopharyngeal carcinoma, 387–388
Neck. *See also specific topic, e.g.,* Head and neck cancer
anatomy related to radical neck dissection, 369, 370, 371–373
cancer
of hypopharynx or cervical esophagus, 400–401
management of metastatic, 387–388
sarcoma, 401–402
Neck – *Continued*
chemical skin peeling on, 421
dissection
bilateral, in tongue cancer, 359
palliative, 388–389
radical, 365–389. *See also* Radical neck dissection
supraomohyoid, 383–385, 386
flaps from, 36, 56
Klippel-Feil syndrome and, 126
lines and folds in aging, 410
obscure primary tumor of, 401
Necrobiosis lipoidica, 542
Necrosis, 542
avascular, of bone grafts, 86
in electrical burns, 491, 492
heat and, 3
postoperative
abdominal dermolipectomy, 842
arm reduction, 850
breast reconstruction, 794, 798
hypospadias repair, 864
mastectomy, 777, 778, 779
reduction mammoplasty, 737, 746–747, 748
thigh reduction, 849
pressure sores and, 818
radiation, 487
omental plus skin grafts in, 787, 791
of skin flaps, 45, 46
in auricle reconstruction, 305
prevention in radical neck dissection, 369–370
Necrotizing vasculitis, 542
Neocolporrhapy, 886–891
complications, 888, 890–891
lining for vagina and vulva formation, 887–888, 889, 890
perineal pocket dissection, 886–887
shortening and repositioning urethra, 887
split-thickness skin grafts in, 888, 889
Nerve(s). *See also* Hand nerves; Nerve grafts; Peripheral nerve(s); *and specific nerve, e.g.,* Facial nerve
block for anesthesia, 228
covering in protection from trauma, 41
crosses and grafts in facial palsy, 338, 339, 343
finger, 569
dissection in amputation, 577
free transfer of, 681
injuries
stump evaluation in, 688
in temporal bone fractures, 267
wrist, 615

Nerve(s) – *Continued*
- regeneration, 688
- repair
  - end-to-end, 689, 690–693. *See also* End-to-end nerve repair
  - microsurgical, 685–695. *See also* Microsurgical, repair of peripheral nerves
  - prosthetic sheath in, 107
  - reexploration after failure of, 695
  - regeneration after primary vs. secondary, 688
- sensory fibers to skin grafts, 35
- skin flaps for bare, 41
- skin grafts for, 17, 21
- tumors
  - intraneural interfascicular dissection in, 686, 688
  - neuromas, 107, 577, 625, 644

Nerve grafts
- advantages and results, 693, 694
- in continuity restoration, end-to-end repairs vs., 689, 693
- in facial palsy, 338, 339, 343
- free, 681
- indications for, 629
- length and fascicular pattern, 694
- microvascular peripheral nerve repair, 685
- after nerve tumor excision, 688
- technique, 693–695
  - distant suture site, 695
  - donor nerves, 694–695
  - tension and, 693–694

Neurectomy in facial palsy, 338, 339, 342, 343, 344
Neurilemomas, 645
Neurinomas, 686, 688
Neurofibromas, 686
- hand, 644
- scalp, 274

Neurofibromatosis, 540
Neurogenic sarcomas of jaw, 361
Neuromas, 107, 625
- excision of, 107
- of hand, 577, 644

Neurovascular flaps
- in fingertip injury, 572, 573, 575
- free, in tissue transfer, 671, 672
- local, in lip reconstruction, 346

Nevus (nevi)
- blue, 531–532, 643
- change into malignant melanoma, 511, 648
- classification, 643
- compound, 530, 643
- excision of, 273, 643
- forehead and scalp, 273
- giant pigmented, 530–531
- hair follicle, 533
- hairy, 273
- hand, 643
- intradermal, 530, 643
- junctional, 273, 530, 643
- organoid, 535
- of Ota, 532
- skin grafts in overgrafting, 19
- treatment related to malignant degeneration of, 643

Nevus flammeus (port-wine stain), 273, 518–519, 560
Nevus sebaceous, 535
Nevus verrucosus, 532
Nipple. *See* Areola-nipple complex
Nipple graft in nipple-areola construction, 791
Nodular hidranenoma, 534
Nodular pseudosarcomatous fascitis, 537
Nodular subepidermal fibrosis, 536–537
Noduli cutanei, 536–537
Noma (cancrum oris), 548
Nonabsorbable sutures
- described, 10, 11
- wound infection and, 12

Nose. *See also* Nasal reconstruction
- aging and, 410
- anatomy, reconstruction and, 321
- bifid with median cleft lip, 122–123
- in bilateral cleft lip
  - described, 198
  - rotation-advancement in correction, 198–199, 200, 201
  - secondary revisions, 203
- cartilage repair, 233
- cavernous hemangiomas, 521
- dacryocystorhinostomy in naso-orbital injury, 232–233, 234
- fractures
  - classification of, 242, 249
  - frontonasoethmoid region, 259–260
  - reduction of, 249–250
- grafts from
  - in lower eyelid reconstruction, 282–283, 284
  - mucosal, 18–19, 215, 216
  - skin, 233
- hematoma of septum, 233
- implants and prostheses for, 100, 321, 322, 323
- mucous membranes
  - cocaine for anesthetizing, 228
  - grafts from, 18–19, 215, 216
  - management in soft palate closure, 215, 216
  - repair of, 233
- packs
  - after fracture reduction, 250
  - to maintain fragment position, 233
- parrot's beak, 120, 145
- perinasal osteotomy, 142
- rhinoplasty, 424–433, 434–439. *See also* Rhinoplasty
- skin
  - excision in rhinophyma, 544–545
  - variations in, 321
- soft tissue injury management, 233
- in unilateral cleft lip, 193, 197
  - rotation-advancement in correction, 194, 195–196, 196–197
  - secondary correction, 198
- wedge excision of nostril, 7

Obesity
- gynecomastia in, 802
- lipectomy in abdominal, 838–839, 840
- medical therapy, 838

Oblique facial clefts, 123
Obwegeser's technique for saggital mandible split, 165, 169–170
Ocular hypertelorism, 259
Ombrédanne hood
- chordee correction and, 856
- penile resurfacing and, 859, 861, 862

Omental flaps
- omentum lengthening for, 58
- in reconstruction in lymphedema, 831–832
- skin grafts plus, 58
  - in breast reconstruction, 787, 791
  - in radiation necrosis, 787, 791
  - survival of, 35

Omentum, free transfer of, 681
Omphalocele, 19
Oral cancer. *See* Mouth, cancer
Orbicularis oculi muscle, 336
Orbicularis oris muscle
- anatomy, 336
- lip function and, 344
  - myomectomy in facial palsy, 343, 344

Orbit
- anatomy, 251, 253
- in anophthalmia, 155
- bone grafts to rims, 134
- in Crouzon's or Apert's syndrome, 145
- dacryocystorhinostomy in nasoorbital injury, 232–233, 234
- edema, 252
- fractures
  - blowout, 251–259. *See also* Blowout fracture(s)

Orbit, fractures – *Continued*
frontonasoethmoid region, 259–260
hypertelorism, 134–138, 145, 148, 149, 259. *See also* Orbital hypertelorism
hypotelorism with median cleft lip, 120–122
implants and prostheses for, 102, 350
in blowout fractures, 255–256, 258
palpation of infraorbital margins, 243
skin grafts from, in eyelid reconstruction, 284
surgery. *See also* Craniofacial surgery; *and specific topic, e.g.,* Orbital osteotomy
anesthetic complications, 138
dystopia, 138
elevation in craniofacial microsomia, 157–158
exenteration, skin graft closure of, 18
hypertelorism correction, 135–138
rim advancement, 143, 144, 153, 154
split of lateral wall, 146
Tessier technique, 139–140
in Treacher Collins syndrome, 139–140
wall deformity in hypertelorism, 135
Orbital hypertelorism, 134–138
in Crouzon's or Apert's syndrome, 145, 148, 149
described, 134–135
etiology, 259
surgical correction, 135–138
combined with Le Fort Types III and I osteotomy, 148, 149
intracranial approach (frontal bar), 135–138
medial wall osteotomy, 135, 136
subcranial orbital correction, 135, 136
wall deformity types in, 135
Orbital osteotomy, 135–138
frontal spur, 137
Le Fort III maxillary advancement with, 146–147
in hypertelorism, 135, 136
median wall, 135, 136
orbital dystopia, 138
orbital size expansion, 155
rim advancement, 143, 144
subcranial, 135, 136
Orchiectomy
in male-to-female surgery, 887
prosthesis in, 106
Organoid nevi, 535
Oroocular clefts, 123
Oropharyngeal cancer, 383
Orthodontia
in cleft palate, 222
maxillary retrusion and collapse and, 173, 174
postoperative, 222
in craniofacial microsomia, 172
in facial asymmetry, 171–172
in maxillary overdevelopment and protrusion, 174, 175
in maxillary retrusion and collapse, 173, 174
in micrognathia, 164
postoperative
alveolar or prepalatal cleft repair, 211–212
bilateral cleft lip closure, 192
cleft palate repair, 222
in prognathism, 167, 168, 170
in temperomandibular joint disorders, 183
Ostectomy
craniofacial
in apertognathia, 172
in maxillary protrusion, 174
in maxillary retrusion and collapse, 174
operative technique in macrogenia, 170–171
in prognathism, 168–169
in pressure sores, 820, 821, 823, 824
Osteoarthrotomy of temperomandibular joint, 187, 188
Osteocutaneous free groin flap
for short bone defects, 678, 680
for tibial defects, 673, 674
Osteogenic sarcoma(s), 401, 402
hand, 648
jaw, 360, 361, 362
prognosis, 362
Osteoid osteomas of hand, 646
Osteoma(s)
hand, 646
jaw, 361
Osteotomy
craniofacial, 155, 186. *See also* Maxillary osteotomy
anterior, 143, 168, 170
apertognathia and, 172
in coronal synostosis, 154–155
in craniofacial microsomia, 156–158
in Crouzon's or Apert's syndrome, 145–148
C-shaped (vertical oblique), 164–165, 172
incisions and exposures in, 133–134
in mandibular asymmetry, 171
in mandibular overdevelopment, 172
Osteotomy, craniofacial, – *Continued*
in maxillary fractures, 176, 248, 249
in maxillary hypoplasia, 173, 174
in maxillary protrusion, 175
in maxillary retrusion and collapse, 173, 174
in microgenia, 166–167
in micrognathia, 165
nasomaxillary osteotomy, 142
orbital osteotomy, 135–138, 143, 144, 146–147, 153, 154. *See also* Orbital osteotomy
perinasal osteotomy, 142
in periorbital correction, 139–140
in prognathism, 168, 169, 170
in retrognathia, 164–165
in retromaxillism, 143
tangential, in skull defects, 493
Tessier technique, 139–140
in Treacher Collins syndrome, 139–141
winged, 143, 144
iliac, in exstrophy of bladder, 867
in rhinoplasty, 429–430, 431
Otoplasty
after auricle construction, 306
in invaginated ears, 446, 448
in lop ears, 446, 447, 448
in prominent ears, 440–446
abnormal conchal depth, 445–446
antihelical fold tubing, 441
conchal cartilage excision, 441
conchal-mastoid sutures, 441, 445, 446
ear cartilage exposure, 442, 443
ear positioning, 442
helical cartilage excision, 444
indications and timing, 441
marsupialization of auricular cartilage, 441–442
mattress sutures in, 441, 443, 444
posterior cartilage thinning, 441
postoperative dressings, 444–445
preoperative preparation and anesthesia, 441
scratching cartilage, 441, 442, 443, 444, 445, 446
skin excision in, 441–442, 443, 444, 445, 446
in satyr ears, 448
in shell ears, 448
Ovary, embryologic development of, 873, 874
Overgrafting
in burns, 272–273
of nevi, 19
in radiation injury, 273

Overtattooing, 562, 563, 565
Oxygen therapy
  in burns, 462, 477
  hyperbaric, skin graft survival and, 31

Pachydermatocele, 274
Padgett electric dermatome, 27
Padgett-Hood dermatome, 25, 26
Pain. *See also* Sensation
  in bladder spasm after hypospadias correction, 864
  in facial injuries, 227
  after fingertip injury repair, 571, 573
  after mastectomy, 775–779
  in radiation injuries, 487
  temperomandibular joint, 180, 181, 182
Palatal obturators
  in fistulas, 350
  in Pierre Robin syndrome, 124
Palate
  anatomy, 205–206
  cleft, 205, 206. *See also* Cleft palate
    classification, 208–209
    repair, 212–218
  in Crouzon's syndrome, 120
  fistulas, 219, 350
  lengthening procedures
    in soft palate closure, 214, 215–217
    in velopharyngeal incompetence, 221
  paresis in hemifacial microsomia, 117, 118
  prostheses
    in fistulas, 350
    lift, after cleft palate repair, 222
    obturators, 124, 350
    in Pierre Robin syndrome, 124
  soft
    closure, 211, 214, 215–217, 222. *See also* Soft palate closure
    speech and movement of, 205, 207
  tumors, 362
Palatopharyngoplasty in velopharyngeal incompetence, 221–222
Palmar artery aneurysms, 645–646
Palmar flaps in fingertip injury, 575
Palmaris longus muscle grafts in facial palsy, 342
Palmaris longus tendon grafts, 612
Palpebral fissure
  antimongoloid slope, 118, 119, 131, 139
    bone grafts for, 119
Palpebral fissure – *Continued*
  widening, in facial palsy, 338, 339
Palpebral ligament separation, 259, 260
Papilloma(s)
  cutaneous, 536
  intraductal breast, 762, 763–764
  jaw, 361
  tongue, 357
Paralysis. *See specific topic, e.g.,* Facial palsy
Paraplegia
  pressure sores in
    prevention, 818–819
    treatment, 819–823
  rehabilitation in, 824
Pardue adjacent flap for cleft earlobes, 316
Paronychia, 548, 580, 581
Parotid gland
  absence, 117
  anatomy of region, 392, 393
  fistulas, 236
  injury, 236
  removal, 392, 393
  transection in radical neck dissection, 370, 375
  tumors, 391–393, 396
    benign, 391–392
    malignant, 391, 392
    prognosis, 392, 393, 394, 396
    treatment, 392–393
Parrots' beak nose, 120, 145
Pectoralis muscle
  anatomy, 777
  breast implant insertion under, 767, 776–778, 785–786, 787
    dissection in mastectomy and, 767
    timing, 785
  subpectoral dissection in breast reconstruction, 785–786, 787
Pectus excavatum, 106
Pedicle flaps
  in avulsion of scalp, 267, 268
  defined, 36
  double, in pressure T, sore closure, 820, 822
  in reconstruction in lymphedema, 830–831, 831–832
  scrotal, in penile avulsion injuries, 870
  subcutaneous in nasal reconstruction, 326, 329
  in wound closure after circular excision, 8
Peninsular flaps
  converting into island flaps, 39
  described, 38, 39, 40
Penis
  amputation in male-to-female surgery, 888
  avulsion injuries, 869–870
Penis, avulsion injuries – *Continued*
    avulsion of scrotal skin with, 871–872
  burns of, 869
  chordee, 856, 864
  circumcision, 864, 875
  corpora cavernosa rupture, 869
  corpus spongiosum stump after male-to-female surgery, 890
  epispadias, 865–866
  erection, 855–856
    in avulsion injuries, 869, 870
    after hypospadias surgery, 864
  exstrophy of bladder with normal, 865
  flaps from, 870
    in epispadias repair, 865–866
    in hypospadias repair, 859, 860, 861, 862
    in neovagina creation, 888
  fractures, 869
  hypospadias, 855–865. *See also* Hypospadias
  implants for stiffening, 894
  lacerations, 869
  phalloplasty, 892–895. *See also* Phalloplasty
  resurfacing in Cecil-Culp technique, 858
  size, sex assignment and, 877, 878
  strangulation injuries, 869
  traumatic amputation, 870–871, 878
Periareolar technique for augmentation mammoplasty, 721, 722, 723–724
Pericardial closure, 19
Perichondrium
  grafts from, in auricle reconstruction, 309
  transplantation as free grafts, 89
Pericranial flaps
  as base for skin grafts, 57
  for dural defects, 493
Perineal hypospadias repair, 861–862, 863
Perinasal osteotomy, 142
Perineum
  avulsion with scrotal loss, 871
  dissection in neovagina formation, 886–887
Perineural sutures in end-to-end nerve repair, 690, 693
Periosteum repair in replantation, 704
Peripheral nerve(s). *See also* Microsurgical repair of peripheral nerves
  anatomy, 618–619
  fascicle groups, 686–687
  hand, 618–629. *See also* Hand nerves

Peripheral nerve(s) – *Continued*
injury. *See* Hand nerves, injury repair; Microsurgical repair of peripheral nerves
in leprosy, 548
preparation in amputated part for replantation, 701–702
prostheses in, 107
repair, 626–629
continuity restoration, 688–689
fascicle alignment, 707
hand, 622–629. *See also* Hand nerves, injury repair
microsurgical. *See* Microsurgical repair of peripheral nerves
in replantation, 707
sutures in, 618, 619, 626, 627, 628, 707
tumors, 644–645
intraneural interfascicular dissection in, 686, 688
Peritoneal closure, 19
Peroneus longus muscle transposition, 814
Peterson reverse abdominoplasty flap in breast reconstruction, 786, 791, 793, 794
Phalanges. *See* Finger(s)
Phalloplasty, 892–895
Davies and Birdsell technique, 892, 894
Durfee and Roland technique, 895
Gillies technique, 892, 893
Horton technique, 894–895
Phaloplethysmography as circulation test, 45
Pharynx. *See also* Hypopharynx
implants and prostheses for, 104–105, 222
pharyngocutaneous fistula, 399
resection in parotid gland tumors, 393
tumors of, 400–401
Philtrum, 344
Pierre Robin syndrome
etiology, 123–124
palate obturator in, 124
physical characteristics in, 123, 163, 209
positioning patient in, 124
tracheotomy in, 125
tongue-to-lip adhesion in, 124–125
Pigmented lesions, differential diagnosis of, 530
Pigmented nevi, 530–531
Pilar cysts of scalp, 274, 536
Pilomatricoma, 536
Pitanguy technique for reduction mammoplasty, 741, 742
Plagiocephaly, jigsaw Type III in, 151–152
Plantar surfaces, grafts vs. flaps for, 18
Plantar warts, 549
Platysma muscle
dissection in rhytidectomy, 413–414
inclusion in radical neck dissection, 365, 369–370, 375, 376, 377
Pleural closure, 19
Plummer-Vinson syndrome, 400
Polyethylene
implants, described, 95, 96, 100, 106
in total hip replacement, 106
Polyglycolic acid absorbable sutures, 10–11
Polyostotic fibrous dysplasia of jaws, 125
Polypropylene sutures, 10, 11
Polyurethane
for covering breast implants, 776
implants, described, 95, 96
Pontes technique for breast reconstruction, 786, 791, 795
Poromas, 534
Port-wine stain, 518–519
medical tattooing for, 560
treatment principles, 273
Postage-stamp-sized skin grafts, 29, 31
Postauricular skin grafts, 19, 20
Postcricoid carcinoma, 400
Posterior pharyngeal flaps in velopharyngeal incompetence, 219–221
Postgravid breast hypertrophy, 738
Pott's puffy tumor, 267
Pregnancy
breast in, 737, 738
sex hormones in
anomalous sexual development and, 878
gender dysphoria and, 884
Pregnancy tumors
of jaw, 361
of tongue, 357
Premaxillary protrusion, 199–200
Prepalatal clefts
alveolus in, 207, 211
classification, 208
embryologic development of, 207
Prepuce
grafts from, 20–21
in epispadias, 866
in hypospadias, 858, 861, 862
splitting, for penile resurfacing, 859, 860, 861
Pressure
hemostasis and, 9–10
skin flaps and, 37, 45
Pressure dressings. *See* Dressing(s)
Pressure sores, 818–824
Pressure sores – *Continued*
causes, 818, 824
closure, 819–824
bony prominence removal, 820, 821
flaps in, 18, 41, 58, 820, 821, 822, 823
grafts in, 18, 820, 822, 824
hemostasis in, 820
ischial, 820, 821, 823, 824
postoperative care, 822
sacral, 820, 822
trochanteric, 820, 822–823
wound suturing, 822–823
locations, 818
preoperative care, 819
prevention, 818–819
resection and excision of ulcer, 819, 820
"Pretranssexuals," gender dysphoria and, 885
Progesterone, breast and, 737, 763
Prognathism, 167
cephalometric analysis in, 162, 163
macrogenia vs., 167
maxillary retroposition in secondary, 173
orthodontia in, 167, 168, 170
surgical management
anterior alveolar osteotomy, 168, 170
complications, 168
osteotomy of mandibular body or ramus, 168–169
preoperative planning, 167–168
sagittal split of mandible, 169–170
true vs. relative, 167
Progressive facial hemiatrophy, 127–128
Prominent ears, otoplasty in, 440–445, 445–446. *See also* Otoplasty, in prominent ears
Proplast implants, described, 95
Prostheses. *See* Breast implants and prostheses; Dentures; Implants and prostheses
Proximal shaft hypospadias repair, 861, 862
Pseudohermaphroditism, 877
Pseudomalignant strawberry hemangioma, 520
Pseudoprognathism, 163, 167
Pseudosarcomatous skin lesions, 537
Pseudoxanthoma elasticum, 541
Psoriasis of fingernails, 548
Psychological factors in plastic surgery
augmentation mammoplasty, 719, 720–721
auricle reconstruction, 299
breast cancer, 765

Psychological factors in plastic
surgery – *Continued*
breast reconstruction, 785
burns, 462, 468
ear deformities, 441
facial soft tissue injuries, 238
gender dysphoria, 883, 884–885
intersex, 878
mastectomy, 765, 785
mastopexy in ptosis, 750
skin cancer resection, 501
treatment of gender identity
problems, 885
vaginal agenesis, 873
Pterygoid muscles
anatomy, 336, 337
myotomy in jaw hypermobility,
186
Ptosis
breast, 720, 750–756. *See also*
Breast ptosis
eyebrow, 416, 417–418
eyelid, 293–298, 404. *See also*
Eyelid ptosis
Ptosis adiposa of Sichel, 404
Puberty
breast hypertrophy in precocious,
738
gynecomastia in, 802
Puncture wounds of face, 229, 238
Pyoderma gangrenosum, 547
Pyogenic granulomas, 520, 521

Quadratus labii muscles
anatomy, 336
myomectomy in facial palsy,
342, 343, 344
Quadrilateral flaps
in cupid's bow construction, 198
in unilateral cleft lip closure, 194

Rabies vaccination in animal bites,
237–238
Radial nerve
for grafts, 694
muscles innervated by, 619–620
Radiation injury, 484–488
acute, 485
chronic, 272, 485–486
histopathology, 485–486, 487
malignancy after, 497–498
pathogenesis, 484
scalp and forehead, 273
treatment, 272, 486–488
excision and resurfacing, 273,
487–488
general principles, 486–487
skin flaps in, 787, 791
skin grafts in, 22, 273
Radical neck dissection, 365–389
anatomy of neck related to technique,
369, 370, 371–373

Radical neck dissection – *Continued*
anterior facial vein and external
maxillary artery, 370, 376, 377
carotid artery and sheath, 375,
378, 379, 380, 381, 382
in cervical esophageal or hypo-
pharyngeal cancer, 400
cervical plexus, 375, 380, 381
closure and suction catheters,
380, 381, 382
continuous vs. discontinuous,
366, 368
digastric muscle, 365, 375, 378,
379, 382
facial nerve, 370, 375, 376, 377
hypoglossal nerve, 365, 380,
381, 382
incisions, 369, 374, 375
indications, 365, 385–386
intraoperative antibiotics, 369
jugular vein, 365, 375, 378,
379, 382
in laryngeal carcinoma, 399
lymphadenectomy and, 365
mandible resection and, 386–387
modifications, 382–383
monoblock technique, 365, 368,
369, 384
morbidity, 366, 368, 385–386
muscle flaps in, 374, 383, 384
in obscure primary tumors, 401
omohyoid muscle, 365, 375, 378,
379, 382
parotid gland transection, 370, 375
patient preparation and intubation,
369
in primary branchiogenic carcinoma,
401
platysma muscle, 365, 369–370,
375, 376, 377
pressure dressings after, 380, 381
after radiotherapy, 383, 384
radiotherapy plus, 366, 367, 368,
369, 388–389
results, 366, 367, 368, 388–389
in salivary gland tumors, 393,
394, 395
in sarcomas, 402
skin flaps in, 368–369, 374, 383,
384
elevation of, 369–370, 376, 377
necrosis prevention, 369–370
skin grafts in, 368
sternocleidomastoid muscle, 365,
375, 378, 379, 380, 381
stylohyoid muscle, 365, 382
submaxillary triangle, 365, 370,
375, 376, 377, 382
thoracic and cervical ducts, 375
in thyroid cancer, 397
trapezius muscle, 375, 380, 381, 382
vagus, 375, 378, 379, 380, 381, 382

Radiodermatitis
histopathology, 485–486, 487
malignant changes, 497–498
management, 486–488
Radioisotopic tests of circulation, 45
Radiotherapy, 368
head and neck cancer, 366, 369,
388–389
chemotherapy plus, 389
metastatic, 388
radical neck dissection after,
383, 384
radical neck dissection plus, 366,
367, 368, 369
history of, thyroid cancer and,
396
of hypertrophic scars and keloids,
555–556
in hypopharyngeal or esophageal
cancer, 400, 401
immune mechanism and, 368
in laryngeal cancer, 399
in mouth cancer, 363
in osteogenic sarcoma etiology, 401
in parotid gland tumors, 393
radiation injury from, 484–488
in sarcomas, 275, 402
in skin cancer, 497
in submaxillary gland tumors, 394
in thyroid cancer, 397, 398
in tongue cancer, 359
in warts, 642
Random pattern flaps
blood supply, 38, 39
described, 46, 48
planning and survival, 38
Ranula of mouth, 362–363
Rectangular flaps in lip recon-
struction, 346
Rectovaginal fistulas, 888, 890,
899
Reduction mammoplasty, 737,
739–750
age criteria for, 749
basis of technique for, 737, 739
Dufourmentel and Mouly technique,
739, 740
Elbaz and Verheeke technique, 740
free nipple grafts in, 744, 746, 747
history of, 737
indications, 738
McKissock technique, 742–746
operative technique, 744, 745,
746
preoperative planning, 742,
743, 744
Meye and Kesselring technique, 740
Pitanguy technique, 741, 742
postoperative care, 746–747
postoperative complications,
747–749
abnormal scarring, 748

Reduction mammoplasty, postoperative complications – *Continued*
hematoma, 746, 748
late shape loss, 749, 750
necrosis, 737, 746–747, 748
recurrent hypertrophy, 749
sensation changes, 748–749
wound dehiscence, 748
Regnault technique, 739–740
result evaluation, 747
aesthetic errors, 749–750
Skoog technique, 741–742
Strömbeck technique, 741
Reese dermatome, 26
Regnault technique for mastopexy, 752
Regnault technique for reduction mammoplasty, 739–740
Relay skin grafts, 29
Replantation, 697–714
amputated part care, 700
blood supply and circulation and, 697, 698
observation and checking, 706, 707, 713
preoperative monitoring, 700–701
bone fixation in, 704, 705, 709, 710
in children, 698–699
contamination and, 698
in digit amputation, 697, 699
vein grafts in, 665, 668
dressings in, 711–712
checking for bleeding, 713
in ear amputation, 303
equipment for, 704–705
extremity growth after, 699
hemostasis in, 703, 704, 713
history of, 697
history taking for, 700
late complications of, 713
lengthy warm ischemia time and, 698
operative technique, 703–711
amputation level and, 709–711
arteries, 705–706, 707
bone, 704, 705, 709, 710
extensor tendons, 704
flexor tendons, 704
microscope introduction, 704–705
nerves, 707
periosteum, 704
positioning for surgery, 705
repair sequence, 704–705
skin closure, 708
tourniquet use, 704
vein grafts, 708–709
veins, 707–708
organization and team, 713–714
in penile amputation, 871
postoperative medications, 712–713
Replantation – *Continued*
preoperative management of arteries, 703, 706
preoperative patient care, 700–701
preoperative preparation of amputated part, 701–703
bone resection, 701, 703
hemostasis, 703
neurovascular preparation, 701–702
skin incisions, 701, 702
tendon exposure, 702
preoperative stump preparation, 703
reexploration, 713
requirements for performing, 682
salvage, 698–699
selection of patients for, 697–799
transport for, 700
Resection and excison
in abdominal dermolipectomy, 838, 839, 840
of abnormal scars, 555
of alveolar tumors, 362
in animal bites, 237
in arm reduction, 849, 850
of bladder mucosa in exstrophy of bladder, 867
of bone, for replantation, 701, 703
in Bowen's disease, 508
of burn wounds, 469, 470, 471–472
electrical burns, 491–492, 493
of carotid body tumors, 401
in chordee, 856
of decorative tattoos, 562, 563
extent in mastectomy, 766–767, 768
in external auditory canal cancer, 502
in eyebrow ptosis, 418
in facial injuries
avulsion, 230–232, 239–240
scars, 238–240
simple lacerations, 229–230
in finger ankylosis
extensor limitation, 599
flexion contracture, 600–601
metacarpophalangeal joint, 602–603
in flexor tendon injury of thumb, 615
in gynecomastia, 803, 804–805, 806
of hand skin, 636
in head and neck cancer, 400, 401, 402
in palliation, 388
of primary lesion, 369
in hidradenitis suppurativa, 546
Resection and excison – *Continued*
in keratoacanthoma, 508
in laryngeal cancer, 399
of lip scars, 345
of lipomas, 644
in lymphedema
staged subcutaneous between flaps, 831, 832–835
total subcutaneous plus skin grafts, 831, 832, 834–835
in malignant melanoma, 512–513, 515, 648
in mastopexy, 755, 756
circumareolar, 752
of nerve tumors, 686, 688
of nevi, 273, 643
in palate cancer, 362
of pressure sores, 819, 820
of radiation injuries, 273, 487–488
in reduction mammoplasty, 739, 740, 741, 742, 744, 745, 746
in rhinophyma, 544–545
in rhinoplasty, 431–432
in rhytidectomy, 413, 414, 415, 416, 417, 148
of salivary gland tumors, 395
parotid glands, 392, 393
submaxillary glands, 394
of sarcomas, 275, 402
of scalp lesions, 274, 275
in skin carcinoma, 499–500, 501–502
basal cell carcinoma, 499, 504, 505
burrowing lesions, 503–504
cytodiagnosis and, 499–500
limits of, 499
squamous cell carcinoma, 499, 506, 507
timing, 500–501
of skin lesions, 3–10. *See also* Excision of skin lesions
of skin in otoplasty, 441–442, 443, 444, 445, 446
in thigh reduction, 843, 844, 846, 847, 848
in thyroid cancer, 397
in tongue cancer, 359
of turban tumors, 274
of xanthomas, 644
Retrognathia
cephalometric analysis in, 162, 163
characteristics, 161, 163
micrognathia vs., 163
in Pierre Robin syndrome, 123, 124
surgical management, 140–141
osteotomy, 164–165
sagittal split of mandible, 170
temperomandibular joint arthritis and, 181–182

Retrognathia – *Continued*
in Treacher Collins syndrome, 140–141
Reverse abdominoplasty in breast reconstruction, 786, 791, 793, 794
Rheumatoid arthritis
of hand, 631–636
athroplasty at metacarpophalangeal joint, 632–634
dermal rhytidectomy, 636
interphalangeal joint reconstruction, 634–635
pathogenesis, 631–632
postoperative care, 636
tendon rupture and wrist deformity, 635–636
thumb reconstruction, 635
temperomandibular joint, 181–182, 185
Rhinophyma, 544–545
Rhinoplasty, 424–433, 434–439
in adolescents, 433
alar base wedge resection in, 431–432
alar cartilage incisions and sculpturing, 424, 426, 427–429, 433
anesthesia in, 424, 427
cartilage grafts in, 434–437, 438
columella management, 427, 431, 432
in elderly, 433
external markings in, 424, 426
implants in, 100, 434, 435
intercartilagenous incisions, 134, 424, 426, 427
nasal bone fractures and osteotomy in, 429–430, 431
nasal bridge (hump) surgery, 429, 430
nasal septum suturing, 431, 432
nasal tip surgery, 424, 426, 427–429, 430
augmentation, 428–429, 433
secondary procedures, 436, 437–438
parrots' beak nose, 120
postoperative packings and dressings, 432
preoperative evaluation and preparation, 424, 425
reduction in, 321
rhytidectomy plus, 433
secondary, 434–439
alloplastic grafts in, 434, 435
cartilage grafts in, 434–437, 438
goals and principles, 434
transfixion incision and sutures in, 427, 431–432
upper lateral cartilage surgery, 430–431
Rhinorrhea, 243, 249
Rhytidectomy, 411–417, 418–419
anesthesia in, 412
chemical face peel plus, 421
complications, 419
dissection in, 413–414
excision of excess skin, 415, 416, 417, 418
forehead lift, 418
identification of excess skin, 414–416
incision planning and techniques, 411, 412, 413
Penrose drain placement, 414, 416, 417
plication and closure, 414–416
postoperative dressings and care, 416–417
preoperative marking, 412–413
preoperative preparation, 411–412
problems in male, 418–419
rhinoplasty plus, 433
suture placement, 414, 415, 416
upper ("temple tuck"), 418
for wrinkled lower lid skin, 404
Ribs, free transfer of, 678, 680. *See also specific topic, e.g.,* Costal cartilages; Split-rib grafts
Riding breeches deformity, 846, 847, 848
Ricketson technique for hypospadias, 857, 858
Rokitansky-Kusher-Hauser syndrome, 783, 876
Romberg's disease (hemifacial atrophy), 103, 127–128, 349
Rotation-advancement flaps. *See also* Advancement flaps; Rotation flaps
in avulsion defects of face, 235
in bilateral cleft lip, 198–203
complete closure, 199–203
forked, 202–203
incomplete closure, 198–199
in fingertip injury, 572
in lip reconstruction, 345
in lower eyelid reconstruction, 281, 282, 283, 284
secondary, after cleft lip closure, 198
in unilateral cleft lip closure, 194–197
complete closure, 195–196
incomplete closure, 196–197
Rotation flaps
in avulsion of scalp, 267, 268
in breast reconstruction, 786, 791, 792
described, 48
dog ears at pivot point of, 48–49
donor site closure, 48
in eyelid reconstruction, 281, 282, 283, 284, 286, 287, 288, 289
Rotation flaps – *Continued*
in forehead defects, 272
in lip reconstruction, 346
in multiple excision of skin lesions, 6
in nasal reconstruction, 325, 326, 327
planning, 46, 47, 49, 50
in pressure sore closure, 820, 821, 822
in radical neck dissection, 368–369, 383, 384
tension on, 47, 48, 49
Z-plasty and, 65–66
Rule of nines in burn area estimation, 456

Sabattini-Stein-Estlander-Abee flap in cleft lip, 198
Sacral ulcers, closures of, 820, 822
Saddle nose, 100
Saline wheal test of circulation, 45
Salivary gland tumors, 361
parotid glands, 391–393
sublingual and accessory glands, 395, 396
submaxillary glands, 393–395
Salpingo-oophorectomy in female-to-male surgery, 892, 894
Saphenous nerve as graft donor, 695
Sarcoidosis, 542
Sarcoma(s), 275
head and neck, 401
Kaposi's, 532, 543, 828
neurogenic of jaw, 361
osteogenic, 360, 361, 362, 401, 402, 648. *See also* Osteogenic sarcoma(s)
scalp, 274, 275
Satyr ears, 448
Scalp
anatomy and embryology, 265, 266
avulsion, 267, 268
burns, 272–273, 493
cirsoid aneurysms of, 274
concealing scars in, 4
congenital defects of, 266
contusions, 267
dissecting cellulitis of, 547
flap use on, 272
for avulsion, 267, 268
in baldness, 276–277
in lesions, 266
flaps from
in alopecia, 276–277, 545–546
for dural defects, 493
free flaps, 676, 677
hair from
in alopecia, 275–277, 545–546
in eyebrow reconstruction, 292, 293

Scalp, hair from – *Continued*
in eyelash provision, 119
incisions
in rhytidectomy, 414
for zygomatic fracture fixation, 250–251
lacerations, 266, 267
lesions
benign tumors, 273–274
bone defects and, 266
malignant tumors, 274–275
multiple excision of, 6–7
pilar cysts, 274, 536
ulcers, 266
radiation injury, 273
skin grafts for, 266, 267, 268, 272
skull defect repair in loss of, 269–272
split-thickness skin grafts from, 20
Scar(s). *See also specific topic, e.g.,* Facial scars
after augmentation mammoplasty, 723, 724
burn
contracture of, 64, 65
enzymatic debridement of, 472
necrotic tissue removal, 471–472
tangential excision of, 472
circular, 64
concealing, 3, 4, 5
contracture
in burns, 64, 65
Y-V advancement flap for, 53–54
Z-plasty for, 62, 64, 65, 66
in excision of skin lesions, 3–5
dermabrasion for, 419
in flexion creases, 64
after hand nerve injury repair, 624, 625
hypertrophic, 552–558. *See also* Hypertrophic scars; Keloids
race and abnormal scarring, 555
after reduction mammoplasty, 739, 740
abnormal, 748
inverted-T pattern, 739, 740–741
revision, 238–239, 240
altering polarity, 239, 240
V-Y plasty for, 238, 239, 240
W-plasty for, 65, 238, 239, 240
Z-plasty for, 62, 64, 65, 66, 238, 239, 240
study before rhytidectomy, 411–412
skin tapes and, 15
suture, 11–12
Scar(s), suture – *Continued*
eversion of skin edges and, 12
overgrafting, 19
unstable, 306
U-shaped
concealing, 5
Z-plasty for, 64, 65, 266
wound healing and normal, 553
Z-plasty in, 62, 64, 65, 66, 238, 239, 240
changing direction, 65
on face, 238, 239, 240, 266
flexion crease scars, 64
lengthening scar contracture, 62, 64, 65, 66
planning and, 63
size and, 60, 62
U-shaped scars, 266
Schwannomas, 538, 645, 686, 688
Scleroderma, 537–538
Sclerosing hemangiomas, 536–537
Scrotal hypospadias repair, 861–862, 863
Scrotum
avulsion of, 871–872
cleft, in hypospadias, 861–862, 863
construction in female-to-male surgery, 894
flaps from
for avulsion injuries of penis, 870
in hypospadias repair, 862
in neovagina construction, 887–888, 889
penetrating wounds of, 871
Sebaceous adenomas, 535
Sebaceous carcinoma, 535
Sebaceous cysts
hand, 642
scalp, 274
skin, 535–536
Sebaceous epitheliomas, 535
Sebaceous hyperplasia, 535
Sebaceous secretion
in skin flaps, 57
in skin grafts, 34
Sebaceous tumors, 535
Seborrheic keratosis, 532, 643
Segmental arteries, 37–38
Semicircular incision for gynecomastia, 803
Semicircular technique for thigh reduction, 843–844, 845
operative technique, 843–844
preoperative planning, 843, 844, 845
Senile keratoses, 532, 643
Senile sebaceous hyperplasia, 535
Sensation
burns and, 458
importance in feet, 811
Sensation – *Continued*
inadequate after replantation, 713
loss
after augmentation mammoplasty, 721, 723, 726–727
after reduction mammoplasty, 748–749
in skin flaps, 42, 57
in skin grafts, 34–35
Seroma(s)
encapsulated of scalp, 267
removal, in skin graft recipient bed, 22, 31
Sex
of assignment and rearing in intersex, 877
defined, 884
gender dysphoria, 883–895. *See also* Gender dysphoria
misdiagnosis before hypospadias repair, 862, 864
Sex change surgery. *See* Gender dysphoria
Sex chromosomes
in gender dysphoria, 884
genital sex development and, 873
in testicular feminization syndrome, 876
in Turner's syndrome, 877
Shell ears, 448
Shock
in burns, 453, 454, 477–478
electrical burns, 490
hypovolemia and, 463
in facial injury, 227
Short face syndrome, 173
Sickle flap in facial reconstruction, 51
Silabrasion in decorative tattoo removal, 563–565
Silastic implants
in chin augmentation, 433
for hand
joints, 636
tendons, 615
in velopharyngeal incompetence, 104–105
Silicone(s)
adhesives, 98
in augmentation mammoplasty, 105, 751. *See also* Breast implants and prostheses
chemical composition, 720
evaluation, 725
fluids, 103
gels, 725
history of, 719–720
implant fixation, 725
injectables, 719, 720
types and manufacturers, 724–725, 731–736
available forms of medical grade, 97–98, 731–736

Silicone(s) – *Continued*
for chin, 100–101
clinical advantages of implants, 98–99
family, described, 96, 97
fluids, 95–96, 98
advantages, 103
approval for clinical injection, 103
for breast, 103
for facial deformities, 103, 104
tissue response to, 104
technique for using, 103–104
handling, 99
inflatable subcutaneous bag, 56
rubber, 97–98, 99
handling, 99
in nasal reconstruction, 100
tube in esophageal reconstruction, 105
in velopharyngeal incompetence, 104–105, 221
toxicity and carcinogenicity of, 99, 102
Silk sutures, 10, 11, 14
Simons-Barraquer syndrome, 846, 847
Simple elliptical excision of skin lesions, 5–6
Simple interrupted sutures, 13–14
Simplex lymphangioma, 518, 523
Single pedicle advancement flap, described, 52, 53
Sistrunk's technique for thyroglossal duct cysts and fistulas, 127
Six-flap Z-plasty, 62
Skeletal tumors, 155–156
Skewer sutures in nerve repair, 628–629
Skin. *See also specific topic, e.g.,* Hypertrophic scars; Necrosis; Skin Carcinoma
abdominal dermochalasis, 838
dermolipectomy for, 839, 840, 841, 842
aging, 410–411
antigenic differences in, 85
benign lesions, 530–538. *See also specific topic, e.g.,* Nevus (nevi)
blood supply of, 36, 37–38
chemical peeling (chemosurgery), 418, 421–422
closure in replantation, 708
decubitus ulcers, 18, 41, 58, 818–824. *See also* Pressure sores
dermabrasion, 419–421
excision. *See also* Resection and excision
in amputated part for replantation, 701, 702
Skin, excision – *Continued*
of excess hand skin, 636
in gynecomastia, 806
in lymphedema, 831, 832–835
excision of lesions, 3–10. *See also* Excision of skin lesions
infections, 546–549
lines, 3–4
loss on lower extremity
traumatic, 812
vascular disease and, 811
massive replacement in skin cancer, 502–503
physical properties
scarring related to, 5, 555
skin flap limitations and, 325
radiation injury, 485–488
sloughs after rhytidectomy, 419
temperature as blood flow indicator, 713
thickness, 16
wound closure, 10–16. *See also* wound closure
Skin carcinoma, 497–498
assessment of, 498–499
basal cell, 504–506
clinical types, 504–505
limits of excision, 499
multiple, congenital anomalies and, 505–506
recurrence, 505
site and incidence, 504
terebrating, 503–504
treatment, 504, 505
contraindications to immediate therapy, 500
cytotoxic therapy, 497, 498
diagnosis, 498
metastases, 497, 499, 506
Mohs' chemosurgery, 497, 498
multiple, 503–504
planning surgery, 503–504
technique of massive skin replacement, 502–503
pathogenesis, 484
prognosis, 497
psychological factors and, 501
radiation injury and, 486, 488
radiotherapy, 497
recurrence, 499, 507
ressection and excision in, 499–500, 501–502
basal cell carcinoma, 499, 504, 505
cytodiagnosis and adequacy of, 499–500
limits of, 499
squamous cell carcinoma, 499, 506, 507
squamous cell, 506–507
clinical signs, 506
treatment, 499, 506–507
Skin carcinoma – *Continued*
susceptibility to, dermabrasion and, 498
treatment aims, 497
Skin clips in wound closure, 15
Skin flaps, 36–57. *See also specific flap or topic, e.g.,* Chest wall, flaps from; Composite flaps; Delayed skin flaps; Radical neck dissection, skin flaps in
adjacent skin expansion by silicone bag, 56
arterialized, advantages of, 35, 36. *See also* Axial pattern flaps
blood supply and flow
area of body related to, 42
classification of flap by, 38–41, 46, 48
design of flap and, 42
maintaining, 45–46
tests of, 44–45
bulkiness of, 57
classification
by blood supply, 38–41, 46, 48
by position transferred to, 48–57
color and texture of, 34, 57
Crane principle and, 56–57
defined, 36
delayed, 36, 38, 42–45. *See also* Delayed skin flaps
distant, 54–56. *See also* Distant flaps
division timing, 36, 44
donor sites. *See* Donor sites, skin flaps, closure of
durability of, 57
free, 675–678, 812. *See also* Free flaps
growth of, 35, 57
hair growth and sebaceous secretion, 57
hematomas in, 37–45
indications for, 41–42
infection of, 37, 45–46
kinking of, 37, 45, 46
local, 48–54. *See also* Local flaps
necrosis, 45, 46, 305
prevention in radical neck dissection, 369–370
for open cavity wounds, 41
operating through, on underlying structure, 41–42
as padding over bony prominences, 41
planning and design, 36, 46, 47, 49
bipedicle vs. single pedicle, 36
blood supply and, 36, 37–38, 42
pattern cutting, 46, 47
rotation about pivot point, 50
safe dimensions, 36
size and location, 42
pressure and, 37, 45

Skin flaps – *Continued*
principles of use, 36
in sensation restoration, 42
sensation and sweating in, 57
skin, physical properties and, 25
subcutaneous tissue carried by, 56–57
survival of
bipedicle vs. single pedicle, 42
blood supply and, 36, 37–38, 42
delay and, 44
patient age and, 36, 42
viability tests, 44–45
surviving length, 36, 42
tension and, 37, 45, 46, 47, 48, 49
thinning, 57
transfer
delayed flaps, 44
distant, 39, 56
indirect, 56
outlining, 46
Z-plasty in tissue rotation in, 65–66
Skin grafts, 16–35. *See also specific topic, e.g.,* Bone, exposed, covering, skin grafts in; Full-thickness skin grafts; Radical neck dissection, skin grafts in; Split-thickness skin grafts
accessory skin structures in, 34
allografts, 75–85, 86
attachment to skin flap margin, 29, 48
basic application technique, 28
on bare bone, 41, 267, 269, 812
blood supply
clinical vascularization, 86
comparative vascularity, 22
survival and, 21–23, 86
vascularization stages, 22–23
bridging phenomenon and, 21
classification, 16–17
in closing deep structures, 19
color of, 34, 86
preventing hyperpigmentation, 34
contraction of
area related to, 31–32
growth and, 35
contracture of
prevention, 18, 31–32, 34
primary vs. secondary, 33–34
sutures and, 32
cutting, 24–28
dermatomes for, 24, 25, 26–27, 86
knives for, 24–26, 28
patterns, 26, 27–28
razors for, 26
thickness control, 24, 27
defined, 16

Skin grafts – *Continued*
dressings for, 10, 23, 28, 29, 30, 31
for immobilization, 23, 31–32, 34
before tourniquet release, 28
durability of, 35
epithelial inlay (stent), 30
fixation of, 16, 29–30
on flexor surfaces, 18
grafting to infected wounds, 24
granulation tissue formation and, 21, 22
growth of, 35
handling for drainage through, 29
hematoma development beneath, 22, 23, 31, 87
hemostasis for, 10, 23, 28
indications for use of, 17–19
infection management, 31
mesh expansion of, 29
in burns, 473
in muscle transposition, 816
in ulcer coverage, 811
muscle flaps plus, 57–58
survival of, 35
omental flaps plus, 35, 58
open technique for, 31
overgrafting
in burns, 272–273
of nevi, 19
in radiation injury, 273
pericranial flap as base for, 57
permanent vs. temporary, 17
postage-stamp-sized, 29, 31
postoperative inspection of, 23, 30
recipient bed
adherence to, 31
arteriosclerotic vasculature as, 22
bacterial growth, 24
contact between, 21, 23–24
hematoma, 22, 23, 31, 87
hemostasis, 10, 23, 28
infected, 29
open wound preparation and evaluation, 23–24
survival and, 16–17, 86
vascularity of, 21–22
relay grafts, 29
sensation in, 34–35
stability and secondary procedures, 41
storage of, 28, 32, 85
survival, 35
hyperbaric oxygen and, 31
recipient bed and, 16–17, 86
tension and, 23
thickness and, 16–17
vascularity and, 21–23, 86
suturing, 29, 32
tension
growth and, 35

Skin grafts, tension – *Continued*
survival and, 23
thickness, 17, 86
control in cutting, 24, 27
tissue culture of, 17
translucency of, 16
Skin lines, 3–4
Skin staples, 15
Skin tapes
in skin graft fixation, 29–30
in wound closure, 14–15
Skoog technique for bilateral cleft lip and nasal repair, 201
Skull. *See also* Calvaria (Calvarium); Forehead; Scalp
bare, management in burns, 493
carcinoma metastases to, 273
congenital deformity of, 120
contour restoration
after cranioplasty, 270
implants and prostheses for, 102
coronal synostosis, 154–155
craniofacial surgery, 131–158. *See also* Craniofacial surgery
defects
alloplastic materials for, 269
bone grafts for, 269–272
decortication in, 267, 269
open wound repair, 41, 267, 269, 272
skin flaps for, 41, 272
skin grafts for, 267, 269, 463
soft tissue closure, 272
fractures
frontonasoethmoid region, 256–260
primary treatment, 267, 269
surgical exposure of, 133. *See also* Craniofacial surgery; Cranioplasty
Smooth muscle tumors, 535
Soft palate closure
intraalveolar veloplasty plus palate lengthening in, 214, 215–217
nasal mucosa management, 215, 216
prostheses in, 211, 222
speech in prosthetic vs. surgical, 211
timing, 211
velopharyngeal competency achievement, 214. *See also* Velopharyngeal incompetence
Soleus muscle transposition for tibial defects, 814–815
Speech
in cleft palate, 207
as consideration in repair, 207, 217
production of normal, 207
soft palate movement and, 205, 207
testing, 207
training after male-to-female surgery, 891

Speech – *Continued*
velopharyngeal incompetence correction and, 222
Spermatic cords
burying in thigh subcutaneous pocket, 871–872
ligation in male-to-female surgery, 887
Spine, pressure sore closure over, 823
Spira technique for modified total mastectomy, 772, 773
Spiradenomas, 534
Split-level eyelid resection in ptosis, 294, 295, 296–297, 298
Split-rib grafts, 87, 88, 134
autogenous, 88
in congenital facial asymmetry, 156, 157, 158
in cranioplasty, 269–270
Le Fort III maxillary advancement plus forehead, 146–147
in mandible augmentation, 118, 166
in maxillary retrusion and collapse, 173, 174
in nasal reconstruction, 322
onlay, in maxillary hypoplasia, 173
in periorbital correction, 139–140
technique of taking, 134, 270–271
in zygoma hypoplasia, 134, 139
Splinting. *See* Immobilization
Split-thickness skin grafts
areola, in nipple-areolar construction, 791
in avulsion injuries
penile, 869–870
perineal, 871
scalp, 267, 268
scrotal skin, 871
skin of leg, 812
burn wound closure, 18, 492, 493
contraction of, 31, 33
in covering donor sites of grafts or flaps, 17, 18, 28, 33, 48, 86, 273
cutting, 24–27
defined, 16
dermal grafts from, 86
donor site bleeding, 21
dressing, 33
durability of, 17–18
in dural defects, 493
after excision in hidradenitis suppurativa, 546
to feet, 812
in fingertip injury, 571–572, 573
in forehead defects, 272
meshed, 811, 816
in mucosa replacement, 18
in muscle flap covering, 58
Split-thickness skin grafts – *Continued*
muscle transposition plus, plan for, 813, 816
in nasal reconstruction, 323–324
in neovagina construction, 888, 889
omentum plus
in breast reconstruction, 787, 791
in radiation necrosis, 787, 791
in omphalocele, 19
overgrafting
in forehead burns, 272–273
graft donor sites, 19
in phalloplasty, 894
in pressure sore closure, 41, 822, 824
in resurfacing radiation injuries, 273, 487, 488
in skull defects, 269, 493
survival of, 16–17, 86
taking in supraclavicular region, 20
temporary application of, 17
thickness in classification of, 16–17
types, 16–17
in vaginal agenesis, 878–879
vascularity of, 22
Squamous cell carcinoma, 507–508, 532–533
congenital branchial cleft cysts and, 401
external ear, 502
floor of mouth, 363
hand, 647
immune mechanism and, 507
lip, 507
lymph node dissection in, 506–507
metastatic neck, 401
scalp, 274, 275
skin, 506–507
clinical signs, 506
radiation in etiology of, 486, 488
treatment, 499, 506–507
Stainless steel
implants, 95
sutures, 10, 11
Staggering in altering scar polarity, 239, 240
Staples in wound closure, 15
Steatocystoma multiplex, 536
Stein technique for lip reconstruction, 346
Stensen's duct injury, 236
Stent in McIndoe technique for vaginal agenesis, 878, 879
Sternal area scars, 4, 12
Steroid therapy. *See* Corticosteroid therapy
Straight line closure of cleft lip, 193, 198
Strangulation injuries of penis, 869
Strawberry hemangiomas, 273, 519–520
Strip grafts in alopecia, 276, 545–546
Strömbeck technique for reduction mammoplasty, 741
Sturge-Weber syndrome, 518–519
Stryker dermabrasion instrument, 420
Stryker dermatome, 27
Subcranial hypertelorism, 148, 149
Subcranial orbital osteotomy, 135
Subcutaneous flaps in nasal reconstruction, 326, 329
Subcutaneous pseudosarcomatous fibromatosis, 537
Subcutaneous tissue
dissection in rhytidectomy, 413
excision in lymphedema, 831, 832–835
staged between flaps, 831, 832–835
total, skin grafts plus, 831, 832, 834–835
infections, 579
pocket for spermatic cord and testes in, 871–872
skin flaps carrying, 56–57
Subcuticular (intradermal) continuous sutures, 13, 14
Sublingual gland tumors, 395, 396
Subluxation of temperomandibular joint, 182, 185, 186, 262
Subluxation-flexion deformity of hand, 632, 635
Submaxillary gland tumors, 393–395
diagnosis, 394
pathology, 393–394, 396
treatment, 395
Submental lipectomy, 417
Submucosal cleft palate, 209
Subpectoral dissection
breast prosthesis insertion and, 767, 776–778, 785–786, 797
in breast reconstruction, 785–786, 787
in mastectomy, 767
Supraclavicular skin grafts, 19–20
Supraomohyoid neck dissection, 383–385
indications, 383–384, 385, 386
technique, 384–385
Sural nerve as donor site, 694
Surgical shaving in rhinophyma, 544, 545
Sutures and suturing, 10–14
in abdominal dermolipectomy, 838–839, 841, 842
absorbable sutures, 10, 11
avoiding suture marks in skin, 11–12

Sutures and suturing – *Continued*
in boutonnière deformity, 605, 606
buried sutures, 12
continuous sutures, 13–14
of distal sites of nerve grafts, 695
in ear reconstruction, 233
eversion of skin edges in, 12
in eyelid repair, 281, 282, 405, 406, 408
in facial wounds, 230
of hand tendons
in arthroplasty of metacarpophalangeal joint, 634
in extensor tendon injury, 606, 607
figure-of-eight sutures, 607
in flexor tendon grafts, 613, 614
in flexor tendon injuries, 608, 614, 615
in primary repair, 608
keloid formation and, 12
knot tying, 14
in microvascular surgery, 655–656
in ligating blood vessels, 9
in lip injuries, 237
in mallet finger, 604, 605
mattress sutures, 12, 13, 14
in microvascular surgery, 653, 661, 662, 663, 668, 685. *See also* peripheral nerves
basic technique, practice in, 655–657, 658
knot tying, 655–656
of veins in replantation, 708
monofilament vs. multiple filament sutures, 10, 11, 12
in mouth wounds, 237
of nasal septum in rhinoplasty, 431, 432
nonabsorbable sutures, 10, 11
operative technique of suturing, 12–14
peripheral nerves, 618, 619, 626, 627, 628–629
end-to-end repair, 690–693
epineural, 618, 619, 627, 628, 690, 691, 692, 707
fascicular, 618, 619, 627, 628–629, 707
guide, 690, 692
intrafascicular, 690, 692
perineural, 690, 693
skewer, 628–629
wrapping suture sites, 693
in penile amputation, 870–871
placement in rhytidectomy, 414, 415, 416
scars from, 11, 12
simple interrupted sutures, 13–14
in skin closure, 12, 13–14
of skin flap donor sites, 49

Sutures and suturing – *Continued*
of skin grafts, 29, 32
tension of, scarring and, 11
of veins in replantation, 708
of wound edges, 11, 12
Swan neck deformity in rheumatoid arthritis, 631, 632, 633, 634
Sweat gland carcinomas, 275
Sweating
excessive, 546
in skin flaps, 57
in skin grafts, 34
Syndactylism, division in, 20
Synostosis, coronal, 154–155. *See also* Apert's syndrome; Crouzon's syndrome
Synovectomy in hand rheumatoid arthritis, 632, 633, 634, 635
Syphilis, 357, 358
Syringocystadenoma papilliferum, 535
Syringomas, 534
Systemic lupus erythematosus, 539
Systemic scleroderma, 539

T excision
in abdominal obesity, 839, 840
of skin lesions, 7–8
Tangential excision of burn wounds, 472
Tanzer technique for total ear reconstruction, 300, 301, 302, 303
Tapes
in skin graft fixation, 29–30
in wound closure, 14–15
Tarsorrhaphy in eyelid suspension, 338, 339–340
Tarsus flaps in eyelid reconstruction, 285, 288
Tattoos, adventitious (traumatic)
defined, 227, 559
on face, 227, 229
treatment, 229, 559–560
dermabrasion, 419
overgrafting, 19
types, 559
Tattoos, decorative
chemical agents to remove, 563, 565
choice of technique of removing, 562
defined, 560–562
dermabrasion or silabrasion for, 563–565
electrical devices in removing, 563, 565
overtattooing, 562, 563, 565
surgical excision of, 562, 563
Tattoos, medical, 560
for areolar formation, 560, 792

Tattoos, medical – *Continued*
in lip scars, 345
Teeth. *See also* Malocclusion; Orthodontia
in alveolar and prepalatal cleft repair, 211–212
care in cleft palate, 222
dentition and terminology, 244
extraction in maxillary overdevelopment, 174
in facial fractures, 242, 244–245
arch bars and wire suspension in maxillary, 249, 267
in fracture line, 244–245
intermaxillary fixation of, 245–246
wiring in occlusion in mandibular, 247–248
preprosthetic surgery, 178, 179
terms for positonal relations, 180
Teflon implants
for chin, 100
described, 95, 96
in velopharyngeal incompetence, 105
Telecanthus, 122
"Temple tuck," 418
Temporal bone
fractures, nerve injuries with, 267
in hemifacial microsomia, 117
Temporalis muscle
anatomy, 336
flaps, use of, 58, 349
transfers in facial palsy, 338, 340, 342
Temperomandibular joint, 179–188
anatomy, 179–180
ankylosis, 182, 183, 186–187
apertognathia and, 182
basic movements of, 180
clinical evaluation of, 180–181
dislocation, 182, 183, 260, 262
management, 185, 186
infections, 182
nonoperative management of disorders, 182–183
osteoarthritis, 181, 185
pain, 180, 181, 182
rheumatoid arthritis, 181–182, 185
subluxation, 182
management, 185, 186, 262
surgical management of disorders, 183–188
anesthesia and intubation in, 183–184
ankylosis, 187–188
arthroplasty, 185, 187, 188
condylectomy, 185, 187
in hypermobility, 185–186
incisions in, 184–185
menisectomy, 185, 186
osteoarthrotomy, 187, 188
postoperative care, 188

Temperomandibular joint
– *Continued*
terms for positional relations, 180
tumors, 182
Temperomandibular joint syndrome, 181, 182–183
Tendon(s)
adhesions, 713
grafts
in adhesions, 713
in boutonnière deformity, 634–635
in flexor tendon injuries, 610, 611–614
palmaris longus use in, 612
hand, injuries of, 604–615. *See also* Hand tendon injuries
prosthetic replacement, 107, 615
in hand, 615
in replantation, 577
amputated part, 702
repair technique, 704
stump, 703
skin flaps for bare, 41, 56–57
skin grafts for, 17, 22
bridging phenomenon and, 21
suturing hand
in arthroplasty of metacarpophalangeal joint, 634
in extensor tendon injuries, 606, 607
figure-of-eight sutures, 607
flexor tendon grafts, 613, 614, 615
flexor tendon injuries, 608, 614, 615
primary repair, 608
on wrist, 615
transfer, in wrist deformity, 636
Tennison-Randall technique for cleft lip closure, 194
Tenosynovitis in hand, 631, 643–644
Tenotomy
in extensor limitation of fingers, 599
in metacarpophalangeal joint ankylosis, 602
Tension
free tissue transfer and, 554–555
in hypertrophic scar etiology, 554–555
on nerve grafts, 693–694
on skin flaps, 37, 45, 46, 49
rotation flaps, 47, 48, 49
on skin grafts
growth and, 35
survival and, 23
of sutures, scarring and, 11
Terebrating (boring) basal cell carcinoma of skin, 503–504
Tessier technique for periorbital correction, 139–140
Testes
burying in subcutaneous pocket in thigh, 871–872
embryologic development of normal, 873, 874
injuries, 871
prostheses for, 106, 894
Testicular feminization syndrome (androgen insensitivity syndrome), 876–877, 878
Tetanus prophylaxis
in burns, 460, 467, 476, 491
in facial injuries, 238
in penile avulsion injuries, 869
in puncture wounds, 229, 238
Textile implants, described, 95–96
Thenar flaps in fingertip injuries, 575
Thermacouple test of circulation, 45
Thermal burns. *See* Burn(s)
Thermography test of circulation, 45
Thigh
burying testes and spermatic cord in, 871–872
indirect flaps from, 56
as skin graft donor site, 21
graft cutting, 25, 26
in neovagina construction, 888, 889
Thigh reduction, 838, 843–849
circular, 844, 845, 846
combined circular and vertical, 846, 847
complications, 848–849
patient selection for, 843
in secondary deformities, 848
semicircular, 843–844, 845
operative technique, 843–844
preoperative planning, 843, 844, 845
trochanteric defatting, 846, 847, 848
vertical, 846, 847
Thoracic duct
embryologic development of, 826
radical neck dissection and, 375
Thoracic nerve palsy, 798
Thoracodorsal axillary flap for scalp defects, 272
Thoracoepigastric flaps
in breast reconstruction, 786 787, 788–789
described, 56
Three-point-sutures, 29
Thrombosis
free flaps and, 676
lymphedema and, 829
pressure sores and, 818
Thumb
amputation
functional loss and, 576
reconstruction from index finger, 42
replantation, 699
bone loss and injury, 572, 573–574
degloving management, 573–574
innervation, 621
joint injuries, 594–597
interphalangeal joints, 595
metacarpophalangeal joints, 595–596
joint stabilization, 635
metacarpal fractures and, 587
prostheses for, 635
reconstruction
from index finger, 42
in rheumatoid arthritis, 635
skin flaps in sensation restoration, 42
tendon injuries, 614–615
Z-plasty for contracted web, 635
Thyroglossal duct cysts and fistulas, 126–127
Thyroid cancer, 395–398
diagnosis, 397
metastatic spread, 396–397
postoperative management, 398
treatment and prognosis, 397–398
Tibial defects
flaps for, 41, 56
disadvantages of cross leg flaps, 812
muscle transposition plus, 813–815
osteocutaneous free groin flaps, 673, 674
skin grafts for, 41
Tie-over dressings for skin grafts, 23, 29, 30
Tissue culture of skin grafts, 17
Tissue transplantation, 75–90
allografts, 75–85. *See also* Allograft(s)
autografts, 85–90
classification in, 75
free tissue transfer, 75, 668, 671–675. *See also* Free tissue transfer
Tissue typing, 82–83
Toe(s)
isolation of donor toe for transfer, 680
toe-to-hand free tissue transfer, 671, 672, 680–681
Toksu technique for hypospadias repair, 858
Tongue. *See also* Glossectomy
atrophy of ipsilateral side, 127
benign changes in, 355–356

Tongue – *Continued*
cancer, 354–355, 357–360
classification and staging, 354–355
diagnosis, 357–358
mandible resection in, 386
metastases, 355, 359
prognosis, 358, 359–360
treatment, 358–359, 386
congenital fissured, 356
flaps from, in vermillion reconstruction, 348
geographic, 356
glossitis rhomboidica medians, 356
glossoptosis, 123
hairy, 355, 356
leukoplakia, 356, 357, 358
mucoceles, 356
syphilitic chancre of, 357, 358
tumors, 354–366. *See also* Tongue, cancer
benign not requiring excision, 356
benign requiring excision, 356–357
ulcers, 356, 357, 358
underdevelopment of, 117
Tongue-to-lip adhesion in Pierre Robin syndrome, 124–125
Tracheotomy
in burns, 462, 475, 477
in cystic hygroma, 523
in facial fractures, 243, 260, 262
indications for, 243
in Pierre Robin syndrome, 125
postoperative, in head and neck cancer, 368
preoperative, in radical neck dissection, 369
superior vs. inferior, 243, 244
Tragus construction, 305, 306
Transaxillary technique for augmentation mammoplasty, 721, 722, 724, 725
Transfusion
in burns, indications and precautions, 463, 464–465
hepatitis and, 464–465
in replantation, 700
Transplantation antigens, 76, 77
Transposition flaps
in avulsion defects of face, 235
in cheek reconstruction, 52, 348, 349
described, 49
donor site closure, 49, 50
examples, 49–51, 52
in fingertip injury, 573, 574, 575
planning, 46, 49, 50
thickness of, 51
in wound closure, 8
Transsexualism. *See also* Gender dysphoria
classic, described, 883–884
gender identity in, 885
use of term, 883
Transverse flaps in breast reconstruction, 786, 787, 788–789, 796
Transvestitism, 884
Trauma. *See specific topic, e.g.,* Facial fractures; Facial soft tissue injury
Traumatic (adventitious) tattooing
defined, 227, 559
on face, 227, 229
treatment, 229, 559–560
dermabrasion in, 419
overgrafting in, 19
types of, 559
Treacher Collins syndrome
etiology, 119
physical signs, 118–119, 138–139
mandibular deformity, 118, 140–141, 163
retrognathia, 140–141
surgical management, 119
complications, 141–142
mandibular deformity and retrognathia, 140–141
Tessier technique for periorbital correction, 139–140
zygoma hypoplasia, 139
Triamcinolone therapy for hypertrophic scars on keloids, 556–557, 806–807, 842–843, 849, 850
Triangular flaps
in distal shaft hypospadias, 859, 860
in unilateral cleft lip closure, 194
Triangular wedge excision in lip reconstruction, 345, 346
Trichilemmal cysts, 536
Trichoepitheliomas, 533–534
Trichofolliculomas, 533
Tricholemmoma, 534
Trifluoroisopropyl as wound adhesive, 15–16
"Trigger finger," 631
Tripartite osteotomy, 143, 144
Trochanter
fat pad correction, 846, 847, 848
pressure sore management, 820, 822–823
True aneurysms on hand, 645–646
True myxomas, 537
True hermaphroditism, 877
Trunk
flaps for wounds of, 41, 58
prosthetic implants for, 106
skin flaps from
direct flaps, 54, 55
Trunk, skin flaps from – *Continued*
indirect flaps, 56
pedicled flaps, 57
skin grafts from, 26
suture scars on, 12
Tubed flaps
arterial, from abdomen, 56
for avulsion defects of face, 235
bipedicle, from thigh, 56
in breast reconstruction, 786
from other breast, 787, 791, 796
in phalloplasty, 892, 893, 894
Tuberculosis, cutaneous, 548
Tuberculosis verrucosa cutis, 549
Tuberous sclerosis complex, 537
Tumbling in flap migration, 56
Tumors. *See specific topic, e.g.,* Condyloma acuminata; Jaw(s), tumors
Turban tumors (cylindromas), 274, 534–535
Turner's syndrome, 877
Turnover flaps in radical neck dissection, 383, 384
Tylosis, 532

Ulcer(s)
decubitus, 18, 41, 58, 818–824. *See also* Pressure sores
leg, 30, 32, 811, 812
radiation and, 485–486, 487
scalp, 266
tongue, 356, 357, 358
Ulnar nerve
injury in tendon laceration, 615
muscles innervated by, 620–622
as nerve graft donor, 695
palsy
in leprosy, 548
test for, 620
Upper extremities. *See* Arms; Finger(s); Hand; Thumb
Umbilicus, abdominal dermolipectomy and, 838, 839, 841, 843
Ureters, embryologic development of, 873
Urethra. *See also* Urethroplasty
conversion of female to male, 892, 893, 894, 895
hypospadias repair and, 865
injuries of male, 872
management in epispadias repair, 865–866
neovagina creation and, 887
rupture of, 872
strictures
dilatation of, 865, 872
hypospadias repair and, 864, 865
trauma and, 872
Urethroplasty
in hypospadias repair, 856, 857, 858
flaps in, 859, 860

Urethroplasty, in hypospadias repair – *Continued*
perineal or scrotal hypospadias, 862, 863
proximal shaft hypospadias, 861, 862
silicone rubber tube use in, 106
Urethrocutaneous fistulas, 865
Urethrovaginal fistulas, 890
Urinary diversion
in exstrophy of bladder, 867
in hypospadias, 862, 864
Urine
incontinence
in epispadias, 865, 866
in exstrophy of bladder, 867
output in burns, 465–466, 476
Uterus, embryologic development of, 873
U-shaped scars
on face, 238, 239–240
forehead, 266
Z-plasty for, 64, 65, 266
Uvula, bifid, 209

Vagina. *See also* Vaginal agenesis
congenital absence of, 873, 876, 878
construction of. *See also* Neocolporrhapy; Vaginal agenesis, treatment
bowel for, 880–881
in male-to-female surgery, 886–891
embryologic development of, 873
flap from, in phalloplasty, 895
stenosis of neovagina, 888
in testicular feminization syndrome, 877
Vaginal agenesis, 873–881
diagnosis, 878
differential diagnosis, 273, 876–878
iatrogenic causes, 878
psychological factors and, 873
treatment
inlay split-thickness skin grafting, 878–879
nonoperative method of Frank, 880
Williams vulovaginoplasty, 880, 881
Vagus in radical neck dissection, 375, 378, 379, 380, 381, 382
"Valise handle" technique for auricle reconstruction, 305–306, 310, 316
Vallis strip grafts in baldness, 276
Vascular gigantism, 524–525
Vasculature. *See* Arteries; Blood vessels; Circulation and blood supply; Vein(s)
Vasculitis
leg ulceration and, 811
Vasculitis – *Continued*
necrotizing, 542
skin lesions and, 541–542
Vasodilation, delayed flaps and, 42, 43
Vein(s). *See also* Blood vessels; Vein grafts
failure after free tissue transfer, 673, 675
lymph node anastomoses in lymphedema, 830, 831
microvascular anastomoses
end-to-end, 663, 664, 665
luminal diameter differences and, 665, 666
in replantation, 707–708
adventitia removal, 708
checking postoperative circulation, 703
localization, 707–708
suturing, 708
stasis, ulceration and, 811
thrombosis, lymphedema and, 827
venography, 829
Vein grafts
in replantation, 708–709
anastomoses, 709
donor sites, 708–709
harvesting and size of, 709
use in microvascular surgery, 665, 668, 669–670
Velopharyngeal closure, defined, 205, 206. *See also* Velopharyngeal incompetence
Velopharyngeal incompetence
in absence of cleft palate, 219
in cleft palate, 218, 219–222
diagnosis, 218
implants in management, 104–105, 221
palatal lengthening in, 221
posterior pharyngeal augmentation in, 221–222
posterior pharyngeal flaps in, 219–221
postoperative care, 222
soft palate closure and, 214
speech and, 207, 222
Veloplasty in soft palate closure, 214, 215–217
Vermillion, 344
classification of defects, 348
realignment after wedge excision, 7
reconstruction, 348
secondary correction in cleft lip closure, 197
Vermillion bordered (Abbe) lip flap, 7, 345–346, 348
division, 44
in lip reconstruction, 348
in secondary correction of cleft lip, 198
Verrucae (warts), 549, 642–643
Verrucous hemangiomas, 522–523
Vertical mattress sutures, 12, 13, 14
Vertical thigh reduction, 846, 847
V-flaps from trunk to arm, 54, 55
Virginal breast hypertrophy, 738
Vitallium implants, described, 95, 96
Volar flaps
in finger amputation, 576, 577
in fingertip injury, 572, 573, 574–575
in flexor tendon grafting, 611, 613
Volkmann's ischemic contracture, 622
Vomer
in cleft palate, 205
flaps, in hard palate repair, 210, 213, 214
Von Recklinghausen's neurofibromatosis, 540
V-wedge in helix mobilization, 314
Vulva
construction in male-to-female surgery, 887–888, 889, 890
deformity after thigh reduction, 849
Vulvovaginoplasty in vaginal agenesis, 880, 881
V-Y advancement flaps
in auricle reconstruction, 313
in Dupuytren's contracture, 53–54
in fingertip injury, 573, 574–575
in helical rim losses, 309, 314
in invaginated ear correction, 446, 448
multiple, 54
in scar contractures, 53–54
in vermillion defects, 348
V-Y plasty
in facial scar revision, 238, 239, 240
in wound closure, 8
V-Y rolldown for mucosal defects, 197

Waltzing in flap migration, 56
Wart virus infections, 549
Warthin's tumor, 391, 393, 395
Warts (verrucae), 549, 642–643
Wasmund technique for mandibular deformity, 141
Waterhouse-Friderichsen syndrome, 542
Webster-Dufourmentel semicircular incision for gynecomastia, 803
Weber-Fergusson incision in palatal malignancies, 362
Webs, Z-plasty for, 62, 63, 64
Weck blade for cutting skin grafts, 24–25

Wedge flaps
  in eyelid reconstruction, 286, 287
  in upper lip defects, 7
Wedge resection
  of alar base in rhinoplasty, 431–432
  of eyelid skin in blepharoplasty, 404, 405, 406
  in full-thickness lip and mouth burns, 492
  in lip reconstruction, 345, 346, 348
  of nostril, 7
  in reduction mammoplasty, 739, 740, 744, 745
  in skin lesion excision, 7, 9
Wegener's syndrome, 542
Weinhold technique for abdominal obesity, 839, 840
Wens, 274, 536
Whiteheads, 536
Wild-fire strawberry hemangiomas, 520
William vulvovaginoplasty technique, 880, 881
Wolffian ducts, development of genitourinary tract and, 873, 874
Wooky technique for hypopharyngeal reconstruction, 399, 401
Wound(s). *See also specific topic, e.g.,* Burn(s), wounds; Contracture(s); Facial soft tissue injury; Scar(s); Wound closure
  dehiscence
    after augmentation mammoplasty, 727
    after hypospadias repair, 864
    after reduction mammoplasty, 748
  healing
    chemical skin peeling and, 421
    after dermabrasion, 420
    in hand tendon injury, 604
    normal vs. abnormal scars and, 552, 553
  infection
    on hand, 579
    hypertrophic scarring and, 552, 553, 554, 555
    in skin grafting, 29
    suture types and, 12
  length, scar concealment and, 5
  microorganism culture in pressure sores, 818, 819
  tension, hypertrophic scarring and, 554–555
Wound closure, 10–16. *See also specific topic, e.g.,* Facial soft tissue injury; Sutures and suturing
  adhesives in, 15–16, 756, 758

Wound closure – *Continued*
  avoiding suture marks in skin, 11–12
  buried sutures in, 12
  after circular excisions, 8
  in cranioplasty, 272
  edges of wounds, 11
    of unequal thickness, 12
  in eyelid loss
    lower lid, 281, 282
    upper lid, 286
  in forehead laceration, 267
  in free tissue transfer, 675
  in mouth, 237
  operative technique, described, 12–14
  in penile lacerations, 869
  in pressure sores, 822–823
  punctate wounds on face, 229, 238
  in radiation injury, 487
  skin flaps for, 41
  skin graft recipient bed, 23–24
    bacterial contamination and, 24
    blood supply and, 24
    in burns, 18, 492, 493
    after circular incisions, 8
    in facial wounds, 18
    after wedge excision of nostril, 7
  skull wounds, 267, 269, 272
  skin staples and clips in, 15
  skin tapes in, 14–15
  sutures and suturing in, 10–14. *See also* Sutures and suturing
W-plasty
  in changing scar direction, 65, 239, 240
  in facial scar revision, 238, 239, 240
Wrinkles, 3, 4
  chemical face peel for, 421
  dermabrasion for, 419–420
  removal of deep forehead, 418
Wrist
  flexor tendon injury, 615
  innervation, 619
  nerve injuries in tendon lacerations, 615
  operative technique in replantation at level of, 710
  rheumatoid arthritis, 632, 635–636
  tendon transfer for deformities, 636
W-technique for abdominoplasty, 839, 840, 841, 842
Wunderer technique for mandibular deformity, 141

Xanthelasma palpebrarum, 538
Xanthoma planum, 538
Xanthoma(s)
  hand, 643–644
  jaw, 361
  skin, 537–538
Xenografts
  bone, 84
  cartilage, 85
  defined, 75
  as donor site coverage, 33
  rejection of, 75
Xeroderma pigmentosum, 489, 540

Y-V advancement
  of eyebrow in hypertelorism, 122
  Z-plasty plus, 62
Y-V advancement flaps. *See* V-Y advancement flaps

Zipper syndrome, 869
Z-plasty, 49, 58–66
  in cleft lip, 64
  defined, 58
  in ear lobule rotation, 305
  in enlargement of urethral meatus, 887
  for eversion of skin edges, 12
  in external auditory canal stenosis, 309
  in eyelid repair, 232
  in facial wounds, 230
  five-flap Y-V advancement, 62, 63
  four-flap, 62
  geometric principles of, 58–62
    gain in length and, 59–60, 61, 62
    variation of angle size, 60–62
  in helix mobilization, 314
  multiple, 6, 62, 65
  of nasal mucosa in soft palate closure, 215, 216
  in oblique facial clefts, 123
  operative technique for
    60 degree–60 degree angled, 59, 66
  planning, 60
    for proper situation, 62–63, 64
  in reduction mammoplasty, 739, 740
  in regional fasciectomy, 638
  rotation of tissue in flaps of, 65–66
  in scars
    direction changing, 65
    on face, 238, 239, 240, 266
    flexion crease scars, 64
    lengthening scar contracture, 62, 64, 65, 66
    planning and, 63
    size and, 60, 62
    U-shaped scars, 266
  six-flap, 62
  skin contraction and, 60
  transposing flaps of, 60

Z-plasty – *Continued*
  uses, summary, 63–66
  in vermillion defects, 348
  for webs, 62, 63, 64
    contracted thumb, 635
Zygoma
  arch construction in craniofacial
      microsomia, 157, 158
  fractures, 242, 250–251
    classification, 242, 250, 251
    management, 250–251, 252
  osteotomy, 143
  palpation over, 243
  rib grafts to, 134, 139
  step cut with Le Fort III
      maxillary advancement, 146
  underdevelopment, 117, 118
Zygomaticus muscle
  anatomy, 336
  myomectomy in facial palsy,
      342, 343